Physiology Terms and Symbols

S0-ALN-070

GENERAL ABBREVIATIONS

General abbreviations include:

P	pressure
V	volume
f	frequency or rate of breathing
t	time

A dash above indicates a mean or average value ($\bar{P}$ = mean pressure). A dot above indicates time factor ($\dot{V}$ = volume per unit time or flow). A percent sign indicates % of predicted normal.

GAS PHASE SYMBOLS

Primary gas phase symbols include:

V	gas volume (pressure, temperature, and water vapor saturation must be stated)
F	fractional concentration (usually dry)

Qualifying symbols used to describe the gas phase (either small capital letters or capital subscripts) include:

A	Alveolar
B	Barometric
E	Expired
DS	Dead space
L	Lung
I	Inspired
T	Tidal

CONDITIONS OF MEASUREMENT

Standard abbreviations describing the conditions of pressure, temperature, and humidity include:

STPD	standard temperature and pressure, dry. These are the conditions of a volume of gas at 0° C, at 760 mm Hg, without water vapor.
BTPS	body temperature (37° C), barometric pressure (at sea level = 760 mm Hg), and saturated with water vapor.
ATPD	ambient temperature, pressure, dry
ATPS	ambient temperature and pressure, saturated with water vapor

BLOOD PHASE SYMBOLS

Primary blood phase symbols include:

Q	Volume of blood
C	Concentration in blood phase
S	Saturation in blood phase

Blood phase qualifying symbols are always in lower case and include the following:

a	arterial
c	capillary
p	pulmonary
v	venous
s	shunt

MECHANICS OF BREATHING SYMBOLS

In addition to pressure (P), other symbols used in pulmonary mechanics include:

C	compliance
G	conductance
R	resistance
W	work

Modifying symbols usually indicate where a measurement is made and include:

A	alveolar (or alv)
ab	abdomen
am	ambient
ao	airway opening
aw	airway
B	barometric
bs	body surface
di	diaphragm
dyn	dynamic
E	expiratory
el	elastic
es	esophageal
L	transpulmonary
m	mouth
max	maximum
pl	pleural
rc	rib cage
rs	respiratory system
st	static
tm	transmural
W	chest wall

RM161 .E37 2003
Egan's fundamentals of
respiratory care//
Northeast Lakeview Colleg
33784000112573

Northeast Lakeview College
33784 0001 1257 3

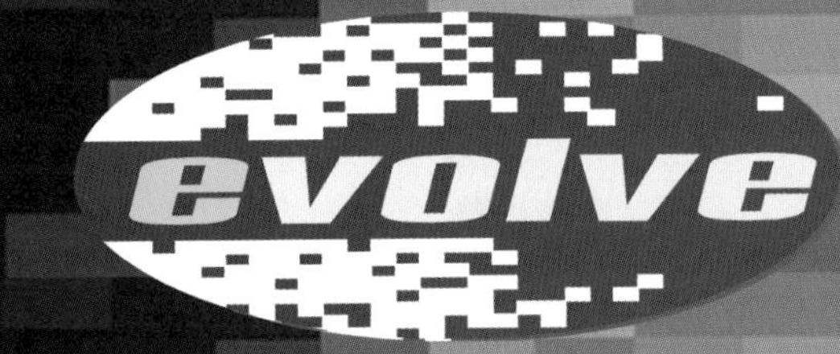

The Latest Evolution in Learning.

Evolve provides online access to free learning resources and activities designed specifically for the textbook you are using in your class. The resources will provide you with information that enhances the material covered in the book and much more.

Visit the Web address listed below to start your learning evolution today!

LOGIN: http://evolve.elsevier.com/Wilkins/Egans

Evolve Online Courseware for *Egan's Fundamentals of Respiratory Care*, 8th Edition offers the following features:

- **WebLinks**
  Links to places of interest on the web specific to respiratory care.
- **Content Updates**
  Find out the latest information about Egan's and the field of respiratory care.
- **Frequently Asked Questions**
  Additional materials to enhance the textbook content.
- **Links to Related Products**
  See what else Elsevier Science has to offer in a specific field of interest.

Think outside the book...evolve.

EGAN'S

Fundamentals *of* Respiratory Care

EGAN'S

Fundamentals *of* Respiratory Care

EIGHTH EDITION

ROBERT L. WILKINS, PhD, RRT, FAARC
Chairman/Professor
Department of Cardiopulmonary Sciences
School of Allied Health Professions
Loma Linda University
Loma Linda, California

JAMES K. STOLLER, MD, MS
Professor and Vice Chairman of Medicine
Head, Section of Respiratory Therapy
Pulmonary and Critical Care Medicine Department
The Cleveland Clinic Foundation
Cleveland, Ohio

CRAIG L. SCANLAN, EdD, RRT, FAARC
Professor and Director
Graduate Programs in Health Sciences
School of Health Related Professions
University of Medicine and Dentistry of New Jersey
Newark, New Jersey

Consulting Editors:

DAVID C. SHELLEDY, PhD, RRT, RPFT
Chairman, Department of Respiratory Care
The University of Texas Health Science Center at San Antonio
San Antonio, Texas

LUCY KESTER, RRT, MBA, FAARC
Education Coordinator
Respiratory Therapy Section
Pulmonary and Critical Care Medicine Department
The Cleveland Clinic Foundation
Cleveland, Ohio

With 45 contributors and 639 illustrations

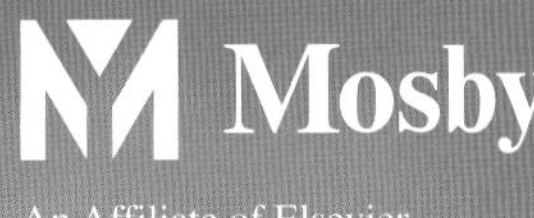

An Affiliate of Elsevier

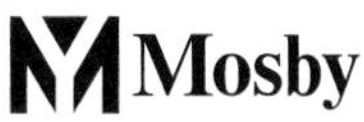

An Affiliate of Elsevier

11830 Westline Industrial Drive
St. Louis, Missouri 63146

Egan's Fundamentals of Respiratory Care, Eighth Edition ISBN 0-323-01813-0
Copyright © 2003, Mosby, Inc. All rights reserved.

No part of this publication may be reproduced or transmitted in any form or by any means, electronic or mechanical, including photocopying, recording, or any information storage and retrieval system, without permission in writing from the publisher. Permissions may be sought directly from Elsevier's Health Sciences Rights Department in Philadelphia, PA, USA: phone: (+1) 215 238 7869, fax: (+1) 215 238 2239, e-mail: healthpermissions@elsevier.com. You may also complete your request on-line via the Elsevier Science homepage (http://www.elsevier.com), by selecting 'Customer Support' and then 'Obtaining Permissions'.

NOTICE

Pharmacology is an ever-changing field. Standard safety precautions must be followed, but as new research and clinical experience broaden our knowledge, changes in treatment and drug therapy may become necessary or appropriate. Readers are advised to check the most current product information provided by the manufacturer of each drug to be administered to verify the recommended dose, the method and duration of administration, and contraindications. It is the responsibility of the licensed prescriber, relying on experience and knowledge of the patient, to determine dosages and the best treatment for each individual patient. Neither the publisher nor the author assumes any liability for any injury and/or damage to persons or property arising from this publication.

Previous editions copyrighted 1969, 1973, 1977, 1982, 1990, 1995, 1999

Acquisitions Editor: Karen Fabiano
Developmental Editor: Mindy Copeland
Publishing Services Manager: Pat Joiner
Senior Project Manager: Karen M. Rehwinkel
Senior Designer: Mark A. Oberkrom
Cover Art: Studio Montage
Interior Designer: Joan Wendt

Printed in China

Last digit is the print number: 9 8 7 6 5 4 3

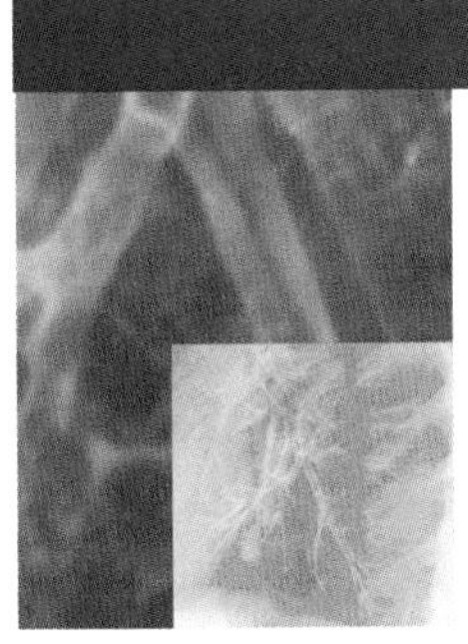

Contributors

ALEXANDER B. ADAMS, MPH, RRT, FAARC
Assistant Professor of Medicine
University of Minnesota
Research Associate
Regions Hospital
St. Paul, Minnesota

ALEJANDRO C. ARROLIGA, MD
Head, Section of Critical Care Medicine
Pulmonary and Critical Care Medicine Department
The Cleveland Clinic Foundation
Cleveland, Ohio

WILL BEACHEY, MEd, RRT
Associate Professor and Director
School of Respiratory Care
St. Alexius Medical Center/University of Mary
Bismarck, North Dakota

KEVIN K. BROWN, MD
Director of Interstitial Lung Disease Program
National Jewish Medical and Research Center
Division of Pulmonary Sciences and Critical Care Medicine
University of Colorado Health Sciences Center
Denver, Colorado

CHARLES CARROLL, EdD, RRT
Vice President, Planning and Development
Daytona Beach Community College
Daytona Beach, Florida

ROBERT L. CHATBURN, BS, RRT-NPS, FAARC
Director, Respiratory Care Department
University Hospitals of Cleveland
Associate Professor
Case Western Reserve University
Cleveland, Ohio

HOWARD A. CHRISTIE, PA-C, RRT
Pulmonary and Critical Care Medicine Department
The Cleveland Clinic Foundation
Cleveland, Ohio

ELLIOT D. CROUSER, MD
Assistant Professor of Medicine
Department of Internal Medicine
Division of Pulmonary and Critical Care Medicine
Ohio State University School of Medicine
Columbus, Ohio

DOUGLAS DEMING, MD
Professor of Pediatrics
Medical Director of Neonatal Respiratory Care
Director of Neonatal/Perinatal Respiratory Care Training Program
Loma Linda University School of Medicine
Loma Linda, California

F. HERBERT DOUCE, MS, RRT-NPS, RPFT
Associate Professor, Allied Medical Professions
Director, Respiratory Therapy Division
The Ohio State University
Columbus, Ohio

RAED DWEIK, MD
Pulmonary and Critical Care Medicine Department
The Cleveland Clinic Foundation
Cleveland, Ohio

JOHN A. EVANS, BS, RRT
Respiratory Care Program Director
Florence-Darlington Technical College
Florence, South Carolina

RUAIRI J. FAHY, MD
Clinical Assistant Professor of Medicine
The Ohio State University
OSU Medical Center
Columbus, Ohio

KARL S. FERNANDES, MD, SCCP
Attending Physician
Pulmonary and Critical Care Specialists
Toledo, Ohio

JIM FINK, MS, RRT, FAARC
Fellow, Respiratory Science
Division of Scientific Affairs
Aerogen, Inc.
Mountain View, California

LAWRENCE S. GOLDSTEIN, MD
Eastern Ohio Pulmonary Consultants
Youngstown, Ohio

ALBERT J. HEUER, PhD, MBA, RRT, RPFT
Associate Professor and Director of Clinical Education
Cardiopulmonary Sciences
University of Medicine and Dentistry of New Jersey
Newark, New Jersey

GEORGIA E. HODGKIN, EdD, RD, FADA
Associate Professor
Department of Nutrition and Dietetics
School of Allied Health Professions
Loma Linda University
Loma Linda, California

W. WILLIAM HUGHES, PhD
Dean, Mathematics and Science
Valley College
San Bernardino, California;
Associate Clinical Professor
of Pathology and Human Anatomy
Loma Linda University
Loma Linda, California

LAURIE A. KILKENNY, MD
Pulmonary, Allergy and Critical Care Medicine
University of Pittsburgh Medical Center
Pittsburgh, Pennsylvania

GLEN R. KUCK, MSEd, RRT
Department of Cardiopulmonary Sciences
School of Allied Health Professions
Loma Linda University
Loma Linda, California

CYNTHIA ANN KWIATKOWSKI, MA, RRT
Clinical Assistant Professor
Department of Primary Care
School of Health Related Professions
University of Medicine and Dentistry of New Jersey
Newark, New Jersey

SUNGCHUL LIM, MD
Department of Internal Medicine
Chonnam National University Hospital,
Kwangju, Korea

DAVID L. LONGWORTH, MD
Chairman, Department of Medicine
Baystate Medical Center
Springfield, Massachusetts;
Vice Chairman
Department of Medicine
Tufts University School of Medicine
Boston, Massachusetts

ARTHUR B. MARSHAK, RRT, RPFT
Department of Cardiopulmonary Sciences
School of Allied Health Professions
Loma Linda University
Loma Linda, California

CYNTHIA MALINOWSKI, MA, RRT
Assistant Professor
Department of Cardiopulmonary Sciences
School of Allied Health Professions
Loma Linda University
Loma Linda, California

†RICK MEYER, MS, RRT
Respiratory Care Program
Mount San Antonio Junior College
Walnut, California

MARY JANE MYSLINSKI, PT, EdD
Associate Professor
Department of Developmental Sciences and Rehabilitation
Physical Therapy Program
University of Medicine and Dentistry of New Jersey
Newark, New Jersey

PETER B. O'DONOVAN, MD
Staff, Section of Chest Radiology
Department of Radiology
The Cleveland Clinic Foundation
Cleveland, Ohio

TIMOTHY B. OP'T HOLT, EdD, RRT
Professor
Cardiorespiratory Care
University of South Alabama
Mobile, Alabama

JAY I. PETERS, MD
Professor and Director, Critical Care Fellowship Program,
Division of Pulmonary and Critical Care Medicine
Medical Director, Department of Respiratory Care
The University of Texas Health Science Center at San Antonio
San Antonio, Texas

†Deceased.

JOSEPH L. RAU, PhD, RRT, FAARC
Professor and Chair
Cardiopulmonary Care Sciences
Georgia State University
Atlanta, Georgia

GREGG L. RUPPEL, MEd, RRT, RPFT, FAARC
Adjunct Professor, Division of Pulmonary, Critical Care, and Occupational Medicine
Director, Pulmonary Function Laboratory
St. Louis University Hospital
St. Louis, Missouri

ROBERT SCHILZ, DO, PhD
Department of Pulmonary and Critical Care Medicine
University Hospitals of Cleveland
Cleveland, Ohio

STEVEN K. SCHMITT, MD
Staff Physician
Department of Infectious Disease
Cleveland Clinic Foundation
Cleveland, Ohio

KIM F. SIMMONS, MHS, RRT
Director of Clinical Education
Department of Cardiopulmonary Science
Louisiana State University Medical Center
School of Allied Health Professions
New Orleans, Louisiana

N. LENNARD SPECHT, MD
Assistant Professor of Medicine
Medical Director
Respiratory Care Program
Loma Linda University
Loma Linda, California

CHARLIE STRANGE, MD
Associate Professor of Pulmonary and Critical Care Medicine
Medical University of South Carolina
Charleston, South Carolina

PATRICK J. STROLLO, Jr., MD
Associate Professor of Medicine
Medical Director, Sleep Disorders Laboratory
Division of Pulmonary, Allergy, and Critical Care Medicine
University of Pittsburgh Medical Center
Pittsburgh, Pennsylvania

EUGENE J. SULLIVAN, MD, FCCP
Division of Pulmonary and Allergy Drug Products
Center for Drug Evaluation and Research
U.S. Food and Drug Administration
Rockville, Maryland

JOHN THOMPSON, RRT
Director Clinical Technology
Children's Hospital;
Associate in Anesthesia
Harvard Medical School
Boston, Massachusetts

DAVID L. VINES, MHS, RRT
Assistant Professor
Department of Respiratory Care
The University of Texas Health Science Center at San Antonio
San Antonio, Texas

THERESA A. VOLSKO, BS, RRT, FAARC
Director, Respiratory Services
Advanced Health Systems, Inc.
Hudson, Ohio

DEBORAH WHITE, RPFT, RRT
Department of Pediatrics/Allergy and Pulmonary Division
Washington University School of Medicine;
Pulmonary Function Laboratory
St. Louis Children's Hospital
St. Louis, Missouri

BARBARA G. WILSON, MED, RRT
Manager, Global Scientific Communications Strategy
GlaxoSmithKline
Research Triangle Park, North Carolina

KENNETH A. WYKA, MS, RRT
Director of Respiratory Marketing
Allied Health Care Services
Orange, New Jersey;
Adjunct Professor
School of Health Professions
Montclair State University
Upper Montclair, New Jersey

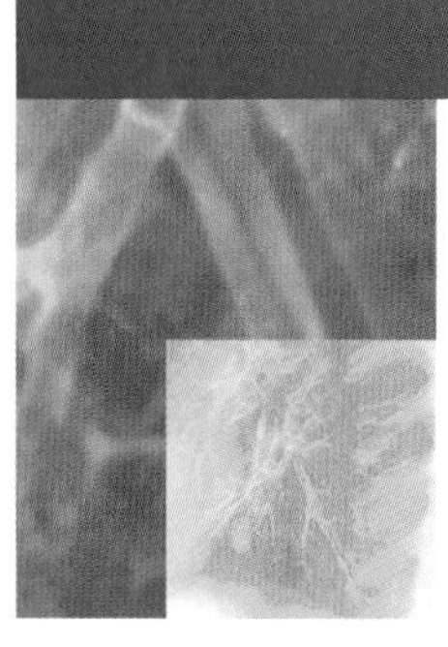

Reviewers

ALLEN W. BARBARO, MS, RRT
Director
Respiratory Care Program
Collin County Community College
McKinney, Texas

NANCY COLLETTI, MS, RRT, RCVT
Clinical Assistant Professor
Respiratory Care Program
School of Health Technology and Management
SUNY at Stony Brook
Stony Brook, New York

MARIE FENSKE, EdD, RRT
Division Chair
Respiratory Care Program
GateWay Community College
Phoenix, Arizona

DONNA JOHNSEY, BS, RRT
Director of Clinical Education
Allied Health
Jackson State Community College
Jackson, Tennessee

LISA M. JOHNSON
Clinical Instructor
Respiratory Care Program
School of Health Technology and Management
Stony Brook University
Stony Brook, New York

SINDEE KALMINSON KARPEL, MPA, RRT, AE-C
Associate Professor
Director of Clinical Education
Department of Allied Health Sciences
Borough of Manhattan Community College
City University of New York
New York, New York

JOE KOSS, RRT, MS
Director of Clinical Education
Respiratory Therapy
Indiana University
Indianapolis, Indiana

DAVID LUCAS, MS, RRT
Program Director
Respiratory Care Program
Cuyahoga Community College
Parma, Ohio

CANDACE SCHLADENHAUFFEN
Program Chair
Respiratory Care Program
Ivy Tech State College
Fort Wayne, Indiana

ROBERT A. SINKIN, MD
Medical Director of the NICU
Associate Chief, Clinical Affairs, Neonatology
Associate Professor of Pediatrics
Department of Pediatrics
University of Rochester Medical Center
Rochester, New York

To my wife Kristi, you are the love of my life.
RLW

To Terry and Jake, for their love, support, and inspiration.
JKS

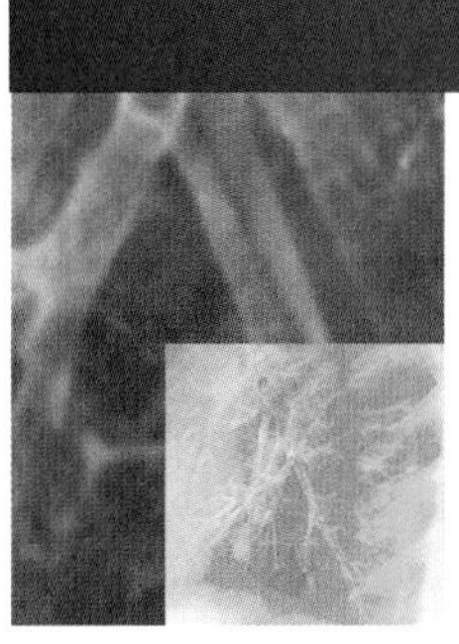

Preface

As in previous editions of "Egan's," the primary goal of this edition is to impart to students the fundamental knowledge needed to perform safe and effective respiratory care. Today's respiratory care student has an enormous amount of information to master before he or she is ready to practice independent patient care. Because the editors recognize this growing body of information, this text continues to expand in size and is now organized into 7 sections and 49 chapters covering a wide range of important topics related to the fundamentals of respiratory care. In order of presentation, the 7 sections are:

I. Foundations of Respiratory Care
II. Applied Anatomy and Physiology
III. Assessment of Respiratory Disorders
IV. Synopsis of Cardiopulmonary Disease
V. Basic Therapeutics
VI. Acute and Critical Care
VII. Preventative and Long-Term Care

All 49 chapters use numerous instructive features to help the reader with learning. Each chapter features learning objectives, a chapter outline, and a list of key terms at the beginning, mini clinis (short, problem-oriented case stories to illustrate key points) and rules of thumb throughout the chapter, and a summary of key points at the end of each chapter. These features have been carefully planned and produced to help the reader focus, absorb, and apply important information to the practice of patient care. Excerpts of the AARC Clinical Practice Guidelines (CPGs) have been updated and have been placed at key points in applicable chapters. The CPGs represent the work of many experts and present important information, such as indications, contraindications, and outcome assessment techniques, associated with specific respiratory care procedures. We thank the AARC for allowing us to place them in this edition.

In addition to substantial updating of all chapters, entirely new chapters for this edition include Chapter 28 (Neonatal and Pediatric Respiratory Disorders) and Chapter 42 (Noninvasive Positive Pressure Ventilation). Chapter 28 is authored by experts in neonatal and pediatric respiratory care and reflects the high level of knowledge and expertise required of respiratory therapists who care for patients in this area of specialty. Adding Chapter 42 was prompted by the increasing interest and use of ventilation without an endotracheal tube. In addition to these two new chapters, each chapter has been carefully reviewed, revised, and edited to reflect current knowledge of respiratory care.

In keeping with the book's long-standing role as a resource for a broad spectrum of health care providers, we believe this text will also be useful to practicing respiratory therapists, physicians, and nurses who care for patients with cardiopulmonary disease. These clinicians will find important information that will improve the quality of their patient care. Sections IV through VII are especially aimed at practitioners in addition to students.

A book of this size and scope requires collaboration among many individuals, whose efforts we wish to graciously acknowledge. First, we heartily thank all the contributors, whose expertise, thoroughness, and craftsmanship make this a truly excellent, authoritative text. Second, we acknowledge the staff at Mosby, whose abiding commitment to excellence allows this book to maintain its long-standing tradition of quality. A special thanks goes to Mindy Copeland, developmental editor at Mosby, for her consistent high-quality input into this project. She is a joy to work with and her skills as a developmental editor are unsurpassed. Finally, we take this opportunity to acknowledge Dr. Donald F. Egan, who authored the first edition of this text. His original words and sentences are gone, but the fire he lit continues to burn brightly.

RLW and JKS

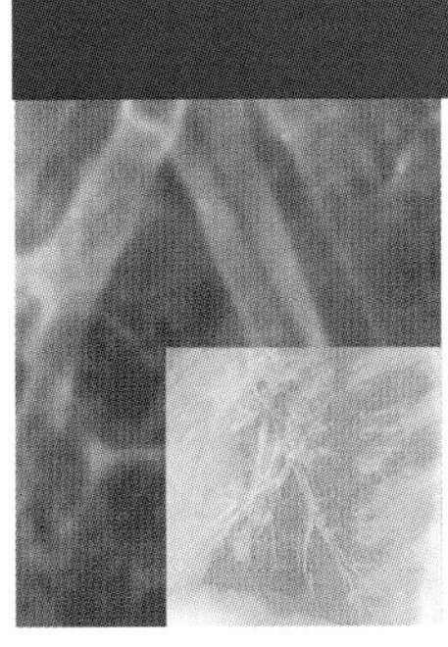

Contents

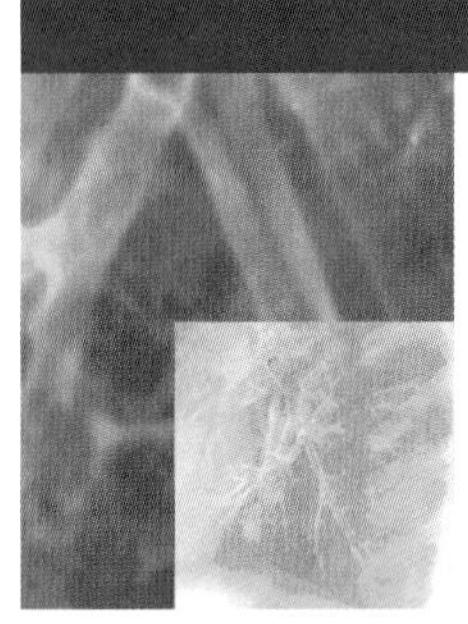

American Association for Respiratory Care Clinical Practice Guideline Excerpts

EGAN'S
Fundamentals *of* Respiratory Care

SECTION I

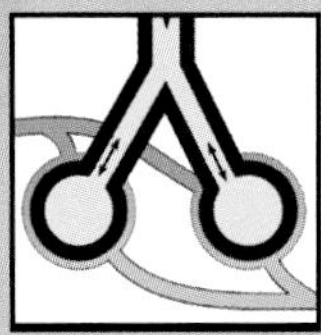

Foundations of Respiratory Care

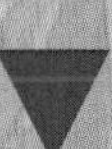
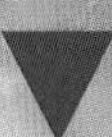
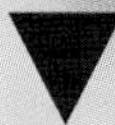

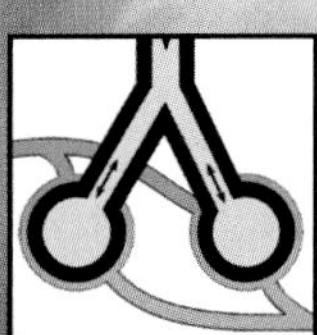

CHAPTER 1

Quality and Evidence-Based Respiratory Care

Lucy Kester and James K. Stoller

In This Chapter You Will Learn:

- What elements constitute quality respiratory care
- What methods are used for monitoring quality of respiratory care delivery
- How respiratory care protocols enhance the quality of respiratory care services
- What disease management is
- What evidence-based medicine is

Chapter Outline

Key Terms

algorithms
Committee on Accreditation for Respiratory Care (CoARC)
Continuous Quality Improvement (CQI)
cross-training
disease management
evidence-based medicine
Joint Commission on Accreditation of Healthcare Organizations (JCAHO)
misallocation
National Board for Respiratory Care (NBRC)
patient-focused care
quality
quality assurance
respiratory care protocols
respiratory therapy consult service
therapist-driven protocols

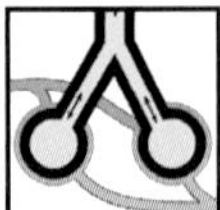

Quality is defined as a characteristic reflecting excellence, fineness, or high grade. John Ruskin, a nineteenth-century British author, once stated, "Quality is never an accident. It is always the result of intelligent effort." Conclusions drawn from the assessment of quality are only temporary because the components of quality are constantly changing. Specifically, quality, as applied to the practice of respiratory care, is multidimensional. It encompasses the personnel who perform respiratory care, the equipment used, and the method or manner in which care is provided. Determining the quality of services provided by a respiratory care department requires intelligent efforts to establish guidelines for delivering quality care and a method for monitoring this care. The conclusions derived from monitoring the care will change as the practice of respiratory care changes along with the expectations of those receiving respiratory care. In the current cost-attentive era of healthcare, quality can be challenged by the pressures of minimizing cost, making measurement of quality all important.

This chapter reviews the issue of quality in respiratory care. First we review the elements of a hospital-based respiratory care program, focusing on medical direction, practitioners, and technical direction. With the objective of quality being the competent delivery of indicated services, we discuss **respiratory care protocols** as one strategy to ensure quality. Methods for monitoring quality are discussed next, with attention to the role of the **Joint Commission on Accreditation of Healthcare Organizations** (**JCAHO**) and peer review organizations (PROs). We then discuss the effect of new healthcare delivery strategies on respiratory care quality and finally review the concept of evidence-based medicine as it applies to the practice of respiratory care.

ELEMENTS OF A HOSPITAL-BASED RESPIRATORY CARE PROGRAM: ROLES SUPPORTING QUALITY CARE

Medical Direction

The medical director of respiratory care is professionally responsible for the clinical function of the department (Box 1-1). Medical direction for respiratory care is usually provided by a pulmonary physician or an anesthesiologist. Whether the role of a respiratory care service medical director is designated as a full- or part-time position, it is a full-time responsibility; the medical director must be available on a 24-hour basis for consultation with and advice to both other physicians and the respiratory care staff. The current philosophy of cost-containment and cost-effectiveness, dictated by the medical care market forces, poses a challenge to both the medical and technical leadership of respiratory care services to provide increasingly high-quality patient care at low cost. Therefore a medical director must possess administrative and medical skills.[1] Perhaps the most essential aspect of providing quality respiratory care is to ensure that the care being provided is indicated and that it is delivered competently and appropriately. Traditionally, it has been the physician who has evaluated patients for respiratory care and has written the specific respiratory therapy orders for the respiratory therapist (RT) to follow.

However, such traditional practices have often been shown to cause **misallocation** of respiratory care.[2-4] This misallocation may consist of ordering therapy that is not indicated, ordering therapy to be delivered by an inappropriate method, or failing to provide therapy that is indicated.[5] Table 1-1 reviews selected studies evaluating the allocation of respiratory care services and the frequency of misallocated care.[3,6-11] These studies provide ample evidence that misallocation of respiratory care occurs frequently. Such misallocation has led to the use of respiratory care protocols that are implemented by RTs (as described under "Methods for Enhancing the Quality of Respiratory Care").

Box 1-1 • Responsibilities of a Medical Director of Respiratory Care

- Medical supervision of respiratory therapists in the following areas:
  - General medical, surgical, and respiratory nursing wards
  - Intensive care units
  - Ambulatory care (including rehabilitation)
  - Pulmonary function laboratory
- Development and approval of departmental clinical policies and procedures
- Supervision of ongoing quality assurance activities
- Medical direction for respiratory care in-service and training programs
- Education of medical and nursing staffs regarding respiratory therapy
- Participation in the selection and promotion of technical staff
- Participation in the preparation of the departmental budget

Respiratory Therapists

In addition to capable medical direction and application of well-constructed respiratory care protocols (see p. 8), capable RTs are an indispensable element of a quality respiratory care program. The quality of RTs depends primarily on their training, education, and experience. Training teaches students to perform tasks at a competent level, whereas clinical education provides

Table 1-1 ▶▶ Frequency of Misallocation of Respiratory Care Services in Selected Series

Type of Service	Author(s)	Date	Patient Type	N Patients	Frequency of Overordering	Frequency of Underordering
Supplemental Oxygen	Zibrak et al[6]	1986	Adults	NS	55% reduction in incentive spirometry after therapist supervision began	NA
	Brougher et al[7]	1986	Adult, non-ICU inpatients	77	38% ordered to receive oxygen despite adequate oxygenation	NA
	Small et al[8]	1992	Adult, non-ICU inpatients	47	72% of those checked had Pao_2 >60 mm Hg or Sao_2 >90% but were prescribed oxygen	NA
	Kester and Stoller[3]	1992	Adult, non-ICU inpatients	230	25.2% overall for five respiratory care services; 28% for supplemental oxygen	10.5% overall for five respiratory care services; 8% for supplemental oxygen
	Albin et al[9]	1992	Adult, non-ICU inpatients	274	61% ordered to receive supplemental oxygen despite Sao_2 ≥92%	21% underordered, including 19% prescribed to receive inadequate O_2 flow rates
Bronchial Hygiene Techniques	Zibrak et al[6]	1986	Adults	NS	55% reduction in incentive spirometry after therapist supervision began	NA
	Shapiro et al[10]	1988	Adult, non-ICU inpatients	3400 evaluators	61% reduction of bronchial hygiene after system implemented	NA
	Kester and Stoller[3]	1992	Adult, non-ICU inpatients	230	32%	8%
Bronchodilator Therapy	Zibrak et al[6]	1986	Adults	NS	50% reduction in incentive aerosolized medication after therapist supervision began	NA
	Kester and Stoller[3]	1992	Adult, non-ICU inpatients	230	12%	12%
Intermittent Positive Pressure Breathing (IPPB)	Zibrak et al[6]	1986	Adults	NS	92% reduction in IPPB after therapist supervision began	NA
	Kester and Stoller[3]	1992	Adult, non-ICU inpatients	230	40%	6.7%
Arterial Blood Gases	Browning et al[11]	1989	SICU Inpatients	724 ABGs	42.7% inappropriately ordered before guidelines implemented	NA

From Stoller JK: Respiratory care clinics of North America: therapist-driven protocols, vol 2, Philadelphia, 1996, WB Saunders.
NA, Not assessed.

students with a knowledge base they can use in evaluating a situation and making appropriate decisions.[12] Clearly, both adequate training and clinical education are required to produce qualified RTs for assessing patients and implementing respiratory care protocols.[13]

Respiratory Therapists' Designations and Credentials

Currently three tiers of practitioners exist in respiratory care: (1) on-the-job trained technicians (OJTs), (2) certified respiratory therapists (CRTs), and (3) registered respiratory therapists (RRTs). As the name implies, OJTs were trained in the hospital with the length of training varying from institution to institution. Although a number of OJTs are currently practicing respiratory therapy under a "grandfather clause," on-the-job training is no longer recognized as an educational pathway to becoming an RT. Students eligible to become CRTs or RRTs are trained and educated in colleges and universities. Following completion of an approved respiratory therapy program, graduates may become credentialed by taking an entry-level examination to become a CRT. The CRT is then eligible to sit for the registry examinations to become a credentialed RRT. Those completing a 2-year program graduate with an associate in science degree, and those graduating from a 4-year program receive a baccalaureate degree.

Respiratory care education programs are reviewed by the **Committee on Accreditation for Respiratory Care (CoARC)**. This committee is sponsored by the following organizations: the American Association for Respiratory Care (AARC), the American College of Chest Physicians (ACCP), the American Society of Anesthesiologists (ASA), and the American Thoracic Society (ATS). The CoARC is responsible for ensuring that respiratory therapy educational programs follow accrediting standards or essentials as endorsed by the American Medical Association (AMA). Members of the CoARC visit respiratory therapy educational programs to judge applications for accreditation and make periodic reviews. An annual listing of accredited respiratory therapy programs is published.

Credentialing is a general term that refers to the recognition of individuals in particular occupations or professions. In general, the two major forms of credentialing in the health fields are state licensure and voluntary certification. Licensure is the process in which a government agency gives an individual permission to practice an occupation. Typically, a license is granted only after verifying that the applicant has demonstrated the minimum competency necessary to protect the public health, safety, or welfare. Licensure laws are normally made by state legislatures and enforced by specific state agencies, such as medical and nursing boards. In states where licensure laws govern an occupation, practicing in the field without a license is considered a crime punishable by fines and/or imprisonment. Licensure regulations are based on a practice act that defines (and limits) exactly what activities the professional can perform. Two other forms of state credentialing are less restrictive. States that use title protection simply safeguard the use of a particular occupational or professional title. Alternatively, states may request or require practitioners to register with a governmental agency (registration). Neither title protection nor state registration necessarily constitute a true practice act, and because both title protection and registration are voluntary, neither provides strong protection against unqualified or incompetent practice.[14]

Certification is a voluntary, nongovernmental process whereby a private agency grants recognition to an individual who has met certain qualifications. Examples of qualifications are graduation from an approved educational program, completion of a specific amount of work experience, and acceptable performance on a qualifying examination(s). The term *registration* is often used interchangeably with the term *certification*, but it may also refer to a type of governmental credentialing. As a voluntary process, certification involves standards that are often higher than the minimum standards specified for entry-level competency. A major difference between certification and licensure is that certification generally does not prevent others from working in that occupation, as do most forms of licensure.[14]

Both types of credentialing apply in respiratory care. The primary method of ensuring quality in respiratory care is voluntary certification or registration conducted by the **National Board for Respiratory Care (NBRC)**. The NBRC is an independent national credentialing agency for individuals who work in respiratory care and related services. The NBRC is cooperatively sponsored by the AARC, the ACCP, the ASA, the ATS, and the National Society for Pulmonary Technology (NSPT). Representatives of these organizations make up the governing board for the NBRC, which assumes the responsibility for all examination standards and policies through a standing committee. The NBRC provides the credentialing process for both the entry-level CRT and the advanced-practitioner RRT. Recently, an additional advanced-practitioner credential, Neonatal/Pediatric Specialist (NPS), has been established for the field of pediatrics. The NBRC also encourages professionals in the field to maintain and upgrade their skills through voluntary recredentialing. Both CRTs and RRTs may demonstrate ongoing professional competence by retaking examinations. Individuals who pass these examinations are issued a certificate recognizing them as "recredentialed" practitioners. In addition to the certification and registration of RTs, the NBRC provides credentialing in the area of pulmonary function testing for Certified Pulmonary Function Technologists (CPFTs) and Registered Pulmonary Function Technologists (RPFTs). Currently, more than 252,000 practitioners are credentialed in the United States and abroad. Table 1-2 shows the distribution of these credentialed individuals, many of whom hold more than one credential.

At the time of publication, 45 states, the District of Columbia, and Puerto Rico have some type of licensure or title protection act regarding respiratory therapy. Many states use the NBRC entry-level respiratory care examination for state licensing, whereas others simply verify NBRC credentials. Most licensure acts require the RT to attain a specified number of continuing education credits to maintain his or her license. Continuing education helps practitioners keep abreast of the changes and advances that take place in their health-care field.[14]

Certification and licensure help ensure that only qualified RTs participate in the practice of respiratory care. Many institutions conduct annual skills checks or

Table 1-2 ▶▶ Distribution of Credentialed Practitioners

Credential Type	Number of Credentialed Practitioners
CRT	156,449
RRT	78,544
CPFT	10,889
RPFT	3771
NPS	6590

As of January 2001.
Note: Practitioners may hold more than one credential (i.e., RRTs are also CRTs and NPS are also CRTs and RRTs).

Box 1-2 • Additional Respiratory Therapist Skills Required for Implementing Protocols

- Assess and evaluate patients regarding indications for therapy and for the most appropriate delivery method
- Be cognizant of age-related issues and how they affect the patient's ability to understand and use various treatment modalities
- Adapt hospital policies and procedures to alternate care sites
- Conduct and participate in research activities to ensure a scientific basis for advances in respiratory care technology
- Communicate effectively with all members of the healthcare team and contribute to the body of literature concerning the field of respiratory care

competency evaluations in compliance with the JCAHO requirements. Beyond JCAHO-required skills checks, experience with respiratory care protocols suggests the need to develop and monitor additional skills among RTs (Box 1-2). Assurance and maintenance of these skills requires ongoing training and quality review programs, which are discussed under the heading "Monitoring Quality Respiratory Care."

Professionalism

By definition, professionalism is a key attribute to which all RTs should aspire and that must guide respiratory care practice. *Webster's New Collegiate Dictionary* defines a profession as "a calling that requires specialized knowledge and often long and intensive academic preparation." A professional is characterized as an individual conforming to the technical and ethical standards of a profession. RTs demonstrate their professionalism by maintaining the highest practice standards, by engaging in ongoing learning, by conducting research to advance the quality of respiratory care, and by participating in organized activities through professional societies. Box 1-3 lists the professional attributes of an RT. We emphasize the importance of these attributes because the continued value and progress of the field depends critically on the professionalism of each practitioner.

Box 1-3 • Characteristics of a Respiratory Therapist

- Completes an accredited respiratory therapy program
- Obtains professional credentials
- Participates in continuing education activities
- Adheres to the code of ethics put forth by his or her institution and/or state licensing board
- Joins professional organizations

Technical Direction

Another important element for delivering quality respiratory care is technical direction. Technical direction is often the responsibility of the manager of a respiratory care department, who must make sure the equipment and the associated protocols and procedures have sufficient quality to ensure the safety, health, and welfare of the patient using the equipment. Medical devices are regulated under the Medical Device Amendment Act of 1976, which comes under the authority of the U.S. Food and Drug Administration (FDA). The FDA also regulates the drugs delivered by RTs. It is the purpose of the FDA to establish safety and effectiveness standards and to ensure that these standards are met by equipment and pharmaceutical manufacturers.

Procedures and protocols related to the use of equipment and medications must be written to provide a guide for the respiratory care staff. In addition, equipment must be safety checked and specific maintenance procedures must be performed on a regular basis. Because of rapidly changing respiratory care technology, the technical director's job poses significant challenges. For example, circuit boards and computers have replaced once relatively simple mechanical devices. New medications and delivery devices for the treatment of asthma and new strategies for treating other respiratory diseases (e.g., low-stretch ventilatory approaches for acute respiratory distress syndrome) continue to evolve. Those responsible for technical direction must be certain that these new devices, methods, and strategies not only are effective but also deliver a benefit commensurate with the cost.

METHODS FOR ENHANCING QUALITY RESPIRATORY CARE

Respiratory Care Protocols

In an effort to enhance the allocation of respiratory care services, respiratory care protocols (also known as **therapist-driven protocols**) have been developed and are currently in use in many hospitals in the United States, Canada, and other countries. Respiratory care protocols are guidelines for delivering appropriate respiratory care treatments and services (i.e., treatments and services that are indicated, delivered by the correct method, and discontinued when no longer needed). Protocols may be written in outline form or may use **algorithms** (an example of which is a branching logic-flow diagram; see Figures 1-1 and 1-2).

A survey conducted by the AARC in 1995 indicated that of 1892 responding hospitals, 40% were using respiratory care protocols and an additional 18% were in the process of implementing protocols.[15] More recently, Gaylin et al.[16] conducted a telephone survey of 371 RT members of the AARC, 51% of whom were practitioners, 26% clinical supervisors, and 23% administrators. When asked if their organizations used guidelines or protocols, 98% of the respondents indicated that they did. Of the 2% that did not, 53% were planning their use.[16] Indeed, the use of respiratory care protocols by qualified RTs is a logical practice based on the premise that well-trained RTs possess extensive knowledge of respiratory care modalities and have the assessment and communication skills required to effectively execute the protocols.[17]

However, the success of a respiratory care protocol program requires several key elements involving medical direction, respiratory therapy, nursing personnel, and the hospital environment (Box 1-4). As further evidence of the widespread acceptance of protocols, the ACCP has identified the elements of an acceptable respiratory care protocol (Box 1-5). This document may serve as a guide for developing protocols. Protocols may be constructed for individual therapies, such as aerosol therapy, bronchopulmonary hygiene, oxygen therapy, hyperinflation techniques, suctioning, and pulse oximetry. Protocols can also be

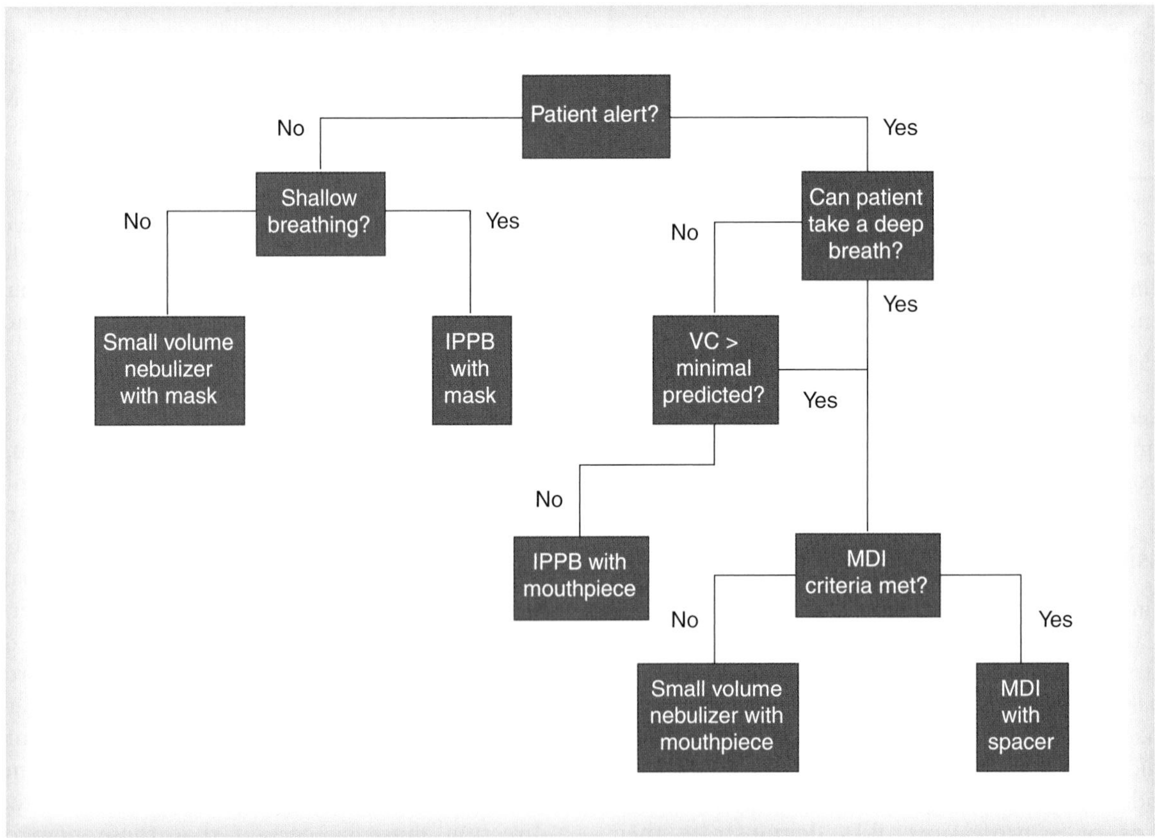

Figure 1-1 · Respiratory Care Protocol

Aerosolized bronchodilator therapy algorithm for current or history of bronchospasm.

Box 1-4 • Key Elements of a Respiratory Care Protocol Program

- Strong and committed medical direction
- Capable therapists
- Active quality monitoring
- Collaborative environment among RTs, physicians, and nurses
- Responsiveness of all elements to address and correct problems

Box 1-5 • Elements of an Acceptable Respiratory Care Protocol as Described by the ACCP

- Clearly stated objectives
- Outline that includes an algorithm
- Description of alternative choices at decision and action points
- Description of potential complications and corrections
- Description of end points and decision points at which the physician must be contacted
- Protocol program

ACCP, American College of Chest Physicians

MINI CLINI

A Specific Treatment Protocol (Aerosolized Bronchodilator Therapy)

PROBLEM

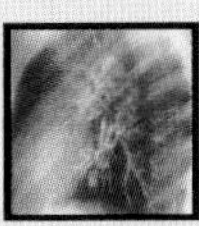

A 54-year-old woman is admitted to the hospital with an exacerbation of chronic obstructive pulmonary disease (COPD). She has a history of smoking one and a half packs of cigarettes a day for 32 years. She is alert and oriented, with a respiratory rate of 32 breaths/min. On auscultation she has bilateral wheezes on inspiration and exhalation. Her vital capacity (1.3 L) is greater than her predicted minimal vital capacity (0.872 L), but she is unable to take in a slow, deep breath and hold it for greater than 5 seconds, which is the criterion sometimes used for appropriate metered-dose inhaler (MDI) use. Following the aerosol therapy protocol algorithm, she would receive an aerosolized bronchodilator treatment via a small-volume nebulizer with a mouthpiece. An algorithm for aerosolized bronchodilator therapy is shown in Figure 1-1.

MINI CLINI

A Specific Purpose Protocol (Oxygen Therapy Titration)

PROBLEM

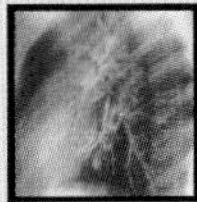

A 42-year-old man has returned to a medical-surgical nursing unit from the recovery room following a cholecystectomy. He has no history of lung disease and is wearing a nasal cannula at 2 L/min. He is alert and oriented, with a respiratory rate of 18 breaths/min and a heart rate of 82 beats/min. When the respiratory therapist arrives to check his oxygen setup and pulse oximeter reading, his SpO_2 (pulse oximeter reading) is 97% on the 2-L nasal cannula. Following the oxygen therapy titration protocol algorithm, the therapist removes the nasal cannula and returns in 15 minutes to recheck the patient's SpO_2 reading, which is now 93% on room air. The therapist discontinues the oxygen therapy. An oxygen therapy titration algorithm is shown in Figure 1-2.

Box 1-6 • Sequence of Events for a Respiratory Therapy Consult Service

1. A physician writes an order for a respiratory care protocol or consult.
2. The nursing unit secretary notifies an RT evaluator.
3. The evaluator assesses the patient using specific guidelines.
4. The evaluator writes a care plan using designated indications and algorithms and documents the care plan in the patient's chart for review by the physician.
5. The RT covering the nursing unit delivers the care.
6. The patient is assessed on a shift-by-shift basis for changes in status and indicated modifications for the care plan, which are also documented.
7. The physician is notified of any deterioration in the patient's status.
8. When indications for respiratory care no longer exist, respiratory care treatment is discontinued and notification is placed in the patient's chart.

written for a specific purpose, such as arterial blood gas sampling, weaning from mechanical ventilation, decannulating a tracheostomy, and titrating oxygen therapy.

A comprehensive approach for using protocols is to combine specific protocols to form a **respiratory therapy consult service** or an evaluate-and-treat program, which is used in institutions such as the University of California at San Diego and the Cleveland Clinic Foundation. With the use of such a service, the sequence of events for a respiratory therapy consult service may occur as shown in Box 1-6.

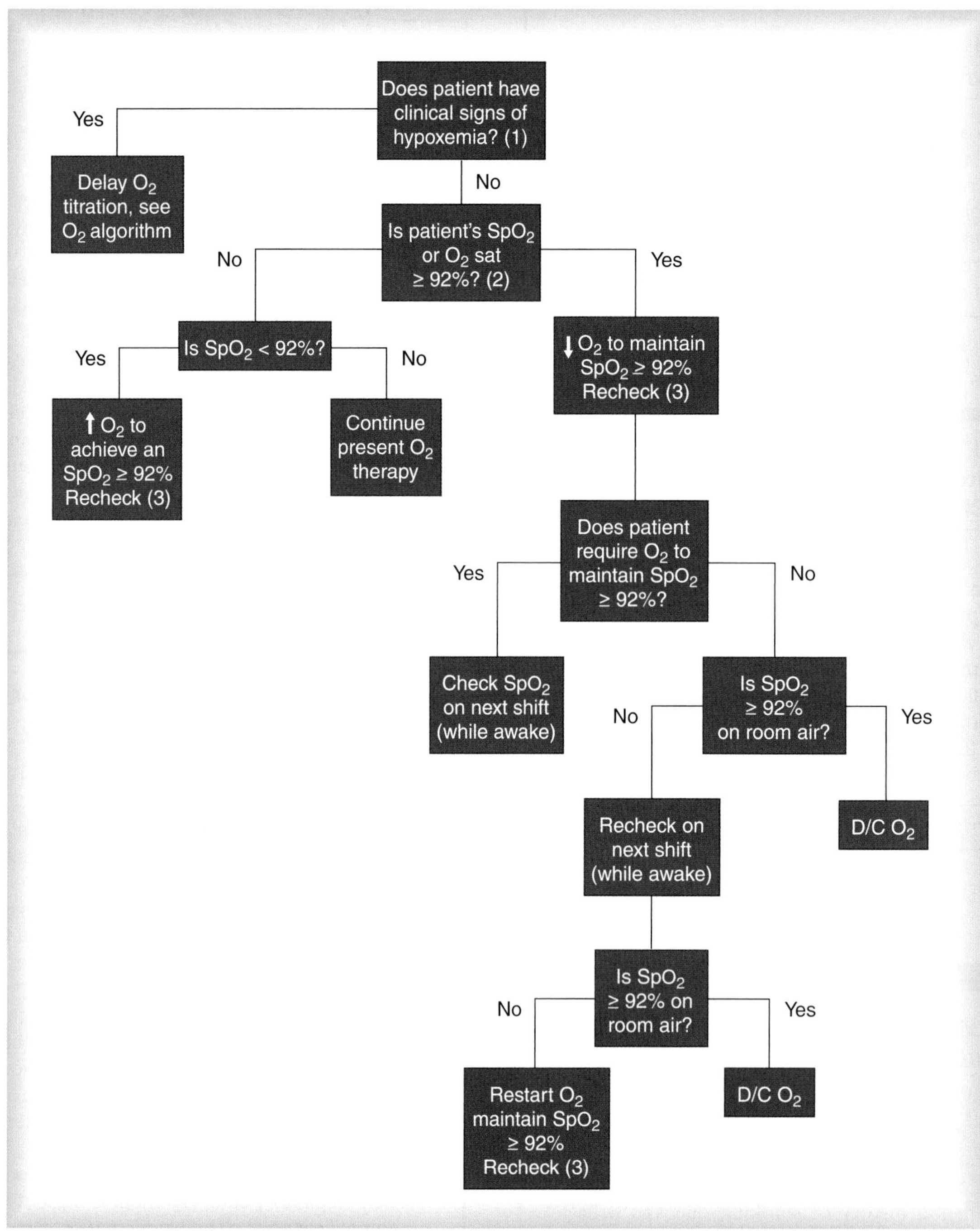

Figure 1-2 · Respiratory Care Protocol

Determining when oxygen concentration should be increased or decreased or when the therapy should be discontinued. *(1)* Shortness of breath (SOB), tachycardia, diaphoresis, confusion. *(2)* SpO_2 criteria may be modified with documented evidence of preexisting chronic hypoxemia. *(3)* Appropriate time lapse for recheck: 10 minutes for patients without pulmonary history; 20 minutes for patients with pulmonary history. *Note:* Oxygen concentration should not be decreased more than once per shift.

A carefully structured assessment tool and care plan form (Figures 1-3 and 1-4) are essential elements for a comprehensive protocol program. Such tools will help ensure consistency among therapist evaluators. The Mini Clini on Writing a Respiratory Care Plan (see p. 13) demonstrates how an assessment tool and care plan document, used in conjunction with corresponding algorithms, can guide therapists in formulating an appropriate respiratory care plan.

Respiratory Therapy Evaluation

Date________ Ht 5′7″

Time________ Age 40

Diagnosis GI dysmotility, history of asthma

Respiratory Therapist ________

Chart Assessment

Points	**0**	**x**	**1**	**x**	**2**	**x**	**3**	**x**	**4**	**x**	**Points**
Pulmonary status	(−) History (−) Smoking		Smoking history <1pk a day		Smoking history ≥1pk a day		Pulmonary impairment (acute or chronic)	X	Severe or chronic with exacerbation		3
Surgical status	No surgery	X	General surgery		Lower abdominal		Thoracic or upper abdominal		Thoracic with pulmonary disease		0
Chest x-ray	Clear or not indicated		Chronic radiographic changes		Infiltrates, atelectasis, or pleural effusions	X	Infiltrates in more than one lobe		Infiltrate + atelectasis and/or pleural effusion		2

Lab Test: Date: WBC 10.2 Hgb 11.6 Plts 260 K	Date:	pH	$PaCO_2$	PaO_2	HCO_3	Sat / FIO_2
		(No	ABG	drawn)		

Pulmonary Function Test: Minimal Pred. VC 0.927 L VC 1.35 L Peak flow____	SpO_2 / FIO_2 96%/RA	Vital Signs: HR 84 BP 110/78 RR 20 Temperature (24 hr. max.) 36.8° C

Points	**0**	**x**	**1**	**x**	**2**	**x**	**3**	**x**	**4**	**x**	**Points**
Respiratory pattern	Regular pattern, RR 12-20	X	Increased RR 21-25		Dyspnea on exertion, irregular pattern RR 26-30		Decreased vital capacity* RR 31-35		Severe SOB, use of accessory muscles RR >35		0
Mental status	Alert, oriented, cooperative	X	Lethargic, follows commands		Confused, does not follow commands		Obtunded		Comatose		0
Breath sounds	Clear to auscultation		Decreased unilaterally		Decreased bilaterally	X	Crackles in the bases		Wheezing and/or rhonchi	X	4
Cough	Strong, spontaneous, nonproductive		Strong, productive		Weak, nonproductive	X	Weak, productive, or weak with rhonchi		No spontaneous cough or may require suctioning		2
Level activity	Ambulatory	X	Ambulatory with assistance		Nonambulatory		Paraplegic		Quadriplegic		0

*VC < or = To minimal predicted:

Predicted Ideal Body Weight
Males: 50 + (2.4 × inches >60)
Females: 45 + (2.4 × inches >60)
Multiply above ideal body wt. × 15 ml for min. pred. VC

Total Points: 11

Triage #: 3

TRIAGE 1	TRIAGE 2	TRIAGE 3	TRIAGE 4	TRIAGE 5
>20	(16-20)	(11-15)	(6-10)	(0-5)

Figure 1-3

An evaluation form for guiding a standardized patient assessment and assigning a severity of respiratory illness score. The score for the greatest degree of dysfunction for each assessment category is written in the right-hand column and then tallied to determine the severity of respiratory illness (triage) score. *(Courtesy Cleveland Clinic Foundation Department of Pulmonary and Critical Care Medicine, Cleveland, Ohio.)*

Respiratory Therapy Consult/Evaluation

Your patient has been evaluated by the Respiratory Therapy Consult Service. Based on the patient's clinical indicators, the Care Plan designated below will be implemented.

IMPRINT/LABEL

Date of Evaluation ____________________

Time of Evaluation ____________________

Diagnosis(es) GI dysmotility

Hx asthma

Post Thoracic Surgery Protocol ☐

Clinical Indications

Aerosol Therapy	**Broncho/Pulm Hygiene**	**Hyperinflation**	**Oxygen Therapy**	**Respiratory Monitoring**	**Suctioning**
☒ Bronchospasm	☐ Productive cough	☒ Atelectasis	☐ SpO_2<92% on room air	☐ O_2 titration (pulse ox.)	☐ Presence of secretions
☒ History of bronchospasm	☐ Rhonchi on auscultation	☒ Decreased breath sounds	☐ PaO_2 <65% on room air	☐ Unstable resp. status	☐ Unable to cough effectively
☐ Inflammation/ mucosal edema	☐ History of mucous prod. disease	☐ Prevent atelectasis	☐ Clinical signs of hypoxemia	☐ SpO_2 <92% on room air or 4 Lpm O_2 (ABGs)	☐ Altered consciousness
☐ Proteinaceous secretions	☐ Patient unable to deep breathe and cough spontaneously			Oximetry sat/FIO_2	Vital capacity
☐ Dried secretions				96%/RA	1.35 l

Care Plan

Aerosol Therapy

	Neb.	MDI	**Frequency**
Albuterol		X	QID and prn
			at night

				Frequency
bph	☐ Pos. drainage	☐ Percussion	☐ Vibration	
Hyperinflation	☒ Incen. spiro.	☐ CPAP/PEP	☐ IPPB	To be used q1 hr
Oxygen Therapy	☐ FIO_2 % ______	☐ Liters/minute________		
Monitoring	☐ Pulse oximetry	☐ ABGs	☐ Resp. mechanics	
Suctioning	☐ Nasal-tracheal	☐ Tracheal		

Comments Patient needs encouragement to cough effectively.

Triage Number 3

Signature: Respiratory Therapy Evaluator

Print Name: ____________________ /Beeper: ____________

Care plan modifications, made in response to changes in the patient's condition, are available for your review through the Phamis Last Word computer system.

Figure 1-4

A care plan form for recording the patient's indications for therapy and the therapeutic modalities for treating the indications. *(Courtesy Cleveland Clinic Foundation Department of Pulmonary and Critical Care Medicine, Cleveland, Ohio.)*

MINI CLINI

Writing a Respiratory Care Plan

PROBLEM

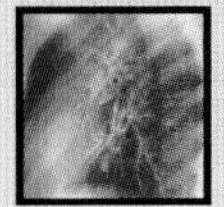

A 40-year-old woman with a history of asthma was admitted to the hospital for gastrointestinal dysmotility with abdominal distension. Her chest x-ray study showed an elevated diaphragm with accompanying atelectasis in the bases of her lung fields. Her laboratory test results were as follows: white blood cell count 10,200; hemoglobin 11.6 g/dL; and platelet count 260,000/mm^3. Her pulse oximetry reading was 96% on room air; no arterial blood gases were drawn. Her heart rate was 84 beats/min, blood pressure 110/78 mm Hg, respiratory rate 20 breaths/min, and temperature 36.8° C. She was alert and oriented, and her vital capacity was 1.35 L. She is 5 feet 7 inches tall and has a predicted minimal vital capacity of 0.927 L. On auscultation her breath sounds were decreased bilaterally and she had slight inspiratory wheezes in the apices of her lung fields. She had a weak, nonproductive cough and was able to ambulate on her own. Her assessment score sheet and her respiratory therapy care plan, using the respiratory therapy consult protocol and treatment algorithms currently in use at the Cleveland Clinic Foundation, are shown (see Figures 1-3 and 1-4).

Demonstrated advantages of respiratory care protocols have included better allocation of respiratory care services without an increased frequency of respiratory care treatments and cost-savings. Other advantages include more dynamic respiratory care, with more adjustment of respiratory care services to keep pace with patients' changing clinical status and more versatile use of respiratory care services.[17-21]

Monitoring Quality Respiratory Care

Beyond ensuring that all elements of a high-quality respiratory care program are in place, quality must be monitored to ensure that it is being maintained. Strategies to monitor quality include intrainstitutional monitoring practices and centralized, governmental monitoring bodies, such as the JCAHO.

Many healthcare organizations, including hospitals, subacute facilities, and outpatient clinics seek voluntary accreditation as a way to improve their service and assure the public that they maintain high standards. In healthcare, no accrediting organization is more important than the JCAHO. The JCAHO was formed in 1951 by the American College of Surgeons, the American Hospital Association, and the AMA. Accreditation by the JCAHO is based on satisfying specific standards established by professional and technical advisory committees.

Box 1-7 • Nine Steps for a Quality Assurance Plan

1. Identify problem(s)
2. Determine cause(s) of problem(s)
3. Rank problem(s)
4. Develop strategy(ies) for resolving problem(s)
5. Develop appropriate measurement techniques
6. Implement problem-resolution strategy(ies)
7. Analyze and compile results of the intervention
8. Report results to appropriate personnel
9. Evaluate intervention outcome

Box 1-8 • The Goals of a Respiratory Care CQI Plan as Delineated by the AARC

Goals of a respiratory care CQI plan should include at least the following:

- Provide a method for ongoing monitoring of both quality and appropriateness of respiratory care
- Ensure that respiratory care methods and procedures are cost-effective
- Ensure that respiratory care methods and procedures are effective
- Identify, rank, and resolve patient care–related problems

AARC, American Association for Respiratory Care.

The JCAHO requires a hospital service to have a **quality assurance** plan to provide a system for controlling quality. Nine generally recognized steps for a quality assurance plan are used as the basis for quality assurance programs (Box 1-7).

Current JCAHO standards for accreditation emphasize organization-wide efforts for **Continuous Quality Improvement (CQI)**. Despite increased emphasis on cost-containment, quality care remains the first goal of hospitals and respiratory care services. CQI is an ongoing process designed to detect and correct factors hindering the provision of quality and cost-effective healthcare.

This process crosses departmental boundaries and follows the continuum of the patient's care. The AARC has delineated four goals that should be included in a CQI plan (Box 1-8).

Beyond general monitoring goals for respiratory care, use of respiratory care protocols creates the need for additional quality monitoring benchmarks regarding correctness, consistency, efficacy, and effectiveness (Box 1-9).

Specific methods to monitor the quality of respiratory care protocol programs include conducting care plan audits in real time and ensuring practitioner training by using case study exercises.

Monitoring correctness of respiratory care plans can be accomplished by using a care plan audit system. Care plan auditors must be therapists who are experienced in providing respiratory care and patient assessment. The auditors must also be practiced in using the institution's protocol system and in writing care plans. With an auditing system, the auditor will write a care plan for a selected patient and compare it with the care plan written by the therapist evaluator to determine correctness. A specified number of audits should be performed monthly, with results tabulated and reported monthly or quarterly, depending on the size of the hospital. Feedback must be provided to the evaluators whose care plans are being audited to demonstrate their proficiency or to indicate areas that require improvement. Figure 1-5 provides an example of a

Stamp Here

Care Plan Audit

Date:____________________
Auditor:____________________
Therapist:____________________

Diagnosis:____________________

A = Auditor
T = Therapist

Triage Score

	0	1	2	3	4
Pulmonary Status					
Surgical Status					
Chest X-Ray					
Respiratory Pattern					
Mental Status					
Breath Sounds					
Cough					
Level of Activity					

The triage score was_________% correct.* Total A___ T___

* "% Correct" defined as the percent of auditor's scores (for each of the eight axes) with which the therapist's score agrees.

Care Plan

	Aerosol	bph	Hyperinflation	Oxygen	Pulse Ox	Suctioning
A = Auditor						
T = Therapist						

The care plan was_____% correct.*

* "% Correct" defined as (number of agreements)/six (total items for therapy).

Care plan complete? Yes No

Evaluation on time? Yes No

Frequencies correct? Yes No

Comments:____

____

Figure 1-5

A form for providing feedback to therapist evaluators on their patient assessment and care plan writing performance. An *A* (auditor) and a *T* (therapist) in the same triage scoring box or therapeutic category indicates agreement. *(Courtesy Cleveland Clinic Foundation Department of Pulmonary and Critical Care Medicine, Cleveland, Ohio.)*

Box 1-9 • Quality Monitoring Benchmarks

- Monitoring the correctness of respiratory care plans
- Monitoring the consistency of formulating respiratory care plans among therapist evaluators
- Evaluating the efficacy of the algorithms or protocols
- Evaluating the overall effectiveness of the protocol program

form used at the Cleveland Clinic to provide feedback to evaluators.

Another monitoring method found useful for respiratory therapy consult services is the case study exercise (or patient-simulation exercise). Case study exercises can help determine the consistency of respiratory care plans among therapist evaluators. The scores of individual therapists may be tracked over time to identify problems and to assess improvement.

Case study exercises consist of a set of three or four patient scenarios. All therapists working under the protocol system, whether or not they are evaluators, complete an assessment sheet and, following the associated algorithms, write a care plan for each scenario. The assessment sheets and the care plans are then compared with the "gold standard," or correct assessments and care plans as determined by the consensus of the education coordinator and the supervisors. Scores are then tabulated for the individual therapists, and the number of errors for each therapy is examined. If a particular therapy consistently has a large number of associated errors, the algorithm is reviewed for errors or vagueness. To facilitate administering and grading case study exercise results, we used a computer-based system with which therapists can complete the assessments and care plans. The program scores the assessments and care plans and provides immediate feedback to the therapist. Individual therapists' performance data can then be added to a database to calculate and track aggregate performance statistics.

Peer Review Organizations

In addition to the voluntary accreditation process that healthcare organizations use to help ensure that patients are receiving quality care, the federal government has established an elaborate system of PROs to evaluate the quality and appropriateness of care given to Medicare beneficiaries. Such PROs evaluate care provided to individual patients in real time to assess and ensure compliance with federal guidelines.

NEW PATIENT CARE DELIVERY MODELS AND QUALITY OF RESPIRATORY CARE

As healthcare organizations strive to improve the quality of patient care while reducing costs, several new healthcare models have evolved. The models that have been most commonly implemented are hospital restructuring and redesign, **patient-focused care**, protocols, and **disease management**. The following sections describe these models and review available information regarding their effect on the quality of patient care and on RTs.

Hospital Restructuring and Redesign

Restructuring and redesign involves changing the basic organization of healthcare services in an attempt to do more with less while increasing value. To accomplish this, an organization may need to flatten its hierarchies (i.e., reduce the number of management tiers) and decentralize some departments. The ultimate goal is to attain greater organizational effectiveness and productivity while preserving or increasing employee satisfaction. Approaches for restructuring commonly include cross-training employees, using unlicensed assistive staff, and decentralizing services by bringing them directly to the patient.[22]

Flattening hierarchies often affects allied health departments such as nursing, physical therapy, pharmacy, and laboratory medicine, as well as respiratory therapy. The larger the hospital and the more tiers of management that exist, the greater the potential for eliminating positions, especially middle management and supervisory positions. Because respiratory care departments are labor-intensive, high-budget departments, they are sometimes targeted for "downsizing" and decentralization.[22] However, restructuring does not always mean that respiratory care departments will be asked to eliminate positions.[23] In a 1995 AARC survey of 4985 hospital respiratory care departments, 31% of 1192 respondents (38% response rate) reported that they lost some positions when their institution participated in restructuring or redesign, whereas 54% did not.[15]

When respiratory care departments are decentralized and respiratory care management is eliminated, RTs are deployed to individual nursing units and report to nursing supervisors. In the aforementioned AARC survey, only 3% of the respondents reported that their departments had been totally decentralized. Some departments reported that, although their RTs had been assigned to specific nursing units, a core group of personnel were maintained for managing equipment, continuing education, and maintaining quality assurance activities. Respiratory care departments with an effective protocol program in place were less likely to be decentralized.[16] When total decentralization occurs, the responsibilities of equipment purchase and maintenance, continuing education, and quality improvement are assigned to nursing personnel, who often are uncomfortable with these additional burdens.[22]

Another aspect of restructuring and redesign is cross-training personnel and using assistive staff. Personnel cross-training is the method most frequently cited as the optimal strategy for decreasing the redundancy of patient care activities, thus reducing the number of healthcare personnel coming into contact with the patient and increasing efficiency. Cross-training among professional healthcare workers is accomplished by teaching activities normally performed by a specific discipline, but not restricted by licensing, to personnel of another discipline. For example, nurses might cross-train RTs to perform phlebotomy, whereas RTs might cross-train nurses to perform metered-dose inhaler (MDI) therapy. By cross-training an RT to perform some nursing skills, it could be possible to keep an RT on a specific nursing unit at all times, performing nursing duties during periods of low respiratory therapy activity, and perhaps decreasing the number of nurses for that unit.

Cross-training assistive personnel involves on-the-job training of unlicensed tasks to personnel who may not have an educational background in healthcare. These multiskilled assistive personnel may learn to perform some nursing functions such as taking vital signs, measuring intake and output, inserting urinary catheters, and so on; laboratory technician activities such as phlebotomy and simple urinalysis; and respiratory therapy activities such as incentive spirometry follow-up and oxygen checks. Again, the use of cross-trained assistive personnel, whose compensation is lower than licensed healthcare workers, may enable an institution to reduce the number of nurses, laboratory technicians, and RTs that they employ, thus reducing costs.

Although little information has been published regarding the effect of hospital redesign and personnel cross-training on the delivery of respiratory care, questions remain concerning monitoring the competence of assistive personnel.[16,22] Who is responsible for ensuring that cross-trained individuals maintain competence in each of the areas for which they have been cross-trained? Who is responsible for the continuing education for these individuals? Evidence validating the effectiveness of assistive personnel as surrogates for RTs is needed before this alternate model can be endorsed.

Patient-Focused Care

Patient-focused care organizes staff and services around the needs of the patient, bringing specific services and resources directly to the patient. This model is designed to enhance the quality and productivity of patient services, thus increasing patient satisfaction. Examples of the types of services include radiology, laboratory, and pharmacy. In addition, patient-focused care addresses the perception that patients prefer to have care provided by fewer people and that coming into contact with a large number of caregivers during a hospital stay is confusing and disturbing to patients and causes unnecessary delays in care delivery.

Providing a true patient-focused care environment requires that each nursing unit have its own admitting service, radiology unit, medical laboratory, pharmacy, and physical therapy facilities, so patients do not have to travel outside the unit for these services. This model also emphasizes the use of cross-trained personnel who are assigned to a specific unit, thus allowing the patient to be cared for by fewer healthcare providers.

Several reports demonstrate that patient-focused care does reduce the number of healthcare workers providing care to an individual patient, and anecdotes report increased patient satisfaction,[22] but the expense of relocating radiology, laboratory facilities, and pharmacy services to individual nursing units has limited the use of this model.

Again, studies reporting the specific effect of patient-focused care on the practice of respiratory care are lacking currently, as are reports describing the purchase and maintenance of respiratory therapy equipment and the continuing education and competence testing for the cross-trained personnel.

Protocols

As described previously, protocols are guided pathways to help direct specific aspects of a patient's treatment regimen. The primary purpose of respiratory care protocols is to provide therapy to patients needing and likely to benefit from therapy, but to avoid delivering services to patients not likely to benefit. The use of a comprehensive protocol program using clinical practice guidelines can provide a dynamic system for modifying the respiratory care regimen in response to a patient's changing clinical status.

The now widespread use and acceptance of respiratory care protocols has been encouraged by studies reporting reduced misallocation of respiratory care and the cost-savings associated with protocols. Indeed, in addition to observational studies, the benefits of RT protocols have been demonstrated in randomized, controlled trials for weaning patients from mechanical ventilation[24-26] and for allocating respiratory therapy to adult non-ICU inpatients.[20,21] Table 1-3 presents selected studies demonstrating the effect of respiratory care protocols on the misallocation of respiratory therapy.[27-32]

Most studies show a significant decrease in over-ordering respiratory care services, whereas only a few

Table 1-3 ▶▶ Changes in Modalities after Protocol Implementation

	Observed Reductions In	
Author and Year Published	**Misallocated Therapy After Implementation of Protocols (%)**	**Change from Preprotocol to Current Status**
Hart et al,[28] 1992	37% (aerosol, hyperinflation)	48%-11%
Walton et al,[29] 1990	49.1% (aerosol, chest physiotherapy)	
Beasley et al,[30] 1992	11.9% (blood gas use)	42.7%-30.8%
Ford,[31] 1994	57% (aerosol, chest physiotherapy)	7000-4000 treatments
Orens,[32] 1993	35% (aerosol, bronchopulmonary, hygiene, hyperinflation oxygen, oximetry)	

From Haney DJ: Respiratory care clinics of North America: therapist-driven protocols, vol 2, Philadelphia, 1996, WB Saunders.

Table 1-4 ▶▶ Cost-Savings Associated With Respiratory Care Protocols

Author	Date	Duration of Study	Cost-savings
Hart et al[28]	1992	3 mo	$4316 (decrease in actual costs)
Walton et al[29]	1990	6 yr	9.7% (decrease in charges)
Orens[32]	1993	1 yr	$81,826 (decrease in costs for one nursing unit)
Ford[31]	1994	1 yr	$150,000 (decrease in costs)
Shrake et al[33]	1994	3 mo	$5318 (departmental savings)
Komara and Stoller[34]	1995	40 patients	53.3% (decrease in costs)
Shrake et al[33]	1994	2 yr, 4420 patients; cost comparisons: 3 mo postprotocol	$15,337 for 3 study months, annualized to $61,348/year
Stoller et al[20]	1998	1 yr, 145 patients	$20 (decrease in true costs/patient)
Kollef et al[21]	2000	9 mo, 694 patients	$186 (decrease in charges/patient)

Modified from Haney DJ: Respiratory care clinics of North America: therapist-driven protocols, vol 2, Philadelphia, 1996, WB Saunders.

address underordering services, a phenomenon that is more difficult to assess. Table 1-4 reviews studies addressing the cost-savings associated with using protocols, which suggest that respiratory care protocols can affect savings by enhancing appropriate allocation of respiratory care services.[27-34] Table 1-5 summarizes the results of the five currently available randomized, controlled trials regarding the effectiveness of respiratory care protocols. These studies establish the efficacy of respiratory care protocols in weaning patients from mechanical ventilation[24-26] and in enhancing the allocation of services to adult non-ICU inpatients.[20,21]

Disease Management

Disease management is a commonly used term in current healthcare and refers to an organized strategy of delivering care to a large group of individuals. Specifically, disease management has been defined as a systematic population-based approach to identify persons at risk, intervene with specific programs of care, and measure clinical and other outcomes.[35,36] Four essential components compose disease management programs: (1) an integrated healthcare system that can provide coordinated care across the full range of patients' needs; (2) a comprehensive knowledge base, regarding the prevention, diagnosis, and treatment of disease, that guides the plan of care; (3) sophisticated clinical and administrative information systems that can help assess patterns of clinical practice; and (4) a commitment to continuous quality improvement. For example, disease management of chronic obstructive pulmonary disease (COPD) might be adopted by an insurance company or by a large health maintenance organization in defining its practice approach to individuals with COPD. The disease management program might contain algorithms addressing when to suspect COPD, tests to perform (e.g., spirometry, α1-antitrypsin level, diffusing capacity), medications to prescribe based on disease severity, management of exacerbations, indications for rehabilitation, and so forth. Such disease management programs are often outlined in documents containing branched logic algorithms, which specify care, much like respiratory care protocols; however, disease management protocols often address large groups and are based on an underlying diagnosis (e.g., diabetes, COPD, asthma) rather than on individual signs and symptoms.

Table 1-5 ▶▶ Summary of Available Randomized Trials Regarding the Effectiveness of Respiratory Care Practitioners

Clinical Activity	Author	Date	*N* Patients	Findings
Weaning From Mechanical Ventilation	Kollef et al[24]	1997	357	Use of protocols was associated with shorter duration of mechanical ventilation
	Ely et al[25]	1996	300	Routine daily trials of spontaneous breathing trials was associated with shorter duration of mechanical ventilation
	Marelich et al[26]	2000	253	Use of protocols shortened duration of mechanical ventilation
Respiratory Care Protocol Service	Stoller et al[20]	1998	145	Use of respiratory therapy consult service was associated with improved allocation of respiratory care service with lower costs and no adverse events
	Kollef et al[21]	2000	694	Use of respiratory protocol service was associated with fewer orders discordant with guidelines and lower charges

From Stoller JK: Are respiratory therapists effective? Assessing the Evidence, Respir Care 46:56, 2001.

Other dimensions of the COPD disease management program include a data collection activity about the number of patients served, the outcomes of care, and perhaps, the associated costs. In addition, ongoing review and periodic updating and revision of the care algorithms is an important dimension of the program.

▶ EVIDENCE-BASED MEDICINE

Another important concept regarding quality care is that of evidence-based medicine. Evidence-based medicine refers to an approach to determining optimal clinical management based on several practices[36-39]: (1) a rigorous and systematic review of available evidence, (2) a critical analysis of available evidence to determine what management conclusions are most sound and applicable, and (3) a disciplined approach to incorporating the literature with personal practice and experience. The tools of evidence-based medicine include systematically reviewing the available literature and meta-analyses regarding a single clinical topic, then analyzing and summarizing the body of literature by assessing the quality of the available evidence and giving greater weight to better-designed, more rigorous studies. For example, a meta-analysis performed as part of an evidence-based approach to determining optimal therapy for COPD might weigh the results of large randomized clinical trials above those of small observational studies. Furthermore, if more than one randomized, controlled trial of a single treatment were available, an evidence-based medicine approach might guide the pooling of data and the collective analysis to determine the most rigorously supported clinical practice.

Although some point out that evidence-based medicine does not differ from prior practice in which clinicians were always called on to carefully analyze available data and make clinical judgments based on the best-quality information available, evidence-based medicine does specify precise methods for analyzing available information and allowing the clinician to best judge the available evidence. Several recent publications in respiratory care have considered the effectiveness of RTs[3] and of various respiratory care treatment modalities using an evidence-based approach.[38,39]

KEY POINTS

Quality respiratory care can be defined as the competent delivery of indicated respiratory care services:

- ➤ Crucial elements for quality respiratory care include the following:
  - Energetic and competent medical direction
  - Method for providing indicated/appropriate respiratory care
  - Educated, competent respiratory care personnel
  - Adequate, well-maintained equipment
  - Intelligent system for monitoring continuous quality improvement
- ➤ Misallocation of respiratory care services, which hinders the delivery of quality respiratory care, can be defined as overordering and/or underordering of respiratory care services and is common in current practice.

KEY POINTS—cont'd

- Respiratory care protocols are guidelines for delivering appropriate respiratory care services and are widely used in current respiratory care practice.
- Available evidence suggests that use of respiratory care protocols can improve allocation of respiratory care services.
- Delivery of quality respiratory care requires the combined activities of a qualified and committed medical director, along with capable RTs, and can be enhanced by well-constructed respiratory care protocols.
- Practitioner credentialing is important in respiratory care, with the RRT representing the highest credential, based on successful completion of the NBRC examination.
- Maintaining and improving quality requires ongoing monitoring, as may be accomplished by quality audits and repeated competence testing of the RTs.
- Other current approaches to enhancing quality respiratory care delivery include patient-focused care models and hospital redesign and restructuring, which often involves cross-training allied healthcare providers.
- Evidence-based medicine is an approach to determining optimal patient management based on critically assessing the available evidence. It is recommended that RTs use this approach as they assess the support for respiratory care management strategies.

References

1. McDonald P, Mathias J: Modern respiratory care services. In Scanlan CL, Spearman C, Sheldon RL, editors: Egan's fundamentals of respiratory care, ed 6, St Louis, 1995, Mosby.
2. Stoller JK: Misallocation of respiratory care services: time for a change, Respir Care 38:263, 1993 (editorial).
3. Kester L, Stoller JK: Ordering respiratory care services for hospitalized patients: practices of overuse and underuse, Cleve Clin J Med 59:581, 1992.
4. Malloy R et al: Reduction of unnecessary care through utilization of a respiratory care plan, Respir Care 37:1277, 1992 (abstract).
5. Stoller JK: Why therapist-driven protocols? A balanced view, Respir Care 39:706, 1994 (editorial).
6. Zibrak JD, Rossetti P, Wood E: Effect of reductions in respiratory therapy on patient outcomes, N Engl J Med 315:292, 1986.
7. Brougher LI et al: Effectiveness of medical necessity guidelines in reducing cost of oxygen therapy, Chest 39:646, 1986.
8. Small D et al: Uses and misuses of oxygen in hospitalized patients, Am J Med 92:591, 1992.
9. Albin RJ et al: Pattern of non-ICU inpatient supplemental oxygen utilization in a university hospital, Chest 102:1672, 1992.
10. Shapiro BA et al: Authoritative medical direction can assure cost-beneficial bronchial hygiene therapy, Chest 93:1038, 1988.
11. Browning JA, Kaiser DL, Durbin CG: The effect of guidelines on the appropriate use of arterial blood gas analysis in the intensive care unit, Respir Care 34:269, 1989.
12. Kester L, Stoller JK: Respiratory care education: current issues and future challenges, Respir Care 41:98, 1996 (editorial).
13. Stoller JK: Are respiratory therapists effective? Assessing the evidence, Respir Care 46:56, 2001.
14. Longest B, Scanlan C: Respiratory care and the healthcare system. In Scanlan CL, Spearman C, Sheldon RL, editors: Egan's fundamentals of respiratory care, ed 6, St Louis, 1995, Mosby.
15. Dubbs W, Weber K: AARC survey measures effects of restructuring on respiratory care nationwide, AARC Times 20:29, 1996.
16. Gaylin DS et al: The role of respiratory care practitioners in a managed healthcare system: emerging areas of clinical practice, Am J Manag Care 5:749, 1999.
17. Stoller JK: The rationale for therapist-driven protocols. In Stoller JK, Kester L, editors: Respiratory care clinics of North America: therapist-driven protocols, vol 2, Philadelphia, 1996, WB Saunders.
18. Stoller JK et al: Physician-ordered respiratory care vs physician-ordered use of a respiratory therapy consult service: early experience at the Cleveland Clinic Foundation, Respir Care 38:1143, 1993.
19. Stoller JK et al: Physician-ordered respiratory care vs physician-ordered use of a respiratory therapy consult service: results of a prospective observational study, Chest 110:422, 1996.
20. Stoller JK et al: Randomized controlled trial of physician-directed versus respiratory therapy consult service-directed respiratory care to adult non-ICU inpatients, Am J Respir Crit Care Med 158:1068, 1998.
21. Kollef MH et al: The effect of respiratory therapist-initiated treatment protocols on patient outcomes and resource utilization, Chest 117:467, 2000.
22. Kester L, Stoller JK: Respiratory care in the adult non-ICU setting, Respir Care 42:101, 1997.
23. Bunch D: Restructuring doesn't always mean downsizing, AARC Times 19(7):22, 1995.
24. Kollef MH et al: A randomized, controlled trial of protocol-directed versus physician-directed weaning from mechanical ventilation, Crit Care Med 25:567, 1997.
25. Ely EW et al: Effect on the duration of mechanical ventilation of identifying patients capable of breathing spontaneously, N Engl J Med 335:1864, 1996.
26. Marelich G et al: Protocol weaning of mechanical ventilation in medical and surgical patients by respiratory care practitioners and nurses, Chest 118:459, 2000.

27. Haney DJ: Therapist-driven protocols for adult non-intensive care unit patients: availability and efficacy. In Stoller JK, Kester L, editors: Respiratory care clinics of North America: therapist-driven protocols, vol 2, Philadelphia, 1996, WB Saunders.
28. Hart SK et al: The effects of therapist-evaluation of orders and interaction with physicians on the appropriateness of respiratory care, Respir Care 37:1279, 1992.
29. Walton JR, Shapiro BA, Harrison EH: Review of a bronchial hygiene evaluation program, Respir Care 35:1214, 1990.
30. Beasley K, Darin J, Durbin C: The effect of respiratory care department management of a blood gas analyzer on the appropriateness of arterial blood gas utilization, Respir Care 37:343, 1992.
31. Ford R: The University of California San Diego experience with patient-driven protocols. From the AARC State-of-the-Art Conference: Therapist-driven protocols, Dallas, May 1994.
32. Orens DK: A manager's perspective on a respiratory therapy consult service, Respir Care 38:884, 1993 (editorial).
33. Shrake K et al: Benefits associated with a respiratory care assessment-treatment program: results of a pilot study, Respir Care 39:715, 1994.
34. Komara JJ, Stoller JK: The impact of a postoperative oxygen therapy protocol on use of pulse oximetry and oxygen therapy, Respir Care 40:1125, 1995.
35. Epstein RS, Sharwood LM: From outcomes research to disease management: a guide for the perplexed, Ann Intern Med 124: 832, 1996.
36. Elrodt G et al: Evidence-based disease management, JAMA 278:1687, 1997.
37. Stoller JK: 2000 Donald F. Egan Scientific Lecture: Are respiratory therapists effective? Assessing the evidence, Respir Care 46:56, 2001.
38. Respiratory Care Special Issue: Evidenced-based medicine in respiratory care, Part I. Respir Care 46(11), 2001.
39. Respiratory Care Special Issue: Evidenced-based medicine in respiratory care, Part II. Respir Care 46(12), 2001.

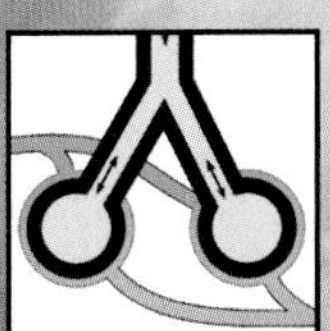

CHAPTER 2

Patient Safety, Communication, and Recordkeeping

Robert L. Wilkins and Craig L. Scanlan

In This Chapter You Will Learn:

- What safety hazards and risks are common among patients receiving respiratory care
- How to minimize common safety hazards and patient risks
- How to apply good body mechanics and posture to move patients
- How to ambulate a patient
- What harmful effects electrical current can have on the body
- How to recognize and avoid electrical shock hazards
- What conditions are needed for fire and how to avoid fire hazards
- How communication can affect patient care
- What factors affect the communication process
- How to improve your effectiveness in health communication
- How to recognize and help resolve interpersonal or organizational sources of conflict
- What constitutes a medical record
- What legal and practical obligations are involved in recordkeeping
- How to maintain a problem-oriented medical record

Chapter Outline

Key Terms

ambulation
ampere
attending
auditory
channel (communication)
feedback
ground (electrical)
macroshock
microshock
nonflammable
POMR
SOAP

Respiratory therapists (RTs) share general responsibilities for providing safe and effective patient care with other members of the healthcare team. These responsibilities include basic patient safety and medical recordkeeping. In addition to performing these technical skills, all health professionals must be able to effectively communicate with each other and with their patients and patients' families. This chapter provides the foundation knowledge skills needed to effectively assume these general aspects of patient care.

SAFETY CONSIDERATIONS

Patient safety is always the first consideration in respiratory care. Although the RT usually does not have full control over the patient's environment, efforts must be made to minimize safety hazards and patient risks whenever possible. The key areas of potential risk common to most patients receiving respiratory care are (1) patient movement and ambulation, (2) electrical hazards, and (3) fire hazards.

Patient Movement and Ambulation

Basic Body Mechanics

Posture involves the relationship of the body parts to each other. Good posture is needed to reduce the risk of injury to the person lifting patients or heavy equipment. Poor posture may place inappropriate stress on certain bones, muscles, and organs. Figure 2-1 illustrates the correct body mechanics for lifting a heavy object. Note that the correct technique calls for a straight spine and use of the leg muscles to life the object. Figure 2-2 applies this concept to lifting and moving a patient.

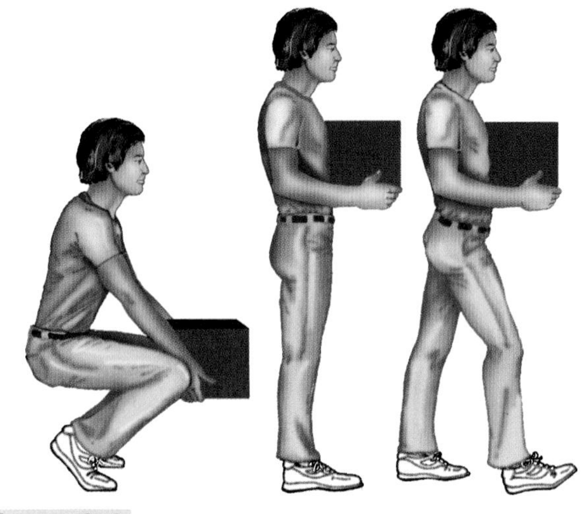

Figure 2-1
Body mechanics for lifting and carrying objects.

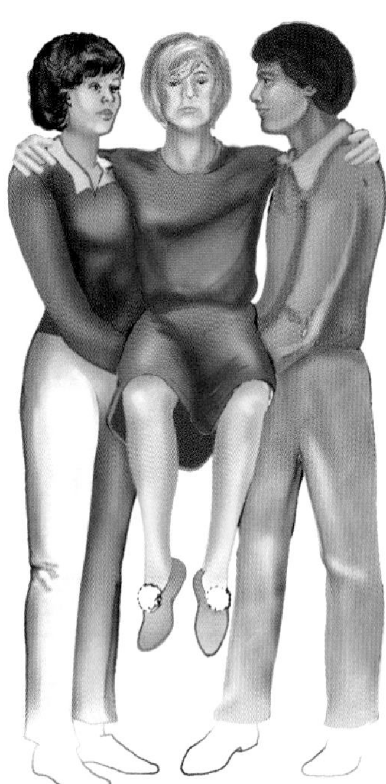

Figure 2-2
Carrying technique for patient able to sit.

Moving the Patient in Bed

Conscious people assume positions that are the most comfortable for them. For example, bedridden patients with acute or chronic respiratory dysfunction often assume a high Fowler's position, with arms flexed and thorax leaning forward. This position helps decrease their work of breathing. However, in other cases patients may have to assume certain positions for therapeutic reasons.

Figure 2-3 demonstrates the correct technique for lateral movement of a bed-bound patient. Figure 2-4 illustrates the ideal method for moving a conscious patient toward the head of a bed. Last, Figure 2-5 shows the proper technique for assisting a patient to the bedside position for dangling of legs or transfer to a chair.

Ambulation

Ambulation (walking) helps maintain normal body function. Bed rest, even with appropriate movement exercises, produces many bad effects. Ambulation should begin as soon as a patient is physiologically stable and free of severe pain. Safe patient movement includes the following steps:

1. Place the bed in a low position and lock its wheels.
2. Place all equipment (e.g., intravenous [IV] equipment, nasogastric tube, surgical drainage tubes) close to the patient to prevent dislodging during ambulation.

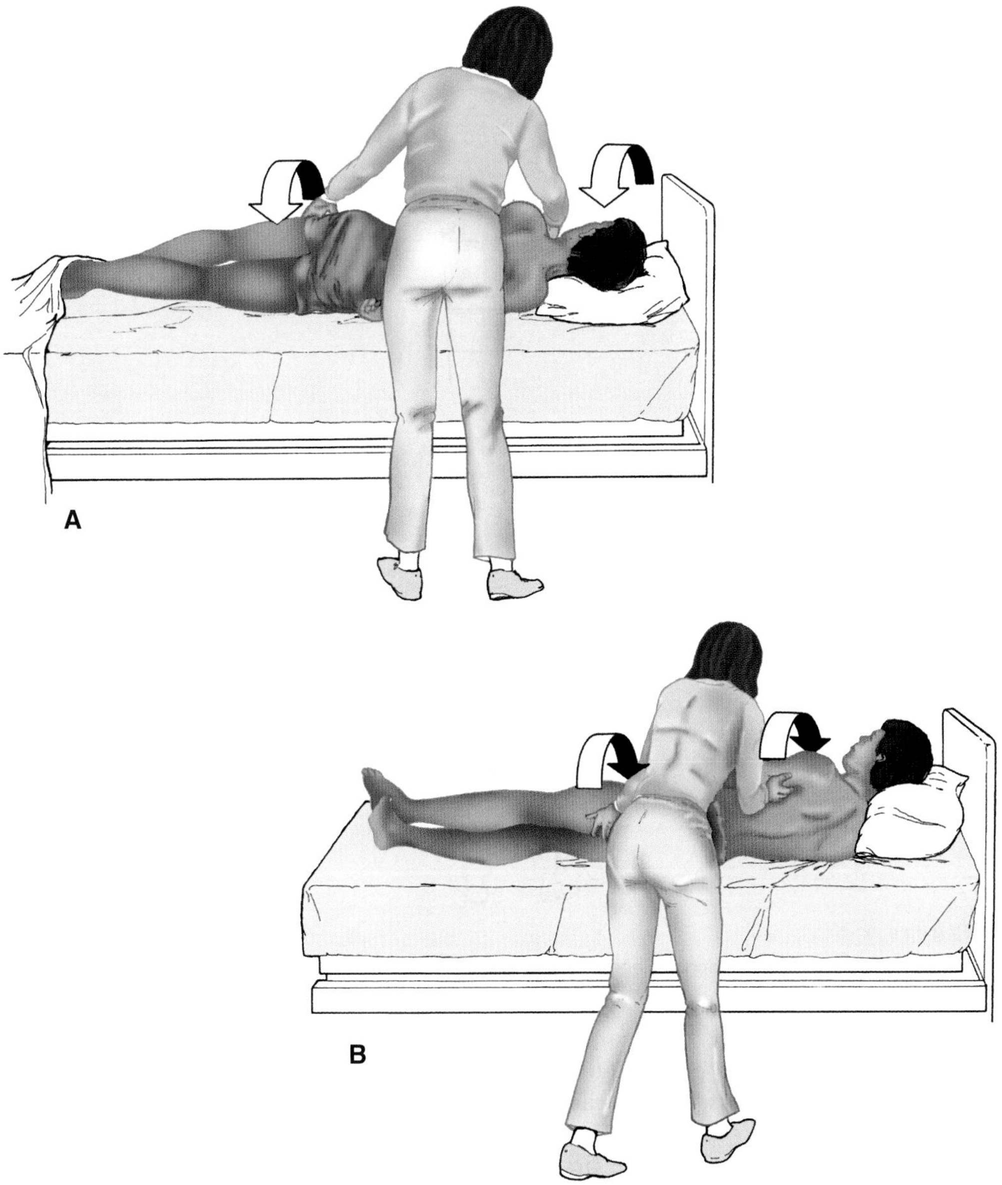

Figure 2-3
A, Method to pull bed-bound patient. **B,** Method to push bed-bound patient.

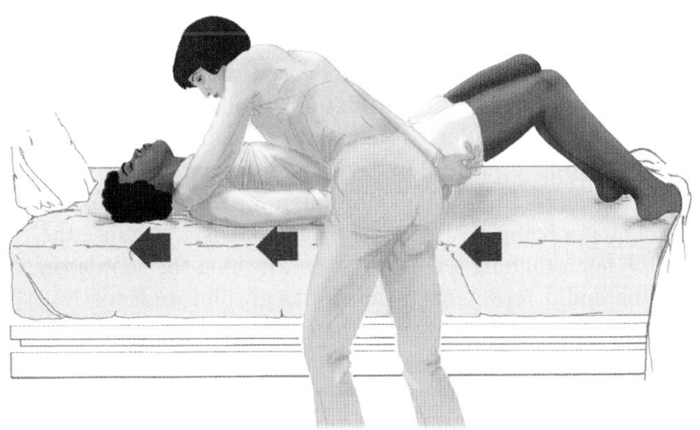

Figure 2-4
Method to move patient up in bed with patient's assistance.

3. Move the patient toward the nearest side of bed.
4. Assist the patient to sit up in bed (i.e., arm under nearest shoulder and one under farthest armpit).
5. Place one hand under the patient's farthest knee and gradually rotate the patient so that the legs are dangling off the bed.
6. Let the patient remain in this dangling position until dizziness or lightheadedness lessens (encouraging the patient to look forward rather than at the floor may help).
7. Assist the patient to a standing position.
8. Encourage the patient to breathe easily and unhurriedly during this initial change to a standing posture.

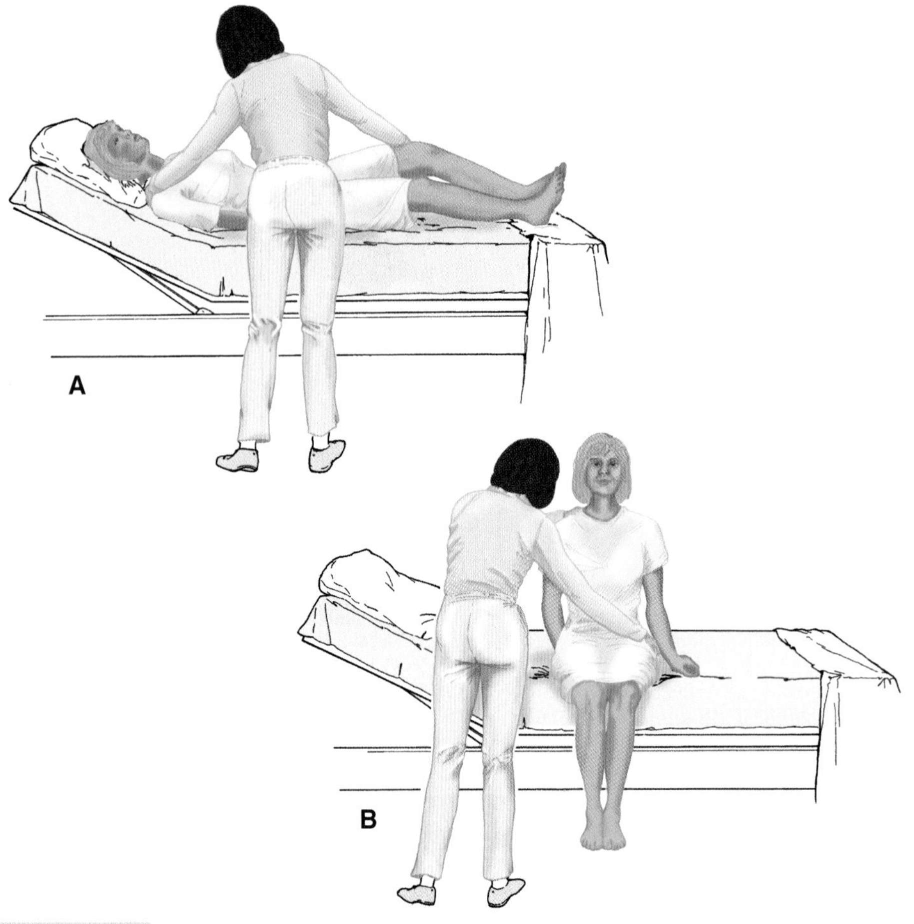

Figure 2-5
Method to assist patient in dangling legs at side of bed.

9. Walk with the patient using no, minimal, or moderate support (moderate support requires the assistance of two practitioners, one on each side of the patient).
10. Limit walking to 5 to 10 minutes for the first exercise.

Monitor the patient during ambulation. Note the patient's level of consciousness, color, breathing, strength or weakness, and complaints throughout the activity. Make sure that chairs are present so emergency seats are available if the patient becomes uncomfortable. Encourage your patient to ambulate frequently until no assistance is required.

Electrical Safety

With the more frequent use of electrical equipment in hospitals, the potential for electrical accidents has increased. The presence of invasive devices, such as internal catheters and pacemakers, only worsens this problem. RTs must understand the fundamentals of electrical safety because respiratory care often involves use of electrical devices.

MINI CLINI

"Tingling" Equipment

PROBLEM

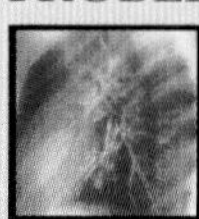

An RT is caring for a patient on a mechanical ventilator that requires both electrical and pneumatic power for operation. When the RT touches the metal housing of the ventilator, a shock is felt. How should the RT handle the situation based on this observation?

DISCUSSION

All therapeutic instruments used in patient care, including mechanical ventilators, should be connected to grounded outlets (three wire). Because the ground wire is only a protection device and not part of the main circuit, equipment may continue to operate without the clinician being aware that a problem exists. Because the RT felt a tingling sensation when touching the ventilator, this could represent an improper ground and possible serious current leakage. In this situation, the RT should immediately take the equipment out of service and get it replaced (while providing back-up ventilation). All electrical equipment used in patient care should be routinely checked for appropriate grounding.

Physiological Effects of Electrical Current

Current is the primary factor determining the effect of a shock. Voltage and resistance are important only because they determine how much current flows.

The harmful effects of electrical current depend on (1) the amount of current flowing through the body, (2) the duration for which this current is applied, and (3) the path the current takes through the body.

For example, as long as a person is insulated by normal clothing and shoes and is in a dry environment, a 120-V shock may hardly be felt. However, if the same person was standing without shoes on a wet floor, the same voltage could be fatal. This difference is a result of differences in resistance to current. In the first case, resistance is high, thus current flow through the body is low. In the second situation, resistance is low, and the current flow is dangerously high.

A shock hazard exists only if the electrical "circuit" through the body is complete. This means that two electrical connections to the body are required for a shock to occur. In electrical devices, these connections typically consist of a "hot" wire and a "neutral" wire. The neutral wire completes the circuit by taking the electrical current to a **ground.** A ground is simply a low-resistance pathway to a point of zero voltage, such as the earth (thus the term *ground*).

Figure 2-6 shows how current can flow through the body. In this case, a piece of electrical equipment is connected to AC line power via a standard three-prong plug. However, unknown to the practitioner, the cord has a broken ground wire. Normally, current leakage from the equipment would flow back to the ground through the ground wire. However, this pathway is not available. Instead, the leakage current finds a path of low resistance through the practitioner to the damp floor (an ideal ground).

Once current begins to flow, its path through the body determines the severity of the shock. Normally, the skin offers high resistance to current flow. However, moisture affects skin resistance. Through dry, intact skin, resistance is high (approximately 1,000,000 Ω); resistance through wet skin is only about 1000 Ω.

Current can readily flow into the body, causing damage to vital organs when the skin is bypassed via conductors such as pacemaker wires or saline-filled intravascular catheters. Even urinary catheters and catheters used to drain fluid from the body can provide a path for current flow. The heart is particularly sensitive to electrical shock. Experiments with dogs have shown that ventricular fibrillation can occur when currents as low as 20 μA (20 microamperes or 20 millionths of an **ampere**) are applied directly to the heart. Although the current is potentially lethal, a current this low is not normally noticed.

Thus the severity of a shock hazard depends on both the amount of current and the path it takes through the body. A **macroshock** exists when a high current (usually greater than 1 mA, or one thousandth of an ampere) is applied externally to the skin. A **microshock**, on the other hand, exists when a small, usually imperceptible current (less than 1 mA) bypasses the skin and follows a direct, low-resistance path into the body. Patients susceptible to microshock hazards are termed *electrically sensitive* or *electrically susceptible*. Table 2-1 summarizes the different effects of these two types of electrical shock.

Preventing Shock Hazards

Most shock hazards are caused by inappropriate or inadequate grounding. Shock hazards can thus be eliminated or minimized if a few basic rules for patient and equipment grounding are followed.

General Precautions. General precautions for all patient situations include never grounding the patient and always ensuring that all patient-related equipment is properly grounded.

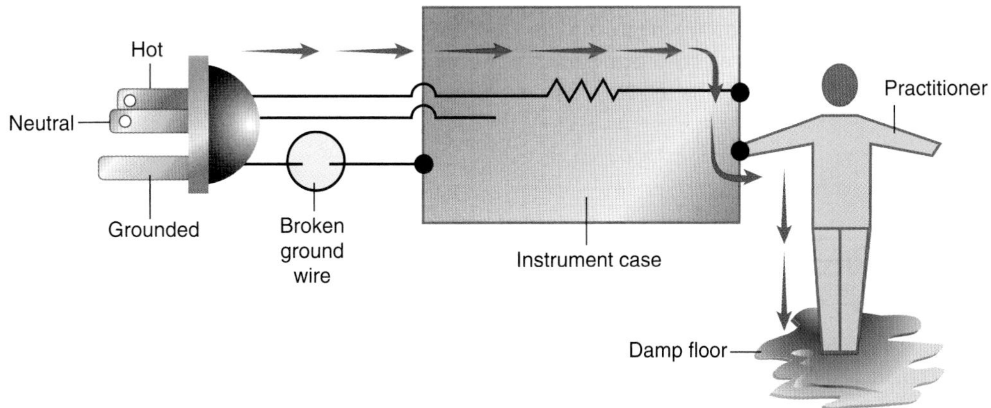

Figure 2-6
Hazard created by broken ground wire.

Table 2-1 ▶▶ Effects of Electrical Shock*

Amperes (A)	Milliamperes (mA)	Microamperes (μA)	Effects
Applied To Skin (Macroshock)			
6 or more	>6000	>6,000,000	Sustained myocardial contraction followed by normal rhythm; temporary respiratory paralysis; burns, if small area of contact
0.1 to 3	100-3000	100,000	Ventricular fibrillation; respiratory center intact
0.050	50	50,000	Pain; fainting; exhaustion; mechanical injury; heart and respiratory function intact
0.016	16	16,000	"Let go" current; muscle contraction
0.001	1	1000	Threshold of perception; tingling
Applied to Myocardium (Microshock)			
0.001	0.1	100	Ventricular fibrillation

*Physiologic effects of AC shocks applied for 1 second to the trunk or directly to the myocardium. Duration of exposure and current pathway are major determinants of human response to electrical shock.

Do Not Ground the Patient. The primary purpose of electrical safety measures is to prevent the patient from becoming part of an electrical circuit. If a patient is grounded, he or she can become part of the circuit. In such cases, patient contact with any source of electricity will cause current flow through the body.

Figure 2-7 shows how a microshock to the heart can occur when a patient is electrically grounded. Current flows normally from the line plug to an electrical amplifier and transducer. However, in this case the equipment line power cord has a broken ground wire. Thus low-ampere leakage current seeks out an alternative low potential ground. In this case, the leakage current finds its ground by flowing through a saline-filled vascular catheter and into the patient's heart. The result is a microshock, with possible ventricular fibrillation and death.

Eliminating the electrical path to ground from the patient would have prevented the current flow. Therefore ensuring that the patient is isolated from electrical ground is the best way to minimize shock hazards.

Unfortunately, isolating the patient from ground is not always easy. For example, older electrocardiogram (ECG) equipment typically uses the right leg lead as a patient ground. Because many patients on continuous ECG monitors have other electrical apparatus in contact with the body, this is an obvious hazard. Modern ECG monitors overcome this problem by the use of isolation transformers, which isolate the patient from ground.

In addition to ECG equipment, other patient devices, such as indwelling catheters, may close an electrical circuit by providing a conducting pathway to ground. For this reason, all devices connected to a patient should be checked to ensure that the patient is in fact isolated from electrical ground.

Ground Electrical Equipment Near the Patient. All electrical equipment (e.g., lights, electrical beds, motors, monitoring or therapeutic instruments) should be connected to grounded outlets with three-wire cords. In these cases, the third (ground) wire prevents the dangerous buildup of voltage that can occur on the metal frames of some electrical equipment.

Modern electrical devices used in hospitals are designed so that their frames are grounded but their connections to the patient are not. In this manner, all electrical devices in reach of the patient are grounded,

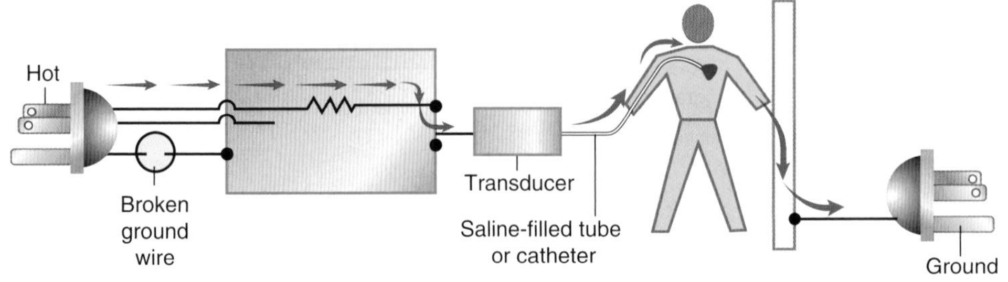

Figure 2-7

Possible microshock hazard caused by patient grounding.

but the patient remains isolated from ground. Unfortunately, because the ground wire is simply a protection device and not part of the main circuit, equipment will continue to operate normally even if the ground wire is broken. Therefore all electrical equipment, particularly those devices used with electrically susceptible patients, must be checked for appropriate grounding on a regular basis by a qualified electrical expert.

Precautions for Electrically Sensitive Patients. Additional precautions should be followed with electrically susceptible patients.

Avoid Contact With Transcutaneous Conductors. Avoid contacting a bare pacemaker wire or the conducting part of a catheter while simultaneously touching any metal object with the other hand, because this action, as shown in Figure 2-8, can close the circuit between a defective instrument with a current leak and a grounded patient. This hazard can be minimized by covering exposed pacemaker wires with a nonconducting material such as plastic or rubber.

Connect All Electrical Equipment to a Common Ground. If two pieces of electrical equipment have different grounds, a malfunction in one can produce a voltage difference between the two instruments and thus current flow. For this reason, all electrical devices used on a microshock-sensitive patient must be connected to wall outlets with a common ground. In most modern hospitals, patient areas have a special electrical panel to which all electrical equipment should be connected. These panels usually provide the safest grounding for equipment and should be used exclusively for connecting equipment to a power source. They are also connected to back-up sources should electrical failure occur.

Great advances in healthcare have occurred because of modern electrical equipment, and the use of such devices will undoubtedly increase. The benefits of these devices can be achieved without shock hazards if clinicians make sure that equipment is properly grounded and that the patient is isolated from hazardous current paths. Keeping track of equipment ground wires, noting frayed wires or other obvious electrical hazards, and strictly following the key precautions just described can help prevent shock hazards.

Fire Hazards

For a fire to start, three conditions must exist: (1) flammable material must be present, (2) oxygen must be present, and (3) the flammable material must be heated to or above its ignition temperature. When all three conditions are present, a fire will start. Conversely, removing any one of the conditions can stop a fire from starting or extinguish it once it has begun. Fire is

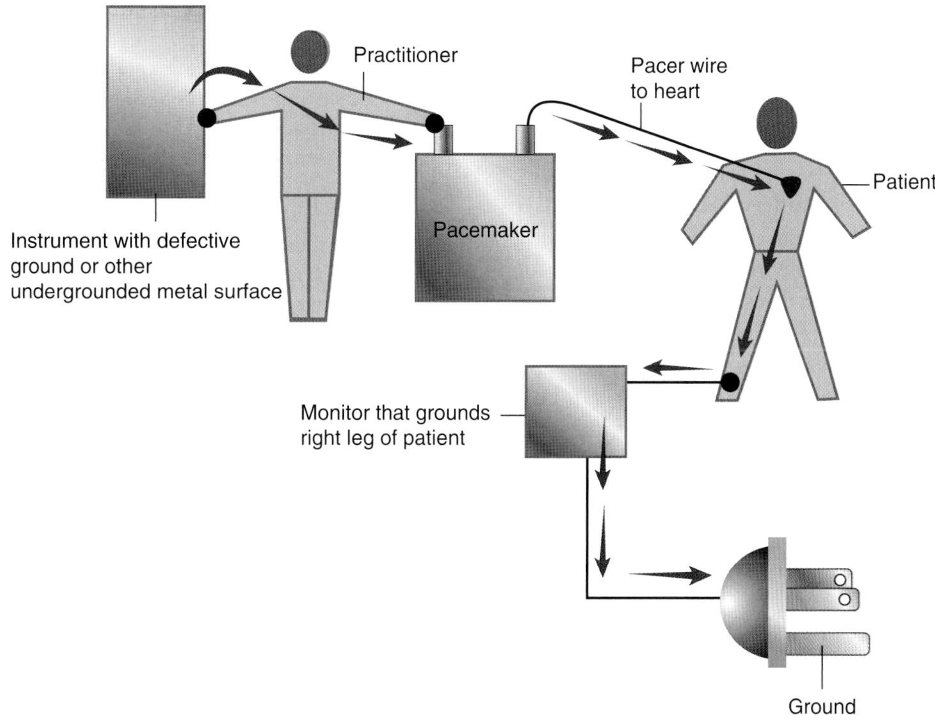

Figure 2-8

Possible hazard through use of certain cardiac monitors and a pacemaker.

a real and serious hazard around respiratory care patients using supplemental oxygen. Although oxygen is **nonflammable**, it greatly accelerates the rate of combustion. Burning speed increases with an increase in either the concentrations or partial pressure of oxygen.

To minimize the fire hazards associated with oxygen use, any flammable material should be removed from the vicinity of use. Flammable materials include cotton, wool, polyester fabrics and bed clothing, paper materials, plastics, and certain lotions or salves such as petroleum jelly. This is particularly important whenever oxygen enclosures, such as tents or Croupettes, are used.

Clinicians must make certain that ignition sources, such as cigarettes, are not allowed in rooms where oxygen is in use. In addition, great care must be taken to avoid the use of electrical equipment capable of generating high-energy sparks, such as exposed switches. All appliances that transmit house current should be kept out of oxygen enclosures.

A frequent source of worry is the presence of static electrical sparks generated by friction. Even in the presence of high oxygen concentrations, the overall hazard from static sparks with the materials in common use is very low. In general, solitary static sparks do not have sufficient heat energy to raise common materials to their flash points. The minimal risk that may be present can be further reduced by maintaining high relative humidity (greater than 60%).

▶ COMMUNICATION

Communication is a dynamic process involving sharing of information, meanings, and rules among people. Communication has five basic components: sender, message, channel, receiver, and feedback (Figure 2-9).

The sender is the individual or group transmitting the message. The message is the information or attitude communicated by the sender. Messages may be verbal or nonverbal. Verbal messages are voiced or written. Examples of different kinds of messages are discussions, letters, and memos. Nonverbal communication is any communication that is not voiced or written. Nonverbal communication includes gesture, facial expression, eye movements and contact, voice tone, space, and touch.

The **channel** of communication is the method used to transmit messages. The most common channels are those involving sight and hearing, such as written and oral messages. However, other sensory input, such as touch, may be used with or for visual or auditory communication. In addition, communication channels may be formal (memos or letters) or informal (conversation).

MINI CLINI

Communication

PROBLEM

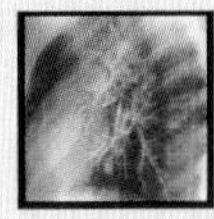

A 73-year-old man with chronic obstructive pulmonary disease (COPD) is admitted to the emergency department for acute shortness of breath that is not relieved with rest. The patient has been admitted more than eight times during the past year for various respiratory problems. The patient's doctor thinks that this episode may reflect a worsening of his disease process and orders an inhaled bronchodilator via a metered-dose inhaler. After the RT enters the room and introduces herself, the patient becomes quite defensive, stating that he doesn't need any assistance with treatments and that she should just leave the medication in the room. The RT has not treated the patient in the past and has to decide how to respond to the patient's request.

DISCUSSION

Although this patient exhibited reluctance in allowing the RT to administer the therapy, enough verbal and perhaps nonverbal communication (message) was expressed by the patient (sender) for the RT (receiver) to determine a plan of action. Because human communication is a two-way process, the RT serves an active role for further messages and interaction. This is a key concept for the RT to master because it helps in identifying a patient's problems, evaluating progress, and recommending further respiratory care. The RT must recognize that when an individual verbalizes disagreement with a treatment order and exhibits defensive behavior, the RT must attempt to understand what the patient is saying and not overreact. For example, the RT could try to put the patient at ease by demonstrating good eye contact, gesturing effectively, and maintaining a safe distance from the patient when talking. The RT should seek feedback from the patient to ensure that the message was understood as it was intended. In this situation, it may be appropriate for the RT to observe the patient self-administer the medication, as long as the patient can demonstrate proper technique. Allowing the patient to actively participate in medical care when feasible may serve to help him maintain a sense of control over his disease process.

The receiver is the target of the communication. Depending on the message being transmitted, the receiver can be an individual or a group.

The last essential part of communication is **feedback**. Human communication is a two-way process in which the receiver serves an active role. Feedback from receiver to sender allows change of later messages and the interaction as a whole. Because of feedback, both sender and receiver are influenced by communication interactions.

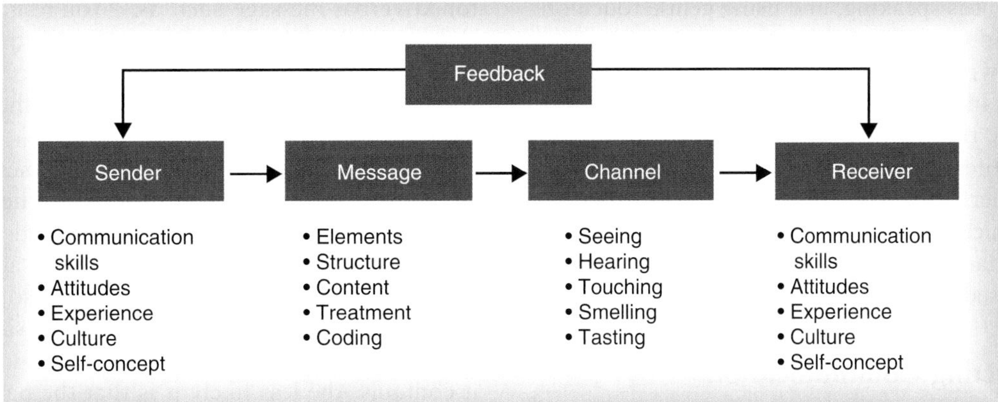

Figure 2-9

Elements of human communication. See text on p. 28 for details.

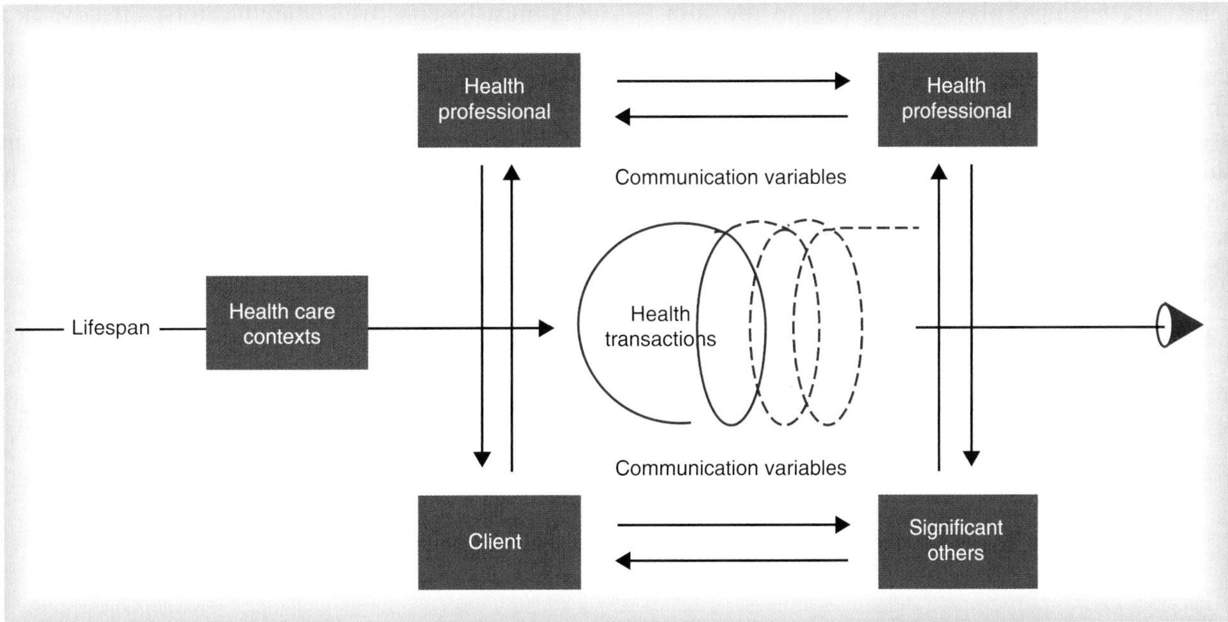

Figure 2-10

Health communication model. *(Modified from Northouse PG, Northouse LL: Health communication: a handbook for health professionals, Englewood Cliffs, NJ, 1985, Prentice-Hall.)*

Health Communication

Health communication is a subset of human communication. Health communication takes place in a healthcare context and involves interactions among healthcare professionals, their patients or clients, and significant others (Figure 2-10).

Communication has a tremendous effect on healthcare. After all, healthcare is a great human undertaking, with social relationships at its core. Communication influences the evaluation and treatment of patients, including their willingness to comply, their satisfaction, and even their emotional well-being. Communication also affects the morale and performance of healthcare professionals.

Communication skills play a key role in the RT's ability to identify a patient's problem, to evaluate the patient's progress, and to make recommendations for respiratory care. Treatment outcomes may also be affected by communication. The RT, through effective communication, can help patients cope with hospitalization and obtain maximal benefit from their care.

RTs can communicate empathy to their patients through the use of key words and eye contact and the proper use of touch. Communicating empathy to your patients is an effective way of letting them know you truly care for their well-being and are willing to provide respiratory care that will help their breathing. Techniques involve asking the patient about his or her breathing on a regular basis, making good eye contact when the patient is speaking, and using gentle touch on the arm or hand when comforting the patient.

Most RTs work in complex healthcare organizations, which can affect morale and job performance. In this setting, the quality of communication among healthcare professionals has a major effect on job satisfaction, performance, and productivity. Indeed, failed communication is the primary source of conflict in complex organizations. Conflict and conflict resolution are discussed on page 33.

Factors Affecting Communication

Many factors affect health communication (Figure 2-11). The uniquely human or "internal" qualities of sender and receiver (including their prior experiences, attitudes, values, cultural backgrounds, and self-concepts and feelings) play a large role in the communication process. Consider, for example, how prior difficulties with uncaring RTs might affect the way in which a patient with chronic obstructive pulmonary disease (COPD) communicates with you. In addition, consider the interaction between a physician who is committed to extending an elderly patient's life, and the family, who values relief of the patient's suffering above all else. Finally, consider an RT with strong negative feelings against homosexuals being assigned to treat a patient with AIDS who happens to be gay.

In general, the verbal and nonverbal components of communication should enhance and reinforce each other. For example, the RT who combines a compassionate-toned verbal message such as, "You're going to be all right now," with a confirming touch of the hand is sending a much stronger message to the anxious patient than the message provided by either component alone.

Finally, both the complexity of the message and the channel of communication used affect the outcomes of health communication. A communicated message consists of more than just content. A message's elements, structure, treatment, and coding can also affect how it is received and interpreted. Consider the simple example of a written patient consent form. The more "legalese" it contains, the less likely it is that the patient will pay attention to its meaning.

Effective Health Communication

RTs must be effective communicators. Effective health communication occurs when the intent or purpose of the interaction is achieved. Several key purposes of health communication are summarized in Box 2-1.

The RT must consider the roles involved, the message, the channel, and the appropriate feedback to help achieve these purposes when communicating.

Roles

In terms of role, the RT may be primarily the sender or the receiver. For example, when the RT is teaching a patient how to perform a lung function test, the RT's role of sender is paramount. On the other hand, when

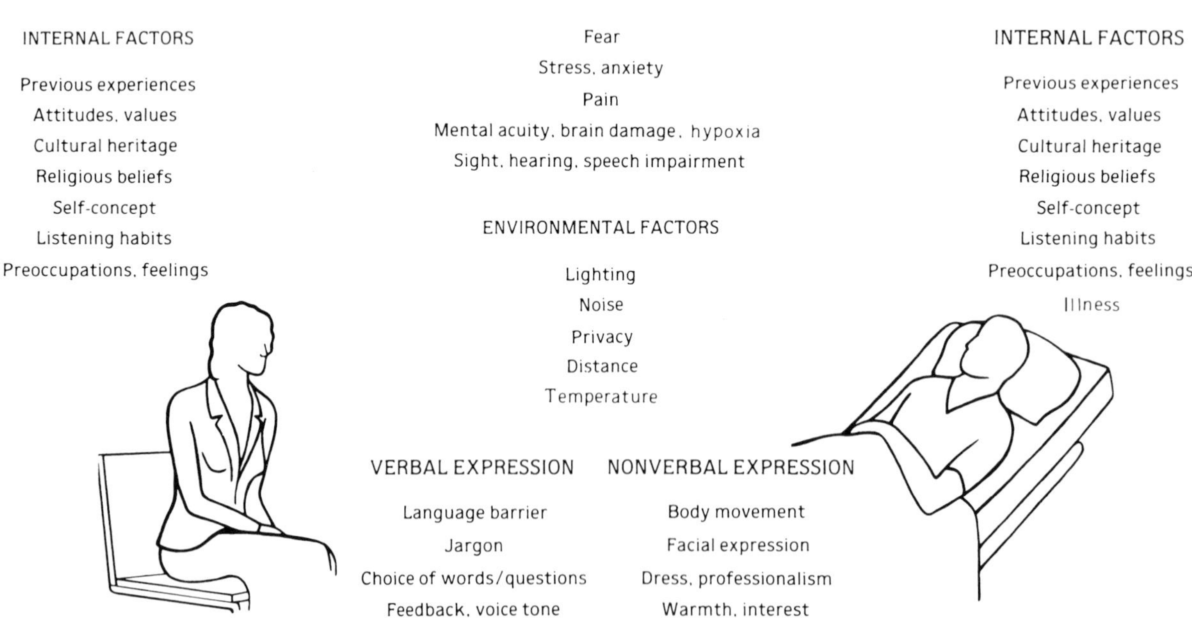

Figure 2-11

Factors influencing communication. *(Modified from Wilkins RL, Sheldon RL, Krider SJ: Clinical assessment in respiratory care, ed 4, St Louis, 2000, Mosby.)*

Box 2-1 • Basic Purposes of Health Communication

- To establish rapport with another individual, such as a colleague, a patient, or a member of the patient's family
- To obtain information, such as during a patient interview
- To relay pertinent information, as when charting the results of a patient's treatment
- To give instructions, as when teaching a patient how to perform a lung function test
- To persuade others to take action, as when attempting to convince a patient to quit smoking

the RT is interviewing a patient to obtain information, the RT's role as receiver is most important.

Message and Channel

In terms of the message and channel, charting the results of a patient's treatment (to inform other health professionals) requires formality, objectivity, brevity, accuracy, and consistency in the use of medical jargon. Obviously, this type of message or channel would not be used to establish rapport with a patient. Instead, a less formal channel would be used; jargon would be avoided; and feelings and feedback, both verbal and nonverbal, would be emphasized.

Feedback

The central role played by feedback is evident in all of the listed purposes of health communication. For example, when instructing a patient to perform a lung function test, it is only by judging the patient's understanding and actual performance that the RT can assess the effectiveness of the teaching effort. Likewise, the feedback received by an RT while trying to establish rapport with a patient's family indicates the success of that effort and can provide clues as to how to improve the relationship.

Improving Communication Skills

To enhance your ability to communicate effectively, focus on improving sending, receiving, and feedback skills. In addition, identify and overcome common barriers to effective communication.

The Practitioner as Sender

Your effectiveness as a sender of messages can be improved in several ways. These suggestions may be applied to the clinical setting as follows.

Share information rather than telling. Health professionals often provide information in an authoritative manner by telling colleagues or patients what to do or say. This approach can cause defensiveness and lead to uncooperative behavior. Conversely, sharing information creates an atmosphere of cooperation and trust.

Seek to relate to people rather than control them. This is of particular significance during communication with patients. Healthcare professionals often attempt to control patients. Few people like to be controlled. Patients feel much more important if they are treated as an equal partner in the relationship. For example, explaining procedures to patients and asking their permission to proceed is a way to make them feel a part of the decision making regarding their care.

Value disagreement as much as agreement. People will often disagree with what you say. When individuals express disagreement, make an attempt to understand what they are saying and do not become defensive. Be prepared for disagreement and be open to the input of others.

Eliminate threatening behavior. The first step in effective communication is to put your listeners at ease. If you appear to be a threat to patients or staff, they will resist communication.

Use effective nonverbal communication techniques. The nonverbal communication that you use is just as important as what you say. Nonverbal techniques include good eye contact, effective gesturing, distance between yourself and others when talking, facial expressions, and voice tone. It is important that your nonverbal communication matches what you are actually saying. For instance, if you are trying to gain the rapport of a patient but do not look him or her in the eye, your communication will not be as effective. Your eye contact and facial expressions help convey what you are trying to say and cause your words to have more impact.

The Practitioner as Receiver and Listener

Receiver skills are just as important as sender skills. Messages sent are of no value unless they are received as intended. This requires active listening on the part of the receiver. Learning to listen requires a strong commitment and great effort. Following a few simple principles can help improve your listening skills.

Work at listening. Listening is often a difficult process. It takes great effort to hear what others are saying. Focus your attention on the speaker and on the message.

Stop talking. Practice silent listening and avoid interrupting the speaker during an interaction. Interrupting the patient is a sure way to diminish effective communication.

Resist distractions. It is easy to be distracted by surrounding noises and conversations. This is particularly true in a busy environment such as a hospital. When you are listening, try to tune out other distractions and give your full attention to the person who is speaking.

Keep your mind open; be objective. Being open-minded is often difficult. All people have their own opinions that may influence what they hear. Try to be objective in your listening so you treat everyone fairly.

Hear the speaker out before making an evaluation. Do not just listen to the first few words of the speaker. This is a common mistake made by listeners. Often, listeners hear the first sentence and tune out the rest, assuming that they know what is being said. It is important to listen to the entire message; otherwise, you may miss important information.

Judge content, not delivery. Many people have difficulty communicating what they are trying to say. When listening to others, listen to what they are saying rather than to their style of delivery.

Maintain composure; control emotions. Allowing emotions, such as anger or anxiety, to distort your understanding or drawing conclusions before a speaker completes his or her thoughts or arguments is a common error in listening.

Active listening is a key component in healthcare communication. Many of the messages being sent are vital to patient care. If you do not listen effectively, important information may be lost and the care of your patients jeopardized.

Providing Feedback

To enhance communication with others, effective feedback needs to be provided. Examples of effective feedback mechanisms in oral communication with patients include attending, paraphrasing, requesting clarification, perception checking, and reflecting feelings.

MINI CLINI

Different Perceptions of the Problem

PROBLEM

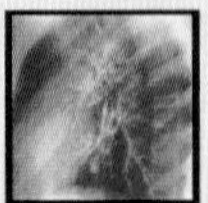

Dr. Thompson became angry at Carol, the pulmonary function technologist, because a test he ordered was not completed by a certain time. Dr. Thompson needed the results of the test before leaving for a conference. He left angrily, without telling Carol why he had needed the test results early.

DISCUSSION

Carol did not see the importance of the problem and assumed that Dr. Thompson would eventually "cool off." In this case, the individual perceptions of the problem were different, and the problem was not resolved.

Attending. **Attending** involves the use of gestures and posture that communicates one's attentiveness. Attending also involves confirming remarks such as, "I see what you mean."

Paraphrasing. Paraphrasing, or repeating the other's response in one's own words, is a technique useful in confirming that understanding is taking place between the parties involved in the interaction. However, overuse of paraphrasing can be irritating.

Requesting clarification. Requesting clarification begins with an admission of misunderstanding on the part of the listener, with the intent being to better understand the message through restating or using alternative examples or illustrations. Overuse of this technique, as with paraphrasing, can hamper effective communication, especially if it is used in a condescending or patronizing manner. Thus requests for clarification should be used only when truly necessary and always be nonjudgmental in nature.

Perception checking. Perception checking involves confirming or disproving the more subtle components of a communication interaction, such as messages that are implied but not stated. As an example, the RT might sense that a patient is unsure of the need for a treatment. In this case, the RT might check this perception by saying, "You don't seem to be sure that you need this treatment. Is that correct?" Of course, by verifying or disproving this perception, both the professional and patient will come to understand each other better.

Reflecting feelings. Reflecting feelings involves the use of statements as "verbal mirrors" to better determine the emotions of the other party. Nonjudgmental statements such as, "You seem to be anxious about (this situation)," provide the opportunity for patients to express and reflect on their emotions and can help them confirm or deny their true feelings.

Minimizing Barriers to Communication

There are many potential barriers to effective communication. The skillful communicator will try to identify and eliminate or minimize the influence of these barriers in all interactions. By minimizing the influence of these barriers, the sender can help ensure that the message will be received as intended. Key barriers to effective communication are detailed below.

Use of symbols or words that have different meanings. Words and symbols (including nonverbal communication) can mean different things to different people. These differences in meaning derive from differences in the background or culture between sender and receiver and the context of the communication. For example, RTs often use the letters "COPD" to refer to patients with chronic obstructive lung disease caused by long-term smoking. Patients may hear the letters "COPD" used in reference to them and be confused about the meaning and interpret COPD to mean a fatal lung disease. Never assume that the patient has the same understanding as you in the interpretation of commonly used symbols or phrases.

Different value systems. Everyone has his or her own value system, and many people do not recognize the values held by others. A large difference between the values held by individuals can interfere with communication. For instance, a clinical supervisor may inform her students of the penalties for being late with clinical assignments. If a student does not value timeliness, he or she may not take seriously what is being said.

Different perceptions of the problem. Problems exist in all organizations. Different individuals perceive these problems in different ways. These perceptual differences often cause a lack of understanding among individuals, which impairs communication.

Emphasis on status. A hierarchy of positions and power exists in most healthcare organizations. If superiority is emphasized by those of higher status, communication can be stifled. Everyone has experienced interactions with professionals who make it clear who is in charge. Emphasis on status can be a barrier to communication not only among health professionals but also between health professionals and their patients.

Conflict of interest. Many people are affected by decisions made in healthcare organizations. If people are afraid that a decision will take away their advantage or invade their territory, they may try to block communication. An example might be a staff member who is unwilling to share expertise with students. This person may feel that a student is invading his or her territory.

Lack of acceptance of differences in points of view, feelings, values, or purposes. Most of us are aware that people have different opinions, feelings, and values. These differences can thwart effective communication. To overcome this barrier, the effective communicator allows others to express their differences. Encouraging individuals to communicate their feelings and points of view is a benefit to all. Most of us think we are always correct. Accepting input from others promotes growth and cooperation.

Feelings of personal insecurity. It is difficult for people to admit feelings of inadequacy. Those who are insecure will not offer information for fear that they appear ignorant, or they may be defensive when criticized, thus blocking clear communication. Many of us have worked with individuals who are insecure, thereby realizing the difficulty in communicating with them.

In summary, to become an effective communicator, you should first identify the purpose of each communication interaction and your role in it. You should also use specific sending, receiving, and feedback skills in each interaction. Last, you should try to minimize any identified barriers to communication with patients or peers, to ensure that messages are received as intended.

Conflict and Conflict Resolution

Conflict is sharp disagreement or opposition among people's interests, ideas, or values. Because no two people are exactly alike in their backgrounds or attitudes, conflict can be found in every organization.

Healthcare professionals experience a great deal of conflict in their jobs. Rapid changes occurring in healthcare have made everyone's jobs more complex and often more stressful. Because conflict is inevitable, all healthcare professionals must be able to recognize its sources and help resolve or manage its effect on people and on the organization.

Sources of Conflict

The first step in conflict management is to identify its potential sources. The four primary sources of conflict in organizations are (1) poor communication, (2) structural problems, (3) personal behavior, and (4) role conflict.

Poor communication. Poor communication is the primary source of conflict in organizations. The previously discussed barriers to communication are all potential sources of conflict. For example, if a supervisor is not willing to accept different points of view for dealing with a difficult patient, an argument may occur. The importance of good communication cannot be overemphasized.

Structural problems. The structure of the organization itself can increase the likelihood of conflict. Conflict tends to grow as the size of an organization increases. Conflict is also greater in organizations whose employees are given less control over their work and in organizations where certain individuals or groups have excessive power. Structural sources of conflict are the most rigid and are often impossible to control.

Personal behavior. Personal behavior factors are a major source of conflict in organizations. Different personalities, attitudes, and behavioral traits create the possibility of great disagreement among healthcare professionals and between healthcare professionals and patients.

Role conflict. Role conflict is the experience of being pulled in several directions by individuals who have different expectations of a person's job functions. For example, a clinical supervisor is often expected to function both as a staff member and as a student supervisor. Trying to fill both roles simultaneously can cause stress and create interpersonal conflict.

Conflict Resolution

Conflict resolution or management is the process by which people control and channel disagreements within an organization. There are five basic strategies for handling conflict: (1) competing, (2) accommodating,

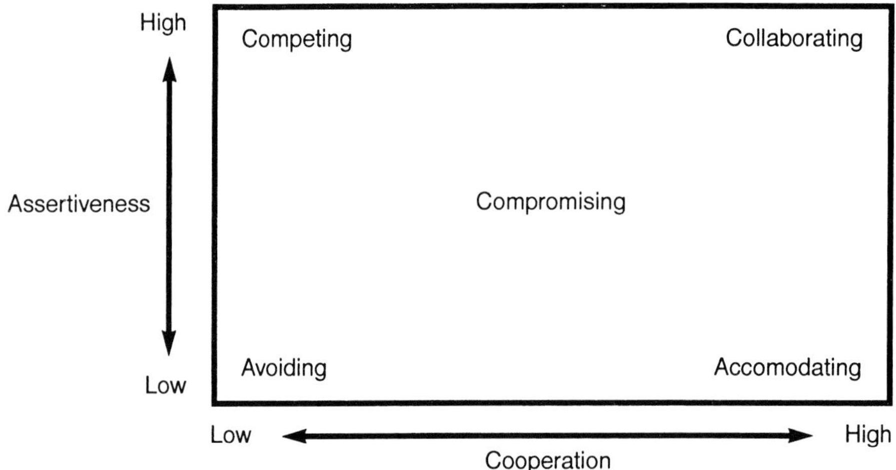

Figure 2-12

Methods of conflict resolution. *(From Marriner A: Managing conflict: comparing strategies and their use, Nurs Manag 13:29, 1982.)*

(3) avoiding, (4) collaborating, and (5) compromising. Figure 2-12 compares these strategies on the dimensions of cooperativeness and assertiveness.

Competing. Competing is an assertive and uncooperative conflict resolution strategy. Competing is a power-oriented method of resolving conflict. For example, the supervisor who uses rank or other forces to attempt to win is using the competing strategy. This strategy may be useful when an unpopular decision must be made or when one must stand up for his or her rights. However, because it often causes others to clam up and feel inferior, competing should be used cautiously.

Accommodating. Accommodating is the opposite of competing. Accommodating is unassertive and cooperative. When people accommodate others involved in conflict, they neglect their own needs to meet the needs of the other party. Accommodation is a useful strategy when it is essential to maintain harmony in the environment. Accommodation is also appropriate when an issue is much more important to one party or the other in a dispute.

Avoiding. Avoiding is both an unassertive and an uncooperative conflict resolution strategy. In avoiding conflict, one or both parties decide not to pursue their concerns. Avoidance may be appropriate if there is no possibility of meeting one's goals. In addition, if one or both of the parties are hostile, avoidance may be a good strategy, at least initially. However, too much avoidance can leave important issues unattended or unresolved.

Collaborating. As a conflict resolution strategy, collaborating is the opposite of avoiding. Collaborating is assertive and cooperative. In collaboration, the involved parties try to find mutually satisfying solutions to their conflict. Collaboration usually takes more time than other methods and cannot be applied when the involved parties harbor strong negative feelings about each other.

Compromising. Compromising is a middle-ground strategy that combines assertiveness and cooperation. Those who compromise give up more than those who compete but give up less than those who accommodate. Compromise is best used when a quick resolution is needed that both parties can live with. However, because both parties often feel they are losing, compromise should not be used exclusively.

Deciding which type of conflict resolution strategy to use requires knowledge of the context, the specific underlying problem(s), and the desires of the involved parties.

▶ RECORDKEEPING

A medical record or chart presents a written picture of occurrences and situations pertaining to a patient throughout his or her stay in a healthcare institution. Medical records are the property of the institution and are strictly confidential. This means that the content of a patient's medical records is not to be read or discussed by anyone except those directly caring for the patient in a hospital or medical-care facility.

Because the law requires that a record be kept of the patient's care, a patient's chart is also a legal document. For this reason, charting or recordkeeping must be done so that it is meaningful for days, months, or years, in case it must be used in court.

Components of a Traditional Medical Record

Each healthcare facility has its own specification for the medical records it keeps. Although the forms

MINI CLINI

Legal Aspects of Recordkeeping

PROBLEM

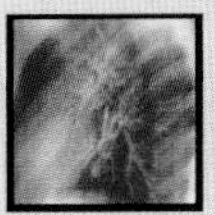

A patient was given a respiratory treatment by a respiratory care student who then forgot to chart that the therapy was given. The student reasoned that because he did not observe any adverse effects during or immediately following the treatment and, furthermore, he knew that the treatment was in fact given, not documenting the treatment in the medical record this one time would be acceptable. What are the problems associated with this student's judgment and subsequent actions?

DISCUSSION

The medical record is a legal document intended to identify types of care given to a patient and to serve as a source of information to the physician, RT (including the student), and other healthcare providers in developing an individualized plan of care. It further serves as a tool for evaluating the effectiveness in reaching the goals of therapy. Hospitals and other healthcare agencies critically evaluate the medical records of patients to maintain high-quality patient care. Failure to document care rendered, such as a respiratory treatment, hinders the process of providing high-quality care in several ways.

First, information that is important to the physician and other caregivers interested in the patient's respiratory status will be missing. In this situation, although the student observed a lack of response by the patient during and immediately following the treatment, a delayed effect could still have taken place. Consequently, the physician or RT would have difficulty in establishing the cause of a condition change in the patient related to the respiratory treatment. From a legal perspective, patient care not documented may be viewed as care not rendered, thus making the hospital or institution vulnerable to charges of patient neglect, which would be difficult to defend in a court of law.

themselves vary among institutions, most acute-care medical records share common sections (Box 2-2).

Figure 2-13 provides an example of a weaning flow sheet form for patients undergoing rapid or slow weaning. Flow sheets are designed to briefly report data and to decrease time spent in documentation. Note how a single time entry can include many measurements and how review of a sequence of entries can reveal trends in patient status.

Legal Aspects of Recordkeeping

Legally, documentation of the care given to a patient means that care was given; no documentation means that care was not given. Hospital accreditation agencies critically evaluate the medical records of patients. Again, if the RT does not document care given (i.e.,

Box 2-2 • General Sections Found in a Patient's Medical Record

ADMISSION SHEET
Records pertinent patient information (e.g., name, address, religion, nearest of kin), admitting physician, and admission diagnosis

HISTORY AND PHYSICAL
Records the patient's admitting history and physical examination, as performed by the attending physician or resident

PHYSICIAN'S ORDERS
Records the physician's orders and prescriptions

PROGRESS SHEET
Keeps a continuing account of the patient's progress for the physician

NURSES' NOTES
Describes the nursing care given to the patient, including the patient's complaints (subjective symptoms), the nurses' observations (objective signs), and the patient's response to therapy

MEDICATION RECORD
Notes drugs and IV fluids that are given to the patient

VITAL SIGNS GRAPHIC SHEET
Records the patient's temperature, pulse, respirations, and blood pressure over time

I/O SHEET
Records patient's fluid intake (I) and output (O) over time

LABORATORY SHEET
Summarizes the results of laboratory tests

CONSULTATION SHEET
Records notes by physicians who are called in to examine a patient to make a diagnosis

SURGICAL OR TREATMENT CONSENT
Records the patient's authorization for surgery or treatment

ANESTHESIA AND SURGICAL RECORD
Notes key events before, during, and immediately after surgery

SPECIALIZED THERAPY RECORDS/PROGRESS NOTES
Records specialized treatments or treatment plans and patient progress for various specialized therapeutic services (e.g., respiratory care, physical therapy)

SPECIALIZED FLOW SHEETS
Records measurement made over time during specialized procedures (e.g., mechanical ventilation, kidney dialysis)

Date: ______________ Weaning Day #______ Patient Name: ____________________________

Current Ventilator Settings		Spont. Resp. Mechanics		Pre-wean ABG	Post-wean ABG
Mode		Min. Volume (V_E)	L	pH	pH
Resp. Rate		Rest. Rate		$PaCO_2$	$PaCO_2$
Tidal Volume	mL	Tidal Volume	mL	PaO_2	PaO_2
Peak Pressure	cmH_2O	Max. Insp. Pressure	cmH_2O	HCO_3	HCO_3
FiO_2		Vital Capacity	mL	BE	BE
PEEP	cmH_2O	f/V_t ratio		SaO_2	SaO_2
PSV	cmH_2O	Static Comp.	mL/cmH_2O	PaO_2/FiO_2	PaO_2/FiO_2
AutoPEEP	cmH_2O	Plateau Pressure	cmH_2O	FiO_2	FiO_2

No Spontaneous Mechanics due to: ☐ Hemodynamic instability ☐ ICP ☐ Paralytics ☐ Sedation Other ________________

No Weaning due to: ☐ Hemodynamic instability ☐ ICP ☐ Paralytics ☐ Sedation ☐ Poor Spont Mechs ☐ Other ______________

Weaning Mode Guidelines			**Weaning Guideline**	**Extubation Guidelines**
	Criteria	Objectives	Reduce PSV to 75%, 50%, 25% of initial setting	Pressure Support
Rapid	Vent < 5 days	Vent adjustment Q 30 mins		Rapid PSV < 5 cm H_2O × 2 hrs ⇨ extubate
Slow	Vent > 5 days	Vent adjustment Q 1 hour		Slow PSV < 5 cm H_2O × 4 hrs ⇨ extubate

Time	Duration	PSV Level	PSV/Spont V_t	V_E	RR	HR	SpO_2/ SaO_2	BP	MAP (mmHg)	PEEP	F_IO_2	RCP initials

Total Weaning Time: ____________________ Last successfully weaned PSV level: ______________ cmH_2O

Weaning Failure Guidelines

1. MAP change ≥ 20 mmHg?	Yes	No
2. HR change ≥ 20 bpm?	Yes	No
3. $PaCO_2$ ⇧ by 10 – 20 mmHg and is 10 over pt. projected baseline?	Yes	No
4. PaO_2 ⇩ by 10 – 20 mmHg despite ⇧ FiO_2 to .45?	Yes	No
5. pH < 7.30?	Yes	No
6. RR > 30 – 35 bpm?	Yes	No
7. SpO_2 < 90% on FiO_2 ≥ .50?	Yes	No
8. f/V_t > 105?	Yes	No

Actions

- Successful wean? Yes No (if No, comment) ______________________________
- Extubated? Yes No (if No, comment) ______________________________

Practitioner #1: ____________________________

Practitioner #2: ____________________________

Loma Linda University Medical Center
Loma Linda University Community Medical Center
Department of Respiratory Care

Figure 2-13

Documentation form for fast or slow weaning tolerance. (*From Loma Linda University Medical Center, Loma Linda, California.*)

patient assessment data, interventions, and evaluation of care rendered), the practitioner and the hospital may be accused of patient neglect.

Adequate documentation of care is valuable only in reference to standards and criteria of care. Respiratory care departments, like all departments in healthcare facilities, must generate their own standards of patient care. For each standard, criteria must be outlined so that the adequacy of patient care can be measured. Documentation must reflect these standards.

Practical Aspects of Recordkeeping

Recordkeeping is one of the most significant duties that you perform. Documentation is required for each medication, treatment, or procedure. Accounts of the patient's condition and activities must be charted accurately and in clear terms. Briefness is essential, although a complete account of each patient encounter is needed. The use of standardized terms and abbreviations is acceptable. Documentation of consultations with the attending physician that include the date and time of the conversation is recommended.

In general, accounts of care and the patient's condition are hand-printed or written. In some institutions, computerized patient information systems also facilitate data entry by selection from menus of choices or direct typing (see Chapter 6). In either case you must document only what is—not an interpretation or a judgment. Assessments of data must be clearly within one's professional domain. When a practitioner cannot interpret the data obtained, he or she should state so in the record and contact another professional for advice or referral and document the referral in the patient's medical record. Other general rules for medical recordkeeping are listed in Box 2-3. Each institution, in addition to these general rules, has its own additional policies governing medical recordkeeping.

Box 2-3 • General Rules for Medical Recordkeeping

- Entries on the patient's chart should be printed or handwritten. After completing the account, sign the chart with one initial and your last name and your title (CRT, RRT, LRT, Resp Care Student; e.g., S. Smith, CRT). Institutional policy may require that supervisory personnel countersign student entries.
- Do not use ditto marks.
- Do not erase. Erasures provide reason for question if the chart is used later in a court of law. If a mistake is made, a single line should be drawn through the mistake and the word "error" printed above it. Then continue your charting in a normal manner.
- Record after completing each task for the patient and sign your name correctly after each entry.
- Be exact in noting the time, effect, and results of all treatments and procedures.
- Chart patient complaints and general behavior. Describe the type, location, onset, and duration of pain. Describe clearly and concisely the character and amount of secretions.
- Leave no blank lines in the charting. Draw a line through the center of an empty line or part of a line. This prevents charting by someone else in an area signed by you.
- Use standard abbreviations.
- Use the present tense. Never use the future tense, as in "Patient to receive treatment after lunch."
- Spell correctly. If you are not sure about the spelling of a word, use a dictionary to look it up.
- Document conversations with the patient or other healthcare providers that you feel are important.

The Problem-Oriented Medical Record

The problem-oriented medical record (**POMR**) is an alternative documentation format used by some healthcare institutions. The POMR contains four basic parts: (1) the database, (2) the problem list, (3) the plan, and (4) the progress notes. The precise forms these records take vary between institutions.

The database contains routine information about the patient, including a general health history, physical examination results, and the results of diagnostic tests.

In the POMR, a problem is something that interferes with a patient's physical or psychological health or ability to function. The patient's problems are identified and listed, based on the information provided by the database. The list of problems is dynamic; new problems are added as they develop and other problems are removed as they are resolved.

The POMR progress notes contain the findings (subjective and objective data), assessment, plans, and orders of the doctors, nurses, and other practitioners involved in the care of the patient. The format used is often referred to as **SOAP**. Figure 2-14 shows a representative SOAP form for respiratory care progress notes. Box 2-4 provides an example of a SOAP entry. Table 2-2 provides a partial listing of common objective data gathered by RTs and examples of applicable assessments and plans. In many institutions, all caregivers chart on the same form, using the SOAP format.

Subjective →	Objective →	Assessment →	Plan →
	Vital signs: RR ___ HR ___ BP ___ Temp. ___ On antipyretic agent? ☐ Yes ☐ No Chest assessment: Insp. ___ Palp. ___ Perc. ___ Ausc. ___		PRESENT PLAN
Anterior R L Posterior L R	Radiography ___ Bedside spir.: PEFR $\bar{a}$ ___ $\bar{p}$ ___ Tx SVC ___ FVC ___ NIF ___		PLAN MODIFICATIONS
Pt. name	Cough: ☐ Strong ☐ Weak Sputum production: ☐ Yes ☐ No Sputum char. ___		
Age / Male / Female Date / Time Admitting diagnosis	ABG: pH ___ $PaCO_2$ ___ HCO_3^- ___ PaO_2 ___ SaO_2 ___ SpO_2 ___ Neg. O_2 transport factors ___		
Therapist Hospital	Other: ___		

Respiratory Assessment Flow Chart

Figure 2-14. Example of a SOAP Form for Respiratory Care Progress Notes

Respiratory care flow sheet. *(From Des Jardins T, Burton GG: Case studies to accompany clinical manifestations and assessment of respiratory disease, St Louis, 2002, Mosby.)*

Box 2-4 • Example of SOAP Entry

6/29/02

PROBLEM 1

Pneumonia

SUBJECTIVE

"My chest hurts when I take a deep breath."

OBJECTIVE

Awake; alert; oriented to time, place, and person; sitting upright in bed with arms leaning over the bedside stand; pale, dry skin; respirations 26 breaths/min and shallow; pulse 98 beats/min, regular and faint to palpation; blood pressure 112/68 mm Hg, left arm, sitting position; body temperature is 101° F; bronchial breath sounds in lower posterior lung fields; occasionally expectorating small volumes of mucopurulent sputum.

ASSESSMENT

Pneumonia continues

PLAN

Therapeutic: Assist with coughing and deep breathing at least every 2 hours; postural drainage and percussion every 4 hours; assist with ambulation as per physician orders and patient tolerance.
Diagnostic: Continue to monitor lung sounds before and after each treatment.
Education: Teach to cough and deep breathe and evaluate return demonstration.

Table 2-2 ▶▶ Common Objective Data, Assessments, and Plans

Objective Data	Assessment	Plan
Airways		
Wheezing	Bronchospasm	Bronchodilator Tx
Inspiratory stridor	Laryngeal edema	Cool mist/racemic epinephrine
Coarse crackles	Secretions in large airways	Bronchial hygiene Tx
Cough		
Weak cough	Poor secretion clearance	Bronchial hygiene Tx, lung volume expansion therapy
Secretions		
Amount: >30 mL/24 hr	Excessive secretions	Bronchial hygiene Tx
Yellow/opaque sputum	Acute airway infection	Treat underlying cause
Frothy secretions	Pulmonary edema	Treat underlying cause (e.g., CHF)
Lung Parenchyma		
Dull percussion note, bronchial breath sounds	Infiltrates, atelectasis, consolidation	Lung expansion Tx, oxygen Tx
Opacity on chest x-ray film	Infiltrates, atelectasis, consolidation	Lung expansion Tx, oxygen Tx
Pleural Space		
Increased resonance to percussion	Pneumothorax	Evacuate air*/lung expansion Tx
Decreased resonance	Pleural effusion, pneumonia	Evacuate fluid*/lung expansion Tx
Thorax		
Barrel chest	Airtrapping (hyperinflation)	Treat underlying cause (e.g., asthma)
Posterior/lateral curvature of spine	Kyphoscoliosis	Lung expansion Tx
Arterial Blood Gases		
↓pH, ↑$Paco_2$, ↔HCO_3^-	Acute ventilatory failure	Mechanical ventilation*
↔pH, ↑$Paco_2$, ↑HCO_3^-	Chronic ventilatory failure	Low flow oxygen, bronchial hygiene Tx
↑pH, ↔$Paco_2$, ↑HCO_3^-	Metabolic alkalosis	Hypokalemia: give potassium* Hypochloremia: give chloride*
↓pH, ↔$Paco_2$, ↓HCO_3^-	Metabolic acidosis	Lactic acidosis: give oxygen
Oxygenation		
Pao_2 <60 mm Hg	Moderate hypoxemia	Oxygen Tx and treat underlying cause
Pao_2 <40 mm Hg	Severe hypoxemia	Oxygen Tx, positive airway pressure Tx

Modified from Des Jardins T, Burton GG, Tietsort J: Respiratory care case studies: the therapist-driven protocol approach, St Louis, 1997, Mosby.
*Physician ordered.

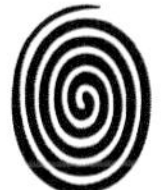

RULE OF THUMB

Charting Progress Notes Using the SOAP Format

SOAP stands for: Subjective, Objective, Assessment, Plan

- *Subjective* information obtained from the patient, his or her relatives, or a similar source
- *Objective* information based on caregivers' observations of the patient, the physical examination, or diagnostic or laboratory tests such as arterial blood gases or pulmonary function tests
- *Assessment,* which refers to the analysis of the patient's problem
- *Plan* of action to be taken to resolve the problem

KEY POINTS

- Begin patient ambulation as soon as a patient is physiologically stable and free of severe pain.
- A microshock is a small, imperceptible current (less than 1 mA) that enters the body through external wires or catheters; microshocks can cause ventricular fibrillation.
- To avoid electrical hazards, never ground the patient and always ground equipment; avoid contact with transcutaneous conductors on electrically sensitive patients.
- Fire hazards can be minimized by removing flammable materials and ignition sources from areas where oxygen is in use.

Continued

KEY POINTS—cont'd

- Communication skills play a key role in the ability to identify a patient's problems, to evaluate the patient's progress, to make recommendations for respiratory care, and to achieve desired patient outcomes.
- Individuals' prior experiences, attitudes, values, cultural backgrounds, self-concepts, and feelings play a large role in the communication process.
- To enhance communication ability, focus on improving sending, receiving, and feedback skills; in addition, be able to identify and overcome common barriers to effective communication.
- One of five basic strategies can be used for handling conflict: competing, accommodating, avoiding, collaborating, and compromising; choosing the best strategy requires knowledge of the context, the specific underlying problem(s), and the desires of the involved parties.
- A medical record is a confidential document that summarizes the care received by a patient; legally, a failure to document care means that care was not given.
- Following accepted standards, each medication, treatment, or procedure provided to the patient, including his or her condition and response to therapy, must be documented in accurate and clear terms.
- When entering notes in a POMR, use a SOAP format (Subjective, Objective, Assessment, Plan).

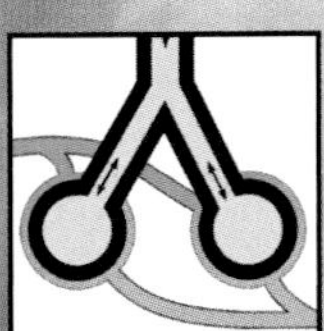

CHAPTER 3

Principles of Infection Control

†Rick Meyer and Craig L. Scanlan

In This Chapter You Will Learn:

- Why infection control is an important fundamental in respiratory care
- How infection spreads between patients and among healthcare personnel
- How to select the best method for processing reusable equipment
- How and when to pasteurize respiratory care equipment
- How to select and apply chemical disinfectants for processing respiratory care equipment
- How to select a method and prepare and sterilize respiratory care equipment
- How to monitor the effectiveness of sterilization procedures
- How to apply barrier and isolation procedures
- How to protect yourself and your patients from infection
- What role you play in bacteriologic surveillance and hospital epidemiology

Chapter Outline

Key Terms

airborne precautions
antiseptics
autogenous infection
bactericidal
bacteriological surveillance
CDC Level
cohorting
colonization
contact precautions
disinfection
droplet nuclei
droplet precautions
fomites
high-efficiency particulate air/aerosol (HEPA) filters

Continued

†Deceased.

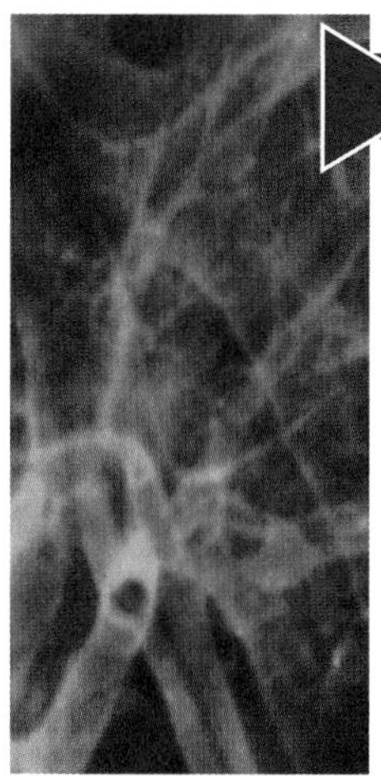

Key Terms—cont'd

high-level disinfectants
immunocompromised host
intermediate-level disinfectants
isolation precautions
latex
low-level disinfectants
multidrug-resistant (MDR) organisms
National Institute for Occupational Safety and Health (NIOSH)
nosocomial infections
opportunistic
OSHA
pasteurization
ppm
processing indicators
respirators
sporicidal
standard precautions
sterilization
surveillance
transmission-based precautions
ventilator-associated pneumonia
vegetative bacteria
virucidal
virulence

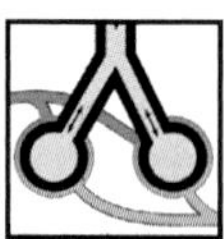

Approximately 10% of all patients admitted to an intensive care unit acquire a nosocomial infection during their hospitalization.[1] In addition, approximately 25% of patients undergoing mechanical ventilation develop pneumonia as a complication and approximately 30% of these patients will die as a result of lung infection.[1] It costs billions of dollars per year to treat hospital-acquired (**nosocomial**) infections, and billions more are spent making up for the lost economic productivity resulting from these illnesses.

Historically, respiratory care equipment and procedures have been identified as a major cause of nosocomial infections. However, as the sophistication of respiratory care procedures has evolved, so too has our understanding of infection control. The plastic industry now makes sterilized, prepackaged, single-patient-use, and inexpensive respiratory equipment, which has caused infections associated with respiratory care equipment to decrease significantly.

Despite this progress, respiratory therapists (RTs) must always be on guard to protect their patients against infection. Moreover, health professionals are now giving increased attention to handwashing and protecting themselves against infection, especially those infections transmitted by blood and body fluids.

Protecting our patients and ourselves against infections requires strict adherence to infection control procedures. Infection control procedures aim to eliminate the sources of infectious agents, create barriers to their transmission, and monitor and evaluate the effectiveness of control.

Infection control is a major and ongoing responsibility of all RTs. To fulfill this responsibility, the RT must be able to select and apply a variety of infection control procedures. This chapter provides the foundation needed to assume these important responsibilities.

SPREAD OF INFECTION

Infection occurs when a pathogen is able to overcome the barriers of the host. Some pathogens only promote an immune response, whereas other pathogens attach themselves and replicate inside the host tissues, causing major clinical manifestations. Three elements must be present for an infection to spread: (1) a source of pathogens, (2) a susceptible host, and (3) a route of transmission[2,3] (Figure 3-1).

Source

In the hospital, the primary sources of pathogens are either people (patients, personnel, or visitors) or contaminated objects (e.g., equipment, linen, medications). A person may have an acute disease, may be in the incubation period of the disease, or may simply be colonized by pathogens, without symptoms. People may also serve as their own source of infection, via endogenous flora. This latter process is called **autogenous infection.**

Microorganisms differ in their relative **virulence.** Highly virulent organisms need be present only in small

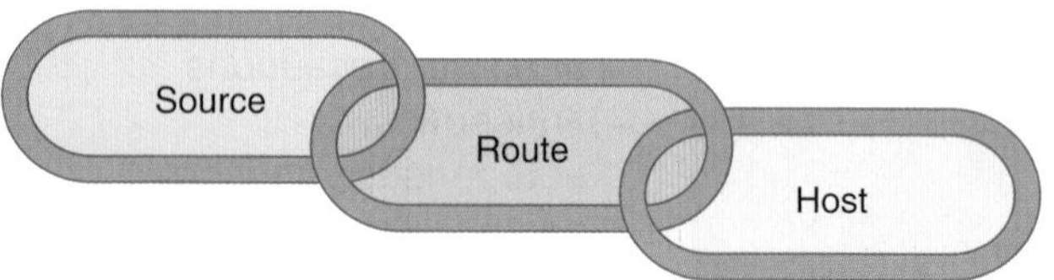

Figure 3-1
Elements that must be present for infection to spread.

numbers to cause infection. On the other hand, microorganisms of low virulence must exist in large numbers to cause infection or be present in an **immunocompromised host.**

Most cases of nosocomial pneumonia are bacterial in origin.[4] Gram-negative bacilli, including *Pseudomonas aeruginosa, Enterobacter species, Klebsiella pneumoniae, Escherichia coli, Serratia marcescens,* and *Proteus species,* are the most common offenders. However, the incidence of nosocomial pneumonias caused by gram-positive cocci, such as *Staphylococcus aureus* (especially the methicillin-resistant strains) and *Streptococcus pneumoniae,* is increasing. In addition, many bacterial pneumonias can be linked to the presence of two or more different organisms at the same time.

Box 3-1 • Conditions Associated With Oropharyngeal Colonization by Gram-Negative Bacilli

- Acidosis
- Azotemia
- Chronic alcohol abuse
- Coma
- Diabetes mellitus
- Endotracheal intubation
- Hypotension
- Nasogastric tube
- Neutralization of gastric secretions
- Respiratory distress syndrome
- Underlying respiratory disease

Host

The mere presence of microorganisms in a host is called **colonization.** Infection results when microorganisms cause cell or tissue damage. Whether a host actually becomes infected depends on both the organism's virulence and the host's resistance.

Resistance to infection varies greatly. Some individuals may be immune to infection or able to resist colonization. Others exposed to the same organism may simply carry it but show no symptoms. Still others may develop clinical disease. Persons with diabetes mellitus, lymphoma, leukemia, neoplasia, or uremia are particularly prone to developing infection, as are those treated with certain antimicrobials, corticosteroids, irradiation, or immunosuppressive agents. Age, chronic disease, shock, coma, traumatic injury, or surgical procedures also increase susceptibility to infection.

The high incidence of nosocomial gram-negative bacterial pneumonias is associated with factors that promote colonization of the pharynx with these organisms. Gram-negative colonization dramatically increases in critically ill patients, which increases the likelihood of developing these pneumonias (Box 3-1). Nosocomial pneumonias indicate failure to prevent cross-transmission of infecting organisms, and the transmitted infecting organisms are normally more virulent and more antibiotic resistant, which is simply a result of some severely infected individuals common to hospital populations.

Most nosocomial pneumonias occur in surgical patients, especially those who have had chest or abdominal procedures. In these patients, normal swallowing and clearance mechanisms are impaired, allowing bacteria to enter and remain in the lower respiratory tract. Intubation, anesthesia, surgical pain, and use of narcotics and sedatives further impair host defenses.

The risk of pneumonia is not the same for all surgical patients. Patients at highest risk include the elderly, the severely obese, those with chronic obstructive pulmonary disease (COPD) or a history of smoking, and those having an artificial airway in place for long periods.[5]

Patients with an artificial tracheal airway are at high risk for nosocomial pneumonia for several reasons. Typically, patients requiring prolonged intubation already have one or more factors predisposing to infection, such as severe COPD. Another risk factor may be increased upper airway colonization with gram-negative bacteria. Moreover, because the tube bypasses the normal protective mechanisms of the upper airway, bacteria have easy access to the lower respiratory tract. Last, handling of these tubes increases the likelihood of cross contamination, particularly during suctioning.

Some pneumonias occur primarily in immunocompromised hosts. Doctors may purposefully suppress a patient's immune response with drugs, as in organ transplant cases. Alternatively, immunosuppression may be a result of underlying disease, as with acquired immunodeficiency syndrome (AIDS). Immunocompromised hosts, regardless of cause, are highly susceptible to infections, especially those caused by **opportunistic** bacteria, fungi, or viruses.

Transmission Route

There are five major routes for transmission of pathogens: contact, droplet, airborne, common vehicle, and vectorborne. For some organisms, transmission may occur via multiple routes. For example, the human immunodeficiency virus (HIV) can spread either by direct contact (sexual intercourse) or by indirect contact with a contaminated inanimate object (needles). Table 3-1 provides examples of the common transmission routes for selected microorganisms.[2]

Table 3-1 ▶▶ Routes of Infectious Disease Transmission

Mode	Type	Examples
Contact	Direct	Hepatitis A Venereal disease HIV *Staphylococcus* Enteric bacteria
	Indirect	*Pseudomonas aeruginosa* Enteric bacteria Hepatitis B and C HIV
Droplet		*Haemophilus influenzae* (type B) pneumonia and epiglottitis *Neisseria meningitidis* pneumonia Diphtheria Pertussis Streptococcal pneumonia Influenza Mumps Rubella Adenovirus
Vehicle	Waterborne	Shigellosis Cholera
	Foodborne	Salmonellosis Hepatitis A
Airborne	Aerosols	Legionellosis
	Droplet nuclei	Tuberculosis Varicella Measles
	Dust	Histoplasmosis
Vectorborne	Ticks and mites	Rickettsia, Lyme disease
	Mosquitoes	Malaria
	Fleas	Bubonic plague

Contact Transmission

Contact transmission is the most important and most common route for spread of nosocomial infections. Contact transmission may occur either directly or indirectly.

Direct contact transmission occurs via direct body-surface-to-body-surface transfer between a host and an infected or colonized person. This occurs by mucus-to-mucus contact (intercourse/kissing) or contacting the skin of a diseased individual or carrier. Sexually transmitted diseases, such as syphilis, spread this way. In the hospital, infection spreads by this route when a worker with contaminated hands touches a patient, changes a dressing, or performs other procedures requiring direct contact. This is the most common route for transmitting *Staphylococcus* and many of the enteric bacterial infections. Direct contact also can occur between patients.

Indirect contact involves contact between a susceptible host and a contaminated object. We call objects that transmit infectious agents **fomites**. Common fomites include clothing, dressings, instruments, and equipment that serve as a contact vehicle for the spread of infection. For example, indirect patient contact with a contaminated nebulizer is a common route for spread of *P. aeruginosa*. Contaminated needles are another common fomite for indirect contact transmission, especially for hepatitis and HIV.

Droplet Transmission

Droplet transmission occurs when individuals discharge large contaminated liquid droplets into the air by coughing, sneezing, or talking. These droplets can travel only short distances, probably no more than approximately 3 feet. However, if they come into contact with a nearby person, they can easily deposit on that host's conjunctivae, nasal mucosa, or mouth. Pneumonia and epiglottitis caused by *Haemophilus influenzae* are transmitted in this manner, as are influenza and rubella. Procedures such as suctioning or bronchoscopy also can generate large contaminated droplets. Because these large droplets do not remain suspended in the air, special air handling procedures are of little help in preventing droplet transmission.

Airborne Transmission

Airborne transmission occurs by the spread of contaminated **droplet nuclei** or dust particles. Droplet nuclei are the residue of evaporated water droplets. Because of their small size (≤ 5 μm), droplet nuclei can remain suspended in the air for long periods. Dust or dirt particles, usually greater than 50 mm in size, act as minute fomites. Tuberculosis (TB) and measles are good examples of infections transmitted via droplet nuclei. Most fungal infections are transmitted via the airborne route on dust particles. Organisms transmitted via the airborne route can be widely dispersed by air currents before contacting a susceptible host. This is why special air handling and ventilation procedures are needed to combat airborne transmission.

Common Vehicle Transmission

Vehicle transmission occurs via host exposure to pathogens in contaminated food or water. Salmonellosis and hepatitis A are examples of foodborne infections. Shigellosis and cholera are examples of waterborne infections.

Vectorborne Transmission

Vectorborne transmission occurs when an animal, especially an insect, transfers an infectious agent from one host to another. Vectorborne transmissions, such as malaria (mosquito vector), are of major concern in tropical countries. Although vectorborne transmissions are also responsible for many serious infections in United States, they are of little significance in hospital-acquired infections.

Spread of Infection to the Lungs

Infectious agents can gain entry into the lungs via three mechanisms. First, a patient may aspirate contaminated oropharyngeal or gastric secretions. Second, a patient may inhale liquid droplets, droplet nuclei, or dust particles containing pathogens. Third, the pathogen may spread to the lungs from a distant site of infection via the blood (hematogenous spread).

Of these three routes, aspiration probably causes most nosocomial bacterial pneumonias. Aspiration occurs most often in persons who cannot swallow normally. These patients usually have one or more of the following risk factors: decreased consciousness, dysphagia, or a nasogastric tube. Endoscopic procedures and bronchoscopy increase the risk of aspiration.

▶ INFECTION CONTROL STRATEGIES

Infection control aims to break the chain of events causing the spread of infection. To do so, one can decrease host susceptibility, eliminate the source of pathogens, and interrupt the transmission routes.

Decreasing Host Susceptibility

Decreasing host susceptibility to infection is the most difficult and least feasible approach to infection control. Hospital efforts to decrease host susceptibility focus mainly on employee immunization. Depending on the relative risks involved, hospital personnel may be immunized against influenza, hepatitis, diphtheria, tetanus, and sometimes, TB (with bacille Calmette-Guérin [BCG] vaccine).

RULE OF THUMB

All RTs, because of frequent contact with contaminated blood and body fluids, should undergo immunization for hepatitis.

Eliminating the Source of Pathogens

It is impossible to eliminate all pathogens from any working environment. Nonetheless, standard infection control procedures always make efforts to eliminate pathogens. Infection control procedures designed to remove environmental pathogens fall into two major categories: general sanitation measures and specialized equipment processing.

If the environment is dirty, all other infection control efforts will be futile. General sanitation measures help keep the overall environment clean. General sanitation aims to reduce the number of pathogens to a safe level. This is achieved through sanitary laundry management,

MINI CLINI

Spread of Infection

PROBLEM

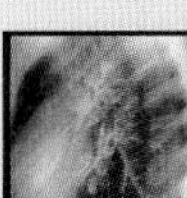

You work in the neonatal intensive care unit of a large urban hospital. Over the last 2 days, a number of infants in the unit have developed serious *Staphylococcus aureus* infections. Identify the most likely source and route of transmission and suggest ways to prevent spread of this serious infection.

DISCUSSION

In hospitals, *S. aureus* commonly colonizes the skin of both health professionals and visitors. Neonates are also very susceptible hosts because of their poor immunity. Staphylococcus infections spread mainly via direct contact transmission (see Table 3-1). To help prevent the spread of this infection to the newborn infants, we should try to disrupt the transmission route. Rigorous handwashing and use of gloves will help. In addition, we might isolate the infected babies from those not infected.

food preparation, and housekeeping. Environmental control of the air (using specialized ventilation systems) and water complement these efforts.

The goal of specialized equipment processing is to decontaminate equipment capable of spreading infection. Equipment processing involves cleaning, disinfection, and sterilization.

Interrupting Routes of Transmission

General sanitation measures and equipment processing have limits. To prevent the spread of infections, healthcare personnel also must take measures to stop infection. The three major approaches used to prevent the spread of infection in healthcare agencies are (1) specialized equipment handling procedures, (2) barrier/isolation precautions, and (3) the use of single-patient-use disposable equipment.

▶ EQUIPMENT PROCESSING

Cleaning

Cleaning is the first step in all equipment processing. Cleaning involves removing dirt and organic material from equipment, usually by washing[6] (Table 3-2). Failure to properly clean equipment can render all subsequent processing efforts ineffective.

Cleaning should take place in a designated facility with separate dirty and clean areas. Before being cleaned, the equipment should be disassembled and examined for worn parts. Complete disassembly helps ensure good exposure to the cleaning agent. After disassembly, the parts should be placed in a clean basin filled with hot water and soap or detergent.

Because water alone cannot dissolve organic matter, soaps or detergents should be used to clean equipment. Soaps act by lowering surface tension and forming an emulsion with organic matter. Unfortunately, soaps have little **bactericidal** activity and work poorly in hard water. Detergents work in hard water but can be inactivated by proteins. Most detergents are weakly bactericidal, but only against gram-positive bacteria. Some commercial products combine a germicide with a detergent, thus providing the dual action of cleaning and disinfection.

Automated cleaning systems can be used as an alternative to manual washing. These devices, which are similar to kitchen dishwashers, use several cycles to wash and rinse equipment. Some automated systems also provide either a pasteurization or chemical disinfection cycle.

Many devices, including most electrical equipment, cannot be immersed in water. In these cases, the surface of the device should be disinfected using a 70% ethyl alcohol solution or the equivalent.

All equipment should be carefully rinsed and dried after cleaning. Good rinsing removes any soap or detergent residues, which can irritate human tissue. These residues also may impair subsequent disinfection or sterilization efforts.

Drying is important because residual water dilutes and alters the pH of disinfectant solutions. In addition, if equipment is to be gas sterilized, residual water may combine with ethylene oxide (EtO) gas to form ethylene glycol, which can be toxic to human tissue. Drying is important even if no further disinfection occurs because a humid environment encourages bacterial growth.

When clean equipment is reassembled before additional processing, care must be taken to avoid recontamination. To avoid recontamination of the processed equipment, it should first be moved to the clean area, then a vigorous hand scrub should be performed before reassembly. Ideally, reassembly should occur in a laminar flow hood that helps prevent recontamination. Although careful cleaning will remove most pathogens from the equipment, it cannot eliminate the risk of infection. For this reason, most equipment must undergo either disinfection or sterilization.

Table 3-2 ▶▶ Equipment Processing Definitions

Term	Definition
Cleaning	The removal of all foreign material (e.g., soil, organic material) from objects
Disinfection (general term)	The inactivation of most pathogenic organisms, excluding spores
Disinfection, low level	The inactivation of most bacteria, some viruses, and fungi, without destruction of resistant microorganisms such as *Mycobacterium tuberculosis* or bacterial spores
Disinfection, intermediate level	The inactivation of all vegetative bacteria, most viruses, most fungi, and *M. tuberculosis,* without destruction of bacterial spores
Disinfection, high level	The inactivation of all microorganisms, *except* bacterial spores (with sufficient exposure times, spores may also be destroyed)
Sterilization	The complete destruction of all forms of microbial life

Disinfection

Disinfection destroys the vegetative form of pathogenic organisms but cannot kill bacterial spores. Disinfection can involve either physical or chemical methods. The most common physical method of disinfection is pasteurization; many chemical methods are used to disinfect respiratory care equipment.

Pasteurization

Pasteurization is the application of moist heat at temperatures below the boiling point of water. Like heat sterilization, pasteurization coagulates cell proteins. However, pasteurization temperatures are too low to kill spores.

The major pathogenic spore-forming bacteria are *Bacillus anthracis*, *Clostridium tetani*, *Clostridium perfringens*, and *Clostridium botulinum*. Although all these bacteria are capable of causing disease, none is a common source of nosocomial infection. For this reason, pasteurization is an efficient and cost-effective way to disinfect respiratory care equipment.[6]

Respiratory care equipment is pasteurized using the batch method. In this process, previously cleaned equipment is immersed in a water bath at 70° C for 30 minutes. This kills all **vegetative bacteria** and most viruses, including HIV.[4] Most equipment can easily withstand these conditions without damage.

The major problem with pasteurization is not the process itself, but the difficulty in avoiding equipment recontamination following immersion. Special filtered dryers, used with laminar flow assembly hoods and scrupulous aseptic technique, can help minimize recontamination.

Chemical Disinfection

Chemical disinfection involves application of chemical solutions to contaminated surfaces or equipment. For disinfection, the equipment is immersed in the solution. After a set time, the equipment is removed, rinsed in sterile water (to remove toxic residues), and then dried. Equipment must be handled aseptically, with sterile gloves and towels, to prevent recontamination during subsequent reassembly and packaging.

Table 3-3 provides a summary of the common chemical disinfectants and their activity against various pathogens. The **CDC Level** specified in Table 3-3 is established by the U.S. Centers for Disease Control and Prevention. What follows is a brief discussion of the most common agents in each category (i.e., low-, intermediate-, and high-level disinfectants).

Low-Level Disinfectants. Low-level disinfectants kill most bacteria and some viruses and fungi but do not eliminate resistant microorganisms such as Mycobacterium tuberculosis, spores, and nonlipid viruses. Agents in this category include acetic acid and the quaternary ammonium compounds.

Acetic acid (found in white vinegar) has been used for disinfection in both the hospital and home. A 1.25% solution, equal to one part white vinegar (5% acetic acid) to three parts water, kills most vegetative bacteria, including *P. aeruginosa*.[7]

Quaternary ammonium compounds, or "quats," are cationic detergents containing ammonium ions.[8] Modern third-generation quats are fungicidal, bactericidal, and virucidal against lipophilic viruses, but not **sporicidal** or tuberculocidal. Quats can retain their disinfectant activity for up to 2 weeks if kept undiluted. However, contact with soaps, anionic detergents, organic material, or hard water all reduce quat activity. Hospital use of quats is limited mainly to surface disinfection of countertops and devices that cannot be soaked (e.g., ventilators). Although quats are popular in the home care setting, most agencies recommend true high-level disinfectants for home infection control.

Intermediate-Level Disinfectants. Intermediate-level disinfectants kill all vegetative bacteria and fungi but

Table 3-3 ▶▶ Common Chemical Disinfectants

Disinfectant	CDC Level	Gram-positive Bacteria	Gram-negative Bacteria	Tubercle Bacillus	Spores	Viruses*	Fungi
Acetic acid	Low	+	+	?	?	?	±
Quaternary ammoniums	Low	+	±	0	0	±	+
Alcohols	Intermediate	+	+	+	0	±	±
Iodophors	Intermediate	+	+	+		±	+
Phenolics	Intermediate	+	+	+	±	±	+
Glutaraldehyde	High	+	+	+	±	+	+
Hydrogen peroxide	High	+	+	+	±	+	+
Peracetic acid	High	+	+	+	+	+	+
Sodium hypochlorite	High	+	+	+	±	+	+

+, Good; ±, fair; ≈, poor; ?, unknown; 0, little or none.
*Viral activity depends on whether the virus is lipophilic or hydrophilic.

have variable activity against spores and certain viruses. Agents in this category include the alcohols, phenolics, and iodophors.

Water solutions of both 70% ethyl and 90% isopropyl alcohol are good intermediate-level disinfectants. Alcohols are inactivated by protein and can damage rubber, plastics, and the shellac mounting of lensed instruments. Alcohol wipes are a good choice for disinfecting small surfaces, such as medication vial tops. Alcohols are also useful as surface disinfectants for stethoscopes, ventilators, manual ventilation bags, and resuscitation mannequins. However, alcohols cannot sterilize medical or surgical materials.

Phenolics (ortho-phenylphenol and ortho-benzyl-para-chlorophenol) are bactericidal, fungicidal, and tuberculocidal but have variable activity against spores and viruses (see Table 3-3). Phenolics retain their activity in the presence of organic matter and can remain effective on surfaces long after application. Unfortunately, phenolics are absorbed easily by porous material, and the residual disinfectant causes tissue irritation. Phenolics are also associated with neonatal hyperbilirubinemia when used in nurseries. For these reasons, phenolics are generally limited to use as surface disinfectants. Manufacturers also add phenolics to detergents to enhance their germicidal activity.

Iodophors are mixtures of iodine with surface-active organic compounds. The most common iodophor is povidone-iodine (polyvinylpyrrolidone with iodine). Unlike iodine tinctures, iodophors are water soluble, nonstaining, and less irritating to tissue. Iodophors are bactericidal, virucidal, and tuberculocidal (see Table 3-3). However, iodophors have limited sporicidal activity and can require prolonged contact to kill fungi. In low concentrations, iodophors are good antiseptics (chemical germicides formulated for use on skin or tissue).

High-Level Disinfectants. High-level disinfectants can destroy all microorganisms except bacterial spores. Some agents are also sporicidal, given sufficient exposure time. Common high-level chemical disinfectants include glutaraldehyde, stabilized hydrogen peroxide, chlorine (sodium hypochlorite), and peracetic acid.

When 2% glutaraldehyde is alkalized to a pH between 7.5 and 8.5, it can kill vegetative bacteria, *M. tuberculosis,* fungi, and viruses in less than 10 minutes and can kill common spores *(Bacillus* and *Clostridium species)* in 3 hours (see Table 3-3). This sporicidal activity qualifies glutaraldehyde as a true sterilizing agent.

Glutaraldehyde, in addition to its broad-spectrum antimicrobial activity, works well in the presence of organic matter and does not damage metals, lensed instruments, rubber, or plastics. This makes it ideally suited for high-level disinfection or sterilization of endoscopes, respiratory and anesthesia equipment, dialyzers, and spirometry tubing. The minimum exposure time for these applications is 20 minutes. Because of its toxicity and high cost, glutaraldehyde should not be used as a disinfectant for either surfaces or noncritical items.

Once alkaline glutaraldehyde is activated, it can retain activity for up to 28 days. However, age is only one factor determining antimicrobial activity; use conditions, such as dilution and organic stress, also affect disinfectant power. Because repeated use of glutaraldehyde results in significant dilution, concentrations must be monitored regularly. Test strips are available for this purpose. Glutaraldehyde solutions should be discarded after 28 days or when the concentration drops below 1.0%, whichever comes first.

Healthcare workers exposed to glutaraldehyde vapors have reported various forms of tissue inflammation, including epistaxis, rhinitis, and asthma. These problems are most likely when vapor levels exceed the **OSHA**-recommended ceiling of 0.2 **ppm**. Vapor levels can become hazardous when processing occurs in a poorly ventilated room, when the disinfectant spills, or when immersion baths remain open. In addition, direct skin contact with glutaraldehyde solutions may cause dermatitis. Use of improved ventilation, exhaust or fume hoods, tight-fitting lids on immersion baths, and gloves and goggles can help minimize these problems. To protect a patient thoroughly, any equipment disinfected with glutaraldehyde should be rinsed before use. Failure to do so can cause inflammatory mucosal reactions, especially when using invasive devices.

MINI CLINI

Selection of a Disinfectant

PROBLEM

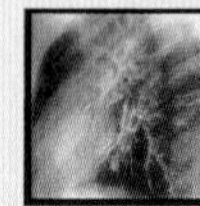

You work in the pulmonary function laboratory of a community hospital. Immediately after performing spirometry on a patient, you learn that he has been admitted and tests positive for pulmonary tuberculosis. You also remember him coughing into the spirometry tubing. You have four more patients scheduled for spirometry testing, beginning in 45 minutes. How should you process the spirometry tubing to prevent transmission of the tuberculosis?

DISCUSSION

Ideally, you would have a back-up set of tubing to deal with this type of problem. If not, you will have to quickly disinfect or sterilize the tubing. Because permanent spirometry tubing is made from heat-liable plastics, you cannot use either steam (damage) or EtO gas (aeration time too long). Instead, you should select a broad-spectrum, quick-acting disinfectant solution that works well in the presence of organic matter and does not damage rubber or plastic. Glutaraldehyde is a good choice, with a minimum exposure time of 20 minutes. A stabilized hydrogen peroxide–based compound or a 1:50 sodium hypochlorite solution might also be considered.

Hydrogen peroxide is a popular wound antiseptic. Recently, stabilized hydrogen peroxide–based compounds have proved themselves as high-level disinfectants (see Table 3-3). At room temperature, a 6% solution is bactericidal, fungicidal, and virucidal in 10 minutes.[4] Sterilization (sporicidal action) occurs in 6 hours at 20° C.[4] Stabilized hydrogen peroxide–based solutions remain active for up to 6 weeks; require no mixing or activation; do not produce harsh fumes; and appear to be safe for use with rubber, plastic, and stainless steel.

Sodium hypochlorite (household bleach) is a fast-acting, inexpensive, broad-spectrum disinfectant. Hypochlorite solutions are stable for up to 1 month when properly stored. Available chlorine levels determine antimicrobial activity. Bleach contains 5.25% sodium hypochlorite, or 52,500 ppm available chlorine. Exposure to a 1:50 dilution (approximately 1000 ppm) for 10 minutes is sufficient to kill vegetative bacteria, bacterial spores, and *M. tuberculosis*.

The CDC recommends a 1:10 dilution of bleach (or an Environmental Protection Agency [EPA]-registered disinfectant) to clean blood spills. Because organic matter inactivates hypochlorites, any contaminated surface should be cleaned before disinfectant application. For decontamination of resuscitation training mannequins, use of at least 500 ppm available chlorine for 10 minutes is recommended. One should avoid mixing any acid solution with bleach, which can result in rapid production of toxic chlorine gas.

Even at low concentrations (0.001% to 0.2%) and in the presence of organic matter, peracetic acid acts rapidly to kill all microorganisms, including spores. The byproducts of peracetic acid (acetic acid, hydrogen peroxide, water, and oxygen) are harmless, and it leaves no residue. Unfortunately, peracetic acid is unstable and corrosive to common metals.[9] A specially formulated 0.35% solution, containing buffers and anticorrosives, has been developed to overcome these problems.[10] This product has excellent sporicidal and tuberculocidal activity and may prove to be a good alternative to glutaraldehyde.

Sterilization

Sterilization is the complete destruction of all forms of microbial life. Both physical and chemical means can achieve sterilization. Physical methods include various forms of heat and ionizing radiation. Chemical methods of sterilization include EtO gas and selected liquid solutions. Table 3-4 compares and contrasts the major methods of sterilization.

For most objects, heat is the quickest and easiest sterilization method.[8] In general, the higher the temperature, the shorter the time needed for sterilization. However, different temperatures and durations are needed to kill various organisms. Common methods of heat sterilization include incineration, dry heat, boiling, and moist heat under pressure (autoclaving).

Incineration, or burning, is used for sterilization only when the object has no further use or is so contaminated that its reuse is prohibited. Dry heat sterilization uses a simple hot-air oven. For items to be sterilized, they are simply placed in the oven for 1 to 2 hours at temperatures between 160° and 180° C. Dry heat is ideal for most glass and metal objects. However, few respiratory care items can withstand this process.

Boiling water at sea level (100° C) kills all vegetative bacteria and most viruses in 30 minutes. However, some spores can withstand boiling for long periods. Thus boiling does not ensure sterilization. Moreover, water boils at lower temperatures at different altitudes, making the process even less effective.

Autoclaving is the application of steam under pressure. Autoclaving is efficient, quick, cheap, clean, and reliable. Unfortunately, most respiratory care equipment is heat labile and can be damaged by autoclaving.

Table 3-4 ▶▶ Comparison of Sterilization Methods

Method	Applicable Equipment	Advantages	Disadvantages
Incineration	Disposables; grossly contaminated articles	Surest method; simple	Limited use; may result in air pollution
Dry heat	Laboratory glassware; metal instruments	Inexpensive; simple; nontoxic	Damages heat-sensitive equipment
Boiling	Metals; heat-resistant plastics	Inexpensive; simple	Time consuming; altitude dependent; may damage some equipment
Autoclave (pressurized steam)	Metal instruments; linens	Inexpensive; fast; nontoxic; prewrapping of items	May damage heat- or moisture-sensitive equipment
Ionizing radiation	Foods; some medical supplies	Fast; effective; prewrapping of items	Expensive; toxic byproducts may be produced
Ethylene oxide	Heat-sensitive items	Effective; prewrapping of items	Time consuming; expensive; toxic residues must be removed by aeration

The higher the temperature and pressure, the shorter the time needed for sterilization. For example, at 15 psi, the temperature of steam is 121° C and full sterilization requires 15 minutes. On the other hand, at 20 psi, steam's temperature increases to 126° C and sterilization takes only 10 minutes. The combination most commonly used for autoclaving is 15 psi at 121° C.

Equipment must be cleaned before autoclaving. Clean equipment is then wrapped in muslin, linen, or paper, all of which steam easily penetrates. Items must be properly packed in the autoclave to ensure exposure. In addition, chamber air must be evacuated before steam is introduced. After sterilization, the packaging prevents recontamination during handling and storage.

Two forms of *ionizing radiation* are used to sterilize medical equipment: x-rays and gamma rays. Although many commercial products are sterilized in this manner, the required equipment and shielding costs are too expensive for hospitals. Moreover, in the dose required for sterilization, ionizing radiation can chemically alter some materials and create toxic byproducts.

Ultraviolet (UV) light is another ionizing source used in infection control. Although UV light kills most bacteria, it poorly penetrates common materials. For this reason, it is not a good choice for equipment disinfection or sterilization. However, UV light is useful in decontaminating the air circulating to or from operating rooms, nurseries, communicable-disease wards, and bacteriologic labs.[11]

Ethylene oxide (EtO) is a colorless, toxic gas and potent sterilizing agent. Because it is active at ambient temperatures and is harmless to rubber and plastics, EtO is a good sterilant for items that cannot be autoclaved. Like steam, EtO penetrates most packaging materials, thereby permitting prewrapping.

Were it not for its many hazards, EtO would be the ideal sterilant.[12] Unfortunately, acute exposure to EtO gas can cause airway inflammation, nausea, diarrhea, headache, dizziness, and even convulsions. Chronic exposure to the gas is associated with respiratory infections, anemia, and altered behavior. Residual EtO left on processed equipment can cause tissue inflammation and hemolysis. When combined with water, EtO forms ethylene glycol, which also can irritate tissues. Other potential problems include carcinogenic, mutagenic, and teratogenic effects. Last, EtO concentrations higher than 3% are explosive.

Safe use of EtO requires special attention to general safety precautions, equipment preparation, and sterilization cycle parameters (Box 3-2). In addition, because of its toxicity, residual EtO must be removed from equipment after sterilization via a process called *aeration*.

Aeration is most important for porous materials, such as plastics or rubber, which retain EtO. Polyvinyl chloride, commonly called PVC, needs the longest aeration time. Other plastics, such as polyethylene and polypropylene, require less aeration time. Nonporous materials such as metal and glass do not absorb EtO and can be used immediately after sterilization.

Box 3-2 • Guidelines For the Safe Use of Ethylene Oxide (EtO)

PRELIMINARY SAFETY PRECAUTIONS

- Ensure proper room ventilation
- Know proper handling, use, storage, labeling, spill, and first-aid procedures
- Locate fire extinguishers, safety showers, and emergency respiratory equipment

EQUIPMENT PREPARATION

- Disassemble, thoroughly clean, and dry all items undergoing sterilization
- Wrap or seal items in muslin, paper, or polyethylene using EtO indicator tape
- Label any items requiring aeration

STERILIZATION PROCESS

- Always wear gloves and goggles when changing EtO cylinders
- Follow sterilizer manufacturer's loading instructions
- Load items loosely (provide space to ensure gas circulation)
- Insert biologic indicator system
- Ensure proper sterilization conditions:
  - Minimum gas concentration of 450 mg/L
  - Relative humidity between 30% and 60%
  - Temperature between 50° and 60° C
  - Time between $1\frac{1}{2}$ and 6 hours
- After cycle is over, open sterilizer and leave area for at least 15 minutes

EQUIPMENT AERATION

- Follow manufacturer's aeration instructions
- Aerate equipment in an approved aeration chamber only
- Transfer sterilized materials to the aerator quickly and with minimal handling
- Ensure proper aeration conditions:
  - 8 hours at 60° C *or*
  - 12 hours at 50° C

MONITORING AND SURVEILLANCE

- Monitor EtO levels periodically per OSHA and JCAHO guidelines:
  - Maximal continuous exposure level is 1 ppm for 8 hours
  - Short-time exposure limit is 5-10 ppm for 15 minutes
- Report adverse symptoms of a patient's treatment immediately

EQUIPMENT HANDLING PROCEDURES

Equipment handling procedures that help prevent the spread of pathogens include maintenance of in-use equipment, processing of reusable equipment, the application of one-patient-use disposables, and fluid and medication precautions.

Maintenance of In-Use Equipment

In-use respiratory care equipment that can spread pathogens includes nebulizers, ventilator circuits, bag-valve-mask devices (BVMs; manual resuscitators), and suction equipment. Oxygen therapy and pulmonary function equipment are also implicated as potential sources of nosocomial infections.

Nebulizers

Large-volume nebulizers are the worst offenders. Contamination occurs via use of nonsterile fluids, entrainment of contaminated air, handling of internal parts, or back-flow of condensate (from the delivery tubing) into the reservoir. Once bacteria are introduced into the reservoir, they can multiply enough within 24 hours to cause infection if nebulized and inhaled.

Small-volume medication nebulizers (SVNs) can also produce bacterial aerosols. SVNs have been associated with nosocomial pneumonia, including Legionnaires' disease, resulting from either contaminated medications or contaminated tap water used to rinse the reservoir. Procedures designed to prevent nebulizers from spreading pathogens appear in Box 3-3.

Box 3-3 • Procedures to Minimize Infection Risk With Nebulizers

LARGE-VOLUME NEBULIZERS AND MIST TENTS

- Always fill nebulizers with sterile distilled water (see the section Fluids and Medications Precautions on p. 56).
- Fill fluid reservoirs immediately before use. Do not add fluid to replenish partially filled reservoirs. If fluid is to be added, discard the remaining old fluid first.
- Drain tubing condensate away from the patient and discard as contaminated waste; do not allow condensate to drain back into reservoir.
- Sterilize or high-level disinfect large-volume nebulizers between patients and after every 24 hours of use on the same patient.
- Use mist-tent nebulizer and reservoirs that have undergone sterilization or high-level disinfection and replace them between patients.
- Do not use large-volume room-air humidifiers that create aerosols unless they can be sterilized or subjected to high-level disinfection at least daily and filled only with sterile water.

SMALL-VOLUME NEBULIZERS (SVNs)

- Between treatments on the same patient, disinfect, rinse with sterile water, or air-dry SVNs.
- Between patients, replace SVNs with sterile or high-level disinfected units.
- Use only sterile fluids for nebulization and dispense these fluids aseptically.
- If using multidose vials, handle, dispense, and store them according to manufacturer's instructions.

Ventilators and Ventilator Circuits

The internal workings of ventilators are not common sources for infection. This is partly a result of the widespread use of **high-efficiency particulate air/aerosol (HEPA) filters**, which have an efficiency rate of 99.97%, and the use of ensheathed suction catheters, which helps reduce endotracheal tube contamination. An inspiratory HEPA filter (placed between the machinery and the external circuit, proximal to any humidifier) can eliminate bacteria from the driving gas and prevent retrograde contamination back into the machine. An expiratory filter using a heated thermistor to prevent condensation performs the same function and still protects the internal ventilator components. Expiratory filters also prevent pathogens from being expelled into the surroundings from the patient's expired air.

The external ventilator circuitry poses the most significant contamination risk, particularly in systems using heated humidifiers. The humidifiers themselves are rarely the problem. Bubble or wick designs produce little or no aerosol, and thus pose minimal infection risk. In addition, heating the humidifier reduces or eliminates growth of most bacterial pathogens. However, because tap or distilled water may harbor heat-resistant pathogens, sterile water should still be used to fill bubble-type humidifiers.

The primary problem stems from contaminated condensate in the inspiratory limb of the ventilator circuit. Most often, the source of this contamination is the patient. Spillage of contaminated condensate into the patient circuit and the patient occurs when moving the tubing or the patient, thereby increasing the risk of autogenous infection. In addition, microorganisms in this condensate can be transmitted to other patients via the hands of the healthcare worker handling the fluid, if he or she is negligent.

One way to address this problem is by reducing or eliminating circuit condensation. This is easily achieved using heated wire circuits or a heat-and-moisture exchanger (HME). Evidence suggests that to prevent bacterial colonization, even if the HME remains free of secretions, the maximal duration it may be used is 96 hours (4 days).[13]

Based on current knowledge, both the CDC and the American Association for Respiratory Care (AARC) developed guidelines addressing ventilator-associated infection control. Box 3-4 provides general procedures for minimizing nosocomial infection associated with ventilator use. Mechanical ventilation exposes the patient to the risk of **ventilator-associated pneumonia** (VAP), and the frequency of circuit changes and its relationship to VAP has been investigated.[14] New evidence shows that changing ventilator circuits every 7 days is safe and keeps them free from bacterial contamination.[15]

VENTILATOR CIRCUIT CHANGES

AARC Clinical Practice Guidelines (Excerpts)*

➤ INDICATIONS

- The decision to change a ventilator circuit should be governed by:
  - Length of time the existing circuit has been in use
  - Type of circuit and humidification device in use
  - Circuit function (presence of a malfunctioning circuit or a circuit that leaks)
  - Appearance of ventilator circuit (circuits that do not appear clean should be replaced)

➤ CONTRAINDICATIONS

- Presence of patient condition that might make tolerance of disconnection hazardous to patient
- Inability to safely and effectively ventilate or maintain patient during the ventilator circuit change
- Absence of a clean and functional circuit to use as a replacement

➤ PRECAUTIONS AND POSSIBLE COMPLICATIONS

- Conditions that may predispose patients to harm during the changing process:
  - Hemodynamic instability
  - Blood gas imbalances
  - Airway obstruction
  - Artificial airway displacement
  - Contamination of patient or staff from exposure to material in circuit
- Failure to adequately support patient during disconnection from the ventilator:
  - Inappropriate or inadequate ventilation
  - Inappropriate or inadequate oxygenation
  - Inappropriate increase in work of breathing
  - Airway obstruction
- Failure to ensure that replacement circuit has been properly disinfected and is operationally sound:
  - Transmission of pathogens to patient and to healthcare personnel
  - Hazards of exposure to residual toxic disinfectants or associated disinfectant byproducts
  - Malfunctioning or suboptimally functioning ventilator or circuit
  - Failure to ensure proper ventilator function with patient reconnection
  - Potential for patient-ventilator disconnection
- Manipulation and disconnection of the ventilator tubing can cause contaminated ventilator condensate to spill into patient's airway, exposing patient to further risk of infection
- Changing circuits more frequently than is necessary may increase the risk of nosocomial pneumonia
- Failure to ensure proper ventilator function before reinstituting mechanical ventilation may endanger patient

➤ ASSESSMENT OF NEED

- To determine the need for ventilator circuit changes, the clinician should assess:
  - The need to limit the transmission of infection (per CDC and/or institutional standards)
  - The need to prevent malfunction and to maintain optimal performance
  - The need to maintain a circuit clean in appearance, as determined by inspection

*For complete guideline see *Respir Care* 39:797, 1994.

Box 3-4 • Procedures to Minimize Infection Risk With Mechanical Ventilators

- Do not routinely sterilize or disinfect the internal workings of ventilators.
- Do not routinely change ventilator circuit more often than every 48 to 72 hours.
- Sterilize or high-level disinfect reusable breathing circuits and humidifiers.
- Periodically drain tubing condensate away from patient and discard.
- Wash hands after draining tubing condensate or handling the fluid.
- Do not place bacterial filters distal to humidifier reservoirs.
- Use sterile water to fill bubble humidifiers.
- Use sterile, distilled, or tap water to fill wick humidifiers.
- Change heat-moisture exchangers (HME) according to manufacturer's recommendation and/or when you observe evidence of gross contamination or mechanical dysfunction.
- Do not routinely change HME breathing circuits while in use.

Bag-Valve-Mask Devices

BVMs are a source for colonizing both the airways of intubated patients and the hands of medical personnel. Obviously, nondisposable BVMs should be sterilized or high-level disinfected between patients. In addition, the exterior surface of any BVM should be cleaned of visible debris and disinfected at least once a day.[16]

Suction Systems

Tracheal suctioning increases the risk of infection. Proper handwashing and gloving help minimize this risk. Although much has been made of the infection control advantages of ensheathed suction systems over open tracheal suction systems, evidence shows neither one to be clearly superior.[4] On the other hand, because they prevent spraying of circuit condensate and secretions into the environment, they reduce endotracheal tube contamination and inhibit the transmission of organisms to healthcare personnel.[3]

To minimize the risk of cross contamination during suctioning with an open system, a fresh, sterile single-use catheter should be used on each patient. In addition, only sterile fluid should be used to remove secretions from the catheter. Last, both the suction collection tubing and collection canister should be changed between patients, except in short-term care units, where only the collection tubing needs to be changed.[4]

Box 3-5 • Procedures to Minimize Infection Risk With Oxygen Therapy Apparatus[4]

- Humidifiers are not needed with flows less than 4 L/min.
- When needed and whenever possible, prefilled, sterile disposable humidifiers should be used.
- With reusable humidifiers, fluid reservoirs should be filled immediately before use with sterile distilled water.
    - Fluid must not be added to replenish partially filled reservoirs. If fluid is to be added, the remaining old fluid must be discarded first.
- The tubing and oxygen delivery device should be changed between patients; prefilled, sterile, disposable humidifiers do not need to be changed between patients in high-use areas such as the recovery room.
- Prefilled, disposable humidifiers can be used safely for up to 30 days.[17]

Oxygen Therapy Apparatus

Oxygen therapy devices pose much less risk than other in-use equipment but are still a potential infection hazard. For example, in-use nondisposable oxygen humidifiers have a contamination rate as high as 33%.[17] Conversely, prefilled, sterile disposable humidifiers present a negligible infection risk.[17,18] Based on this knowledge, procedures that can help prevent oxygen therapy apparatus from spreading pathogens are outlined in Box 3-5.

Pulmonary Function Equipment

The inner parts of pulmonary function testing equipment are not a major source for spread of infection. However, contamination of external tubing, connectors, rebreathing valves, and mouthpieces can occur during testing. These components should be cleaned and subjected to high-level disinfection or sterilization between patients.[4] The common practice of using HEPA filters to isolate the spirometer from the patient makes logical sense but has yet to be proven either effective or necessary in preventing nosocomial infection.[4]

Other Respiratory Care Devices

Use of other respiratory care equipment, including oxygen analyzers, the handheld bedside respirometer, and circuit probes, has been linked with hospital outbreaks of gram-negative bacterial infections.[4] Direct patient-to-patient contact via either the device itself or the contaminated hands of caregivers are the most likely transmission routes. Proper handwashing and sterilization or high-level disinfection of these devices between patients is the way to get control of this problem.

Processing Reusable Equipment

Improperly processed reusable equipment is another potential source for pathogens. General principles for cleaning, disinfection, and sterilization were previously provided. This section provides specific guidelines for processing reusable respiratory care equipment and a special section on bronchoscope disinfection.

Respiratory Care Equipment

Several factors must be considered in selecting a processing method for reusable respiratory care equipment (Box 3-6). First, because the infection potential of equipment varies according to use, devices should be categorized by their infection risk. Medical devices fall into three infection risk categories: critical, semicritical, and noncritical (Table 3-5).

Once a device's risk category is known, its composition must be matched to the resources available for hospital disinfection and sterilization. Noncritical items, such as ventilators, need undergo only low- to intermediate-level disinfection. Semicritical items, or those that directly or indirectly contact mucous membranes, must undergo at least high-level disinfection. Most respiratory care equipment falls into this category. Last, critical items (invasive devices) must undergo true sterilization.

In this manner, each reusable device will undergo the most effective and least costly processing approach available. Box 3-7 provides further guidance on processing reusable respiratory care equipment.

Box 3-6 • Factors to Consider in Processing Reusable Equipment

- Infection risk (critical, semicritical, noncritical)
- Material and equipment configuration
- Available hospital disinfection resources
- Relative cost (both labor and materials)

Bronchoscopes and Endoscopes

RTs often assist the physician during the bronchoscopy. In this capacity, they must ensure proper infection control, including equipment preparation and processing.

As many as one in four endoscopes remain contaminated after cleaning and disinfection.[4] *M. tuberculosis*, atypical mycobacteria, and *P. aeruginosa* are the most common organisms found in contaminated bronchoscopes. Inadequate preliminary cleaning, improper use of disinfectants, and failure to follow recommended procedures contribute to this problem. In addition, flexible bronchoscopes are particularly difficult to disinfect and easy to damage. Box 3-8 outlines the proper procedure for cleaning and disinfecting endoscopes, as promoted by the Association for Professionals in Infection Control and Epidemiology.[19]

Disposable Equipment

An important alternative to continually reprocessing equipment is the use of single-patient-use disposables. In the past, only oxygen therapy devices, suction apparatus, and supply items were disposable. Today,

Table 3-5 ▶▶ Processing of Medical Equipment According to Infection Risk Categories

Category	Description	Examples	Processing
Critical	Devices introduced into the bloodstream or other parts of the body	Surgical devices Intravascular catheters Implants Heart-lung bypass components Dialysis components Bronchoscope forceps/brushes	Sterilization
Semicritical	Devices that directly or indirectly contact mucous membranes	Endoscopes/bronchoscopes Oral, nasal, and tracheal airways Ventilator circuits/humidifiers PFT mouthpieces and tubing Nebulizers and their reservoirs Resuscitation bags Laryngoscope blades/styles Pressure, gas, or temp probes	High-level disinfection
Noncritical	Devices that touch only intact skin or do not contact patient	Face masks Blood pressure cuffs Ventilators	Detergent washing Low- to intermediate-level disinfection

Modified from Chatburn RL: Respir Care 34:98, 1989.

Box 3-7 • Guidelines for Processing Reusable Respiratory Care Equipment

- All reusable respiratory care equipment should undergo low- or intermediate-level disinfection as part of the initial cleaning.
- All reusable breathing circuit components (including tubing and exhalation valves, medication nebulizers and their reservoirs, large-volume nebulizers and their reservoirs, and humidifiers and their reservoirs) should be considered semicritical items.
- Semicritical items should be sterilized between patients; heat-stable items should be autoclaved and heat-liable items should undergo EtO sterilization.
- If sterilization is not feasible, semicritical items should undergo high-level disinfection or pasteurization.
- The inner parts of ventilators need not be routinely sterilized or disinfected between patients.
- Respirometers, oxygen analyzer probes, and other equipment used to monitor multiple patients should not directly touch any part of a ventilator circuit or patient's mucous membranes. Rather, disposable extension pieces and HEPA filters should be used to isolate the device. If the device cannot be isolated from the patient or circuit, it must be sterilized or receive high-level disinfection before use on other patients.
- Once nondisposable resuscitation bags have been used on a patient, they should be sterilized or receive high-level disinfection before use on other patients.

Box 3-8 • Procedure for Cleaning and Disinfecting Endoscopes[19]

- External surfaces, ports, and internal channels are mechanically cleaned with water and a detergent.
- Biopsy forceps and specimen brushes are separated out and sterilized.
- The external surface and all endoscope channels are rinsed and drained.
- Endoscope is immersed in high-level disinfectant.
- Disinfectant solution is perfused through all channels for at least 20 minutes.
- The endoscope and all channels are rinsed with sterile water; if this is not feasible, tap water can be used, followed with an alcohol rinse.
- The endoscope and inner channels are completely dried using clean, forced air.
- The endoscope is stored in a way that prevents recontamination.

MINI CLINI

Selection of Equipment Processing Methods

PROBLEM

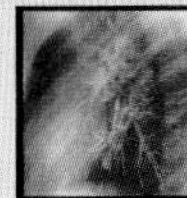

A patient is discharged from the intensive care unit after extubation from mechanical ventilatory support. The following contaminated nondisopsable items are returned to the respiratory care department for processing: the ventilator, the ventilator circuit and humidifier, a resuscitation bag, a mechanical (vane-type) respirometer, and a laryngoscope with blades. Outline what processing you would select for each item and why.

DISCUSSION

First, the circuit, humidifier, and resuscitation bag should be disassembled and cleaned, using a soap or detergent combined with a low- or intermediate-level disinfectant. Because the ventilator, respirometer, and laryngoscope/blades cannot be immersed in water, they should immediately undergo surface disinfection, using 70% ethyl alcohol or the equivalent.

After cleaning and initial disinfection, you should sort the items according to risk category and heat sensitivity. No items from this patient are a critical infection risk. The ventilator circuit, humidifier, resuscitation bag, respirometer, and laryngoscope are semicritical items, whereas the ventilator itself is a noncritical item. The ventilator circuit, humidifier, and resuscitation bag are also plastic and probably heat labile. The respirometer and laryngoscope are heat stable.

When possible, semicritical items should be sterilized between use on patients; the heat-stable items should be autoclaved and heat-labile items should undergo EtO sterilization. The ventilator (a noncritical item) need undergo only low- to intermediate-level surface disinfection (already done). The inner parts of the ventilator need not be sterilized or disinfected between patients.

manufacturers provide a whole range of disposables, including humidifiers, nebulizers, incentive spirometers, ventilator circuits, BVMs, and monitoring transducers.

Three major issues are involved in using disposables: cost, quality, and reuse. Cost issues boil down to straightforward dollar comparisons between purchasing and processing reusables versus stocking and distributing disposables. Good comparisons take into account both direct and indirect costs (e.g., personnel, inventory, maintenance) and risk factors. Most recent findings support the cost-effectiveness of disposables over reusables in respiratory care.

Cost savings notwithstanding, many quality issues persist. Although disposable devices generally perform well, poor quality control remains a problem.[20] Respiratory care managers need to carefully evaluate disposable devices being considered for bulk purchase before actual clinical use.[21] To ensure reliability, this

Box 3-9 • Patient Body Fluids

- Amniotic fluid
- Blood
- Cerebrospinal fluid
- Pericardial fluid
- Peritoneal fluid
- Perspiration
- Pleural fluid
- Semen
- Saliva
- Synovial fluid
- Vaginal secretions
- Vitreous humor

Box 3-10 • Fluids and Medications Precautions[4]

- Sterile fluids should always be used for tracheal suctioning and to fill nebulizers and bubble humidifiers. These fluids should be dispensed aseptically.
- Sterile water should be used when rinsing equipment. If tap water must be used, either an alcohol rinse must follow or the equipment must thoroughly air dry before use.
- If a large stock bottle of sterile fluid must be reused, the container must be resealed and dated after opening. Remaining fluid should be discarded within 24 hours.
- When multidose medication vials are being used, they must be handled, dispensed, and stored according to manufacturers' instructions (on the label or package insert). Medication must not be used after its expiration date.

evaluation should include physical testing of multiple units of each model being assessed. Last, bedside clinicians need to carefully inspect and confirm the operation of any disposable device before use.

Reusing high-cost, high-volume disposable equipment saves hospitals money. The unsafe practice of reusing devices labeled by the manufacturer for "single-use only" raises significant safety concerns and issues of negligence.[22] The CDC recommends that single-use items be considered for reuse only if there is hard evidence that reprocessing poses no threat to the patient and does not alter the device's function.[4] Those responsible for reusing disposable equipment bear a significant burden of proof. Without such proof, users of reprocessed single-use items may be transferring legal liability for the product's safe performance from the manufacturer to themselves or their employer.[23]

Fluids and Medications Precautions

Because of the hospital workplace, occupational exposure to blood and body fluids is evident. This repeated exposure means reasonably anticipated skin, eye, mucous membrane, or parenteral contact with blood or other potentially infectious body fluids. Box 3-9 lists patient body fluids capable of contamination. Unit dosing has decreased but has not eliminated the infection hazard associated with medications. Box 3-10 outlines several simple procedures designed to help prevent cross contamination while using fluids and medications.

▶ BARRIER MEASURES AND ISOLATION PRECAUTIONS

A major route for the spread of infections is by contact with infected persons. Thus measures that place "barriers" between the source and the host can help prevent the spread of infection. General barrier methods include handwashing, the use of personal protective equipment (PPE) (gloves, masks, goggles, gowns), and patient placement and transport procedures. Other barrier-related protective procedures involve the handling of contaminated articles and equipment, the use of needles and syringes, and the handling of laboratory specimens. Combinations of these methods designed to help reduce the spread of infection are called **isolation precautions.**

General Barrier Measures

Handwashing

The importance of handwashing with the liberal application of soap and scrubbing with strong friction cannot be overstressed. Because the most common route for transmission of nosocomial infection is hand contact, careful, methodical handwashing before and after patient care is the single most effective way to reduce exposing patients to contagious disease. The patient's bed and bed linen is one of the foulest and dirtiest places in a hospital. Prompt and thorough washing of hands before and after any patient contact is imperative, even when gloves have been used. Efficient handwashing means cleaning the palms of the hands, around the wrists and forearms, between the fingernails, around the cuticles, and between the digits for no less than 15 seconds (Figure 3-2). Rinsing is from forearm to fingertips and the water faucet is turned off with a clean towel. Drying of the hands can be by cloth towels, paper towels, warm forced air, or a hand-activated dryer, of which none has proven to be more efficient than the others.[24]

A
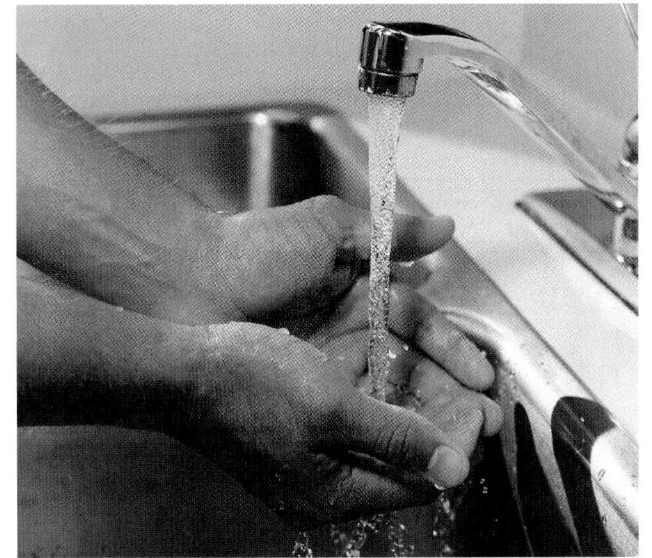

B
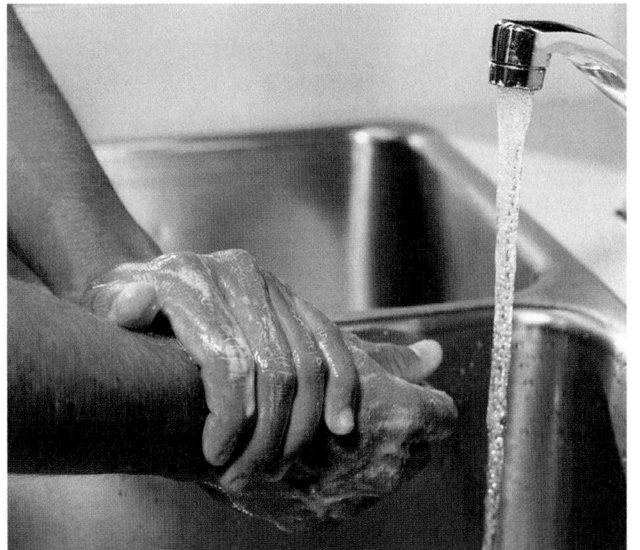

C
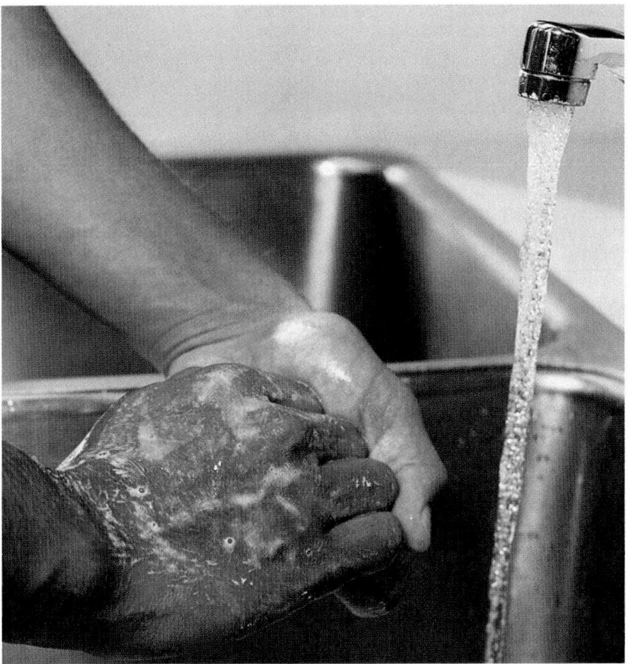

D
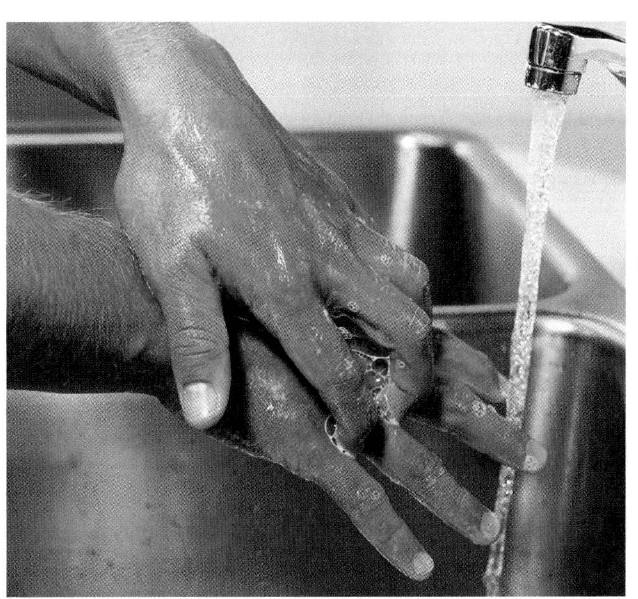

Figure 3-2 · Steps to Handwashing Demonstrated

A, Thorough wetting of hands. **B,** Washing around wrist and forearm. **C,** Scrubbing palm of hand. **D,** Washing between digits on back of hand.

Continued

Gloves

There are three major reasons for wearing gloves. First, gloves protect caregivers from contamination when contacting patients' blood, body fluids, secretions, excretions, mucous membranes, or nonintact skin. The use of gloves is also mandated by OSHA. Second, gloves protect patients from acquiring infections from colonized health personnel during invasive procedures. Last, gloves reduce the likelihood of cross contamination between patients via caregivers' hands.

Caregivers should wear sterile gloves whenever performing invasive procedures. Clean gloves are satisfactory for all other uses. Gloves should be changed, regardless of use, between each patient contact and after any direct contact with infectious material, even if in the middle of a procedure. After removing the gloves, caregivers must always wash their hands. Gloves may have small, invisible defects or may be torn during use. Moreover, the hands can be contaminated during removal of the gloves. For these reasons, the wearing of gloves should never be used as a substitute for handwashing.

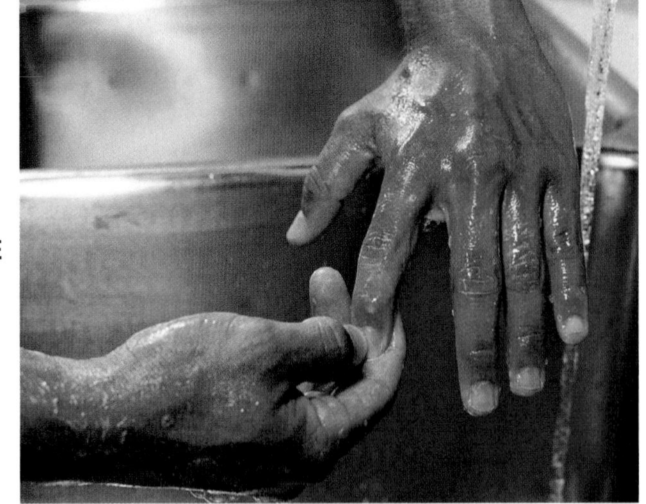

E

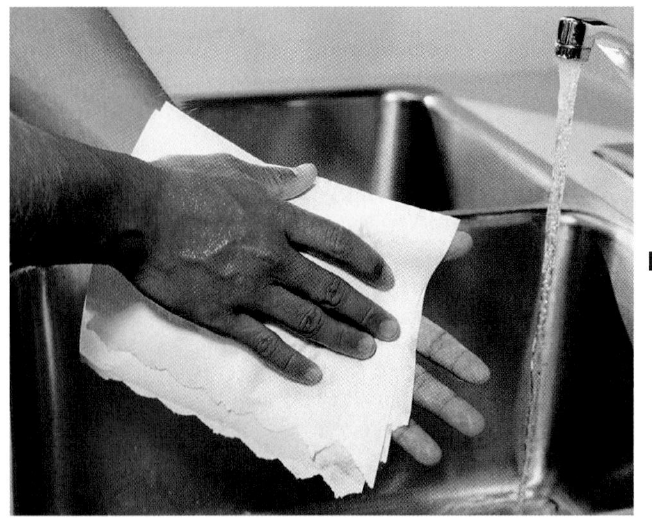

F

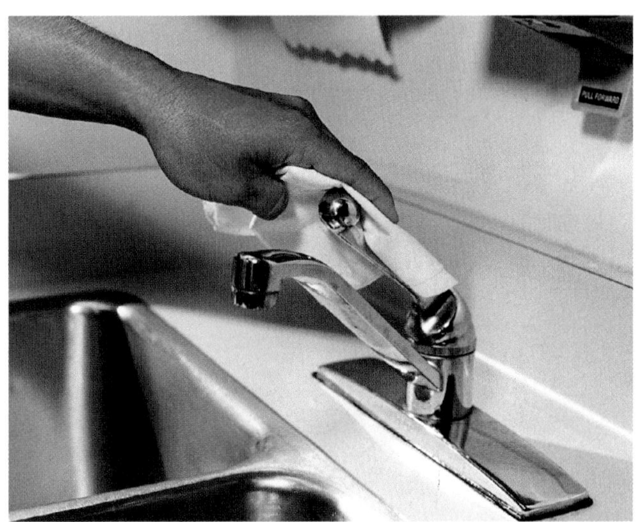

G

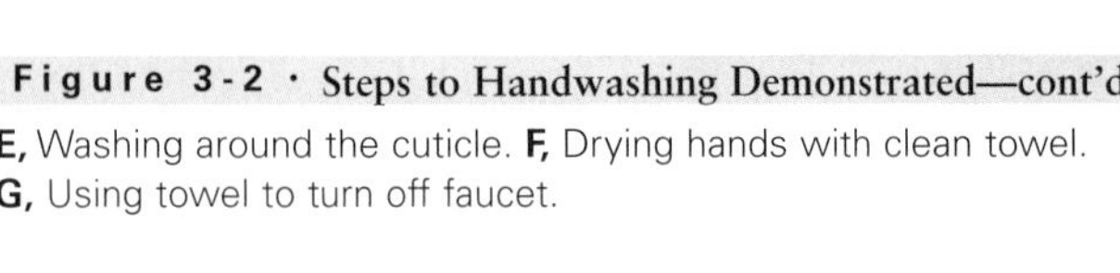

Figure 3-2 · Steps to Handwashing Demonstrated—cont'd

E, Washing around the cuticle. **F,** Drying hands with clean towel. **G,** Using towel to turn off faucet.

Because gloving reduces acquisition of vancomycin-resistant *Enterococcus* species on the hands,[25] wearing gloves should be considered routine for inpatient care.

Frequent use of latex products including gloves can place the caregiver at greater risk for developing latex allergies, which results from repeated exposures to proteins in the natural rubber latex through the skin. The amount of exposure needed to sensitize an individual to the natural rubber latex is not known.

Some body lotions can actually cause a breakdown of the latex in a glove, thereby diminishing protection against blood and body fluids. Oil-based hand creams and lotions cause a reaction between the hydrocarbons and the latex itself in a matter of minutes. This may not be enough to cause a pinhole but may be enough to weaken the glove to the point of barrier penetration or breakage.

Masks, Goggles, Face Shields, and Respiratory Protection

Masks, goggles, and face shields provide barrier protection for the eyes, nose, and mouth against contact transmission of pathogens. The mucous membranes surrounding the eyes are capable of absorbing fluids. Eye shields should be worn along with other protective devices during any procedure that can generate splashes or sprays of blood, body fluids, secretions, or excretions. In addition, a surgical mask needs to be worn whenever contacting infected patients who are coughing or sneezing.

All masks should fully cover both the nose and the mouth. Because masks become ineffective when moist, they should be discarded after each use. Masks should not be reused or lowered around the neck.

Recently, the spread of TB has become a major area of concern in hospitals.[26] Although surgical masks can prevent the spread of infection by large-particle aerosols, they are not very effective against TB, which spreads via small droplet nuclei. Currently, the **National Institute for Occupational Safety and Health (NIOSH)** recommends particulate filter **respirators** that meet its N95 (*N* category at 95% efficiency) performance criteria for protective use with TB.[27]

Gowns, Aprons, and Protective Apparel

Gowns and other protective apparel (aprons, leg coverings, boots or shoe covers) also provide barrier protection and can help reduce the spread of infection. Gowns, as with gloves, serve multiple purposes. First, a gown should be worn to prevent clothing from contamination and to protect the skin from blood and body fluid exposure. For this purpose, either a gown treated to make it impermeable to liquids or a splash apron should be worn.

A gown also should be worn when caring for patients with contagious disorders that cause serious illness. This may help reduce cross contamination between patients. When a gown is worn for this purpose, it should be removed before leaving the patient's environment and then the hands should be washed.

As with gloves and masks, a gown should be worn only once and then be discarded. In most situations, aseptically clean, freshly laundered, or disposable gowns are satisfactory. RTs may need to wear sterile gowns in some instances, as when caring for patients with extensive burns or wounds.

Patient Placement

Private rooms help prevent contact transmission. For this reason, any patient with a serious infection spread via the contact route should be placed in a private room with its own handwashing and toilet facilities. Private rooms are also recommended for patients who have poor hygiene, contaminate the environment, or cannot be expected to help maintain infection control precautions (infants, children, and patients with altered mental status). A private room with appropriate ventilation is also needed to reduce airborne transmission, as when caring for patients with TB.[26]

When a private room is not available, patients infected with the same organism (and no other) can share a room. The term used to describe this approach is called **cohorting**. If a private room is not available and cohorting is not possible, caregivers should consult with infection control personnel before placing patients. If an infected patient must share a room with noninfected patients, all patients, personnel, and visitors must be required to use applicable infection control precautions.

Transport of Infected Patients

By limiting the transport of patients with contagious disease, the risk of cross infection can be reduced. However, infected patients do need to be transported, and when that occurs the patient needs to wear appropriate barrier protection (masks, gowns, impervious dressings). All personnel receiving the patient need to be notified of the patient's impending arrival and what infection control measures are required.

Handling Contaminated Articles and Equipment

Contaminated items, whether reusable or disposable, should be enclosed in an impervious bag before removal from a patient's room. Bagging helps prevent accidental exposure of both personnel and the environment to contaminated articles. A single bag is satisfactory if (1) the bag is strong and impervious and (2) the contaminated items can be bagged without contaminating the bag's outer surface. Otherwise, the contaminated items should be double bagged. Bags used for contaminated articles or waste materials should be clearly labeled or color-coded for this purpose.

After bagging, reusable patient-care equipment must be returned to the applicable processing area. Contaminated reusable equipment should remain bagged until ready for decontamination or sterilization. When contaminated waste is being discarded, both the agency's procedures and any applicable local, state, or federal regulations must be followed.

Using Needles and Syringes

Needlestick injuries are a growing area of concern among healthcare personnel. This is because accidental skin puncture with a contaminated sharp can transmit blood-borne pathogens such as hepatitis and HIV to the worker.[28] Obviously, all personnel should exercise extreme caution when handling any sharp instruments, including needles and syringes. Methods to prevent needlestick injuries are covered in the following discussion on Standard Precautions.

Handling Laboratory Specimens

When gathering laboratory specimens (such as sputum), extreme care needs to be taken to prevent contamination of the external surface of the container. If the outside of the container is contaminated, the caregiver must either disinfect it or place it in an impervious bag. To minimize the likelihood of laboratory specimens leaking during transport, they should always be placed in a sturdy container with a secure lid. When gathering a specimen from a patient on isolation precautions, the container must be placed in an appropriately labeled, impervious bag before it is removed from the room.

Isolation Precautions

Isolation precautions represent specific combinations of the barrier methods just discussed. There are two levels of isolation precautions. The first and most general level is **standard precautions** (Box 3-11). Healthcare professionals should use standard precautions in caring for all patients, regardless of their diagnosis or presumed infection status. The second level of isolation measures is **transmission-based precautions.** Transmission-based precautions are added to standard precautions when

Box 3-11 • Standard Precautions

HANDWASHING

- Wash hands after touching blood, body fluids, secretions, excretions, and contaminated items, even if wearing gloves.
- Wash hands immediately after removing gloves, between patient contacts, and when otherwise indicated to avoid cross contamination.
- Wash hands between tasks and procedures on the same patient if cross contamination of different body sites is possible (e.g., tracheostomy care following assistance with a bedpan).
- Use plain soap for routine handwashing; use an antimicrobial soap or a waterless antiseptic if specified by the infection control program.

GLOVES

- Wear clean gloves when touching blood, body fluids, secretions, excretions, and contaminated items.
- Put on clean gloves just before touching mucous membranes and nonintact skin.
- Change gloves between tasks and procedures on the same patient after contact with infections material.
- Remove gloves promptly after use, before touching noncontaminated items and environmental surfaces, and before going to another patient.
- Wash hands immediately after removing gloves.

MASKS, EYE PROTECTION, FACE SHIELDS

- Wear a mask and eye protection or a face shield to protect mucous membranes of the eyes, nose, and mouth during procedures and patient care activities that are likely to generate splashes or sprays of blood, body fluids, secretions, and excretions.

GOWNS

- Wear a clean gown to protect skin and to prevent soiling of clothing during procedures and patient care activities that are likely to generate splashes or sprays of blood, body fluids, secretions, or excretions.
- Remove a soiled gown as promptly as possible and wash hands to avoid transfer of microorganisms to other patients or environments.

PATIENT CARE EQUIPMENT

- Handle used patient care equipment soiled with blood, body fluids, secretions, and excretions in a manner that prevents skin and mucous membrane exposures, contamination of clothing, and transfer of microorganisms to other patients and environments.
- Do not use reusable equipment to care for another patient unless it has been cleaned and reprocessed appropriately.
- Properly discard single-use items.

OCCUPATIONAL HEALTH AND BLOODBORNE PATHOGENS

- Exercise extreme caution when handling needles, scalpels, and other sharp instruments or devices; when cleaning used instruments; and when disposing of used needles.
- Never recap used needles, handle them using both hands, or point toward any part of the body; rather, use either a one-handed "scoop" technique or a mechanical device designed for holding the needle sheath.
- Do not remove used needles from disposable syringes by hand and do not bend, break, or otherwise manipulate used needles by hand.
- Place used disposable syringes and needles, scalpel blades, and other sharp items in appropriate puncture-resistant containers; place reusable syringes and needles in a puncture-resistant container for transport to the reprocessing area.
- Use mouthpieces, resuscitation bags, or other ventilation devices as an alternative to mouth-to-mouth resuscitation methods in areas where the need for resuscitation is predictable.

PATIENT PLACEMENT

- Place patients who contaminate the environment or who do not (or cannot be expected to) assist in maintaining appropriate hygiene or environmental control in a private room.
- If a private room is not available, consult with infection control specialists regarding patient placement.

Box 3-12 • Airborne Precautions (used *in addition to* Standard Precautions)

PATIENT PLACEMENT

- Place the patient in a private negative-pressure room that has 6 to 12 air changes per hour and either safe external air discharge or HEPA filtration of recirculated air.
- Keep the room door closed and the patient in the room.
- If a private room is not available, cohorting is acceptable.
- If a private room is not available and cohorting is not feasible, consult with infection control professionals before patient placement.

RESPIRATORY PROTECTION

- Wear respiratory protection when entering the room of a patient with known or suspected infectious pulmonary tuberculosis.
- Susceptible persons should not enter the room of patients known or suspected to have measles (rubeola) or varicella (chickenpox) if other immune caregivers are available.
- If susceptible persons must enter the room of a patient known or suspected to have measles or varicella, they should wear respiratory protection.
- Persons immune to measles or varicella need not wear respiratory protection.

PATIENT TRANSPORT

- Limit the transport of the patient from the room to essential purposes only.
- If transport or movement is necessary, minimize patient dispersal of droplet nuclei by having the patient wear a surgical mask.

dealing with patients known or suspected to be infected by pathogens spread by either the airborne, droplet, or contact route.

Standard Precautions

Standard precautions help reduce the general risk of infection from both recognized and unrecognized sources. Standard precautions apply to (1) blood; (2) all body fluids, secretions, and excretions *(except sweat)*, regardless of whether or not they contain visible blood; (3) nonintact skin; and (4) mucous membranes. Standard precautions should be used when caring for all patients. Box 3-11 outlines the key elements constituting standard precautions.

Transmission-Based Precautions

Transmission-based precautions are used with patients documented or suspected to have severe contagious infections for which standard precautions alone are insufficient. Thus transmission-based precautions are always applied in addition to standard precautions. There are three types of transmission-based precautions: airborne, droplet, and contact. Two or more of these types can be combined for diseases having multiple transmission routes.

Airborne precautions help reduce airborne transmission of infectious agents. Common examples of diseases transmitted via this route include legionellosis, TB, varicella, measles, and histoplasmosis. Organisms transmitted via this route can be dispersed over long distances by air currents. For this reason, special air handling and ventilation are required to prevent airborne transmission. Box 3-12 outlines the key elements constituting airborne precautions.

Additional guidelines apply in managing patients with known or suspected TB. Box 3-13 lists the major guidelines directly applicable to RTs, as promoted by the CDC.[26] RTs who work extensively with TB patients should be familiar with the full scope of all CDC recommendations.

Droplet precautions help reduce droplet transmission of infectious agents. Common examples of respiratory diseases transmitted via this route include *H. influenzae* meningitis, streptococcal pneumonia, epiglottitis, diphtheria, pertussis, influenza, mumps, rubella, and adenovirus infections. Box 3-14 outlines the key elements constituting droplet precautions.

Contact precautions help reduce the risk of transmission of microorganisms by direct or indirect contact. Common examples of diseases transmitted via these routes include hepatitis, venereal disease, AIDS, and staphylococcal and enteric bacterial infections. Box 3-15 outlines the key elements constituting contact precautions.

A number of organisms responsible for these infections are becoming resistant to common antibiotics. For this reason, the Hospital Infection Control Practices Advisory Committee provides additional precautions to help prevent the spread of antibiotic-resistant organisms.[29]

Box 3-13 • Selected Guidelines for Preventing Transmission of Tuberculosis (TB)

GENERAL GUIDELINES

- Triage of patients in ambulatory-care and emergency settings should include vigorous efforts to promptly identify patients suspected of having active TB.
- In the ambulatory-care setting, patients suspected of having active TB should (1) be placed in a separate area apart from other patients (ideally in a room or enclosure designed for airborne isolation); (2) wear surgical masks; and (3) be instructed to cover their mouths and noses with tissues when coughing or sneezing.
- Promptly start any patient with suspected or confirmed TB on appropriate drug therapy.
- If a TB patient does not respond to therapy within 2 to 3 weeks, the most likely reasons are noncompliance with the drug regimen or the presence of **multi drug-resistant TB (MDR-TB)**.
- Outpatients with diagnosed active TB should have appointments scheduled to avoid exposing HIV-infected or otherwise severely immunocompromised persons to *M. tuberculosis*.
- In hospitals and other inpatient facilities, any patient with suspected or confirmed active TB should immediately be placed in a room meeting airborne isolation standards.
- The number of persons entering the isolation room should be minimal. All persons, including visitors, who enter the room should wear respiratory protection.
- TB patients should remain in their isolation rooms with the door closed. When possible, special procedures should be performed in the isolation room.
- Treatment and procedure rooms in which patients with suspected or confirmed TB must receive care should meet the ventilation recommendations for airborne isolation rooms.
- Isolation should be discontinued only when the patient is on effective therapy, is improving clinically, and has had three consecutive negative sputum AFB smears collected on different days; patients with MDR-TB should be retained in isolation throughout their stay.
- Hospitalized patients who have active TB should be monitored for relapse by having sputum AFB smears examined regularly (e.g., every 2 weeks).
- Discharge planning for TB patients should include (1) a confirmed outpatient appointment with the provider who will manage the patient until the patient is cured, (2) sufficient medication to last until the outpatient appointment, and (3) placement into case-management or outreach programs of the public health department.
- Patients who may be infectious should be discharged only to facilities that have isolation capability or to their homes. If such a patient is sent home, the infection status of all household members must be determined. If the household includes uninfected persons at high risk for active TB (e.g., young children or immunocompromised persons), arrangements must be made to prevent their exposure until the patient is noninfectious.

GUIDELINES FOR COUGH-INDUCING AND AEROSOL-GENERATING PROCEDURES

- Cough-inducing procedures include endotracheal intubation and suctioning, diagnostic sputum induction, aerosol treatments (e.g., pentamidine therapy), and bronchoscopy.
- Cough-inducing procedures should not be performed on patients who may have infectious TB unless the procedures are essential and can be performed with appropriate precautions.
- If clinically practical, patients with suspected or confirmed active TB should receive oral prophylaxis for PCP (as opposed to aerosolized pentamidine).
- All cough-inducing procedures performed on patients who may have infectious TB should be performed using booths or special enclosures; if this is not feasible, a room that meets the ventilation requirements for airborne isolation can be used.
- After completion of cough-inducing procedures, patients who may have infectious TB should remain in their isolation rooms or enclosures until coughing subsides. They should be required to cover their mouths and noses with tissues when coughing.
- Before the enclosure or room is used for another patient, enough time should be allowed to pass for at least 99% of airborne contaminants to be removed (this time varies according to the efficiency of the ventilation or filtration system).

MINI CLINI

Isolation Methods

PROBLEM

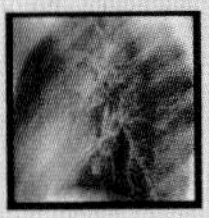

A serious influenza outbreak occurs in a local long-term care facility. You are called to the emergency department as four of the sickest patients are being admitted together to your hospital for treatment. Currently no private rooms are available for these patients. Outline the key isolation methods you would apply to help prevent the spread of influenza in your institution.

DISCUSSION

Influenza spreads via the droplet route. Therefore, we must apply *both* standard and droplet precautions for these patients. When transporting these patients out of the emergency department, you must be sure that they wear a surgical mask. Because private rooms are not available, these patients will have to be cohorted. If this is not feasible, the patients must be separated from other patients by at least 3 feet. Special air handling and ventilation are not necessary, and the door may remain open. In addition to following standard precautions, all caregivers and visitors should wear a surgical mask when within 3 feet of these patients (or entering the room).

Box 3-14 • Droplet Precautions (used *in addition to* Standard Precautions)

PATIENT PLACEMENT

- Place the patient in a private room.
- If a private room is not available, cohorting is acceptable.
- If a private room is not available and cohorting is not feasible, separate the infected patient from other patients and visitors by at least 3 feet.
- Special air handling and ventilation are not necessary, and the door may remain open.

MASK

- Wear a surgical mask within 3 feet of the patient.
- Some hospitals may want to implement the wearing of a mask to enter the room.

PATIENT TRANSPORT

- Limit the movement and transport of the patient from the room to essential purposes only.
- If transport or movement is necessary, minimize droplet transmission by having the patient wear a surgical mask.

Box 3-15 • Contact Precautions (used *in addition to* Standard Precautions)

PATIENT PLACEMENT

- Place the patient in a private room.
- If a private room is not available, cohorting is acceptable.
- If a private room is not available and cohorting is not feasible, consult with infection control specialists before patient placement.

GLOVES AND HANDWASHING

- Wear clean gloves when entering the room.
- During the course of providing care for a patient, change gloves after having contact with infectious material such as feces or wound drainage.
- Remove gloves before leaving the patient's environment and wash hands immediately with an antimicrobial agent or a waterless antiseptic agent.
- After glove removal and handwashing, ensure that hands do not touch potentially contaminated environmental surfaces or items in the patient's room.

GOWNS

- Wear a clean gown when entering the room if you anticipate that your clothing will contact the patient, environmental surfaces, or items in the patient's room.
- Wear a clean gown when entering the room if the patient is incontinent or has diarrhea, an ileostomy, a colostomy, or wound drainage not contained by a dressing.
- Remove the gown before leaving the patient's room.
- After gown removal, ensure that clothing does not contact potentially contaminated environmental surfaces.

PATIENT TRANSPORT

- Limit the transport of the patient from the room to essential purposes only.
- If the patient must be transported, ensure that precautions are maintained to minimize the risk of disease transmission to other patients or contamination of the environment.

PATIENT-CARE EQUIPMENT

- When possible, dedicate the use of noncritical patient care equipment to a single patient or patient cohort.
- If use of common equipment or items cannot be avoided, ensure that it is adequately cleaned and disinfected before use on another patient.

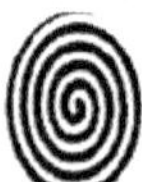

RULE OF THUMB

Apply standard precautions when caring for *all* patients.

1. Wash your hands after touching blood, body fluids, or contaminated items (even if wearing gloves).
2. Wear fresh, clean gloves for all tasks and procedures involving potential contact with blood, body fluids, and/or contaminated items.
3. Exercise extreme caution when handling "sharps."
4. Handle soiled equipment in a manner that prevents skin and mucous membrane exposures, contamination of clothing, and transfer of microorganisms to other patients and environments.

Immunocompromised and Burn Patients

Patients with leukemia, cancer, and severe burns, or patients receiving immunosuppressive therapies are highly susceptible to infection. In the past, these patients were placed in "protective isolation." Recent evidence indicates that this approach is no more useful in preventing infection than vigorous handwashing. This is because the most common source of infection in immunocompromised patients is their own (endogenous) flora.

Obviously, immunocompromised patients should be separated from those with infectious diseases, preferably by placement in a private room. Under these conditions, careful adherence to routine standards for asepsis is generally all that is needed to minimize the risk of infection. The CDC provides specific guidelines for preventing legionellosis and pulmonary aspergillosis in immunocompromised patients.[4]

In regard to burn patients, their wounds usually become infected within 48 to 72 hours after the initial incident. For this reason, care of patients with severe burns must always involve efforts to minimize wound colonization and to prevent infection. Although procedures for major burns vary, most burn centers enforce strict contact isolation procedures.

▶ SURVEILLANCE

Surveillance is an ongoing process designed to ensure that infection control procedures work. Surveillance generally involves three components: (1) equipment processing quality control, (2) routine sampling of in-use equipment, and (3) microbiological identification. During major outbreaks of nosocomial infections, surveillance also involves epidemiological investigation.

Normally, an infection control committee establishes surveillance policies and an infection control nurse or epidemiologist administers them. The surveillance program may be centralized or decentralized (to the various service departments). In the latter case, RTs work directly with an infection control nurse or epidemiologist to implement departmental surveillance procedures.

Equipment Processing Quality Control

The first step in equipment processing quality control is ensuring that personnel adhere to established procedures. Supplementing this evaluation involves assessing how well the sterilization procedures actually work. To make this determination, either special processing indicators or culture sampling are used.

Processing Indicators

As the name implies, **processing indicators** show whether a sterilization or disinfection process worked. There are two types of processing indicators: chemical and biological.

Chemical indicators are usually impregnated on packaging tape. These indicators change color when exposed to specific conditions. Steam autoclave indicators change color after exposure to a given temperature for a specific time. Likewise, EtO indicators change color after exposure to a given concentration of the gas. Because neither autoclave nor EtO processing changes the appearance of packaging, indicator tape also helps one distinguish between processed and unprocessed items.

Although a chemical indicator can tell us that a package has been through a sterilizer cycle, it cannot ensure that the contents are actually sterile. Only biological indicators can provide that information. Biological indicators consist of strips of paper impregnated with bacterial spores. These spore strips are

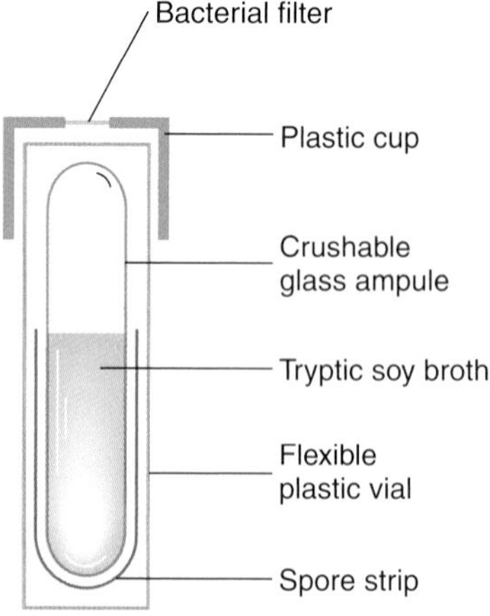

Figure 3-3

Biological sterilization indicator.

housed in a plastic capsule with a glass ampule that contains a growth medium (Figure 3-3). To prevent contamination with other organisms, the capsule cap contains a gas-permeable bacterial filter.

For the capsule to be used, it must be wrapped in packaging material and placed in a relatively inaccessible location inside the sterilizer. After sterilization, the ampule should be crushed and the spores exposed to the growth medium. The capsule is then incubated according to the manufacturer's instructions. After the incubation period, turbidity or a color change indicates bacterial growth and failure of the sterilization process.

Unfortunately, the incubation period needed to verify sterility ranges from 1 to 3 days. This requires processed equipment to be held from use until its sterility is ensured. Obviously, this "down time" adds to the cost of care by demanding larger inventories of reusables. For this reason, the CDC recommends that sterilizers be checked with biological indicators at least once a week.

Culture Sampling

For procedures such as pasteurization and chemical disinfection to be evaluated, bacteriological samples from processed equipment must be obtained and cultured. When culture sampling is performed correctly, it determines how much residual bacteria remains on equipment. This provides essential information about the efficacy of the disinfection process.

Unfortunately, contamination during sampling procedures is common, making equipment culture results difficult to interpret. Moreover, if adherence to disinfection protocols is carefully monitored, regular culture sampling is not needed. Thus in the absence of a nosocomial epidemic, regular culturing of processed equipment is not warranted.

However, culturing is useful in assessing packaging adequacy and material shelf life and for determining disinfectant action. Last, sampling of in-use equipment is a normal component of **bacteriological surveillance**.

Sampling of In-Use Equipment

Surveillance procedures usually involve random sampling and culturing of in-use equipment. The purpose of sampling in-use equipment is twofold: (1) it helps establish how often in-use items should be removed from use and reprocessed and (2) it can help identify the source of nosocomial epidemics before they become widespread.

Three common methods are used to sample respiratory care equipment: (1) swab sampling, (2) liquid broths, and (3) aerosol impaction. Each method aids sample collection from particular equipment or equipment locations.

Swab Sampling

Swab sampling is used to obtain cultures from easily accessible equipment surfaces. A specially prepared sterile swab is rubbed on the equipment surface at a single location. Each location requires a new swab. Using aseptic technique, a swab is placed inside the tube of sterile liquid broth or is used to inoculate a plate of growth media. A record of the date, time, equipment source, and location from which each sample was taken must be maintained. After collection, samples are sent to the microbiology laboratory for incubation and identification.

Liquid Broths

Swab sampling cannot reach inside all equipment tubing. In these situations, a sterile liquid broth may be used to obtain a sample. When using aseptic technique, the broth is poured into the tubing and "swished" back and forth, then is poured into a sterile container for culturing. Labeling protocol is the same as with swab sampling.

Aerosol Impaction

Because nebulizers may be a major source for the spread of infection, the actual particulate output of these devices may need to be sampled. Liquid particle aerosols can be sampled using inertial impaction devices. These range in complexity from simple funnel/culture plate systems to multichamber devices that separate aerosol particles according to size. Regardless of the device used, asepsis must be maintained during both equipment setup and sample collection. Labeling protocol is the same as with other sample collection methods.

Microbiological Identification

The hospital microbiology laboratory fulfills a central role in bacteriological surveillance. The laboratory cultures, isolates, stains, and identifies organisms according to a variety of specialized procedures.

Microbiology personnel work closely with the infection control professionals in support of the surveillance program; regular diagnostic activities often reveal patterns of infection with certain microorganisms that can precede widespread outbreaks. The combination of diagnostic activities with ongoing surveillance can help prevent or minimize large-scale in-hospital epidemics.

When the surveillance program is decentralized to the departmental level, RTs work with the microbiology laboratory staff to develop, maintain, and evaluate the methods and procedures used to gather and interpret bacteriological samples.

KEY POINTS

- Between 10% and 40% of all nosocomial infections affect the respiratory system, resulting in high patient mortality.
- There are five major routes for transmission of pathogens: contact, droplet, airborne, common vehicle, and vectorborne.
- Infection control procedures involve (1) eliminating the sources of infectious agents, (2) creating barriers to their transmission, and (3) monitoring and evaluating the effectiveness of control.
- Failure to properly clean equipment can render all subsequent processing efforts ineffective.
- Physical or chemical disinfection destroys the vegetative form of pathogenic organisms but cannot kill bacterial spores.
- Intermediate-level disinfectants (e.g., alcohols, phenols, iodophors) are best used as surface disinfectants or antiseptics.
- Glutaraldehyde (20 minutes) is the best choice for high-level disinfection of semicritical respiratory care equipment.
- For all microbial life to be destroyed completely, equipment must be sterilized.
- For sterilization of critical heat-labile items, EtO should be used; heat-stable critical items should be autoclaved.
- Among respiratory care equipment, large-volume nebulizers have the greatest potential to spread infection.
- The patient's bed and bed linen are among the dirtiest places in the hospital.
- Ventilator circuits may be used up to 7 days before they need to be changed.
- HMEs may be used up to 96 hours before they need to be changed.
- Single-use items should be reused only if there is hard documented evidence that reprocessing poses no threat to the patient and does not alter the device's function.
- Sterile fluids must always be used for tracheal suctioning and for filling nebulizers and humidifiers.
- Hands need to be thoroughly washed after any patient contact, even when gloves are used.
- Standard precautions must be used in caring for all patients, regardless of their diagnosis or infection status.

KEY POINTS—cont'd

- The use of gloves is part of routine basic care when there is skin contact with a patient.
- Masks, goggles, and/or a face shield must be worn during any procedure that can generate splashes or sprays of blood, body fluids, secretions, or excretions.
- Petroleum-based lotions and hand creams must be avoided when latex gloves are being worn.
- When infected patients are being transported, appropriate barrier protection must be used.
- Contaminated items should be bagged before removal from a patient's room.
- Extreme caution must be exercised when handling or disposing of all "sharps."
- In the management of patients with known or suspected TB, the CDC guideline must be followed.
- Familiarity with the agency's overall infection control program, including surveillance policies and procedures, is a must.

References

1. Marik PE: Fever in the ICU, Chest 117:855, 2000.
2. Garner JS: Guideline for isolation precautions in hospitals, Infect Control Hosp Epidemiol 17:53, 1996.
3. Schaberg DR: How infections spread in the hospital, Respir Care 34:81, 1989.
4. Centers for Disease Control and Prevention, Infection Control Practices Advisory Committee: Guideline for prevention of nosocomial pneumonia, Respir Care 39:1191, 1994.
5. Stephen F: Pulmonary complications following lung resection, Chest 118:1263, 2000.
6. Rutala WA: APIC guideline for selection and use of disinfectants, Am J Infect Control 24:313, 1996.
7. Chatburn RE, Kallstrom TJ, Bajaksouzian MS: A comparison of acetic acid with a quaternary ammonium compound for disinfection of hand-held nebulizers, Respir Care 33:179, 1988.
8. Crow S: Sterilization processes: meeting the demands of today's health care technology, Nurs Clin North Am 28:687, 1993.
9. Crow S: Peracetic acid sterilization: a timely development for a busy healthcare industry, Infect Control Hosp Epidemiol 13:111, 1992.
10. Malchesky PS: Peracetic acid and its application to medical instrument sterilization, Artif Organs 17:147, 1993.
11. Riley RL, Nardell EA: Clearing the air: the theory and application of ultraviolet air disinfection, Am Rev Respir Dis 139:1286, 1989.

12. Haney PE, Raymond BA, Lewis LC: Ethylene oxide: an occupational health hazard for hospital workers, AORN J 51:480, 1990.
13. Thomachot L et al: Changing heat and moisture exchangers after 96 hours rather than after 24 hours: a clinical and microbiological evaluation, Crit Care Med 28:714, 2000.
14. Kollef MH: The prevention of ventilator-associated pneumonia, N Engl J Med 340:627, 1999.
15. Jiang NH et al: Effects of decreasing the frequency of ventilator circuit changes to every 7 days on the rate of ventilator-associated pneumonia in a Beijing hospital, Respir Care 46:891, 2001.
16. Weber DJ et al: Manual ventilation bags as a source for bacterial colonization of intubated patients, Am Rev Respir Dis 142:892, 1990.
17. Golar SD, Sutherland LL, Ford GT: Multipatient use of prefilled disposable oxygen humidifiers for up to 30 days: patient safety and cost analysis, Respir Care 38:343,1993.
18. Seto WH et al: Evaluating the sterility of disposable wall oxygen humidifiers, during and between use on patients, Infect Control Hosp Epidemiol 11:604, 1990.
19. Martin MA, Reichelderfer M: APIC guideline for infection prevention and control in flexible endoscopy, Am J Infect Control 22:19, 1994.
20. Alvine GF et al: Disposable jet nebulizers. How reliable are they? Chest 101:316, 1992.
21. Kissoon N et al: Evaluation of performance characteristics of disposable bag-valve resuscitators, Crit Care Med 19:102, 1991.
22. Ball CK, Schafer EM, Thorne D: Reusing disposables: same old story—more characters added, Insight 21:77, 1996.
23. Medical Devices Agency: The reuse of medical devices supplied for single use only (MDA DB 9501), London, 1995, Department of Health.
24. Gustafson DR et al: Effects of 4 hand-drying methods for removing bacteria from washed hands: a randomized trial, Mayo Clin Proc 75:705, 2000.
25. Tenorio AR et al: Effectiveness of gloves in the prevention of hand carriage of vancomycin-resistant enterococcus species by health care workers after patient care, Clin Infect Dis 32:826, 2001.
26. Centers for Disease Control and Prevention: Guidelines for preventing the transmission of Mycobacterium tuberculosis in health-care facilities, 1994, MMWR Recomm Rep 43(RR-13):1, 1994.
27. U.S. Department of Health and Human Services, Department of Labor: Respiratory protective devices: final rule and notice, Federal Register 60:30336, 1995.
28. Emergency Care Research Institute: Needlestick injuries, Technol Respir Care 11:1, 1991.
29. Hospital Infection Control Practices Advisory Committee: Recommendations for preventing the spread of vancomycin resistance, Infect Control Hosp Epidemiol 16:105, 1995.

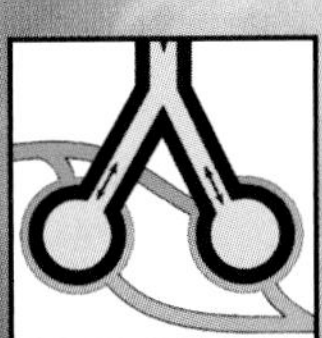

CHAPTER 4

Ethical and Legal Implications of Practice

Charles Carroll

In This Chapter You Will Learn:

- Philosophical foundations of ethics
- What constitutes an ethical dilemma and how they arise in healthcare
- How professional codes of ethics apply to ethical decision making
- How traditional ethical principles are useful in resolving ethical dilemmas
- What information should be gathered before making an ethical decision
- How the systems of civil and criminal law differ
- What constitutes professional malpractice and negligence
- How a respiratory therapist can become liable for wrongful acts
- What elements constitute a practice act
- How licensing affects legal responsibility and liability
- How changes in healthcare delivery have shaped the ethical and legal aspects of practice

Chapter Outline

Key Terms

assault
autonomy
battery
beneficence
benevolent deception
breach of contract
compensatory justice
confidentiality
consequentialism
defendant
distributive justice
double effect
formalism
informed consent
intuitionism
justice
libel
malpractice
negligence
nonmaleficence
plaintiff

Continued

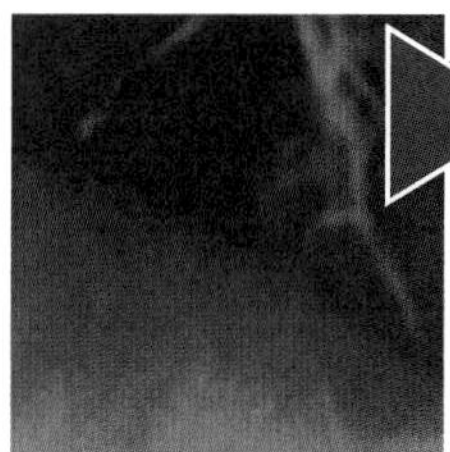

Key Terms—cont'd

res ipsa loquitur
respondeat superior
role fidelity
rule utilitarianism
scope of practice
slander
strict liability
tort
veracity
virtue ethics

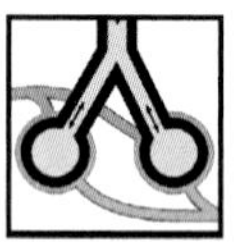

The effective respiratory therapist (RT) must possess excellent clinical skills and an understanding of the business of healthcare. The healthcare industry, like all industries, must deliver services in an atmosphere in which ethical and legal considerations are an integral part of the organizational culture. RTs regularly encounter circumstances that require them to make choices or take actions that have ethical and legal implications. In society, ethics and law help maintain order and stability. In professional practices, ethics guide RTs in carrying out their duties in a morally defensible way. Law establishes the minimum legal standards to which practitioners must adhere. Although not always the case, ethical practice may require a standard above that of legal practice.

The force behind law is statutory punishment, ranging from reparations and fines to licensure suspension and incarceration. On the other hand, sanctions for ethical misconduct involve censorship or expulsion from the profession. In some cases, ethical misconduct and legal misbehavior may result from the same incident. The distinction between illegal acts and unethical behavior is not always straightforward. A given act may fit any one of the following categories, depending on the circumstances and the ethical orientation of the person involved: ethical and legal, unethical but legal, ethical but illegal, or unethical and illegal. This chapter provides a foundation of principles related to the ethical and legal practice of respiratory care.

PHILOSOPHICAL FOUNDATIONS OF ETHICS

Although an in-depth discussion of philosophy is beyond the scope of this chapter, it is important to note that ethics has its origins in philosophy. Philosophy may be defined as the love of wisdom and the pursuit of knowledge concerning humankind, nature, and reality.[1] Ethics is one of the philosophical disciplines of philosophy, which includes law, religion, economics, and etiquette. Although ethics share a common origin with these disciplines, they are clearly different from these disciplines.[1]

ETHICAL DILEMMAS OF PRACTICE

The growth of respiratory care has paralleled the development of advanced medical technology and treatment protocols. At the same time, during the 1970s through the 1990s, an ever-growing and sophisticated patient population, fueled by medical benefit packages from the government and employers, developed rising expectations about acceptable standards of care. In the latter part of the 1990s, managed care strategies and other cost-containment methods, adopted by most third-party payers, slowed the growth of the healthcare industry. The ethical and legal issues faced by practitioners, although changed in many cases, continued to grow. In the earlier growth period, RTs faced ethical dilemmas and legal issues associated with patient expectations, staffing, and quality of care, among others. In the later period, RTs continued to face ethical dilemmas and legal issues; however, they may now be more related to rationing of care, dealing with conflicts associated with third-party standards of care, and what the RT believes to be the appropriate standard of care, among others. Staffing issues continue to be a problem and are at the root of many of the ethical and legal concerns faced by RTs. As respiratory care continues to mature as a profession, these challenges are likely to increase.

RTs continue to work in complex healthcare settings, making it difficult to predict definitively the range of ethical dilemmas likely to be experienced on a regular basis. The clinical aspects and the management aspects of healthcare are rife with possibilities for ethical dilemmas. In addition, the ethical orientation of the RT plays a role in recognition and identification of ethical dilemmas. The healthcare industry continues to be in a period of dynamic change. New technological and management methodologies are continuously being introduced to accomplish the missions and goals of healthcare organizations. Over the past decade, there has been an almost complete change from a relatively open fee-for-service system to one in which care is managed in some fashion and the fees are in some form of capitation. These changes are the source for many questions and for both perceived and real ethical dilemmas.

For example, managed care uses a concept known as "restrictive gate keeping." Restrictive gate keeping requires patients to obtain prior approval from their third-party payer, usually an insurance company, before hospitalization and before certain procedures. When the hospital admission or procedure is approved, specific requirements or limitations are usually associated with the patient's care. As a result, healthcare workers, RTs included, may find themselves engaged in clinical processes that are dictated more by the third-party payers than by patient needs. Under these circumstances, healthcare workers may feel frustrated and helpless if they believe that a patient needs care beyond that approved by the third-party payer.

The rationing of care continues to be a side effect of staffing patterns created by managed care. Although all businesses must carefully balance staffing patterns against productivity, managed care has brought this concept home in a major way to healthcare facilities. For example, the RT working in an understaffed department may decide that Patient A can really forego therapy because the department is short staffed and Patient A is really not going to get better anyway. Although this may at first sound like a case of simple neglect of duty, it is in fact also an ethical dilemma.

The approaches used to address ethical issues in healthcare range from the specific to the general. Specific guidance in resolving ethical dilemmas is usually provided by a professional code of ethics. General approaches involve the use of ethical theories and principles to reach a decision.[2]

MINI CLINI

Conflicting Obligations

PROBLEM

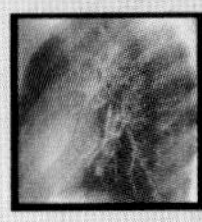

Therapist H, a registered RT with 18 years' experience, has worked for a large regional medical center for the past 10 years. She is generally happy with her work but is concerned about the financial stability of the hospital. As a result, she has signed on with a temporary agency to ensure that she will have work if the hospital decides to initiate a reduction in force. On one of her scheduled days off, Therapist H agrees to work a shift for the temporary agency at another hospital. Two hours before her shift is scheduled to begin, she receives a phone message from the medical center where she is employed. Her supervisor asks Therapist H to report to work at the medical center because the only experienced therapist on the shift has been in an automobile accident. Therapist H is torn between her obligation to the medical center where she has worked for 10 years and the agency.

DISCUSSION

Professionalism and ethics generally require a commitment to one's duties. In this situation, Therapist H must consider not only her duty, but also the consequences of each decision that she might make. In either case, there is the possibility that her decision will leave a staffing shortage at one of the hospitals.

DISCUSSION QUESTIONS

Should Therapist H cancel her shift with the agency although she has agreed to give the agency a 4-hour notice except in an emergency? Should she work the shift at the agency as scheduled, using the rationale that she did not create the staffing problem at the medical center? Should she call her supervisor and explain the situation and ask for help in making the right decision, realizing that the final decision would still be hers? Should she call her supervisor and tell him that she is ill and cannot come in and report to the agency job?

▶ CODES OF ETHICS

A code of ethics is an essential part of any profession that claims to be self-regulating. The adoption of a code of ethics is one way in which an occupational group establishes itself as a profession. A code may try to limit competition, restrict advertisement, or promote a particular image in addition to setting forth rules for conduct.[3]

The first American medical code of ethics (established in 1847) was as much concerned with separating orthodox practitioners from nontraditional ones as it was with regulating behavior. Even modern codes tend to be vague regarding what is prescribed and what is to be avoided.

The American Association for Respiratory Care (AARC) has also adopted a Statement of Ethics and Professional Conduct. The current code appears in Box 4-1. This code represents a set of general principles and rules that have been developed to help ensure that the health needs of the public are provided in a safe, effective, and caring manner. Codes for different professions might differ from those governing respiratory care because they may seek different goals. However, they all seek to establish parameters of behavior for members of the chosen profession. Unfortunately, professional codes of ethics often represent overly simplistic or prohibitive notions of how to deal with open misbehavior or flagrant abuses of authority over which few would disagree.

The really difficult ethical decisions stem from situations in which two or more right choices are incompatible, in which the choices represent different priorities, or in which limited resources exist to achieve a desired end. Ethicists readily admit that reducing these issues to simple formulations is no easy task. Indeed, the number and complexity of ethical dilemmas continues to grow as the complexity of life increases in this new millennium. For healthcare, the difficult ethical dilemmas continue to involve concerns about the practical limits

Box 4-1 • AARC Statement of Ethics and Professional Conduct (EP.1294)

The Respiratory Care Practitioner, in the conduct of their professional activities, shall be bound by the following ethical and professional principles. Respiratory Care Practitioners shall:

- Demonstrate behavior that reflects integrity, supports objectivity, and fosters trust in the profession and its professionals.
- Actively maintain and continually improve their professional competence and represent it accurately.
- Perform only those procedures or functions in which they are individually competent and which are within the scope of accepted and responsible practice.
- Respect and protect the legal and personal rights of patients they treat, including the right to informed consent and refusal of treatment.
- Divulge no confidential information regarding any patient or family unless disclosure is required for responsible performance of duty or required by law.
- Provide care without discrimination on any basis, with respect for the rights and dignity of all individuals.
- Promote disease prevention and wellness.
- Refuse to participate in illegal or unethical acts and shall refuse to conceal illegal, unethical, or incompetent acts of others.
- Follow sound scientific procedures and ethical principles in research.
- Comply with state or federal laws that govern and relate to their practice.
- Avoid any form of conduct that creates a conflict of interest and shall follow the principles of ethical business behavior.
- Promote the positive evolution of the profession and healthcare in general through improvement of the access, efficacy, and cost of patient care.
- Refrain from indiscriminate and unnecessary use of resources, both economic and natural, in their practice.

on financial resources, the growing emphasis on individual autonomy, and research advances such as cloning and stem cell research. Resolution of these more complex problems requires a more general approach than that provided by a code of ethics. This more general perspective is provided by ethical theories and principles.

ETHICAL THEORIES AND PRINCIPLES

Ethical theories and principles provide the foundation for all ethical behavior. Contemporary ethical principles have evolved from many sources. These include Aristotle and Aquinas' natural law, Judeo-Christian morality,

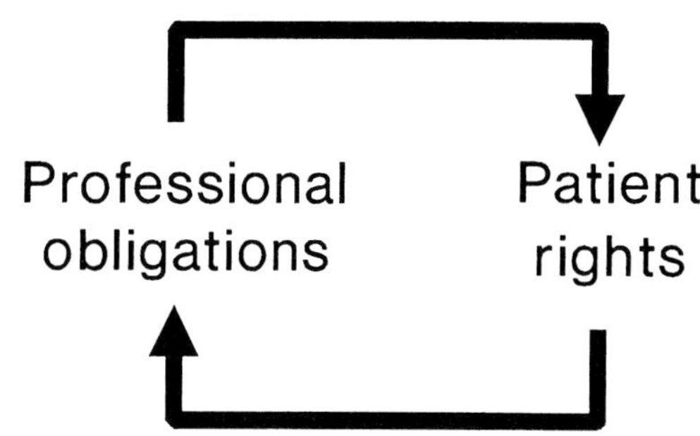

Figure 4-1

Reciprocal relationship between professional obligations and patient rights.

Kant's universal duties, and the values characterizing modern democracy.[4,5] Although some controversy exists, most ethicists agree that **autonomy, veracity, nonmaleficence, beneficence, confidentiality, justice,** and **role fidelity** are the primary guiding principles in contemporary ethical decision making.[1,4]

Each of these ethical principles, as applied to professional practice, consists of two components: a professional duty and a patient right (Figure 4-1). For example, the principle of autonomy obliges health professionals to uphold others' freedom of will and freedom of action. The principle of beneficence obliges us to further the interests of others, either by promoting their good or by actively preventing their harm. The principle of justice obliges us to ensure that others receive what they rightfully deserve or legitimately claim.

Expressed in each duty is a reciprocal patient right. Reciprocal patient rights include the right to autonomous choice, the right not to be harmed, and the right to fair and equitable treatment. More specific rules can be generated from these general principles of rights and obligations, such as those included in a code of ethics.

Autonomy

The principle of autonomy acknowledges patients' personal liberty and their right to decide their own course of treatment and follow through a plan on which they freely agree. It is from this principle that rules about **informed consent** are derived.

Under the principle of autonomy, an RT's use of deceit or coercion to get a patient to reverse the decision to refuse a treatment is considered unethical. Likewise, it is unethical, and illegal, to threaten a patient who is unwilling to sign a consent form.

Veracity

The principle of veracity is often linked to autonomy, especially in the area of informed consent. In general, veracity binds the healthcare provider and the patient

MINI CLINI

Patient Rights

PROBLEM

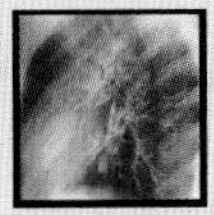

An RT working at a hospital receives a physician order to administer an aerosolized bronchodilator treatment to a 26-year-old female asthmatic patient admitted for suspected pneumonia. The patient refuses the treatment on entering the room, stating that she is having a "bad day" today and does not want to be bothered by anyone. The patient is regarded as being competent and fully capable of making healthcare decisions for herself. How could the RT handle this situation?

DISCUSSION

The RT must acknowledge and respect the patient's right to freely decide whether or not to allow the respiratory care treatment. According to the principles of ethical theory and conduct, healthcare professionals have an obligation to promote patient autonomy by permitting freedom of will and freedom of action. An additional requirement on the part of the practitioner is that coercion or deceit not be used to get a patient to reverse his or her decision to refuse a treatment. Indeed, according to the American Hospital Association Patient's Bill of Rights, the patient has the right to refuse treatment to the extent permitted by law and to be informed of the medical consequences of her action.

The RT could talk to the patient and explore what the term "bad day" meant to her. It might be that she is not feeling well because of breathing problems from her asthma condition and worsening symptoms of possible pneumonia. The RT has an important role in ensuring that the patient understands the benefits of the respiratory treatment, as well as the health consequences of refusal. Thus the patient can make a well-informed decision. By the RT approaching the patient in a professional, nonthreatening manner, she may feel more at ease and be willing to discuss in greater depth why she does not want to take the treatment. It is not uncommon for patients to initially refuse therapy only to change their mind following communication with the RT. Should the patient still refuse the treatment following discussion with the RT, the RT should remain nonjudgmental, even if he or she disagrees with the patient's decision. Appropriate documentation in the medical record and physician notification should then occur.

to tell the truth. The nature of the healthcare delivery process is such that both parties involved are best served in an environment of trust and mutual sharing of all information. Problems with the veracity principle revolve around such issues as **benevolent deception**. In actions of benevolent deception, the truth is withheld from the patient for his or her own good.

When the physician decides to withhold the truth from a conscious, well-oriented adult, the decision affects the interactions between healthcare providers and the patient and has a chilling effect on the rapport that is so necessary for good care. In a poll conducted by the Louis Harris group, 94% of Americans surveyed indicated that they wanted to know everything about their cases, even the dismal facts. Other than with pediatrics and rare cases in which there is evidence that the truth would lead to a harm (such as suicide), the truth, provided in as pleasant a manner as possible, is probably the best policy.[6]

Truth-telling can also involve documentation and medical recordkeeping. This type of dilemma is occurring more and more frequently under strict managed care reimbursement protocols. The Mini Clini on this page provides a good example of this type of dilemma.

Nonmaleficence

The principle of nonmaleficence obligates healthcare providers to avoid harming patients and to actively prevent harm where possible. It is sometimes difficult to uphold this principle in modern medicine because, in many cases, drugs and procedures have secondary effects that may be harmful in varying degrees. For example, we might ask whether it is ethical to give a high dose of steroids to an asthmatic patient, knowing the many harmful consequences of these drugs. One solution to these dilemmas is based on the understanding that

MINI CLINI

Veracity

PROBLEM

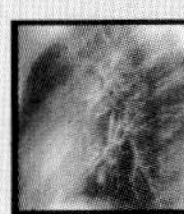

Jon performs pulmonary function testing, including blood gases, for his hospital. Many of the patients he sees are attempting to qualify or requalify for continuous reimbursement for home oxygen use. To qualify, the patient's Pa_{O_2} must be less than 60 mm Hg. Patient A, who has home oxygen therapy, is attempting to requalify although her condition has improved from what it was a year earlier. Her blood gas results show a Pa_{O_2} of 63 mm Hg. The patient's husband asks Jon if there is anything he can do, while relating how greatly his wife benefits from the oxygen. Jon tells the husband that there is nothing that he can do and assists the husband in taking the patient out to her car. At the car, the husband pulls out his wallet, shows it to Jon and repeats the question.

DISCUSSION POINT

RTs have an obligation to carry out their duties in the most competent and professional manner possible. Failure to do so may constitute both an ethical dilemma and a legal issue.

DISCUSSION QUESTIONS

What is the potential ethical dilemma in this situation? What other ways could Jon have chosen to handle this situation?

many helping actions inevitably have both a good and a bad effect, or **double effect**. The key is the first intent. If the first intent is good, then the harmful effect is viewed as an unintended result. The double effect brings us to the essence of the definition of the word dilemma. The word comes from the Greek "di," or "two," and "lemma," or "assumption" or "proposition."[7]

Beneficence

The principle of beneficence raises the "do no harm" requirement to an even higher level. Beneficence requires that health providers go beyond doing no harm and actively contribute to the health and well-being of their patients. In this dictum lies many quality-of-life issues. Practitioners of medicine today possess the technology to keep some individuals alive well beyond any likelihood of meaningful recovery. This presents real dilemmas for those who are confronted with the ability to prolong life but not the ability to restore any uniquely human qualities.

In these cases, some interpret the principle of beneficence to mean that they must do everything to promote a patient's life, regardless of how useful the life might be to that individual. Other professionals in the same situation might believe they are allowing the principle to be better served by doing nothing and allowing death to occur without taking heroic measures to prevent it. In an attempt to allow patients to participate in resolving this dilemma, legal avenues, called *advanced directives*, have been developed. The two types of advanced directives currently available and relatively widely used are the living will and the durable power of attorney for healthcare. Because of the Patient Self-Determination Act of 1990, most states require that all healthcare agencies receiving federal reimbursement under Medicare/Medicaid legislation provide adult clients with information on advanced directives.[8]

Confidentiality

The principle of confidentiality is founded in the Hippocratic Oath; it was later reiterated by the World Medical Association in 1949. It obliges healthcare providers to "respect the secrets which are confided even after the patient has died." Confidentiality, as with the other axioms of ethics, must often be balanced against other principles, such as beneficence.

The main ethical issue surrounding confidentiality is whether more harm is done by occasionally violating its mandate or by always upholding it, regardless of the consequences. This limitation to confidentiality is known as the *Harm Principle*. This principle requires that practitioners refrain from acts or omissions in which foreseeable harm to others could result, especially when the others are vulnerable to risk. For example, this principle would require that confidentiality be maintained for a patient with acquired immunodeficiency syndrome (AIDS) in matters involving his or her landlord. In this case, confidentiality is justified because the landlord is not particularly vulnerable. However, if the patient were planning to marry, the Harm Principle would require that confidentiality be broken because of the special vulnerability of the spouse.

Confidentiality is usually considered a qualified, rather than an absolute, ethical principle in most healthcare provider-patient relationships. These qualifications are often written into codes of ethics. For example, the American Medical Association Code of Ethics, Section 9, provides the following guidelines: "A physician may not reveal the confidences entrusted to him in the course of medical attendance or the deficiencies he may observe in the character of patients, unless he is required to do so by law or unless it becomes necessary in order to protect the welfare of the community or a vulnerable individual." Under the requirements of public health and community welfare there is often a legal requirement to report such things as child abuse, poisonings, industrial accidents, communicable diseases, blood transfusion reactions, narcotic use, and injuries caused with knives or guns.[9] In many states, child abuse statutes protect the practitioner from liability even if the report should prove false, as long as the report was made in good faith. Failure to report a case of child abuse can leave that practitioner legally liable for additional injuries that the child may sustain after being returned to the hostile environment.

Unfortunately, breaches of confidentiality more often result from careless slips of the tongue than from rational decision making. Such social trading in gossip about patients is unprofessional, unethical, and in certain cases, illegal.

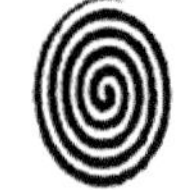

RULE OF THUMB

Patient information should be discussed only in private and with persons who have a legitimate reason and need to know.

Because of the widespread use of computerized databases, confidential information, once highly protected, is now relatively easy to obtain. Clinical data are available for close scrutiny by the clerical staff, laboratory personnel, and other healthcare providers. The widespread use of these data systems represents a real threat to patient confidentiality. In an attempt to reduce this threat, most clinical databases are restricted to use by only those healthcare workers who have a need to know. Therefore, in addition to being unethical,

MINI CLINI

Confidentiality

PROBLEM

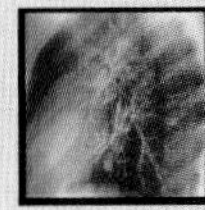

Mary, an RT, is working the evening shift at a large urban medical center when she receives a phone call from a friend telling her that her next door neighbor has been admitted to the medical center. Mary's first thought is to check the neighbor's file on the computer system to see why her neighbor has been hospitalized.

DISCUSSION POINT

Mary knows that the medical center has a policy that employees are to access only those charts for which they have a reason to do so.

DISCUSSION QUESTIONS

Should Mary access this chart via the computer system? If she does, what kind of violation will she be committing, ethical, legal, or both? What ethical principles, if any, would apply here? What is the harm in simply checking the computer on this patient? Is anyone likely to know if Mary accesses this patient's information?

an RT who reads the file of a patient who he or she is not treating will likely be in violation of institutional policy. The Mini Clini above provides an example.

Despite medical and sociological advances, potential violations of the individual's right to privacy in populations such as patients with AIDS pose a special threat because disclosure may result in economic, psychological, or physical harm to the patient. RTs would do well to adhere to the dictum found in the Hippocratic Oath: "What I may see or hear in the course of the treatment or even outside of treatment of the patient in regard to the life of men, which on no account one must spread abroad, I will keep to myself, holding such things to be shameful to be spoken about."[10]

Justice

The principle of justice involves the fair distribution of care. Rising healthcare expectations, coupled with the decreased availability of care because of cost, is making this principle an important one for healthcare workers. Population trends and the financial shortfalls in programs such as Medicaid and Medicare will continue to contribute to the importance of this principle.

The United States is rapidly approaching the point at which a balance must be found between healthcare expenses and the revenue available to pay for them. Efforts to achieve this balance will inevitably lead to some form of rationing of the delivery of healthcare services. This type of justice is properly referred to as **distributive justice**.

A second form of justice seen in healthcare is **compensatory justice**. This form of justice calls for the recovery for damages that were incurred as a result of the action of others. Damage awards in civil cases of medical malpractice or negligence are examples of compensatory justice. Ironically, compensatory justice has played a major role in increasing the cost of healthcare. The cost of malpractice insurance and the practice of defensive medicine both contribute significantly to the total cost of treating patients.

Role Duty

Modern healthcare is a team effort by necessity. This is because no single individual can be solely responsible for providing all of a patient's healthcare needs. Today there are more than 100 specialties under the heading of allied health. These professions, along with nursing, provide more than 80% of all patient care. Each of these specialties has its own practice niche, defined by tradition or by licensure law. Practitioners have a duty to understand the limits of their role and to practice with fidelity. For example, because of differences in role duty, an RT might be ethically obliged not to tell a patient's family how critical the situation is, instead having the attending physician do so.[2] The Mini Clini below presents another example of the ethics of role duty.

MINI CLINI

Role Duty

PROBLEM

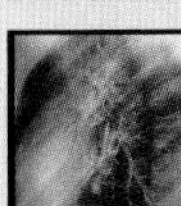

Sue, an RT, receives a request to perform a blood gas analysis for a patient on a ventilator because, as reported by the nurse, the patient's oxygen saturation is only 61%. The patient has an order for blood gases as needed. As the nurse and RT look at the results, they both are surprised because the saturation is now 93%. The nurse suggests repeating the blood gases. The RT is about to comply until she notes that the monitor display on which the nurse is relying shows the patient with an oxygen saturation of 93% and a pulse rate of 61 beats/min.

DISCUSSION POINT

Teamwork and role delineation are both essential components of good patient care. Each practitioner also has an obligation to perform his or her duties in the most competent and professional manner possible.

DISCUSSION QUESTIONS

What kind of issue or dilemma exists here, legal, ethical, or both? What should the RT do at this point? Should an incident report be written, and if so, by whom?

ETHICAL VIEWPOINTS AND DECISION MAKING

In deciding ethical issues, some practitioners try to adhere to a strict interpretation of one or more ethical principles (such as those just described). Others seek to decide the issue solely on a case-by-case basis, considering only the potential good (or bad) consequences. Still others would appeal to the image of a "good practitioner," asking themselves what a virtuous person would do in a similar circumstance. Finally, many practitioners acknowledge that they largely follow their intuition for making ethical decisions. These different viewpoints represent the four dominant theories underlying modern ethics.[4,11,12] The viewpoint that relies on rules and principles is called **formalism** or duty-oriented reasoning. The viewpoint in which decisions are based on the assessment of consequences is called **consequentialism**. The viewpoint that asks what a virtuous person would do in a similar circumstance is called **virtue ethics**. When intuition is involved in the decision-making process, the approach is called **intuitionism**.

Formalism

Formalist thought asserts that certain features of an act itself determine its moral rightness. In this framework, ethical standards of right and wrong are described in terms of rules or principles. These rules function apart from the consequences of a particular act. An act is considered morally justifiable only if it upholds the rules or principles that apply.

The major objection to this duty-oriented approach lies in its potential for inconsistency. Critics of formalist reasoning insist that no principle or rule can be framed that does not have exceptions. Moreover, these critics claim that no principle or rule can be framed that does not conflict with other rules.

Consequentialism

For the consequentialist, an act is judged to be right or wrong based on its consequences. Each possible act is assessed in terms of the relative amount of good (over evil) that it will bring into being. The most common application of consequentialism judges acts according to the principle of utility. The principle of utility, in its simplest form, aims to promote the greatest general good for most people.

Critics of this approach claim that it has two fundamental flaws. First, the "calculus" involved in projecting and weighing the amount of good over evil that might occur is not always possible. Second, reliance on the principle of utility to the exclusion of all else can result in actions that are incompatible with ordinary judgments about right and wrong. A classic example of this problem can be seen in the true World War II case of the battle for North Africa. In this scenario, there were two groups of soldiers but only enough antibiotics for one group. One group required the medication for syphilis contracted in the local brothels; the other group needed antibiotics for wounds sustained in battle. Thus the dilemma arose as to who should receive the antibiotics.

Formalist or duty-oriented reasoning would base the decision about who should receive the antibiotics on some concept of justice, such as giving priority to the sickest or to those most in need. However, the actual decision in this case was a consequentialist one, based not on the desire to justly distribute the drug, but rather on the need to obtain a quick victory with as few casualties as possible. Therefore the scarce medication was given to those who were "wounded" in the brothels rather than in battle because these soldiers could be restored quickly and returned to the front lines to aid the war effort.

Mixed Approaches

Mixed approaches to moral reasoning try to capitalize on the strengths inherent in these two major lines of ethical thought. One approach, called **rule utilitarianism**, is a variation of consequentialism. Under this framework, the question is not which act has the greatest utility, but which rule would promote the greatest good if it were generally followed.

For example, the rule utilitarian would agree with the formalist that truth-telling is a necessary ethical principle, but for a different reason. To the rule utilitarian, truth-telling is a needed principle not because it has any underlying moral rightness, but because it promotes the greatest good in professional-patient relationships. Specifically, if truth-telling were not followed consistently, trusting relationships between patients and health professionals would be impossible.

The rule utilitarian approach is probably the most appealing and useful to health professionals. It is appealing because it addresses both human rights and obligations and the consequences of our actions. Moreover, rule utilitarianism seems best able to account for the modern realities of human experience that so often affect the day-to-day practice of healthcare.

Virtue Ethics

A theory of virtue ethics has evolved based in part on the limits of both formalism and consequentialism. Virtue ethics is founded not in rules or consequences but in personal attributes of character or virtue. Under this formulation, the first question is not, "How do I act in this situation?" but, rather, "How should I carry out my life if I am to live well?" or "How would the good RT act?"

Virtue-oriented theory holds that professions have historical traditions. Thus individuals entering a profession enter into a relationship not only with current practitioners but also with those who have come before them. With these traditions comes a history of character standards set by those who have previously distinguished themselves in that profession.

According to this perspective, the established practices of a profession can give guidance, without an appeal to either the specific moral principles or consequences of an act.[2] Thus when the professional is faced with an ethical dilemma, he or she need only envision what the "good practitioner" would do in a similar circumstance. For instance, it is hard to imagine the good RT stealing from the patient, charging for services not provided, or smothering a patient with a pillow.

Rapidly changing fields such as respiratory care do pose some problems for virtue ethics. What might be considered good ethical conduct at one time might be deemed wrong the next time. An example of this change over time is the RT who is asked not only to disconnect a brain-dead patient from a ventilator but also to remove the feeding tubes and intravenous lines.

In addition to virtue ethic's difficulty with changing values, it provides no specific directions to aid decision making. Moreover, the heavy reliance of virtue ethics on experience rather than on reason makes creative solutions less likely. Last, practitioners often find themselves in conflicting role situations for which virtue ethics has no answers. A good example is the RT who practices the virtue of being a good team player but is confronted with the need to "blow the whistle" on a negligent or incompetent team member.[2] Despite these limitations, virtue ethics is probably the way most practitioners make their ethical decisions.

Intuitionism

Intuitionism is an ethical viewpoint that holds that there are certain self-evident truths, usually based on moral maxims such as "treat others fairly." The easiest way to understand intuitionism is to think of as many timeless maxims as you can and you will have the basis for intuitionism. These maxims may range from "do not kill" to "look before you cross the street."[5]

Comprehensive Decision-Making Models

To aid in the process of decision making in bioethics, several comprehensive models have developed. Figure 4-2 depicts one example of a comprehensive decision-making model that combines the best elements of formalism, consequentialism, and virtue ethics.

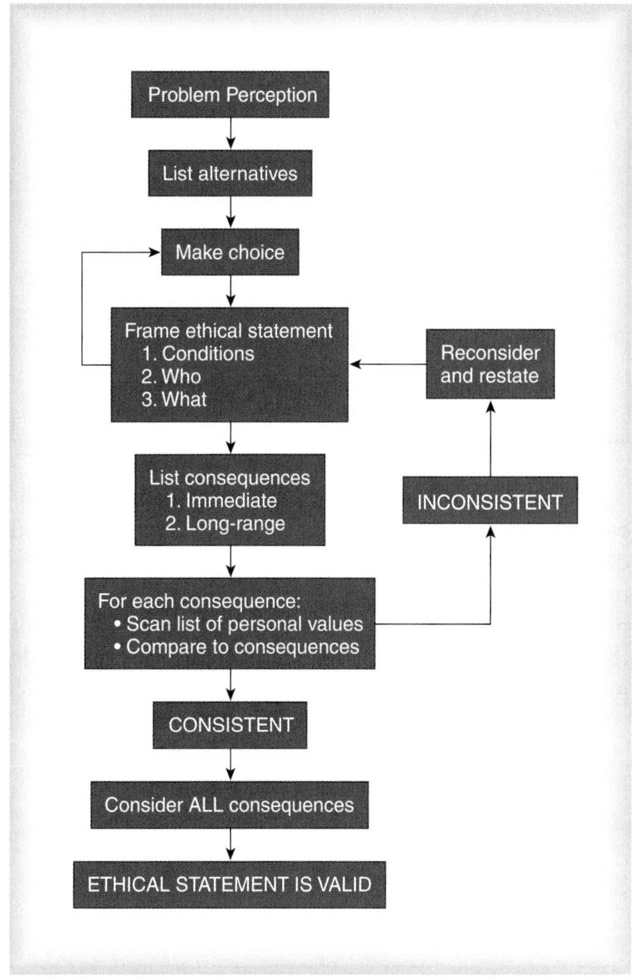

Figure 4-2

A comprehensive ethical decision-making model. *(Redrawn from Brody H: Ethical decisions in medicine, ed 2, Boston, 1981, Little, Brown & Co.)*

As is evident in this approach, the ethical problem is framed in terms of the conditions and who is affected. Initially, an action is chosen based on its predicted consequences. Then the potential consequences of this decision are compared with the human values underlying the problem. The short test of this comparison is a simple restatement of the Golden Rule that is, "Would I be satisfied to have this action performed on me?" The initial decision is considered ethical if, and only if, it passes this test of human values.

A somewhat simpler but nonetheless comprehensive model is used by many ethicists. The model uses eight key steps (Box 4-2).

With or without these models, RTs are often at a double disadvantage in ethical decision making. This is because RTs not only must live with their own decisions but must also support (and act on) the decisions of their physician colleagues. Unless excellent communication exists, misunderstandings can occur. Such misunderstandings may be an essential factor in the high job stress, burnout, and attrition in respiratory care.

Box 4-2 • Ethical Decision-Making Model

1. Identify the problem or issue.
2. Identify the individuals involved.
3. Identify the ethical principle or principles that apply.
4. Identify who should make the decision.
5. Identify the role of the practitioner.
6. Consider the alternatives (long-term and short-term consequences).
7. Make the decision (including the decision not to act).
8. Follow the decision to observe its consequences.

Classes in ethics, decision making, and communication skills are critical components of the preparation of RTs for the often confusing and frustrating practice in today's medical settings. The specialty requires practitioners who can go beyond simple assertions of their beliefs of being right or wrong and provide justifications that are both right and reasoned.

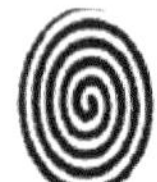

RULE OF THUMB

Never attempt to make ethical decisions for others. You can only make them for yourself.

LEGAL ISSUES AFFECTING RESPIRATORY CARE

Unfortunately, there are times when decisions cannot be made in the confines of the medical community and with the help of the patients it serves. These problems often find their way to the courts. The problem of professional liability in the delivery of healthcare is immense and plays a key role in skyrocketing healthcare costs. Limits on medical liability have been key factors in recent legislation.

Practitioners are caught in the middle. On one hand, they are required to hold down costs by avoiding overuse of technology and therapeutics. On the other hand, they are faced with a level of consumerism that holds them accountable as never before. Clearly the costs, losses, frustration, and distraction brought about by the current level of legal intervention in healthcare practice are a national crisis.

Systems of Law

Under our legal system, the law is divided into two broad classes: public and civil law. Public law deals with the relationships of private parties and the government. Civil law is concerned with the recognition and enforcement of the rights and duties of private individuals and organizations.

Public (Criminal and Administrative) Law

The two major divisions of public law are criminal law and administrative law. Criminal law deals with acts or offenses against the welfare or safety of the public. Offenses against criminal law are punishable by fines, imprisonment, or both. In these cases, the accuser is the state and the person prosecuted is the defendant.

Administrative law is the second major branch of public law. Administrative law consists of the countless regulations set by governmental agencies. Healthcare facilities are inundated by a host of administrative and agency rules that affect almost every aspect of operation. RTs are obligated to abide by these rules and regulations.

Civil Law

Private or civil law protects private citizens and organizations from others who might seek to take unfair and unlawful advantage of them. If an individual feels that his or her rights have been compromised, he or she can seek redress in the civil courts. In these cases, the individual bringing the complaint is known as the **plaintiff**, and the individual accused of wrong is the **defendant**. Civil courts decide between the two parties, with regard to the degree of wrong and the level of reparation required. The category of civil law best related to respiratory care is tort law.

Tort Law. A **tort** is a civil wrong, other than a breach of contract, committed against an individual or property, for which a court provides a remedy in the form of an action for damages. Causes for the complaints may range from assault and battery to invasion of privacy. The basic functions of torts are to keep the peace between individuals and to substitute a remedy for personal injury instead of vengeance.

There are three basic forms of torts: negligent torts, intentional torts, and torts in which liability is assessed regardless of fault (as in the case of manufacturers of defective products). The basic difference between negligent and intentional torts is the element of intent. An intentional tort always involves a willful act that violates another's interest. A negligent tort does not have to involve any action at all. Instead, a negligent tort can consist of an omission of an action.

Professional Negligence. **Negligence**, in its simplest terms, is the failure to perform one's duties competently. Negligence may involve acts of commission or omission. The tort of negligence is concerned with the compensation of an individual for loss or damages arising from the unreasonable behavior of another. The normal standard for the claim is the duty imposed on individuals not to cause risk or harm to others, the standard being what a reasonable and prudent person should have foreseen and avoided.

In negligence cases, the breach of duty often involves the matter of foreseeability. Cases in which the patient falls, is burned, is given the wrong medication, or is harmed by defects in an apparatus often revolve around the healthcare provider's duty to anticipate the harm. Duty can be defined as an obligation to do a thing, a human action exactly conformable to the law that requires us to obey.

For the tort of negligence to be a valid claim, the four conditions listed in Box 4-3 must be met.

The assessment of what is reasonable and prudent for an RT can be determined by guidelines established by a professional group (e.g., the AARC), by direct expert testimony, or by circumstantial evidence. In the latter case, the legal principle **res ipsa loquitur** (the thing speaks for itself) may apply. *Res ipsa loquitur* is sometimes invoked to show that the harm would not ordinarily have happened if those in control had used appropriate care. In these cases, negligence is established by inference.

For a claim of *res ipsa loquitur* to be supported, three basic conditions must be met: (1) the harm was such that it would not normally occur without someone's negligence, (2) the action responsible for the injury was under the control of the defendant, and (3) the injury did not result from any contributing negligence or voluntarily assumed risk on the part of the injured party.

An example of *res ipsa loquitur* might be the failure to recognize that a patient's right mainstem bronchus had been intubated with a resultant pneumothorax. For negligence to occur, the breach in duty must also cause actual damage or injury to the individual. The injured party must file the lawsuit within the time frame set by the statute of limitations. The term *injury*, in this sense, may include not only physical harm but also mental anguish and other invasions of the patient's rights and privileges. The claim must be supported by a preponderance of evidence to prevail.

Last, for the tort of negligence to be sustained, the breach of duty must be shown to be the direct or "proximate" cause of the injury. A causal relationship must exist between the negligent action and the resulting damage. The mere failure to provide the appropriate standard of care is insufficient to necessitate payment of damages unless injury occurs as a direct result of the action or omission.

Box 4-3 • The "Four Ds" of Negligence

- The practitioner owes a *D*uty to the patient.
- The practitioner was *D*erelict with that duty.
- The breach of duty was the *D*irect cause of damages.
- *D*amage or harm came to the patient.

MALPRACTICE. **Malpractice**, as a form of negligence, can involve professional misconduct, unreasonable lack of skill or fidelity in professional duties, evil practice, or unethical conduct. There are three classifications of malpractice: (1) criminal malpractice, including such crimes as assault and battery or euthanasia (handled in criminal court); (2) civil malpractice, such as negligence or practice below a reasonable standard (handled in civil court); and (3) ethical malpractice, which includes violations of professional ethics and may result in censure or disciplinary actions by licensure boards.

Intentional Torts. An intentional tort is a wrong perpetrated by one who intends to break the law. This is in contrast to negligence, in which the professional fails to exercise adequate care in doing what is otherwise permissible. The acts must be intentionally performed to produce the harm or must be performed with the belief that the result was likely to follow.

These torts are more serious than the tort of negligence, in that the defendant intended to commit the wrong. Consequently, punitive, as well as actual, damages may be awarded. Examples of intentional torts are those that involve defamation of character, invasion of privacy, deceit, infliction of mental distress, and **assault** and **battery**.

In the hospital, the unwarranted discussion of the patient's condition, diagnosis, or treatment for purposes other than the exchange of information is always deemed suspect in regard to defamation of character. Under the general title of defamation of character are the torts of **libel** and **slander**. Slander is the verbal defamation of an individual by false words by which his or her reputation is damaged. Libel is printed defamation by written words, cartoons, and such representations to cause the individual to be avoided or held in contempt. Libel and slander do not exist unless they are seen or heard by a third person. If the practitioner directed such remarks only to the individual involved, it would not be slanderous. On the other hand, if the remark was made in the presence of a third party, it might constitute slander.

Caution in regard to unauthorized disclosure of patient information is especially critical in cases involving such diseases as AIDS, which often carries a high degree of medical and social stigma. Patients have the legal right to expect that all information about their illness will be held in strict confidence. Several states now have civil liability and criminal penalties for the release of confidential HIV test results in which the breach of confidence results in economic, psychological, or bodily harm to the patient.

An assault is an intentional act that places another person in fear of immediate bodily harm. Threatening to injure someone is considered an act of assault. Battery, on the other hand, represents unprivileged, nonconsensual physical contact with another person. In the classic act of assault and battery, one individual threatens and actually injures another.

Although battery is an unusual charge against a clinician (because of the nature of the work), it is one that creates special problems. The major element of battery is physical contact without consent. When a practitioner performs a procedure without the patient's consent, this contact may be considered battery. In most instances, there is an implied consent, created when the patient solicits care from the physician. This implied consent allows the performance of ordinary procedures without written consent. In all cases of unusual, difficult, or dangerous procedures, such as surgery, the courts require written consent. For this reason, to avoid being accused of battery, RTs should always explain all procedures involving physical contact to their patients before they proceed.

There are two general defenses against intentional torts. The first defense is that there was a lack of intent to harm and that only clinicians who engage in intentional conduct are liable. For example, if a practitioner fainted during a procedure and thereby caused the patient injury, he or she would not be liable because the action was not voluntary. The second defense is that the patient gave consent to the procedure. If the patient consented to the action, knowing the risks involved, the practitioner would not be liable. Thus consent by the patient for both nonroutine and routine procedures should be obtained before care is rendered.

Strict Liability. **Strict liability** is a theory in tort law that can be used to impose liability without fault, even in situations where injury occurs under conditions of reasonable care. The most common cases of strict liability are those involving the use of dangerous products or techniques. Courts have imposed this principle on medical equipment manufacturers, as well as on hospitals. However, strict liability generally has not been extended to professional services.

Breach of Contract. **Breach of contract** is a much rarer malpractice claim than negligence. This claim is based on the theory that when a healthcare professional renders care, an implicit or explicit professional-patient "contract" is established. Essentially, the contract binds the healthcare professional to place the patient's welfare as the foremost concern, to act only in the patient's behalf, to protect the patient's life, to preserve the patient's health, to relieve suffering, and to protect privacy. When the patient is injured as a result of the services rendered under this contract, the patient may claim that the failure of the healthcare professional to competently perform the service is a breach of the contract.

RTs are responsible for their actions, as are members of all other professions. When these actions result in the injury of another, the injured party may turn to the courts for redress. If the RT, while acting for the physician, injures the patient through some negligent act, the patient may sue both the practitioner and the physician.

Civil Suits. Civil action can be brought for many reasons, such as to challenge a law or to enjoin an activity. However, as in the case of malpractice suits, most seek monetary damages. The following scenario is an example of a situation that might involve the RT: The physician intends to order 0.5 mL of a bronchodilator for a 3-year-old asthmatic patient but inadvertently prescribes 5.0 mL of the drug. Because of the overdose given by the RT the child dies.

A clearly articulated legal principle in negligence is that the duty owed to the patient is commensurate with the patient's needs. In short, the more vulnerable the patient, the greater the caregiver's duty to protect. When the order is not clear or seems inappropriate under this principle, clinicians have an obligation to clarify rather than risk harm.

The suit could be brought against the physician for negligence for ordering the overdose, against the nurses and RT for failing to recognize that the dose was incorrect for the child, and possibly, against the pharmacist for failing to gain adequate information as to the nature of the patient so that an appropriate dosage could be calculated. The plaintiff would base the secondary charges against the nurses and allied health practitioners on the theory that liability would be incurred by those who missed an opportunity to correct the first wrongdoer's mistake. The hospital's risk management department and legal counsel will provide direction and counsel to the RT in the case of a civil suit. It is extremely important that the RT adhere to this professional advice.

Medical Supervision

RTs are required by their **scope of practice** to work under competent medical supervision. This requirement creates not only a professional relationship but also a legal one. If the RT is employed by the physician, the physician is liable for his or her actions. The legal framework for this liability is found in the principle **respondeat superior** (let the master answer).

Under this doctrine, the physician assumes responsibility for the wrongful actions of the RT as long as such negligence occurred in the course of the employer-employee relationship. For this liability to be incurred, two conditions must be met: (1) the act must be within the scope of employment and (2) the injury caused must be the result of an act of negligence.

If the RT acted outside of his or her scope of practice, as outlined by licensure laws or by institutional regulations, the court would have to decide whether the physician would still be liable. For instance, if the RT, while in the patient's room to deliver an aerosol treatment, went beyond the normal scope of practice and adjusted cervical traction, thereby causing injury, it is doubtful that the physician could be held fully responsible. However, under the principle of *respondeat superior*, the hospital, as a corporate entity, could be held responsible for the actions of its employees.

Historically, RTs have not been named individually as defendants in malpractice cases because the law generally has not focused on their role as specialized healthcare providers separate from the healthcare facility. Either the hospital or the physician is usually named as the defendant for the acts of the practitioner. RTs in these cases have been viewed simply as employees, merely carrying out the orders of a superior. However, with the increased application of state licensure regulations governing respiratory care, this relative protection from liability is changing rapidly.

Scope of Practice

One measure of professionalism is the extent to which the group is willing to direct its own development and regulate its own activities. This self-direction is carried out mainly through professional associations and state licensure boards, which attempt to ensure that professionals exhibit minimum levels of competence.

Basic Elements of a Practice Act. Some practice acts emphasize one area over another but most acts address the following elements:

- Scope of professional practice
- Requirements and qualifications for licensure
- Exemptions
- Grounds for administrative action
- Creation of examination board and processes
- Penalties and sanctions for unauthorized practice

Licensure Laws and Regulations. In licensure legislation there is always a clause specifying a scope of practice. The scope-of-practice statutes give general guidelines and parameters for the clinician's practice. Deviation from these statutes could be a source of legal problems as the specialty seeks to add new duties. Practitioners must know the limits of their scope of care and seek amendments to the licensure regulations as they expand their practice. Ideally, the original language of a licensure law should be broad enough to account for changes in practice without requiring continual amendment. Continuing education and regular review of the practice act is essential to ensure compliance with both the statute and evolving rules of the practice act.

Providing Emergency Care Without Physician Direction. One unique area that allows practice without the direction of a competent physician is that of rendering emergency medical care to injured persons. Good Samaritan laws protect citizens from civil or criminal liability for any errors they make while attempting to give emergency aid. Most states have legislated Good Samaritan statutes to encourage individuals to give needed emergency medical assistance. It is necessary for this aid to be given in good faith and free of gross negligence or willful misconduct. However, it is unlikely that the RT would be protected for giving aid that clearly went beyond the expected skills of the individual or aid that went beyond that which could be defined as first aid, such as performing a tracheostomy. Good Samaritan rules in general apply only to roadside accidents and emergency situations outside the hospital.

▶ INTERACTION OF ETHICS AND THE LAW

A good example of the interaction of ethics and the law in respiratory care is the diversification of the field into home care and durable medical equipment supply. This diversification has led to new relationships between these elements of the healthcare system and has created real potential for unethical and unlawful activity. For example, if the practitioner accepts some remuneration, such as a finder's fee or percentage of the total lease costs for referring patients to a particular home care company or equipment service, he or she should be prepared to face charges of unethical and perhaps illegal practice.

Several federal statutes address the legality of these types of transactions. Many states also have statutes. Generally, these statutes state that anyone who knowingly or willfully solicits, receives, offers, or pays directly or indirectly any remuneration in return for Medicare business is guilty of a criminal offense. Violation of these statutes carries the potential for prison and/or a substantial fine. If the practitioner is aware of others who are engaged in these practices, he or she should report these activities to the appropriate state or federal Medicare agency.

To aid the clinician in maintaining an ethical stance on these new issues, the AARC has established a position statement about ethical performance of respiratory home care.

HEALTHCARE AND CHANGE

The healthcare industry is experiencing rapid change relating to how services are funded and how patients and healthcare workers interact. This is happening at the same time that ethical considerations are reemerging as significant components of how healthcare should be structured and delivered. It is no secret that managed care, in its strongest forms, affects the ethical decision-making process. Although the effect is not necessarily negative, it forces healthcare workers to take a new look at ethical dilemmas to arrive at both the best ethical and managed care outcome. Patients no longer freely choose who will deliver healthcare services to them. Healthcare practitioners not only must consider the best services to deliver to patients; they must also consider the best managed care outcome.

Regardless, in this atmosphere, if ethical reasoning is to be of any value, it must continue to account for the reality of human experience and needs and take its rightful place among the many considerations that compete for the practitioners' attention. These considerations include (1) factual premises and beliefs, such as the definition of death; (2) legal concepts, such as tort laws; (3) externally imposed mandates or expectations, such as hospital accreditation standards; and (4) the best managed care outcome.

In many instances, such considerations uphold our underlying moral convictions and strengthen support for a given action. The real challenge to RTs arises when moral principles dictate one course of action and factual knowledge, legal concepts, or external expectations dictate another.

Long ago, Socrates demanded that professionals acknowledge the social context of their activities and that they recognize their obligations toward the segment of society that they profess to serve. As our analysis of ethical reasoning and the law has made clear, only by identifying, justifying, and prioritizing basic principles of human values can the RT resolve the difficult questions of professional behavior consistently. To the extent that clearly articulated principles guide our choices and actions, all involved will be well served.

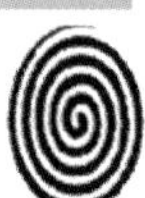

RULE OF THUMB

The letters RCP are used to indicate Respiratory Care Practitioner. They also suggest three important characteristics for the RT to follow when confronted with ethical dilemmas:

*R*espect
*C*ompassion
*P*rofessionalism

KEY POINTS

- Ethical dilemmas occur when there are either two equally desirable or equally undesirable choices. Ethical dilemmas may involve situations that are either legal or illegal.
- Common ethical dilemmas in respiratory care include determining the scope of practice, confidentiality, working within levels of professional responsibility, professional development issues, staffing patterns, and recordkeeping.
- Professional codes of ethics are general guidelines established to identify ideal behavioral parameters by members of a professional group. These codes are often simplistic and tend to deal with flagrant behavior over which there is little disagreement.
- The traditional ethical principles are rooted in philosophical thought and include autonomy, beneficence, confidentiality, role fidelity, justice, nonmaleficence, and veracity. These principles are used in various ways in the ethical decision-making process.
- There are two basic ethical theories: formalism and consequentialism. The most commonly used ethical decision-making model is the mixed approach. The mixed approach combines components of formalism, consequentialism, and modern decision-making theory.
- The basic information that must be identified before a reasoned ethical decision is made includes the problem or issue, the individuals involved, and the ethical principle or principles that apply, as well as a determination of who should make the decision and the role of the practitioner.
- Public law deals with the relationships of private parties and the government. Civil law is concerned with the recognition and enforcement of the rights and duties of private individuals and organizations.
- Professional malpractice is negligence in which a professional has failed to provide the care expected, resulting in harm to someone. Examples of situations that RTs might encounter include attempting procedures beyond the practitioner's skill level, failure to perform a duty as assigned, or failure to perform the duty correctly.

Continued

KEY POINTS—cont'd

- RTs, like members of other professions, are responsible for their actions. If their actions result in injury to others, the injured party or parties are entitled to seek redress in the courts.
- A professional license provides a framework under which a licensee carries out his or her duties. Because licensure acts define who can perform specified duties, it is expected that the duties will be performed in a responsible manner, and the professional will be responsible for his or her actions. The purpose of licensure is to provide for the public's safety.
- Patients are increasingly more educated and hold higher expectations from healthcare practitioners. Many patients are assuming responsibility for their own healthcare, placing the healthcare practitioner into the role of consultant. Therefore practitioners must carry out their duties with an eye toward defending themselves in the case of legal action.

References

1. Brincat CA, Wike VS: Morality and the professional life: values at work, Upper Saddle River, NJ, 2000, Prentice Hall.
2. Carroll C: Legal issues and ethical dilemmas in respiratory care, Philadelphia, 1996, FA Davis.
3. Edge R, Groves R: The ethics of health care: a guide for practice, Albany, 1994, Delmar.
4. Beauchamp TL, Childress JF: Principles of biomedical ethics, ed 4, New York, 1994, Oxford University Press.
5. Boylan M: Business ethics: basic ethics in action, Upper Saddle River, NJ, 2001, Prentice Hall.
6. Husted GL, Husted JH: Ethical decision making in nursing, St Louis, 1991, Mosby.
7. Pickett JP et al: The American Heritage Dictionary of the English Language, ed 4, Boston, Houghton Mifflin Company, 2000.
8. Logue B: Rights: death control and the elderly in America, New York, 1993, Macmillan.
9. Hill TP, Shirley D: A good death: taking more control at the end of your life, Reading, Mass, 1992, Addison-Wesley.
10. Pozgar G: Legal aspects of health care administration, Gaithersburg, Md, 1990, Aspen Publishers.
11. Hippocrates: The oath. In The Loeb classical library: Hippocrates, no. 147-150, Cambridge, Mass, 1948, Harvard University Press (Translated by WHS Jones).
12. Ross WD: The right and the good, Oxford, 1930, Clarendon Press.

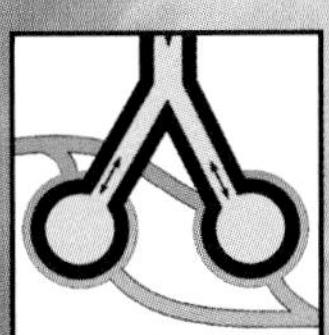

CHAPTER 5

Physical Principles of Respiratory Care

Craig L. Scanlan and Robert L. Wilkins

In This Chapter You Will Learn:

- What properties characterize the three states of matter
- How heat transfer occurs among substances
- How to use the three common temperature scales
- How substances undergo change of state
- What factors influence the vaporization of water
- How water vapor capacity, absolute humidity, and relative humidity are related
- How to predict gas behavior under changing conditions, including at extremes of temperature and pressure
- What principles govern the flow of fluids

Chapter Outline

States of Matter
- Internal energy of matter
- Internal energy and temperature
- Heat and the First Law of Thermodynamics
- Heat transfer

Change of State
- Liquid-solid phase changes (melting and freezing)
- Properties of liquids
- Liquid-vapor phase changes
- Properties of gases

Gas Behavior Under Changing Conditions
- Gas laws
- Effect of water vapor
- Properties of gases at extremes of temperature and pressure
- Critical temperature and pressure

Fluid Dynamics
- Pressures in flowing fluids
- Patterns of flow
- Flow, velocity, and cross-sectional area
- The Bernoulli effect
- Fluid entrainment
- The Venturi and Pitot tubes
- Fluidics and the Coanda effect

Key Terms

absolute humidity
adhesion
ATPS
Avogadro's law
BTPS
Coanda effect
cohesion
condensation
conduction
convection
critical temperature
Dalton's law
evaporation
flow resistance
fluid entrainment
Graham's law
Henry's law
kinetic energy
laminar flow
Laplace's law
latent heat of fusion
latent heat of vaporization
Law of continuity
Pascal's principle

Continued

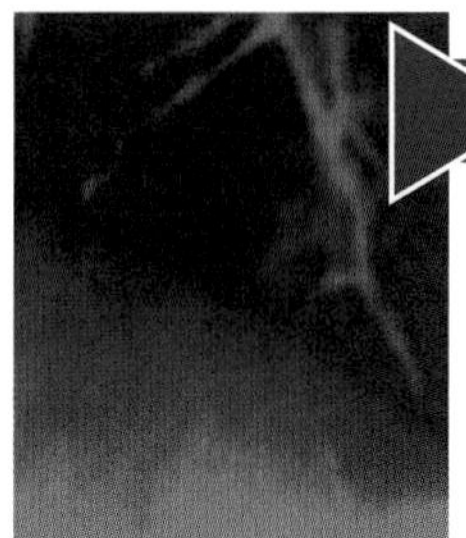

Key Terms—cont'd

Poiseuille's law
potential energy
radiation
relative humidity (RH)
Reynold's number
solubility coefficient
STPD
strain-gauge pressure transducers
surface tension
thermal conductivity
turbulent flow
vaporization
viscosity
water vapor pressure

STATES OF MATTER

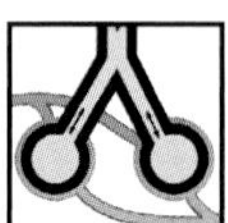

There are three primary states of matter: solid, liquid, and gas. Figure 5-1 depicts simplified models of these states of matter.

Solids have a high degree of internal order; their atoms or molecules are limited to back-and-forth motion about a central position, as if held together by springs (Figure 5-1, *A*). Solids maintain their shape because their atoms are kept in place by strong mutual attractive forces, called *van der Waals forces*.

Liquid molecules also exhibit mutual attraction. However, because these forces are much weaker in liquids than in solids, liquid molecules can move about freely (Figure 5-1, *B*). This freedom of motion explains why liquids take the shape of their containers and are capable of flow. However, like solids, liquids are dense and cannot easily be compressed.

In a gas, molecular attractive forces are very weak. Thus gas molecules, which lack restriction to their movement, exhibit rapid, random motion with frequent collisions (Figure 5-1, *C*). Gases have no inherent boundaries and are easily compressed and expanded. Moreover, like liquids, gases can flow. For this reason, both liquids and gases are considered fluids.

Internal Energy of Matter

All matter possesses energy. The energy matter possesses is called *internal energy*. There are two major types of internal energy: (1) the energy of position, or **potential energy**, and (2) the energy of motion, or **kinetic energy**.

The atoms of all matter, at ordinary temperatures, are in constant motion. Thus all matter has some kinetic energy. However, most internal energy in solids and liquids is potential energy. This potential energy is a result of the strong attractive forces between molecules. These intermolecular forces cause rigidity in solids and cohesiveness and viscosity in liquids. In contrast, because these attractive forces are so weak in gases, most of their internal energy is kinetic energy.

Internal Energy and Temperature

Temperature and kinetic energy are closely related. The temperature of a gas, with most of its internal energy spent keeping molecules in motion, is directly proportional to its kinetic energy. In contrast, the temperatures of solids and liquid represent only part of their total internal energy.

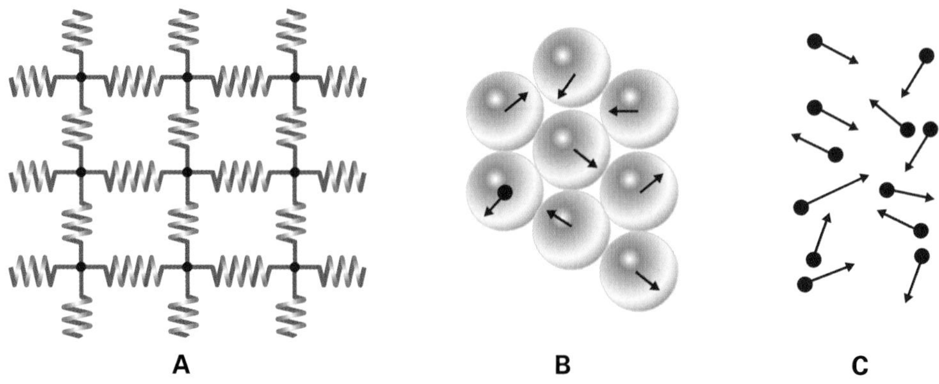

Figure 5-1 · Simplified Models of the Three States of Matter

A, Solid. **B,** Liquid. **C,** Gas.

Absolute Zero

In concept, a temperature should exist at which there is no kinetic energy. This temperature is absolute zero. Although researchers have come close to absolute zero, no one has actually achieved it.

Temperature Scales

Absolute zero provides a logical zero point on which to build a temperature scale. The SI units for temperature are degrees Kelvin, with a zero point equal to absolute zero (0° K). Because the Kelvin scale has 100 degrees between the freezing and boiling points of water, it is a centigrade, or 100-step, temperature scale.

The centimeter-gram-second (cgs) temperature system is based on Celsius units (° C). Like the Kelvin scale, the Celsius scale is a centigrade scale (100 degrees between the freezing and boiling points of water). However, 0° C is not absolute zero, but instead is the freezing point of water.

In Celsius units, kinetic molecular activity stops at approximately –273° C. Therefore 0° K equals –273° C, and 0° C equals 273° K. Thus to convert degrees Celsius to degrees Kelvin, you simply add 273:

$$°K = °C + 273$$

For example:

$$25°C = 25 + 273 = 298°K$$

Conversely, to convert degrees Kelvin to Celsius, you simply subtract 273. For example:

$$310°K = 310 - 273 = 37°C$$

The Fahrenheit scale is the primary temperature scale in the fps or British system of measurement. Absolute zero on the Fahrenheit scale equals –460° F.

To convert degrees Fahrenheit to degrees Celsius, use the following formula:

$$°C = \frac{5}{9}(°F - 32)$$

For example:

$$°F = 98.6$$

$$°C = \frac{5}{9}(98.6 - 32)$$

$$°C = 37$$

To convert degrees Celsius to degrees Fahrenheit, simply reverse this formula:

$$°F = \left(\frac{9}{5} \times °C\right) + 32$$

For example:

$$°C = 100$$

$$°F = \left(\frac{9}{5} \times 100\right) + 32$$

$$°F = 212$$

Figure 5-2 shows the relationship between the kinetic activity of matter and temperature on all three common temperature scales. For ease of reference, five key points are defined. These include the zero point of each scale, the freezing point of water (0° C), body temperature (37° C), and the boiling point of water (100° C).

Heat and the First Law of Thermodynamics

According to the First Law of Thermodynamics, energy can neither be created nor destroyed, only transformed in nature. Thus any energy a substance gains must exactly equal the energy lost by its surroundings. Conversely, if a substance loses energy, this loss must

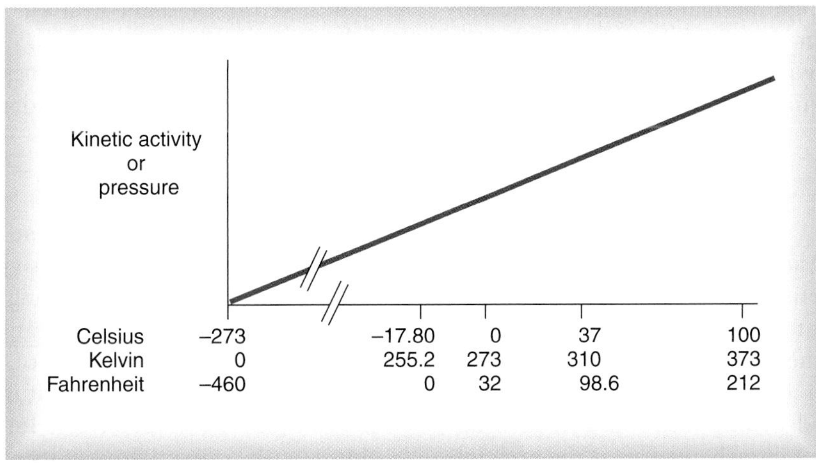

Figure 5-2

Linear relationship between gas molecular activity, or pressure, and temperature. The graph shows comparable readings on three scales for five temperature points.

be offset by an equal gain in the energy of its surroundings. This is stated as a simple formula:

$$U = E + W$$

U is the internal energy of an object, *E* is the energy transferred to or from the object, and *W* is the external work performed on the object. In this sense, the quantity *E* is equivalent to heat. Heating is the transfer of internal energy from a high-temperature object to a low-temperature object.

Based on this formula, you can increase the internal energy of an object by heating it or by performing work on it.

Heat Transfer

When two objects exist at different temperatures, the First Law of Thermodynamics tells us that heat will move from the hotter object to the cooler object until the objects' temperatures are equal. Two objects with the same temperature exist in thermal equilibrium.

This heat transfer can be affected in four ways: (1) **conduction**, (2) **convection**, (3) **radiation**, and (4) **evaporation/condensation**.

Conduction

Heat transfer in solids occurs mainly via conduction. Conduction is the transfer of heat by direct contact between hot and cold molecules. How well heat transfers by conduction depends on both the number and force of molecular collisions between adjoining objects.

Heat transfer between objects is quantified by using a measure called **thermal conductivity**. Table 5-1 lists the thermal conductivities of selected substances in cgs units. As is evident, solids, particularly metals, tend to have high thermal conductivity. This is why metals feel cold to the touch, even when at room temperature. In this case, the metal's high thermal conductivity quickly draws heat away from the skin, creating a feeling of "cold." In contrast, with fewer molecular collisions than in solids and liquids, gases exhibit low thermal conductivity.

Table 5-1 ▶▶ Thermal Conductivities in (cal/sec)/(cm^2 × ° C/cm)

Material	Thermal Conductivity (k)
Silver	1.01
Copper	0.99
Aluminum	0.50
Iron	0.163
Lead	0.083
Ice	0.005
Glass	0.0025
Concrete	0.002
Water at 20° C	0.0014
Asbestos	0.0004
Hydrogen at 0° C	0.0004
Helium at 0° C	0.0003
Snow (dry)	0.00026
Fiberglass	0.00015
Cork board	0.00011
Wool felt	0.0001
Air at 0° C	0.000057

From Nave CR, Nave BC: Physics for the health sciences, ed 3, Philadelphia, 1985, WB Saunders.

Convection

Heat transfer in both liquids and gases occurs mainly by convection. Convection involves the mixing of fluid molecules at different temperatures. For example, although air is a poor heat conductor (see Table 5-1), it can efficiently transfer heat by convection. To do so, the air is first warmed in one location and then circulated to carry the heat elsewhere. This is the principle behind forced-air heating in houses and convection heating in infant incubators. Fluid movements carrying heat energy are called *convection currents*.

Radiation

Radiation is another mechanism for heat transfer. Whereas conduction and convection require direct contact between two substances, radiant heat transfer occurs without direct physical contact. Indeed, heat transfer by radiation occurs even in a vacuum, as when the sun warms the earth.

Thus the concept of radiant energy is similar to that of light. Radiant energy given off by objects at room temperature is mainly in the infrared range, which is invisible to the human eye. On the other hand, objects such as an electrical stove burner or a kerosene heater radiate some of their energy as visible light. In the clinical setting, radiant heat energy is commonly used to keep newborn infants warm.

The following formula defines the rate at which an object gains or loses heat by radiation:

$$\frac{E}{t} = ekA(T_2 - T_1)$$

In this formula, *E/t* is the heat loss or gain per unit time. The symbol e is the emissivity of the object, or its relative effectiveness in radiating heat. The constant *k* is the Stefan-Boltzmann constant (based on mass and surface area). *A* is the area of the radiating object, and T_1 and T_2 are the temperatures of the environment and the object, respectively. In simple terms, for an object with a given emissivity, the larger the surface area (relative to mass) and the lower the surrounding temperature, the greater the radiant heat loss per unit time.

Evaporation/Condensation

Vaporization is the change of state from liquid to gas. Vaporization requires heat energy. According to the First Law of Thermodynamics, this heat energy must come from the surroundings. In one form of vaporization, called **evaporation**, heat is taken from the air surrounding the liquid, thereby cooling the air. In warm weather or during strenuous exercise, the body takes advantage of this principle of *evaporation cooling* by producing sweat. The liquid sweat evaporates and thus cools the skin.

Condensation is the opposite of evaporation. During condensation, a gas turns back into a liquid. Because vaporization takes heat from the air around a liquid (cooling), condensation must give heat back to the surroundings (warming). The next section expands on the concept of change of state and provides more detail on the processes of vaporization and condensation.

▶ CHANGE OF STATE

All matter can change state. Because respiratory therapists (RTs) work extensively with both liquids and gases, they must have a good understanding of both the key characteristics of these states and basic processes underlying their phase changes.

Liquid-Solid Phase Changes (Melting and Freezing)

When a solid is heated, its kinetic energy increases. This added internal energy increases molecular vibrations. If enough heat is applied, these vibrations eventually weaken the intermolecular attractive forces. At some point, molecules will break free of their rigid structure and the solid will change into a liquid.

Melting

The changeover from the solid to liquid state is called *melting*. The temperature at which this changeover occurs is the melting point. The range of melting points is considerable. For example, water (ice) has a melting point of 0° C, carbon has a melting point of more than 3500° C, and helium has a melting point of less than –272.2° C.

Figure 5-3 depicts the phase change caused by heating water. At the left origin of –50° C, water is solid ice. As the ice is heated, its temperature rises. At its melting point of 0° C, the ice begins to change into liquid water. However, the full change to liquid water requires additional heat. Notice that this additional heat energy changes the state of water, but does not immediately change its temperature.

The extra heat needed to change a solid to a liquid is the **latent heat of fusion**. In cgs units, the latent heat of fusion is defined as the number of calories required to change 1 g of a solid into a liquid without changing its temperature. For example, the latent heat of fusion of ice is 80 cal/g, whereas that of oxygen is 3.3 cal/g. This change of state, compared with simply heating a solid, requires enormous energy.

Freezing

Freezing is the opposite of melting. Because melting requires large amounts of externally applied energy, you would expect freezing to return this energy to the surroundings. This is exactly what occurs. During freezing, heat energy is transferred from a liquid back to the environment, usually by exposure to cold.

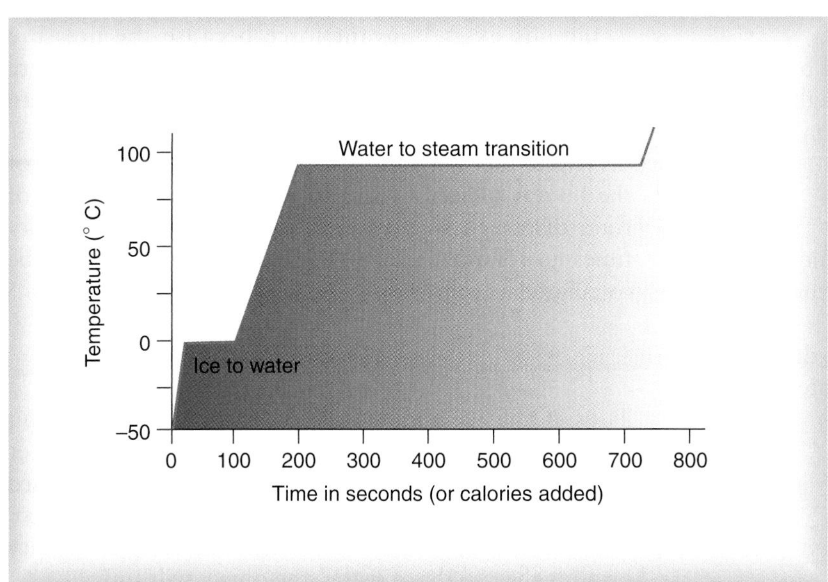

Figure 5-3
Temperature as a function of time for 1 g of water heated at the rate of 1 cal/sec. *(Modified from Nave CR, Nave BC: Physics for the health sciences, ed 3, Philadelphia, 1985, WB Saunders.)*

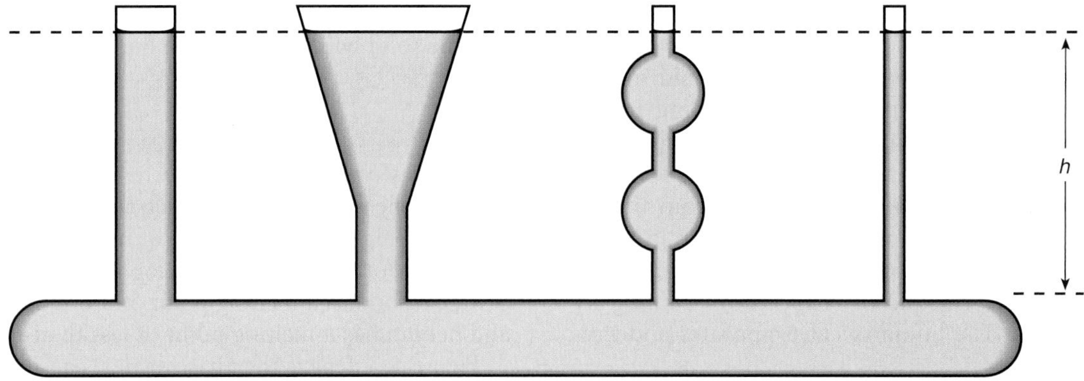

Figure 5-4 · **Pascal's Principle**

Liquid pressure depends only on the height (*h*) and not on the shape of the vessel or the total volume of liquid. *(Modified from Nave CR, Nave BC: Physics for the health sciences, ed 3, Philadelphia, 1985, WB Saunders.)*

As a substance's kinetic energy decreases, its molecules begin to regain the stable structure of a solid. According to the First Law of Thermodynamics, the energy required to freeze a substance must equal that needed to melt it. Thus the freezing and melting points of a substance are the same.

Properties of Liquids

Liquids exhibit flow and assume the shape of their container. Liquids also exert pressure, which varies with depth and density. Variations in liquid pressure within a container produce an upward supporting force, called *buoyancy*.

Although melting weakens intermolecular bonding forces, liquid molecules still attract one another. The persistence of these cohesive forces among liquid molecules helps explain the physical properties of viscosity, capillary action, and surface tension.

Pressure in Liquids

Liquids exert pressure. The pressure exerted by a liquid depends on both its height (depth) and weight density (weight per unit volume), which is shown in equation form:

$$P_L = h \times d_w$$

P_L is the static pressure exerted by the liquid, h is the height of the liquid column, and d_w is the liquid's weight density.

For example, to compute the pressure at the bottom of a 33.9-foot (1034-cm)–high column of water (density = 1 g/cm^3), you would use this equation:

$$P_L = h \times d_w$$
$$= 1034 \text{ cm} \times (1 \text{ g/cm}^3)$$
$$= 1034 \text{ g/cm}^2$$

The answer (1034 g/cm^2) also equals 1 atmosphere of pressure, or approximately 14.7 lb/in^2. Of course, this figure does not account for the additional atmospheric pressure (P_B) acting on the top of the liquid. The total pressure at the bottom of the column equals the sum of the atmospheric and liquid pressures. In this case, the total pressure is 2068 g/cm^2, equal to 29.4 lb/in^2, or 2 atmospheres.

As shown in Figure 5-4, a given liquid's pressure is the same at any specific depth (h), regardless of the container's shape. This is because a liquid's pressure acts equally in all directions. This concept is called **Pascal's principle.**

Buoyancy (Archimedes' Principle)

Thousands of years ago, Archimedes showed that an object submersed in water appeared to weigh less than in air. This effect, called *buoyancy*, explains why certain objects float in water.

Liquids exert buoyant force because the pressure below a submerged object always exceeds the pressure above it. This difference in liquid pressure creates an upward or supporting force. According to Archimedes' principle, this buoyant force must equal the weight of the fluid displaced by the object. Because the weight of fluid displaced by an object equals its weight density times its volume (d_w = V), the buoyant force (B) may be calculated as follows:

$$B = d_w \times V$$

Thus if the weight density of an object is less than water (1 g/cm^3), it will displace a weight of water greater than its own weight. In this case, the upward buoyant force will overcome gravity, and the object will float. Conversely, if an object's weight density exceeds the weight of water, the object will sink.

Clinically, Archimedes' principle is used to measure the specific gravity of certain liquids. Figure 5-5 shows the use of a hydrometer to measure the specific gravity of urine. The specific gravity of gases also can be measured. In this case, oxygen or hydrogen is used as the standard instead of water.

Gases also exert buoyant force, although much less than that provided by liquids. For example, buoyancy helps keep solid particles suspended in gases. These suspensions, called aerosols, play an important role in respiratory care. More detail on the characteristics and use of aerosols is provided in Chapter 33.

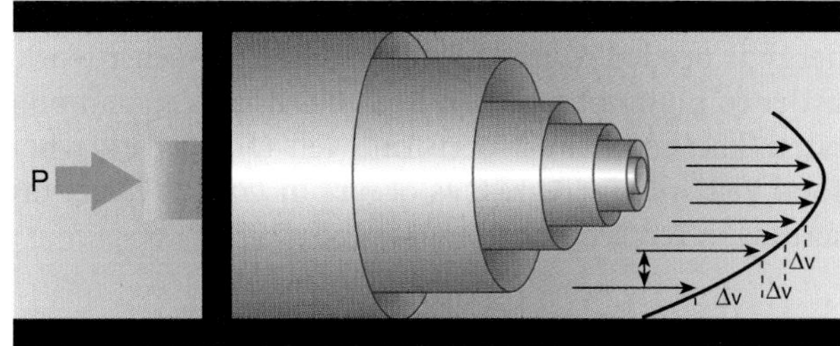

Figure 5-6

The effects of shear stress or pressure (P) on shear rate (velocity gradient [v]) in a Newtonian fluid. *(Modified from Winters WL, Brest AN, editors: The microcirculation, Springfield, Ill, 1969, Charles C Thomas.)*

Viscosity

Viscosity is the force opposing a fluid's flow. Viscosity in fluids is like friction in solids. A fluid's viscosity is directly proportional to the cohesive forces between its molecules. The stronger these cohesive forces, the greater the fluid's viscosity. The greater a fluid's viscosity, the greater its resistance to deformation and the greater its opposition to flow.

Viscosity is most important when fluids move in discrete cylindrical layers, called *streamlines*. This pattern of motion is called **laminar flow**. As shown in Figure 5-6, frictional forces between the streamlines and the tube wall impede movement of a fluid's outer layers. Each layer, moving toward the center of the tube, hinders the motion of the next inner layer less and less. Thus laminar flow consists of concentric layers of fluid flowing parallel to the tube wall at velocities that increase toward the center.

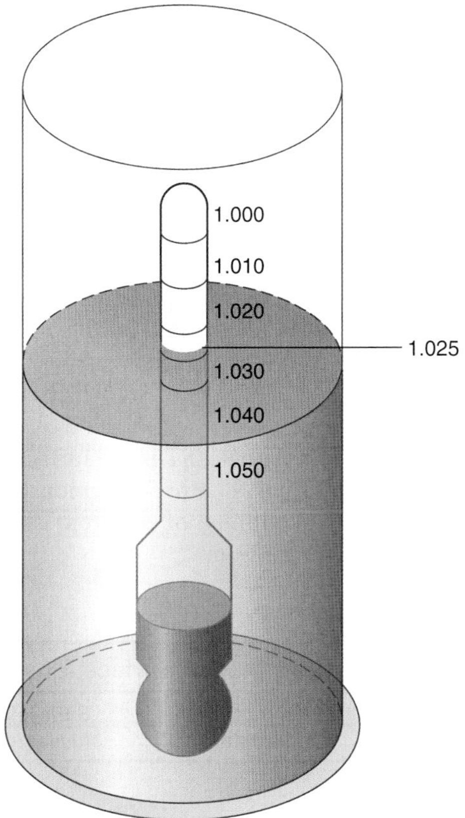

Figure 5-5

Using a hydrometer to measure the specific gravity of a urine specimen. The scale value of 1.025 indicates that this urine sample has a weight density 1.025 times greater than water.

The difference in the velocity among these concentric layers is called the shear rate. The shear rate is simply a measure of how easily the layers separate. How easily the layers separate depends on two factors: (1) the pressure pushing or driving the fluid, called the *shear stress*, and (2) the viscosity of the fluid. Shear rate is directly proportional to shear stress and inversely proportional to viscosity:

$$\text{shear rate} \approx \frac{\text{shear stress}}{\text{viscosity}}$$

Rearranging the equation to solve for viscosity:

$$\text{viscosity} \approx \frac{\text{shear stress}}{\text{shear rate}}$$

The cgs unit for viscosity is the poise. A poise equals the force of 1 dyne over an area of 1 cm^2 for a period of 1 second (dyne-sec/cm^2). The viscosity of liquids is measured in centipoises (10^{-2} poises), and that of gases is measured in micropoises (10^{-6} poises). The SI unit for viscosity is the Pascal-second (Pa-s); 1 Pa-s is equal to 10 poises.

In uniform fluids such as water or oil, viscosity varies with temperature. Because higher temperatures weaken the cohesive forces between molecules, heating a uniform fluid lowers its viscosity. Conversely, cooling a fluid increases its viscosity. This is why a car's engine is so hard to start on a cold winter morning. The oil becomes so viscous that it impedes movement of the engine's parts.

Blood, unlike water or oil, is a complex fluid. This is because blood contains not only water (plasma) but also cells in suspension. For this reason, blood has a viscosity approximately five times greater than that of water. The greater the viscosity of a fluid, the more energy is needed to make it flow. Thus the heart works harder to pump blood than it would if it were pumping water. The heart must perform even more work when blood viscosity increases, as occurs in *polycythemia* (an increase in red blood cell mass).

Cohesion and Adhesion

The attractive force between like molecules is called **cohesion**. The attractive force between unlike molecules is **adhesion**.

These forces can be observed at work by placing a liquid in a small-diameter tube. As shown in Figure 5-7, the top of the liquid forms a curved surface, or *meniscus*. When the liquid is water, the meniscus is concave (Figure 5-7, *A*). This is because water molecules at the surface adhere to the glass more strongly than they cohere to each other. In contrast, a mercury meniscus is convex (Figure 5-7, *B*). In this case, the cohesive forces pulling the mercury atoms together exceed the adhesive forces trying to attract the mercury to the glass.

Surface Tension

Surface tension is a force exerted by like molecules at a liquid's surface. A small drop of fluid provides a good illustration of this force. As shown in Figure 5-8, cohesive forces affect molecules inside the drop equally from all directions. However, only inward forces affect molecules on the surface. This imbalance in forces causes the surface film to contract into the smallest possible area, usually a sphere or curve (meniscus). This phenomenon explains why liquid droplets and bubbles retain a spherical shape.

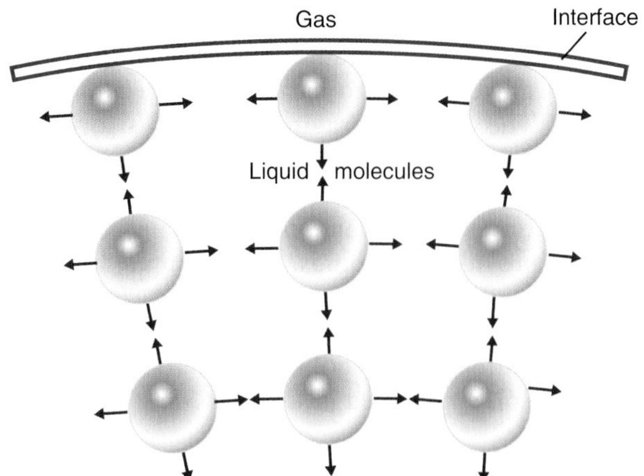

Figure 5-8 · The Force of Surface Tension in a Drop of Liquid

Cohesive force *(arrows)* attracts molecules inside the drop to one another. Cohesion can pull the outermost molecules inward only, creating a centrally directed force that tends to contract the liquid into a sphere.

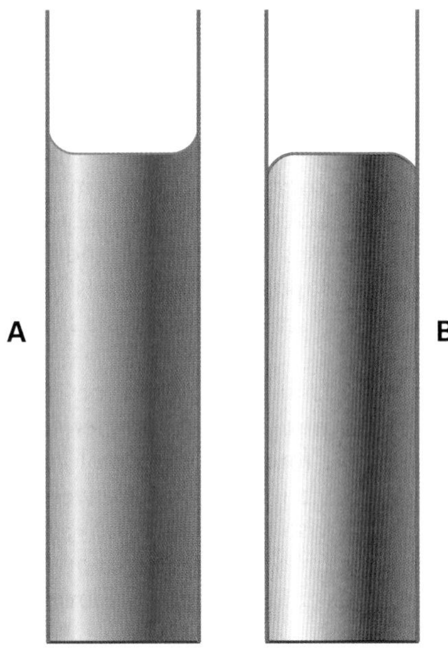

Figure 5-7

The shape of the meniscus depends on the relative strengths of adhesion and cohesion. **A,** Water; adhesion stronger than cohesion. **B,** Mercury; cohesion stronger than adhesion.

Surface tension is quantified by measurement of the force needed to produce a "tear" in a fluid surface layer. Table 5-2 lists the surface tensions of selected liquids in dynes/cm (cgs). For a given liquid, surface tension varies inversely with temperature. Thus the higher the temperature, the lower the surface tension.

Surface tension, like a fist compressing a ball, increases the pressure inside a liquid drop or bubble. According to **Laplace's law**, this pressure varies directly with the surface tension of the liquid and inversely with its radius. The equation for a liquid bubble follows:

$$P = \frac{4ST}{r}$$

P is the pressure in the bubble, *ST* is the surface tension, and *r* is the bubble radius. Figure 5-9 demonstrates this relationship for two bubbles of different sizes, each with the same surface tension.

Table 5-2 ▶▶ Examples of Surface Tension

Substance	Temperature (° C)	Surface Tension (dynes/cm)
Water	20°	73
Water	37°	70
Whole blood	37°	58
Plasma	37°	73
Ethyl alcohol	20°	22
Mercury	17°	547

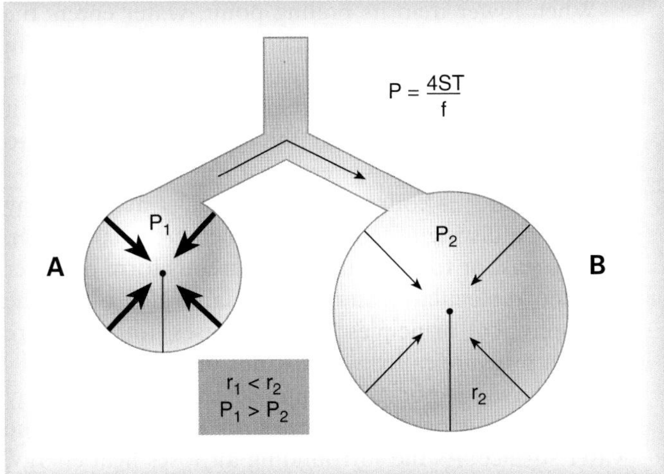

Figure 5-9 · Laplace's Relationship

Two bubbles of different sizes with the same surface tension. Bubble *A*, with the smaller radius, has the greater inward or deflating pressure and is more prone to collapse than the larger bubble *B*. Because the two bubbles are connected, bubble *A* would tend to deflate and empty into bubble B. Conversely, because of bubble *A*'s greater surface tension, it would be harder to inflate than bubble *B*.

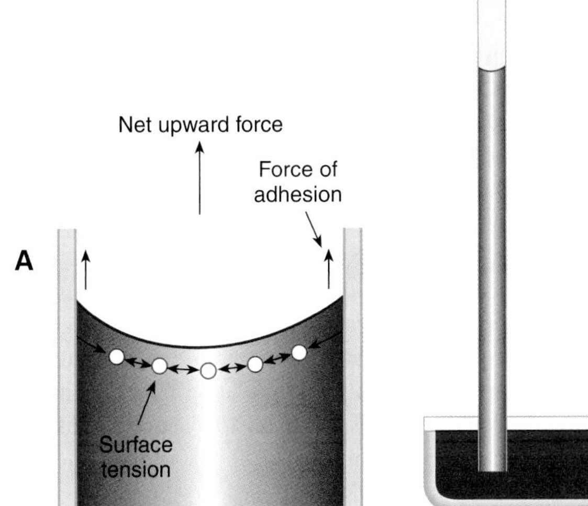

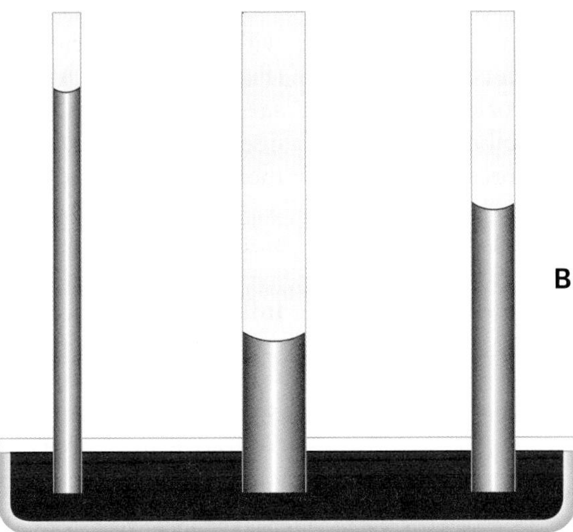

Figure 5-10 · Capillary Action

A, Adhesion and surface tension contribute to capillarity. **B,** The liquid rises highest in the smallest tube. *(Modified from Nave CR, Nave BC: Physics for the health sciences, ed 3, Philadelphia, 1985, WB Saunders.)*

Because the lungs' alveoli resemble clumps of bubbles, it follows that surface tension plays a key role in the mechanics of ventilation (see Chapter 9). Moreover, alveolar surface tension abnormalities occur in certain clinical conditions, such as infant respiratory distress syndrome. The role of surface tension in disease is addressed in Chapters 24 and 28.

Capillary Action

Capillary action is a phenomenon in which a liquid in a small tube moves upward, against gravity. Capillary action involves both adhesive and surface tension forces. As shown in Figure 5-10, *A*, the adhesion of water molecules to the walls of a thin tube causes an upward force on the liquid's edges and produces a concave meniscus.

Because surface tension acts to maintain the smallest possible liquid-gas interface, instead of just the edges of the liquid moving up, the whole surface is pulled upward. How strong this force is depends on the amount of liquid that contacts the tube's surface. Because a small capillary tube creates a more concave meniscus and thus a greater area of contact, liquid will rise higher in tubes with smaller cross-sectional areas (Figure 5-10, *B*).

Capillary action is the basis for "capillary-stick" blood samples. The absorbent wicks used in some gas humidifiers are also an application of this principle, as are certain types of surgical dressings.

Liquid-Vapor Phase Changes

Only after ice completely melts does additional heat raise the temperature of the newly formed liquid (Figure 5-3 on p. 89). As the water temperature reaches 100° C, a new change of state begins, from liquid to vapor. This change of state is called *vaporization*. There are two different forms of vaporization: boiling and evaporation.

Boiling

Boiling occurs at the *boiling point.* The boiling point of a liquid is the temperature at which its vapor pressure equals atmospheric pressure. When a liquid boils, its molecules must have enough kinetic energy to force themselves into the atmosphere against its opposing pressure. Because the weight of the atmosphere retards the escape of vapor molecules, the greater the ambient pressure, the greater the boiling point. Conversely, when atmospheric pressure is low, liquid molecules escape more easily, and boiling occurs at lower temperatures. This is why cooking times must be increased at higher altitudes.

Although boiling is associated with high temperatures, the boiling points of most liquefied gases are very low. For example, at 1 atmosphere pressure, oxygen boils at −183° C.

Energy is also needed to vaporize liquids, as with other phase changes. The energy required to vaporize a liquid is the **latent heat of vaporization.** In cgs units, the latent heat of vaporization is the number of calories required to vaporize 1 g of a liquid at its normal boiling point.

Whereas melting weakens attractive forces between molecules, vaporization eliminates them. Elimination of these forces converts essentially all of a substance's internal energy into kinetic energy. For this reason, vaporization requires substantially more energy than does melting. As shown in Figure 5-3 on p. 89, almost seven times more energy is needed to convert water to steam (540 cal/g) than is needed to melt ice.

Evaporation, Vapor Pressure, and Humidity

Boiling is only one type of vaporization. A liquid also can change into a gas at temperatures lower than its boiling point through a process called *evaporation.* Water is a good example (Figure 5-11).

When lower than its boiling point, water enters the atmosphere by evaporation. The liquid molecules are in constant motion, as in the gas phase. Although this kinetic energy is less intense than in the gaseous state, it allows some molecules near the surface to escape into the surrounding air as water vapor (Figure 5-11, *A*).

After water is converted to a vapor, it acts like any gas. To be distinguished from visible particulate water, such as mist or fog, this invisible gaseous form of water is called molecular water. Molecular water obeys the same physical principles as other gases and therefore exerts a pressure called **water vapor pressure.**

Of course, evaporation requires heat. The heat energy required for evaporation comes from the air next to the water surface. As the surrounding air loses heat energy, it cools. This is the principle of *evaporation cooling,* which was previously described.

If the container is covered, water vapor molecules will continue to enter the air until it can hold no more (Figure 5-11, *B*). At this point, the air over the water is saturated with water vapor. However, vaporization does not stop once saturation occurs. Instead, for every molecule escaping into the air another returns to the water reservoir. These conditions are referred to as a *state of equilibrium.*

Influence of Temperature. No other factor influences evaporation more than temperature. Temperature affects evaporation in two ways. First, the warmer the air, the more vapor it can hold. Specifically, the capacity of air to hold water vapor increases with temperature. Thus the warmer the air contacting a water surface, the faster the rate of evaporation.

Second, if water is heated, its kinetic energy is increased and thus more molecules are helped to escape from its surface (Figure 5-11, *C*). Last, if the container of heated water is covered, the air will again become

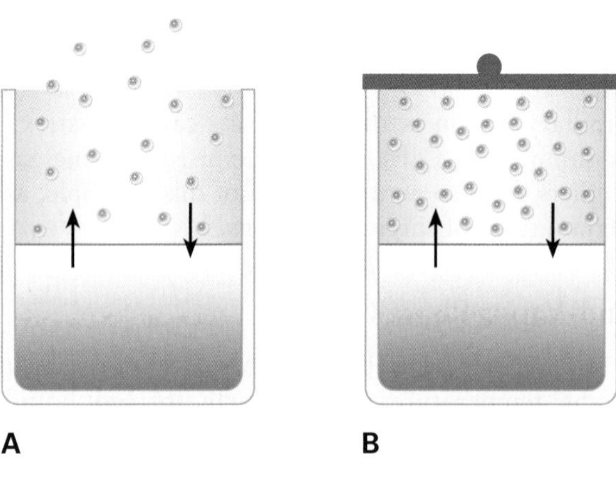

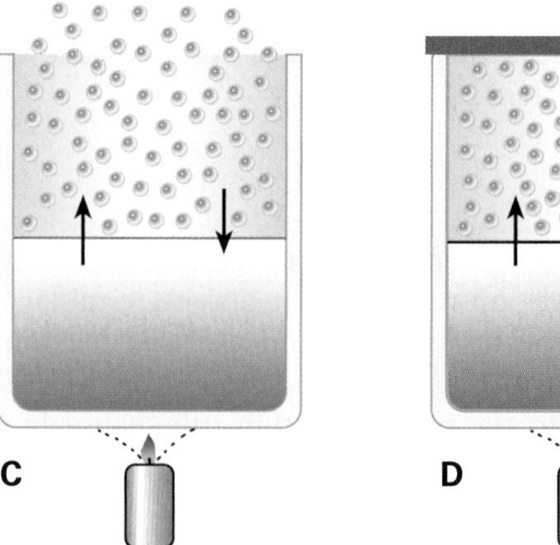

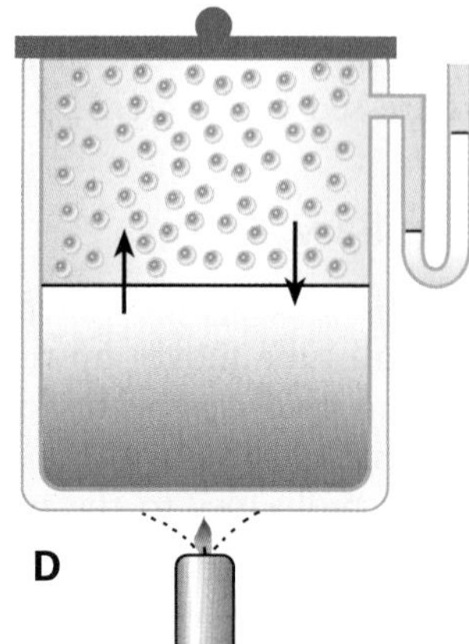

Figure 5-11
Factors influencing vaporization of water. See text for details.

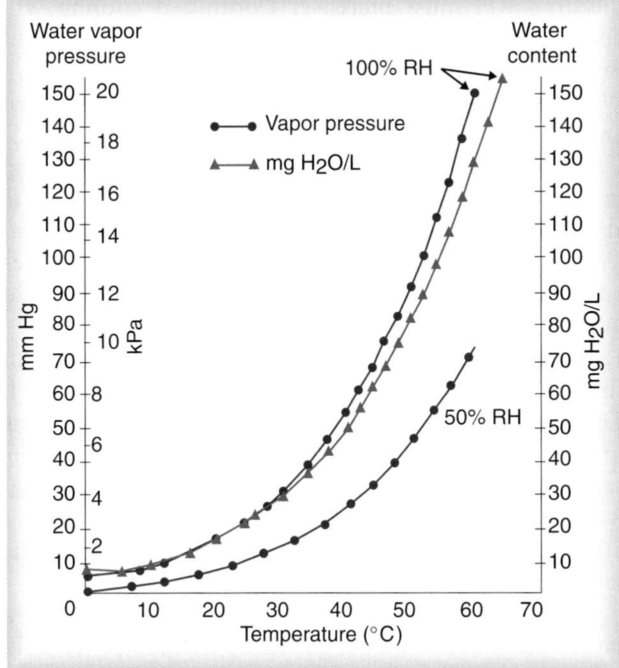

Figure 5-12

Water vapor pressure (P_{H_2O}) and absolute humidity (mg H_2O/L) curves for gas that is fully saturated (relative humidity [RH] = 100%) and gas that is half saturated (RH = 50%).

saturated (Figure 5-11, *D*). However, the heated saturated air, compared with the unheated air (Figure 5-11, *B*), now contains more vapor molecules and thus exerts a higher vapor pressure (as shown by the manometer in Figure 5-11, *D*). Therefore the temperature of a gas affects both its capacity to hold molecular water and the water vapor pressure.

The relationship between water vapor pressure and temperature is graphed in Figure 5-12. The left vertical axis plots water vapor pressure in both mm Hg and kPa (kilopascal). The horizontal axis plots temperatures between 0° and 70° C. This graph shows that the greater the temperature, the greater the saturated water vapor pressure *(bold black dots)*. Table 5-3 lists actual water vapor pressures in saturated air in the clinical range of temperatures (20° to 37° C).

Humidity. Water vapor pressure represents the kinetic activity of water molecules in air. For the actual amount or weight of water vapor in a gas to be found, the water vapor content or **absolute humidity** must be measured.

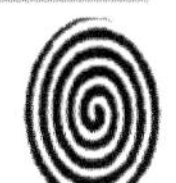

RULE OF THUMB

Gases in the lungs exist under conditions known as body temperature and pressure, saturated (BTPS), equivalent to 37° C and 100% relative humidity. Under these conditions, the water vapor content is approximately 44 mg/L, and the water vapor pressure is 47 torr.

Absolute humidity can be measured by weighing the water vapor extracted from air using a drying agent. Alternatively, absolute humidity can be computed with meteorological data according to the techniques of the U.S. Weather Bureau. The common unit of measure for absolute humidity is milligrams of water vapor per liter of gas (mg/L).

Table 5-3 ▶▶ Water Vapor Pressures and Contents at Selected Temperatures

Temperature (°C)	Vapor Pressure (mm Hg)	Water Vapor Content (mg/L)	ATPS to BTPS Correction Factor*
20	17.50	17.30	1.102
21	18.62	18.35	1.096
22	19.80	19.42	1.091
23	21.10	20.58	1.085
24	22.40	21.78	1.080
25	23.80	23.04	1.075
26	25.20	24.36	1.068
27	26.70	25.75	1.063
28	28.30	27.22	1.057
29	30.00	28.75	1.051
30	31.80	30.35	1.045
31	33.70	32.01	1.039
32	35.70	33.76	1.032
33	37.70	35.61	1.026
34	39.90	37.57	1.020
35	42.20	39.60	1.014
36	44.60	41.70	1.007
37	47.00	43.80	1.000

ATPS, Ambient temperature, pressure, dry; *BTPS*, body temperature, barometric pressure, and saturated with water vapor.
*Correction factors are based on 760 mm Hg pressure.

Absolute humidity values for saturated air at various temperatures are plotted against the right vertical axis of Figure 5-12, using "x" hash marks. The middle column of Table 5-3 lists these absolute humidity values for saturated air between 20° and 37° C.

A gas does not need to be fully saturated with water vapor. If a gas is only half saturated with water vapor, its water vapor pressure and absolute humidity are only half that in the fully saturated state. For example, air that is fully saturated with water vapor at 37° C and 760 mm Hg has a water vapor pressure of 47 mm Hg and an absolute humidity of 43.8 mg/L (see Table 5-3). However, if the same volume of air were only 50% saturated with water vapor, its water vapor pressure would be 0.50×47 mm Hg, or 23.5 mm Hg, and its absolute humidity would be 0.50×43.8 mg/L, or 21.9 mg/L.

When a gas is not fully saturated, its water vapor content can be expressed in relative terms using a measure called **relative humidity (RH)**. The RH of a gas is the ratio of its actual water vapor content to its saturated capacity at a given temperature. RH is expressed as a percentage and is derived with the following simple formula:

$$\%RH = \frac{\text{content (absolute humidity)}}{\text{saturated capacity}} \times 100$$

For example, saturated air at a room temperature of 20° C has the capacity to hold 17.3 mg/L water vapor (see Table 5-3). If the absolute humidity is 12 mg/L, then the RH is calculated as follows:

$$\%RH = \frac{\text{content (absolute humidity)}}{\text{saturated capacity}} \times 100$$

$$\%RH = \frac{12}{17.3} \times 100$$

$$\%RH = 69\%$$

In reality, actual water vapor content does not have to be measured for RH to be computed. Simple instruments called *hygrometers* allow direct measurement of RH without extracting and weighing the water in air.

When the water vapor content of a volume of gas equals its capacity, the RH is 100%. When the RH is 100%, a gas is fully saturated with water vapor. Under these conditions, even slight cooling of the gas causes its water vapor to turn back into the liquid state, a process called *condensation*.

Condensed moisture deposits on any available surface, such as on the walls of a container or delivery tubing, or even on particles suspended in the gas. Condensation returns heat to and warms the surrounding environment, whereas vaporization of water cools the adjacent air.

If air that is at an RH of 90% is cooled, its capacity to hold water vapor will decrease. Although the air's water vapor capacity decreases, its content remains constant. With a lower capacity but the same content, the air's RH must increase. Continued cooling will decrease the air's water vapor capacity until it eventually equals the water vapor content (RH = 100%). When content equals capacity, the air is fully saturated and can hold no more water vapor.

Because RH never exceeds 100%, any further drop in temperature causes condensation. The temperature at which condensation begins is called the *dew point*. Cooling a saturated gas below its dew point causes increasingly more water vapor to condense into liquid water droplets.

Figure 5-13 provides a useful analogy of the relationship between water vapor content, capacity, and RH. The various-sized glasses represent the capacity of a gas to hold water vapor. The bigger the glass, the greater its capacity. The water in the glasses represents the actual water vapor content. Thus a glass that is half full is at 50% capacity, or 50% RH. A full glass represents the saturated state, which is equivalent to 100% RH.

Figure 5-13, *A*, shows what happens when we heat a saturated gas. Warming a gas raises its capacity to hold water vapor but does not necessarily change its content. This is equivalent to pouring the contents of the full glass on the left into progressively larger glasses. The amount of water does not change, but as the glasses get bigger, they become less full. We started with a full glass (100% RH) but end up with one that is only one-third full (33% RH).

Of course, a decrease in capacity would have the opposite effect. In Figure 5-13, *B*, we start with a large glass, which is half full (50% RH). We decrease the

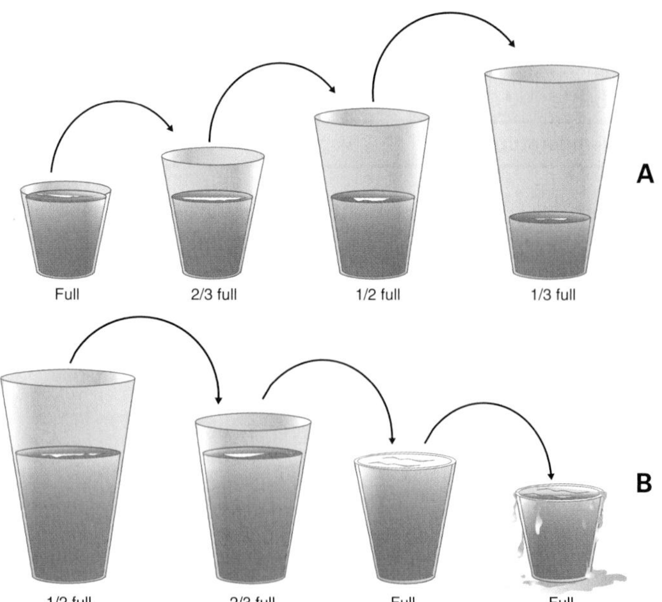

Figure 5-13 · Relative Humidity Analogy

A, The effect of increasing capacity without changing content, as when heating a saturated gas. **B,** The effect of decreasing capacity, as when cooling a gas. See text for details.

MINI CLINI

Condensation/Evaporation

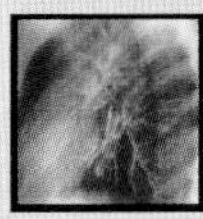

A good clinical example of condensation and evaporation is the hygroscopic condenser humidifier, a form of artificial nose (Figure 5-14). These devices consist of layers of water-absorbent material encased in plastic. When a patient exhales into an artificial nose, the warm, saturated expired gas cools, causing condensation on the absorbent surfaces. As condensation occurs, heat is generated in the device. When the patient inhales through the device, the inspired gases are warmed, and the previously condensed water now evaporates, aiding in airway humidification. Chapter 32 provides more detail on humidification devices, including the artificial nose.

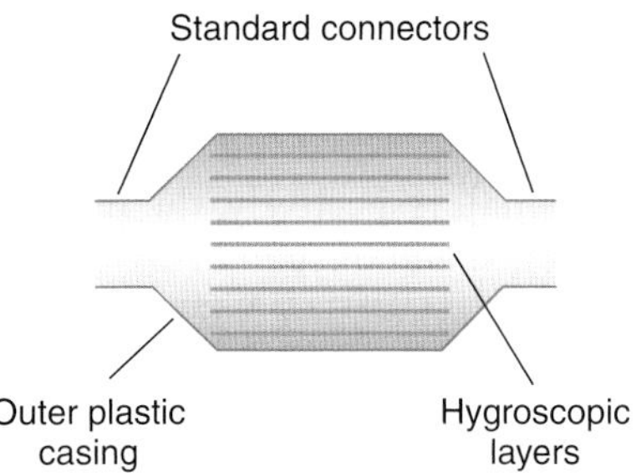

Figure 5-14
Hygroscopic condenser humidifier.

capacity by pouring the water into progressively smaller glasses (equivalent to decreasing the gas temperature). Eventually, the water volume is enough to fill a smaller glass (100% RH). What happens if we try to empty this full glass into an even smaller one? Because the smaller glass has less capacity, the excess content must spill over. This spillover is analogous to the condensation occurring when a saturated gas cools below its dew point. However, it should be noted that although condensation has removed the excess moisture from the air, the smaller glass is still full (100% RH).

In clinical practice, two additional measures of humidity are used: *percent body humidity* (%BH) and *humidity deficit.*

The %BH of a gas is the ratio of its actual water vapor content to the water vapor capacity in saturated gas at body temperature (37° C). Thus %BH is the same as RH, except that the capacity (or denominator) is fixed at 43.8 mg/L:

$$\%BH = \frac{\text{content (absolute humidity)}}{\text{capacity at } 37^\circ \text{ C}} \times 100$$

or

$$\%BH = \frac{\text{content (absolute humidity)}}{43.8 \text{ mg/L}} \times 100$$

For example, saturated air at 20° C contains approximately 17.3 mg/L water vapor, whereas saturated air at body temperature contains 43.8 mg/L. In this case, the air is providing approximately 40% ([17.3 ÷ 43.8] × 100) body humidity.

The humidity deficit represents the amount of water vapor the body must add to the inspired gas to achieve saturation at body temperature (37° C). To compute the humidity deficit, simply subtract the actual water vapor content from its capacity at 37° C (43.8 mg/L). In the previous example, the humidity deficit would be computed as follows:

$$\text{humidity deficit} = \text{content} - \text{capacity } (37^\circ \text{ C})$$

$$\text{humidity deficit} = 43.8 \text{ mg/L} - 17.3 \text{ mg/L}$$

$$\text{humidity deficit} = 26.5 \text{ mg/L}$$

This means that under these conditions, 26.5 mg of water vapor must be added to every liter of inspired gas to achieve full saturation at 37° C.

Influence of Pressure. Whereas high temperatures increase vaporization, high pressures impede this process. Remember that water molecules trying to escape from a liquid surface must push their way out against the opposing air molecules. If the surrounding air pressure is high, there will be more opposing air molecules, and vaporization will decrease. Conversely, low atmospheric pressures increase vaporization.

Influence of Surface Area. The greater the available surface area of the gas in contact with air, the greater the rate of liquid evaporation. This can be easily proved by comparing how quickly equal volumes of water evaporate under dry conditions from a flat plate versus a tall, narrow glass. The water spread over a flat plate will evaporate more quickly as compared with the same amount of liquid in a tall, narrow glass. This principle is applied to the design of certain humidifiers to increase their ability to put water vapor in the passing gas.

Properties of Gases

Gases share many properties with liquids. Specifically, gases exert pressure, are capable of flow, and exhibit the property of viscosity. However, unlike liquids, gases are readily compressed and expanded and fill the spaces available to them by diffusion.

Kinetic Activity of Gases

Because a gas's intermolecular forces of attraction are so weak, most of a gas's internal energy is kinetic energy. Kinetic theory says that gas molecules travel about randomly at very high speeds and with frequent collisions.

The velocity of gas molecules is directly proportional to temperature. As a gas is warmed, its kinetic activity increases, its molecular collisions increase, and its pressure rises. Conversely, when a gas is cooled, molecular activity decreases, particle velocity and collision frequency decline, and the pressure drops.

Molar Volume and Gas Density

A major principle governing chemistry is **Avogadro's law**. This law states that the 1-g atomic weight of any substance contains exactly the same number of atoms, molecules, or ions. This number, 6.023×10^{23}, is *Avogadro's constant*. In SI units, this quantity of matter equals 1 *mole*.

Molar Volume. Avogadro's law states that equal volumes of gases under the same conditions must contain the same number of molecules. Thus 1 mole of a gas, at a constant temperature and pressure, should occupy the same volume as 1 mole of any other gas. This ideal volume is termed the *molar volume*.

At standard temperature and pressure, dry (STPD), the ideal molar volume of any gas is 22.4 L. In reality, there are small deviations from this ideal. For example, although the molar volumes of both oxygen and nitrogen are 22.4 L at STPD, that of carbon dioxide is closer to 22.3 L. These values will be used later to calculate gas densities and convert dissolved gas volumes into moles per liter.

Density. Density is the ratio of a substance's mass to its volume. A dense substance has heavy (high atomic weight) particles packed closely together. Uranium is a good example of a dense substance. Conversely, a low-density substance has a low concentration of light atomic particles per unit volume. Hydrogen gas is a good example of a low-density substance.

In clinical practice, weight is often substituted for mass and thus weight density (weight per unit volume or d_w) is actually measured. Solid or liquid weight density is commonly measured in grams per cubic centimeter (cgs). For gases, the most common unit is grams per liter.

Because weight density equals weight divided by volume, the density of any gas at STPD can be computed easily by dividing its molecular weight (gmw) by the universal molar volume of 22.4 L (22.3 for CO_2). Box 5-1 provides examples of gas density calculations.

For the density of a gas mixture to be calculated, the percentage or fraction of each gas in the mixture must be known. For example, to calculate the density of air at STPD, the following equation is used:

Box 5-1 • Examples of Gas Densities d_w at STPD

$$d_wO_2 = \frac{gmw}{22.4} = \frac{32}{22.4} = 1.43 \text{ g/L}$$

$$d_wN_2 = \frac{gmw}{22.4} = \frac{28}{22.4} = 1.25 \text{ g/L}$$

$$d_wHe = \frac{gmw}{22.4} = \frac{4}{22.4} = 0.179 \text{ g/L}$$

$$d_wCO_2 = \frac{gmw}{22.3} = \frac{44}{22.3} = 1.97 \text{ g/L}$$

$$d_w\text{air} = \frac{(FN_2 \times \text{gmw } N_2) + (FO_2 \times \text{gmw } O_2)}{22.4 \text{ L}}$$

$$d_w\text{air} = \frac{(0.79 \times 28) + (0.21 \times 32)}{22.4 \text{ L}}$$

$$d_w\text{air} = 1.29 \text{ g/L}$$

FN_2 and FO_2 equal, respectively, the fractional concentrations of nitrogen and oxygen in air.

Gaseous Diffusion

Diffusion is the process whereby molecules move from areas of high concentration to areas of lower concentration. Kinetic energy is the driving force behind diffusion. Because gases have high kinetic energy, they diffuse most rapidly. However, diffusion also occurs in liquids and can even take place in solids. Gas diffusion rates are quantified using **Graham's law**. Mathematically, the rate of diffusion of a gas *(D)* is inversely proportional to the square root of its gram molecular weight:

$$D_{gas} \propto \frac{1}{\sqrt{gmw}}$$

According to this principle, lighter gases diffuse rapidly, whereas heavy gases diffuse more slowly. Moreover, because diffusion is based on kinetic activity, anything that increases molecular activity will quicken diffusion. Thus heating and mechanical agitation speed diffusion.

Gas Pressure

Whether free in the atmosphere, enclosed in a container, or dissolved in a liquid such as blood, all gases exert pressure. In physiology, the term *tension* is often used to refer to the pressure exerted by gases when dissolved in liquids.

A gas's pressure or tension depends mainly on its kinetic activity. In addition, gravity affects gas pressure. Gravity increases gas density, thereby increasing the rate of molecular collisions and gas tension. This explains why atmospheric pressure decreases with altitude.

Pressure is a measure of force per unit area. The SI unit of pressure is the N/m^2, or pascal (Pa). Pressure in the cgs system is measured in $dynes/cm^2$, whereas pounds per square inch (lb/in^2) or "psi" is the British fps pressure unit. Pressure can also be measured indirectly as the height of a column of liquid, as is commonly done to determine atmospheric pressure.

Measuring Atmospheric Pressure. Atmospheric pressure is measured with a barometer. A barometer consists of an evacuated glass tube approximately 1 m long. This tube is closed at the top end, with its lower, open end immersed in a mercury reservoir (Figure 5-15). The pressure of the atmosphere on the mercury reservoir forces the mercury up the vacuum tube a distance equivalent to the force exerted.

In this manner, the height of the mercury column (measured in either inches [British] or millimeters [cgs]) represents the downward force of atmospheric pressure. Thus barometer pressure is reported with readings such as 30.4 inches of mercury (Hg) or 772 mm Hg. This means that the atmospheric pressure is great enough to support a column of mercury 30.4 inches or 772 mm high.

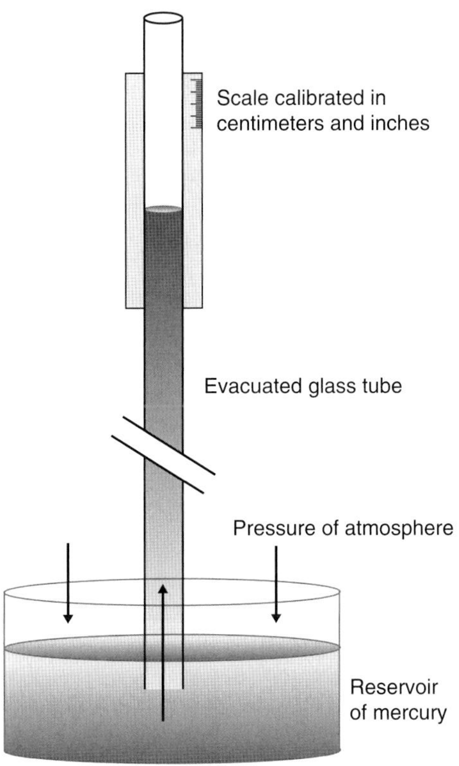

Figure 5-15

The major components of a mercury barometer.

Alternatively, the term *torr* may be used in pressure readings. Torr is short for Torricelli, the seventeenth century inventor of the mercury barometer. At sea level, 1 torr equals 1 mm Hg. Thus a pressure reading of 772 torr is the same as 772 mm Hg.

Of course, the height of a column of mercury is not a true measure of pressure. Height is a linear measure, whereas pressure represents force per unit area. We already know that the pressure exerted by a liquid is directly proportional to its depth (or height) times its density:

$$\text{pressure} = \text{height} \times \text{density}$$

At sea level, the average atmospheric pressure will support a column of mercury 76 cm (760 mm) or 29.9 inches high. If we also know that mercury has a density of 13.6 g/cm^3 (0.491 lb/in^3), then the average atmospheric pressure (P_B) is calculated as follows:

$$\text{cgs units: } P_B = 76 \text{ cm} \times 13.6 \text{ g/cm}^3 = 1034 \text{ g/cm}^2$$

$$\text{fps units: } P_B = 29.9 \text{ in} \times 0.491 \text{ lb/in}^3 = 14.7 \text{ lb/in}^2$$

These two measures, 1034 g/cm^2 and 14.7 lb/in^2, are considered standards in the cgs and British fps systems, each being equivalent to one atmosphere of pressure (1 atm).

Like any solid material, a barometer's housing reacts to temperature changes by expanding and contracting. In addition, the mercury column acts like a large thermometer. Thus both pressure *and* temperature affect a barometer's mercury level. Therefore, for accuracy, the reading must be corrected for temperature changes. The U.S. Weather Bureau provides temperature correction factors for barometric readings (Appendix 1). To correct the reading, subtract the applicable table value from the observed reading. For pressures between those listed in the table, use simple linear interpolation.

Clinical Pressure Measurements. Mercury is the most common fluid used in pressure measurements, both in barometers and at the bedside. Because of mercury's high density (13.6 g/cm^3), it assumes a height that is easy to read for most pressures in the clinical range. Water columns can also be used to measure pressure (in cm H_2O), but only low pressures. Because water is 13.6 times less dense than mercury, 1 atm of pressure would support a water column 33.9 feet high, or about as tall as a two-story building!

Both mercury and water columns are still used in clinical practice, especially when vascular pressures are being measured. However, these traditional tools are rapidly being replaced by mechanical or electronic pressure-measuring devices. Even so, these new instruments must still be calibrated against a mercury or water column before making measurements.

The simplest mechanical pressure gauge is the

aneroid barometer, which is common in homes. An aneroid barometer consists of a sealed evacuated metal box with a flexible, spring-supported top that responds to external pressure changes (Figure 5-16). This motion activates a geared pointer, which provides a scale reading analogous to pressure.

This same concept underlies the simple mechanical *manometers* used to measure blood or airway pressure at the bedside (Figure 5-17). However, rather than the pressure acting externally on the sealed chamber, the inside is connected to the pressure source. In this manner, the flexible chamber wall expands and contracts as pressure increases or decreases.

A flexible chamber can also be used to measure pressure electronically. These devices are called **strain-gauge pressure transducers**. In these devices, pressure changes expand and contract a flexible metal diaphragm connected to electrical wires (Figure 5-18). The physical strain on the diaphragm changes the amount of electricity flowing through the wires. By measuring this change in electrical flow, we are indirectly measuring changes in pressure.

Although mm Hg and cm H_2O are still the most common pressure units used at the bedside, they do not represent the SI standard. The SI unit of pressure is the kilopascal (kPa). One kPa equals approximately 10.2 cm H_2O or 7.5 torr. To accurately convert between these pressure units, use the factors provided in the rear inside cover of this book.

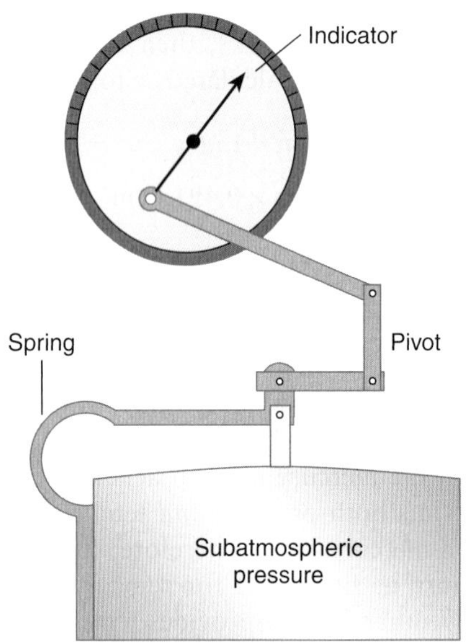

Figure 5-16

Aneroid barometer.

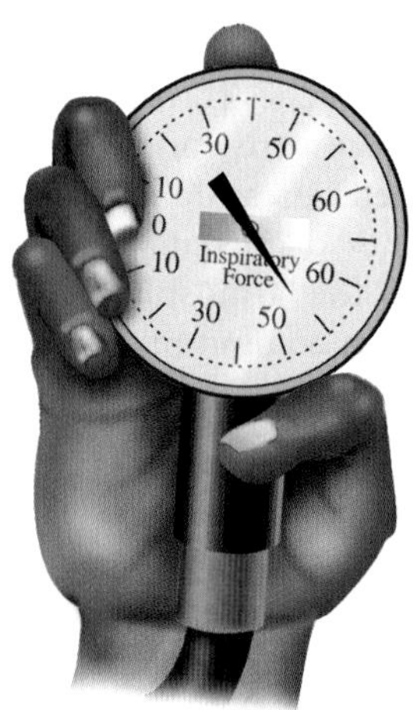

Figure 5-17

A mechanical manometer used to measure a patient's airway pressure.

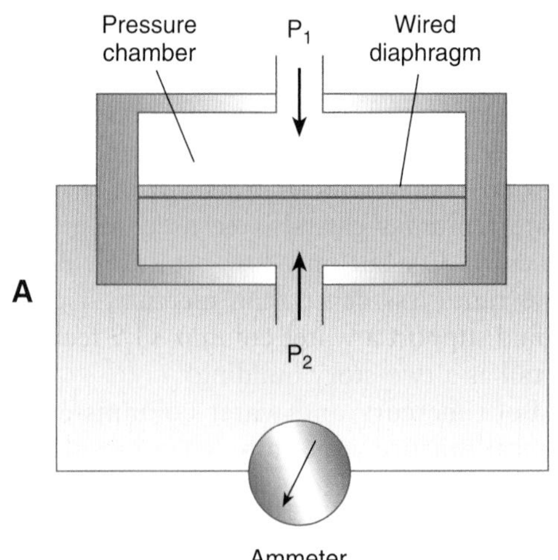

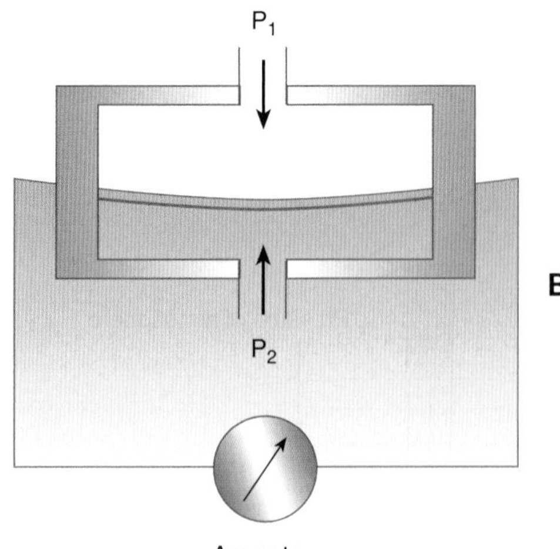

Figure 5-18 · Strain-gauge Pressure Transducer

A, No pressure is applied. **B,** Pressure is applied to the transducer. An ammeter shows a change in electrical current proportional to the magnitude of pressure applied.

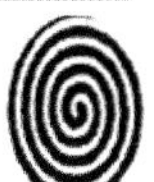

RULE OF THUMB

One kPa equals approximately 10 cm H_2O. Thus a pressure of 10 kPa equals approximately 100 H_2O. Conversely, a pressure of 60 cm H_2O equals approximately 6 kPa.

Partial Pressures (Dalton's Law)

Many gases exist together as mixtures. Air is a good example of a gas mixture, consisting mainly of oxygen and nitrogen. A gas mixture, like a solitary gas, exerts pressure. The pressure exerted by a gas mixture must equal the sum of the kinetic activity of all its component gases. The pressure exerted by a single gas in a mixture is called its *partial pressure*.

Dalton's law describes the relationship among the partial pressure and the total pressure in a gas mixture. According to this law, the total pressure of a mixture of gases must equal the sum of the partial pressures of all component gases. Moreover, the principle states that the partial pressure of a component gas must be proportional to its percentage in the mixture.

Thus a gas making up 25% of a mixture would exert 25% of the total pressure. For consistency, the percentage of a gas in a mixture is usually expressed in decimal form, using the term *fractional concentration*. Therefore a gas that is 25% of a mixture has a fractional concentration of 0.25.

For example, air consists of approximately 21% O_2 and 79% N_2. To compute the partial pressure of each component, simply multiply each component's fractional concentration by the total pressure. Assuming a normal atmospheric pressure of 760 torr, the individual partial pressure is computed as follows:

partial pressure = fractional concentration × total pressure

$$Po_2 = 0.21 \times 760 \text{ torr} = 160 \text{ torr}$$

$$Pn_2 = 0.79 \times 760 \text{ torr} = \underline{600 \text{ torr}}$$

$$760 \text{ torr}$$

As predicted by Dalton's Law, the sum of these partial pressures equals the total pressure of the gas mixture.

What if the total pressure changed? Barometric pressure changes, in addition to minor fluctuations caused by weather, are mainly a function of altitude. Considering only oxygen, we know that its fractional concentration, or FIO_2, remains constant at approximately 0.21. At a P_B of 760 torr, the Po_2 is equal to 0.21 × 760, or 160 torr. At 25,000 feet, the FIO_2 of air is still 0.21. However, the PB is only 282 torr, and the resulting Po_2 is 0.21 × 282, or 59 torr, just more than one third of that available at sea level! Because the Po_2 (not its percentage) determines its physiological activity, high altitudes can impair oxygen uptake by the lungs. This explains why mountain climbers must sometimes use extra oxygen at high altitudes. By increasing the amount of O_2 above 0.21, we can raise its partial pressure and ensure adequate uptake by the lungs. For a practical application of this principle, see the accompanying Mini Clini above.

In contrast, high atmospheric pressures increase the PIO_2 in an air mixture. Pressures above atmospheric are called *hyperbaric* pressures. Hyperbaric pressures commonly occur only in underwater diving and in special hyperbaric chambers.

For example, at a depth of 66 feet under the sea, water exerts a pressure of 3 atm, or 2280 mm Hg (3 × 760). At this depth, the oxygen in an air mixture breathed by a diver exerts a Po_2 of 0.21 × 2280, or approximately 479 mm Hg. This is nearly three times the Po_2 at sea level!

The same conditions can be created on dry land in a hyperbaric chamber. For example, the navy uses hyperbaric chambers for controlled depressurization of deep-sea divers and to treat certain types of diving accidents. Clinically, hyperbaric chambers and oxygen are used

MINI CLINI

Why Are Oxygen Masks Needed on Airplanes?

PROBLEM

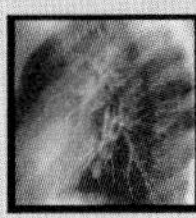

People who have traveled by air are familiar with the safety instructions given by the crew before flight. Instructions are included on how to use the oxygen masks. When and why are these masks needed?

DISCUSSION

At a typical cruising altitude of 30,000 feet, the P_B outside the airplane cabin is approximately 226 torr. Thus the inspired partial pressure of oxygen, or PIO_2, is calculated as follows:

$$PIO_2 = 0.21 \times 226 \text{ torr} = 47 \text{ torr}$$

If the cabin were to depressurize, travelers inside would be exposed to this low PIO_2. At this PIO_2, most people become unconscious within seconds and will eventually die of lack of oxygen (anoxia).

To overcome this problem, emergency oxygen masks are available when the cabin depressurizes. These masks, assuming a tight fit, probably provide approximately 70% oxygen, or an FIO_2 of 0.70. The PIO_2 of a person wearing a mask under these conditions is calculated as follows:

$$PIO_2 = 0.70 \times 226 \text{ torr} = 158 \text{ torr}$$

This PIO_2 (about the same as at sea level) is sufficient to keep the passengers alive until the crew can bring the plane to a safe altitude.

together to treat a variety of conditions, including carbon monoxide poisoning and gangrene. Chapter 35 provides more details on this use of high-pressure oxygen.

Solubility of Gases in Liquids (Henry's Law)

Gases can dissolve in liquids. Carbonated water and soda pop are good examples of a gas (CO_2) dissolved in a liquid (water).

Henry's law predicts how much of a given gas will dissolve in a liquid. According to this principle, at a given temperature, the volume of a gas that dissolves in a liquid is equal to its solubility coefficient times its partial pressure:

$$V = \alpha \times P_{gas}$$

V is the volume of dissolved gas, α is the solubility coefficient of the gas in the given liquid, and P_{gas} is the partial pressure of the gas above the liquid. The solubility of gases in liquids is compared by using a measure called the **solubility coefficient**. The solubility coefficient equals the volume of a gas that will dissolve in 1 mL of a given liquid at standard pressure and specified temperature. For example, the solubility coefficient of oxygen in plasma, at 37° C and 760 torr pressure, is 0.023 mL/mL. Under the same conditions, 0.510 mL of CO_2 can dissolve in 1 mL of plasma.

Temperature plays a major role in gas solubility. High temperatures decrease solubility and low temperatures increase solubility. This is why an open can of soda pop may still fizz if left in the refrigerator but quickly goes flat when left out at room temperature.

Temperature's effect on solubility is a result of changes in kinetic activity. As a liquid is warmed, the kinetic activity of any dissolved gas molecules is increased. This increase in kinetic activity increases the molecules' escaping tendency and partial pressure. As an increasing number of gas molecules escape, the amount left in a solution decreases rapidly. For a practical application of this principle, see the Mini Clini, which discusses blood gases and patient temperature.

MINI CLINI

Blood Gases Versus Patient Temperature

PROBLEM

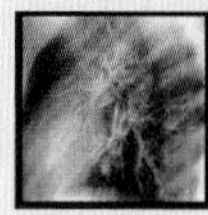

RTs frequently need to sample and measure the partial pressures of oxygen and carbon dioxide in patients' arterial blood. These samples are called arterial blood gases, or ABGs.

Typically, ABG samples are measured in analyzers kept at a normal body temperature of 37° C. However, not all patients have normal body temperatures. Many will be feverish (hyperpyrexia) and some will have low body temperatures (*hypothermia*). What effect does this have on the measurements?

DISCUSSION

The direct relationship between temperature and partial pressure causes higher arterial Po_2 and Pco_2 readings at higher temperatures. At 37° C, the normal adult's arterial Po_2 is approximately 100 torr. However, at 47° C the Po_2 would be nearly twice as high. A smaller increase from 37° to 39° C increases the arterial Po_2 less markedly from 100 to approximately 110 torr. Likewise, a rise in temperature raises the arterial Pco_2. Arterial Pco_2 values increase approximately 5% per degree Celsius. Thus an increase in temperature from 37° to 39° C increases the Pco_2 by approximately 10%, from 40 to 44 torr.

Of course, the reverse is also true. Decreased temperatures decrease the arterial partial pressures of oxygen and carbon dioxide. Nomograms are available to help compute these corrections; however, they only correct for the relationship between temperature and pressure. Nomograms do not take into account metabolic and cardiovascular changes that accompany a change in a patient's temperature. For this reason, the use of corrected Po_2 and Pco_2 readings remains controversial.

▶ GAS BEHAVIOR UNDER CHANGING CONDITIONS

Gases, with large distances between their molecules, are easily compressed and expanded. When a gas is pressurized, the molecules are squeezed closer together. On the other hand, if a gas-filled container could be enlarged, the gas would expand to occupy the new volume. Figure 5-19 illustrates the concepts of gas compression and expansion.

Gas Laws

Several laws help define the relationship among gas pressure, temperature, mass, and volume (Table 5-4). Using these laws, the behavior of gases under changing conditions can be predicted.

Underlying all these laws are three basic assumptions: (1) No energy is lost during molecular collisions, (2) the volume of the molecules themselves is negligible, and (3) no forces of mutual attraction exist between these molecules. These three assumptions describe the behavior of an "ideal gas." Under normal conditions, most gases exhibit ideal behavior.

Effect of Water Vapor

In clinical practice, most gas law calculations must take into account the presence of water vapor. Water vapor, like any gas, occupies space. Thus the dry volume of a

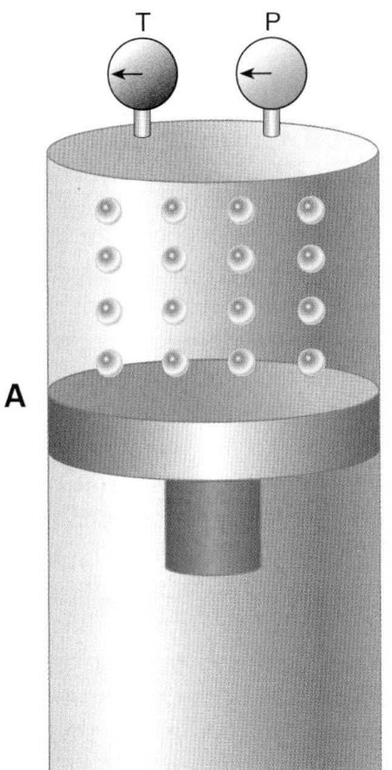

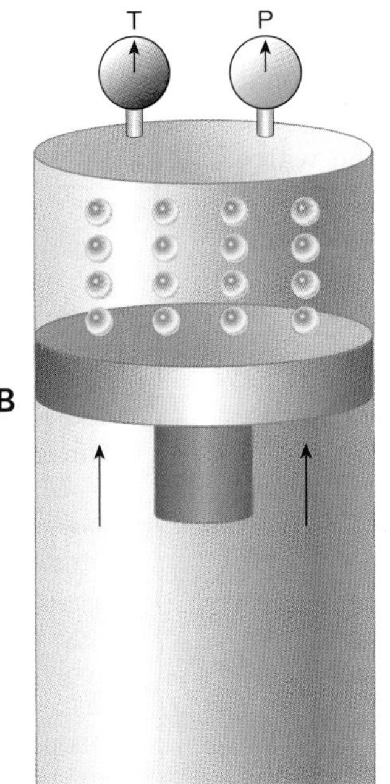

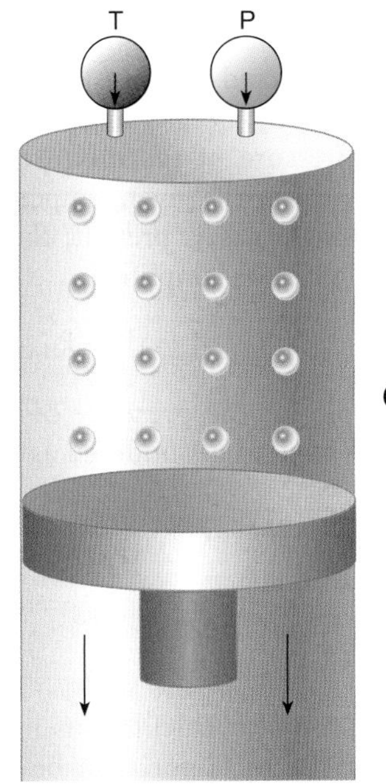

Figure 5-19

A mass of gas in the resting state exerts a given pressure *(P)* at a given temperature *(T)* in cylinder **A.** In cylinder **B,** as the piston compresses the gas, the molecules are crowded closer together, and the increased energy of molecular collisions increases both the temperature and pressure. Conversely, as the gas expands in cylinder **C,** molecular interaction decreases, and the temperature and pressure fall.

Table 5-4 ▶▶ Laws Describing Gas Behavior Under Changing Conditions

Gas Law	Basic Relationship	Constants	Description	Working Formula*	Clinical Applications
Boyle's law	$P \times V = k$	Temperature, mass	The volume of a gas varies inversely with its pressure	$P_1V_1 = P_2V_2$	Ventilation (Chapter 9) Body plethysmography (Chapter 17) Compressed volume (Chapter 40)
Charles' law	$\frac{V}{T} = k$	Pressure, mass	The volume of gas varies directly with changes in its temperature (° K)	$\frac{V_1}{T_1} = \frac{V_2}{T_2}$	ATPS to BTPS corrections (this chapter; Chapter 17)
Gay-Lussac's law	$\frac{P}{T} = k$	Volume, mass	The pressure exerted by a gas varies directly with its absolute temperature	$\frac{P_1}{T_1} = \frac{P_2}{T_2}$	Cylinder pressures (Chapter 33)
Combined Gas law	$PV = nRT$	—	Interaction of above (none held constant)	$\frac{P_1V_1}{nT_1} = \frac{P_2V_2}{nT_2}$	Complex interactions of variables

P, Pressure; *V*, volume; *T*, temperature (° Kelvin); *n*, mass; *R*, the gas constant (a combined constant of proportionality).
*Use the working formulas to calculate the new value of a parameter when a gas undergoes a change in P, V, n, or T. For example, to solve for a new volume (V_2) using Boyle's law, you would simply rearrange its working equation as follows:

$$V_2 = V_1 \times \frac{P_1}{P_2}$$

gas at a constant pressure and temperature is always smaller than its saturated volume. The opposite is also true. Correcting from the dry state to the saturated state always yields a larger gas volume.

On the other hand, the pressure exerted by water vapor is independent of the other gases with which it mixes, depending only on the temperature and RH. Therefore the addition of water vapor to a gas mixture always lowers the partial pressures of the other gases present. This fact becomes relevant when discussing the partial pressure of gases in the lung where the gases are saturated with water vapor at body temperature.

Corrected Pressure Computations

To compute the new or corrected partial pressure of a gas after saturation with water vapor, the following formula is applied:

$$P_C = F_{gas} \times (P_T - P_{H_2O})$$

P_C is the corrected gas pressure, F_{gas} is the fractional concentration of the gas in the gas mixture, P_T is the total gas pressure of the mixture, and P is the water vapor pressure at the given temperature (see Table 5-3). If only a single gas is present, then F_{gas} equals 1, and the formula can be simplified:

$$P_C = (P_T - P_{H_2O})$$

For example, in the presence of water vapor, Boyle's law would have to be modified as follows:

$$V_2 = V_1 \times \frac{(P_1 - P_{H_2O} \text{ at } T_1)}{(P_2 - {H_2O} \text{ at } T_2)}$$

Correction Factors

Instead of complex calculations involving water vapor, simple correction factors can be used. In gas volume conversions, the three most common computations are as follows:

- Correction from ambient temperature and pressure saturated (**ATPS**) to body temperature and pressure, saturated (**BTPS**)
- Correction from ATPS to standard temperature and pressure (0° C and 760 torr), dry (**STPD**)
- Correction from STPD to BTPS

The values in the third column of Table 5-3, when multiplied by V_1, will convert a gas volume from ATPS to BTPS. Appendix 2 provides the factors needed to convert a gas volume from ATPS to STPD. To use Appendix 2, simply multiply the ATPS volume by the factor corresponding to the specified temperature and *uncorrected* barometric pressure. Last, Appendix 3 provides the factors needed to correct volumes from STPD to BTPS. To use Appendix 3, simply multiply the STPD volume by the factor corresponding to the ambient pressure.

MINI CLINI

Variations From Ideal Gas Behavior: Expansion Cooling and Adiabatic Compression

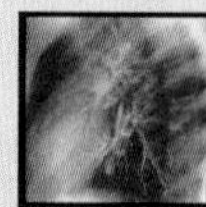

Boyle's law describes gas behavior under constant temperature, or isothermal conditions. During isothermal conditions, the temperature of an ideal gas should not change with either expansion or contraction. For example, if an ideal gas were to rapidly escape from a high-pressure cylinder into the atmosphere, its temperature should not change. In fact, the rapid expansion of real gases causes substantial cooling. This phenomenon of expansion cooling is called the *Joule-Thompson Effect.*

A rapidly expanding gas cools because the attractive force between its molecules is broken. Because the energy needed to break these forces must come from the gas itself, the temperature of the gas must decrease. This drop in temperature, depending on the pressure drop that occurs, can be large enough to actually liquefy the gas. This is the primary method used to liquefy air for the production of oxygen, as described in Chapter 33.

Whereas isothermal processes keep gas temperature constant, *adiabatic compression* and expansion have no such restrictions. During an adiabatic process, a gas's heat energy is allowed to rise or fall as it undergoes changes in pressure or volume.

Adiabatic compression of a gas can cause rapid increases in temperature. A diesel engine uses this principle to ignite fuel without a spark. Adiabatic compression can also occur in gas delivery systems where rapid compression occurs within a fixed container. The rise in temperature caused by this rapid compression can ignite any combustible material in the system. It is for this reason that RTs must take care to clear any combustible matter from high-pressure gas delivery systems before pressurization.

Properties of Gases at Extremes of Temperature and Pressure

As previously described, most gases exhibit ideal behavior under normal conditions. However, gases can deviate from these expectations, especially at the extremes of pressure and temperature. The Mini Clini on this page provides two good clinical examples of how gas behavior can deviate from the ideal.

As previously discussed, weak attractive forces (van der Waals forces) between gas molecules oppose their kinetic activity. Both temperature and pressure affect these forces. For example, at high temperatures, the increased kinetic activity of gas molecules far overshadows these forces. However, at very low temperatures kinetic activity lessens and these forces become more important. Likewise, very low pressures permit gas molecules to move freely about with little mutual attraction. In contrast, high pressures crowd molecules together, increasing the influence of these forces.

The actual space occupied by gas molecules also can influence their behavior. At low pressure, the total mass of matter in a gas is a negligible fraction of the total volume. However, at very high pressures molecular density becomes important, altering the expected relationship between pressure and volume.

Critical Temperature and Pressure

For every liquid there is a temperature above which the kinetic activity of its molecules is so great that the attractive forces cannot keep them in a liquid state. This temperature is called the **critical temperature.**

The critical temperature is the highest temperature at which a substance can exist as a liquid. The pressure needed to maintain equilibrium between the liquid and gas phases of a substance at this critical temperature is the *critical pressure*. Together, the critical temperature and pressure represent the *critical point* of a substance.

For example, the critical temperature of water is 374° C. At this temperature, a pressure of 218 atm is needed to maintain equilibrium between water's liquid and gaseous forms. No pressure can return water vapor to its liquid form above 374° C.

Gases, compared with liquids, have much lower critical points. Table 5-5 lists the critical points of four gases used in clinical practice: oxygen, helium, carbon dioxide, and nitrous oxide. Note that the critical temperatures of oxygen and helium are well below the normal room temperature of 20° C (68° F), whereas those of carbon dioxide and nitrous oxide are above room temperature.

The concept of critical temperature can be applied to distinguish between a true gas and a vapor. A true gas, like oxygen, has a critical temperature so low that at room temperature and pressure it cannot exist as a liquid. In contrast, a vapor is the gaseous state of a substance coexisting with its liquid or solid state at room temperature and pressure. This is why molecular water is referred to as *water vapor*.

The concept of critical temperature and pressure also helps explain how gases are liquefied. Of course, a gas can be liquefied by being cooled to below its boiling point. Alternatively, a gas could be liquefied by being cooled to below its critical temperature and then being compressed. The more a gas is cooled below its critical temperature, the less pressure will be needed to liquefy it. However, under no circumstances can pressure alone liquefy a gas existing above its critical temperature.

According to these principles, any gas with a critical temperature above ambient should be able to be liquefied simply by having pressure applied. Both CO_2 and N_2O have critical temperatures above normal room temperature (see Table 5-5). Thus both gases can be liquefied by simple compression and stored as liquids at room temperature without cooling. However, both liquefied gases still need to be stored under pressure, usually in strong metal cylinders.

Table 5-5 ▶▶ Critical Points of Three Gases

Gas	°C	°F	Atmosphere
Helium (He)	−267.9	−450.2	2.3
Oxygen (O_2)	−118.8	−181.1	49.7
Carbon dioxide (CO_2)	31.1	87.9	73.0
Nitrous oxide (N_2O)	36.5	97.7	71.8

Liquid oxygen is produced by separating it from a liquefied air mixture at a temperature below its boiling point (−183° C or −297° F). After it is separated from air, the oxygen must be maintained as a liquid by being stored in insulated containers below its boiling point. As long as the temperature does not exceed −183° C, the oxygen will remain liquid at atmospheric pressure. If higher temperatures are needed, higher pressures must be used. If at any time the liquid oxygen exceeds its critical temperature of −118.8° C, it will convert immediately to a gas.

▶ FLUID DYNAMICS

So far, liquids and gases have been presented under static, or nonmoving, conditions. However, both liquids and gases can flow. *Flow* is the bulk movement of a substance through space.

The study of fluids in motion is called *hydrodynamics*. Because many respiratory care devices use hydrodynamic principles, the RT must have a good understanding of the basic concepts governing fluids in motion.

Pressures in Flowing Fluids

As we have seen, a static liquid's pressure depends solely on the depth and density of the fluid. In contrast, the pressure exerted by a liquid in motion depends on the nature of the flow itself.

As shown in Figure 5-20, *A*, the pressure exerted by a static fluid is the same at all points along a horizontal tube, depending only on the height *(h)* of the liquid column. However, when the fluid flows out through the bottom tube, the pressure progressively falls all along the tube length (Figure 5-20, *B*). In addition, we observe that the decrease in pressure between each of the equally spaced vertical tubes is the same.

This decrease in fluid pressure along the tube reflects a cumulative energy loss, as predicted by the Second Law of Thermodynamics. In simple terms, this law states that in any mechanical process, there will always be a decrease in the total energy available to do work.

Available energy decreases because frictional forces oppose fluid flow. Frictional resistance to flow exists both within the fluid itself (viscosity) and between the fluid and the tube wall. In general, the greater the viscosity of the fluid and the smaller the cross-sectional area of the tube, the greater the drop in pressure along the tube.

For any given tube length, **flow resistance** equals the difference in pressure between the two points along the tube divided by the actual flow. This is expressed as a formula:

$$R = \frac{(P_1 - P_2)}{\dot{V}}$$

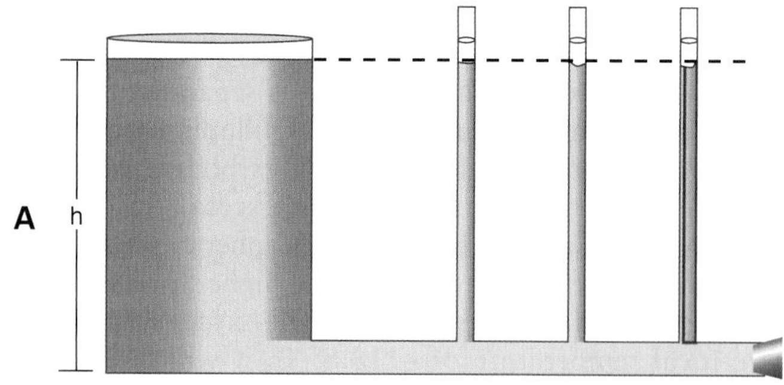

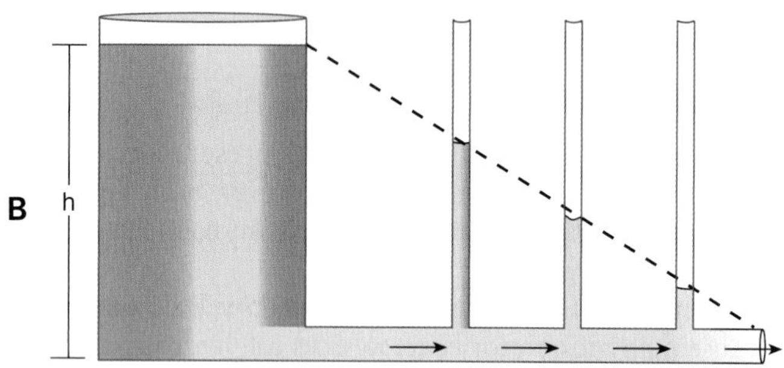

Figure 5-20

A, The pressure is the same at all points along the horizontal tube when there is no flow. **B,** A progressive decrease in pressure occurs as the fluid flows. *(Modified from Nave CR, Nave BC: Physics for the health sciences, ed 3, Philadelphia, 1985, WB Saunders.)*

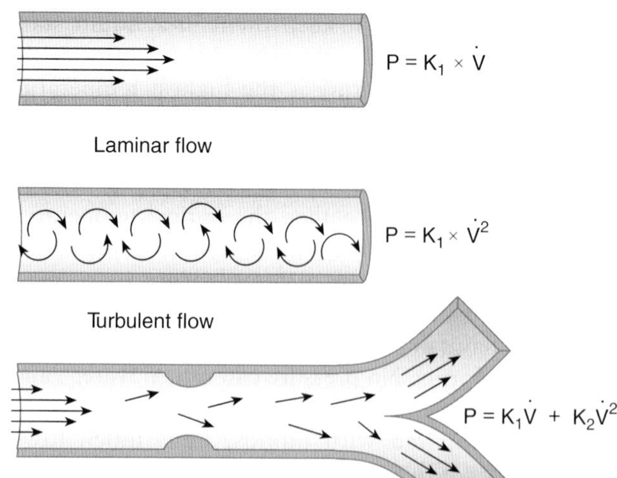

Figure 5-21

The three patterns of flow: laminar, turbulent, and transitional. *(Modified from Moser KM, Spragg RG: Respiratory emergencies, ed 2, St Louis, 1982, Mosby.)*

R is the total flow resistance, P_1 is the pressure at the upstream point (point 1), P_2 is the pressure at the downstream point (point 2), and $\dot{V}$ is the flow (volume per unit time). This formula has wide application in pulmonary physiology and respiratory care. The Mini Clini at right provides a good example of such application.

Patterns of Flow

The pressure difference that results from flow also varies with the pattern of flow. There are three primary patterns of flow through tubes: laminar, turbulent, and transitional (Figure 5-21).

Laminar Flow

As discussed earlier, during laminar flow a fluid moves in discrete cylindrical layers or streamlines. The difference in pressure required to produce a given flow, under conditions of laminar flow through a smooth tube of fixed size, is defined by Poiseuille's Law:

$$\Delta P = \frac{8nl\dot{V}}{\pi r^4}$$

ΔP is the driving pressure gradient, n is the viscosity of the fluid, l is the tube length, $\dot{V}$ is the fluid flow, r is the tube radius, and π and 8 are constants.

MINI CLINI

A Differential Pressure Pneumotachometer

PROBLEM

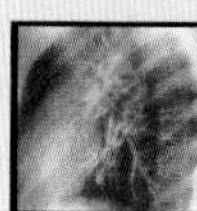

It is often necessary to measure and record changes in air flow as a patient breathes. How can we apply the formula for resistance to measure and record air flow?

DISCUSSION

Air flow can be measured by using a device called a pneumotachometer. One of the simplest designs is the differential pressure *pneumotachometer*. A differential pressure pneumotachometer incorporates a flow tube with a known and constant resistance (R = K). If the formula for resistance is rearranged to solve for flow, it appears as follows:

$$\dot{V} = \frac{(P_1 - P_2)}{K}$$

Thus flow through a tube with constant resistance is directly proportional to the pressure difference across the tube. By measuring this pressure difference (using a strain-gauge transducer, like that described in Figure 5-18), we can measure flow. To ensure linearity between pressure and flow, the flow pattern through the tube must remain laminar.

According to this formula, for fluids flowing in a laminar pattern, the driving pressure will increase whenever the fluid viscosity, tube length, or flow increases. In addition, greater pressure will be required to maintain a given flow if the tube radius decreases.

Turbulent Flow

Under certain conditions, the pattern of flow through a tube changes significantly, with a loss of regular streamlines. Instead, fluid molecules form irregular eddy currents in a chaotic pattern called **turbulent flow** (see Figure 5-21).

This changeover from laminar to turbulent flow depends on several factors, including fluid density *(d)*, viscosity *(h)*, linear velocity *(v)*, and tube radius *(r)*. In combination, these factors determine **Reynold's number** (N_R):

$$N_R = \frac{v \times d \times 2r}{\eta}$$

In a smooth-bore tube, laminar flow becomes turbulent when N_R exceeds 2000 (the number is dimensionless). According to the previous formula, conditions favoring turbulent flow include increased fluid velocity, increased fluid density, increased tube radius, or decreased fluid viscosity. In the presence of irregular tube walls, turbulent flow can occur when N_R is less than 2000.

When flow becomes turbulent, Poiseuille's law no longer applies. Instead, the pressure difference across a tube is defined as follows:

$$\Delta P = \frac{fl\dot{V}^2}{4\pi^2 r^5}$$

ΔP is the driving pressure, f is a friction factor based on the fluid's density and viscosity and the tube wall roughness, l is the tube length, and $\dot{V}$ is the fluid flow.

Figure 5-22 compares the relationship between pressure and flow under laminar and turbulent conditions. As can be seen, when flow is laminar (Poiseuille's law), the relationship between driving pressure and flow is linear. However, when flow becomes turbulent, driving pressure varies with the square of the flow ($\dot{V}^2$). Thus to double flow under laminar conditions, we need only double the driving pressure. To double flow under turbulent conditions, we would have to increase the driving pressure fourfold.

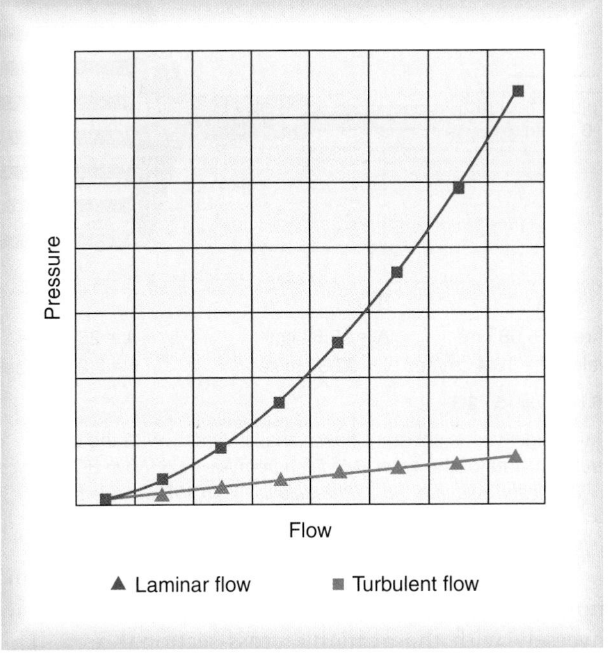

Figure 5-22
The relationship between driving pressure and flow under laminar and turbulent conditions.

Transitional Flow

Transitional flow is a mixture of laminar and turbulent flow. Flow in the respiratory tract is mainly transitional in nature. When flow is transitional, the total driving pressure equals the sum of the pressures resulting from laminar and turbulent flow:

$$\Delta P = (k_1 \times \dot{V}) + (k_2 \times \dot{V}^2)$$

Here, k_1 and k_2 are factors indicating the respective contribution of laminar and turbulent flow to overall driving pressure. When flow is mainly laminar, the pressure varies linearly with the flow. When flow is mainly turbulent, driving pressure varies exponentially with the flow. With all else equal, pressures generated during laminar flow are most affected by fluid viscosity, whereas fluid density is the key factor when flow is turbulent.

Flow, Velocity, and Cross-Sectional Area

Flow is the bulk movement of a volume of fluid per unit of time. Clinically, the most common units of flow are liters per minute (L/min) or liters per second (L/sec). In contrast, velocity is a measure of linear distance traveled by the fluid per unit of time. Centimeters per second (cm/sec) is a common velocity unit used in pulmonary physiology.

Although fluid flow and velocity are different measures, the two concepts are closely related. The key factor relating velocity to flow is the cross-sectional area of the conducting system. Figure 5-23 demonstrates this relationship.

Throughout the tube, the fluid flows at a constant rate of 5 L/min. At point *A*, with a cross-sectional area of 5.08 cm^2, the velocity of the fluid is 16.4 cm/sec. At point *B*, the cross-sectional area of the tube decreases to 2.54 cm^2, half its prior value. At this point, the velocity of the fluid doubles to 32.8 cm/sec. At point *C*, the passage divides into eight smaller tubes. Although each tube is smaller than its "parent," together they provide a tenfold increase in the cross-sectional area available for flow, compared with point *B*. Thus the velocity of the fluid decreases proportionately, from 32.8 to 3.28 cm/sec.

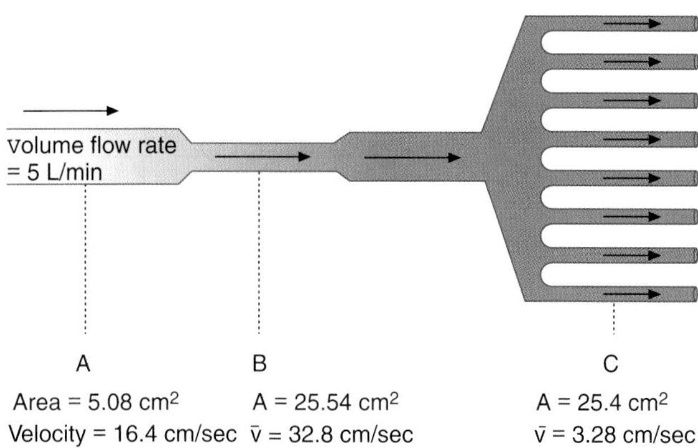

Figure 5-23

Fluid velocity, at a constant flow, varies inversely with the cross-sectional area of the tube. *(Modified from Nave CR, Nave BC: Physics for the health sciences, ed 3, Philadelphia, 1985, WB Saunders.)*

These observations show that the velocity of a fluid moving through a tube at a constant flow varies inversely with the available cross-sectional area. This relationship is called the **Law of Continuity.** Mathematically, the equation is as follows:

$$(A_1 \times v_1) + (A_2 \times v_2) + (A_n \times v_n) = k$$

A is the cross-sectional area of the tube; *v* is the velocity of the fluid; *1*, *2*, and *n* are different points in the tube; and *k* is a constant value.

Although the principle holds true only for incompressible liquids, the qualitative features are similar for gas flow. This principle also underlies the application of nozzles or jets in fluid streams. Nozzles and jets are simply narrow passages in a tube designed to increase fluid velocity. A garden-hose nozzle is a good example of this principle in action. Clinically, jets are used in many types of respiratory care equipment, including pneumatic nebulizers (see Chapter 32) and gas entrainment or mixing devices (see Chapter 35).

The Bernoulli Effect

When a fluid flows through a tube of uniform diameter, pressure decreases progressively over the tube length. The first three water columns in Figure 5-24 demonstrate this continuous pressure drop. However, when the fluid passes through a constriction, the pressure drop is much greater. This large pressure drop can be observed in the fourth water column in Figure 5-24.

The eighteenth-century scientist Daniel Bernoulli was the first to carefully study this effect, which now bears his name. Bernoulli explained the pressure drop depicted in Figure 5-24 by showing how a moving fluid's potential, kinetic, and pressure energies interact.

A fluid's position determines its potential energy. The common adage that "water always seeks its lowest level" is actually an expression of potential energy. At the top of a tilted tube, gravity gives any fluid the potential energy to flow "downhill." In this case, the fluid's potential energy is proportional to the difference between the height of the tube's inlet and outlet. If a tube is level, the fluid's potential energy remains constant and can be disregarded.

Kinetic energy is the amount of work performed by matter in motion. The kinetic energy of a moving fluid is directly proportional to both its velocity and mass. The greater the velocity and mass (density) of a fluid, the greater its kinetic energy. If mass is constant, kinetic energy varies directly with velocity only.

Whereas potential and kinetic energy are common physical concepts, the principle of pressure energy is unique to fluid flow. A fluid's pressure energy is the radial or outward force exerted by the moving fluid. This radial force is measured as the fluid's *lateral pressure.*

According to the First Law of Thermodynamics, the total energy at any given point in a fluid stream must be the same throughout the tube. If potential energy is held constant (a level tube), then the sum of the kinetic and pressure energies at any given point in a fluid stream must equal their sum at any other point.

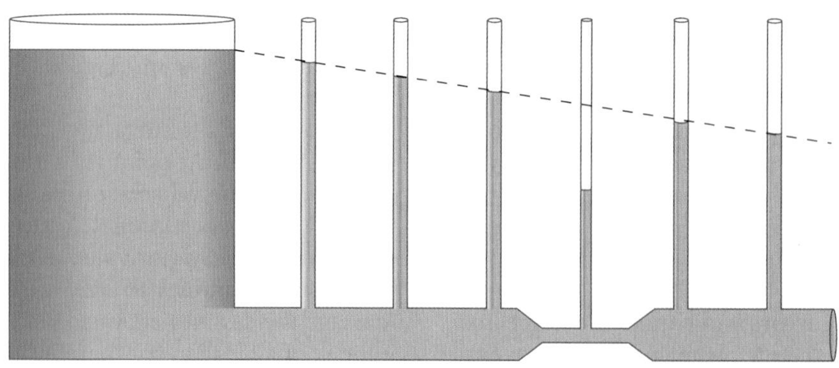

Figure 5-24

The Bernoulli effect. *(Modified from Nave CR, Nave BC: Physics for the health sciences, ed 3, Philadelphia, 1985, WB Saunders.)*

Velocity is equivalent to the kinetic energy of a fluid, whereas lateral force equates to pressure energy. Because a moving fluid's velocity and lateral pressure sum must always be equal, they must vary inversely with each other. In other words, if additional energy is applied to increase velocity, then the energy available to exert pressure must decrease. As velocity increases, lateral pressure decreases. Conversely, as velocity decreases, lateral pressure increases.

Figure 5-25 demonstrates this relationship. Fluid is flowing through a tube at a point with a certain velocity (v_a) and a lateral pressure (P_a). According to the Law of Continuity, as the fluid moves into the narrow or constricted portion of the tube, its velocity must increase ($v_b > v_a$). According to the Bernoulli theorem, the higher velocity at point b should result in a lower lateral pressure at that point ($P_b < P_a$). Thus as a fluid flows through the constriction, its velocity increases and its lateral pressure decreases.

Fluid Entrainment

When a flowing fluid encounters a very narrow passage, its velocity can increase greatly. In some cases, the rise in velocity can be so great as to cause the fluid's lateral pressure to fall below that exerted by the atmosphere (i.e., to become negative).

If an open tube is placed distal to such a constriction, this negative pressure can actually pull another fluid into the primary flow stream (Figure 5-26). This effect is called **fluid entrainment**. In Figure 5-26, air is the entrained fluid. This use is common in the home where faucet aerators mix air into the water stream. In the laboratory, a similar faucet attachment, called a *water aspirator*, is used to create negative pressure or vacuum.

In respiratory care, the most common application of fluid entrainment is the *air injector*. An air injector is a device designed to increase the total flow in a gas stream. In this case, a pressurized gas, usually oxygen, serves as the primary flow source. This pressurized gas passes through a nozzle or jet, beyond which is an air entrainment port. The negative lateral pressure created at the jet orifice entrains air into the primary gas stream, thereby increasing the total flow output of the system.

The amount of air entrained depends on both the diameter of the jet orifice and the size of the air entrainment ports (Figure 5-27). For a fixed jet size, the larger the entrainment ports, the greater the volume of air entrained and the higher the total flow (Figure 5-27, *B*). The entrained volume can still be altered, with fixed entrainment ports, by changing the jet diameter (Figure 5-27, *C*). A large jet results in a lower gas velocity and less entrainment, whereas a small jet boosts velocity, entrained volume, and total flow.

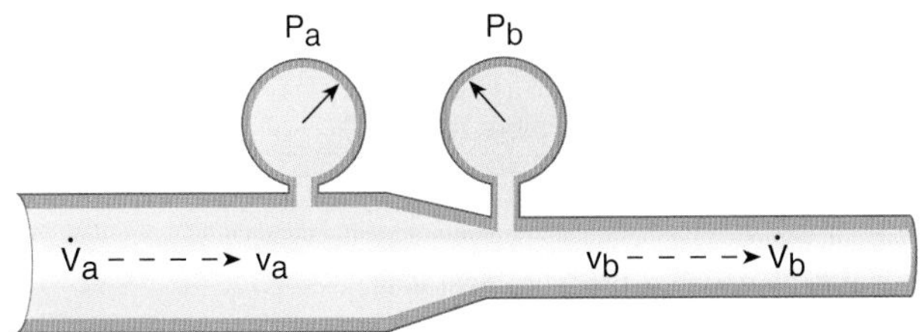

Figure 5-25

According to the Bernoulli theorem, a flowing fluid's lateral pressure must vary inversely with its velocity. $\dot{V}_a$, Flow in tube "a"; v_a, velocity in tube "a"; v_b, velocity in tube "b"; $\dot{V}_b$, flow in tube "b"; P_a, lateral wall pressure in tube "a"; P_b, lateral wall pressure after restriction (see text).

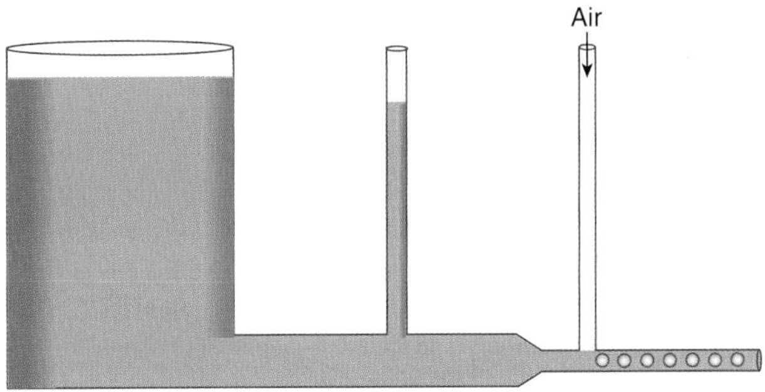

Figure 5-26

Fluid entrainment based on the Bernoulli effect. *(Modified from Nave CR, Nave BC: Physics for the health sciences, ed 3, Philadelphia, 1985, WB Saunders.)*

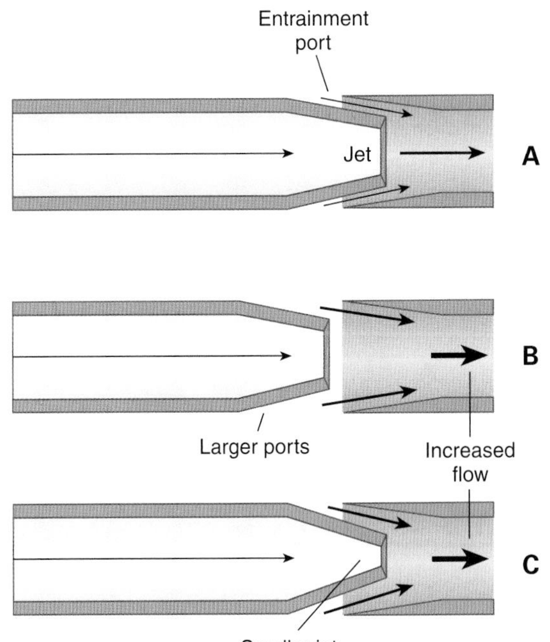

Figure 5-27 · **Air Injector**

A, The basic design. **B,** Greater entrainment and total flow occurs with larger entrainment ports. **C,** Alternatively, a smaller jet increases source gas velocity and entrains more air.

The Venturi and Pitot Tubes

A Venturi tube is a modified entrainment device, developed approximately 200 years ago by Giovanni Venturi. A Venturi tube widens just after its jet or nozzle (Figure 5-28). As long as the angle of dilation is less than 15 degrees, this widening helps restore fluid pressure back toward prejet levels.

The Venturi tube, as compared with a simple air injector, provides greater entrainment. Moreover, this design helps keep the percentage of entrained fluid constant, even when the total flow varies. However, the Venturi tube has one major drawback. Any buildup of pressure downstream from the entrainment port decreases fluid entrainment.

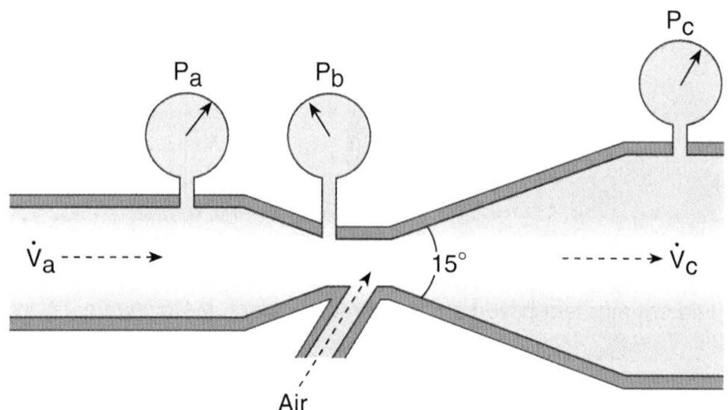

Figure 5-28 · A Venturi Tube

The original lateral pressure at point (P_a) falls at the restriction (P_b). Pressure is almost completely restored distal to the restriction (P_c), if the angle of tube dilation does not exceed 15 degrees. $\dot{V}_a$, Flow before restriction; $\dot{V}_c$, flow from entrainment plus driving flow.

An alternative design, called a Pitot tube, partly overcomes this problem. Rather than restoring fluid pressure, a Pitot tube restores fluid velocity. This lessens the effect of downstream pressure on fluid entrainment.

Fluidics and the Coanda Effect

Fluidics is a branch of engineering that applies hydrodynamic principles in flow circuits for purposes such as switching, pressure and flow sensing, and amplification. Because fluidic devices have no moving parts, they are very dependable and require little maintenance.

The primary principle underlying most fluidic circuitry is a phenomenon called wall attachment, or the **Coanda effect**. This effect is observed mainly when a fluid flows through a small orifice with properly contoured downstream surfaces.

Based on the Bernoulli effect, we know that the negative pressure created at a jet or nozzle will entrain any surrounding fluid, such as air, into the primary flow stream (Figure 5-29, *A*). If a carefully contoured curved wall is added to one side of the jet (Figure 5-29, *B*), the pressure near the wall becomes negative relative to atmospheric. Thus the atmospheric pressure on the other side of the gas stream pushes it against the wall, where it remains "locked" until interrupted by some counterforce. By carefully extending the wall contour, we can actually deflect the fluid stream through a full 180-degree turn!

A variety of fluidic devices can be designed using this principle, including on/off switches, pressure and flow sensors, and flow amplifiers. These individual components can be combined into integrated fluidic logic circuits, which function much like electronic circuit boards but without the need for electrical power.

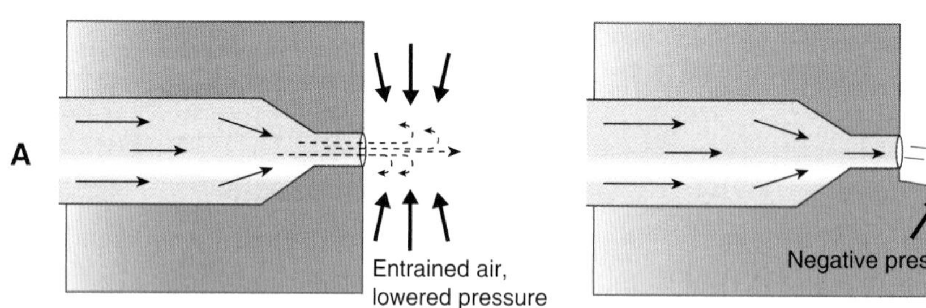

Figure 5-29 · The Coanda Wall Effect

A, Entrainment into the fluid stream. **B**, Wall attachment initiated by negative pressure near wall.

KEY POINTS

- Gases have no inherent boundary, are readily compressed and expanded, and can flow.
- Three temperature scales are in common use: Kelvin (SI), Celsius (cgs), and Fahrenheit (fps); conversion among these scale units can be done by using simple formulas.
- Transfer of heat energy can occur by conduction, convection, radiation, and evaporation.
- Liquids exert pressure and exhibit the properties of flow, buoyant force, viscosity, capillary action, and surface tension.
- The pressure exerted by a liquid depends on both its height (depth) and weight density.
- Surface tension forces increase the pressure inside a liquid drop or bubble; this pressure varies directly with the surface tension of the liquid and varies inversely with the radius.
- A liquid can vaporize by either boiling or evaporation; in evaporation, the required heat energy is taken from the air surrounding the liquid, thereby cooling the air.
- Vaporization causing cooling and condensation causes warming of the surroundings.
- The capacity of air to hold water vapor increases with temperature.
- RH is the ratio of water vapor content (absolute humidity) to saturated water vapor capacity; for a constant content, cooling increases RH and warming decreases RH.

KEY POINTS—cont'd

- The rate of diffusion of a gas is inversely proportional to its molecular weight.
- The total pressure of a mixture of gases must equal the sum of the partial pressures of all component gases.
- The volume of a gas that dissolves in a liquid equals its solubility coefficient times its partial pressure; high temperatures decrease gas solubility and low temperatures increase gas solubility.
- A gas's volume and pressure vary directly with temperature; however, with constant temperature, gas volume and pressure vary inversely.
- A substance's critical temperature is the highest temperature at which it can exist as a liquid; gases with critical temperatures above room temperature can be stored under pressure as liquids without cooling.
- Under conditions of laminar flow, the difference in pressure required to produce a given flow is defined by Poiseuille's law.
- The velocity of a fluid flowing through a tube at a constant rate of flow varies inversely with the available cross-sectional area; this allows entrainment of other fluids at jets or nozzles.

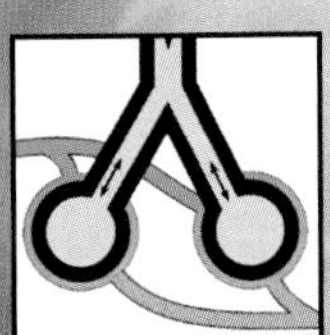

CHAPTER 6

Computer Applications in Respiratory Care

Glen R. Kuck and Craig L. Scanlan

In This Chapter You Will Learn:

- How computers work
- Which application program to use for a given task
- How computers communicate with each other
- How computers are used to manage patient information
- How computers aid in patient monitoring and diagnostic testing
- How computers control instrument or device function
- How computers are used to assist in data interpretation and diagnosis
- How to use the Internet to access quality clinical and professional information
- What nontechnical issues computer usage raises in healthcare delivery

Chapter Outline

Key Terms

algorithm
analog-to-digital converter (ADC)
application program
arithmetic logic control unit (ALC)
bandwidth
browser
byte
cathode ray tubes (CRTs)
central processing unit (CPU)
CD-R
CD-ROM
CD-RW
closed-loop systems
communication protocols
data communication
database management system (DBMS)
DVD
e-mail
expert system
external memory
floppy disk
gigabyte (Gb)
hard disks
hospital information systems (HIS)
hypertext links
hypertext markup language (HTML)
hypertext transfer protocol (HTTP)
internal memory
Internet
kilobyte (Kb)
local area network (LAN)

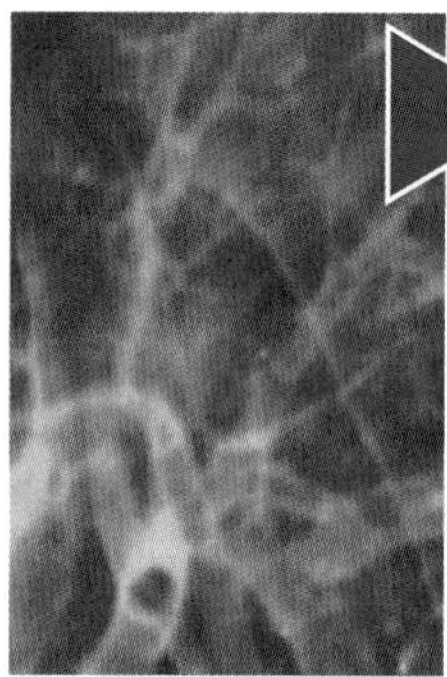

Key Terms—cont'd

liquid crystal displays (LCDs)
megabyte (Mb)
modem
network
newsgroup
open-loop systems
operating system
program
programming languages
random access memory (RAM)
read only memory (ROM)
servers
software
transmission control protocol/Internet protocol (TCP/IP)
universal resource locator (URL)
wide area network (WAN)

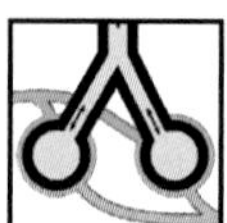

Computers are becoming an increasingly valuable tool in the delivery and management of respiratory care. From bedside care and department management to personal professional development, computers are facilitating and enhancing the way respiratory therapists (RTs) practice their profession. For RTs to efficiently function in the modern healthcare setting, they must possess a working knowledge of how computers, computer programs, computer networks, and the Internet can be used to improve patient care and advance the profession.

HOW COMPUTERS WORK

RTs should have a basic understanding of both computer hardware and software. This section provides an overview of computer equipment and programs.

Hardware

Modern computers consist of four key hardware components: a central processing unit, memory to store data and instructions, input devices, and output devices.

Central Processing Unit

The **central processing unit** (**CPU**) is the "brain" or "calculator" of the computer. All computers need a CPU in order to work. The CPU is usually located inside the system unit with many support devices and tools for storing and retrieving information. The CPU is what makes sense of all the information that passes through a computer. It carries out instructions and tells the rest of the computer system and its devices what to do. It performs much like a traffic light, controlling the flow of information throughout the computer system. It reads and stores information on storage devices such as hard drives, floppy disks, and compact discs; performs calculations; makes decisions; and enables programs to function (Figure 6-1).

CPUs have a subcomponent known as the **arithmetic logic control unit** (**ALC**). The purpose of the ALC is to carry out the calculations and data manipulations necessary for the CPU to make sense of the information it stores and retrieves. In this chapter, the term CPU will be used to refer to both the CPU and its subprocessors.

Memory

Computers use many different types of memory to carry out their functions and enable users to move their information from one computer to another. Two general classes of memory are **internal memory** and **external memory**. Internal memory is immediately available to the CPU, whereas external memory is provided by mass storage devices such as disk drives. First, this discussion considers what memory is and how it is stored, retrieved, and processed.

Memory is the electronic "space" where computers store data or instructions. Information is stored in the form of binary digits, or bits, symbolized as either a 0 or a 1. Eight bits combine to form a **byte**. One byte can represent a character, such as the letter A. For computers to work with larger numbers, they must be able to handle combinations of 32 or 64 bits at one time. It is the CPU that reads, stores, and interprets the information in memory.

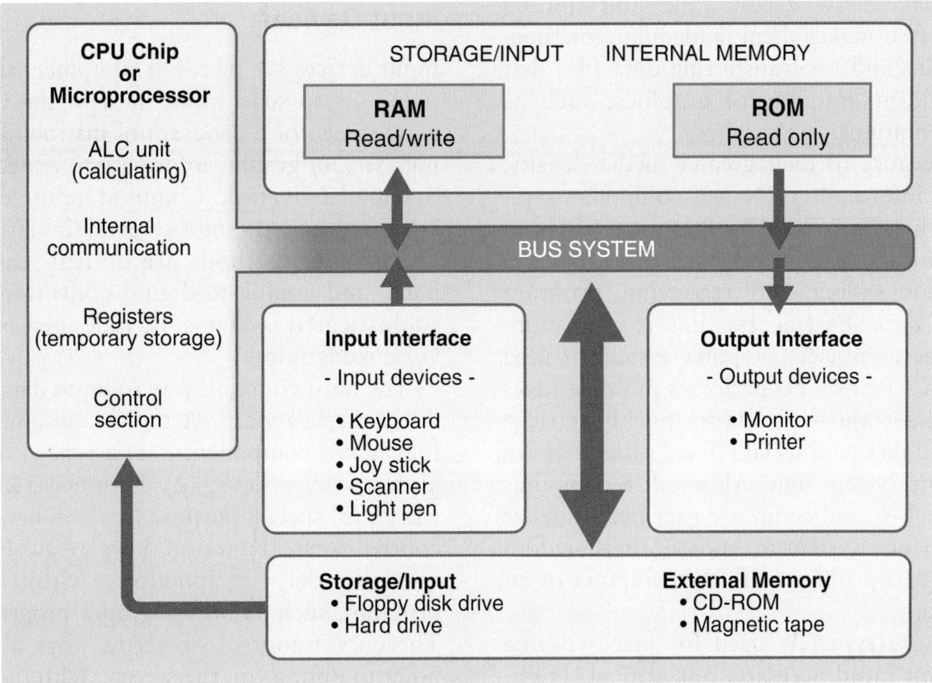

Figure 6-1

Components of a computer system. *(Microsoft Corporation © 1993. Reproduced with permission.)*

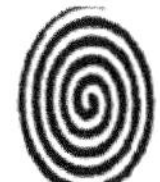

RULE OF THUMB

One **kilobyte (Kb)** equals 1024 bytes. A **megabyte (Mb)** equals 1024 Kb, or approximately a million bytes. A **gigabyte (Gb)** equals 1024 Mb, or approximately a billion bytes. On average, a page of double-spaced typed text contains approximately 2000 characters, including spaces (to a computer, a space is a character). This is equivalent to approximately 2 Kb of raw data. Thus 100 Kb equals approximately 50 pages of text, whereas 1 Mb (1000 Kb) is equivalent to approximately 500 pages. The addition of formatting codes and graphics, as used in modern word processors, increases this Kb-per-page ratio by as much as tenfold.

Internal Memory. Internal memory consists of two types: **read only memory (ROM)** and **random access memory (RAM)**. Typically, ROM contains the basic instructions that get a computer up and operating once it is turned on. ROM instructions are stored in battery-powered semiconductor chips. For this reason, ROM instructions remain in memory even when the computer loses AC power.

RAM consists of semiconductor chips that store data or instructions for use by the CPU. RAM, unlike ROM, is normally empty unless "filled" by a program or data. Loading a program causes the CPU to store instructions in RAM for subsequent use. Because data are stored in RAM electronically, loss of power causes loss of data. If information is essential to either start-up or function of a computer, it must be stored in a battery-powered chip.

As the demand for computer technology has increased, so has the amount of memory necessary to store and enable the software to run. Historically, computers used to require as little as 64 Kb of RAM. To work efficiently, modern computers need at least 32 Mb of main memory, with 64 Mb becoming the standard.

External Memory. Computers use external memory or mass storage to enable users to store, retrieve, and transfer much larger amounts of information from one computer to another. These devices include hard and floppy disks, magnetic tapes, and optical memory such as compact discs.

The storage capacity of magnetic media varies according to the density of its surface material. For example, a typical 3.5-inch **floppy disk** can store approximately 1.44 Mb of data (although there are some newer and more expensive "Superdisks" that can store up to 120 Mb of data; however, they require a special "Superdisk drive"), which equals 700 double-spaced pages of typewritten information. Although floppy disks are the most commonly used external memory, they have slow access time and limited capacity, which often makes them inadequate for time-critical applications and for transferring data files that may have significant amounts of graphics, such as Powerpoint presentations.

Hard disks, because of their greater media density, hold much more information. (Newer computers typically have as much as 15 to 80 Gb!) Because a CPU can quickly read from and write to a hard disk, it is the ideal medium for saving and retrieving program instructions and data. Fast access time is even more important in large multiuser computer systems, called **servers**. Because a server's CPU performs multiple tasks for multiple users, it must be able to quickly retrieve needed data. Hard disks are usually fixed disks that are installed inside the system unit. Although a computer technician or a well-versed computer user may transfer a hard disk from one system to another, it is seldom done unless there is a problem with the computer or an upgrade is desired.

Tape systems are typically used for large-volume data storage when rapid access is not critical. High-capacity tape drives can be used for backing up data stored on hard drives. Data backup is required because hard disks can fail. The tape backup can restore the data or programs after repair or replacement of the hard drive. Although tapes are still used, optical disks are typically the preferred backup method and have started to replace tape backup systems.

Optical disks, similar to audio compact discs, are another common form of mass storage. Currently, the most common type of optical disk is the **CD-ROM**, which can hold approximately 650 Mb of data. A CD-ROM contains readable information only, unlike a magnetic hard disk. A CD-ROM player simply reads prerecorded instructions or data on the disc. Increasingly popular are the **CD-R** and **CD-RW**. Both the CD-R and CD-RW require a special CD-writer drive. These optical disks allow users to transfer up to 650 Mb of information onto them. The difference between the two types of disks is that the CD-R allows users to transfer information onto them only once. Once CD-Rs have the information stored on them, the information can be transferred from one computer to another as many times as the user likes; however, the user can never add any additional information to the CD-R. With CD-RWs, information can be added or deleted as often as the user likes. More recent formats such as the **DVD** can hold as much as 17 Gb of data; however, the DVD medium tends to be expensive and the special drives required to transfer the information onto the DVD medium can be many times more expensive than a CD-writer drive. Because of optical disks' large storage capacity, they are ideal for archiving (storing) large volumes of textual and graphic data, such as medical records or electrocardiograms (ECGs).

Input Devices

Input devices are pieces of equipment that the computer user uses to send input data to the CPU. Input data may consist of a program of instructions or the words, numbers, or graphic information needed by the program to complete its task. Common input devices include the keyboard and the mouse or a similar pointing device. Other input methods are optical scanners, digitizing pads, and analog-to-digital converters (ADCs). Some sophisticated systems include pen-based input and voice recognition.

The most common way to input data into a computer is via the keyboard. A typical computer keyboard has four major components: (1) a typewriter-like section of alphanumeric keys, (2) a numeric keypad (for data entry), (3) special-purpose function keys, and (4) cursor-control keys. Function keys (e.g., F1, F2) perform specially defined functions within an application program, such as bringing up a program's help screen. The cursor-control or arrow keys allow the user to point to options on the screen. With these input devices, the user interacts with the computer by simply pointing to a screen item and clicking a button (mouse/trackball) or touching the screen (touch screen). The touch screen is more practical for many bedside applications (i.e., bedside monitors), whereas the mouse is ideal for desktop use. In fact, well-designed touch screens can eliminate the need for both the keyboard and mouse.

When a computer must acquire and store or analyze physical data, such as pressure or flow, a special input device is needed. This is because most physical measurements are made using analog devices. A good example of an analog measurement device is an electronic pneumotachometer, used to measure respiratory airflow. The output signal from the pneumotachometer (either a voltage or a current change) is analogous to the flow. Although this analog signal can be displayed on an electronic X-Y recorder, it cannot be directly analyzed by a digital computer.

Because a computer deals with only binary data, the analog signal must be converted to digital format. This is accomplished by using a special input device called an **analog-to-digital converter (ADC)**. An ADC transforms the analog input (e.g., changing voltage) into a series of pulses by sampling the signal at known intervals. By sampling at a rapid rate (thousands of times per second), the digital value can closely approximate the analog signal. After the analog signal has been converted to digital form, the computer can manipulate the data. ADCs are used in modern ECG machines, pulse oximeters, gas analyzers, hemodynamic monitors, spirometers, and most laboratory instruments.

Other input devices used in medical applications include optical scanners, bar code readers, pen-based (handwriting) systems, and voice recognition systems.

Optical scanners translate images (e.g., radiographic films) into digital form for computer input. Bar code readers scan and input bar codes for items such as patient supplies, pharmaceuticals, and laboratory specimens. Pen-based systems allow the user to input data using printed letters and words, and voice recognition converts the human voice into input commands or words.

Output Devices

Common output devices include the computer monitor or screen, a variety of printers, and plotters. Output data may also consist of digital or analog signals designed to activate or control specialized equipment.

The computer monitor is the most common output device and is used to display both the user interface and the events associated with various program functions. Most computer monitors are simple **cathode ray tubes (CRTs)**. Most monitors range from 15 to 19 inches and are capable of producing millions of colors for crisp, picture-quality images. New technologies, such as **liquid crystal displays (LCDs)**, provide alternatives to the CRT; however, they tend to be much more expensive.

The printer is the primary means for converting computer output into "hard copy." Several types of printers are used in medical applications. These include (1) dot-matrix, (2) thermal, (3) ink-jet, and (4) laser printers.

Dot-matrix printers use a moving print head that creates printed output via a pattern of pins impacting on paper through an inked ribbon. These devices are good for simple-text, low-resolution graphic output and for printing on forms with carbon copies, but they are noisy. Thermal printers are small, lightweight, quiet devices that use special heat-sensitive paper for printed output. Ink-jet printers form images by spraying small dots of black or multicolored ink on paper. Current ink-jet technology can produce near photo-quality color images. Laser printers use electrophotographic technology to rapidly print a full page of characters or graphics (as fast as 50 pages per minute).

A digital plotter is a specialized X-Y display device. Digital plotters are used to produce complex graphic images. A plotter translates digital computer output into the motion of a drawing pen on paper. Special codes sent to the plotter can cause it to switch pens; this ability allows for different line thicknesses and colors.

Output data may also consist of digital or analog signals designed to activate or control specialized equipment. In respiratory care, a microprocessor-based ventilator can take an input signal, such as flow, and convert it to volume and send an output signal that tells the exhalation valve to open when the desired volume is achieved.

Software

Software instructs the computer what to do and how to do it. A complete set of software instructions is called a **program.** Most computer programs are based on algorithms. An algorithm is a clearly defined, step-by-step procedure for solving a specific problem. From the algorithm, the actual sequence of program instructions is developed.

Software exists at various "levels." The lowest level of computer instruction occurs within the microprocessor itself. This level consists of binary coded instructions (i.e., 1s and 0s) called *machine language.* Although programs are still written in machine language, most modern software is developed using high-level **programming languages** such as BASIC, C++, or JAVA. Common applications of software are described subsequently.

Operating System

The next functional level of software is the computer **operating system.** An operating system oversees the basic functions of the computer, including command and program execution, basic input and output control, memory management, file management, multitasking, and the applications interface. Operating systems may have text-based or graphics-based user interfaces (GUIs). Operating systems such as MS-DOS or UNIX use a text-based interface with English-like commands such as "COPY" (to copy a file) or "EXEC" (to execute a program). Operating systems such as Microsoft Windows 2000 rely on a graphic user interface, with icons used to represent programs and functions (Figure 6-2). The user can instruct the operating system to perform a specific task by pointing and clicking on an icon. Most modern consumer computers use the GUI interface as opposed to the text-based interface.

Application Programs

An operating system is of little use by itself. To perform other tasks, a computer needs application programs. An **application program** is a set of preprogrammed instructions that allow a computer to perform a specific function. Generic functions provided by application programs include word processing, database management, and statistical computation. Specific medical or health application programs include those designed to monitor patients and control diagnostic or therapeutic equipment.

Word Processing Programs. Word processors are application programs that deal primarily with text and documents. A word processor is used to create, edit, store, and retrieve text files or documents. Multipurpose

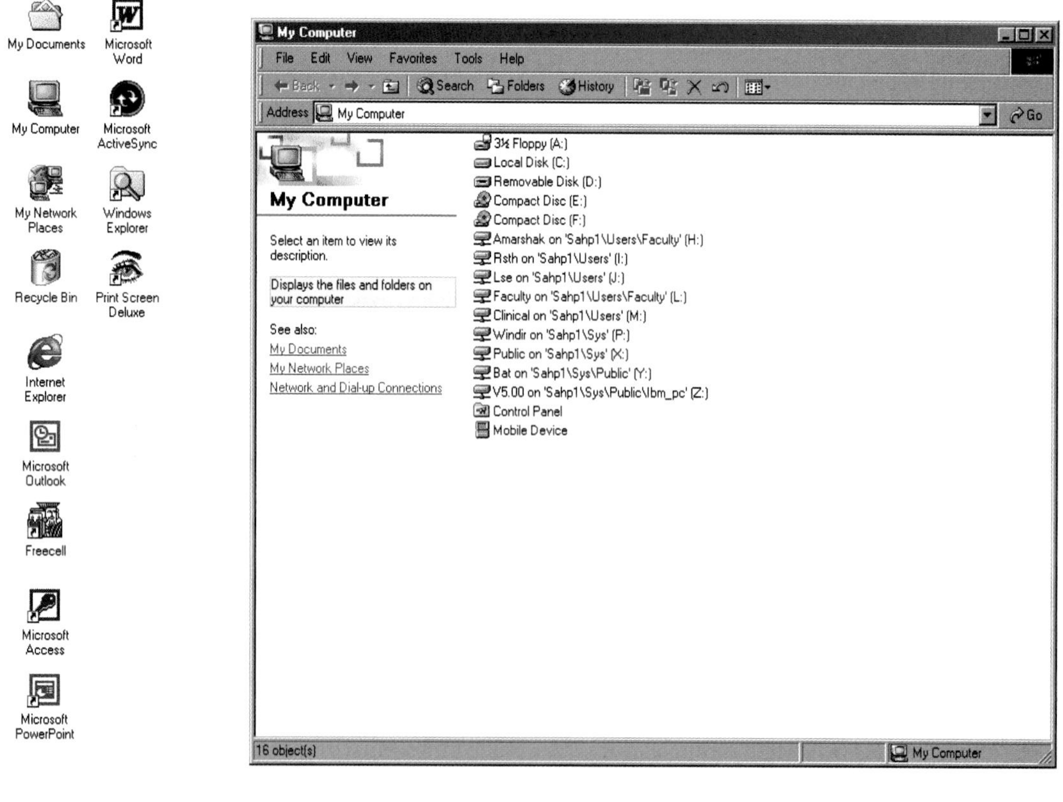

Figure 6-2 · A Graphics-Based User Interface (Windows 2000)

Programs and functions appear on the desktop *(left)*. A "Start" icon *(bottom)* provides a cascading menu of options. Windows (e.g., My Computer) provide functionality, in this case icon-based access to the hard disk files and file structure.

word processing software generally includes a variety of editing and formatting functions, including text justification, text searching and replacement, copy and move operations, and spell checking.

Word processing programs are particularly good for creating or maintaining documents that must be updated periodically. In respiratory care, such documents include policy and procedure manuals, monthly reports, and department forms. A word processor can also be used to generate reports of tests or procedures. Some respiratory care application programs have built-in text editing capacity.

Spreadsheets. A spreadsheet is a numeric analysis program based on a tabular format of rows and columns. The intersection of a row and column represents a cell. A cell may contain a number, a formula, or a text label. A formula can apply a mathematical operation to any data in the spreadsheet by referencing other cells. Once a formula is set up, it can be copied, reused, or modified for application to other column or row data. Complex spreadsheets can look up data from another source, perform statistical operations, and provide "what if" modeling of numerical data to predict the effect of changing assumptions. Most popular spreadsheet programs include sophisticated report formatting and graphing capabilities. This allows the user not only to perform complicated calculations but also to display the data in multiple formats.

Database Management Systems. A **database management system (DBMS)** is a software program used to organize, store, retrieve, and manipulate textual, numerical, and/or graphical data. A DBMS consists of two related components: an underlying program of computer instructions that provides the storage, retrieval, and manipulation functions and one or more databases.

A database is simply a collection of records. A record contains data describing a single person, object, or event. Each piece of datum in a record is called a *field*. The power of a DBMS lies in its ability to search for, sort, and report on specific categories of information quickly and accurately. For example, a DBMS could be used to report on the respiratory care procedures for patients admitted within a given time period.

First, the DBMS would be queried to search for all patients who received respiratory care services between the two specified dates. The resulting list of patients can then be sorted according to diagnosis, age, admitting physician, or any other field in the database.

The most sophisticated database systems are relational systems. A relational DBMS allows the user to work with more than one database at a time. This is accomplished by linking data in one file with relevant data in another file, such as the patient's name or identification. Fields from any linked database can be combined when organizing a report. Once these linkages are established, they not only minimize the need to reenter data but also decrease the likelihood of input error.

MINI CLINI

Selecting the Appropriate Application Program

PROBLEM

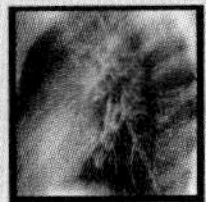

Three shift supervisors need to accomplish three different tasks. Paul has to prepare a written justification to the medical staff for applying protocol-based weaning in the cardiac recovery unit. Darshana has to find and report on the mortality of all patients admitted with a diagnosis of asthma for the past calendar year. Wilson has to prepare a budget request for new capital equipment for the coming year. Which computer application programs should they select?

DISCUSSION

Paul's written justification for a protocol would best be supported by a word processing program. Darshana should use either the Department or Hospital Information System's database management application to find, organize, and report on her data. Wilson would do well to use a spreadsheet to help figure the cost of his budget plan.

HOW COMPUTERS COMMUNICATE

Data communication is the process of sharing data among computers. Two components are needed for computers to "talk" to each other. First, there must be a connection for transmitting data between systems. Second, there must be a common "language" that allows each computer to understand the other's actions and commands.

Computers can be connected using telephone lines, digital wires or cables, and radio waves. Because telephone transmission uses analog acoustic signals, computers connected over telephone lines must use modems to communicate (Figure 6-3). A **modem** (modulator-demodulator) is a special type of ADC designed to work with acoustic signals. Standard telephone modems can transmit data at rates as fast as 56 Kb/sec. Digital wires or cables have greater **bandwidth**, or transmission capacity; 10 Mb/sec is common; 100 Mb/sec is possible. Radio waves provide wireless connections, including satellite data communication.

Communication protocols provide the common language needed for computers to talk to one another. Typically, a communication protocol includes both a mechanism to "package" data and a common set of status signals. Computers, using status signals, can notify each other when a data packet has been sent, where it is going, when it has been accepted, and if needed, how to reassemble it. In addition, most communication protocols provide an automatic error-correction mechanism. If an error is detected, the protocol will retransmit the data until accuracy is verified.

Computer Networks

A computer **network** consists of two or more computers that are connected to one another and that are capable of communicating with each other (Figure 6-4). If the computers are in close physical proximity to each other (e.g., in an office or building), the system is called a **local**

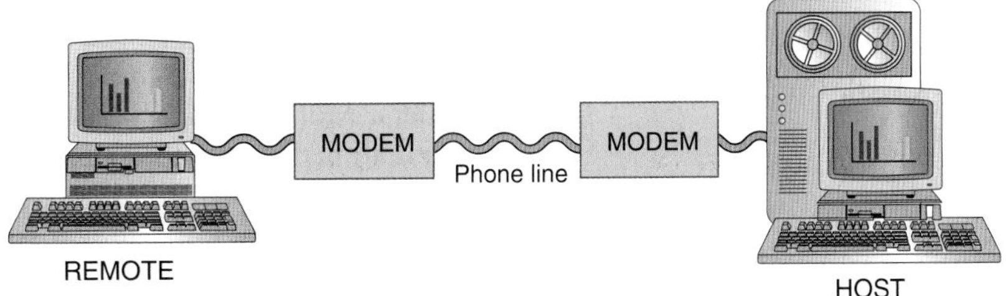

Figure 6-3

Host-remote data communications over standard telephone lines. A remote computer accesses a host system using a simple communication protocol. Input from the remote computer controls software running on the host. Output from the host computer is sent back to the remote's screen, printer, or disk drive.

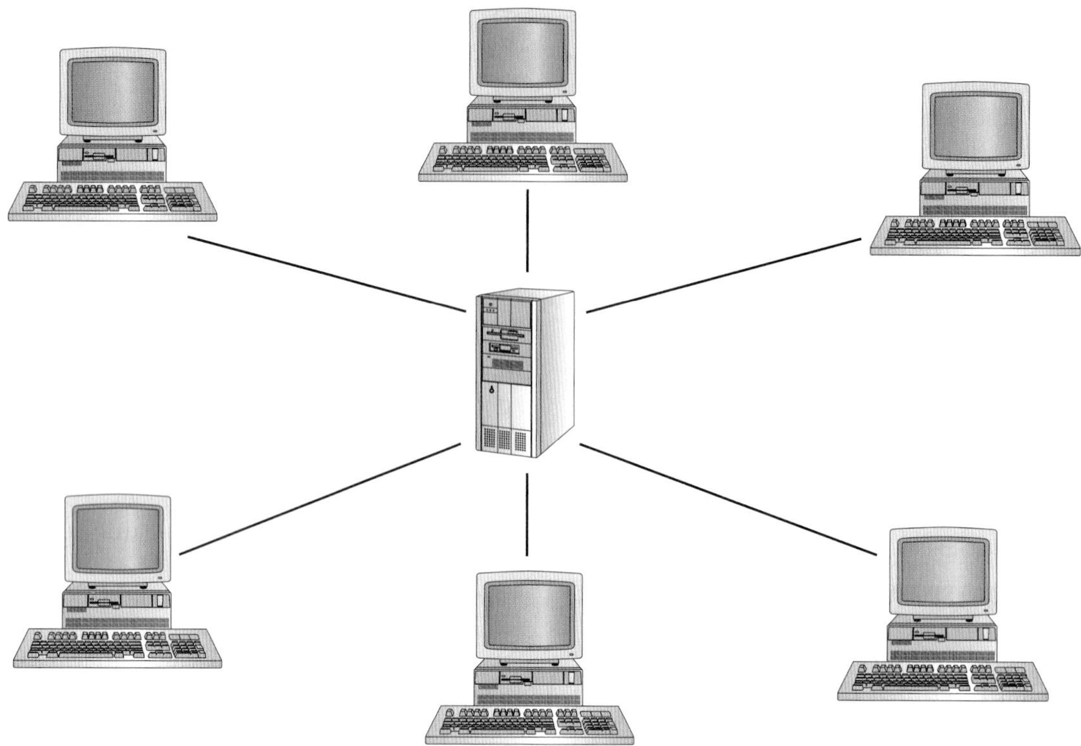

Figure 6-4 · A Computer Network

Illustrated is a series of client workstations or personal computers connected to a network server, a common configuration in the healthcare setting. The server manages network traffic, provides file storage and retrieval, and allows shared access to peripheral devices such as printers. In addition, client-server software can allow distributed processing of information, such as that provided by a modern hospital information system.

area network (**LAN**). In a **wide area network** (**WAN**), computers are connected across long distances, such as between cities. The **Internet** is a global WAN, literally consisting of a network of computer networks.

COMPUTER APPLICATIONS IN RESPIRATORY CARE

Information Management

Healthcare is an information-intensive enterprise. The massive data processing capacity of computers make them an ideal tool for managing healthcare information.

Hospital-wide Information Systems

The first use of computers in the hospital setting was limited to business applications. Hospitals developed and computerized patient billing systems to replace manual bookkeeping methods. Direct involvement of clinicians with such systems was minimal.

The next logical step was to incorporate clinical data as components of the hospital information system. This was accomplished after patient discharge. Selected elements of patient data, such as the admitting diagnosis and discharge status, were incorporated into the database. Such information was used primarily for reimbursement reporting. In the late 1970s, advances in technology resulted in the creation of interactive patient information management systems. These systems incorporate a large host or server database with remote terminal or client access. The remote or client workstations provide simultaneous access to relevant patient data by hospital staff and clinicians (Figure 6-5).

Basic patient information management systems allow access to commonly needed data elements, such as admitting diagnosis, attending physician, or physician orders. More sophisticated systems replace some or all manual medical recordkeeping functions. For example, some patient information systems not only provide physician order entry but also allow users to enter progress notes, chart data such as vital signs, and maintain a cumulative record of diagnostic test results. To minimize user training and aid in data input, such systems are often menu driven. This format allows the user to select common treatment options or data needs. Clinicians can quickly enter information into the record with specialized input devices, such as bar code readers.

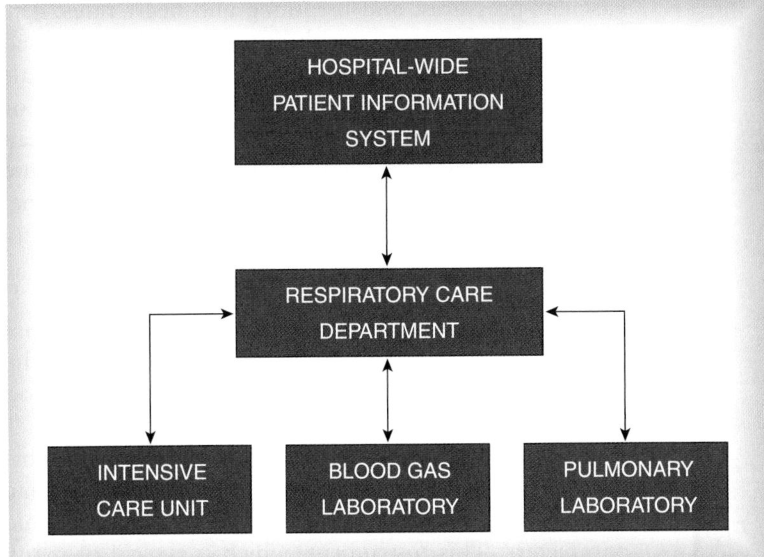

Figure 6-5
Schematic of an integrated clinical information system, combining clinical areas with the respiratory care department and the hospital information system.

Locating terminals in most hospital departments give easy access to patient records.

The next step was to broaden the function of the system beyond management of patient data. **Hospital information systems** (**HIS**) integrate a number of functions beyond medical recordkeeping. These functions include laboratory information management, nursing care documentation, and resource scheduling. Many HIS support interfaces to laboratory instruments and other diagnostic equipment. Because many instruments use microcomputers, software and hardware capacity for communicating with the hospital server or host is essential. Management of very busy departments such as pharmacy, radiology, and respiratory care often requires dedicated modules within the HIS.

Departmental Information Management

Many respiratory care departments use computer-based management systems. As noted, HIS often provide specialized departmental modules to streamline department functions. In the absence of a hospital-wide patient information system, departmental computing can be used to track physician orders, to record patient treatments, and to create billing and procedure summaries. When a hospital-wide patient information system is used, departmental computing may focus on personnel management and material resources. Departmental computing may be used to facilitate scheduling of staff, to monitor productivity, to maintain inventory, and to keep track of equipment maintenance schedules.

Two methods are commonly used to track physician orders and record patient treatments. In the first method, RTs enter relevant data into a department computer after completing their rounds. This process may be time-consuming. It requires both transcription of treatment notes and their transfer into the computer. When the number of computers or terminals is limited, access by a large staff may be problematic.

Instead of manually recording notes on the hospital wards, practitioners can use handheld computers for point-of-care data entry (Figure 6-6). Selected patient information, new orders, treatment times, and even ventilator settings can be logged directly into the handheld unit. This information can be downloaded into a central workstation or off loaded to a printer. Software operating on the central station combines each therapist's report with those downloaded by other practitioners. This allows all data for a given shift to be compiled. Automation of day-to-day procedures enhances standardization of care and ensures accuracy in charting and billing.

In addition to dedicated respiratory care management systems, many general-purpose software packages can be used to improve department management. Spreadsheets are readily adapted to report everything from department statistics to actual diagnostic test results. Word processing can be used for procedure manuals, reports, correspondence, and intradepartmental communications. Statistics and financial packages designed for small businesses often lend themselves to improved departmental recordkeeping and management.

It should be noted that the problems of a poorly organized department are seldom remedied by converting to a computer-based system. Careful planning by both caregivers and managers is needed to effectively implement an automated system. Well-defined objectives should be the starting point for setting up either a hospital-wide or a departmental information management system.

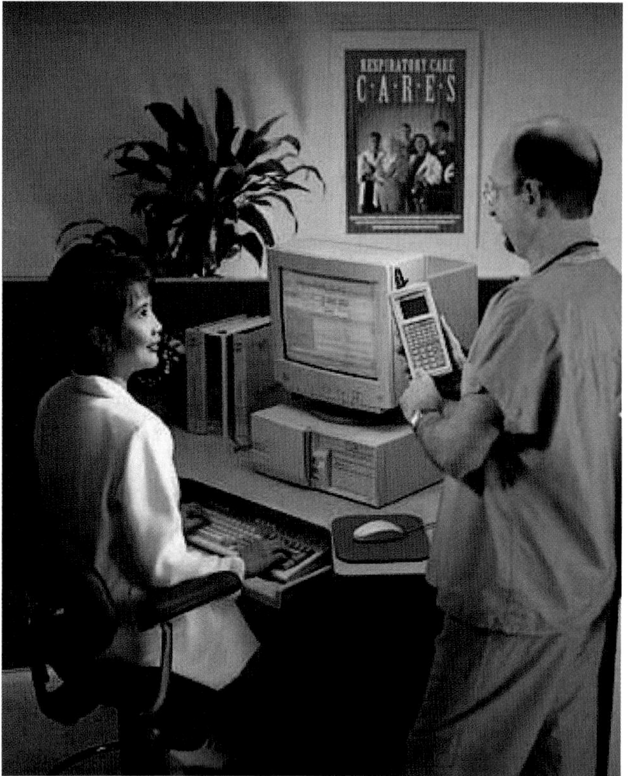

Figure 6-6

Handheld computers make it possible to capture and control information in respiratory care departments and other clinical ancillary departments. Mobile point-of-care clinical documentation can help increase staff productivity and help improve clinical documentation and the monitoring and tracking of clinical outcomes. In addition, they can integrate cost and billing information, improve resource allocation, and control and optimize workflow. *(Courtesy Nellcor Puritan Bennett Inc, Pleasanton, Calif.)*

Clinical Applications

The use of computers to measure and/or interpret clinical data and to diagnose patient conditions represents a natural extension of computers' unique capabilities. Simple algorithms are satisfactory for data acquisition, retrieval, and computation. Computer-based interpretation and diagnosis necessarily uses artificial intelligence (AI) software. Common AI applications in respiratory care provide pulmonary function testing (PFT), arterial blood gas (ABG) and ECG interpretation, hemodynamic assessment, and diagnosis of patient conditions.

Computer-aided Monitoring

Perhaps the most common application of computers encountered in respiratory care is their use in bedside monitoring equipment.

Ventilation Monitors. Simple electronic integrators and timers have long been used to process analog signals. These devices compute tidal volumes, airway and vascular pressures, and breathing and heart rates. The use of microprocessors with appropriate ROM-based software to store, display, and interpret these signals has become commonplace in the past 20 years. For example, the tidal volume signal from a ventilator can be combined with breathing rates and used to compute minute ventilation. The combination of flow, volume, and pressure signals permit monitoring of airway resistance and static and dynamic compliance.

Hemodynamic Monitors. Dedicated microprocessors are also used to monitor hemodynamic data at the bedside. The indwelling reflective oximeter is a good example of such an instrument. The reflective oximeter measures mixed venous oxygen saturation in vivo. This information is combined with thermodilution cardiac output measurements to derive several hemodynamic parameters. This instrument, which is typical of many computerized bedside monitors, combines data acquired "online" with external parameters entered by the user (Figures 6-7 and 6-8).

Electrocardiographic Monitoring. Monitoring ECG signals is often computer assisted (Figure 6-9). The ECG signal is sampled using ADCs. The resulting digital data can then be stored for later review. Digital storage allows interpretation of rate, rhythm, and axis, along with signs of hypertrophy or infarction. Another advantage of digital ECG storage is that individual tracings can be managed in a database. Database storage permits comparison of electrocardiographic changes over time. Digital storage also lends itself to easy access to ECG data. ECGs can be displayed on remote computers or terminals, or can even be transferred by facsimile.

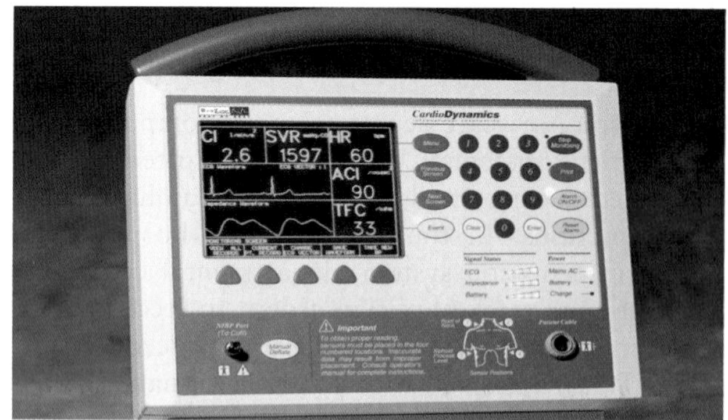

Figure 6-7

Modern noninvasive hemodynamic monitors are capable of providing a wealth of important information, including stroke volume (SV), cardiac output (CO), systemic vascular resistance (SVR), velocity index (VI), thoracic fluid content (TFC), systolic time ration (STR), left ventricular ejection time (LVET), preejection period (PEP), left cardiac work/index (LCW/LCWI), heart rate (HR), and mean arterial pressure (MAP). *(Courtesy CardioDynamics International Corporation, San Diego, Calif.)*

Hemodynamic Status Report

Name:		**Age:** 68	**Height:** 5 ft 7 in
ID:		**Sex:** Female	**Weight:** 155 lb
			BSA: 1.82 m²

10 Beat Average **Page 1 of 1**

Parameter	Description	Value	Low Normal High
HR	Heart Rate	70	58 86
SBP	Systolic Blood Pressure	142	100 140
DBP	Diastolic Blood Pressure	77	60 90
MAP	Mean Arterial Pressure	95	84 100
CI	Cardiac Index	2.5	2.5 4.7
CO	Cardiac Output	4.5	4.5 8.5
SI	Stroke Index	36	24 57
SV	Stroke Volume	65	44 103
SVRI	Systemic Vascular Res. Index	2833	1337 2483
SVR	Systemic Vascular Resistance	1564	742 1378
ACI	Acceleration Index	104	90 170
VI	Velocity Index	47	33 65
TFC	Thoracic Fluid Content	31.5	21.0 37.0
LCWI	Left Cardiac Work Index	3.1	3.0 5.5
LCW	Left Cardiac Work	5.6	5.4 10.0
STR	Systolic Time Ratio	0.44	0.30 0.50
PEP	Pre-Ejection Period	120	
LVET	Left Ventricular Ejection Time	269	

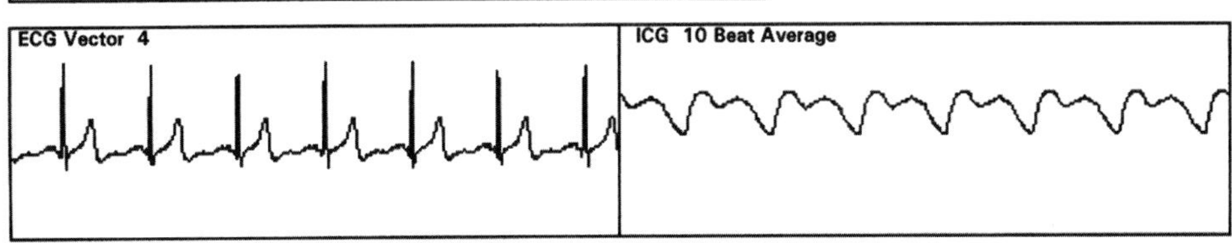

Clinical Note:____________________

Data Collection: 09/22/00 at 15:36
Report Generated: 09/22/00 at 15:37 **Signature:**________________

Figure 6-8

Some hemodynamic monitors have the ability to print out spot-status reports.

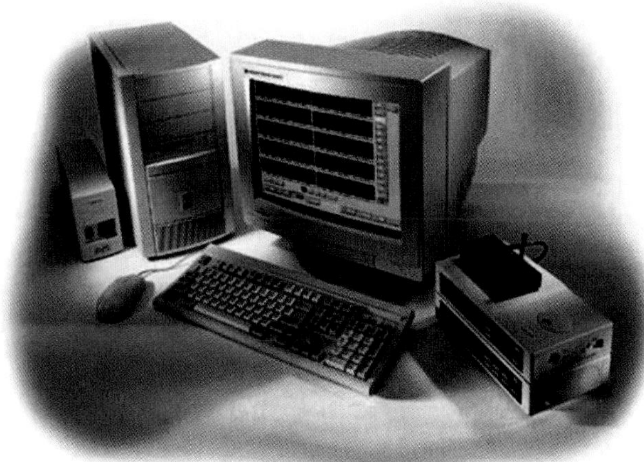

Figure 6-9

Computer technology enables healthcare providers to monitor up to 30 or more patients from a centralized location. Such technology provides reliable, remote access to critical patient data. Visual and audible alarms continuously indicate patient and equipment status. Some centralized monitoring equipment can even identify and reject artifacts that could otherwise be mistaken for a pulse. Touch screens and printable trend and waveform data add to the flexibility of such systems. *(Courtesy Nellcor Puritan Bennett Inc, Pleasanton, Calif.)*

Laboratory Information Systems

Because of the large volumes of data produced, most clinical laboratories use computers to store data and report results. Blood gas laboratories are often interfaced to either a hospital-wide system or a dedicated laboratory computer. Laboratory systems may be categorized as one of three types: (1) a module in a larger hospital-based system, (2) a stand-alone computer laboratory system, or (3) a desktop computer interfaced to one or more instruments.

Blood gas analyzers, like many other instruments, can communicate with computers. This allows the analyzer to be interfaced to any of these three systems. Many manufacturers supply both software and hardware so that patient results can be stored by computer. Some blood gas analyzers include disk drives or other computer components, so an external microcomputer is not needed. Vendors of hospital and laboratory information systems typically provide interface hardware and software that can be adapted to a wide range of analyzers (Figure 6-10).

Laboratory information systems have many advantages over manual methods. Patient data can be stored and retrieved systematically. Reports can be generated in multiple formats to meet specific needs. Trend reports can be generated to track a patient's progress. Billing information and department reports can be maintained with greater accuracy than is possible with most manual systems. Quality assurance data, such as daily quality controls or proficiency test results, can be stored as well.

One disadvantage of automated instrumentation is the large volume of data that must be maintained. A year's worth of blood gas test results can quickly fill several hundred Mb of disk space. In addition, some means of data backup must be provided. A backup system usually involves both an archive copy of stored data and a manual system to report results in the event of computer downtime. Tape backup or

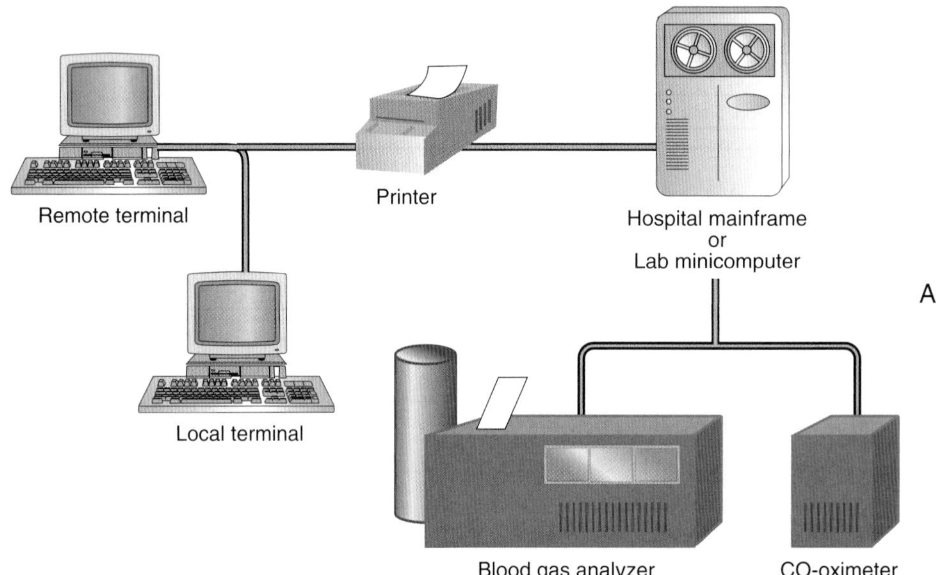

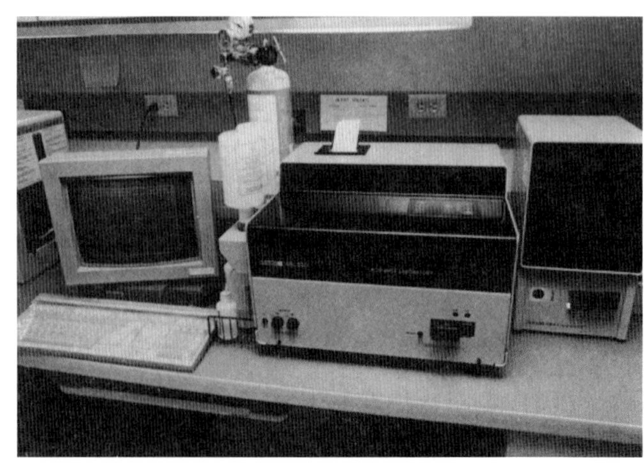

Figure 6-10 · Laboratory Information System for Blood Gas Reporting

A, Schematic representation of the components of a laboratory information system in which a blood gas analyzer and CO oximeter are interfaced. The blood gas devices communicate with the hospital or laboratory computer through standard serial ports. The system then makes the data available to all terminals and printers. **B,** An automated blood gas system using the type of interface described. The blood gas analyzer and CO oximeter are linked to the hospital mainframe, which echoes results back to the local terminal.

optical storage is often used if a large database of results must be maintained.

Pulmonary Function Testing

Most PFT systems are computerized. Two levels of automation are common: the dedicated microprocessors or the desktop computer systems (Figure 6-11).

Most portable or bedside PFT devices use a dedicated microprocessor. The PFT software itself is coded into ROM. Data storage may occur during power-on only, or limited data may be stored in battery-powered RAM. Many portable systems can "dump" stored data to an external printer or to a desktop computer. These systems often include a miniature keypad equipped with function keys.

Most laboratory PFT systems now use desktop computers. A typical system includes an IBM-compatible personal computer (PC) with a high-resolution graphics display interfaced to a spirometer, gas analyzers, and associated equipment. The pulmonary function software is loaded from disk. Patient data are stored on hard disk, with floppy disk or tape used for backup. Some systems support a database format for data storage. Hard copy reports and spirograms are provided by printer.

Some hospitals interface their PFT system with either the hospital-wide or laboratory information systems. This arrangement requires significant expertise not only in interfacing but also in programming. More commonly, PC-based PFT systems are networked in a LAN, with data stored on the server. This allows reports and graphics to be accessed from multiple workstations. Cardiopulmonary exercise and metabolic measurement systems are two other types of equipment that use desktop computers in the pulmonary function laboratory.

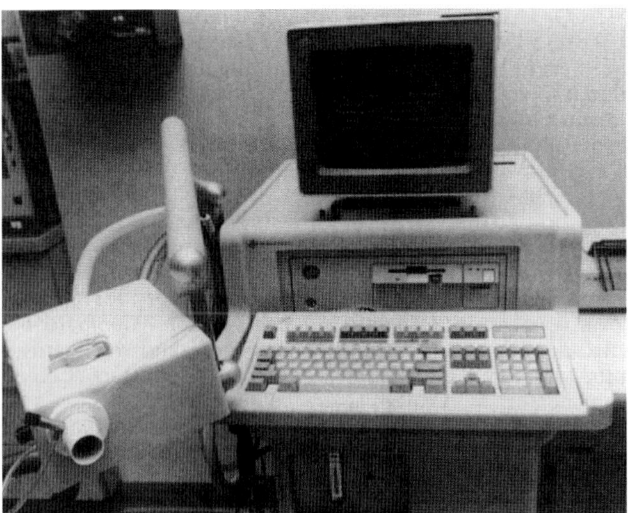

Figure 6-11 · Computer-Based Pulmonary Function Testing (PFT) System

A typical PFT system interfaced to a personal computer. Signals from a flow sensor and various gas analyzers are digitized and processed by the computer. Spirograms and related tracings are displayed directly on the computer screen and can be printed if needed. Patient data are stored as hard disk files. Interfacing with standard desktop computers permits various components (e.g., memory, disk drives, printers) to be upgraded as needed.

Mechanical Ventilation

As noted previously, most mechanical ventilators also use microprocessors for monitoring and control. Systems designed for monitoring and control can assess complex data and either suggest appropriate actions (**open-loop systems**) or take such actions automatically (**closed-loop systems**). The systems already described are open-loop computer systems. They provide clinical data or advice but defer to the user to take appropriate actions. Closed-loop computerized control systems use input data provided by one or more sensors. The data from the sensors are the basis for predefined actions; there is no need for user input. A predetermined result is achieved by monitoring one or more responses continuously and making adjustments to achieve the desired end.

A relatively simple example of a closed-loop control system used in respiratory care is the servo-controlled heated humidifier. The RT sets a desired gas temperature, and the controller, based on input from a temperature sensor, increases or decreases the power output to the heating element. This feedback maintains the desired gas temperature. This type of closed-loop control can be accomplished without a microprocessor, by using a simple electromechanical relay. The humidifier, by incorporating a microprocessor circuit with software stored in ROM, becomes an "intelligent" system. This provides additional functions such as default temperature control in the event of sensor failure or recognition of operational problems (i.e., automated troubleshooting).

Computer-assisted Interpretation and Diagnosis

Pulmonary Function Test Interpretation. A number of computer algorithms are currently used to aid in PFT interpretation. These algorithms examine data obtained from standard pulmonary function studies, including spirometry, lung volume, diffusing capacity, and bronchodilator response. In most instances, the patient's measured values are compared with reference values based on age, height, gender, and race. Generalized statements about the patient data can be derived by applying statistical standards of normality or abnormality. Computer-assisted PFT interpretation focuses on pattern recognition. Obstructive and restrictive lung diseases display characteristic changes in lung volumes and flows. The computer can classify these patterns just as a trained observer would.

Computer-assisted interpretation is ideal for screening purposes. Patients who may require more sophisticated testing can be identified. Because of the variability of "normal" pulmonary function parameters in healthy individuals and because of the effect of patient effort on test results, computer-assisted interpretation should be reviewed by a qualified interpreter.

Arterial Blood Gas Interpretation. Interpretation of ABG test results by both physicians and RTs may be unreliable. Because blood gas interpretation uses a fixed set of rules, **expert system** software (AI) has been developed and applied in this area. Blood gas values, including the patient's temperature and F_{IO_2}, are input by the user. Standard algorithms are used to derive values such as the A-a gradient, hemoglobin saturation, and HCO_3^- level. Both acid-base status and oxygenation status are interpreted using a knowledge base of known rules. Some interpretive systems allow the user to compare results with expected acid-base responses to specific conditions, such as chronic hypercapnia. The results of computer-assisted analyses are highly consistent with the interpretations provided by experts. All computer-assisted interpretations should be reviewed by a qualified clinician, preferably before therapeutic intervention.

Hemodynamic Assessment. The number and complexity of hemodynamic measurements make their interpretation difficult. Hemodynamic assessment represents an ideal area for applying clinical expert systems. Pertinent data are input by the user. The system outputs a standard hemodynamic profile for the patient based on these data (Figure 6-12). The system then consults a knowledge base to provide a hemodynamic interpretation. If the system cannot make a definitive assessment, it alerts the clinician. Alternatively, the system may provide suggestions to help refine the diagnosis.

Other Applications of Computer-assisted Interpretation. Expert systems may be used in other applications of interest to the RT. These include general diagnostic systems, computer-assisted ECG interpretation, and cardiopulmonary fitness profiles.

Expert systems designed to support general clinical diagnosis have a broad scope. They must deal with a large number of clinical disorders by examining extensive lists of clinical signs and symptoms. Patient data are used to predict plausible hypotheses, similar to differential diagnoses. The preliminary hypotheses are then used to predict other clinical manifestations that must be confirmed or used to alter the original hypotheses. The output of these general diagnostic systems is usually a ranked list, with the most likely diagnoses listed in order of probability.

Computer-assisted ECG interpretation uses an extensive set of rules applied to numerous measurements taken from standard 12-lead ECG signals. In most systems, the rule-based software is encoded in a ROM chip inside the electrocardiograph instrument. After the software digitizes and stores appropriate samples of all 12 ECG leads, it applies its rules. The output consists of the standard ECG measurements (i.e., rate, intervals, axis) and a list of interpretive statements. The interpretation is stored as a series of acronyms, which can be edited as necessary by the user.

Cardiopulmonary data, derived from an exercise test, can be used to assess the level of fitness of an individual. An expert system can examine variables stored during an exercise test. These variables include oxygen consumption, ventilation, heart rate, and blood pressure responses. The system, by comparing the observed patterns with those known to occur in various diseases or conditions, can suggest which factors might limit the subject's ability to perform exercises. Such systems can also suggest the frequency and intensity of training appropriate for rehabilitation or conditioning.

Integrated Approaches

Some individuals argue that computers may actually make patient care more difficult. Large volumes of patient data made available by computers can be overwhelming. Data from multiple sources are seldom integrated into a unified package. In many cases, the HIS maintains one type of information and the departmental database and intensive care unit (ICU) monitoring systems focus on other relevant but separate data.

Because certain elements of this diverse information may be pertinent to providing high-quality care to the patient, some hospitals are beginning to develop integrated approaches to acquisition, storage, and retrieval of relevant clinical data. For example, a respiratory care department's computer may be linked to both the HIS and selected clinical patient management systems. These might include blood gas and pulmonary function laboratories and the ICU monitoring system. By using such a framework, both general patient information and pertinent clinical data can be integrated. The patient record can be continuously updated across all systems. This gives clinicians full access to the information needed to plan, provide, and evaluate patient care.

Such systems are beginning to appear. Many HIS vendors offer subsystems that allow specialization on a departmental level. For example, results of PFT studies or blood gas analyses can be uploaded into a patient care database. Unfortunately, total systems integration

EXAMPLE OF INTERACTION WITH A HEMODYNAMIC MONITORING EXPERT SYSTEM

What is the patient's first name?
→Mary
What is the patient's last name?
→Smith
What is Mary Smith's patient number?
→123456789
There is no record of Mary Smith, #123456789, on file. Do you wish to establish a file for this patient (Y/N)?
→Y
What is Mary Smith's height (in inches)?
→65
What is Mary Smith's weight (in pounds)?
→160
What is Mary Smith's heart rate (in beats/min)?
→90
What is Mary Smith's cardiac output (in L/min)?
→3.0
What is Mary Smith's central venous pressure or right atrial pressure (in mm Hg)?
→−1
What is Mary Smith's mean pulmonary artery pressure (in mm Hg)?
→10
What is Mary Smith's mean pulmonary wedge pressure (in mm Hg)?
→5
What is Mary Smith's mean arterial pressure (in mm Hg)?
→50
Which of the following clinical signs does Mary Smith exhibit?
(check all that apply):

postural hypotension	altered sensorium
skin pallor*	cool skin*
oliguria	concentrated urine*
weak pulse*	flat neck veins*

A

```
The following is a summary of the patient's hemodynamic parameters:

                         HEMODYNAMIC PROFILE
          Lastname: Smith  Firstname: Mary  ID# 123456789

     Cardiac Index ........................... 1.7 L/min/meter sq
     Stroke Volume ........................... 33.3 ml/beat
     Stroke Index ............................ 18.5 ml/beat/meter sq
     LV Stroke Work Index .................... 11.3 gm-m/meter sq
     RV Stroke Work Index .................... 2.8 gm-m/meter sq
     Pulmonary Vascular Resistance ........... 133 dynes/sec/cm-5
     Systemic Vascular Resistance ............ 1359 dynes/sec/cm-5
     Pulmonary Vascular Resistance Index ..... 240 dynes/sec/cm-5/m sq
     Systemic Vascular Resistance Index ...... 2446 dynes/sec/cm-5/m sq

     These data are indicative of a patient
     with hypovolemic shock

     Press any key to conclude this consultation...
1H
```

B

Figure 6-12 · Expert System for Hemodynamic Assessment

A, Script of the input required for hemodynamic assessment as entered by the practitioner. **B,** Output of the consultation with the expert system. Calculated data are presented along with diagnostic statements reflecting the expert system's interpretation of the data.

is not yet a reality because of the lack of standards for communicating among different computer systems.

Using the Internet

Over the past decade, no technological change has had a greater effect on the computer industry than the rapid growth and use of the Internet. Today, healthcare is among the fastest growing content areas on the Internet. With this growth comes significant promise, but also major problems. Clearly, RTs need to understand how best to use this new and evolving resource.

The Internet is a global network of computer networks. It was designed originally in the 1950s as a U.S. Department of Defense project and began as a linkage between just four western research centers. Today, the Internet is the largest and most accessible single source of information and communication in existence, consisting of thousands of interconnected computer networks with tens of thousands of linked computers. Today, more than 200 million people are using the Internet.

Internet Capabilities

Electronic Mail. Internet **e-mail** is a major mechanism for exchange of information and ideas among both the lay public and professionals. E-mail is now handled internally by many World Wide Web browsers. E-mail can provide one-on-one professional consultation among health professionals on matters such as case management or use of technology. Targeted mailing lists (LISTSERVs) extend this concept and allow quick communication about rapidly evolving aspects of clinical practice (e.g., a new medical device found to be hazardous).

An e-mail message, like a letter sent through the mail, must be sent to a specific address. The format for an e-mail address is name@site. The name portion of the address is the recipient's e-mail account name. The site portion of the address is the domain name of the mail server used by the recipient. For example, "sdjones@medicalcenter.org" is the proper addressing for S.D. Jones (with an e-mail account name of sdjones) at the organization (org) whose domain name is "medicalcenter." If you do not know someone's e-mail address, there is a variety of "white page" services on the Internet.

Group Discussion (Usenet Newsgroups). A logical extension of the mailing list is the interactive discussion group or **newsgroup**. Usenet (originally the AT&T UNIX User Network) enables tens of thousands of people throughout the world to participate in ongoing discussion groups. These newsgroups are organized into hierarchies by subject matter and are recognizable by a system of prefix coding. For example, newsgroups beginning with the prefix "sci.," which are at the highest level of the hierarchy, are involved in discussions on scientific topics. A subcategory of these groups is "sci.med," consisting of all newsgroups dealing with medicine and its related products and regulations. Deeper into the hierarchy one might find "sci.med.cardiology," a specific newsgroup discussing all aspects of cardiovascular diseases. It is important to note that newsgroups may or may not be moderated; in a moderated newsgroup a moderator determines what is or is not appropriate to post. Unmoderated newsgroups are much freer flowing, with readers posting whatever they please. Most current Web browsers have built-in newsreader capability.

Hypertext Browsing (World Wide Web). Most content on the Internet is accessed via the World Wide Web, or Web for short. Physically, the Web consists of thousands of network computer servers using the **hypertext transfer protocol (HTTP)** to deliver content to client computers over **transmission control protocol/Internet protocol (TCP/IP)** connections. Content is stored on these computers in a special format called **hypertext markup language (HTML)**. Because HTML is text based, any computer with the appropriate software can read the stored information, making it somewhat of a universal language. There are more than 100 million "pages" of HTML information online, with few areas of content not covered.

To access this huge source of information, the following is needed:

- A computer
- **Browser** software
- A modem or network connection
- An Internet service provider (ISP)

Because HTML is universal, the Web can be accessed by using any computer platform that runs a Web browser (e.g., Apple, IBM-compatible, UNIX). A Web browser is the client software that interprets and displays HTML pages. Netscape's Navigator (Communicator) and Microsoft's Internet Explorer are good browsers. If a computer is already on a network connected to the Internet then it is ready to go. Otherwise, a modem and a telephone line are needed to connect to an ISP. For a fee, an ISP provides private parties (individuals and organizations) with dial-up access to the Internet. Most ISPs also provide the needed software and technical support; some have their own content areas. Selection of an ISP should always be guided by the precept "let the buyer beware," because of the rapid changes occurring in the Internet marketplace. In any case, monthly fee payment is probably a good choice until these services become more reliable.

Once a browser is up and running and the computer is connected to the Internet, the user will want to start accessing content. Content on the Web is accessed by using an addresslike location specifier called a **universal resource locator** or **URL** (similar to e-mail). Fortunately, once the user starts accessing desired locations that he or she will want to revisit, browsers allow URLs to be easily saved under simple names the user chooses. To avoid having to write down or memorize long and sometimes illogical URLs, the user should use these "bookmarks" (Netscape Navigator) or "Favorites" (Microsoft Internet Explorer) frequently. If the user forgets to save a URL that he or she wants to access later, several search sites on the Web can help.

Once a user is at a Web site, he or she will find many areas of potential interest included as **hypertext links** (Table 6-1). Typically, a hypertext link appears in an HTML document as either underlined text or a graphic icon. Clicking on a hypertext link evokes the TCP/IP protocol needed to find, transmit, and display the linked HTML document on the computer. The linked document could be on the server currently being accessed or on another computer halfway around the world.

Of course, the physical location of the linked document is generally unimportant to the user; ready access to the information is what matters. However, against this advantage of ready access is the very real complexity of millions of potential links across tens of thousands of computers. Given that there are no road maps on the Web, finding the proper information quickly can be a difficult task indeed. A subsequent section on finding information on the Internet provides some guidance.

Finding Information on the Internet

Most new Internet users find themselves randomly following interesting links or "surfing" for information. Although this can be fun, it is an extremely inefficient process, much like randomly browsing the book stacks in a large library. For greater efficiency and better results, users should apply a systematic search process.

MINI CLINI

Universal Resource Locator (URL)

PROBLEM

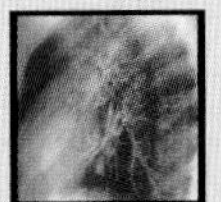

What does all that stuff in a URL mean?

DISCUSSION

A URL has three major components: (1) the protocol, (2) the server's domain name, and (3) the document location. The following URL (the Web "address" for the AARC's Clinical Practice Guidelines [CPG]) helps explain these components:

http://www.aarc.org/cpgs/cpg_index.html

The "http://" portion of the URL indicates that the Web browser has requested a Web page transfer (the HTTP protocol). The "www.aarc.org" is the domain name of the server being queried. The "/cpgs/cpg_index.html" portion of the URL is the actual path name on the server's hard drive for the CPG index document. For the user to avoid having to write down or remember the URLs of sites he or she wishes to revisit, this information should be saved in the browser's Bookmarks or Favorites.

Table 6-1 ▶▶ Representative Web Home Pages of Interest to Respiratory Care Practitioners

Organization	Home Page URL
American Association for Respiratory Care	www.aarc.org
American Academy of Allergy, Asthma, and Immunology	www.aaaai.org
American Academy of Pediatrics	www.aap.org
American College of Allergy, Asthma, and Immunology	www.allergy.mcg.edu
American College of Chest Physicians	www.chestnet.org
American Heart Association	www.americanheart.org
American Lung Association	www.lungusa.org
American Medical Association	www.ama-assn.org
American Sleep Disorders Association	www.asda.org
American Society for Testing and Materials	www.astm.org
American Society of Anesthesiologists	www.asahq.org
American Thoracic Society	www.thoracic.org
Centers for Disease Control and Prevention	www.cdc.gov
Joint Commission on Accreditation of Healthcare Organizations	www.jcaho.org
Merck & Co (access the Merck Manual)	www.merck.com
National Association for Medical Direction of Respiratory Care	www.namdrc.com
National Board for Respiratory Care	www.nbrc.org
National Committee for Clinical Laboratory Standards	www.nccls.org
National Heart, Lung, and Blood Institute	www.nhlbi.nih.gov
National Library of Medicine (Access MedLine)	www.nlm.nih.gov
Society of Critical Care Medicine	www.sccm.org

Systematic searching involves two complementary approaches: Web link pages and search tools. Web link pages are collections of relevant links to sites found useful by the page developer. In general, the link-page strategy works best when the source of the links is a recognized organization or institution.

Users should always complement their usage of link pages with Internet search tools. Search tools provide much wider access to Internet resources, including Web, Usenet, and Gopher information. There are three primary types of Internet search tools: indices, search engines, and metasearch tools.

Search Engines. Search engines continually search Internet sites, capture and evaluate relevant text, and store the information in a searchable database. Users search the database by entering keywords or phrases or by using Boolean operators (Table 6-2). Popular sites that provide Internet search engines include AltaVista, Excite, HotBot, Lycos, Go, and Webcrawler (Figure 6-13; Table 6-3).

AltaVista uses natural language queries, as do most search engines. For a simple search, users type in a word, phrase, or question (e.g., *asthma causes or what causes asthma?*), then click *Search*. To refine a simple search, users can require or exclude words or request that the search be conducted on an exact phrase (usually by surrounding it in quotation marks). To broaden a search, most search engines allow use of "wildcards." For example, in AltaVista, an asterisk (*)

Table 6-2 ▶▶ Boolean Operators Used in Advanced Internet Searches

Keyword	Action
AND	Finds only pages containing all of the specified words or phrases. Mary AND lamb finds pages with both the word *Mary* and the word *lamb*. Most search engines assume the AND operator when two or more words are entered without quotes.
OR	Finds pages containing at least one of the specified words or phrases. Mary OR lamb finds pages containing either *Mary* or *lamb*, or both.
NOT	Excludes pages containing the specified word or phrase. Mary NOT lamb finds pages with *Mary* but not containing lamb (some search engines require the AND when using NOT [e.g., Mary AND NOT lamb]).
NEAR	Finds pages containing both specified words or phrases within a certain proximity to each other (e.g., 10 words). Mary NEAR lamb would find the nursery rhyme but likely not religious or Christmas-related pages.

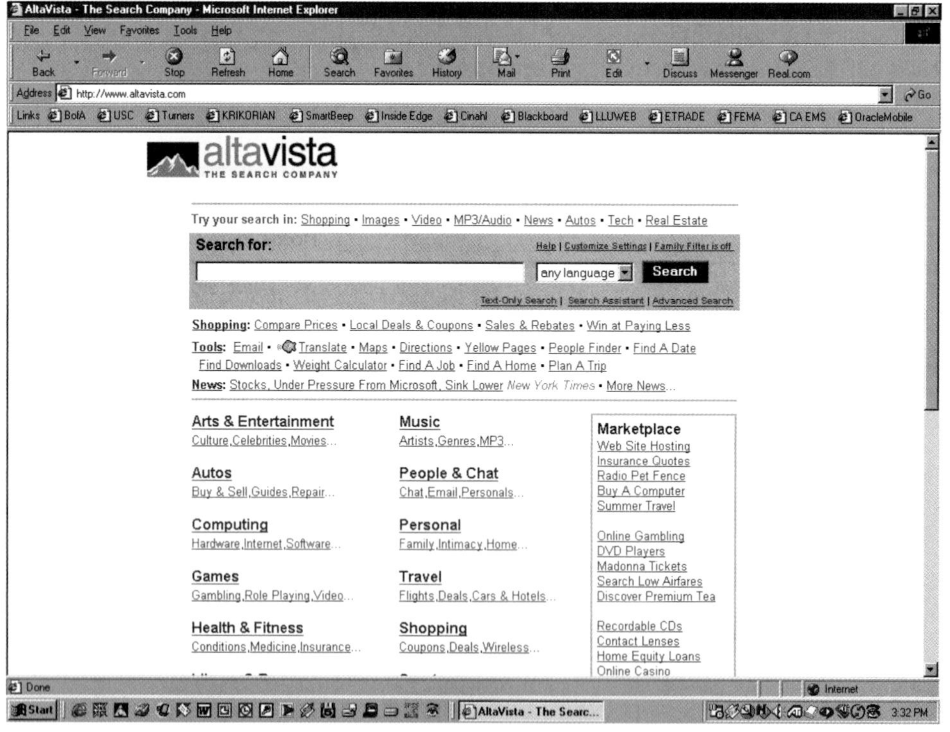

Figure 6-13 · User Interface for AltaVista Search Engine

To search, users type in a word, phrase, or question and click the *Search* button. Advanced searching requires knowledge, AltaVista's search syntax, and use of Boolean operators. *(Reproduced with the permission of AltaVista.)*

Table 6-3 ▶▶ Popular Internet Search Sites

Internet Search Site	URL
AltaVista	www.altavista.com
Excite	www.excite.com
HotBot	www.hotbot.com
Overture	www.overture.com
Lycos	www.lycos.com
WebCrawler	www.webcrawler.com

added to the end of a text string finds Web pages containing any words that start with those letters (asthma* finds asthma, asthmatic, asthmatics, asthmaticus). For more detail on specific search strategies, users should consult the help pages at the applicable search site.

Evaluating Internet Resources

Although narrowing an Internet search to just the right content can be difficult, the most challenging task when using Internet resources is ensuring their quality. Most Internet information resources, unlike published books and journal articles, do not undergo quality review. Moreover, because anyone can place information on the Internet, the potential for false, misleading, or out-of-date information (and plain old charlatanism) is very real. For now, it is up to the user to determine what is and is not valid. Box 6-1 offers a checklist for evaluating Internet resources.

Box 6-1 • Checklist for Evaluating Internet (Web) Information

Note: The greater the number of questions answered "yes", the more likely the source is of high quality. Questions in **bold type** must be answered "yes" for the source to be of value in your research.

CRITERION #1: AUTHORITY

1. **Is it clear who is sponsoring the page?**
2. Is there a link to a page describing the purpose of the sponsoring organization?
3. **Is there a way to verify the legitimacy of the page's sponsor? That is, is there a phone number or address contact for more information? (Simply an e-mail address is not enough.)**
4. Is it clear who wrote the material, and are the author's qualifications for writing on this topic clearly stated?
5. If the material is protected by copyright, is the name of the copyright holder given?

CRITERION #2: ACCURACY

1. Are the sources for any factual information clearly listed so they can be verified in another source?
2. Is the information free of grammatical, spelling, and other typographical errors? (These kinds of errors not only indicate a lack of quality control but also can actually produce inaccuracies in information.)
3. Is it clear who has the ultimate responsibility for the accuracy of the content of the material?
4. If statistical data are presented in graphs and/or charts, are they clearly labeled and easy to read?

CRITERION #3: OBJECTIVITY

1. Is the information provided as a public service?
2. Is the information free of advertising?
3. If there is any advertising on the page, is it clearly differentiated from the informational content?

CRITERION #4: CURRENCY

1. Are there dates on the page to indicate:
   a. When the page was written?
   b. When the page was first placed on the Web?
   c. When the page was last revised?
2. Are there any other indications that the material is kept current?
3. If material is presented in graphs and/or charts, is it clearly stated when the data were gathered?
4. If the information is published in different editions, is it clearly labeled what edition the page is from?

CRITERION #5: COVERAGE

1. Is there an indication that the page has been completed and is not still under construction?
2. If there is a print equivalent to the Web page, is there a clear indication of whether the entire work is available on the Web or only parts of it?
3. If the material is from a work that is out of copyright (as is often the case with a dictionary or thesaurus), has there been an effort to update the material to make it more current?

Modified from *Checklist for an informational web page*, ©Wolfgram Memorial Library, Widener University, Chester, Pa, 1996.

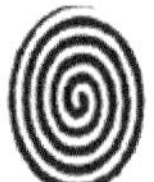

RULE OF THUMB

The first rule in evaluating Internet resources is to "consider the source." A more in-depth evaluation of the source should include assessment of its authority, accuracy, objectivity, currency, and coverage. If the source providing the Internet information is not listed directly on the page, check out the URL. If it ends in ".edu" or ".gov" it is sponsored by an educational institution or a U.S. government agency. In general, these are reliable sources.

NONTECHNICAL ISSUES RELATED TO COMPUTERS

Several concerns become apparent as computers are used for storing patient information and automating data reduction. These concerns include confidentiality, technical skills, software errors, and lay access to medical information.

Confidentiality

Computer storage of patient records raises several concerns in regard to sensitive data. Most HIS regulate access to patient data by means of passwords. Individuals using the system must "log on" by using a password that identifies them and determines their level of access. Comprehensive algorithms are available to manage various levels of access. The greatest concern is how to apply these algorithms so that appropriate personnel can view or edit patient data.

Implementing a password system requires policies that define who may access patient demographic, clinical, and billing information. These policies should define not only levels of access but also the way data are to be handled. This may include regulations for printing of patient information versus simple screen viewing. Most systems provide utilities for auditing, which help users perform specific functions. The use of such audit functions can help ensure observance of hospital policies.

HIS generally provide capabilities for "blacking out" selected patient information. Departmental computer systems or PC-based equipment may not offer the same capability. In these cases, it is important that policies be established to regulate how patient data are to be handled.

Technical Skills

The use of computers interfaced to spirometers, blood gas analyzers, and ventilators can promote a false sense of complacency. This complacency occurs when the user has an incomplete understanding of the technical aspects of the instrument-computer interface. This phenomenon has been termed the *black box mentality*.

Many tasks previously performed by a technologist or therapist are now managed by computer. Calculations and measurements that were performed manually are now executed by the computer. This promotes a tendency to teach individuals to use the computerized instrument without a detailed understanding of the process involved. In effect, the computer allows an individual with minimal understanding of a technical procedure (such as blood gas analysis) to perform the task. Serious problems can arise when a computerized system malfunctions and the user fails to detect an irregularity. Users of computerized instruments (such as monitors and ventilators) need a greater understanding of the technical process than does someone using a similar instrument in the manual mode. Computer-based equipment requires that the user be knowledgeable not only about the specific device but also about the computer itself and how it is interfaced.

Software Errors and Risk of Patient Harm

As clinical software applications increase in number, so too has the concern over the potential for software errors causing patient harm. In 1997, the U.S. Food and Drug Administration's medical device quality system regulation became fully effective. This quality system includes requirements for validation of component or accessory software used in medical devices.

Lay Access to Medical Information

An increasing number of lay people are using the Internet as a source of information on health and disease. Although a well-informed healthcare consumer is a good thing, the variable quality of Internet information can result in misinformed consumers. To help address this growing problem, the Health On the Net Foundation (http://www.hon.ch) has established a Code of Conduct (HONcode) designed to help ensure the quality of medical and health information available on the Web. There are eight key principles in the HONcode, addressing the source, currency, supporting evidence, use of information, confidentiality, and advertising. Sites complying with the HONcode display an identifying logo and a link to the Health On the Net Foundation.

KEY POINTS

- A computer has four major hardware components: (1) a CPU, (2) input devices, (3) memory to store data and instructions, and (4) output devices.
- The CPU is the "brain" or "calculator" of the computer. All computers need a CPU in order to work.
- For a computer to process analog information, such as physiological data, it must first be converted to digital form using an ADC.
- A software program is a set of instructions (written by humans) that tell a computer what to do and how to do it; application programs can accomplish specific tasks, such as word processing, mathematical manipulations, and database management.
- Computers share information via a process called *data communication;* communication protocols provide the common language needed for computers to communicate with one another.
- Hospital-wide computer systems provide a means to store, retrieve, and report on both financial and patient-related clinical information.
- Clinicians use computers to help interpret data, reach diagnoses, and automate certain aspects of patient care; most pulmonary function systems, blood gas analyzers, bedside monitors, and ventilators now incorporate microprocessor technologies.
- The Internet is a global network of computer networks that provides e-mail, newsgroups, remote access, file transfer, and information retrieval services.
- To find information on the Internet, users can use link sites, search engines, and indices.
- Because there are few quality controls on Internet information, users are responsible for critically evaluating its authority, accuracy, objectivity, currency, and coverage.
- Major issues raised in using computer technology in healthcare include confidentiality, technical skills, software errors, and lay access to medical information.

Bibliography

Brunner JX, Thompson JD: Computerized ventilation monitoring, Respir Care 38:110, 1993.

Clemmer TP, Gardner RM: Medical informatics in the intensive care unit: state of the art, Int J Clin Monit Comput 8:237, 1991.

Cohen T et al: Information technology in tomorrow's health care, Biomed Instrum Technol 28:441, 1994.

East TD: Role of the computer in the delivery of mechanical ventilation. In Tobin MJ, editor: Principles and practice of mechanical ventilation, New York, 1994, McGraw-Hill.

East TD: Computers in the ICU: panacea or plague? Respir Care 37:170, 1992.

East TD, Morris AH: Decision support systems for management of mechanical ventilation, Respir Care 41:327, 1996.

East TD, Young WH, Gardner RM: Digital electronic communication between ICU ventilators and computers and printers, Respir Care 37:1113, 1992.

East TD et al: A successful computerized protocol for clinical management of pressure control inverse ratio ventilation in ARDS patients, Chest 101:697, 1992.

Elliott CG: Quality assurance for respiratory care services: a computer-assisted program, Respir Care 38:54, 1993.

Gardner RM, Elliott CG, Greenway L: The computer for charting and monitoring. In Kacmarek RM, Hess D, Stoller JK, editors: Monitoring in respiratory care, St Louis, 1993, Mosby.

Greenway L, Jeffs M, Turner K: Computerized management of respiratory care, Respir Care 38:42, 1993.

Henderson S et al: Performance of computerized protocols for the management of arterial oxygenation in an intensive care unit, Int J Clin Monit Comput 8:271, 1991.

Korst RJ et al: Validation of respiratory mechanics software in microprocessor-controlled ventilators, Crit Care Med 20:1152, 1992.

Lampotang S: Microprocessor-controlled ventilation systems and concepts. In Kirby RR, Banner MJ, Downs JB, editors: Clinical application of ventilatory support, New York, 1990, Churchill Livingstone.

Peters R, Sikorski R: Navigating to knowledge: tools for finding information on the Internet, JAMA 277:505, 1997.

Sanborn WG: Microprocessor-based mechanical ventilation, Respir Care 38:72, 1993.

Sikorski R, Peters R: Medical literature made easy: querying databases on the Internet, JAMA 277:959, 1997.

Silberg WM, Lundberg GD, Musacchio RA: Assessing, controlling, and assuring the quality of medical information on the Internet: caveat lector et viewor—let the reader and viewer beware, JAMA 277:1244, 1997 (editorial).

Sittig DF et al: Clinical evaluation of computer based respiratory care algorithms, Int J Clin Monit Comput 7:177, 1990.

Snowden S et al: An advisory system for artificial ventilation of the newborn utilizing a neural network, Med Inf (Lond) 18:367, 1993.

Thomsen GE et al: Clinical performance of a rule-based decision support system for mechanical ventilation of ARDS patients. In Safran C, editor: Proceedings of the 17th Annual Symposium on Computer Applications in Medical Care, New York, 1993, McGraw-Hill.

Woodward B: The computer-based patient record and confidentiality, N Engl J Med 333:1419, 1995.

SECTION II

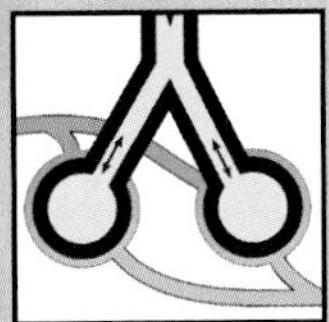

Applied Anatomy and Physiology

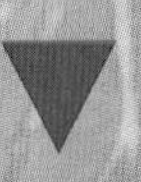
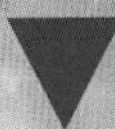
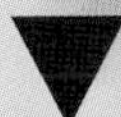

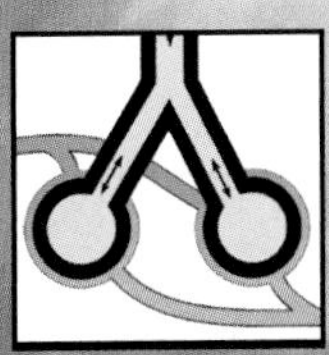

CHAPTER 7

The Respiratory System

Gregg L. Ruppel and Deborah White

In This Chapter You Will Learn:

- What the major events are in the development of the respiratory system in the prenatal, perinatal, and postnatal periods, and how they relate to neonatal pathology
- What the key elements of normal fetal circulation and anatomy are
- What happens to the respiratory system at birth
- How to identify the main structures in the thorax and describe their functions
- How the primary and accessory ventilatory muscles function during various levels of activity in healthy subjects
- How somatic and autonomic innervation of the lungs and thoracic musculature relate to loss of function as occurs with disease
- Which major structures are part of the upper respiratory tract and how they function
- How gas is conducted through the lower respiratory tract during spontaneous breathing
- How to identify the lobes and segments of the right and left lungs as they might be described from a chest x-ray, computed tomography (CT) scan, bronchoscopy, or physical examination
- How to compare the function of the large airways and small airways
- What structures in the respiratory bronchioles and alveoli are involved in asthma and emphysema

Chapter Outline

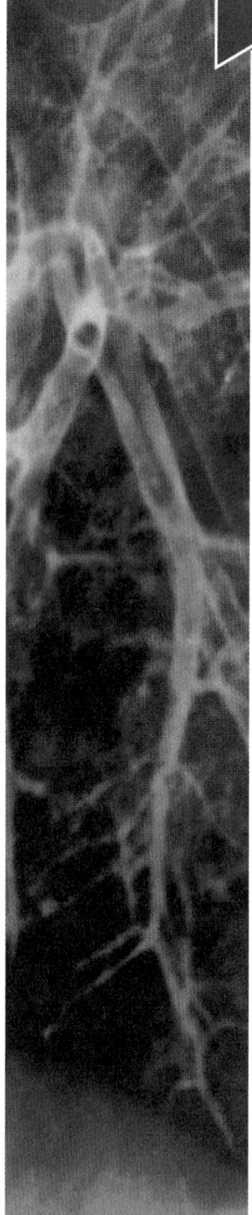

Key Terms

acinus
airway resistance
alveolar macrophage
alveolar-capillary membrane
angle of Louis
anterior nares
apices
apnea
autonomic nervous system
bronchi
bronchioles
carina
chromosomes
compliance
costal cartilages
costophrenic angle
cricoid cartilage
deoxyribonucleic acids (DNA)
diaphragm
dichotomous branching
differentiation
ductus arteriosus
dysynapsis
epiglottis
epithelium
Eustachian tubes
external oblique
fissures
foramen ovale
functional residual capacity (FRC)
gene expression
genotype
glottis
goblet cells
hemidiaphragms
hilum
human genome
hypopharynx
inflation reflex
intercostal nerves
intercostals
internal oblique
irritant receptors
J receptors
L/S ratio
laminar flow
laryngeal braking
lingula
lobes
manubrium
mast cells
mediastinum
mesenchyme
morphogenesis
mucosa
nasopharynx
oropharynx
ossification
palate
parietal pleura
pectoralis major
pericardium
phenotype
phrenic nerves
pleura
pneumocytes
pores of Kohn
pulmonary surfactant
rebreathing
rectus abdominis
recurrent laryngeal nerves
retractions
scalenes
secondary lobules
segments
septum
specific compliance
sternomastoids
sternum
stretch receptors
supernumerary arteries
time constant
trachea
transversus abdominis
turbinates
vagovagal reflex
vagus nerve
vertebra
visceral pleura
xiphoid process

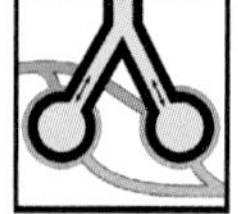

The respiratory system functions primarily to exchange oxygen and carbon dioxide between the atmosphere and the cells of the body. These functions begin early in fetal development and change dramatically at the time of birth. From the moment of conception, the human body, including the respiratory system, embarks on a journey of tremendous growth and development, from embryo and fetus to infant and toddler, through the pubertal years, and into young adulthood. The mature lung experiences a relatively quiescent period through midlife and then begins a gradual loss of lung tissue and function that continues through the elderly years. The fully developed respiratory system, together with the cardiovascular system, sustains the body in both normal and stressful conditions (see Chapter 8).

In infants, children, and adults, the respiratory system must move gas in and out of the lungs with a minimal amount of work. The system filters out inhaled contaminants while warming and humidifying inspired gas. The respiratory system brings inspired gas into contact with pulmonary capillary blood flow, ensuring rapid and efficient exchange of oxygen and carbon dioxide. The system responds to changing demands in the body, as occurs during exercise or in disease states.

The list of potential interventions for treating respiratory diseases is endless, and the role of the respiratory therapist (RT) in providing these treatment modalities is both exciting and challenging. Competent clinical practice in this area requires knowledge of the many pathophysiological differences among infants, children, and adults. Understanding these differences can assist the RT in providing quality care to patients of any age.

▶ THE GENETIC FRAMEWORK

The master plan for the amazing transition from embryo to infant to adult is encoded in the genetic material present at conception. The expression of the genes of the embryo is the framework for every anatomical, cellular, and physiological function of the body. Modification of gene expression, either from natural environmental phenomena or from those artificially imposed, will have an enormous impact on future strategies in treating respiratory diseases.

The Human Genome Project was initiated in the early 1990s as an international effort to map all human genes. Genetic material within all living creatures is the framework on which all molecular and physiological functions are based. Units of genetic material, referred to as *genes*, are composed of a helical arrangement of **deoxyribonucleic acids (DNA)**. A variable number of genes compose the rod-shaped structures called **chromosomes** found in the nuclei of each cell. The **human genome** contains 23 pairs of these chromosomes, with one of each pair inherited from the mother and the other from the father. Identifying the location (locus) and sequencing the DNA of each gene provides a unique road map of the human genome. It has become increasingly evident that altering the genetic structure of cells has far-reaching implications in treating, preventing, or reversing potential life-threatening heritable diseases.

Cystic fibrosis (CF) is one of the most notable inheritable diseases that almost always affects the respiratory system. In 1989, the gene responsible for developing CF, ΔF508, was cloned on chromosome 7. Since then, more than 700 mutations of this gene have been described.[1] The inheritance pattern of CF follows that of a classic Mendelian recessive trait; that is, CF requires a defective gene from both the mother and the father to manifest the disease (Figure 7-1). If the mother and father are carriers of the CF gene (but do not have CF themselves), the odds are 1 in 4 (25%) that each child will have CF. The odds are 2 in 4 (50%) that each child will be a carrier of CF. The chance of each child being completely normal is 1 in 4. Individuals with only one affected gene are carriers of CF but do not have the disease. Unfortunately, the picture of most genetically inherited diseases is not this simple. The actual genetic composition of a gene is referred to as the **genotype**. The clinical manifestation caused by morphological, physiological, or biochemical alterations of that genetic mutation is called the **phenotype**. The phenotypic picture of a child with CF is highly variable, depending on the particular CF mutation inherited. The disease may affect any secretory organ of the body (e.g., lungs, liver, pancreas, sweat glands). The degree of involvement of each organ system may range from negligible to life threatening. Therefore identification of the "CF gene" has been only the first step in understanding the complex mechanisms of gene expression and their implications for molecular and physiological functions.

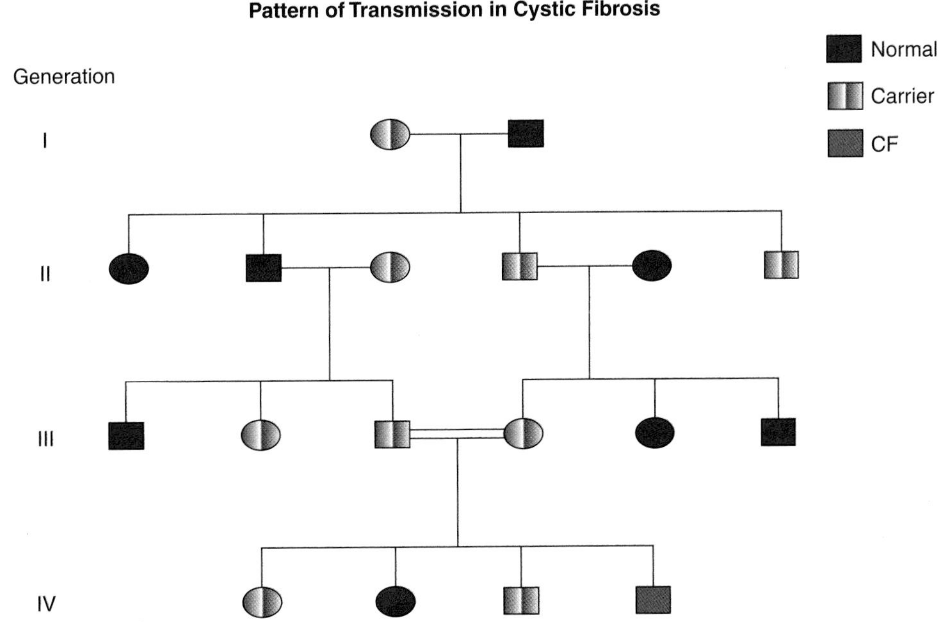

Figure 7-1

Generation I represents the marriage of a female carrier for cystic fibrosis (CF) to a normal male. Generation II includes the couple's four children—2 of 4 carry the CF gene. Generation III depicts the offspring of two couples, both of whom have one spouse who carries the CF gene. Generation IV represents the four children of the marriage of two CF carriers—2 children (50%) are carriers for CF, 1 child (25%) is normal, 1 child (25%) has CF.

Several other examples of respiratory disorders involve heritable factors. Asthma affects at least 10% of the general population. It is likely that the development and severity of asthma involves multiple genes that are inherited and that interact in complicated pathways.[2] As in an electrical circuit with many separate switches, each switch has to be turned on in a particular sequence for the circuit to be complete. Similarly, **gene expression** may be turned "on" or "off" and may require specific stimuli to switch genes "on," leading to the development of asthma. Mounting evidence indicates that mothers who smoke during pregnancy subject their fetuses to increased risk of developing asthma early in childhood. Second-hand smoke places infants and young children at increased risk, as can other environmental pollutants.[3] Viral infections, especially respiratory syncytial virus, may play a role in young infants who develop wheezing and later become asthmatics. The phenotypic picture of asthma covers a spectrum from very mild disease that is easily amenable to treatment to life-threatening, severe bronchospasm and sudden death.

Another respiratory disorder that recently has been genetically identified, and that affects infants in the neonatal period, is surfactant-B deficiency. As discussed subsequently, surfactant B is one of several important phospholipids that spread over the alveolar surface and stabilize the air sacs shortly after birth. Lack of surfactants may lead to respiratory distress and, ultimately, death in the perinatal period. Having advance knowledge of a genetic disorder before birth enhances the potential for rapid intervention at birth and may improve the infant's chance of survival.

As the Human Genome Project continues, the number of genetic disorders and mutations described will increase dramatically. Early detection of a genetic disease may lend itself to intervention in utero or shortly after birth. Parents may choose to use amniocentesis as a tool to identify genetic disorders and to help make decisions regarding their unborn child. Early detection, intervention, and genetic manipulation may alter the phenotypic expression and ultimate consequences of a genetic disorder in the future.

▶ DEVELOPMENT OF THE RESPIRATORY SYSTEM

Unlike other major organs that begin working early in fetal life, the lungs are not afforded any practice for their role. Embryonic development must be sufficient to allow the respiratory system to take on a new role at birth, much different from the previous role of the fetal respiratory system. Respiratory system development is an ongoing process that begins in the early embryonic period and extends for years after birth. Developmental **morphogenesis** of the human respiratory system parallels that of all mammals. It can be categorized into five stages, divided into two periods, based on the predominant tissue characteristics.[4,5] Table 7-1 summarizes these major developmental events. The first period, termed the *embryonic period*, begins at approximately day 26 after conception as an outpouching of the primitive foregut. This ventral bud eventually develops into the entire respiratory system, whereas the dorsal extension is destined to develop into the esophagus. All human cells originate from one of three embryological germ tissues: endoderm, mesoderm, or ectoderm. The **epithelium**, or lining cells, of the entire respiratory system are endodermal in origin. The supporting structures of the tracheobronchial tree, such as muscle and connective tissue, form as the lung bud extends into surrounding **mesenchyme** (mesoderm). The tracheal bud soon bifurcates into two mainstem bronchi, which continue to grow and branch into segmental and subsegmental bronchi. Concurrently, the vascular components of the respiratory system emerge. The pulmonary arteries form as buds off the sixth pair of aortic arches, and rudimentary pulmonary veins emerge from the developing heart. Injury to the embryo during this critical phase of development can lead to many congenital anomalies, including tracheoesophageal fistulas, choanal atresia, pulmonary hypoplasia, and complex heart and vascular anomalies.

At approximately 6 weeks' gestation, the lung has the appearance of a glandular structure, hence the name of the second stage of development, the *pseudoglandular stage*. For the next 10 weeks, the growth and branching of the tracheobronchial tree is accelerated, with formation of smaller and smaller airways, both respiratory and nonrespiratory bronchioles. The distinction between these two types of bronchioles is important. Nonrespiratory bronchioles, like bronchi and the trachea, are conducting airways only. Respiratory bronchioles eventually participate in gas exchange.

Branching and dividing of the tracheobronchial tree occurs in several ways. A single bud that develops off of an existing structure is termed a *monopodial bud*. Airways that divide into two or more airways do so by dichotomous branching. Most of the divisions of airways occur in a nonsymmetrical fashion termed *irregular* **dichotomous branching**.[6,7] The epithelial lining of the airways begin to differentiate into tall, columnar epithelium in the proximal airways and evolve into cuboidal epithelium in the more distal bronchioles. The appearance of cilia, mucous glands, and goblet cells complete the major constituents of the epithelial lining and are of tremendous importance to the functioning of the mucociliary escalator after birth. Absence and/or dysfunction of cilia, as seen in Kartagener's syndrome and primary cilia dyskinesia, compromise the ability of the respiratory system to eliminate inhaled organisms and pollutants. Likewise, abnormal mucus production

Table 7-1 ▶▶ Summary of Cardiopulmonary Development

Approximate Gestational Age	Developmental Event
Embryonic Period	
21 days	Primitive foregut outpouches
23 days	Single heart tube appears
26 days	Lung bud identified
4 wk	Mainstem bronchi formed Pharynx formed
5 wk	Lobar bronchi formed Pulmonary artery identified
6 wk	Segmental bronchi formed Subsegmental bronchi appear
Fetal Period	
Pseudoglandular Stage	
7 wk	Diaphragm complete
8 wk	Heart formation complete
10 wk	Lymphatics present in lung Cilia develop
12 wk	Conventional and supernumerary arteries present
13 wk	Columnar and cuboidal epithelium present Goblet cells and mucous glands present
14 wk	Principle arterial pathways present
16 wk	Terminal bronchioles form All conducting airways finished
Canalicular Stage	
17 wk	Respiratory bronchioles develop Rudimentary acini forming
20-22 wk	Types I and II cells identified Immature surfactants (sphingomyelin and lecithin) seen
24-26 wk	Pulmonary capillaries develop
Saccular Stage	
26-28 wk	Saccules developing Alveolar capillary surface sufficient for extrauterine life Type I and type II cells further differentiated
29-36 wk	Early alveoli developing
Alveolar Stage	
36-40 wk	Lecithin production rises rapidly Phosphatidylglycerol (PG) present Alveoli mature and increase rapidly
Birth-2 yr	Alveoli continue to increase in number and size Arterial development parallels alveolar growth

can lead to devastating pulmonary disorders, as seen in bronchiectasis, chronic bronchitis, and CF. Other cells found embedded within the epithelium, including Clara cells, brush cells, and Kulchitsky's cells, all with uncertain functions, arise during the pseudoglandular stage.

Below the epithelium, smooth muscle cells continue to differentiate from mesenchyme, and vascular growth parallels that of the branching airways. Mesoderm-derived cartilage provides rigidity, especially for the trachea and mainstem bronchi. Beginning with the trachea and moving distally, the amount of cartilage supporting the airway decreases as smooth muscle cells increase in number and assume the role of maintaining airway patency. Once again, events that alter the morphogenesis of smooth muscle, cartilage, and vascular structures can lead to pulmonary disorders encountered early in infancy, including tracheomalacia or bronchomalacia and congenital lobar emphysema.

The third stage of development begins at week seventeen and is known as the *canalicular stage*. Terminal nonrespiratory bronchioles undergo 2 to 4 more generations of branching into respiratory bronchioles. Several more divisions of alveolar ducts lead to rudimentary blind tubules. The prominent feature of this stage is the formation of the **acinus**, or basic gas-exchanging unit of the lung supplied by a terminal bronchiole. In addition, early **differentiation** into two distinct types of **pneumocytes** is evident.

By weeks 24 to 26, the fetus is potentially viable if born prematurely; however, during the *saccular stage*, the acinus continues to perfect its structure and function. From this point until birth, there is a rapid proliferation of alveolar ducts and sacs from the rudimentary tubular extensions of the respiratory bronchioles. The type I pneumocytes of the saccule walls thin and elongate, dramatically increasing the surface area available for gaseous exchange. Type I cells are destined to become the primary gas-exchange cells in the lung with close approximation to developing capillaries. Type II pneumocytes, containing specialized lamellar bodies, soon manufacture and secrete the vital pulmonary surfactants necessary to alter surface tension and keep the lungs inflated.

The further differentiation into hexagonal-shaped alveoli, accompanied by capillary proliferation within alveolar walls, begins the final stage of fetal lung development, known as the *alveolar stage*. Type I pneumocytes contain few organelles and their purpose is chiefly gas exchange. Type II cells contain abundant organelles, most notably lamellar inclusion bodies. Conversely, type II pneumocytes serve several important functions, including pulmonary surfactant production, repair following lung injury, and ion balance and fluid control. These cuboidal cells actually outnumber type I cells. However, they occupy only approximately 5% of the total alveolar surface area.

The mechanisms that control differentiation of type II pneumocytes and synthesis of **pulmonary surfactants** in the fetal lung are understood only partially. Human pulmonary surfactant consists of 90% phospholipid, 10% protein, and trace carbohydrates. Early research in pulmonary surfactants centered on the phospholipid components, mainly phosphatidylcholine (lecithin and sphingomyelin [L/S]) and phosphatidylglycerol (PG). Quantification of these phospholipids, known as the **L/S ratio** and PG level, provides an index to the relative lung maturity of the infant before birth. Corticosteroids may be given to women in preterm labor to enhance rapid maturation of type II pneumocytes and pulmonary surfactants. Insufficient surfactants in a premature infant can lead to the development of a membrane that lines the alveolar cells and progressively interferes with gas exchange and lung expansion. This condition is known as *hyaline membrane disease* and often develops into infant respiratory distress syndrome.

Research into surface-active agents has led to development of exogenous surfactants. These substances are used to treat premature infants with insufficient pulmonary surfactants. Recently, attention has turned to the protein constituent of pulmonary surfactants. Four families of surfactant proteins (SP) have been identified in pulmonary surfactant: SP-A, SP-B, SP-C, and SP-D.[8] Together these proteins play a complex biochemical role at the molecular level in the synthesis, regulation, and degradation of pulmonary surfactant. Lack of these proteins is now known to also cause respiratory failure, even in full-term infants.

Fetal lung fluid is a unique combination of pulmonary surfactants, aspirated amniotic fluid, and plasma ultrafiltrate from the fetal microcirculation. This fluid helps establish the functional residual capacity (FRC) of the lung during intrauterine life. It also helps maintain a critical electrolyte balance and electrochemical gradient so that fluid is not absorbed until birth.

▶ TRANSITION FROM UTERINE TO EXTRAUTERINE LIFE

At birth, the lungs undergo a rapid and dramatic transition from fluid-filled, nonrespiratory structures to ones that fill with air, increase blood flow twentyfold, and assume the role of gas exchange for the newborn infant.[9] It is important to understand the complex physiological changes that must occur to allow a smooth transition to extrauterine life.

Placental Circulation

Survival of the fetus requires a circulatory link between the mother and embryo. Within a week of uterine implantation, fingerlike projections called *chorionic villi* arise from the embryo's aorta and invade the uterine endometrium. As the villi increase in size and number, they further erode the endometrium, creating irregular pockets, and ultimately maternal blood fills these spaces, continually bathing the fetal capillaries in an oxygen- and nutrient-rich environment (Figure 7-2). As gestation progresses, the villi decrease in size but increase in number. This increases the surface area for maternal-fetal gas exchange.

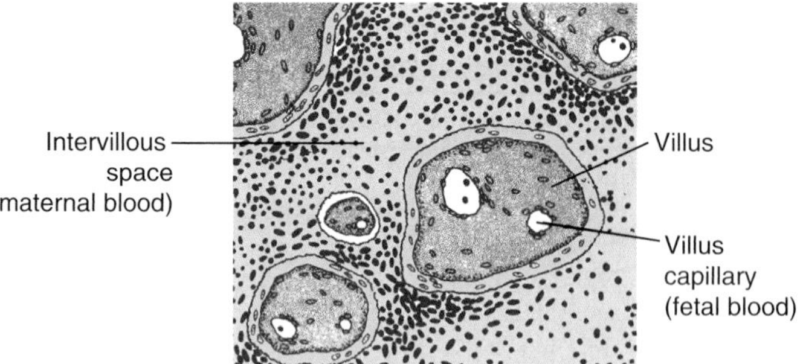

Figure 7-2

Microscopic appearance of the villi in an intervillous space. Fetal capillaries permeate the villi, which are immersed in maternal blood within the intervillous spaces.

The maternal uterine tissues and blood vessels of the fetal chorionic villi make up the placenta. Figure 7-3 shows a cross section of a well-developed placenta. Maternal blood flows into the intervillous space through the spiral arteries. Here, maternal and fetal blood come into close proximity, aiding diffusion of O_2, CO_2, and metabolic products. After exchange takes place, maternal blood exits through venous channels and returns to the maternal circulation. Oxygenated fetal blood leaves the chorionic villi capillaries to join placental venules, which merge to form a single umbilical vein.[9]

On the fetal side of the placenta, the chorionic and amnionic layers give rise to the umbilical cord. The umbilical cord contains a single umbilical vein (returning blood to the fetus) and two umbilical arteries (carrying blood to the placenta). The umbilical vein is generally larger than the arteries but with thinner walls. For a short time after birth, the umbilical vessels remain open and can be used for infusion or blood sampling.

Abnormal implantation of the placenta, tearing of the placenta from the uterine wall, or decreased placental blood flow can retard intrauterine growth or cause fetal asphyxia. Prenatal asphyxia places the newborn (neonate) at higher risk for respiratory distress in the immediate postnatal period.

Maternal and fetal circulations are generally separate, but small communications can exist. This has been verified by the findings of maternal cells in fetal blood and fetal cells in maternal blood. Drugs, bacteria, and viruses can cross the intervillous space and cause a

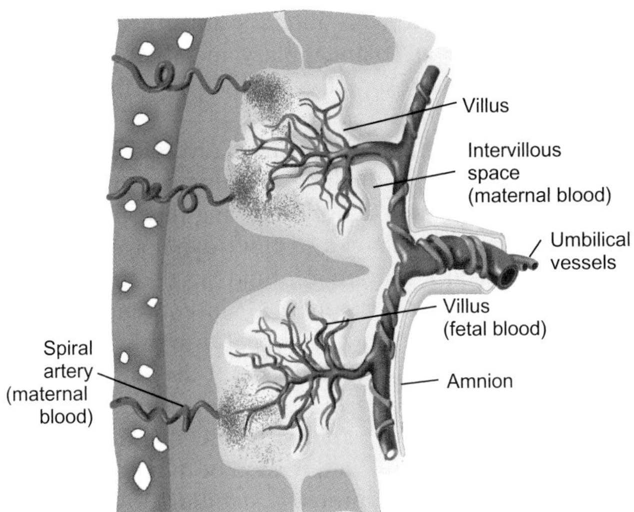

Figure 7-3
Section through the placenta showing the spiral arteries that supply maternal blood to the intervillous space, the branching villi immersed in the intervillous space, and the umbilical vessels that branch repeatedly to terminate as villous capillaries.

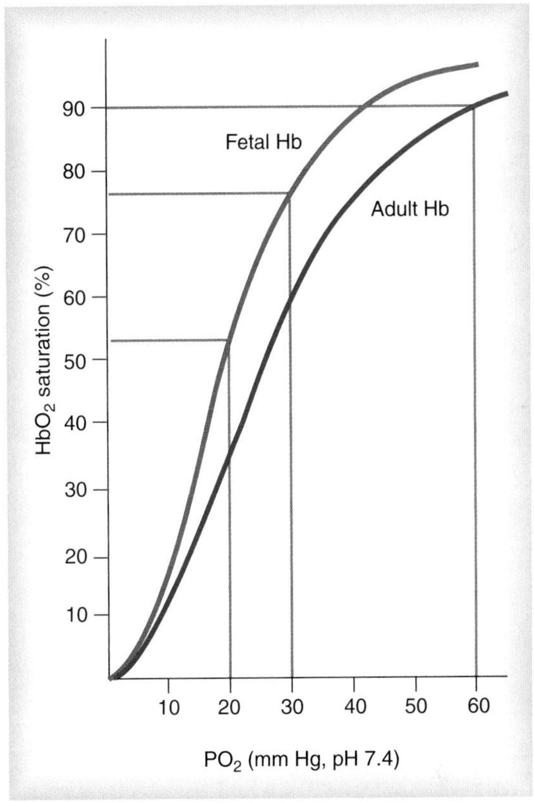

Figure 7-4
Fetal hemoglobin (Hb) produces a left shift of the oxyhemoglobin (HbO_2) curve. *(Modified from Koff PB, Eitzman DV, Neu J: Neonatal and pediatric respiratory care, St Louis, 1988, Mosby.)*

variety of problems. Various factors favor diffusion of oxygen to the fetus. The partial pressure gradient for oxygen (Pao_2) between maternal blood and fetal blood allows for oxygen to diffuse into chorionic villi capillaries. The maternal blood in the intervillous space has a mean Pao_2 of approximately 50 mm Hg.[10] Fetal blood returning to the placenta has a Pao_2 of approximately 19 mm Hg. The Bohr effect also aids oxygen uptake by the fetus. In addition, fetal hemoglobin (HbF) has increased O_2-carrying capacity and is a major factor responsible for fetal survival in this relatively hypoxic environment. As seen in Figure 7-4, increased oxygen affinity is manifested by a left shift of the fetal oxyhemoglobin dissociation curve. P_{50} is 6 to 8 mm Hg less than adult hemoglobin (HbA). At birth, 75% of circulating hemoglobin is HbF. HbA gradually replaces HbF. By the first 4 to 6 months of life, most of the infant's hemoglobin is HbA. Because of the left shift of the HbF dissociation curve, cyanosis will appear at lower Po_2 values than in adults. The Po_2 in blood returning to the fetus through the umbilical vein is only approximately 30 mm Hg. Table 7-2 summarizes the normal values of both the umbilical arteries and vein in a term fetus.

Table 7-2 ▶▶ Approximate Normal Blood Gases in a Term Fetus

Value	Umbilical Artery	Umbilical Vein
pH	7.36	7.39
$Paco_2$ mm Hg	47	43
Pao_2 mm Hg	19	30

Fetal Circulation

Oxygenated blood from the placenta is carried in the umbilical vein to the fetal circulation by the hepatic system (Figure 7-5). Approximately one third of this blood flows to the lower trunk and extremities. The other two thirds is shunted past the liver through the ductus venosus into the inferior vena cava. This freshly oxygenated blood mixes with the venous blood returning from the lower trunk and extremities and enters the right atrium. Approximately 50% of this blood is shunted from the right atrium into the left atrium through the **foramen ovale.** Left atrial blood goes to the left ventricle, then to the ascending aorta, where it continues on to the brain, brachiocephalic trunk, and descending aorta.

Venous blood from the superior vena cava is directed downward through the right atrium into the right ventricle, then into the main pulmonary artery. Because of the low Po_2 in the fetal environment, pulmonary vascular resistance is high. For this reason, the mean pulmonary artery pressure in the fetus is higher than in the aorta. Because blood follows the path of least resis-

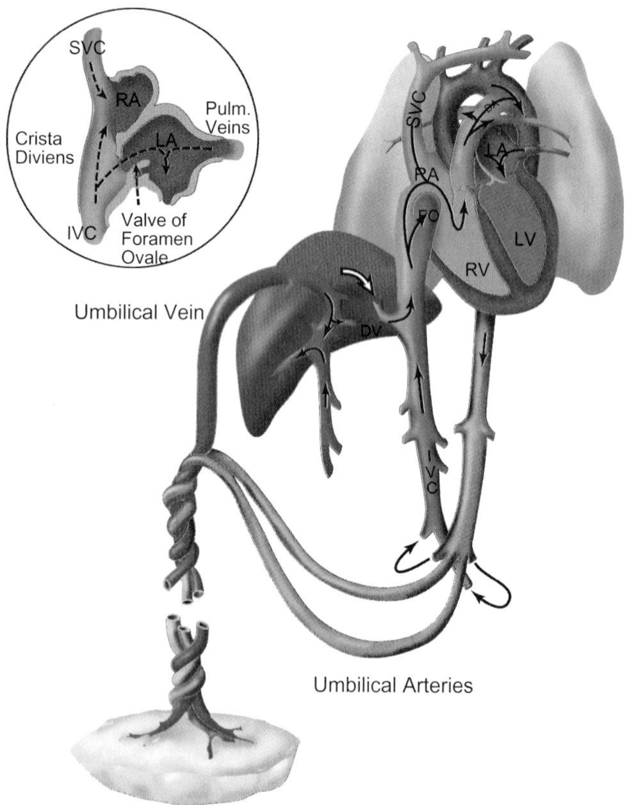

Figure 7-5

Fetal circulation. *DA*, Ductus arteriosus; *DV*, ductus venosus; *FO*, foramen ovale; *IVC*, inferior vena cava; *LA*, left atrium; *LV*, left ventricle; *RA*, right atrium; *RV*, right ventricle; *SVC*, superior vena cava.

tance, less than 10% of the blood entering the pulmonary artery actually flows into the lungs.[11] The rest is shunted from the main pulmonary artery to the descending aorta by the **ductus arteriosus.** The ductus arteriosus remains open because of the volume of blood flowing through it, the reduced fetal $Pa{O_2}$, and circulating prostaglandins (from maternal sources). Shunted flow from the ductus arteriosus then mixes with the blood ejected from the left ventricle. A portion of this less oxygenated blood circulates to the gut and lower extremities, with the rest returning to the placenta for reoxygenation by the two umbilical arteries.

Cardiopulmonary Events at Birth

Before birth, the placenta provides nutrition and respiratory, digestive, and renal functions for the fetus. When the fetus and placenta separate at birth, rapid and dramatic changes must occur before breathing can begin. The fetal lung is normally filled with a volume of fluid equal to the FRC, or approximately 30 mL/kg. The fluid in the fetal lung is a liquid ultrafiltrate of the plasma and is manufactured in the microcirculation of the developing lung.[12] Fetal lung fluid moves from the microcirculation to the interstitium, then through openings in the alveolar-capillary membrane into the airways, into the oropharynx, and then out of the mouth and into the amniotic fluid.

At birth, lung fluid movement is reversed and liquid must be cleared from the lungs to allow air inflation. A few days before labor (if at term), lung fluid production stops, favoring the change of fluid dynamics. Because the protein concentration of fluid in the pulmonary capillaries is higher than the protein concentration of fluid in the alveolus, lung fluid begins to move into the circulation. Labor also helps drying of the lung, through an increase in circulating catecholamines. During normal vaginal delivery, approximately one third of the lung fluid is cleared by compression of the thorax in the birth canal. The pulmonary capillaries clear the remaining fluid through the lymphatics.

The newborn must develop very high transpulmonary pressure gradients during the first few breaths to replace the remaining lung fluid with air and establish a stable FRC. These large pressure gradients overcome the opposing forces of fluid viscosity in the airways and surface tension in the alveoli. The stimulus for these initial respiratory efforts is both peripheral and central in origin.

First, the newborn infant is bombarded by new tactile and thermal stimuli, all of which stimulate breathing. In addition, as placental gas transfer is suddenly interrupted, the newborn quickly becomes hypoxemic, hypercapnic, and acidotic. As shown in Figure 7-6, essentially no air enters the newborn lung until the transpulmonary pressure gradient exceeds 40 cm H_2O. As lung volume increases in a stepwise fashion with each breath, less and less pressure is needed to overcome the opposing forces. Normally, the resting FRC is achieved within three to four breaths.

As shown in Figure 7-7, when the lung expands and breathing begins, the $Pa{O_2}$ increases, the $Pa{CO_2}$ decreases, and the pH rises back toward normal. This decreases pulmonary vascular resistance and allows blood flow to increase to the lung. The ductus arteriosus closes as a result of the decreased blood flow through it (because of increased blood flow through the pulmonary arteries), the direct constriction effect of a higher $Pa{O_2}$, and the removal of maternal prostaglandin sources.

Constriction of the ductus arteriosus promotes increased blood flow through the lungs. Cessation of umbilical flow causes a rapid rise in systemic vascular resistance. As systemic vascular resistance increases, left-sided heart pressures rise. Left atrial pressures also rise because of the increase in blood volume coming back from the lungs. With left-sided heart pressures now higher than right-sided pressures, the foramen ovale closes. When this last right-to-left shunt closes, the transition between the fetal and extrauterine circulations is functionally complete. Full transition

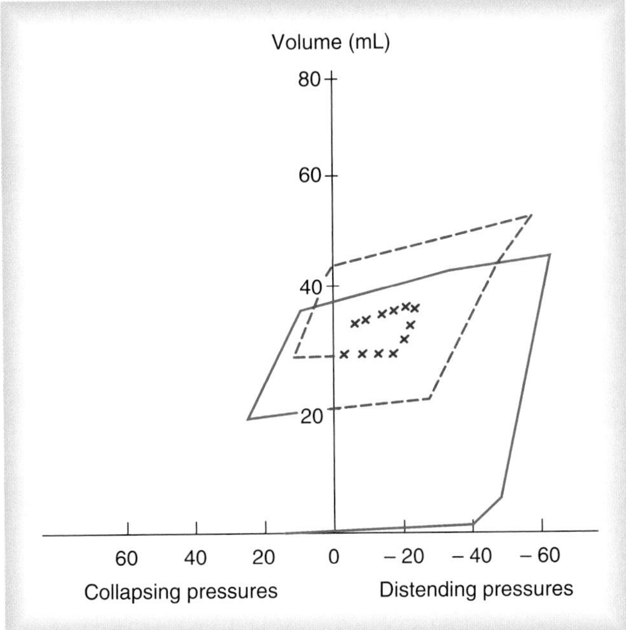

Figure 7-6

Transpulmonary pressures develop in the human neonate during the first three breaths after birth. *(Modified from Avery ME: The lung and its disorders in the newborn infant, ed 2, Philadelphia, 1964, WB Saunders.)*

occurs later, as the ductus arteriosus and foramen ovale close anatomically. Anatomical closure of the ductus, through fibrosis, normally occurs within 3 weeks of birth. Permanent closure of the tissue flap covering the foramen ovale may take several months.

All of these changes normally occur during the first few minutes after birth and allow the newborn infant to achieve normal gas exchange. A number of abnormal conditions can interfere with these transition events and lead to failure of the respiratory or cardiovascular systems.

POSTNATAL LUNG DEVELOPMENT

The infant lung is a unique structure and not merely a miniaturization of the adult lung. The airways, distal lung tissue, and pulmonary capillary bed all continue to grow and develop after birth. However, growth is asymmetrical, with each of the five lobes, their supporting airways, and blood supply developing independently and uniquely from child to child. An understanding of the key anatomical and physiological differences between pediatric and adult patients is essential for RTs caring for all age-groups.

Head and Upper Airway

As shown in Figure 7-8, relative to the body, the head of an infant is larger than that of an adult. The weight of the head can cause acute flexion of the cervical spine in infants with poor muscle tone. Infant neck flexion causes acute airway obstruction. Although the head is larger, an infant's nasal passages are proportionately smaller than are an adult's. These small nasal passages make nasal intubation more difficult and risky in

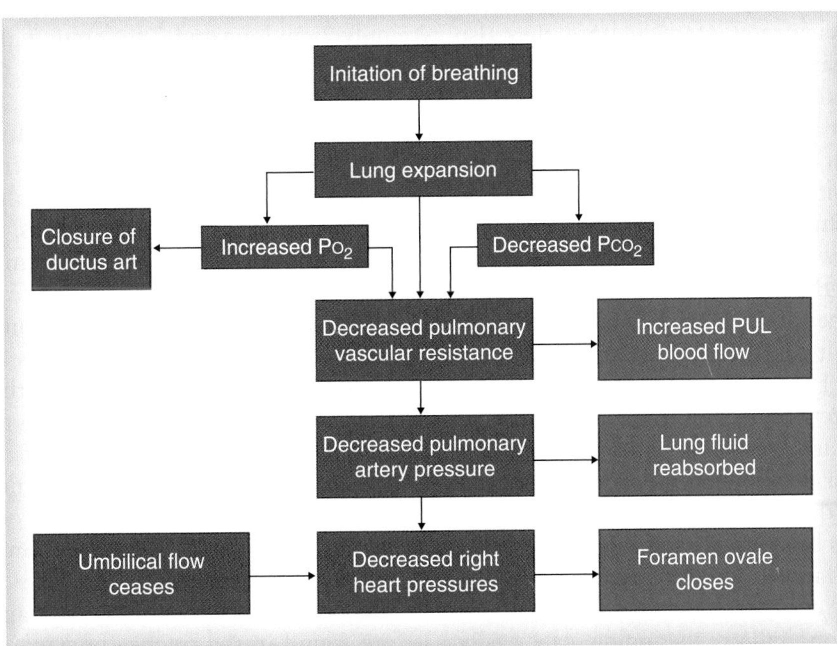

Figure 7-7

Newborn respiratory and circulatory changes. *(Modified from Kirby RR, Smith RA, Desautels DD, editors: Mechanical ventilation, New York, 1985, Churchill-Livingstone.)*

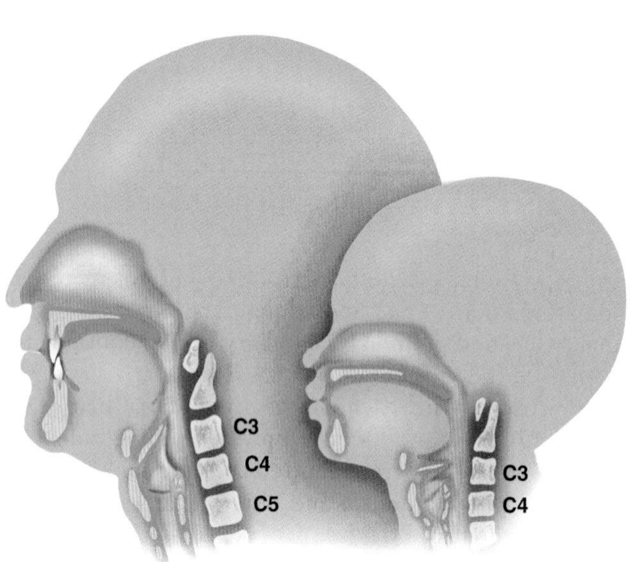

Figure 7-8

Comparison of adult and pediatric airways.

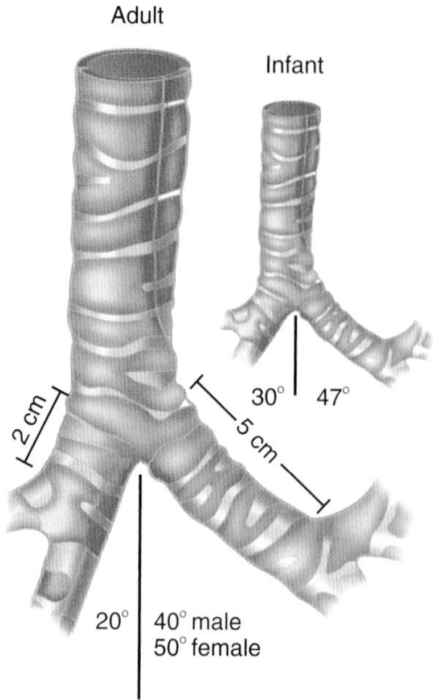

Figure 7-9

Comparison of adult and pediatric tracheas. *(Modified from Finucane BT, Santora AH: Principles of airway management, Philadelphia, 1988, FA Davis.)*

infants. In addition, the infant's jaw is much rounder and the tongue is much larger relative to the oral cavity.[13] This increases the likelihood of airway obstruction with loss of muscle tone.

Most infants breathe exclusively through the nose. However, 30% to 40% of newborn infants will sometimes breathe through the mouth, both spontaneously and in response to nasal occlusion.[14] If a preterm infant is breathing orally, he or she may be more prone to airway obstruction. As normal infants mature, they also do more oral breathing, especially when nasal obstruction is present.[15] At approximately 4 to 5 months of age, most infants are capable of full oral ventilation. An infant's larynx lies higher in the neck than in later years, with the glottis located between C3 and C4, and is more funnel-shaped than an adult's. For this reason, the narrowest passage is through the cricoid cartilage, rather than the glottis, as in adults.

The epiglottis of the infant is longer and less flexible than that of the adult and lies higher and in a more horizontal position. During swallowing, the infant's larynx provides a direct connection to the nasopharynx. This creates two nearly separate pathways, one for breathing and one for swallowing, allowing infants to breathe and suckle at the same time. Anatomical descent of the epiglottis begins between 2½ and 3 months of age. The mucosa of the infant's upper airway, especially the larynx, is thin and easily traumatized. Continuous attempts at intubation and/or suctioning can easily cause swelling and obstruction in these areas. In addition, mechanical stimulation of the neonatal larynx may result in prolonged apnea.[16]

Conducting Airways and Peripheral Airway Growth

The large conducting airways of infants are shorter and narrower than those of adults. The normal newborn trachea is approximately 5 to 6 cm long and 4 mm in diameter, whereas in small preterm infants it may be only 2 cm long and 2 to 3 mm wide. Because of smaller airways, a newborn's anatomical dead space is proportionately smaller than an adult's, being approximately 0.75 mL/lb of body weight. As shown in Figure 7-9, the mainstem bronchi branch off the trachea in the infant at less acute angles than in the adult, particularly on the right. However, as with adults, the right mainstem bronchus of the infant is still more in line with the trachea than the left.

Mean airway diameter, from main bronchi to respiratory bronchioles, increases 200% to 300% from birth through adulthood.[4] Smooth muscle is present in the airways of the neonate down to the level of the respiratory bronchioles and continues to increase until the child is approximately 8 months of age. After this age, smooth muscle proliferation occurs primarily in the proximal airways, while chondrocytes producing connective tissue and cartilage predominate in the proximal airways. Distinct C-shaped rings of cartilage are found in the trachea and mainstem bronchi of the neonate. The amount of cartilage progressively decreases in the more distal bronchi and eventually disappears in airways smaller than 2 mm in diameter.

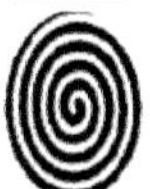

RULE OF THUMB

In the adult, the distinction between bronchi and bronchioles is (1) size and (2) presence of cartilage. Airways greater than 2 mm in diameter that contain cartilage are bronchi. Airways less than 2 mm in diameter without cartilage are bronchioles.[5,9]

Despite the presence of cartilage in the central airways of the infant, the trachea and larger bronchi of the neonate lack the rigidity of the adult central airways. The compliant nature of these airways makes them prone to compression and/or collapse. Tracheomalacia and bronchomalacia are relatively common problems in infants. These conditions, which may cause noisy or stridorous breathing, are alarming to parents. The malacia may be self-limiting and resolve without treatment over time or may lead to serious complications, including ventilatory failure.

Development of the lower tracheobronchial tree also has implications for respiratory problems in the newborn. Recent studies have shown that some male infants have proportionately smaller airways than females of the same age.[3] In addition, hyperresponsiveness of airway smooth muscle in young infants has been clearly demonstrated. The combination of anatomical differences and airway smooth muscle reactivity may account for a significant percentage of wheezy illnesses in young infants.

Alveolar and Vascular Growth

Estimates of alveolar surface at birth place the number of alveoli from 20 million to possibly as many as 150 million, covering an area of 1 to 4 m^2. Controversy exists regarding how long after birth alveoli continue to grow. Recent studies suggest that the alveolarization process is complete by only 1 to 2 years of age.[4,5] Estimates of alveolar numbers at maturity range between 200 and 600 million.

Associated pulmonary capillary growth at the alveolar level is rapid during the first 2 months of the infant's life. Subsequently, capillaries continue to develop in unison with alveoli. However, the ratio of alveoli to arteries decreases with age (20:1 in a newborn, 12:1 in a 2-year old, 8 to 10:1 in older children).[5] This expansion of the pulmonary capillary bed eventually makes it the largest vascular bed in the body, covering 70 to 80 m^2 in the adult. The pulmonary capillary bed receives its blood supply from the left and right pulmonary arteries. The pulmonary arteries (and branches), arising from the right ventricle, transport venous or deoxygenated blood to the lung to participate in gaseous exchange.

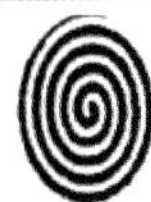

RULE OF THUMB

The pulmonary artery and its branches are the only "arteries" in the body to carry deoxygenated blood. Similarly, the pulmonary veins are the only "veins" that carry oxygenated blood back to the left side of the heart.

The pulmonary artery and its branches are classified as either conventional arteries or **supernumerary arteries.** Pulmonary artery development begins during the embryonic stage and simply follows the branching of the bronchial tree. Each time an airway divides, the accompanying blood vessel also divides. Postnatally, conventional arteries continue to branch until approximately 18 months of age.[5] Supernumerary artery development is established in the early pseudoglandular period. These are the arteries that branch from the conventional arteries; however, they do not follow the pattern of airway division, nor do they divide in any regular pattern. These arteries supply the gas-exchange units of the lung. Growth, in number and size, of supernumerary arteries continues after birth until approximately 8 years of life and, ultimately, far outnumber conventional arteries.

The respiratory system is a unique organ in that it receives blood supply from both the left and right sides of the heart. The bronchial arteries arise from the aorta (left ventricle) and supply oxygenated blood to the tracheobronchial tree. Like other systemic arteries, the bronchial arteries supply oxygen to the airway tissue, blood vessels, nerves, lymphatics, and visceral pleura. In addition, oxygen is directly absorbed across the airway lumen. Although the pulmonary and bronchial circulations have entirely different purposes, they are not mutually exclusive. There is mixing of the bronchial and pulmonary circulation at the level of the acinus. This is important because it provides a means of collateral circulation and shunting of blood. Dual circulation benefits both blood supplies and helps compensate for deficiencies or disease processes affecting either circulation.

Lymphatic Circulatory System

Paralleling the development of the pulmonary vascular circulation is the vast network of the lymphatic circulation. The lymphatic vessels occupy and traverse the same connective tissue spaces around the bronchi, bronchioles, blood vessels, and pleura. The close approximation of the vascular circulation and lymphatic circulation permit the lymphatics to control fluid and protein balance within the lung. The lymphatic system also serves a key role in lung defense mechanisms.

Nervous Pathways and the Control of Breathing

The development and interaction of nervous pathways in the lung is not completely understood. The phrenic and intercostal nerves are the primary components of the somatic (motor) nervous system. They innervate the diaphragm and intercostal muscles, respectively, which are largely responsible for the excursion and relaxation of the chest cage during breathing.

The response of the pulmonary vasculature to either sympathetic or parasympathetic innervation is not clear cut and is influenced by age and vascular tone.[5] The **vagus nerve** is also the origin for several sensory nerves. In newborns, the Hering-Breuer reflex (inhibition of inspiration) serves to promote short breath-hold periods when expiration is prevented. Head's paradoxical reflex results in a rapid lung inflation and may be related to "gasping" in infants or, perhaps, sighing in later life.[10,17] Other stretch receptors, known as J receptors, are located near the pulmonary capillaries in the acinus. Congestion and stretch of the walls of the capillaries stimulate these receptors, promoting a more rapid, shallow breathing pattern.[5] Irritant receptors, located throughout the tracheobronchial tree, are also vagal in origin. These receptors respond to a variety of unpleasant irritants, such as smoke, gas fumes, and aspirated stomach contents and foreign bodies. Gasping, cough, and spasms of the bronchi and/or larynx may result.

The development of these sensory vagal responses on control of breathing in the infant is not completely understood, but has gained significance in recent years. Lung transplantation was first performed in 1963 and has become an accepted and viable treatment for severe incurable lung diseases such as CF and pulmonary fibrosis.[10,17] Lung transplantation is now being performed on young infants with pulmonary hypertension and pulmonary surfactant deficiencies. Excision and removal of the diseased lungs severs all nervous innervation. Implanting denervated lungs into the recipient might be expected to have serious consequences in breathing control. Remarkably, lung transplantation in humans has little effect on respiratory rate and pattern of breathing. However, disruption of airway mechanics, vascular supply, lymphatics, ventilation/perfusion ($\dot{V}/\dot{Q}$) relationships, and immunological defense mechanics continue to plague lung transplant recipients.

Neonates, especially preterm infants, have frequent short periods of **apnea** and periodic breathing. Apneic spells are usually a longer than normal duration of breathing cessation and may be accompanied by bradycardia. Sepsis, anemia, gastric reflux, and lung disease can cause apnea. Apnea episodes occur most often during sleep or oral feeding. Apnea and periodic breathing, in the absence of other pathologic conditions, may be caused by immature respiratory responses.[10,17]

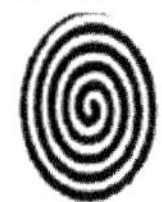

RULE OF THUMB

Apnea in the newborn is characterized by short periods of respiratory cessation (10 seconds or less) that do not result in adverse physiological changes.

Extensive research continues into sleep patterns seen in premature infants and in full-term newborns. Discerning normal mechanisms of arousal from sleep from those experienced by infants with near-death or apparent life-threatening episodes (ALTEs) and sudden infant death syndrome (SIDS) is a challenge. Interrelated are issues of prematurity and neuronal control of breathing, arousal responses, and circadian rhythms and thermal regulation in the newborn. The effects of socioeconomic factors, race, maternal smoking, and bottle feeding have all been implicated in cases of ALTEs and SIDS. Sleep position (prone versus supine) has been rigorously investigated. Pediatricians now recommend that infants be placed on firm mattresses on their backs (supine) or sides. Sleeping in the prone position, on soft bedding, has been shown to cause **rebreathing**[18] and has been identified as a significant risk factor for SIDS. Objects under or surrounding the baby (e.g., blankets and pillows) currently are being investigated as a potential cause of rebreathing, as is bedsharing.

Central and peripheral chemoreceptors are active in the neonate. However, they differ in presence and level of response. By late fetal life, response to carbon dioxide, via the central chemoreceptors, is present. Newborns respond to hypercarbia in a fashion similar to adults, but their ventilatory response is not as pronounced. Tidal volumes in adults can increase tenfold to twentyfold, whereas infants challenged with inhaled CO_2 increase their minute ventilation no more than threefold to fourfold. In addition, unlike adults, the response to hypoxia via peripheral chemoreceptors is paradoxical in both premature and full-term infants. A newborn exposed to severe hypoxemia (PaO_2 less than 30 to 40 mm Hg) responds with a short period of hyperventilation, followed by apnea.[19] Central nervous system (CNS) depression is the best explanation for this phenomenon.[20]

Metabolic and Ventilatory Requirements

The basal metabolic rate of a full-term 3-kg infant is approximately 2 kcal/kg/hr, which is nearly twice that of an adult. This means that the infant's oxygen requirement and CO_2 production (per kilogram) are also double that of an adult. This high metabolic rate demands twice as much ventilation per minute per kilogram. When adjusted for body weight, infant tidal volumes are approximately the same as those in adults

(6 to 7 mL/kg). Therefore to meet the greater ventilatory demand, the infant must increase his or her breathing rate to an average of 30 to 40 breaths/min. This high rate of breathing, in turn, wastes more ventilation per minute than in the adult. This occurs despite the fact that the anatomical dead space of an infant is proportionately smaller than that of the adult.

Chest Wall Development and Lung Volumes

Substantial differences exist between the "respiratory pump" of the infant and of the adult. The **functional residual capacity (FRC)** of the lung represents a volume that is in reserve. This "stored" lung capacity is called into play when respiratory demands to increase ventilation or oxygenation cannot be met by normal tidal breathing. The resting FRC is a volume determined by the passive, static balance between chest wall and lung tissue. The chest wall force, expanding the lung, is markedly reduced in the infant. Also reduced, but to a lesser degree, is lung tissue recoil. The resultant balance of the static forces in the infant favors a reduced FRC and total lung capacity (TLC).[4] Low lung volumes seem to be a significant disadvantage. They can lead to airway closure, atelectasis, $\dot{V}/\dot{Q}$ mismatch, shunting, and resultant hypoxemia. A small FRC means that changes in ventilation will rapidly change blood gas values.[21,22] The combination of a small FRC and high oxygen consumption in an infant deprived of oxygen can quickly lead to profound hypoxemia. Infants possess a remarkable ability to dynamically elevate their FRC above static, resting levels. Infants do not passively exhale to FRC as adults do. Passive exhalation is interrupted while expiratory flow rates are still relatively high.[4] The infant actively ends expiration and begins the next inspiratory phase (Figure 7-10). This is accomplished through several important mechanisms. Adults empty their lungs through elastic recoil of lung tissue, without significant use of any muscles. However, infants actively use their diaphragms to slow expiration. In addition, they adduct (close) the vocal cords and narrow the larynx. The combination of these two maneuvers effectively regulates volume in the lung and dynamically elevates the FRC. RTs can identify this as a method of maintaining auto positive end-expiratory pressure (autoPEEP). The narrowing of the glottis or larynx is referred to as **laryngeal braking**. Infants in respiratory distress commonly grunt, a manifestation of laryngeal braking. Because of the lack of rigidity of the chest wall, suprasternal, substernal, intercostal, and subcostal **retractions** are easily seen in distressed infants. Physiologically, the PEEP that is created through diaphragmatic and laryngeal braking improves oxygenation.

Unlike an adult's, an infant's thoracic muscles are immature, providing little structural or ventilatory support. The infant thoracic cage is more boxlike, with the ribs being horizontally orientated, or elevated (Figure 7-11). In addition, the diaphragm inserts into the thoracic cage in a horizontal plane, decreasing the ability to effectively contract.[4]

The infant diaphragm moves mainly up and down, having little effect on lateral chest dimensions. Therefore the anteroposterior (AP) diameter of the infant thorax changes little during inspiration. Compounding the situation is a proportionately larger abdominal viscera restricting vertical motion. The ribs take on a progressively downward slope as the child grows, and by 10 years of age the rib cage has the configuration seen in adults. **Ossification** of the ribs and sternum continues to approximately age 25 years, whereas costal cartilage calcification may continue into old age. In general, muscle mass increases throughout childhood and into early adulthood.[5]

Compliance, Airway Resistance, and Pressure-Volume Relationships

The rib cage and muscles of the respiratory system develop around and in unison with airways and alveoli. An incredibly complicated relationship develops between lung volume, compliance of the lung and chest wall, airway resistance, and the pressure-volume relationships that are created. Table 7-3 reviews changes in anatomical structures and physiological parameters

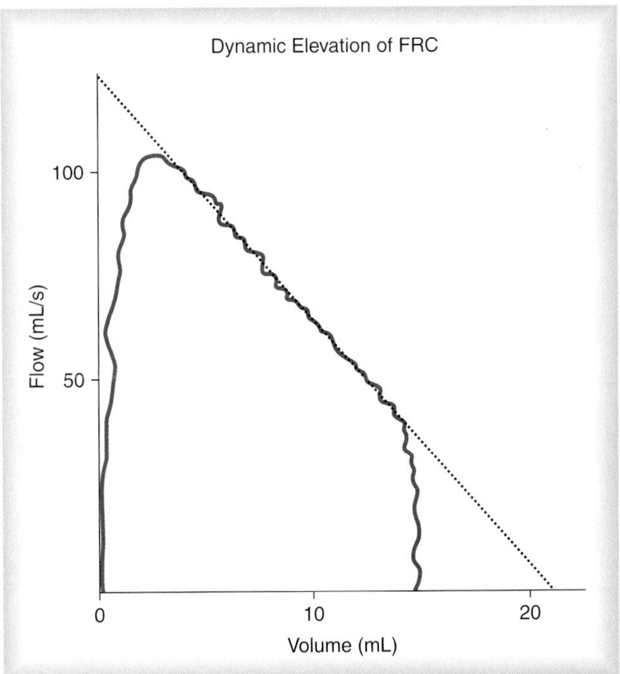

Figure 7-10

Passive flow-volume curve in an infant, showing abrupt inspiration substantially above passive functional residual capacity (FRC). *(Modified from Taussig LM, Landau LI, editors: Pediatric and respiratory medicine, St Louis, 1999, Mosby.)*

from newborns to adults. It is important to understand the changing mechanics of breathing from infancy to adulthood (see also Mechanics of Ventilation in Chapter 9). RTs are often responsible for altering these mechanics through ventilator manipulations.

Compliance

The infant's chest wall is very compliant; it deforms easily. Chest wall compliance decreases after 1 year of age, and by adulthood the chest wall is rigid and much less compliant. Less straightforward are the pressure-volume relationships and changes in compliance and elastic recoil. Lung compliance increases with age, likely related to the number and maturity of alveoli present at various ages. Respiratory system **compliance** is a parameter often measured in a pediatric pulmonary function laboratory, along with lung volume, specifically FRC. Compliance expressed per unit of lung volume (FRC) is termed **specific compliance.** This is an

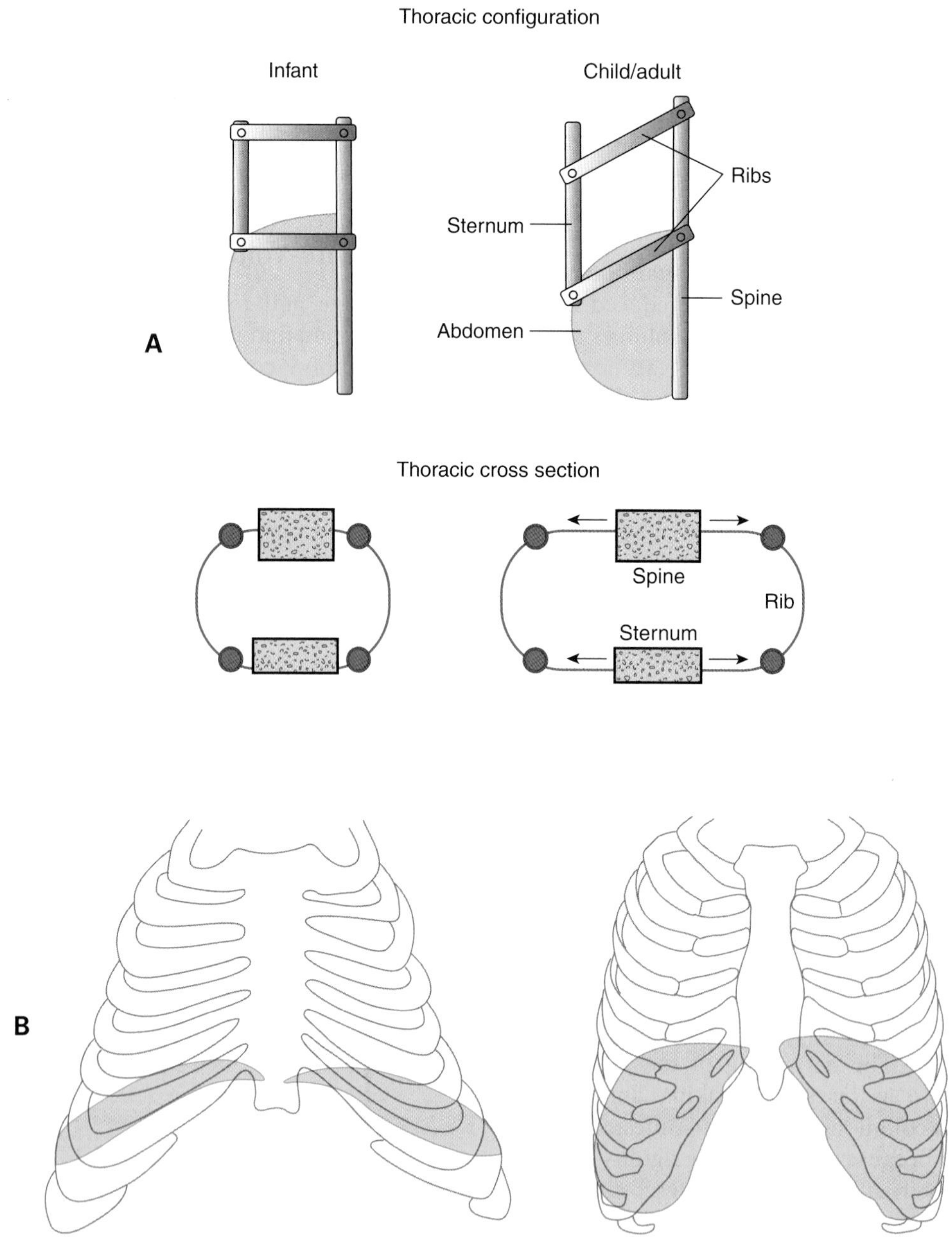

Figure 7-11

A, Changes in configuration and cross-sectional shape of the thorax from infancy to early childhood. **B,** Newborn *(left)* and adult *(right)* ribcages. The shaded areas represent the anterior projection of the diaphragm. *(Modified from Taussig LM, Landau LI, editors: Pediatric and respiratory medicine, St Louis, 1999, Mosby.)*

Table 7-3 ▶▶ Anatomical and Physiological Comparisons in Children Versus Adults

	Infant	Child 8-20 yr	Adult
Anatomical			
Body weight, kg	3	Variable	70
Lung weight, g	50	350	800
Lung tissue, % total	28	15	9
Number of alveoli × 10	20-150	300	300-600
Diameter of alveoli, μm	50	150	300
Number of respiratory airways × 10^6	1.5	14	14
Pulmonary capillary bed surface area, m^2	3	32	70
Physiological			
Tidal volume, mL/kg	6		6
Respiratory rate, breaths/min	35		15
Heart rate, beats/min	>100		70
V_D/Vt ratio	0.3		0.33
O_2 consumption, mL/kg/min	6.4		3.5
CO_2 production, mL/kg/min	6		3
Calories, kcal/kg/hr	2		1
Vital capacity, mL/kg	35		70
FRC, mL/kg	30		35
TLC, mL/kg	63		86
Lung compliance, mL/cm H_2O	7.9		150
Specific lung compliance, C_L/FRC	0.038		0.05

V_D/Vt, Dead space to tidal volume ratio.

extremely useful way to compare changing compliance, especially in infants experiencing rapid lung growth. Specific lung compliance is relatively unchanged with increasing age. Average values for specific lung compliance (C_L/FRC) are as follows: newborns 1 day old (0.055), infants 1 month to 2 years old (0.038), children 9 years old (0.063), young adults 25 years old (0.050), and adults older than 60 years (0.041).[5]

Airway Resistance

Airway resistance can be defined as the pressure gradient required to produce flow through an airway (see Pressure Differences during Breathing in Chapter 9). Airway resistance differs dramatically in all humans from the upper airways (nose, pharynx, and larynx) to the lower peripheral airways. Upper airway resistance accounts for at least 50% of total resistance through the respiratory system.[7] Growth and changes in proportions of the upper and lower airways alter airway resistance from infancy to adulthood.

The newborn lung has relatively large airways compared with distal lung tissue. Airway resistance is low, and the lungs empty rapidly. The rate at which the lungs and airways empty is termed the **time constant** (flow/volume or 1/time) of the lung. Infants have high or increased time constants because their airways empty rapidly. As the child grows, alveolar multiplication slows, but the alveoli expand tremendously in volume. There is essentially little change in airway number. However, the conducting and peripheral airways lengthen and dilate extensively, with a resultant increase in absolute airway resistance. When corrected for the increasing lung volume from infant to adult, specific airway resistance increases, thereby increasing exhalation time. The time constant, which is 1/time, decreases.[7]

It is important to recognize the role of individual variability in airway versus alveolar growth. Measurements of compliance and airway resistance can vary greatly. This disparity in airway versus lung growth is termed **dysynapsis**. It may be present early in life and is theorized to be genetically determined. An example of this phenomenon can be seen in young infants who wheeze early in life. Some go on to develop asthma later in childhood and adulthood, whereas others appear to outgrow their symptoms, as airway growth "catches up" to alveolar growth. These children may have difficult early years, with wheeze and frequent infections, but be free of disease as adults. With so much variability in the normal lung, understanding the mechanics of breathing in the diseased lung is a challenge for RTs.

▶ THE RESPIRATORY SYSTEM IN THE ADULT

The Thorax

The rib cage, thoracic vertebrae, and sternum form the thorax. It contains the esophagus, trachea, lungs, heart, and great vessels (Figure 7-12). The thorax is cone shaped, bounded by the diaphragm at its base, with a narrow opening at the top. The first ribs and the upper sternum form this opening, called the *thoracic inlet* or *operculum.*

The thorax consists of three compartments: the mediastinum and the left and right pleural cavities. The centrally located mediastinum contains the trachea, esophagus, heart, and great vessels of the circulatory system. The left and right pleural cavities contain the lungs.

The thoracic "cage" serves two purposes. First, its bony structures protect the vital organs inside. Second, the thoracic bones and muscles interact to increase and decrease chest volume. This action generates the pressure differences that allow gas to flow into and out of the lungs.

Gross Structure and Function

Lung Topography

A series of *imaginary lines* can be drawn to establish reference points and identify landmarks on the thorax. These lines and points help identify the location of underlying structures. The imaginary lines can also be used to describe the location of abnormal findings during physical examination (see Chapter 14).

On the anterior chest, the midsternal line divides the thorax into equal halves. The left and right midclavicular lines are parallel to the midsternal line. These are drawn through the midpoints of the left and right clavicles, respectively (Figure 7-13).

The midaxillary line divides the lateral chest into equal halves. The anterior axillary line is parallel to the

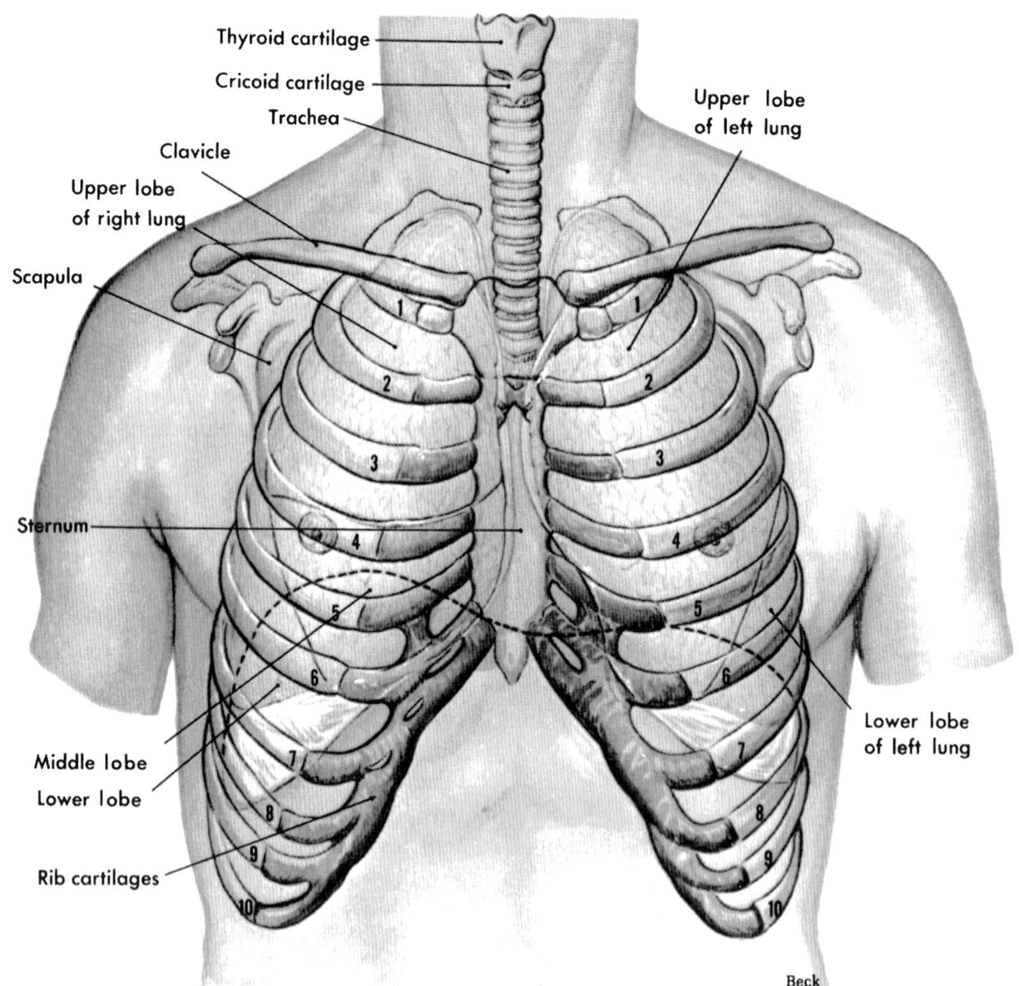

Figure 7-12

Projection of the lungs and trachea in relation to the rib cage and clavicles. The *dotted line* indicates the location of the dome-shaped diaphragm at the end of expiration and before inspiration. Note that the apex of each lung projects above the clavicle. Ribs 11 and 12 are not visible in this view. *(From Anthony CO, Thibodeau GA: Textbook of anatomy and physiology, ed 13, St Louis, 1990, Mosby.)*

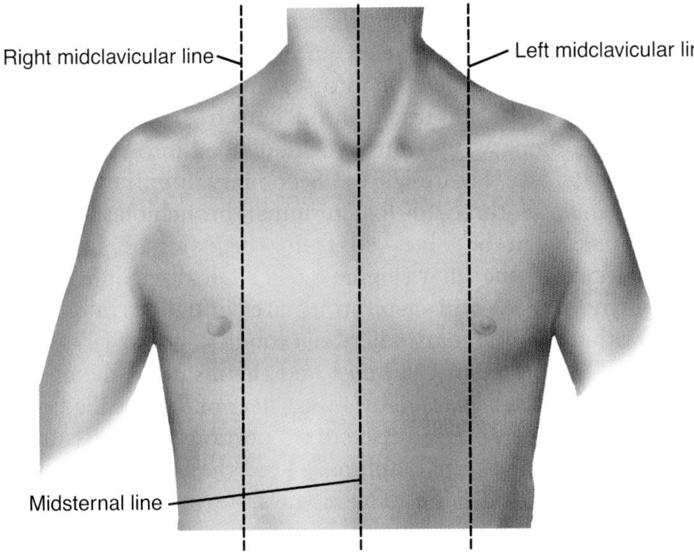

Figure 7-13

Imaginary lines on anterior chest wall.

midaxillary line. It is situated along the anterolateral chest. The posterior axillary line is also parallel to the midaxillary line. It is located on the posterolateral chest wall (Figure 7-14).

Three imaginary vertical lines are described on the posterior thorax. The midspinal line divides the posterior chest into two equal halves. The left and right midscapular lines are parallel to the midspinal line. They pass through the inferior angles of the scapulae in the relaxed upright subject (Figure 7-15).

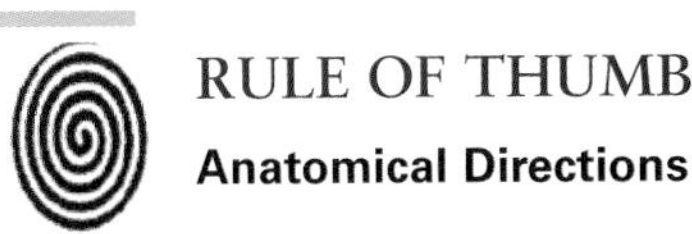

RULE OF THUMB

Anatomical Directions

Descriptions of various anatomical structures often use the following terms:

Anterior, anteriorly The front of the body, toward the front
Posterior, posteriorly The back of the body, toward the back
Anteroposterior (AP) In a direction from the front to the back
Lateral, laterally The side of the body, toward the side
Medial, medially The midline of the body, toward

Mediastinum

The **mediastinum** divides the thorax vertically, separating the left and right pleural cavities. The mediastinum is bounded on either side by the pleural cavities, anteriorly by the sternum, posteriorly by the thoracic vertebrae, inferiorly by the diaphragm, and superiorly by the thoracic inlet.

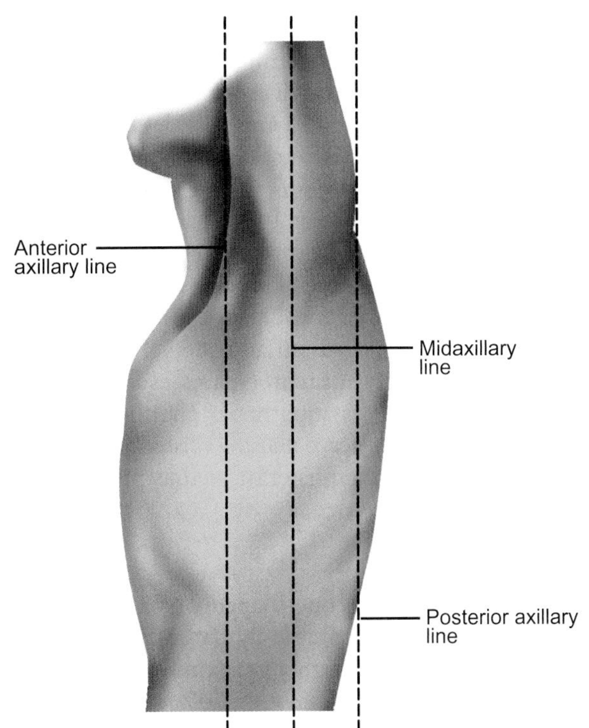

Figure 7-14

Imaginary lines on lateral chest wall.

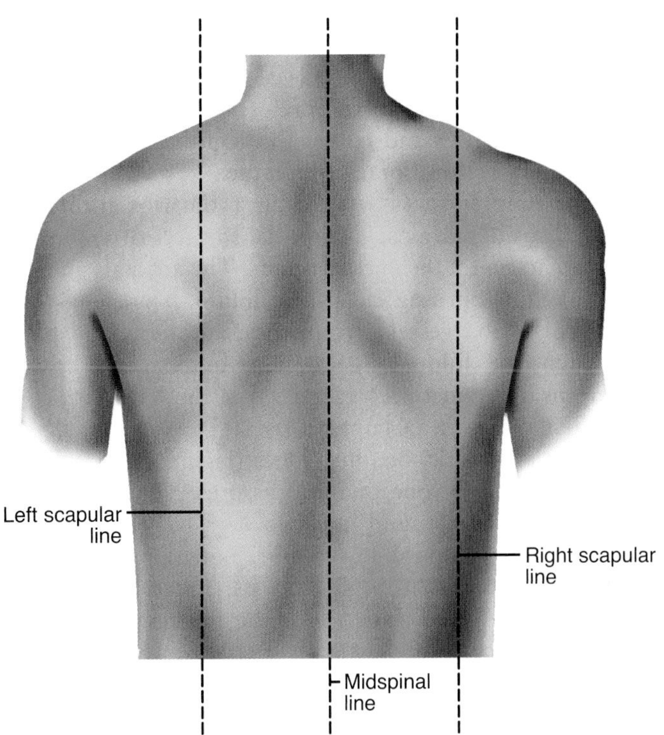

Figure 7-15

Imaginary lines on posterior chest wall.

The mediastinum is subdivided into three subcompartments.[23] Between the sternum and **pericardium** is an anterior compartment, which contains the thymus gland and anterior mediastinal lymph nodes. The middle compartment contains the pericardium and heart. This compartment also contains the great vessels. The phrenic and upper portions of the vagus nerves, along with the trachea and portions of the right and left mainstem bronchi, and their associated lymph nodes are in the middle compartment. The posterior compartment lies between the pericardium and the vertebral column and contains the thoracic aorta, esophagus, and thoracic duct. The sympathetic chains and lower portions of the vagus nerve and the posterior mediastinal lymph nodes are in the posterior mediastinum.

Lungs and Pleura

The lungs are paired, cone-shaped organs. They lie in the pleural cavities, separated by the mediastinum. The average adult lungs weigh approximately 800 g, but their volume is 90% gas and only 10% tissue. The heart and mediastinum protrude to the left. As a result, the left lung is somewhat narrower than the right. The liver elevates the right hemidiaphragm, making the right lung shorter than the left.

The lungs extend from the diaphragm to a point 1 to 2 cm above the clavicles (see Figure 7-12). The tops of the lungs are called the **apices**. At end-expiration, the anterior lower lung borders extend to approximately the sixth rib at the midclavicular line. Laterally, the lower lung border is at the eighth rib at the maxillary line. The top of the lungs, viewed posteriorly, extend to the first thoracic **vertebra**. The inferior border (posteriorly) rises and falls with breathing between the ninth and twelfth thoracic vertebrae.

The lung surfaces lying against the ribs form the curved costal margins. The medial surfaces of the lungs are adjacent to the mediastinum. The medial surface contains an opening called the **hilum**. The mainstem bronchi, blood vessels, lymphatics, and nerves all pass through the hilum. The apices, hilum, and costal margins are sometimes referenced in the interpretation of chest x-rays (see Chapter 18).

Each lung is divided into **lobes** (Figure 7-16), which are separated by one or more **fissures**. The right lung has upper, middle, and lower lobes. The left lung has only an upper and a lower lobe. Both lungs have an oblique fissure that begins on the anterior chest at approximately the sixth rib at the midclavicular line. These fissures extend laterally and upward until they cross the fifth rib on the lateral chest in the midaxillary line. The fissures continue on the posterior chest to approximately the third thoracic vertebra. The right lung also has a horizontal fissure that separates the upper and middle lobes. This horizontal fissure extends from the fourth rib at the sternal border around to the fifth rib at the midaxillary line.

Each lobe is divided into **segments** according to the branches of the tracheobronchial tree. These bronchopulmonary segments are subdivided into **secondary lobules** (see Figure 7-16). Secondary lobules contain clusters of three to five terminal bronchioles. These lobules can be observed from the external and cut surface of the lung (Figure 7-17). Localized infection, hemorrhage, and aspiration are initially contained within the boundaries between lobules.

The surface of the lungs and the inside of the chest walls are each covered by a thin layer of tissue called the **pleura**. Pleural tissue also covers portions of the fissures between lobes, the diaphragm, and the lateral portions of the mediastinum. The tissue covering the lungs is called the **visceral pleura**. The visceral pleura extends onto the hilar bronchi and vessels and into the major fissures. The deeper portions of the visceral pleura contain elastic and fibrous tissue, small venules, and lymphatics. The septa between lobes are continuous with this layer. Veins and lymphatics follow these septa, starting as small vessels in the visceral pleura.

The pleura covering the inner surface of the chest wall and the mediastinum is called the **parietal pleura** (Figure 7-18). Portions of the parietal pleura are named according to the structures that they contact. The costal pleura lines the inner surface of the rib cage. The medi-

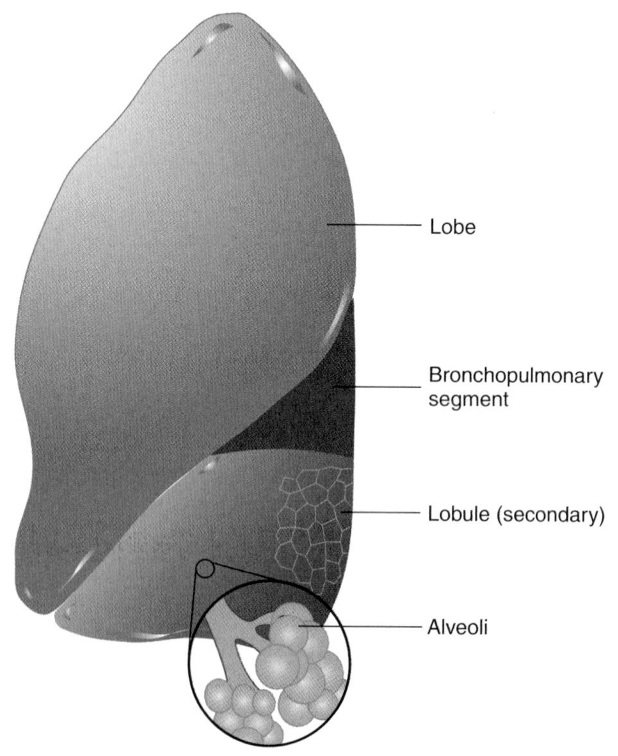

Figure 7-16

Units of the lung. Alveoli are actually microscopic in size.

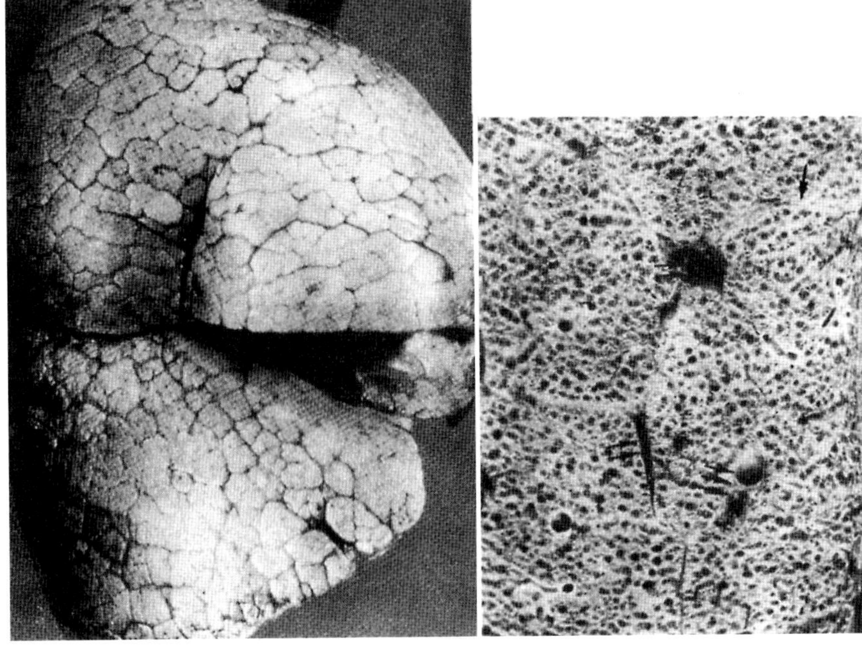

Figure 7-17

A, Outer surface of lung. **B,** Cut surface of lung, showing interlobular septum *(one arrow)*, small veins in these septa *(two arrows)*, and a pulmonary artery and bronchiole near the center of the secondary lobule *(three arrows)*. *(From Heitzman ER: The lung: radiologic-pathologic correlations, ed 2, St Louis, 1984, Mosby.)*

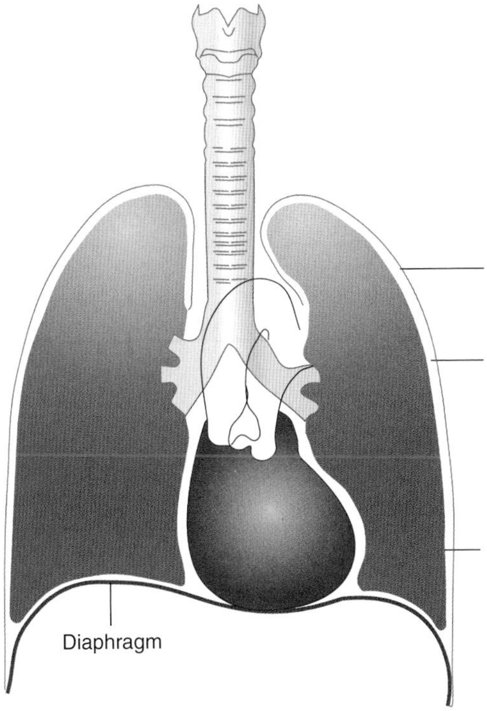

astinal pleura covers the mediastinum. The diaphragmatic pleura covers the diaphragm. The acute angle where the costal pleura joins the diaphragmatic pleura is known as the **costophrenic angle**. This area contains no lung tissue and is clearly visible on normal chest x-rays. Excess fluids between the visceral and parietal pleura tend to pool here in an upright individual. This causes the angle to appear blunted or flattened on the chest x-ray (see Chapter 18).The upper dome of the parietal pleura extends above the first rib and encloses the thoracic inlet. At the hilum, parietal pleura becomes continuous with the visceral pleura. Although the two portions of the pleura are described by different names, they form one continuous lining.

Between the visceral and parietal pleura is the pleural cavity. This "cavity" is really a potential space, occupied by a thin layer of serous fluid. This fluid forms a thin film of uniform thickness that couples the visceral and parietal pleural surfaces. The fluid allows the pleura to slip easily over one another[24]; it also permits chest wall forces to be transmitted to the lungs. If air, blood, or other fluids are introduced into this space, the two pleural surfaces can separate. When this happens, the parietal pleura remains fixed against the inner wall of the thorax, and the lung and the visceral pleura are displaced inward, away from the chest wall.

Figure 7-18

Overall relationship of chest organs, cavities, and investments. The mediastinum occupies space between the lungs and contains the trachea, mainstem bronchi, heart, and great vessels. Each lung sits within its chest cavity. This cavity is lined by parietal pleura, which covers the chest cage, diaphragm, and lateral mediastinum, and is also lined by visceral pleura, which covers the lungs.

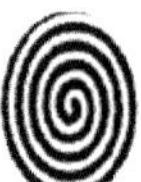

RULE OF THUMB

A number of procedures require entry into the pleural cavity. These include thoracentesis to drain fluid or pus and placement of chest tubes to treat pneumothorax. Incisions or punctures made during such procedures are always done immediately above a selected rib. The intercostal nerves, veins, and arteries all lie in a groove below each rib. To avoid these structures, needles and tubes are placed above a rib.

MINI CLINI

Penetrating Chest Injury

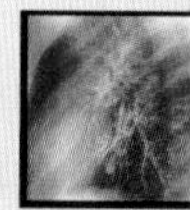

Normally, the parietal and visceral pleura are in physical contact with one another and are separated only by a thin, liquid film or fluid. This liquid film allows these two pleural membranes to slide over one another with little friction. This film also provides a cohesive force that resists separation of the membranes. When the respiratory muscles move the rib cage outward in an inspiratory effort, the lung is literally pulled by the cohesive forces between the parietal and visceral pleura. The elastic recoil forces of the lung resist this outward movement.

PROBLEM

A person suffers a traumatic penetrating wound to the chest. The chest wall and parietal pleura are punctured, leaving the visceral pleura intact. What happens to the lungs and chest wall?

ANSWER

The lung on the affected side collapses. Air is drawn (sucked) into the chest with an inspiratory effort, separating the parietal and visceral pleura. The chest wall expands outward. (Air in the pleural space is called *pneumothorax*.) The elastic recoil of the lung normally creates a subatmospheric intrapleural pressure. In the intact chest, the lung is expanded above its resting volume, while the chest wall is pulled inward below its resting volume. Both structures recoil in opposite directions but are held in position by the other's equal and oppositely directed recoil force. If the chest wall is punctured, as in this problem, air rushes into the pleural space. Elastic recoil of the lungs is unopposed. The lung collapses, pulling more air into the chest. The thorax, unopposed, recoils outward. Treatment of pneumothorax involves sealing the puncture, inserting a tube into the chest cavity (a "chest tube") and applying vacuum to re-expand the lung.

The lung itself has elastic properties. This elasticity results from surface tension forces in the alveoli and from tissue forces. The presence of elastin fibers in the alveolar walls, around the small airways, and in pulmonary capillaries produces elastic recoil. Collagen fibers probably contribute little to the elastic properties of the lungs, acting primarily to limit expansion at high lung volumes.[25] Because of the healthy lung's elasticity, it tends to recoil to a lower volume. When a lung is removed from the chest cavity, it quickly collapses to a smaller size. The same occurs if air or fluid enters into the pleural space. This tendency of the lung to contract results in development of subatmospheric intrapleural pressure (see Chapter 9). It is possible for individual lobes of the lung to collapse. The most common cause of a lobar collapse is obstruction of its bronchus.

Bones of the Thoracic Cage

The thoracic cage includes the thoracic vertebrae, the sternum, and the ribs and costal cartilages (Figure 7-19). These structures provide support and protection for the contents of the thorax. They also serve as points of origin and insertion for the respiratory muscles.

Vertebrae

The 12 thoracic vertebrae share a common structure with their cervical and lumbar counterparts' entire vertebral column. Each vertebra has a body with pedicles, laminas, and spinous and transverse processes. Thoracic vertebrae differ in that their transverse processes have facets that serve as points of articulation for the head of each rib. The orientation of these facets allows the rotation and elevation that characterize rib movement.

Sternum

The **sternum** is a dagger-shaped bony structure in the median line at the front of the chest. It serves as the point of attachment for the **costal cartilages** and numerous muscles. It also provides protection for the underlying organs. The adult sternum averages 18 cm in length. It consists of three portions: the upper triangular manubrium; the long, narrow body; and the pointed lower xiphoid process.

The **manubrium** articulates with the first and second ribs and the clavicle. The upper surface of the manubrium forms an easily identified depression between the clavicles called the suprasternal notch. The manubrium is a point of attachment for portions of the pectoralis major muscle. It also serves as the sternal origin of the sternomastoid muscle (see the section, Muscles, on p. 159). The manubrium articulates with the body of the sternum and second costal cartilages (second ribs), forming a slightly oblique angle called the **angle of Louis.** The angle of Louis is an important external landmark.

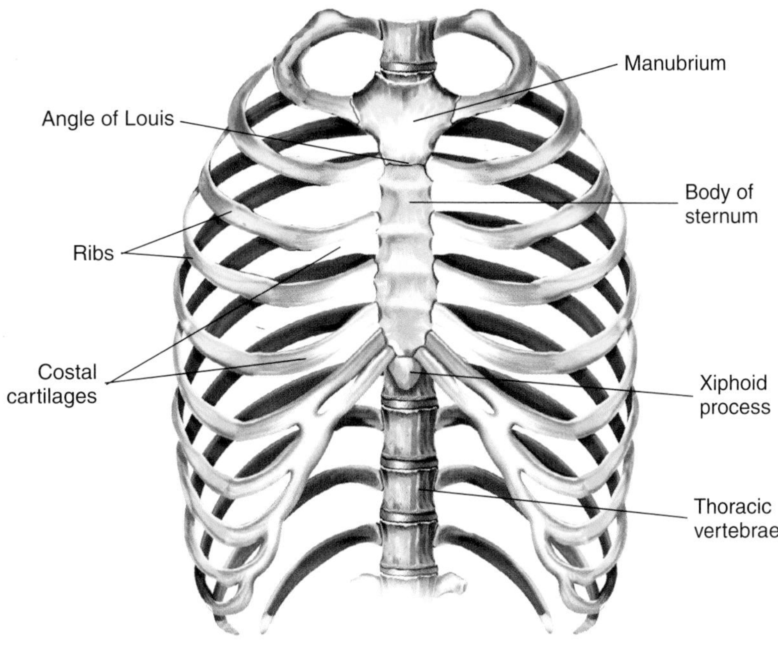

Figure 7-19

Chest cage. Ribs arch around from vertebral column, joining the sternum through cartilaginous extensions.

It marks the point at which the **trachea** divides into left and right mainstem bronchi and also marks the upper margin of the heart. In adults, the body of the sternum is a single bone, articulating with the second through seventh ribs via the costal cartilages (see Figure 7-19).

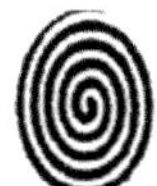

RULE OF THUMB

Where the manubrium and body of the sternum meet, the anterior chest wall shows a slight depression that forms an oblique angle (when viewed from the side). This depression is referred to as the *angle of Louis*. Beneath this important landmark, *the trachea divides into the right and left mainstem bronchi.*

The **xiphoid process** is a cartilaginous structure, located approximately at the level of the tenth thoracic vertebra. The xiphoid process is the smallest portion of the sternum, and its shape varies. It articulates with the seventh rib pair. The xiphoid process serves as an attachment point for portions of the diaphragm and abdominal muscles.

Ribs

Twelve pairs of ribs correspond to the twelve thoracic vertebrae. The first seven rib pairs connect directly to the sternum via the costal cartilages (see Figure 7-19). Ribs 8 through 10 connect to the ribs above and indirectly to the sternum through costal cartilages. This cartilage is soft and moderately flexible during childhood and adolescence. The cartilages become calcified with age, and the rib cage then becomes less flexible. The eleventh and twelfth rib pairs have no connection to the other rib pairs or sternum. These ribs are often referred to as *floating ribs*. The floating ribs terminate in cartilaginous-free ends in the wall of the abdomen.

Each rib consists of a *head*, a *neck*, and a *body* (Figures 7-20 and 7-21). Except for ribs 10 through 12, the rounded head has two facets for articulation with corresponding facets on the thoracic vertebrae. The flattened neck is approximately 2.5 cm long and extends outward from the head. On the posterior surface of the neck is a tubercle, which is most prominent in the upper ribs. The tubercle articulates with the transverse process of the lower of the two vertebrae to which the head of the rib is connected. The rib shaft is thin and curved, with numerous ridges and grooves. The ridges serve as points of attachment for muscles. The costal groove on the underside of each rib contains an intercostal artery, a vein, and a nerve (see Figures 7-20 and 7-22). To prevent damage to these structures, when needles or tubes are placed into the intercostal space, contact with the inferior margin of the rib above must be avoided.

Rib Movement

The first rib moves slightly, raising and lowering the sternum. Its small motion increases the AP diameter of

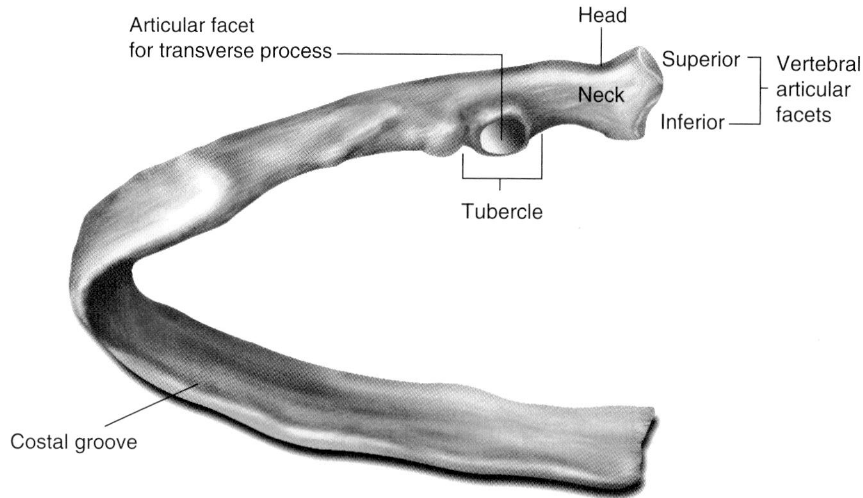

Figure 7-20

A typical middle rib, from the left side of the body, viewed posteriorly (from the back). The head end (and tubercle) articulates with the vertebral column, whereas the shaft articulates with the sternum.

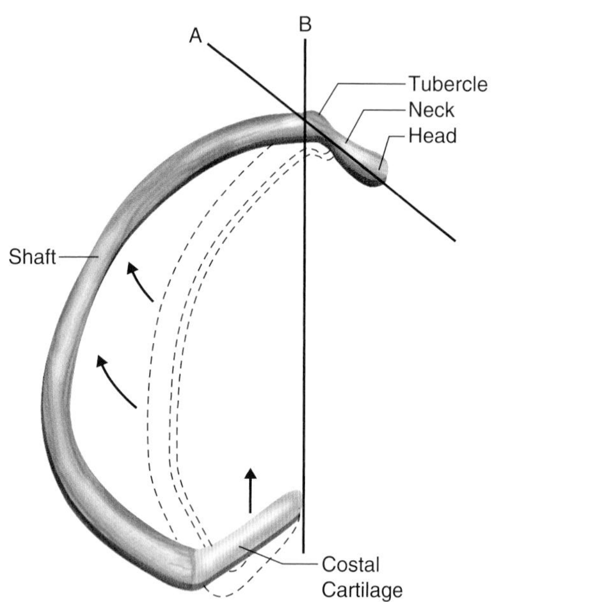

Figure 7-21

The two axes, about which the vertebrosternal ribs rotate during ventilation, are indicated by lines *A* and *B*. The former axis passes through the length of the rib head and neck; the latter axis follows an anteroposterior direction from the tip of the costal cartilage to the tubercle. The rib undergoes a compound movement from its starting positions *(dotted outline)*, with the shaft swinging upward and laterally about axis *B* and the anterior end moving upward about axis *A*.

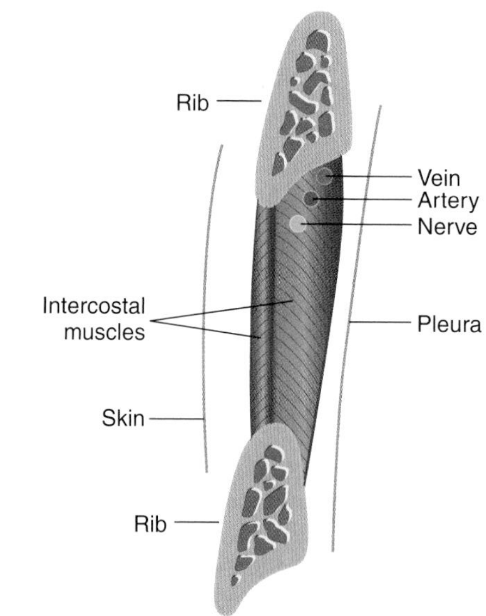

Figure 7-22

Intercostal muscles fill spaces between ribs. An intercostal artery, vein, and nerve run in a groove just beneath the lower edge of each rib.

the chest. This action is not used during quiet breathing. It becomes important under conditions that require increased ventilation, such as exercise.

Ribs 2 through 7 play an important role in ventilation. These ribs move simultaneously about two axes (see Figure 7-21). As each rib rotates about the axis of its neck, its sternal end rises and falls. This movement increases the AP thoracic diameter. This action is described as a "pump handle" motion. At the same time, the rib moves about its long axis from its angle at the sternum. This motion causes the middle part of the rib to move up and down. This "bucket handle" motion increases and decreases the transverse diameter of the chest. The compound action of ribs 2 through 7 changes both the AP and transverse diameters smoothly and evenly.

Ribs 8 through 10 rotate in a pattern similar to that of ribs 2 through 7. However, elevation of the anterior ends of these ribs produces a backward movement of the lower sternum. This reduces the thoracic AP diameter (Figure 7-23). Outward rotation of the middle section of the ribs, as with ribs 2 through 7, increases the transverse diameter of the thorax. Ribs 11 through 12 do not participate in changing the contour of the chest but act as muscle insertion points and to protect the contents of the upper abdomen.

Muscles

Various muscles contribute to the flow of gas into and out of the lungs. These muscles may be divided into the *primary* and *accessory* muscles of ventilation.[26] The diaphragm and intercostal muscles are the primary muscles of ventilation. They are active during both quiet breathing and exercise. The accessory muscles of ventilation assist the diaphragm and **intercostals** when ventilatory demand increases. The scalenes, sternomastoid, pectoralis major, and abdominals are the predominant accessory muscles. Other abdominal and chest wall muscles may also function as accessory muscles.

Diaphragm. The **diaphragm** is a large muscle that arises from the lumbar vertebrae, the costal margin, and the xiphoid process. Its fibers converge into a broad connective sheet called the *central tendon*. The diaphragm is configured like a dome and divides the thorax from the abdomen. The central tendon combines with the pericardium to divide the dome into two "leaves." These leaves are referred to as the right and left hemidiaphragms. Because the liver is located immediately below the right hemidiaphragm, the right hemidiaphragm is approximately 1 cm higher than the left **hemidiaphragm** at the end of a quiet breath. The right dome is positioned at the ninth thoracic vertebra posteriorly and at the fifth rib anteriorly. On the left, the diaphragm comes to rest at end-expiration at the tenth thoracic vertebra posteriorly and the sixth rib anteriorly. Movements of the hemidiaphragms are synchronous in healthy subjects.[27] However, innervation by separate phrenic nerves allows each hemidiaphragm to function independently. Many clinical situations arise in which the hemidiaphragms move asynchronously.

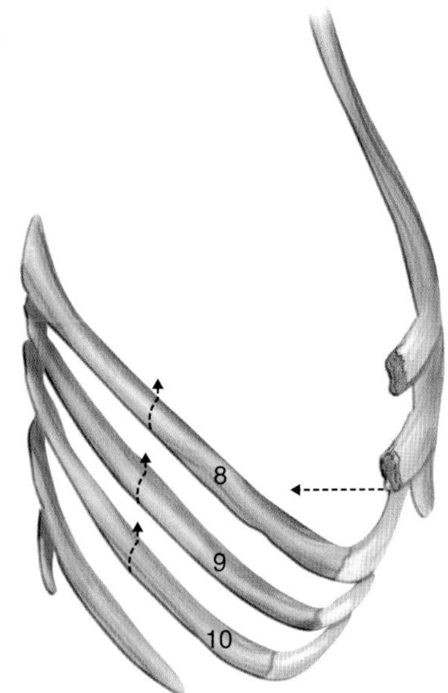

Figure 7-23

The vertebrochondral ribs, *8* to *10*, have laterosuperior movement, but elevation of their anterior ends retracts the lower end of the sternum, shortening the anteroposterior diameter of the thorax in that plane.

The diaphragm accounts for approximately 75% of the change in thoracic volume during quiet inspiration. During tidal breathing, the diaphragm moves approximately 1.5 cm. In an average-sized adult, each centimeter of vertical movement results in a volume change of approximately 350 mL. At high levels of ventilation, the diaphragm may move 6 to 10 cm. The ability of the diaphragm to change thoracic volume may be altered when either obstructive or restrictive lung disease is present (see Chapter 9).

During quiet breathing, the excursion of each hemidiaphragm is about equal. With deep inspiration, the right diaphragm may descend more than the left diaphragm. In healthy subjects, diaphragm movement is approximately the same in the erect and supine positions. However, in a head-down (i.e., 45-degree) tilt, the resting level of the diaphragm rises approximately 6 cm into the thorax. This reduces the FRC and the expiratory reserve volume (see Chapter 17). When a subject lies in a lateral position, the lower hemidiaphragm tends to rise into the chest.

The diaphragm produces two important mechanical effects. First, contraction draws the central tendon down. This flattens the diaphragm, increasing thoracic volume and lowering intrathoracic pressure. As the diaphragm descends, intraabdominal pressure increases. The muscles of the abdominal wall relax, allowing the upper abdomen to balloon outward. The second mechanical action of the diaphragm is achieved by contraction of its costal fibers. This raises the lateral costal margins (Figure 7-24, *A*). Increasing abdominal pressure during inspiration acts as a fulcrum. Continued contraction of the diaphragmatic fibers pulls up and outward on the costal margin. This further increases thoracic volume.

Various pulmonary diseases may disturb this dual action of the diaphragm. For example, in advanced emphysema, air is trapped in the lungs. The trapped gas displaces the diaphragm to an abnormally low and flat position. When this happens, there is less vertical excursion during inspiration. Contraction of the costal fibers in this case pulls the lower chest boundary *inward*. This results in *narrowing* rather than expansion of the lateral dimensions of the thorax (Figure 7-24, *B*). Nonpulmonary diseases can also affect diaphragm

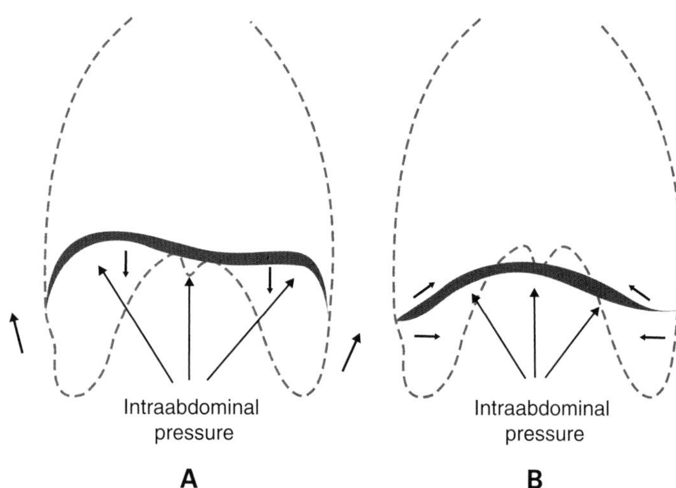

Figure 7-24

A, When a normal diaphragm contracts, it descends, gradually building up pressure in the abdomen until the intraabdominal pressure acts as a fulcrum against which continued contraction everts the costal margin, further enlarging the thorax. **B,** If the diaphragm is abnormally low at the start of inspiration, contraction can only pull in the costal margin, reducing the lower thoracic diameters.

MINI CLINI

Lung Hyperinflation and Lung Reduction in Emphysema

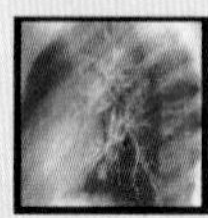

Emphysema is a disease characterized by the destruction of elastic lung tissue. This causes the emphysematous lung to have less elastic recoil than a normal lung.

PROBLEM

Why do patients with severe emphysema have enlarged, overinflated lungs? How does hyperinflation interfere with breathing? What can be done to alleviate the problem?

ANSWER

Emphysema destroys elastic fibers in the lung. This causes the lung to lose some of its natural tendency to recoil. As the disease progresses, the inward recoil force of the lung becomes less than the normal outward recoil force of the chest wall. The two oppositely directed recoil forces are no longer in balance. The stronger outward recoil force of the chest wall pulls the lung outward to a new enlarged volume. The results are an expanded chest wall and an overinflated lung at the end of a normal, quiet exhalation. Hyperinflation "flattens" the diaphragm for similar reasons, making it less effective during inspiration. Loss of elastic tissue allows small airways to collapse, resulting in "air trapping," exaggerating hyperinflation even more. Therapy for emphysema is directed at reducing the effects of air trapping. Bronchodilators may improve ventilation, reducing trapped gas and lessening the work of breathing. Maneuvers such as pursed-lip breathing may also assist in reducing gas trapping, especially during exertion. Surgical removal of overdistended lung tissue ("bullae") is known as lung volume reduction surgery. By removing nonfunctional tissue, the remaining lung may assume a more normal size and improve gas exchange at the alveolar level. The chest wall is returned to a more normal configuration and the mechanics of breathing are improved.

function. Splinting or rigidity of the abdominal wall can interfere with diaphragmatic descent during inspiration.

Although the diaphragm is the primary ventilatory muscle, it is not essential for survival. Adequate ventilation is possible using accessory muscles, even if the diaphragm is paralyzed. If either or both of the diaphragm leaves are paralyzed, the affected component(s) remains in its resting position. During deep inspiration, the paralyzed diaphragm rises as other ventilatory muscles reduce the intrathoracic pressure. During quiet breathing, the paralyzed diaphragm may remain immobile or may move in either direction. The pressures above and below a paralyzed diaphragm tend to make it rise during inspiration. The outward movement of the lower ribs tends to stretch and flatten it.

The diaphragm does not actively participate in exhalation. It returns to its resting position during the passive recoil of the thorax. During forced exhalation or against resistance, the diaphragm acts like a piston. It expels gas from the lung as it is pushed upward by increased abdominal pressure. Abdominal pressure increases because of contraction of abdominal muscles. The diaphragm performs important functions other than ventilation. It aids in generating high intraabdominal pressures by remaining fixed while the abdominal muscles contract. This facilitates vomiting, coughing and sneezing, defecation, and parturition.

Intercostal Muscles. The intercostal muscles consist of two sets of fibers located between each rib pair (Figures 7-21 and 7-25). The *external intercostal* muscles arise from the lower edge of each rib, from the tubercle to the costochondral junction. The fibers pass down and anteriorly to insert into the upper edge of the rib below. These muscles are thicker than the internal intercostals.

The *internal intercostal* muscles lie beneath the external intercostals. They arise from the lower edge of each rib from the anterior end of the intercostal space to the rib angles. The fibers pass downward and posteriorly to insert into the upper edge of the rib below.

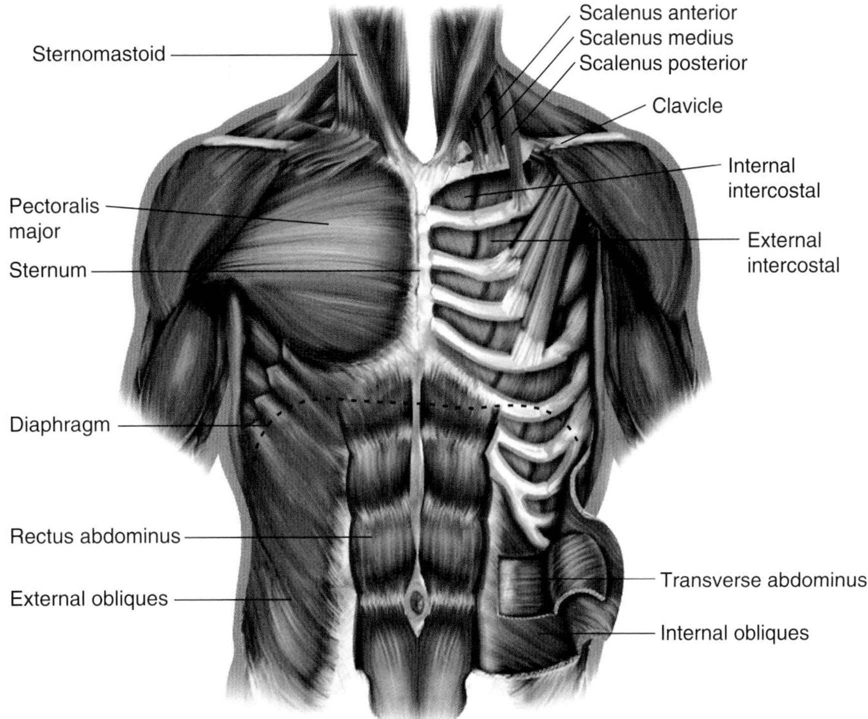

Figure 7-25

The muscles of ventilation.

MINI CLINI

Significance of Intercostal Retractions

Intercostal retractions are inward movements of the tissues between the ribs of the chest wall during inspiration. This causes the ribs to stand out prominently during inspiratory efforts.

PROBLEM

Why do infants and adults in respiratory distress with severe airway obstruction or noncompliant ("stiff") lungs exhibit inspiratory intercostal retractions?

ANSWER

The intrapleural space (i.e., space between the lungs and chest wall) normally exhibits a subatmospheric pressure. This is caused by the tendency of the lung to recoil inward while the chest wall tends to recoil outward. The magnitude of this subatmospheric pressure increases with inspiration. During inspiration, ventilatory muscles enlarge the chest, the diaphragm descends, and the intrathoracic volume increases. During normal, quiet breathing with unobstructed airways, the drop in intrathoracic pressure during inspiration is relatively small. However, if the airways become severely obstructed (e.g., foreign body aspiration or asthmatic bronchoconstriction), much greater inspiratory effort is required because of the high resistance to airflow. This increased effort translates into a much greater drop in intrathoracic pressure as the thorax enlarges and tries to pull air through obstructed airways. The drop in intrathoracic pressure "sucks" the soft tissues between the ribs inward, causing intercostal retractions. Abnormally stiff lungs (e.g., in pneumonia, atelectasis, or fibrotic lung diseases) may also cause intercostal retractions. In this case, the lungs themselves have an abnormally high recoil force that resists inflation. Again, increased inspiratory efforts reduce intrapleural pressure more than normal and intercostal retractions occur, signaling greatly increased work of breathing. Retractions may also be seen in the soft tissue above the clavicles. Retractions may not be visible in obese or muscular patients, even though abnormal pulmonary pressures are generated.

Controversy exists regarding the function of the intercostal muscles. Studies of the muscles indicate that the external intercostals and the portion of the internal intercostals between the costal cartilages are active during breathing. Contraction of these muscles during inspiration elevates the ribs, increasing thoracic volume. This action occurs primarily near the resting expiratory level. At high lung volumes, the intercostals actually lower the ribs.[28] Absence of this function is documented during paralysis. Intercostal muscles probably stabilize the chest wall and prevent intercostal bulging or retraction during large intrathoracic pressure changes. Myographic studies also reveal intercostal activity continuing from quiet inspiration into early exhalation. This expiratory activity may limit high air flows and reduce airway turbulence during exhalation. The intercostals of the lower ribs, at flows greater than 50 L/min or during maximal voluntary exhalation, also contract at end-expiration. This presumably stabilizes the chest in the presence of powerful abdominal contractions.

Retractions occur when the patient generates a large subatmospheric pressure during inspiration. This phenomenon usually occurs in the presence of severe airway obstruction or markedly stiff lungs. The best place to look for evidence of retractions is *the "notch" above the clavicles*. This is where the apices of the lungs are located and where the intrapleural pressure is lowest in an upright patient.

Scalene Muscles. The anterior, medial, and posterior scalene muscles make up a functional unit (see Figure 7-25). The **scalenes** are primarily skeletal muscles of the neck. They also function as important accessory muscles of ventilation. The scalenes arise from the transverse processes of the lower five cervical vertebrae. The anterior and medial scalenes insert into the upper surface of the first rib. The posterior scalene inserts into the upper surface of the second rib. The scalenes elevate and fix the first and second ribs. Their most important function is to assist in inspiration when the diaphragm and intercostal muscles cannot meet ventilatory demands. Such instances may occur in healthy subjects during exercise or in patients who have pulmonary disease. In healthy subjects, inspiratory efforts against a closed glottis or obstructed airway activate the scalenes. When alveolar pressure falls to –10 cm H_2O, scalenes are active in all subjects. The scalene muscles are inactive during expiratory efforts until alveolar pressure reaches ±40 cm H_2O. The function of the scalene muscles during expiration is fixation of the ribs as abdominal muscles contract. This action may prevent herniation at the apices of the lung during coughing.

Sternomastoid Muscles. The **sternomastoids** are another important accessory muscle group (see Figure 7-25). The sternomastoids help rotate and support the head. They arise bilaterally from the manubrium of the sternum and the medial end of the clavicle. Each sternomastoid courses upward and slightly posteriorly. Sternomastoids insert into the mastoid process and occipital bone of the skull. These muscles are prominent on either side of the neck. They are especially noticeable as the head turns from side to side.

When the sternomastoids function to move the head, they pull from their sternoclavicular origin. This rotates the head to the opposite side, turning it slightly upward. When the head and neck are held fixed by other muscles, the sternomastoids act as ventilatory muscles. They pull from their skull insertions to elevate the first rib and the sternum. This motion increases the AP diameter of the chest. In all subjects, the sternomastoids contract when alveolar pressures reach –10 cm H_2O. These muscles are inactive during exhalation. The sternomastoids become active at high lung volumes or with high ventilatory demands, such as during exercise.[29]

In chronic obstructive pulmonary disease (COPD) with hyperinflation, the sternomastoids may become active during inspiration. The loss of lung recoil in COPD causes the thorax to become enlarged as the lung hyperinflates. The diaphragm assumes a low, flat position and fails to function effectively, as discussed previously. The sternomastoids contract and pull up on the sternum. The ribs rotate about their neck axes but not about the rib angle–sternal junction axes. This produces an up-and-down motion but little side expansion. In severe hyperinflation, AP expansion of the thorax may cause the lower ribs to draw in, partially negating any increase in lung volume.

Pectoralis Major Muscle. A third important accessory muscle of ventilation is the **pectoralis major**. The pectoralis is a powerful bilateral anterior chest muscle. Its primary function is pulling the upper arms into the body in a hugging motion (see Figure 7-25). It arises from the clavicle, the sternum, the first six costal cartilages, and a fibrous sheath enclosing muscles of the abdominal wall. The muscle fibers converge into a thick tendon, which inserts into the upper part of the humerus. The pectoralis major forms the anterior fold of the axilla. In muscular subjects, its outlines are plainly visible beneath the skin.

When the pectoralis is used as an accessory muscle of ventilation, it pulls in a direction opposite that of its primary function. If the arms and shoulders are fixed, the pectoralis can use its insertion as an origin. Patients leaning on the elbows or firmly grasping a wide object fix the arms and shoulders. The pectoralis can then pull on the anterior chest. This motion lifts the ribs and sternum, increasing AP diameter of the thorax. Patients who have COPD often lean on their elbows or support their arms to allow use of the pectoralis. In advanced COPD, the action of this accessory muscle may provide most of the ventilation. It aids inspiration only, taking no part in exhalation.

Abdominal Muscles. Several muscles make up the abdominal wall, providing support for the abdominal contents (see Figure 7-25). Four abdominal muscle groups play an indirect but important role in ventilation.[30] These include the external and internal

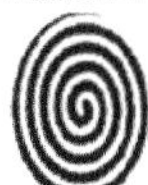

RULE OF THUMB

Patients with advanced COPD often use accessory muscles to assist the flattened diaphragm. The muscle groups used include shoulder and neck muscles normally used to move the arms and head. To use these muscles, the "shoulder girdle" must be stabilized. COPD patients often do this by *supporting their arms* on a stationary object in front of them. The back of a chair, a shopping cart, or any similar object allows the shoulders to be immobilized so that the accessory muscles can raise the anterior

obliques, the transverse abdominals, and the rectus abdominis groups.

The **external oblique** muscle arises from the lower eight ribs. Its posterior fibers insert into the iliac crest. The remaining fibers course downward and forward. They insert into a fibrous sheath (aponeurosis) with their counterparts from the other side. The **internal oblique** arises from the iliac crest and the inguinal ligament. Its posterior fibers pass upward to insert onto the last three ribs. The remaining fibers slope upward and forward to a fibrous aponeurosis.

The **transversus abdominis** arises from the costal cartilages of the lower ribs, iliac crest, and lateral part of the inguinal ligament. It courses horizontally forward to an aponeurosis. The **rectus abdominis** arises from the pubic bones. It passes upward in a sheath and inserts into costal cartilages 5 through 7.

The abdominal muscles function mainly in expiration. Their action is twofold. Contraction of the rectus abdominis decreases the distance from the xiphoid to the pubis. Contraction of the external oblique decreases the transverse diameter of the rib cage. Both actions normally decrease rib cage diameter, and hence deflate the lungs. These muscles are normally inactive during quiet breathing. They become active when the elastic recoil of the lung and thorax cannot provide the needed expiratory flow. This happens when expiratory flows reach 40 L/min (e.g., coughing, sneezing), significant resistance impedes exhalation, or gas is forcibly exhaled below the resting expiratory level. Contraction of the abdominals increases intraabdominal pressure, driving the diaphragm upward.

The abdominals can also contribute to inspiration by contracting at end-exhalation. This reduces end-expiratory lung volume, so the chest wall can recoil outward assisting the next inspiratory effort.[31] Elevating abdominal pressure increases both the length and radius of curvature of the diaphragm. Both of these effects result in greater transdiaphragmatic pressure for a given contractile tension. In COPD patients, any increase in ventilatory demand significantly increases the use of the abdominal muscles. Loss of effective use of the abdominals places patients with airway obstruction at a disadvantage.

The abdominal muscles are also used for voluntary maneuvers such as forceful expiration. Forced expiration is used in various pulmonary function tests (see Chapter 17). Such maneuvers are performed in measuring the FVC, forced expiratory flow, and maximal expiratory pressure. High intraabdominal pressures are transmitted to the lungs to generate maximal transpulmonary pressures. This results in maximal expiratory airflow, measured to assess the status of the airways. Subjects with weak or dysfunctional abdominal muscles are often unable to generate normal maximal expiratory flows.

Actions of the primary and secondary muscles of ventilation are summarized in Table 7-4.

Table 7-4 ▶▶ Summary of Respiratory Muscle Action

Level	Inspiration	Expiration
Quiet ventilation	Diaphragm in all subjects Intercostals in most subjects Scalenes in some subjects	Some persistence of inspiratory muscle contraction in expiration
Modest increase in ventilation (<50 L/min)	Diaphragm in all subjects Intercostals in most subjects Scalenes in some subjects	Some persistence of inspiratory muscle contraction in expiration
Moderate increase in ventilation (50-100 L/min)	Diaphragm in all subjects Intercostals in most subjects Scalenes in most subjects Sternomastoid action toward end of inspiration	Some persistence of inspiratory muscle contraction Abdominal and intercostals at end of expiration
Significant increase in ventilation (>100 L/min)	All inspiratory accessories active	Abdominals active throughout inspiration

INNERVATION OF THE LUNG AND THORACIC MUSCULATURE

The lung is innervated by both the autonomic and somatic nervous systems. The **autonomic nervous system** provides both motor and sensory pathways to the lung. The somatic system provides only motor innervation to the respiratory muscles.[32]

Somatic Innervation

Somatic innervation of the respiratory system consists of efferent motor stimulation of the diaphragm and intercostals (Figure 7-26).

Paired **phrenic nerves** innervate the diaphragm. The phrenic nerves originate as branches of spinal nerves C3 to C5 in the cervical plexuses. They enter the chest in front of the subclavian arteries, lateral to the carotid arteries. The phrenic nerves run down each side of the mediastinum in front of the hilar structures. The left phrenic nerve travels a longer course than the right phrenic nerve and extends around the heart. Injury to the phrenic nerves may result in paralysis of the diaphragm. Such injuries include neck trauma and chest wounds.

The intercostal muscles receive their motor innervation via the **intercostal nerves**. The intercostal nerves (T2 to T11) leave the vertebral column between adjacent vertebrae. The intercostals, unlike other spinal nerves, do not form plexuses. They go directly to the structures they innervate. The ventral rami (branches) of the intercostal nerves provide motor innervation to the intercostal muscles. The dorsal rami innervate the muscles and skin of the back.

Autonomic Innervation

Autonomic innervation is via branches of the paired vagus nerves and the upper four or five thoracic sympathetic ganglia.[33] Both contribute fibers to the anterior and posterior pulmonary plexuses at the roots of the lung (see Figure 7-26).

Efferent Pathways

Each vagus nerve, on entry into the chest, sends a branch that curves back up to the larynx. These branches are the **recurrent laryngeal nerves.** Each vagus nerve also gives off a branch called the *superior laryngeal nerve.* The external branch of this nerve supplies the cricothyroid muscle. The internal branch provides sensory

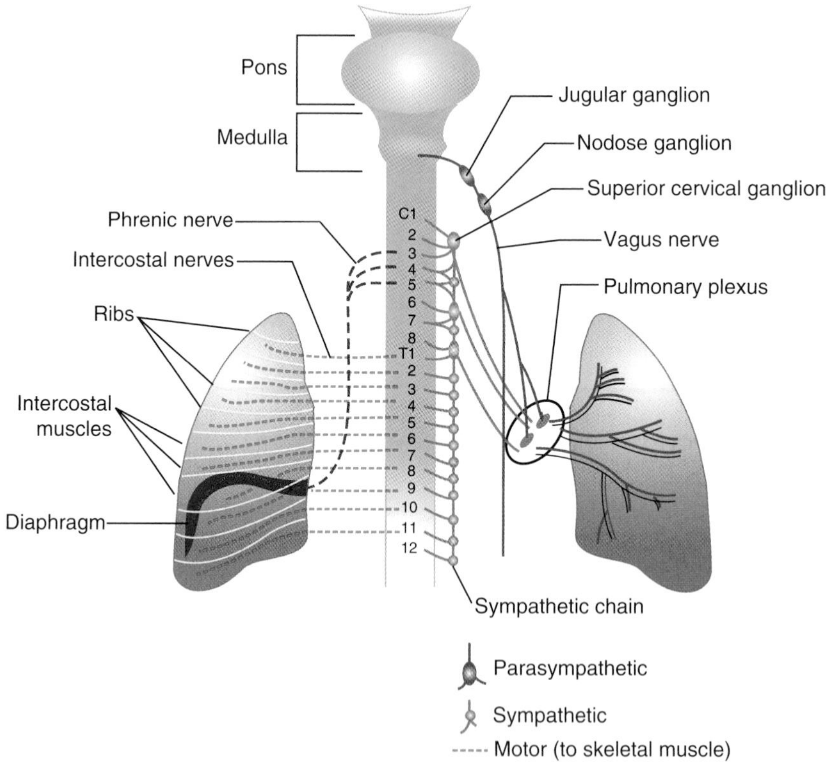

Figure 7-26

Schema of the autonomic innervation (motor and sensory) of the lung and the somatic (motor) nerve supply to the intercostal muscles and diaphragm. *(Modified from Murray JF: The normal lung, ed 2, Philadelphia, 1986, WB Saunders.)*

fibers to the larynx. The recurrent laryngeal nerves provide the primary motor innervation to the larynx. Damage to laryngeal nerves can cause unilateral or bilateral vocal cord paralysis, depending on which branches are involved. This may result in hoarseness, loss of voice, and an ineffective cough. The most common causes of laryngeal nerve damage are trauma and thoracic or mediastinal tumors.

Entering at the hilum, autonomic nerve fibers subdivide with the airways. The largest branches accompany the **bronchi**. The smallest nerve fibers parallel the pulmonary veins. Both sympathetic and parasympathetic efferents innervate the smooth muscle and glands of the airways. Anatomical and physiological evidence indicates that the parasympathetic system predominates.[3] Autonomic motor fibers from both systems combine to influence the caliber of the airways. Both systems affect the volume of the terminal respiratory units, the activity of the bronchial glands, and the diameter of the pulmonary blood vessels.[34]

Afferent Pathways

Most afferent fibers from the lungs to the CNS are vagal in origin. Important sensory paths are associated with well-defined receptors in both the airways and lung tissue. Three of these vagal receptor sites are the bronchopulmonary stretch receptors, the irritant receptors, and the J receptors. Additional receptors are located outside the lung. The muscle proprioceptors and the peripheral chemoreceptors are involved in the control of ventilation (see Chapter 13).

Characteristics of the pulmonary vagal receptors are summarized in Table 7-5.[25] Pulmonary **stretch receptors** are located in the smooth muscle of the bronchi and bronchioles. They progressively discharge during lung inflation up to the end of inspiration. This **inflation reflex** is thought to adjust the depth of inspiration. Animal studies indicate that these receptors influence the duration of the expiratory pause between breaths. The inflation reflex is probably very weak or absent during quiet breathing in healthy adults. There appears to be a strong inflation reflex only in newborn infants.[25,34]

A special reflex thought to be associated with the stretch receptors is *Head's paradoxical reflex*. This reflex stimulates a deeper breath rather than inhibiting further inspiration. It may be the basis for occasional deep breaths. Deep breaths or sighs occur with normal breathing, presumably preventing alveolar collapse. Head's reflex may also be responsible for gasping in newborn infants as they progressively inflate their lungs.[34,35]

Irritant or mechanical receptors are located in the subepithelial tissues of the larger airways.[36] They are found mainly in the posterior wall of the trachea and at bifurcations of the larger bronchi. These receptors respond to a variety of mechanical, chemical, and physiological stimuli. The stimuli include physical manipulation or irritation, inhalation of noxious gases, histamine-induced bronchoconstriction, asphyxia, and microembolization of the pulmonary arteries.[33,34]

Stimulation of the **irritant receptors** can result in bronchoconstriction, hyperpnea, glottic closure, and cough. Stimulation of these receptors can also cause a reflex slowing of the heart rate (bradycardia). This response is referred to as the **vagovagal reflex.** It may occur during tracheobronchial suctioning, intubation, or bronchoscopy. These procedures may cause significant mechanical irritation of the airway. Applying local anesthetics can blunt the vagovagal reflex.

J receptors are so named because they are found primarily in "juxtaposition" to the pulmonary capillaries. The primary role of the J receptors is their response to increases in pulmonary capillary pressures.[33,34] When capillary pressure increases, as in congestive heart failure, stimulation of the J receptors results in rapid, shallow

Table 7-5 ▶▶ Characteristics of the Three Pulmonary Vagal Sensory Reflexes

Receptor	Location	Fiber Type	Stimulus	Responses
Pulmonary stretch, slowly adapting	Association with smooth muscle of intrapulmonary airways	Medullated	Lung inflation Increased transpulmonary pressure	Hering-Breuer inflation reflex Bronchodilation
Irritant, rapidly adapting	Epithelium of (mainly) extra pulmonary airways	Medullated	Irritants Mechanical stimulation Anaphylaxis Pneumothorax Hyperpnea Pulmonary congestion	Bronchoconstriction Hyperpnea Expiratory constriction of the larynx Cough Bradycardia
Type I	Alveolar wall	Nonmedullated	Increased interstitial volume (congestion)	Rapid shallow breathing Severe expiratory constriction of larynx Hypotension, bradycardia Spinal reflex inhibition

breathing. J receptor stimulation can also cause bradycardia, hypotension, and expiratory narrowing of the glottis. Stimulation of these receptors may contribute to the sensation of dyspnea, which accompanies pulmonary edema, pulmonary embolism, and pneumonia.[25]

▶ VASCULAR SUPPLY

The vascular supply of the lungs is composed of the pulmonary and bronchial circulations. The pulmonary circulation carries mixed venous blood from the tissues through the lungs to restore its oxygen content and remove carbon dioxide. The bronchial circulation provides arterial blood to the lungs to meet their metabolic requirements. A network of lymphatics is also involved in fluid transport from the lungs. The lymphatic system removes fluid from the lung tissue and pleural space and returns it to the systemic circulation.

Pulmonary Circulation

The pulmonary circulation originates on the right side of the heart. Oxygen-depleted mixed venous blood returns to the heart via the inferior and superior vena cavae. This blood is pumped to the lungs by the right ventricle through the pulmonary artery. The main pulmonary artery exits the right ventricle and passes upward (Figure 7-27). The pulmonary artery divides into right and left pulmonary arteries just below the point of tracheal division (the carina). The pulmonary arteries accompany the right and left mainstem bronchi. This symmetry continues as the bronchi divide into the distal air spaces with the pulmonary arteries adjacent to the bronchi and bronchioles. Pulmonary arterioles extend to the terminal lung units, where they subdivide into a bed of alveolar capillaries (Figure 7-28). The alveolar capillaries provide a large surface area to exchange O_2 and CO_2 with the alveoli.[37] Arterialized blood is collected from the alveoli by the pulmonary venules, which combine into larger veins. Four to five major pulmonary veins return arterialized blood to the left atrium of the heart for delivery to the systemic circulation.

Pressures in the normal pulmonary circulatory system are only approximately one sixth of those in the systemic circulation.[37,38] Although the entire cardiac output passes through both systems, the pulmonary circulation offers a much lower resistance. The pulmonary circulation, including the right ventricle, is a

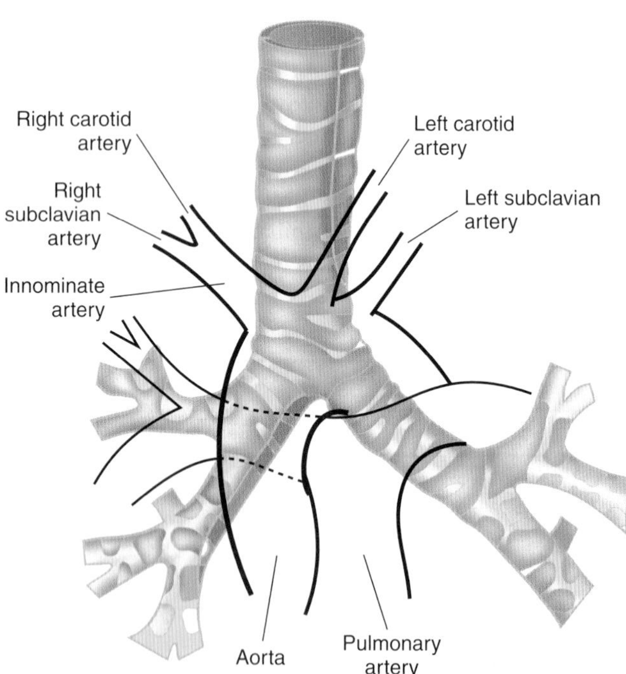

Figure 7-27

Relative positions of the trachea and mainstem bronchi with the main pulmonary artery and aorta (with their main branches) as they leave the right and left ventricles of the heart. The aorta arches over the main pulmonary artery, which divides into right and left branches that enter the lungs. The aorta supplies oxygenated blood to the remainder of the body.

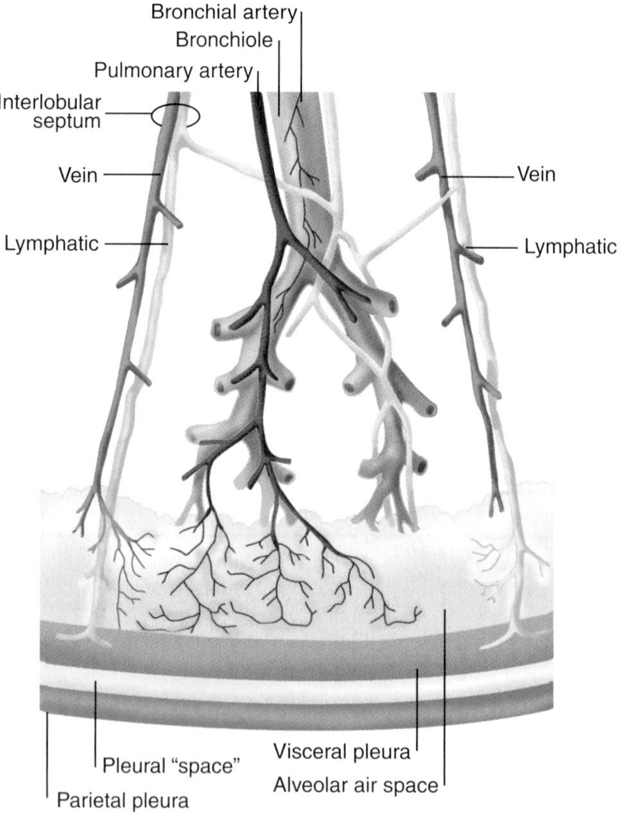

Figure 7-28

Distal pulmonary arteries, bronchioles, and air spaces with their associated bronchial arteries. Pulmonary veins lie in fibrous tissue septa between these paired pulmonary arteries and airway. Note that lymphatic channels travel with both sets of structures.

low-pressure, low-resistance system. These low vascular pressures are essential in maintaining fluid balance at the alveolar-capillary interface. Increased pressure in the pulmonary circulation, as occurs in congestive heart failure, can disrupt fluid balance. Rising backpressure from the left side of the heart can cause fluid leaks into the interstitial spaces and alveoli, impairing gas exchange.

Because the pulmonary circulation is a low-pressure system, blood flow is highly dependent on gravity. In the upright lung, hydrostatic pressure in the pulmonary vessels decreases approximately 1 cm H_2O per centimeter distance from the base to the apex.[37] Blood flow is very low at the apex of the lung in resting subjects. Perfusion increases linearly down the lung in proportion to the hydrostatic pressure, which results in the lung bases receiving nearly *20 times* as much blood flow as the apices.[13] Gravity-related effects also occur in recumbent positions, but are less pronounced. The distribution of pulmonary blood flow is closely related to pulmonary gas exchange (see Chapter 9).

Bronchial Circulation

Mixed venous blood in the pulmonary arteries lacks sufficient oxygen for the metabolic needs of the lung. A separate arterial supply called the *bronchial circulation* (see Figure 7-28) also accompanies the bronchi.[39] The metabolic needs of the lung are comparatively low, and much of the lung parenchyma is oxygenated by direct contact with inspired gas. Because of this, blood flow through the bronchial circulation is only 1% to 2% of the total cardiac output.

A single right artery arises from an upper intercostal, right subclavian, or internal mammary artery. Two bronchial arteries supply the left lung, and they branch directly from the upper thoracic aorta. Bronchial arteries follow their respective bronchi. Two or three branches accompany each subdivision of the conducting airway. The bronchial arterial circulation terminates in a plexus of capillaries that anastomose with the alveolar capillary bed.

The bronchial and pulmonary circulations share an important compensatory relationship.[25] Decreased perfusing pressure in the pulmonary arterial circulation tends to cause an increase in bronchial artery blood flow to the affected area. This minimizes the danger of pulmonary infarction, as sometimes occurs when a blood clot (pulmonary embolus) enters the lung. Similarly, loss of bronchial circulation can be partially offset by increases in pulmonary arterial perfusion. This may occur after lung transplantation. When such compensatory pathways are blocked, tissue necrosis of the affected area often results.

Lymphatics

The lymphatic system consists of a network of lymphatic vessels, lymph nodes, the tonsils, the thymus gland, and the spleen. Its primary function is to clear fluid from the interstitial spaces. The lymphatic system also plays an important role in the body's immune system. It removes

MINI CLINI

Blood Pressure in the Lung

The pulmonary circulation is a low-pressure, low-resistance system that is able to accept the entire cardiac output.

PROBLEM

How is the pressure in the pulmonary circulation measured? There are no arteries that can be easily accessed, as is the case when systemic blood pressure is measured with a blood cuff and stethoscope.

ANSWER

Blood pressure in the pulmonary circulation can be measured only by inserting a catheter into the lungs through the heart. A long catheter is usually inserted into a large systemic vein and passed through the right atrium and ventricle into the pulmonary artery. This invasive technique is complicated because the catheter, which must be small and flexible, has to get through the tricuspid and pulmonic valves in the heart. The introduction of a balloon-tipped catheter makes placement much easier. A small balloon on the end of the catheter may be inflated or deflated as necessary. The catheter is inserted with the balloon deflated. When the tip reaches the right atrium, the balloon is inflated so that it "floats" through the heart, carried along by the blood flow. Once the catheter is in the pulmonary artery, the balloon is deflated and a pressure transducer can be used to measure the systolic and diastolic pressures. The balloon-tipped catheter can also be advanced into a pulmonary arteriole so that when the balloon is inflated, backpressure from the left atrium can be measured through the pulmonary capillaries. When the balloon-tipped catheter is inflated in this position, it is said to be *wedged* into a pulmonary arteriole. The pressure from the left side of the heart is referred to as the *pulmonary capillary wedge pressure* (PCWP), or sometimes just as *wedge pressure*. Modern pulmonary artery catheters have multiple channels that permit sampling of mixed venous blood, as well as measurement of pressures, oxygen saturation, and cardiac output.

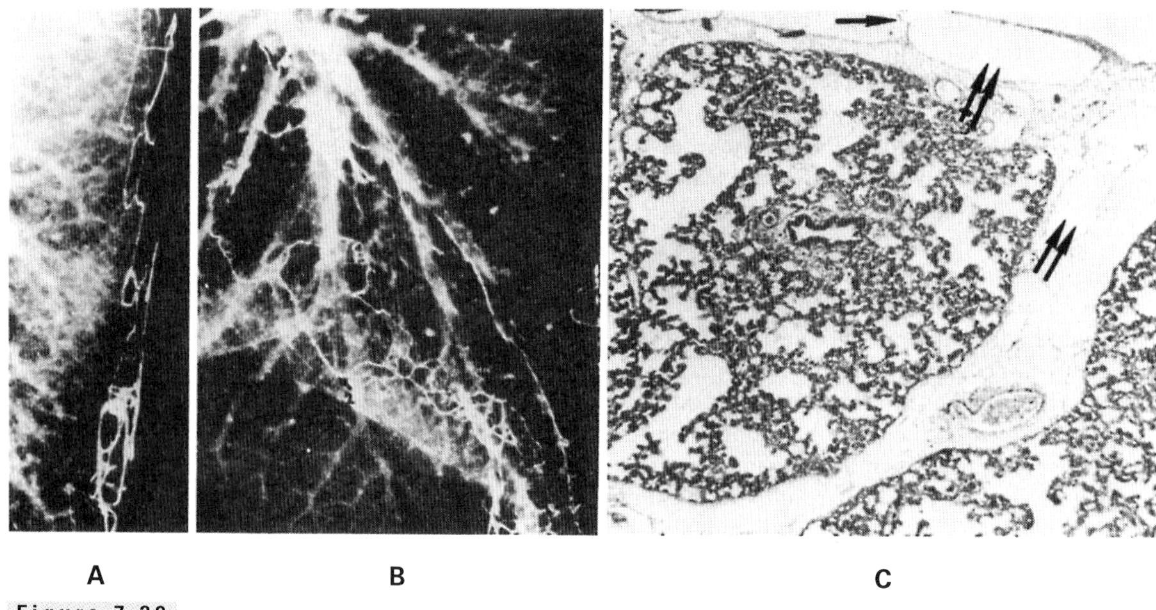

Figure 7-29

Radiographs of lymphatic channels following their infection with contrast material. **A,** The pleural lymphatics are seen in the profile. **B,** One lymphatic channel (fine structure) following a pulmonary vein. **C,** Tissue section shows pleural lymphatics *(one arrow)* and septal lymphatics *(two arrows)*. *(**A** from Trapnell DH: Br J Radiol 36:660, 1963. **B** and **C** from Heitzman ER: The lung: radiologic-pathologic correlations, ed 2, St Louis, 1984, Mosby.)*

bacteria, foreign material, and cell debris via the lymph fluid. It also produces lymphocytes and plasma cells to aid in defense. Both roles are essential for maintaining normal function of the respiratory system.

The pulmonary lymphatic system consists of superficial and deep vessels.[40] The superficial (pleural) network drains the lung surface and pleura. The deep (peribronchovascular) network drains the lung tissue. Both originate as dead-end lymphatic capillaries in their respective regions. Deep lymph vessels are closely associated with the terminal lung units. However, they do not extend to the level of the alveolar-capillary membrane. The lymphatic system works with phagocytic cells in the alveoli to provide defense against foreign material able to penetrate to the alveolar level.

Lymph fluid returns to the circulatory system through lymphatic channels that course toward the hilum.[41] These channels join in the pleura. They travel toward the hilum in the septa accompanying veins and in the bronchopulmonary artery complexes (Figures 7-28 and 7-29). Lymph flow is directed through one or more lymph nodes clustered about each hilum. From there, lymph travels through the mediastinum. It rejoins the general circulation via either the right lymphatic or the thoracic duct.

Lymphatic channels are usually not visible on chest radiographs. They may be detected if they are distended or thickened by disease (see Chapter 18). Pulmonary edema and pleural effusion become evident on chest radiographs when the lymphatic system is unable to remove excess fluid in the lung.

ANATOMY OF THE RESPIRATORY TRACT

Upper Respiratory Tract

The upper respiratory tract consists of the nasal and oral cavities, the pharynx, and the larynx (Figure 7-30). It performs four important respiratory functions.[42,43] The nose, pharynx, and larynx *conduct respiratory gases* to and from the lungs. These structures serve as frontline *defense mechanisms* for the lungs. The nasal passages also *humidify inspired air* and *exchange heat* for the respiratory system and body as a whole.

The Nose

Adults normally breathe through their noses. Conditions such as nasal polyps or mucosal edema sometimes prohibit nasal breathing. High ventilatory flows, as occur during strenuous exercise, may require mouth breathing, especially in persons with excessive nasal resistance. This resistance to flow is often caused by inflammation of the structures of the nose that heat, humidify, and filter inspired gas.

The frontal process of the maxilla, two nasal bones, cartilage, and fatty connective tissue form the external nose (see Figure 7-30). There are two flared openings called *alae*. The alae enclose a space on each side called the *vestibule*. The vestibules have hairs that act as a gross

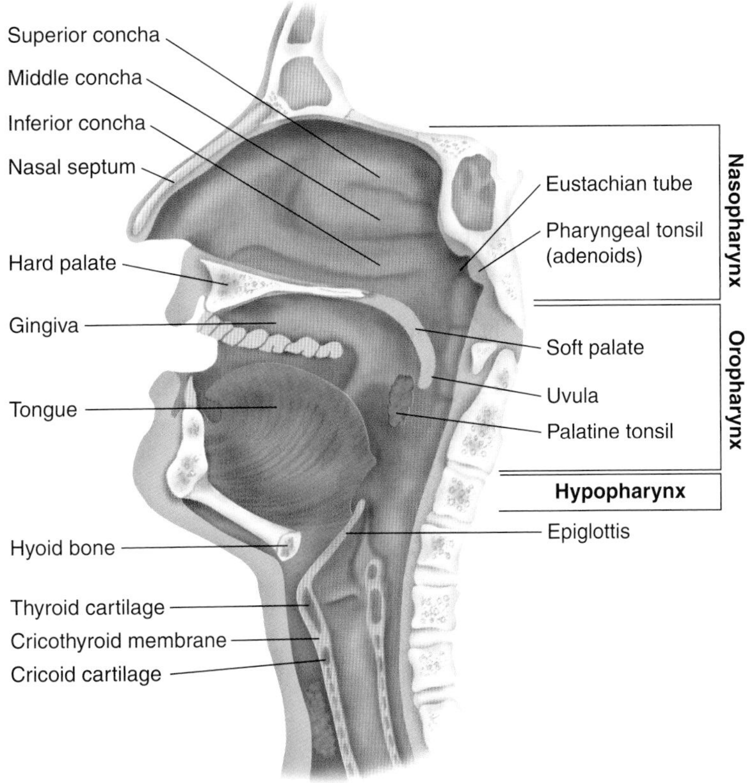

Figure 7-30

Structures of upper airway and oral cavity. The larynx is the landmark for separation of upper and lower airway.

filter. Located posterior to the vestibules are the openings to the internal nose, or the **anterior nares.** These openings have the smallest cross-sectional area in the adult respiratory tract.[42]

The internal nasal passages are separated in the midline by a **septum.** The septum is formed anteriorly by cartilage. The nasal septum commonly deviates to one side or the other. Three bony shelves project into the nasal cavity from the superior, middle, and inferior conchae. These **turbinates** divide the nasal cavities into superior, middle, and inferior passages. The olfactory receptors providing the sense of smell lie above the superior turbinates on each side.

The turbinates are lined by highly vascularized tissue. This lining consists of *pseudostratified, ciliated columnar epithelium.* This epithelium is interspersed with mucus-secreting goblet cells. These structures provide a large surface area for heat and water exchange. Both inspired and expired gases are conditioned.

The nose warms inspired air close to body temperature (37° C) and saturates inspired gas with water vapor when it reaches the nasopharynx.[42] During expiration, water vapor condenses in the nose, which retains heat and moisture for the next inhalation. The nasal mucosa functions unimpaired even in very dry environmental conditions. Bypassing the nose can severely compromise the respiratory system's ability to warm and humidify inspired gas. This occurs with endotracheal intubation or tracheostomy (see Chapter 30).

The defense function of the nose involves several mechanisms. Hairs in the vestibules act as a filter for large particles. Filtration is enhanced by the flow pattern through the nasal cavity. Inspired gas is accelerated to a high velocity through the anterior nares. It then changes direction sharply as it enters the internal nasal cavity. This pattern causes particles larger than a few microns to impact on the nasal mucosa. Ciliary action or nose blowing then clears these particles. Past the external nares, the cross-sectional area increases. This results in a decrease in gas velocity. Turbulence increases because of the narrow convolutions of the passages. Low velocity and turbulence combine to remove any remaining particles. Filtration is based on impaction, sedimentation, and diffusion.

Surface fluids originate from the goblet cells and submucosal glands. This fluid lining has mild antibacterial properties. Mucosal fluids also remove water-soluble irritant gases such as sulfur dioxide. Ciliary activity (see Figure 7-41) transports surface fluids backward. Foreign matter is then cleared by swallowing. These defense mechanisms ensure that inspired air is free from inanimate or bacterial contamination and common air pollutants.

Paranasal Sinuses

The paranasal sinuses are symmetrically paired spaces adjacent to the nasal cavity. The paranasal sinuses consist of the frontal, maxillary, ethmoid, and posterior sphenoid sinuses (Figure 7-31, *A*). All the paranasal sinuses are named for the bones in which they occur. Most of the sinuses open into the nasal cavity between the turbinates (Figure 7-31, *B* and *C*). The purposes of the sinuses are unclear, but they may provide temperature insulation, strengthen the skull without additional weight, or enhance voice resonance.[35] Problems can develop when drainage of the paranasal sinuses becomes impaired. Chronic sinus infections are a source of contaminated materials that may be aspirated into the lower respiratory tract.

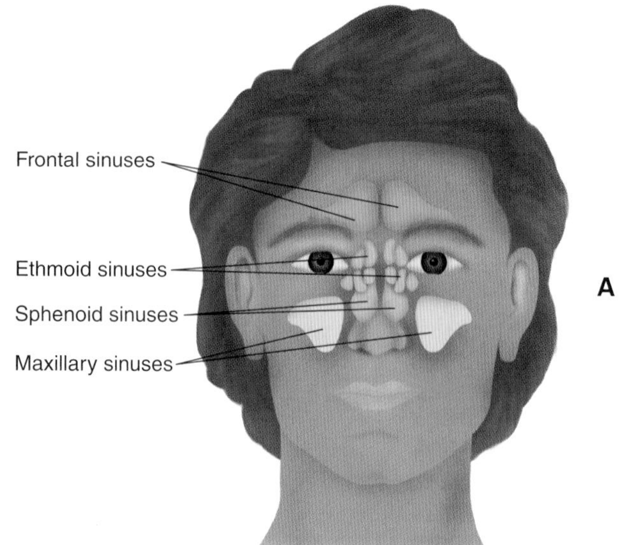

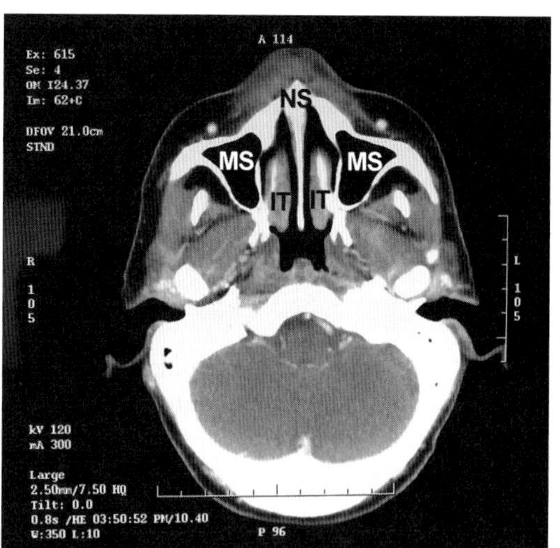

Figure 7-31

A, Positions of the frontal, maxillary, sphenoid, and ethmoid sinuses; the nasal sinuses are named for the bones in which they occur. **B,** Axial computed tomography (CT) scan at the approximate level of the inferior turbinates (IT) and maxillary sinuses (MS). The nasal septum (NS) is also well defined. **C,** Coronal CT scan showing the anterior ethmoid sinuses (AE) and the middle turbinates (MT) in addition to the structures seen in **B**.

Oral Cavity

The oral cavity serves multiple purposes. It is involved in digestion, speech, and respiration. The oral cavity is considered to be an accessory respiratory passage. In adults, mouth breathing is used mainly during speech and strenuous exercise. It also is used when upper respiratory tract infections or foreign materials obstruct the nose.

The **palate** separates the nasal cavity from the oral cavity (Figures 7-31, *B*, and 7-32). The anterior two thirds of the palate has a bony skeleton and is called the *hard palate*. The posterior third of the palate does not have such support and is called the *soft palate*. The *uvula* extends from the midline of the soft palate at the back of the mouth (see Figure 7-32). The uvula and the surrounding walls control flow in eating, drinking, sneezing, coughing, and vomiting.

The tongue is involved in mechanical digestion, taste, and phonation. The posterior surface of the tongue is supplied with many sensory nerve endings. These nerves produce a vagal gag reflex when stimulated, which protects the lungs from aspiration. This reflex must be considered when passing tubes or instruments through the mouth in conscious or semiconscious patients. The *lingual tonsils* are located at the base of the tongue.

The mucosal surfaces of the oral cavity also provide humidification and warming of inspired air. These surfaces are much less efficient than those provided by the nose. Saliva is produced by major and minor salivary glands. Saliva functions primarily as a wetting and digestive agent for food, but provides some humidification of inspired gas. The oral cavity ends at a double web on each side, called the *palatine folds*. The palatine tonsils sit between these folds on each side (see

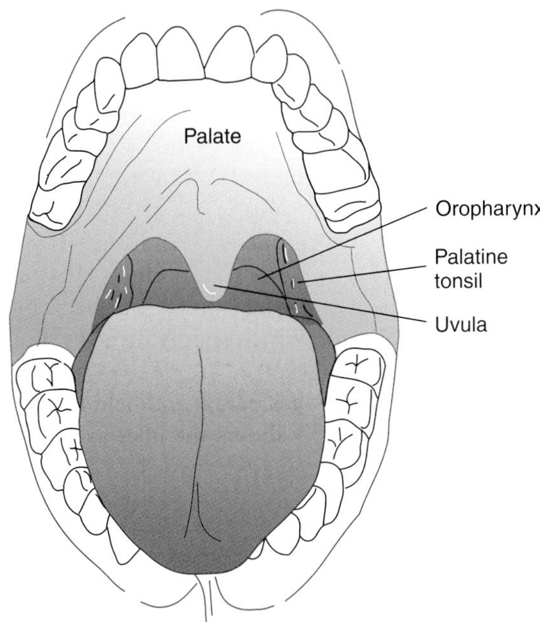

Figure 7-32

View into opened mouth. Soft midline uvula is seen hanging from fleshy palatine pillars. The pharynx is seen at the back of the mouth.

Figure 7-32). The palatine tonsils are vascularized lymphoidal tissues that play an immunological role, especially in childhood.

Reflexes from the mouth, pharynx, and larynx protect the lower respiratory tract during swallowing.[44] These protective functions can be severely compromised during anesthesia or unconsciousness. Poor oral hygiene may expose the lower respiratory tract to pathogenic bacteria, thus increasing the risk of infection.

Pharynx

The pharynx extends from the nasal cavities and mouth to the point where the airway and the digestive tract separate. It is divided into three sections: the nasopharynx, the oropharynx, and the hypopharynx (see Figure 7-30). The entire pharynx is lined with stratified squamous epithelium.

The nasopharynx lies behind the nasal cavities. The muscles of the palate occlude the nasopharynx during swallowing and coughing. The **eustachian tubes** open into the lateral nasopharynx. These tubes connect the nasopharynx with each middle ear and with the mastoid sinuses. The adenoid tonsils are located on the posterior wall of the nasopharynx.

In back of the oral cavity is the **oropharynx**. It extends from the uvula to the epiglottis and base of the tongue. Nasotracheal and nasogastric tubes must turn inferiorly at the nasopharynx to reach the trachea, lungs, or stomach.

The inferior portion of the pharynx between the epiglottis and the larynx is called the **hypopharynx**.

MINI CLINI

Opening the Airway: Snoring and Resuscitation

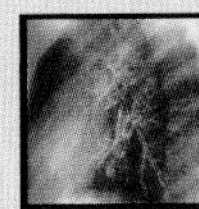

The upper airway in adults and children serves a protective role. Reflexes from the airway prevent foreign material from entering the trachea during eating and sleeping. The position, size, and shape of the upper airway also contribute to "protect" the lower airways.

PROBLEM

What are the similarities between snores and unconscious victims needing to be resuscitated?

ANSWER

Both groups may exhibit upper airway obstruction. Snoring is often associated with obstructive sleep apnea (OSA). Snorers usually exhibit narrowing of the oropharyngeal, retropalatal, and/or hypopharyngeal airways. This narrowing is often observed in obese subjects or in those with thick necks. During sleep, pressure gradients across the upper airways exaggerate the narrowing and can result in complete collapse. Sleep studies document inspiratory efforts with little or no airflow. Management of OSA includes weight loss (to reduce anatomical narrowing of the airway), nasal continuous positive airway pressure to hold the airway open, surgical correction (uvulopalatopharyngoplasty) to remove obstructing tissue, medications that alter sleep or modify neural control of breathing, and oral appliances that modify the shape of the oropharynx. Individuals who lose consciousness (such as during a heart attack) usually flex their necks. The head slumps forward, forcing anterior structures (such as the tongue) backward against the posterior pharynx. This action protects but may also completely block the airway. Opening the airway in unconscious victims is much simpler than in patients with OSA. The head is tilted back, extending the lower jaw and opening the airway. This simple maneuver is the first step in resuscitation of those suffering either a respiratory or cardiac arrest.

Immediately below the hypopharynx, the digestive and respiratory tracts separate. The shape of the hypopharynx changes dramatically during swallowing and speech.

The relative positions of the oral cavity, pharynx, and larynx are critical to the patency of the upper airway in unconscious patients. In upright subjects, the head and neck form a 90-degree angle with the axis of the pharynx and larynx (Figure 7-33, *B*). With loss of consciousness, the head flexes forward and decreases this angle (Figure 7-33, *A*). This positional change can partially or completely obstruct the upper airway. Extension of the head and lower jaw alleviates this obstruction (Figure 7-33, *C*). Extension of the head moves the tongue away from the rear of the pharynx. This technique is used to maintain the airway in unconscious patients and facilitates placement of artificial airways.

Larynx

The larynx is a complex structure located immediately below the pharynx. The larynx "hangs" from the hyoid bone at the base of the tongue. It can be palpated (felt) at the thyroid cartilage, or "Adam's apple." The larynx consists of nine cartilages and numerous muscles and ligaments (Figure 7-34). These structures combine to protect the lower airway during breathing and swallowing.[43] The major function of the larynx is sound production.

The **epiglottis** is a flat cartilage that extends from the base of the tongue backward and upward (see Figures 7-30 and 7-34). It is attached anteriorly to the hyoid bone by ligaments. Its pointed stalk attaches to the thyroid cartilage below. The epiglottis is 2 to 4 cm in length, 2 to 3 cm in width, and 2 to 5 mm in depth. It is not easily visualized in adults but it can be seen in small children and crying babies because of its higher position. The epiglottis does not occlude the airway during swallowing. It is pushed down and back by the tongue and rising larynx, which simply diverts food into the esophagus.[43]

The inlet to the larynx lies below and behind the base of the tongue. Figure 7-35 shows the inlet as it appears

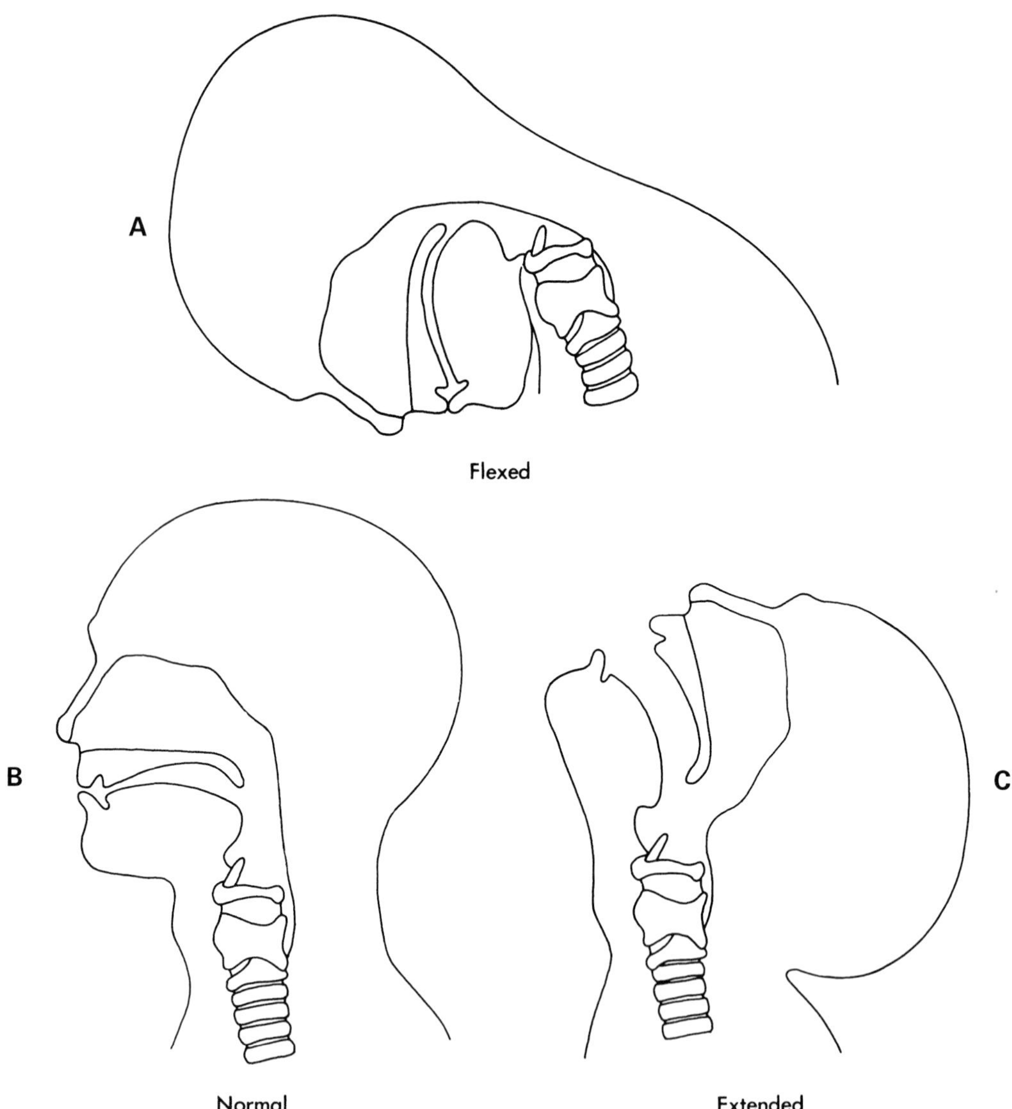

Figure 7-33

The position of the head affects patency of airway. **A,** With the head flexed, airway may be kinked, making breathing or intubation difficult. **B,** Normal upright relationship of the head and neck to the chest. **C,** Extension of the head straightens airway, making breathing, clearance of material, or intubation easier.

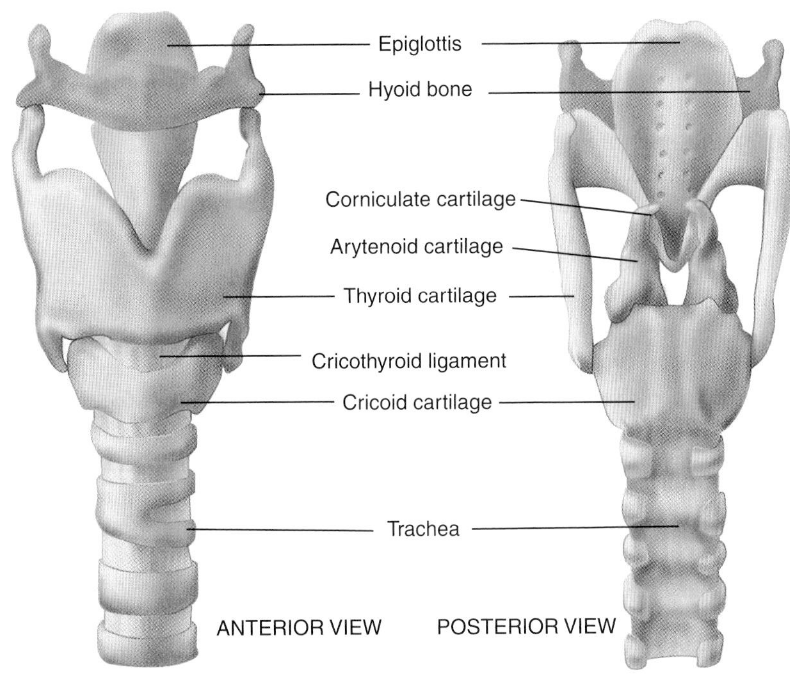

Figure 7-34

Anterior and posterior views of the laryngeal cartilages and trachea.

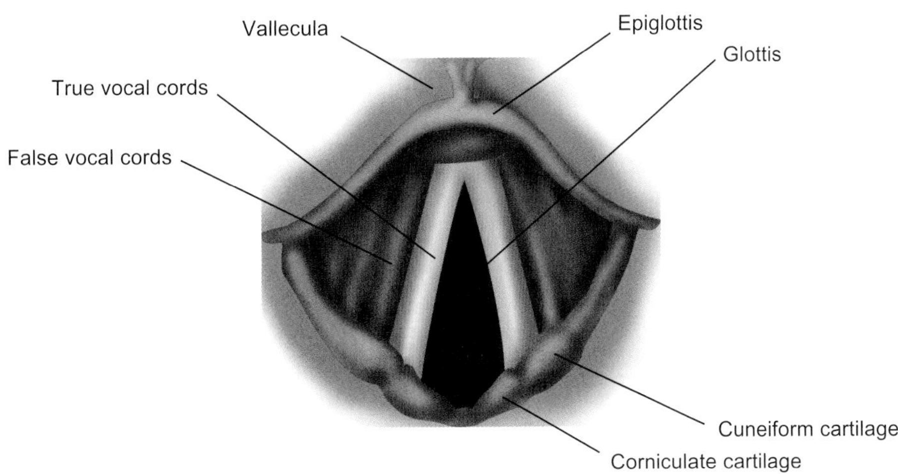

Figure 7-35

Interior of larynx.

when viewed with a laryngoscope. The base of the tongue is attached to the epiglottis by three folds. These folds form a space between the tongue and the epiglottis called the *vallecula*, which is a key landmark in oral intubation.

Above the true vocal cords are the false vocal cords. These vestibular folds can act together with the true cords to close off the lower airway, which is needed to generate an increased intrathoracic pressure. This action is essential for an effective cough. Patients who have artificial airways cannot produce an effective cough, because the artificial airway prevents the true and false cords from sealing the airway. The false cords can also completely obscure the view of the true cords, especially during reflex contraction of the laryngeal muscles. The true vocal cords appear as white-bordered veils, separated by a space known as the **glottis**. The vocal cords are composed of muscle, ligament, and submucosal soft tissue. They have a mucous-membrane covering. The tissue below this mucous membrane readily accumulates fluid. Because the lymphatic drainage to this area is sparse, swelling caused by the fluid resolves slowly.

The vocal cords project from the paired arytenoid cartilages. Sound is produced by vibration of the cords in the air stream. The distance between the vocal cords changes with adduction or abduction of the arytenoids. These movements alter the pitch produced by varying the tension on the vocal cords. Varying the volume of air passing the cords varies the sound intensity. The cords may flutter during normal breathing. They are drawn apart during inspiration by active muscular contraction and relax toward the midline during expiration (Figure 7-36).

The lower border of the larynx is formed by a ring called the **cricoid cartilage** (see Figure 7-34). The cricoid cartilage is the only rigid structure that completely encircles the airway. Its inner diameter sets the limit for the size of endotracheal tubes passed through the larynx. The cricoid ring is the narrowest portion of the airway in infants.

Between the thyroid and cricoid cartilages, a membranous space can be palpated. This space is called the *cricothyroid ligament* (see Figure 7-34). Emergency opening of the airway, called a *cricothyrotomy*, may be performed through this ligament. Catheters for removal of secretions, supply of supplementary oxygen, or ventilation can be inserted through the cricothyroid ligament. Because of the proximity of the laryngeal nerves and vocal cords, extreme caution must be used in these procedures. True surgical tracheostomy is usually placed 1 to 3 cm below the cricoid cartilage.

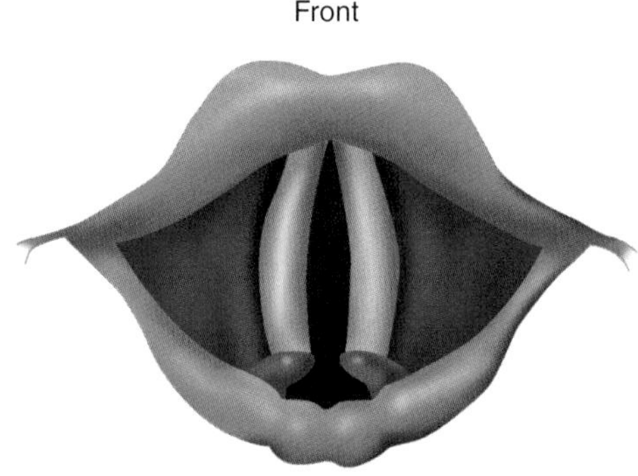

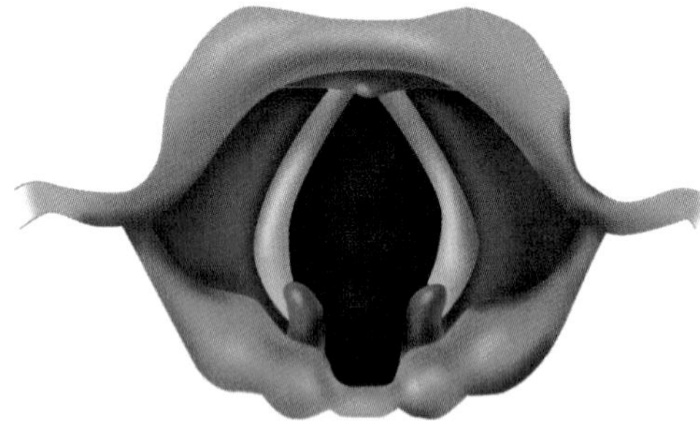

Figure 7-36

View into larynx from the back of the mouth to the front. Vocal cords vary in tension, length, and relationship to one another. Note open (abducted) inspiratory position *(top)* versus expiratory or resting closed (adducted) position *(bottom)*. The inside of the trachea with its cartilaginous rings can usually be seen through the opening between the vocal cords.

Lower Respiratory Tract

Trachea

The trachea marks the beginning of the conducting system, often called the *tracheobronchial tree*. The trachea is a tubular structure that begins at the cricoid cartilage. It proceeds through the neck into the mediastinum. The trachea extends to the articulation between the manubrium and body of the sternum (angle of Louis). At this point it divides into two mainstem bronchi.

The adult trachea averages 2.0 to 2.5 cm in diameter, ranging from 10 to 12 cm in length. The trachea's support comes from 16 to 20 C-shaped cartilaginous rings. Each tracheal ring is 4 to 5 mm high. At the back of the trachea, a thin tracheal muscle (the *musculus trachealis*) extends between the ends of the cartilages (Figure 7-37). This structure provides support, yet allows variation in diameter. The portion of the trachea within the thorax is particularly affected by pressure differences across its walls. The most dramatic compression occurs during coughing.[43] High intrathoracic pressures cause the posterior wall to "collapse" inward. This narrows the tracheal lumen and generates very high flows.

The trachea is almost midline in the neck. In the upper mediastinum it deviates slightly to the right, which allows room for the aorta to pass by on its left side (Figure 7-38). There is a sharp cartilage at the point of tracheal bifurcation. This cartilage, called the **carina**, divides flow to the right or left side. The right mainstem bronchus angles off at 20 to 30 degrees from the midline. The left mainstem bronchus deflects more sharply at 45 to 55 degrees (see Figure 7-38). Objects aspirated in upright subjects have a tendency to follow the straighter course into the right mainstem bronchus. In supine subjects, aspiration goes into the dependent lung units.

Airway Divisions and Segmental Anatomy

Each mainstem bronchus divides into branches that supply the lung lobes. The right mainstem bronchus gives rise to the upper lobe bronchus, then divides into the middle and lower lobe bronchi. The left mainstem bronchus divides into upper and lower lobe bronchi. The left lung lacks a middle lobe. A division of the left upper lobe, the **lingula**, corresponds to the right middle lobe. Its bronchus arises from the left upper lobe bronchus.

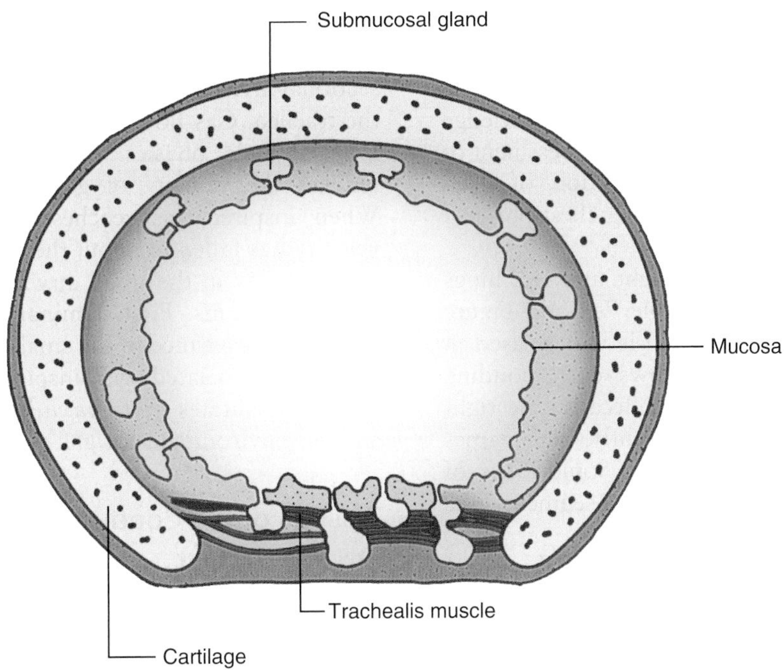

Figure 7-37

The trachea is composed of C-shaped cartilaginous rings connected posteriorly by a membrane-covering thin tracheal muscle. This arrangement allows variation in tracheal caliber. Note mucosal and submucosal glands lining the airway.

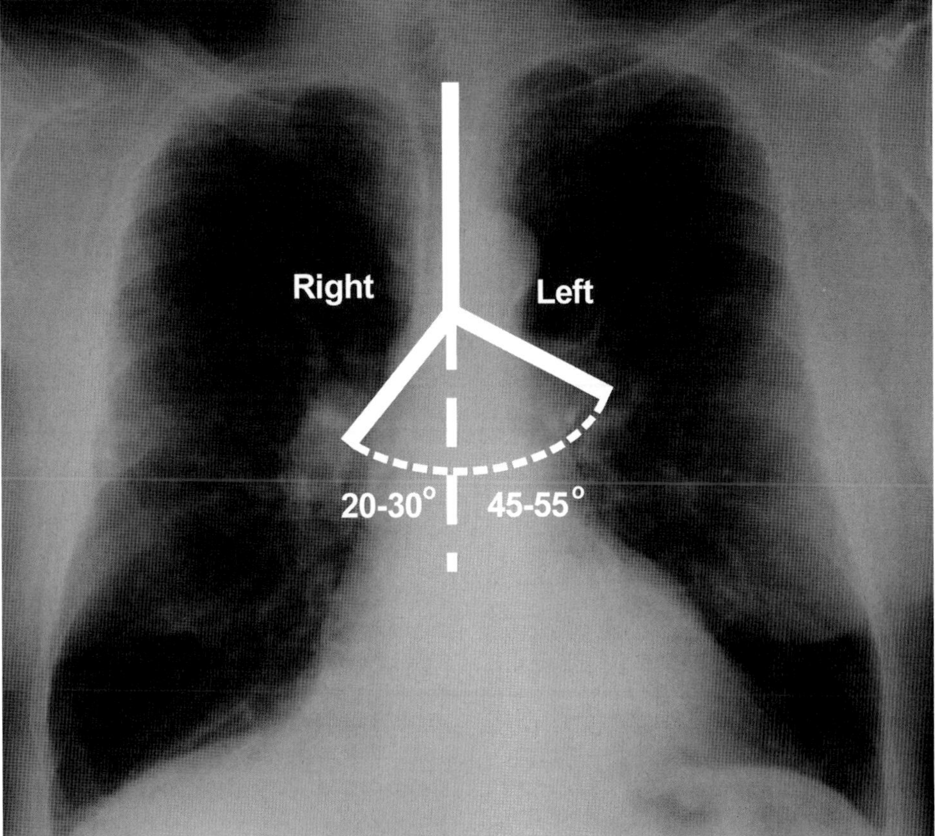

Figure 7-38

Course of trachea and right and left mainstem bronchi, superimposed on a standard chest x-ray. Notice that the right mainstem bronchus continues on a straighter course from midline than does the left mainstem bronchus.

The lobes are divided into anatomical units called *bronchopulmonary segments*. There are normally 10 segments in the right lung and 8 segments in the left lung (Table 7-6 and Figure 7-39). Detailed knowledge of segmental anatomy is useful in physical assessment of the thorax. Understanding the orientation of each segment is necessary for those providing chest physical therapy (see Chapter 37).

The segmental patterns of the right and left lungs are similar, except as noted in Table 7-6 and Figure 7-39. A standardized naming system is widely used in North America.[45] This system shows corresponding segments on the left and right lung. Because the right middle lobe and the lingula differ slightly, their names describe their segmental relationships. Some lobes of the left lung are combined to form single segments (see Table 7-6).

The bronchi continue to divide into smaller, but more numerous airways.[46] Each branch gives rise to two lower "generations" (Table 7-7). Lobar bronchi divide into segmental bronchi, which divide into subsegmental bronchi. These divisions continue until airways, called the **bronchioles**, arise. Bronchioles begin 5 to 14 generations below the segmental bronchi. They are 1 to 2 mm in diameter and are referred to as the *small airways*. Bronchioles are the smallest "conducting" airways of the lower respiratory tract. They differ from the larger airways in that they lack cartilage in their walls.

With further divisions, the number of airways increases tremendously. The cross-sectional area of the conducting system increases exponentially (see Table 7-7). At the level of the terminal bronchioles, the cross-sectional area is approximately 20 times greater than at the trachea. Gas flow in these airways conforms to the laws of fluid physics. Increased cross-sectional area reduces the velocity of gas flow during inspiration. When inspired gas reaches the alveoli, its average velocity has fallen to about the same rate as diffusion.[47] Low velocity in the small airways and alveoli is useful for two reasons. First, **laminar flow** develops, which minimizes resistance in the small airways and decreases the work associated with inspiration. Second, low gas velocity facilitates *rapid mixing* of gases. This provides a stable environment for gas exchange.[48]

Tissues of the Conducting Airways

The walls of all the conducting airways share a similar gross structure. However, they vary considerably in the number and types of cellular elements (Figure 7-40). All conducting airways have three major tissue layers. These layers are the mucosa, the submucosa, and a connective tissue envelope called the *adventitia*.[49]

The **mucosa** is composed of an epithelial lining and a layer of connective tissue known as the *lamina propria*. Between these tissues is a basement membrane. The primary cell type of the mucosa in the larger airways is *pseudostratified, ciliated columnar epithelium*. Between these ciliated cells are mucus-secreting goblet cells. Basal cells are also found on the basement membrane

Table 7-6 ▶▶ Bronchopulmonary Segments*

Segment	Number	Segment	Number
Right Upper Lobe		**Left Upper Lobe**	
Apical	1	Upper division	
Posterior	2	Apical-posterior	1 and 2†
Anterior	3	Anterior	3
Right Middle Lobe		Lower division (lingula)	
Lateral	4	Superior lingula	4
Medial	5	Inferior lingula	5
Right Lower Lobe		**Left Lower Lobe**	
Superior	6	Superior	6
Medial basal	7	Anterior basal	7 and 8
Anterior basal	8	Lateral basal	9
Lateral basal	9	Posterior basal	10
Posterior basal	10		

*The subdivisions of the lung and bronchial tree are fairly constant. Slight variations between right and left sides are noted by combined names and numbers.
†**Note:** Some authors feel that the left lung should be numbered so that there are eight segments, where the apical-posterior is numbered 1 and the anteromedial is numbered 6.

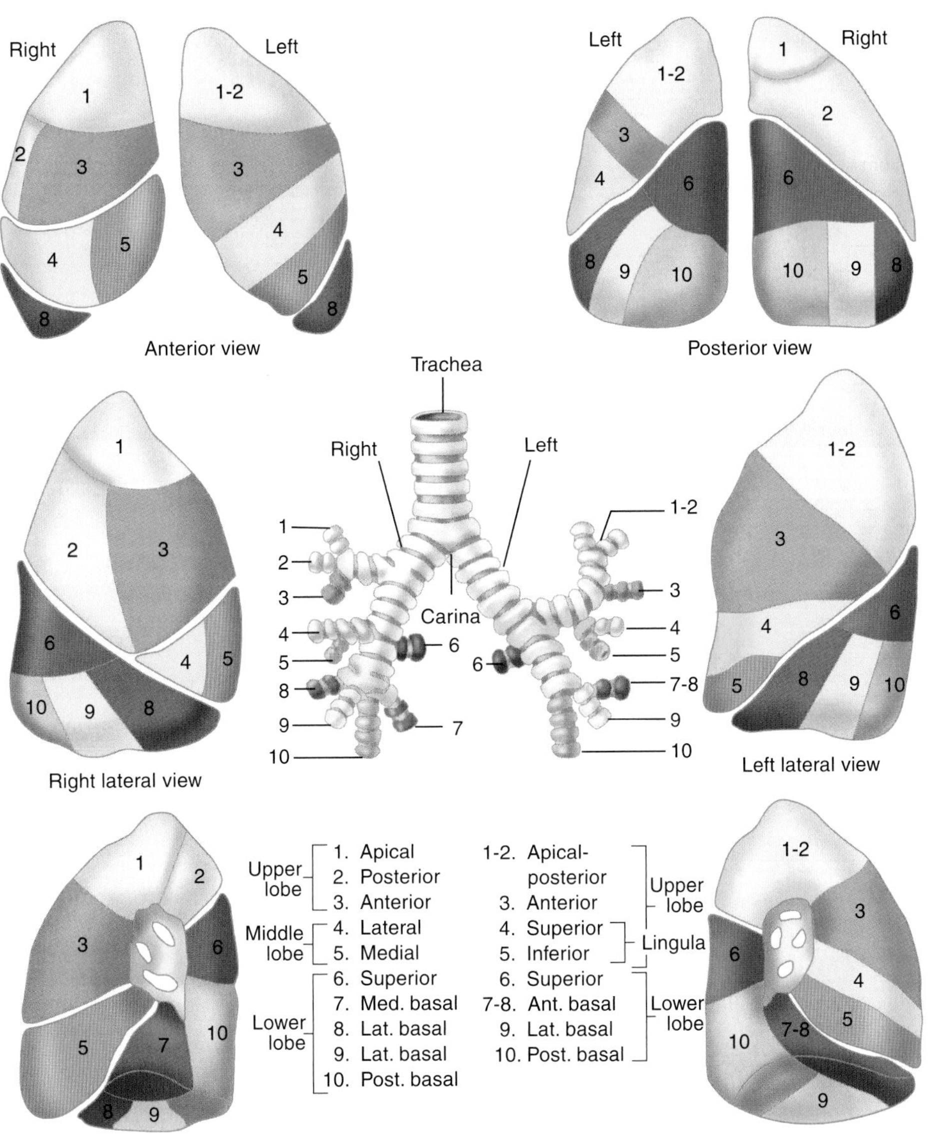

Figure 7-39 Bronchopulmonary segments diagrammed in different views (anterior, posterior, lateral, medial). Note similarities with minor variations between the right and left lungs.

Table 7-7 ▶▶ Bronchial and Bronchiolar Divisions

Structure	Trachea	Segmental Bronchus	Terminal Bronchiole	Number	Diameter of Individual Structures	Total Cross-sectional Area
Cartilaginous Conducting Structures						
Trachea	0			1	2.5 cm	5.0 cm^2
Main bronchi	1			2	11-19 mm	3.2 cm^2
Lobar	2-3			5	4.5-13.5 mm	2.7 cm^2
Segmental	3-6	0		19	4.5-6.5 mm	3.2 cm^2
Subsegmental	4-7	1		38	3-6 mm	6.6 cm^2
Bronchi		2-6		Varies	Varies	Varies
Terminal bronchi		3-7		1000	1.0 mm	7.9 cm^2
No Cartilage in Walls						
Bronchioles		5-14		Varies	Varies	Varies
Terminal bronchioles		6-15	0	35,000	0.65 nn	116 cm^2
Respiratory bronchioles			1-8	Varies	Varies	Varies
Terminal respiratory bronchioles			2-9	630,000	0.45 mm	1000 cm^2
Alveolar ducts/sacs			4-12	4×10^6	0.40 mm	1.71 m^2
Alveoli				300×10^6	0.25-0.30 mm	70 m^2

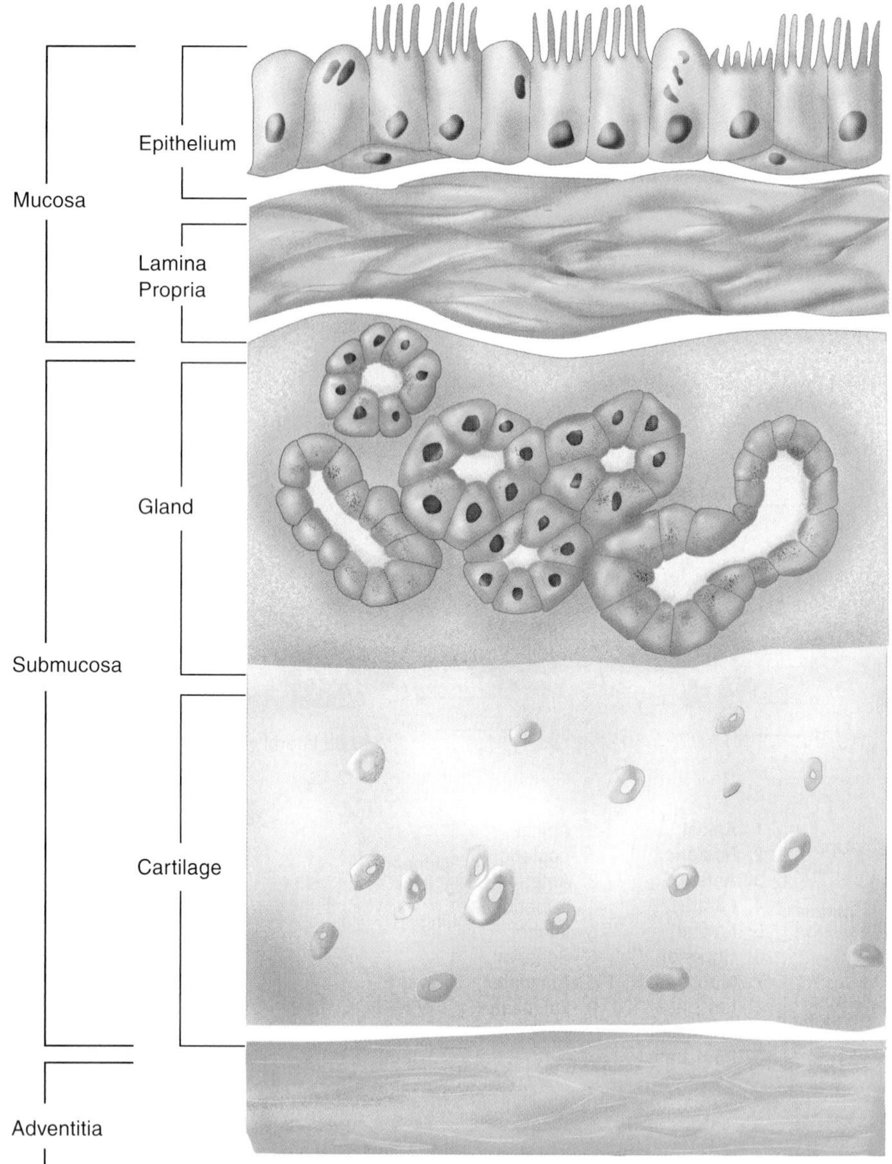

Figure 7-40

Various tissue layers in the trachea, illustrating not only the epithelium but also the underlying lamina propria and submucosal glands. Ducts from these glands (not shown) reach the tracheal lumen and allow secretions to be added to the mucus layer. Incomplete rings (cartilage layer) ensure a noncollapsible tube for airflow.

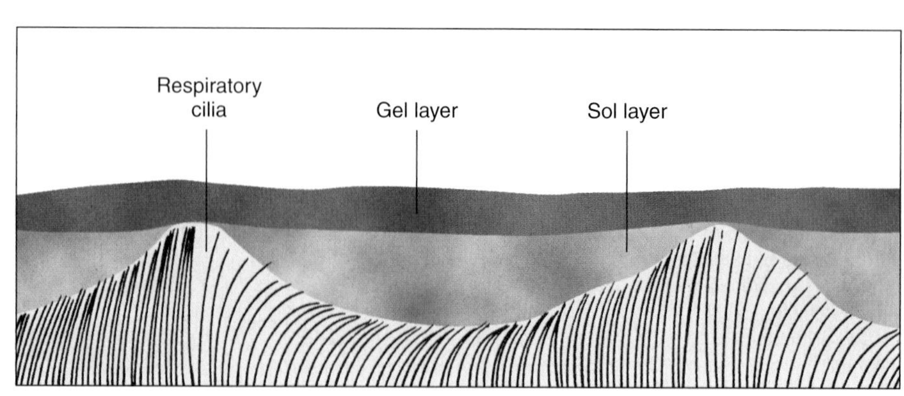

Figure 7-41

Respiratory cilia are bathed in the sol portion of the mucus layer above them. Their power strokes allow mucus movement in the viscous gel layer, always in the same direction.

MINI CLINI

Exercise-Induced Bronchospasm

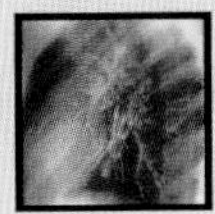

The upper airway, along with the trachea and mainstem bronchi, plays a critical role in conditioning the air that people breathe. These airways not only conduct gas from the atmosphere to the lower airways, but they also warm, humidify, and filter it.

PROBLEM

Some individuals experience shortness of breath, wheezing, and coughing when they exercise. How are many of the same subjects able to swim vigorously with few asthmalike symptoms?

ANSWER

Exercise-induced asthma (EIA) or bronchospasm (EIB) appears to be triggered by reflexes from the large airways (upper airway, trachea, bronchi). These airways warm and humidify inspired gas. Water vapor is absorbed from the fluid lining of the airways and is replenished from the cells lining the airways. As gas is expired, it cools and some of the water vapor is reabsorbed. Only a small amount of water is lost from the body via this mechanism. Exercise (with its increased ventilatory demands) causes an increase in the heat and water loss from the airways. The airways of some individuals are especially sensitive ("hyperresponsive"). When these subjects exercise and increase their ventilation, the loss of heat and/or water from the large airways can trigger an asthmatic reaction (i.e., coughing, wheezing, and shortness of breath). The phenomenon is especially noticeable when susceptible subjects exercise in cold, dry conditions. Asthma is sometimes diagnosed by having patients hyperventilate breathing cold, dry gas and then measuring how much airflow decreases. Swimming usually involves exercise in a warm, high-humidity environment. The preconditioned air breathed during swimming often reduces or eliminates EIB. Many asthmatic children can swim vigorously with few symptoms, even though other sports trigger their bronchospasm. For activities other than swimming, bronchodilators may provide protection from EIB.

beneath these primary cell types. Basal cells are thought to differentiate into ciliated and goblet cells. This occurs in the normal growth process and in mucosal repair.[50]

The ciliated cells of the mucosa clear and defend the respiratory tract. Each of these cells has approximately 200 cilia. Consequently, there are 1 to 2 billion cilia per square centimeter of mucosa.[49] Each cilium is approximately 6 to 7 mm long. These cilia "beat" in a rhythmic manner approximately 20 times each second, which produces a sequential motion of the cilia called a *metachronal wave* (Figure 7-41). The metachronal "wave length" is approximately 20 mm and propels surface material in a specific direction. In the nose, this motion propels material back to the pharynx. From the bronchioles up to the larynx, it moves material toward the pharynx. In healthy lungs, this mechanism allows inhaled particles to be removed within 24 hours.[51]

The effectiveness of ciliary action depends on the fluid layer above the mucosal epithelium.[52] Inhaled particles are carried on a mucous blanket on top of the cilia. The cilia beat in a less viscous *sol* layer (see Figure 7-41). Drying of the respiratory mucosa inhibits ciliary action. Excessive mucous production and certain drugs also alter ciliary clearance. Anticholinergic agents, such as atropine, slow the rate of movement of the mucous blanket, which may be a result of their drying effects on the production of secretions. Drugs that stimulate the parasympathetic nervous system can increase ciliary activity.

Beneath the lamina propria of the mucosa is the submucosa (see Figure 7-40). The submucosa of large airways contains *bronchial glands*, a capillary network, smooth muscle, and elastic tissue. Bronchial glands vary in size up to a millimeter in length and connect to the bronchial surface by long, narrow ducts. These glands are the major source of respiratory tract secretions in healthy lungs. The number of these glands increases significantly in diseases such as chronic bronchitis. **Mast cells** are also found in the submucosa and release potent vasoactive substances such as histamine.[53] Histamine causes vasodilation and bronchoconstriction, acting directly on smooth muscle. This type of inflammatory reaction is characteristic of diseases such as asthma.

The smooth muscle of the airways varies in location and structure. In the large airways (e.g., the trachea) smooth muscle is bundled in sheets. In smaller airways, smooth muscle forms a helical pattern. Muscle fibers crisscross and spiral around the airway walls. This placement reduces the diameter of the airway and shortens it when the muscle contracts. This pattern of smooth muscle continues into the terminal lung units, even to the alveolar ducts.

Between the submucosa and adventitia of the large airways are incomplete rings or plates of cartilage, which provide structural support for the larger airways (see Figure 7-40). The small airways depend on transmural pressure gradients and the "traction" of surrounding elastic tissues to remain open. During a forced expiration, pressures across the walls of the small airways exceed the supporting forces of the elastic tissues. As a result, the small airways can collapse. The cartilage in the larger airways prevents their collapse during such maneuvers.

The adventitia is a sheath of connective tissue that surrounds the airways. It is interspersed with bronchial arteries, veins, nerves, lymph vessels, and adipose tissue.

The cells of the respiratory mucosa change as they progress into the smaller airways (Figure 7-42). As the thickness of the airway walls decreases, bronchial

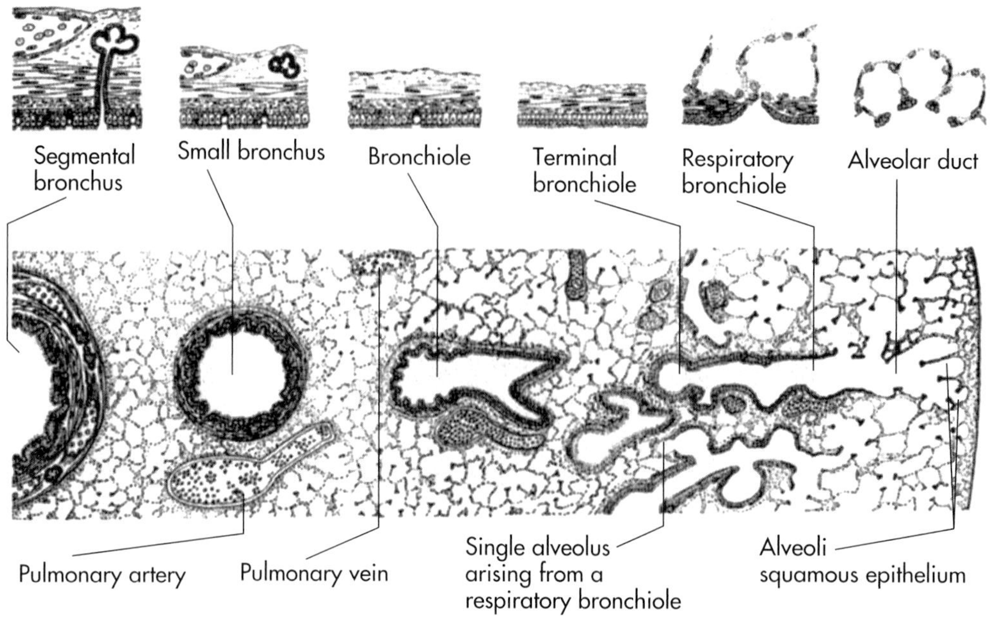

Figure 7-42

Histological diagram of airways from the segmental bronchus to the alveolus. *(From Freeman WH, Bracegridle B: An atlas of histology, London, 1966, Heinemann Educational.)*

glands become fewer in number. At the bronchiolar level, the number of ciliated cells decreases. Simple columnar and cuboidal epithelial cells begin to predominate, which are interspersed with goblet cells.

Transitional and Respiratory Zones

The terminal bronchioles begin about 17 generations beyond the trachea. All of the airways above the terminal bronchioles simply condition and/or conduct gases. Further subdivisions below the terminal bronchioles are unique passageways called *respiratory bronchioles* (Figures 7-43 and 7-44).

Respiratory bronchioles have a dual function. Like conducting airways, not only do they move gas but they also have alveolar pouches on their surfaces that allow gas exchange. The respiratory bronchioles constitute the *transitional zone* in the lung. They lie between zones dedicated purely to conduction and gas exchange.

The primary function of the lung—gas exchange—takes place in the *terminal respiratory unit*.[25] Terminal respiratory units begin at approximately the seventeenth division of bronchi and consist of all structures distal to a terminal bronchiole (see Figure 7-43). Terminal units have two to five orders of respiratory bronchioles. These are followed by a similar number of generations of *alveolar ducts*. Alveolar ducts are only as long as they are wide and terminate in clusters of 10 to 16 alveoli.

The alveolus is the final anatomical unit in the respiratory system and is the primary site of gas exchange. Adult lungs have approximately 300 million alveoli. The surface area for gas exchange ranges from 40 to 100 m^2, averaging 70 m^2. By comparison, the lung has 35 times more surface area than the skin in the average adult. The architecture of the alveolar region is essentially a pocket of air surrounded by a thin membrane containing an extensive capillary network (see Figures 7-44 and 7-45).

Scanning electron microscopy of the alveoli provides a detailed view of their various structures (Figure 7-46). The two principal cells found in the alveolus are type I, *squamous pneumocytes*, and type II, *granular pneumocytes* (see Figure 7-45). Type I cells are the very thin, flat cells that line the alveoli. Openings between type I cells (called the **pores of Kohn**) provide communication between adjacent alveoli. Type II cells are cuboidal, are also called *septal cells*, and are more numerous than type I cells. Because of their shape they occupy less than 5% of the alveolar surface. These cells are thought to be the source of the surface-active substance called pulmonary surfactant.[54] Type II cells proliferate in cases of injury. They may also give rise to new type I cells.

A third cell type found in the alveoli is the **alveolar macrophage** (see Figure 7-46). These are phagocytic

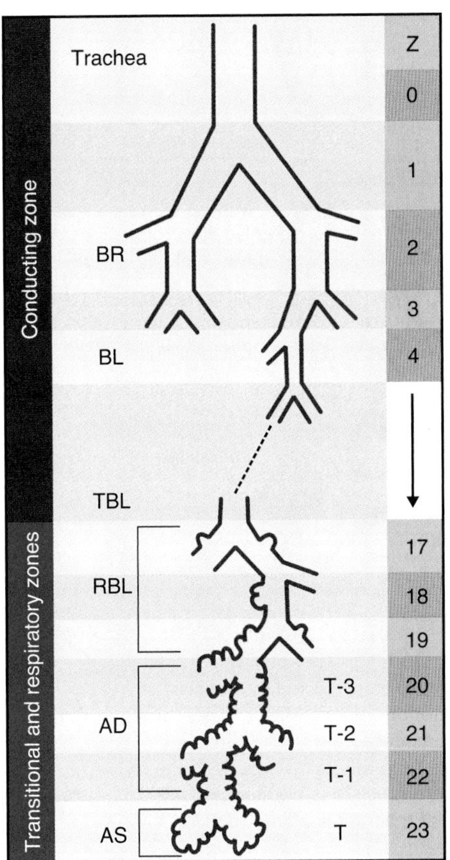

Figure 7-43

The airways that only conduct gases back and forth are designated the conducting zone of the lung. These include approximately the first 17 divisions of the tracheobronchial tree. The unit where gas exchange occurs, from respiratory bronchiole to alveolar space, is called the *respiratory zone. AD,* Alveolar duct; *AS,* alveolar space; *BL,* bronchiole; *BR,* bronchus; *RBL,* respiratory bronchiole; *TBL,* terminal bronchiole; *Z,* order of airway division. *(Modified from Weibel ER: Morphometry of the human lung, Heidelberg, 1963, Springer-Verlag.)*

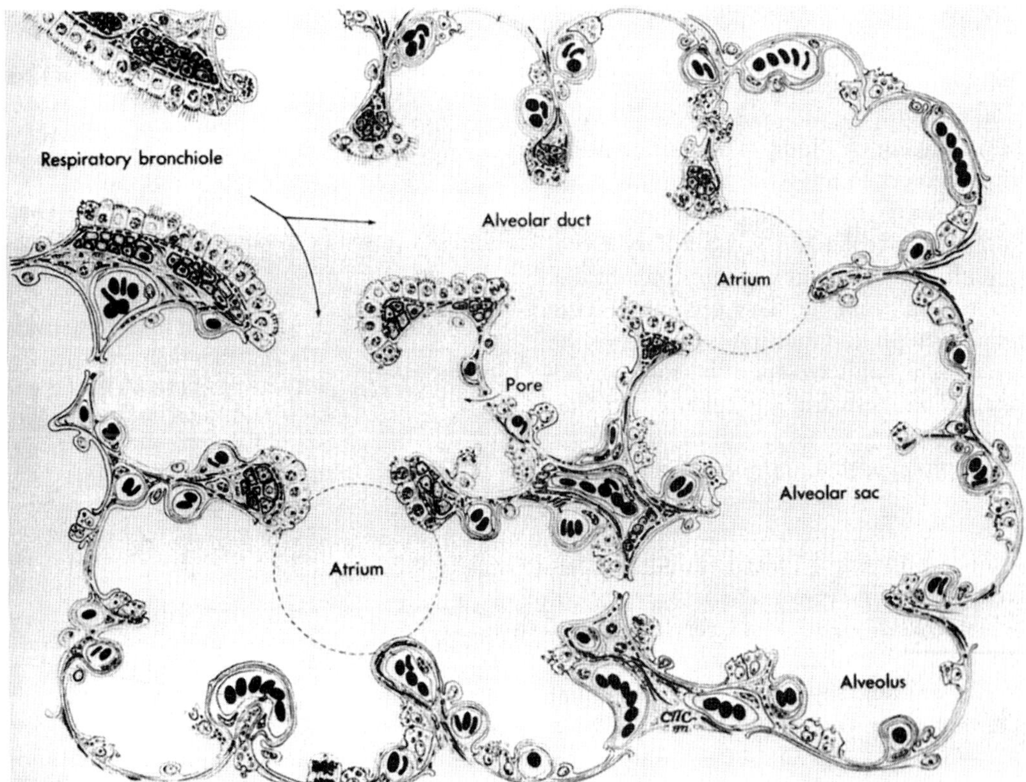

Figure 7-44

Microscopic view of terminal airways. These units compose the respiratory zone of the lung. *(From Sorokin SP: The respiratory system. In Greep RO, Weiss L, editors: Histology, New York, 1973, McGraw-Hill.)*

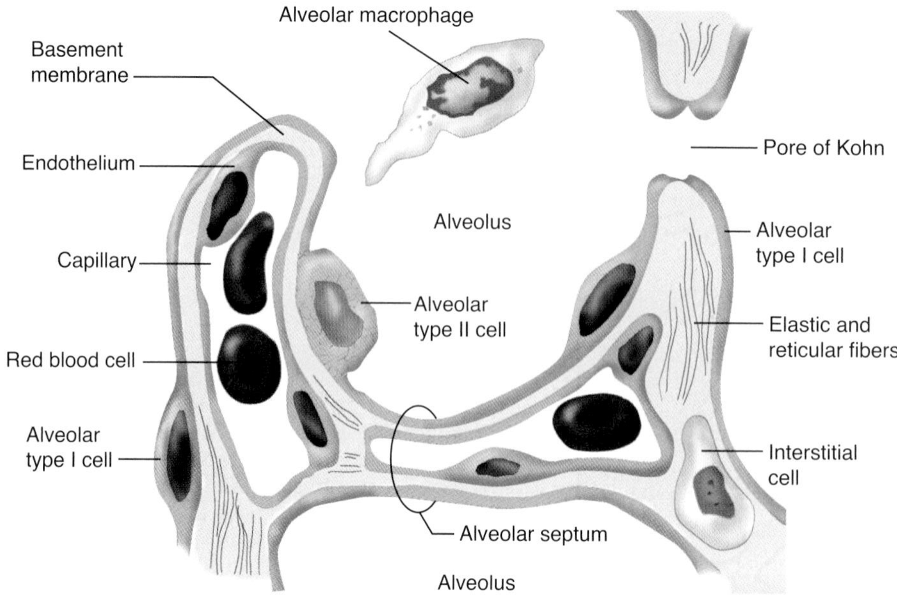

Figure 7-45

Magnified view of an alveolus. Alveolar walls, or septa, are occupied mainly by capillaries. The basement membrane of the capillary is fused with that of the alveolar lining. The interstitium contains a few interstitial fibers, composed mostly of reticular support fibers, elastic fibers, and one interstitial cell. An incomplete portion of the alveolar septum, called a *pore of Kohn*, is shown (see also Figure 7-46). Type I lining cells are very flat. The small distance between blood and air makes gas exchange remarkably efficient. Type II cells are much less numerous than type I cells. Type II cells are the source of surfactant. The alveolar macrophages are mobile phagocytic cells that migrate into the alveoli from the bloodstream.

cells that clear bacteria and other material invading the alveoli.[55] Alveolar macrophages, unlike types I and II cells, do not originate in the lung. They differentiate from stem cell precursors in the bone marrow and are transported to the lung by the circulatory system.[25]

The tissue between alveolar air and capillary blood is the *alveolar septum* or **alveolar-capillary membrane.** Each septum contains a dense capillary network (Figure 7-47, *A*). The short length and multiple branches of the capillaries around the alveolus present a sheetlike surface for gas exchange. This network is structured so that 100 to 300 mL of capillary blood is spread over 70 m^2 of surface. For example, each square meter of alveolar surface would be covered by just a teaspoon of blood.

In addition to the large surface area for gas exchange, the distance between alveolar gas and blood is small. The alveolar-capillary membrane is only approximately 0.2 μm (Figure 7-47, *B*). Only very thin tissue and fluid layers must be crossed for gas exchange to occur (Figure 7-47, *C*). These short distances are essential for efficient gas exchange. Transfer of O_2 and CO_2 in the lung depends on diffusion gradients across this membrane. The red blood cell spends less than 1 second in transit through the pulmonary capillaries. Gas exchange is so efficient in the healthy lung that it is complete before the blood reaches the end of the capillary.

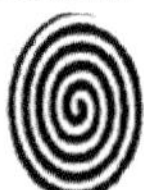

RULE OF THUMB

The right lung is slightly larger than the left lung because of the location of the heart. The right lung has a sizable middle lobe, and the left lung has the smaller lingula of the left upper lobe. For purposes of estimating the contribution of the right and left lungs to ventilation and to gas exchange, the *60-to-40 rule* is sometimes used. The right lung is assumed to have 60% of the ventilation/gas-exchange capacity, and the left lung is assumed to have the remaining 40%. For example, if a patient required removal of the entire left lung (pneumonectomy), a 40% decrease in lung volume would be expected.

Intercommunicating Channels

Gas-exchange lung units are not "dead-end" passages. Several forms of intercommunicating channels exist throughout the lung. Such channels may be found at the alveolar level, between bronchioles and alveoli, and among bronchioles.[56]

The pores of Kohn (see Figures 7-45 and 7-46) vary from 5 to 15 μm in diameter with breathing. They allow collateral air movement between adjacent alveoli.

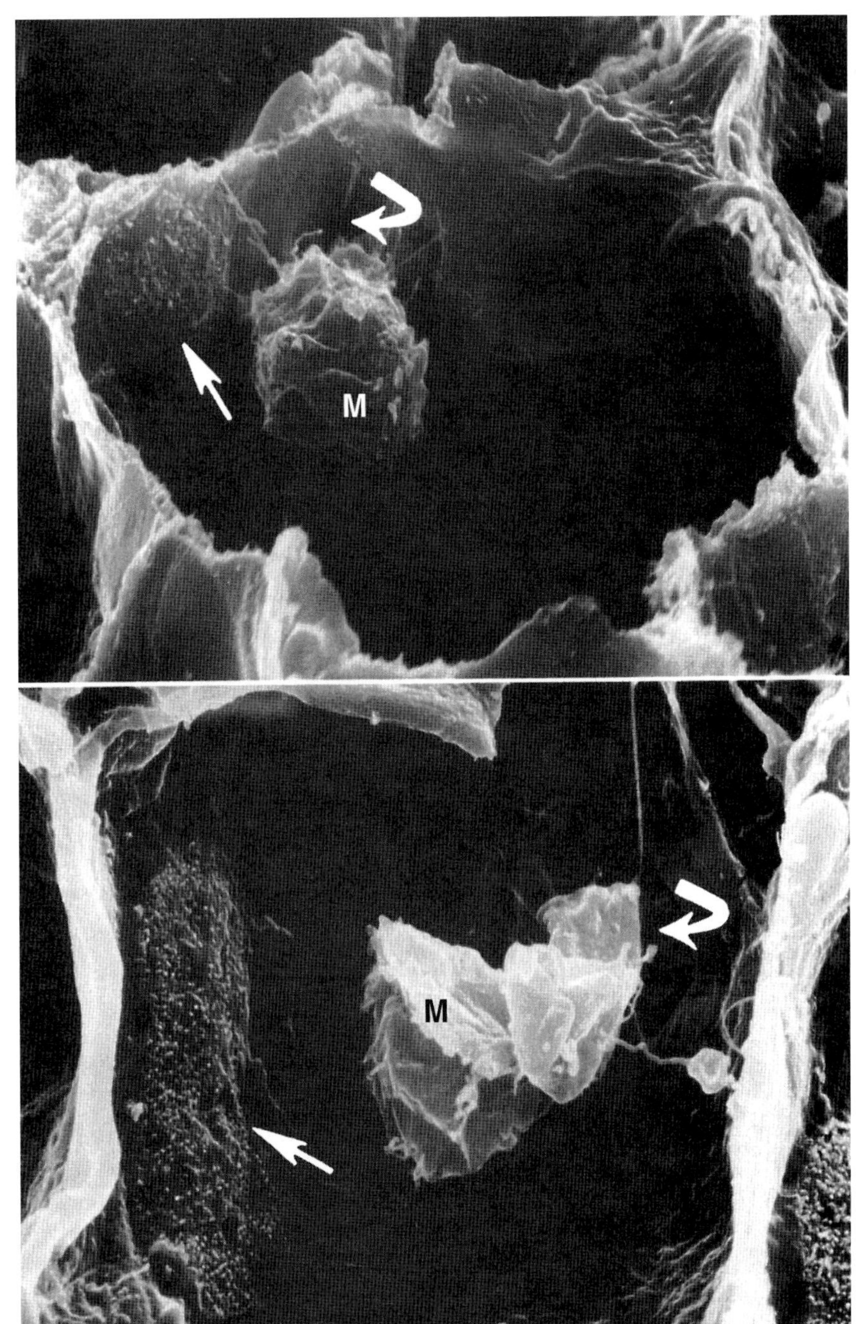

Figure 7-46 · Scanning Electron Micrographs of Alveolar Air Spaces

A, Note thin partitions or septa between adjacent alveoli. The thin, platelike type I cells compose most of these. Type II cells have projections off their surfaces that appear dotted or hairy *(straight arrow)*. Alveolar macrophage *(M)* is seen at the back, partially covering the pore of Kohn *(curved arrow)*. **B,** A similar view with two or three macrophages passing through the pore of Kohn. *(Courtesy Mike Wagner, San Diego, Calif.)*

These pores may explain why a lobule beyond an obstructed bronchiole remains partially inflated. Alveolar pores are not present during early postnatal lung development and they increase in size and number throughout life by an unknown mechanism.

Other types of intercommunicating channels between terminal bronchioles are the *canals of Lambert*. These openings are approximately 30 µm in size. They appear to remain open even when bronchiolar smooth muscle contracts. The canals of Lambert provide for gas movement between primary lobules.

A third, larger pathway for collateral ventilation may also exist. *Intersegmental respiratory bronchioles* have been demonstrated in normal human lungs. These channels are found in airways with diameters of 80 to 150 mm, especially in the lower lobes.[57] Such channels may represent a major source for collateral gas exchange and facilitate even distribution of ventilation during breathing. They may also contribute to the lung's ability to respond to structural damage caused by disease.

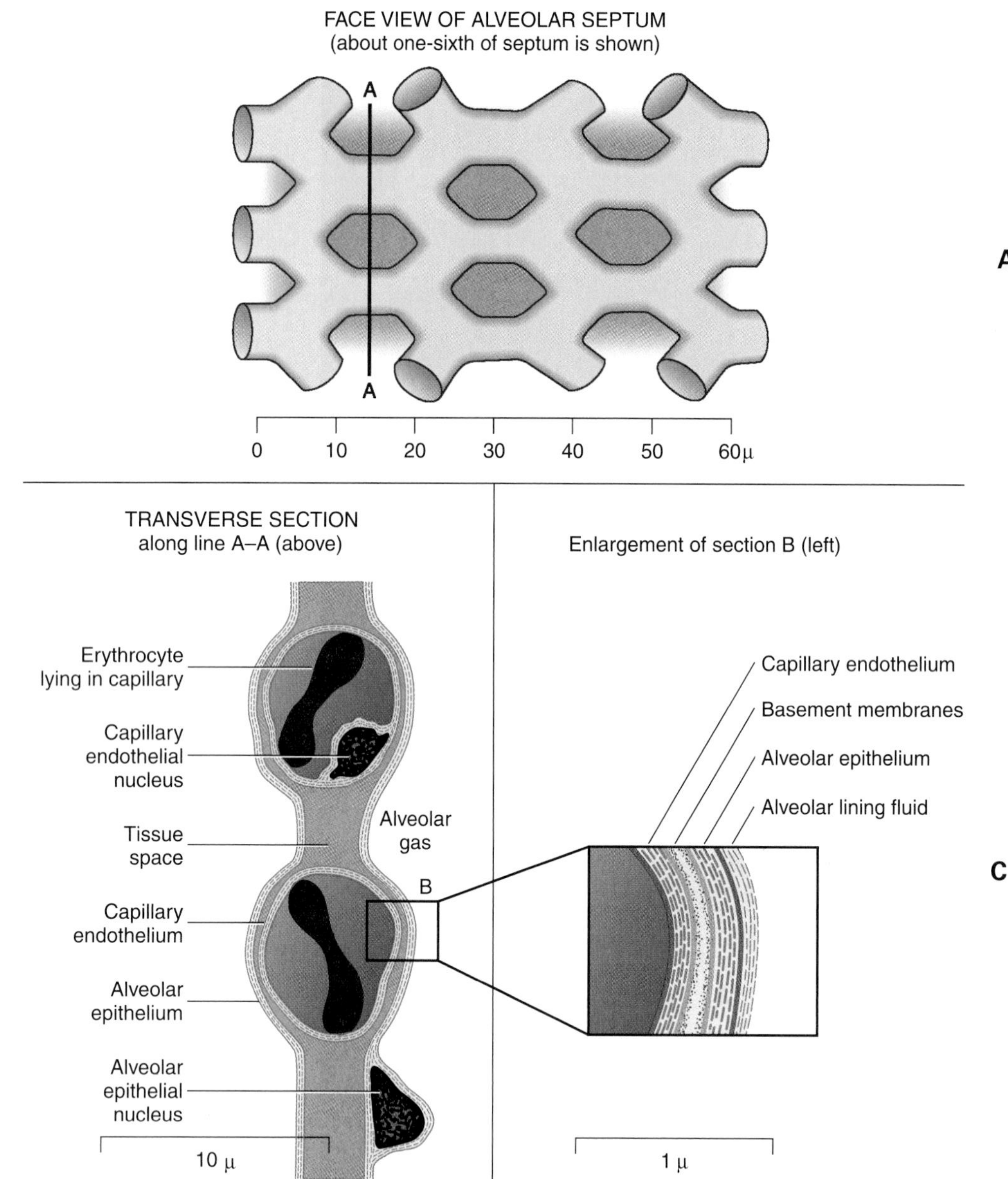

Figure 7-47

A, Face view of an alveolar septum (of which approximately one sixth is shown). The capillary network is dense, with the spaces between the capillaries being less than the diameter of the capillaries. **B,** Section (A–A) through two capillaries, demonstrating the very thin membrane through which gas exchange takes place. **C,** Enlargement of **B.** *(Modified from Nunn JF: Applied respiratory physiology, ed 2, London, 1977, Butterworth.)*

▶ OTHER FUNCTIONS OF THE LUNG

The lungs, in addition to gas exchange, perform other functions related to homeostasis. These functions are anatomical and metabolic in nature.

The pulmonary circulation serves as a blood reservoir for the left ventricle. This reservoir maintains stable left ventricular volumes despite small changes in cardiac output. The pulmonary blood volume (approximately 600 mL) is sufficient to maintain normal left ventricle filling for several cardiac cycles. This is important if filling of the right heart is temporarily decreased or interrupted.

The pulmonary circulation also acts as a filter for the systemic circulation. It traps particles before they enter the systemic circulation, where blockages could be life-threatening. This filtering mechanism prevents particles from reaching the coronary and cerebral circulations. Harmful particles that are filtered include fibrin and blood clots, fat cells, platelet aggregates, and debris found in stored blood or intravenous fluids.

The lungs play an active role in metabolism. They are responsible for synthesis, activation, inactivation, and detoxification of many bioactive substances.[58] Heparin, histamine, bradykinin, serotonin, and certain prostaglandins are stored or synthesized in the lung. The lung releases these substances in response to physiological or immunological challenges.[59] Angiotensin is converted to its active form by the lung. Adenosine triphosphate and norepinephrine are partially removed from the blood and inactivated by the lungs.

KEY POINTS

- Various structures of the respiratory system accomplish gas exchange by integrating their respective forms and functions.
- The genetic framework of each individual determines the development of his or her respiratory system from conception and on through adult life.
- The development of the respiratory system follows a well-defined schedule; interruptions or insults in the course of development can result in respiratory disease at birth and in adulthood.
- Fetal circulation and respiration differ markedly from those functions in the postnatal period.
- The transition from intrauterine to extrauterine life involves the nonaerated, fluid-filled lung converting to an efficient organ of gas exchange. Closure of the foramen ovale and ductus arteriosus are important events in this transition.
- The thorax houses and protects the lungs; it is also the mechanical bellows that makes ventilation possible.
- The diaphragm is the primary muscle of ventilation; together with the accessory muscles and thoracic structures, it provides the ability to move large volumes of gas into and out of the lungs.
- Motor and sensory neurons innervate the muscles of ventilation and various lung tissues. They provide feedback for responding to changing ventilatory demands.

KEY POINTS—cont'd

- The upper respiratory tract heats and humidifies inspired air. Its various structures also protect the lungs against foreign substances.
- The lower respiratory tract conducts respired gases from the upper airway to the respiratory zones of the lung. It contains many structures that help clear and defend the lung.
- The airways branch into lobes in both the right and left lungs; these lobes consist of various segments. This structural arrangement provides for efficient gas exchange in both health and disease states.
- The respiratory bronchioles and alveoli provide a large surface that facilitates gas exchange. Disruption of these structures occurs with many types of pulmonary diseases.

References

1. Wilfond BS, Taussig LM: Cystic fibrosis: general overview. In Taussig LM, Landau LI, editors: Pediatric respiratory medicine, St Louis, 1999, Mosby.
2. Le Souef PN: Molecular genetics and pediatric respiratory medicine. In Taussig LM, Landau LI, editors: Pediatric respiratory medicine, St Louis, 1999, Mosby
3. Martinez FD et al: Asthma and wheezing in the first six years of life, N Engl J Med 332:133, 1995.
4. Gaultier C: Developmental anatomy and physiology of the respiratory system. In Taussig LM, Landau LI, editors: Pediatric respiratory medicine, St Louis, 1999, Mosby.
5. O'Brodvich HM, Haddad GG: The functional basis of respiratory pathology and disease. In Cherniak V, Boat TF, editors: Kendig's disorders of the respiratory tract in children, ed 6, Philadelphia, 1998, WB Saunders.
6. Murray JF: Postnatal growth and development of the lung. In Murray JF, editor: The normal lung, ed 2, Philadelphia, 1986, WB Saunders.
7. Wohl ME: Developmental physiology of the respiratory system. In Cherniak V, Boat TF, editors: Kendig's disorders of the respiratory tract in children, ed 6, Philadelphia, 1998, WB Saunders.
8. Hamvas A: Inherited surfactant protein-B deficiency. In Barnes L, editor: Advances in pediatrics, vol 44, St Louis, 1997, Mosby.
9. Schnapf B, Kirley S: Fetal lung development. In Barnhart S, Czervinske M, editors: Perinatal and pediatric respiratory care, Philadelphia, 1995, WB Saunders.
10. Longo L: Fetal gas exchange. In Crystal R, West J, editors: The lung: scientific foundations, New York, 1991, Raven.
11. Koff PB, Eitzman DV, Neu J: Neonatal and pediatric respiratory care, ed 2, St Louis, 1993, Mosby.

12. Bland R: Fetal lung liquid and its removal near birth. In Crystal R, West J, editors: The lung: scientific foundations, New York, 1991, Raven.
13. Hazinski, M, van Stralen D: Physiological and anatomical differences between children and adults. In Levin D, Morriss F, editors: Essentials of pediatric intensive care, St Louis, 1990, Quality Medical Publishing.
14. Miller MJ et al: Oral breathing in newborn infants, J Pediatr 107:465, 1985.
15. Miller MJ et al: Effect of maturation on oral breathing in sleeping premature infants, J Pediatr 109:515, 1986.
16. Harding R: Function of the larynx in the fetus and newborn, Annu Rev Physiol 46:645, 1984.
17. Lumb AB: Control of breathing. In Lumb AB, editor: Nunn's applied respiratory physiology, ed 5, Oxford; Boston, 2000, Butterworth-Heinemann.
18. Kemp JS et al; Softness and potential to cause rebreathing: differences in bedding used by infants at high and low risk for sudden infant death syndrome, J Pediatr 132:234, 1998.
19. Rigatto H, Brady JP: Periodic breathing and apnea in preterm infants: I. Evidence of hypoventilation possible because of central respiratory depression, Pediatrics 50:202, 1972.
20. Rigatto H, Brady JP, de la Torre Verduzco R: Chemoreceptor reflexes in preterm infants: I. The effect of gestational age and postnatal age on the ventilatory response to inhalation of 100% and 15% oxygen, Pediatrics 55:604, 1975.
21. Carlo WA, Martin RJ: Principles of neonatal assisted ventilation, Pediatr Clin North Am 33:221, 1986.
22. Greenough A, Roberton NR: Neonatal ventilation, Early Hum Dev 13:127, 1986.
23. Fraser RG, Pare JA: Structure and function of the lung with emphasis on roentgenology, Philadelphia, 1971, WB Saunders.
24. Lai-Fook SJ: Mechanics of the pleural space: fundamental concepts, Lung 165:249, 1987.
25. Murray JF: The normal lung: the basis for diagnosis and treatment of pulmonary disease, ed 2, Philadelphia, 1986, WB Saunders.
26. Epstein SK: An overview of respiratory muscle function, Clin Chest Med 15:619, 1994.
27. Celli B: The diaphragm and respiratory muscles, Chest Surg Clin North Am 8:207, 1998.
28. De Troyer A: Mechanics of intercostal space and actions of external and internal intercostal muscles, J Clin Invest 75:850, 1985.
29. Celli BR: Clinical and physiologic evaluation of respiratory muscle function, Clin Chest Med 10:199, 1989.
30. Iscoe S: Control of abdominal muscles, Prog Neurobiol 56:433, 1998.
31. Mier A et al: Action of the abdominal muscles on the ribcage in humans, J Appl Physiol 58:1438,1985.
32. Richardson JB: Nerve supply to the lung, Am Rev Respir Dis 119:785, 1979.
33. Barnes PJ: Neural control of human airways in health and disease, Am Rev Respir Dis 134:1289, 1986.
34. Coleridge HM, Coleridge JC: Pulmonary reflexes: neural mechanisms of pulmonary defense, Ann Rev Physiol 56:69, 1994.
35. Crofton J, Douglas A: Respiratory diseases, ed 3, Oxford, England, 1981, Blackwell Scientific.
36. Karlsson JA, Sant'Ambrogio G, Widdicombe JG: Afferent neural pathways in cough and reflex bronchoconstriction, J Appl Physiol 65:1007, 1988.
37. Green JF: The pulmonary circulation. In Zelis R, editor: The peripheral circulation, New York, 1975, Grune & Stratton.
38. Milnor WR: Pulmonary hemodynamics. In Bergel DH, editor: Cardiovascular fluid dynamics, vol 2, New York, 1972, Academic Press.
39. Charan NB: The bronchial circulatory system: structure, function and importance, Respir Care 29:1226, 1984.
40. Nagaishi C: Functional anatomy and histology of the lung, Baltimore, 1972, University Park Press.
41. Bhattacharya J: The microphysiology of lung liquid clearance, Adv Exp Med Biol 381:95, 1995.
42. Proctor DF: The upper airways: I. Nasal physiology and defense of the lung, Am Rev Respir Dis 115:97.
43. Proctor DF: The upper airways: II. The larynx and trachea, Am Rev Respir Dis 115:315, 1977.
44. Wheatey JR, Amis TC: Mechanical properties of the upper airway, Curr Opin Pulm Med 4:363, 1998.
45. Boyden EA: Segmental anatomy of the lungs, New York, 1955, McGraw-Hill.
46. Weibel ER: Morphometry of the human lung, New York, 1962, Academic Press.
47. Foster RE et al: The lung: physiologic basis of pulmonary function tests, ed 3, St Louis, 1986, Mosby.
48. Engle LA: Gas mixing within the acinus of the lung, J Appl Physiol 54:609, 1983.
49. Rhodin JAG: Ultrastructure and function of the human tracheal mucosa, Am Rev Respir Dis 93(Suppl):1, 1966.
50. Breeze RG, Wheeldon EB: The cells of the pulmonary airways, Am Rev Respir Dis 116:705, 1977.
51. Pavia D et al: General review of tracheobronchial clearance, Eur J Respir Dis Suppl 153:123,1987.
52. Widdicombe JG: Control of secretions of tracheobronchial mucus, Br Med Bull 34:57, 1978.
53. Schulman ES: The role of mast cells in inflammatory responses in the lung, Crit Rev Immunol 13:35, 1993.
54. Clements JA et al: Pulmonary surface tension and alveolar stability, J Appl Physiol 16:444, 1972.
55. Fels AO, Cohn ZA: The alveolar macrophage, J Appl Physiol 60:353, 1986.
56. Menkes HA, Traysman RJ: Collateral ventilation, Am Rev Respir Dis 116:287, 1977.
57. Anderson JB, Jespersen W: Demonstration of intersegmental respiratory bronchioles in normal human lungs, Eur J Respir Dis 61:337, 1980.
58. Toews GB: Pulmonary defense mechanisms, Semin Respir Infect 8:160, 1993.
59. Thompson AB et al: Immunologic functions of the pulmonary epithelium, Eur Respir J 8:127, 1995.

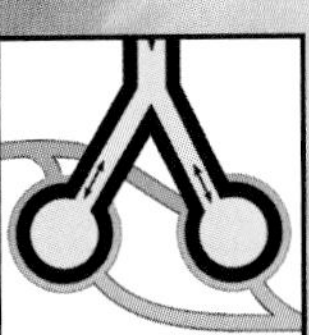

CHAPTER 8

The Cardiovascular System

W. William Hughes

In This Chapter You Will Learn:

- How the anatomy of the heart and vascular systems relate to their function
- What key properties are characteristic of cardiac tissue
- How local and central control mechanisms regulate the heart and vascular systems
- How the cardiovascular system coordinates its functions under normal and abnormal conditions
- How the electrical and mechanical events of the heart relate to a normal cardiac cycle

Chapter Outline

Key Terms

afterload
arteriovenous anastomosis
automaticity
baroreceptors
cardiac output
chemoreceptors
contractility
end-diastolic volume (EDV)
Frank-Starling law
heart rate
negative feedback loop
negative inotropism
pericardium
positive inotropism
preload
regurgitation
stenosis
stroke volume
vasoconstriction
vasodilation

▶ FUNCTIONAL ANATOMY

The Heart

Anatomy of the Heart

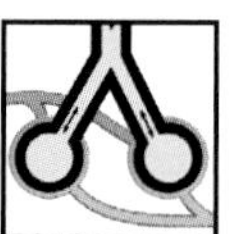

The heart is a hollow, muscular organ approximately the size of a fist. It is positioned obliquely in the middle compartment of the mediastinum of the chest, just behind the sternum (Figure 8-1). Approximately two thirds of the heart lies to the left of the sternum's midline. The apex of the heart is formed by the tip of the left ventricle and lies just above the diaphragm at the level of the fifth intercostal space. The base of the heart is formed by the atria. It projects to the right and lies just below the second rib. Surface grooves called *sulci* mark the boundaries of the heart chambers. The coronary sulcus lies between the atria and the ventricles, and the anterior and posterior longitudinal sulci mark the boundaries between the ventricles themselves.

The heart resides within a loose, membranous sac called the parietal **pericardium**. The outer fibrous layer consists of tough connective tissue. The inner serous layer is thinner and more delicate, being continuous with a similar visceral layer called the *visceral pericardium*, or *epicardium*, which is on the outer surface of the heart and great vessels. The pericardial fluid that separates these two layers helps minimize friction as the heart contracts and expands within the pericardium. Inflammation of the pericardium results in a clinical condition called *pericarditis*.

The heart wall consists of three layers: (1) the outer epicardium, (2) the middle myocardium, and (3) the inner endocardium. The endocardium is a thin layer of tissue, continuous with the inner layer of blood vessels. The myocardium composes the bulk of the heart and consists of bands of involuntary striated muscle fibers. It is the contraction of these muscle fibers that creates the pumplike action needed to move blood throughout the body.

Support for the heart's four interior chambers and valves is provided by four atrioventricular (AV) rings, which form a fibrous "skeleton." Each ring is composed of dense connective tissue termed *anuli fibrosi cordis*. The two atrial chambers are thin-walled "cups" of myocardial tissue, separated by an interatrial septum. On the right side of the interatrial septum is an oval depression called the *fossa ovalis cordis*, which is the remnant of the fetal foramen ovale. In addition, each atrium has an appendage, or auricle, the function of which is unknown.

The two lower heart chambers, or ventricles, make up the bulk of the heart's muscle mass and do most of the pumping that circulates the blood (Figure 8-2). The mass of the left ventricle is approximately two thirds larger than that of the right ventricle and has a spherical appearance when viewed in anteroposterior cross section. The right ventricle is thin walled and oblong, forming a pocketlike attachment to the left ventricle. Because of this relationship, contraction of the left

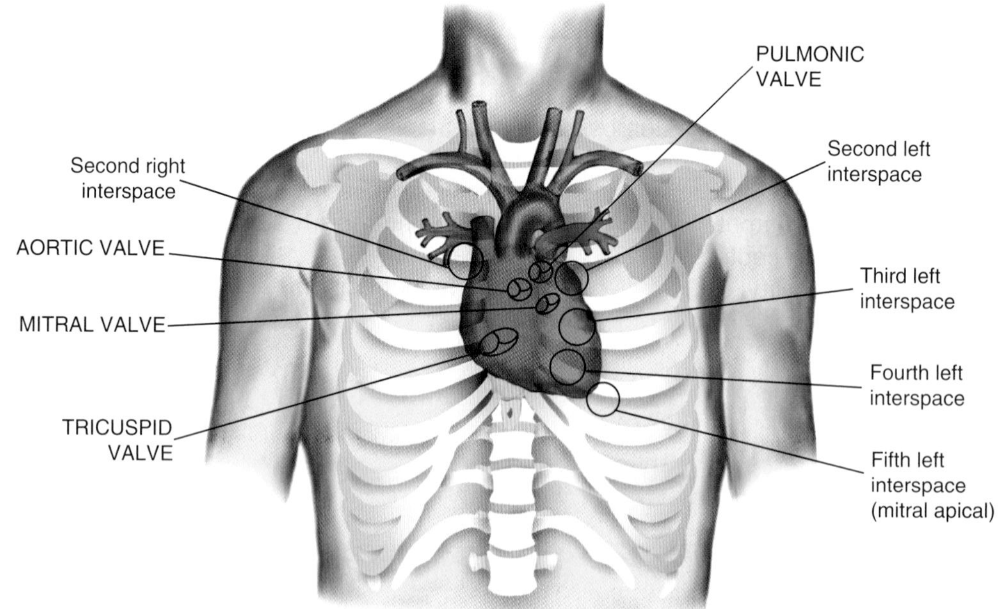

Figure 8-1

Anterior view of the thorax showing the position of the heart in relationship to the ribs, sternum, diaphragm, and the position of the heart valves. *(From Seidel HM et al: Mosby's guide to physical examination, ed 2, St Louis, 1991, Mosby.)*

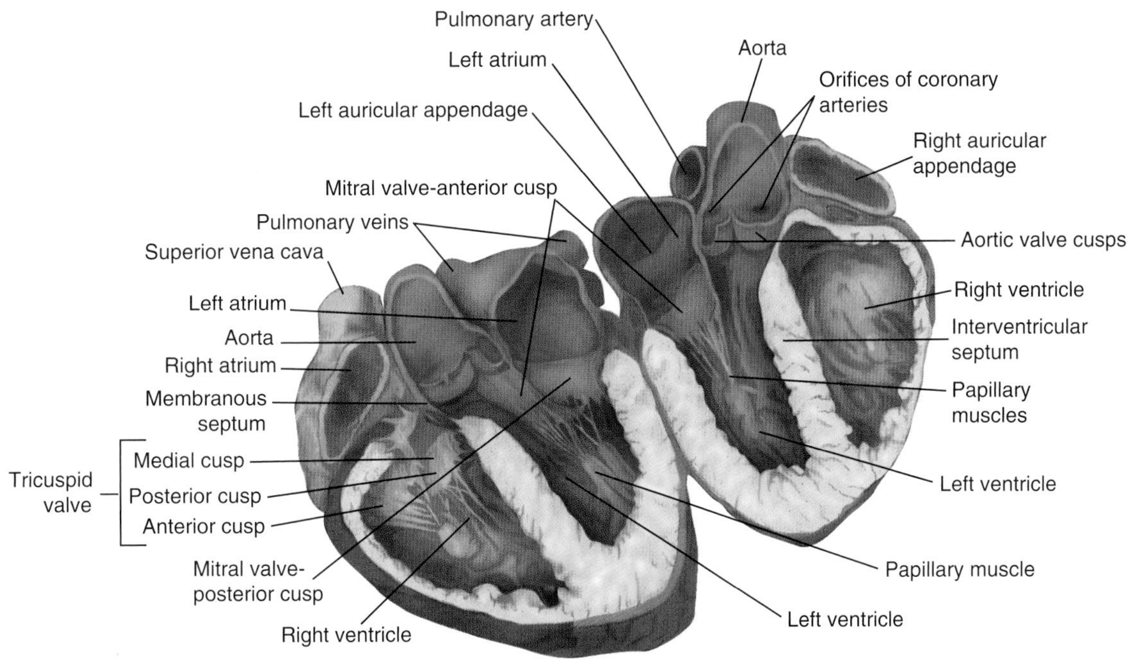

Figure 8-2

Drawing of the heart split perpendicular to the interventricular septum to illustrate anatomical relationships of the heart. *(From Berne RM, Levy MN, editors: Physiology, ed 3, St Louis, 1993, Mosby.)*

ventricle actually pulls in the right ventricular wall, aiding its contraction. The effect, termed *left ventricular aid*, explains why some forms of right ventricular failure are less harmful than might be expected.

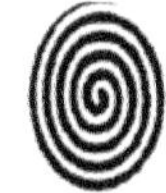

RULE OF THUMB

Left ventricular contraction aids right ventricular contraction.

The right and left ventricles are separated by a muscle wall called the interventricular septum (see Figure 8-2). Ventricular muscle fibers are arranged in an overlapping spiral fashion. Contractions of these fibers results in a wringing action that helps eject blood from the ventricles.

The valves of the heart are flaps of fibrous tissue firmly anchored to the anuli fibrosi cordis. Those located between the atria and ventricles are called *AV valves*. The valve between the right atrium and ventricle is called the *tricuspid valve* (see Figure 8-2). The valve between the left atrium and ventricle is called the *bicuspid*, or *mitral, valve*. The AV valves close during systole (contraction of the ventricles), thereby preventing backflow of blood into the atria. Closure of these valves provides a critical period of isovolemic contraction, during which chamber pressures quickly rise just before ejection of the blood.

The free ends of the AV valves are anchored to papillary muscles of the endocardium by the *chordae tendineae cordis*. During systole, papillary muscle contraction prevents the AV valves from swinging upward into the atria. Damage to either the chordae tendineae cordis or the papillary muscles can impair function of the AV valves.

Common valve problems include regurgitation and stenosis. **Regurgitation** is the backflow of blood through an incompetent or damaged valve. **Stenosis** is a pathological narrowing or constriction of a valve outlet, which causes increased pressure in the affected chamber and vessels. Both conditions affect cardiac performance. For example, in mitral stenosis, high pressures in the left atrium back up into the pulmonary circulation. This can cause pulmonary edema.

A set of semilunar valves separates the ventricles from their arterial outflow tracts (Figure 8-3). Consisting of three half-moon–shaped cusps attached to the arterial wall, these valves prevent backflow of blood into the ventricles during diastole (or when the heart's chambers fill with blood). The pulmonary valve is at the outflow tract of the right ventricle. During systole, blood flows through the open pulmonary valve from the right ventricle into the pulmonary artery. The aortic valve is located at the outflow tract of the left ventricle. During systole, blood flows through the open aortic valve from the left ventricle into the aorta. As with the AV valves, the semilunar valves can leak (regurgitation) or become obstructed (stenosis).

Like the lung, the heart has its own circulatory system, which is called *coronary circulation*. However,

MINI CLINI

Mitral Stenosis, Poor Oxygenation, and Increased Work of Breathing

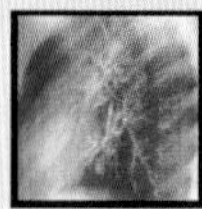

The mitral valve separates the left atrium and ventricle. A stenotic mitral valve is one that is narrowed and that offers high resistance to the blood flowing through it into the ventricle. Pulmonary edema is a condition in which fluid collects in the spaces between the alveolar and capillary walls, known as the *interstitial spaces*.

PROBLEM

Why does a patient with mitral stenosis have poor oxygenation of the blood and increased work of breathing?

DISCUSSION

Blood flows from the lungs into the left atrium, where it may encounter high resistance through a narrowed, stenotic mitral valve. This causes high pressure to build in the left atrium. Pressure in the pulmonary veins and, eventually, in the pulmonary capillaries also increases. This high pressure within the capillaries engorges them and forces fluid components of the blood plasma out of the vessels into the interstitial spaces, creating pulmonary edema. This collection of fluid interferes with oxygen diffusion from the lung into the blood. Engorged capillaries surrounding the alveoli create a stiff "web" around each alveolus, which makes expanding the lungs difficult. Some areas of the lung expand more easily than do others. This causes inhaled air to be preferentially directed into these compliant regions, whereas "stiffer," more noncompliant regions are underventilated. The underventilated regions do not properly oxygenate the blood as perfusing them. Thus mitral stenosis, a cardiac problem, has significant pulmonary consequences.

unlike the lung, the heart has a high metabolic rate, which requires more blood flow per gram of tissue weight than any other organ except the kidney. To meet these needs, the coronary circulation provides an extensive network of branches to all myocardial tissue (Figure 8-4).

Two main coronary arteries, a left and a right, arise from the root of the aorta. Because of their position, the coronary arteries get the maximal pulse of pressure

MINI CLINI

Heart Rate and Coronary Perfusion

PROBLEM

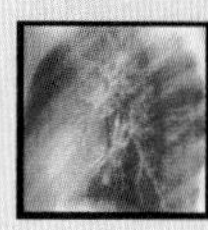

Why might an extremely high heart rate decrease blood flow through the coronary arteries?

DISCUSSION

Blood flow through the coronary arteries occurs only during ventricular diastole. During systole, the myocardium contracts with such force that coronary artery pressures actually rise above aortic pressures. Thus myocardial perfusion occurs only during diastole. As heart rate increases, both systolic and diastolic times must necessarily decrease. As diastolic time decreases, less and less time is available for coronary artery perfusion, until finally coronary blood flow can be significantly reduced. This is critically important in the individual who already has compromised coronary circulation caused by arteriosclerotic heart disease. Not only is coronary artery perfusion compromised with severe tachycardia, but also decreased ventricular filling time causes decreased stroke volume and decreased cardiac output.

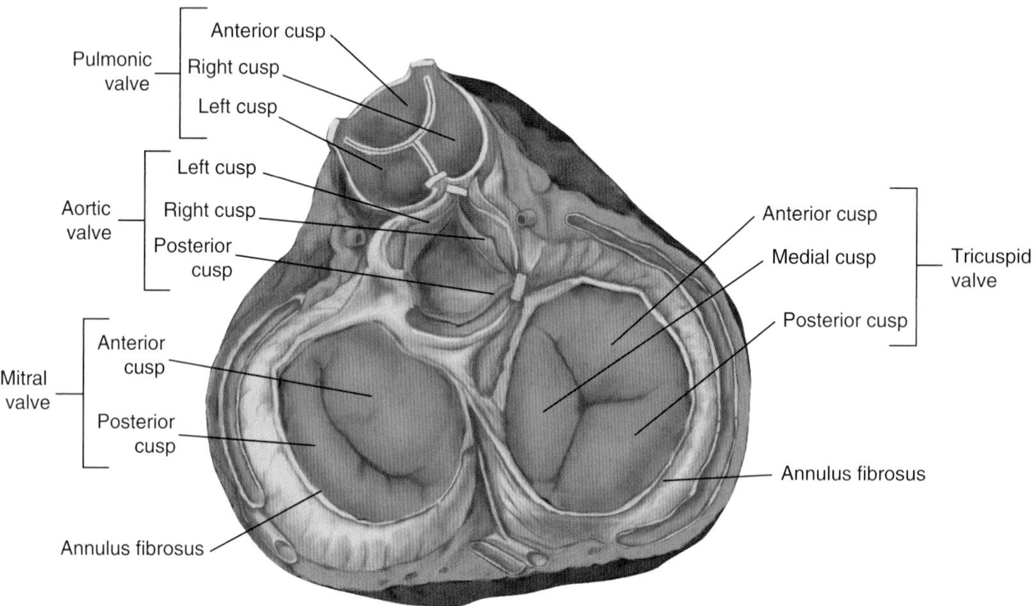

Figure 8-3

Four cardiac valves as viewed from the base of the heart. Note how the leaflets overlap in the closed valves.

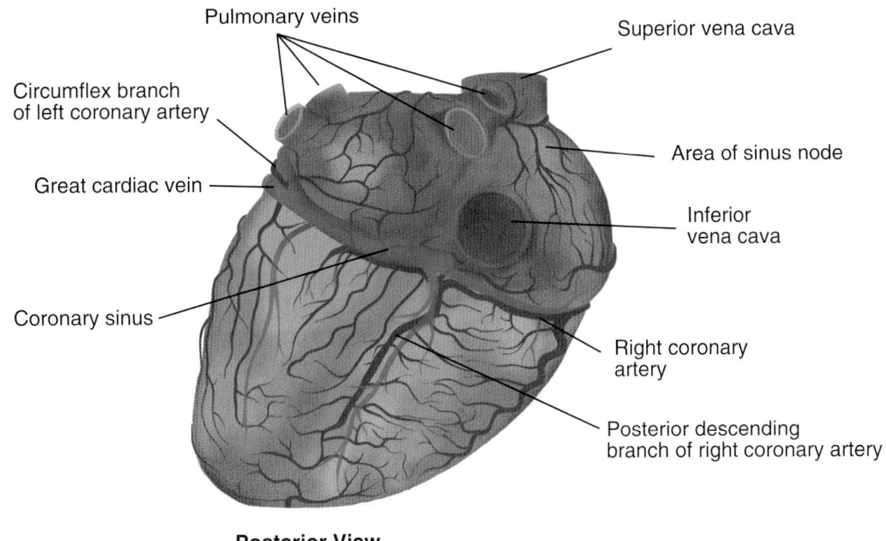

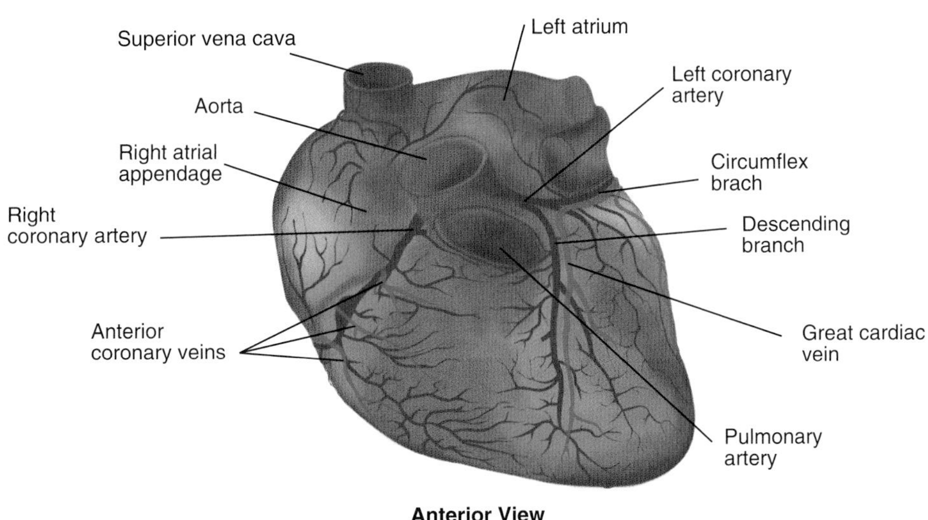

Figure 8-4

Coronary circulation as seen on anterior and posterior surfaces of the heart, illustrating the location and distribution of the principal coronary vessels.

generated by contraction of the left ventricle. However, only during ventricular diastole (relaxation) will blood flow through the coronary arteries. Although there can be major individual differences in the branching of the coronary circulation, the basic layout is similar in all humans.

The left coronary artery divides into two branches between the pulmonary artery and the tip of the left atrial appendage. An *anterior descending branch* courses down the anterior sulcus to the apex of the heart. A *circumflex branch* moves along the coronary sulcus toward the back and around the left atrial appendage. The circumflex branch subdivides into smaller arteries, which feed the back side of the left ventricle. In combination, the branches of the left coronary artery normally supply most of the left ventricle, the left atrium, the anterior two thirds of the interventricular septum, the lower half of the interatrial septum, and part of the right atrium.

The right coronary artery also begins at the aorta, where it proceeds diagonally to the right across the coronary sulcus. As it moves across the front surface of the right ventricle, it divides into many small branches. The right coronary artery ends in its *posterior descending branch*, which descends within the posterior interventricular sulcus (see Figure 8-4). Approximately one in five people have a predominant left coronary artery system, which results when the posterior descending branch arises from the terminal branch of the left circumflex coronary artery. Together, the branches of the right coronary artery supply the anterior and posterior portions of the right ventricular myocardium, the right atrium, the sinus node, the posterior third of the interventricular septum, and a portion of the base of the right ventricle.

The coronary veins closely parallel the arteries (see Figure 8-4). The great cardiac vein follows the anterior descending artery in the anterior interventricular sulcus. The small cardiac vein accompanies the right coronary artery in the coronary sulcus. The left posterior coronary vein follows a branch of the circumflex artery, and the middle cardiac vein parallels the posterior descending artery. These veins gather together into a large vessel called the *coronary sinus*, which passes left to right across the posterior surface of the heart. The coronary sinus empties into the right atrium between the opening of the inferior vena cava and the tricuspid valve.

In addition to these major routes for return blood flow, some coronary venous blood flows back into the heart through the *thebesian veins*. The thebesian veins empty directly into all the heart chambers. Thus any blood coming from the thebesian veins that enters the left atrium or ventricle will mix with arterial blood coming from the lungs. Whenever venous blood mixes with arterial blood, the overall oxygen content falls. Because the thebesian veins bypass, or shunt, around the pulmonary circulation, this phenomenon is called an *anatomical shunt*. When combined with a similar bypass in the bronchial circulation (see Chapter 7), these normal anatomical shunts account for approximately 2% to 3% of the total cardiac output.

Properties of the Heart Muscle

The heart's performance as a pump depends on its ability to initiate and conduct electrical impulses and to synchronously contract its muscle fibers quickly and efficiently. These actions are possible only because myocardial tissues possess four key properties: (1) excitability, (2) inherent rhythmicity, (3) conductivity, and (4) contractility.

The myocardial property of *excitability* is the same as that exhibited by other muscles and tissues. Excitability is the ability of cells to respond to electrical, chemical, or mechanical stimulation. Electrolyte imbalances and certain drugs can increase myocardial excitability and produce abnormalities in electrical conduction.

The unique ability of the cardiac muscle to initiate a spontaneous electrical impulse is called *inherent rhythmicity*, or **automaticity**. Although such impulses can arise from any cardiac tissue, this ability is highly developed in specialized areas called *pacemaker*, or *nodal tissues*. The sinoatrial (SA) node and the AV node are good examples of specialized heart tissues that are designed to initiate electrical impulses (see Chapter 15). An electrical impulse from any source other than a normal pacemaker is considered abnormal and represents one of the many causes of what are called *cardiac arrhythmias*.

Conductivity is the ability of myocardial tissue to spread, or radiate, electrical impulses. This property is similar to that of smooth muscle in that it allows the myocardium to contract without direct neural innervation (as required by skeletal muscle). The rate with which electrical impulses spread throughout the myocardium is extremely variable. In the nodal areas, impulses move as slowly as 5 cm/sec. In comparison, the Purkinje fibers conduct impulses at 300 to 400 cm/sec. These differences in conduction velocity are needed to ensure synchronous contraction of the cardiac chambers. Abnormal conductivity can affect the timing of chamber contractions and thus decrease cardiac efficiency.

Contractility, in response to an electrical impulse, is the primary function of the myocardium. Unlike those of other muscle tissues, however, cardiac contractions cannot be sustained or tetanized because myocardial tissue exhibits a prolonged period of inexcitability after contraction. The period during which the myocardium cannot be stimulated is called the *refractory period*.

Microanatomy of Heart Muscle

Understanding of how cardiac muscle contracts requires knowledge of the heart's microanatomy. As seen under the microscope, myocardium tissue consists of an arrangement of striated, cylindrically shaped muscle fibers approximately 15 μm wide and 100 μm long. Individual fibers are enclosed in a membrane called the *sarcolemma*, surrounded by a rich capillary network (Figure 8-5). Cardiac fibers are separated by irregular transverse thickenings of the sarcolemma called *intercalated disks*. These disks provide structural support and aid in electrical conduction between fibers.

Each muscle fiber consists of many smaller units called *myofibrils*, which contain repeated structures approximately 2 μm in size called *sarcomeres*. Within the sarcomeres are contractile protein filaments responsible for shortening the myocardium during systole. These proteins are of two types. The thick filaments are composed mainly of myosin, and the thin filaments consist mostly of actin.

According to the sliding filament theory, myocardial cells contract when actin and myosin combine to form reversible bridges between these thick and thin filaments. These bridges cause filaments to slide over one another, shortening the sarcomere and thus muscle fibers as a whole.

In principle, the tension developed during myocardial contraction is directly proportional to the number of crossbridges between the actin and myosin filaments. In turn, the number of crossbridges is directly pro-

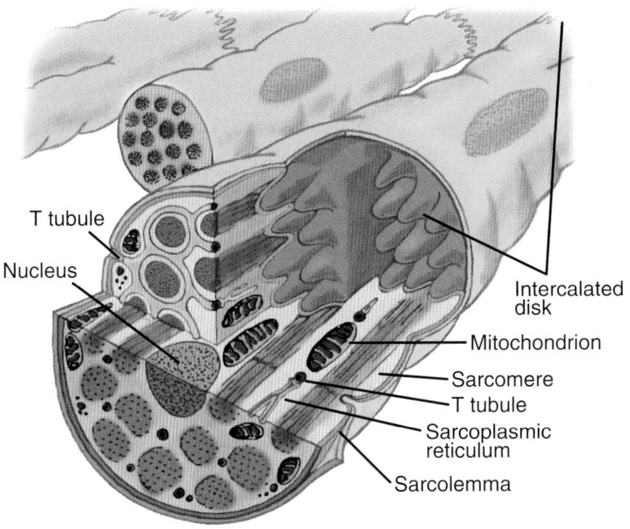

Figure 8-5

The major structural features of cardiac muscle fibers. Note the presence of intercalated disks connecting successive sarcomeres. *(Modified from Moffett DF, Moffett SB, Schauf CL: Human physiology: foundations & frontiers, ed 2, St Louis, 1993, Mosby.)*

portional to the length of the sarcomere. This principle underlies Starling's law of the heart, also known as the **Frank-Starling law**. According to this law, the more a cardiac fiber is stretched, the greater the tension it generates when contracted.

The Frank-Starling law holds true only up to a sarcomere length of 2.2 μm. Beyond this length, the actin and myosin filaments become partially disengaged, and fewer crossbridges can be formed. With fewer crossbridges, the overall tension developed during contraction is less. This relationship is of major importance and will be explored later in the discussion of the heart as a pump.

The Vascular System

The blood flow to and from the heart is depicted in Figure 8-6. Venous, or deoxygenated, blood from the head and upper extremities enters the right atrium from the superior vena cava, and blood from the lower body enters from the inferior vena cava. From the right atrium, blood flows through the tricuspid valve into the right ventricle. The right ventricle pumps the blood through the pulmonary valve, into the pulmonary arteries, and on to the lungs. Arterial, or oxygenated, blood returns to the left atrium through the pulmonary veins. The left atrium pumps blood through the mitral valve into the left ventricle. The blood is then pumped through the aortic valve and into the aorta. From the aorta, the blood flows out to the tissues of the upper and lower body. From the capillary network of the various body tissues, venous blood returns to the vena cava.

Systemic Vasculature

The systemic vasculature consists of three major components: (1) the arterial system, (2) the capillary system, and (3) the venous system. Although all three components are responsible for circulating blood to and from the tissues and lungs, these various vessels are more than just passive conduits. In fact, they regulate not only the amount of blood flow per minute (**cardiac output**) but also its bodily distribution. To achieve this function, each component has a unique structure and plays a somewhat different role in the circulatory system as a whole.

The *arterial system* consists of large, highly elastic, low-resistance arteries and small, muscular, variable-resistance arterioles. With their high elasticity, the large arteries help transmit and maintain the head of pressure generated by the heart. Together, the large arteries are called *conductance vessels.*

Just as faucets control the flow of water into a sink, the smaller arterioles control blood flow into the capillaries. Arterioles provide this control by varying their flow resistance. For this reason, arterioles are often referred to as *resistance vessels.*

The vast *capillary system,* or microcirculation, maintains a constant environment for the body's cells and tissues by the transport and exchange of nutrients and waste products. For this reason, the capillaries are commonly referred to as *exchange vessels.*

Figure 8-7 shows the structure of a typical capillary network. Blood flows into the network by an arteriole and out through a venule. A direct communication between these vessels is called an **arteriovenous anastomosis**. When open, an arteriovenous anastomosis allows arterial blood to shunt around the capillary bed and flow directly into the venules. Downstream from the arteriovenous anastomosis, the arteriole divides into terminal arterioles, which further branch into thoroughfare channels and true capillaries. Capillaries have smooth muscle rings at their proximal ends, called *precapillary sphincters.* Contraction of these sphincters decreases blood flow in that area, whereas relaxation increases perfusion. In combination, these various channels, sphincters, and bypasses allow precise control over the direction and amount of blood flow to a given area of tissue.

The *venous system* consists of small, expandable venules and veins, as well as larger, more elastic veins. Besides conducting blood back to the heart, these vessels act as a reservoir for the circulatory system. At any given time, the veins and venules hold approximately three fourths of the body's total blood volume. Moreover, the volume held in this reservoir can be quickly changed simply by altering the tone of these vessels. By quickly changing its holding capacity, the venous system can match the volume of circulating

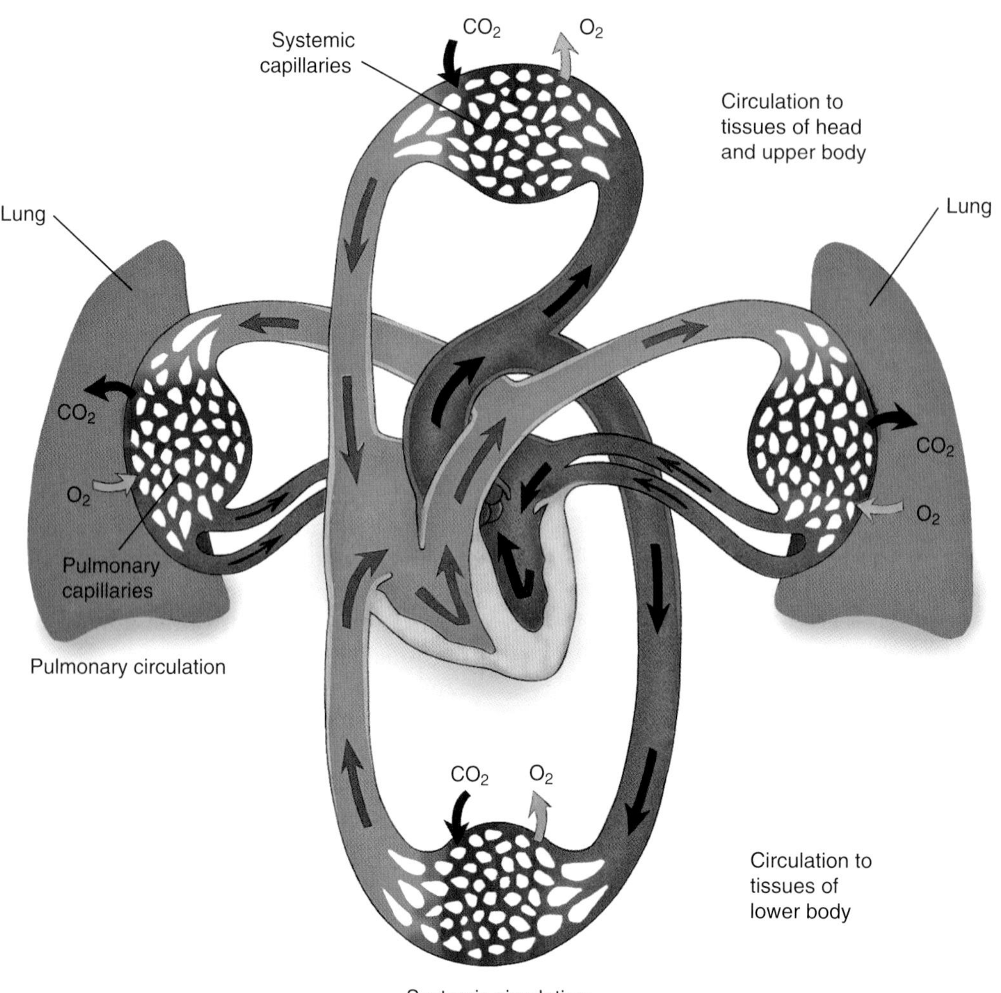

Figure 8-6

Generalized circulatory pathways between the heart, lung, and extremities.

blood to that needed to maintain adequate perfusion. Accordingly, the components of the venous system, especially the small, expandable venules and veins, are termed *capacitance vessels*.

As the part of the circulation with the lowest pressures, the venous system must overcome gravity to return blood to the heart. The following four mechanisms combine to aid venous return to the heart: (1) sympathetic venous tone; (2) skeletal muscle pumping, or "milking" (combined with venous one-way valves); (3) cardiac suction; and (4) thoracic pressure differences caused by respiratory efforts.

This last mechanism is often called the *thoracic pump*. As an aid to venous return, the thoracic pump is particularly important to respiratory therapists (RTs). This is because artificial ventilation with positive pressure reverses normal thoracic pressure gradients. Positive pressure ventilation thus impedes, rather than assists, venous return. Fortunately, as long as blood volume, cardiac function, and vasomotor tone are adequate, positive pressure ventilation has a minimal effect on venous return.

Although the heart is a single organ, it functions as two separate pumps. The right side of the heart provides the pressures needed to drive blood through the low-resistance, low-pressure pulmonary circulation. The left side of the heart generates enough pressure to propel blood through the higher-pressure systemic circulation.

Vascular Resistance

Like the movement of any fluid through tubes, blood flow through the vascular system is opposed by frictional forces. The sum of all frictional forces opposing blood flow through the systemic circulation is called *systemic vascular resistance* (SVR). SVR must equal the difference in pressure between the beginning and the end of the circuit, divided by the flow. The beginning pressure for the systemic circulation is the mean aortic

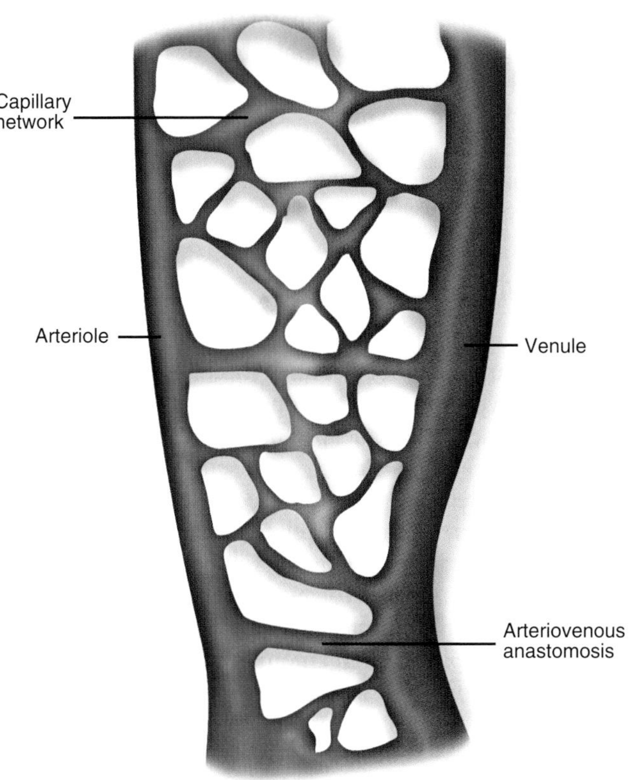

Figure 8-7

Components of a microcirculatory network. Blood flows from arteriolar to venular vessels through a network of capillaries. Opening of the arteriovenous anastomosis directs blood flow out of the capillary network. *(Modified from Stevens A, Lowe J: Human histology, ed 2, St Louis, 1997, Mosby.)*

pressure; ending pressure equals right atrial pressure. Flow for the system as a whole equals the cardiac output. Thus SVR can be calculated by the following formula:

$$\text{SVR} = \frac{\text{Mean aortic pressure} - \text{Right atrial pressure}}{\text{Cardiac output}}$$

Given a normal mean aortic pressure of 90 mm Hg, a mean right atrial pressure of approximately 4 mm Hg, and a normal cardiac output of 5 L/min, the normal SVR is computed as follows:

$$\text{SVR} = \frac{90\text{ mm Hg} - 4\text{ mm Hg}}{5\text{ L/min}}$$

$$= 17.2\text{ mm Hg/L/min}^*$$

The same concepts can be used to compute flow resistance in the pulmonary circulation. Beginning pressure for the pulmonary circulation is the mean pulmonary artery pressure; ending pressure equals left atrial pressure. Flow for the pulmonary circulation is the same as it is for the systemic system, which equals the cardiac output. Thus *pulmonary vascular resistance* (PVR) can be calculated by using the following formula:

*Multiply times 80 to convert to dynes-sec/cm^5.

$$\text{PVR} = \frac{\text{Mean pulmonary artery pressure} - \text{Left atrial pressure}}{\text{Cardiac output}}$$

Given a normal mean pulmonary artery pressure of approximately 16 mm Hg and a normal mean left atrial pressure of 8 mm Hg, the normal PVR is computed as follows:

$$\text{PVR} = \frac{16\text{ mm Hg} - 8\text{ mm Hg}}{5\text{ L/min}}$$

$$= 1.6\text{ mm Hg/L/min}^*$$

Note that resistance to blood flow in the pulmonary circulation is normally much less than it is in the systemic circulation. Indeed, the pulmonary vasculature is characterized as a low-pressure, low-resistance circulation.

Determinants of Blood Pressure

The cardiovascular system maintains sufficient pressure to propel blood throughout the body. In fact, the cardiovascular system's first priority is to keep perfusion pressures normal, even under changing conditions.

If the equation for computing vascular resistance is rearranged by deleting the normally low atrial pressure, then the average blood pressure in the circulation is directly related to both cardiac output and flow resistance.

$$\text{Mean arterial pressure} = \text{Cardiac output} \times \text{Vascular resistance}$$

With a constant rate and force of cardiac contractions, cardiac output (blood flow per minute) is approximately equal to the circulating blood volume. Under similar conditions, vascular resistance varies inversely with the size of the blood vessels (i.e., the capacity of the vascular system). All else being constant, mean arterial pressure is directly related to the volume of blood in the vascular system and inversely related to its capacity.

$$\text{Mean arterial pressure} = \frac{\text{Volume}}{\text{Capacity}}$$

Based on this relationship, it is seen that mean arterial pressure can be regulated by the following: changing the volume of circulating blood, changing the capacity of the vascular system, or changing both. Volume changes can reflect absolute changes in total blood volume, such as those resulting from shock or blood transfusion. Alternatively, changes in "relative" volume can occur when cardiac output rises or falls. Changes in system capacity occur mainly with changes in the smooth muscle tone of the blood vessels, particularly the expandable venules and veins.

To maintain adequate perfusion pressures under changing conditions, the cardiovascular system balances

*Multiply times 80 to convert to dynes-sec/cm^5.

relative volume and resistance. In exercise, for example, the circulating blood volume undergoes a relative increase. However, blood pressure remains near normal. This is because the skeletal muscle vascular beds dilate, causing a large increase in system capacity. However, when blood loss occurs, as with hemorrhage, system capacity is decreased by constricting the venous vessels. Thus perfusing pressures can be kept near normal until the volume loss overwhelms the system.

Remember that regulation of blood flow and pressure is much more complex than is suggested by these simplified equations. Cardiovascular control is accomplished by a complex array of integrated functions.

CONTROL OF THE CARDIOVASCULAR SYSTEM

The cardiovascular system is responsible for transporting metabolites to and from the tissues under a variety of conditions and demands. It must act in a highly coordinated fashion. Coordination is achieved by integrating the functions of the heart and vascular system. The goal is to maintain adequate perfusion to all tissues according to their needs.

It may seem strange, but the heart plays only a secondary role in regulating blood flow. The cardiovascular system regulates blood flow mainly by altering the capacity of the vasculature and the volume of blood it holds. In essence, the vascular system tells the heart how much blood it needs, rather than the heart dictating what volume the vascular system will receive.

These integrated functions involve both *local* and *central* control mechanisms. Local, or *intrinsic*, controls operate independently, without central nervous control. Intrinsic control alters perfusion under normal conditions to meet metabolic needs. Central, or *extrinsic*, control involves both the *central nervous system* (CNS) and circulating *humoral agents*. Extrinsic control mechanisms maintain a basal level of vascular tone. However, central control mechanisms will take over when the competing needs of local vascular beds must be coordinated.

Knowledge of vascular regulatory mechanisms and factors controlling cardiac output is essential to understanding how the cardiovascular system responds under both normal and abnormal conditions.

Regulation of Peripheral Vasculature

A basal level of vascular muscle tone is normally maintained throughout the vascular system at all times. Basal muscle tone must be present to allow for effective regulation. If blood vessels remained in a completely relaxed state, further dilation would be impossible, and local increases in perfusion could not occur.

Local vascular tone is maintained by the smooth muscle of the precapillary sphincters of the microcirculation and can function independently of neural control. Central control of vasomotor tone involves either direct CNS innervation or circulation hormones. Central control mainly affects the high-resistance arterioles and capacitance veins.

Local Control

Local regulation of tissue blood flow involves both myogenic and metabolic control mechanisms. Myogenic control involves the relationship between vascular smooth muscle tone and perfusing pressure. Increased perfusing pressures increase vascular muscle tone, whereas decreased pressures decrease vascular tone. *Myogenic control* ensures relatively constant flows to the capillary beds despite changes in perfusion pressures.

Metabolic control involves the relationship between vascular smooth muscle tone and the level of local cellular metabolites. High amounts of carbon dioxide or lactic acid, low pH levels, low partial pressures of oxygen, histamines (released during inflammatory response), endothelium-derived relaxing factor, and some prostaglandins all cause relaxation of the smooth muscle, thereby increasing flow to the affected area.

The influence of myogenic and metabolic control mechanisms varies in different organ systems, with the brain being the most sensitive to changes in the local metabolite levels, particularly those of CO_2 and pH. The heart, on the other hand, shows a strong response to both myogenic and metabolic factors.

Central Control

Central control of blood flow is achieved mainly by the sympathetic division of the autonomic nervous system. Again, the level of central control varies among organs and tissues. Although mainly skeletal muscle and skin are regulated by central control, the brain also is minimally regulated by this mechanism.

Smooth muscle contraction and increased flow resistance are mainly caused by adrenergic stimulation and the release of norepinephrine. Smooth muscle relaxation and vessel dilation occur as a result of stimulation of either *cholinergic* or specialized *adrenergic* β-receptors. Whereas the contractile response is distributed throughout the entire vascular system, dilation response appears to be limited to the precapillary vessels.

Regulation of Cardiac Output

The heart, like the vascular system, is regulated by both intrinsic and extrinsic factors. These mechanisms act together, along with vascular control, to ensure that the heart's output matches the different needs of the tissues.

The total amount of blood pumped by the heart per minute is called the *cardiac output*. Cardiac output is simply the product of the *heart rate* and the volume ejected by the left ventricle on each contraction, or *stroke volume*.

$$\text{Cardiac output} = \text{Heart rate} \times \text{Stroke volume}$$

A normal resting cardiac output of approximately 5 L/min can be calculated by substituting a normal heart rate (70 contractions/min) and stroke volume (75 mL, or 0.075 L, per contraction).

$$\text{Cardiac output} = 70 \text{ beats/min} \times 0.075 \text{ L/beat}$$
$$= 5.25 \text{ L/min}$$

Of course, this is a hypothetical average, because actual cardiac output varies considerably in both health and disease states.

Regardless of an individual's state of health or disease, a change in cardiac output must involve a change in stroke volume, a change in rate, or both. Stroke volume is affected mainly by intrinsic control of three factors: (1) preload, (2) afterload, and (3) contractility. Rate is affected primarily by extrinsic, or central, control mechanisms.

Changes in Stroke Volume

Stroke volume is the volume of blood ejected by the left ventricle during each contraction, or systole. The heart does not eject all the blood it contains during systole. Instead, a small volume, called the *end-systolic volume* (ESV), remains behind in the ventricles. During the resting phase, or diastole, the ventricles fill back up to a volume called the **end-diastolic volume** (EDV).

Therefore, stroke volume equals the difference between the end-diastolic volume and the end-systolic volume.

$$\text{Stroke volume} = \text{EDV} - \text{ESV}$$

In a healthy male at rest, the EDV ranges between 110 and 120 mL. Given a normal stroke volume of approximately 70 mL, a normal ejection fraction *(EF)*, or proportion of the EDV ejected on each stroke, can be computed as follows:

$$\text{EF} = \frac{\text{SV}}{\text{EDV}}$$
$$= \frac{70}{110}$$
$$= 0.64, \text{ or } 64\%$$

Thus on each contraction, the normal heart ejects approximately two thirds of its stored volume. Decreases in ejection fraction are normally associated with a weakened myocardium and decreased contractility.

As shown in Figure 8-8, an increase in stroke volume occurs when either the EDV increases or the ESV decreases. Conversely, a decrease in stroke volume occurs when either the EDV decreases or the ESV increases.

The heart's ability to change stroke volume solely according to the EDV is an intrinsic regulatory mechanism based on the Frank-Starling law. Because the EDV corresponds to the initial stretch, or tension, placed on the ventricle, the greater the EDV (up to a point), the greater the tension developed on contraction,

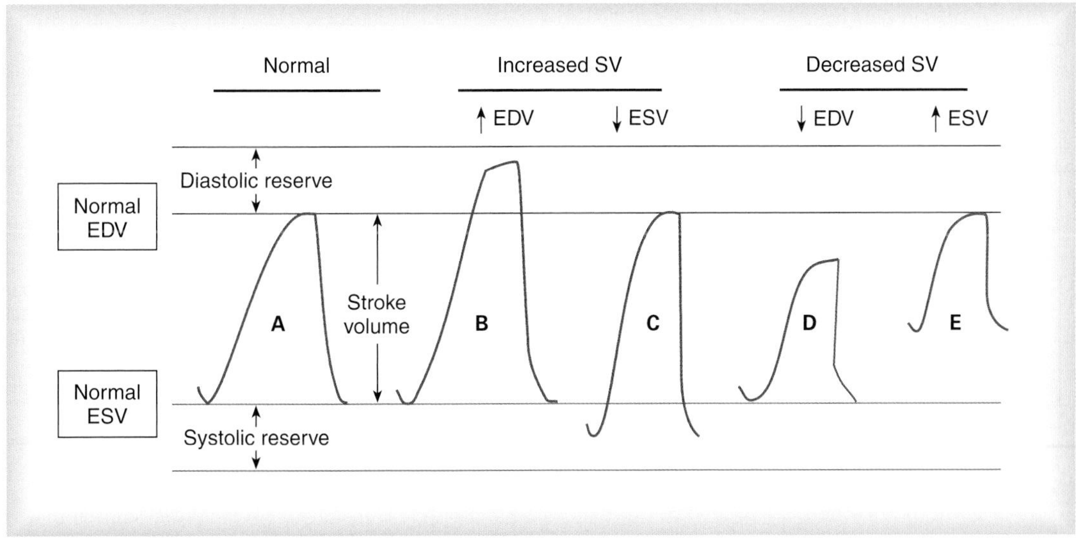

Figure 8-8

Relationship between stroke volume *(SV)*, end-diastolic volume *(EDV)*, and end-systolic volume *(ESV)*. **A,** Normal relationship between EDV, ESV, and SV; **B,** increased SV resulting from increased EDV; **C,** increased SV resulting from decreased ESV; **D,** decreased SV resulting from decreased EDV (hypovolemia) and; **E,** decreased SV resulting from increased ESV (poor contractility).

and vice versa. This concept is similar to stretching a rubber band—the greater the stretch (up to a point), the greater the contractile force.

In clinical practice, this initial ventricular stretch is called **preload,** while the tension of contraction is equivalent to stroke volume. Figure 8-9 applies the Frank-Starling law to ventricular function by plotting ventricular stretch against stroke volume. Ventricular stretch is directly proportional to EDV, and EDV in turn is directly related to the pressure difference across the ventricle wall. Thus preload can be measured indirectly as the ventricular end-diastolic pressure.

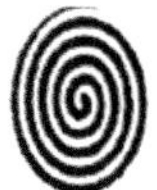

RULE OF THUMB

Increases in preload result in increased stroke volume in the healthy heart.

Another major factor affecting stroke volume is the force against which the heart must pump. This is called **afterload.** In clinical practice, left ventricular afterload equals the SVR. In other words, the greater the resistance to blood flow, the greater the afterload.

All else being constant, the greater the afterload on the ventricles, the harder it is for them to eject their volume. Thus for a given EDV, an increase in afterload causes the volume remaining in the ventricle after systole (the ESV) to increase. Of course, if the EDV remains constant while the ESV increases, the stroke volume (EDV − ESV) will decrease (see Figure 8-8). Normally, however, the heart muscle responds to increased afterload by altering its contractility.

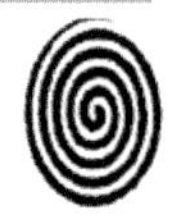

RULE OF THUMB

Increases in afterload can decrease stroke volume, especially in the failing heart.

Contractility represents the amount of systolic force exerted by the heart muscle at any given preload. At a given preload (EDV), an increase in contractility results in a higher EF, a lower ESV, and thus a higher stroke volume. Conversely, a decrease in contractility results in a lower EF, higher ESV, and decreased stroke volume.

Changes in contractility affect the slope of the ventricular function curve (see Figures 8-9 and 8-10). Higher stroke volumes for a given preload (increased slope) indicate a state of increased contractility, often referred to as **positive inotropism.** The opposite is also true. Lower stroke volumes for a given preload indicate decreased contractility, referred to as **negative inotropism.**

In addition to local mechanisms, cardiac contractility is influenced by neural control, circulating hormonal factors, and certain drugs.

Whether local or central in origin, all of these factors influence the reactivity of contractile proteins, mainly by affecting calcium metabolism in the sarcomere. Typically, neural or drug-mediated *sympathetic* stimulation has a positive inotropic effect. Conversely, *parasympathetic* stimulation exerts a negative inotropic effect. Profound *hypoxia* and *acidosis* impair myocardial metabolism and decrease cardiac contractility.

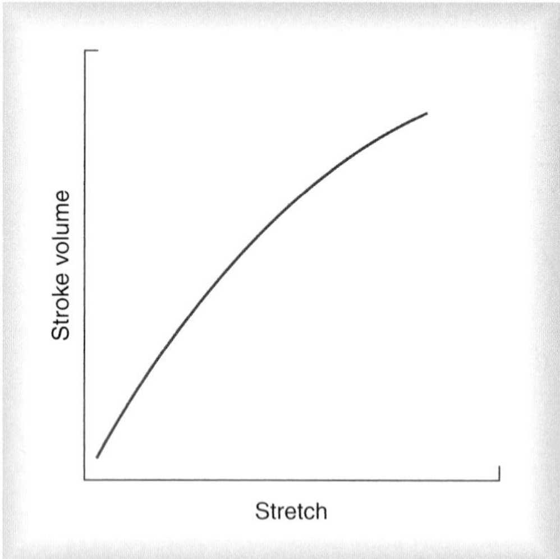

Figure 8-9

The Frank-Starling law—stroke volume as a function of ventricular end-diastolic stretch. An increase in the stretch of the ventricles immediately before contraction (end-diastole) results in an increase in stroke volume. Note that ventricular end-diastolic stretch is synonymous with the concept of preload.

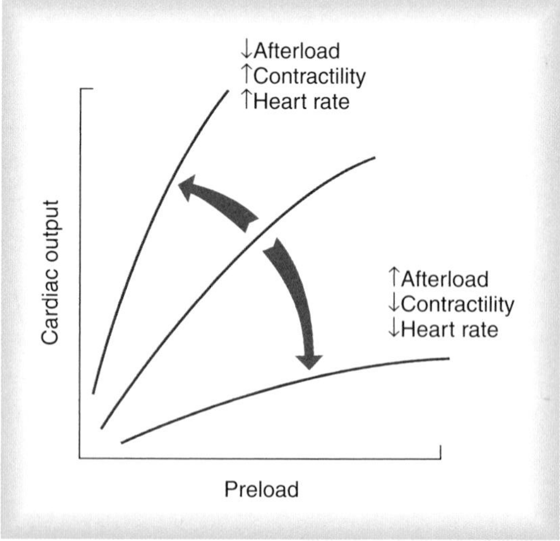

Figure 8-10

Effects of preload, afterload, contractility, and heart rate on cardiac output function curve. *(Modified from Green JF: Fundamental cardiovascular and pulmonary physiology, ed 2, Philadelphia, 1987, Lea & Febiger.)*

MINI CLINI

The Effect of Increased Afterload on Cardiac Output in the Normal Heart

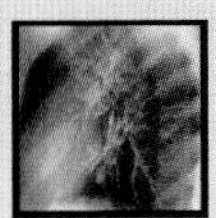

Afterload is the force against which the heart works to eject its stroke volume. Afterload can be thought of as outflow resistance. It is apparent that as afterload increases, the stroke volume ejected by the ventricle decreases, assuming that the heart's contractility (force with which the heart contracts) remains constant.

PROBLEM

During exercise, the healthy person's blood pressure rises considerably, indicating that the afterload has increased. Yet the healthy heart's stroke volume and cardiac output do not decrease. Why is this so?

DISCUSSION

When afterload increases, the initial ventricular contractions that experience the increased afterload produce smaller stroke volumes. This in turn causes more blood to be left in the ventricle at the end of systole (i.e., the ESV is increased). During the subsequent diastole, blood rushes in from the atria to fill the ventricle, and because of the higher than normal ESV, the ventricle becomes more distended and stretched than before. The healthy heart muscle responds to increased stretch in a way described by the Frank-Starling law; that is, the heart now contracts with greater force than before, ejecting a greater stroke volume. By increasing contractility in this fashion, stroke volume and cardiac output are not compromised by increased afterload in the healthy heart.

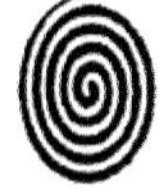

RULE OF THUMB

Hypoxia and acidosis decrease cardiac contractility and output.

Changes in Heart Rate

The last factor influencing cardiac output is **heart rate.** Unlike the factors controlling stroke volume, those affecting rate are mainly of central origin (i.e., neural or hormonal).

As expected, cardiac output rises and falls with like changes in heart rate. However, this relationship is maintained only up to approximately 160 to 180 beats/min in a healthy heart. At higher heart rates, there is not enough time for the ventricles to fill completely. This causes a drop in EDV, a decrease in stroke volume, and a fall in cardiac output. The drop in EDV associated with an elevated heart rate usually occurs well below 160 beats/min in the diseased heart.

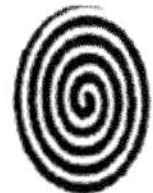

RULE OF THUMB

Increase in heart rate will increase cardiac output in the healthy heart up to a rate of 160 to 180 beats/min.

The combined effects of preload, afterload, contractility, and heart rate on cardiac performance are graphically portrayed in Figure 8-10. The middle ventricular function curve represents the normal state. The upper, steeper curve represents a hypereffective heart. In the hypereffective heart, a given preload results in a greater than normal cardiac output. Factors contributing to this state include decreased afterload, increased contractility, and increased heart rate. The bottom curve has less slope than normal, indicating a hypoeffective heart. Factors contributing to this state include increased afterload, decreased contractility, and decreased rate.

Cardiovascular Control Mechanisms

Cardiovascular control is achieved by integrating local and central regulatory mechanisms that affect both the heart and the vasculature. The goal is to ensure that all tissues receive sufficient blood flow to meet their metabolic needs. Under normal resting conditions, this goal is achieved mainly by local regulation of the heart and vasculature. However, when demands are increased or abnormal, such as during exercise or massive bleeding, central mechanisms take over primary control.

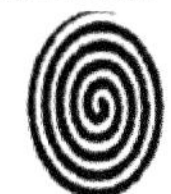

RULE OF THUMB

Blood flow to a specific vascular bed is primarily regulated by local mechanisms.

Central control of cardiovascular function occurs by interaction between the brainstem and selected peripheral receptors. The brainstem constantly receives data from these receptors about the pressure, volume, and chemical status of the blood. The brainstem also receives input from higher brain centers, such as the hypothalamus and cerebral cortex. These inputs are integrated with those coming from the heart and blood vessels to maintain adequate blood flow and pressure under all but the most abnormal conditions.

Cardiovascular Control Centers

Figure 8-11 provides a simplified diagram of the cardiovascular regulatory centers.

MINI CLINI

Heart Rate and the Administration of Bronchodilator Drugs

PROBLEM

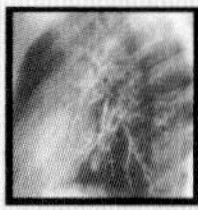

You are giving a bronchodilator aerosolized drug to a patient, and you notice a significant increase in the patient's heart rate. Would you expect increased heart rate to be a common side effect of drugs that cause bronchodilation?

DISCUSSION

The discharge rate of the sinus node, and thus the heart rate, is increased by sympathetic nervous stimulation and decreased by parasympathetic nervous stimulation. The airways of the lung are dilated by sympathetic nervous stimulation and constricted by parasympathetic stimulation. Drugs that cause bronchodilation either mimic sympathetic stimulation (sympathomimetic) or block parasympathetic stimulation (parasympatholytic). Both of these drug actions also cause the heart rate to increase, as noted. Parasympatholytic drugs bring about effects similar to sympathetic stimulation because by inhibiting parasympathetic activity, they allow sympathetic impulses to predominate, ultimately causing a sympathetic-like response.

Areas in the medulla receive input from higher brain centers, peripheral pressure, and chemical receptors. Stimulation of the vasoconstrictor area within the medulla increases output to adrenergic receptors in the vascular smooth muscle, causing **vasoconstriction** and increased vascular resistance. A vasodepressor area works mainly by inhibiting the vasoconstrictor center.

Closely associated with the vasoconstrictor center is a cardioaccelerator area. Stimulation of this center increases heart rate by increasing sympathetic discharge to the heart's SA and AV nodes. A cardioinhibitory area plays the opposite role. Stimulation of this center decreases heart rate by increasing vagal (parasympathetic) stimulation to the heart. The vascular and cardiac centers also interact among themselves. For example, stimulation of the vasoconstrictor area tends to excite the cardioaccelerator center, causing a rise in both blood pressure and heart rate. Conversely, excitation of the vasodepressor area inhibits both the vasoconstrictor and cardioinhibitory areas. This causes vasodilation and an increase in heart rate.

Higher brain centers also influence the cardiovascular system, both directly and through the medulla. Signals coming from the cerebral cortex in response to exercise, pain, or anxiety pass directly through the

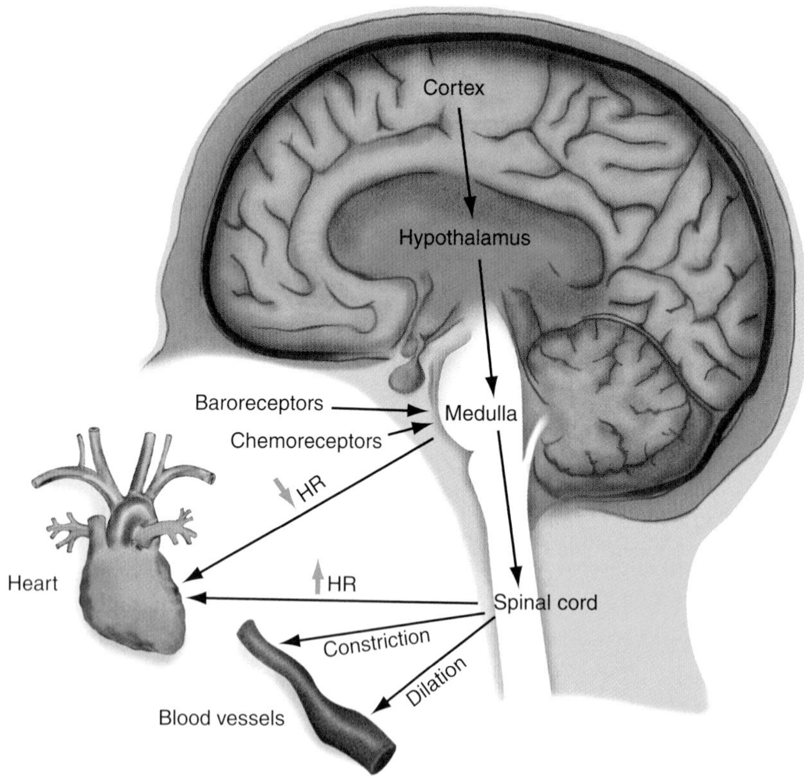

Figure 8-11

Schematic summarizing major known neural pathways involved in central regulation of cardiovascular function. This design is oversimplified to illustrate the major relationships between higher brain centers and peripheral receptors.

cholinergic fibers to the vascular smooth muscle, causing **vasodilation**. Signals from the hypothalamus, particularly its heat-regulating areas, indirectly affect heart rate and vasomotor tone through the cardiovascular centers.

The cardiovascular centers also are affected by local chemical changes in the surrounding blood and cerebral spinal fluid. For example, decreased levels of carbon dioxide tend to inhibit the medullary centers. General inhibition of these centers causes a decrease in vascular tone and thus a fall in blood pressure. A local decrease in oxygen tension has the opposite effect. Mild hypoxia in this area tends to increase sympathetic discharge rates. This tends to elevate both heart rate and blood pressure. Severe hypoxia has a depressant effect.

Peripheral Receptors

In addition to high-level and local input, the cardiovascular centers receive signals from peripheral receptors (see Figure 8-11). There are two types of peripheral cardiovascular receptors: baroreceptors and chemoreceptors. Baroreceptors respond to pressure changes, whereas chemoreceptors respond to changes in blood chemistry.

The cardiovascular system has two different sets of **baroreceptors**. The first set is located in the aortic arch and carotid sinuses. These receptors monitor arterial pressures generated by the left ventricle. The second set is located in the walls of the atria and the large thoracic and pulmonary veins. These low-pressure sensors respond mainly to changes in vascular volumes. Baroreceptor output is directly proportional to the stretch on the vessel wall. The greater the blood pressure, the greater the stretch and the higher the rate of neural discharge to the cardiovascular centers in the medulla.

Together with the cardiovascular regulatory centers, these receptors form a **negative feedback loop**. A negative feedback system is designed to stabilize a controlled variable, in this case blood pressure. In a negative feedback loop, stimulation of a receptor causes an opposite response by the effector. In the case of the arterial receptors, a rise in blood pressure increases aortic and carotid and receptor stretch, and thus the discharge rate. The increased discharge rate causes an opposite response by the medullary centers (i.e., a depressor response). Venomotor tone decreases, blood vessels dilate, and heart rate and contractility both decrease. Decreased blood pressure (decreased baroreceptor output) has the opposite effect, causing vessel constriction and increased heart rate and contractility.

Whereas the high-pressure arterial receptors constantly control blood pressure, the low-pressure sensors are responsible for long-term regulation of plasma volume. The low-pressure atrial and venous baroreceptors regulate plasma volume mainly through their effects on the following:

- Renal sympathetic nerve activity
- Release of antidiuretic hormone (ADH), which is also called *vasopressin*
- Release of atrial natriuretic factor (ANF)
- The renin-angiotensin-aldosterone system

The major pathways for plasma volume control are outlined in Figure 8-12. As indicated, an increase in blood volume stimulates the atrial and venous baroreceptors. This causes a decrease in ADH and aldosterone levels and an increase in the ANF level. ADH and aldosterone cause sodium and water retention, whereas ANF is a potent diuretic. Thus decreases in ADH and aldosterone and increases in ANF all promote sodium and water excretion. Combined with a CNS-mediated rise in renal filtration, these humoral mechanisms decrease the overall plasma volume. A decrease in blood volume has the opposite effect (i.e., sodium and water retention and an increase in plasma volume).

Chemoreceptors are small, highly vascularized tissues located near the high-pressure sensors in the aortic arch and carotid sinus. Whereas baroreceptors respond to pressure changes, chemoreceptors are sensitive to changes in blood chemistry. They are strongly stimulated by decreased oxygen tensions, although low pH or high levels of carbon dioxide also can increase their discharge rate. The major cardiovascular effects of chemoreceptor stimulation are vasoconstriction and increased heart rate.

Because these changes occur only when the cardiopulmonary system is overtaxed, the chemoreceptors probably have little influence under normal conditions. Their influence on respiration, however, is clinically important. For this reason, the peripheral chemoreceptors are discussed in greater detail in Chapter 7.

Response to Changes in Overall Volume

The coordinated response of the cardiovascular system is best demonstrated under abnormal conditions. Among the most common clinical conditions in which all essential regulatory mechanisms come into play is the large blood loss that occurs with hemorrhage. Figure 8-13 illustrates changes in these key factors during progressive blood loss in an animal model.

With 10% blood loss, the immediate drop in the *central venous pressure* (CVP) causes a 50% decrease in the discharge rate of the low-pressure (atrial) baroreceptors. There is little change in the activity of the high-pressure (arterial) receptors. The initial response, mediated through the medullary centers, is an increase in sympathetic discharge to the sinus node. This causes a progressive rise in heart rate. At the same time, plasma levels of ADH (vasopressin) begin to rise. These two initial changes are sufficient to maintain normal arterial blood pressure.

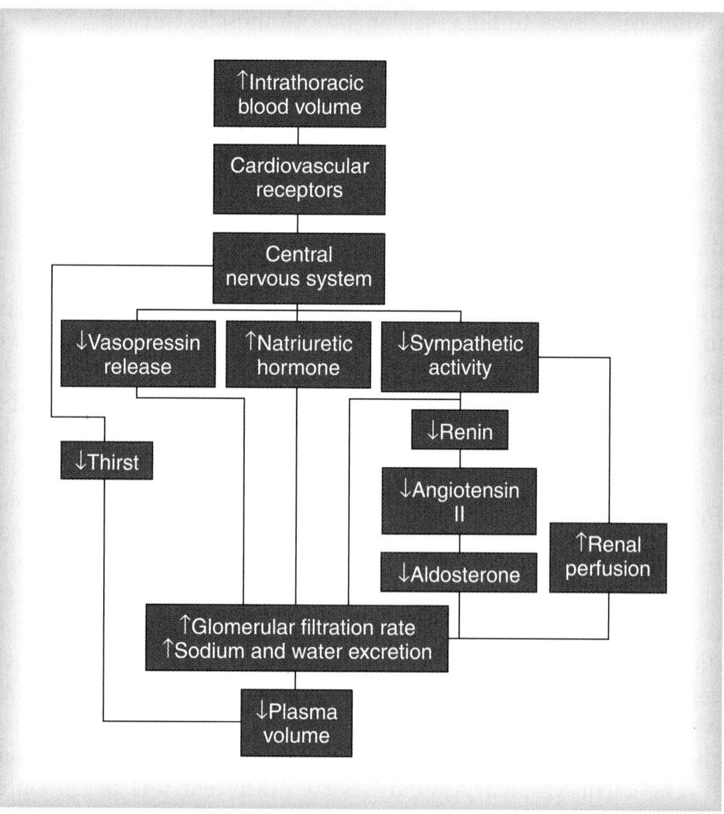

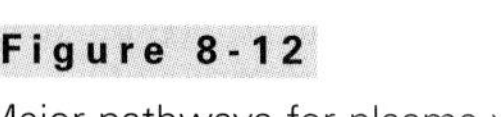

Figure 8-12

Major pathways for plasma volume control. See text for details. *(Modified from Smith JJ, Kampine JP: Circulatory physiology: the essentials, ed 3, Baltimore, 1990, Williams & Wilkins.)*

As the blood loss becomes more severe (20%), atrial receptor activity decreases further. This increases the intensity of sympathetic discharge from the cardiovascular centers. Plasma ADH and heart rate continue to climb, as does peripheral vasculature tone. An increase in vascular tone occurs mainly through constriction of the capacitance vessels in the venous system, thereby slowing the drop in CVP.

Not until blood loss approaches 30% does the arterial pressure start to drop. At this point, arterial receptor activity begins to decrease, resulting in a marked rise in systemic vascular tone. Despite the magnitude of blood loss, CVP levels off. As long as no further hemorrhage occurs, blood pressure, and therefore tissue perfusion, can be maintained at adequate levels.

If blood loss continues, then central control mechanisms begin to take over. Massive vasoconstriction occurs in the resistance vessels, shunting blood away from skeletal muscle to maintain blood flow to the brain and heart. Rising levels of local metabolites in these areas, especially CO_2 and other acids, override central control and cause further vessel dilation and increased blood flow. Unfortunately, as these metabolites build up, and as the tissues become hypoxic, cardiac function becomes impaired and vasodilation occurs throughout the body. This signals the onset of a state of irreversible shock, after which death ensues.

▶ EVENTS OF THE CARDIAC CYCLE

Up to this point, this chapter has focused on the heart's mechanical properties, and in Chapter 15 the electrical activities of the heart are discussed. Although they are discussed separately, keep in mind that the mechanical and electrical events are interdependent. Given the critical role of RTs in dealing with cardiovascular problems, an in-depth knowledge of how these events relate is essential.

The events of the cardiac cycle are portrayed in Figure 8-14. The top of the figure shows a time axis scaled in tenths of a second. Next are the timing bars for ventricular systole and diastole and pressure events in the atria, ventricles, and aorta. These are followed by an electrocardiogram (ECG), heart sounds, and ventricular flow (see Chapter 15 for an explanation of the ECG waves).

Going from left to right, the P wave (atrial depolarization) begins the ECG (equivalent to late diastole). Before this point, the ventricles have been passively filling with blood through the open AV valves. The P wave signals atrial depolarization. Within 0.1 second, the atria contract, causing a slight rise in both atrial and ventricular pressures (the *a waves*). This atrial contraction helps preload the ventricles, increasing their volume

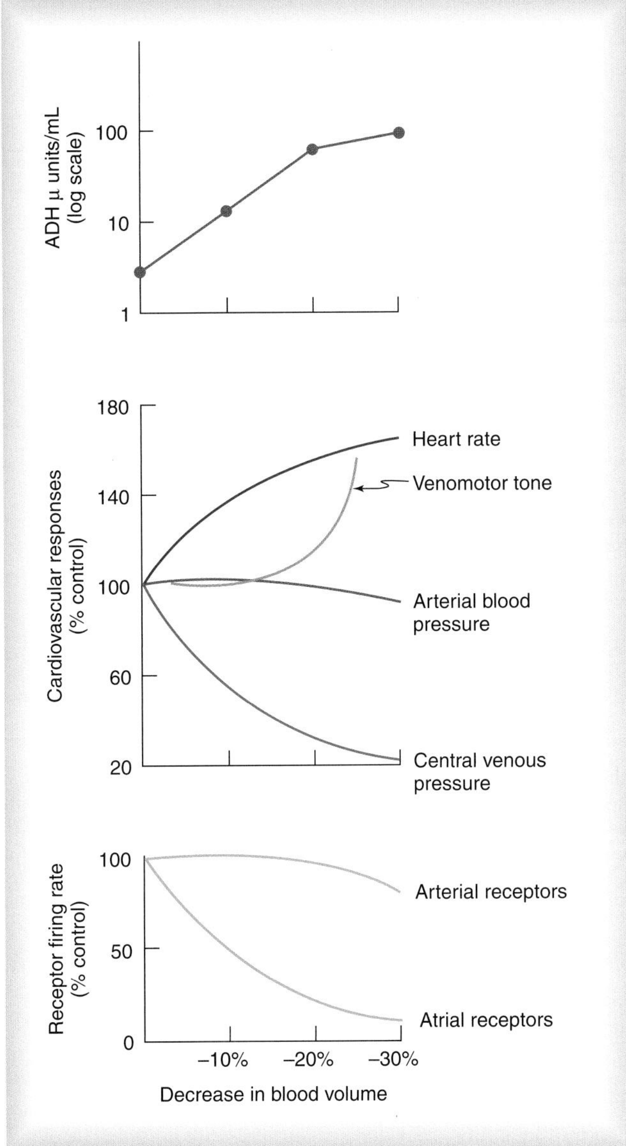

Figure 8-13

Plasma levels of antidiuretic hormone (ADH), cardiovascular responses, and receptor firing rates in response to graded hemorrhage in the dog. See text for details. *(Modified from Richardson DR: Basic circulatory physiology, Boston, 1976, Little, Brown & Co. Venomotor tone data are those of WJ Sears as cited in Gauer OH, Henry JP, Behn C: Annu Rev Physiol 32:547, 1970. All other data are from Henry JP et al: Can J Physiol Pharmacol 46:287, 1968.)*

by as much as 25%. Toward the end of diastole, the electrical impulses from the atria reach the AV node and bundle branches. This initiates ventricular depolarization (the QRS complex). Within a few hundredths of a second after depolarization, the ventricles begin to contract. As soon as ventricular pressures exceed those in the atria, the AV valves close. Closure of the mitral valve occurs first, followed immediately by closure of the tricuspid valve. This marks the end of ventricular diastole, producing the first heart sound on the phonocardiogram.

Immediately after AV valve closure, the ventricles become closed chambers. During this short isovolemic phase of contraction, ventricular pressures rise rapidly. Upward bulging of the AV valves during this phase causes a slight upswing in atrial pressure graphs, called the *c wave*. Within 0.05 seconds, ventricular pressures rise to exceed those in the aorta and pulmonary artery. This opens the semilunar valves.

Toward the end of systole, as repolarization starts (indicated by the T wave), the ventricles begin to relax. Consequently, ventricular pressures drop rapidly. When arterial pressures exceed those in the relaxing ventricles, the semilunar valves close. Closure of the semilunar valves generates the second heart sound.

Rather than immediately dropping off, aortic and pulmonary pressures rise again after the semilunar valves close. Note the feature termed the *dicrotic notch*, which is caused by the elastic recoil of the arteries. This recoil provides the extra "push" that helps maintain the head of pressure created by the ventricles.

As the ventricles continue to relax, their pressures drop below those in the atria. This reopens the AV valves. As soon as the AV valves open, the blood collected in the atria rushes to fill the ventricles, causing a rapid drop in atrial pressures (the *v wave*). Thereafter, ventricular filling slows as the heart prepares for a new cycle.

Knowledge of these normal events helps one understand many of the diagnostic and monitoring procedures used for patients with cardiopulmonary disorders. Among the most common are the measurement of CVP, balloon-directed pulmonary artery catheterization, and direct arterial pressure monitoring.

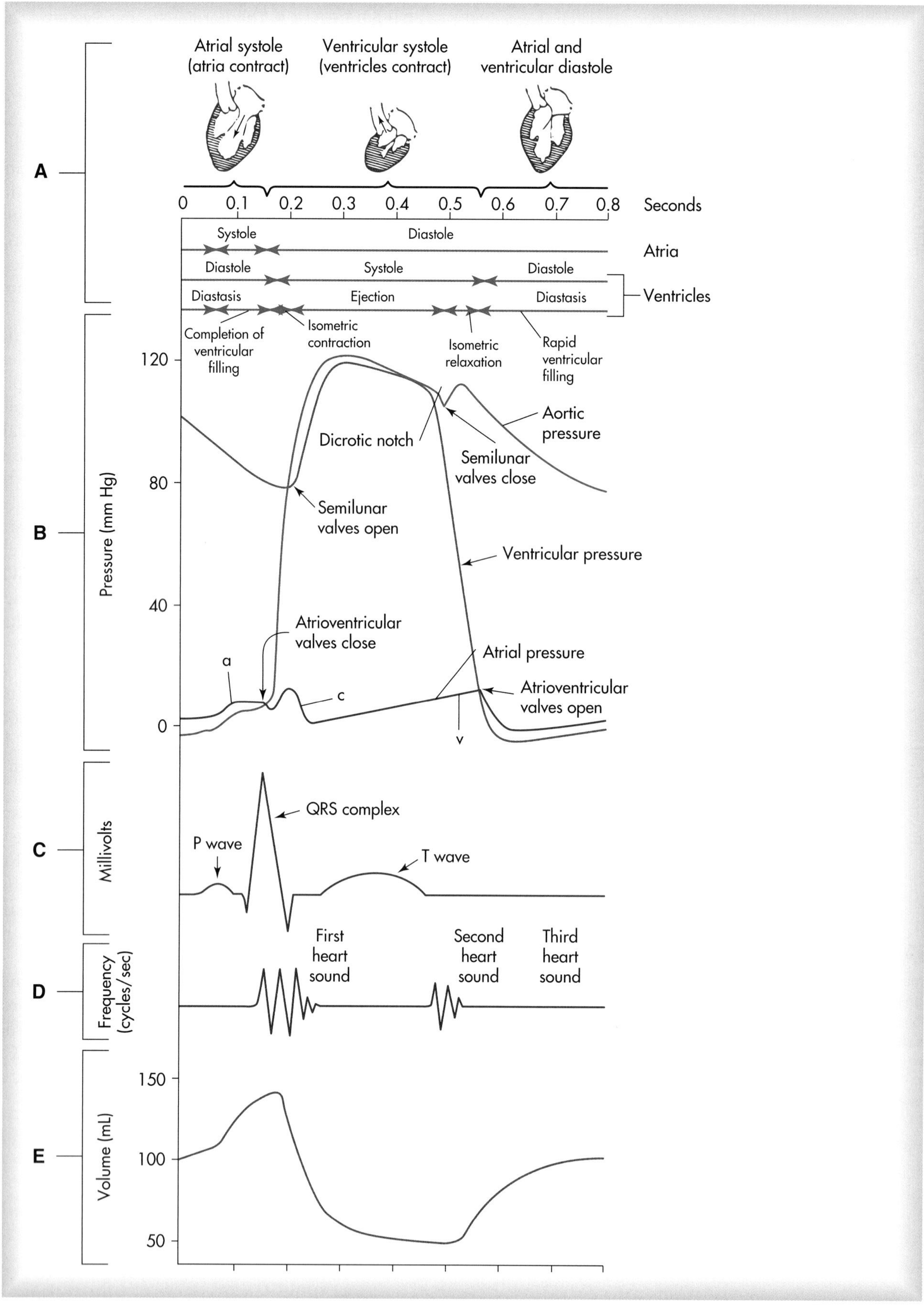

Figure 8-14

The cardiac cycle. **A,** Timing of cardiac events; **B,** simultaneous pressures created in the aorta, left ventricle, and right atrium during the cardiac cycle; **C,** electrical activity during the cardiac cycle; **D,** heart sounds corresponding to the cardiac cycle; **E,** ventricular blood volume during the cardiac cycle. *(Modified from Moffett DF, Moffett SB, Schauf CL: Human physiology: foundations & frontiers, ed 2, St Louis, 1993, Mosby.)*

KEY POINTS

- The cardiovascular system consists of the heart and a complex vascular network, which work together to maintain homeostasis by continually distributing and regulating blood flow throughout the body.
- Specialized mechanical and electrical properties of cardiac tissue, combined with internal and external control mechanisms, provide the basis for coordinated cardiac function.
- The vascular system is regulated by both local and central control mechanisms.
- Cardiac output is primarily determined by four factors: preload, afterload, contractility, and heart rate.
- The vascular network assumes an active role in the control and distribution of blood flow.
- The heart and the vascular systems work together in a coordinated fashion to ensure that all body tissues receive sufficient blood to meet their metabolic needs.
- Under conditions of increased demand, special compensatory mechanisms are called on to maintain stable blood flow.
- Failure of cardiovascular control mechanisms often requires the intervention of RTs to help restore and maintain normal function.

Bibliography

Andreoli CC et al: Cecil essentials of medicine, ed 5, Philadelphia, 2001, WB Saunders.

Berne RM, Levy MN, editors: Physiology, ed 4, St Louis, 1998, Mosby.

Brody TM, Larner J, Minneman KP: Human pharmacology: molecular to clinical, ed 3, St Louis, 1998, Mosby.

Ganong WF: Review of medical physiology, ed 20, New York, 2001, Lange Medical Books/McGraw-Hill.

Guyton AC, Hall JE: Textbook of medical physiology, ed 10, Philadelphia, 2000, WB Saunders.

Mathers LH et al: Clinical anatomy principles, St Louis, 1996, Mosby.

Moore KL, Dalley AF: Clinically oriented anatomy, ed 4, Baltimore, 1999, Williams & Wilkins.

Stevens A, Lowe J: Human histology, ed 2, St Louis, 1997, Mosby.

Thibodeau GA, Patton KT: Anthony's textbook of anatomy & physiology, ed 15, St Louis, 1996, Mosby.

Woods SL, Froelicher ESS, Motzer SA: Cardiac nursing, ed 4, Philadelphia, 2000, Lippincott.

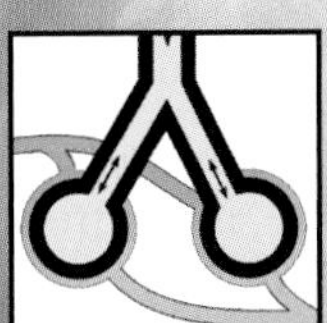

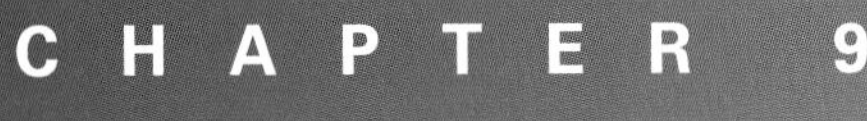

CHAPTER 9

Ventilation

Gregg L. Ruppel

In This Chapter You Will Learn:

- What physiological purposes ventilation serves
- What pressure gradients are responsible for gas movement and lung inflation
- What forces oppose gas movement into and out of the lungs
- How surface tension contributes to lung recoil
- How lung, chest wall, and total compliance are related
- What factors affect airway resistance
- How various lung diseases affect the work of breathing
- Why ventilation is not evenly distributed throughout the lung
- How the time constants affect alveolar filling and emptying
- What factors affect alveolar ventilation and why they are important
- How to calculate alveolar ventilation, dead space, and the V_D/V_T

Chapter Outline

Key Terms

acidemia
ankylosing spondylitis
ascites
cartilaginous
collagen
distensible
embolism
endotracheal
interface
intrapulmonary
kyphoscoliosis
parenchyma
plethysmograph
pneumotachometer
pulmonary fibrosis
sepsis
spirometer

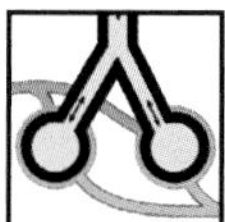

The primary functions of the lungs are to supply the body with oxygen (O_2) and to remove carbon dioxide (CO_2). To accomplish this, the lungs must be adequately ventilated. Ventilation is the process of moving air in and out of the lungs. This distinguishes ventilation from respiration, which involves complex chemical and physiological processes at the cellular level.

In health, ventilation is regulated to meet the body's needs under varying conditions. However, in disease, this process can be disrupted. Inadequate ventilation or increased work of breathing often results. Respiratory care is often directed toward restoring adequate and efficient ventilation. Respiratory care modalities reduce the work of breathing and provide artificial ventilation if necessary. Providing effective respiratory care requires an understanding of normal ventilatory processes, as well as how various diseases may affect ventilation.

MECHANICS OF VENTILATION

Normal ventilation is a cyclical activity that has two phases: inspiration and expiration. During each cycle, a volume of gas moves in and out of the respiratory tract. This volume, measured during either inspiration or expiration, is called the *tidal volume* or V_T. The normal V_T removes CO_2 and supplies O_2 to meet metabolic needs. There must be sufficient reserve to meet increased ventilatory demands, such as during exercise. The *vital capacity* (VC) and its subdivisions provide the necessary reserves for increasing ventilation (see Chapter 17).

Ventilation can be related to the following equation of motion for the respiratory system:

$$\text{Pressure} = \frac{\text{Volume}}{\text{Compliance}} + (\text{Resistance} \times \text{Flow})$$

where:

Pressure = Force generated by the respiratory muscles during inspiration

Volume = Volume change (e.g., V_T)

Compliance = Distensibility of the lungs and thorax

Resistance = Airflow and tissue resistance

Flow = Volume change per unit of time

The compliance and resistance of the lungs and thorax make up the load against which the respiratory muscles must work to ventilate the lungs. In healthy lungs, this work is performed during the inspiratory phase. Expiration is normally a passive maneuver.

Pressure Differences During Breathing

Ventilation occurs because of pressure gradients created by expansion and contraction of the thorax. Figure 9-1 shows the key pressures and gradients involved in ventilation. These pressures usually are measured in centimeters of water (cm H_2O). Respiratory pressures are often expressed relative to atmospheric pressure. A respiratory pressure of 0 is equivalent to 1 atmosphere (i.e., 1034 cm H_2O, or 760 mm Hg). A positive pressure is one that is greater than atmospheric pressure. The term *negative pressure* is sometimes used to describe subatmospheric pressures (i.e., less than 1 atmosphere).

Mouth pressure, at the opening of the airway, is abbreviated by the term P_{ao}. Unless positive or negative pressure is applied to the airway, P_{ao} is always 0 (i.e., atmospheric pressure). Pressure at the body surface (P_{bs}), equal to atmospheric pressure, is also usually 0. Alveolar pressure (P_{alv}), often referred to as **intrapulmonary** pressure, varies during the breathing cycle. Pleural pressure (P_{pl}) is usually negative (i.e., subatmospheric) during quiet breathing. P_{pl} also varies during the breathing cycle.

The difference between two pressures is called a *pressure gradient.* Three important pressure gradients are involved in ventilation: (1) transrespiratory, (2) transpulmonary, and (3) transthoracic. The transrespiratory pressure gradient (P_{rs}) represents the difference in pressure between the atmosphere (body surface) and the alveoli:

$$P_{rs} = P_{alv} - P_{bs}$$

In a spontaneously breathing subject, the pressures at the body surface and at the airway opening (mouth) both equal atmospheric pressure. The following equation substitutes P_{ao} for P_{bs}:

$$P_{rs} = P_{alv} - P_{ao}$$

The transrespiratory pressure gradient causes gas to flow into and out of the alveoli during breathing. The transpulmonary pressure gradient, or P_L, equals the pressure difference between the alveoli and the pleural space, as shown in the following equation:

$$P_L = P_{alv} - P_{pl}$$

P_L is the pressure difference that maintains alveolar inflation. Changes in P_L during breathing result in corresponding changes in alveolar volume. The transthoracic pressure gradient, or P_w, represents the difference in pressure between the pleural space and the body surface, as shown in the following equation:

$$P_w = P_{pl} - P_{bs}$$

P_w is the pressure across the chest wall. It represents the total pressure necessary to expand or contract the lungs and chest wall together.

During a normal breathing cycle, the glottis remains open. P_{bs} and P_{ao} remain at 0 (i.e., atmospheric) throughout the cycle; therefore only changes in P_{alv} and

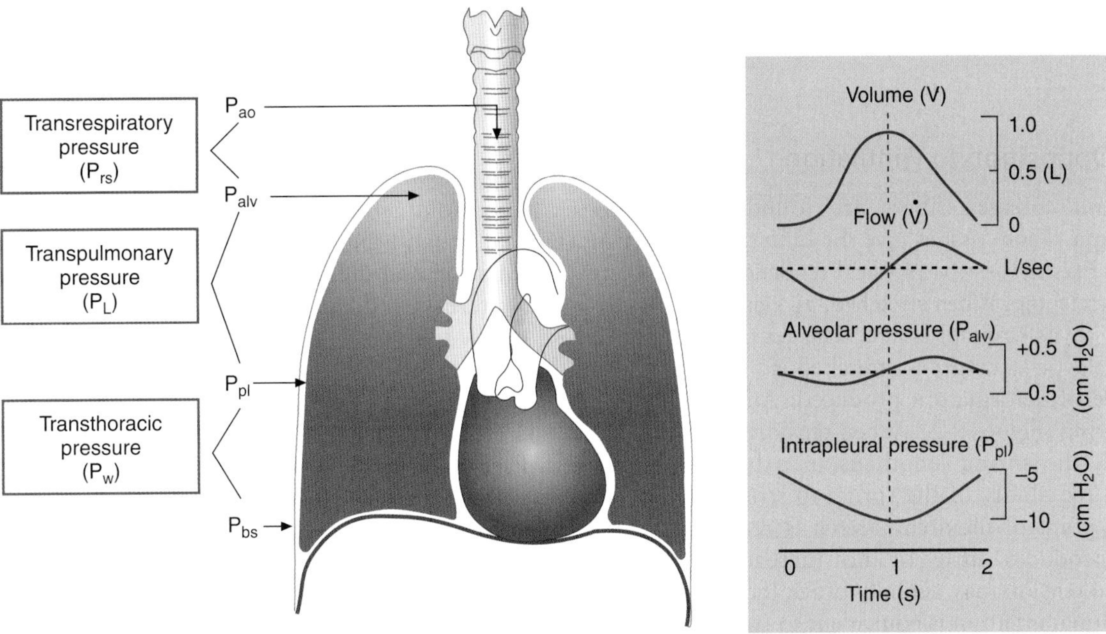

Figure 9-1

Pressures, volumes, and flows involved in ventilation. P_{alv}, Pressure in the alveoli (intrapulmonary pressure); P_{ao}, pressure at the airway opening (mouth pressure); P_{bs}, pressure at the body surface; P_{pl}, pressure in the pleural space (intrapleural pressure). The transrespiratory pressure gradient ($P_{rs} = P_{alv} - P_{ao}$) is responsible for gas flow into and out of the lungs. The transpulmonary pressure gradient ($P_L = P_{alv} - P_{pl}$) is responsible for the degree of alveolar inflation. The transthoracic pressure gradient ($P_w = P_{pl} - P_{bs}$) is the difference in pressure across the chest wall, or the total pressure necessary to expand or contract the lungs and chest wall together. Changes in flow and volume are related to changes in these pressure gradients, as depicted in the graphs on the right. Flow ($\dot{V}$) and P_{alv} are biphasic during a single breath; alveolar volume (V) increases as P_{pl} falls. *(Modified from Martin L: Pulmonary physiology in clinical practice: the essentials for patient care and evaluation, St Louis, 1987, Mosby.)*

P_{pl} are of interest. Before inspiration, pleural pressure is approximately −5 cm H_2O, and alveolar pressure is 0 cm H_2O. Therefore the transpulmonary pressure gradient is also approximately −5 cm H_2O in the resting state. This pressure gradient maintains the lung at its resting volume. Alveolar and airway opening pressures are both 0, so the transrespiratory pressure gradient also is 0. No gas moves into or out of the respiratory tract.

Inspiration begins when muscular effort expands the thorax. Thoracic expansion causes a *decrease* in pleural pressure. As the pleural pressure drops, the transpulmonary pressure gradient widens, causing the alveoli to expand. As the alveoli expand, their pressures fall below the pressure at the airway opening. This "negative" transrespiratory pressure gradient causes air to flow from the airway opening to the alveoli, increasing their volume.

P_{pl} continues to decrease until the end of inspiration. Alveolar pressure approaches equilibrium with the atmosphere. Alveolar filling slows, and inspiratory flow decreases to 0 (see Figure 9-1). At this point, called *end-inspiration*, alveolar pressure has returned to 0 and the transpulmonary pressure gradient reaches its maximal value (for a normal breath) of approximately −10 cm H_2O.

As expiration begins, the thorax recoils and P_{pl} starts to rise. As pleural pressure rises, the transpulmonary pressure gradient narrows and alveoli begin to deflate. As the alveoli become smaller, alveolar pressure exceeds that at the airway opening. This positive transrespiratory pressure gradient causes air to move from the alveoli toward the airway opening. When alveolar pressure has fallen back to atmospheric pressure, flow ceases and a new cycle begins.

These events occur during normal tidal volume excursions. Similar pressure changes accompany deeper inspiration and expiration. The magnitude of the pressure changes is greater with deeper breathing. During a forced expiration, pleural pressure may actually rise above atmospheric pressure.

Forces Opposing Inflation of the Lung

To generate the pressure gradients just described, the lungs must be distended. This distension requires several opposing forces to be overcome for inspiration to occur. Normal expiration is passive, using the energy stored during inspiration. The forces opposing lung inflation may be grouped into two categories: *elastic forces* and *frictional forces*. Elastic forces involve the tissues of the lungs and thorax, along with surface tension in the alveoli. Frictional forces include resistance caused by gas flow and tissue movement during breathing.

Elastic Opposition to Ventilation

Elastic and **collagen** fibers are found in the lung **parenchyma.** These tissues give the lung the property of elasticity. *Elasticity* is the physical tendency of an object to resist stretching. When stretched, an elastic body tends to return to its original shape. The tension developed when an elastic structure is stretched is proportional to the degree of deformation produced. An example is a simple spring (Figure 9-2). When tension on a spring is increased, the spring lengthens in a linear manner. However, the ability of the spring to stretch is limited. Once the point of maximal stretch is reached, further tension produces little or no increase in length. Additional tension may actually break the spring.

In the lung, inflation is equivalent to stretching. Lung elastic forces oppose inflation. To increase lung volume, pressure must be applied. This property may be demonstrated by subjecting a lung that has been removed from the body to different pressures and measuring the changes in volume (Figure 9-3). To simulate the pressures during breathing, the lung is placed in an airtight jar. The force to inflate the lung is provided by a pump that varies the pressure around the lung inside the jar. This action mimics thoracic expansion and contraction. The amount of stretch (inflation) is measured as volume by a **spirometer.** Changes in volume for a given pressure are plotted on a graph.

During inspiration, greater and greater negative pressures are required to stretch the lung to a larger volume. As the lung is stretched to its maximum, the inflation "curve" becomes flat. This flattening indicates *increasing* opposition to expansion.

As with a spring when tension is removed, deflation occurs passively as pressure in the jar is allowed to return toward atmospheric. Deflation of the lung does not follow the inflation curve exactly. During deflation, lung volume at any given pressure is slightly greater than it is during inflation. This difference between the inflation and deflation curves is called *hysteresis.*[1] This hysteresis indicates that factors other than simple elastic tissue forces are present.

Surface Tension Forces

Part of the hysteresis exhibited by the lung is a result of surface tension forces in the alveoli. If a lung is filled with fluid such as saline, the pressure-volume curves look much different from those of an air-filled lung (Figure 9-4). Less pressure is needed to inflate a fluid-filled lung to a given volume. Only a lung filled with air exhibits hysteresis. This phenomenon indicates that a gas-fluid **interface** in the air-filled lung changes its inflation-deflation characteristics. Lung elasticity varies with lung volume.

A lung filled with air is more difficult to inflate than one filled with fluid, because of surface tension at the gas-fluid interface in the alveoli. The lung contains millions of alveoli, each lined with a thin film of fluid. This gas-fluid interface causes surface tension forces, so the alveoli resemble bubbles (see Chapter 5).

The recoil of the lung is a combination of tissue elasticity and these surface tension forces in the alveoli. During inflation, additional pressure is needed to overcome surface tension forces. During deflation, surface tension forces are reduced, resulting in altered

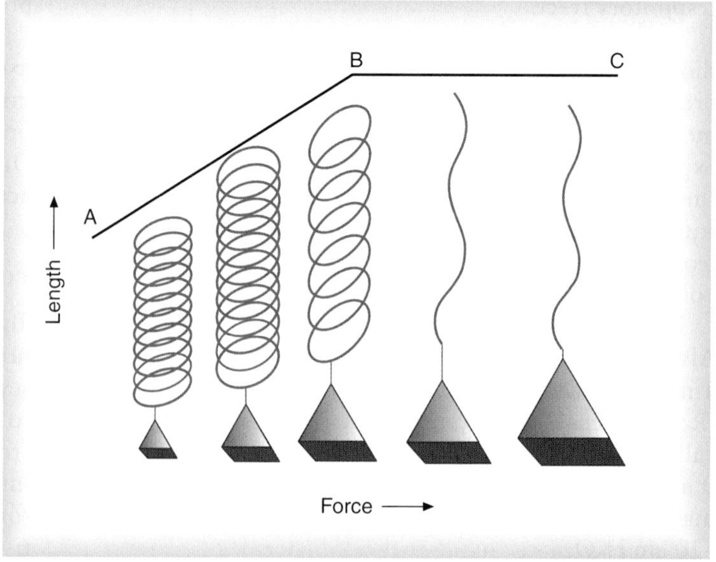

Figure 9-2

Graphic representation of the force-length relationship applied to a simple spring (increase in length with increase in force). With increasing force, or weight in this example, the spring lengthens in a linear manner, from *A* to *B*, but at the point of maximal stretch, further force produces no additional increase in length (*B* to *C*).

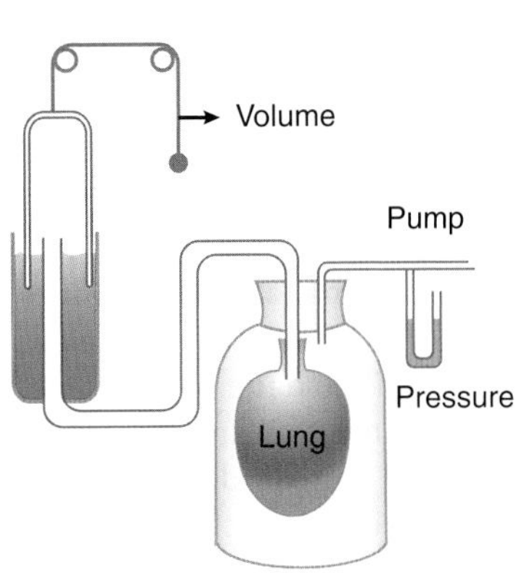

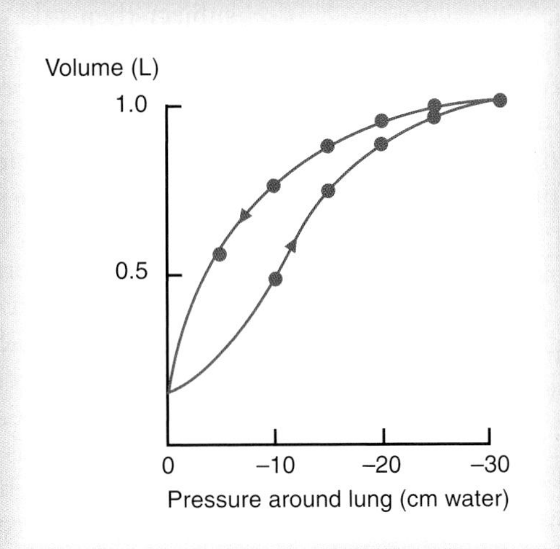

Figure 9-3

Measurement of the pressure-volume curve of an excised lung. The lung is held at various subatmospheric pressures for a few seconds while its volume is measured. The curve is nonlinear and flattens at high expanding pressures (subatmospheric). Note that the inflation and deflation curves are not the same. This difference is called *hysteresis. (Modified from West JB: Respiratory physiology: the essentials, ed 6, Baltimore, 2000, Williams & Wilkins.)*

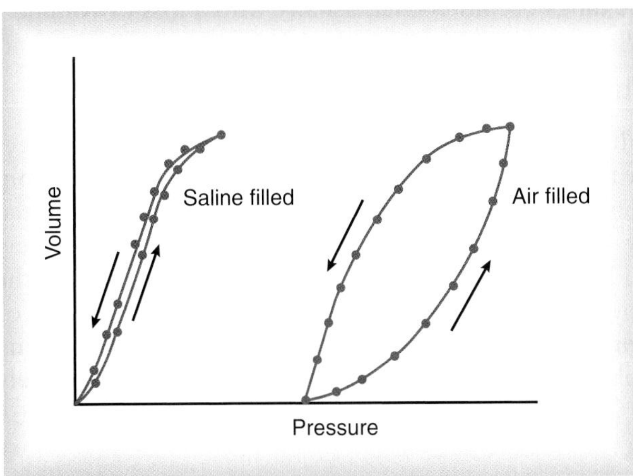

Figure 9-4

Static pressure-volume curves of saline- and air-filled excised lungs, demonstrating the effects of elastic forces *(left)* and elastic plus surface tension forces *(right)* on static compliance of the lung. *(Modified from Slonim NB, Hamilton LH: Respiratory physiology, ed 5, St Louis, 1987, Mosby.)*

pressure-volume characteristics. A substance called *pulmonary surfactant* lowers surface tension in the lung. Alveolar type II cells probably produce pulmonary surfactant (see Chapter 7). Unlike typical surface-active agents, pulmonary surfactant changes surface tension according to its area.[1] Pulmonary surfactant's ability to lower surface tension decreases as surface area (i.e., lung volume) increases. Conversely, when surface area decreases, the ability of pulmonary surfactant to lower surface tension increases. This property of changing surface tension to match lung volume helps stabilize the alveoli. Any disorder that alters or destroys pulmonary surfactant can cause significant changes in the work of distending the lung.

MINI CLINI

Surfactant Replacement Therapy and Lung Mechanics

PROBLEM

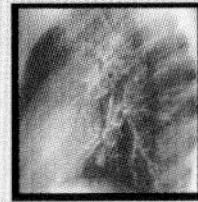

If an infant is born prematurely, the lungs may be unable to synthesize adequate amounts of pulmonary surfactant. How does this condition affect lung mechanics, and what effect will surfactant replacement therapy have on lung compliance and the work of breathing?

DISCUSSION

The liquid molecules that line each alveolus attract one another. This attraction creates a force called *surface tension,* which tends to shrink the alveolus. Pulmonary surfactant molecules have weak intramolecular attractive forces. When surfactant molecules are mixed with other liquid molecules that have higher intramolecular attraction, the surfactant molecules are pushed to the surface of the liquid, where they form the air-liquid interface. Because of the weak intramolecular attraction between these surfactant molecules at the surface, the liquid lining of the alveoli exhibits much less surface tension than it would in the absence of pulmonary surfactant. The premature infant with inadequate surfactant has abnormally high intraalveolar surface tension. This produces a collapsing force that increases lung recoil and reduces lung compliance. Greater muscular effort is required to overcome increased recoil during inspiration, and the work of breathing is increased. The infant may eventually become fatigued and develop ventilatory failure. Instillation of surfactant into the lungs reduces surface tension to its normal level. This increases lung compliance, reduces elastic recoil, and reduces the muscular work required to inflate the lung.

Lung Compliance

Tissue elastic forces and surface tension oppose lung inflation. Compliance measures the distensibility of the lung, whereas elastance is the property of resisting deformation. Compliance is the reciprocal of elastance:

$$\text{Compliance} = \frac{1}{\text{Elastance}}$$

Compliance of the lung (C_L) is defined as volume change per unit of pressure change. It is usually measured in liters per centimeter of water, as follows:

$$C_L = \frac{\Delta V\ (\text{liters})}{\Delta P\ (\text{cm } H_2O)}$$

The volume in this equation is measured simply as the inspired volume at a known inflation pressure. The inflation pressure is the difference between alveolar and pleural pressures (the transpulmonary pressure gradient [see Figure 9-1]). Compliance of a healthy adult lung averages 0.2 L/cm H_2O.

Compliance is usually measured under static conditions (i.e., no airflow). When there is no airflow, alveolar pressure equals 0. Under static conditions, the transpulmonary pressure gradient equals intrapleural pressure. Therefore lung compliance (C_L) can be expressed as follows:

$$C_L = \frac{\Delta V\ (\text{liters})}{\Delta P_{pl}\ (\text{cm } H_2O)}$$

Measurement of pulmonary compliance requires placement of a balloon in the esophagus. The balloon is connected to a sensitive pressure transducer. The subject then takes a deep breath and exhales, holding his or her breath at different lung volumes. The esophageal balloon measures intrapleural pressure at each volume. A graph of change in lung volume versus change in intrapleural pressure (Figure 9-5, *A*) is the compliance curve of the lung.

Figure 9-5, *B*, compares a normal compliance curve with those observed in emphysema and **pulmonary fibrosis**. The curve from a subject with emphysema is steeper and displaced to the left. The shape of this curve represents large changes in volume for small pressure changes (increased compliance). Increased compliance results from loss of elastic fibers, which occurs in emphysema. The lungs become more **distensible**, usually resulting in hyperinflation. The compliance curve of the patient with pulmonary fibrosis is flatter than the normal curve, shifted down and to the right. This indicates smaller changes in volume for any given pressure change (decreased compliance). Interstitial fibrosis is characterized by an increase in connective tissue. Consequently, the lungs become stiffer, usually with a loss of volume.

Chest Wall Compliance

Inflation and deflation of the lung occur with changes in the dimensions of the chest wall. The relationship between the lungs and the chest wall can be illustrated by plotting their relaxation pressure curves separately and combined (Figure 9-6). In the intact thorax, the lungs and chest wall recoil to a resting volume, or *functional residual capacity* (FRC). The normal resting volume of the intact thorax (FRC) is approximately

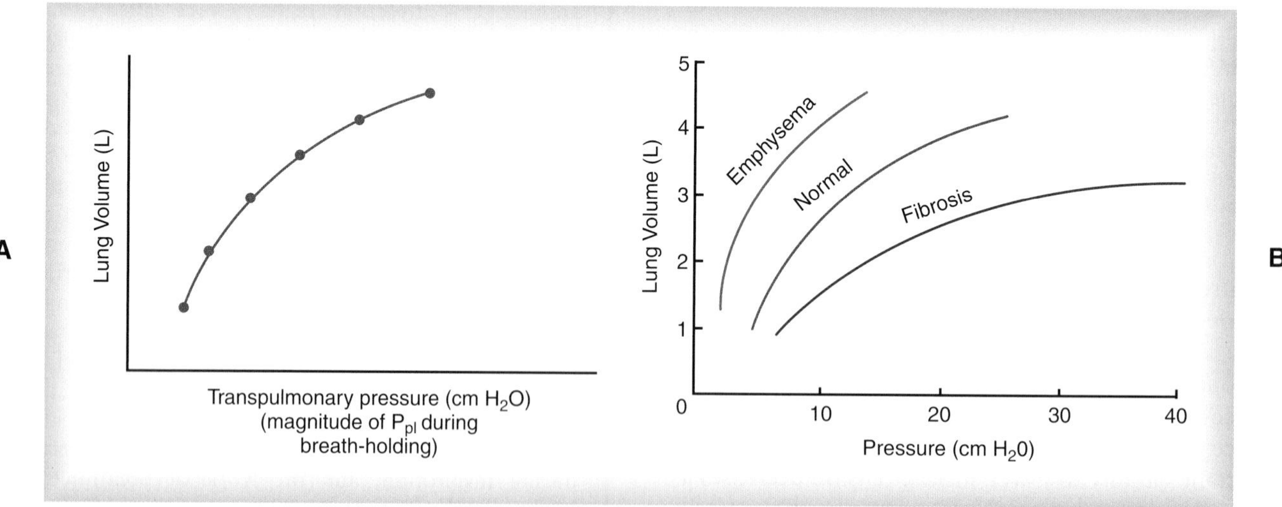

Figure 9-5

A, Compliance measurement. After swallowing an esophageal balloon, the subject inhales a full breath, then exhales slowly. At specific lung volumes, he holds his breath with the glottis open, ensuring an alveolar pressure of 0. Lung volume is plotted against esophageal pressure, generating a compliance curve. **B,** Compliance curves. Normal lung compliance is approximately 0.2 L/cm H_2O (measured from the lower portion of the curve, near resting lung volume). Compliance is high in emphysema because of the destruction of elastic tissue; conversely, it is low in pulmonary fibrosis because of increased elastic recoil. *(Modified from Martin L: Pulmonary physiology in clinical practice: the essentials for patient care and evaluation, St Louis, 1987, Mosby.)*

40% of the total lung capacity (TLC). If the normal lung–chest wall relationship is disrupted, the lung tends to collapse to a volume less than the FRC, and the thorax expands to a volume larger than the FRC.

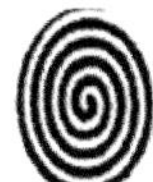

RULE OF THUMB

The lungs and chest wall each have their own compliance, or distensibility. In healthy adults, the compliance of the lungs and chest wall are approximately equal at *0.2 L/cm H_2O*. However, because the lungs are contained within the thorax, the two systems act as springs pulling against each other. This reduces the compliance of the system to approximately half that of the individual components, or *0.1 L/cm H_2O*. This has many practical implications, particularly for mechanical ventilation of the lungs. Any disease process that alters the compliance of the lungs or chest wall can seriously disrupt the normal mechanics of ventilation.

The chest wall, like the lung, has elastic properties. The elastic properties of the chest wall result from its bones and muscles, as described in Chapter 7. Unlike the lungs, which only collapse, the chest wall may recoil either inward or outward. The direction in which the chest wall moves depends on the volume of lung inflation.

The lung–chest wall system may be compared with two springs pulling against each other. The chest wall spring tends to expand, whereas the lung spring tends to contract. At the resting level, the forces of the chest wall and lungs balance. The tendency of the chest wall to expand is offset by the contractile force of the lungs. This balance of forces determines the resting lung volume, or FRC. The opposing forces between the chest wall and lungs are partially responsible for the subatmospheric pressure in the intrapleural space. Diseases that alter the compliance of either the chest wall or lung disrupt the balance point, usually with a change in lung volume.

Inhalation occurs when the balance between the lungs and chest wall shifts. Energy from the respiratory muscles overcomes the contractile force of the lungs. At

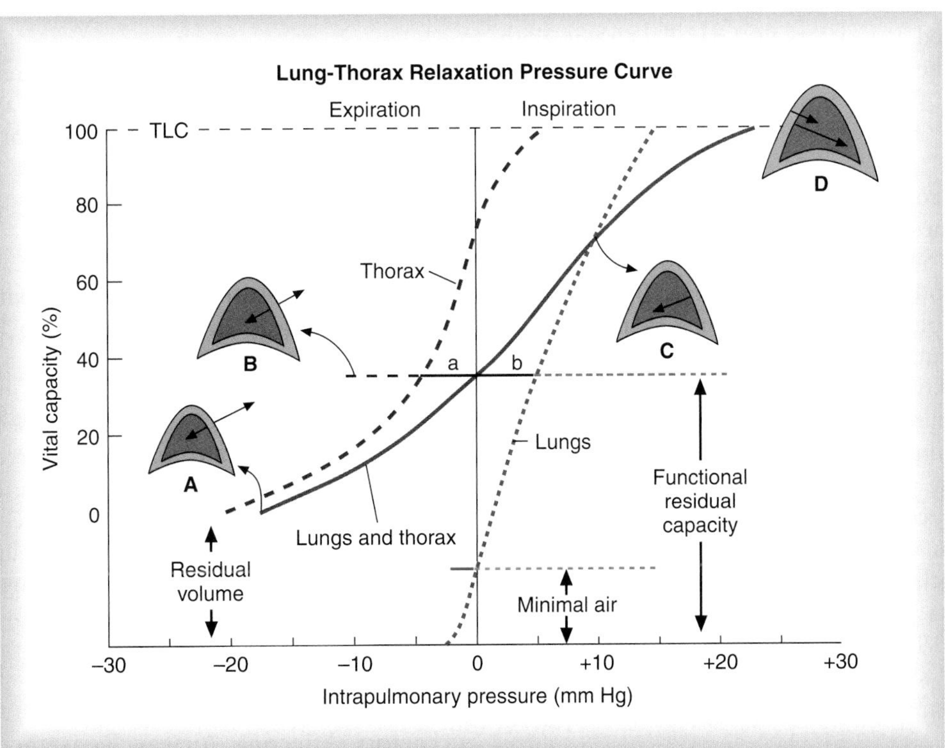

Figure 9-6

Relationship between the lungs and chest wall. Lung volume, as a percentage of vital capacity, is plotted against recoil pressure (plotted as a positive value). The combined lung-thorax relaxation curve *(solid line)* is the summation of the individual lung and thorax curves. Equilibrium (zero pressure) occurs where the lung and thoracic recoil forces balance (a + b = 0). This point is the functional residual capacity (lung *B*). Lung *A* represents low lung volume with greater recoil pressure exerted by the chest wall. Lung *C* shows a chest wall recoil of 0 at approximately 70% of the total lung capacity *(TLC)*. When TLC is higher than 70%, greater pressures are required to distend both the lungs and the thorax (lung *D*). *(Modified from Beachey W: Respiratory care anatomy and physiology, St Louis, 1998, Mosby.)*

the beginning of the breath, the tendency of the chest wall to expand facilitates lung expansion. When lung volume nears 70% of the VC, the chest wall reaches its natural resting level. When lung volume is higher than 70%, it resists further expansion. Inspiratory muscle effort must overcome the recoil of both the lungs and the chest wall to reach TLC.

During exhalation, potential energy "stored" in the stretched lung (and chest wall at high volumes) causes passive deflation. Exhalation below the resting level (FRC) requires muscular effort to overcome the tendency of the chest wall to expand. The expiratory muscles (see Chapter 7) provide this energy.

Compliance of the chest wall, like lung compliance, is a measure of distensibility. The compliance of the normal chest wall is similar to that of the lungs (0.2 L/cm H_2O). Obesity, **kyphoscoliosis**, and **ankylosing spondylitis** can reduce chest wall compliance and lung volumes.

Total Compliance

The total compliance of the respiratory system equals lung compliance (C_L) plus the compliance of the thorax (C_T). Total compliance of the lung-thorax system (C_{LT}) may be calculated as resistors in a parallel circuit, with C_{LT} less than either individual component:

$$\frac{1}{C_{LT}} = \frac{1}{C_L} + \frac{1}{C_T}$$

Lung-thorax compliance (C_{LT}) is difficult to measure. A relaxed or anesthetized subject may be placed in a body respirator. Subatmospheric pressure applied to the surface of the body produces ventilation. By measuring pressures and volumes as the patient is ventilated, the C_{LT} can be calculated. The C_{LT} of healthy individuals measured this way is approximately 0.1 L/cm H_2O. C_{LT} also can be measured in a patient intubated with a cuffed **endotracheal** tube. The lungs are inflated to various levels by positive pressures. By measuring the resulting volume changes, compliance data can be obtained. This method is often used for patients who are receiving mechanical ventilation (see Chapter 41). The C_{LT} of healthy patients measured by this method also is approximately 0.1 L/cm H_2O. The total compliance of the respiratory system can be altered by disorders affecting compliance of the lungs, chest wall, or both.

Frictional (Nonelastic) Opposition to Ventilation

Frictional forces also oppose ventilation. Frictional opposition is unrelated to the elastic properties of the lungs and thorax. It occurs only when the system is in motion. Frictional opposition to ventilation has the following two components: tissue viscous resistance and airway resistance.

Tissue Viscous Resistance

Tissue viscous resistance is the impedance of motion caused by displacement of tissues during ventilation. The tissues displaced include the lungs, rib cage, diaphragm, and abdominal organs. The energy to displace these structures is comparable with the impedance caused by friction in any dynamic system. Tissue resistance accounts for only approximately 20% of the total resistance to lung inflation. Obesity, fibrosis, and **ascites** can alter tissue viscous resistance, increasing the total impedance to ventilation.

Airway Resistance

Gas flow through the airways also causes frictional resistance. Impedance to ventilation by the movement of gas through the airways is called *airway resistance*. Airway resistance accounts for approximately 80% of the frictional resistance to ventilation.

Airway resistance (Raw) is the ratio of driving pressure responsible for gas movement to the flow of the gas, calculated as follows:

$$\text{Raw} = \frac{\Delta P}{\dot{V}}$$

Driving pressure (ΔP) is the pressure difference between the alveoli and the airway opening (i.e., transrespiratory pressure gradient, or $P_{alv} - P_{ao}$). The following equation substitutes for ΔP:

$$\text{Raw} = \frac{P_{alv} - P_{ao}}{\dot{V}}$$

Driving pressure is measured in centimeters of water (cm H_2O), and flow is measured in liters per second (L/sec). Airway resistance is written cm H_2O/L/sec. Airway resistance in healthy adults ranges from approximately 0.5 to 2.5 cm H_2O/L/sec.

Airway resistance is usually measured in a pulmonary function laboratory (see Chapter 17). Flow ($\dot{V}$) is measured with a **pneumotachometer.** Alveolar pressures are determined in a body **plethysmograph**, an airtight box in which the patient sits. Pressure changes in the plethysmograph reflect alveolar pressures. By measuring flow and alveolar pressure, airway resistance can be calculated.

Factors Affecting Airway Resistance. Two patterns characterize the flow of gas through the respiratory tract: *laminar flow* and *turbulent flow*.[2] A third pattern, called *tracheobronchial flow*, is a combination of laminar and turbulent flow (see Figure 5-21). In laminar flow, gas moves in discrete layers, or streamlines. Layers near the center of an airway move faster than those close to the tube wall. This results from friction between gas molecules and the wall. Gas

MINI CLINI

HeO_2 Therapy for Airway Obstruction

PROBLEM

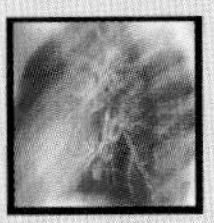

Patients with significant obstruction in the upper airway, trachea, or mainstem bronchi expend a large amount of energy overcoming the resistance to breathing. What type of gas therapy would be most advantageous in this situation?

DISCUSSION

Because most (approximately 80%) of the resistance to breathing occurs in the upper and large airways, disease processes that increase resistance in these airways cause tremendous increases in the work of breathing. Traumatic injuries to the vocal cords or trachea, along with tumors or foreign bodies in the trachea or mainstem bronchi, are good examples of the types of clinical problems that can markedly increase the work of breathing. Patients who must breathe against high levels of resistance are prone to respiratory muscle fatigue and failure. Gas flow in the upper and large airways is predominantly turbulent. Turbulent flow is highly influenced by gas density. Patients with large airway obstruction can often be treated with a mixture of helium and oxygen. HeO_2, usually an 80%-to-20% mixture, can be administered to reduce the work of breathing until the obstructive process can be treated. Unfortunately, a HeO_2 mixture does little for patients with small airway obstruction, as occurs in emphysema or asthma. Flow in the small airways is mainly laminar and largely independent of the density of the gas breathed.

flowing in a laminar pattern consists of concentric layers parallel to the tube wall. Flows increase toward the center of the tube.

Poiseuille's law (see Chapter 5) defines laminar flow through a smooth, unbranched tube of fixed dimension. The pressure required to cause a specific flow of gas through a tube is calculated as follows:

$$\Delta P = \frac{\eta 81\dot{V}}{\pi r^4}$$

where:

ΔP = Driving pressure (dynes/cm^2)

η = Coefficient of viscosity of the gas

l = Tube length (cm)

$\dot{V}$ = Gas flow (mL/sec)

r = Tube radius (cm)

(π and 8 are constants)

By eliminating factors that remain constant, such as viscosity, length, and known constants, this equation can be rearranged as follows to solve for $\dot{V}$:

$$\Delta P \approx \frac{\dot{V}}{r^4}$$

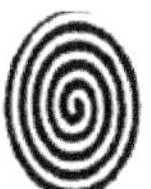

RULE OF THUMB

A change in the caliber of an airway by a factor of 2 causes a sixteenfold change in resistance. This applies to human airways, as well as artificial airways (i.e., endotracheal and tracheostomy tubes). If the size of a patient's airway is reduced from 2 mm to 1 mm, airway resistance increases by a *factor of 16*! Similarly, if a 4.5-mm endotracheal tube is replaced with a 9-mm tube, the pressure required to cause a flow of 1 L/sec through the tube will decrease sixteenfold. This rule has many practical consequences. It is the basis for bronchodilator therapy and for using the largest practical size of artificial airway.

This equation can be rearranged as follows to solve for $\dot{V}$:

$$\dot{V} \approx \Delta P r4$$

This equation is significant when applied to the following clinical situations involving the airways:

1. For gas flow to remain constant, delivery pressure must vary *inversely* with the fourth power of the airway's radius. Reducing the radius of a tube by half requires a sixteenfold pressure increase to maintain a constant flow. To maintain ventilation in the presence of narrowing airways, large increases in driving pressure may be needed.
2. If the gas delivery pressure ventilating the lung remains constant, gas flow will vary directly with the fourth power of the airway's radius. Reducing the airway radius by half will decrease the flow sixteenfold at a constant pressure. Small changes in bronchial caliber can markedly change gas flow through an airway.

Under certain conditions, gas flow through a tube changes significantly. The orderly pattern of concentric layers is no longer maintained. Gas molecules form irregular currents. This pattern is called turbulent flow (see Figure 5-21). Transition from laminar to *turbulent flow* depends on the following factors: gas density (d), viscosity (h), linear velocity (v), and tube radius (r). Table 9-1 compares changes in flow and pressure resulting from laminar and turbulent flow.

Table 9-1 ▶▶ Comparison of Driving Pressures, Laminar Versus Turbulent Flow

Flow	Laminar	Turbulent
	Driving Pressure (DP)	
1	1	1
2	2	4
4	4	16
8	8	64
16	16	256

Values are nondimensional units demonstrating proportional effect.

Table 9-2 ▶▶ Distribution of Airway Resistance

Location	Total Resistance (%)
Nose, mouth, upper airway	50
Trachea and bronchi	30
Small airways (<2 mm)	20

Distribution of Airway Resistance

Approximately 80% of the resistance to gas flow occurs in the nose, mouth, and large airways. Only approximately 20% of the total resistance to flow is attributable to airways smaller than 2 mm in diameter. This appears to contradict the fact that resistance is inversely related to the radius of the conducting tube.

Branching of the tracheobronchial tree increases the cross-sectional area with each airway generation (Figure 9-7). As gas moves from the mouth to the alveoli, the combined cross-sectional area of the airways increases exponentially (see Chapter 7). According to the laws of fluid dynamics, this increase in cross-sectional area causes a decrease in gas velocity. The decrease in gas velocity promotes a laminar flow pattern, particularly in the smaller (i.e., less than 2 mm) airways.

Turbulent flow predominates in the mouth, trachea, and primary bronchi (Table 9-2). Gas velocity is high, favoring turbulent flow patterns. At the level of the terminal bronchioles, the cross-sectional area increases more than thirtyfold. Gas velocity is very low here. In normal small airways, flow is laminar. The driving pressure across these airways is less than 1% of the total driving pressure for the system.

The diameter of the airways is not constant. During inspiration, the stretch of surrounding lung tissue and widening transpulmonary pressure gradient increase the diameter of the airways. The higher the lung volume, the more these factors influence airway caliber (Figure 9-8). The increase in airway diameter with increasing lung volume decreases airway resistance. As lung volume decreases toward residual volume, airway diameters also decrease. Airway resistance rises dramatically at low lung volumes.

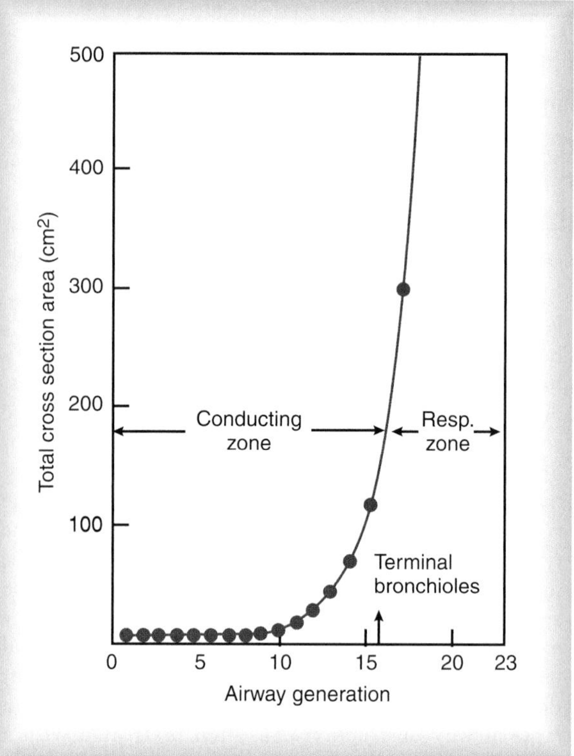

Figure 9-7

Because no gas exchange takes place in the conducting zone, this region is called the *anatomical dead space* (see Chapter 7). The gas exchange surface increases markedly at the level of the terminal bronchiole. *(Modified from West J: Respiratory physiology: the essentials, ed 6, Baltimore, 2000, Williams & Wilkins.)*

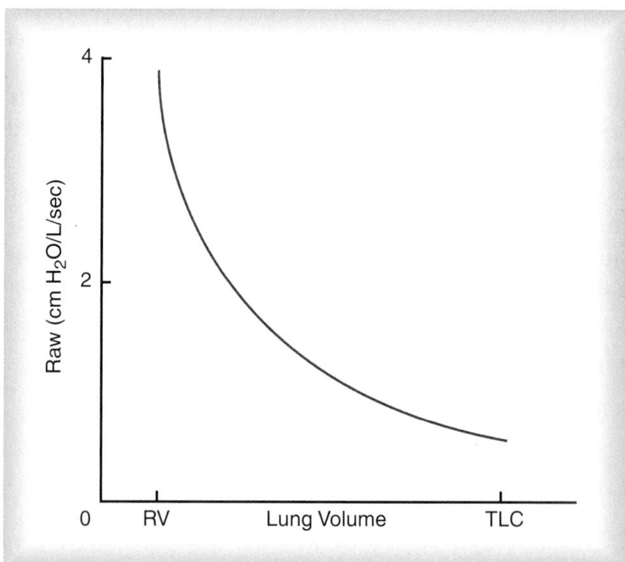

Figure 9-8

Change in airway resistance (Raw) with change in lung volume. Resistance to airflow is highly dependent on lung volume. At low lung volumes, near residual volume *(RV)*, the airways are compressed and resistance increases markedly. At high lung volumes, near total lung capacity *(TLC)*, the airways are distended and resistance falls. See text for discussion.

MECHANICS OF EXHALATION

Airway caliber is determined by several factors, which include anatomical support provided to the airways and pressure differences across their walls. Anatomical (i.e., physical) support comes from cartilage in the wall of the airway and from "traction" provided by surrounding tissues. The larger airways depend mainly on **cartilaginous** support. Because smaller airways lack cartilage, they depend on support provided by surrounding lung parenchyma.[3]

The airways are also supported by the pressure difference across their walls. This transpulmonary pressure gradient helps stabilize the airways, particularly the small ones. The difference between the pleural pressure and the pressure inside the airway is called the *transmural pressure gradient.*

During quiet breathing, pleural pressure is normally subatmospheric. Airway pressure varies minimally and is usually close to 0 (see Figure 9-1). The transmural pressure gradient during normal quiet breathing is negative, even during exhalation. It ranges between –5 and –10 cm H_2O. This negative transmural pressure gradient helps maintain the caliber of the small airways.

During a forced exhalation, contraction of expiratory muscles can increase pleural pressure above atmospheric pressure. This reverses the transmural pressure gradient, making it positive. If the positive transmural pressure gradient exceeds the supporting force provided by the lung parenchyma, the small airways may collapse. In healthy airways, this occurs only with forced exhalation and at low lung volumes. In diseased airways, it may occur with normal breathing.

Forceful contraction of the expiratory muscles causes pressure across the thorax to rise. This increases pleural pressure from its normal negative value to above atmospheric (Figure 9-9). Alveolar pressure during forced exhalation equals the sum of pleural pressure and the elastic recoil pressure of the lung itself.

The pressure along the airway drops as gas flows from the alveoli toward the mouth. Moving "downstream" (toward the mouth), transmural pressure drops continually. At some point along the airway, the pressure inside equals the pressure outside in the pleural space. This point is referred to as the *equal pressure point* (EPP). Downstream from this point, pleural pressure exceeds the airway pressure. The resulting positive transmural pressure gradient causes airway compression and can lead to actual collapse. Airway compression increases expiratory airway resistance and limits flow. At the EPP, greater expiratory effort only increases pleural pressure, further restricting flow.[4] Dynamic compression is responsible for the characteristic flow patterns observed in forced expiratory tests of pulmonary function (see Flow-Volume Curves in Chapter 17).

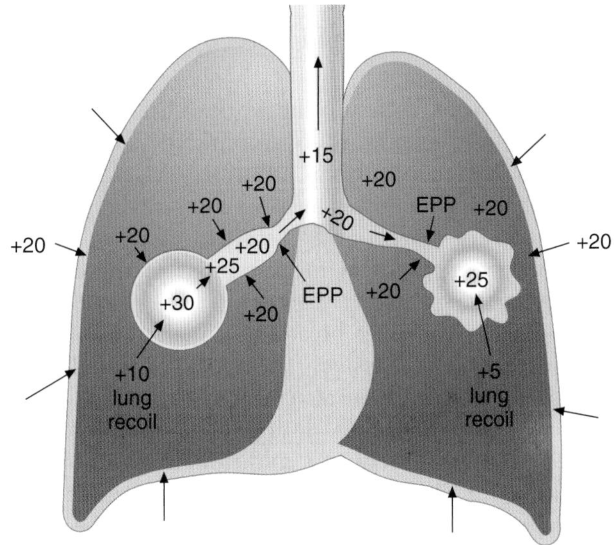

Figure 9-9

Generation of equal pressure point (*EPP*) in normal and diseased lungs during a forceful exhalation. In a normal lung *(left)*, pleural pressure (P_{pl}) rises to approximately +20 cm H_2O. Alveolar pressure is the sum of P_{pl} (+20 cm H_2O) and lung elastic recoil pressure (+10 cm H_2O), or +30 cm H_2O. Airway pressure falls along the airway from the alveolus to the mouth. At the EPP, pressure within the airway equals P_{pl}. Further toward the mouth, airway pressure falls below P_{pl}, resulting in a narrowed airway and limitation of airflow. This normally occurs in healthy individuals only during forced exhalation. The EPP moves "upstream" from larger airways toward smaller airways as the lung empties. In lung diseases such as emphysema *(right)*, the same forces come into play. P_{pl} is still +20 cm H_2O, but lung elastic recoil pressure is only +5 cm H_2O. As a result, driving pressure is only +25 cm H_2O. This causes the EPP to occur in smaller airways than normal; thus airways narrow or collapse at a higher lung volume than in healthy lungs. In patients with emphysema, airway collapse is further complicated by loss of support for the small airways. *(Modified from Martin L: Pulmonary physiology in clinical practice: the essentials for patient care and evaluation, St Louis, 1987, Mosby.)*

In healthy individuals, dynamic compression occurs only at lung volumes well below the resting expiratory level. Additional anatomical support is provided by the surrounding lung parenchyma. This tissue support opposes the collapsing force created by negative transmural pressure gradients. In pulmonary emphysema, the elastic tissue responsible for supporting the small airways is destroyed. Destruction of elastic tissue has multiple outcomes. It increases the compliance of the lung (i.e., elastic recoil decreases; see Figure 9-9). Emphysema also obliterates the anatomical structures responsible for small airway support.[4] Reduced compliance allows lung volume to increase. Expiratory flow is limited by airway collapse during exhalation.

WORK OF BREATHING

The respiratory muscles do the work of breathing. This work requires energy to overcome the elastic and frictional forces opposing inflation. Assessment of mechanical work involves measurement of the physical parameters of force and distance. Assessment of metabolic work involves measurement of the oxygen cost of breathing.

During normal quiet breathing, inhalation is active and exhalation is passive. The work of exhaling is recovered from potential energy "stored" in the expanded lung and thorax during inhalation. However, forced exhalation requires additional work by the expiratory muscles. The actual work of forced expiration depends on the mechanical properties of the lungs and thorax.

Mechanical

Work done on an object is the product of the force exerted on the object times the distance it is moved. Work may be measured in either dyne-centimeters (dyne-cm)* or joules (J),† as follows:

$$\text{Work} = \text{Force} \times \text{Distance}$$

Pressure equals force per unit area (distance^2). Volume is the cube of length (distance^3). The product of pressure (P) and volume (V) has the same dimension as work, as demonstrated by the following:

$$P \times V = \frac{\text{Force}}{\text{Area}} \times \text{Volume}$$

$$P \times V = \frac{\text{Force}}{\text{Distance}^2} \times \text{Distance}^3$$

or

$$P \times V = \frac{\text{Force}}{\text{Distance}^2} \times (\text{Distance} \times \text{Distance}^2)$$

Canceling out distance^2 in both numerator and denominator yields the following equation:

$$P \times V = \text{Force} \times \text{Distance}$$

The mechanical work of breathing can be calculated as the product of the pressure across the respiratory system and the resulting change in volume:

$$\text{Work of breathing} = \Delta P \times \Delta V$$

The mechanical work of breathing cannot be measured easily during spontaneous breathing. This is because the respiratory muscles contribute to the resistance offered by the chest wall. Total mechanical work can be measured during artificial ventilation, if the respiratory muscles are completely at rest. Change in lung volume may be related to the pressure difference between the airway opening and the body surface.

Work of breathing is calculated by integrating the pressure and volume. This is equivalent to determining the area under a volume-pressure curve of the lung (Figure 9-10). Change in pressure is plotted on the x-axis. Change in volume is plotted on the y-axis. The product of pressure and volume represents an area on the graph. The larger the area, the greater the amount of work.

If the lung is inflated slowly, with airflow interrupted to plot volume and pressure changes, a straight line is obtained (see Figure 9-10, *solid line AB*). Because conditions during these measurements are static, the straight line represents the change in volume for a given change in pressure, caused solely by the elastic properties of the lung. The slope of the line is the compliance of the lung. The work done overcoming purely elastic forces opposing inflation is represented by the triangular area 1 in Figure 9-10. Lung pressure and volume changes also may be measured during dynamic inflation. During airflow, a curvilinear relationship develops between end-expiration and end-inspiration (see Figure 9-10, *line ACB*). This curve represents the additional resistance produced by the friction of tissue

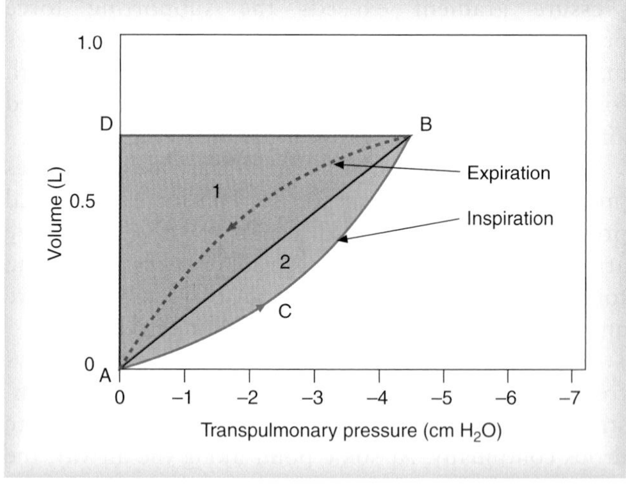

Figure 9-10

Factors involved in the work of breathing. Point A is the resting level (FRC), and B is end-inspiration. The *straight solid A-B* represents the pressure required to overcome simple elastic forces, and the *curved line A-C-B* represents the additional pressure required to overcome frictional resistance (airway and tissue). At B, where airflow momentarily ceases, frictional resistance is inactive. Area 1 represents the work required to overcome elastic forces; area 2 represents the work required to overcome frictional forces. The work of breathing is the sum of these two areas. The *curved dashed line* within area 1 represents the pressure-volume curve of passive exhalation using energy stored during inspiration.

*A centimeter-gram-second (CGS) unit of measurement.

†An international system (SI) unit of measurement.

and gas flow, most of which is airway resistance. At points of zero flow (see Figure 9-10, *A* and *B*), there is no airway or tissue resistance, and the curve rejoins the static compliance line. The work required to overcome these frictional forces is represented by the loop labeled as area 2 in Figure 9-10.

The total mechanical work for one breath is the sum of the work overcoming both the elastic and frictional forces opposing inflation. This is represented as the sum of areas 1 and 2 in Figure 9-10. In healthy adults, approximately two thirds of the work of breathing can be attributed to elastic forces opposing ventilation. The remaining third is a result of frictional resistance to gas and tissue movement.

In the presence of pulmonary disease, work of breathing can increase dramatically (Figure 9-11). The areas of the volume-pressure curves for patients with obstruction or restriction are greater than they are in healthy subjects.[5] The reasons for these increases in the mechanical work are quite different. In restrictive lung disease, the area of the volume-pressure curve is greater because the slope of the static component (compliance) is less than normal. The area of the volume-pressure curve in obstructive lung disease is increased because the portion associated with frictional resistance is markedly widened. The leftward "bulge" of the loop indicates positive pleural pressure during expiration (see Figure 9-11, *C*).

In healthy individuals, the mechanical work of breathing depends on the pattern of ventilation. Large tidal volumes increase the elastic component of work. High breathing rates (and hence, high flows) increase frictional work. When changing from quiet breathing to exercise ventilation, healthy subjects adjust their tidal volumes and breathing frequencies to minimize the work of breathing.

Similar adjustments occur in individuals who have lung disease (Figure 9-12). Patients with "stiff lungs" (i.e., increased elastic work of breathing), such as in pulmonary fibrosis, assume a rapid, shallow breathing pattern. This pattern minimizes the mechanical work of distending the lungs. Patients who have airway obstruction assume a ventilatory pattern that reduces the

MINI CLINI

Optimal Breathing Pattern in Obstructive Airway Diseases

PROBLEM

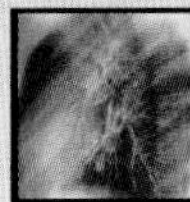

Patients with advanced emphysema have lost elastic tissue and have reduced elastic recoil (i.e., lung compliance is abnormally high). The lack of elastic fibers also reduces radial "traction" around the outside circumference of small airways. This makes the small airways without cartilage support prone to collapse. When the patient exhales, especially during forced exhalation, airway resistance is abnormally high because small airways collapse prematurely. The EPP migrates distally to this point, as extra luminal pressure exceeds intraluminal pressure. (See Mechanics of Exhalation, p. 217) This greatly increases the work of breathing.

What instructions should be given to this type of patient to help minimize the work of breathing?

DISCUSSION

This type of increased work of breathing arises from increased airway resistance during exhalation. (The work required to overcome elastic resistance is actually less than normal because lung compliance is high.) In addition, many lung units may have longtime constants because of high resistance and high compliance. This results in mismatching of ventilation and pulmonary blood flow, often resulting in hypoxemia. To minimize the work of breathing and maldistribution of ventilation, airflow should be slow. Slow breaths reduce turbulence and increase the laminar flow characteristics of the gas stream. Low flows also minimize the effects of lung units with longtime constants. To keep airways patent and prevent premature closure, exhaling against a slight resistance may be helpful. This increases pressure in the airways throughout the expiratory phase and counteracts the collapsing effect of extraluminal pressure surrounding the airways. Patients should be instructed to breathe slowly and deeply and to exhale slowly through pursed lips to create a slight expiratory resistance. This should reduce the frictional work of breathing while promoting more even distribution of ventilation.

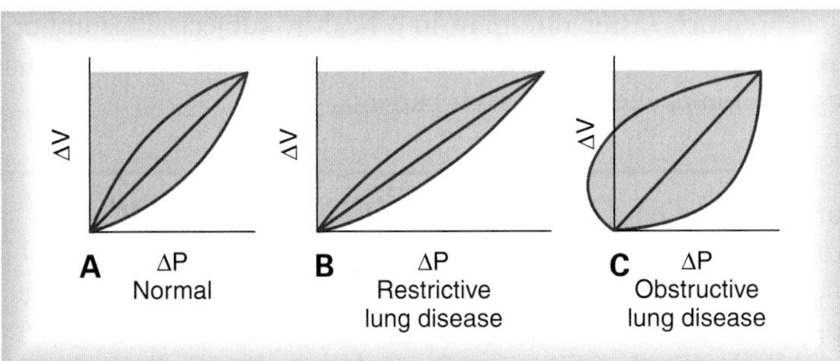

Figure 9-11

Comparison of the work of breathing *(shaded areas)* for a healthy subject **(A)**; a patient with restrictive ventilatory impairment (such as pulmonary fibrosis) **(B)**; and a patient with airway obstruction (such as emphysema) **(C)**.

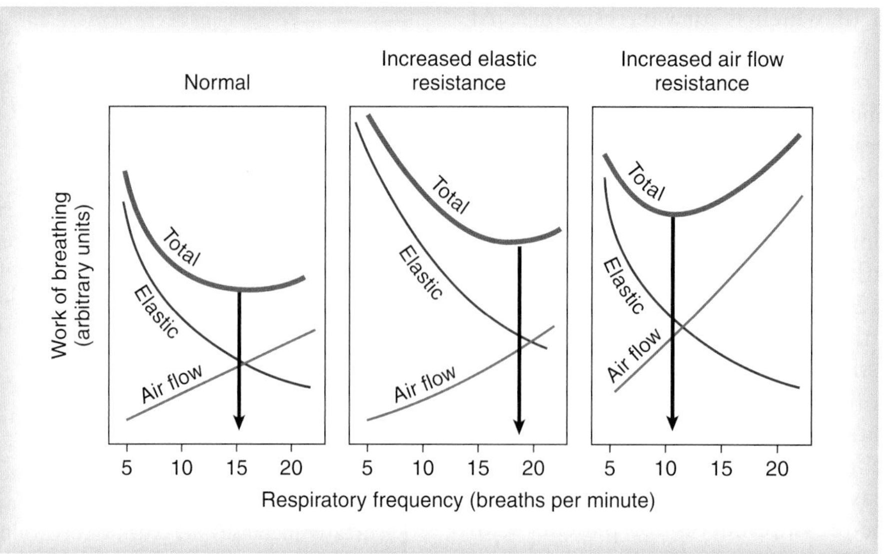

Figure 9-12

Work required to overcome airflow plus elastic resistance equals total work. In healthy lungs, total work of breathing is minimal at approximately 15 breaths/min *(left)*. To achieve the same minute volume with stiff lungs (increased elastic resistance), minimum work is performed at higher frequencies *(middle)*. However, with increased airflow resistance (obstructive lung disease), minimum work requires lower rates of breathing *(right)*. *(Modified from Nunn JF: Applied respiratory physiology, ed 2, London, 1977, Butterworth.)*

frictional work of breathing. Breathing slowly and deeply minimizes tissue and airway resistance.

Increased work of breathing is often complicated by *respiratory muscle weakness*, which may result from electrolyte imbalance, **acidemia**, shock, or **sepsis**.[5] When increased work of breathing occurs with respiratory muscle weakness, inspiratory muscles can fatigue. Tidal volume decreases, and respiratory rate increases as the muscles fatigue. Gas exchange may be compromised by ventilation-perfusion imbalances and increased dead space resulting from the combination of low tidal volume and increased dead space (see Efficiency and Effectiveness of Ventilation, p. 224).

Metabolic

To perform work, the respiratory muscles consume oxygen. The rate of oxygen consumption ($\dot{V}O_2$) by the respiratory muscles reflects their energy requirements. It also provides an indirect measure of the work of breathing.

The oxygen cost of breathing is assessed by measuring the $\dot{V}O_2$ at rest and at increased levels of ventilation. If no other factors increase oxygen consumption, then the additional oxygen uptake is a result of respiratory muscle metabolism. The oxygen cost of breathing in healthy individuals averages from 0.5 to 1.0 mL of oxygen per liter of increased ventilation. This represents less than 5% of the oxygen consumption of the body. At high levels of ventilation (i.e., higher than approximately 120 L/min), the oxygen cost of breathing increases tremendously.

The $\dot{V}O_2$ of the respiratory muscles is closely related to the inspiratory pressures generated by the diaphragm. This *transdiaphragmatic* pressure (P_{di}) can be measured by a technique similar to that used for measuring intrapleural pressure (see Lung Compliance, p. 212). A thin catheter with two small balloons is advanced into the esophagus. One balloon remains in the esophagus while the balloon at the tip is placed in the stomach. The pressure difference between the balloons measures the pressure across the diaphragm. The greater the pressure required in overcoming inspiratory resistance, the higher the oxygen consumption of the respiratory muscles.

In the presence of pulmonary disease (either obstructive or restrictive), the oxygen cost of breathing may increase dramatically with increasing ventilation (Figure 9-13). In an obstructive disease such as emphysema, increased ventilation causes the oxygen consumption of the respiratory muscles to increase at a much faster rate than in a healthy subject. This abnormally high oxygen cost of breathing is one factor that limits exercise in such patients.

▶ DISTRIBUTION OF VENTILATION

Ventilation is not distributed evenly in healthy lungs. Regional and local factors account for this unevenness in the distribution of ventilation. Uneven ventilation

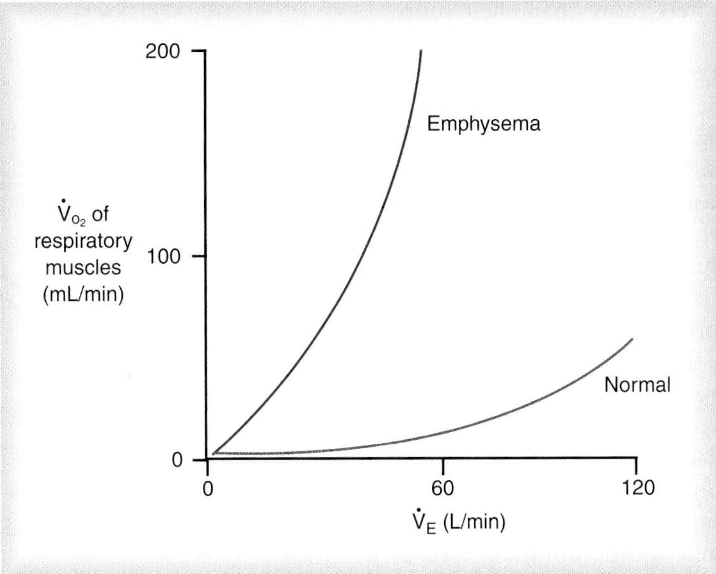

Figure 9-13

Relationship of oxygen cost of breathing to expiratory minute volume for a healthy subject and for a patient with emphysema.

helps explain why the lung is less than perfect for gas exchange (see Chapter 10). In disease, the distribution of ventilation can worsen dramatically. The resulting deficiencies in gas exchange can be life-threatening. The maldistribution of ventilation in disease represents a primary cause of impaired oxygen and carbon dioxide exchange (see Chapter 10).

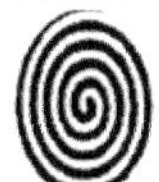

RULE OF THUMB

Gravity, to a large extent, determines where ventilation goes in the lungs. In the upright lung, the weight of the lung tissues causes alveoli at the bases to be smaller but more easily distended. Alveoli at the top of the lung are larger but distend less easily. Gravity also causes most blood flow through pulmonary capillaries to go to the bases. The pressure-volume characteristics of the upright lung direct most ventilation to these dependent portions, thus matching ventilation and blood flow to promote gas exchange. This phenomenon can be useful clinically when localized lesions (e.g., lobar pneumonia) cause ventilation-perfusion abnormalities. By placing the patient in a position in which functional lung units are dependent and diseased units are elevated, the matching of ventilation and perfusion can be optimized and gas exchange often improves.

Regional Factors

Two factors affect regional distribution of gas in the healthy lung: (1) relative differences in thoracic expansion and (2) regional transpulmonary pressure gradients. In upright individuals, these factors direct more ventilation to the bases and periphery of the lungs than to the apices and central zones.

Differences in Thoracic Expansion

The configuration of thoracic bony structures and the action of the respiratory muscles cause proportionately greater expansion at the lung bases than at the apices (see Chapter 7). Expansion of the lower chest is approximately 50% greater than that of the upper chest.[6] The action of the diaphragm preferentially inflates the lower lobes of the lung.

Transpulmonary Pressure Gradients

The transpulmonary pressure gradient (see Mechanics of Ventilation, this chapter) is not equal throughout the thorax. It varies substantially within the lung, as well as from the top to the bottom of the lung.

At a given level of alveolar inflation, the transpulmonary pressure gradient is directly related to the pleural pressure. Pleural pressure represents the pressure on the outer surface of the lung. Its effect lessens toward more centrally located alveoli. Changes in the transpulmonary pressure gradient are greatest in peripheral alveoli (i.e., near the lung's surface). The changes are least in the alveoli of the central zones. Peripheral alveoli expand proportionately more than their more central counterparts.

Top-to-bottom differences in pleural pressure have an even greater effect on the distribution of ventilation, especially in the upright lung.[1] Pleural pressure increases by approximately 0.25 cm H_2O for each centimeter, from the lung apex to its base. This increase in pressure is a result of the weight of the lung and the effect of gravity. In an adult-sized lung, pleural pressure at the apex is approximately –10 cm H_2O. At the base, pleural pressure is only approximately –2.5 cm H_2O. Because of these differences, the transpulmonary pressure gradient at the top of the upright lung is greater than it is at the bottom. Alveoli at the apices have a higher volume than alveoli at the bases.

Despite their higher volume, alveoli at the apices expand less during inspiration than alveoli at the bases. Apical alveoli rest on the upper portion of the pressure-volume curve (Figure 9-14). This part of the curve is relatively flat. Each unit of pressure change causes only a small change in volume. Alveoli at the lung bases are positioned on the middle portion of the pressure-volume curve. That part of the curve is relatively steep. For each unit of pressure change there is a larger change in volume (greater compliance). For a given transpulmonary pressure gradient, alveoli at the bases expand more than alveoli at the apices. The bases of the upright lung receive approximately four times as much ventilation as do the apices.

These gravity-dependent differences also are observed in recumbent individuals. The magnitude of the differences is less than in the upright lung because the height is less. Ventilation is still greatest in the dependent zones of the lung. In recumbent subjects, the posterior regions are dependent. Lying on the side causes more ventilation to go to whichever lung is lower.

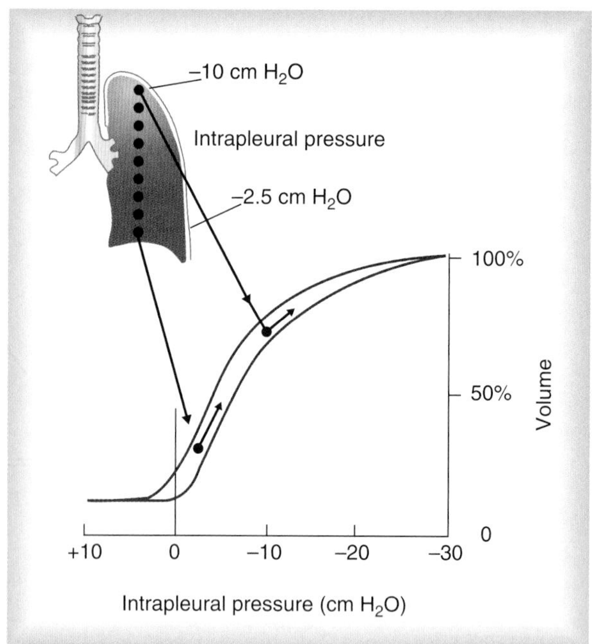

Figure 9-14

Causes of regional differences in ventilation from the apex to the base of an upright lung. Because of the lung's weight and the influence of gravity, intrapleural pressure at the apex is more negative (subatmospheric) than at the base. Alveoli at the apex are maintained at a higher resting inflation volume than are those at the base. However, alveoli at the apex reside on the flatter upper portion of the pressure-volume curve. Alveoli at the base are positioned on the lower, steeper portion. Thus for an equal change in intrapleural pressure, alveoli at the base expand more during inspiration than do those at the apex. This causes more ventilation to go to the bases in the upright lung. *(Modified from West JB: Respiratory physiology: the essentials, ed 6, Baltimore, 2000, Williams & Wilkins.)*

Local Factors

Alveolar filling and emptying is affected by local factors. Individual respiratory units and their associated airways may differ from each other. These local factors contribute to uneven ventilation in healthy lungs. Their influence on gas distribution becomes particularly important in disease.

Each respiratory unit has an elastic element, the alveolus, and a resistive element, the airway. Change in alveolar volume and the time required for the change to occur depend on the compliance and resistance of each respiratory unit.[1]

In terms of compliance, the more distensible the unit, the greater the volume change at a given transpulmonary pressure will be. Lung units with high compliance have less elastic recoil than normal. These units fill and empty more slowly than normal units. Lung units with low compliance (high elastic recoil) increase their volume less. They fill and empty faster than normal.

Airway resistance also affects emptying and filling. The size of the airway influences how much driving pressure reaches distal lung units. In healthy airways, the pressure drop between the airway opening (i.e., the mouth) and the alveolus is minimal. Most of the driving pressure is available for alveolar inflation. If the airway is obstructed, high resistance to gas flow can occur. The pressure drop across the obstruction may be substantial. Less driving pressure is available for alveolar inflation; thus there is less alveolar volume change.

Time Constants

Compliance and resistance determine local rates of alveolar filling and emptying. The relationship between the compliance and resistance of a lung unit can be measured. This property of each lung unit is called its *time constant*. The time constant is simply the product of each unit's compliance and resistance:

$$\text{Time Constant} = C \times R$$

where:

C = Compliance (L/cm H_2O)

R = Resistance (cm H_2O/L/sec)

The pressure and volume units (cm H_2O and L, respectively) cancel out. The time constant is expressed in seconds.

A lung unit will have a long time constant if resistance or compliance is high. Units with long time constants take longer to fill and empty than units with normal compliance and resistance (Figure 9-15). Lung units have a short time constant when resistance or compliance is low. Lung units with short time constants fill and empty more rapidly than those with normal compliance and resistance.

Time constants affect local distribution of ventilation in the lung. When the time available for inflation is fixed, units with long time constants fill less and empty more slowly than normal units. Units with short time constants also fill less than normal because of low compliance. The ventilation going to lung units with either long or short time constants is less than that received by units with normal compliance and resistance.

Frequency Dependence of Compliance

Variations in time constants can affect ventilation throughout the lung. Abnormal ventilation is characteristic of obstruction in the small airways. This type of obstruction occurs in emphysema, asthma, and chronic bronchitis. The time constants of many lung units are increased. These long time constants are mainly caused by increased resistance to flow in the small airways. Loss of normal tissue elastic recoil, such as in emphysema, also contributes to slowed filling and emptying.

At increased breathing rates, units with long time constants fill less and empty more slowly than units with normal compliance and resistance. More and more inspired gas goes to lung units with relatively normal time constants. When more inspired volume goes to a smaller number of lung units, higher transpulmonary pressures must be generated to maintain alveolar ventilation. Compliance of the lung appears to decrease as breathing frequency increases.

This phenomenon is called *frequency dependence of compliance*. Compliance measured during breathing is

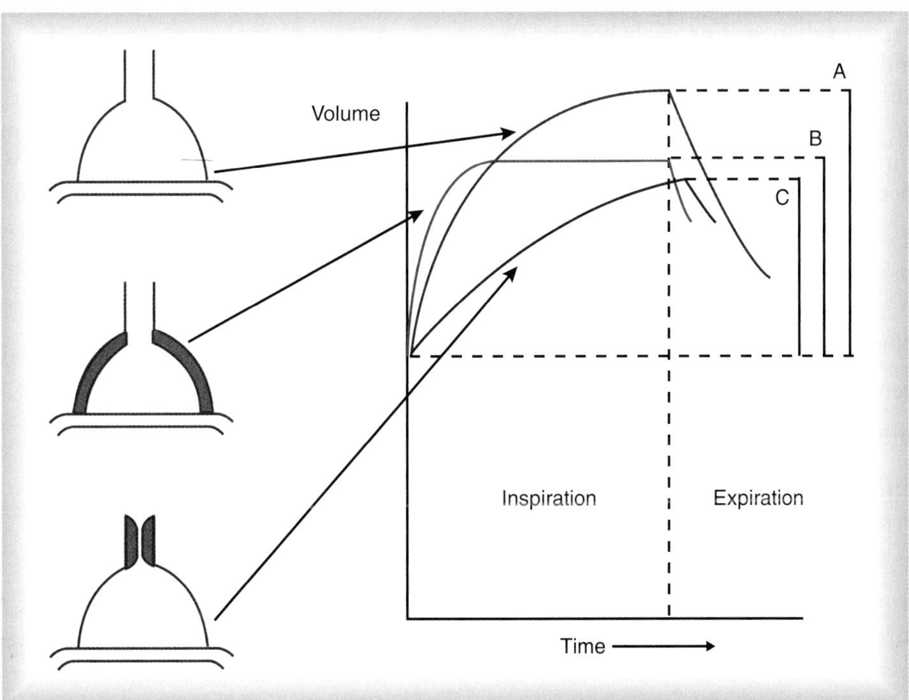

Figure 9-15

Effect of changes in resistance and compliance on time constants of lung units inflated with equal pressures. Lung unit *A* has normal resistance and compliance, and it fills and empties at a normal rate (normal time constant). Lung unit *B* has normal resistance but low compliance. It fills and empties faster than normal (low time constant), but at a lower volume. Lung unit *C* has normal compliance but high resistance. It fills and empties slower than normal (high time constant) and at a lower volume. *(Modified from West JB: Respiratory physiology: the essentials, ed 6, Baltimore, 2000, Williams & Wilkins.)*

not static (see Work of Breathing, Mechanical, p. 218); it includes pressure changes created by resistance to airflow. The term *dynamic compliance* is used to assess pressure-volume relationships during breathing. If dynamic compliance decreases as the respiratory rate increases, some lung units must have abnormal time constants. Any stimulus to increase ventilation, such as exercise, may redistribute inspired gas. Mismatching of ventilation and perfusion can result in hypoxemia, severely limiting an individual's ability to perform daily activities.

▶ EFFICIENCY AND EFFECTIVENESS OF VENTILATION

To be effective, ventilation must meet the body's needs for oxygen uptake and carbon dioxide removal. To be efficient, ventilation should consume little oxygen and should produce the minimum amount of carbon dioxide.

Efficiency

Even in healthy lungs, ventilation is not entirely efficient. A substantial volume of inspired gas is wasted with each breath; this wasted ventilation is referred to as *dead space*. Gases must move in and out through the same airways leading to the exchange area. This volume does not participate in gas exchange. For each breath, the gas left in the conducting tubes is wasted. Similarly, regional or local differences in ventilation cause some gas that reaches the alveoli to be wasted. This occurs in alveoli that have little or no perfusion. This relationship can be described by the following equation:

$$\dot{V}_E = \dot{V}_A + \dot{V}_D$$

where:

$\dot{V}_E$ = Total volume per minute, or minute ventilation

$\dot{V}_A$ = Alveolar ventilation per minute

$\dot{V}_D$ = Wasted ventilation per minute, or dead space

Similarly, the efficiency of ventilation for a single breath can be expressed as follows:

$$V_T = V_A - V_D$$

where:

V_T = Tidal volume

V_A = Alveolar volume

V_D = Dead space volume

Minute Ventilation

Ventilation is usually assessed in liters per minute (L/min). The total volume moving in or out of the lungs per minute is called *minute ventilation*. Minute ventilation (exhaled) is denoted by $\dot{V}_E$, which is calculated as the product of frequency of breathing (f) times the expired tidal volume:

$$\dot{V}_E = f \times V_T$$

For example, for a healthy adult breathing at a rate of 12 breaths/min and having a Vt of 500 mL:

$$\dot{V}_E = 12 \times 500 \text{ mL}$$

$$= 6000 \text{ mL/min, or } 6 \text{ L/min}$$

Minute ventilation depends on the size of the subject and his or her metabolic rate. $\dot{V}_E$ values range from 5 to 10 L/min in healthy adult subjects.

Alveolar Ventilation

The efficiency of ventilation depends on the volume of fresh gas reaching the alveoli (V_A). Rearranging the previously presented equation for calculating tidal volume yields the following:

$$V_A = V_T - V_D$$

Alveolar ventilation is usually expressed per minute as $\dot{V}_A$, which is the product of breathing rate (f) and alveolar volume per breath (V_A):

$$\dot{V}_A = f \times V_A$$

Alveolar ventilation depends on tidal volume, dead space, and breathing rate. For example, in a healthy adult with a respiratory rate of 12, V_T of 500 mL, and V_{DS} of 150 mL, alveolar ventilation is calculated as follows:

$$\dot{V}_A = 12 \times (500 \text{ mL} - 150 \text{ mL})$$

$$= 12 \times 350 \text{ mL}$$

$$= 4200 \text{ mL/min}$$

Compare this volume with that described for minute ventilation. $\dot{V}_A$ is always less than $\dot{V}_E$ because of the effect of dead space.

Dead Space Ventilation

Estimation of wasted ventilation is essential in assessing the efficiency of ventilation. Dead space can be subdivided into the following two components: anatomical dead space and alveolar dead space. When these are considered together, they often are referred to as *physiological dead space*.

Anatomical Dead Space

The volume of the conducting airways is called the *anatomical dead space*, or V_{Danat}. V_{Danat} averages approximately 1 mL per pound of body weight (2.2 mL/kg). For a subject who weighs 150 lb, V_{Danat} is approximately 150 mL.

V_{Danat} does not participate in gas exchange because it is rebreathed. During exhalation of a 500-mL tidal breath, the first 150 mL of gas comes from the anatomical dead space. The remaining 350 mL is alveolar gas. At the end of exhalation, the airways contain 150 mL of alveolar gas. During the next inhalation, this 150-mL volume is rebreathed. Only approximately 350 mL of fresh gas reaches the alveoli per breath.

Alveolar Dead Space

In addition to the ventilation wasted on the conducting airways, some alveoli may not participate in gas exchange. These alveoli are ventilated but not perfused with mixed venous blood. Without perfusion, gas exchange cannot occur. Any gas that ventilates unperfused alveoli also is wasted (dead space).

The volume of gas ventilating unperfused alveoli is called *alveolar dead space,* or V_{Dalv}. Significant amounts of V_{Dalv} are pathological. V_{Dalv} is usually related to defects in the pulmonary circulation. A clinical example of such a defect is a pulmonary **embolism.** A pulmonary embolus blocks a portion of the pulmonary circulation. This obstructs perfusion to ventilated alveoli, creating alveolar dead space. Alveolar dead space occurs in addition to the anatomical dead space.

Physiological Dead Space

The sum of anatomical and alveolar dead space is called *physiological dead space* (V_{Dphy}):

$$V_{DSphy} = V_{Danat} + V_{Dalv}$$

The total volume of wasted ventilation, or physiological dead space, equals the sum of the conducting airways and the alveoli that are ventilated but not perfused (Figure 9-16).

Physiological dead space includes both the normal and abnormal components of wasted ventilation. V_{Dphy} is the preferred clinical measure of ventilation efficiency. Measuring V_{Dphy} more accurately assesses alveolar ventilation:

$$\dot{V}_A = f \times (V_T - V_{Dphy})$$

or

$$\dot{V}_A = \dot{V}_E - V_{Dphy}$$

Physiological dead space is measured clinically by using a modified form of the *Bohr equation.*

Dead Space/Tidal Volume Ratio

In clinical practice, V_{Dphy} is often expressed as a ratio to tidal volume. This ratio (V_D/V_T), provides an index of the wasted ventilation (anatomical plus alveolar dead space) per breath. The V_D/V_T ratio represents the *efficiency* of ventilation. In the healthy adult, physio-

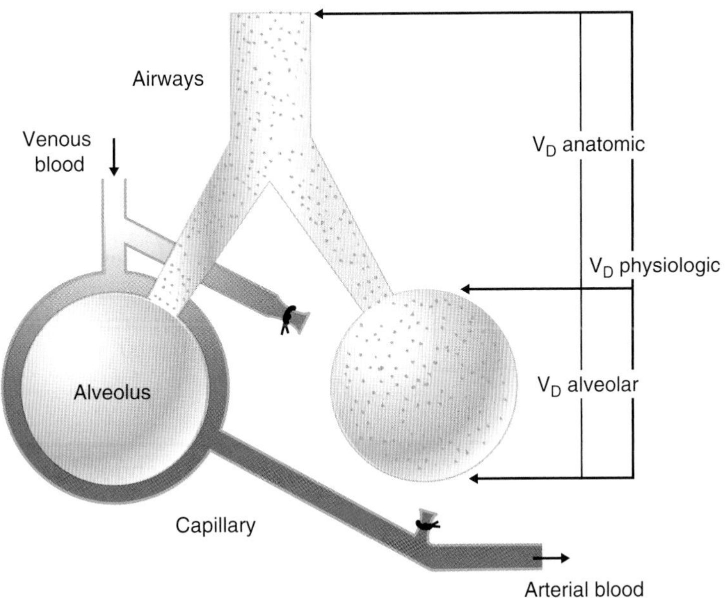

Figure 9-16

Three types of dead space. The alveolus on the left is normally perfused and ventilated. The alveolus on the right is ventilated but not perfused. Anatomical dead space is composed of the conducting tubes leading to both alveoli. The volume of the alveolus on the right represents alveolar dead space. Physiological dead space is the sum of the two components.

MINI CLINI

Minute Ventilation, Dead Space, and $PaCO_2$

PROBLEM

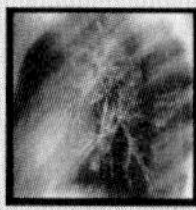

A patient breathing at a rate of 12 breaths/min has a tidal volume of 600 mL and a measured physiological dead space (V_{Dphy}) of 200 mL. This ventilatory pattern produces a $PaCO_2$ of 40 mm Hg. Several hours later, the patient has a breathing rate of 24 breaths/min, but the minute ventilation ($\dot{V}_E$) has remained the same as before. Arterial blood gas analysis reveals a $PaCO_2$ of 72 mm Hg. Why has the $PaCO_2$ increased even though the $\dot{V}_E$ remained constant?

DISCUSSION

The initial minute ventilation ($\dot{V}_E$) and alveolar ventilation ($\dot{V}_A$) were as follows:

$$\dot{V}_E = 600 \times 12$$
$$= 7200 \text{ mL/min}$$
$$\dot{V}_A = (600 - 200) \times 12$$
$$= 4800 \text{ mL/min}$$

This $\dot{V}_A$ of 4800 mL/min was responsible for maintaining a $PaCO_2$ of 40 mm Hg. When respiratory rate increased to 24 breaths/min and $\dot{V}_E$ remained at 7200 mL/min, tidal volume (V_T) must have decreased:

$$V_T = 7200 \div 24$$
$$= 300 \text{ mL}$$

However, if dead space remained at 200 mL, then alveolar ventilation subsequently decreased:

$$\dot{V}_A = (300 - 200) \times 24$$
$$= 2400 \text{ mL/min}$$

The reduction in $\dot{V}_A$ (from 4800 mL/min to 2400 mL/min) explains the increase in $PaCO_2$ from 40 mm Hg to 72 mm Hg. $PaCO_2$ is inversely proportional to alveolar ventilation. Because $\dot{V}_A$ was reduced by half, $PaCO_2$ should have doubled. This approximates the data actually observed. Normally, increased CO_2 tension in the blood causes acidemia and results in increased alveolar ventilation. This patient, although tachypneic, is hypoventilating.

logical dead space is approximately one third of the tidal volume, with a normal range of 0.2 to 0.4. The V_D/V_T ratio normally decreases with exercise. Both V_T and V_D increase with increased ventilation during exertion, but the tidal volume normally increases to a greater degree; thus the ratio decreases (in healthy subjects). V_D/V_T increases with diseases that cause significant dead space, such as pulmonary embolism.

Clinical Significance

Table 9-3 lists the effects of changes in various parameters that determine alveolar ventilation ($\dot{V}_A$). In healthy individuals, $\dot{V}_A$ depends on the rate of breathing and Vt. High respiratory rates and low tidal volumes result in a high proportion of wasted ventilation per minute (low $\dot{V}_A$). The most efficient breathing pattern is slow, deep breathing.

In pulmonary disease, an increased V_{Dphy} causes a decrease in $\dot{V}_A$, unless compensation occurs. An increased breathing rate by itself worsens the problem. Effective compensation for increased V_{Dphy} requires an increased tidal volume. Elevating V_T increases the elastic work of breathing. This increases oxygen consumption by the respiratory muscles. In some patients, these increased demands cannot be met. In such cases, $\dot{V}_A$ may not be adequate to meet body needs.

Effectiveness

Ventilation is effective when it removes carbon dioxide at a rate that maintains a normal pH. Under resting metabolic conditions, the body produces approximately 200 mL of CO_2 per minute. Alveolar ventilation must match carbon dioxide production per minute to ensure homeostasis.

The balance between CO_2 production ($\dot{V}CO_2$) and $\dot{V}_A$ determines the PCO_2 in the lungs and arterial blood. This balance also helps determine the pH of arterial blood. The partial pressure of CO_2 in the alveoli and blood is directly proportional to its production ($\dot{V}CO_2$) and inversely proportional to its rate of removal by alveolar ventilation ($\dot{V}_A$):

Table 9-3 ▶▶ Changes in Alveolar Ventilation (mL) Associated With Changes in Rate, Volume, and Physiological Dead Space

Ventilatory Pattern	Rate of Breathing (Breaths/min)	Tidal Volume (mL)	Minute Ventilation (mL)	Physiological Dead Space (mL)	Alveolar Ventilation (mL)
Normal	12	500	6000	150	4200
High rate, low volume	24	250	6000	50	2400
Low rate, high volume	6	1000	6000	150	5100
Increased dead space	12	500	6000	300	2400
Compensation for increased dead space	12	650	7800	300	4200

$$P_{CO_2} \cong \frac{\dot{V}_{CO_2}}{\dot{V}_A}$$

Alveolar and arterial partial pressures of carbon dioxide are normally in equilibrium at approximately 40 mm Hg. If $\dot{V}_A$ falls, $\dot{V}_{CO_2}$ will exceed its rate of removal. The Pa_{CO_2} will rise above its normal value of 40 mm Hg, and the arterial pH level will fall. Ventilation that does not meet metabolic needs (i.e., does not maintain a normal pH) is termed *hypoventilation*. Hypoventilation is indicated by the presence of an elevated Pa_{CO_2} and a pH level below the normal range (7.35 to 7.45).

If alveolar ventilation increases, the $\dot{V}_{CO_2}$ will be less than its rate of removal. Pa_{CO_2} will fall below its normal value of 40 mm Hg, and pH will rise. Ventilation in excess of metabolic needs is termed *hyperventilation*. Hyperventilation is indicated by a lower than normal Pa_{CO_2} and a pH above the normal range.

Sometimes hyperventilation is confused with the increased ventilation that occurs in response to increased metabolism. A good example is the changes observed during low or moderate levels of exercise. Ventilation rises in proportion to the increased $\dot{V}_{CO_2}$ from exercise. The Pa_{CO_2} remains in the normal range of 35 to 45 mm Hg, and the pH level remains near 7.40. The increase in ventilation that occurs with increased metabolic rates is termed *hyperpnea*.

Effectiveness of ventilation is determined by the partial pressure of carbon dioxide and the resulting pH, specifically in arterial blood. Ventilation is effective when the Pa_{CO_2} is maintained at a level that keeps the pH within normal limits.

Ineffective ventilation occurs when carbon dioxide production and alveolar ventilation are out of balance. Hypoventilation is ineffective because carbon dioxide removal is inadequate to meet metabolic needs. Hyperventilation is ineffective because excessive energy is expended needlessly. There is no direct or consistent correlation between measures of ventilation ($\dot{V}_E$, V_T, f) and effectiveness of ventilation. Hypoventilation or hyperventilation must be determined by arterial blood gas analysis (see Chapters 12 and 16).

KEY POINTS

- Ventilation occurs because of pressure differences across the lung during breathing. Gas flows into the lung when the diaphragm creates a subatmospheric pressure in the lung; gas flows out of the lung when the recoil properties of the lung create a slight positive pressure.

KEY POINTS—cont'd

- The forces that oppose lung inflation may be grouped into two categories: elastic forces and frictional forces.
- Frictional forces opposing ventilation include airway and tissue resistance.
- Airway resistance accounts for 80% of the frictional resistance to ventilation in the healthy adult lung.
- Exhalation is normally passive but becomes active when airway resistance is abnormally high.
- The work of breathing is performed by the muscles of breathing; respiratory muscle fatigue causes a drop in the tidal volume and an increase in the respiratory rate.
- Even a healthy lung does not distribute ventilation evenly throughout the lungs; greater ventilation normally occurs in the bases.
- The total volume of gas moving in and out of the lungs each minute is called the *minute volume*.
- Homeostasis is present when the alveolar ventilation matches carbon dioxide production.

References

1. West JB: Respiratory physiology: the essentials, ed 6, Baltimore, 2000, Lippincott Williams & Wilkins.
2. Beachey W: Respiratory care anatomy and physiology: foundations for clinical practice, St Louis, 1998, Mosby.
3. Lumb AB: Nunn's applied respiratory physiology, ed 5, London, 1999, Butterworth-Heinemann Medical.
4. Thurlbeck WM: Pathophysiology of chronic obstructive pulmonary disease, Clin Chest Med 11:389, 1990.
5. Rochester DF: Respiratory muscles and ventilatory failure: 1993 perspective, Am J Med Sci 305:394, 1993.
6. Martin L: Pulmonary physiology in clinical practice: the essentials for patient care and evaluation, St Louis, 1987, Mosby.

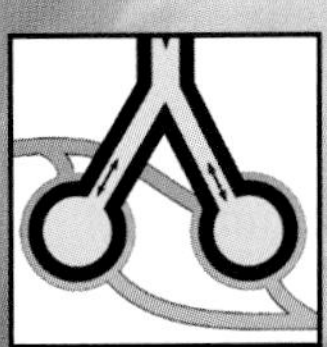

CHAPTER 10

Gas Exchange and Transport

Craig L. Scanlan and Robert L. Wilkins

In This Chapter You Will Learn:

- How oxygen and carbon dioxide move between the atmosphere and tissues
- What determines alveolar oxygen and carbon dioxide pressures
- How to compute the alveolar partial pressure of oxygen
- What effect normal regional variations in ventilation and perfusion have on gas exchange
- How to compute total oxygen contents for arterial blood
- What causes the arteriovenous oxygen content difference to change
- What factors affect oxygen loading and unloading from hemoglobin
- How carbon dioxide is carried in the blood
- How oxygen and carbon dioxide transport are interrelated
- What factors impair oxygen delivery to the tissues and how to distinguish among them
- What factors impair carbon dioxide removal

Chapter Outline

Key Terms

alveolar air equation
anemia
Bohr effect
carbamino compound
carboxyhemoglobin (HbCO)
dysoxia
fetal hemoglobin (Hb F)
Fick formula
Fick's first law of diffusion
hypoxemia
hypoxia
ischemia
methemoglobinemia
P50
respiratory exchange ratio (R)
right-to-left shunts
sickle cell
venous admixture
ventilation/perfusion ratio ($\dot{V}/\dot{Q}$)

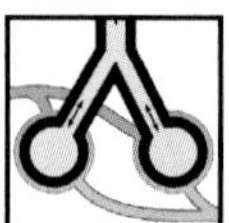

Respiration is the process of getting oxygen into the body for tissue utilization and removal of carbon dioxide into the atmosphere. This complex process involves both gas exchange (at the lungs and at the cellular level) and transport of those gases. Oxygen must be moved into the lungs, where it diffuses into the pulmonary circulation and is transported in the blood to the tissues. Carbon dioxide builds up in the tissues because of metabolism and diffuses into the capillary blood before being carried to the lung for exchange with alveolar gases. Normally, these processes are well integrated. However, in disease states, impaired gas exchange or transport can cause physiological imbalances, which can alter function or threaten survival. At such times, respiratory care intervention may be the only way to maintain or restore a level of function consistent with life. This chapter provides the background knowledge that respiratory therapists (RTs) need to understand and treat patients with diseases that affect gas exchange.

▶ DIFFUSION

Whole-Body Diffusion Gradients

Gas movement between the lungs and tissues occurs by simple diffusion (see Chapter 5). Figure 10-1 shows the normal diffusion gradients for oxygen and carbon dioxide. For oxygen, there is a stepwise downward "cascade" of partial pressures from the normal atmospheric inspired partial pressure of oxygen (P_{IO_2}) of 159 mm Hg to a low point of 40 mm Hg or less in the capillaries. The intracellular P_{O_2} (approximately 5 mm Hg) provides the final gradient for oxygen diffusion into the cell.

The diffusion gradient for carbon dioxide is the opposite of that for oxygen. The partial pressure of carbon dioxide (P_{CO_2}) is highest in the cells (approximately 60 mm Hg) and lowest in room air (1 mm Hg). This reverse cascade causes CO_2 movement from the tissues into the venous blood, which is transported to the lungs and—with the aid of ventilation—out to the atmosphere.

Determinants of Alveolar Gas Tensions

Alveolar Carbon Dioxide

The *alveolar partial pressure of carbon dioxide*, or P_{ACO_2}, varies directly with the body's production of carbon dioxide ($\dot{V}_{CO_2}$) and inversely with alveolar ventilation ($\dot{V}_A$). Using a factor of 0.863 to convert $\dot{V}_{CO_2}$ from standard temperature and pressure, dry (STPD) to body temperature and pressure, saturated (BTPS), the relationship is expressed by the following formula:

$$P_{ACO_2} = \frac{\dot{V}_{CO_2}}{0.863 \times \dot{V}_A}$$

Given a normal $\dot{V}_{CO_2}$ of 200 mL/min and a normal alveolar ventilation of 5.8 L/min, application of this formula yields a P_{ACO_2} of approximately 40 mm Hg:

$$P_{ACO_2} = \frac{200 \text{ mL/min}}{(0.863 \times 5.8 \text{ L/min})} \cong 40 \text{ mm Hg}$$

The P_{ACO_2} will increase above this level if carbon dioxide production increases while alveolar ventilation remains constant or when alveolar ventilation decreases while V_{CO_2} remains constant. Likewise, the P_{ACO_2} will fall if carbon dioxide production decreases or alveolar ventilation increases. Normally, complex respiratory control mechanisms maintain the P_{ACO_2} within a range of 35 to 45 mm Hg under a variety of conditions (see Chapter 13). For example, if CO_2 production increases,

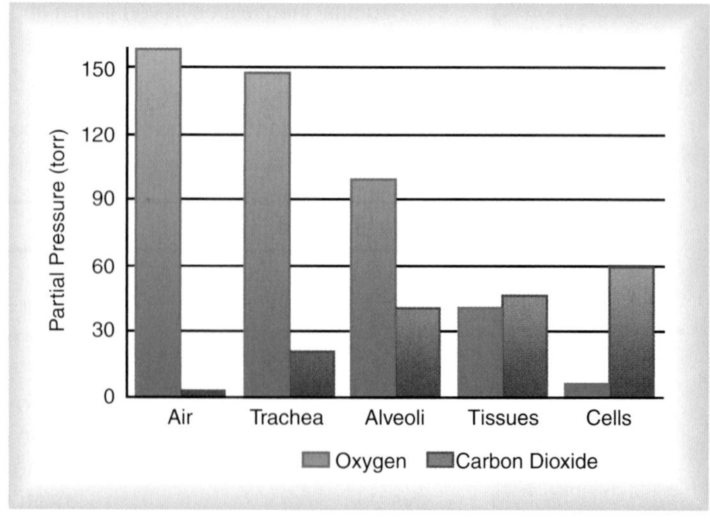

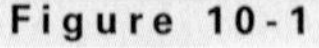
Figure 10-1

Normal diffusion gradients for oxygen and carbon dioxide. Note the downward cascade for oxygen from air to cells, with a reverse gradient for carbon dioxide.

as with exercise or fever, ventilation automatically increases to maintain a P_{ACO_2} within normal range.

Alveolar Oxygen Tensions

Many factors determine the *alveolar partial pressure of oxygen (P_{AO_2})*. Most important is the *inspired partial pressure of oxygen, or P_{IO_2}*. In addition, once in the lungs, oxygen is diluted by both water vapor and carbon dioxide. To account for all these factors, the following alveolar air equation is applied:

$$P_{AO_2} = F_{IO_2} \times (P_B - 47) - \frac{P_{ACO_2}}{0.8}$$

where:

F_{IO_2} = Fraction of inspired oxygen

P_b = Barometric pressure

47 = Water vapor tension (in mm Hg) at 37° C

P_{ACO_2} = Alveolar P_{CO_2}

0.8 = Normal respiratory exchange ratio (R)

The equation component $F_{IO_2} \times (P_B - 47)$ is a simple application of Dalton's law:

Partial pressure = Fractional concentration × Total pressure

However, under BTPS conditions in the lungs, the total pressure available for oxygen is reduced by an amount equal to the saturated water vapor pressure at 37° C, or 47 mm Hg.

The equation component $P_{ACO_2} \div 0.8$ accounts for the alveolar carbon dioxide. However, the Pa_{CO_2} cannot simply be subtracted, as was done for water vapor. Instead, the equation must be corrected for the difference between O_2 and CO_2 movement into and out of the alveoli. This is done by dividing the P_{ACO_2} by the **respiratory exchange ratio (R)**. R is the ratio of carbon dioxide excretion to oxygen uptake, which normally averages 0.8 throughout the lung. In addition, because the arterial P_{CO_2} nearly equals the alveolar P_{CO_2}, the Pa_{CO_2} can be substituted for the P_{ACO_2}.

For example, if the F_{IO_2} is 0.21, the P_B is 760 mm Hg, and the Pa_{CO_2} is 40 mm Hg, the normal alveolar partial pressure of oxygen can be estimated as follows:

$$P_{AO_2} = 0.21 \times (760 \text{ mm Hg} - 47) - \frac{40 \text{ mm Hg}}{0.8}$$

$$= 99.73 \text{ mm Hg}$$

In clinical practice, if a patient is breathing 60% or more oxygen ($F_{IO_2} \geq 0.60$), the correction for R can be dropped. This yields the following simplified form of the alveolar air equation:

$$P_{AO_2} = F_{IO_2} (P_B - 47) - Pa_{CO_2}$$

MINI CLINI

The Alveolar-Arterial P_{O_2} Difference and the a/A Ratio

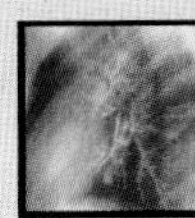

Not all of the oxygen from the alveoli gets into the blood. Why this occurs is discussed later in this chapter. This Mini Clini considers how the *efficiency* of oxygen transfer from the alveoli to the blood can actually be computed.

Several bedside computations can be used to compute the efficiency of pulmonary oxygen transfer. The most common is the difference between the alveolar and arterial P_{O_2}, called the *A-a gradient,* written as $P(A - a)O_2$. Normally this difference is small—only 5 to 10 mm Hg when air is breathed and no more than 65 mm Hg when 100% oxygen is breathed.

Another common bedside computation is the ratio of arterial to alveolar P_{O_2}, called the *a/A ratio*. The a/A ratio should be thought of as the proportion of oxygen getting from the alveoli to the blood. Normally this proportion is at least 90% (a ratio of 0.9).

PROBLEM

Compute and interpret the $P(A - a)O_2$ and a/A ratio for a 45-year-old woman breathing 70% oxygen at sea level, with the following blood gases: Pa_{O_2}, 50 mm Hg; Pa_{CO_2}, 50 mm Hg.

DISCUSSION

1. Compute the P_{AO_2} as follows:
   $P_{AO_2} = F_{IO_2} \times (Pb - 47) - P_{ACO_2}$ (patient breathing more than 60% oxygen)
   $P_{AO_2} = 0.7 \times (760 \text{ mm Hg} - 47 \text{ mm Hg}) - 50 \text{ mm Hg}$
   $P_{AO_2} = 449$ mm Hg
2. Compute the $P(A - a)O_2$ as follows:
   $P(A - a)O_2 = P_{AO_2} - Pa_{O_2}$
   $P(A - a)O_2 = 449 \text{ mm Hg} - 50 \text{ mm Hg}$
   $P(A - a)O_2 = 399$ mm Hg
3. Compute the a/A as follows:
   a/A = Pa_{O_2}/P_{AO_2}
   a/A = 50 mm Hg/449 mm Hg
   a/A = 0.11

Both the $P(A - a)O_2$ and the a/A ratio are abnormal. Compared with a normal of 65 mm Hg or less, the $P(A - a)O_2$ of nearly 400 mm Hg is very high. This indicates a large difference between the alveolar and arterial P_{O_2} values (i.e., inefficient oxygen transfer). Likewise, the a/A ratio of 0.11 indicates that only approximately 11% of the oxygen in the alveoli is getting into the blood.

Although the patient is receiving a high F_{IO_2} (0.70), she has a severe problem getting oxygen into her blood.

The accompanying Mini Clini provides an example of how to use the alveolar air equation.

Changes in Alveolar Gas Partial Tensions

In addition to carbon dioxide, oxygen, and water vapor, alveoli normally contain nitrogen. Nitrogen is inert and plays no role in gas exchange. However, nitrogen does occupy space and exert pressure. According to Dalton's law (see Chapter 5), the partial pressure of alveolar nitrogen must equal the pressure it would exert if it alone were present. Thus to compute the partial pressure of alveolar nitrogen, subtract the pressures exerted by all the other alveolar gases, as follows:

$$P_{AN_2} = P_B - (P_{AO_2} + P_{ACO_2} + P_{H_2O})$$

$$P_{AN_2} = 760 \text{ mm Hg} - (100 \text{ mm Hg} + 40 \text{ mm Hg} + 47 \text{ mm Hg})$$

$$P_{AN_2} = 760 \text{ mm Hg} - 187 \text{ mm Hg}$$

$$P_{AN_2} = 573 \text{ mm Hg}$$

Because both water vapor tension and P_{AN_2} remain constant, the only partial pressures that change in the alveolus are O_2 and CO_2. Based on the alveolar air equation, if the F_{IO_2} remains constant, then the P_{AO_2} must vary inversely with the P_{ACO_2}.

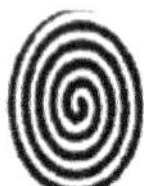

RULE OF THUMB

Because the total combined partial pressures of oxygen and carbon dioxide in room air are approximately 140 mm Hg (100 mm Hg + 40 mm Hg, respectively), the impact of a change in P_{ACO_2} on P_{AO_2} can be estimated with the following simple equation:

$$P_{AO_2} = 140 \text{ mm Hg} - P_{ACO_2}$$

For example, if the P_{ACO_2} of a patient breathing room air rises from 40 to 60 mm Hg (an increase of 20 mm Hg), then the P_{AO_2} should fall by approximately 20 mm Hg. This equation assumes a constant value for R.

Of course, the P_{ACO_2} itself varies inversely with the level of alveolar ventilation. Thus for a constant CO_2 production, a decrease in $\dot{V}_A$ simultaneously raises the P_{ACO_2} and lowers the P_{AO_2}, whereas an increase in $\dot{V}_A$ has the opposite effect (Figure 10-2). However, ventilation can be increased only so much. Neural control mechanisms and the increased of work breathing prevent decreases in P_{ACO_2} much below 15 to 20 mm Hg. Thus whenever a patient is breathing room air at sea level, the RT should not expect to see a P_{aO_2} any higher than 120 to 130 mm Hg during hyperventilation. P_{O_2} values higher than 120 to 130 mm Hg with a reduced P_{aCO_2} indicate that the patient is breathing supplemental oxygen. See the accompanying Mini Clini for a clinical application of these principles.

MINI CLINI

Assessing Arterial Gas Partial Pressures

PROBLEM

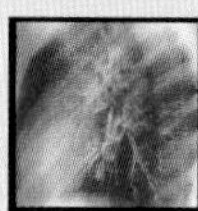

The RT is given the following arterial blood gas report for a patient who was just admitted to the emergency department: P_{aO_2} = 170 mm Hg; P_{aCO_2} = 23 mm Hg. Without additional data, what conclusions can the RT draw about the F_{IO_2} in this case?

DISCUSSION

In room air, the total pressure exerted by oxygen and carbon dioxide in the alveoli (and blood) should be approximately 140 mm Hg. In this case, the total is 170 mm Hg (P_{aO_2}) + 23 mm Hg (P_{aCO_2}), or 193 mm Hg. Whenever total pressure significantly exceeds 140 mm Hg and the P_{aO_2} is higher than 120 to 130 mm Hg, the RT can be ensured that the patient is breathing supplemental oxygen.

Mechanism of Diffusion

As described in Chapter 5, diffusion is the process whereby gas molecules move from an area of high partial pressure to an area of low partial pressure. To diffuse into and out of the lung and tissues, oxygen and carbon dioxide must move through significant barriers.

Barriers to Diffusion

The barrier to gaseous diffusion in the lung is the alveolar-capillary membrane. For carbon dioxide or oxygen to move between the alveoli and the pulmonary capillary blood, the following three barriers must be penetrated: (1) alveolar epithelium, (2) interstitial space, and (3) capillary endothelium. In addition, to pass into and out of the red blood cells (RBCs), these gases also must traverse the erythrocyte membrane.

Fick's First Law of Diffusion

The bulk movement of a gas through a biological membrane ($\dot{V}_{gas}$) is described by **Fick's first law of diffusion:**

$$\dot{V}_{gas} = \frac{A \times D}{T}(P_1 - P_2)$$

In this formula, *A* is the cross-sectional area available for diffusion, *D* is the diffusion coefficient of the gas, *T* is the thickness of the membrane, and $(P_1 - P_2)$ is the partial pressure gradient across the membrane.

According to Fick's law, the greater the surface area, diffusion constant, and pressure gradient, the more diffusion will occur. Conversely, the greater the distance across the membrane, the less diffusion will occur.

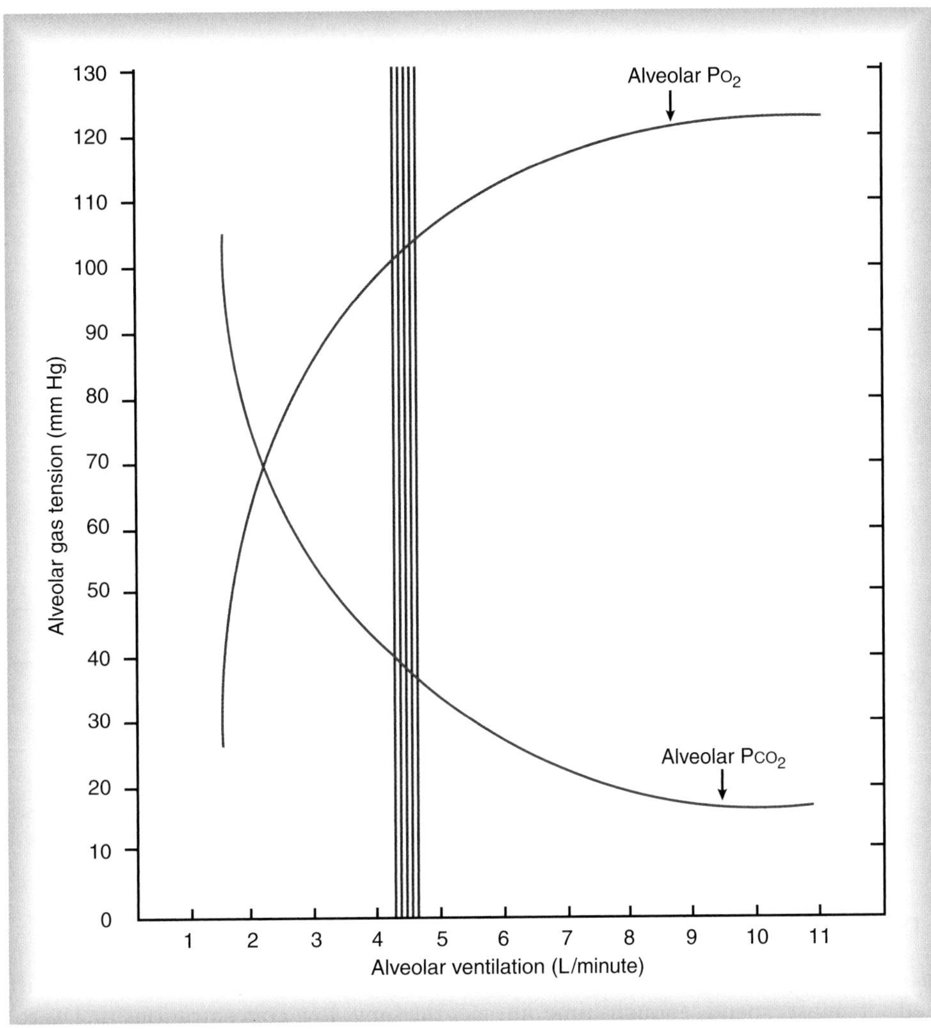

Figure 10-2

The effect of alveolar ventilation on alveolar gases. *(From Pilbeam SP: Mechanical ventilation, ed 3, St Louis, 1998, Mosby.)*

Given that the area of and distance across the alveolar-capillary membrane are relatively constant in healthy people, diffusion in the normal lung mainly depends on gas pressure gradients.

Pulmonary Diffusion Gradients

For gas exchange to occur between the alveoli and pulmonary capillaries, a difference in partial pressures $(P_1 - P_2)$ must exist. Figure 10-3 shows the size and direction of these gradients for oxygen and carbon dioxide.

In the normal lung, the alveolar PO_2 averages approximately 100 mm Hg, whereas the mean PCO_2 is approximately 40 mm Hg. Venous blood returning to the lungs has a lower PO_2 (40 mm Hg) than alveolar gas. Thus the pressure gradient for O_2 diffusion into the blood is approximately 60 mm Hg (100 mm Hg–40 mm Hg). Therefore as blood flows past the alveolus, it takes up oxygen, leaving the capillary with a PO_2 close to 100 mm Hg.

Because venous blood has a higher PCO_2 than alveolar gas (46 mm Hg versus 40 mm Hg), the pressure gradient for CO_2 causes diffusion of CO_2 in the opposite direction, from the blood into the alveolus. This continues until the capillary PCO_2 equilibrates with the alveolar level, approximately 40 mm Hg.

Although the pressure gradient for carbon dioxide is approximately one tenth of that for oxygen, CO_2 has little difficulty diffusing across the alveolar-capillary membrane. CO_2 diffuses approximately 20 times faster across the alveolar-capillary membrane than does oxygen, because of its much higher solubility in plasma. On the other hand, disorders that impair the lung's diffusion capacity can affect oxygen movement into the blood. This is true especially when blood flow through the lung is rapid, because this reduces the time in which the RBCs are in contact with the alveoli.

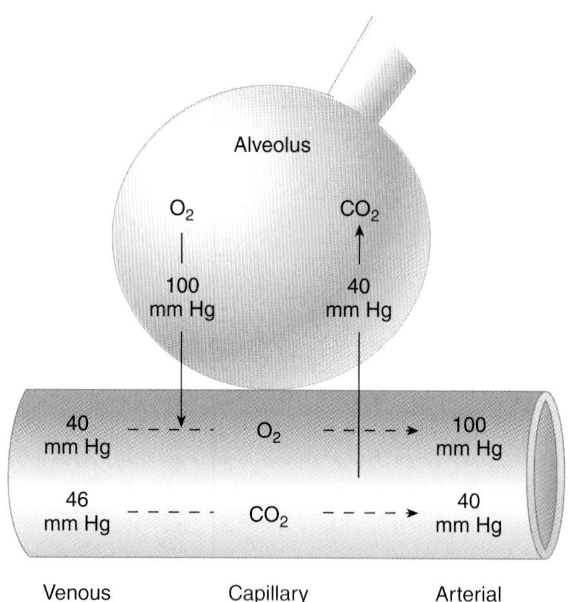

Figure 10-3

Ventilation maintains the mean alveolar gas pressures for O_2 and CO_2 at approximately 100 and 40 mm Hg, respectively. As blood enters the venous end of the capillary it gives up CO_2 and loads O_2 until these two gases are in equilibrium with alveolar pressures. At this point the blood is "arterialized."

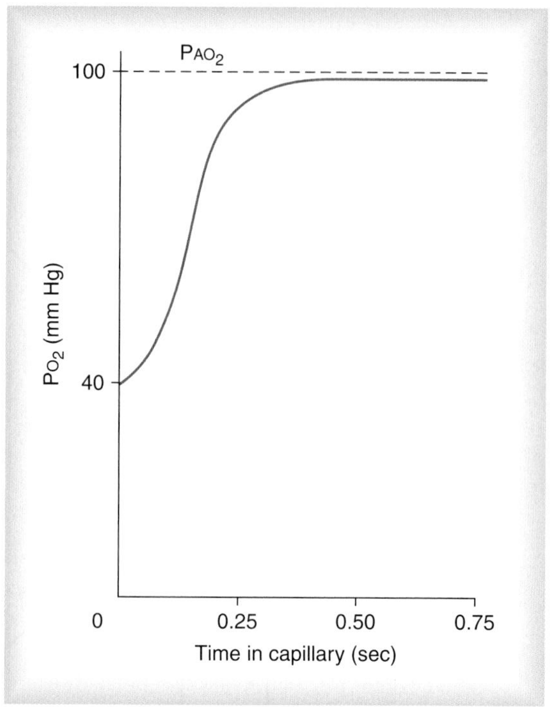

Figure 10-4

Alveolar-capillary P_{O_2} gradient. Normal transit time for a red blood cell in the pulmonary capillary is approximately 0.75 seconds. Normally, the blood P_{O_2} equilibrates with the alveolar P_{O_2} well before it reaches the end of the capillary.

Time Limits to Diffusion

For blood leaving the pulmonary capillary to be adequately oxygenated, it must spend enough time in contact with the alveolus to allow equilibration. If the time available for diffusion is inadequate, blood leaving the lungs may not be fully oxygenated. The diffusion time in the lung depends on the rate of pulmonary blood flow. As depicted in Figure 10-4, blood normally takes approximately 0.75 seconds to pass through the pulmonary capillary. This is more than enough time to ensure complete diffusion of oxygen across the alveolar-capillary membrane.

If blood flow increases, such as during heavy exercise, capillary transit time can decrease to as low as 0.25 seconds. Even this short time frame is adequate to ensure that equilibration takes place, as long as no other factors impair diffusion. However, in the presence of a diffusion limitation, rapid blood flow through the pulmonary circulation can result in inadequate oxygenation. Fever and septic shock, which cause increased cardiac output, are good examples of conditions that limit diffusion time because of increased blood flow.

In clinical practice, knowledge of the lung's diffusing capacity can be helpful in evaluating certain diseases. The diffusing capacity of the lung (D_L) is the bulk flow of gas (mL/min) that diffuses into the blood for each 1–mm Hg difference in the pressure gradient. Although oxygen can be used to measure the diffusion capacity of the lung, low concentrations (0.1% to 0.3%) of carbon monoxide are used more commonly. Chapter 17 provides details on the technique for measuring diffusing capacity, as well as its diagnostic use.

Systemic Diffusion Gradients

The partial pressure gradients in the tissues are the opposite of those in the lung. As cellular metabolism depletes its oxygen, the intracellular P_{O_2} drops below that of the blood entering the tissue capillary. Oxygen diffuses from the tissue capillary blood (P_{O_2} = 100 mm Hg) to the cells (P_{O_2} <40 mm Hg). Simultaneously, carbon dioxide diffuses from the cells (P_{CO_2} >46 mm Hg) into the capillary blood (P_{CO_2} = 40 mm Hg). After equilibration, blood leaves the tissue capillaries as venous blood, with a P_{O_2} of approximately 40 mm Hg and a P_{CO_2} of approximately 46 mm Hg.

Just as arterial blood reflects pulmonary gas exchange, venous blood reflects events occurring in the tissues. To assess tissue gas exchange, the RT must consider venous blood parameters. The use of venous blood to assess tissue oxygenation also is discussed in Chapter 43.

NORMAL VARIATIONS FROM IDEAL GAS EXCHANGE

Up to this point, this chapter has focused almost entirely on gas pressures in a perfect alveolus (i.e., one with ideal ventilation and blood flow). In reality, however, the normal lung is an imperfect organ of gas exchange. Clinically, this becomes clear when the Pa_{O_2} is measured in the average individual. Rather than equaling the alveolar P_{O_2} of 100 mm Hg, the Pa_{O_2} of healthy individuals breathing air at sea level is always approximately 5 to 10 mm Hg less than the calculated Pa_{O_2}.

Two factors account for this difference: (1) right-to-left shunts in the pulmonary and cardiac circulation and (2) regional differences in pulmonary ventilation and blood flow.

Anatomical Shunts

Two right-to-left anatomical shunts exist in the normal human being: (1) the bronchial venous drainage and (2) the thebesian venous drainage (see Chapters 7 and 8). A right-to-left shunt diverts poorly oxygenated venous blood directly into the arterial circulation, thereby lowering the oxygen content of arterial blood. Together, these normal shunts account for approximately three fourths of the normal difference between the P_{AO_2} and the Pa_{O_2}. The remaining difference is a result of normal inequalities in pulmonary ventilation and perfusion.

Regional Inequalities in Ventilation and Perfusion

The normal respiratory exchange ratio of 0.8 assumes that both ventilation and perfusion in the lung are in balance, with every liter of alveolar ventilation ($\dot{V}_A$) matched by approximately 1 L of pulmonary capillary blood flow ($\dot{Q}c$).

Any variation from this perfect balance will alter gas tensions in the affected alveoli. As previously discussed, changes in $\dot{V}_A$ affect the alveolar P_{CO_2}, which in turn alters the alveolar P_{O_2}. Changes in blood flow also alter alveolar gas pressures. For example, if blood flow to an area of lung increases, CO_2 coming from the tissues will be delivered faster than it can be removed, causing a rise in alveolar P_{CO_2}. At the same time, oxygen will be taken up by the capillaries faster than it can be restored by ventilation, causing a fall in alveolar P_{O_2}. A decrease in pulmonary capillary blood flow will have the opposite effect (i.e., a fall in alveolar P_{CO_2} and a rise in alveolar P_{O_2}).

Ventilation/Perfusion Ratio

Changes in $\dot{V}_A$ and $\dot{Q}c$ are expressed as a ratio called the **ventilation/perfusion ratio** ($\dot{V}/\dot{Q}$). An ideal ratio of 1.0 indicates that ventilation and perfusion are in perfect balance. A high $\dot{V}/\dot{Q}$ indicates that ventilation is greater than normal, perfusion is less than normal, or both. In areas with a high $\dot{V}/\dot{Q}$, the P_{O_2} is higher and the P_{CO_2} is lower than normal. Conversely, a low $\dot{V}/\dot{Q}$ indicates that ventilation is less than normal, perfusion is greater than normal, or both. In areas with a low $\dot{V}/\dot{Q}$, the alveolar P_{O_2} is lower and the P_{CO_2} is higher than normal.

Effect of Alterations in the $\dot{V}/\dot{Q}$

Figure 10-5 shows graphs of the effect of $\dot{V}/\dot{Q}$ changes on the respiratory exchange ratio (R), plotting all possible values of alveolar P_{O_2} and P_{CO_2}. Note that when ventilation and perfusion are in perfect balance ($\dot{V}/\dot{Q}$ = 0.99), R equals 0.8. At this point, the alveolar

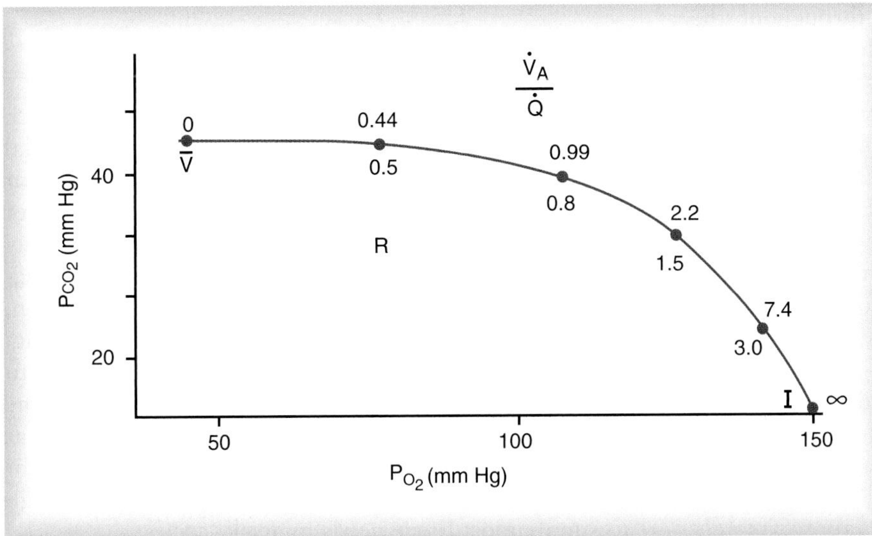

Figure 10-5
The relationship between alveolar P_{O_2} and P_{CO_2} with changes in the ratio of ventilation to perfusion and the respiratory exchange ratio. *(From Cherniak RM, Cherniak L: Respiration in health and disease, ed 3, Philadelphia, 1983, Saunders.)*

P_{O_2} and P_{CO_2} values equal the ideal values of 100 and 40 mm Hg, respectively.

As the $\dot{V}/\dot{Q}$ rises above 1.0 (following the curve to the right), R increases. The result is a higher alveolar P_{O_2} and a lower alveolar P_{CO_2}. At the extreme right of the graph, perfusion is 0 ($\dot{V}/\dot{Q} = \infty$). Areas with ventilation but no blood flow represent alveolar dead space, as defined in Chapter 9. The makeup of gases in these areas is similar to that of inspired air (P_{O_2} = 150 mm Hg; P_{CO_2} = 0 mm Hg).

As the $\dot{V}/\dot{Q}$ falls below 1.0 (following the curve to the left), R decreases. The result is a lower alveolar P_{O_2} and a higher alveolar P_{CO_2}. At the extreme left of the graph, there is perfusion but no ventilation ($\dot{V}/\dot{Q} = 0$). With no ventilation to remove CO_2 and restore fresh oxygen, the makeup of gases in these areas is like that of mixed venous blood ($P\bar{v}_{O_2}$ = 40 mm Hg; $P\bar{v}_{CO_2}$ = 46 mm Hg).

Venous blood entering areas with $\dot{V}/\dot{Q}$ ratios of 0 cannot pick up oxygen or unload carbon dioxide, leaving the lungs unchanged. As this venous blood returns to the left side of the heart, it mixes with well-oxygenated arterial blood, diluting its oxygen contents in a manner similar to that described for a right-to-left anatomical shunt. For such areas to be distinguished from true anatomical shunts, exchange units with $\dot{V}/\dot{Q}$ values of 0 are called *alveolar shunts*. Although small anatomical shunts are normal, alveolar shunts are not.

Causes of Regional Differences in $\dot{V}/\dot{Q}$

Regional variations in $\dot{V}/\dot{Q}$ in the normal lung are mainly caused by gravity and thus are most evident in the upright posture. Because the pulmonary circulation is a low-pressure system, blood flow in the upright lung varies considerably from top to bottom (see Chapter 7). Farther down the lung, perfusion increases linearly in proportion to the hydrostatic pressure so the lung bases receive nearly 20 times as much blood flow as do the apexes.

Regional differences in ventilation throughout the lung also occur, but they are less drastic than the differences in perfusion. Like perfusion, ventilation also is increased in the lung bases, with approximately four times as much ventilation going to the bases than to the apexes of the upright lung. These regional differences in ventilation are caused by gravity's effect on pleural pressures (see Chapter 9).

Table 10-1 summarizes the relationships between ventilation and perfusion by lung region. At the lung apexes, ventilation exceeds blood flow, resulting in a high $\dot{V}/\dot{Q}$ (approximately 3.3), high P_{O_2} (132 mm Hg), and low P_{CO_2} (32 mm Hg). Farther down the lung, blood flow increases more than ventilation, so toward the middle, the two are approximately equal ($\dot{V}/\dot{Q}$ = 1.0). At the bottom of the lung, blood flow is greater than ventilation, resulting in a low $\dot{V}/\dot{Q}$ (approximately 0.66), low P_{O_2} (89 mm Hg), and slightly higher P_{CO_2} (42 mm Hg).

Table 10-1 ▶▶ Summary of Variations in Gas Exchange in the Upright Lung, by Region

Lung Region	$\dot{V}/\dot{Q}$ Ratio	Mean P_{AO_2} (mm Hg)	Mean P_{ACO_2} (mm Hg)	Blood Flow
Apexes	3.3	132	32	Low
Middle	1.0	100	40	Moderate
Bases	0.66	89	42	High

As shown in Table 10-1, most blood flows to the lung bases, where the P_{O_2} is lower and the P_{CO_2} is higher than normal. After leaving the lung, this relatively large volume of blood combines with the smaller volume coming from the middle and apical regions. The result is a mixture with less oxygen and more carbon dioxide than would come from an ideal gas exchange unit.

▶ OXYGEN TRANSPORT

Blood carries oxygen in two forms. A small amount of oxygen exists in a simple physical solution, dissolved in the plasma and erythrocyte intracellular fluid. However, the majority of oxygen is carried in a reversible chemical combination with hemoglobin inside the RBC.

Physically Dissolved Oxygen

As gaseous oxygen diffuses into the blood, it immediately dissolves in the plasma and erythrocyte fluid. By applying Henry's law (Chapter 5), the amount of dissolved oxygen in the blood (at 37° C) can be computed with the following simple formula:

$$\text{Dissolved oxygen (mL/dL)} = P_{O_2} \times 0.003$$

This equation is plotted in Figure 10-6, which demonstrates that the relationship between partial pressure and dissolved oxygen is direct and linear. For example, in normal arterial blood with a Pa_{O_2} of approximately 100 mm Hg, there is approximately 0.3 mL/dL of dissolved oxygen. However, if an individual with normal arterial blood breathes pure oxygen, the arterial P_{O_2} increases to approximately 670 mm Hg. In this case, the dissolved oxygen would increase to approximately 2.0 mL/dL. The blood of someone breathing pure oxygen in a hyperbaric chamber at 3 atm (2280 mm Hg) would carry nearly 6.5 mL/dL of dissolved oxygen in the plasma. This amount is enough to supply most tissue needs by itself!

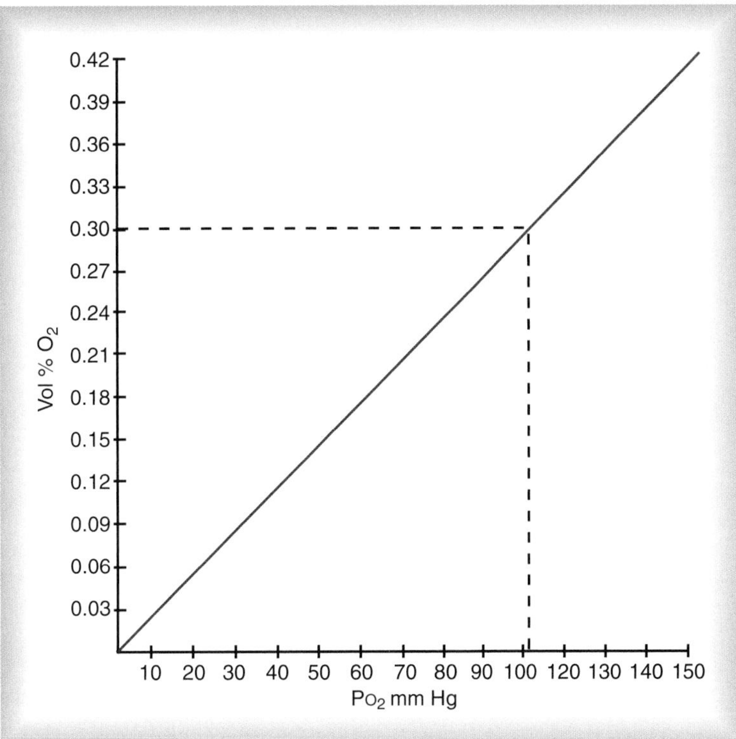

Figure 10-6

The relationship between Po_2 and dissolved oxygen contents of plasma at 37° C. The *dashed line* emphasizes the fact that arterial blood, with an average Po_2 of 100 mm Hg, has 0.3 mL of oxygen dissolved in each deciliter (100 mL).

Chemically Combined Oxygen (Oxyhemoglobin)

Hemoglobin and Oxygen Transport

Most blood oxygen is transported in chemical combination with hemoglobin (Hb) in the erythrocytes. Hb is a conjugated protein, consisting of four linked polypeptide chains (the globin portion), each of which is combined with a porphyrin complex called *heme*. The four polypeptide chains of Hb are coiled together into a ball-like structure, the shape of which determines its affinity for oxygen.

As shown in Figure 10-7, each heme complex contains a centrally located ferrous iron ion (Fe^{2+}). When hemoglobin is not carrying oxygen, this ion has four unpaired electrons. In this deoxygenated state, the molecule exhibits the characteristics of a weak acid. As such, deoxygenated hemoglobin (abbreviated as *Hb*) serves as an important blood buffer for hydrogen ions, a factor critically important in CO_2 transport.

Oxygen molecules bind to hemoglobin by way of the ferrous iron ion, one for each protein chain. With complete oxygen binding, all electrons become paired, and the Hb is converted to its oxygenated state (referred to as *oxyhemoglobin* and abbreviated HbO_2).

In whole blood, each gram of Hb can carry approximately 1.34 mL of oxygen. Given an average blood Hb content of 15 g/dL, the oxygen-carrying capacity of the blood can be computed from its chemical combination with Hb:

$$1.34 \text{ mL/g} \times 15 \text{ g/dL} = 20.1 \text{ mL/dL}$$

Compared with the blood's limited ability to carry dissolved oxygen (0.3 mL/dL), the addition of hemoglobin increases the oxygen-carrying capacity nearly seventyfold! The amount of the oxygen-carrying capacity of hemoglobin actually used depends on its saturation with oxygen.

Hemoglobin Saturation

Saturation is a measure of the proportion of available hemoglobin that is actually carrying oxygen. Saturation is computed as the ratio of HbO_2 (content) to total hemoglobin (capacity). Hb saturation (Sao_2) is always expressed as a percentage of this ratio and calculated according to the following formula:

$$Sao_2 = \frac{[HbO_2]}{\text{Total Hb}} \times 100$$

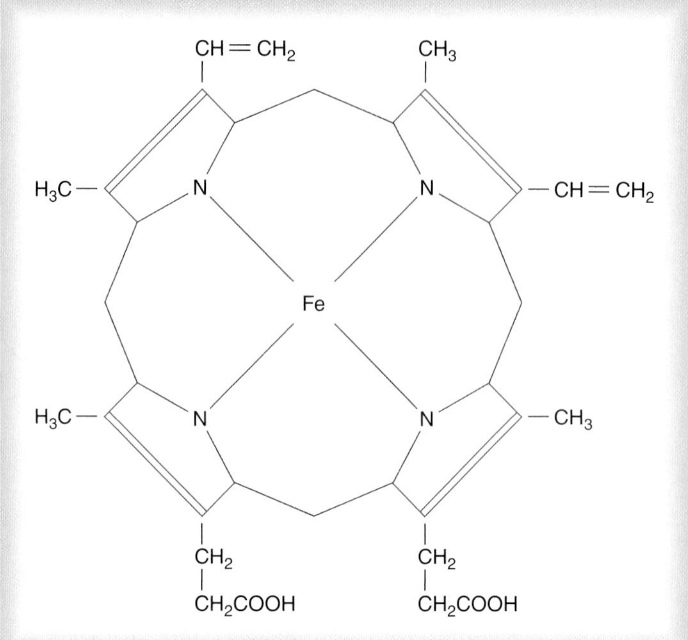

Figure 10-7
Structure of heme.

where $[HbO_2]$ equals the oxyhemoglobin content. For example, if there were a total of 15 g/dL Hb in the blood, of which 7.5 g was HbO_2, the Sao_2 would be calculated as follows:

$$Sao_2\ (\%) = \frac{7.5}{15} \times 100 = 50\%$$

In this example, the hemoglobin is said to be 50% saturated. This means that only half the available hemoglobin is actually carrying oxygen, and the remainder is unoxygenated. In actual clinical practice, both Sao_2 and total Hb content are measured directly to derive the $[HbO_2]$.

HbO_2 Dissociation Curve

Hemoglobin saturation with oxygen varies with changes in Po_2. Plotting the saturation (y-axis) against the Po_2 (x-axis) yields the HbO_2 dissociation curve (Figure 10-8).

Unlike dissolved O_2, hemoglobin saturation is not linearly related to Po_2. Instead, the relationship forms an S-shaped curve. The relatively flat upper part of this curve represents the normal operating range for arterial blood. Because the slope is minimal in this area, minor changes in Pao_2 have little effect on Sao_2, indicating a strong affinity of hemoglobin for oxygen. For instance, with a normal arterial Po_2 of 100 mm Hg, the Sao_2 is approximately 97%. If some abnormality reduced the Pao_2 to 65 mm Hg, the Sao_2 would still be approximately 90%.

However, with a Po_2 lower than 60 mm Hg, the curve steepens dramatically. Here, in the normal operating range of the tissues, even a small drop in Po_2 causes a large drop in Sao_2, indicating a lessening affinity for oxygen. This normal decrease in the affinity of hemoglobin for oxygen helps release large amounts of oxygen to the tissue, where the Po_2 is low. This also explains why it is necessary to keep the Pao_2 higher than 60 mm Hg in clinical practice.

Total Oxygen Content of the Blood

The total oxygen content of the blood equals the sum of that dissolved and chemically combined with hemoglobin. For total oxygen content to be calculated, the following three values must be known: (1) Po_2, (2) total hemoglobin content (g/dL), and (3) hemoglobin saturation. Given these values, the following equation can be applied:

$$Cao_2 = (0.003 \times Po_2) + (Hb_{tot} \times 1.34 \times So_2)$$

where Cao_2 equals the total oxygen content, Po_2 equals the partial pressure of oxygen in the blood, Hb_{tot} equals the total hemoblobin content in g/dL, and So_2 equals the hemoglobin saturation with oxygen (as a decimal). Typically, clinicians want to know the oxygen content of arterial blood (Cao_2). The $(0.003 \times Po_2)$ component of the equation represents the dissolved oxygen, whereas the $(Hb_{tot} \times 1.34 \times So_2)$ component represents the chemically combined oxyhemoglobin.

For example, assume that the RT obtains a sample of normal arterial blood with a Po_2 of 100 mm Hg

MINI CLINI

Relating Hemoglobin Saturation and $Pa{O_2}$

PROBLEM

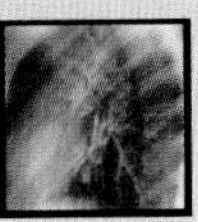

Pulse oximeters are simple bedside devices that measure Hb saturation by way of a noninvasive probe taped to the patient's finger or forehead. Although oximeters measure Hb saturation percentage, blood oxygenation still tends to be quantified according to arterial $P{O_2}$. Is there a simple way to relate these two measures without carrying around an oxyhemoglobin dissociation curve?

DISCUSSION

First, although extremely useful, pulse oximeters are not very accurate (4%), and they measure only normal hemoglobin saturation. For this reason, their use should be limited to following trends or warning of significant changes in hemoglobin saturation with oxygen.

Even so, RTs will often need to estimate arterial $P{O_2}$ from oximeter readings. The following simple rule should be helpful. It is called the *40-50-60/70-80-90* rule. Assuming normal pH, $P{CO_2}$, and Hb values, saturations of 70%, 80%, and 90% are roughly equivalent to $P{O_2}$ values of 40, 50, and 60 mm Hg, respectively:

Hemoglobin saturation	Approximate $Pa{O_2}$
70%	40 mm Hg
80%	50 mm Hg
90%	60 mm Hg

Thus a patient with a pulse oximeter reading of 90% has a $Pa{O_2}$ of approximately 60 mm Hg. Should the saturation drop to 80%, the $Pa{O_2}$ will fall to approximately 50 mm Hg. Note that this rule works only in the middle range of $P{O_2}$ values, where the curve is most linear; it should not be applied with saturations higher than 90%. For example, a saturation of 100% may represent a $Pa{O_2}$ of 200 mm Hg.

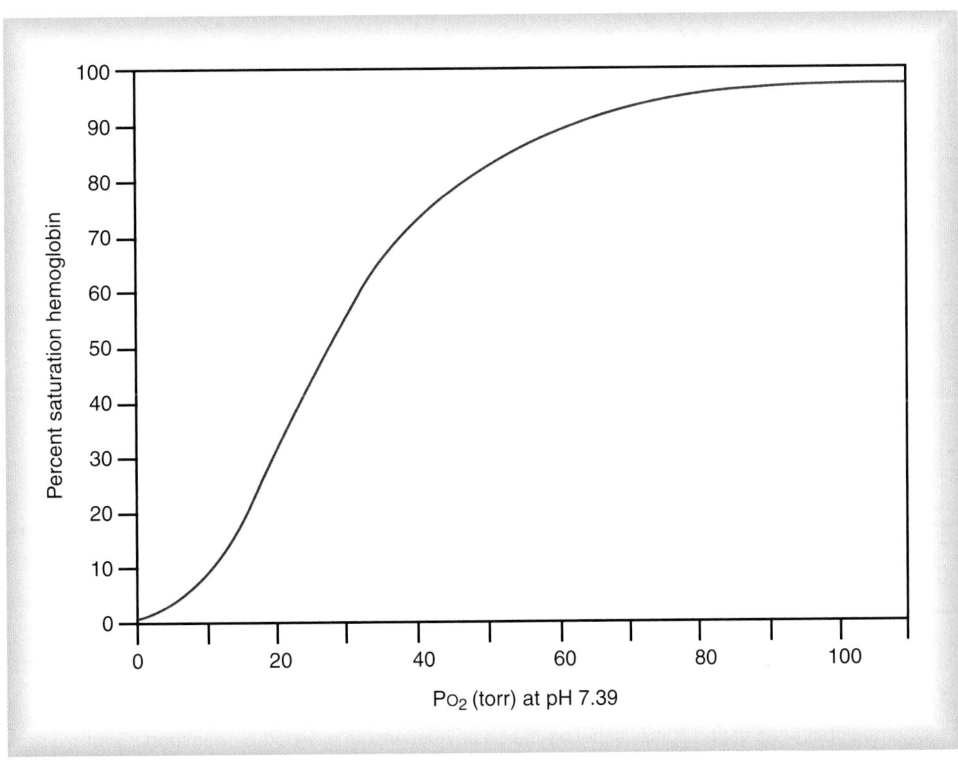

Figure 10-8

The oxygen dissociation curve plots the relationship between plasma $P{O_2}$ (x-axis) and hemoglobin saturation (y-axis).

containing 15 g/dL of hemoglobin that is 97% saturated with oxygen. To compute the total oxygen content, the RT should apply the aforementioned equation as follows:

$$Cao_2 = (0.003 \times Pao_2) + (Hb_{tot} \times 1.34 \times Sao_2)$$

$$Cao_2 = (0.003 \text{ mL} \times 100 \text{ mm Hg}) + (15 \text{ g/dL} \times 1.34 \times 0.97)$$

$$Cao_2 = (0.3 \text{ mL}) + (19.5 \text{ g/dL})$$

$$Cao_2 = 19.8 \text{ mL/dL}$$

Normal Loading and Unloading of Oxygen (Arteriovenous Differences)

Figure 10-9 uses the oxyhemoglobin dissociation curve to demonstrate the effects of oxygen loading and unloading in the lungs and tissues. Point Ⓐ represents freshly arterialized blood leaving the lungs, with a Po_2 of approximately 100 mm Hg and a hemoglobin saturation of approximately 97%.

As blood perfuses body tissues, oxygen uptake causes a fall in both Po_2 and saturation, such that venous blood leaving the tissues (point Ⓥ) has a Po_2 of approximately 40 mm Hg, with a hemoglobin saturation of approximately 73%.

Using a normal Hb content of 15 g/dL, and knowing the saturation at each possible Po_2, the RT can calculate total oxygen content at any Po_2 in the manner previously described. The y-axis of Figure 10-9 provides this information, in Sao_2 increments of 10%. Table 10-2 summarizes the difference between the oxygen content of these normal arterial and venous points.

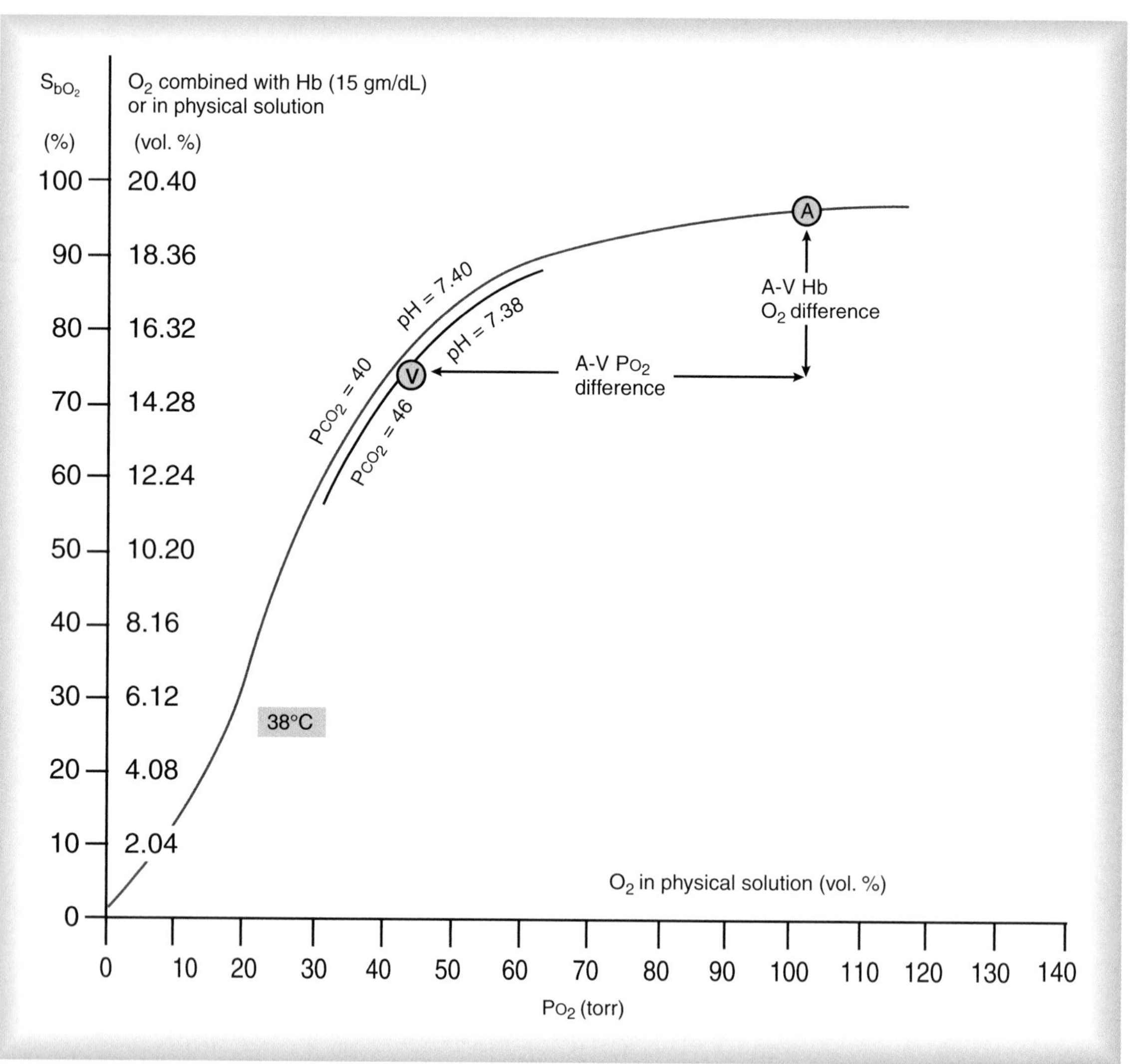

Figure 10-9

The normal oxyhemoglobin dissociation curve, showing the basic relationship of blood O_2 transport. Point Ⓐ represents normal values for arterial blood leaving the lungs (the loading point). Point Ⓥ represents normal values for venous blood leaving the tissues (the unloading point). The slight difference in curve position resulting from pH and CO_2 changes helps oxygen unloading at the tissues. Differences between the oxygen content at these two points represent the amount of oxygen taken up by the tissues on one pass through the systemic circulation. *(Modified from Slonim NB, Hamilton LH: Respiratory physiology, ed 5, St Louis, 1987, Mosby.)*

Table 10-2 ▶ ▶ Oxygen Content of Arterial and Venous Blood

Oxygen Content	Arterial O_2 (mL/dL)	Venous O_2 (mL/dL)
Combined O_2 ($1.34 \times 15 \times SO_2$)	19.5	14.7
Dissolved O_2 ($PO_2 \times 0.003$)	0.3	0.1
Total O_2 content	19.8	14.8

As indicated in Table 10-2, the difference between the arterial and venous oxygen contents is normally approximately 5 mL/dL. This is the *arteriovenous oxygen contents difference,* abbreviated as $C(a-\bar{v})O_2$. $C(a-\bar{v})O_2$ is the amount of oxygen given up by every 100 mL of blood on each pass through the tissues.

Fick Formula

The $C(a-\bar{v})O_2$ indicates oxygen extraction in proportion to blood flow. If this measure is combined with total-body oxygen consumption, cardiac output can be calculated. The basis for this calculation is the classic **Fick formula:**

$$\dot{Q}_t = \frac{\dot{V}O_2}{C(a-\bar{v})O_2 \times 10}$$

In this equation, $\dot{Q}_t$ is cardiac output (L/min), $\dot{V}O_2$ is the whole-body oxygen consumption (mL/min), and $C(a-\bar{v})O_2$ is the arteriovenous oxygen contents difference (mL/dL). The factor of 10 converts mL/dL to mL/L. Given a normal $\dot{V}O_2$ of 250 mL/min and a normal $C(a-\bar{v})O_2$ of 5 mL/dL, a normal cardiac output is calculated as follows:

$$\dot{Q}_t = \frac{250 \text{ mL/min}}{5 \text{ mL/dL} \times 10}$$

$$\dot{Q}_t = \frac{250 \text{ mL/min}}{5 \text{ mL/L}}$$

$$\dot{Q}_t = 5.0 \text{ L/min}$$

Significance of the $C(a-\bar{v})O_2$

According to the Fick formula, if the oxygen consumption remains constant, a decrease in cardiac output will increase the $C(a-\bar{v})O_2$. Conversely, if the cardiac output rises and oxygen consumption remains constant, the $C(a-\bar{v})O_2$ will fall proportionately. Although the Fick formula for calculating cardiac output has been replaced by other techniques, the principle relating $C(a-\bar{v})O_2$ to perfusion is used to monitor tissue oxygenation at the bedside. More details on these methods are provided in Chapter 43.

Factors Affecting Oxygen Loading and Unloading

In addition to the shape of the HbO_2 curve, many other factors affect oxygen loading and unloading. The following are among those most important in clinical practice: blood pH, body temperature, and erythrocyte concentration of certain organic phosphates. Variations in the structure of Hb also affect oxygen loading and unloading. Chemical combinations of Hb with substances other than oxygen, such as carbon monoxide, also can affect oxygen loading and unloading.

pH (Bohr Effect)

The impact of changes in blood pH on hemoglobin affinity for oxygen is called the **Bohr effect.** As shown in Figure 10-10, the Bohr effect alters the position of the HbO_2 dissociation curve. A low pH (acidity) shifts the curve to the right, whereas a high pH (alkalinity) shifts it to the left. These changes are a result of variations in the shape of the Hb molecule caused by fluctuations in pH.

As blood pH drops and the curve shifts to the right, the Hb saturation for a given PO_2 falls (decreased Hb affinity for oxygen). Conversely, as blood pH rises and the curve shifts to the left, the Hb saturation for a given PO_2 rises (increased affinity of Hb for oxygen).

These changes enhance oxygen loading in the lungs and oxygen unloading in the tissues. As blood in the tissues picks up CO_2, its pH falls from 7.40 to approximately 7.37. Thus the HbO_2 curve shifts to the right, lowering the affinity of Hb for oxygen. With lower affinity for oxygen, Hb more readily gives up its oxygen, thus aiding its unloading at the tissues. Conversely, when venous blood returns to the lungs, the pH goes back up to 7.40. This change in pH shifts the HbO_2 curve back to the left, thereby increasing the affinity of Hb for oxygen and enhancing its uptake from the alveoli.

Body Temperature

Variations in body temperature also affect the HbO_2 dissociation curve. As shown in Figure 10-11, a drop in body temperature shifts the curve to the left, increasing Hb affinity for oxygen. Conversely, as body temperature rises, the curve shifts to the right, and the affinity of Hb for oxygen decreases. As with the Bohr effect, these changes enhance normal oxygen uptake and delivery. At the tissues, temperature changes are directly related to metabolic rate, such that areas of high metabolic activity have higher temperatures. In areas such as exercising muscle, higher temperatures decrease Hb affinity for oxygen, thereby enhancing its release to the tissues. Conversely, in hypothermia, the oxygen demands of the tissues are greatly reduced, and Hb need not give up as much of its oxygen.

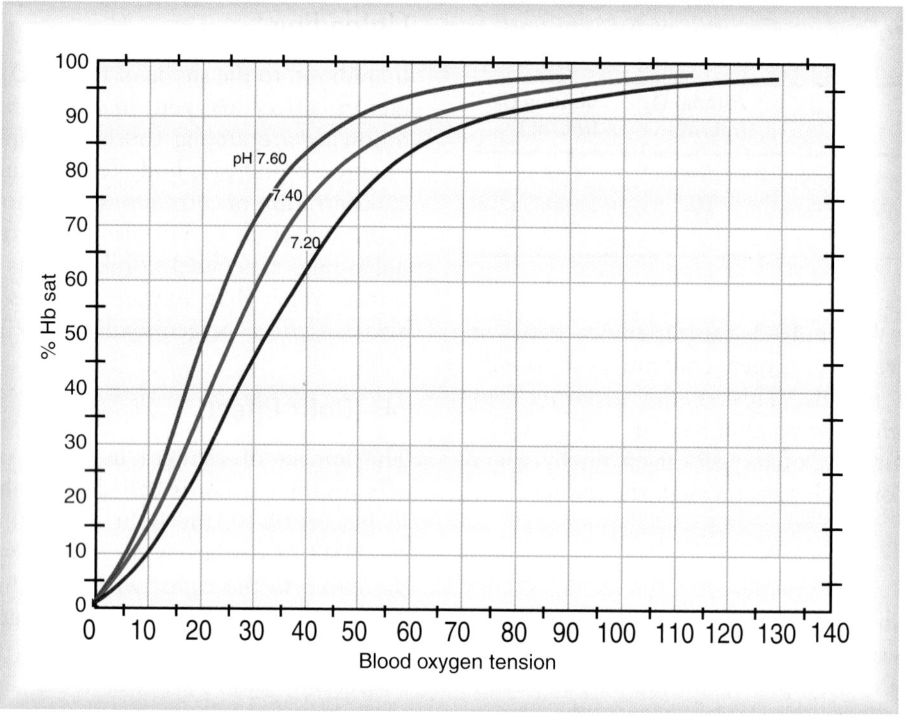

Figure 10-10

Oxygen dissociation curve of blood at 37° C, showing variations at three pH levels. A right shift (lower pH) decreases hemoglobin (Hb) affinity for oxygen, whereas a left shift (higher pH) increases Hb affinity for oxygen.

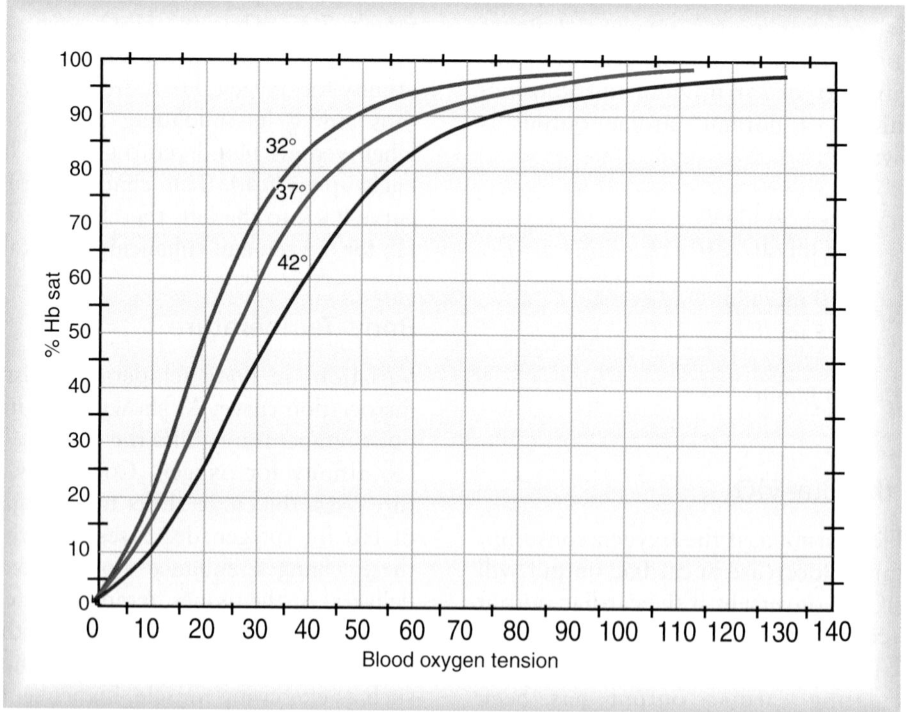

Figure 10-11

Oxygen dissociation curve of blood at a pH of 7.40, showing variations at three temperatures. For a given oxygen tension, the lower the temperature, the more the hemoglobin (Hb) holds onto its oxygen, maintaining a higher saturation.

Organic Phosphates (2,3-DPG)

The organic phosphate 2,3-diphosphoglycerate (2,3-DPG) is found in abundance in the RBCs, where it forms a loose chemical bond with the globin chains of deoxygenated Hb. In this configuration, 2,3-DPG stabilizes the molecule in its deoxygenated state, thereby reducing its affinity for oxygen. Indeed, without 2,3-DPG, Hb affinity for oxygen would be so great that normal oxygen unloading would be impossible.

Increased 2,3-DPG concentrations shift the HbO_2 curve to the right, promoting oxygen unloading. Conversely, low 2,3-DPG concentrations shift the curve to the left, increasing Hb affinity for oxygen.

Alkalosis, chronic **hypoxemia,** and **anemia** all tend to increase 2,3-DPG concentrations and promote oxygen unloading. Conversely, acidosis results in a lower intracellular level of 2,3-DPG and a greater affinity of Hb for oxygen.

Erythrocyte concentrations of 2,3-DPG in banked blood decrease over time. After a week of storage, the 2,3-DPG level may be less than one third of the normal value. This change shifts the HbO_2 curve to the left, thereby decreasing the availability of oxygen to the tissues. Large transfusions of banked blood that is more than a few days old can severely impair oxygen delivery, even in the presence of a normal Po_2.

Abnormal Hemoglobins

Abnormalities in the hemoglobin molecule also can affect oxygen loading and unloading. Structural abnormalities occur when the amino acid sequence in the molecule's polypeptide chains varies from normal. Changes in the amino acid sequences alter the shape of the molecule, thereby increasing or decreasing its oxygen affinity. More than 120 abnormal hemoglobins have been identified. Even in healthy individuals, between 15% and 40% of the circulating Hb may be abnormal.

Hb S (**sickle cell** hemoglobin) is a special form of abnormal Hb. Although Hb S has less affinity for oxygen than does normal hemoglobin, changes in Hb S solubility are what do the most harm. Deoxygenated Hb S is less soluble than either oxygenated Hb S or normal hemoglobin. In its deoxygenated form, Hb S can actually crystallize inside the erythrocyte, causing the characteristic deformation in cell shape. This increases erythrocyte fragility (leading to hemolysis) and increases the risk of thrombus formation.

Methemoglobin (metHb) is an abnormal form of the molecule, in which the heme-complex normal ferrous iron ion (Fe^{2+}) loses an electron and is oxidized to its ferric state (Fe^{3+}). In the ferric state, the iron ion cannot combine with oxygen. The result is a special form of anemia called **methemoglobinemia.** The most common cause of methemoglobinemia is nitrite poisoning. The presence of metHb turns the blood brown, which can produce a slate-gray skin coloration that is often confused with cyanosis. The presence of metHb is confirmed by spectrophotometry (see Chapter 16). Methemoglobinemia is treated with reducing agents such as methylene blue or ascorbic acid.

Carboxyhemoglobin (HbCO) is the chemical combination of hemoglobin with carbon monoxide (CO). Hemoglobin's affinity for CO is more than 200 times greater than it is for oxygen. Thus even extremely low concentrations of carbon monoxide quickly displace oxygen from hemoglobin, forming HbCO. A carbon monoxide partial pressure as low as 0.12 mm Hg can displace as much as half the oxygen from hemoglobin. Because HbCO cannot carry oxygen, each gram of Hb saturated with carbon monoxide represents a loss in carrying capacity. Moreover, the combination of carbon monoxide with hemoglobin shifts the HbO_2 curve to the left, further impeding oxygen delivery to the tissues. Treatment for carbon monoxide poisoning involves giving the patient as much oxygen as possible, because oxygen reduces the half-life of HbCO (Table 10-3). Sometimes a hyperbaric chamber is required to rapidly reverse the binding of CO with the hemoglobin.

During fetal life and for up to 1 year after birth, the blood has a high proportion of a hemoglobin variant called **fetal hemoglobin (Hb F).** Hb F has a greater affinity for oxygen than does normal adult Hb, as manifested by a leftward shift of the HbO_2 curve. Given the low Po_2 values available to the fetus in utero, this leftward shift aids oxygen loading at the placenta. Because of the relatively low pH of the fetal environment, oxygen unloading at the cellular level is not greatly affected. However, after birth, this enhanced oxygen affinity is less advantageous. Over the first year of life, Hb F is gradually replaced with normal Hb.

Measurement of Hemoglobin Affinity for Oxygen

Variations in the affinity of Hb for oxygen are quantified by a measure called the $\mathbf{P_{50}}$. The $\mathbf{P_{50}}$ is the partial pressure of oxygen at which the Hb is 50% saturated, standardized to a pH level of 7.40. A normal P_{50} is approximately 26.6 mm Hg. Conditions that cause a decrease in Hb affinity for oxygen (a shift of the HbO_2

Table 10-3 ▶▶ Half-life of Carboxyhemoglobin (HbCO) at Different Oxygen Exposures

HbCO Half-life (min)	Inhaled Fio_2	Pao_2 (mm Hg)
280-320	0.21 at 1 atm	100
80-90	1.0 at 1 atm	673
20-30	1.0 at 3 atm	2193

curve to the right) increase the P_{50} to higher than normal. Conditions associated with an increase in affinity (a shift of the HbO_2 curve to the left) decrease the P_{50} to lower than normal. For example, with 15 g/dL Hb, a 4–mm Hg increase in P_{50} results in approximately 1 to 2 mL/dL more oxygen being unloaded in the tissues than when the P_{50} is normal. Figure 10-12 shows the effect of changes in P_{50} and summarizes how the major factors previously discussed affect Hb affinity for oxygen.

▶ CARBON DIOXIDE TRANSPORT

Figure 10-13 shows the physical and chemical events of gas exchange at the systemic capillaries. In the pulmonary capillaries, all events occur in the opposite direction. Although the primary focus is on carbon dioxide transport, Figure 10-13 also includes the basic elements of oxygen exchange. Oxygen exchange is included here for completeness, as well as to show that the exchange and transport of these two gases are closely related.

Transport Mechanisms

Approximately 45 to 55 mL/dL of carbon dioxide is normally carried in the blood in the following three forms: (1) dissolved in physical solution, (2) chemically combined with protein, and (3) ionized as bicarbonate.

Dissolved in Physical Solution

As with oxygen, carbon dioxide produced by the tissues dissolves in the plasma and erythrocyte intracellular fluid. However, unlike oxygen, dissolved carbon dioxide plays an important role in transport, accounting for approximately 8% of the total released at the lungs. This is because of carbon dioxide's high solubility in plasma.

Chemically Combined With Protein

Molecular carbon dioxide has the capacity to chemically combine with free amino groups (NH_2) of protein molecules (Prot), forming a **carbamino compound:**

$$\text{Prot-NH}_2 + \text{CO}_2 \Leftrightarrow \text{Prot-NHCOO}^- + \text{H}^+$$

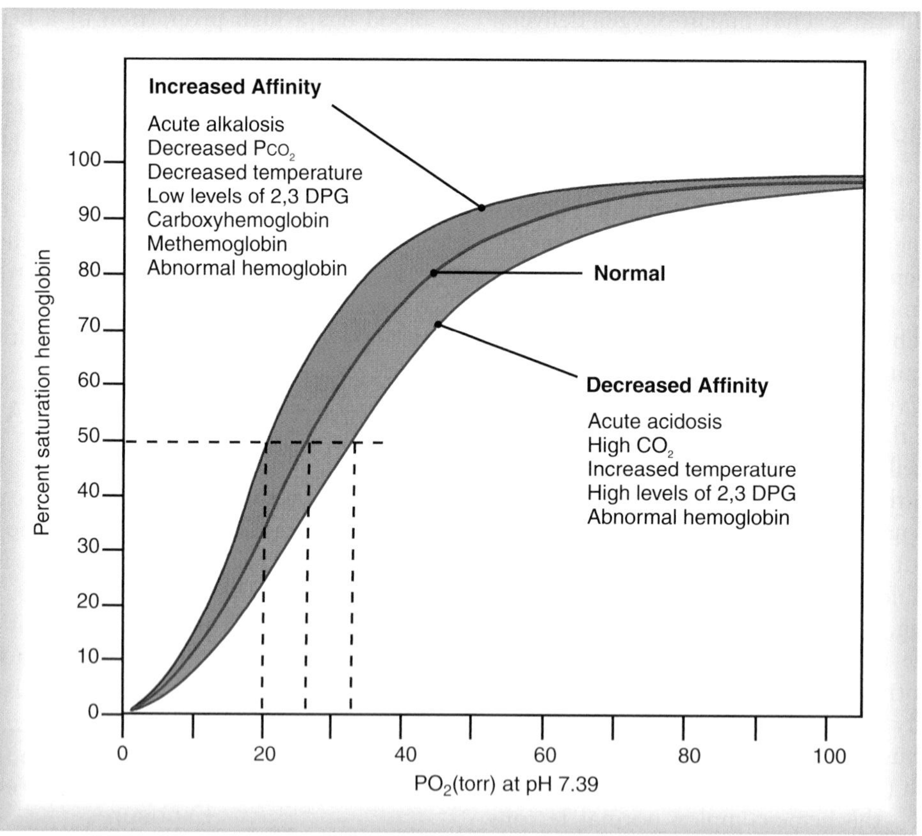

Figure 10-12

Conditions associated with altered affinity of hemoglobin for O_2. P_{50} is the Pa_{O_2} at which hemoglobin is 50% saturated (normally 26.6 mm Hg). A lower than normal P_{50} represents increased affinity of hemoglobin for O_2. A high P_{50} is seen with decreased affinity. *(Modified from Lane EE, Walker JF: Clinical arterial blood gas analysis, St Louis, 1987, Mosby.)*

A small amount of the carbon dioxide leaving the tissues combines with plasma proteins to form these carbamino compounds. A larger fraction of the CO_2 combines with erythrocyte Hb to form a carbamino compound called *carbaminohemoglobin*. As indicated in the previous equation, this reaction produces H^+ ions. These H^+ ions are buffered by the reduced Hb, which is made available by the concurrent release of oxygen.

The availability of additional sites for H^+ buffering increases the affinity of Hb for CO_2. Moreover, because reduced Hb is a weaker acid than HbO_2, pH changes associated with the release of the H^+ ions in the formation of carbaminohemoglobin are minimized. Carbaminohemoglobin constitutes approximately 12% of the total carbon dioxide transported.

Ionized as Bicarbonate

Approximately 80% of the blood carbon dioxide is transported as bicarbonate. Of the carbon dioxide that dissolves in plasma, a small portion combines chemically with water in a process called *hydrolysis*. Hydrolysis of carbon dioxide initially forms carbonic acid, which quickly ionizes into hydrogen and bicarbonate ions:

$$CO_2 + H_2O \Leftrightarrow H_2CO_3 \Leftrightarrow HCO_3^- + H^+$$

The H^+ ions produced in this reaction are buffered by the plasma proteins, in much the same way as hemoglobin buffers H^+ in the RBC. However, the rate of this plasma hydrolysis reaction is extremely slow, producing minimal amounts of H^+ and HCO_3^-.

Most carbon dioxide undergoes hydrolysis inside the erythrocyte. This reaction is greatly enhanced by an enzyme catalyst called *carbonic anhydrase (CA)*. The resulting H^+ ions are buffered by the imidazole group (R-NHCOO$^-$) of the reduced Hb molecule. Again, the concurrent conversion of HbO_2 to its deoxygenated form helps buffer H^+ ions, thereby enhancing the loading of carbon dioxide as carbaminohemoglobin.

As the hydrolysis of carbon dioxide continues, HCO_3^- ions begin to accumulate in the erythrocyte. To maintain a concentration equilibrium across the cell membrane, some of these anions diffuse outward into the plasma. Because the erythrocyte is not freely permeable by cations, electrolytic equilibrium must be maintained by way of an inward migration of anions. This is achieved by the shifting of chloride ions (Cl^-) from the plasma into the erythrocyte, a process called the *chloride shift*, or the *Hamburger phenomenon*.

Carbon Dioxide Dissociation Curve

As with oxygen, carbon dioxide has a dissociation curve. The relationship between blood P_{CO_2} and carbon dioxide content is depicted in Figure 10-14.

The first point to note is the effect of Hb saturation with oxygen on this curve. As previously discussed,

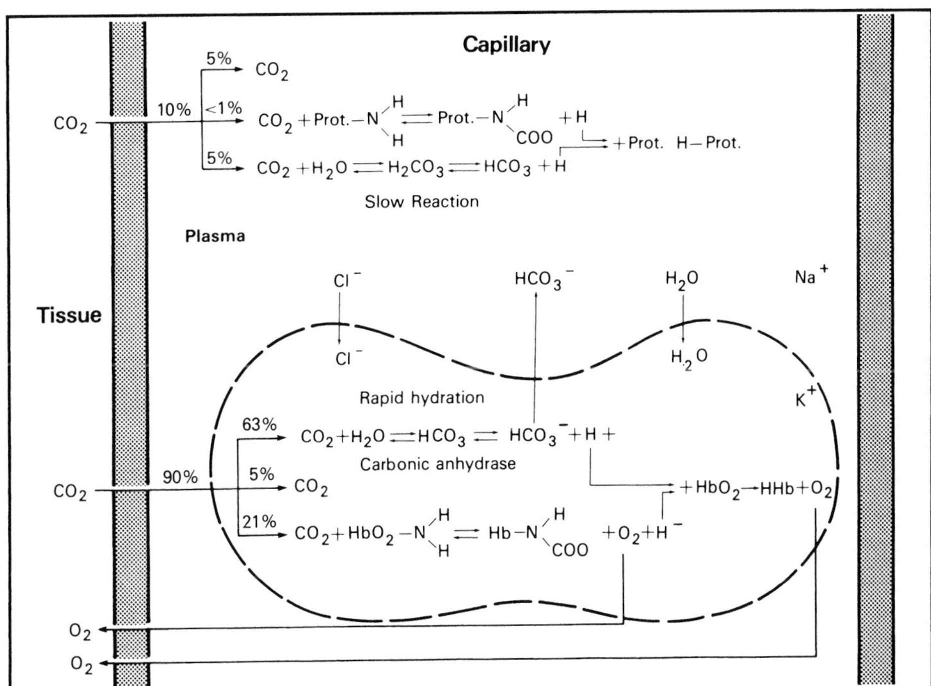

Figure 10-13

Summary diagram of the various fates of CO_2 as it diffuses from the cells and interstitial spaces into the peripheral capillaries before its transport toward the venous circulation. *(Modified from Martin DE, Youtsey JW: Respiratory anatomy and physiology, St Louis, 1988, Mosby.)*

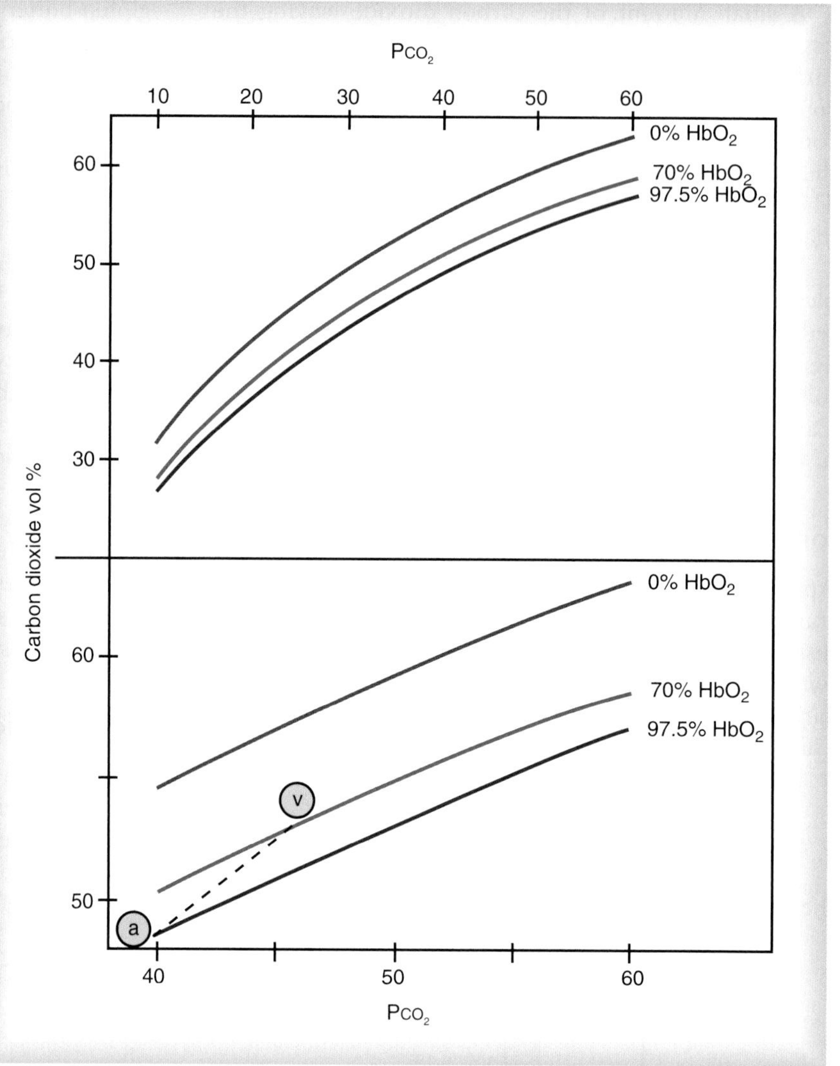

Figure 10-14

Carbon dioxide dissociation curves. **A,** The relationship between carbon dioxide content and tension at three levels of hemoglobin saturation. **B,** Close-up of the curves between P_{CO_2} of 40 and 60 mm Hg.

CO_2 levels, through their influence on pH, modify the oxygen dissociation curve (Bohr effect). Figure 10-14 shows that oxyhemoglobin saturation also affects the position of the CO_2 dissociation curve. The influence of oxyhemoglobin saturation on CO_2 dissociation is called the *Haldane effect*. As previously explained, this phenomenon is a result of changes in the affinity of hemoglobin for CO_2, which occur as a result of its buffering of H^+ ions.

Figure 10-14, *A*, shows the carbon dioxide dissociation curves for three levels of blood oxygen saturation. The first two are physiological values, and the third extreme value is provided for contrast. Figure 10-14, *B*, amplifies selected segments of these curves in the physiological range of P_{CO_2}. Note first the arterial point ⓐlying on the curve representing an Sa_{O_2} of 97.5%. At this point, the P_{CO_2} is 40 mm Hg and the carbon dioxide content is approximately 48 mL/dL. The venous point ⓥ falls on the curve representing an Sa_{O_2} of approximately 70%. At this point, the P_{CO_2} is 46 mm Hg and the carbon dioxide content is approximately 52 mL/dL. Because oxygen saturation changes from arterial to venous blood, the true physiological CO_2 dissociation curve must lie somewhere between these two points. This physiological curve is represented as the *dashed line* in Figure 10-14, *B*.

At point ⓐ, the high Sa_{O_2} decreases the blood's capacity to hold carbon dioxide, thus helping unload this gas at the lungs. At point ⓥ, the lower Sv_{O_2} (venous oxygen saturation) increases the blood's capacity for CO_2, thus aiding uptake at the tissues.

The total carbon dioxide content of arterial and venous blood is compared in Table 10-4. Note that the amounts of CO_2 are expressed in gaseous volume equivalents (mL/dL) and as millimoles per liter (mmol/L). This latter measure of the chemical combining power of CO_2 in solutions is critical in understanding the role of this gas in acid-base balance.

ABNORMALITIES OF GAS EXCHANGE AND TRANSPORT

Gas exchange is abnormal when either tissue oxygen delivery or carbon dioxide removal is impaired.

Impaired Oxygen Delivery

Oxygen delivery ($\dot{D}O_2$) to the tissues is a function of arterial oxygen content (CaO_2) times cardiac output. ($\dot{Q}_t$):

$$\dot{D}O_2 = CaO_2 \times \dot{Q}_t$$

When oxygen delivery falls short of cellular needs, **hypoxia** occurs. According to the preceding equation, hypoxia occurs if (1) the arterial blood oxygen content is decreased (hypoxemia), (2) cardiac output or perfusion is decreased (shock or **ischemia**), or (3) abnormal cellular function prevents proper uptake of oxygen (**dysoxia**). Table 10-5 summarizes causes, common clinical indicators, mechanisms, and examples of hypoxia.

Table 10-4 ▶▶ Carbon Dioxide Content of Arterial and Venous Blood

Unit of Measure	Arterial	Venous
mmol/L	21.53	23.21
mL/dL	48.01	51.76

Hypoxemia

Hypoxemia occurs when the PaO_2 is decreased to lower than the predicted normal based on the age of the patient. Impaired oxygen delivery also occurs in the presence of abnormalities that prevent saturation of the hemoglobin with oxygen (see subsequent discussion).

Decreased PaO_2. A decreased PaO_2 may be caused by a low ambient PO_2, hypoventilation, impaired diffusion, ($\dot{V}/\dot{Q}$) imbalances, and right-to-left anatomical or physiological shunting. The PO_2 also decreases normally with aging. In fact, the normal predicted PaO_2 falls steadily with age, and the average is approximately 85 mm Hg at the age of 60 years (see later discussion).

Breathing gases with a low O_2 concentration at sea level or breathing air at pressures less than atmospheric

Table 10-5 ▶▶ Causes of Hypoxia

Cause	Primary Indicator	Mechanism	Example
Hypoxemia			
Low PIO_2	Low PAO_2 Low PaO_2	Reduced Pb	Altitude
Hypoventilation	High $PaCO_2$	Decreased $\dot{V}_A$	Drug overdose
$\dot{V}/\dot{Q}$ imbalance	Low PaO_2 High $P(A\text{–}a)O_2$ on air; resolves with O_2	Decreased $\dot{V}_A$ relative to perfusion	COPD, aging
Anatomical shunt	Low PaO_2 High $P(A\text{–}a)O_2$ on air; does not resolve with O_2	Blood flow from right to left side of heart	Congenital heart disease
Physiological shunt	Low PaO_2 High $P(A\text{–}a)O_2$ on air; does not resolve with O_2	Perfusion without ventilation	Atelectasis
Diffusion defect	Low PaO_2 High $P(A\text{–}a)O_2$ on air; resolves with O_2	Damage to alveolar-capillary membrane	Interstitial lung disease
Hemoglobin Deficiency			
Absolute	Low Hb content Reduced CaO_2	Loss of Hb	Hemorrhage
Relative	Abnormal SaO_2 Reduced CaO_2	Abnormal Hb	Carboxyhemoglobin
Low Blood Flow	Increased $C(a\text{–}\bar{v})O_2$	Decreased perfusion	Shock, ischemia
Dysoxia	Normal CaO_2 Decreased $C(a\text{–}\bar{v})O_2$	Disruption of cellular enzymes	Cyanide poisoning

COPD, Chronic obstructive pulmonary disease.

lowers the alveolar O_2 tension, thereby decreasing the PaO_2. A common example of this problem occurs during travel to high altitudes, where the visitor often suffers the ill effects of hypoxia for several days. This condition is called *mountain sickness*. In such cases, although the PaO_2 is reduced, the pressure gradient between the alveolar and the arterial blood for oxygen [abbreviated as $P(A - a)O_2$] remains normal.

Assuming a constant FIO_2, the alveolar PO_2 varies inversely with the alveolar PCO_2. Thus a rise in the alveolar PCO_2 (hypoventilation) is always accompanied by a proportionate fall in alveolar PO_2. The $P(A - a)O_2$ is normal in such cases. Conversely, hyperventilation will lower the $PACO_2$ and help compensate for hypoxemia.

Even when the alveolar PO_2 is normal, disorders of the alveolar-capillary membrane may limit diffusion of O_2 into the pulmonary capillary blood, thereby lowering the PaO_2. Examples of this are pulmonary fibrosis and interstitial edema. However, as previously noted, a pure diffusion limitation is a relatively uncommon cause of hypoxemia at rest.

Ventilation-perfusion ($\dot{V}/\dot{Q}$) imbalances are the most common cause of hypoxemia in patients with lung disease. A $\dot{V}/\dot{Q}$ imbalance is an abnormal deviation in the distribution of ventilation to perfusion in the lung. The normal lung has some $\dot{V}/\dot{Q}$ mismatch; however, in disease states, the range of $\dot{V}/\dot{Q}$ imbalances becomes much greater.

Figure 10-15 shows the possible range of $\dot{V}/\dot{Q}$ ratios. As shown in the top two units, when ventilation is greater than perfusion (a high $\dot{V}/\dot{Q}$), there is wasted ventilation, or alveolar dead space. Conversely, when ventilation is less than perfusion, the $\dot{V}/\dot{Q}$ ratio is low (bottom two lung units). In this case, blood leaves the lungs with an abnormally low oxygen content. In lung disease, $\dot{V}/\dot{Q}$ imbalances usually cause both excess wasted ventilation and poor oxygenation. Because a $\dot{V}/\dot{Q}$ imbalance impairs oxygen exchange, the PaO_2 is reduced.

To understand how a $\dot{V}/\dot{Q}$ imbalance causes hypoxemia, reinspect the normal oxyhemoglobin dissociation curve, with PO_2 plotted against oxygen content (Figure 10-16). Note that the curve is nearly flat in the physiological range of PaO_2 (higher than 70 mm Hg) but falls steeply when lower than 60 mm Hg. Points representing the oxygen content of three separate lung units also are shown. These units have $\dot{V}/\dot{Q}$ ratios of 0.1, 1.0, and 10.0.

Blood leaving the normal unit ($\dot{V}/\dot{Q} = 1$) has a normal oxygen content (19.5 mL/dL). Blood leaving the unit with poor ventilation ($\dot{V}/\dot{Q} = 0.1$) has a low oxygen content (16.0 mL/dL). Because hemoglobin is almost fully saturated at a normal PO_2 of 100 mm Hg, blood leaving the overventilated unit ($\dot{V}/\dot{Q} = 10$) has an oxygen content that is just slightly higher than normal (20.0 mL/dL). When the blood from all three units mixes together, the result is an oxygen content that is lower than normal (18.5 mL/dL). Thus *the decrease in oxygenation caused by the poorly ventilated unit is not compensated for by the high $\dot{V}/\dot{Q}$ unit.*

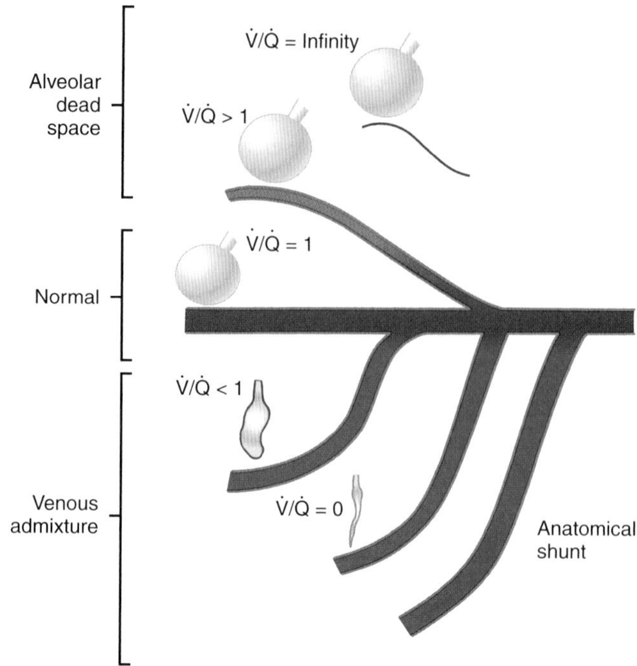

Figure 10-15

The range of $\dot{V}/\dot{Q}$ ratios. *(Modified from Martin L: Pulmonary physiology in clinical practice: the essentials for patient care and evaluation, St Louis, 1987, Mosby.)*

A $\dot{V}/\dot{Q}$ of 0 represents a special type of imbalance. When the $\dot{V}/\dot{Q}$ is 0, there is blood flow but no ventilation. The result is equivalent to a right-to-left anatomical shunt, shown at the bottom of Figure 10-15. Venous blood bypasses ventilated alveoli and mixes with freshly oxygenated arterial blood, resulting in what is called a **venous admixture**. Right-to-left physiological shunting results in a more severe form of hypoxemia than does a simple $\dot{V}/\dot{Q}$ imbalance, as seen in conditions such as pulmonary edema, pneumonia, and atelectasis.

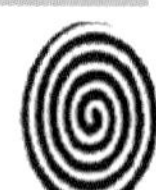

RULE OF THUMB

Although $\dot{V}/\dot{Q}$ imbalances are the most common cause of hypoxemia in patients with respiratory diseases, physiological shunting also can occur commonly, especially in patients who are critically ill. To differentiate between hypoxemia caused by a $\dot{V}/\dot{Q}$ imbalance and hypoxemia caused by shunting, apply the following 50/50 rule: If the oxygen concentration is more than 50 (%) and the PaO_2 is less than 50 (mm Hg), significant shunting is present; otherwise the hypoxemia is mainly caused by a simple

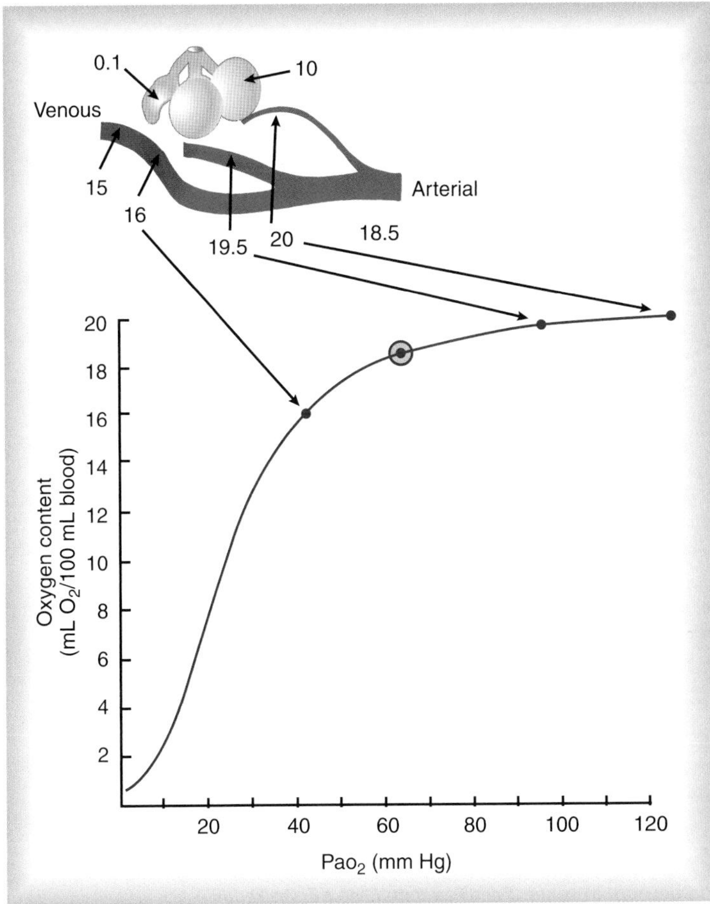

Figure 10-16

Oxygen dissociation curve: Pa_{O_2} versus oxygen content. Oxygen content from alveolar-capillary units with $\dot{V}/\dot{Q}$ ratios of 0.1, 1, and 10 are 16, 19.5, and 20.0 mL/dL, respectively. Lines are drawn for each content to its point on the dissociation curve. The average oxygen content, 18.5 mL/dL, is represented by a *circle* on the dissociation curve. *(Modified from Martin L: Pulmonary physiology in clinical practice: the essentials for patient care and evaluation, St Louis, 1987, Mosby.)*

When a low Pa_{O_2} is observed, the RT must take into account the normal decrease in arterial oxygen tensions that occurs with aging. As shown in Figure 10-17, for an individual breathing air at sea level, the "normal" $P(A - a)O_2$ increases in a near-linear fashion with increasing age *(shaded area)*. This results in a gradual decline in the Pa_{O_2} over time and is probably caused by reduced surface area in the lung for gas exchange and increases in $\dot{V}/\dot{Q}$ mismatching. Thus a Pa_{O_2} of 85 mm Hg in a 60 year old would be interpreted as normal, but the same Pa_{O_2} in a 20 year old would indicate hypoxemia. One may estimate the expected Pa_{O_2} in older adults by using the following formula:

$$\text{Expected } Pa_{O_2} = 100.1 - (0.323 \times \text{Age in years})$$

Hemoglobin Deficiencies. A normal Pa_{O_2} does not guarantee either adequate arterial oxygen content or delivery. For the arterial oxygen content to be adequate, there also must be enough normal hemoglobin in the blood. If the blood hemoglobin is low—even when the Pa_{O_2} is normal—hypoxia can occur because of low oxygen content in the arterial blood.

Hemoglobin deficiencies, or anemias, can be either absolute or relative. An absolute hemoglobin deficiency occurs when the hemoglobin concentration is lower than normal. Relative hemoglobin deficiencies are caused by either the displacement of oxygen from normal hemoglobin or the presence of abnormal hemoglobin variants. A low blood hemoglobin concentration may be caused by either a loss of RBCs, as with hemorrhage, or by inadequate erythropoiesis. Regardless of the cause, a low hemoglobin content can seriously impair the oxygen-carrying capacity of the blood, even in the presence of a normal supply (Pa_{O_2}) and adequate diffusion.

Figure 10-18 plots the relationship between arterial oxygen content and Pa_{O_2} as a function of hemoglobin concentration. As can be seen, progressive falls in blood hemoglobin content cause large drops in arterial oxygen content (Ca_{O_2}). In fact, a 33% decrease in hemoglobin content (from 15 to 10 g/dL) reduces the Ca_{O_2} as much as would a drop in Pa_{O_2} from 100 to 40 mm Hg.

Relative hemoglobin deficiencies are caused by abnormal forms of hemoglobin. As previously discussed, both carboxyhemoglobinemia and methemoglobinemia can cause abnormal oxygen transport, as can abnormal hemoglobin variants. In carboxyhemoglobinemia and methemoglobinemia, each gram of affected hemoglobin is comparable with the loss of a gram of normal hemoglobin. Abnormal hemoglobins have variable

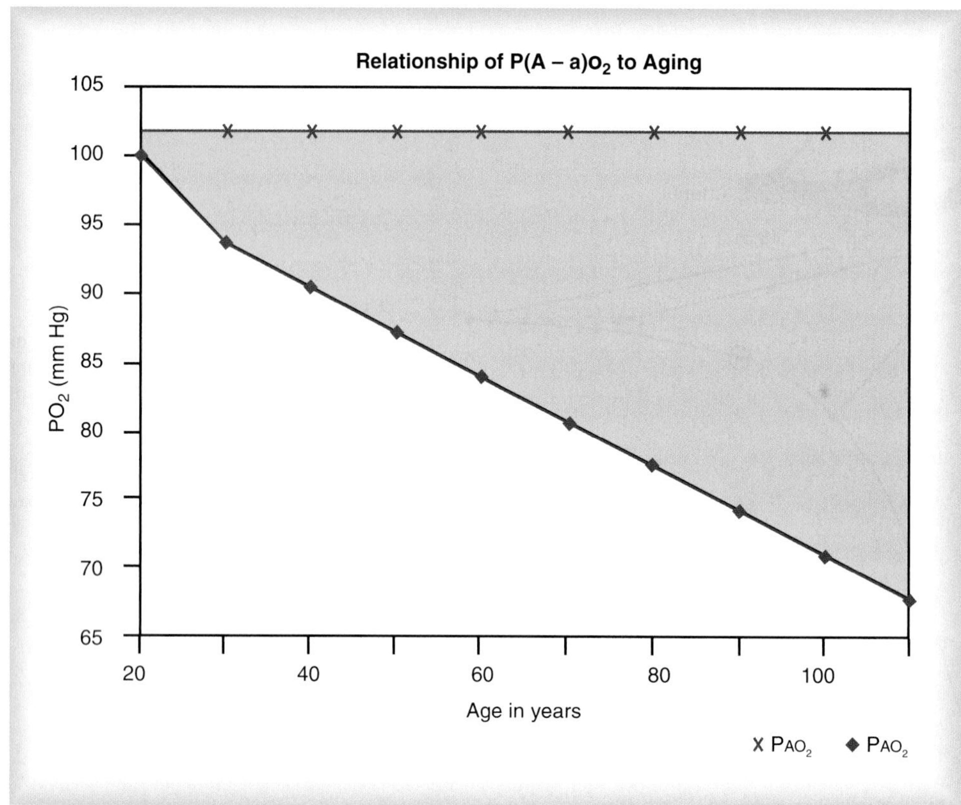

Figure 10-17

The relationship between $P(A - a)O_2$ and aging. As Pao_2 naturally falls with age, $P(a - a)O_2$ increases at the rate of approximately 3 mm Hg each decade beyond 20 years. *(Modified from Lane EE, Walker JF: Clinical arterial blood gas analysis, St Louis, 1987, Mosby.)*

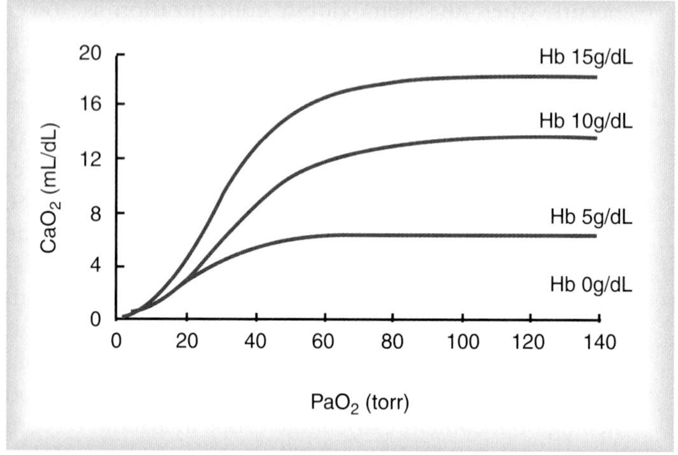

Figure 10-18

The relationship between Cao_2 and Pao_2 as a function of blood hemoglobin (Hb) concentration. Progressive decreases in Hb cause large drops in Cao_2.

effects on oxygen transport. Those causing left shifts in the dissociation curve impede oxygen unloading and thus are most likely to cause hypoxia.

Reduction in Blood Flow (Shock or Ischemia)

Because oxygen delivery depends on both arterial oxygen content and cardiac output, hypoxia can still occur when the Cao_2 is normal if blood flow is reduced. There are two types of reduced blood flow: (1) circulatory failure (shock) and (2) local reductions in perfusion (ischemia).

Circulatory Failure (Shock). In circulatory failure, tissue oxygen deprivation is widespread. Although the body tries to compensate for the lack of oxygen by directing blood flow to vital organs, this response is limited. Thus prolonged shock ultimately causes

MINI CLINI

Effect of Anemia on Oxygen Content

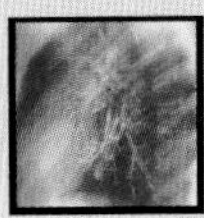

In its most common form, anemia is a clinical disorder in which the number of red blood cells is decreased. Because the red blood cells carry hemoglobin, anemia decreases the amount of this oxygen-carrying protein.

PROBLEM

What effect will anemia that causes a progressive drop in hemoglobin from (1) 15 g/dL to (2) 12 g/dL to (3) 8 g/dL to (4) 4 g/dL have on the amount of oxygen carried in a patient's blood? Assume that the Po_2 and saturation stay normal at 100 mm Hg and 97%, respectively.

DISCUSSION

1. Calculate dissolved oxygen the same way for all four examples as follows:

$$\text{Dissolved } O_2 = 100 \times 0.003 = 0.30 \text{ mL/dL}$$

2. Compute chemically combined oxygen as follows:

$$\text{Chemically combined } O_2 = \text{Hb (g/dL)} \times 1.34 \text{ mL/g} \times Sao_2$$

   a. 15 g/dL × 1.34 mL/g × 97% = 19.50 mL/dL
   b. 12 g/dL × 1.34 mL/g × 97% = 15.60 mL/dL
   c. 8 g/dL × 1.34 mL/g × 97% = 10.40 mL/dL
   d. 4 g/dL × 1.34 mL/g × 97% = 5.20 mL/dL

3. Compute total oxygen content as follows:

$$Cao_2 = \text{Dissolved } O_2 + \text{Chemically combined } O_2$$

   a. 0.30 + 19.50 = 19.80 mL/dL
   b. 0.30 + 15.60 = 15.90 mL/dL
   c. 0.30 + 10.40 = 10.70 mL/dL
   d. 0.30 + 5.20 = 5.50 mL/dL

Loss of hemoglobin decreases the amount of oxygen carried in a patient's blood, even though the Po_2 and saturation remain normal. For example, with a hemoglobin concentration of 4 g/dL, the amount of oxygen carried in a patient's blood is only approximately one fourth the normal concentration (5.50 versus 19.80 mL/dL).

irreversible damage to the central nervous system and eventual cardiovascular collapse.

Local Reductions in Perfusion (Ischemia). Even when whole-body perfusion is adequate, local reductions in blood flow can cause localized hypoxia. Ischemia can result in anaerobic metabolism, metabolic acidosis, and eventual death of the affected tissue. Myocardial infarction and stroke (cerebrovascular accident) are good examples of ischemic conditions that can cause hypoxia and tissue death.

Dysoxia

Dysoxia is a form of hypoxia in which the cellular uptake of oxygen is abnormally decreased. The best example of dysoxia is cyanide poisoning. Cyanide disrupts the intracellular cytochrome oxidase system, thereby preventing cellular use of oxygen.

Dysoxia also may occur when tissue oxygen consumption becomes dependent on oxygen delivery. Figure 10-19 plots tissue oxygen consumption ($\dot{V}o_2$) against oxygen delivery ($\dot{D}o_2$) in both normal and pathological states.

Normally, the tissues extract as much oxygen as they need from what is delivered, and oxygen consumption equals oxygen demand *(flat portion of solid line)*. However, if delivery falls, conditions begin to change *(solid line)*. At a level called the *point of critical delivery*, tissue extraction reaches a maximum. Further decreases in delivery then result in an oxygen "debt," which occurs when oxygen demand exceeds oxygen delivery. Under conditions of oxygen debt, oxygen consumption becomes dependent on oxygen delivery *(sloped line)*. This in turn leads to lactic acid accumulation and metabolic acidosis.

In pathological conditions such as septic shock and adult respiratory distress syndrome *(dotted line)*, this critical point may occur at levels of oxygen delivery considered normal. In addition, the slope of the curve

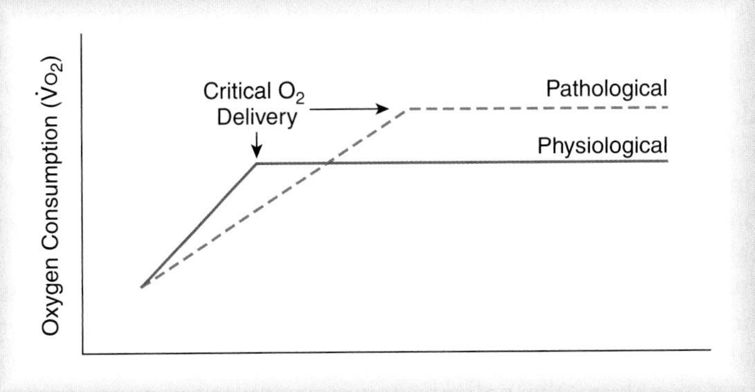

Figure 10-19
Physiological versus pathological O_2 consumption-delivery relationship. Note that critical O_2 delivery occurs at higher O_2 delivery in pathological state. The slope of the pathological consumption curve below the critical delivery point reflects the decrease in the O_2 extraction ratio that exists in these situations. *(Modified from Pasquale MD, Cipolle MD, Cerra FB: Oxygen transport: does increasing supply improve outcome? Respir Care 38:800, 1993.)*

below the point of critical delivery may be less than normal, indicating a decreased extraction ratio ($\dot{V}O_2$/$\dot{D}O_2$). In combination, these findings indicate that oxygen demands are not being met and that a defect exists in the cellular mechanisms regulating oxygen uptake.

Impaired Carbon Dioxide Removal

Any disorder that lowers alveolar ventilation ($\dot{V}_A$) relative to metabolic need impairs carbon dioxide removal. Impaired carbon dioxide removal by the lung causes hypercapnia and respiratory acidosis (see Chapter 12).

A decrease in alveolar ventilation occurs when (1) the minute ventilation is inadequate, (2) the dead space ventilation per minute is increased, or (3) a $\dot{V}/\dot{Q}$ imbalance exists.

Inadequate Minute Ventilation

Clinically, an inadequate minute ventilation usually is caused by decreased tidal volumes. This occurs in restrictive conditions, such as atelectasis, neuromuscular disorders, or impeded thoracic expansion (e.g., kyphoscoliosis). A decrease in respiratory rate is less common but may be present with respiratory center depression, as in drug overdose.

Increased Dead Space Ventilation

An increase in dead space ventilation is caused by either (1) rapid, shallow breathing (an increase in anatomical dead space per minute) or (2) increased physiological dead space (($\dot{V}/\dot{Q}$ = 0). In either case, the proportion of wasted ventilation increases. Without compensation, this lowers alveolar ventilation per minute and impairs carbon dioxide removal.

$\dot{V}/\dot{Q}$ Imbalances

In theory, any $\dot{V}/\dot{Q}$ imbalance should cause a rise in $PaCO_2$. However, the $PaCO_2$ does not always increase in these cases. Indeed, many patients who are hypoxemic because of a $\dot{V}/\dot{Q}$ imbalance have a low or normal $PaCO_2$. This common clinical finding suggests that $\dot{V}/\dot{Q}$ imbalances have a greater effect on oxygenation than on carbon dioxide removal.

Careful inspection of the oxygen and carbon dioxide dissociation curves supports this finding. The oxygen and carbon dioxide dissociation curves are plotted on the same scale in Figure 10-20. The upper carbon dioxide curve is nearly linear in the physiological range. The lower oxygen curve is almost flat in the physiological range. Point a on each curve is the normal arterial point for both content and partial pressure. To the *right of the graph* are two lung units, one with a low $\dot{V}/\dot{Q}$, the other with a high $\dot{V}/\dot{Q}$. The blood oxygen and carbon dioxide contents from each unit are plotted on the curves.

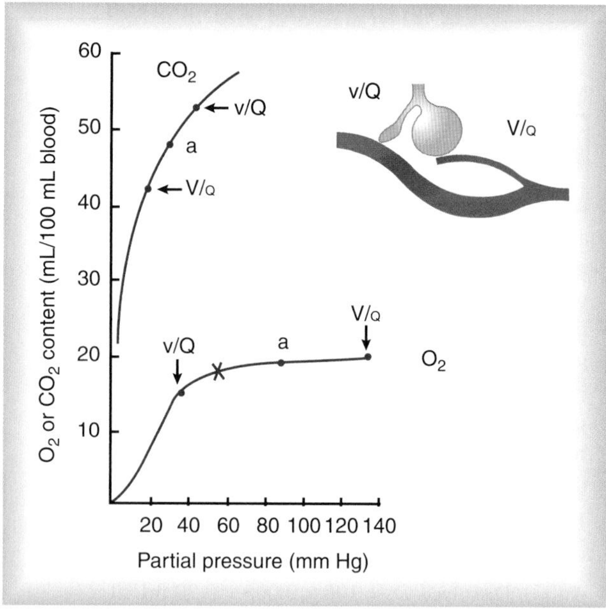

Figure 10-20

$\dot{V}/\dot{Q}$ imbalance and the dissociation curves for carbon dioxide and oxygen. *v/Q* represents low $\dot{V}/\dot{Q}$ units, and *V/Q* represents high $\dot{V}/\dot{Q}$units. See text for discussion.

The final carbon dioxide content, arrived at by averaging the high and low $\dot{V}/\dot{Q}$ points, is shown as point a on the carbon dioxide curve. Note that this is the same as the normal arterial point for carbon dioxide.

The final oxygen content, also arrived at by averaging the high and low $\dot{V}/\dot{Q}$ points, is shown as point X on the oxygen curve. Whereas the averaged value for carbon dioxide was normal, the PaO_2 resulting from averaging the oxygen content of the high and low $\dot{V}/\dot{Q}$ units is well below normal (point a on the oxygen curve).

Thus the effect of low $\dot{V}/\dot{Q}$ units is a decreased PaO_2 and an increased $PaCO_2$. The effect of high $\dot{V}/\dot{Q}$ units is the opposite (i.e., an increased PO_2 and a decreased PCO_2). However, the shape of the dissociation curves dictates that a high $\dot{V}/\dot{Q}$ unit can reverse the high PCO_2 but not the low PO_2. *Thus any increase in PCO_2 from low $\dot{V}/\dot{Q}$ units can be corrected by a reduction in PCO_2 from high $\dot{V}/\dot{Q}$ units.* However, these same high $\dot{V}/\dot{Q}$ units cannot compensate for the reduced oxygen content because the oxygen curve is nearly flat when the PO_2 is higher than normal.

Of course, patients with $\dot{V}/\dot{Q}$ imbalances still must compensate for the high PCO_2 coming from underventilated units. To compensate for these high PCO_2 values, the patient's minute ventilation must increase

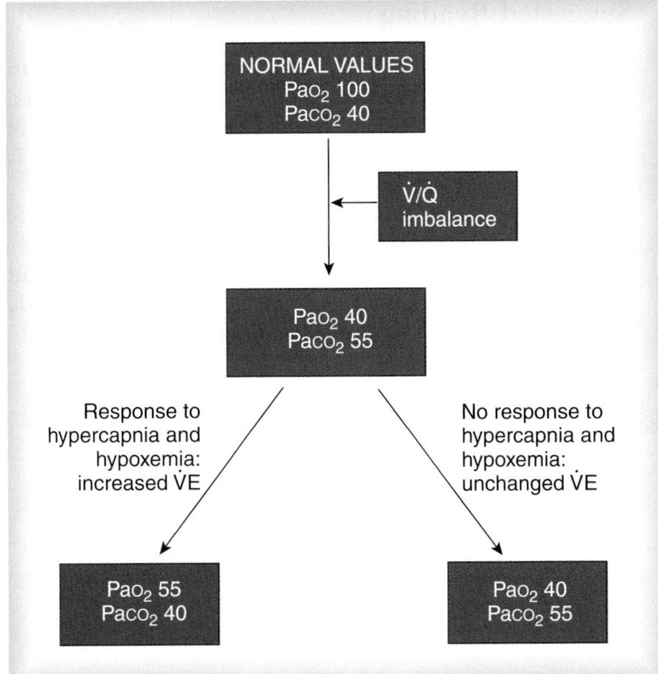

Figure 10-21

Changes in Pa_{O_2} and Pa_{CO_2} caused by a $\dot{V}/\dot{Q}$ imbalance. All values are given in millimeters of mercury (mm Hg).

(Figure 10-21). Patients who can increase their minute ventilation tend to have either a normal or a low Pa_{CO_2}, combined with hypoxemia.

Conversely, patients with a $\dot{V}/\dot{Q}$ imbalance who cannot increase their minute ventilation are hypercapnic. In general, this occurs only when the $\dot{V}/\dot{Q}$ imbalance is severe and chronic, as in chronic obstructive pulmonary disease. Such a patient must sustain a higher than normal minute ventilation just to maintain a normal Pa_{CO_2}. If the energy costs required to sustain a high minute ventilation are prohibitive, the patient will opt for less work and hence an elevated Pa_{CO_2}.

KEY POINTS

- The movement of gases between the lungs and the tissues depends mainly on diffusion.
- The alveolar P_{CO_2} varies directly with carbon dioxide production and inversely with alveolar ventilation.
- The alveolar P_{O_2} is computed using the alveolar air equation.
- With a constant F_{IO_2}, the alveolar P_{O_2} varies inversely with the alveolar P_{CO_2}.
- Normal alveolar P_{O_2} averages 100 mm Hg, with a mean alveolar P_{CO_2} of approximately 40 mm Hg.

KEY POINTS—cont'd

- Mixed venous blood has a P_{O_2} of approximately 40 mm Hg and a P_{CO_2} of approximately 46 mm Hg.
- Ventilation and perfusion must be in balance for pulmonary gas exchange to be effective.
- Because of normal anatomical shunts and $\dot{V}/\dot{Q}$ imbalances, pulmonary gas exchange is less than perfect.
- In disease, the $\dot{V}/\dot{Q}$ ratio can range from zero (perfusion without ventilation or physiological shunting) to infinity (pure alveolar dead space).
- Blood carries a small amount of oxygen in physical solution, of which most is carried in chemical combination with erythrocyte hemoglobin.
- Hemoglobin saturation is the ratio of oxyhemoglobin to total hemoglobin, expressed as a percentage.
- To compute total oxygen contents of the blood, add the dissolved oxygen content ($0.003 \times P_{O_2}$) to the product of Hb content × Hb saturation × 1.34.
- The arteriovenous oxygen content difference $C(a-\bar{v})O_2$ is the amount of oxygen given up by every 100 mL of blood on each pass

KEY POINTS—cont'd

through the tissues. All else being equal, the $C(a-\bar{v})O_2$ varies inversely with cardiac output.

- Hemoglobin affinity for oxygen increases with high P_{O_2}, high pH, low temperature, and low levels of 2,3-DPG.
- Hemoglobin abnormalities can affect oxygen loading and unloading and can cause hypoxia.
- Most carbon dioxide is transported in the blood as ionized bicarbonate; other forms include carbamino compounds in physical solution.
- Changes in carbon dioxide levels modify the oxygen dissociation curve (Bohr effect). Changes in hemoglobin saturation affects the carbon dioxide dissociation curve (Haldane effect). These changes are mutually beneficial.
- Hypoxia occurs if (1) the arterial blood oxygen content is decreased, (2) blood flow is decreased, or (3) abnormal cellular function prevents proper uptake of oxygen.
- A decreased Pa_{O_2} level may be a result of a low ambient P_{O_2}, hypoventilation, impaired diffusion, ventilation-perfusion ($\dot{V}/\dot{Q}$) imbalances, and right-to-left anatomical or physiological shunting.
- A decrease in alveolar ventilation occurs when (1) the minute ventilation is inadequate, (2) dead space ventilation is increased, or (3) a $\dot{V}/\dot{Q}$ imbalance exists.

Suggested Reading

Crapo RO, Campbell EG: Aging of the respiratory system. In Fishman AP: Fishman's pulmonary diseases and disorders, ed 3, New York, 1998, McGraw-Hill.

West JB: Respiratory physiology: the essentials, ed 5, Baltimore, 1995, Williams & Wilkins.

West JB: Pulmonary pathophysiology: the essentials, ed 5, Philadelphia, 1998, Lippincott Williams & Wilkins.

West JB: Pulmonary physiology and pathophysiology: an integrated, case-based approach, Philadelphia, 2001, Lippincott Williams & Wilkins.

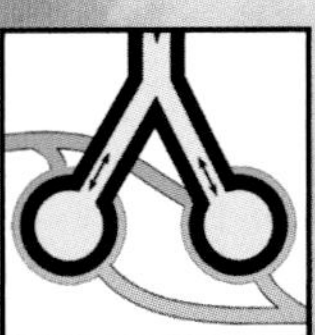

CHAPTER 11

Solutions, Body Fluids, and Electrolytes

Gregg L. Ruppel

In This Chapter You Will Learn:

- What the characteristics of solutions are, including concentrations of solutes
- How osmotic pressure functions and what its action is in relation to cell membranes
- How to calculate the solute content of a solution using ratio, weight/volume, and percent methods
- What the ionic characteristics of acids, bases, and salts are
- How proteins can function as bases
- How to calculate the pH of a solution when given the $[H^+]$ in nanomoles per liter
- Where fluid compartments are located in the body and what their volumes are
- How water loss and replacement occur
- What roles are played by osmotic and hydrostatic pressure in edema
- What clinical findings are associated with excess or deficiency of the seven basic electrolytes

Chapter Outline

Solutions
- Definition of a solution
- Concentration of solutions
- Osmotic pressure of solutions
- Quantifying solute content and activity
- Calculating solute content
- Quantitative classification of solutions

Electrolytic Activity and Acid-Base Balance
- Characteristics of acids, bases, and salts
- Designation of acidity and alkalinity

Body Fluids and Electrolytes
- Fluids
- Electrolytes

Key Terms

acid
active transport
anions
base
cations
colloid
edema
humidity deficit
hydrostatic pressure
hypercalcemia
hyperchloremia
hyperkalemia
hypermagnesemia
hypernatremia
hyperphosphatemia
hypertonic
hypocalcemia
hypochloremia
hypokalemia
hypomagnesemia
hyponatremia
hypophosphatemia
hypotonic
interstitial fluid
ionic
isotonic
nano
nonpolar covalent
osmotic pressure
plasma
polar covalent
protein bases
solution

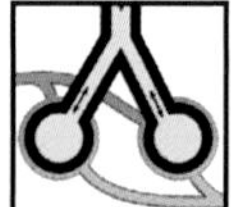

In healthy individuals, body water and various chemicals are regulated to maintain an environment in which biochemical processes continue. Imbalances in the amount or concentration of chemicals in the body occur in many diseases. The nature and importance of body fluids and electrolytes require an understanding of physiological chemistry. This chapter provides the reader with the background knowledge needed to understand body chemistry.

▶ SOLUTIONS

Definition of a Solution

The body is a watery medium, which holds chemical substances and particles in **solution** or suspension. These substances and particles combine with water in the following three ways: as (1) *colloids,* (2) *suspensions,* or (3) *solutions.*

Colloids (sometimes called dispersions or gels) consist of large molecules that attract and hold water. These molecules are uniformly distributed throughout the dispersion and they tend not to settle. The protoplasm inside cells is a common example of a **colloid.**

Suspensions are composed of large particles that float in a liquid. Suspensions do not behave like the solvent and solute found in a true solution. Red blood cells in **plasma** are an example of a suspension. Dispersion of suspended particles depends on physical agitation. Particles settle when the suspension is allowed to stand.

A solution is a stable mixture of two substances. One substance is evenly dispersed throughout the other. The substance that dissolves is called the *solute.* The medium in which it dissolves is called the *solvent.*

The ease with which a solute dissolves in a solvent is its *solubility,* which is influenced by four factors:

1. *Nature of the solute.* The ease with which substances go into a solution in a given solvent is a physical characteristic of matter and varies widely.
2. *Nature of the solvent.* Solvents vary widely in their ability to dissolve substances.
3. *Temperature.* Solubility of most solids increases with increased temperature. However, the solubility of gases varies inversely with temperature.
4. *Pressure.* Solubility of gases in liquids varies directly with pressure.

The effects of temperature and pressure on the solubility of gases are important. Oxygen and carbon dioxide transport can change markedly with changes in body temperature or the pressure to which the body is exposed (see Chapters 9 and 10).

Concentration of Solutions

A solution is *dilute* if the amount of solute is relatively small in proportion to the solvent (Figure 11-1, *A*). A *saturated* solution has the maximal amount of solute that can be held in a given volume of a solvent at a constant temperature. If there is an excess of solute (Figure 11-1, *B*), then the dissolved solute is in equilibrium with the undissolved solute. Solute particles precipitate into the solid state at the same rate that other particles go into solution. This equilibrium characterizes a saturated solution.

A solution is *supersaturated* when it contains more solute than does a saturated solution at the same temperature and pressure. If a saturated solution is heated, the solute equilibrium is upset and more solute goes into solution. If undissolved solute is removed and the solution is cooled gently, there will be an excess of dissolved solute (Figure 11-1, *C*). The excess solute of supersaturated solutions may be precipitated out of the solution by physical stimuli such as shaking or vibrating. Precipitation also may occur if more solute is added.

Osmotic Pressure of Solutions

Most of the solutions of physiological importance in the body are dilute. Solutes in dilute solution demonstrate many of the properties of gases. This behavior results from the relatively large distances between the

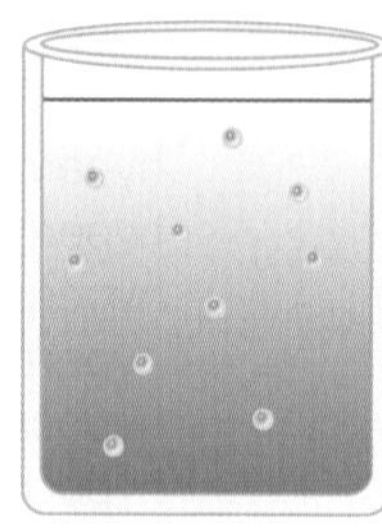

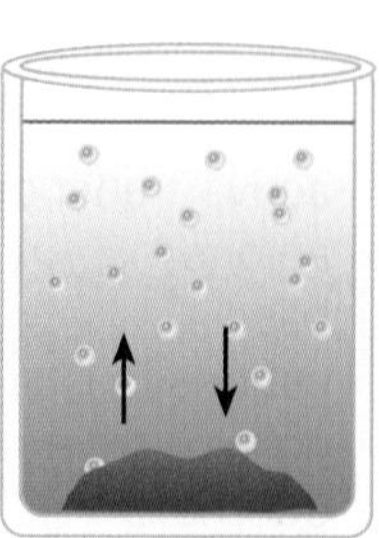

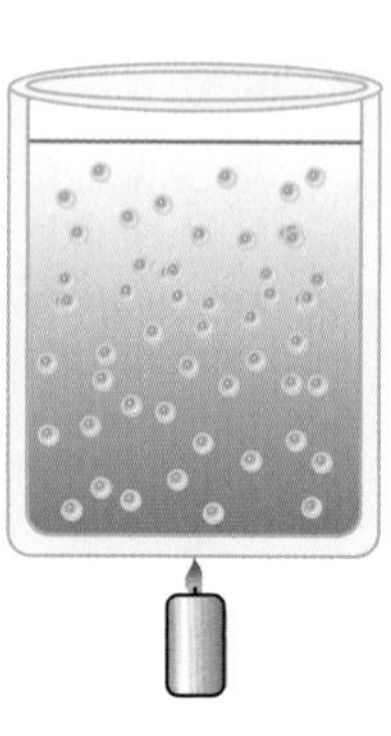

Figure 11-1
In the dilute solution **(A),** there are relatively few solute particles. In the saturated solution **(B),** the solvent contains all the solute it can hold in the presence of excess solute. Heating the solution **(C)** dissolves more solute particles, which may remain in the solution if cooled gently, creating a state of supersaturation.

molecules in dilute solutions. The most important physiological characteristic of solutions is their ability to exert pressure.

Osmotic pressure is the force produced by solvent particles under certain conditions. A membrane that permits passage of solvent molecules, but not solute, is called a *semipermeable membrane*. If such a membrane divides a solution into two compartments, molecules of solvent can pass through it from one side to the other (Figure 11-2, *A*). The number of solvent molecules passing (or diffusing) in one direction must equal the number of solute molecules passing in the opposite direction. An equal ratio of solute to solvent particles (i.e., the concentration of the solution) is maintained on both sides of the membrane.

If a solution is placed on one side of a semipermeable membrane and pure solvent on the other, solvent molecules will move through the membrane into the solution. The force driving solvent molecules through the membrane is osmotic pressure. Osmotic pressure may be measured by connecting a manometer to the expanding column of the solution (Figure 11-2, *B* and *C*). Osmotic pressure tries to distribute solvent molecules so that the same concentration exists on both sides of the membrane.

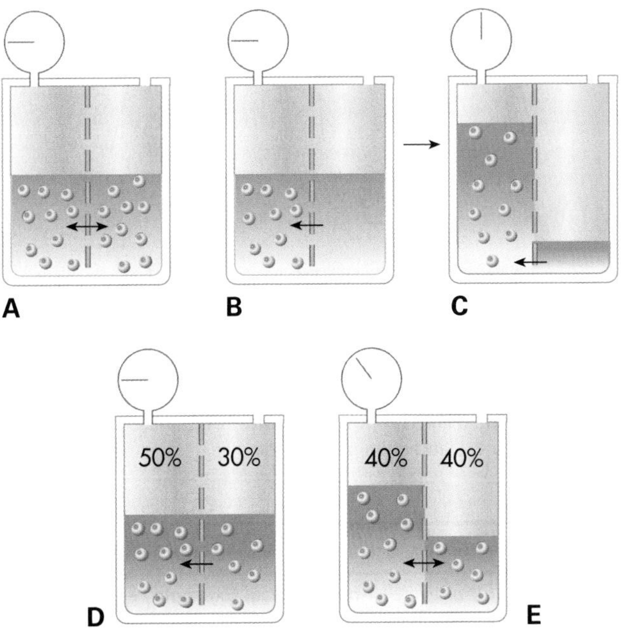

Figure 11-2

Osmotic pressure is illustrated by the solutions in the five containers. Each container is divided into two compartments by a semipermeable membrane, which permits passage of solvent molecules but not solute *(circles)*. The number of solute particles represents relative concentrations of the solutions. Solute particles are fixed in number and are confined by the membranes. Volume changes are a function of the diffusible solvent. Solvent movement is indicated by arrows through the membranes. The *arrows* between containers *B* and *C*, and between *D* and *E*, indicate how osmotic pressure progresses.

Osmotic pressure can also be visualized as an attractive force of solute particles in a concentrated solution. If 100 mL of a 50% solution is placed on one side of a membrane and 100 mL of a 30% solution is placed on the other side, solvent molecules will move from the dilute to the concentrated side (Figure 11-2, *D* and *E*). The particles in the concentrated solution attract solvent molecules from the dilute solution until equilibrium occurs. Equilibrium exists when the concentrations (i.e., ratio of solute/solvent) in both compartments are equal (40% in Figure 11-2).

Osmotic pressure depends on the number of particles in solution. A 2% solution has twice the osmotic pressure of a 1% solution. For a given amount of solute, osmotic pressure is inversely proportional to the volume of solvent. Osmotic pressure varies directly with temperature, increasing by $\frac{1}{273}$ for each 1° C.

Most cell walls are semipermeable membranes. Through osmotic pressure, water is distributed throughout the body within certain physiological ranges. *Tonicity* describes how much osmotic pressure is exerted by a solution. Average body cellular fluid has a tonicity equal to a 0.9% solution of sodium chloride (NaCl; sometimes referred to as *physiological saline*). Solutions with similar tonicity are called **isotonic.** Those with more tonicity are **hypertonic,** and those with less tonicity are **hypotonic.** Some cells have *selective permeability*, allowing passage not only of water, but also of specific solutes. Through these mechanisms, nutrients and physiological solutions are distributed throughout the body.

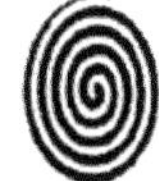

RULE OF THUMB

Solutions that have osmotic pressures equal to the average intracellular pressure in the body are called *isotonic*. This is roughly equivalent to a saline solution (NaCl) of 0.9%. Solutions with higher osmotic potential are called *hypertonic*, whereas those with lower osmotic pressure are called *hypotonic*. Administration of isotonic solutions usually causes no net change in cellular water content. Hypertonic solutions draw water out of cells. Hypotonic solutions usually cause water to be absorbed from the solution into cells.

In electrochemical terms, there are three basic types of physiological solutions. Depending on the solute, solutions are **ionic** (electrovalent), **polar covalent,** or **nonpolar covalent** (Table 11-1). In ionic and polar covalent solutions, some of the solute ionizes into separate particles known as *ions*. A solution in which this dissociation occurs is called an *electrolyte solution*

(Figure 11-3). If an electrode is placed in such a solution, positive ions migrate to the negative pole of the electrode. These ions are called **cations**. Negative ions migrate to the positive pole of the electrode; they are called **anions**. In nonpolar covalent solutions, molecules of solute remain intact and do not carry electrical charges; these solutions are referred to as *nonelectrolytes*. These nonelectrolytes are not attracted to either the positive or negative pole of an electrode (hence the designation *nonpolar*). All three types of solutions coexist in the body. These solutions also serve as the media in which colloids and simple suspensions are dispersed.

Quantifying Solute Content and Activity

The amount of solute in a solution can be quantified in two ways: (1) by *actual weight* (grams or milligrams) and (2) by *chemical combining power*. The weight of a solute is relatively easy to measure and specify. However, it does not indicate chemical combining power. For example, the sodium ion (Na^+) has a gram ionic weight of 23. The bicarbonate ion (HCO_3^-) has a gram ionic weight of 61. Because the gram atomic weight of every substance has 6.023×10^{23} particles, these ions have the same chemical combining power in solution. The number of chemically reactive units is more meaningful than their weight.

Equivalent Weights

In medicine it is customary to refer to physiological substances in terms of chemical combining power. The measure commonly used is *equivalent weight*. Equivalent weights are amounts of substances that have equal chemical combining power. For example, if chemical A reacts with chemical B, one equivalent weight of A will react with exactly one equivalent weight of B. No excess reactants of A or B will remain.

The following two magnitudes of equivalent weights are used to calculate chemical-combining power: the gram equivalent weight (gEq) and the milligram equivalent weight, or milliequivalent (mEq). One milliequivalent is $\frac{1}{1000}$ of a gEq.

Gram Equivalent Weight Values. A gEq of a substance is calculated as its gram atomic (formula) weight divided by its valence. The valence signs (+ or –) are disregarded.

$$\text{gEq} = \frac{\text{Gram atomic (formula) weight}}{\text{Valence}}$$

For example, the gEq of sodium (Na^+), with a valence of 1, equals its gram atomic weight of 23 g. The gEq of calcium (Ca^{2+}) is its atomic weight divided by 2, or 20 g. The gEq of ferric iron (Fe^{3+}) is its atomic weight divided by 3, or approximately 18.6 g.

For radicals such as sulfate (SO_4^{2-}), the formula for sulfuric acid (H_2SO_4) shows that one sulfate group combines with two atoms of hydrogen. Half (0.5) of a mole of sulfate is equivalent to 1 mole of hydrogen

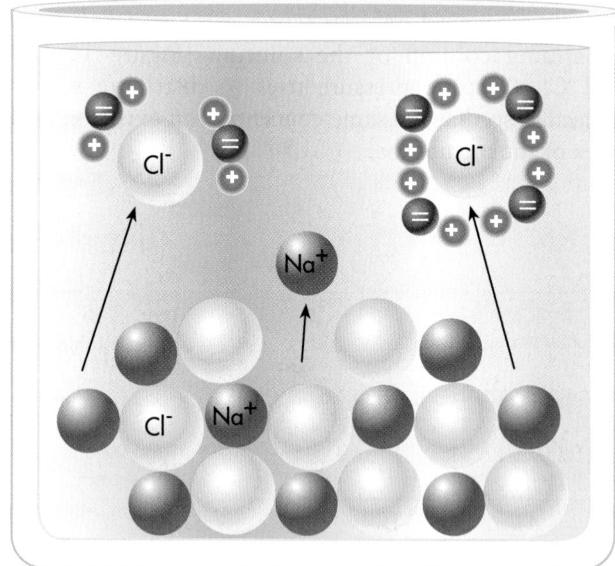

Figure 11-3
Sodium chloride (NaCl) is shown as a crystalline mass of ions being dissociated by the attraction of water dipoles.

Table 11-1 ▶▶ Types of Physiological Solutions

Type	Characteristics	Physiological Example
Ionic (electrovalent)	Ionic compounds dissolved from crystalline form, usually in water (hydration); form strong electrolytes with conductivity dependent on concentration of ions	Saline solution (0.9% NaCl)
Polar covalent	Molecular compounds dissolved in water or other solvents to produce ions (ionization); electrolytes may be weak or strong, depending on degree of ionization; solutions polarize and are good conductors	Hydrochloric acid (HCl) (strong electrolyte); acetic acid (CH_3COOH) (weak electrolyte)
Nonpolar covalent	Molecular compounds dissolved into electrically neutral solutions (do not polarize); solutions are not good conductors; nonelectrolytes	Glucose ($C_6H_{12}O_6$)

atoms. The gEq of SO_4^{2-} is half its gram formula weight, or 48 g. If an element has more than one valence, the valence must be specified or must be apparent from the observed chemical combining properties.

Gram Equivalent Weight of an Acid. The gEq of an acid is the weight of the acid (in grams) that contains 1 mole of replaceable hydrogen. The gram equivalent weight of an acid may be calculated by dividing its gram formula weight by the number of hydrogen atoms in its formula, as shown in the following reaction:

$$HCl + Na^+ \rightarrow NaCl + H^+$$

The single H^+ of hydrochloric acid (HCl) is replaced by Na^+. One mole of HCl has one mole of replaceable hydrogen. By definition, the gEq of HCl must be the same as its gram formula weight, or 36.5 g. The two hydrogen atoms of sulfuric acid (H_2SO_4) are both considered to be replaceable. Therefore 1 mole of sulfuric acid contains 2 mole of replaceable hydrogen. Therefore the gram equivalent weight of H_2SO_4 is half its gram formula weight, or 49 g.

Those acids in which hydrogen atoms are not completely replaceable are exceptions to the rule. In some acids, H+ replacement varies according to specific reactions. Carbonic acid (H_2CO_3) and phosphoric acid (H_3PO_4) are examples of such exceptions. Their equivalent weights are determined by the conditions of their chemical reactions.

For example, H_2CO_3 has two hydrogen atoms. In physiological reactions, only one is considered replaceable:

$$H_2CO_3 + Na^+ \rightarrow NaHCO_3 + H^+$$

Only one hydrogen atom is released; the other remains bound. Therefore 1 mole of carbonic acid contains only 1 mole of replaceable hydrogen. The gram equivalent weight of carbonic acid is the same as its gram formula weight, or 62 g.

Gram Equivalent Weight of a Base. The equivalent weight of a base is its weight (grams) containing 1 mole of replaceable hydroxyl (OH^-) ions. Like acids, the gEq of bases is calculated by dividing gram formula weight by the number of OH^- groups in its formula.

Conversion of Gram Weight to Equivalent Weight. To determine the number of gram equivalent weights in a substance, the gram weight is divided by its calculated equivalent weight, as shown in the following example:

$$\frac{58.5 \text{ g NaCl}}{\text{gEq } 58.5 \text{ g}} = 1 \text{ gEq}$$

$$\frac{29.25 \text{ g NaCl}}{\text{gEq } 58.5 \text{ g}} = 0.5 \text{ gEq}$$

Milligram Equivalent Weights. The concentrations of most chemicals in the body are quite small. The term *milligram equivalent weight* (milliequivalent), or mEq, is preferred. A milliequivalent is simply 0.001 gEq:

$$\text{mEq} = \frac{\text{gEq}}{1000}$$

For example, the normal concentration of potassium (K^+) in the plasma ranges between 0.0035 and 0.005 gEq/L. These values may be converted to milliequivalents by multiplying by a factor of 1000. The normal concentration of K^+ in the plasma ranges between 3.5 and 5.0 mEq/L.

Solute Content by Weight

The measurement of many electrolytes is based on actual weight rather than on milliequivalents. This weight is expressed as milligrams per 100 mL of blood or body fluid. The units for this measurement are abbreviated as mg% or mg/dL (milligrams per deciliter). This text uses the modern designation mg/dL.

Values stated in mg/dL may be converted into their corresponding equivalent weights and reported as mEq/L. Conversion between mEq/L and mg/dL may be calculated as follows:

$$(1)\ \text{mEq/L} = \frac{\text{mg/dL} \times 10}{\text{Equivalent weight}}$$

$$(2)\ \text{mg/dL} = \frac{\text{mEq/L} \times \text{Equivalent weight}}{10}$$

For example, to convert a serum value of 322 mg/dL of Na^+ to mEq/L, the equation is used as follows:

$$\text{mEq/L} = \frac{\text{mg/dL} \times 10}{\text{Equivalent weight}}$$

$$= 322 \times 10/23$$

$$= 140 \text{ mEq/L}$$

In clinical practice, electrolyte replacement is common when a laboratory test identifies a significant deficiency. The electrolyte content of intravenous solutions is usually stated in milligrams per deciliter or in mEq per liter. Lactated Ringer's solution is one such infusion used for electrolyte replacement (Table 11-2).

Calculating Solute Content

In addition to gEq, mEq, and mg/dL, several other methods of calculating solute content exist. These common chemical standards are used to compute solute content and dilution of solutions.

Quantitative Classification of Solutions

The amount of solute in a solution may be quantified by the following six methods:

1. *Ratio solution.* The amount of solute to solvent is expressed as a proportion (e.g., 1:100). Ratio solutions are used commonly in describing concentrations of drugs.
2. *Weight per volume solution (W/V).* The W/V solution is commonly used for solids dissolved in liquids. It is defined as weight of solute per volume of solution. This method is sometimes erroneously referred to as a *percent solution.* W/V solutions are commonly expressed in grams of solute per 100 mL of solution. For example, 5 g of glucose dissolved in 100 mL of solution is properly called a *5% solution*, according to the weight-per-volume scheme. A liquid dissolved in a liquid is measured as volumes of solute to volumes of solution.
3. *Percent solution.* A percent solution is weight of solute per weight of solution. Five grams of glucose dissolved in 95 g of water is a true percent solution. The glucose is 5% of the total solution weight of 100 g.
4. *Molal solution.* A molal solution contains 1 mole of solute per kilogram of solvent, or 1 mmol/g solvent. The concentration of a molal solution is independent of temperature.
5. *Molar solution.* A molar solution has 1 mole of solute per liter of solution, or 1 mmol/mL of solution. Solute is measured into a container, and solvent is added to produce the solution volume desired.
6. *Normal solution.* A normal solution has 1 gEq of solute per liter of solution, or 1 mEq/mL of solution. For all monovalent solutes, normal and molar solutions are the same. The equivalent weights of their solutes equal their gram formula weights. Equal volumes of solutions of the same normality contain chemically equivalent amounts of their solutes. If the solutes react chemically with one another, then equal volumes of the solutions will react completely. Neither substance will remain in excess. In the analytical process of titration, normal solutions are often used as standards to determine the concentrations of other solutions.

Dilution Calculations

Dilute solutions are made from a stock preparation. Preparation of medications often involves dilution. Dilution calculations are based on the weight per unit volume principle (the aforementioned W/V solution method).

Table 11-2 ▶▶ Concentration of Ingredients in Lactated Ringer's Solution

Substance	mg/dL	Approximate mEq/L
NaCl (Sodium chloride)	600 Na	130
	310 Cl	109
$NaC_3H_5O_3$ (Sodium lactate)	30 $C_3H_5O_3$	28
KCl (Potassium chloride)	30 K	4
$CaCl_2$ (Calcium chloride)	20 Ca	27

MINI CLINI

Gas Dilution and Lung Volume

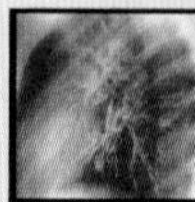

The dilution equation ($V_1C_1=V_2C_2$) is commonly used to calculate volumes or concentrations of medications when a specific dosage needs to be administered to a patient. If three of the variables are known, the fourth can be determined. This technique also can be applied to other areas of medicine.

PROBLEM

The residual volume (RV) is the volume of gas left in the lungs after a patient has exhaled completely. Since it cannot be removed without completely collapsing the lungs, is there any way to measure this volume?

SOLUTION

Residual volume can be measured indirectly using a variation of the dilution equation. If a known volume (V_1) and concentration (C_1) of a test gas are placed in a container, and the patient is allowed to breathe this gas, the gas concentration will fall (C_2), allowing calculation of the new volume (V_2). In this case the new volume is the old volume (V_1) plus the unknown volume in the patient's lungs (RV). This method is widely used in pulmonary function laboratories. In practice, helium (He) is used as the test gas because the patient can rebreathe it without absorbing or metabolizing it. A spirometer is used as the container to hold the test gas. A mixture of approximately 10% helium is prepared in a volume of 8 to 10 L. The exact values are the C_1 and V_1 of the dilution equation. The patient then rebreathes from the spirometer. Oxygen is added and carbon dioxide removed to keep the spirometer volume constant. The He concentration falls as the gas in the spirometer and patient's lungs mix. After a few minutes of rebreathing, the He concentration reaches equilibrium (C_2). The new volume (V_2) is calculated by simple rearrangement of the dilution equation:

$$V_2 = \frac{V_1C_1}{C_2}$$

Because the volume in the spirometer (V1) was known, it can be subtracted from V_2 to obtain the patient's RV. (See Chapter 17 for further discussion of lung volume measurements.)

Diluting a solution increases its volume without changing the amount of solute it contains. This reduces the concentration of the solution. The amount of solute in a solution can be expressed as volume times concentration. For example, 50 mL of a 10% solution (10 g/dL) contains 50 × 0.1, or 5 g. In the dilution of a solution, initial volume (V_1) multiplied by initial concentration (C_1) equals final volume multiplied by final concentration. This can be expressed as follows:

$$V_1C_1 = V_2C_2$$

This equation is sometimes referred to as the *dilution equation*. Whenever three of the variables are known, the fourth can be calculated as follows:

1. Diluting 10 mL of a 2% (0.02) solution to a concentration of 0.5% (0.005) requires finding the new volume (V_2) by rearranging the dilution equation as follows:

$$V_2 = \frac{V_1C_1}{C_2}$$

$$V_2 = \frac{10 \text{ mL} \times 0.02}{0.005}$$

$$V_2 = 40 \text{ mL}$$

2. If 50 mL of water is added to 150 mL of a 3% (0.03) solution, the new concentration is calculated by rearranging the dilution equation to find C_2 as follows:

$$C_2 = \frac{V_1C_1}{V_2}$$

$$C_2 = \frac{150 \text{ mL} \times 0.02}{(50 \text{ mL} + 150 \text{ mL})}$$

$$C_2 = 0.0225\ (2.25\%)$$

3. Given 50 mL of a 0.33 normal (N) solution, dilute it to a 0.1 N concentration. Here, concentration is given as normality, but it can be used similarly to a percent. The new volume (V_2) can be calculated by rearranging the dilution equation as follows:

$$V_2 = \frac{V_1C_1}{C_2}$$

$$V_2 = \frac{50 \text{ mL} \times 0.33}{0.1}$$

$$V_2 = 165 \text{ mL}$$

▶ ELECTROLYTIC ACTIVITY AND ACID-BASE BALANCE

Acid-base balance depends on the concentration and activity of electrolytic solutes in the body. Clinical application of acid-base homeostasis is covered in detail in Chapter 12.

Characteristics of Acids, Bases, and Salts

Acids

An *acid* is a compound that yields hydrogen ions when placed in an aqueous solution. Such substances consist of hydrogen atoms covalently bonded to a negative valence nonmetal or radical. An example of such a compound is hydrochloric acid (HCl).

Another definition of an acid is that of Brönsted-Lowry, in which an acid is any compound that is a proton (H^+) donor. By this definition, many substances other than traditional acids can be included. For example, an ammonium ion (NH_4^+) qualifies as an acid because it donates a proton (H^+) in reactions such as the following:

$$NH_4Cl + NaOH \rightarrow NH_3 + NaCl + HOH$$

In this reaction, sodium and chloride ions are not involved in the proton transfer. The equation can be rewritten ionically as follows to demonstrate the acidity of the ammonium ion:

$$NH_4^+ + OH^- \rightarrow NH_3 + HOH$$

The ammonium ion donates a hydrogen ion (proton) to the reaction. The H^+ combines with the hydroxide ion (OH^-). This converts the former into ammonia gas and the latter into water.

Acids With Single Ionizable Hydrogen. Simple compounds such as HCl ionize into one cation and one anion:

$$HCl \rightarrow H^+ + Cl^-$$

Acids With Multiple Ionizable Hydrogens. The H^+ ions in an acid may become available in stages. The degree of ionization increases as an electrolyte solution becomes more dilute. Concentrated sulfuric acid ionizes only one of its two hydrogen atoms per molecule, as follows:

$$H_2SO_4 \rightarrow H^+ + HSO_4^-$$

With further dilution, second-stage ionization occurs:

$$H_2SO_4 \rightarrow H^+ + H^+ + SO_4^-$$

Bases

A *base* is a compound that yields hydroxyl ions (OH^-) when placed into aqueous solution. A substance capable of inactivating acids is also considered a base. These compounds, called *hydroxides*, consist of a metal that is ionically bound to a hydroxide ion or ions. The hydroxide also may be bound to an ammonium cation (NH_4^+). A good example of this type of base is sodium hydroxide (NaOH). The Brönsted-Lowry definition of a base is *any compound that accepts a proton.* This includes substances other than hydroxides, such as ammonia, carbonates, and certain proteins.

Hydroxide Bases. In aqueous solution, the following are typical dissociations of hydroxide bases:

$$Na^+OH \rightarrow Na^+ + OH^-$$

$$K^+OH \rightarrow K^+ + OH^-$$

$$Ca^{2+}(OH^-)_2 \rightarrow Ca^{2+} + 2(OH^-)$$

Inactivation of an acid is part of the definition of a base. This is accomplished by OH- reacting with H^+ to form water:

$$NaOH + HCl \rightarrow NaCl + HOH$$

Nonhydroxide Bases. Ammonia and carbonates are good examples of nonhydroxide bases. Proteins, with their amino groups, also can serve as nonhydroxide bases.

Ammonia. Ammonia qualifies as a base because it reacts with water to yield OH^-:

$$NH_3 + HOH \rightarrow NH_4^+ + OH^-$$

and neutralizes H^+ directly:

$$NH_3 + H^+ \rightarrow NH_4^+$$

In both instances, NH_3 accepts a proton to become NH_4^+. Ammonia plays an important role in renal excretion of acid (see Chapter 12).

Carbonates. The carbonate ion, CO_3^{2-}, can react with water in the following way to produce OH-:

$$(1) \quad Na_2CO_3 \Leftrightarrow 2Na^+ + CO_3^{2-}$$

$$(2) \quad CO_3^{2-} + HOH \Leftrightarrow HCO_3^- + OH^-$$

In this reaction, the carbonate ion accepts a proton from water, becoming the bicarbonate ion. It simultaneously produces a hydroxide ion. The carbonate ion also can react directly with H^+ to inactivate it:

$$CO_3^{2-} + H^+ \Leftrightarrow HCO_3^-$$

Protein Bases. Proteins are composed of amino acids bound together by peptide links. Physiological reactions in the body occur in a mildly alkaline environment. This allows proteins to act as H^+ receptors, or bases. Cellular and blood proteins acting as bases are transcribed as *prot⁻*.

The imidazole group of the amino acid histidine serves as an H^+ acceptor on a protein molecule (Figure 11-4). Their ability to accept hydrogen ions limits their activity in solution, which is called *buffering.* The buffering effect of hemoglobin is produced by imidazole groups in the protein. Each hemoglobin molecule contains 38 histidine residues. The oxygen-carrying component (heme group) of hemoglobin is attached to a histidine residue. The ability of hemoglobin to accept H^+ ions depends on the oxygenation state of the molecule. Deoxygenated (reduced) hemoglobin is a stronger base (i.e., a better H^+ acceptor) than oxygenated hemoglobin. This difference partially accounts for the ability of reduced hemoglobin to buffer more acid than can oxygenated hemoglobin (see Chapter 12). Plasma proteins also act as buffers, but with less buffering power than hemoglobin, which contains more histidine.

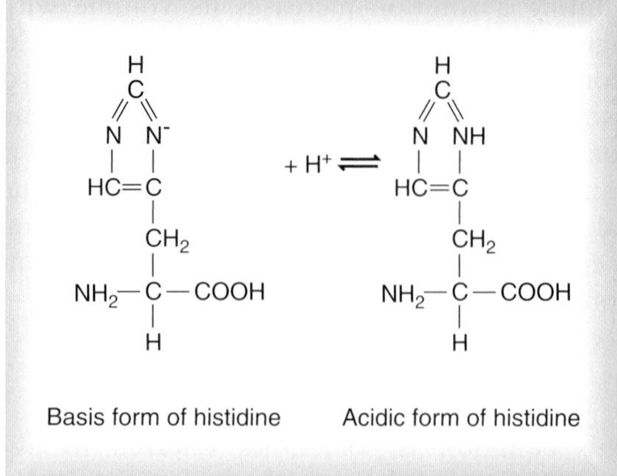

Figure 11-4

Histidine portion of a protein molecule serving as a proton acceptor (base).

Designation of Acidity and Alkalinity

Pure water can be used as a reference point for determining acidity or alkalinity. The concentration of both H^+ and OH^- in pure water is 10^7 mmol/L. A solution that has a greater H^+ concentration or lower OH^- concentration than water acts as an acid. A solution that has a lower H^+ concentration or a greater OH^- concentration than water is *alkaline,* or basic.

The H^+ concentration $[H^+]$ of pure water has been adopted as the standard for comparing reactions of other solutions. Electrochemical techniques are used to measure the $[H^+]$ of unknown solutions. Acidity or alkalinity is determined by variation of the $[H^+]$ above or below 1×10^{-7}. For example, a solution with a $[H^+]$ of 89.2×10^{-4} has a higher $[H^+]$ than water and therefore is acidic. A solution with a $[H^+]$ of 3.6×10^{-8} has fewer hydrogen ions than water and is, by definition, alkaline.

Two related techniques are used for expressing the acidity or alkalinity of solutions using the $[H^+]$ of water as a neutral factor: (1) the *$[H^+]$ in nanomoles per liter* and (2) the *logarithmic pH scale.*

Nanomolar Concentrations

The acidity or alkalinity of solutions may be reported using the molar concentration of H^+ compared with that of water. The $[H^+]$ of water is 1×10^{-7} mol/L, or 0.0000001 (one ten-millionth of a mole). The prefix for billionths is **nano**. The $[H^+]$ of water can be designated as 100 nanomoles per liter (100 nmol/L). A solution that has a $[H^+]$ of 100 nmol/L is neutral. One with more than 100 nmol/L is acidic; one with less than 100 nmol/L is alkaline.

This system is limited because of the wide range of possible $[H^+]$. The system is applicable in clinical medicine because the physiological range of $[H^+]$ is narrow. $[H^+]$ in healthy individuals is usually between 30 and 50 nmol/L.

pH Scale

pH is the negative logarithm of the $[H^+]$ used as a positive number. pH is derived by converting the value for $[H^+]$ to a negative exponent of 10 and calculating its logarithm. For example, the $[H^+]$ of water is 1×10^{-7} mol/L. Because the negative logarithm of 1×10^{-7} is 7, the pH of water is 7. Similarly:

$$[H^+] = 4.0 \times 10^{-8} \text{ mol/L}$$

$$\begin{aligned} pH &= -\log (4.0 \times 10^{-8}) \\ &= -\log 4.0 + -\log 10^{-8} \\ &= -\log 4.0 + \log 10^{8} \\ &= -0.602 + 8 \\ &= 7.40 \end{aligned}$$

In this scheme, any solution with a pH of 7.00 is neutral, corresponding to the $[H^+]$ of pure water. For pH values below 7.00, the $[H^+]$ increases logarithmically, becoming more acidic. For pH values above 7.00, the $[H^+]$ decreases logarithmically, becoming more alkaline. A change of 1 pH unit is equivalent to a tenfold change in $[H^+]$ (Figure 11-5). A pH of 7.00 is equivalent to a $[H^+]$ of 100 nmol. A pH of 8.00 is equivalent to a $[H^+]$ concentration of 10 nmol. Similarly, a change in pH of 0.3 units equals a twofold change in $[H^+]$.

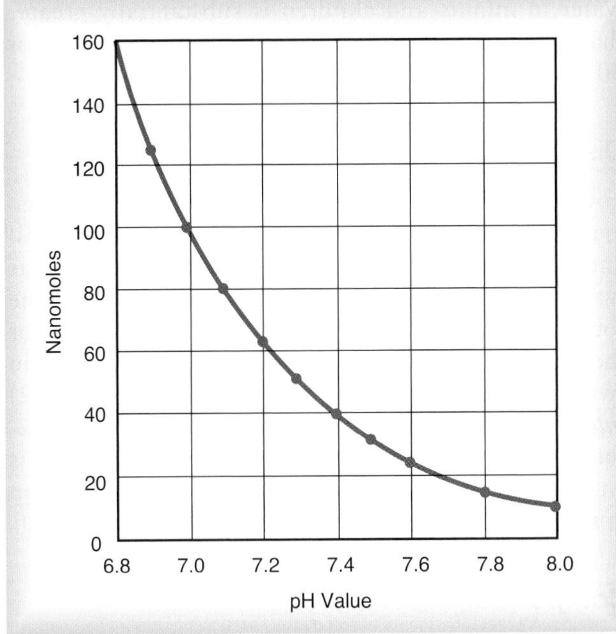

Figure 11-5

Relationship between pH and nmol $[H^+]$ concentrations. A pH of 7.00 equals 100 nanomoles/L of H^+.

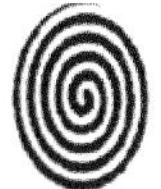

RULE OF THUMB

The pH scale is logarithmic. pH is a positive number representing the negative log of the hydrogen ion concentration $[H^+]$ of a solution. To visualize changes in acidity or alkalinity, the following two rules are helpful:

1. A pH change of *0.3 units equals a twofold change* in $[H^+]$.
2. A pH change of *1 unit equals a tenfold change* in $[H^+]$.

For example, if a patient's blood pH fell from 7.40 (normal) to 7.10, the $[H^+]$ concentration would be twice as high. If a patient's urine pH fell from 7.00 to 6.00, the $[H^+]$ would have increased by 10 times.

BODY FLUIDS AND ELECTROLYTES

Fluids

Water is a major component of the body. It makes up 45% to 80% of an individual's body weight, depending on that person's weight, gender, and age. Leanness is associated with higher body water content. Obese individuals have a lower percentage of body water (as much as 30% less) than normal-weight individuals. Men have a slightly higher percentage of total body water than women have. Total percentage of body water in infants and children is substantially greater than it is in adults. In the newborn, water accounts for 80% of the total body weight (Table 11-3).

Distribution

Total body water is divided into the following two major compartments: (1) *intracellular* (within the cells) and (2) *extracellular* (outside the cells). Intracellular water accounts for approximately two thirds of the total body water, and extracellular water accounts for the remaining one third. Extracellular water is found in two subcompartments: (1) *intravascular water* and (2) *interstitial water*. Intravascular water makes up approximately 5% of the body weight. Interstitial water is water in the tissues between the cells. It makes up approximately 15% of the body weight.

Composition

The concentration of solutes in intracellular and extracellular fluids differs significantly. Sodium (Na^+), chloride (Cl^-), and bicarbonate (HCO^{3-}) are predominantly extracellular electrolytes. Potassium (K^+), magnesium (Mg^{2+}), phosphate (PO_4^{3-}), sulfate (SO_4^{2-}), and protein constitute the main intracellular electrolytes. Intravascular and **interstitial fluid** have similar electrolyte compositions. However, plasma contains substantially more protein than interstitial fluid. Proteins, chiefly albumin, account for the high osmotic pressure of plasma. Osmotic pressure is an important determinant of fluid distribution between vascular and interstitial compartments.

Regulation

Movement of certain ions and proteins between body compartments is restricted. However, water diffuses freely. Control of total body water occurs through regulation of water intake (thirst) and water excretion (urine production, insensible loss, and stool water). The kidneys are mainly responsible for water excretion. If water intake is low, the kidneys reduce urine volume. This can concentrate solutes in the urine up to four times those in the plasma. If water intake is high, the kidneys can excrete large volumes of dilute urine.

The kidneys maintain the volume and composition of body fluids by two related mechanisms. First, filtration and reabsorption of sodium adjust urinary sodium excretion to match changes in dietary intake. Second, water excretion is regulated by secretion of *antidiuretic hormone* (ADH, or vasopressin). These mechanisms allow the kidneys to maintain the volume and concentration of body fluid despite variations in salt and water intake. Analysis of the urine (urinalysis) often provides diagnostic clues in disorders of body fluid volume.

Water Losses. Water may be lost from the body through the skin, lungs, kidneys, and gastrointestinal (GI) tract. Water loss can be *insensible*, such as vaporization of water from the skin and lungs, or *sensible*, such as losses from urine and the GI tract (Table 11-4). Other fluid losses from the body are called *additive* losses. Such losses may occur during vomiting, diarrhea, or suctioning from the stomach. Fever, in conjunction with sweating, also can cause additive losses. For each degree of body temperature higher than 99° F that persists for 24 hours, an additional 1000 mL of fluid is required.

The GI tract manufactures 8 to 10 L of fluid per day. More than 98% of this volume is reclaimed in the large intestine. In patients who are vomiting or have diarrhea, water losses through the GI tract can be considerable. Individuals with severe burns or open wounds can also lose large quantities of water.

Other causes of abnormal fluid loss include certain renal and respiratory disorders. Patients with renal disease may have to excrete larger quantities of urine to get rid of extra nitrogenous wastes. Patients with

Table 11-3 ▶▶ Distribution of Body Fluids

Body Water	Adult Male (% body weight)	Adult Female (% body weight)	Infant (% body weight)
Total Body Water	60 ± 15	50 ± 15	80
Intracellular	45	40	50
Extracellular	15-20	15-20	30
Interstitial	11-15	11-15	24
Intravascular	4.5	4.5	5.0

Table 11-4 ▶▶ Daily Water Exchange

Regulation	Average Daily Volume (mL)	Maximum Daily Volume
Water Losses		
Insensible		
Skin	700	1500 mL
Lung	200	
Sensible		
Urine	1000-1200	2000+ mL/hr
Intestinal	200	8000 mL
Sweat	0	2000+ mL/hr
Water Gain		
Ingestion		
Fluids	1500-2000	1500 mL/hr
Solids	500-600	1500 mL/hr
Body metabolism	250	1000 mL

increased ventilation also have increased water losses through increased evaporation from the respiratory tract. Patients with artificial airways are prone to evaporative water loss if inspired air is not adequately humidified. Artificial airways bypass the normal heat and water exchange processes of the nose (see Chapter 7). The lower airway must make up the difference between the low water content of inspired air and the saturated conditions in the lung. This difference, called the **humidity deficit**, can result in large evaporative water losses. A patient with a tracheostomy may lose an additional 700 mL of water per day if humidification is inadequate. Water loss can be minimized by providing adequate humidification to the inspired air (see Chapter 32).

Infants have a greater proportion of body water than do adults, particularly in the extracellular compartments (see Table 11-3). Water loss in infants may be twice that of adults. Infants also have a greater body surface area (in proportion to body volume) than adults, making their basal heat production twice as high. Higher metabolic rates in infants necessitate greater urinary excretion. Infants turn over approximately half of their extracellular fluid volume daily; adults turn over approximately one seventh. Fluid loss or lack of intake can rapidly deplete an infant of water.

Water Replacement. Water is replenished in two major ways: ingestion and metabolism (see Table 11-4).

Ingestion. Water is replaced mainly by ingestion, through the consumption of liquids. The average adult drinks 1500 to 2000 mL of water per day. Another 500 to 600 mL of water are ingested from solid food.

Metabolism. Water also is gained from the oxidation of fats, carbohydrates, and proteins in the body. The destruction of cells also releases some water. During total starvation, 2000 mL of water can be produced daily by the metabolism of 1 kg of fat. Recovery after surgery or trauma may be similar to starvation. Under such conditions, approximately 500 mg of protein and a similar amount of fat are metabolized. This yields approximately 1 L of water per day.

Transport Between Compartments

Homeostasis depends largely on the total volume of body fluids and on fluid transport between body compartments.

The first stage of homeostasis is fluid exchange between systemic capillaries and interstitial fluid by passive diffusion. Capillary walls are permeable to crystalline electrolytes. This allows equilibrium between the two extracellular compartments to occur quickly. Plasma, except for the large protein molecules, can also move through capillary walls into the tissue spaces.

Movement of fluid and solutes from capillary blood to interstitial spaces is enhanced by the difference in **hydrostatic pressure** between compartments. Hydrostatic pressure difference depends on blood pressure, blood volume, and the vertical distance of the capillary from the heart (i.e., the effect of gravity). Hydrostatic pressure tends to cause fluid to leak out of capillaries into the interstitial spaces.

Osmotic pressure differences between interstitial and intravascular compartments oppose hydrostatic pressure. Proteins in colloidal suspension in the plasma cause this difference in osmotic pressure. Proteins such as albumin are too large to pass through the pores of the capillary. Instead, these proteins remain in the intravascular compartment and exert osmotic pressure, which draws water and small solute molecules back into the capillaries.

For example, in a typical capillary, blood pressure is approximately 30 mm Hg at the arterial end and approximately 20 mm Hg at the venous end (Figure 11-6). Colloid osmotic pressure of the intravascular fluid remains constant at approximately 25 mm Hg. Hydrostatic pressure along the capillary continually decreases. At the arterial end, hydrostatic pressure normally exceeds osmotic pressure and water flows out of the vascular space into the interstitial space. At the venous end, colloidal osmotic pressure exceeds hydrostatic forces. Water is pulled back into the vascular compartment.

The outflow of water and electrolytes from the capillary at the arterial end is not completely balanced by the return on the venous end. Slightly more water diffuses out than is reabsorbed. This slight outward excess is balanced by fluid return through the lymphatic circulation. Fluid return by lymphatic channels also depends on pressure differences. The pressure in the interstitial space is determined by the volume of interstitial fluid and its electrolyte content. Interstitial fluid moves from a region of higher pressure (the interstitial space) to a region of lower pressure (the lymphatic channels). This lymph moves into larger lymphatic spaces, where the pressure is continuously decreasing.

These relationships may be expressed by the Starling equilibrium equation:

$$Q_f = K_1(P_{ch} - P_{ih}) - K_2(P_{co} - P_{io})$$

where:

Q_f = Bulk flow of fluid between intravascular and interstitial compartments

P_{ch} = Capillary hydrostatic pressure

P_{ih} = Interstitial fluid hydrostatic pressure

P_{co} = Capillary osmotic pressure

P_{io} = Interstitial osmotic pressure

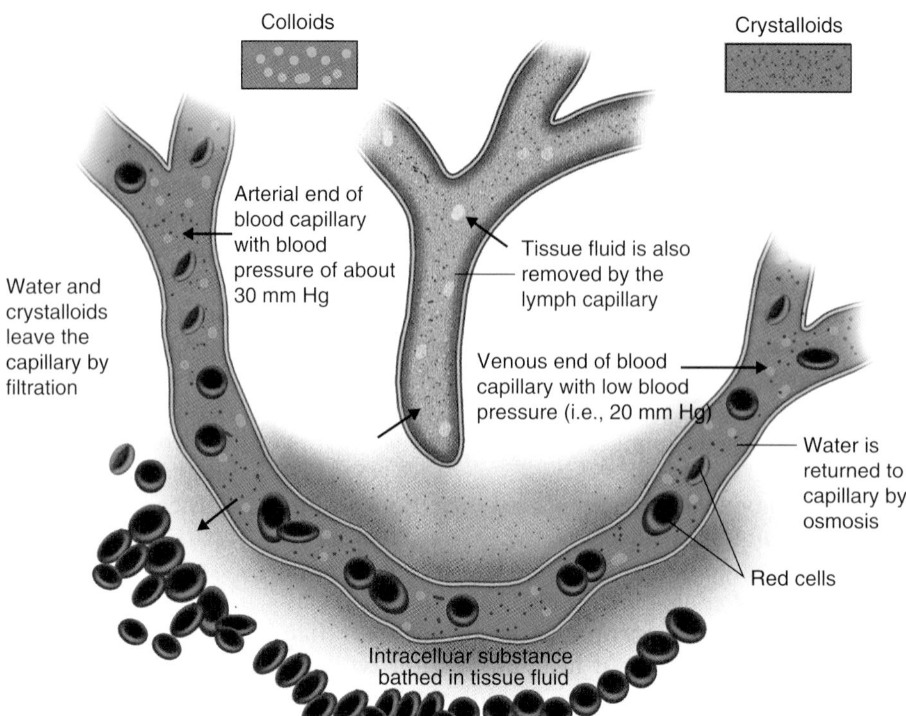

Figure 11-6

Tissue fluid is formed by a process of filtration at the arterial end of the blood capillary *(left)*, where blood pressure exceeds colloid osmotic pressure. The fluid is absorbed by the blood capillaries and lymphatic vessels. It will return to the venous end of the capillary *(right)* when colloid osmotic pressure exceeds blood pressure. Fluid is absorbed into the lymphatic capillary system when interstitial fluid pressure is greater than the pressure within the lymphatic capillary. Normally, little colloid escapes from the blood capillary. Colloid that does escape is returned to the blood circulation by the lymphatic vessels. *(Modified from Burke SR: The composition and function of body fluids, ed 3, St Louis, 1980, Mosby.)*

K_1 = Capillary permeability coefficient for fluids and electrolytes

K_2 = Capillary permeability coefficient for proteins

Three examples of the forces in this equation are fluid return from gravity-dependent areas of the body, fluid exchange in the lung, and tissue **edema**.

Because of hydrostatic effects, capillary pressure in the feet can be as high as 100 mm Hg when an individual is standing. Reabsorption of tissue fluid can be accomplished although hydrostatic pressure greatly exceeds colloidal osmotic pressure. Three factors favor reabsorption under these circumstances. First, high intravascular hydrostatic pressure is somewhat balanced by a proportionally greater interstitial pressure. Second, the "pumping" action of the skeletal muscles surrounding leg veins lowers venous pressures. Third, lymph flow back to the thorax is enhanced by a similar mechanism. This facilitates clearance of excess interstitial fluid.

The lungs present a somewhat different situation. In systemic tissues, a constant exchange of interstitial fluid is essential. In the lungs, the alveoli must be kept relatively dry. Otherwise, interstitial fluid in the alveolar-capillary spaces would impede the diffusion of gas. Colloid osmotic pressure in pulmonary blood vessels is the same as it is in the systemic circulation. To minimize interstitial fluid in the alveolar-capillary region, the hydrostatic pressure difference must be kept low. The pulmonary circulation is in fact a low-pressure system. The mean pulmonary vascular pressures are approximately one sixth of those in the systemic circulation. Colloid osmotic pressure exceeds hydrostatic forces across the entire length of the pulmonary capillaries in healthy individuals. Therefore the alveoli are relatively free of excess interstitial water.

If hydrostatic pressure increases in the pulmonary circulation, this balance can be upset. This causes fluid movement into the alveolar-capillary spaces. Excess fluid in the interstitial space is called *edema*. In the lungs, edema caused by increased hydrostatic pressure often is a result of backpressure from a failing left ventricle (e.g., in congestive heart failure).

Edema can be caused by other factors. The Starling equilibrium equation shows that edema can be caused by a decrease in colloid osmotic pressure or an increase in capillary permeability. For example, if albumin is depleted in the blood, the balance of forces is upset, favoring increased movement of fluid into the interstitium. Likewise, an increase in the capillary permeability results in more fluid leaving the capillaries. Increased capillary permeability is a major factor in certain types of acute lung injuries (see Chapter 24).

Electrolytes

Electrolytes in the various body fluids are not passive solutes. They maintain the internal environment while making essential chemical and physiological events possible. There are seven major electrolytes: sodium, chloride, bicarbonate, potassium, calcium, magnesium, and phosphorus (phosphate).

Sodium (Na^+)

Regulation of sodium concentration in plasma and urine is related to regulation of total body water. Fifty percent of the total body stores of sodium are extracellular. The remainder is found in bone (40%) and in cells (10%). The normal serum concentration of sodium ranges from 136 to 145 mEq/L. In cells, the sodium concentration is much lower, averaging only 4.5 mEq/L.

The average adult ingests and excretes approximately 100 mEq of sodium every 24 hours. Children require approximately half this amount, and infants typically exchange 20 mEq of sodium per day. Most sodium is reabsorbed through the kidney. Approximately 80% of the body's sodium is reclaimed passively in the proximal tubules. The remainder is actively reabsorbed in the distal tubules. Sodium reabsorption in the kidneys is governed mainly by the level of aldosterone, which is secreted by the adrenal cortex. Na^+ reabsorption in the distal tubules of the kidney occurs in exchange for other cations. Sodium balance is involved in acid-base homeostasis (i.e., H^+ exchange) and the regulation of potassium (K^+). Abnormal losses of sodium may occur for a number of reasons, as shown in Table 11-5.

Chloride (Cl–)

Chloride is the most prominent anion in the body. Two thirds of the body's store of chloride is extracellular. The remainder is intracellular. Intracellular chloride is present in significant amounts in red and white blood cells. It also is present in cells that have excretory functions, such as the GI mucosa.

Normal serum levels of chloride (Cl^-) range between 98 and 106 mEq/L. The concentration of extracellular

Table 11-5 ▶▶▶ Electrolyte Disorders and Clinical Findings

Electrolyte	Imbalance	Causes	Symptoms
Sodium (Na^+)	**Hyponatremia**	Gastrointestinal loss, sweating, fever, diuretics, ascites, congestive heart failure, kidney failure	Weaknesses, lassitude, apathy, headache, orthostatic hypotension, tachycardia
	Hypernatremia	Net sodium gain, net water loss, increased aldosterone, steroid therapy	Tremulousness, irritability, ataxia, confusion, seizures, coma
Chloride (Cl^-)	**Hypochloremia**	Gastrointestinal loss, diuretics	Metabolic alkalosis, muscle spasm, coma (severe cases)
	Hyperchloremia	Dehydration, metabolic acidosis, respiratory alkalosis	(Minimal)
Potassium (K^+)	**Hypokalemia**	Diuretics, steroid therapy, renal tubular disease, vomiting, diarrhea, malnutrition, trauma	Muscle weakness, paralysis, ECG abnormalities, supraventricular arrhythmias, circulatory failure, cardiac arrest
	Hyperkalemia	Chronic renal disease, hemorrhage, tissue necrosis, nonsteroidal antiinflammatory drugs, ACE inhibitors, cyclosporine, K^+-sparing diuretics	ECG changes, ventricular arrhythmias, cardiac arrest
Calcium (Ca^{2+})	**Hypocalcemia**	Hyperparathyroidism, pancreatitis, renal failure, trauma	Hyperactive tendon reflexes, muscle twitching, spasm, abdominal cramps, ECG changes, convulsions (rarely)
	Hypercalcemia	Hyperthyroidism, hyperparathyroidism, metastatic bone cancer, sarcoidosis	Fatigue, depression, muscle weakness, anorexia, nausea, vomiting, constipation
Magnesium (Mg^{2+})	**Hypomagnesemia**	Inadequate intake/impaired absorption of Mg^{2+}, pancreatitis, alcoholism	Muscle weakness, irritability, tetany, ECG changes, arrhythmias, delirium, convulsions
	Hypermagnesemia	Dehydration, renal insufficiency, tissue trauma, lupus erythematosus	ECG changes (along with hyperkalemia, cardiac arrest, respiratory muscle paralysis)
Phosphate (HPO_4^{2-})	**Hypophosphatemia**	Starvation, malabsorption, hyperparathyroidism, hyperthyroidism, uncontrolled diabetes mellitus	Diaphragmatic weakness
	Hyperphosphatemia	Endocrine disorders, acromagaly, chronic renal insufficiency, acute renal failure, tissue trauma	(Minimal)

ACE, Angiotensin-converting enzyme; *ECG*, electrocardiogram.

MINI CLINI

Water, Salt, and Congestive Heart Failure

PROBLEM

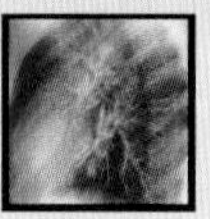

Why do patients who have congestive heart failure (CHF) need to adhere to a low-salt diet?

SOLUTION

CHF occurs when the left ventricle cannot pump all of the blood presented to it. This leads to pooling of blood in the lungs and venous circulation and an increase in peripheral venous pressure. Normally, the ventricle pumps the majority of the blood entering it. This volume is the "preload" of the heart. The volume of extracellular water partially determines the preload of the ventricle.

The ventricle can fail as a pump either because of intrinsic heart disease, such as infarction or ischemia, or because of elevated distal pressures against which it must pump (hypertension). In addition to pooling of blood in the systemic venous circulation, blood also can back up in the lungs, resulting in congestion and edema.

The most important determinant of the extracellular water volume is its sodium (Na^+) content. Changes in extracellular water are dictated by the net gain or loss of sodium, with an accompanying gain or loss of water. To reduce the work of the heart, fluid volume must be carefully regulated. By restricting salt intake, extracellular fluid volume can be reduced, allowing the heart to function more effectively as a pump. Treatment of CHF must address not only excess fluid volume but also the underlying cause.

Diuretics are often used to help reduce fluid volume. Many diuretics cause the kidney to excrete sodium, causing water to follow and reducing the extracellular fluid load. Because some diuretics also cause potassium (K^+) to be excreted, care must be taken in the management of CHF not to cause electrolyte imbalances. Potassium supplements may be used so that diuresis does not result in hypokalemia. Because of the central role of extracellular water in CHF, weighing the patient is a simple yet sensitive means of detecting excess fluid volume.

chloride is inversely proportional to that of the other major anion, bicarbonate (HCO_3^-). Cl- is regulated by the kidney in much the same manner as Na+ (80% reabsorbed in the proximal tubules and 20% reabsorbed in the distal tubules). Chloride is usually excreted with potassium in the form of KCl. Thus an imbalance in one of these electrolytes usually affects both. Replacement therapy usually includes both K^+ and Cl^-. The stomach and the small bowel also affect the balance of Cl^-, and sweat contains hypotonic quantities of chloride. Abnormal chloride levels may occur for a variety of reasons (see Table 11-5).

Bicarbonate (HCO_3^-)

Next to chloride, bicarbonate (HCO_3^-) is the most important body fluid anion. It plays an important role in acid-base homeostasis and is the strong base in the bicarbonate-carbonic acid buffer pair (see Chapter 12). HCO_3^- is the primary means for transporting carbon dioxide from the tissues to the lungs. The ratio of HCO_3^- to carbonic acid in healthy individuals is maintained near 20:1. This results in a pH of close to 7.40. Bicarbonate stores are evenly divided between intracellular and extracellular compartments. Normal serum HCO_3^- levels in arterial blood range from 22 to 26 mEq/L. Bicarbonate levels are slightly higher in venous blood as CO_2 is being transported to the lungs.

In acid-base disorders, the kidneys regulate bicarbonate levels to maintain a near normal pH. In healthy individuals, more than 80% of blood HCO_3^- is reabsorbed in the proximal tubules of the kidney. The remainder is reclaimed in the distal tubules. In respiratory acidosis, the kidneys retain or produce HCO_3^- to buffer the additional acid caused by CO_2 retention. In respiratory alkalosis, the opposite occurs. A reciprocal relationship exists between Cl^- and HCO_3^- concentrations. Bicarbonate retention is associated with chloride excretion, and vice versa (see Chapter 12).

Potassium (K^+)

Potassium is the main cation of the intracellular compartment. Most of the body's K^+ (98%) is found in cells. **Active transport** of K^+ into the cells occurs through an ionic pump mechanism. An electrical differential across the cell membrane also facilitates K^+ movement into the cell. For every three K^+ ions that enter a cell, two Na^+ ions and one H^+ ion must leave. This transfer maintains electrical neutrality in the cell.

The difference in K^+ distribution is evident when comparing concentrations between fluid compartments. Intracellular K^+ concentration is approximately 150 mEq/L, whereas serum K^+ concentration normally ranges between only 3.5 and 5.0 mEq/L. Serum K^+ is only an indirect indicator of the total body potassium. Serum potassium is usually analyzed by assessing both its intake and excretion.

The average adult excretes 40 to 75 mEq of potassium in the urine every 24 hours. An additional 10 mEq is excreted in the stool. The average dietary intake of potassium is 50 to 85 mEq/day. Patients who have undergone surgery, have sustained trauma, or have renal disease often have greater K^+ losses. Consequently, they need K^+ replacement averaging 100 to 120 mEq/day.

Serum K^+ concentration is determined primarily by the pH of extracellular fluid and the size of the intracellular K^+ pool. In extracellular acidosis, excess H^+ ions are exchanged for intracellular K^+. Movement of K^+ from intracellular to extracellular spaces may produce dangerous levels of hyperkalemia. Alkalosis has just the opposite effect. When pH rises, K+ moves into cells. In the absence of acid-base disturbances, serum K^+ reflects total body potassium. With excessive loss of K^+ from the GI tract, serum K^+ falls. A 10% loss of total body K^+ drops the serum K^+ level approximately 1 mEq/L.

Renal excretion of K^+ is controlled by aldosterone levels. Aldosterone inhibits the enzyme responsible for K^+ transport in the distal renal tubular cells of the kidney. Metabolic acidosis also inhibits the transport system. Na^+ and H^+ ions enter cells at the expense of increased K^+ excretion. Alkalosis has the reverse effect. It stimulates cellular retention of potassium. Kidney failure results in potassium retention and hyperkalemia.

Hypokalemia disturbs cellular function in a number of organ systems. These include the GI, neuromuscular, renal, and cardiovascular systems (see Table 11-5). Management of hypokalemia involves replacement of K+ losses and treatment of the underlying disorder. To manage the associated Cl^- deficit, K^+ is given with Cl^-. Caution is required in the administration of intravenous K^+, because cardiac muscle is very sensitive to extracellular concentrations of this electrolyte.

Hyperkalemia is most common in renal insufficiency (see Table 11-5). The primary treatment of hyperkalemia is restriction of K^+ intake. The processes that precipitated the hyperkalemia also must be controlled. Temporary measures for reducing serum K^+ levels include administration of insulin, calcium gluconate, sodium salts, or large volumes of hypertonic glucose. Cation exchange resins may be given orally or rectally. If these measures fail, peritoneal or renal dialysis can aid in K^+ removal.

Calcium

Calcium is an important mediator of neuromuscular function and cell enzyme processes. Most of the body's calcium is contained in the bones. The normal serum calcium is 9.0 to 10.5 mg/L, or 4.5 to 5.25 mEq/L. This concentration is maintained by substances such as vitamin D and parathyroid hormone.

Calcium is present in the blood in the following three forms: ionized, protein bound, and complex. The proportion of calcium in each form is affected by blood pH, concentration of plasma proteins, and presence of calcium-combining anions (e.g., HCO_3^- and HPO_4^{2-}). Approximately 50% of serum calcium is not ionized and is bound to plasma albumin. Another 5% forms calcium anion complexes. The remaining 45% is ionized Ca^{2+}. Ionized calcium is physiologically active in processes such as enzyme activity, blood clotting, neuromuscular irritability, and bone calcification. Acidemia increases, and alkalemia decreases, the concentration of Ca^{2+} in the serum.

Abnormal levels of calcium can cause a range of serious symptoms (see Table 11-5). Treatment of **hypocalcemia** consists of correcting the underlying cause and replacing Ca^{2+}, either orally or intravenously. Acute **hypercalcemia** requires emergency treatment because death may occur quickly if serum Ca^{2+} rises higher than 17 mg/L (8.5 mEq/L). In such cases, there is usually an associated deficit of extracellular fluid. Volume replacement lowers serum Ca^{2+} by dilution. Steroids and chelating agents, such as EDTA,* are sometimes helpful in lowering serum calcium.

Magnesium

Magnesium is an important electrolyte for muscle function. It also is related to neural conduction, particularly in the cardiac conduction system (see Table 11-5). Normal values for serum Mg^{2+} range from 1.3 to 2.1 mEq/L in healthy adults. Serum levels of magnesium may remain normal even if total body stores are depleted by up to 20%. Fatty acids and excess phosphates impair magnesium uptake. At least 65% to 70% of Mg^{2+} is in a diffusible state. Approximately 35% of serum magnesium is bound to proteins.

Phosphorus

Approximately 80% of body phosphorus is contained in bones and teeth. Of this, 10% is combined with proteins, carbohydrates, and lipids in muscle tissue and blood, and the remainder is incorporated into complex organic compounds. Organic phosphate (HPO_4^{2-}) is the main anion within cells. Inorganic phosphate plays a primary role in the metabolism of cellular energy, being the source from which adenosine triphosphate is synthesized. In acid-base homeostasis, phosphate is the main urinary buffer for titratable acid excretion (see Chapter 12). The serum phosphate level (1.2 to 2.3 mEq/L) is only an approximate indicator of total body phosphorus. Serum phosphate levels are influenced by several factors (see Table 11-5), including the serum calcium concentration and the pH of blood.

*Ethylenediaminetetraacetic acid

KEY POINTS

- The body is a water-based organism in which chemical substances and particles exist in solution or suspension.
- The concentration of solutes in a solution may be quantified (1) by actual weight (grams or milligrams) or (2) by chemical combining power (equivalents or milliequivalents). The weight of a solute does not necessarily give an indication of its chemical combining power, but gram equivalent weights do.
- Solutions involve the action of osmotic pressure. Body cell walls are semipermeable membranes, and osmotic pressure maintains the distribution of water in physiological ranges.
- Concentrations of solutions may be calculated using ratio, weight/volume, or percent methods. These techniques are useful in the preparation of medications and therapeutic fluids.
- Physiologically active compounds in the body are mostly weak electrolytic covalent substances. In aqueous solutions, some molecules ionize, leaving the remainder intact. Equilibrium is maintained between the ions and un-ionized molecules.
- Proteins made up of amino acids can function as bases in the mildly alkaline environment of the body. This makes hemoglobin and plasma proteins excellent buffers.
- Acidity or alkalinity is determined by variation of $[H^+]$ above or below 1×10^{-7} mol/L. Two methods for recording acidity or alkalinity use H^+ concentration of water as the neutral standard: (1) the actual measured molar concentration of H^+ in nanomoles per liter and (2) the logarithmic pH scale.
- Water makes up 45% to 80% of an individual's body weight. Percentage of total body water depends on weight, gender, and age. Total body water is divided into intracellular and extracellular water. Extracellular water is further divided into intravascular and interstitial water.
- Control of total body water is regulated by water intake and excretion. The kidneys maintain the volume and composition of body fluids by two related mechanisms: (1) filtration and reabsorption of sodium and (2) regulation of water excretion in response to changes in secretion of ADH.
- A balance between hydrostatic and osmotic pressure keeps water in the appropriate body compartments. Plasma proteins account for the high colloid osmotic pressure of plasma. Colloid osmotic pressure determines distribution of fluid between vascular and interstitial compartments. Imbalances in osmotic and hydrostatic pressures can result in edema.
- Electrolytes help maintain the internal environment and make important chemical and physiological events possible. The concentrations of electrolytes in the intracellular and extracellular fluid compartments differ markedly. Sodium, chloride, bicarbonate, potassium, calcium, magnesium, and phosphorus are essential to homeostasis. Increased or decreased concentrations of any of these can result in disease and sometimes death.

Bibliography

Abraham WT, Schrier RW: Body fluid volume regulation in health and disease, Adv Intern Med 39:23, 1994.

Arsenian MA: Magnesium and cardiovascular disease, Prog Cardiovasc Dis 35:271, 1993.

Gettes LS: Electrolyte abnormalities underlying lethal and ventricular arrhythmias, Circulation 85(Suppl):I70, 1992.

Grobbee DE: Electrolytes and hypertension: results from recent studies, Am J Med Sci 307(Suppl 1):S17, 1994.

Laski ME, Kurtzman NA: Acid-base disorders in medicine, Dis Mon 42:51, 1996.

Leier CR, Dei Cas L, Metra M: Clinical relevance and management of the major electrolyte abnormalities in congestive heart failure: hyponatremia, hypokalemia, and hypomagnesia, Am Heart J 128:564, 1994.

Keyes JL: Fluid, electrolyte, and acid-base regulation, 2000, iUniverse.com.

Martin GS: Fluid balance and colloid osmotic pressure in acute respiratory failure: emerging clinical evidence, Crit Care, 4(Suppl 2):S21, 2000.

McPherson RA: Tietz clinical guide to laboratory tests, ed 4, Philadelphia, 2001, WB Saunders.

Metheny NM: Fluid and electrolyte balance: nursing considerations, ed 4, Philadelphia, 2000, Lippincott Williams & Wilkins.

Oster JR, Preston RA, Materson BJ: Fluid and electrolyte disorders in congestive heart failure, Semin Nephrol 14:485, 1994.

Plante GE et al: Disorders of body fluid balance: a new look into the mechanisms of disease, Can J Cardiol 11:788, 1995.

Puschett JB: Disorders of fluid and electrolyte balance: diagnosis and management, New York, 1985, Churchill-Livingstone.

Rasool A, Palevsky PM: Treatment of edematous disorders with diuretics, Am J Med Sci, 319:25, 2000.

Sica DA: Renal disease, electrolyte abnormalities, and acid-base imbalance in the elderly, Clin Geriatr Med 10:197, 1994.

Terry J: The major electrolytes: sodium, potassium, and chloride, J Intraven Nurs 17:240, 1994.

Webster PO: Electrolyte balance in heart failure and the role for magnesium ions, Am J Cardiol 70:44S, 1992.

Wierner-Kronish JP, Broaddus VC: Interrelationships of pleural and pulmonary interstitial liquid, Annu Rev Physiol 55:209, 1993.

Williams ME: Endocrine crises: hyperkalemia, Crit Care Clin 7:155, 1991.

Williamson JC: Acid-base disorders: classification and management strategies, Am Fam Physician 52:584, 1995.

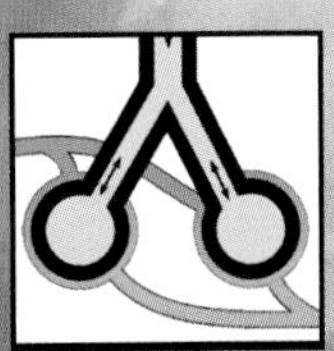

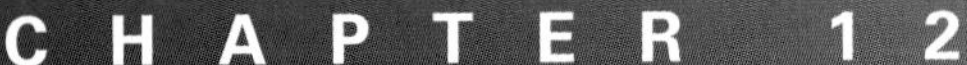

Acid-Base Balance

Will Beachey

In This Chapter You Will Learn:

- How the lungs and kidneys regulate volatile and fixed acids
- How an acid's equilibrium constant is related to its ionization and strength
- What constitutes open and closed buffer systems
- Why open and closed buffer systems differ in their ability to buffer fixed and volatile acids
- How to use the Henderson-Hasselbalch equation in hypothetical clinical situations
- How the kidneys and lungs compensate for each other when the function of one is abnormal
- How renal absorption and excretion of electrolytes affect acid-base balance
- How to classify and interpret arterial blood acid-base status
- How to use arterial acid-base information to decide on a clinical course of action
- Why acute changes in the blood's carbon dioxide level affect the blood's bicarbonate ion concentration
- How to calculate the anion gap and use it to determine the cause of metabolic acidosis
- How standard bicarbonate and base excess measurements are used to identify the nonrespiratory component of acid-base imbalances

Chapter Outline

Key Terms

acidemia
alkalemia
anion gap
base excess (BE)
buffer base
closed buffer system

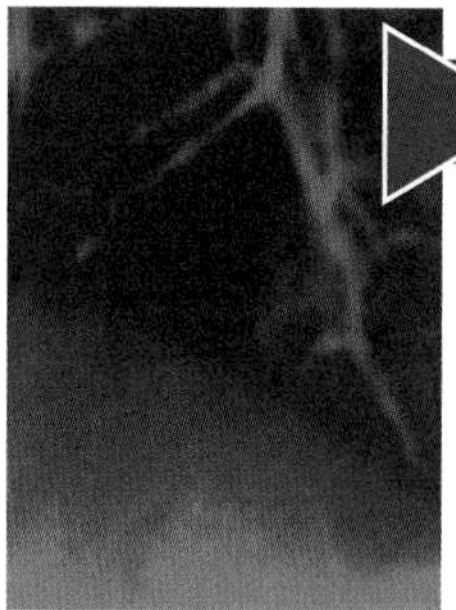

Key Terms—cont'd

conjugate base
equilibrium constant
fixed acids
Henderson-Hasselbalch (H-H) equation
hyperventilation
hypoventilation
isohydric buffering
Kussmaul's respiration
metabolic acidosis
metabolic alkalosis
open buffer system
reabsorption
respiratory acidosis
respiratory alkalosis
standard bicarbonate
volatile acids

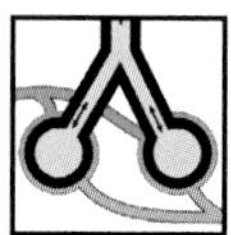

The body's metabolic processes continually generate hydrogen ions; thus their regulation is of utmost biological importance. Even small hydrogen ion concentration changes can cause vital metabolic processes to fail. Various physiological mechanisms work together to keep the hydrogen ion concentration of body fluids in a range that is compatible with life. This chapter helps the clinician understand how these mechanisms work and how to detect abnormalities in their function. With this knowledge, the clinician can make informed decisions about treating the underlying causes of acid-base disturbances.

HYDROGEN ION REGULATION IN BODY FLUIDS

Acid-base balance refers to physiological mechanisms that keep the hydrogen concentration of body fluids in a range that is compatible with life. Hydrogen ions react readily with the protein molecules of vital cellular catalytic enzymes. Such reactions change the protein molecule's shape and may render the enzyme inactive. To sustain life, the body must maintain the pH of fluids within a narrow range, from 7.35 to 7.45 ($[H^+]$ of 45 to 35 nmol/L).

Hydrogen ions formed in the body come from either *volatile* or *fixed* (nonvolatile) acids. **Volatile acids** in the blood arise from and are in equilibrium with a dissolved gas. The only volatile acid of physiological significance in the body is carbonic acid (H_2CO_3), in equilibrium with dissolved CO_2. Normal aerobic metabolism generates approximately 13,000 mmol/L of CO_2 each day, producing an equal amount of H^+:

$$\begin{array}{l} CO_2 + H_2O \longrightarrow H_2CO_3 \longrightarrow HCO_3^- + H^+ \\ \uparrow \\ \text{Aerobic metabolism} \end{array}$$

In a process called **isohydric buffering**,[1] most of the H^+ produced causes no change in pH at the tissue level, because newly forming deoxygenated hemoglobin immediately combines with it. When blood reaches the lungs, hemoglobin releases hydrogen ions to form CO_2 as shown:

$$\begin{array}{l} \text{Ventilation} \\ \uparrow \\ CO_2 + H_2O \longleftarrow H_2CO_3 \longleftarrow HCO_3^- + H^+ \\ \hfill \uparrow \\ \hfill HHb \longrightarrow H^+ + Hb^- \end{array}$$

In this way, ventilation eliminates carbonic acid, keeping pace with its production. Isohydric buffering and ventilation are the two major mechanisms responsible for maintaining a stable pH in the face of massive CO_2 production.[1]

Catabolism of proteins continually produces **fixed acids** such as sulfuric and phosphoric acids. In addition, anaerobic metabolism produces lactic acid. Unlike carbonic acid, these fixed acids are nonvolatile and are not in equilibrium with a gaseous component. Therefore the H^+ of fixed acids must be buffered by bases in the body or eliminated in the urine by the kidneys. Compared with daily CO_2 production, fixed acid production is small, averaging only approximately 50 to 70 milliequivalents (mEq) per day.[2] Certain diseases, such as untreated diabetes, increase fixed acid production. H^+ ions so produced stimulate respiratory centers in the brain. The resulting increase in ventilation eliminates more CO_2, pulling the hydration reaction to the left:

$$\begin{array}{l} \text{Increased } \dot{V}_A \\ \uparrow \\ CO_2 + H_2O \longleftarrow H_2CO_3 \longleftarrow HCO_3^- + H^+ \\ \hfill \uparrow \\ \hfill \text{Fixed acid } H^+ \end{array}$$

In this way, the respiratory system compensates for fixed acid accumulation, preventing a significant increase in $[H^+]$.

Strong and Weak Acids and Bases: Equilibrium Constants

Strong acids and bases ionize almost completely in an aqueous solution. Weak acids and bases ionize only to a small extent. An example of a strong acid is hydrochloric acid. Nearly 100% of the HCl molecules dissociate to form H^+ and Cl^-:

(1) $$HCl \longrightarrow H^+ + Cl^-$$

At *equilibrium,* the concentration of HCl is extremely small, compared with either $[H^+]$ or $[Cl^-]$. There is no arrow pointing to the left in reaction (1), emphasizing that HCl ionizes almost totally in solution.

In contrast, carbonic acid is an example of a relatively weak acid:

(2) $$H_2CO_3 \underset{\rightarrow}{\longleftarrow} HCO_3^- + H^+$$

The long arrow pointing to the left indicates that at *equilibrium* the concentration of undissociated H_2CO_3 molecules is far greater than that of HCO_3^- or H^+.

The **equilibrium constant** of an acid is a measure of the extent to which the acid molecules dissociate (ionize). At equilibrium, the number of dissociating H_2CO_3 molecules in reaction (2) is equal to the number of associating HCO_3^- and H^+ ions, even though the concentrations of reactants and products are unequal. In this state, no further change will occur in $[H_2CO_3]$, $[HCO_3^-]$, or $[H^+]$. Therefore at equilibrium the following is true:

(3) $$\frac{[HCO_3^-] \times [H^+]}{[H_2CO_3]} = K_A \textit{ (Small)}$$

where K_A is the equilibrium constant for H_2CO_3. (K_A is also known as the acid's *ionization* or *dissociation* constant.)

The K_A is small because the H_2CO_3 concentration is quite large with respect to the numerator of reaction (3). The value of K_A is always the same for H_2CO_3, regardless of its initial concentration.

A strong acid, such as HCl, has a *large* K_A because the denominator [HCl] is extremely small, compared with the numerator ($[H^+] \times [Cl^-]$):

(4) $$\frac{[H^+] \times [Cl^-]}{[HCl]} = K_A \text{ (Large)}$$

As shown by equations (3) and (4), K_A indicates an acid's strength.

Buffer Solution Characteristics

A buffer solution resists changes in pH when an acid or a base is added to it. Buffer solutions are mixtures of acids and bases. The acid component is the H^+ cation, formed when a weak acid dissociates in solution. The base component is the remaining anion portion of the acid molecule, known as the conjugate base. An important blood buffer system is a solution of carbonic acid and its conjugate base, bicarbonate ion (HCO_3^-):

$$H_2CO_3 \text{ (Acid)} \underset{\rightarrow}{\longleftarrow} HCO_3 \text{ (Conjugate base)} + H^+$$

In the blood, bicarbonate ions (HCO_3^-) combine with sodium ions (Na^+) to form sodium bicarbonate ($NaHCO_3$). If hydrogen chloride, a strong acid, is added to the $H_2CO_3/NaHCO_3$ buffer solution, bicarbonate ions react with the added hydrogen ions to form more weak carbonic acid molecules and a neutral salt:

$$HCl + H_2CO_3/Na^+HCO_3^- \longrightarrow 2H_2CO_3 + NaCl$$

The strong acidity of HCl is converted to the relatively weak acidity of H_2CO_3, preventing a large decrease in pH.

Similarly, if sodium hydroxide, a strong base, is added to this buffer solution, it reacts with the carbonic acid molecule to form the weak base, sodium bicarbonate, and water:

$$NaOH + H_2CO_3/NaHCO_3 \longrightarrow 2NaHCO_3 + H_2O$$

The strong alkalinity of NaOH is changed to the relatively weak alkalinity of $NaHCO_3$. Again, pH change is minimized.

Bicarbonate and Nonbicarbonate Buffer Systems

Blood buffers are classified as bicarbonate or nonbicarbonate buffer systems. The bicarbonate buffer system consists of carbonic acid (H_2CO_3) and its conjugate base, bicarbonate ion (HCO_3^-). The nonbicarbonate buffer system consists mainly of phosphates and proteins, including hemoglobin. The blood **buffer base** is the sum of bicarbonate and nonbicarbonate bases measured in mmol/L of blood.[3]

The bicarbonate system is an **open buffer system** because H_2CO_3 is in equilibrium with dissolved CO_2, which is readily removed by ventilation. That is, when H^+ is buffered by HCO_3^-, the product, H_2CO_3, is continually broken down into water and carbon dioxide. Ventilation removes carbon dioxide from the reaction, preventing it from reaching equilibrium with the reactants. Therefore buffering activity can continue without being slowed or stopped:

$$HCO_3^- + H^+ \longrightarrow H_2CO_3 \longrightarrow H_2O + CO_2 \text{ (Exhaled gas)}$$

A nonbicarbonate buffer system is a **closed buffer system** because all the components of acid-base reactions remain in the system. (In the following discussions, nonbicarbonate buffer systems are collectively represented as *Hbuf/Buf*$^-$, where *Hbuf* is the weak acid, and *Buf*$^-$ is the conjugate base.)

When H^+ is buffered by Buf^-, the product, HBuf, accumulates and eventually reaches equilibrium with the reactants, preventing further buffering activity:

$$Buf^- + H^+ \leftrightarrow Hbuf$$

Box 12-1 summarizes the characteristics and components of bicarbonate and nonbicarbonate buffer systems.

Open and closed buffer systems differ in their ability to buffer fixed and volatile acids. They also differ in their ability to function in wide-ranging pH environments. Both systems are physiologically important, each playing a unique and essential role in maintaining pH homeostasis. Table 12-1 summarizes the approximate contributions of various blood buffers to the total buffer base. Bicarbonate buffers have the greatest buffering capacity because they function in an open system.

Bicarbonate and nonbicarbonate buffer systems do not function in isolation from one another. They are intermingled in the same solution (whole blood) and are in equilibrium with the same hydrogen ion concentration (Figure 12-1). Increased ventilation increases the CO_2 removal rate, causing nonbicarbonate buffers (Hbuf) to release hydrogen ions. Decreased ventilation ultimately causes Hbuf to accept more hydrogen ions.

pH of a Buffer System: Henderson-Hasselbalch Equation

Buffer solutions in body fluids consist of mostly undissociated acid molecules and only a small amount of H^+

Box 12-1 • Classification of Whole Blood Buffers

OPEN SYSTEM
BICARBONATE
Plasma
Erythrocyte

CLOSED SYSTEM
NONBICARBONATE
Hemoglobin
Organic phosphates
Inorganic phosphates
Plasma proteins

From Beachey W: Respiratory care anatomy and physiology: foundations for clinical practice, St Louis, 1998, Mosby.

Table 12-1 ▶▶ Individual Buffer Contributions to Whole Blood Buffering

Buffer Type	Total Buffering (%)
Bicarbonate	
Plasma bicarbonate	35
Erythrocyte bicarbonate	18
Total Bicarbonate Buffering	53
Nonbicarbonate	
Hemoglobin	35
Organic phosphates	3
Inorganic phosphates	2
Plasma proteins	7
Total Nonbicarbonate Buffering	47
Total	100

From Beachey W: Respiratory care anatomy and physiology: foundations for clinical practice, St Louis, 1998, Mosby.

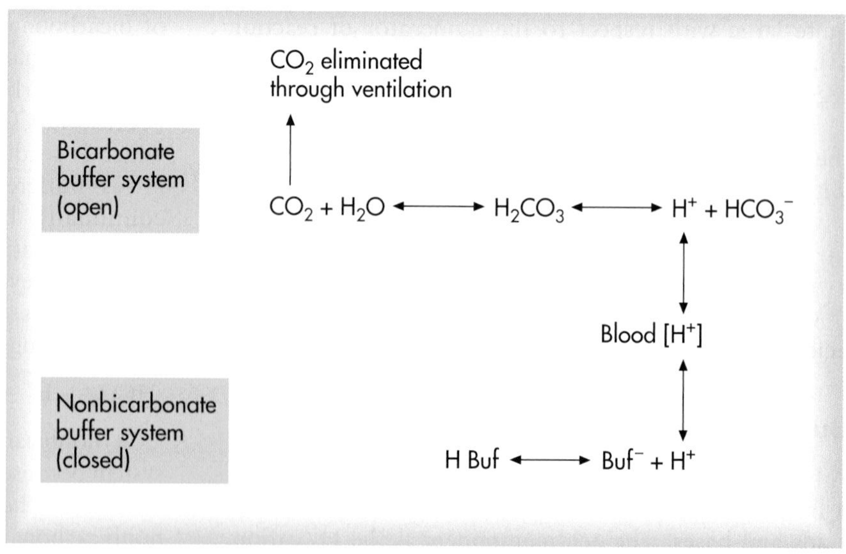

Figure 12-1
The bicarbonate and nonbicarbonate buffer systems exist in equilibrium in the plasma. *(Modified from Beachey W: Respiratory care anatomy and physiology: foundations for clinical practice, St Louis, 1998, Mosby.)*

and conjugate base anions. A buffer solution's hydrogen ion concentration $[H^+]$ can be calculated if the concentrations of the buffer's components and the acid's equilibrium constant are known. Consider the bicarbonate buffer system. As described earlier, the equilibrium constant (K_A) for H_2CO_3 is as follows:

$$K_A = \frac{[H^+] \times [HCO_3^-]}{[H_2CO_3]}$$

$[H^+]$ can be calculated by algebraic rearrangement of this equation, as follows:

$$[H^+] = K_A \times \frac{[H_2CO_3]}{[HCO_3^-]}$$

Thus $[H^+]$ is determined by the ratio between undissociated acid molecules $[H_2CO_3]$ and base anions $[HCO_3^-]$. This equation is the basis for deriving the **Henderson-Hasselbalch (H-H) equation:**

$$pH = 6.1 + \log \frac{[HCO_3^-]}{PCO_2 \times 0.03}$$

pH is a logarithmic expression of $[H^+]$, and the term 6.1 is the logarithmic expression of the H_2CO_3 equilibrium constant. Because dissolved carbon dioxide ($P_{CO_2} \times 0.03$) is in equilibrium with and directly proportional to blood $[H_2CO_3]$, and because blood P_{CO_2} is more easily measured than $[H_2CO_3]$, dissolved CO_2 is used in the denominator of the H-H equation. The H-H equation is specific for calculating the pH of the blood's bicarbonate buffer system. Calculating this pH is important because it equals blood plasma pH. Because all buffer systems in the blood are in equilibrium with the same pH, the pH of one buffer system is the same as the pH of the entire plasma solution (the isohydric principle).[1]

Clinical Use of the Henderson-Hasselbalch Equation

The H-H equation allows the pH, $[HCO_3^-]$, or P_{CO_2} to be computed if two of these three variables are known (shown as follows for P_{CO_2} and HCO_3^-):

$$[HCO_3^-] = \text{antilog } (pH - 6.1) \times (P_{CO_2} \times 0.03)$$

$$P_{CO_2} = \frac{[HCO_3^-]}{(\text{antilog } [pH - 6.1] \times 0.03)}$$

Blood gas analyzers *measure* pH and P_{CO_2}, but *compute* $[HCO_3^-]$. Assuming a normal arterial pH of 7.40 and a Pa_{CO_2} of 40 mm Hg, arterial $[HCO_3^-]$ can be calculated as follows:

$$pH = 6.1 + \log ([HCO_3^-]/[P_{CO_2} \times 0.03])$$

$$7.40 = 6.1 + \log ([HCO_3^-]/[40 \times 0.03])$$

$$7.40 = 6.1 + \log ([HCO_3^-])/1.2)$$

Solving for $[HCO_3^-]$:

$$[HCO_3^-] = \text{antilog } (7.40 - 6.1) \times 1.2$$

$$= \text{antilog } (1.3) \times 1.2$$

$$= 20 \times 1.2$$

$$= 24 \text{ mEq/L}$$

MINI CLINI

Applying the Henderson-Hasselbalch Equation Clinically

PROBLEM

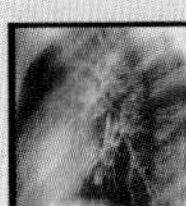

The respiratory therapist (RT) is caring for a patient who is being mechanically ventilated. The patient has a tidal volume (V_T) of 800 mL at a frequency of 10/min, yielding a minute ventilation ($\dot{V}_E$) of 8 L/min. The patient's Pa_{CO_2} is 55 mm Hg, the pH is 7.30, and the bicarbonate is 26 mEq/L, and he wishes to maintain a pH of 7.35. How much does he need to change the Pa_{CO_2} to achieve this desired pH, and what change in the patient's V_T does the require?

SOLUTION

First, the RT needs to calculate the Pa_{CO_2} required to achieve a pH of 7.35 using the known values:

$$Pa_{CO_2} = \frac{26 \text{ mEq/L}}{0.03 \times \text{antilog } (7.35 - 6.1)}$$

$$Pa_{CO_2} = \frac{26}{0.53}$$

$$Pa_{CO_2} = 49 \text{ mm Hg}$$

Next, he must calculate the $\dot{V}_E$ required to produce a Pa_{CO_2} of 49 mm Hg. Because $\dot{V}_E$ is inversely proportional to Pa_{CO_2}, the following can be stated:

$$(\dot{V}_E)_1 \times (Pa_{CO_2}) = (\dot{V}_E)2 \times (Pa_{CO_2})_2$$

where 1 and 2 represent current and future values respectively. The RT then solves for $(\dot{V}_E)_2$ as follows:

$$(8 \text{ L/min}) \times 55 \text{ mm Hg} = (\dot{V}_E)_2 \times 49 \text{ mm Hg}$$

$$\frac{(8 \times 55)}{49} = (\dot{V}_E)_2$$

$$8.98 \text{ L/min} = (\dot{V}_E)_2$$

Increasing the patient's $\dot{V}_E$ from 8 L/min to approximately 9 L/min will yield a Pa_{CO_2} of 49 mm Hg and a pH of approximately 7.35. Now the RT simply divide's the new $\dot{V}_E$ of 9 L/min by the respiratory frequency to calculate the new V_T required.

$$9 \text{ L/min}/10 = 900 \text{ mL}$$

A V_T of 900 mL at a rate of 10 breaths/min should produce an arterial pH of 7.35, according to the H-H equation.

The H-H equation is useful for checking a clinical blood gas report to see if the pH, P_{CO_2}, and $[HCO_3^-]$ values are compatible with one another. In this way, transcription errors and analyzer inaccuracies can be detected.

It is also clinically useful to predict what effect changing one H-H equation component will have on the other components. For example, the respiratory therapist (RT) may want to know how low the arterial blood pH will fall for a given increase in Pa_{CO_2}.

Physiological Roles of Bicarbonate and Nonbicarbonate Buffer Systems

The functions of bicarbonate and nonbicarbonate buffer systems are summarized in Table 12-2.

Bicarbonate Buffer System

The bicarbonate buffer system is particularly effective in the body because it is an open system—one of its components (CO_2) is continually removed through ventilation:

$$HCO_3^- + H^+ \rightarrow H_2CO_3 \rightarrow H_2O + CO_2 \uparrow \text{ (Exhaled gas)}$$

This allows HCO_3^- to continue buffering H^+ as long as ventilation continues. Hypothetically, this buffering activity can continue until all body sources of HCO_3^- are used up in binding H^+ ions[3] (i.e., the aforementioned reaction is continually pulled to the right by ventilation).

The bicarbonate buffer system can buffer only fixed acid. An increased fixed acid load in the body (e.g., lactic acid) reacts with HCO_3^- of the bicarbonate buffer system:

$$\begin{array}{c} \quad\quad\quad\quad\quad\quad\quad\quad\quad\quad\quad\quad \text{Ventilation} \\ \quad\quad\quad\quad\quad\quad\quad\quad\quad\quad\quad\quad \uparrow \\ H^+ + HCO_3^- \longrightarrow H_2CO_3 \longrightarrow H_2O + CO_2 \\ \uparrow \quad\quad\quad\quad\quad\quad\quad\quad\quad\quad\quad\quad\quad\quad \\ \text{Fixed acid} \quad\quad\quad\quad\quad\quad\quad\quad\quad\quad \end{array}$$

As shown, the process of buffering fixed acid produces CO_2, which is eliminated in exhaled gas. Large amounts of acid are buffered in this fashion. It should be apparent that if ventilation capability is inadequate, this type of buffering is hindered.

Table 12-2 ▶▶ Buffering Functions

Buffer	Type of System	Acids Buffered
Bicarbonate	Open	Fixed (nonvolatile)
Nonbicarbonate	Closed	Volatile (carbonic) Fixed

From Beachey W: Respiratory care anatomy and physiology: foundations for clinical practice, St Louis, 1998, Mosby.

Of course, the bicarbonate buffer system cannot buffer carbonic (volatile) acid, which accumulates in the blood whenever ventilation fails to eliminate CO_2 as fast as it is produced (hypoventilation). The resulting accumulation of CO_2 drives the hydration reaction in the direction that produces more carbonic acid, hydrogen, and bicarbonate ions, as shown:

$$\begin{array}{l} \text{Hypoventilation} \\ \quad\downarrow \\ CO_2 + H_2O \longrightarrow H_2CO_3 \longrightarrow HCO_3^- + H^+ \end{array}$$

The H^+ produced by dissociating H_2CO_3 molecules cannot be buffered by HCO_3^-, because hypoventilation prevents the reaction from reversing its direction. Therefore carbonic acid must be buffered by closed nonbicarbonate buffer systems.

Nonbicarbonate Buffer System

Table 12-1 lists the nonbicarbonate buffers in the blood. Of these, hemoglobin (Hb) is the most important because it is the most abundant. These buffers are the only ones available to buffer carbonic acid. However, they can buffer H^+ produced by any acid, fixed or volatile. Because nonbicarbonate buffers (Buf-/HBuf) function in closed systems, the products of their buffering activity accumulate, slowing or stopping further buffering activity:

$$H^+ + Buf^- \leftrightarrow HBuf$$

This means that not all of the Buf^- is available for buffering activity. Note that at equilibrium (denoted by the *double arrow*), Buf^- still exists in solution but cannot combine further with H^+. In contrast, most all of the HCO_3^- in the bicarbonate buffer system is available for buffering activity because it functions in an open system where equilibrium between reactants and products does not occur. Both open and closed systems function in a common fluid compartment (blood plasma) as illustrated in the following equation:

$$\begin{array}{l} \quad\quad\quad\quad\text{(Removed by ventilation)} \quad (HCO_3^- \text{ stores}) \\ \quad\quad\quad\quad\quad\quad\quad\quad\uparrow \quad\quad\quad\quad\quad\quad\quad\quad \downarrow \\ \text{Open system: } CO_2 + H_2O \longleftarrow H^+ + HCO_3^- \\ \quad\quad\quad\quad\quad\quad\quad\quad\quad\quad\quad\quad\quad \uparrow \\ \quad\quad\quad\quad\quad\quad\quad\quad\quad\quad\text{Added fixed acid} \\ \quad\quad\quad\quad\quad\quad\quad\quad\quad\quad\quad\quad\quad \downarrow \\ \text{Closed system: } HBuf \leftrightarrow H^+ + Buf^- \\ \quad\quad\quad\quad\quad\quad\quad\quad\quad\quad\quad\quad\quad\quad\quad \uparrow \\ \quad\quad\quad\quad\quad\quad\quad\quad\quad\quad\quad\quad (Buf^- \text{ stores}) \end{array}$$

Most of the added fixed acid is buffered by HCO_3^- because ventilation continually pulls the reaction to the left. Smaller amounts of H^+ react with Buf^- because equilibrium is approached, slowing the reaction.

▶ ACID EXCRETION

Bicarbonate and nonbicarbonate buffer systems are the immediate defense against the accumulation of hydrogen ions. However, if the body failed to eliminate the remaining acids, these buffers would soon be exhausted, and the pH of body fluids would quickly drop to life-threatening levels.

The lungs and kidneys are the primary acid-excreting organs. The lungs can excrete only volatile acid (i.e., the CO_2 from dissociating H_2CO_3). However, as discussed previously, bicarbonate buffers effectively buffer the H^+ originating from fixed acid, converting it to H_2CO_3 and, in turn, to CO_2 and H_2O. By eliminating the CO_2, the lungs can rapidly remove large quantities of fixed acid from the blood. The kidneys also remove fixed acids, but at a relatively slow pace. In healthy individuals, the acid excretion mechanisms of lungs and kidneys are delicately balanced. In diseased individuals, failure of one system can be partially offset by a compensatory response of the other.

Lungs

Because the volatile acid H_2CO_3 is in equilibrium with dissolved CO_2, the lungs can lower blood H_2CO_3 concentration through ventilation. Eliminating CO_2 is extremely important because the H_2CO_3 formed by the reaction between CO_2 and H_2O is more than 500 times that of all other acids combined.[3] H_2CO_3 also is produced by the reaction between fixed acids and bicarbonate buffers. The H_2CO_3 generated by both pathways is eliminated as CO_2 through the lungs. Approximately 24,000 mmol/L of CO_2 is removed from the body daily through normal ventilation. The carbon dioxide excretion of the lungs does not actually remove hydrogen ions from the body. Instead, the chemical reaction that breaks down H_2CO_3 to form CO_2 binds hydrogen ions in the harmless water molecule:

$$H^+ + HCO_3^- \longrightarrow H_2CO_3 \longrightarrow H_2O + CO_2$$

Kidneys

The kidneys physically remove H^+ from the body. The following terms refer to certain kidney functions:

- *Excretion* is the elimination of substances from the body in the urine.
- *Secretion* is the process by which renal tubule cells actively transport substances into the tubule lumen's fluid, or *filtrate*.
- **Reabsorption** is the active or passive transport of filtrate substances back into the tubule cell and then into the blood of nearby capillaries.

The amount of H^+ the kidney tubules secrete into the filtrate depends on the blood's pH. Secreted H^+ ions may originate from H_2CO_3 (when the blood PCO_2 is high) or from fixed acids. The kidneys excrete less than 100 mEq of fixed acid per day, a relatively small amount compared with volatile H_2CO_3 elimination by the lungs.[4] Besides excreting H^+, the kidneys also influence blood pH by retaining or excreting HCO_3^-. For example, if the blood PCO_2 is high, creating high levels of H_2CO_3, then the kidneys excrete greater amounts of H^+ and reabsorb all of the tubule filtrate's HCO_3^- back into the blood. The opposite happens when the blood PCO_2 is low. The kidneys excrete less H^+ and more HCO_3^-. Compared with the ability of the lungs to change blood PCO_2 in seconds, the renal process is slow, requiring hours to days.

Basic Kidney Function

To understand how the kidneys determine whether to excrete acidic or basic urine, some fundamental facts about renal function must be understood. The *glomerulus* is the component of the renal nephron responsible for filtering the blood. Hydrostatic blood pressure forces water, electrolytes, and other nonprotein substances through semipermeable glomerular capillaries. The resulting filtrate is greatly modified in both volume and composition as it flows through the nephron tubules. Excreted filtrate is called *urine*.

Bicarbonate ion is one of the electrolytes filtered from the blood at the glomerulus to become part of the tubular filtrate. This filtration removes base from the blood. At the same time, the nephron's tubular epithelium actively secretes hydrogen ions into the tubular lumen to join the filtrate. This secretion removes acid from the blood. Under normal conditions, the rate of hydrogen ion secretion is almost the same as the rate of bicarbonate ion filtration.[5] This means that the kidneys titrate hydrogen and bicarbonate ions against each other to form carbon dioxide and water.

Hydrogen ion secretion begins with the diffusion of blood carbon dioxide into the tubule cell (Figure 12-2). Aided by the enzyme, carbonic anhydrase, carbon dioxide reacts with water to form carbonic acid, which breaks down into bicarbonate and hydrogen ions. The tubule cell actively secretes hydrogen ions into the filtrate by means of *countertransport*, in which sodium ions (Na^+) and H^+ ions are simultaneously transported in opposite directions. That is, Na^+ and H^+ ions combine with opposite ends of a carrier protein in the luminal border of the tubule cell membrane. Na^+ moves into the cell down its high concentration gradient, providing the energy to secrete H^+ into the tubular filtrate (see Figure 12-2).[6]

The rate of hydrogen ion secretion increases as the concentration of hydrogen ions in the blood plasma

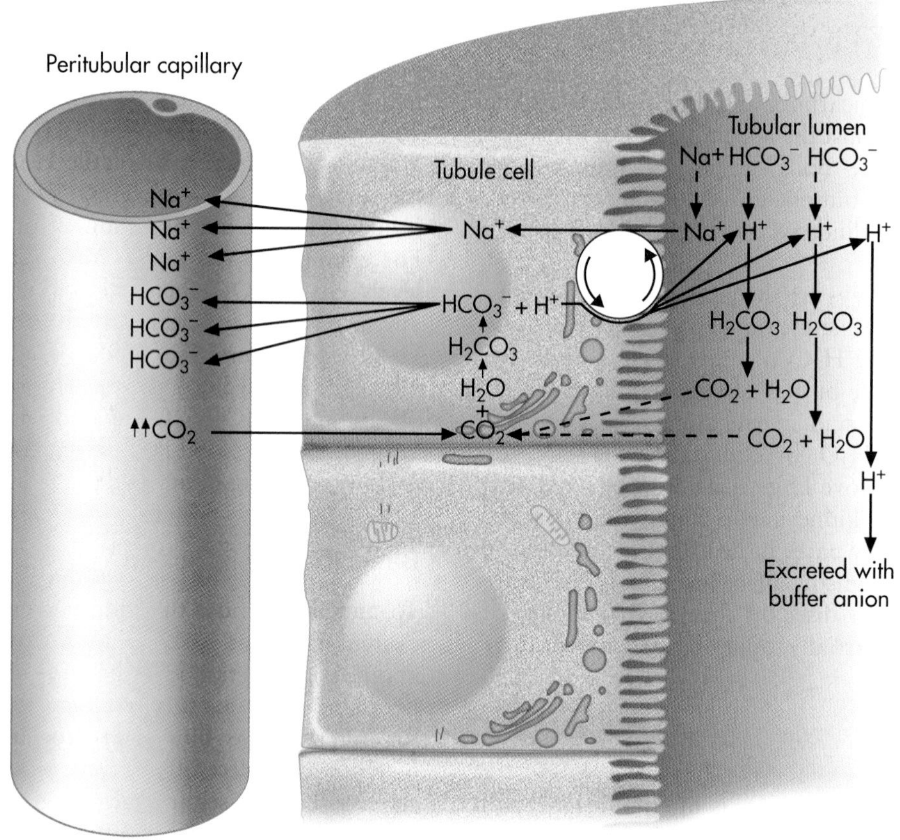

Figure 12-2

Renal response to respiratory acidosis. Filtrate HCO_3^- ions are reabsorbed by first reacting with secreted H^+ ions. *(Modified from Beachey W: Respiratory care anatomy and physiology: foundations for clinical practice, St Louis, 1998, Mosby.)*

rises. Likewise, the rate of hydrogen ion secretion decreases as blood plasma hydrogen ion concentration falls (Figure 12-3). Therefore any factor that raises the $Pa{CO_2}$, such as hypoventilation, increases H^+ secretion, and any factor that lowers the $Pa{CO_2}$, such as hyperventilation, decreases H^+ secretion.

The bicarbonate ion formed in the tubule cell from the reaction between carbon dioxide and water (see Figure 12-2) diffuses back into the blood plasma because the luminal side of the tubule cell is relatively impermeable to bicarbonate ions. Therefore both bicarbonate ions and sodium ions are reabsorbed whenever hydrogen ions are secreted into the tubular filtrate.

Reabsorption of HCO_3^-

Because the renal tubule lumen is relatively impermeable to bicarbonate ions, these ions are reabsorbed indirectly, as shown in Figure 12-2. The bicarbonate ions in the filtrate react with the hydrogen ions secreted by the tubular cells. The resulting carbonic acid breaks down into carbon dioxide and water. Because carbon dioxide is extremely diffusible through biological membranes, it diffuses instantly into the tubule cell. There, carbon dioxide reacts rapidly with water in the presence of carbonic anhydrase, forming HCO_3^- and H^+. The HCO_3^- ion diffuses back into the blood. Thus the reabsorbed HCO_3^- ion is not the same HCO_3^- ion that existed in the tubular fluid. If the tubule cells secrete sufficient H^+, all HCO_3^- in the tubular fluid is reabsorbed in this manner.

The net effect of secreting H^+ (caused by high blood CO_2, as shown in Figure 12-2) is to reabsorb all filtrate HCO_3^-, increasing the quantity of HCO_3^- in the blood. According to the H-H equation, this brings blood pH up toward the normal range.

On the other hand, if blood CO_2 is low, as is the case in a state of **hyperventilation** (see Figure 12-3), the ratio of bicarbonate ions to dissolved CO_2 molecules increases. Consequently, the renal filtrate has more bicarbonate ions than hydrogen ions. Because HCO_3^- cannot be reabsorbed without first reacting with H+, the excess HCO_3^- ions are excreted in the urine, carrying with them some other positive ions such as sodium or potassium. Therefore the net effect of secreting fewer hydrogen ions is to increase the quantity of HCO_3^-

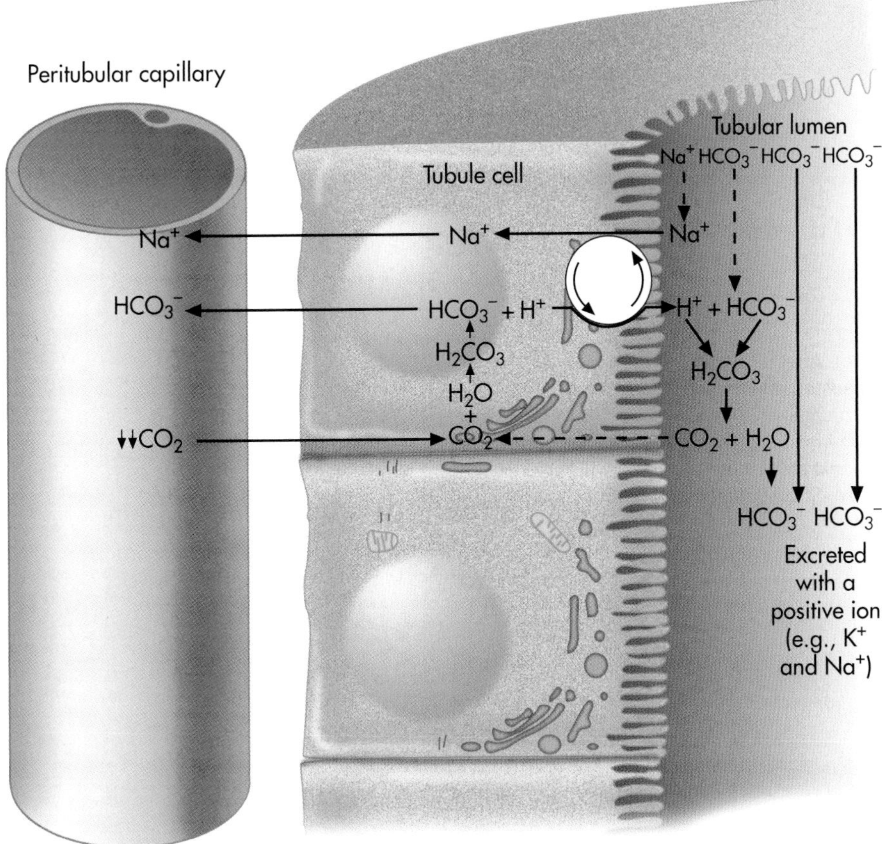

Figure 12-3

Renal response to respiratory alkalosis. Excess HCO_3^- ions are excreted in the urine with a positive ion. *(Modified from Beachey W: Respiratory care anatomy and physiology: foundations for clinical practice, St Louis, 1998, Mosby.)*

(base) lost in the urine. According to the H-H equation, this brings blood pH down toward the normal range. These renal responses to high and low blood P_{CO_2} are the mechanisms by which the kidneys compensate for respiratory acid-base disturbances.

Excess Hydrogen Ion Excretion and the Role of Urinary Buffers

If no buffers existed in the filtrate to react with H^+, the H^+ secreting mechanism would soon cease to function, because when filtrate pH falls to 4.5, H^+ secretion stops.[6] Buffers in the tubular fluid are essential for the secretion and elimination of excess hydrogen ions in acidotic states.

In Figure 12-2, more H^+ ions than HCO_3^- ions are present in the filtrate. After all available HCO_3^- ions react with H^+ ions, the remaining H^+ ions react with two other filtrate buffers, phosphate and ammonia, as illustrated in Figures 12-4 and 12-5. In Figure 12-4, phosphate and hydrogen ions react to form $H_2PO_4^-$, which must be excreted with a positive ion to maintain tubular electroneutrality. Figure 12-5 illustrates tubular ammonia synthesis, which occurs in response to low filtrate pH. The NH_3 molecule reacts with H^+ to form the ammonium ion (NH_4^+). To maintain electroneutrality, the kidney excretes a negatively charged ion to accompany NH_4^+. This negative ion is chloride (Cl^-), the most abundant filtrate anion.

When NH_4^+ reacts with H^+, a HCO_3^- ion diffuses from the tubule cell into the blood (see Figure 12-5). The net effect of ammonia buffer activity is to cause more bicarbonate to be reabsorbed into the blood, counteracting the acidic state of the blood. Figure 12-5 shows that when a chloride ion is excreted in combination with an ammonium ion, the blood gains a bicarbonate ion. Thus blood chloride and bicarbonate ion concentrations are reciprocally related (i.e., when one is high, the other is low). This explains why people with chronically high blood P_{CO_2} tend to have low blood Cl^- concentrations. Activation of the ammonia buffer system enhances Cl^- loss and HCO_3^- gain.

▶ ACID-BASE DISTURBANCES

In healthy individuals, the body buffer systems, the lungs, and the kidneys work together to maintain acid-base homeostasis under a variety of conditions.

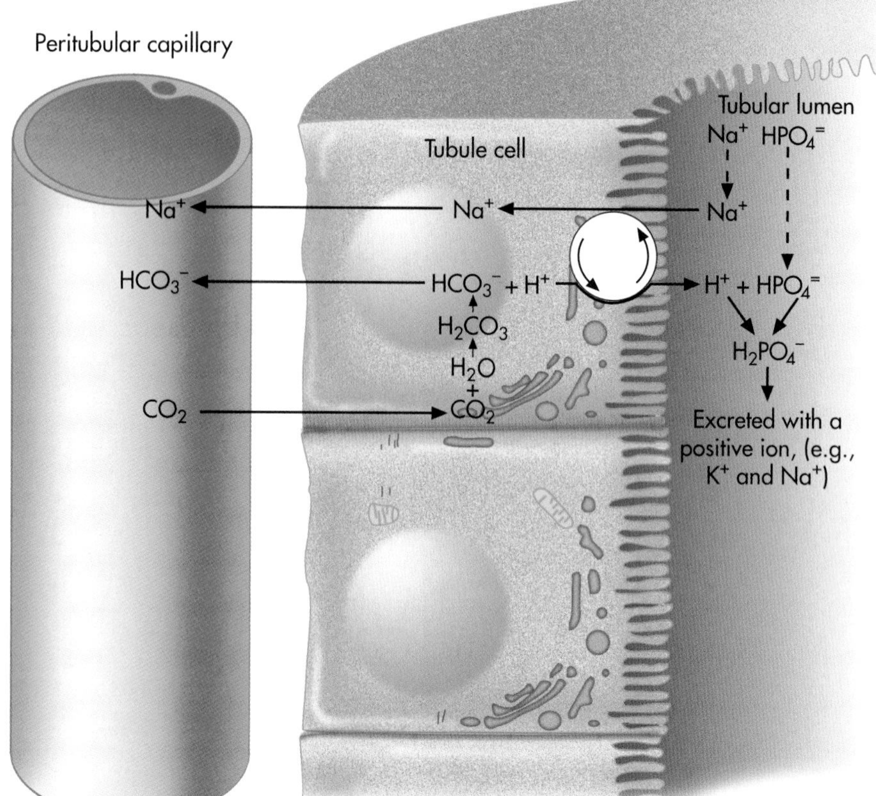

Figure 12-4

The phosphate buffer system. After bicarbonate buffers are exhausted, the remaining H^+ ions react with urinary phosphate buffers. *(Modified from Beachey W: Respiratory care anatomy and physiology: foundations for clinical practice, St Louis, 1998, Mosby.)*

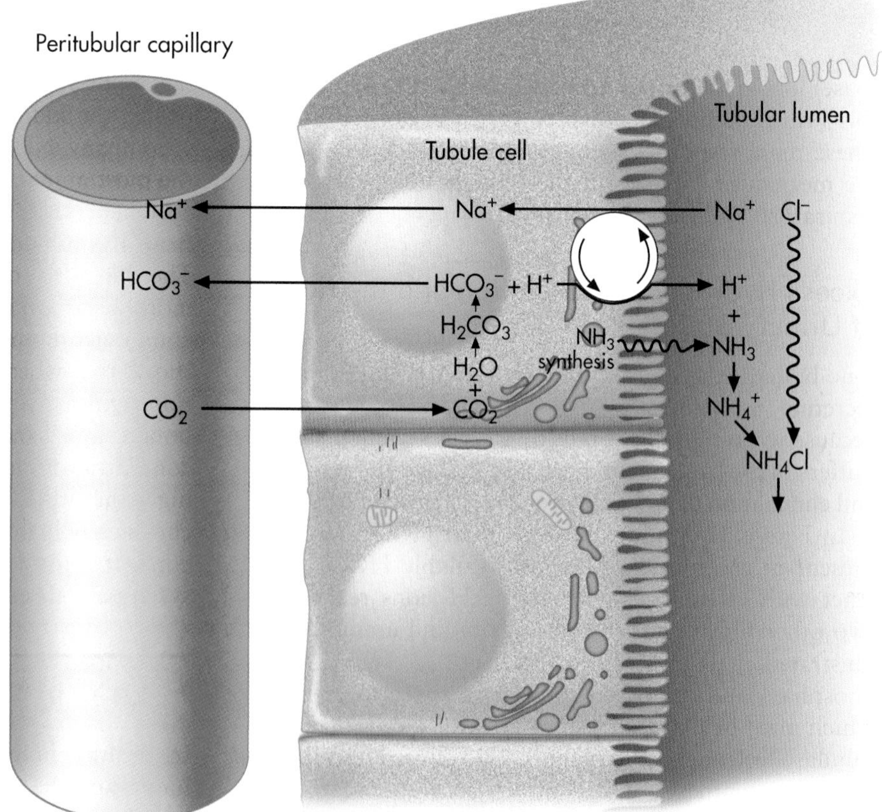

Figure 12-5

Tubule cells secrete ammonia in response to low-filtrate pH. NH_3 molecules buffer H^+ ions, forming NH_4^+ ions, which are excreted with Cl^- ions. *(Modified from Beachey W: Respiratory care anatomy and physiology: foundations for clinical practice, St Louis, 1998, Mosby.)*

Normal Acid-Base Balance

Normally, the kidneys maintain an arterial bicarbonate concentration of approximately 24 mEq/L, whereas lung ventilation maintains an arterial P_{CO_2} of approximately 40 mm Hg. These normal values produce an arterial pH of 7.40, as shown by the H-H equation as follows:

$$pH = 6.1 + \log \frac{[HCO_3^-]}{PCO_2 \times 0.03}$$

$$pH = 6.1 + \log \frac{24}{1.2}$$

$$pH = 6.1 + \log [20]$$

$$pH = 7.40$$

Note that the pH is determined by the *ratio* of $[HCO_3^-]$ to dissolved CO_2, rather than by the absolute values of these components. As long as the ratio of HCO_3^- buffer to dissolved CO_2 is 20:1, the pH will be normal, or 7.40. Because the kidneys control blood $[HCO_3^-]$ and the lungs control blood CO_2 levels, the H-H equation can be conceptually rewritten as follows:

$$pH \propto \frac{\text{Kidney control of } [HCO_3^-]}{\text{Lung control of } P_{CO_2}}$$

Therefore an increase in $[HCO_3^-]$ or a decrease in P_{CO_2} will raise the pH, leading to **alkalemia.** This produces a $[HCO_3^-]/(P_{CO_2} \times 0.03)$ ratio greater than 20:1 (e.g., 25:1). A decreased $[HCO_3^-]$ or an increased P_{CO_2} decreases the pH, leading to **acidemia.** This produces a $[HCO_3^-]/(P_{CO_2} \times 0.03)$ ratio less than 20:1 (e.g., 15:1). The normal ranges for arterial pH, P_{CO_2}, and $[HCO_3^-]$ are as follows:

$$pH = 7.35 \text{ to } 7.45$$

$$Pa_{CO_2} = 35 \text{ to } 45 \text{ mm Hg}$$

$$[HCO_3^-] = 22 \text{ to } 26 \text{ mEq/L}$$

Alkalemia is defined as a blood pH greater than 7.45. Acidemia is defined as a blood pH less than 7.35. *Hyperventilation* is defined as a Pa_{CO_2} less than 35 mm Hg. *Hypoventilation* exists if the Pa_{CO_2} is greater than 45 mm Hg.

Primary Respiratory Disturbances

Abnormal arterial pH levels caused by changes in Pa_{CO_2} are *primary respiratory disturbances*, because the lungs control Pa_{CO_2}. Respiratory disturbances affect the denominator of the H-H equation. A high Pa_{CO_2} increases dissolved CO_2, lowering the pH:

$$\downarrow pH \propto \frac{\rightarrow HCO_3^-}{\uparrow Pa_{CO_2}}$$

where ↓ means *decreased,* → means *no change,* and ↑ means *increased.* Respiratory disturbances causing acidemia are called **respiratory acidosis.** A low Pa_{CO_2} decreases dissolved CO_2, raising the pH. This is called **respiratory alkalosis:**

$$\uparrow pH \propto \frac{\rightarrow HCO_3^-}{\downarrow Pa_{CO_2}}$$

*Hypo*ventilation causes respiratory acidosis, whereas *hyper*ventilation causes respiratory alkalosis.

Primary Metabolic (Nonrespiratory) Disturbances

Nonrespiratory processes change arterial pH by changing $[HCO_3^-]$. They are called *primary metabolic disturbances*. In this context, the term *metabolic* is arbitrary, but by convention, it refers to all nonrespiratory acid-base disturbances. These kinds of disturbances involve a gain or loss of fixed acids or HCO_3^-. Such processes affect the numerator of the H-H equation. For example, an accumulation of fixed acid in the body is buffered by bicarbonate, lowering the plasma $[HCO_3^-]$ and decreasing the pH:

$$\downarrow pH \propto \frac{\downarrow HCO_3^-}{\rightarrow Pa_{CO_2}}$$

The same effect is created by a loss of HCO_3^-. Such nonrespiratory processes causing acidemia are called **metabolic acidosis.**

In contrast, ingesting too much alkali (e.g., sodium bicarbonate or other antacids) raises $[HCO_3^-]$, increasing pH:

$$\uparrow pH \propto \frac{\uparrow HCO_3^-}{\rightarrow Pa_{CO_2}}$$

Plasma $[HCO_3^-]$ can be increased by its *addition*, as in the previous example, or by its *generation*, as occurs when fixed acid is lost from the body.[5] For example, an individual may lose HCl from the body by vomiting large amounts of gastric juice. This loss generates HCO_3^-, as discussed later in Figure 12-8.

Processes that increase arterial pH by losing fixed acid or gaining HCO_3^- produce a condition called **metabolic alkalosis.** Table 12-3 shows the four primary acid-base disturbances causing alkalemia and acidemia.

Compensation: Restoring pH to Normal

When any primary acid-base defect occurs, the body immediately initiates a compensatory response. For example, in hypoventilation (respiratory acidosis), the kidneys restore the pH toward normal by reabsorbing HCO_3^- into the blood. In contrast, the compensatory renal response to hyperventilation (respiratory alkalosis) is urinary elimination of HCO_3^- (bicarbonate diuresis).

Table 12-3 ▶▶ Primary Acid-Base Disorders and Compensatory Responses

Acid-base Disorder	Primary Defect	Compensatory Response
Respiratory acidosis	$\left[\frac{\rightarrow HCO_3^-}{\uparrow \mathbf{Paco_2}}\right] = \downarrow pH$	$\left[\frac{\uparrow HCO_3^-}{\uparrow \mathbf{Paco_2}}\right] = \rightarrow pH$
Respiratory alkalosis	$\left[\frac{\rightarrow HCO_3^-}{\uparrow \mathbf{Paco_2}}\right] = \uparrow pH$	$\left[\frac{\downarrow HCO_3^-}{\uparrow \mathbf{Paco_2}}\right] = \rightarrow pH$
Metabolic acidosis	$\left[\frac{\downarrow \mathbf{HCO_3^-}}{\rightarrow Paco_2}\right] = \downarrow pH$	$\left[\frac{\downarrow HCO_3^-}{\downarrow \mathbf{Paco_2}}\right] = \rightarrow pH$
Metabolic alkalosis	$\left[\frac{\uparrow \mathbf{HCO_3^-}}{\rightarrow Paco_2}\right] = \uparrow pH$	$\left[\frac{\uparrow HCO_3^-}{\uparrow \mathbf{Paco_2}}\right] = \rightarrow pH$

From Beachey W: Respiratory care anatomy and physiology: foundations for clinical practice, St Louis, 1998, Mosby.
→, No change, ↓, decrease; ↑, increase.
Primary defects and compensatory responses appear in boldface type.

Similarly, if a nonrespiratory (metabolic) process lowers or raises [HCO_3^-], the lungs compensate by hyperventilating (eliminating CO_2) or hypoventilating (retaining CO_2), restoring the pH to near normal. Consider the following example of pure (uncompensated) respiratory acidosis in which the PCO_2 level increases to 60 mm Hg.

$$pH = 6.1 + \log \frac{(24\ mEq/L)}{(60\ mm\ Hg \times 0.03)}$$

$$pH = 6.1 + \log (13.3)$$

$$pH = 7.22$$

The kidneys compensate by retaining HCO_3^-, returning the plasma HCO_3^-/dissolved CO_2 ratio to almost 20:1, as shown:

$$pH = 6.1 + \log \frac{(34\ mEq/L)}{(60\ mm\ Hg \times 0.03)}$$

$$pH = 6.1 + \log (18.9)$$

$$pH = 7.38$$

Thus pH is restored to the normal range of 7.35 to 7.45, although the PCO_2 level remains abnormally high. This compensatory response of the kidney produces a high plasma [HCO_3^-], *not to be misconstrued as metabolic alkalosis*. Compensatory renal HCO_3^- retention is a normal secondary response to the primary event of respiratory acidosis.

The lungs normally compensate quickly for metabolic acid-base defects because ventilation can change the $PaCO_2$ within seconds. The kidneys require more time to retain or excrete significant amounts of HCO_3^-, and thus compensate for respiratory defects at a much slower pace. Table 12-3 summarizes the four primary acid-base disturbances and the body's compensatory responses.

The CO_2 Hydration Reaction's Effect on [HCO_3^-]

In the previous examples of pure (uncompensated) respiratory acidosis and alkalosis, it was assumed that the [HCO_3^-] did not change as the $PaCO_2$ level increased or decreased. Arterial [HCO_3^-] does increase slightly as the $PaCO_2$ rises, because the CO_2 hydration reaction generates HCO_3^-. This reaction occurs primarily in the red blood cell because the catalytic enzyme, carbonic anhydrase, is present:

$$CO_2 + H_2O \text{—Carbonic anhydrase} \longrightarrow H_2CO_3 \longrightarrow H^+ + HCO_3^-$$

As H^+ and HCO_3^- are rapidly produced, hemoglobin immediately buffers H^+, generating HCO_3^- in the process:

$$CO_2 + H_2O \rightarrow H_2CO_3 \rightarrow H^+ + HCO_3^- \ \textit{(}HCO_3^- \textit{ generation)}$$

$$\downarrow$$

$$Hb^- + H^+ \rightarrow HHb \ \textit{(Hb buffering of } H^+\textit{)}$$

The amount of HCO_3^- increase depends on the amount of nonbicarbonate buffer that is available to accept the H^+ produced by the hydration reaction. In general, when the nonbicarbonate buffer concentration is normal and the PCO_2 rise is acute, the hydration reaction raises the plasma [HCO_3^-] approximately 1 mEq/L for every 10 mm Hg increase in PCO_2 higher than 40 mm Hg. Figure 12-6 illustrates this hydration reaction effect. Normal status is represented by point A: a $PaCO_2$ of 40 mm Hg, a pH of 7.40, and a plasma HCO_3^- of 24 mEq/L. An acute rise in $PaCO_2$ from 40 to 80 mm Hg proceeds from point A, moving to the left, up the normal blood buffer line (line BAC) to point D, where the buffer line intersects the $PaCO_2$ = 80 mm Hg isopleth. Point D indicates a HCO_3^- of approximately 28.5 mEq/L and a pH of approximately 7.18. This small change in [HCO_3^-] should not be erroneously interpreted as early renal compensation.

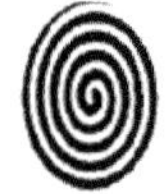

RULE OF THUMB

If PCO_2 increases acutely, the plasma [HCO_3^-] rises by 1 mEq/L for every 10 mm Hg increase in PCO_2 higher than 40 mm Hg.

▶ CLINICAL ACID-BASE STATES

Systematic Acid-Base Classification

In analyzing an acid-base problem, it is helpful to use a series of systematic steps. Consistently applying them to all acid-base disturbances helps avoid the tendency to

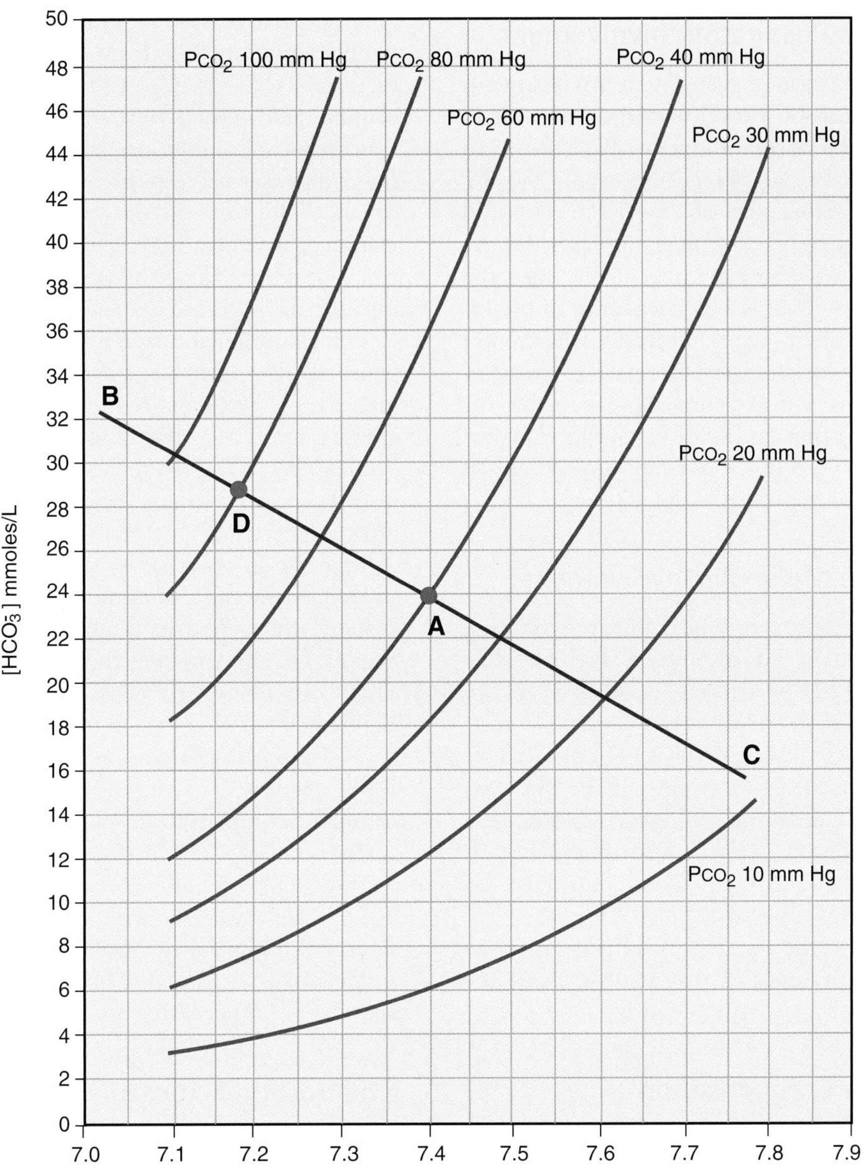

Figure 12-6

The pH-PCO_2 diagram. Because of the hydration reaction between CO_2 and H_2O, acute increases in PCO_2 raise the plasma HCO_3^- concentration along line *CADB*. An acute rise in PCO_2 from 40 to 80 mm Hg (point *A* to point *D*) increases the HCO_3^- concentration from 24 to approximately 29 mEq/L. *(Modified from Masoro EJ, Siegel PD: Acid-base regulation: its physiology and pathophysiology, Philadelphia, 1971, WB Saunders.)*

jump to conclusions. Four steps in acid-base classification are outlined in Box 12-2. The order of the steps is not as important as following the same procedure for each situation.

Step 1: Categorize the pH

If the pH is greater than 7.45, a state of alkalosis exists. If the pH is less than 7.35, a state of acidosis exists. Steps 2 through 4 will help the clinician determine whether an acid-base abnormality is of respiratory or metabolic (nonrespiratory) origin.

Box 12-2 • Systematic Acid-Base Classification

- Inspect the pH (acidemia, alkalemia, or normal).
- Inspect the $Paco_2$ (respiratory component). Can it explain the pH?
- Inspect the HCO_3^- (metabolic component). Can it explain the pH?
- Check for compensation. Did the noncausative component respond appropriately?

From Beachey W: Respiratory care anatomy and physiology: foundations for clinical practice, St Louis, 1998, Mosby.

Step 2: Determine Respiratory Involvement

The $Pa{CO_2}$ is the indicator of respiratory involvement, because the lungs control the level of carbon dioxide in the arterial blood. (The normal range for $Pa{CO_2}$ is 35 to 45 mm Hg.) If the arterial pH is abnormal, the RT should determine whether the observed $Pa{CO_2}$ could cause the abnormality by itself. For example, if the pH was lower than 7.35 (denoting an acidosis) and the $Pa{CO_2}$ was higher than 45 mm Hg, according to the H-H equation, the high $Pa{CO_2}$ would indeed lower the pH (i.e., produce an acidosis). Therefore the respiratory system is at least in part, if not entirely, responsible for the acidosis. On the other hand, if the pH level is less than 7.35 and the $Pa{CO_2}$ is in the normal range, then the acidosis probably is of metabolic origin.

Step 3: Determine Metabolic Involvement

Plasma $[HCO_3^-]$ is the metabolic indicator because $[HCO_3^-]$ is controlled by nonrespiratory factors. (The normal plasma $[HCO_3^-]$ of arterial blood is 22 to 26 mEq/L.) If the arterial pH is abnormal, the RT must determine whether the observed $[HCO_3^-]$ could cause the abnormality by itself. For example, if the pH level was less than 7.35 (denoting an acidosis) and the $[HCO_3^-]$ was lower than 22 mEq/L, according to the H-H equation, the low $[HCO_3^-]$ would produce an acidosis. Thus nonrespiratory factors are in part, if not entirely, responsible for the acidosis. If $[HCO_3^-]$ is in the normal range in the presence of this acidosis, then the acidosis probably is of respiratory origin.

Step 4: Assess for Compensation

The system that is not primarily responsible for the acid-base imbalance usually attempts to return the pH to the normal range. Compensation may be complete (pH is brought into the normal range) or partial (pH is still out of the normal range, but is in the process of moving toward the normal range). In a pure respiratory acidosis, the kidneys compensate by increasing the plasma $[HCO_3^-]$, restoring the pH to normal. Similarly, respiratory alkalosis elicits a compensatory decrease in plasma $[HCO_3^-]$. A pure metabolic acidosis normally stimulates a compensatory increase in ventilation, lowering the $Pa{CO_2}$. A pure metabolic alkalosis causes a compensatory decrease in ventilation, raising the $Pa{CO_2}$. All compensatory responses work to restore the pH to the normal range.

In cases in which compensation has occurred, if the pH is on the acidic side of 7.40 (7.35 to 7.39), the component that would cause an acidosis (either increased $Pa{CO_2}$ or decreased plasma HCO_3^-) is generally the primary cause of the original acid-base imbalance. If compensation is present, but pH is on the alkalotic side of 7.40 (7.41 to 7.45), the component that would cause an alkalosis (either decreased $Pa{CO_2}$ or increased HCO_3^-) is generally the primary cause of the original acid-base disturbance.

Complete compensation refers to any case in which the compensatory response returns the pH to the normal range (7.35 to 7.45). *Partial compensation* refers to instances in which the expected compensatory response has begun but has not had enough time to return the pH into the normal range.

For example, suppose a patient has a partially compensated respiratory acidosis. This is characterized by a high $Pa{CO_2}$, a pH less than 7.35, and a plasma $[HCO_3^-]$ greater than 26 mEq/L. The compensatory response (increased HCO_3^-) is not yet sufficient to return the pH into the normal range, although the expected compensatory activity has clearly begun. By comparison, a completely compensated respiratory acidosis is demonstrated by the same patient several hours later, when the kidneys have had enough time to retain sufficient plasma HCO_3^- to bring the pH into the normal range. This completely compensated respiratory acidosis is characterized by the same originally observed high $Pa{CO_2}$, a pH that is now in the 7.35 to 7.39 range, and a plasma $[HCO_3^-]$ that is greater than it was before complete compensation took place. The pH is on the acidic side of 7.40 because the primary disturbance (high $Pa{CO_2}$) originally created an acidotic environment. In general, the body does not *overcompensate* for an acid-base disturbance. Table 12-4 summarizes acid-base and ventilatory classification. Table 12-5 classifies the degree of compensation for acid-base disturbances.

Respiratory Acidosis

Any physiological process that raises the arterial $P{CO_2}$ (more than 45 mm Hg) and lowers arterial pH (less than 7.35) produces respiratory acidosis. Increased $Pa{CO_2}$

Table 12-4 ▶▶ Acid-Base and Ventilatory Classification

Component	Classification	Range
pH (arterial)	Normal status	7.35-7.45
	Acidemia	<7.35
	Alkalemia	>7.45
$Pa{CO_2}$ (mm Hg)	Normal ventilatory status	35-45
	Respiratory acidosis (hypoventilation)	>45
	Respiratory alkalosis (hyperventilation)	<35
HCO_3^- (mEq/L)	Normal metabolic status	22-26
	Metabolic acidosis	<22
	Metabolic alkalosis	26

From Beachey W: Respiratory care anatomy and physiology: foundations for clinical practice, St Louis, 1998, Mosby.

Table 12-5 ▶▶ Degrees of Acid-Base Compensation

Compensating (Noncausative Component)	pH	Classification
Within normal range	Abnormal	Noncompensated (acute)
Out of normal range in the expected direction	Abnormal	Partially compensated
Out of normal range in the expected direction	Normal	Compensated (chronic)

From Beachey W: Respiratory care anatomy and physiology: foundations for clinical practice, St Louis, 1998, Mosby.

MINI CLINI

Acute (Uncompensated) Respiratory Acidosis

PROBLEM

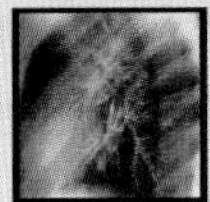

A 35-year-old woman was admitted to the emergency department with a diagnosis of heroin overdose. Her breathing was shallow and slow. Arterial blood gas analysis revealed a pH of 7.30, a P_{CO_2} of 55 mm Hg, and a HCO_3^- of 27 mEq/L. How would the RT assess her respiratory condition?

SOLUTION

The RT should follow these steps:

1. Categorize the pH. The pH is below normal, indicating the presence of acidemia.
2. Determine respiratory involvement. The Pa_{CO_2} is elevated above normal, consistent with a low pH, indicating hypoventilation as a contributing factor to acidemia (respiratory acidosis).
3. Determine metabolic involvement. The HCO_3^- is elevated slightly above normal. However, this is in the expected range for acute respiratory acidosis (1 mEq for each 10–mm Hg increase in P_{CO_2}).
4. Assess for compensation. As explained in step 3, the HCO_3^- is within the expected range for acute respiratory acidosis. Therefore there is no evidence of metabolic compensation.

(hypercapnia) lowers the arterial pH because dissolved CO_2 produces carbonic acid:

$$CO_2 + H_2O \longrightarrow H_2CO_3 \longrightarrow HCO_3^- + H^+$$

Therefore hypercapnia is synonymous with respiratory acidosis.

Causes

Any process in which alveolar ventilation fails to eliminate CO_2 as rapidly as the body produces it causes respiratory acidosis. This could occur in different ways. A person's ventilation may be decreased from a drug-induced central nervous system depression, or a person with limited ventilatory reserve may have a normal Pa_{CO_2} at rest but cannot accommodate the increased CO_2 production associated with increased physical activity. Box 12-3 summarizes causes of respiratory acidosis.

If hypercapnia is uncompensated, respiratory acidosis occurs with a low pH, a high Pa_{CO_2}, and a normal or *slightly* high $[HCO_3^-]$. In this instance, the slightly high $[HCO_3^-]$ is not a sign that the kidneys have started compensatory activity; it merely reflects the effect of CO_2 hydration reaction on $[HCO_3^-]$.

Compensation

Renal compensation for respiratory acidosis begins as soon as the Pa_{CO_2} level rises. The kidney reabsorbs HCO_3^- from the renal tubular filtrate, bringing the arterial pH into the normal range (see Figure 12-2). However, this process cannot keep pace with an acutely rising Pa_{CO_2}. Full compensation may take several days.

Partly compensated respiratory acidosis has a high Pa_{CO_2}, a high $[HCO_3^-]$, and an acid pH—still not quite up in the normal range. A *fully compensated* respiratory acidosis is characterized by a pH on the acidic side of the normal range (less than 7.40 but in excess of 7.35), a high Pa_{CO_2}, and a high $[HCO_3^-]$. The high $[HCO_3^-]$ in

Box 12-3 • Common Causes of Respiratory Acidosis

NORMAL LUNGS

CENTRAL NERVOUS SYSTEM DEPRESSION

Anesthesia
Sedative drugs
Narcotic analgesics

NEUROMUSCULAR DISEASE

Poliomyelitis
Myasthenia gravis
Guillain-Barré syndrome

TRAUMA

Spinal cord
Brain
Chest wall

SEVERE RESTRICTIVE DISORDERS

Obesity (Pickwickian syndrome)
Kyphoscoliosis

ABNORMAL LUNGS

Chronic obstructive pulmonary disease
Acute airway obstruction (late phase)

the presence of a high Pa_{CO_2} is a sign that the Pa_{CO_2} has been high for a considerable time (i.e., the kidneys have had sufficient time to compensate). The underlying pathological process producing hypercapnia is still present. The kidneys simply mask the problem by maintaining a normal-range pH. Because of the hypercapnia, the term *acidosis* is retained in classifying this condition (compensated respiratory acidosis). This emphasizes that lung function is still abnormal, and, if unopposed, it would produce an acidosis.

Correction

The main goal in correcting respiratory acidosis is to improve alveolar ventilation. This may entail various respiratory care modalities ranging from bronchial hygiene and lung expansion techniques to endotracheal intubation and mechanical ventilation. If hypoventilation is chronic and compensation has restored pH within the normal range, corrective action aimed at lowering the Pa_{CO_2} is inappropriate and possibly harmful. In this instance, rapidly lowering the Pa_{CO_2} to normal would induce an alkalosis because of the compensatory $[HCO_3^-]$ retention by the kidneys (Table 12-6).

Respiratory Alkalosis

Any physiological process that lowers the arterial P_{CO_2} (less than 35 mm Hg) and raises the arterial pH (more than 7.45) produces respiratory alkalosis. A low Pa_{CO_2} (hypocapnia) forces the hydration reaction to the left, decreasing carbonic acid concentration and increasing the pH:

$$CO_2 + H_2O \longleftarrow H_2CO_3 \longleftarrow HCO_3^- + H^+$$

Therefore hypocapnia is synonymous with respiratory alkalosis.

Table 12-6 ▶▶ Expected Effect of Acute Changes in Pa_{CO_2} on Arterial pH

Pa_{CO_2} Change	pH Change
Decrease	**Increase**
1 mm Hg	0.01
10 mm Hg	0.10
Increase	**Decrease**
1 mm Hg	0.006
10 mm Hg	0.06
Expected pH when measured Pa_{CO_2} <40 mm Hg:	
Expected pH = 7.40 + (40 mm Hg − Measured Pa_{CO_2})0.01	
Expected pH when measured Pa_{CO_2} >40 mm Hg:	
Expected pH = 7.40 − (Measured Pa_{CO_2} − 40 mm Hg)0.006	

Causes

Any process in which ventilatory elimination of CO_2 exceeds its production causes respiratory alkalosis. The most common cause of hyperventilation in patients with pulmonary disease is probably a low arterial P_{O_2} (hypoxemia). Hypoxemia causes specialized neural structures to signal the brain, increasing ventilation (see Chapter 13). Anxiety, fever, stimulatory drugs, pain, and central nervous system injuries are possible causes of hyperventilation. Other causes may include stimulation of irritant receptors in the lung parenchyma, which may occur in pneumonia or pulmonary edema.

Hyperventilation and respiratory alkalosis also may be *iatrogenically* induced (induced by medical treatment). Such hyperventilation is most commonly associated with overly aggressive mechanical ventilation. It may also be associated with aggressive deep breathing and lung expansion respiratory care procedures. A low Pa_{CO_2}, a high pH, and a normal-range $[HCO_3^-]$ characterize acute respiratory alkalosis. A

MINI CLINI

Chronic (Compensated) Respiratory Acidosis

PROBLEM

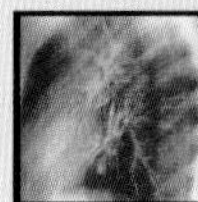

A 73-year-old man is being treated on an outpatient basis for pulmonary emphysema, which was diagnosed 7 years ago. His breathing is labored at rest, with marked use of accessory muscles. Arterial blood gas analysis revealed a pH of 7.36, a P_{CO_2} of 64 mm Hg, and a HCO_3^- of 35 mEq/L. How would the RT assess his respiratory condition?

SOLUTION

The RT should follow these steps:

1. Categorize the pH. The pH is on the acidic side of the normal range, but it is still normal.
2. Determine respiratory involvement. The Pa_{CO_2} is higher than normal, indicating hypoventilation as a contributing factor to the low-normal pH (respiratory acidosis).
3. Determine metabolic involvement. The HCO_3^- is substantially elevated. By itself, this would cause alkalemia, but because pH is on the acidic side of normal, primary metabolic alkalosis is ruled out. Compensation for the respiratory acidosis has occurred.
4. Assess for compensation. The HCO_3^- is approximately 8 to 10 mEq higher than normal. This is consistent with a compensatory response by the kidneys. In addition, the expected pH for a Pa_{CO_2} of 64 mm Hg is [7.40 − (64 mm Hg − 40 mm Hg)0.006], or 7.26 (see Table 12-6). Because the actual pH is 7.36, metabolic compensation (retention of HCO_3^-) must have occurred.

slight drop in $[HCO_3^-]$ is expected from the effect of the hydration reaction. Box 12-4 summarizes causes of respiratory alkalosis.

Clinical Signs

An early sign of respiratory alkalosis is *paresthesia* (numbness or a tingling sensation in the extremities). Severe hyperventilation is associated with hyperactive reflexes and possibly tetanic convulsions. The low Pa_{CO_2} may constrict cerebral vessels enough to impair cerebral circulation, causing light-headedness and dizziness.

Compensation

The kidneys compensate for respiratory alkalosis by excreting HCO_3^- in the urine (bicarbonate diuresis; see Figure 12-3). This activity brings arterial pH down into the normal range. As with respiratory acidosis, renal compensation is a relatively slow process. Complete compensation may take days.

Partly compensated respiratory alkalosis is characterized by a low Pa_{CO_2}, a low $[HCO_3^-]$, and an alkaline pH—still not quite down in the normal range. *Fully compensated* respiratory alkalosis is characterized by a low Pa_{CO_2}, low $[HCO_3^-]$, and a pH on the alkaline side of normal (pH more than 7.40 but not more than 7.45). Compensated respiratory alkalosis is sometimes called *chronic* respiratory alkalosis. The underlying hyperventilation and hypocapnia are still present. Thus the term *alkalosis* is used in classifying this condition, although the pH is within the normal range.

Box 12-4 • Common Causes of Respiratory Alkalosis

NORMAL LUNGS
Anxiety
Fever
Stimulant drugs
Central nervous system lesion
Pain
Sepsis

ABNORMAL LUNGS
Hypoxemia-causing conditions
Acute asthma
Pneumonia
Stimulation of vagal lung receptors
Pulmonary edema
Pulmonary vascular disease

EITHER NORMAL OR ABNORMAL LUNGS
Iatrogenic hyperventilation

Correction

Correcting respiratory alkalosis involves removing the stimulus causing the hyperventilation. For example, if hypoxemia is the stimulus, oxygen therapy is needed.

Alveolar Hyperventilation Superimposed on Compensated Respiratory Acidosis

Consider a patient with a compensated respiratory acidosis who has an arterial pH of 7.38, a Pa_{CO_2} of 58 mm Hg, and a HCO_3^- of 33 mEq/L. If this patient becomes severely hypoxic, the hypoxia may stimulate increased alveolar ventilation if lung mechanics are not too severely deranged. This would acutely lower the Pa_{CO_2}, possibly raising the pH to the alkalotic side of normal. For example, the patient's blood gas values might now be as follows: a pH of 7.44, a Pa_{CO_2} of 50 mm Hg, and a HCO_3^- of 33 mEq/L.

The novice might erroneously interpret these values as compensated metabolic alkalosis. This example demonstrates that blood gas data alone are not a sufficient basis for rational acid-base assessment. The patient's medical history and the nature of the current problem are essential components in accurately evaluating this problem. The blood gas values in this

MINI CLINI

Acute (Uncompensated) Respiratory Alkalosis

PROBLEM

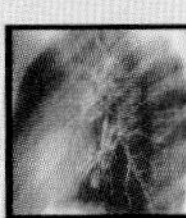

A distraught 77-year-old man experiencing anxiety of apparent psychosomatic origin was brought to the hospital by his wife. The patient exhibited rapid and deep breathing, had slurred speech, and complained about tingling in his extremities. Arterial blood gas analysis revealed a pH of 7.57, a P_{CO_2} of 23 mm Hg, and a HCO_3^- of 21 mEq/L. How would the RT assess his acid-base condition?

SOLUTION

The RT should follow these steps:

1. Categorize the pH. The pH is substantially higher than normal, indicating the presence of an alkalemia.
2. Determine respiratory involvement. The Pa_{CO_2} is well below normal, which is consistent with the high pH, indicating hyperventilation as a contributing factor in the alkalemia (respiratory alkalosis).
3. Determine metabolic involvement. The HCO_3^- is slightly lower than normal. However, this is within the expected range for acute respiratory alkalosis (hydrolysis effect).
4. Assess for compensation. The drop in HCO_3^- is within the expected range for acute respiratory alkalosis (1 mEq for each 5–mm Hg decline in P_{CO_2}).

example are described as acute hyperventilation (although $PaCO_2$ is greater than 45 mm Hg) superimposed on compensated respiratory acidosis.

Metabolic Acidosis

Any process that lowers plasma [HCO_3^-] causes metabolic acidosis. Reducing the [HCO_3^-] decreases blood pH because it decreases the amount of base relative to the amount of acid in the blood.

Causes

Metabolic acidosis can occur in one of the following two ways: (1) fixed (nonvolatile) acid accumulation in the blood or (2) an excessive loss of HCO_3^- from the body. An example of fixed acid accumulation is a state of low blood flow in which tissue hypoxia and anaerobic metabolism produce lactic acid. The resulting hydrogen ions accumulate and react with bicarbonate ions, lowering blood HCO_3^- concentration. An example of bicarbonate loss is severe diarrhea, in which large stores of HCO_3^- are eliminated from the body, also producing a nonrespiratory acidosis.

Because these two kinds of metabolic acidosis are treated differently, it is important to identify the underlying cause. Analysis of the plasma electrolytes is helpful in distinguishing between these two types of metabolic acidosis. Specifically, measuring the **anion gap** is helpful in making this distinction.

MINI CLINI

Compensated (Chronic) Respiratory Alkalosis

PROBLEM

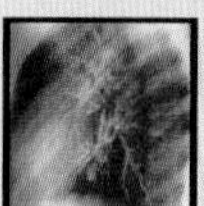

A 27-year-old man was admitted to the hospital with a persistent case of bacterial pneumonia, which had not responded to 6 days of ambulatory care with antimicrobial drugs. He exhibited mild cyanosis and labored breathing. Arterial blood gas analysis (with the patient breathing room air) revealed a pH of 7.44, a $PaCO_2$ of 26 mm Hg, a HCO_3^- of 17 mEq/L, and a PaO_2 of 53 mm Hg. How would the RT assess this patient's acid-base condition?

SOLUTION

The RT should follow these steps:

1. Categorize the pH. The pH is on the alkalotic side of the normal range, but it is still normal.
2. Determine respiratory involvement. The PCO_2 is well below normal, indicating hyperventilation as a contributing factor to the high-normal pH (respiratory alkalosis).
3. Determine metabolic involvement. The HCO_3^- is substantially lower than normal, but because the pH is on the alkalotic side of normal, primary metabolic acidosis is ruled out. Compensation for the respiratory alkalosis has occurred.
4. Assess for compensation. The HCO_3^- is approximately 7 mEq below normal. This is consistent with a compensatory response by the kidneys. In addition, the expected pH for a $PaCO_2$ of 26 mm Hg is [7.40 + (40 mm Hg – 26 mm Hg)0.01], or 7.54 (see Table 12-6). Because the actual pH is 7.44, metabolic compensation (excretion of HCO_3^-) must have occurred.

Anion Gap

The *law of electroneutrality* states that the total number of positive charges must equal the total number of negative charges in the body fluids. Thus *cations* (positively charged ions) in the plasma produce a charge exactly balanced by plasma *anions* (negatively charged ions). The plasma electrolytes (cations and anions) *routinely* measured in clinical medicine are Na^+, K^+, Cl^-, and HCO_3^-. Normal plasma concentrations of these electrolytes are such that the cations (Na^+ and K^+) outnumber the anions (Cl^- and HCO_3^-), leading to the so-called anion gap. In general, K^+ is ignored in calculating the anion gap:

$$\text{Anion gap} = [Na^+] - ([Cl^-] + [HCO_3^-])$$

Figure 12-7, *A*, shows that normal concentrations of these ions in the plasma are as follows: 140 mEq/L for Na^+, 105 mEq/L for Cl^-, and 24 mEq/L for HCO_3^-, yielding an anion gap of 11 mEq/L (140 mEq/L – [105 mEq/L + 24 mEq/L] = 11 mEq/L). The normal anion gap range is 9 to 14 mEq/L.[7]

An increased anion gap (more than 14 mEq/L) is caused by metabolic acidosis in which fixed acids accumulate in the body. The H^+ of these acids react with plasma HCO_3^-, lowering its concentration. This leads to an increased anion gap (i.e., an increase in *unmeasured anions*) (Figure 12-7, B). (When the H^+ ions of fixed acids are buffered by HCO_3^- ions, the anion portion of the fixed acid remains in the plasma, increasing unmeasured anion concentration.) Therefore a high anion gap indicates that fixed acid concentration in the body has increased.

A metabolic acidosis caused by HCO_3^- loss from the body does not cause an increased anion gap. Bicarbonate loss is accompanied by chloride ion gain, which keeps the anion gap within normal limits (Figure 12-7, C). The law of electroneutrality helps explain the reciprocal nature of [HCO_3^-] and [Cl^-] in this instance. With a constant cation concentration, losing HCO_3^- means that another anion must be gained to maintain electroneutrality. In this case, the kidney increases its reabsorption of the most abundant anion in the tubular filtrate, the Cl^- ion. The kind of metabolic acidosis in which HCO_3^- is lost from the body is sometimes called

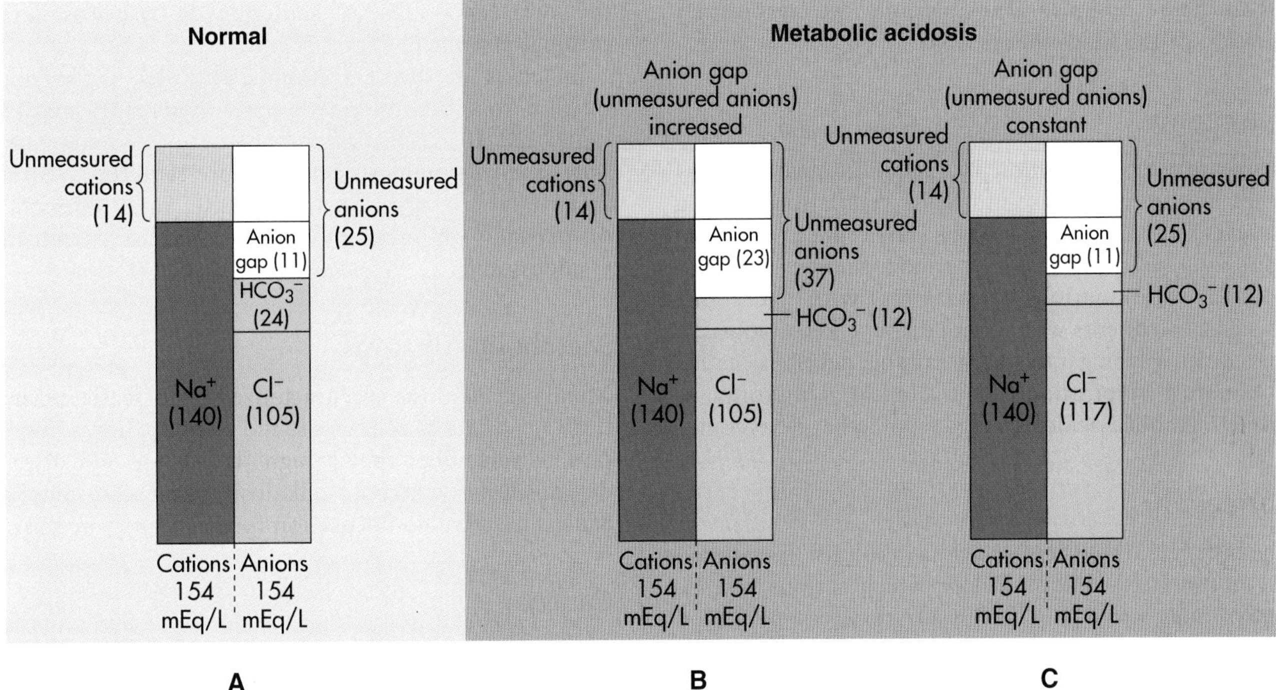

Figure 12-7

The anion gap in normal **(A)** and metabolic acidosis **(B** and **C)**. Fixed acid accumulation increases the anion gap **(B)**, whereas bicarbonate ion loss is accompanied by an equal chloride ion gain, keeping the anion gap within the normal range. *(Modified from Beachey W: Respiratory care anatomy and physiology: foundations for clinical practice, St Louis, 1998, Mosby.)*

hyperchloremic acidosis, because of the characteristic increase in plasma [Cl^-]. Box 12-5 summarizes causes of anion gap and nonanion gap metabolic acidosis.

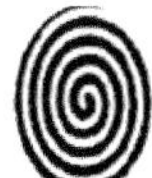

RULE OF THUMB

Metabolic acidosis accompanied by a high anion gap means that the body has accumulated an unusual fixed acid. A metabolic acidosis accompanied by a normal anion gap means that the body has lost a greater than normal number of bicarbonate ions.

Compensation

Hyperventilation is the main compensatory mechanism for metabolic acidosis. The increased plasma [H^+] of metabolic acidosis is buffered by plasma HCO_3^-, reducing the plasma [HCO_3^-], and thus the pH. A low pH activates sensitive receptors in the brain, signaling the respiratory muscles to increase ventilation. This lowers the blood's volatile acid (H_2CO_3) and dissolved CO_2 levels, returning pH toward the normal range. Uncompensated metabolic acidosis suggests that a ventilatory defect must exist. Metabolic acidosis accompanied by a Pa_{CO_2} of 40 mm Hg means that something prevents the lungs from responding appropriately to the brain's stimulation. The defect may

Box 12-5 • Causes of Anion Gap and Nonanion Gap Metabolic Acidosis

HIGH ANION GAP

METABOLICALLY PRODUCED ACID GAIN

Lactic acidosis
Ketoacidosis
Renal failure (e.g., retained sulfuric acid)

INGESTION OF ACIDS

Salicylate (aspirin) intoxication
Methanol (formic acid)
Ethylene glycol (oxalic acid)

NORMAL ANION GAP (HYPERCHLOREMIC ACIDOSIS)

GASTROINTESTINAL LOSS OF HCO_3^-

Diarrhea
Pancreatic fistula

RENAL TUBULAR LOSS: FAILURE TO REABSORB HCO_3^-

Renal tubular acidosis

INGESTION

Ammonium chloride
Hyperalimentation intravenous nutrition

From Beachey W: Respiratory care anatomy and physiology: foundations for clinical practice, St Louis, 1998, Mosby.

lie in nerve impulse transmission, the respiratory muscles, or the lungs themselves.

Symptoms

Respiratory compensation in metabolic acidosis may result in a great increase in minute ventilation, causing patients to complain of dyspnea. Hyperpnea (increased tidal volume depth) is a common finding during a physical examination of patients with metabolic acidosis. In patients with severe diabetic ketoacidosis, a very deep, gasping type of breathing develops, called **Kussmaul's respiration**. Neurological symptoms of severe metabolic acidosis range from lethargy to coma.

Correction

The initial goal in severe acidemia is to raise the arterial pH above 7.20, a level below which serious cardiac arrhythmias are likely.[7] If respiratory compensation maintains the pH at or above this level, immediate corrective action is usually not indicated. Treatment of the underlying cause of acid gain or base loss is the rational approach.

In cases of severe metabolic acidosis, intravenous infusion of sodium bicarbonate ($NaHCO_3$) may be indicated. If respiratory compensation is underway, only small amounts of $NaHCO_3$ are required to attain an arterial pH of 7.20. In any case, rapid correction of arterial pH above 7.20 by $NaHCO_3$ infusion is undesirable.

Metabolic Alkalosis

Metabolic alkalosis is characterized by increased plasma $[HCO_3^-]$ or a loss of H^+ ions, and a high pH. It is important to remember that a high $[HCO_3^-]$ is not always diagnostic of metabolic alkalosis because it may be caused by renal compensation for respiratory acidosis.

Causes

Metabolic alkalosis can occur in one of the following two ways: (1) loss of fixed acids or (2) gain of blood buffer base. Both processes increase plasma $[HCO_3^-]$. To explain why losing fixed acid raises the plasma $[HCO_3^-]$, consider a situation in which vomiting

MINI CLINI

Partially Compensated Metabolic Acidosis

PROBLEM

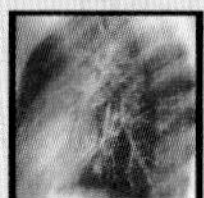

A 42-year-old woman in a diabetic coma was taken to the emergency department. She exhibited gasping and deep respirations. Arterial blood gas analysis revealed a pH of 7.22, a P_{CO_2} of 20 mm Hg, a HCO_3^- of 8 mEq/L, and a base excess (BE) of –16 mEq/L. How would the RT assess her acid-base condition?

SOLUTION

The RT should follow these steps:

1. Categorize the pH. The pH is below the normal range, indicating the presence of acidemia.
2. Determine respiratory involvement. The Pa_{CO_2} is well below normal, indicating severe hyperventilation. By itself, this would cause alkalosis, but the presence of acidemia rules out primary respiratory alkalosis. The low Pa_{CO_2} is probably a compensatory response to primary metabolic acidosis, although this response is insufficient to restore pH to the normal range.
3. Determine metabolic involvement. The HCO_3^- is severely reduced, consistent with the low pH. In the presence of low pH and low Pa_{CO_2}, a low HCO_3^- signals primary metabolic acidosis. This is confirmed by the large BE.
4. Assess for compensation. The severe hyperventilation represents a compensatory response to the primary metabolic acidosis, although compensation is far from complete. Nevertheless, the pH level would be even lower if the Pa_{CO_2} were normal.

MINI CLINI

Compensated Metabolic Acidosis

PROBLEM

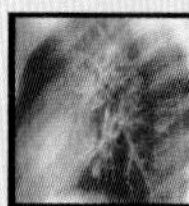

A 38-year-old man suffered for weeks from severe diarrhea without receiving medical attention. Arterial blood gas analysis revealed a pH of 7.36, a P_{CO_2} of 24 mm Hg, a HCO_3^- of 13 mEq/L, and a base excess (BE) of –11 mEq/L. How would the RT assess his acid-base condition?

SOLUTION

The RT should follow these steps:

1. Categorize the pH. The pH is on the acidic side of the normal range, but it is still normal.
2. Determine respiratory involvement. The Pa_{CO_2} is below normal, indicating hyperventilation. By itself, this would cause alkalosis; however, because the pH is on the acidic side of normal, the presence of primary respiratory alkalosis is ruled out. The low Pa_{CO_2} is likely a compensatory response to a primary metabolic problem (possible metabolic acidosis).
3. Determine metabolic involvement. The HCO_3^- level is substantially lower than normal, consistent with a low pH. Given that the pH level is on the acidic side of normal, the low HCO_3^- level signals a possible metabolic acidosis. This is confirmed by the large BE.
4. Assess for compensation. The hyperventilation previously described must represent a compensatory response to primary metabolic acidosis. The pH is in the normal range.

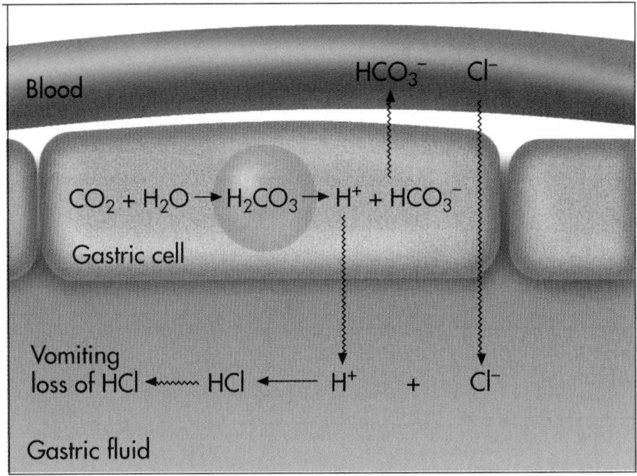

Figure 12-8

Gastric H^+ loss generates HCO_3^-, creating metabolic alkalosis. *(Modified from Beachey W: Respiratory care anatomy and physiology: foundations for clinical practice, St Louis, 1998, Mosby.)*

removes gastric hydrochloric acid (HCl) from the body (Figure 12-8). In response to HCl loss, H^+ diffuses out of the gastric cell into the gastric fluid, where Cl^- accompanies it. This forces the CO_2 hydration reaction in the gastric cell to the right, which generates HCO_3^-. The HCO_3^- ion enters the blood in exchange for the Cl^- ion. Thus the plasma gains a bicarbonate ion for each chloride ion (or hydrogen ion) that is lost[6] (see Figure 12-8).

The causes of metabolic alkalosis are summarized in Box 12-6. Metabolic alkalosis is common in acutely ill patients and is probably the most complicated acid-base imbalance to treat because it involves fluid and electrolyte imbalances. Often, metabolic alkalosis is iatrogenic, resulting from the use of diuretics, low-salt diets, and gastric drainage.[6]

To understand how the loss of chloride, potassium, and fluid volume may cause alkalosis, it is important to understand how the kidney regulates sodium. Approximately 26,000 mEq of Na^+ ions pass through the glomerular membrane daily, yet the body's daily Na^+ intake averages only approximately 150 mEq.[5] Therefore the kidney's main job is to reabsorb sodium, not excrete it. For this reason, and because sodium has a major role in maintaining fluid balance, the kidney places a greater priority on reabsorbing Na^+ than on maintaining chloride, potassium, or acid-base balance.

Normally, sodium is reabsorbed by *primary active transport* (Figure 12-9), in which the sodium-potassium–adenosine triphosphatase (Na^+-K^+-ATPase) pump actively transports Na^+ out of the renal tubule cell into the blood. This process causes Na+ ions to continually diffuse from the filtrate into the tubule cell. Cl^- ions must accompany Na^+ to maintain electroneutrality in the filtrate. If blood chloride concentration is low (hypochloremia), fewer chloride ions are present in the filtrate, which means that the kidney relies more on other mechanisms to reabsorb Na^+. These mechanisms, called *secondary active secretion*, require the kidney to secrete H^+ or K^+ into the filtrate in exchange for Na^+. In this way, Na^+ is reabsorbed and filtrate electroneutrality is preserved. Figures 12-10 and 12-11 illustrate this secondary active secretion process for H^+ and Na^+, respectively. In this way, hypochloremia leads to depletion of blood H^+ (alkalemia) and K^+ (hypokalemia). Preexisting hypokalemia (e.g., from inadequate K^+ intake) in the presence of hypochloremia places an even greater demand on the kidney to secrete H^+ to reabsorb Na^+; thus hypokalemia produces alkalosis. Dehydration (fluid volume depletion, or hypovolemia) further aggravates alkalosis and hypokalemia, because hypovolemia profoundly increases the kidney's stimulus to reabsorb Na^+.

Box 12-6 • Causes of Metabolic Alkalosis (Increased Plasma HCO_3^-)

LOSS OF HYDROGEN IONS

GASTROINTESTINAL

Vomiting
Nasogastric drainage

RENAL

Diuretics (loss of chloride, potassium fluid volume)
Hypochloremia (increased H^+ secretion and HCO_3^- reabsorption)
Hypokalemia (increased H^+ secretion and HCO_3^- reabsorption)
Hypovolemia (increased H^+)

RETENTION OF BICARBONATE ION

$NaHCO_3$ infusion or ingestion

From Beachey W: Respiratory care anatomy and physiology: foundations for clinical practice, St Louis, 1998, Mosby.

Compensation

The expected compensatory response to metabolic alkalosis is hypoventilation (CO_2 retention). Traditionally, it was thought that the hypoxemia accompanying hypoventilation greatly limited respiratory compensation for metabolic alkalosis (i.e., hypoxemia stimulates ventilation and should prevent compensatory hypoventilation). However, more recent evidence does not support this theory.[8] Metabolic alkalosis apparently blunts hypoxemic stimulation to ventilation. Individuals with PaO_2 levels as low as 50 mm Hg may still hypoventilate to $PaCO_2$ levels as high as 60 mm Hg to compensate for metabolic alkalosis. Nevertheless, significant

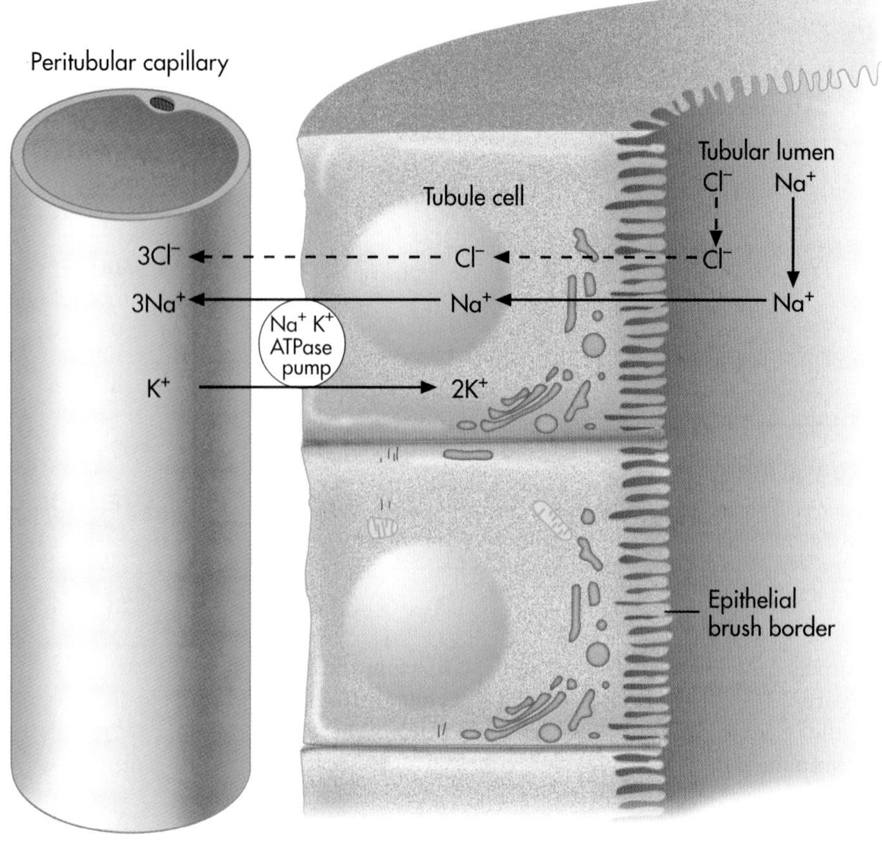

Figure 12-9

Sodium reabsorption through primary active transport. The sodium-potassium–adenosine triphosphatase (Na^+-K^+-ATPase) pump generates tubular cell electronegativity by pumping out more Na^+ ions than it pumps in K^+ ions. This creates both electrostatic and concentration gradients favoring Na^+ diffusion from the filtrate into the tubular cell. Normally, negatively charged chloride ions passively follow sodium ions (cotransport). *(Modified from Beachey W: Respiratory care anatomy and physiology: foundations for clinical practice, St Louis, 1998, Mosby.)*

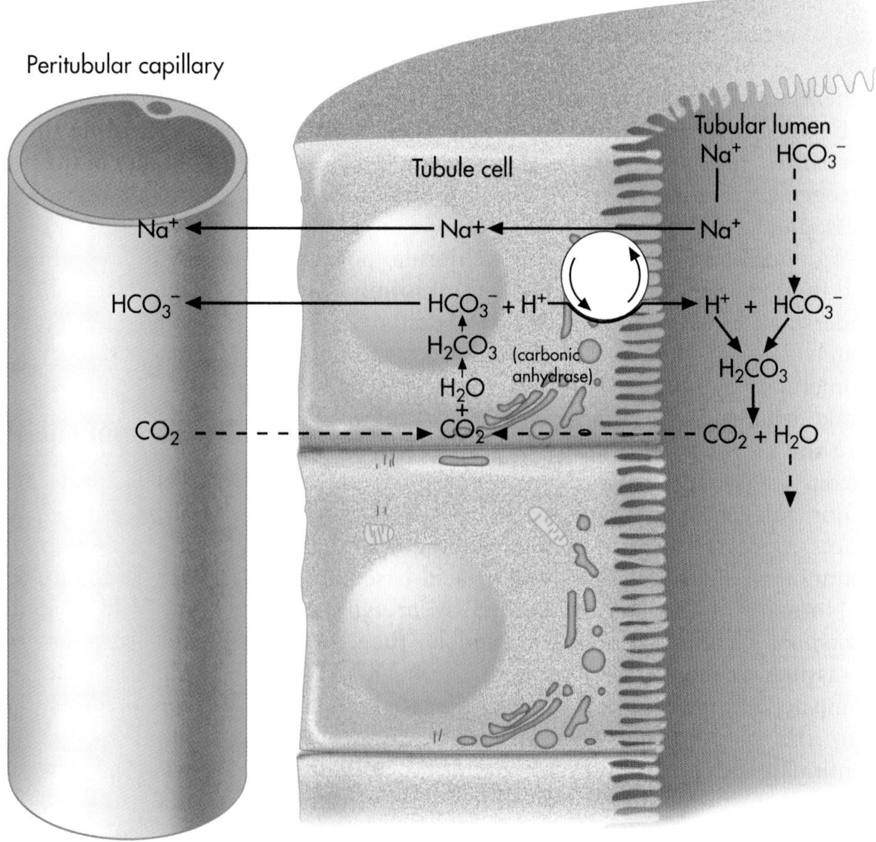

Figure 12-10

Sodium reabsorption through secondary active H^+ ion secretion. Through the counter-transport process, a Na^+ ion is reabsorbed as a H^+ ion is secreted into the filtrate. A HCO_3^- ion is reabsorbed with Na^+ instead of a Cl^- ion. This process becomes more predominant when Cl^- ions are scarce, and it leads to alkalosis. *(Modified from Beachey W: Respiratory care anatomy and physiology: foundations for clinical practice, St Louis, 1998, Mosby.)*

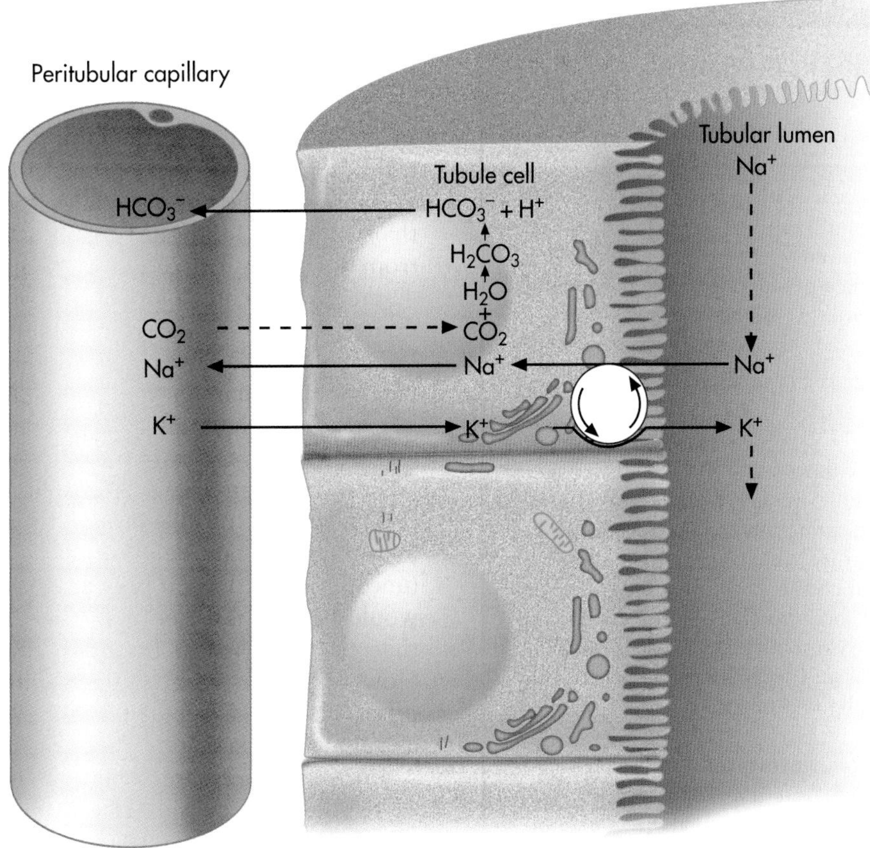

Figure 12-11

Sodium reabsorption through secondary active K^+ ion secretion. This mechanism is more likely to occur when Cl^- ions are scarce and an alkalemia (low H^+) exists. In such instances, hypokalemia develops. *(Modified from Beachey W: Respiratory care anatomy and physiology: foundations for clinical practice, St Louis, 1998, Mosby.)*

CO_2 retention is not often seen in cases of metabolic alkalosis, probably because metabolic alkalosis commonly coexists with other conditions that may cause hyperventilation, such as anxiety, pain, infection, fever, or pulmonary edema.

Correction

Correction of metabolic alkalosis is aimed at restoring normal fluid volume and electrolyte concentrations, especially potassium and chloride levels. Inadequate fluid volume, especially if coupled with hypochloremia, causes excessive secretion and loss of hydrogen and potassium ions because of the great need to reabsorb sodium ions. Thus in treating this type of alkalosis, it is important to supply adequate fluids containing chloride ions. If hypokalemia is a primary factor, then KCl is the preferred corrective agent. In cases of severe metabolic alkalosis, acidifying agents, such as dilute hydrochloric acid, or ammonium chloride may be infused directly into a large central vein.[9]

Metabolic Acid-Base Indicators

Standard Bicarbonate

To eliminate the influence of the hydration reaction on plasma bicarbonate concentration, some laboratories report **standard bicarbonate.** The standard bicarbonate is the plasma concentration of HCO_3^- (in mEq/L) obtained from a blood sample that has been equilibrated (at body temperature) with a P_{CO_2} of 40 mm Hg. This HCO_3^- measurement reflects strictly the metabolic component of acid-base balance, unhampered by the influence of CO_2 on HCO_3^-. However, the process of standardizing the bicarbonate under in vitro laboratory conditions creates an artificial situation not present in the patient's body. Consider the fact that the blood in the patient's vascular system is separated from the extravascular fluid (fluid outside of the vessels) by a thin capillary endothelial membrane, readily permeable to HCO_3^-. When a patient hypoventilates and the blood Pa_{CO_2} level rises, the plasma HCO_3^- also rises

MINI CLINI

Metabolic Alkalosis

PROBLEM

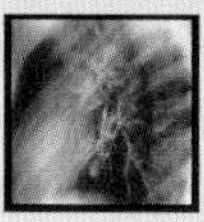

An 83-year-old woman with heart disease had been taking a powerful diuretic to remove excess edematous fluid from her legs and to help keep her free of pulmonary edema. Her blood gas and serum electrolyte analyses revealed the following: a pH of 7.58, a Pa_{CO_2} of 48 mm Hg, a HCO_3^- of 44 mEq/L, a base excess (BE) of +19 mEq/L, a serum K^+ of 2.5 mEq/L, and a serum Cl^- of 95 mEq/L. How would the RT assess her acid-base condition?

SOLUTION

The RT should follow these steps:

1. Categorize the pH. The pH level is substantially above normal, indicating the presence of alkalemia.
2. Determine respiratory involvement. The Pa_{CO_2} is slightly higher than normal, indicating mild hypoventilation. However, because alkalemia is present, the existence of primary respiratory acidosis is ruled out. The elevated Pa_{CO_2} may be a compensatory response to a primary metabolic problem (possible metabolic alkalosis).
3. Determine metabolic involvement. The HCO_3^- is substantially higher than normal. Given the high pH, this elevated HCO_3^- signals a metabolic alkalosis. This is confirmed by the large BE. In addition, the low serum K^+ and Cl^- values indicate hypokalemic/hypochloremic metabolic alkalosis.
4. Assess for compensation. Although the Pa_{CO_2} is slightly elevated, compensation for metabolic alkalosis is minimal. This lack of compensation is consistent with the presence of hypokalemic metabolic alkalosis.

because of the hydration reaction. Consequently, plasma HCO_3^- diffuses into the extravascular fluid until HCO_3^- equilibrium is established between the blood and extravascular fluid. If the patient were now to hyperventilate so that the Pa_{CO_2} is again 40 mm Hg, blood HCO_3^- would decrease and extravascular HCO_3^- would diffuse back into the blood until a HCO_3^- equilibrium is again established. This movement of HCO_3^- cannot occur in a laboratory blood sample when the blood P_{CO_2} of a hypercapnic patient is artificially lowered to 40 mm Hg. Therefore even the standard bicarbonate is not a perfect measure of purely nonrespiratory factors that influence blood pH.

Base Excess

Base excess (BE) is determined by equilibrating a blood sample in the laboratory to a P_{CO_2} of 40 mm Hg (at 37° C) and recording the amount of acid or base needed to titrate 1 L of blood to a pH of 7.40.

A normal BE is ±2 mEq/L. A "positive BE" (greater than +2 mEq/L) indicates a gain of base or loss of acid from nonrespiratory causes. A "negative BE" (less than −2 mEq/L) indicates a loss of base or a gain of acid from nonrespiratory causes. The BE suffers from the same limitation as the standard bicarbonate in that it is an in vitro, rather than in vivo, measurement. That is, in hypercapnia, the buffer base that diffused into the extravascular fluid in vivo cannot be recovered during laboratory in vitro titrations.

The reliance on BE to quantify metabolic acid-base abnormalities can be misleading. In cases of acute (uncompensated) respiratory acidosis, the BE commonly would be within the normal range, indicating correctly that the disturbance is purely respiratory in origin. However, when renal compensation has occurred to offset chronic hypercapnia, the BE measurement is elevated above the normal range because of the compensatory increase in plasma HCO_3^-.

To illustrate, consider the Mini Clini on p. 286, in which the patient has respiratory acidosis for which the body has compensated by renal retention of HCO_3^-. If this patient's blood is equilibrated in vitro to a Pa_{CO_2} level of 40 mm Hg, the HCO_3^- will fall by only 2 or 3 mEq/L to 32 to 33 mEq/L, and the pH will rise well above 7.45. Thus this patient's BE will be well above normal. The high BE may lead the RT to incorrectly conclude that this patient suffers from a primary metabolic alkalosis. However, in this instance, the high BE merely points out that compensation has occurred for the respiratory acidosis and does not mean that the patient has a primary metabolic alkalosis.

Mixed Acid-Base States

Combinations of acid-base disorders may occur in the same patient. A combined disturbance is one in which both respiratory and metabolic disturbances exist, which promote the same acid-base disturbance. For example, consider the following arterial blood gas results: a pH value of 7.62, a Pa_{CO_2} value of 32 mm Hg, and a HCO_3^- value of 29 mEq/L.

The pH indicates alkalemia, consistent with both the low Pa_{CO_2} and the elevated HCO_3^-. This is a combined alkalosis, indicating that the patient has two primary acid-base problems (i.e., respiratory and metabolic alkalosis combined). Therefore compensation is not possible.

KEY POINTS

- The lungs regulate the volatile acid content (CO_2) of the blood, whereas the kidneys control the fixed acid concentration of the blood.
- The larger an acid's equilibrium constant, the more the acid molecule dissociates and yields H^+.
- In the *open* bicarbonate buffer system, H^+ ions are buffered to form the volatile acid, H_2CO_3, which is exhaled into the atmosphere as CO_2. In the *closed* nonbicarbonate buffer system, H^+ ions are buffered to form fixed acids, which accumulate in the body.
- Bicarbonate buffers can buffer only fixed acids, but nonbicarbonate buffers can buffer both fixed and volatile acids.
- The ratio between the plasma [HCO_3^-] and dissolved CO_2 determines the blood pH, according to the H-H equation; a 20:1 [HCO_3^-]/dissolved CO_2 ratio always yields a normal arterial pH of 7.40.
- The kidneys respond to hypoventilation by reabsorbing bicarbonate, and they respond to hypoventilation by excreting bicarbonate.
- The lungs respond to metabolic acidosis by hyperventilating, and they respond to metabolic alkalosis by hypoventilating.
- Pa_{CO_2} abnormalities characterize respiratory acid-base disturbances, and [HCO_3^-] abnormalities characterize metabolic acid-base disturbances.
- Hypochloremia forces the kidneys to excrete increased amounts of H^+ and K^+ ions to reabsorb sodium ions, causing alkalosis and hypokalemia.
- Hypokalemia forces the kidneys to excrete increased amounts of H^+ to reabsorb sodium ions, causing alkalosis.
- Standard bicarbonate and BE measurements are made under conditions of a normal Pa_{CO_2} (40 mm Hg), which means that any abnormality in these measurements reflects only nonrespiratory influences.

References

1. Masoro EJ, Siegel PD: Acid-base regulation: its physiology and pathophysiology, Philadelphia, 1971, WB Saunders.
2. Comroe JH: Physiology of respiration, ed 2, Chicago, 1974, Year Book.
3. Murray JF: The normal lung, ed 2, Philadelphia, 1986, WB Saunders.
4. West JB: Respiratory physiology: the essentials, ed 4, Baltimore, 1990, Williams & Wilkins.
5. Filley GF: Acid-base and blood gas regulation, Philadelphia, 1971, Lea & Febiger.
6. Guyton AC: Textbook of medical physiology, ed 8, Philadelphia, 1991, WB Saunders.
7. Rose BD: Clinical physiology of acid-base and electrolyte disorders, ed 3, New York, 1989, McGraw-Hill.
8. Javaheri S, Kazemi H: Metabolic alkalosis and hypoventilation in humans, Am Rev Respir Dis 136:1011, 1987.
9. Malley WJ: Clinical blood gases: applications and noninvasive alternatives, Philadelphia, 1990, WB Saunders.

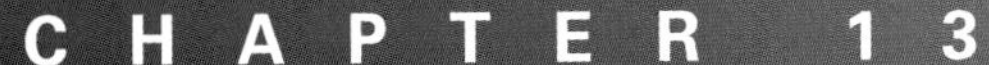

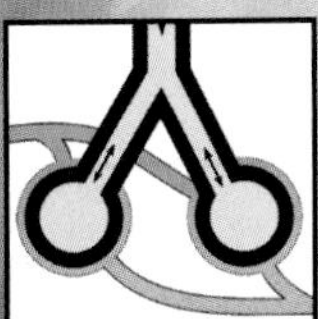

CHAPTER 13

Regulation of Breathing

Will Beachey

In This Chapter You Will Learn:

- Where the structures regulating breathing are located
- How the inspiratory and expiratory neurons in the medulla establish the basic pattern of breathing
- What effect the impulses from the pneumotaxic and apneustic centers in the pons have on the medullary centers of breathing
- The effect various reflexes have on breathing
- How the central and peripheral chemoreceptors differ in the way they regulate breathing
- Why the central chemoreceptors respond differently to respiratory and nonrespiratory acid-base conditions
- How the regulation of breathing in individuals with chronic hypercapnia differs from the regulation of breathing in healthy persons
- Why administering oxygen to patients with chronic hypercapnia poses a special risk that is not present in healthy individuals
- Why ascending to a high altitude has different immediate and long-term effects on ventilation
- Why mechanically ventilated patients with head injuries may benefit from deliberate hyperventilation
- How to characterize abnormal breathing patterns

Chapter Outline

Key Terms

apnea
apneustic breathing
apneustic center
Biot's respiration
blood-brain barrier
chemoreceptors

Continued

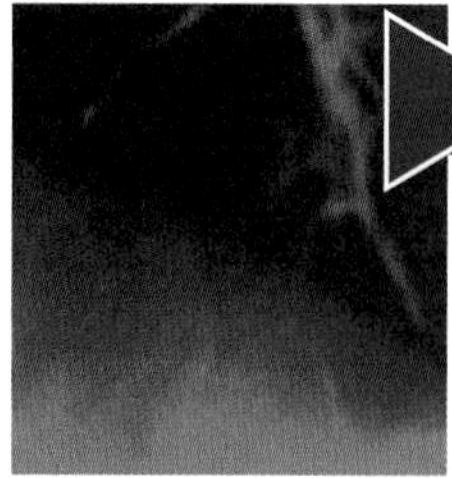

Key Terms—cont'd

Cheyne-Stokes respiration
dorsal respiratory groups (DRG)
Hering-Breuer inflation reflex
J receptors
pneumotaxic center
vagovagal reflexes
ventral respiratory groups (VRG)

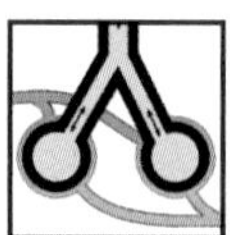

Like the heartbeat, breathing is an automatic activity requiring no conscious awareness. Unlike the heartbeat, breathing patterns can be consciously changed, although voluntary control is limited. Powerful neural control mechanisms overwhelm conscious control soon after one willfully stops breathing. The normal unconscious cycle of breathing is regulated by complex mechanisms that continue to elude our complete understanding. The rhythmic cycle of breathing originates in the brainstem, mainly from neurons located in the medulla. Higher brain centers and many systemic receptors and reflexes modify the medulla's output. These different structures function in an integrated manner, precisely controlling ventilatory rate and depth to accommodate the body's gas exchange needs. This chapter helps the clinician understand basic physiological mechanisms that regulate breathing; with this knowledge, the clinician can anticipate the effects that various therapeutic interventions and disease processes have on ventilation.

MEDULLARY RESPIRATORY CENTER

Animal experiments show that transecting the brainstem just below the medulla (Figure 13-1, *level IV*) stops all ventilatory activity. However, breathing continues rhythmically after the brainstem is transected just above the pons (Figure 13-1, *level I*). Until recently, physiologists thought that separate inspiratory and expiratory neuron "centers" in the medulla were responsible for the cyclical pattern of breathing. Researchers believed that inspiratory and expiratory neurons fired by self-excitation and that they mutually inhibited one another. Recent evidence shows that inspiratory and expiratory neurons are anatomically intermingled and do not necessarily inhibit one another.[1] No clearly separate inspiratory and expiratory centers exist. Instead, the medulla contains several widely dispersed respiratory-related neurons, as shown in Figure 13-1. The **dorsal respiratory groups (DRG)** contain mainly inspiratory neurons, whereas the **ventral respiratory groups (VRG)** contain both inspiratory and expiratory neurons.

Dorsal Respiratory Groups

As shown in Figure 13-1, DRG neurons are mainly inspiratory neurons that are located bilaterally in the medulla. These neurons send impulses to the motor nerves of the diaphragm and external intercostal muscles, providing the main inspiratory stimulus.[1]

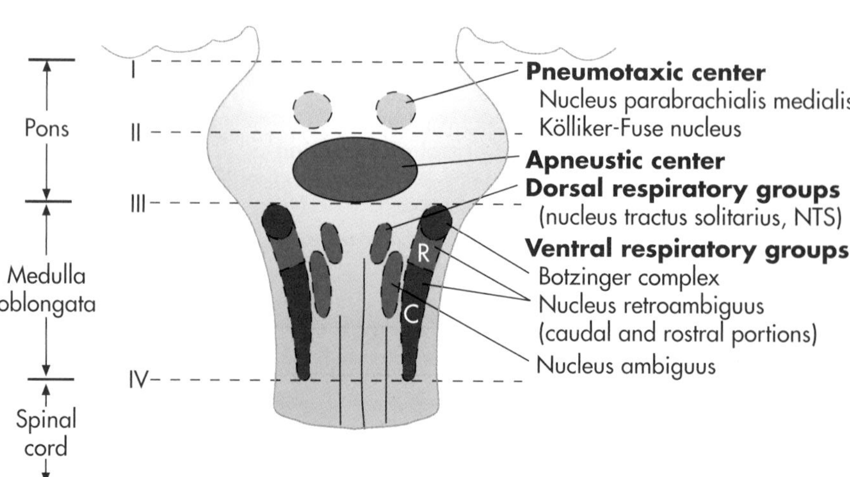

Figure 13-1 Dorsal view of the brainstem. Dashed lines *I* to *IV* refer to transections at different levels. *(Modified from Beachey W: Respiratory care anatomy and physiology: foundations for clinical practice, St Louis, 1998, Mosby.)*

Many DRG nerves extend into the VRG, but few VRG fibers extend into the DRG. Thus reciprocal inhibition is an unlikely explanation for rhythmic, spontaneous breathing.[1]

The vagus and glossopharyngeal nerves transmit many sensory impulses to the DRG from the lungs, airways, peripheral chemoreceptors, and joint proprioceptors. These impulses modify the basic breathing pattern generated in the medulla.

Ventral Respiratory Groups

VRG neurons are located bilaterally in the medulla in two different nuclei and contain both inspiratory and expiratory neurons (see Figure 13-1). Some inspiratory VRG neurons send motor impulses through the vagus nerve to the laryngeal and pharyngeal muscles, abducting the vocal cords and increasing the diameter of the glottis.[2] Other VRG inspiratory neurons transmit impulses to the diaphragm and external intercostal muscles. Still other VRG neurons have mostly expiratory discharge patterns and send impulses to the internal intercostal and abdominal expiratory muscles.

The exact origin of the basic rhythmic pattern of ventilation is not known. No single group of *pacemaker* cells has been identified. Recently, pacemaker-like bursts of activity have been identified in neurons associated with the Botzinger complex (see Figure 13-1). These neurons, forming a structure called the *pre-Botzinger complex*, may function as the respiratory rhythm generator.[3]

Inspiratory Ramp Signal

The inspiratory muscles do not receive an instantaneous burst of signals from the dorsal and ventral inspiratory neurons. Rather, the firing rate of DRG and VRG inspiratory neurons increases gradually at the end of the expiratory phase, creating a *ramp signal* (Figure 13-2). Thus the inspiratory muscles contract steadily and smoothly, gradually expanding the lungs rather than filling them in an abrupt inspiratory gasp. During exercise, various reflexes and receptors influence the medullary neurons, steepening the ramp signal, filling the lungs more rapidly.

During quiet breathing, inspiratory neurons fire with increasing frequency for approximately 2 seconds and then abruptly switch off, allowing expiration to proceed for approximately 3 seconds.[4] At the start of expiration, inspiratory neurons again fire briefly, retarding the early phase of expiration (see Figure 13-2). The inhibitory neurons that switch off the inspiratory ramp signal are controlled by the pneumotaxic center and pulmonary stretch receptors, which are discussed later in this chapter.

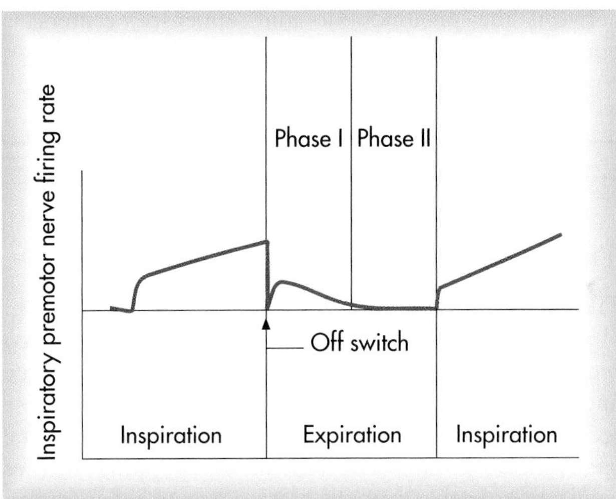

Figure 13-2

Inspiratory neural activity during breathing. Note the inspiratory ramp signal (left) and the braking action of inspiratory signals in the early part *(phase I)* of expiration. *(Redrawn from Leff AR, Shumacher PT: Respiratory physiology: basics and applications, Philadelphia, 1993, WB Saunders.)*

PONTINE RESPIRATORY CENTERS

If the brainstem is transected above the medulla (see Figure 13-1, *level III*), spontaneous respiration continues, although in a more irregular pattern. Thus the pons does not promote rhythmic breathing; rather, it modifies the output of the medullary centers. Figure 13-1 shows two groups of neurons in the pons: (1) the **apneustic center** and (2) the **pneumotaxic center.**

Apneustic Center

The apneustic center is ill defined because its existence and function can be demonstrated only if its connections to the higher pneumotaxic center and vagus nerves are severed. Under such circumstances, the DRG inspiratory neurons fail to switch off, causing prolonged inspiratory gasps interrupted by occasional expirations (apneustic breathing). Apparently, vagal and pneumotaxic center impulses hold the apneustic center's stimulatory effect on DRG neurons in check.

Pneumotaxic Center

The pneumotaxic center is a bilateral group of neurons located in the upper pons (see Figure 13-1). The pneumotaxic center controls the "switch-off" point of the inspiratory ramp, thus controlling inspiratory time. Strong pneumotaxic signals increase the respiratory rate, and weak signals prolong inspiration and increase tidal volumes. The exact nature of the interaction between the pneumotaxic and apneustic centers is poorly understood. Apparently, they work together to control the depth of inspiration.

▶ REFLEX CONTROL OF BREATHING

The Hering-Breuer Inflation Reflex

The **Hering-Breuer inflation reflex**, described by H.E. Hering and Josef Breuer in 1868, is generated by *stretch receptors* located in the smooth muscle of both large and small airways. When lung inflation stretches these receptors, they send inhibitory impulses through the vagus nerve to the DRG neurons, stopping further inspiration. In this way, the Hering-Breuer reflex has an effect similar to that of the pneumotaxic center. In adults, the Hering-Breuer reflex is activated only at large tidal volumes (800 to 1000 mL or more) and, apparently, it is not an important control mechanism in quiet breathing.[1] However, this reflex *is* important in regulating respiratory rate and depth during moderate to strenuous exercise.[2]

Deflation Reflex

Sudden collapse of the lung stimulates strong inspiratory efforts. This may be the result of decreased stretch receptor activity, or it may be caused by the stimulation of other receptors, such as the irritant receptors and J receptors (discussed later in this chapter). Although it is not clear which receptors are involved, it is clear that the vagus nerve is the pathway (as it is for the Hering-Breuer reflex), and that the effect is hyperpnea.[1] The deflation reflex is probably responsible for the hyperpnea observed with pneumothorax.

Head's Paradoxical Reflex

In 1889, Sir Henry Head observed that if the Hering-Breuer reflex is blocked by cooling the vagus nerve, then hyperinflating the lungs causes a further increase in inspiratory effort, which is the opposite of the Hering-Breuer reflex. The receptors for this reflex are called *rapidly adapting receptors*, because they stop firing promptly after a volume change occurs. Head's reflex may help maintain large tidal volumes during exercise and may be involved in periodic deep sighs during quiet breathing. Periodic sighs help prevent alveolar collapse, or atelectasis. Head's reflex also may be responsible for the first breaths of a newborn baby.[1]

Irritant Receptors

Rapidly adapting irritant receptors in the epithelium of the larger conducting airways have vagal sensory nerve fibers. Their stimulation, whether by inhaled irritants or by mechanical factors, causes reflex bronchoconstriction, coughing, sneezing, tachypnea, and narrowing of the glottis. Some of these reflexes have both sensory and motor vagal components and are called **vagovagal reflexes**. Such reflexes are responsible for laryngospasm, coughing, and slowing of the heartbeat. Endotracheal intubation, airway suctioning, and bronchoscopy readily elicit vagovagal reflexes.

Physical stimulation of the conducting airways, as with suctioning or bronchoscopy, may cause a severe case of bronchospasm, coughing, and laryngospasm.

J Receptors

C fibers in the lung parenchyma near the pulmonary capillaries are called *juxtacapillary receptors*, or **J receptors**. Alveolar inflammatory processes (pneumonia), pulmonary vascular congestion (congestive heart failure), and pulmonary edema stimulate these receptors. This stimulation causes rapid, shallow breathing; a sensation of dyspnea; and expiratory narrowing of the glottis.

Peripheral Proprioceptors

Proprioceptors in muscles, tendons, and joints, as well as pain receptors in muscles and skin, send stimulatory signals to the medullary respiratory center. Such stimuli increase medullary inspiratory activity and cause hyperpnea.[2] For this reason, moving the limbs, slapping or splashing cold water on the skin, and other painful stimuli stimulate ventilation in patients with respiratory depression.

Proprioceptors in joints and tendons may be important in initiating and maintaining increased ventilation at the beginning of exercise. Passive limb movement around a joint increases breathing rate in both anesthetized animals and unanesthetized humans.[5]

Muscle Spindles

Muscle spindles in the diaphragm and intercostal muscles are part of a reflex arc that helps the muscles adjust to an increased load. Muscle spindles are sensing elements located on *intrafusal muscle fibers*, arranged parallel to the main *extrafusal muscle fibers* (Figure 13-3). The extrafusal fibers that elevate the ribs are innervated by different motor fibers (alpha fibers) than the intrafusal spindle fibers (gamma fibers). When the main extrafusal muscle fiber and the intrafusal fibers contract simultaneously, the intrafusal muscle fiber's sensing element (spindle) stretches and sends impulses over spindle afferent nerves directly to the spinal cord (see Figure 13-3). The spindle's afferent (sensory) nerve synapses directly with the alpha motor neuron in the spinal cord, sending impulses back to the main extrafusal muscle. This creates a single synapse reflex arc. Alpha motor neuron impulses then cause the main extrafusal muscle fibers to contract with greater force, shortening the nearby intrafusal fibers. The stretch-sensitive spindle is thus unloaded, and its impulses cease. In this way, inspiratory muscle force adjusts to the load imposed by decreased lung compliance or increased airway resistance.

CHEMICAL CONTROL OF BREATHING

The body maintains the proper amounts of oxygen, carbon dioxide, and hydrogen ions in the blood mainly by regulating ventilation. Physiological mechanisms monitoring these substances in the blood allow ventilation to respond appropriately to maintain homeostasis. Hypercapnia, acidemia, and hypoxemia stimulate specialized nerve structures called **chemoreceptors**. Consequently, the chemoreceptors transmit impulses to the medulla, increasing ventilation. Centrally located chemoreceptors in the medulla respond to hydrogen ions, which normally arise from carbon dioxide dissolving in the cerebrospinal fluid (CSF). Peripherally located chemoreceptors in the fork of the common carotid arteries and the aortic arch respond to hypoxia, carbon dioxide, and hydrogen ions.

Central Chemoreceptors

Hydrogen ions, not CO_2 molecules, stimulate highly responsive chemosensitive nerve cells, located bilaterally in the medulla. Nevertheless, these central chemoreceptors are extremely sensitive to CO_2 in an indirect fashion. The chemoreceptors are not in direct contact with arterial blood (Figure 13-4). Instead, they are bathed in the CSF, separated from the blood by a semipermeable membrane called the **blood-brain barrier**. This membrane is almost impermeable to hydrogen and bicarbonate ions, but it is freely permeable to carbon dioxide. When arterial P_{CO_2} rises, CO_2 diffuses rapidly through the blood-brain barrier into the CSF. In the CSF, CO_2 reacts with H_2O to form H^+ and HCO_3^- (see Figure 13-4). The H^+ ions generated in this reaction stimulate the central chemoreceptors, which in turn stimulate the medullary inspiratory neurons. Therefore arterial P_{CO_2} is indirectly the primary minute-to-minute controller of ventilation.

Carbon dioxide diffusing from the blood into the CSF increases the $[H^+]$ almost instantly, exciting the chemoreceptors within seconds. Alveolar ventilation increases by approximately 2 to 3 L/min for each mm Hg rise in Pa_{CO_2}.[6]

The stimulatory effect of chronically high CO_2 on the central chemoreceptors gradually declines over 1 or 2 days, because the kidneys retain bicarbonate ions in response to respiratory acidosis (see Chapter 12), bringing the blood pH level back toward normal. The increased number of bicarbonate ions in the blood eventually diffuses across the blood-brain barrier into

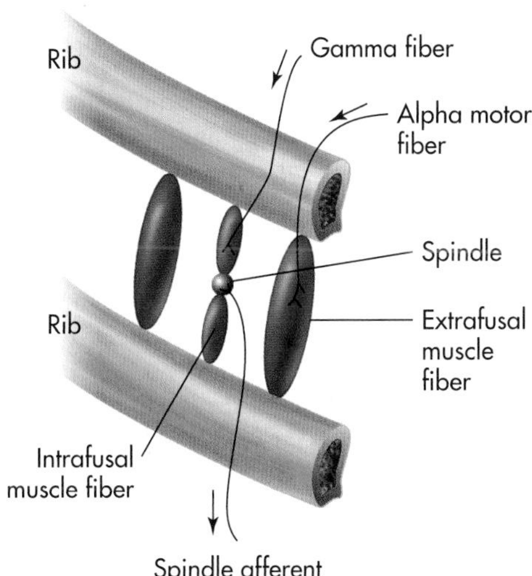

Figure 13-3
Stretch-sensitive muscle spindle located on the intrafusal fibers of intercostal muscles. Motor innervation for intrafusal fibers *(gamma nerve fibers)* is different than for extrafusal fibers *(alpha nerve fibers)*. Spindle afferent nerve fibers synapse with alpha motor neurons in the spinal cord, creating a single synapse reflex arc.

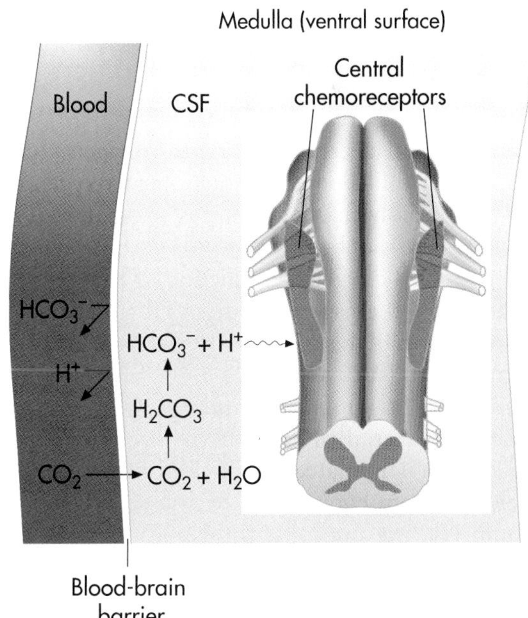

Figure 13-4
Carbon dioxide stimulates the medullary chemoreceptors by forming hydrogen ions in the cerebrospinal fluid (CSF). The blood-brain barrier is almost impermeable to hydrogen and bicarbonate ions, but is freely permeable to CO_2. *(Modified from Beachey W: Respiratory care anatomy and physiology: foundations for clinical practice, St Louis, 1998, Mosby.)*

the CSF, where they buffer H^+ and bring the CSF pH level back to normal. This removes the stimulus to the chemoreceptors, and ventilation decreases. Thus acute increases in $Paco_2$ have a powerful effect on ventilation, which is greatly weakened after a day or two of adaptation.

Peripheral Chemoreceptors

The peripheral chemoreceptors are small, highly vascular structures known as the *carotid* and *aortic bodies*. The carotid bodies are located bilaterally in the bifurcations of the common carotid arteries. The aortic bodies are found in the arch of the aorta. These neural structures are stimulated by decreased Pao_2, increased $Paco_2$, and decreased arterial pH. The carotid bodies send their impulses to the respiratory centers in the medulla by the glossopharyngeal nerve, whereas the aortic bodies send their impulses over the vagus nerve. The carotid bodies exert much more influence over the respiratory centers than the aortic bodies do, especially with respect to arterial hypoxemia and acidemia.[1]

Because the carotid bodies receive an extremely high rate of blood flow, they have little time to remove oxygen from the blood. Consequently, venous blood leaving the carotid bodies has almost the same oxygen content as the arterial blood entering them. This means that the carotid bodies are exposed at all times to *arterial* blood, not venous blood, and they sense *arterial*, not venous, Po_2.

Response to Decreased Arterial Oxygen

The carotid bodies respond to decreased Pao_2 rather than to an actual decrease in arterial oxygen content. That is, the carotid bodies' extraction of oxygen from each unit of rapidly flowing blood is so small that their oxygen needs are met by dissolved oxygen in the plasma. Because dissolved oxygen is a function of Po_2, decreased Pao_2 stimulates the carotid bodies. This explains why conditions associated with low arterial oxygen content but normal Pao_2 (such as anemia and carbon monoxide poisoning) do not stimulate ventilation.

At normal arterial pH and Pco_2 levels, the carotid bodies are not stimulated significantly until the Pao_2 falls below 60 mm Hg.[1] As the Pao_2 level falls from 60 to 30 mm Hg, the rate of carotid body nerve impulse transmission increases sharply and linearly. This Pao_2 fall corresponds to the range in which the oxygen saturation of hemoglobin decreases most rapidly. Because arterial hypoxemia does not significantly stimulate ventilation until the Pao_2 falls below 60 mm Hg, oxygen plays no role in the drive to breathe in healthy individuals at sea level. However, ascending to high altitudes increases ventilation because the low barometric pressure decreases both inspired and arterial Po_2 levels, exciting the peripheral chemoreceptors. However, the resulting increase in ventilation is less than might be expected, because hyperventilation induces a respiratory alkalosis, depressing the medullary respiratory center. This effect may not occur when hypoxemia is caused by severely deranged lung mechanics (e.g., in individuals with severe obstructive lung disease). In such persons, the stimulatory effect of hypoxemia on ventilation may not lower the $Paco_2$ level significantly, regardless of breathing effort.

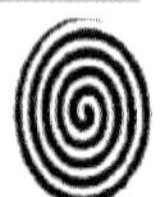

RULE OF THUMB

Hypoxemia does not increase the drive to breathe until the Pao_2 drops below 60 mm Hg, after which the drive to breathe increases proportionally with the fall in Pao_2.

MINI CLINI

Delayed Hyperventilation at High Altitude

PROBLEM

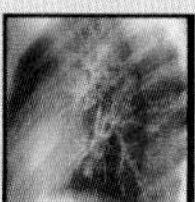

If someone ascends to an elevation of 10,000 feet above sea level, his or her inspired Po_2 falls because of low barometric pressure. Consequently, the peripheral chemoreceptors become excited and stimulate an increase in ventilation. Why must a day or so pass at this altitude before ventilation increases to its maximal level?

SOLUTION

When the peripheral chemoreceptors stimulate ventilation, $Paco_2$ falls, creating alkalemia. This produces an alkalotic CSF, because the blood-brain barrier is nearly impermeable to bicarbonate ions. That is, as CO_2 diffuses out of the CSF in response to the low arterial blood Pco_2, HCO_3^- ions remain behind in the CSF. This exposes the central chemoreceptors to an alkalotic environment, diminishing the effect of the hypoxic ventilatory stimulus. In other words, respiratory alkalosis limits the extent to which ventilation increases. Over the next 24 hours or so, HCO_3^- ions gradually diffuse out of the CSF across the blood-brain barrier, restoring the CSF pH level to normal. In addition, the kidneys excrete HCO_3^- ions to compensate for the respiratory alkalemia. Consequently, the blood pH level falls toward normal, while the hypoxic ventilatory stimulus keeps the $Paco_2$ low. As the CSF pH level returns to normal, the progressively unrestrained hypoxic stimulus further increases ventilation. Thus it takes approximately 24 hours of high altitude exposure before ventilation increases to its maximal level.

Response to Increased Arterial PCO_2 and Hydrogen Ions

For a given increase in $PaCO_2$ or hydrogen ion concentration, the carotid bodies are less responsive than the central chemoreceptors. The peripheral chemoreceptors account for only 20% to 30% of the ventilatory response to hypercapnia.[2] However, they respond to increased arterial hydrogen ion concentration more rapidly than do the central chemoreceptors. This is explained by the fact that the carotid bodies are exposed directly to arterial blood, unlike the central chemoreceptors. Thus the initial ventilatory response to metabolic acidosis is fairly quick, even though H^+ ions cross the blood-brain barrier with difficulty.

The responsiveness of the peripheral chemoreceptors to $PaCO_2$ and hydrogen ions is enhanced by hypoxemia. Conversely, responsiveness to hypoxemia is greatly enhanced by acidemia and hypercapnia. If PaO_2 is held constant at 60 mm Hg, a rise in $PaCO_2$ from 40 to 60 mm Hg and a fall in pH from 7.40 to 7.20 increase the carotid body firing rate by approximately 25%.[2]

People with chronic hypercapnia secondary to advanced chronic obstructive pulmonary disease (COPD) have depressed ventilatory responses to carbon dioxide, partly because of their altered acid-base status, and partly because their deranged lung mechanics prevents them from increasing their ventilation normally.[1] Their altered acid-base status arises from their high levels of blood buffer base, a compensatory response to respiratory acidosis (see Chapter 12).

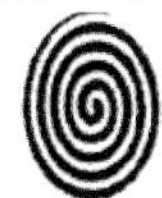

RULE OF THUMB

The ventilatory response to hypoxemia is greatly enhanced by hypercapnia and acidemia.

Control of Breathing During Chronic Hypercapnia

If $PaCO_2$ rises very slowly because of gradually deteriorating lung mechanics (as may occur in severe COPD), the kidneys compensate by gradually increasing plasma bicarbonate concentration, maintaining arterial pH within normal limits (see Chapter 12). As plasma bicarbonate levels increase, these ions slowly diffuse across the blood-brain barrier, keeping CSF pH in its normal range. Thus medullary chemoreceptors sense a normal pH environment, even though the $PaCO_2$ is abnormally high. (Keep in mind that the medullary chemoreceptors respond to hydrogen ions, not the CO_2 molecule.) This explains why the chronically high $PaCO_2$ of severe COPD patients does not have a stimulatory effect on their ventilation. Instead, hypoxemia becomes the minute-to-minute breathing stimulus. These patients are hypoxemic when breathing room air because their lungs have severe mismatches in ventilation and blood flow. It stands to reason that breathing supplemental oxygen might decrease or remove this hypoxemic stimulus, which would further decrease ventilation and raise the $PaCO_2$.

Indeed, the $PaCO_2$ of chronically hypercapnic COPD patients often does rise acutely after these patients are given oxygen. The traditional explanation for this phenomenon is that oxygen removes the hypoxic ventilatory stimulus and induces hypoventilation, but several investigators have questioned this explanation.[7-10]

Several studies have shown that the reduction in minute ventilation following oxygen breathing is not always severe enough to account for the increased $PaCO_2$. Some investigators suggest that oxygen breathing worsens the ventilation-perfusion ($\dot{V}/\dot{Q}$) relationships in the lungs and is responsible for the increase in $PaCO_2$.[7,8] Most investigators agree that oxygen-induced hypercapnia is caused by a combination of factors, the most important of which are (1) removal of the hypoxic stimulus and (2) redistribution of $\dot{V}/\dot{Q}$ in the lungs.[8-10]

Oxygen breathing may worsen $\dot{V}/\dot{Q}$ relationships in chronically hypercapnic patients because oxygen relieves hypoxic pulmonary vasoconstriction in poorly ventilated regions, increasing their blood flow (Figure 13-5, *A* and *B*). At the same time, these poorly ventilated regions may become even less ventilated as oxygen-rich inspired gas "washes out" resident nitrogen gas, making these regions more subject to *absorption atelectasis* (notice the further decreased $\dot{V}$ in Figure 13-5, *B*). Subsequently, inspired gas flows preferentially to already well-ventilated alveoli (see Figure 13-5, *B*), increasing their $\dot{V}/\dot{Q}$ ratios.[7,11] The increased $\dot{V}/\dot{Q}$ in these alveoli is further exaggerated as some cardiac output is redirected to poorly ventilated alveoli, whose vascular resistance was reduced by oxygen breathing.[8] To summarize, breathing supplemental oxygen may further decrease ventilation in low $\dot{V}/\dot{Q}$ regions, shifting more ventilation to the high $\dot{V}/\dot{Q}$ areas (compare Figure 13-5, *A*, with Figure 13-5, *B*). The end-result is an increased level of arterial PCO_2 that could occur without a fall in overall minute ventilation.

Although some investigators believe that the mechanisms just described explain how oxygen induces additional hypercapnia in patients with COPD, recent studies support an equally important role for oxygen suppression of the hypoxic ventilatory stimulus.[10] Whatever the mechanism, the clinically important fact is that uncontrolled oxygen therapy can lead to acute hypercapnia and acidemia in individuals who are already chronically hypercapnic. Therefore it is important to initially give alert, acutely hypoxemic patients with chronic hypercapnia low concentrations of oxygen

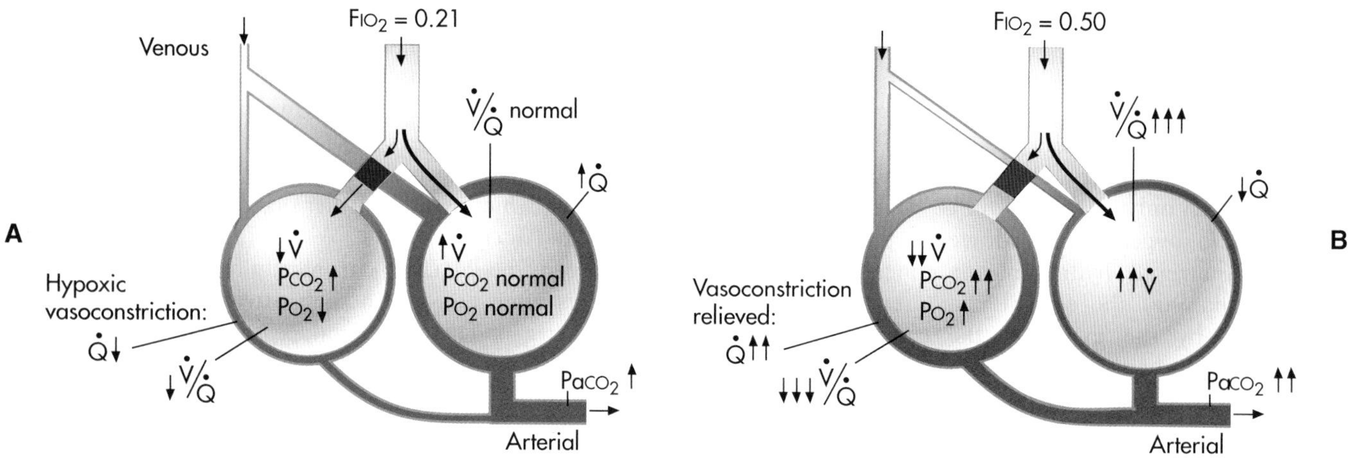

Figure 13-5

Proposed mechanism whereby oxygen administration in chronically hypercapnic people induces further hypercapnia by creating $\dot{V}/\dot{Q}$ mismatches: **A,** Low $\dot{V}/\dot{Q}$ unit *(left)* is hypoxic and hypercapnic while breathing ambient air; this induces pulmonary vasoconstriction. **B,** Breathing 50% oxygen predisposes the poorly ventilated unit to absorption atelectasis, further decreasing its ventilation, and simultaneously relieves hypoxic vasoconstriction, increasing its blood flow. These events (1) further lower the poorly ventilated unit's $\dot{V}/\dot{Q}$ ratio and (2) divert blood flow away from and ventilation toward already well-ventilated units. The latter increases alveolar dead space (high $\dot{V}/\dot{Q}$). *(Modified from Beachey W: Respiratory care anatomy and physiology: foundations for clinical practice, St Louis, 1998, Mosby.)*

(24% to 28%) and to monitor oxygen therapy closely with arterial blood gas analysis, watching for acute CO_2 retention and acidemia. Low levels of oxygen often increase arterial oxygen content quite effectively in these patients, because their arterial blood PaO_2 falls on the steep part of the O_2-Hb equilibrium curve (i.e., small increases in PaO_2 produce relatively large increases in oxygen content) (see Chapter 10).

It is important to note that the diagnosis of COPD on a patient's medical record does not automatically imply the presence of chronic hypercapnia or the potential for oxygen-induced hypercapnia. These characteristics are present in only the severe, end-stage forms of the disease, which comprises only a small percentage of patients with COPD. Therefore concern about oxygen-induced hypercapnia and acidemia is not warranted in most patients with a diagnosis of COPD. Oxygen should never be withheld from acutely hypoxemic COPD patients suffering exacerbations of their disease. Tissue oxygenation is of overriding importance and must not be sacrificed because of undue concern about hypercapnia and acidemia. The clinician must be prepared to mechanically support ventilation if oxygen administration induces severe acidemia.

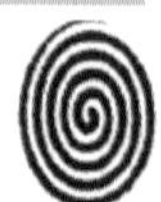

RULE OF THUMB

Tissue oxygenation is of overriding importance and must not be sacrificed because of undue concern about hypercapnia and acidemia in the patient with exacerbated COPD.

VENTILATORY RESPONSE TO EXERCISE

Strenuous exercise increases carbon dioxide production and oxygen consumption by as much as twentyfold.[4] Ventilation normally keeps pace with CO_2 production, keeping $PaCO_2$, PaO_2, and arterial pH constant. Because arterial blood gases do not change, elevated carbon dioxide or hypoxia does not stimulate ventilation in healthy individuals during exertion.

The exact mechanisms responsible for increasing ventilation during exercise is not well understood. Especially mysterious is the abrupt increase in ventilation at the *onset* of exercise long before any chemical or humoral changes can occur in the body. Two predominating theories for this phenomenon are (1) when the cerebral motor cortex sends impulses to exercising muscles, it apparently sends collateral excitatory impulses to the medullary respiratory centers, and (2) exercising limbs moving around their joints stimulate proprioceptors, which transmit excitatory impulses to the medullary centers.[1,12] Evidence also suggests that the sudden increase in ventilation at the onset of exercise is a *learned* response.[1,12] With repeated experience, the brain may learn to anticipate the proper amount of ventilation required to maintain normal blood gases during exercise.

ABNORMAL BREATHING PATTERNS

Commonly described abnormal breathing patterns include **Cheyne-Stokes respiration, Biot's respiration,**

apneustic breathing, and central neurogenic hypoventilation and hyperventilation.

In Cheyne-Stokes respiration, respiratory rate and tidal volume gradually increase and then gradually decrease to complete **apnea** (absence of ventilation), which may last several seconds. Then tidal volume and breathing frequency gradually increase again, repeating the cycle. This pattern occurs when cardiac output is low, as in congestive heart failure, delaying the blood transit time between the lungs and the brain.[4] In this instance, changes in respiratory center P_{CO_2} lag behind changes in arterial P_{CO_2}. For example, when an increased Pa_{CO_2} from the lungs reaches the respiratory neurons, ventilation is stimulated, which then lowers the arterial P_{CO_2} level. By the time this reduced Pa_{CO_2} reaches the medulla to inhibit ventilation, hyperventilation has been in progress for an inappropriately long time. When blood from the lung finally does reach the medullary centers, the low Pa_{CO_2} greatly depresses ventilation to the point of apnea. Arterial P_{CO_2} then rises, but a rise in respiratory center P_{CO_2} is delayed because of low blood flow rate. The brain eventually does receive the high Pa_{CO_2} signal, and the cycle is repeated. Cheyne-Stokes respiration may also be caused by brain injuries in which the respiratory centers over-respond to changes in the P_{CO_2} level.

Biot's respiration is similar to Cheyne-Stokes respiration, except that tidal volumes are of identical depth. It occurs in patients with increased intracranial pressure, but the mechanism for this pattern is unclear.[5]

Apneustic breathing indicates damage to the pons. Central neurogenic hyperventilation is characterized by persistent hyperventilation driven by abnormal neural stimuli. It is related to midbrain and upper pons damage associated with head trauma, severe brain hypoxia, or lack of blood flow to the brain.[13] Conversely, central neurogenic hypoventilation means the respiratory centers do not respond appropriately to ventilatory stimuli, such as carbon dioxide. It also is associated with head trauma and brain hypoxia, as well as narcotic suppression of the respiratory center.[13]

▶ EFFECT OF CARBON DIOXIDE ON CEREBRAL BLOOD FLOW

High levels of arterial carbon dioxide dilate cerebral blood vessels, increasing the normal brain's blood flow. Low Pa_{CO_2} has the opposite effect. In severe head injuries, the brain tissue swells, and carbon dioxide does not necessarily increase cerebral blood flow. As brain tissues swell within the rigid skull, intracranial pressure may rise above cerebral arterial pressure, stopping blood flow to the brain. Hypoventilation in such instances aggravates the problem, because the resulting hypercapnia dilates cerebral vessels, further increasing intracranial pressure.

MINI CLINI

Deliberate Hyperventilation of the Patient With Head Trauma

PROBLEM

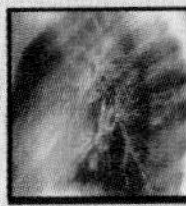

A patient has suffered a head injury and is being supported on a mechanical ventilator in the intensive care unit. The patient's arterial blood gas values are as follows:

$$pH = 7.50$$

$$P_{CO_2} = 28 \text{ mm Hg}$$

$$HCO_3^- = 22 \text{ mEq/L}$$

$$P_{O_2} = 90 \text{ mm Hg}$$

A special pressure-monitoring device indicates a slightly high intracranial pressure. A co-worker assigned to this patient is concerned about the alkalotic acid-base status, but the respiratory therapist (RT) suggests that the alkalosis is appropriate in this instance. How does the RT justify this position?

SOLUTION

Deliberately hyperventilating this patient to keep the Pa_{CO_2} moderately low creates a mild respiratory alkalosis. This lowers the hydrogen ion concentration in the cerebral blood vessels, constricting normal, undamaged vessels. Consequently, cerebral blood flow diminishes, the brain's vascular volume decreases, and intracranial pressure subsides. The lowered intracranial pressure offers less opposition to blood flowing into the brain through cerebral arteries, improving cerebral perfusion. However, the kidneys eventually compensate for this artificially induced alkalosis after several days. As arterial pH returns to the normal range, the vasoconstrictive effect of hypocapnia is diminished.

KEY POINTS

- The DRG and VRG of neurons in the medulla generate the basic cyclical breathing pattern.
- Apneustic center impulses prevent medullary inspiratory neurons from switching off, creating a prolonged, gasping inspiration.
- Impulses from the pneumotaxic center inhibit the apneustic center, shortening inspiratory time and increasing respiratory rate.
- Various reflexes from peripheral sources affect the breathing pattern by altering the medullary center's output.
- Central chemoreceptors in the medulla are bathed in the CSF, separated from arterial blood by a semipermeable membrane called the blood-brain barrier.
- The blood-brain barrier is almost impermeable to arterial hydrogen and bicarbonate ions, but it is freely permeable to arterial carbon dioxide.
- Central chemoreceptors stimulate increased ventilation in response to the hydrogen ions formed in the CSF by the reaction between arterial CO_2 and water.
- Peripheral chemoreceptors, located mainly in the carotid bodies, respond to arterial hypoxemia, hypercapnia, and acidosis.
- The primary stimulus for breathing in healthy individuals is arterial carbon dioxide.
- The secondary stimulus for breathing in healthy individuals is arterial hypoxemia, which is not present until PaO_2 falls below 60 mm Hg.
- The breathing of patients with chronic, compensated hypercapnia is mainly driven by the hypoxic stimulus rather than the CO_2 stimulus.
- Oxygen therapy can induce hypoventilation, acute arterial CO_2 retention, and acidosis in patients with chronic hypercapnia.
- Oxygen should never be withheld for any reason from patients suffering severe hypoxemia.
- Carbon dioxide dilates cerebral blood vessels and raises intracranial pressure; reducing arterial CO_2 constricts cerebral vessels and lowers intracranial pressure.

References

1. Levitzky MG: Pulmonary physiology, ed 5, New York, 1999, McGraw-Hill.
2. Taylor AE et al: Clinical respiratory physiology, Philadelphia, 1989, WB Saunders.
3. Feldman JL, Smith JC: Neural control of respiratory pattern in mammals: an overview. In Dempsey JA, Pack AI, editors: Regulation of breathing, ed 2, New York, 1995, Marcel Dekker.
4. Guyton AC: Textbook of medical physiology, ed 8, Philadelphia, 1991, WB Saunders.
5. Comroe JH: Physiology of respiration, ed 2, Chicago, 1974, Year Book.
6. West JB: Respiratory physiology: the essentials, ed 6, Philadelphia, 2000, Lippincott Williams & Wilkins.
7. Aubier M et al: Effects of administration of O2 on ventilation and blood gases in patients with chronic obstructive pulmonary disease during acute respiratory failure, Am Rev Respir Dis 122:747, 1980.
8. Sassoon CSH, Hassell KT, Mahutte CK: Hypoxic-induced hypercapnia in stable chronic obstructive pulmonary disease, Am Rev Respir Dis 135:907, 1987.
9. Rebuck AS, Slutsky AS: Control of breathing in diseases of the respiratory tract and lungs. In Fishman AP et al, editors: Handbook of physiology, section 3, The respiratory system, vol II, Control of breathing, Bethesda, Md, 1986, American Physiological Society.
10. Dunn WF, Nelson SB, Hubmayr RD: Oxygen-induced hypercapnia in obstructive pulmonary disease, Am Rev Respir Dis 144:526, 1991.
11. Guenard H et al: Effects of oxygen breathing on regional distribution of ventilation and perfusion in hypoxemic patients with chronic lung disease, Am Rev Respir Dis 125:12, 1982.
12. Leff AR, Schumacker PT: Respiratory physiology: basics and applications, Philadelphia, 1993, WB Saunders.
13. Burton GG, Hodgkin JE, Ward JJ: Respiratory care: a guide to clinical practice, ed 4, Philadelphia, 1997, JB Lippincott.

SECTION III

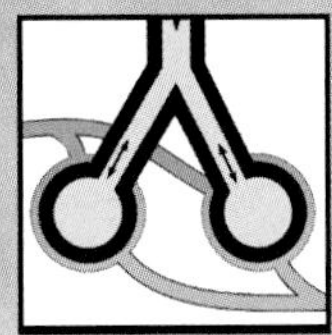

Assessment of Respiratory Disorders

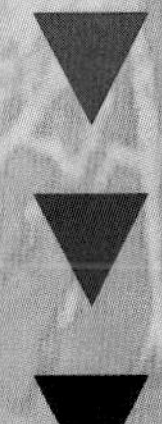

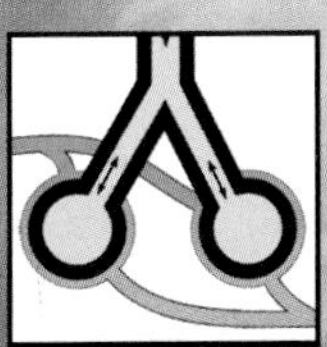

CHAPTER 14

Bedside Assessment of the Patient

Robert L. Wilkins

In This Chapter You Will Learn:

- Why patient interviews are necessary and what techniques are used for conducting a patient interview
- What abnormalities in lung function are associated with common pulmonary symptoms
- What abnormal breathing patterns indicate about underlying pulmonary pathological conditions
- What terms are used to describe normal and abnormal lung sounds
- What mechanisms are responsible for normal and abnormal lung sounds
- Why it is necessary to examine the precordium, abdomen, and extremities in the patient with cardiopulmonary disease

Chapter Outline

Key Terms

abdominal paradox
adventitious lung sounds (ALS)
barrel chest
bradycardia
bradypnea
bronchophony
cough
crackles
cyanosis
diaphoresis
diastolic pressure
dyspnea
febrile
fetid
fever
hemoptysis
hepatomegaly
hypotension
hypothermia
mucoid
orthopnea
pedal edema
phlegm
platypnea
pulse pressure
pulsus alternans
pulsus paradoxus
purulent
respiratory alternans
retractions
rhonchi
rhonchial fremitus
sputum
stridor
subcutaneous emphysema
syncope
systolic pressure
tachycardia
tachypnea
wheezes

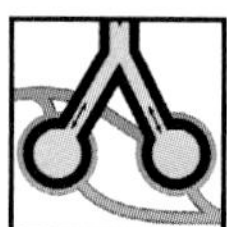

Progress in the field of respiratory care has placed increasing demands on respiratory therapists (RTs) to develop competent bedside assessment skills. Decisions regarding when to begin, change, or end therapy must be based on accurate clinical evidence. Although the physician has the ultimate responsibility for these decisions, RTs often participate in the clinical decision-making process. To fulfill this role effectively, the RT must assume responsibility for gathering and interpreting relevant bedside patient data.

Two key sources of patient data are the medical history and the physical examination. Data gathered initially by interview and physical examination help identify the need for subsequent diagnostic tests. After a tentative diagnosis is made, these assessment procedures also help clinicians select the best treatment approaches. Once a treatment regimen begins, these procedures are again used to monitor patient progress toward predefined goals.

Bedside assessment is the process of interviewing and examining the patient for the signs and symptoms of disease and the effects of treatment. It is a cost-effective way of obtaining pertinent information about the patient's health status. In many cases, it provides the initial evidence that something is wrong and often helps establish the severity of the problem. Unlike some diagnostic tests, bedside assessment techniques are of little risk to the patient.

The patient initially is assessed to identify the correct diagnosis. This initial assessment is most often performed by a physician. Exceptions may occur in emergency situations in which a physician is not available. In such cases, other healthcare personnel such as nurses and RTs may need to rapidly evaluate the patient to implement appropriate life-saving treatment (e.g., cardiopulmonary resuscitation). Once a tentative diagnosis is reached and the physician orders specific treatment, subsequent evaluations are made by healthcare personnel to monitor the patient's hospital stay and evaluate treatment results.

The skills of bedside assessment described here are not difficult to learn; however, mastery requires practice. Initially, students should practice the skills on healthy individuals. This helps improve technique and provides an understanding of normal variations. The ability to discriminate abnormal from the range of possible normal findings is an important skill that requires experience to obtain.

MINI CLINI

Bedside Assessment of the Postoperative Patient

PROBLEM

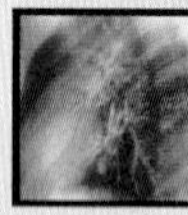

The respiratory therapist (RT) is called to the surgical ward to see a 54-year-old woman who had abdominal surgery 2 days ago. She is currently afebrile, alert, and oriented, but is complaining of dyspnea. Her resting respiratory rate is 34 breaths/min, and the breaths are shallow. Her heart rate is 110 beats/min. She is 5 feet tall and weighs approximately 185 lb. During the brief interview, the RT identifies that the dyspnea has gradually increased over the last 12 hours and increases with exertion. During auscultation, the RT identifies diminished breath sounds in the bases, with some fine, late inspiratory crackles. The remainder of the physical examination is normal. What is the most likely cause of this patient's dyspnea, and what should be done?

SOLUTION

The findings indicate a loss of lung volume as the cause of the sudden dyspnea. The rapid, shallow breathing; fine, late inspiratory crackles; and history of recent abdominal surgery suggest atelectasis. Patients who undergo abdominal surgery are prone to developing atelectasis in the postoperative period.

Other concerns include congestive heart failure and pulmonary thromboembolism. The RT should ask the attending physician to order a chest x-ray examination and begin hyperinflation therapy if the chest film confirms the presence of atelectasis.

▶ INTERVIEWING THE PATIENT AND TAKING A MEDICAL HISTORY

Interviewing furnishes unique information because it provides the patient's perspective. It serves the following three related purposes:

1. To establish a rapport between clinician and patient
2. To obtain essential diagnostic information
3. To help monitor changes in the patient's symptoms and response to therapy

For these reasons, interviewing is a crucial aspect of general patient assessment.

Principles of Interviewing

Interviewing is a way of "connecting" with the patient, which is especially important for the patient who is under the stress of an illness. As depicted in Figure 2-11 on p. 30, the factors that affect communication between the RT and the patient include the following:

- Sensory and emotional factors
- Environmental factors
- Verbal and nonverbal components of the communication process

- Internal factors of values, beliefs, feelings, habits, and preoccupations of both the healthcare professional and the patient

For these reasons, no two interviews are the same.

Although developing interviewing skills takes time and experience, beginners can get a head start by following a few basic guidelines and being knowledgeable about the causes and characteristics of the more common cardiopulmonary symptoms. The following discussion provides some of the guidelines for interviewing and then discusses the more common symptoms associated with diseases of the chest.

Structure and Technique for Interviewing

The ideal interview is one in which the patient feels secure and free to talk about important personal matters. Each interview should begin with a brief introduction by the clinician and the purpose of his or her visit. This is done in the *social space*, approximately 4 to 12 feet from the patient. This begins the process of establishing a rapport with the patient and helps the patient feel more comfortable about answering personal questions. Pulling the curtain between the beds of a semiprivate room also may be helpful in making the patient feel more at ease with the interview (Box 14-1).

Next, the interviewer should move to the *personal space* (2 to 4 feet from the patient) to begin the interview. In this space, the patient does not have to speak loudly in response to questions. The interviewer should assume a physical position at the same level with the patient. This is usually accomplished by pulling up a nearby chair before beginning the formal interview, which helps the interviewer avoid standing over the patient and making him or her feel inferior. Appropriate eye contact with the patient is essential for a quality interview. This aids in better assessment of the patient and gives the patient more confidence in the interviewer. Eye contact allows the interviewer to see confusion, anger, frustration, and other emotions that may be expressed by the patient in response to questions.

Using neutral questions and avoiding leading questions during the interview is important. Asking the patient: "Is your breathing better now?" leads the patient toward a desired response and may elicit false information. Asking the patient, "How is your breathing now?" is a better way to get accurate information about the patient's breathing (Box 14-2).

Common characteristics of symptoms can be identified by asking questions such as the following during the interview:

- When did it start?
- How severe is it? (Rated on a scale of 1 to 10)

Box 14-1 • Guidelines for Effective Patient Interviewing

1. Project a sense of undivided interest in the patient:
   - Provide for privacy and do not permit interruptions.
   - Review records and prepare materials before entering the room.
   - Listen and observe carefully.
   - Be attentive and respond to the patient's priorities, concerns, feelings, and comfort.
2. Establish your professional role during the introduction:
   - Dress and groom professionally.
   - Enter the room with a smile and unhurried manner.
   - Make immediate eye contact.
   - If the patient is well enough, introduce yourself with a firm handshake.
   - State your role and the purpose of your visit, and define the patient's involvement in the interaction.
   - Address adult patients by title (e.g., Mr., Mrs., Ms.) and their last name. Using these formal terms of address alerts the patient to the importance of the interaction.
3. Show your respect for the patient's beliefs, attitudes, and rights:
   - Be sure the patient is appropriately covered.
   - Position yourself so that eye contact is comfortable for the patient. (Ideally, patients should be sitting up, with their eye level at or slightly above yours.)
   - Avoid standing at the foot of the bed or with your hand on the door, because this may send the nonverbal message that you do not have time for the patient.
   - Ask the patient's permission before moving any personal items or making adjustments in the room.
   - Remember that the patient's dialog with you and his or her medical record are confidential.
   - Be honest; never guess at an answer or information that you do not know; do not provide information beyond your scope of practice; providing new information to the patient is the privilege and responsibility of the attending physician.
   - Make no moral judgments about the patient; set your values for patient care according to the patient's values, beliefs, and priorities.
   - Expect the patient to have an emotional response to illness and the healthcare environment.
   - Listen, then clarify and teach, but never argue.
   - Adjust the time, length, and content of the interview to your patient's needs.
4. Use a relaxed, conversational style:
   - Ask questions and make statements that communicate empathy.
   - Encourage the patient to express his or her concerns.
   - Expect and accept some periods of silence.
   - Close even the briefest interview by asking whether there is anything the patient needs or wants to discuss.
   - Tell the patient when you will return.

Box 14-2 • Types of Questions Used in Patient Interviews

1. Open-ended questions encourage patients to describe events and priorities as they see them, helping bring out concerns and attitudes and promote understanding. Questions such as "What brought you to the hospital?" or "What happened next?" encourage conversational flow and rapport, while giving patients enough direction to know where to start.
2. Closed questions such as "When did your cough start?" or "How long did the pain last?" focus on specific information and provide clarification.
3. Direct questions can be open-ended or closed and always end in a question mark. Although they are used to obtain specific information, a series of direct questions or frequent use of the question "Why?" can be intimidating.
4. Indirect questions are less threatening than direct questions, because they sound like statements (e.g., "I gather your doctor told you to take the treatments every 4 hours."). Inquiries of this type also work well to confront discrepancies in the patient's statements (e.g., "If I understood you correctly, it is harder for you to breathe now than it was before your treatment.").
5. Neutral questions and statements are preferred for all interactions with the patient. "What happened next?" and "Can you tell me more about ...?" are neutral, open-ended questions. A neutral, closed question may give the patient a choice of responses, while focusing on the type of information desired (e.g., "Would you say there was a teaspoon, a tablespoon, or a half cup?"). Leading questions, such as "You didn't cough up blood, did you?" should be avoided, because they imply an answer.

- Where on the body is it? (Especially important for chest pain)
- What seems to make it better or worse?
- Has it occurred before? (If so, how long did it last?)

Identifying these characteristics of any new symptom can be helpful in recognizing the cause and potential therapy. This is primarily the role of the attending physician but sometimes falls to other clinicians in certain settings. Once the symptom(s) is established and therapy is started, other questions are used to evaluate the changes in the symptom(s) over the course of the hospital stay. For example, the clinician may ask, "Has the symptom changed in any way since admission?" "Does the therapy seem to make a difference?"

The best interview techniques are of no value if the interviewer is not knowledgeable about the pathophysiology and characteristics of the more common cardiopulmonary symptoms. The interview is a series of focused questions that pursue specific information related to a tentative diagnosis. The ability to ask the key questions at the right time comes from experience and familiarity with the signs and symptoms of lung disease.

Common Cardiopulmonary Symptoms

Dyspnea

Dyspnea is defined as shortness of breath as perceived by the patient. It is a complex symptom that occurs in a variety of settings. The exact mechanisms responsible for dyspnea are not well understood, but it does occur most often when patients sense that their work of breathing is excessive for their level of activity. In general, shortness of breath becomes a concern when the drive to breathe is excessive or when the work of breathing increases. Increases in the drive to breathe occur with hypoxemia, acidosis, fever, exercise, or anxiety. An increase in the work of breathing occurs when the airways become narrowed (e.g., with asthma or bronchitis) or when the lung becomes difficult to expand (e.g., with pneumonia, pulmonary edema, or chest wall abnormality). In some patients, both an increase in the work of breathing and an increase in the drive to breathe may be present, resulting in severe dyspnea.

Dyspnea may be present only when the patient assumes the reclining position, in which case it is referred to as **orthopnea.** Orthopnea is common in patients with congestive heart failure (CHF) and appears to be caused by the sudden increase in venous return that occurs with reclining. The failing left ventricle is unable to accommodate the increased venous return, resulting in pulmonary vascular congestion and dyspnea. Orthopnea is also a symptom of bilateral diaphragmatic paralysis.

Shortness of breath in the upright position is known as **platypnea.** This unusual symptom may accompany arteriovenous malformations in the lung, such as occurs in chronic liver disease (hepatopulmonary syndrome) or some hereditary conditions. Platypnea may be accompanied by *orthodeoxia*, which is oxygen desaturation on assuming an upright position.

It is important to identify and document the degree of dyspnea because it helps determine the severity of the problem. The more severe the illness, the more short of breath the patient becomes at lower and lower levels of exertion in most cases. It also is important to identify at what level of exertion the patient must stop to catch his or her breath. Does the patient need to stop after walking up one flight of stairs or after walking half a block on a flat surface? Obviously, the patient who gets short of breath after walking up several flights of stairs is not nearly as ill as is the patient who is short of breath at rest. In the latter case, the initial examination should be brief and the problem should be treated as soon as possible.

Not all patients with shortness of breath use similar terms or phrases to describe their dyspnea. In fact, studies have shown that patients tend to describe their dyspnea according to the underlying pathophysiolgy[1-3]; for example, patients with asthma tend to use the phrase "my chest is tight," patients with interstitial lung disease tend to state "my breathing is too rapid," and patients with CHF often qualify their dyspnea with the phrase "I feel like I am suffocating." In addition, there may be ethnic differences in the way patients describe their shortness of breath.[4] Clinicians should ask specific questions about the quality and characteristics of the patient's dyspnea to better assess the cause and find appropriate treatment.[5]

The degree of dyspnea at rest should be documented using a numeric intensity or visual analog scale (Figure 14-1). Such scales are important because they provide a way to trend the patient's response to treatment over time. In addition, they are needed because physiological measures of lung function (e.g., pulmonary function tests, PaO_2) do not correlate with the degree of dyspnea in many patients.[6] For example, patients who appear healthy, as evidenced by a normal PaO_2 or forced expiratory volume in 1 second (FEV_1), may be experiencing significant dyspnea that is disruptive to their overall quality of life.

Patients who are receiving mechanical ventilation, and who are alert and oriented, can be evaluated for the presence and degree of dyspnea, although they are intubated, by using the aforementioned scales. Because dyspnea is common in mechanically ventilated patients, it is important for RTs to routinely assess the level of dyspnea in these patients.[7] RTs may need to consult with the attending physician and adjust the ventilator settings (e.g., increase pressure support) when patients communicate the presence of moderate or severe dyspnea during mechanical ventilation.

Modified Borg Scale

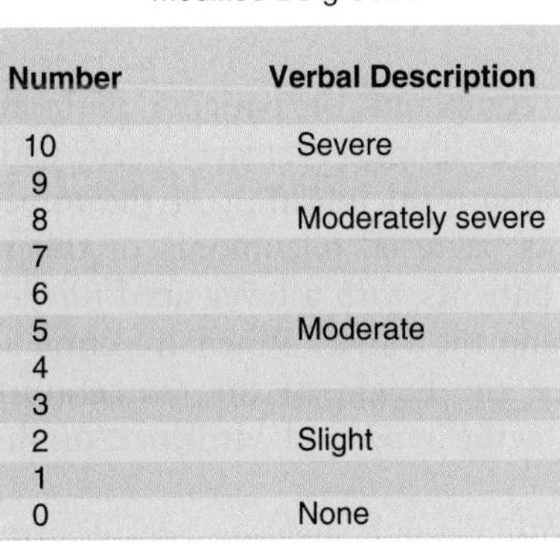

Number	Verbal Description
10	Severe
9	
8	Moderately severe
7	
6	
5	Moderate
4	
3	
2	Slight
1	
0	None

A

Visual Scale

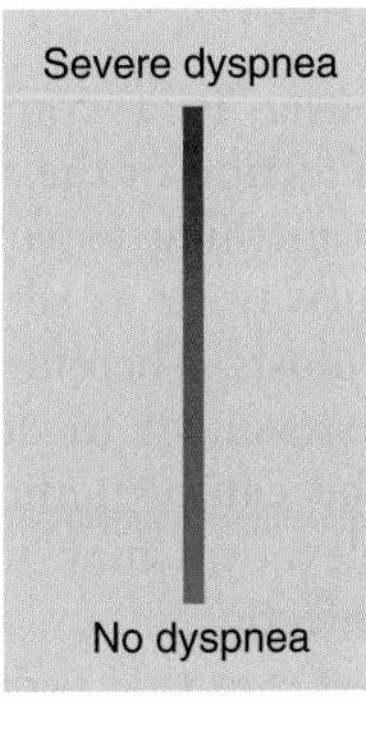

B

{AU: Is legend okay?} **Figure 14-1**
A, Modified Borg scale. **B**, Visual analog scale for measuring the degree of dyspnea.

Cough

A **cough** is one of the most common symptoms seen in patients with pulmonary disease. Coughing is a forceful expiratory maneuver, which expels mucus and foreign material from the airways. It usually occurs when the cough receptors are stimulated by inflammation, mucus, foreign materials, or noxious gases. The cough receptors are located primarily in the larynx, trachea, and larger bronchi.

The effectiveness of a cough depends on the individual's ability to take a deep breath, his or her lung recoil, the strength of his or her expiratory muscles, and the level of airway resistance. The ability to take a deep breath or exhale forcefully is often impaired in patients with neuromuscular disease. Expiratory flow is often limited by factors such as bronchospasm (e.g., asthma) and reduced lung recoil (as in emphysema). Patients with an inadequate ability to cough because of impairment of these factors often have problems with retained secretions and therefore are more prone to pneumonia.

Important characteristics of the patient's cough to identify include whether it is dry or loose, productive or nonproductive, and acute or chronic, as well as its time of occurrence during the day or night. Knowledge of such details may help in determining the cause of the cough. For example, a dry, nonproductive cough is typical for restrictive lung diseases such as CHF or pulmonary fibrosis. A loose, productive cough is more often associated with inflammatory obstructive diseases such as bronchitis and asthma. The most common cause of an acute, self-limited cough is a viral infection of the upper airway. Common causes of chronic coughing include asthma, postnasal drip, chronic bronchitis, and gastroesophageal reflux, although combinations of these often exist.[8]

Sputum Production

Healthy airways produce mucus daily. Normally, however, the quantity of this mucus is minimal, and it certainly is not enough to stimulate the cough receptors. Mucus is gradually moved to the hypopharynx by the mucociliary escalator, where it is either swallowed or expectorated. Disease of the airways may cause the mucous glands, which line the airways, to produce an abnormally increased amount of mucus, which usually stimulates the cough receptors and causes the patient to generate a loose, productive cough. This is seen in acute bronchitis or asthma attacks brought on by airway infection.

RTs need to be aware of the terminology associated with sputum. Technically, mucus from the tracheobronchial tree that has not been contaminated by oral secretions is called **phlegm**. Mucus that comes from the lung but passes through the mouth as it is expectorated is **sputum**. Because this is how most mucus samples from the lung are obtained, the term *sputum* is used in this chapter. Sputum that contains pus cells is said to be **purulent**, suggesting a bacterial infection. Purulent sputum appears thick, colored, and sticky. Sputum that is foul smelling is said to be **fetid**. Sputum that is clear and thick is **mucoid** and is commonly seen in patients with airways disease. Recent changes in the color, viscosity, or quantity of sputum produced are often signs of infection and must be documented and reported to the physician.

Hemoptysis

Coughing up blood or blood-streaked sputum from the lungs is referred to as **hemoptysis**. Hemoptysis is characterized as either massive (more than 300 mL of blood over 24 hours), which is a medical emergency, or nonmassive. Hemoptysis must be distinguished from *hematemesis*, which is vomiting blood from the gastrointestinal tract. Blood from the lung is often seen in patients with a history of pulmonary disease and may be mixed with sputum. Blood from the stomach may be mixed with food particles and occurs most often in patients with a history of gastrointestinal disease.

Nonmassive hemoptysis is caused most often by infection of the airways but also is seen in lung cancer, tuberculosis, trauma, and pulmonary embolism. Hemoptysis associated with infection usually is seen as blood-streaked, purulent sputum. Hemoptysis from bronchogenic carcinoma often is chronic and may be associated with a monophonic wheeze. Common causes of massive hemoptysis include bronchiectasis, lung abscess, and acute or old tuberculosis.

Chest Pain

Most chest pain can be categorized as either *pleuritic* or *nonpleuritic*. Pleuritic chest pain usually is located laterally or posteriorly. It worsens when the patient takes a deep breath, and it is described as a sharp, stabbing type of pain. It is associated with diseases of the chest that cause the pleural lining of the lung to become inflamed, such as pneumonia or pulmonary embolism.

Nonpleuritic chest pain is located typically in the center of the anterior chest and may radiate to the shoulder or back. It is not affected by breathing, and it is described as a dull ache or pressure type of pain. A common cause of nonpleuritic chest pain is angina, which classically is a pressure sensation with exertion or stress and results from coronary artery occlusion. Other common causes of nonpleuritic chest pain include gastroesophageal reflux, esophageal spasm, chest wall pain (e.g., costochondritis), and gallbladder disease.

MINI CLINI

Sudden Onset of Chest Pain

PROBLEM

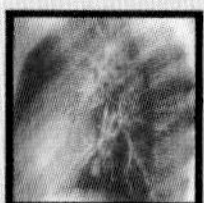

The RT is called to the emergency department to see a 47-year-old man who came to the local hospital with anxiety and chest pain. He is certain he is having a heart attack and demands immediate treatment. The attending physician is on the way to the hospital but has asked the nurse to call the RT in the interim.

The RT places the patient on oxygen and asks him for details about the chest pain. She identifies that the pain is located laterally on the left side and increases with each inspiratory effort.

The patient's vital signs are normal (including respiratory rate) except for a slight increase in heart rate. What is the most likely cause of this patient's chest pain, given its characteristics? What should be done until the patient's physician arrives?

SOLUTION

Chest pain is a worrisome symptom because it can indicate either a life-threatening or a less serious problem. Among the most serious problems are acute heart attack, pulmonary embolism, aortic dissection, and pneumothorax. In this case, the pain is pleuritic. Therefore angina, acute myocardial infarction, and aortic dissection are not likely causes. The pleuritic character of the pain is consistent with pulmonary embolism and pneumothorax, but the normal respiratory rate suggests that pulmonary embolism is not the likely cause of the chest pain. If pneumothorax is present, it must be small.

The RT should continue oxygen therapy and monitor the patient until the attending physician arrives. The RT should ask the nurse to attach chest leads to monitor the patient's heart rate and rhythm just in case the chest pain is related to heart disease. In addition, the RT should try to comfort the patient as much as possible.

Fever

Fever is a common complaint of patients with an infection of the airways or lungs. Fever may occur with something as simple as a viral infection of the upper airway or as serious as bacterial pneumonia or tuberculosis. Therefore all patients with a fever need further assessment to determine the cause. When infection is the cause of the fever, the height of the temperature elevation may indicate the type and virulence of the infection.

Fever that occurs with a cough suggests a respiratory infection. An infection is even more likely to be the cause of the fever if the patient is producing purulent sputum. However, the absence of coughing or sputum production does not necessarily rule out lung infection.

Patients with significant fever will have an increased

metabolic rate and thus an increased oxygen consumption and carbon dioxide production. The increased need for oxygen intake and carbon dioxide removal may cause tachypnea. The increased ventilatory demand in patients with fever complicating severe chronic cardiopulmonary disease may cause acute respiratory failure.

Pedal Edema

Swelling of the lower extremities is known as **pedal edema.** It most often occurs with heart failure, which causes an increase in the hydrostatic pressure of the blood vessels in the lower extremities. This causes fluid to leak into the interstitial spaces and leads to pedal edema, the degree of which depends on the level of heart failure. Patients with chronic hypoxemic lung disease are especially prone to right-sided heart failure (cor pulmonale) because of the heavy demands placed on the right ventricle when hypoxemia causes severe pulmonary vasoconstriction. Eventually, the right side of the heart begins to fail and results in a backup of pressure into the venous blood vessels, especially in the dependent regions such as the lower extremities. This promotes high intravascular venous hydrostatic pressures and pedal edema. The patient will often complain of "swollen ankles" in such cases.

Format for the Medical History

All healthcare practitioners must be familiar with the medical history of the patients they are treating, even if their reason for contact is simply to provide intermittent therapy. The medical history familiarizes clinicians with the signs and symptoms the patient exhibited on admission and the reason the therapy is being administered.

The clinician should begin reviewing the patient's chart by reading about the patient's current medical problems. This information is found under the headings of *chief complaint* (CC) and *history of present illness* (HPI). This section of the medical history represents a detailed account of each of the patient's major complaints. It is written by the physician after his or her interview with the patient at admission to the hospital.

The next step is to review the patient's *past medical history* (PMH), which describes all past major illnesses, injuries, surgeries, hospitalizations, allergies, and health-related habits. This information provides a basic understanding of the patient's previous experiences with illness and healthcare.

Next, the clinician should review the *family and social/environmental history*. This part of the medical history focuses on potential genetic or occupational links to disease and the patient's current life situation. A detailed occupational history is particularly important in assessing pulmonary disorders that may result from inhaling dusts in the workplace, either organic (i.e., containing protein) or nonorganic (e.g., asbestos, silica).

Finally, the clinician should look at the *review of systems*, which is designed to uncover problem areas the patient forgot to mention or omitted. Usually, this information is obtained in a head-to-toe review of all body systems. For each body system, the interviewer obtains information about current, pertinent symptoms. For example, during a review of the respiratory system, questioning would determine the presence or history of cough, hemoptysis, sputum production, chest pain, shortness of breath, and fever (Box 14-3).

▶ PHYSICAL EXAMINATION

A careful physical examination of the patient is essential for evaluating the patient's problem and determining the effects of therapy. The physical examination consists of the following four general steps: (1) inspection (visually examining), (2) palpation (touching), (3) percussion (tapping), and (4) auscultation (listening with a stethoscope).

General Appearance

The first few seconds of an encounter with the patient usually helps reveal both the acuity and severity of the current problem. For an experienced clinician, these initial impressions determine the course of subsequent assessment. For example, if the patient's general appearance indicates an acute problem, the rest of the examination may be abbreviated and focused until the patient's condition is stabilized. On the other hand, if the initial impressions indicate that the patient is stable and not in immediate danger, a more complete assessment can be conducted (Box 14-4).

Several indicators are important in assessing the patient's overall appearance. These include the patient's facial expression, level of anxiety or distress, positioning, and personal hygiene.

In observing the body as a whole, the clinician should look for specific characteristics. Does the patient appear well nourished or emaciated? Weakness and emaciation (cachexia) are signs of general ill health and malnutrition. Is the patient sweating? **Diaphoresis** (sweating) can indicate fever, pain, severe stress, increased metabolism, or acute anxiety.

The general facial expression may help reveal pain or anxiety. Facial expression also can help in evaluating alertness, mood, general character, and mental capacity. More specific facial signs also can indicate respiratory distress. Simple observation of the patient's anxiety level can indicate the severity of the current problem and whether cooperation can be expected. The patient's position also may be useful in assessing the severity of

Box 14-3 • Outline of a Complete Health History

1. Demographic data (obtained from admission interview): name, address, age, birth date, place of birth, race, nationality, marital status, religion, occupation, and source of referral
2. Date and source of history and estimate of the reliability of the historian
3. Brief description of the patient's condition at the time the history or patient profile was taken
4. Chief complaint and reason for seeking treatment
5. History of present illness: chronological description of each symptom
   - Onset: time, type, source, setting
   - Frequency and duration of symptoms
   - Location and radiation of pain
   - Severity (quantity)
   - Quality (character)
   - Aggravating and alleviating factors
   - Associated manifestations
6. Past medical history
   - Childhood diseases and development
   - Hospitalizations, surgeries, injuries, accidents, and major illnesses
   - Allergies
   - Medications
7. Family history
   - Familial disease history
   - Marital history
   - Family relationships
8. Social and environmental history
   - Education
   - Military experience
   - Occupational history
   - Religious and social activities
   - Living arrangements
   - Hobbies and recreation
   - Satisfaction with and stresses of life situation, finances, and relationships
   - Recent travel or other event that might impact health
9. Review of systems (e.g., the respiratory system)
   - Cough
   - Hemoptysis
   - Sputum (amount and consistency)
   - Chest pain
   - Shortness of breath
   - Hoarseness or changes in voice
   - Dizziness or fainting
   - Fever or chills
   - Peripheral edema
10. Patient's printed name and signature

the problem and the patient's response to it. For example, the patient with severe pulmonary hyperinflation tends to sit upright while bracing his or her elbows on a table. This helps the accessory muscles gain a

Box 14-4 • Typical Format for Recording the Physical Examination

INITIAL IMPRESSION
- Age, height, weight, sensorium, and general appearance

VITAL SIGNS
- Pulse rate, respiratory rate, temperature, and blood pressure

HEAD, EARS, EYES, NOSE, AND THROAT (HEENT)
- Inspection findings

NECK
- Inspection and palpation findings

THORAX
- Inspection, palpation, percussion, and auscultation findings of the lungs
- Inspection, palpation, and auscultation findings of the heart

ABDOMEN
- Inspection, palpation, percussion, and auscultation findings

EXTREMITIES
- Inspection and palpation findings

mechanical advantage for breathing. Finally, personal hygiene indicators can help determine both the duration and the impact of the illness on the patient's daily activities.

Level of Consciousness

After observing the patient's overall appearance, the clinician should quickly assess the patient's level of consciousness (alertness). Evaluating the patient's alertness is a simple but important task. If the patient appears conscious, assess the patient's orientation to time, place, and person. This often is called *evaluating the sensorium*. The alert patient who is well oriented to time, place, and person is said to be "oriented × 3," and sensorium is considered normal.

However, if the patient is not alert, the level of consciousness should be assessed. The simple rating scale shown in Box 14-5 allows clinicians to describe the patient's level of consciousness objectively, using common clinical terms.

Depressed consciousness may occur with poor cerebral blood flow or when poorly oxygenated blood perfuses the brain. As cerebral oxygenation falls acutely, the patient initially becomes restless, confused, or disoriented. If hypoxia worsens, the patient may become

Box 14-5 • Levels of Consciousness

CONFUSED
The patient
- Exhibits slight decrease of consciousness
- Has slow mental responses
- Has decreased or dulled perception
- Has incoherent thoughts

DELIRIOUS
The patient
- Is easily agitated
- Is irritable
- Exhibits hallucinations

LETHARGIC
The patient
- Is sleepy
- Arouses easily
- Responds appropriately when aroused

OBTUNDED
The patient
- Awakens only with difficulty
- Responds appropriately when aroused

STUPOROUS
The patient
- Does not awaken completely
- Has decreased mental and physical activity
- Responds to pain and exhibits deep tendon reflexes
- Responds slowly to verbal stimuli

COMATOSE
The patient
- Is unconscious
- Does not respond to stimuli
- Does not move voluntarily
- Exhibits possible signs of upper motor neuron dysfunction, such as Babinski's reflex or hyperreflexia
- Loses reflexes with deep or prolonged coma

comatose. Abnormal consciousness also may occur in chronic degenerative brain disorders, as a side effect of certain medications, and in cases of drug overdose. However, patients with chronic hypoxia may adapt well and may have normal mental status despite significant hypoxemia.

Vital Signs

Vital signs, comprising the body temperature, pulse rate, respiratory rate, and blood pressure, are the most frequently used clinical measurements because they are easy to obtain and provide useful information about the patient's clinical condition. Abnormal vital signs may reveal the first clue of adverse reactions to treatment. In addition, improvement in a patient's vital signs is strong evidence that a given treatment is having a positive effect. For example, a decrease in the patient's breathing and heart rate toward normal after the application of oxygen therapy suggests a beneficial effect.

MINI CLINI

Evidence of Tissue Hypoxia

PROBLEM

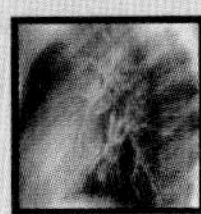

The RT is called to the intensive care unit to see a recently admitted patient who has septic shock. The patient complains of having dyspnea and fever for the last 3 days. His vital signs are as follows: pulse rate, 100 beats/min; respiratory rate, 24 breaths/min; blood pressure, 80/65 mm Hg; and body temperature, below normal.

The patient is alert but confused, and his sensorium has deteriorated over the last 12 hours. Auscultation reveals fine crackles in the bases bilaterally and no murmurs or gallop rhythm. There is no evidence of cyanosis, pedal edema, or jugular vein distension. Capillary refill is 3 seconds, and his extremities are warm to the touch. What suggests that this patient has hypoxia?

SOLUTION

Hypoxia represents a serious problem to the tissues. Any evidence suggesting that this complication may be occurring must be documented and addressed as soon as possible. In this case, the most striking evidence of tissue hypoxia is the abnormal sensorium, which means that the brain may not be getting adequate oxygenation. Appropriate treatment must be initiated soon.

In this patient, the reason the brain is not getting adequate oxygen is that circulation is inadequate, the blood is not well oxygenated, or both. The patient's condition needs to be evaluated further, but it is most likely that the patient needs therapy to correct the circulatory problem.

Body Temperature

The average body temperature for adults is approximately 98.6° F (37° C), with daily variations of approximately 1° F (0.5° C). Recent research suggests that the normal body temperature may be slightly lower than the values traditionally accepted.[9] Body temperature normally varies over a 24-hour day and usually is lowest in the early morning and highest in the late afternoon. Metabolic functions occur optimally when the body temperature is normal.

Body temperature is kept normal by balancing heat production with heat loss. If the body were not able to discharge the heat generated by metabolism, the temperature would rise approximately 2° F per hour. The hypothalamus plays an important role in regulating heat loss and can initiate peripheral vasodilation and sweating (diaphoresis) to dissipate body heat. The respiratory system also helps remove excess heat through ventilation by warming the inspired air, which is subsequently exhaled.

An elevated body temperature (hyperthermia, or hyperpyrexia) can result from disease or from normal activities such as exercise. Temperature elevation caused by disease is called *fever*, and the patient is said to be **febrile**. Fever increases the body's metabolic rate, thereby increasing both oxygen consumption and carbon dioxide production. This increase in metabolism must be matched by an increase in both circulation and ventilation to maintain homeostasis. This is why febrile patients often have increased heart and breathing rates. However, not all patients can easily accommodate the need for increased circulation and ventilation, and respiratory failure can result.

A body temperature below normal is called **hypothermia**. The most common cause of hypothermia is prolonged exposure to cold, to which the hypothalamus responds by initiating shivering (to generate heat) and vasoconstriction (to conserve heat). Other less common causes of hypothermia include head injury or stroke, causing dysfunction of the hypothalamus; decreased thyroid activity; and overwhelming infection, such as sepsis.

Because hypothermia reduces oxygen consumption and carbon dioxide production, patients with hypothermia may exhibit slow, shallow breathing and reduced pulse rate. Mechanical ventilators in the control mode may need appropriate adjustments in the depth and rate of delivered tidal volumes as the body temperature of the patient varies above and below normal.

Body temperature is measured most often at one of the following three sites: mouth, axilla, or rectum. The oral site is the most acceptable for the alert, adult patient, but it cannot be used with infants, comatose patients, or orally intubated patients. Oxygen therapy administered by nasal cannula or simple face mask does not alter the oral temperature reading, although rapid mouth breathing may lower the oral temperature. If a patient ingests hot or cold liquid or has been smoking, oral temperature measurement should be delayed for 10 to 15 minutes for accuracy. The axillary site is acceptable for infants or small children who do not tolerate rectal thermometers, but this site may underestimate core temperature by 1° to 2° C. More recently, the body temperature has been assessed accurately with the use of a handheld device to measure the temperature of the eardrum (tympanic membrane). Rectal temperatures are closest to actual core body temperature.

Pulse Rate

The peripheral pulse should be evaluated for rate, rhythm, and strength (Box 14-6). The normal adult pulse rate is 60 to 100 beats/min, with a regular rhythm. A condition in which the pulse rate exceeds 100 beats/min is called **tachycardia**. Common causes of tachycardia are exercise, fear, anxiety, low blood pressure, anemia, fever, reduced arterial blood oxygen levels, and certain medications. A condition in which the pulse rate is less than 60 beats/min is called **bradycardia**. Bradycardia is less common than tachycardia but can occur with hypothermia, as a side effect of medications, or with certain cardiac arrhythmias.

The amount of oxygen delivered to the tissues depends on the heart's ability to pump oxygenated blood. The amount of blood circulated per minute (cardiac output) is a function of heart rate and stroke volume. When the arterial oxygen content falls below normal, usually because of lung disease, the heart tries to maintain adequate oxygen delivery to the tissues by increasing cardiac output. Cardiac output is increased primarily by increasing the heart rate.

The radial artery is the most common site used to palpate the pulse. The second and third finger pads (but not the thumb) should be used to palpate the radial pulse. Ideally, the pulse rate should be counted for 1 minute. Essential pulse characteristics that should be noted and documented are described in Box 14-6.

Spontaneous ventilation can influence pulse strength, or amplitude. Normally, a slight drop in pulse pressure is present with each inspiratory effort. The slight drop in pulse pressure with inspiration may or may not be noticeable with palpation. A significant decrease in pulse strength during spontaneous inhalation is called **pulsus paradoxus**, or *paradoxical pulse*. Pulsus paradoxus can be quantified with a blood pressure cuff and is common in patients with acute obstructive pulmonary disease, especially those suffering an asthma attack. Pulsus paradoxus also may signal a mechanical restriction of the heart's pumping action, as can occur with constrictive pericarditis or cardiac tamponade. Actual measurement of the paradoxical pulse is discussed further on p. 320.

Pulsus alternans is an alternating succession of strong and weak pulses. Pulsus alternans suggests left-sided heart failure and usually is not related to respiratory

Box 14-6 • Key Characteristics of the Pulse

- Is the pulse *rate* normal, high, or low?
- Is the *rhythm* regular, consistently irregular, or irregularly irregular?
- Are there any changes in the *amplitude* (strength) of the pulse in relation to respiration? Are there changes in amplitude from one beat to another?
- Are there any *other abnormalities*, such as palpable vibrations (thrills or bruits)?

disease. The pulse also may be assessed by palpating the carotid, brachial, femoral, temporal, popliteal, posterior tibial, and dorsalis pedis pulses. The more centrally located pulses (such as the carotid and femoral) should be used when the blood pressure is abnormally low. If the carotid site is used, great care must be taken to avoid the carotid sinus area. Pressure on the carotid sinus area can evoke a strong parasympathetic response and cause bradycardia or even asystole.

Respiratory Rate

The normal resting adult rate of breathing is 12 to 18 breaths/min. **Tachypnea** is an abnormally high respiratory rate. Rapid respiratory rates are associated with exertion, fever, arterial hypoxemia, metabolic acidosis, anxiety, and pain. A slow respiratory rate is called **bradypnea**. Although uncommon, bradypnea may occur in patients who have head injuries or hypothermia, as a side effect of certain medications such as narcotics, with severe myocardial infarction, and in cases of drug overdose. Along with respiratory rate, the pattern of breathing (see p. 322) should be assessed.

The respiratory rate is counted by watching the abdomen or chest wall move in and out. With practice, even the subtle breathing movements of the healthy individual at rest can be identified easily. In some cases, the examiner may need to place his or her hand on the patient's abdomen to confirm the breathing rate.

Ideally, the patient should be unaware that the respiratory rate is being counted. One successful method for accomplishing this is to count the respiratory rate immediately after evaluating the patient's pulse, while keeping your fingers on the patient's wrist, thus giving the impression that the pulse rate is being counted.

Blood Pressure

The arterial blood pressure is the force exerted against the wall of the arteries as the blood moves through them. Arterial **systolic pressure** is the peak force exerted in the major arteries during contraction of the left ventricle. The normal blood pressure varies with age. In general, the normal range for systolic blood pressure in the adult is 90 to 140 mm Hg. **Diastolic pressure** is the force in the major arteries remaining after relaxation of the ventricles; it is normally 60 to 90 mm Hg. **Pulse pressure** is the difference between the systolic and diastolic pressures. A normal pulse pressure is 35 to 40 mm Hg. When the pulse pressure is less than 30 mm Hg, the peripheral pulse is difficult to detect.

Blood pressure is determined by the interaction of the force of left ventricular contraction, the systemic vascular resistance, and the blood volume (see Chapter 8). The blood pressure is recorded by listing systolic pressure over diastolic pressure (e.g., 120/80 mm Hg).

A condition in which the blood pressure is persistently higher than 140/90 mm Hg is called *hypertension* and usually is caused by high systemic vascular resistance. An increased force of ventricular contraction is a less common cause. Sustained hypertension can cause central nervous system abnormalities, such as headaches, blurred vision, and confusion. Other potential consequences of hypertension include uremia (renal insufficiency), CHF, and cerebral hemorrhage, leading to stroke. Acute, severe elevation of blood pressure can cause acute neurological, cardiac, and renal failure and is called *acute hypertensive crisis*.

Hypotension is defined as a blood pressure less than 95/60 mm Hg. The usual causes are left ventricular failure, low blood volume, and peripheral vasodilation. With hypotension, vital body organs may not receive adequate blood flow (underperfusion). Oxygen delivery to the tissues can be impaired, and tissue hypoxia may occur without adequate circulation. For this reason, prolonged hypotension must be prevented.

When healthy individuals sit or stand up, their blood pressure changes little. However, similar postural changes may produce an abrupt fall in the blood pressure in hypovolemic patients. This condition is called *postural hypotension* and can be confirmed by measuring the blood pressure in both the supine and sitting positions or on standing up.

A rapid drop in arterial blood pressure caused by postural hypotension can reduce cerebral blood flow and lead to **syncope** (fainting). In general, postural hypotension is treated by administration of fluid or vasoactive drugs.

Auscultation is the most common technique for measuring arterial blood pressure and requires a blood pressure cuff (sphygmomanometer) and a stethoscope (Figure 14-2). When the cuff is applied to the upper arm and pressurized to exceed systolic blood pressure, the brachial artery blood flow stops. As the cuff pressure is slowly released to a point just below the systolic pressure, blood flows intermittently past the obstruction. Partial obstruction of the blood flow creates turbulence and vibrations called *Korotkoff sounds*. Korotkoff sounds can be heard with a stethoscope over the brachial artery distal to the obstruction.

To measure the blood pressure, the clinician wraps a deflated cuff snugly around the patient's upper arm, with the lower edge of the cuff 1 inch above the antecubital fossa. While palpating the brachial pulse, the clinician inflates the cuff to approximately 30 mm Hg above the point at which the pulse can no longer be felt. He or she then places the diaphragm of the stethoscope over the artery and deflates the cuff at a rate of 2 to 3 mm Hg/sec while observing the manometer.

The *systolic pressure* is recorded at the point at which the first Korotkoff sounds are heard. The point at which the sounds become muffled is the *diastolic pressure*.

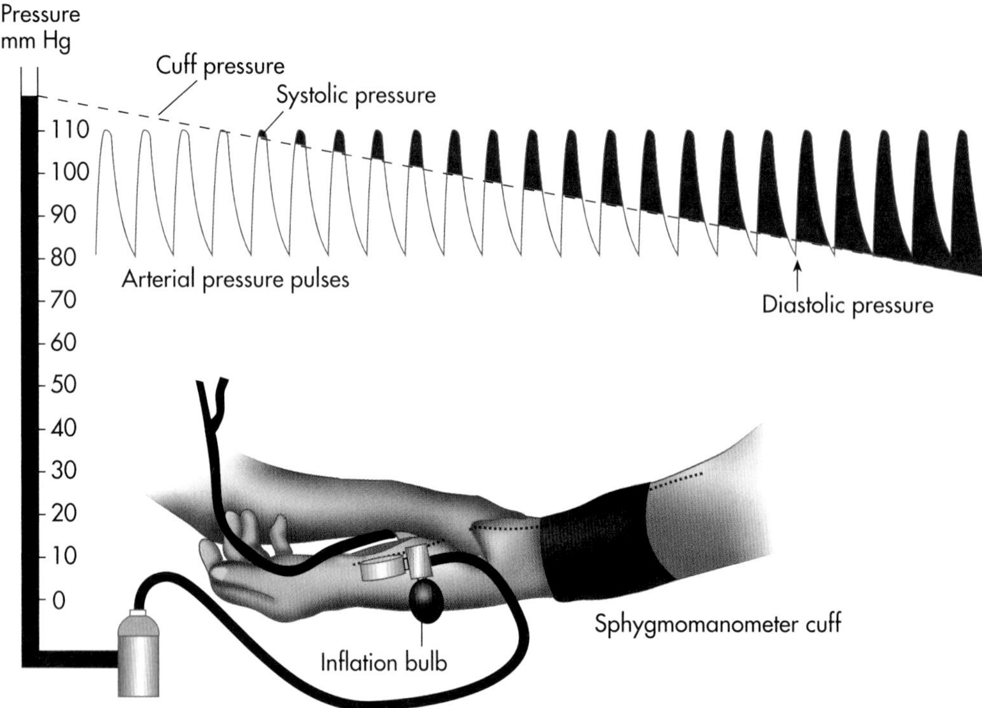

Figure 14-2
Auscultatory method for measuring arterial blood pressure, using a sphygmomanometer and a stethoscope. *(Redrawn from Rushmer RR: Structure and functions of the cardiovascular system, ed 2, Philadelphia, 1976, WB Saunders.)*

This muffling is the final change in the Korotkoff sounds just before they disappear. At this point, cuff pressure equals diastolic pressure, and turbulence ceases. When muffling begins and the sounds disappear at a wide interval, all three pressures are recorded (e.g., 120/80/60 mm Hg). The clinician must perform the procedure rapidly, because the pressurized cuff impairs circulation to the forearm and hand.

The systolic blood pressure usually decreases slightly with normal inhalation. However, a drop in systolic pressure of more than 6 to 8 mm Hg during a resting inhalation is abnormal and is called *paradoxical pulse* (pulsus paradoxus).

A paradoxical pulse is caused by intrathoracic pressure swings created by the respiratory muscles during breathing. Negative intrathoracic pressure during inspiration aids venous return to the right ventricle but impedes arterial outflow from the left ventricle. In addition, increased venous return increases right ventricle pressures, thus constricting left ventricle filling. This briefly reduces left ventricle stroke volume and decreases systolic blood pressure during inhalation.

Although simple palpation may be adequate to signal the presence of paradoxical pulse, it can be quantified only by auscultatory measurement. To obtain this measurement, the clinician inflates the cuff until the radial or brachial pulse can no longer be palpated. Then he or she slowly deflates the cuff until sounds are heard on exhalation only (point 1). Then the clinician reduces the cuff pressure until sounds are heard throughout respiration (point 2). The difference between points 1 and 2 indicates the degree of paradoxical pulse.

Examination of the Head and Neck

Head

The patient's face should be inspected for abnormal signs that indicate respiratory problems. The most common facial signs are nasal flaring, **cyanosis**, and pursed-lip breathing. Nasal flaring occurs when the external nares flare outward during inhalation. This occurs especially in neonates with respiratory distress and indicates an increase in the drive to breathe, which occurs with a variety of problems such as acidosis and hypoxemia.

When respiratory disease reduces arterial oxygen content, cyanosis may be detected, especially around the lips and in the oral mucosa of the mouth (central cyanosis). Cyanosis may be difficult to detect, especially in a poorly lit room. Although central cyanosis suggests inadequate oxygenation (respiratory failure), further investigation is indicated. However, the absence of cyanosis does not necessarily ensure that oxygenation is adequate, because a sufficient amount of desaturated hemoglobin (5 g) must exist before cyanosis can be identified.

Patients with chronic obstructive pulmonary disease (COPD) may use pursed-lip breathing during exhalation. Although this is often taught to patients, many develop this technique on their own. Breathing through pursed lips during exhalation creates resistance to flow. The increased resistance causes development of a slight backpressure in the small airways during exhalation, which prevents their premature collapse.

Neck

Inspection and palpation of the neck helps the clinician determine the position of the trachea and the jugular venous pressure (JVP). Normally, when the patient faces forward, the trachea is located in the middle of the neck. The midline of the neck can be identified by palpating the suprasternal notch. The midline of the trachea should be directly below the center of the suprasternal notch.

The trachea can shift away from the midline in certain thoracic disorders. In general, the trachea shifts toward an area of collapsed lung. Conversely, the trachea shifts away from areas with increased air, fluid, or tissue (e.g., in tension pneumothorax or large pleural effusion). In general, abnormalities in the lung bases do not shift the trachea.

JVP is estimated by examining the height of the blood column in the jugular veins. The JVP reflects the volume and pressure of venous blood in the right side of the heart. Both the internal and external jugular veins can be assessed, although the internal vein is more reliable. Individuals with obese necks may not have visible neck veins, even when the veins are distended.

When lying in a supine position, a healthy individual has neck veins that are full. When the head of the bed is elevated gradually to a 45-degree angle, the level of the blood column descends to a point no more than a few centimeters above the clavicle. With elevated venous pressure, the neck veins may be distended as high as the angle of the jaw, even when the patient is sitting upright.

The degree of venous distension is estimated by measuring the distance the veins are distended above the sternal angle. The sternal angle is used because its distance above the right atrium remains nearly constant (approximately 5 cm) in all positions. With the head of the bed raised 45 degrees, venous distension greater than 3 to 4 cm above the sternal angle is abnormal (Figure 14-3).

Precise measurement (in centimeters) of the jugular pressure is difficult and probably exceeds the accuracy needed for most observers. A simple grading scale of *normal*, *increased*, and *markedly increased* is acceptable.

Jugular pressure may vary with breathing. Under normal circumstances, the blood column descends toward the thorax during inhalation and rises back up with exhalation. For this reason, JVP should always be estimated at the end of exhalation. Under abnormal conditions (e.g., cardiac tamponade), the JVP may rise during inhalation. This is called *Kussmaul's sign*.

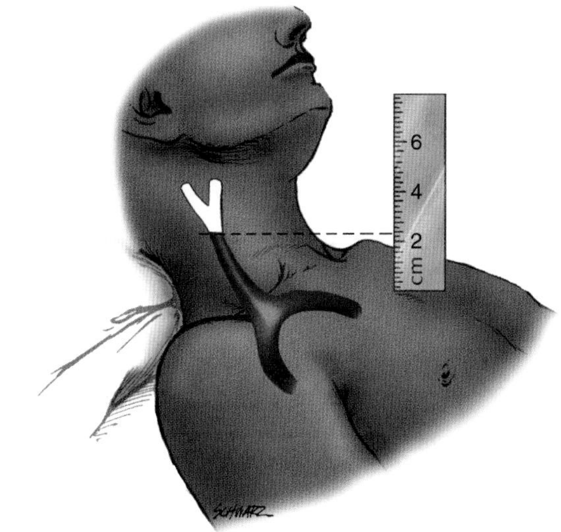

Figure 14-3
Estimation of jugular venous pressure.

The most common cause of jugular venous distension is the failure of the right side of the heart. Right-sided heart failure may occur secondary to left-sided heart failure or chronic hypoxemia. Hypoxemia causes pulmonary vasoconstriction, which increases flow resistance through the pulmonary vasculature. Increased pulmonary vascular resistance increases right ventricular workload. Persistent lung disease with hypoxemia may result in right-sided heart failure and jugular venous distension. Jugular venous distension also may occur with hypervolemia and when venous return to the right atrium is obstructed by mediastinal tumors.

Examination of the Thorax and Lungs

Inspection

The clinician should inspect the chest visually to assess the thoracic configuration and the pattern and effort of breathing. For adequate inspection, the room must be well lighted and the patient should be sitting upright. When the patient is too ill to sit up, the clinician should carefully roll the patient to one side to examine the posterior chest. Inspection, palpation, percussion, and auscultation of the patient's chest require that the patient be disrobed. Consequently, the clinician should make every effort to respect the patient's modesty by covering the chest when possible.

Thoracic configuration. The anteroposterior (AP) diameter of the average adult thorax is less than the transverse diameter. Normally, the AP diameter increases gradually with age but may prematurely increase in

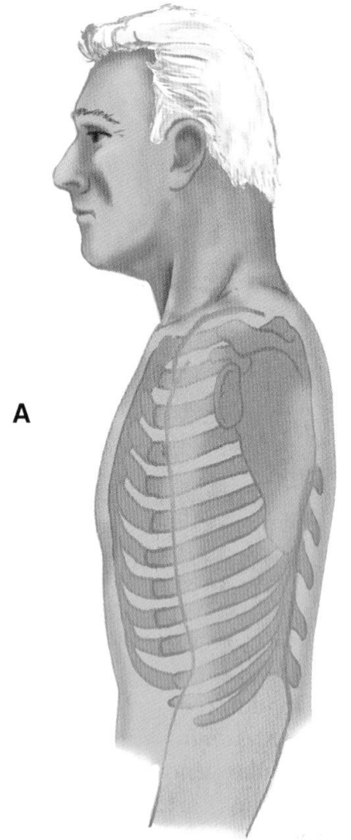

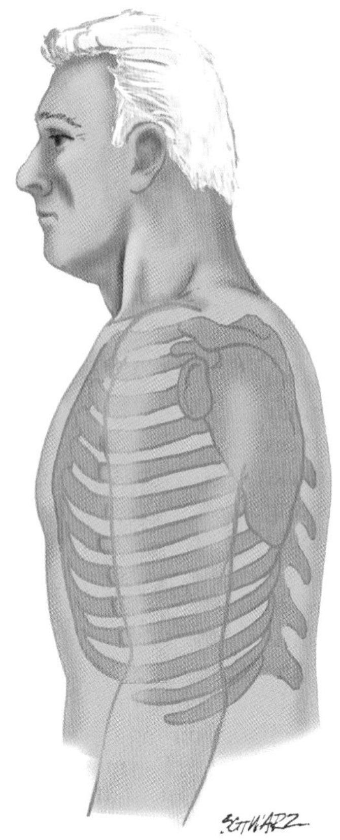

Figure 14-4
A, Patient with normal thoracic configuration. **B**, Patient with increased anteroposterior diameter. Note contrasts in angle of slope of ribs and development of accessory muscles.

patients with COPD. This abnormal increase in AP diameter is called **barrel chest** and is associated with emphysema. When the AP diameter increases, the normal 45-degree angle of articulation between the ribs and spine is increased, becoming more horizontal (Figure 14-4).

Other abnormalities of the thoracic configuration include the following:

Pectus carinatum	Abnormal protrusion of the sternum
Pectus excavatum	Depression of part or all of the sternum, which can produce a restrictive lung defect
Kyphosis	Spinal deformity in which the spine has an abnormal AP curvature
Scoliosis	Spinal deformity in which the spine has a lateral curvature
Kyphoscoliosis	Combination of kyphosis and scoliosis, which may produce a severe restrictive lung defect as a result of poor lung expansion

Breathing Pattern and Effort. At rest, the healthy adult has a consistent rate and rhythm of breathing. Breathing effort is minimal on inhalation and passive on exhalation. Table 14-1 describes some of the common abnormal patterns of breathing.

Any respiratory abnormalities that increase the work of breathing may cause the accessory muscles of ventilation to become active, even at rest in more severe cases. Common causes of an increase in the work of breathing include narrowed airways, as with asthma, and stiff lungs, as with severe pneumonia. Increased work of breathing also can result in **retractions.** Retractions are an intermittent sinking inward of the skin overlying the chest wall during inspiration. They occur when the ventilatory muscles contract forcefully enough to cause a large drop in the intrathoracic pressure. Retractions may be seen between the ribs, above the clavicles, or below the rib cage. These are called *intercostal*, *supraclavicular*, or *subcostal retractions*, respectively.

The patient's breathing pattern often provides reliable clues about the underlying pulmonary problem. A significant reduction in lung volume, such as that which occurs with atelectasis, usually results in rapid, shallow breathing. In general, the greater the loss of lung volume, the higher the patient's respiratory rate will be. Obstruction of the intrathoracic airways (as occurs with asthma) results in a prolonged exhalation time because

Table 14-1 ▶▶ Abnormal Breathing Patterns

Pattern	Characteristics	Causes
Apnea	No breathing	Cardiac arrest
Biot's respiration	Irregular breathing with long periods of apnea	Increased intracranial pressure
Cheyne-Stokes respiration	Irregular type of breathing; breaths increase and decrease in depth and rate with periods of apnea	Diseases of the central nervous system; congestive heart failure
Kussmaul's respiration	Deep and fast respirations	Metabolic acidosis
Apneustic breathing	Prolonged inhalation	Brain damage
Paradoxical respiration	Part or all of the chest wall moves in with inhalation and out with exhalation	Chest trauma; diaphragm paralysis; muscle fatigue
Asthmatic breathing	Prolonged exhalation	Obstruction to airflow out of the lungs

airways within the chest tend to narrow more on exhalation. This alters the normal ratio of inspiratory to expiratory time from 1:1 to 1:3 or 1:4 or more. Obstruction of the extrathoracic upper airway (as with epiglottitis or croup) usually results in a prolonged inspiratory time because airways outside the thorax tend to narrow more on inhalation.

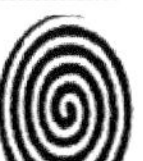

RULE OF THUMB

Lung diseases that cause loss of lung volume (e.g., pulmonary fibrosis, atelectasis) will cause the patient to take rapid, shallow breaths. The increase in respiratory rate is typically proportional to the degree of lung volume reduction.

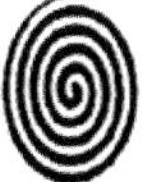

RULE OF THUMB

Lung diseases that cause intrathoracic airways to narrow (e.g., asthma, bronchitis) will cause the patient to breathe with a prolonged expiratory phase.

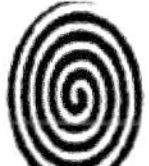

RULE OF THUMB

Lung diseases that cause the upper airway to narrow (e.g., croup, epiglottitis) will cause the patient to breathe with a prolonged inspiratory phase.

The diaphragm may be nonfunctional in patients with spinal injuries or neuromuscular disease and may be severely limited in patients with COPD. When this occurs, the accessory muscles of ventilation become active to maintain adequate gas exchange. Heavy use of accessory muscles is reliable evidence of significant cardiopulmonary disease.

In patients with emphysema, the lungs lose their elastic recoil and become hyperinflated. Over time, the diaphragm assumes a low, flat position because the natural contractile state of the diaphragm is no longer opposed by the normal lung recoil. Contraction of a flat diaphragm tends to draw in the lateral costal margins, instead of expanding them (Hoover's sign) and does little to help move air into the thorax. Ventilation eventually must be achieved by other means such as the use of accessory muscles. The accessory muscles then must assist ventilation by raising the anterior chest in an effort to increase thoracic volume. In fact, the severity of lung disease is directly related to the magnitude of activity of these accessory muscles.

In some patients with COPD, the diaphragm is overworked and underfed. Thus the diaphragm is prone to severe fatigue. Diaphragm fatigue usually results in a distinctive breathing pattern. The fatigued diaphragm is flaccid and is drawn upward into the thoracic cavity with each inspiratory effort of the accessory muscles. This is recognized by inward movement of the anterior abdominal wall during inspiratory efforts and is seen best with the patient in the supine position. This sign is called **abdominal paradox.**[10] In addition, patients with diaphragm fatigue may assume a pattern of breathing in which they alternate between having the accessory muscles dominate for a brief period (a few minutes) followed by a period in which the accessory muscles rest and the diaphragm takes over. This pattern of breathing is known as **respiratory alternans.**

Palpation

Palpation is the art of touching the chest wall to evaluate underlying structure and function. It is used in selected patients to confirm or rule out suspected problems suggested by the history and initial examination findings. Palpation is performed to evaluate vocal fremitus, estimate thoracic expansion, and assess the skin and subcutaneous tissues of the chest.

Vocal fremitus. The term *vocal fremitus* refers to the vibrations created by the vocal cords during speech. These vibrations are transmitted down the tracheobronchial tree and through the lung to the chest wall. When these vibrations are felt on the chest wall, it is called *tactile fremitus*. Assessing vocal fremitus requires a conscious, cooperative patient.

To assess for tactile fremitus, the clinician asks the patient to repeat the word "ninety-nine" while he or she systematically palpates the thorax. The palmar aspect of the fingers or the ulnar aspect of the hand can be used for palpation. If one hand is used, it should be moved from one side of the chest to the corresponding area on the other side. The anterior, lateral, and posterior chest wall should be evaluated.

The vibrations of tactile fremitus may be increased, decreased, or absent. Increased tactile fremitus is caused by the transmission of vibrations through a more solid medium. The normal lung structure is a combination of solid and air-filled tissue. Any condition that increases the density of the lung, such as the consolidation (or alveolar filling) that occurs in pneumonia, increases the intensity of fremitus. However, if an area of consolidation is not in communication with an open airway, speech cannot be transmitted to that area, and fremitus will be absent or decreased.

Tactile fremitus is reduced most often in patients who are obese or overly muscular. In addition, when the pleural space lining the lung becomes filled with air (pneumothorax) or fluid (pleural effusion), fremitus is significantly reduced or absent.

In patients with emphysema, the lungs become hyperinflated, which reduces the density of lung tissue. Because the density is low, speech vibrations transmit poorly through the lung, resulting in a bilateral reduction in fremitus.

Thoracic expansion. The normal chest wall expands symmetrically during deep inhalation. This expansion can be evaluated on the anterior and posterior chest.

To evaluate expansion anteriorly, the clinician places his or her hands over the anterolateral chest, with the thumbs extended along the costal margin toward the xiphoid process. To evaluate posteriorly, he or she positions the hands over the posterolateral chest with the thumbs meeting at the T8 vertebra (Figure 14-5). The patient is instructed to exhale slowly and completely. When the patient has exhaled maximally, the clinician gently secures his or her fingertips against the sides of the patient's chest and extends the thumbs toward the midline until the tip of each thumb meets at the midline. Next, the patient is instructed to take a full, deep breath, and the clinician notes the distance the tip of each thumb moves from the midline. Normally, each thumb moves an equal distance of approximately 3 to 5 cm.

Diseases that affect the expansion of both lungs cause a bilateral reduction in chest expansion. Reduced expansion commonly is seen in neuromuscular disorders and COPD. Unilateral reduction in chest expansion occurs with respiratory diseases that reduce the expansion of one lung or a major part of one lung. This can occur with lobar consolidation, atelectasis, pleural effusion, or pneumothorax.

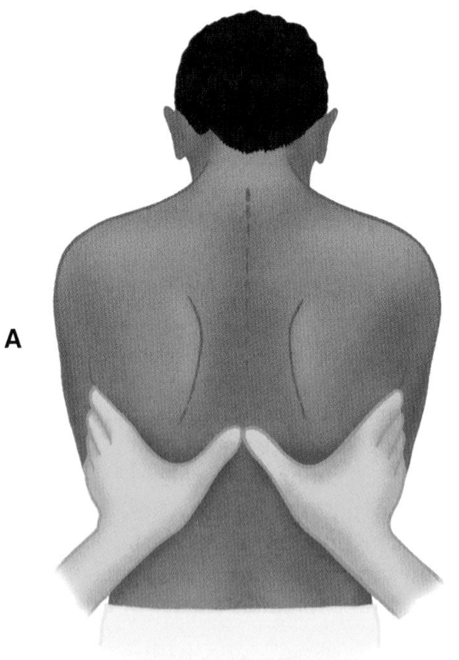

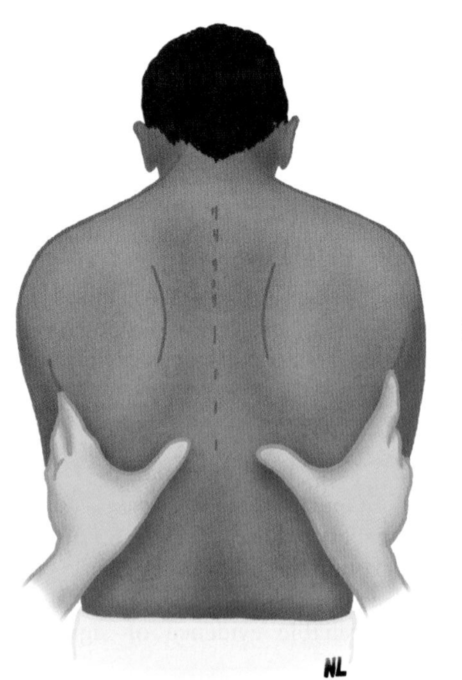

Figure 14-5
Estimation of thoracic expansion. **A**, Exhalation. **B**, Maximal inhalation.

Skin and subcutaneous tissues. The chest wall can be palpated to determine the general temperature and condition of the skin. When air leaks from the lung into the subcutaneous tissues, fine bubbles produce a crackling sound and sensation when palpated. This condition is referred to as **subcutaneous emphysema.** The sensation produced on palpation is called *crepitus.*

Percussion of the Chest

Percussion is the art of tapping on a surface to evaluate the underlying structure. Percussion of the chest wall produces a sound and a palpable vibration useful in evaluating underlying lung tissue. The vibration created by percussion penetrates the lung to a depth of 5 to 7 cm below the chest wall. This assessment technique is not performed routinely on all patients but is reserved for those with suspected conditions for which percussion could be helpful (e.g., pneumothorax).

The technique most often used in percussing the chest wall is called *mediate,* or *indirect,* percussion. If the clinician is right-handed, he or she should place the middle finger of the left hand firmly against the chest wall, parallel to the ribs, with the palm and other fingers held off the chest. The clinician uses the tip of the middle finger of the right hand or the lateral aspect of the right thumb to strike the finger against the chest near the base of the terminal phalanx with a quick, sharp blow. Movement of the hand striking the chest should be generated at the wrist, not at the elbow or shoulder.

The percussion note is clearest if the clinician remembers to keep the finger on the patient's chest firmly against the chest wall and to strike this finger and then immediately withdraw. The two fingers should be in contact for only an instant. As clinicians gain experience in percussion, the feel of the vibration becomes as important as the sound in evaluating lung structures.

Percussion over lung fields. Percussion of the lung fields should be performed systematically, consecutively testing comparable areas on both sides of the chest. Percussion over the bony structures and over the breasts of female patients has no diagnostic value and should not be performed. Asking patients to raise their arms above their shoulders will help move the scapulae laterally and minimize their interference with percussion on the posterior chest wall.

The sounds generated during percussion of the chest are evaluated for intensity (loudness) and pitch. Percussion over normal lung fields produces a moderately low-pitched sound that can be heard easily. This sound is best described as *normal resonance.* When the percussion note is louder and lower than normal, resonance is said to be *increased.* Percussion may produce a sound with characteristics just the opposite of resonance, referred to as *decreased resonance.*

Clinical implications. By itself, percussion of the chest is of little value in making a diagnosis. However, when considered along with other findings, percussion can provide essential information.

Any abnormality that increases lung tissue density, such as pneumonia, tumor, or atelectasis, results in a loss of resonance and decreased resonance to percussion over the affected area. Pleural spaces filled with fluid, such as blood or water, also produce decreased resonance to percussion.

Increased resonance can be detected in patients with hyperinflated lungs. Hyperinflation can result from acute bronchial obstruction, such as asthma, or COPD, such as emphysema. The percussion note also can increase in resonance when the pleural space contains large amounts of air (pneumothorax).

Unilateral problems are easier to detect than bilateral problems, because the normal side provides a normal standard for immediate comparison. The decreased resonance heard when percussing an area of consolidation is easier to detect than the subtle increase in resonance heard with hyperinflation or pneumothorax.

Percussion of the chest has clinically important limitations. Abnormalities that are small or deep below the surface are not likely to be detected during percussion of the chest. This may explain why many clinicians do not routinely use chest percussion to evaluate lung resonance.[11]

Auscultation of the Lungs

Auscultation is the process of listening for bodily sounds. Auscultation over the thorax is performed to identify both normal and abnormal lung sounds. It is used by RTs to assess a patient's condition and subsequently to evaluate the effects of therapy.[12] Because auscultation can be performed quickly, is inexpensive, and represents low risk to the patient, it can be used in many clinical situations. Auscultation is a valuable diagnostic tool.[13] The clinician uses a stethoscope during auscultation to enhance sound transmission and ensures that the room is as quiet as possible whenever performing auscultation.

Stethoscope. A stethoscope has the following four basic parts: (1) a bell, (2) a diaphragm, (3) tubing, and (4) earpieces (Figure 14-6). The bell detects a broad spectrum of sounds and is particularly useful for listening to low-pitched sounds, such as those produced by the heart. It also can be used to auscultate the lungs in certain situations, such as when emaciation causes rib protrusion that restricts placement of the diaphragm flat against the chest. The clinician presses the bell lightly against the chest when trying to hear low-frequency sounds. If the bell is pressed too firmly, the patient's skin will be stretched under the bell, which may act as a diaphragm, filtering out many low-frequency sounds.

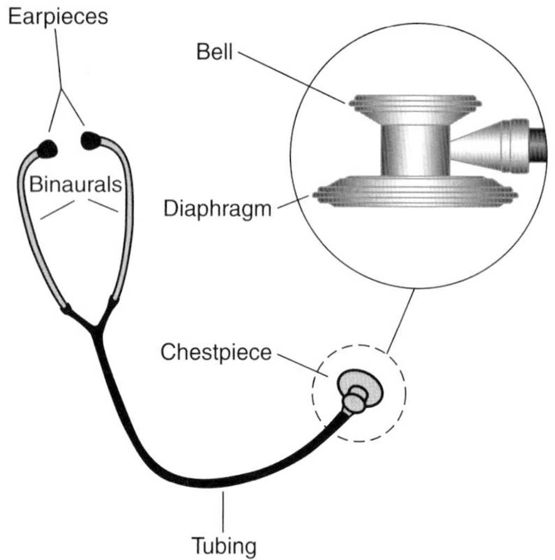

Figure 14-6
Acoustic stethoscope.

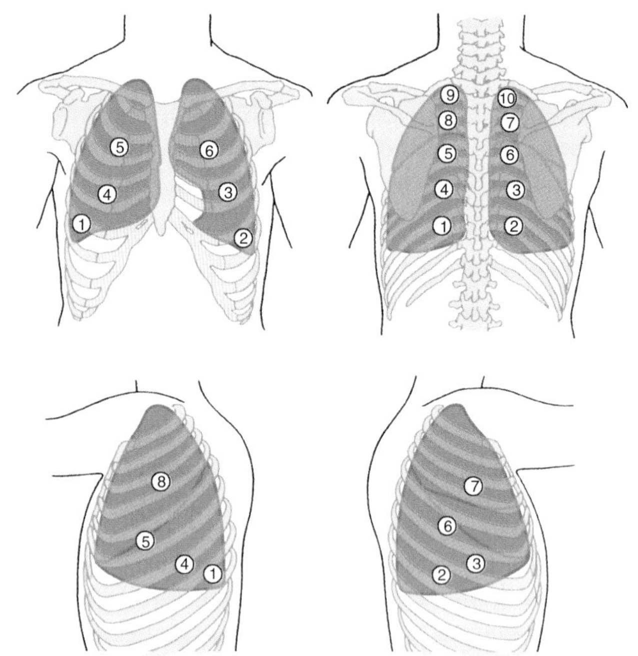

Figure 14-7
Sequencing for auscultation technique. *(Modified from Wilkins RL, Dexter JR, editors: Respiratory diseases: a case study approach to patient care, Philadelphia, 1997, FA Davis.)*

The diaphragm is preferred for auscultation of the lungs because most lung sounds are high frequency. The diaphragm also is useful for listening to high-frequency heart sounds and should be pressed somewhat firmly against the chest to minimize interference with external noises in the room. The ideal tubing should be thick enough to exclude external noises and approximately 25 to 35 cm (11 to 16 inches) long. Longer tubing may impair sound transmission, and shorter tubing makes it difficult to reach the patient's chest.

The stethoscope should be examined regularly for cracks in the diaphragm, wax or dirt in the earpieces, and other defects that may interfere with the transmission of sound. It should be wiped clean with alcohol on a regular basis to prevent a buildup of microorganisms.

Technique. When possible, the patient should be sitting upright in a relaxed position. The patient is instructed to breathe a little more deeply than normal through an open mouth. Inhalation should be active, with exhalation passive. The bell or diaphragm is placed directly against the chest wall when possible, because clothing may produce distortion (although auscultating through a light gown does not appear to influence the normal vesicular breath sound intensity).[14] The tubing must not be allowed to rub against any objects, because this may produce extraneous sounds, which could be mistaken for **adventitious lung sounds (ALS)**. These are discussed further on p. 327.

Auscultation of the lungs must be systematic, including all lobes on the anterior, lateral, and posterior chest. The clinician begins at the bases, comparing side to side, and works toward the lung apexes (Figure 14-7). It is important to begin at the bases because certain abnormal sounds that occur only in the lower lobes may be altered by several deep breaths. At least one full ventilatory cycle should be evaluated at each stethoscope position.

The clinician listens for and distinguishes among the key features of breath sounds. First, he or she identifies the pitch (vibration frequency). Second, he or she notes the amplitude, or intensity (loudness). Third, the clinician identifies the duration of the sound's inspiratory and expiration components. The acoustic characteristics of breath sounds can be illustrated in breath sound diagrams (Figure 14-8). The features of the normal breath sounds are described in Table 14-2. Examiners must be familiar with normal breath sounds before they can expect to identify the subtle changes that may signify respiratory disease.

Terminology. In healthy individuals, the sounds heard over the trachea have a loud, tubular quality. These are

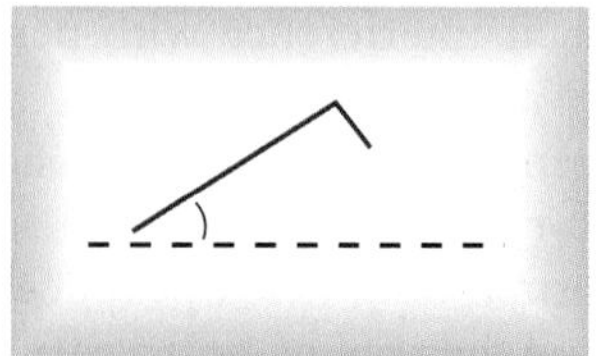

Figure 14-8
Diagram of normal breath sound. Upstroke represents inhalation, and downstroke represents exhalation; length of upstroke represents duration; thickness of stroke represents intensity; angle between upstroke and horizontal line represents pitch.

Table 14-2 ▶▶ Characteristics of Normal Breath Sounds

Breath sound	Pitch	Intensity	Location	Diagram
Vesicular	Low	Soft	Peripheral lung areas	
Bronchovesicular	Moderate	Moderate	Around upper part of the sternum, between the scapulae	
Tracheal	High	Loud	Over the trachea	

referred to as *tracheal breath sounds*. Tracheal breath sounds are loud, high-pitched sounds with an expiratory component equal to or slightly longer than the inspiratory component.

A variation to the tracheal breath sounds can be heard around the upper half of the sternum on the anterior chest and between the scapulae on the posterior chest. These sounds are not as loud as tracheal breath sounds, are slightly lower in pitch, and have equal inspiratory and expiratory components. They are referred to as *bronchovesicular breath sounds*.

When auscultating over the lung parenchyma of a healthy individual, the clinician will hear soft, muffled sounds. These normal breath sounds, referred to as *vesicular breath sounds*, are lower in pitch and intensity than bronchovesicular breath sounds. Vesicular sounds are heard primarily during inhalation, with only a minimal exhalation component (see Table 14-2).

Respiratory disease may alter the intensity of normal breath sounds heard over the lung fields. A slight variation in intensity is difficult to detect, even for experienced clinicians. Breath sounds are described as *diminished* when the intensity decreases and as *absent* in extreme cases. They are described as *harsh* when the intensity increases. When the expiratory component of harsh breath sounds equals the inspiratory component, they are described as *bronchial breath sounds*.

Added sounds or vibrations produced by the movement of air through abnormal airways are termed *adventitious lung sounds (ALS)*. Most ALS can be classified as either *continuous* or *discontinuous*. Continuous ALS have a duration longer than 25 ms.* Discontinuous ALS are intermittent, crackling, or bubbling sounds of short duration, usually less than 20 ms.*

In the past, a variety of terms have been used to describe abnormal lung sounds, and the lack of standardization has limited communication among clinicians.[15,16] A pulmonary nomenclature committee from the American Thoracic Society and the American College of Chest Physicians has published recommendations in an attempt to standardize the terminology used in documenting abnormal lung sounds (Table 14-3). To be consistent with these recommendations, this text uses the term **crackles** to indicate discontinuous abnormal sounds; **wheezes** for high-pitched, continuous sounds; and **rhonchi** for low-pitched, continuous sounds.

*This definition is derived from recording and spectral analysis of lung sounds. Examiners are not expected to time the lung sounds.

Table 14-3 ▶▶ Terminology for Lung Sounds

Suggested Term*	Classification	Outdated Term(s)
Crackles	Discontinuous	Rales/crepitations
Wheezes	High pitched, continuous	Sibilant rales Musical rales Sibilant rhonchi
Rhonchi	Low pitched, continuous	Sonorous rales Low-pitched wheeze

*According to the American Thoracic Society and the American College of Chest Physicians Joint Committee on Pulmonary Nomenclature.

Another continuous type of abnormal sound heard in certain situations, primarily over the larynx and trachea during inhalation, is **stridor**. Stridor is a loud, high-pitched sound, which sometimes can be heard without a stethoscope. Most common in infants and small children, stridor is a sign of obstruction in the trachea or larynx.

When abnormal lung sounds are heard, their location and specific features should be documented. Abnormal lung sounds may be high or low pitched, loud or faint, scanty or profuse, and inspiratory or expiratory (or both).

Using adjectives based on acoustical features, such as *fine*, *coarse*, or *loud*, is the most logical way to document the specific characteristics of ALS. Using adjectives not based on acoustical characteristics, such as *sibilant* or *sonorous*, which have been passed on from one generation of clinicians to the next, only adds to the confusion because their exact meaning is unclear. The timing during the respiratory cycle also should be noted (e.g., late inspiratory).

Mechanisms and significance of lung sounds. The exact mechanisms that produce normal and abnormal lung sounds are not fully known. However, there is enough agreement among investigators to allow a general description.

MINI CLINI

Terminology for Adventitious Lung Sounds

PROBLEM

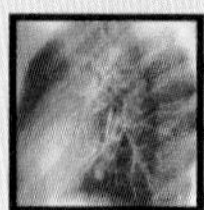

The RT is auscultating a patient who has severe pneumonia in the intensive care unit. He hears low-pitched, discontinuous sounds with inspiration and exhalation. He documents this as "coarse crackles," but his supervisor instructs him to describe them as "rales and rhonchi." Who is right, and what pathological condition is indicated by these sounds?

SOLUTION

The American Thoracic Society and American College of Chest Physicians Joint Committee on Pulmonary Nomenclature has endorsed the term *crackles* for discontinuous abnormal lung sounds. The same committee also has suggested that the term *rhonchi* be used to describe low-pitched, continuous sounds. The term *rhonchi* is not to be used to describe discontinuous sounds. Unfortunately, many clinicians have been trained to describe all secretion sounds as "rales and rhonchi," but this terminology is outdated and inaccurate. The RT's supervisor is mistaken, but diplomacy probably is needed in this case.

Coarse inspiratory and expiratory crackles indicate that excessive airway secretions are present.

Normal breath sounds. Lung sounds heard over the chest of a healthy individual are generated primarily by turbulent airflow in the larger airways. Turbulent airflow creates audible vibrations in the airways, producing sounds that are transmitted through the lungs and chest wall. As the sound travels to the lung periphery and the chest wall, it is altered by the filtering properties of normal lung tissue. Normal lung tissue acts as a low-pass filter, which means it preferentially passes low-frequency sounds. If the clinician places a stethoscope over the chest wall of a friend and listens while he or she speaks, this filtering effect will be evident. The voice sounds will be muffled and difficult to understand because of low-pass filtering. This filtering explains the characteristic differences between tracheal breath sounds, heard directly over the trachea, and vesicular sounds, heard over the lung periphery. Normal vesicular lung sounds essentially are filtered tracheal breath sounds.

Bronchial breath sounds. Bronchial breath sounds are considered abnormal when they are heard over peripheral lung regions. They may replace the normal vesicular sound when lung tissue increases in density, as in atelectasis and pneumonia. When the normal air-filled lung tissue becomes consolidated, the filtering effect is lost, and similar sounds are heard over large upper airways and the consolidated lung.

Diminished breath sounds. Diminished breath sounds occur when the sound intensity at the site of generation (larger airways) is reduced or when the sound transmission through the lung or chest wall is decreased. Sound intensity is reduced with shallow or slow breathing patterns. This type of breathing causes less turbulence in the larger airways and results in diminished breath sounds over the entire chest. Airways plugged with mucus and hyperinflated lung tissue inhibit normal transmission of sounds through the lungs. Air or fluid in the pleural space and obesity reduce sound transmission through the chest wall.

In patients with chronic airflow obstruction, normal breath sound intensity often is reduced significantly throughout all lung fields. This is the result of poor sound transmission through hyperinflated lung tissue, such as occurs with emphysema. Shallow breathing patterns also contribute to decreased breath sounds in patients with COPD.[17]

Wheezes, stridor, and rhonchi. Wheezes, stridor, and rhonchi represent vibrations caused when air flows at a high velocity through a narrowed airway. Airway diameter can be reduced by bronchospasm, mucosal edema, inflammation, tumors, and foreign bodies. The pitch of a wheeze is directly related to the degree of narrowing but is independent of airway length. The greater the narrowing, the higher the pitch.

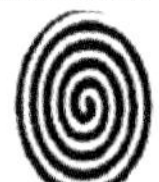

RULE OF THUMB

In general, expiratory wheezes and rhonchi indicate obstruction of intrathoracic airways such as that which occurs with lung diseases (e.g., bronchitis and asthma).

It also is useful to monitor the pitch and duration of wheezing. Improved expiratory flow is associated with a decrease in the pitch and length of the wheezing. For example, if wheezing is present during both inspiration and expiration before treatment, but occurs only late in exhalation after therapy, then the degree of airway obstruction has decreased.

Wheezing may be *monophonic* (single note) or *polyphonic* (multiple notes). A monophonic wheeze indicates that a single airway is partially obstructed. Monophonic wheezing may be heard during inhalation and exhalation or only during exhalation. Polyphonic wheezing suggests that many airways are obstructed, such as with asthma, and is heard only during exhalation. Bronchitis and CHF can also cause polyphonic wheezing. Wheezing during infancy is not predictive of asthma later in life.[18]

Stridor is a serious adventitious lung sound that indicates that the upper airway is compromised. It may occur in patients of any age, but most often is heard from the neck of children. In children, laryngomalacia is the most common cause of chronic stridor, whereas croup is the most common cause of acute stridor.[19] In general, inspiratory stridor is consistent with narrowing above the glottis, whereas expiratory stridor indicates narrowing of the lower trachea. Stridor has been reported to occur in patients with no organic pathological process who have psychological stress.[20] The lack of stridor should never be interpreted to indicate a patent upper airway in patients with labored breathing.

Crackles. Crackles can occur when airflow causes movement of excessive secretions or fluid in the airways. In this situation, crackles are usually coarse (low pitched) and heard during inspiration and expiration. These crackles often clear when the patient coughs and may be associated with **rhonchial fremitus.**

Crackles also may be heard in patients without excess secretions. These crackles occur when collapsed airways pop open during inspiration. Airway collapse or closure can occur in peripheral bronchioles or in larger, more proximal bronchi.

Larger, more proximal bronchi may close during expiration when there is an abnormal increase in bronchial compliance or when the retractile pressures around the bronchi are low. In this situation, crackles usually occur early in the inspiratory phase and are referred to as *early inspiratory crackles* (Figure 14-9). Early inspiratory crackles are usually scanty but may be loud or faint. They often are transmitted to the mouth and are not silenced by a cough or a change in position. They most often occur in patients with COPD, such as chronic bronchitis, emphysema, or asthma, and usually indicate a severe airway obstruction.

Peripheral airways may close during exhalation when the surrounding intrathoracic pressure increases. Crackles produced by the sudden opening of peripheral airways usually occur late in the inspiratory phase. They are high pitched and are referred to as *fine, late inspiratory crackles.* They are more common in the dependent lung regions, where the peripheral airways are most prone to collapse during exhalation. They often are identified in several consecutive respiratory cycles, producing a recurrent rhythm. They may clear with changes in posture or if the patient performs several deep inspirations. Coughing or maximal exhalation by the patient may cause late inspiratory crackles to reappear. Late inspiratory crackles are most common in patients with respiratory disorders that reduce lung volume. These disorders include atelectasis, pneumonia, pulmonary edema, and fibrosis (Table 14-4).

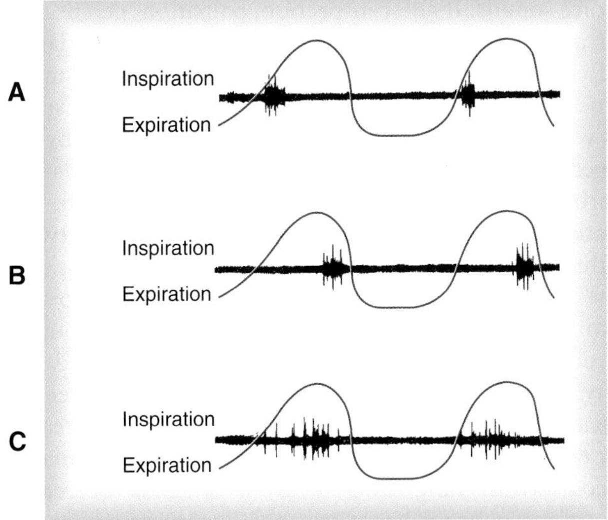

Figure 14-9
Timing of inspiratory crackles. **A**, Early inspiratory crackles. **B**, Late inspiratory crackles. **C**, Paninspiratory crackles.

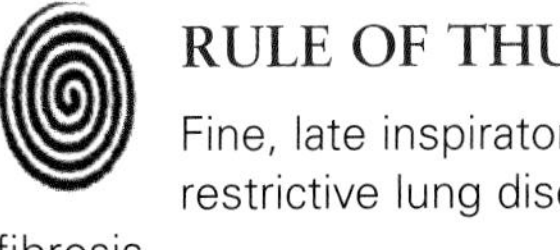

RULE OF THUMB

Fine, late inspiratory crackles suggest restrictive lung diseases such as pulmonary fibrosis.

Pleural friction rub. A pleural friction rub is a creaking or grating sound that occurs when the pleural surfaces become inflamed and the roughened edges rub together during breathing, as in pleurisy. It may be heard only during inhalation but often is identified during both phases of breathing. The rub usually is localized to a certain site on the chest wall. It sounds similar to coarse crackles but is not affected by coughing. The intensity of pleural rubs may increase with deep breathing.

Table 14-4 ▶▶ Application of Adventitious Lung Sounds

Lung Sound	Possible Mechanism	Characteristics	Causes
Wheezes	Rapid airflow through obstructed airways	High pitched, usually expiratory	Asthma, congestive heart failure
Stridor	Rapid airflow through obstructed upper airway	High pitched, monophonic	Croup, epiglottitis, postextubation
Coarse crackles	Excess airway secretions moving through airways	Coarse, inspiratory and expiratory	Severe pneumonia, bronchitis
Fine crackles	Sudden opening of peripheral airways	Fine, late inspiratory	Atelectasis, fibrosis, pulmonary edema

Voice sounds. If chest inspection, palpation, percussion, or auscultation suggest a lung abnormality, evaluation of vocal resonance may be useful in further assessment. Vocal resonance is produced by the same mechanism as is vocal fremitus (see p. 323). Vibrations created by the vocal cords during speech travel down the airways and through the peripheral lung units to the chest wall. The patient is instructed to repeat the words "one," "two," "three," or "ninety-nine" while the clinician listens over the chest wall with a stethoscope, comparing side to side. Normal, air-filled lung tissue filters the voice sounds, producing a significant reduction in intensity and clarity. Pathological abnormalities in lung tissue alter the transmission of voice sounds, causing either increased or decreased vocal resonance. Increased vocal resonance occurs with lung consolidation, whereas decreased vocal resonance is heard over the hyperinflated lung or with pneumothorax.

Bronchophony. An increase in intensity and clarity of vocal resonance produced by enhanced transmission of vocal vibrations is called **bronchophony**. Bronchophony indicates increased lung tissue density, such as occurs in the consolidation phase of pneumonia. Bronchophony is easier to detect when it is unilateral. It often accompanies bronchial breath sounds, a dull percussion note, and increased vocal fremitus.

Vocal resonance is reduced when the transmission of voice sounds through the lung or chest wall is impeded. Hyperinflation, pneumothorax, bronchial obstruction, and pleural effusion all impede transmission of voice sounds and decrease vocal resonance. Decreased vocal resonance usually occurs together with reduced breath sounds and decreased tactile fremitus.

Cardiac Examination

Chronic diseases of the lungs are often associated with other body system abnormalities. Recognition of these other abnormalities can help clinicians identify both the respiratory disorder and its severity. Because of the close relationship between the heart and lungs, the heart is especially at risk in developing problems caused by lung disease.

The techniques for physical examination of the chest wall overlying the heart (precordium) include inspection, palpation, and auscultation. Percussion is of little value. Most clinicians examine the precordium at the same time they assess the lungs.

Inspection and Palpation

Inspection and palpation of the precordium help in identifying normal or abnormal pulsations. Pulsations on the precordium are created by ventricular contraction. Detection of the pulsations depends on the force of ventricular contraction, the thickness of the chest wall, and the quality of the tissue through which the vibrations must travel.

Normally, left ventricular contraction is the most forceful and generates a visible, palpable pulsation during systole. This pulsation is called the *point of maximal impulse (PMI)*. In healthy individuals who are not obese or overly muscular, the PMI can be felt and visualized near the left midclavicular line in the fifth intercostal space.

Right ventricular hypertrophy, a common manifestation of chronic lung disease, often produces a systolic thrust called a *heave* that is felt and possibly visualized near the lower left sternal border. To identify the PMI, the clinician places the palmar aspect of his or her right hand over the lower left sternal border. Right ventricular hypertrophy may be the result of chronic hypoxemia, pulmonary valve disease, or primary pulmonary hypertension.

In patients with chronic pulmonary hyperinflation (emphysema), the PMI may be difficult to locate. Because of the increase in AP diameter and the changes in lung tissue, systolic vibrations are not well transmitted to the chest wall.

The PMI may shift either left or right, following deviations in the position of the lower mediastinum, which may be caused by pneumothorax or lobar collapse. Typically, the PMI shifts toward lobar collapse but away from a tension pneumothorax. The PMI in patients with emphysema and low flat diaphragms may be shifted centrally to the epigastric area.

The second left intercostal space near the sternal border is referred to as the *pulmonic area* and is palpated in an effort to identify accentuated pulmonary valve closure. Strong vibrations may be felt in this area with the presence of pulmonary hypertension or valvular abnormalities (Figure 14-10).

Auscultation of Heart Sounds

Normal heart sounds are created by closure of the heart valves (see Chapter 8). The first heart sound (S_1) is produced by closure of the mitral and tricuspid (atrioventricular, or AV) valves during contraction of the ventricles. When systole ends, the ventricles relax, and the pulmonic and aortic (semilunar) valves close, creating the second heart sound (S_2). Because of the higher pressures in the left side of the heart, mitral valve closure is louder and contributes more to S_1 than closure of the tricuspid valve. For the same reason, closure of the aortic valve usually is more significant in producing S_2. If the two AV or semilunar valves do not close together, a split heart sound is heard. A slight splitting of S_2 is normal and occurs in association with breathing. The normal splitting of S_2 is increased during inhalation because of the decrease in intrathoracic pressure, which

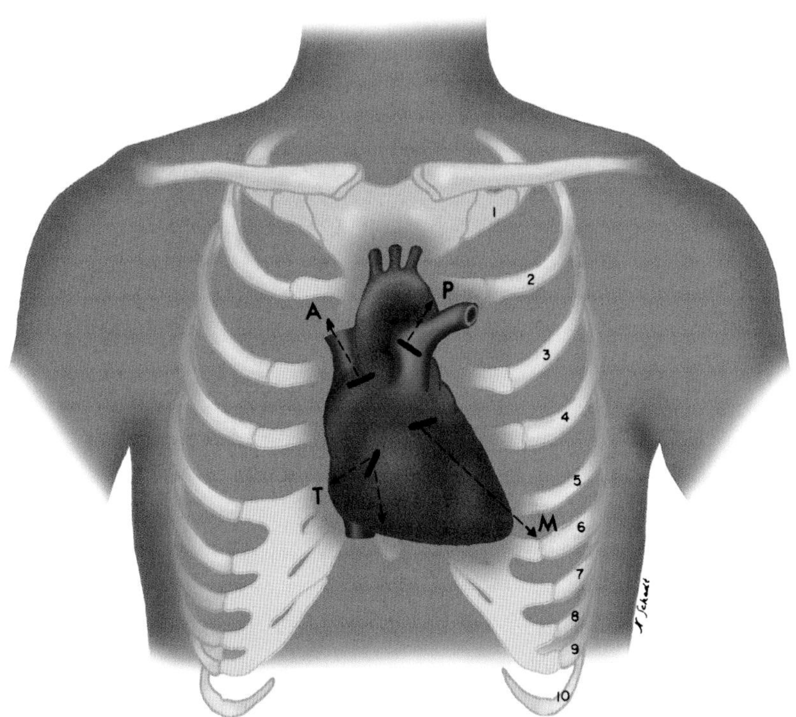

Figure 14-10

Anatomical and auscultatory valve area. Location of anatomical valve sites is represented by *solid bars*. *Arrows* designate transmission of valve sounds to their respective auscultatory valve areas. *A*, Aortic valve; *M*, mitral valve; *P*, pulmonic valve; *T*, tricuspid valve.

improves venous return to the right side of the heart and further delays pulmonic valve closure.

A third heart sound (S_3) can be heard during diastole. It is thought that the S_3 is produced by rapid ventricular filling immediately after systole. The rapid distension of the ventricles causes the walls of the ventricles to vibrate and produce a sound of low intensity and pitch, which is best heard over the apex of the heart. In young, healthy children, an S_3 is considered normal and is called a *physiological* S_3. Otherwise, an S_3 is abnormal. For example, in an older patient with a history of heart disease, an S_3 may signify CHF.

A fourth heart sound (S_4) is produced by mechanisms similar to those that produce S_3. S_4 may occur in healthy individuals or may be considered a sign of heart disease. The S_4 is different from the S_3 only in its timing during the cardiac cycle. S_4 occurs later, just before S_1, whereas S_3 occurs just after S_2.

During auscultation of the heart, alterations in the loudness of either S_1 or S_2 may occur. Reduced intensity of heart sounds may be a result of cardiac or extracardiac abnormalities. Extracardiac factors include alteration in the tissue between the heart and the surface of the chest. Pulmonary hyperinflation, pleural effusion, pneumothorax, and obesity make identification of both S_1 and S_2 difficult. The intensity of S_1 and S_2 also decreases when the force of ventricular contraction is poor, as in heart failure, or when valvular abnormalities exist.

Pulmonary hypertension produces an increased intensity of S_2. This sound is referred to as a *loud* P_2 and is a result of more forceful closure of the pulmonic valve. A lack of S_2 splitting with inhalation also may be the result of pulmonary hypertension. An increased P_2 is identified best over the pulmonic area of the chest (see Figure 14-10).

Cardiac murmurs are identified whenever the heart valves are incompetent or stenotic. Murmurs usually are classified as either *systolic* or *diastolic*. Systolic murmurs are produced by an incompetent AV valve or a stenotic semilunar valve. An incompetent AV valve allows a backflow of blood into the atrium, usually producing a high-pitched "whooshing" noise simultaneously with S_1. A stenotic semilunar valve produces a crescendo-decrescendo sound created by an obstruction of blood flow out of the ventricle during systole.

Diastolic murmurs are created by an incompetent semilunar valve or a stenotic AV valve. An incompetent semilunar valve allows a backflow of blood into the ventricle simultaneously with, or immediately after, S_2. A stenotic AV valve obstructs blood flow from the atrium into the ventricles during diastole and creates a turbulent murmur.

A murmur also may be created by rapid blood flow across normal valves, such as occurs with heavy exertion. In summary, murmurs are created by the following: (1) a backflow of blood through an incompetent valve, (2) a forward flow of blood through a stenotic valve, and (3) a rapid flow of blood through a normal valve.

The heart sounds should be auscultated just before or after the lung sounds, with the use of the bell and diaphragm pieces of the stethoscope. The heart sounds may be easier to identify by requesting that the patient lean forward or lie on his or her left side. This moves the heart closer to the chest wall. When the peripheral pulses are difficult to identify, auscultation over the precordium may provide an easier method of identifying the heart rate. In addition, the rate as heard over the precordium (the apical rate) sometimes must be compared with the palpated peripheral pulse. Normally, these two rates are the same. However, at times the apical rate is higher than the peripheral pulse. This sign, called a *pulse deficit*, is common in atrial fibrillation. Because atrial fibrillation causes an irregular rhythm, some ventricular contractions are too weak to be felt at peripheral locations.

Abdominal Examination

An in-depth discussion of abdominal examination is beyond the scope of this text; however, a review of the findings associated with respiratory diseases is presented here.

The abdomen should be inspected and palpated for evidence of distension and tenderness. Abdominal distension and pain impair diaphragm movement and contribute to respiratory insufficiency or failure. They also may inhibit coughing and deep breathing, which are extremely important in preventing postoperative respiratory complications.

When cor pulmonale is suspected, the clinician should palpate the right upper quadrant of the patient's abdomen and percuss to estimate the size of the liver (Figure 14-11). Right-sided heart failure causes a backup of pressure into the major veins such as the inferior vena cava. The hepatic vein, which empties into the inferior vena cava, may become engorged in this situation, increasing the size of the liver. An enlarged liver is called **hepatomegaly** and may be caused by right-sided heart failure, although many other causes exist.

To assess hepatomegaly, the clinician identifies the superior and inferior borders of the liver by percussion. Normally, the liver spans approximately 10 cm at the midclavicular line. If the liver extends more than 10 cm, it is considered enlarged.

In addition, the clinician should examine the abdominal wall motion with the patient in the supine position. Patients with bilateral diaphragm weakness or paralysis may experience orthopnea and may show abdominal paradox (see p. 323).

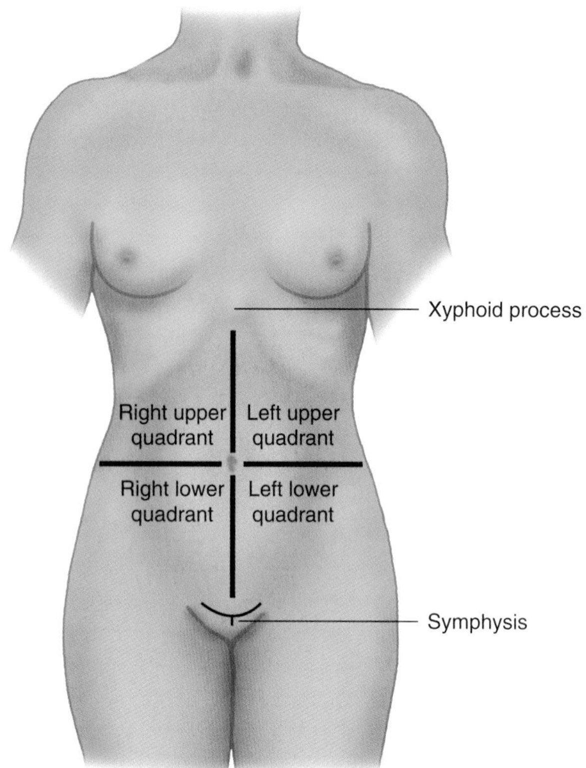

Figure 14-11
Division of the abdomen into quadrants.

Examination of the Extremities

Respiratory disease may cause several abnormalities of the extremities, including digital clubbing, cyanosis, and pedal edema.

Clubbing

Clubbing of the digits is a significant manifestation of cardiopulmonary disease. Clubbing is a painless enlargement of the terminal phalanges of the fingers and toes, which develops over time. As the process advances, the angle of the fingernail to the nail base increases, and the base of the nail feels "spongy." The profile view of the digits allows easier recognition of clubbing (Figure 14-12), but sponginess of the nail bed is the most important sign. Many causes of clubbing exist, including infiltrative or interstitial lung disease, bronchiectasis, various cancers (including lung cancer), congenital heart problems that cause cyanosis, chronic liver disease, and inflammatory bowel disease. COPD alone, even when hypoxemia is present, does not lead to clubbing. Clubbing of the digits in the patient with COPD indicates that something other than obstructive lung disease is occurring.

Cyanosis

The digits also should be examined for cyanosis. Because of the transparency of the fingernails and skin, cyanosis can be detected easily here.

Cyanosis becomes visible when the amount of unsaturated hemoglobin in the capillary blood exceeds 5 to 6 g/dL. This may be caused by a reduction in either arterial or venous oxygen content, or both. Cyanosis of the digits is referred to as *peripheral cyanosis* and is mainly the result of poor blood flow, especially in the

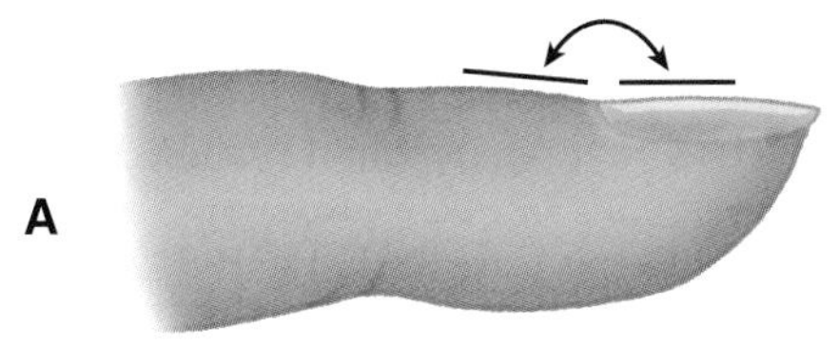

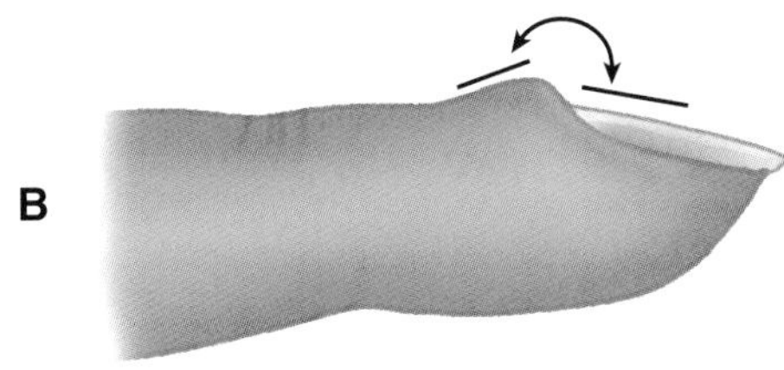

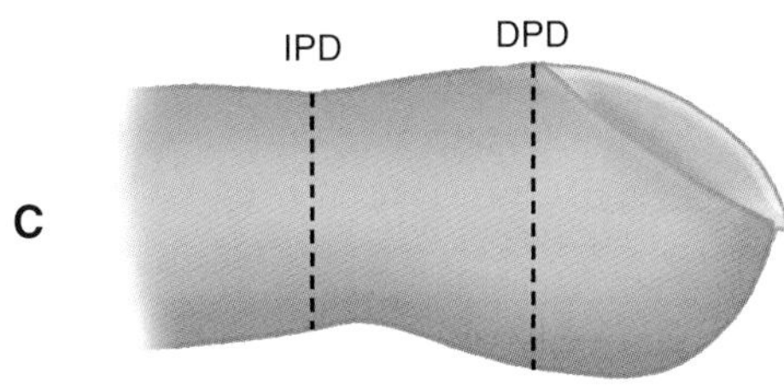

Figure 14-12
A, Normal digit configuration. **B**, Mild digital clubbing with increased hyponychial angle. **C**, Severe digital clubbing; the depth of finger at base of nail (DPD) is greater than the depth of the interphalangeal joint (IPD) with clubbing.

extremities. When capillary blood flow is poor, the tissues extract more oxygen, lowering the venous oxygen content and raising the amount of reduced hemoglobin. Together with coolness of the extremities, peripheral cyanosis is a sign of poor perfusion.

Pedal Edema

Pedal edema most often results from right-sided heart failure, which causes an increase in the hydrostatic pressure of the venous system and leaking of fluid from the vessels into the surrounding tissues. The ankles are affected most often, because they are in a gravity-dependent position throughout most of the day. The edematous tissues "pit," or indent, when pressed firmly with a finger. The height at which pitting edema occurs can indicate the severity of right-sided heart failure. For example, pitting edema that extends to above the knee signifies a more significant problem than edema limited to around the ankles does. Any patient who is suspected of having cor pulmonale or right-sided heart failure caused by chronic left-sided heart failure should be examined for pedal edema.

Capillary Refill

Clinicians assess capillary refill by pressing briefly but firmly on the patient's fingernail and noting the speed at which the blood flow returns. When cardiac output is reduced and digital perfusion is poor, capillary refill is slow, taking several seconds to complete. In healthy individuals with good cardiac output and digital perfusion, capillary refill time is less than 3 seconds. Abnormal refill also may indicate poor vascular supply.

Peripheral Skin Temperature

When perfusion is poor (as in heart failure or shock), compensatory vasoconstriction in the extremities helps shunt blood to the vital organs. This reduction in peripheral perfusion causes the extremities to become cool to the touch. The extent to which the coolness to touch extends toward the body is an indication of the degree of circulatory failure.

KEY POINTS

- The interview is used to identify important diagnostic information and to build a rapport between the healthcare provider and the patient.
- Dyspnea occurs when the work of breathing is excessive for the level of exertion. The work of breathing increases with reduced lung compliance and narrowed airways.
- A cough is one of the most common symptoms of lung disease and occurs when the cough receptors that line the larger airways are stimulated by foreign material, mucus, noxious gases, or inflammation.
- The most common cause of hemoptysis (spitting up blood from the lung) is infection.
- Vital signs provide reliable assessment information about the general condition of the patient and his or her response to therapy.
- Rapid, shallow breathing indicates pathological changes in the lung consistent with a reduction in lung volume.
- A prolonged expiratory phase suggests that the intrathoracic airways are narrowing.
- Normal breath sounds are generated by turbulent airflow in the larger airways.
- Crackles are generated by the sudden opening of closed airways or by the movement of excessive airway secretions.

Continued

KEY POINTS—cont'd

- Wheezes and rhonchi are produced by the rapid vibration of narrow airways as gas passes through at high velocity.
- Cor pulmonale causes jugular venous distension, hepatomegaly, and pedal edema.
- Central cyanosis is a sign of hypoxemia, whereas peripheral cyanosis indicates circulatory failure.

References

1. Simon PM et al: Distinguishable types of dyspnea in patients with shortness of breath, Am Rev Respir Dis 142:1009, 1990.
2. Mahler DA et al: Descriptors of breathlessness in cardiorespiratory diseases, Am J Respir Crit Care Med 154:1357, 1996.
3. O'Donnell DE, Chau LKL, Webb KA: Qualitative aspects of exertional dyspnea in patients with interstitial lung disease, J Appl Physiol 84:2000, 1998.
4. Hardie GE, Janson S, Gold WM: Ethnic difference: word descriptors used by African-American and white asthma patients during induced bronchoconstriction, Chest 117:935, 2000.
5. Mahler DA, Harver A: Do you speak the language of dyspnea? Chest 117:928, 2000.
6. Power J, Bennett SJ: Measurement of dyspnea in patients treated with mechanical ventilation, Am J Crit Care 8:254, 1999.
7. Hansen-Flaschen JH: Dyspnea in the ventilated patient: a call for patient-centered mechanical ventilation, Respir Care 45:1460, 2000.
8. Palombini BC et al: A pathogenic triad in chronic cough: asthma, postnasal drip syndrome, and gastroesophageal reflux disease, Chest 116:279, 1999.
9. Mackowiak PA, Wasserman SS, Levine MM: A critical appraisal of 98.6 degrees F, the upper limit of the normal body temperature, and other legacies of Carl Reinhold August Wunderlich, JAMA 268:1578, 1992.
10. Mier-Jedrzejowicz A et al: Assessment of diaphragm weakness, Am Rev Respir Dis 137:877, 1988.
11. Wilkins RL, Olfert M, Specht L: Chest percussion for resonance is not routinely used by respiratory care practitioners, Respir Care 38:1218, 1993 (abstract).
12. Wilkins RL, Olfert M, Specht L: Survey of respiratory care practitioners for the perceived value of chest auscultation, Respir Care 38:1218, 1993 (abstract).
13. Bettencourt PE et al: Clinical utility of chest auscultation in common pulmonary diseases, Am J Respir Crit Care Med 150:1291, 1994.
14. Wilkins RL et al: Does auscultating through the patient's gown make a difference in the perceived intensity of the vesicular breath sound? Respir Care 45:1004, 2000.
15. Wilkins RL et al: Lung sound nomenclature survey, Chest 98:886, 1990.
16. Wilkins RL, Dexter JR: Comparing RCPs to physicians for the description of lung sounds: are we accurate and can we communicate? Respir Care 35:969, 1990.
17. Schreur HJW et al: Lung sound intensity in patients with pulmonary emphysema and normal subjects at standard flow, Thorax 47:674, 1992.
18. Martinez FD, Wright AL, Taussig LM: Asthma and wheezing in the first six years of life, N Engl J Med 332:133, 1995.
19. Leung AK, Cho H: Diagnosis of stridor in children, Am Fam Physician 60:2289, 1999.
20. Carbone J, Litman RS: Psychogenic stridor: a cause of acute upper airway obstruction, J Am Osteopath Assoc 99:209, 1999.

Bibliography

Bickley LS, Hoekelman RA: Bate's guide to physical examination and history taking, ed 7, Philadelphia, 1999, Lippincott.

Bowers AC, Thompson JM: Clinical manual of health assessment, ed 4, St Louis, 1992, Mosby.

Seidel HM et al: Mosby's guide to physical examination, ed 4, St Louis, 1999, Mosby.

Wilkins RL, Sheldon RL, Krider SJ: Clinical assessment in respiratory care, ed 4, St Louis, 2000, Mosby.

Wilkins RL, Hodgkin JE, Lopez B: Lung sounds: a practical guide, ed 2, St Louis, 1996, Mosby.

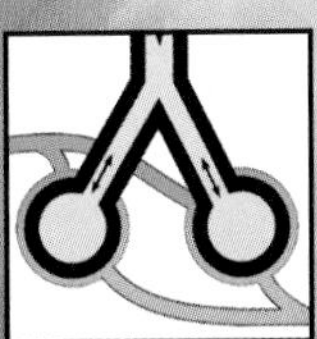

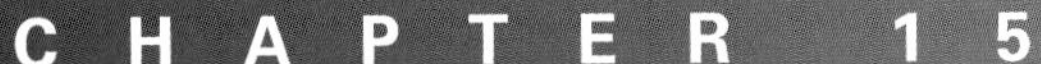

CHAPTER 15

Electrocardiogram and Laboratory Test Assessment

Robert L. Wilkins

In This Chapter You Will Learn:

- Why the electrocardiogram (ECG) is valuable and its limitations
- How to describe the electrophysiology of cardiac cells
- How the cardiac impulse is conducted through the different structures of the heart
- How to recognize normal and abnormal ECG recordings
- How to interpret the complete blood count and other hematology tests
- How to interpret blood chemistry tests such as electrolytes, renal function, serum enzymes, and serum glucose
- How the sputum Gram stain and culture are used

Chapter Outline

The Electrocardiogram
- Basic principles of electrophysiology
- The conduction system
- Basic ECG waves
- Interpreting the ECG

Interpreting Clinical Laboratory Tests
- Complete blood count
- Blood chemistry tests
- Microbiology tests

Key Terms

anemia
automaticity
ectopic foci
hyperglycemia
hyperkalemia
hypernatremia
hypoglycemia
hypokalemia
hyponatremia
leukocytosis
leukopenia
polycythemia

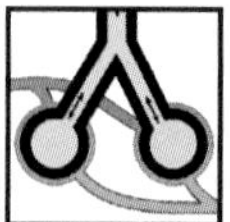

Electrocardiography and clinical laboratory testing are important tools used by healthcare practitioners. Clinical laboratory tests can help healthcare practitioners determine the initial diagnosis of the patient's ailment, quantify the severity of the problem, and monitor the patient's response to therapy. Electrocardiograms (ECGs) often are obtained by respiratory therapists (RTs), which places them at the bedside in prime position to respond to life-threatening arrhythmias. In addition, continuous ECG monitoring is common in the intensive care unit (ICU), and because of their value in determining the general health status of a patient, certain clinical laboratory tests are performed on most patients, regardless of the diagnosis.

For these reasons, RTs must be familiar with the ECG and clinical laboratory results and must be able to interpret them accurately. This chapter facilitates the clinician in reading ECGs and interpreting laboratory tests. Other important assessment tools, such as arterial blood gas (ABG) analysis, pulmonary function tests, and the chest radiograph are discussed in Chapters 17 and 18.

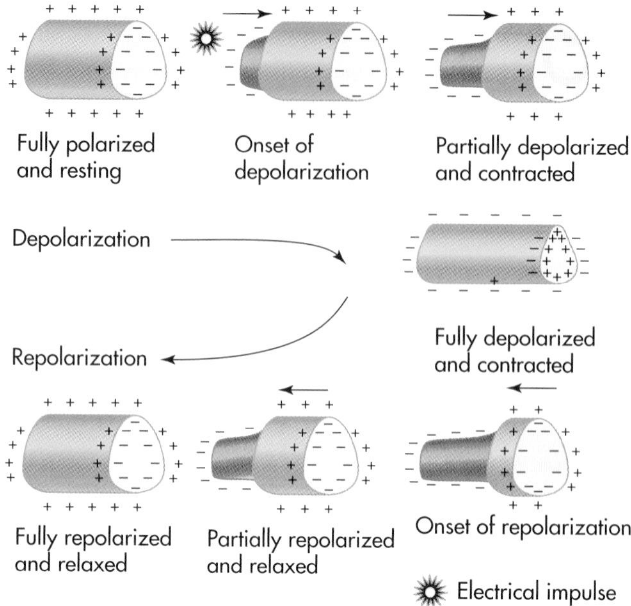

Figure 15-1
Depolarization and repolarization of a cardiac cell. *(Modified from Huszar RH: Basic dysrhythmias: interpretation and management, ed 2, St Louis, 1994, Mosby.)*

▶ THE ELECTROCARDIOGRAM

The ECG is a popular evaluation tool because it is inexpensive, noninvasive, and easy to obtain. It is used primarily to evaluate the patient with an acute clinical condition suggestive of myocardial disease. For example, the adult patient complaining of chest pain is a classic clinical case for which the ECG is used. In addition, the ECG is routinely used by physicians for evaluating the general health status of the middle-aged or older patient before major surgery or for periodic health screening.

However, it is important to point out that the resting ECG has no value as a predictor of future heart problems. It is useful only for detecting abnormalities that have already occurred, such as a recent myocardial infarction (MI). In addition, certain abnormalities, such as valvular defects, cannot be identified directly by the ECG.

Basic Principles of Electrophysiology

Understanding the ECG requires a basic knowledge of physiology related to the contraction and relaxation of the heart muscle. The muscle cells of the heart normally are stimulated and paced by the electrical activity of the cardiac conduction system. The conduction system cells have the ability to stimulate the heart without the influence of the nervous system. However, the autonomic nervous system normally plays a major role in controlling heart function (see the discussion on p. 337).

The cardiac muscle cells normally generate an electrical imbalance across the cell membrane with a positive charge on the outside and a negative charge on the inside. Stimulation of the "polarized" cells causes an influx of sodium into the interior portion of the cell; this is called *depolarization* (Figure 15-1). Depolarization causes the cardiac muscle cells to contract momentarily, which is seen as a shortening of the muscle. This is immediately followed by *repolarization*, which is a rapid return of the cell to the "polarized" position in which the electrical imbalance across the membrane is reestablished.

Cardiac cells have the ability to depolarize without stimulation from a nerve, although the conduction system most often controls the heart rate. The ability to depolarize without stimulation is known as **automaticity** and is an important characteristic of conduction system cells and cardiac muscle cells. Each portion of the conduction system has its own degree of automaticity.

The Conduction System

The conduction system is responsible for controlling the rate at which the heart muscle contracts. It also is responsible for causing the heart chambers to contract in a coordinated fashion, which is essential to move blood effectively. A faulty conduction system could lead to an inappropriate heart rate or to an uncoordinated contraction of the heart. In either case, the patient may not be able to maintain an adequate cardiac output.

Normally, the sinoatrial (SA) node, which is located in the upper portion of the right atrium, has the greatest degree of automaticity and therefore normally paces the

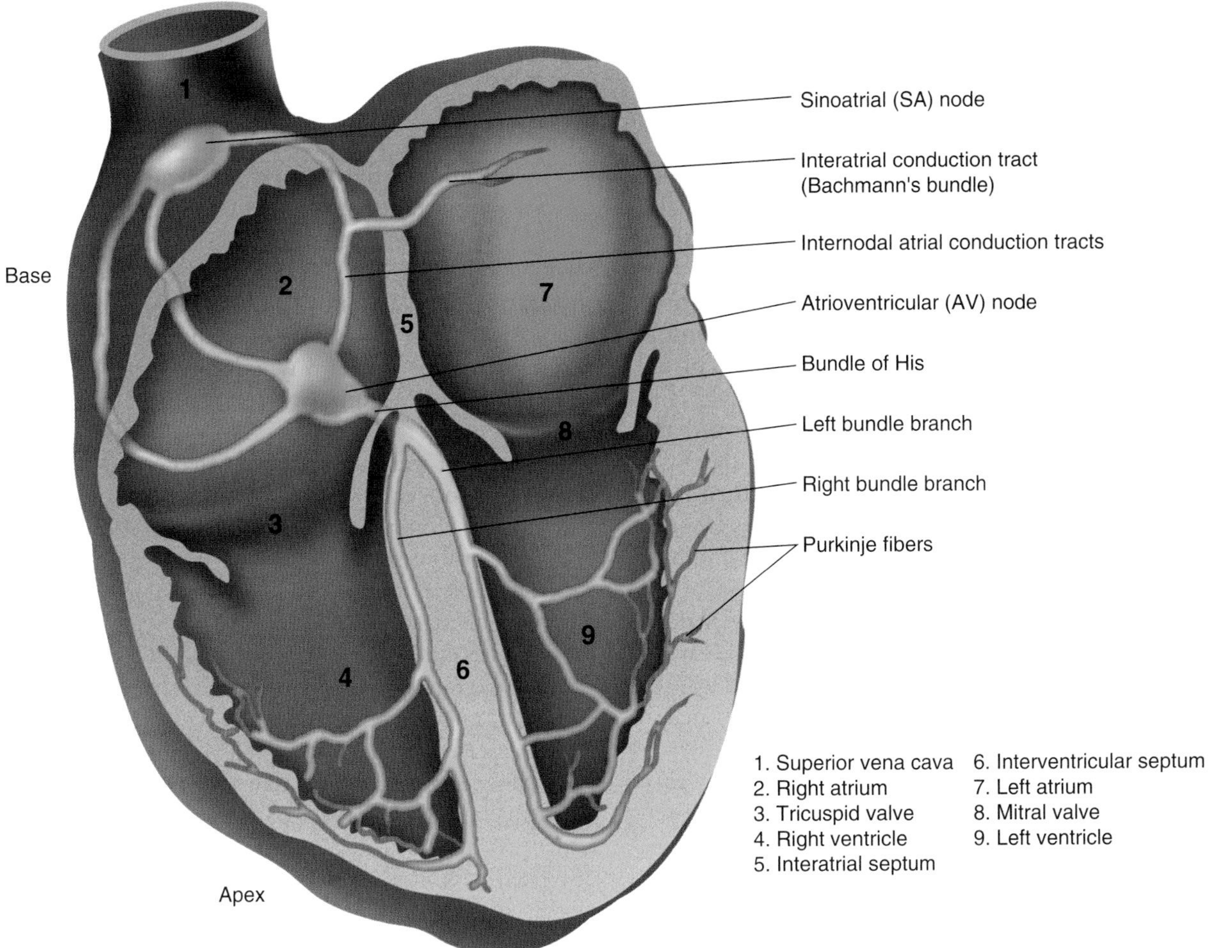

Figure 15-2
Anatomy of the electrical conduction system of the human heart.

heart (Figure 15-2). Any heartbeat originating outside the SA node is considered an **ectopic** beat. The SA node is innervated by the autonomic nervous system, which allows the sympathetic and parasympathetic nervous systems to influence heart rate. Stimulation of the sympathetic nervous system causes an increase in heart rate, whereas activation of the parasympathetic nervous system slows the heart rate by influencing the degree of automaticity within the SA node.

The electrical impulse generated by the SA node travels rapidly across the right atrium, through intraatrial pathways, to the left atrium by way of Bachmann's bundle. This causes a wave of depolarization to occur over the atria, producing atrial contraction. Next, the impulse moves to the atrioventricular (AV) node, located in the intraventricular septum in the inferior aspect of the right atrium (see Figure 15-2). The AV node is the "backup" pacemaker because it has the second greatest degree of automaticity in the healthy heart. In most cases, if the SA node fails to function properly, the AV node will pace ventricular activity and maintain adequate cardiac output.

The impulse is temporarily delayed at the AV node to allow better filling of the ventricles with the blood entering from the atria. The brief delay of the impulse at the AV node also protects the ventricles against excessively fast atrial rates that would lead to inadequate cardiac output if passed on to the ventricles. Excessively fast ventricular rates cause the cardiac output to fall because ventricular filling does not have sufficient time in such circumstances.

The impulse exits the AV node and enters the bundle of His and then rapidly moves to the bundle branches. The bundle branches rapidly carry the impulse into the right and left ventricles. The bundle branches terminate in the Purkinje fibers, which are fingerlike projections that penetrate the myocardium (see Figure 15-2). These fibers stimulate contraction from the apex of the heart upward toward the base of the heart, causing a coordinated contraction of the ventricles, which normally is effective in moving blood. The impulse travels the most rapidly in the Purkinje fibers, which is essential if contraction of the ventricles is to occur in a coordinated fashion. Immediately following depolarization of the ventricles, repolarization occurs in preparation for the next impulse.

Basic ECG Waves

The wave of depolarization occurring in the atria is seen as the *P wave* on the ECG (Figure 15-3). The normal P wave is no more than 2.5 mm high or 3 mm long. Atrial hypertrophy may cause the P wave to enlarge to a height and length beyond the normal parameters. Atrial repolarization is not seen on the ECG tracing because it is obscured by the electrical activity occurring in the ventricles at the same time.

The wave of depolarization occurring over the ventricles is seen as the *QRS complex* on the ECG tracing. The QRS complex is normally larger than the P wave because the muscle mass of the ventricles is much greater than that of the atria. The normal QRS complex is not wider than 3 mm (0.12 second) because of the rapid movement of the impulse through the ventricles by the bundle branches and Purkinje fibers. Abnormalities in the ventricular conduction system may lead to irregular QRS complexes that are wider than normal.

The QRS complex usually consists of several distinct waves, each of which has a letter assigned to it as a label. If the first wave of the complex is negative (downward), it is labeled the *Q wave*. The initial positive (upward) deflection is referred to as the *R wave*, and the next negative deflection after the R wave is labeled the *S wave*. Not all QRS complexes have all three components present, but the waves making up ventricular depolarization are referred to as the *QRS complex*, regardless of its exact makeup. The wave of repolarization occurring in the ventricles immediately after depolarization is the *T wave* (see Figure 15-3).

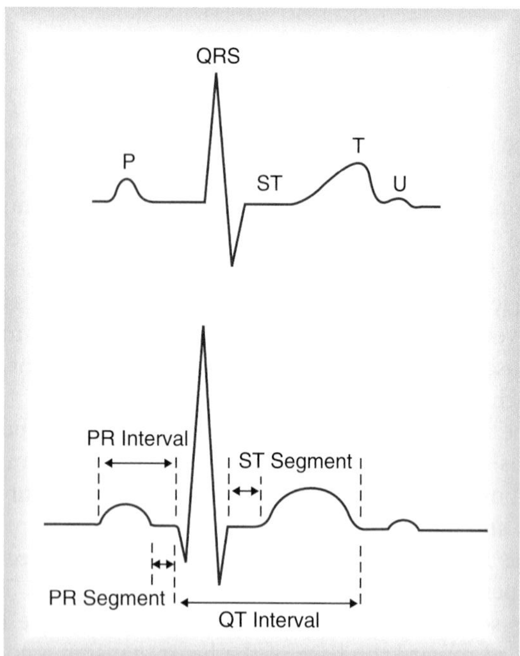

Figure 15-3

Normal configuration of ECG waves, segments, and intervals. *(Modified from Wilkins RL, Krider SJ, Sheldon RL: Clinical assessment in respiratory care, ed 4, St Louis, 2000, Mosby.)*

Two important segments of the ECG pattern must be observed and measured. The first is the PR interval, which refers to the distance (time) between the start of atrial depolarization and the start of ventricular depolarization. This represents the time in which the impulse begins in the SA node and travels across the atria to the AV node, where it is held briefly before passing on to the ventricles. Normally, the PR interval represents a period no longer than 0.20 second. PR intervals longer than 0.20 second suggest that the impulse is abnormally delayed at the AV node and a "block" is present. This may mean that there is a serious defect in the conduction system, which needs immediate attention.

The second important part of the ECG to evaluate is the ST segment, which represents the time from the end of ventricular depolarization to the start of ventricular repolarization. The normal ST segment is isoelectric, which is seen as a flat line that is not above or below the neutral baseline. Certain pathological abnormalities in the myocardium will cause the ST segment configuration to become abnormal. This is seen as an elevated or depressed ST segment and is common in MI (Figure 15-4). Because this represents a potentially life-threatening arrhythmia, abnormal ST segments must be identified as soon as possible.

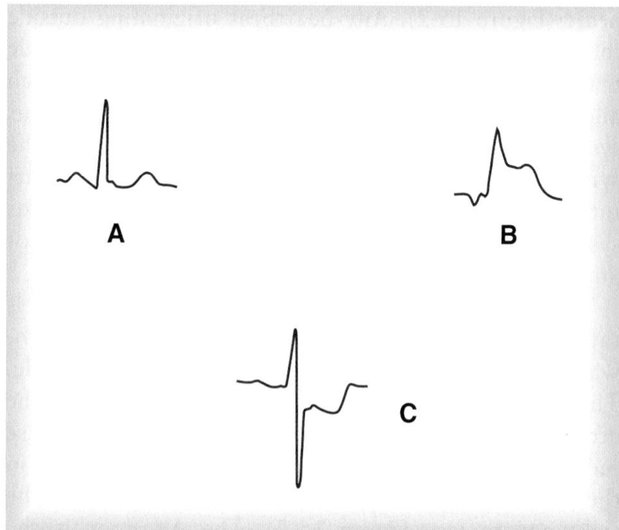

Figure 15-4

ST segments. **A**, Normal. **B**, Abnormal elevation. **C**, Abnormal depression. *(Modified from Wilkins RL, Krider SJ, Sheldon RL: Clinical assessment in respiratory care, ed 4, St Louis, 2000, Mosby.)*

Axis Evaluation

Axis evaluation is used to determine the general direction of current flow during ventricular depolarization. This is helpful to know when hypertrophy of one of the ventricles is suspected, which would cause the direction of current flow to deviate from normal. Normally, the mean QRS axis (vector) points leftward (patient's left) and downward, between 0 and +90 degrees in the frontal plane (Figure 15-5). The normal position of the QRS axis results from the slight tilt of the heart to the left and from the large muscle mass of the left ventricle compared with the right ventricle.

The clinician identifies the mean QRS axis by using the hexaxial reference circle (see Figure 15-5) with the position of each limb lead labeled on the circle. Next, the clinician identifies the limb lead with the most voltage (either positive or negative) from the ECG being evaluated. If the lead with the most voltage is positive (upright), the clinician locates the position of that lead on the hexaxial reference circle. The mean axis must be very close to that position on the circle. If the lead with the most voltage is negative (downward), the mean axis points in the opposite direction from that lead. For example, if the lead with the most voltage is lead II and it is positive, the mean QRS axis must be approximately +60 degrees, because this is where lead II is located on the hexaxial reference circle (see Figure 15-5). This is considered a normal axis because it falls between 0 and +90 degrees.

In some situations, the most voltage may be equally present in two leads. The mean axis must fall equally between the two leads if they are both upright QRS complexes. For example, if the QRS complexes in leads II and aV_F are equally positive in voltage, the mean axis must be at approximately +75 degrees and is considered normal. This is not an uncommon situation.

If the mean QRS axis is between +90 and +180 degrees, the patient has right axis deviation. This is quickly identified by looking at lead I. If lead I is negative, right axis deviation is present. This is commonly seen in patients with chronic obstructive pulmonary disease with cor pulmonale. Left axis deviation is

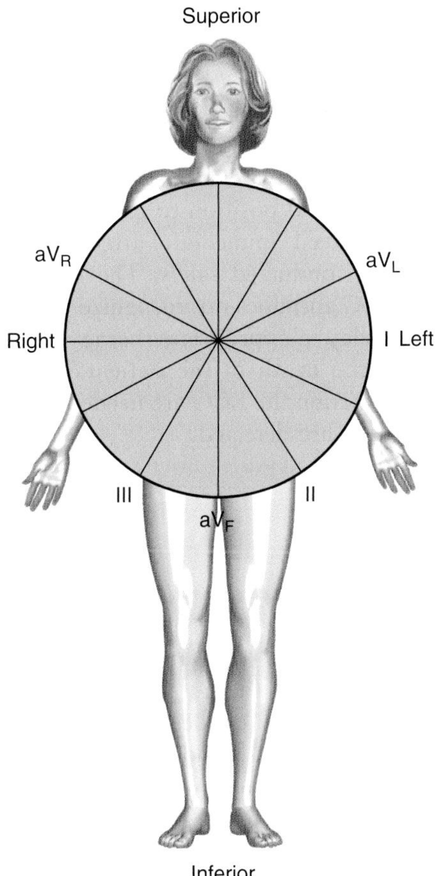

Figure 15-5

Hexaxial reference circle. *(Modified from Goldberger AL: Clinical electrocardiography: a simplified approach, ed 6, St Louis, 1999, Mosby.)*

MINI CLINI

Right Axis Deviation on ECG

PROBLEM

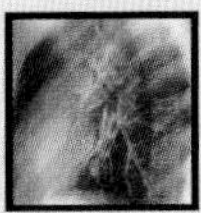

A 54-year-old man with a long history of cigarette smoking has been admitted to the hospital for abdominal surgery. His chest x-ray examination and routine laboratory data are normal. Chest auscultation reveals bilateral expiratory wheezing. The ECG shows a normal sinus rhythm with a right axis deviation. What does the right axis deviation suggest, and is there any connection between it and the long smoking history? How is the right axis deviation detected on the ECG?

SOLUTION

Normally, the mean axis (summary of electrical activity) of the heart travels from top to bottom and from right to left. This results in the mean axis of 0 to +90 in the healthy heart. The slight leftward shift of the normal axis results from the angle at which the heart is situated in the chest and the fact that the left ventricle is normally larger than the right one.

Right axis deviation indicates that the electrical activity of the heart has been abnormally shifted to the patient's right side, between +90 and +180 degrees. This is most commonly the result of right ventricle enlargement, such as occurs with cor pulmonale (right heart failure caused by chronic hypoxic lung disease).

In this patient, the long history of cigarette smoking provides more evidence that he may have cor pulmonale. Further investigation of the patient's respiratory system with pulmonary function testing is needed before surgery is performed. Right axis deviation is detected by noting a negative deflection of the QRS in lead I.

present when the mean axis is between +90 and −90 degrees on the hexaxial reference circle. This is common in patients with left ventricular hypertrophy.

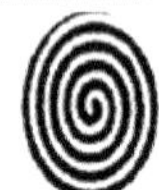

RULE OF THUMB

A negative QRS complex in lead I is consistent with right axis deviation.

ECG Paper and Measurements

ECG paper is made up of gridlike boxes that define time on the horizontal axis and voltage on the vertical axis. Dark lines circumscribe larger boxes that are 5 mm × 5 mm, whereas lighter lines define smaller boxes that are 1 mm × 1 mm (Figure 15-6). Because the paper passes through the electrocardiograph at a set speed of 25 mm/sec, each large box represents 0.20 second, and each small box represents 0.04 second on the horizontal axis. The standard ECG is calibrated so that 1 mV will cause an upward deflection of 10 small boxes or 2 large boxes on the vertical axis. This allows measurement of the exact voltage occurring during depolarization of the cardiac muscle fibers.

MINI CLINI

Weaning Complications

PROBLEM

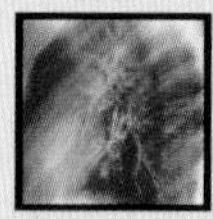

The clinician is in the ICU, attending to a 65-year-old woman who is being weaned from the ventilator after 2 weeks of mechanical ventilation. After 15 minutes of T-piece weaning, she complains of mild shortness of breath, and the bedside ECG shows an increase in heart rate, inverted T waves, and acute elevation of the ST segment. What do the inverted T waves and ST segment elevation indicate? What should be done?

SOLUTION

The inverted T waves and elevated ST segment suggests that the heart is experiencing acute hypoxia, probably caused by the stress of weaning. Changes in $\dot{V}/\dot{Q}$ matching in the lung are probably causing acute hypoxemia and inadequate tissue oxygenation. T wave inversion and ST segment elevation are serious signs indicating that the patient is not tolerating the weaning. She should be put back on the ventilator at an elevated F_{IO_2} and monitored closely. Weaning should not be attempted again until the patient's clinical condition improves significantly. The attending physician should be notified.

Interpreting the ECG

Official ECG interpretation is always performed by a cardiologist or by the patient's attending physician. Unfortunately, the official interpretation is not always rendered in a timely fashion. In some circumstances, RTs will need to recognize serious arrhythmias and respond appropriately. For example, the RT performing a routine ECG on a patient scheduled for surgery the next day is in a good position to recognize an arrhythmia that may need immediate attention before the surgery can be conducted safely. The RT who simply obtains the ECG and does not recognize the arrhythmia may cause a delay in appropriate therapy and indirectly contribute to the death of the patient. The following steps for interpreting the ECG are needed to ensure that all abnormalities are detected.

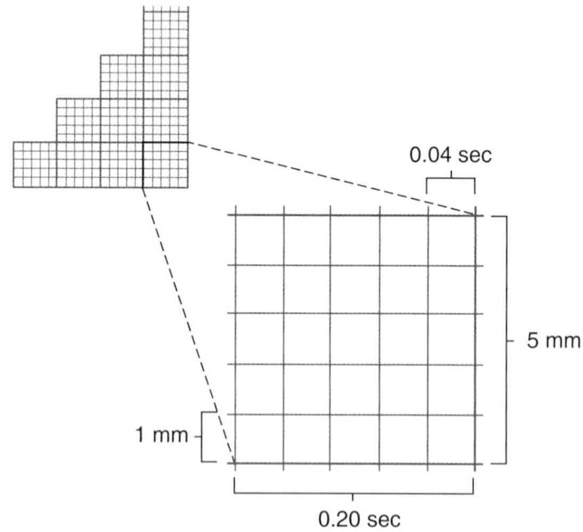

Figure 15-6

Gridlike boxes of ECG paper illustrating the 1- × 1-mm and 5- × 5-mm boxes. *(Modified from Wilkins RL, Krider SJ, Sheldon RL: Clinical assessment in respiratory care, ed 4, St Louis, 2000, Mosby.)*

Steps to Follow

Step 1. *Identify the atrial and ventricular rates.* Normally, the rate of the atria and ventricles is the same, but they may differ when a defect in the conduction system is present. The clinician can identify the heart rate by counting the number of QRS complexes (for the ventricular rate) or the number of P waves (for the atrial rate) in 6 seconds and multiplying this number by 10. He or she also can count the number of large boxes between two successive complexes and divide this number into 300 to obtain the heart rate. This is a reasonable technique when the heart rate is regular.

Step 2. *Measure the PR interval.* This is done by determining the number of small boxes between the start of the P wave and the start of the QRS complex. Normally, this interval is less than 0.20 second (5 small boxes) and is consistently the same for each complex. PR intervals that are longer than 0.20 second or that vary from one complex to the next indicate an abnormality in the conduction system.

Step 3. *Evaluate the QRS complex.* Normally, the QRS complex is shorter than 0.12 second. If it is longer, then there is an abnormality in the conduction system within the ventricles, which often leads to a drop in cardiac output and blood pressure and may cause the patient to experience symptoms such as fainting spells.

Step 4. *Evaluate the T wave.* Normally, the T wave is upright and rounded. Inverted T waves suggest ischemia of the heart muscle, and abnormal configuration of the T wave occurs with electrolyte abnormalities such as **hyperkalemia**.

Step 5. *Evaluate the ST segment.* The ST segment should be flat or at least no more than 1 mm above or below baseline. As stated earlier, significant elevation or depression of the ST segment indicates serious problems with oxygenation of the myocardium and must be recognized as soon as possible.

Step 6. *Identify the R to R interval.* The R to R interval is identified to assess regularity of the rhythm. The distance, in millimeters or time, is measured between the R waves of several successive QRS complexes. Normally, there is little variance in the R to R interval between QRS complexes, but if it exceeds 0.12 second, an abnormal rhythm exists.

Step 7. *Identify the mean QRS axis.* The clinician identifies the limb lead demonstrating the largest amount of voltage. If the lead demonstrates a positive QRS complex, the axis is very close to the position on the hexaxial reference circle where that limb lead is labeled. If the QRS complex with the most voltage is negative, the mean axis is moving in the opposite direction from where that lead is labeled on the hexaxial reference circle.

Recognizing Arrhythmias

Normal Sinus Rhythm. Recognizing abnormal rhythms from an ECG strip is easier if the clinician has an appreciation for the normal tracing. The normal sinus rhythm begins with an upright P wave that is identical from one complex to the next. The PR interval is consistent throughout the rhythm strip and is 0.12 to 0.20 second. The QRS complexes are identical and no longer than 0.12 second. The ST segment is flat. The R to R interval is regular and does not vary more than 0.12 second between QRS complexes. The heart rate is between 60 and 100 beats/min (Figure 15-7).

Sinus Tachycardia. Heart rates exceeding 100 beats/min are abnormal in resting adult patients and are referred to as *sinus tachycardia* when a P wave is appropriately present before each QRS complex (Figure 15-8). Other than the rate exceeding 100 beats/min, sinus tachycardia does not differ from a normal sinus rhythm. This abnormality is common and can be caused by numerous problems. Most often, sinus tachycardia is caused by anxiety, pain, fever, or hypoxemia, or it may be a side effect of certain medications such as bronchodilators. Treatment typically involves eliminating the underlying cause.

Sinus Bradycardia. A heart rate of less than 60 beats/min is referred to as *sinus bradycardia*. Other than the rate being too slow, sinus bradycardia does not differ from a normal sinus rhythm (Figure 15-9). This abnormal rhythm is not as common as is sinus tachycardia, but it represents a significant clinical problem if it causes the

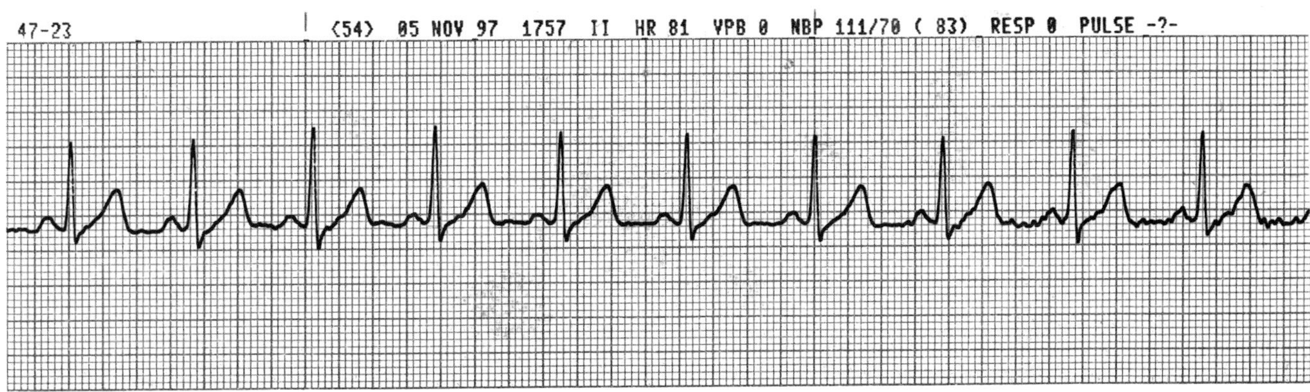

Figure 15-7

ECG tracing demonstrating a normal sinus rhythm.

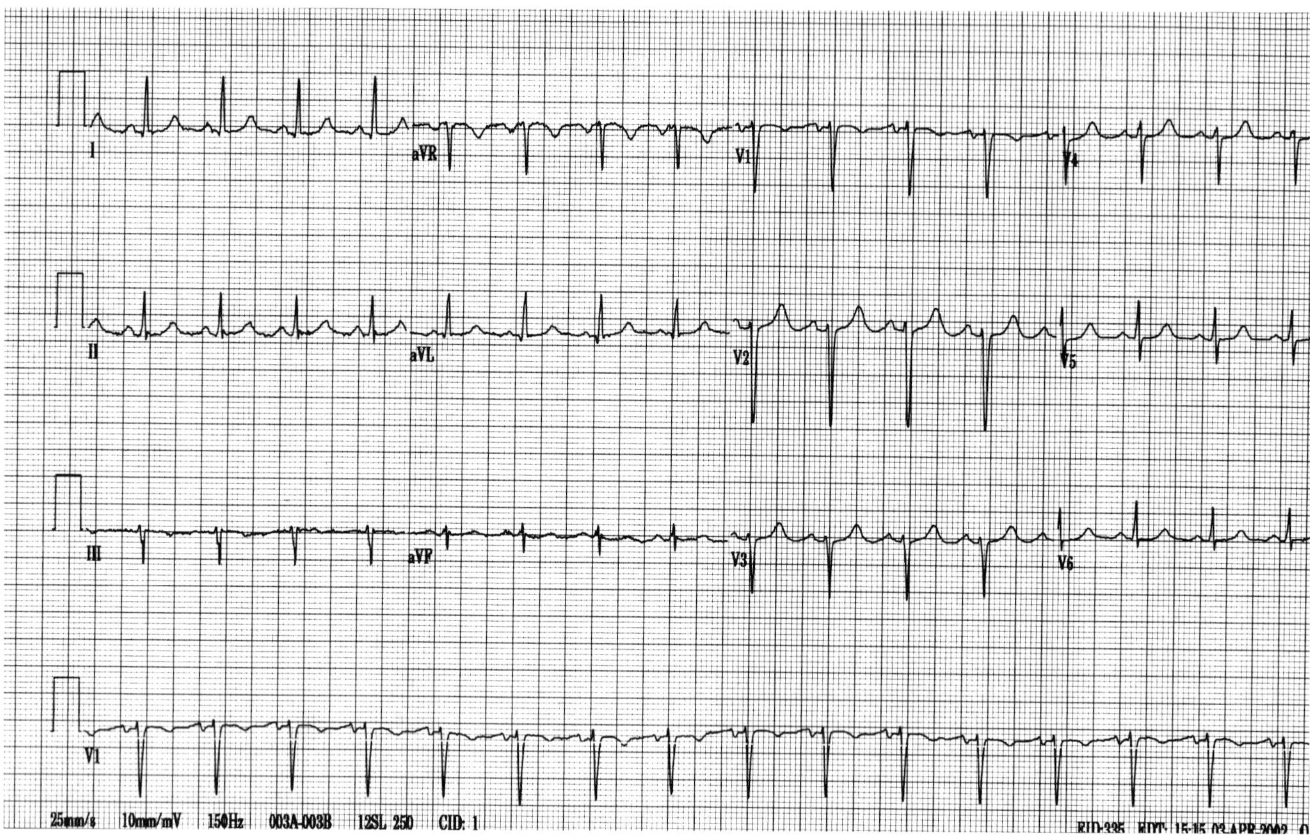

Figure 15-8
ECG tracing demonstrating sinus tachycardia.

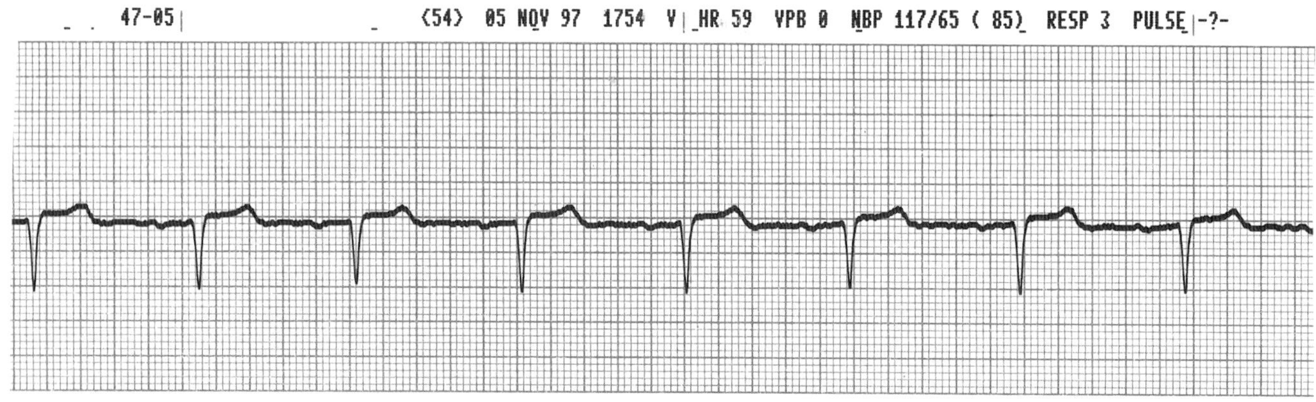

Figure 15-9
ECG tracing demonstrating sinus bradycardia with first-degree heart block.

patient's blood pressure to drop significantly. It is most often caused by hypothermia or abnormalities in the SA node. Numerous medications, such as atropine, are available to stimulate the heart rate when clinical bradycardiac symptoms occur.

Sinus Arrhythmia. Sinus arrhythmia is a common arrhythmia and is recognized by the irregular spacing between QRS complexes. The spacing is measured by identifying the intervals between the R waves of successive QRS complexes, which are normally consistent. When the R to R interval varies more than 0.12 second throughout the rhythm strip, sinus arrhythmia is present (Figure 15-10). This may occur with the effects of breathing on the heart or as a side effect of medications such as digoxin. Most cases of sinus arrhythmia

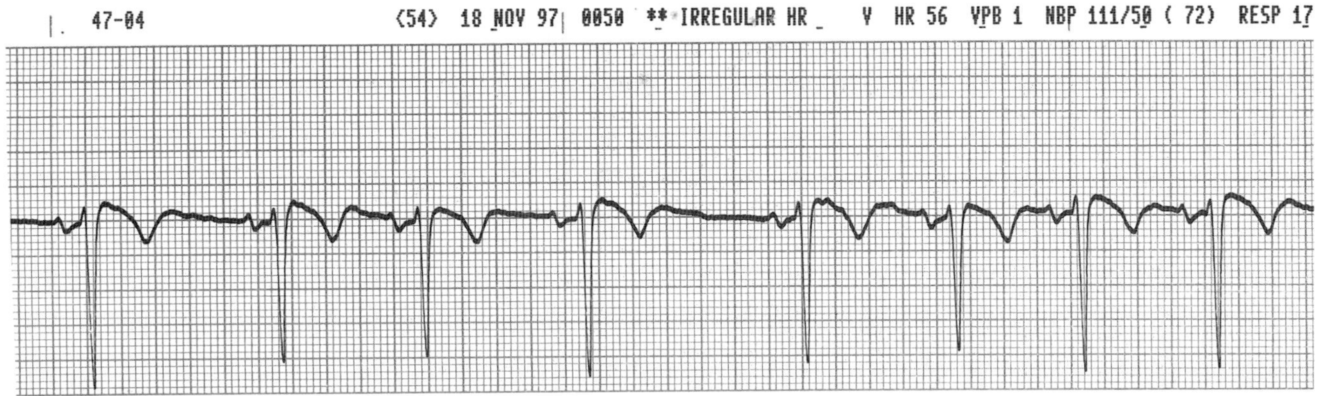

Figure 15-10
ECG tracing demonstrating sinus arrhythmia.

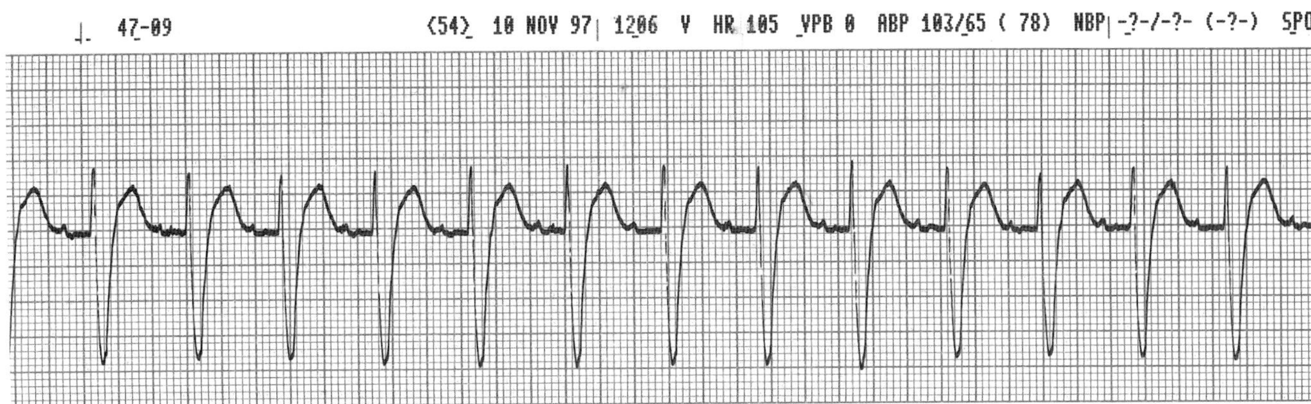

Figure 15-11
ECG tracing demonstrating first-degree heart block.

are benign and do not need treatment. If the arrhythmia is severe, the underlying cause must be identified and eliminated.

First-Degree Heart Block. In first-degree heart block, the PR interval is longer than 0.20 second. In addition, there is one P wave before each QRS complex (Figure 15-11). This indicates that the impulse from the SA node is getting through to the ventricles but is abnormally delayed in passing through the AV node or bundle of His. Typically, the QRS complex has a normal configuration, and the R to R intervals are regular. First-degree heart block is common following an MI that damages the AV node, or it may be a complication of certain medications such as digoxin or β-blockers. Treatment usually is not needed for first-degree heart block if the patient is able to maintain an adequate blood pressure.

Second-Degree Heart Block. Second-degree heart block comes in two different types. Type I (Wenckebach or Mobitz type I) block is a relatively benign and often transient arrhythmia. It occurs when an abnormality in the AV junction delays or blocks conduction of some of the impulses through the AV node. It can be recognized by progressive prolongation of the PR interval until one impulse does not pass on to the ventricles at all (seen as a P wave not followed by a QRS complex). The cycle then repeats itself.

Second-degree heart block type II (Mobitz type II) is less common and is more often the result of serious problems such as MI or ischemia. Type II heart block is seen as a series of nonconducted P waves followed by a P wave that is conducted to the ventricles (Figure 15-12). Sometimes the ratio of nonconducted to conducted P waves is fixed at 3:1 or 4:1. The PR interval for the conducted impulses is consistent.

Treatment for type I second-degree heart block is not needed, because it usually does not impair cardiac output or cause symptoms. Type II second-degree heart block requires treatment in most cases, because the resulting reduction in ventricular rate causes a drop in blood pressure. Medications such as atropine will provide a better cardiac output until a pacemaker can be inserted.

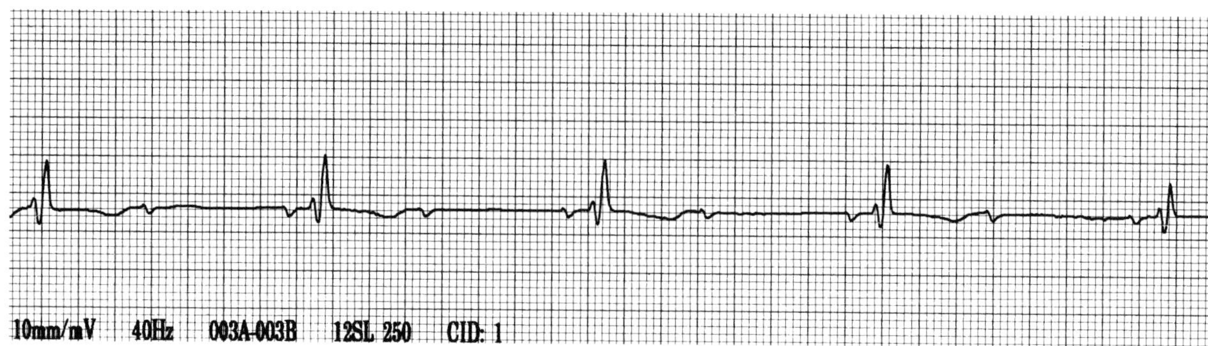

Figure 15-12
ECG demonstrating second-degree heart block type II.

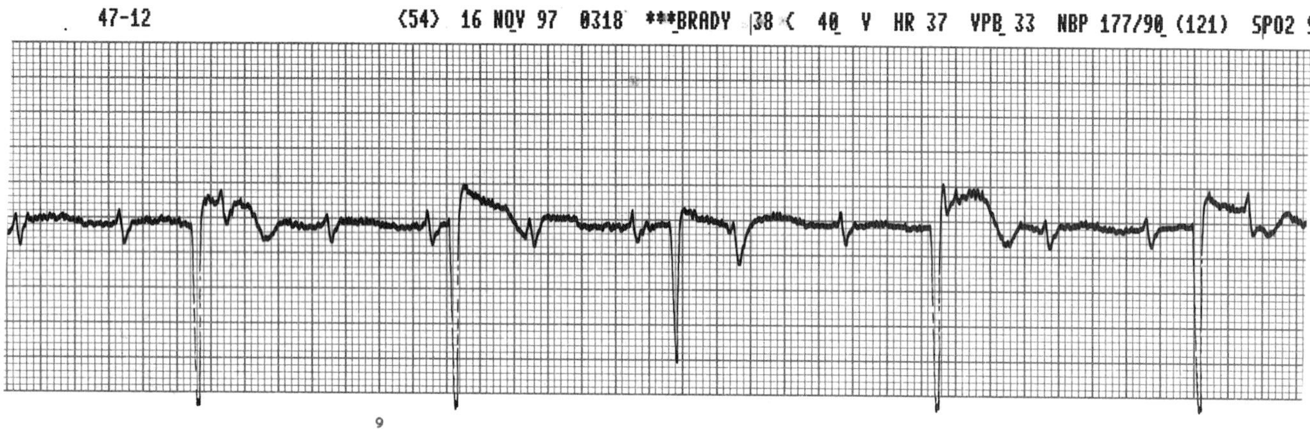

Figure 15-13
ECG tracing demonstrating third-degree heart block.

Third-Degree Heart Block. Third-degree heart block is the most serious of the different types of heart block. It indicates that the conduction system between the atria and ventricles is completely blocked, and impulses generated in the SA node are not conducted to the ventricles. Therefore the atria and ventricles are paced by independent sources. Most commonly, the atria are paced by the SA node and the ventricles by the AV node. This arrhythmia can be recognized when it is established that there is no relationship between the P waves and the QRS complexes. The P to P and R to R intervals are steady and the QRS complexes are normal in configuration if the ventricles are paced by the AV node (Figure 15-13). If the ventricles are paced by an ectopic site in the myocardium, the QRS complexes may be abnormally wide. Typically, the ventricular rate is slower than the atrial rate, because the automaticity of the AV node or other latent points is much slower than the automaticity of the SA node.

Third-degree heart block is a serious arrhythmia because it often is caused by an MI, and it may render the heart unable to meet the normal metabolic demands of the body. Treatment usually includes medication to speed up the ventricles. Eventually, a permanent pacemaker will need to be placed in the patient's heart.

Atrial Flutter. Atrial flutter is the rapid depolarization of the atria resulting from an ectopic focus that depolarizes at a rate of 250 to 350 times per minute. Typically, only one ectopic focus is causing the arrhythmia, which results in each P wave appearing similar. The result is a characteristic sawtooth pattern (Figure 15-14). Numerous P waves are present for every QRS complex, and the QRS complexes are normal in configuration. The R to R interval may be regular or it may vary, depending on the ability of the atrial impulse to pass through the AV node.

A larger variety of conditions can produce atrial flutter, including rheumatic heart disease, coronary heart disease, stress, renal failure, or hypoxemia. This arrhythmia is not considered life-threatening, but it may lead to atrial fibrillation if untreated. Treatment usually includes medications such as digoxin or β-blockers or cardioversion at low voltage.

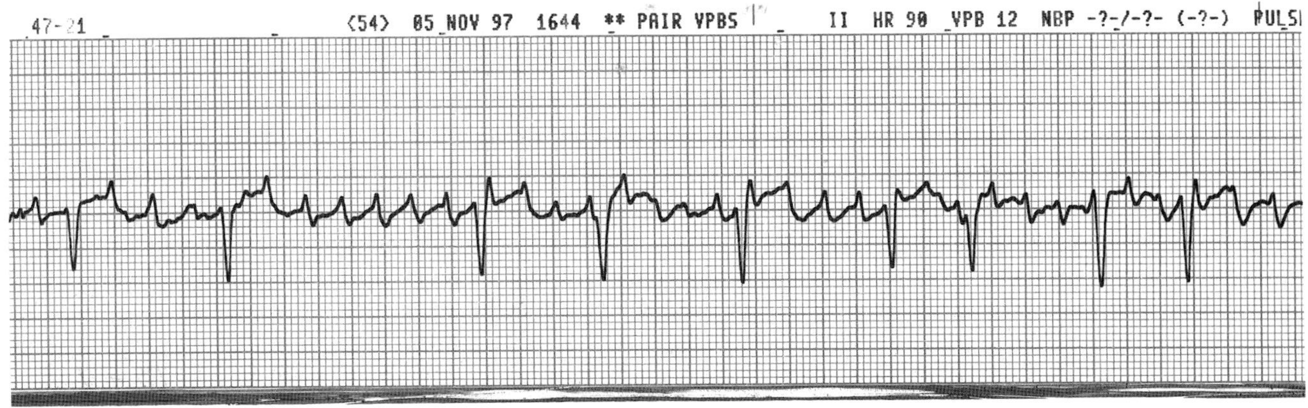

Figure 15-14
ECG tracing demonstrating atrial flutter.

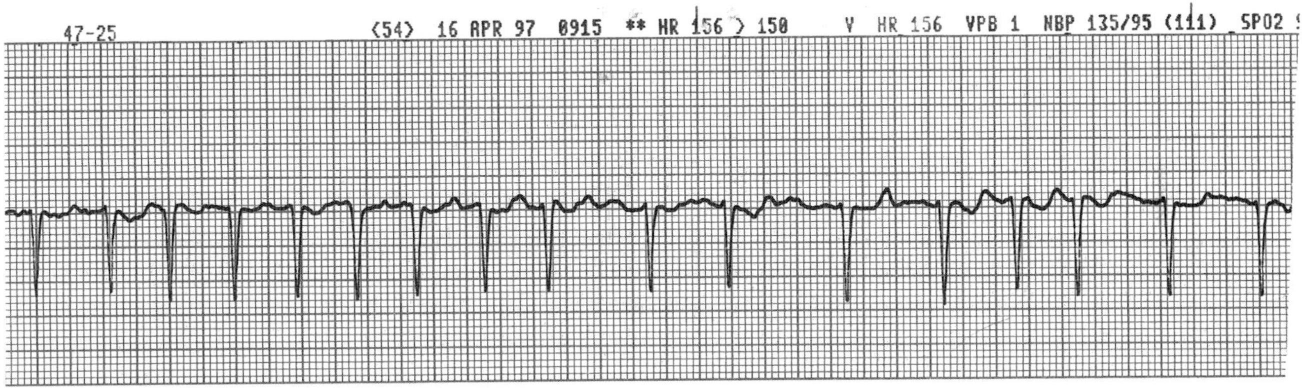

Figure 15-15
ECG tracing demonstrating atrial fibrillation.

Atrial Fibrillation. Atrial fibrillation is present when the atrial muscle quivers in an erratic pattern that does not result in a coordinated contraction. No true P waves are seen in atrial fibrillation (Figure 15-15). The AV node determines the ventricular response to the atrial activity by controlling which impulses pass through and which do not. The ventricular rate may be very irregular and result in an abnormal R to R interval.

The causes of atrial fibrillation are similar to the causes of atrial flutter. However, atrial fibrillation is a more serious arrhythmia, because it can lead to a significant reduction in cardiac output resulting from the loss of the atrial kick that helps fill the ventricles before systole. It also can lead to thrombi formation in the atria caused by the stagnation of blood. Emboli may occur if the thrombi break free and enter the pulmonary artery or aorta. Treatment for atrial fibrillation is similar to that for atrial flutter.

Premature Ventricular Contractions. Premature beats can occur when a portion of the conduction system or myocardium other than the SA node becomes diseased and triggers depolarization of the surrounding cardiac cells. Sources for the impulse outside the SA node are called **ectopic foci.** Ectopic foci occur when hypoxia, acid-base imbalances, or electrolyte abnormalities are present and cause the cardiac cells to become abnormally excited. Premature ventricular contractions (PVCs) are an example of ectopic foci that originate in the ventricles. PVCs are easy to recognize because they cause a unique and bizarre QRS complex, which is much wider than normal (Figure 15-16). The QRS complex of a PVC is wider than normal, because the ectopic focus is using channels outside the normal conduction system to move the impulse throughout the myocardium. PVCs have no P wave preceding them and may occur as a singular event or, more commonly, as a temporary run of PVCs. They also may occur at every other beat. This is known as *bigeminy*.

An occasional PVC is not of major concern and may occur as a result of stress, caffeine or nicotine use, or electrolyte imbalance. However, frequent PVCs are more serious and most often occur in response to ischemia of the myocardium. They also are commonly seen as a

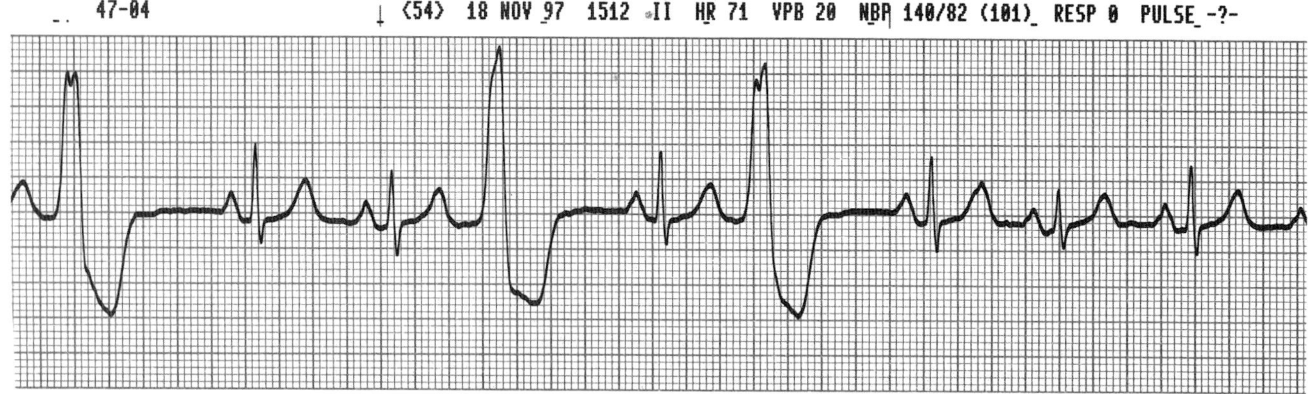

Figure 15-16
ECG tracing demonstrating premature ventricular contractions.

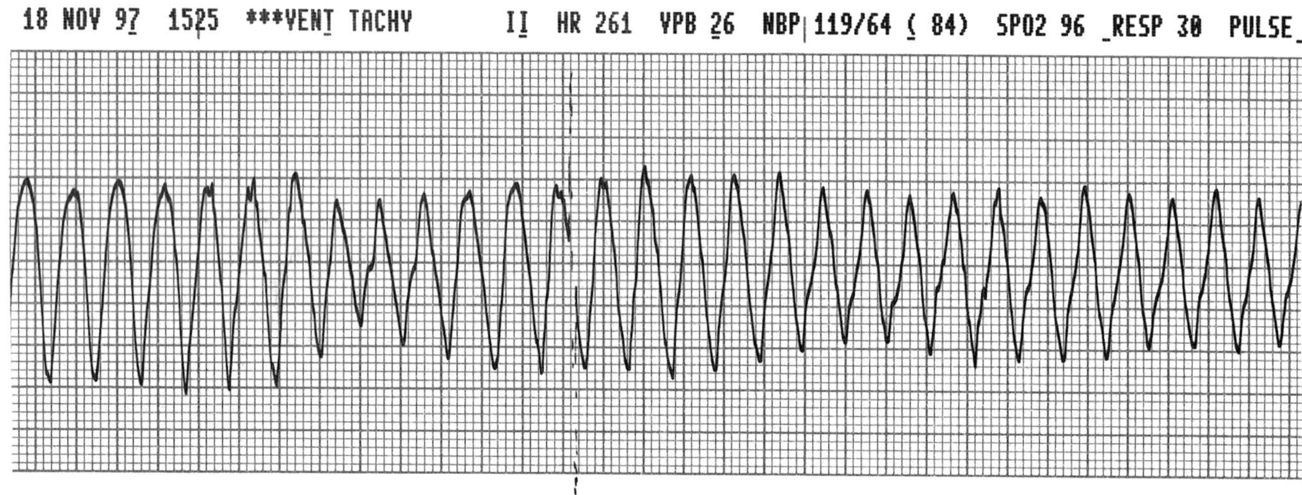

Figure 15-17
ECG tracing demonstrating ventricular tachycardia.

side effect of some medications. Treatment is based on the frequency and cause of the PVCs and is needed when the PVCs are frequent (more than 6 per minute), paired together, or multifocal (come from more than one ectopic focus), or when they land directly on the T wave. In such cases, treatment must be prompt because the problem may progress rapidly to ventricular tachycardia and fibrillation (see subsequent discussion). A complete cardiac evaluation is usually needed to identify the appropriate plan of action. Antiarrhythmic medications (such as lidocaine) may offer a temporary solution until the underlying cause can be identified and treated.

Ventricular Tachycardia. Ventricular tachycardia is a run of three or more PVCs. It usually is easy to recognize as a series of wide, bizarre QRS complexes that have no preceding P wave. The ventricular rate is usually between 100 and 250 beats/min (Figure 15-17).

Ventricular tachycardia is a serious arrhythmia, because it indicates that an ectopic focus is rapidly firing from the ventricles, which results from increased automaticity. It suggests a significant pathological defect in the myocardium and often leads to ventricular fibrillation if untreated. MI, coronary artery disease, and hypertensive heart disease are the most common causes.

Treatment must be prompt and specific. Use of medications, such as lidocaine or procainamide, or cardioversion (defibrillation) are the most useful treatment methods until the underlying cause can be corrected. Ventricular tachycardia is considered a medical emergency, and the patient must be treated and monitored continuously in the ICU until his or her condition is stabilized.

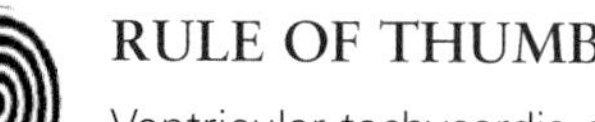

RULE OF THUMB

Ventricular tachycardia causes the cardiac output to drop significantly and places the patient in danger of cardiac arrest.

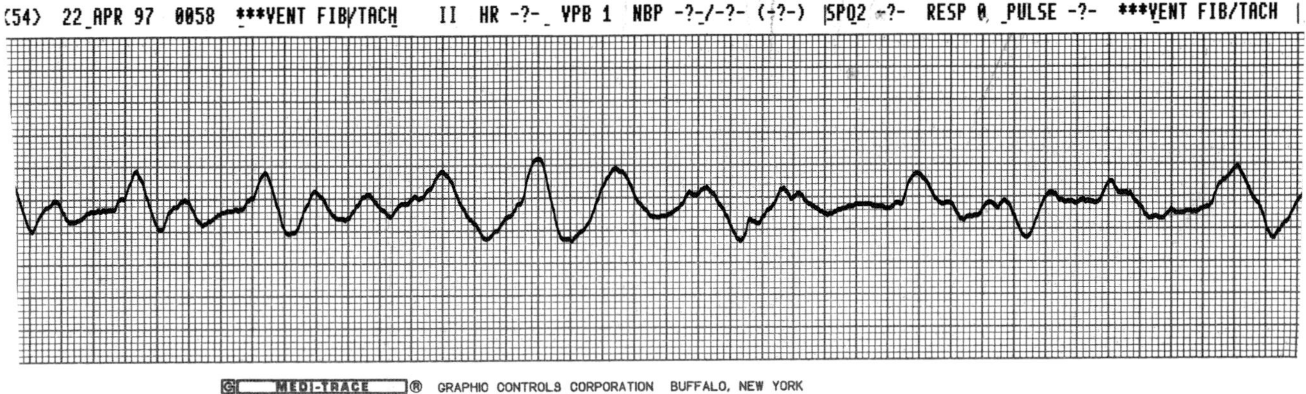

Figure 15-18
ECG tracing demonstrating ventricular fibrillation.

Ventricular Fibrillation. Ventricular fibrillation is defined as erratic quivering of the ventricular muscle mass. It causes the cardiac output to drop to zero and therefore represents a true medical emergency. The ECG tracing of ventricular fibrillation shows grossly irregular fluctuations with a zigzag pattern (Figure 15-18). This pattern is caused by the same problems associated with ventricular tachycardia. Treatment calls for rapid defibrillation, cardiopulmonary resuscitation, and administration of oxygen and antiarrhythmic medications, as well as treatment of the underlying cause of the ischemia.

Table 15-1 ▶▶ Normal Values for the Complete Blood Count in the Adult

Test	Normal Values
Red Blood Cell Count	
Men	4.6-6.2 × 10^6/mm^3
Women	4.2-5.4 × 10^6/mm^3
Hemoglobin (Hb)	
Men	13.5-16.5 g/dL
Women	12-15 g/dL
Hematocrit (Hct)	
Men	40%-54%
Women	38%-47%
Erythocyte Index	
Mean cell volume (MCV)	80-96 μ/mm^3
Mean cell hemoglobin (MCH)	27-31 pg
Mean cell hemoglobin concentration (MCHC)	32%-36%
White Blood Cell Count	**4500-11,500/mm^3**
Differential of White Blood Cells	
Segmented neutrophils	40%-75%
Bands	0%-6%
Eosinophils	0%-6%
Basophils	0%-1%
Lymphocytes	20%-45%
Monocytes	2%-10%
Platelet Count	*150,000-400,000/mm^3*

From Wilkins RL, Krider SJ, Sheldon RL: Clinical assessment in respiratory care, ed 4, St Louis, 2000, Mosby.

▶ INTERPRETING CLINICAL LABORATORY TESTS

Complete Blood Count

The complete blood count (CBC) is routinely performed from a venous blood sample. It provides a detailed description of the number of circulating white blood cells (WBCs), called *leukocytes*, and red blood cells (RBCs), called *erythrocytes*. The WBC count is made up of five different types of cells and is reported under the differential. RBCs are evaluated for size and hemoglobin content. In some cases, this information is useful in determining the diagnosis, but it is most useful for assessing the general health of a patient. Table 15-1 lists the normal CBC results for adults.

White Blood Cell Count

Elevation of the WBC count is known as **leukocytosis.** It results from any number of problems, including stress, infection, and trauma. The degree of leukocytosis is a function of the severity of the problem and the condition of the patient's immune system. For example, a significantly elevated WBC (more than 20,000/mm^3) suggests that a serious infection may be present but that the patient's immune system is generating a significant response.

A WBC below normal is described as **leukopenia.** Leukopenia is not as common as is leukocytosis, but it does occur when the patient's immune system is overwhelmed by an infection or suppressed by disease or therapy. Diseases of the bone marrow, such as lymphoma;

chemotherapy; and radiation therapy for cancer are common causes of leukopenia. Leukopenia commonly is seen in elderly patients with severe pneumonia that is overwhelming the immune system. The prognosis usually is not optimistic in such situations.

Differential of the White Blood Cell Count

The clinical laboratory also performs a differential of the WBC count to determine the exact number of each type of WBC present in the circulating blood. See Table 15-2 for a list of the normal differential counts in the adult patient and common causes for elevation of each cell type. Table 15-2 shows that most circulating WBCs are either neutrophils or lymphocytes. Because leukocytosis usually results from only one of the five cell types responding to a problem, significant elevation of the WBC count (more than 15,000/mm^3) will occur only when either neutrophils or lymphocytes are responding to an abnormality. Because the basophils, eosinophils, and monocytes make up such a small proportion of the circulating WBCs, they are not likely to cause a major increase in the WBC count when responding to disease.

The WBC count differential is best interpreted by determining the absolute count of each WBC. This is calculated by multiplying the percentage of the WBC under study by the total WBC count. This prevents misinterpretation of the WBC count differential when any one cell type changes in absolute numbers and causes a relative change in the percentage of the other four cell types. For example, if the WBC count doubles because of an increase in neutrophils, the relative value of the other four cells will drop in half, although their absolute value did not change. Many laboratories are now reporting the absolute value for each of the five WBCs to avoid this confusion.

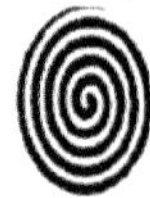

RULE OF THUMB

Elevation of the WBC count is usually caused by an increase in one of the five types of leukocytes.

MINI CLINI

WBC Count Differential

PROBLEM

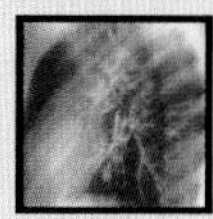

A patient has been admitted to the hospital for acute shortness of breath. A chest x-ray examination reveals pneumonia, and the patient's temperature is elevated. The CBC shows an increased WBC count of 15,000/mm^3, with 75% neutrophils but only 10% lymphocytes. Given that the normal lymphocyte differential is 20% to 45%, does the value of 10% suggest a problem with lymphocyte production by the immune system? What type of pneumonia is probably present in this case?

SOLUTION

The 10% differential for the lymphocytes represents a relative value. Because the total WBC count is markedly elevated, the 10% in relative terms represents 1500 lymphocytes in absolute value, which is well within normal range. If the total WBC count were reduced to less than normal and the differential demonstrated a lymphocyte count of 10%, an abnormal absolute value would be present and would suggest an immunological problem. This patient probably has bacterial pneumonia, given the elevated number of neutrophils.

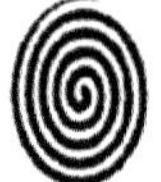

RULE OF THUMB

When bacterial pneumonia is present, the severity of the infection can be assessed by evaluation of the degree of increase in neutrophils. The condition of the patient's immune system can be evaluated by assessment of the total increase in WBCs.

Red Blood Cell Count

The RBC count helps determine the ability of the blood to carry oxygen. An abnormally low RBC count is referred to as **anemia** and suggests that either RBC production by the bone marrow is inadequate or excessive loss of blood has occurred. In either case, the oxygen-carrying capacity of the blood is reduced, and the patient is more likely to experience hypoxia. A

Table 15-2 ▶▶ Normal Values for the White Blood Cell Count Differential and Common Causes for Abnormalities

Cell Type	Relative Value	Absolute Value	Causes for Abnormalities
Neutrophils	40%-75%	1800-7500	Increased with bacterial infection and trauma; reduced with bone marrow diseases
Eosinophils	0%-6%	0-600	Increased with allergic reactions and parasitic infections
Basophils	0%-1%	0-100	Increased with allergic reactions
Monocytes	2%-10%	90-1000	Increased with invasion of foreign material
Lymphocytes	20%-45%	900-4500	Increased with viral and other infections; reduced with immunodeficiency problems

blood transfusion may be needed if the RBC count is too low.

An abnormally elevated RBC count is known as **polycythemia.** It most often occurs when the bone marrow is stimulated to produce extra RBCs in response to chronically low blood oxygen levels, which is referred to as *secondary polycythemia.* Polycythemia helps prevent the negative side effects of reduced PO_2 in the blood by increasing the oxygen-carrying capacity. Patients who live at a high altitude and those with chronic lung disease are most likely to experience chronic hypoxia and to develop secondary polycythemia.

In addition to the RBC count, the clinical laboratory will report the hemoglobin and hematocrit levels. Hemoglobin is a protein substance with the unique ability to bind with oxygen. Each healthy RBC contains 200 to 300 million molecules of hemoglobin, for a hemoglobin level of 12 to 16 g/dL in a healthy adult. Patients with an inadequate hemoglobin concentration will have RBCs that are smaller than normal (microcytic) and lack normal color (hypochromic). Microcytic, hypochromic anemia suggests that the oxygen-carrying capacity of the blood is reduced because of an inadequate hemoglobin concentration. The size of the RBCs is reflected by the mean cell volume and the color of the RBCs is reflected by the mean cell hemoglobin concentration, which are reported in the CBC.

The hematocrit level is the ratio of RBC volume to that of whole blood. It is determined by centrifuging a blood sample to separate the blood cells from the plasma. The proportion of the sample represented by the packed cells is the hematocrit. A low hematocrit reading occurs with anemia, and a high hematocrit reading is common with polycythemia. The hematocrit level is also a reflection of the hydration status of the patient. Dehydration causes it to increase, whereas overhydration causes it to decrease.

RULE OF THUMB

The ratio of hematocrit to hemoglobin is generally approximately 3:1.

Platelet Count

The CBC also reports the number of circulating platelets, which are the smallest formed elements in the blood and are important for coagulation. A significant reduction in the platelet count occurs with bone marrow diseases or with disseminated intravascular coagulation. A low platelet count causes the patient to bruise easily and puts him or her at greater risk of hemorrhage. Other coagulation studies, such as the prothrombin time (PT), provide additional information about the clotting ability of the blood.

RTs need to evaluate the clotting ability of the blood in patients who are to have ABG testing or who are to undergo nasotracheal suctioning. For ABG testing, patients with an abnormally low platelet count or an elevated PT will need to have the puncture site compressed for a longer time after the arterial sample is obtained to prevent hemorrhage. Patients with an extremely low platelet count should have an arterial puncture performed or undergo nasotracheal suctioning only when it is essential because of the risk of bleeding.

Blood Chemistry Tests

Electrolyte Concentrations

The concentrations of numerous electrolytes dissolved in the plasma are determined for most patients with cardiopulmonary disease. They are not measured to make a specific diagnosis, but rather to identify the general health status of the patient and the side effects of certain medications such as diuretics. Electrolytes are essential for homeostasis, and many different abnormalities can occur when their concentration deviates from normal. Cardiac arrhythmias, muscle weakness, and confusion are possible side effects of abnormal electrolyte concentrations. The most common electrolytes reported in the chemistry panel are sodium (Na^+), potassium (K^+), chloride (Cl^-), and total CO_2. The normal values for these electrolytes are listed in Table 15-3.

A low sodium level is referred to as **hyponatremia,** and it may occur with diuretic therapy, diarrhea, or certain kidney problems. Excessive retention of water leads to dilution of the sodium that is present and causes its concentration to be reported as low, although the absolute quantity of sodium in the body may be normal. Patients with severe hyponatremia may develop confusion, decreased mental alertness, muscle twitching, and possible seizures.

Table 15-3 ▶▶ Normal Values for Blood Chemistry Tests

Test	Normal Value
Sodium	137-147 mEq/L
Potassium	3.5-4.8 mEq/L
Chloride	98-105 mEq/L
Carbon dioxide	25-33 mEq/L
Blood urea nitrogen	7-20 mg/dL
Creatinine	0.7-1.3 mg/dL
Total protein	6.3-7.9 g/dL
Albumin	3.5-5.0 g/dL
Cholesterol	150-220 mg/dL
Glucose	70-105 mg/dL

From Wilkins RL, Krider SJ, Sheldon RL: Clinical assessment in respiratory care, ed 4, St Louis, Mosby.

Elevation of the serum sodium level is known as **hypernatremia**. It occurs with renal diseases and excessive water loss. It is not as common as is hyponatremia, but it also leads to significant clinical problems if it is severe.

An abnormally low serum potassium level is known as **hypokalemia**. It occurs when potassium-containing fluids are lost in excessive amounts, such as with the administration of diuretics, vomiting, or diarrhea. Hypokalemia often leads to weakening of the cardiac muscle, which reduces cardiac output. For this reason, hypokalemia must be corrected as soon as possible, especially in the patient with borderline cardiac function.

Abnormal elevation of the serum potassium level is referred to as *hyperkalemia*. It occurs with a variety of ailments, such as renal disease, and tissue trauma, which cause a release of intracellular potassium into the plasma. Hyperkalemia may cause the patient to feel tired, weak, and nauseated. The potassium level is of particular interest in the patient being weaned from mechanical ventilation, because both hyperkalemia and hypokalemia may render the diaphragm weak and less effective.

Chloride is the primary extracellular anion. Hypochloremia (reduced serum chloride) occurs with prolonged vomiting, resulting in the loss of HCl, chronic respiratory acidosis, and certain renal diseases. Hyperchloremia (increased serum chloride) occurs with prolonged diarrhea, certain kidney diseases, and some cases of hyperthyroidism.

The total CO_2 represents the level of HCO_3^- in venous blood. Because the CO_2 concentration is higher in venous blood than it is in arterial blood, the normal venous HCO_3^- level is slightly higher than that seen in the ABG analysis. Any abnormality that causes the arterial HCO_3^- level to increase (e.g., chronic respiratory acidosis) will lead to elevation of the total CO_2 on the venous chemistry panel. Metabolic alkalosis and compensation for respiratory acidosis represent such abnormalities. Disorders that cause the blood HCO_3^- to decrease, such as metabolic acidosis, will lead to abnormally low total CO_2.

Sweat Chloride

Patients with cystic fibrosis have increased levels of chloride in their sweat because of their inability to reabsorb it. Thus these patients will have abnormally elevated chloride levels in their sweat (more than 60 to 80 mEq/L). Although the sweat electrolyte test is an important tool for diagnosing cystic fibrosis, it must be combined with other tests because some patients with the disease may have minimally elevated or normal sweat chloride levels.

Anion Gap

A balance normally exists between cations and anions in the serum. Evaluation of this balance is done by determining the anion gap, which is the difference between the concentration level of the primary cation (Na^+) and the primary anions (HCO_3^- and Cl^-). Because potassium is minimally present in the serum, it is not considered in the calculation of the anion gap. The anion gap is calculated by adding the HCO_3^- and Cl^- values and subtracting this total from the serum sodium. The normal anion gap is 8 to 16 mEq/L. Elevation of the anion gap suggests that a metabolic acidosis is present, and further evaluation of the patient's acid-base status is necessary.

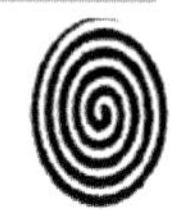

RULE OF THUMB

An anion gap greater than 16 is consistent with the presence of metabolic acidosis.

Renal Function

The most common tests performed to evaluate kidney function are the blood urea nitrogen (BUN) and creatinine. Urea is a waste product of metabolism that is excreted by healthy kidneys. Renal disease often leads to an abnormal elevation of blood urea above 20 mg/dL. Unfortunately, the BUN level also can increase when renal perfusion is not optimal, as in heart failure. It is also influenced by protein intake, various hormones, and hydration status and therefore is not specific to kidney problems.

Creatinine is a waste product that is formed by muscle metabolism and filtered out of the body by the kidneys.

MINI CLINI

Anion Gap

PROBLEM

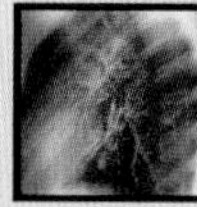

A patient in the ICU is being treated for shock and acute renal failure. No ABGs have been drawn yet, but the RT suspects a respiratory problem because the patient has been breathing more rapidly over the last 12 hours. The electrolyte panel reveals a serum sodium level of 146 mEq/L, a total CO_2 of 20 mEq/L, and a serum chloride level of 100 mEq/L. Does the electrolyte panel suggest any problems, and what should be done if there are any?

SOLUTION

The electrolytes are normal except for a decrease in the serum CO_2. The anion gap is calculated by subtracting the total of the CO_2 and Cl^- from the Na^+ (146 – 120 = 26). The anion gap is elevated (26) in this case, which is consistent with a metabolic acidosis. An ABG analysis is needed to further evaluate the acid-base status of the patient. The patient's rapid breathing probably is related to the metabolic acidosis, because increasing CO_2 removal by hyperventilation will help compensation.

Normal levels are 0.7 to 1.3 mg/dL in the blood serum. Diseases of the kidney that result in a significant proportion of the renal nephrons becoming dysfunctional cause the creatinine level to increase.

Serum Enzymes

Enzymes are present in most body cells (e.g., liver, heart, skeletal muscle). Damage to these tissues causes the release of certain enzymes into the circulating blood. Measurement of the serum enzymes can be helpful in confirming a suspected diagnosis. For example, in a patient with chest pain, MI may be suspected. Elevation of certain serum enzymes supports the diagnosis of MI. The absence of an increase in serum enzymes suggests that the chest pain has another origin. Common enzymes that are measured are described in the subsequent sections.

Aspartate Aminotransferase. Aspartate aminotransferase (AST), formerly known as SGOT (serum glutamic-oxaloacetic transaminase), is found in many tissues. The highest concentrations of AST are found in patients with liver disease, such as hepatitis, and during the second day after an MI. Because an elevated AST may occur with a variety of ailments, evaluating the AST is of little value without results from the medical history and other evaluation tools.

Alanine Aminotransferase. Alanine aminotransferase (ALT), formerly known as SGPT (serum glutamate pyruvate transaminase), is a liver enzyme that increases with liver diseases such as hepatitis. ALT does not exist in heart tissue and therefore does not increase with heart problems unless a secondary liver problem also exists.

Alkaline Phosphatase. Alkaline phosphatase (ALP) also is useful in evaluating the liver function. Because ALP is present in the bones, kidneys, spleen, and intestine, damage to these tissues can increase the serum ALP. For example, patients with bone marrow disease may have a marked elevation of serum ALP.

L-Lactate Dehydrogenase. L-Lactate dehydrogenase (LDH) is an enzyme that occurs in high concentrations in the heart, liver, skeletal muscle, brain, kidney, and RBCs. Elevated LDH levels may occur in a variety of conditions such as hepatitis, renal disease, shock, MI, trauma, widespread carcinoma, and megaloblastic anemia. Electrophoresis can be used to separate LDH into five different isoenzymes. Measuring the level of a specific isoenzyme may help in identifying a more specific location for the source of the problem.

Creatine Kinase. Creatine kinase (CK), also known as *creatine phosphokinase (CPK)*, occurs in the brain, skeletal muscles, and heart. CK from the brain does not cross the blood-brain barrier and does not appear in the serum. Consequently, elevated CK levels are indicative of heart or skeletal muscle disorders. CK can be identified by electrophoresis as either the type from the heart or the type from skeletal muscle. Elevation of the serum CK type that is found only in the heart (CK-MB) is suggestive of an MI.

Serum Glucose

The breakdown of carbohydrates results in the production of serum glucose, which is metabolized by the cells for energy. Insulin is necessary for cells to utilize the glucose circulating in the blood. Patients with diabetes mellitus have reduced insulin production and therefore do not use glucose normally. The lack of insulin leads to abnormal elevation of the serum glucose, which is known as **hyperglycemia**. Severe hyperglycemia occurring simultaneously with metabolic acidosis is consistent with diabetic ketoacidosis and represents a potentially life-threatening condition if not recognized and treated immediately.

An abnormally reduced serum glucose level is known as **hypoglycemia** and may be drug induced, associated with digestive problems, or related to inadequate dietary intake of carbohydrates. The patient with hypoglycemia often complains of weakness, shaking, headache, lethargy, and excessive sweating. Weaning from a ventilator is not likely to be successful in the patient with hypoglycemia.

The normal fasting blood glucose level is approximately 70 to 105 mg/dL. The blood glucose level in any patient must be interpreted in light of when the patient last ate. Recent intake of carbohydrates causes the blood glucose level to rise temporarily for 60 to 90 minutes, until it is metabolized by cells. The normal fasting level should be evaluated approximately 2 hours after the patient has ingested food.

Microbiology Tests

Sputum Gram Stain

The patient who is suspected of having an infection in the lungs or airways may benefit from analysis of a sputum sample. The purpose of such an analysis is to determine the specific microorganism causing the infection, which will indicate the most appropriate antibiotic to be given. The first step in evaluating the sputum sample is the Gram stain, which is performed in the clinical laboratory by a technician who smears the sputum sample on a glass slide, applies a staining solution, and examines it through a microscope.

Initially, the technician uses the Gram stain to determine the quality of the sputum sample. Some patients have difficulty producing an adequate sputum sample from the lung and may actually expectorate only saliva into the sputum cup. In such cases, the Gram stain will demonstrate few (less than 25 per low-power field) or no pus cells and numerous epithelial cells. This indicates that the sample is merely saliva and should be discarded. The sample with numerous pus cells and few or no epithelial cells is most likely a true sample from the lung and is reflective of the infection source.

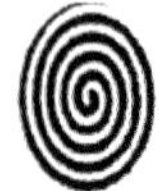

RULE OF THUMB

A legitimate sputum sample has few epithelial cells and many pus cells (leukocytes).

Once the sample has been verified, the laboratory technician identifies the Gram stain reaction (either positive or negative) and the shape of any bacteria present (rods versus cocci). Such results are presumptive, and a definitive diagnosis is made only by isolation and culture of the specific organism present. For example, *Streptococcus pneumoniae*, a common bacterium associated with pneumonia, stains as encapsulated, lancet-shaped, gram-positive diplococci. These results are consistent with the diagnosis of streptococcal pneumonia and allow the physician to begin an appropriate course of antibiotic therapy before the results of the sputum culture are available, perhaps days later.

Sputum Culture

If the Gram stain reveals a legitimate sample, the technician prepares a portion of the sputum for culture. This requires placement of the sputum sample in a medium consistent with growth of the organism. Once the organism has matured, it is examined microscopically to determine its exact type and sensitivity to antibiotic therapy. This allows the physician to prescribe the most effective antibiotic. These same procedures for Gram staining and culturing can be applied to samples of blood, pleural fluid, or any other body fluid involved in an infection.

KEY POINTS

- The ECG is most useful for identifying abnormal cardiac rhythms and evidence of acute myocardial ischemia. It does not evaluate the pumping ability of the heart or structural defects such as valvular abnormalities. The resting ECG cannot predict the likelihood of MI.
- Normally, cardiac cells are polarized with a strong positive charge on the outside of the cell membrane and a negative charge on the inside. Stimulation of these cells causes depolarization by allowing sodium ions to rush inside the cell.
- Most cardiac cells have the ability to depolarize without stimulation from outside sources. This is known as *automaticity*.
- Normally, the cardiac contraction rate and pattern are controlled by the conduction system. The normal impulse begins with the SA node, which initiates cardiac contractions in the healthy heart. If the SA node fails to pace the heart, the AV node serves as the backup pacemaker.
- The normal ECG recording consists of a P wave, QRS wave, and T wave. The P wave represents atrial depolarization, the QRS wave represents ventricular depolarization, and the T wave represents ventricular repolarization.
- Abnormalities in the ST segment of the ECG are of concern because they usually indicate myocardial ischemia.
- The hypoxic heart that is in trouble often starts signaling distress by demonstrating PVCs. If the problem is not corrected, the PVCs become more frequent and may progress to ventricular tachycardia, which may progress to ventricular fibrillation and death if not corrected.

KEY POINTS—cont'd

- Elevation of the WBC count is known as *leukocytosis*. It often occurs with infection, stress, or trauma. A reduced WBC count is known as *leukopenia*.
- Abnormal elevation of the RBC count is known as *polycythemia*, and an abnormal reduction in the RBC count is referred to as *anemia*.
- Normal electrolyte concentrations in the blood plasma are essential for the proper function of all body systems. Abnormal electrolyte counts may cause muscle weakness, confusion, and abnormal cardiac rhythms, among other problems.
- The sputum Gram stain is useful for determining the quality of the sample and the type of organism present. Samples with many epithelial cells and few pus cells are of no value and probably are saliva from the mouth.

Bibliography

Goldberger AL: Clinical electrocardiography: a simplified approach, ed 6, St Louis, 1999, Mosby.

Wilkins RL, Krider SJ, Sheldon RL: Clinical assessment in respiratory care, ed 4, St Louis, 2000, Mosby.

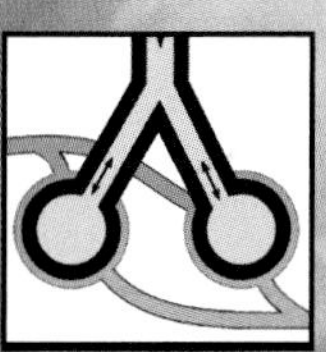

CHAPTER 16

Analysis and Monitoring of Gas Exchange

Craig L. Scanlan and Robert L. Wilkins

In This Chapter You Will Learn:

- What techniques are used to assess gas exchange and when they are indicated
- What equipment to select for a monitoring procedure and how to ensure its proper operation
- How to measure the inspired oxygen concentration (FIO_2)
- How to obtain, process, and analyze blood gas samples
- When and how to perform co-oximetry
- How to obtain and interpret capillary blood samples
- What quality control procedures apply to blood gas analysis
- How to interpret pulse oximetry results
- How and when to perform transcutaneous oxygen and carbon dioxide monitoring
- How to perform capnometry and interpret capnograms

Chapter Outline

Key Terms

analyte
analyzer
arterialized blood
bias
calibration media
capnography
capnometry
collateral circulation
cuvette
electrochemical
ex vivo
fluorescence
imprecision
in vivo
inaccuracy
invasive
modified Allen test
monitor
needle capping device
noninvasive
optode
photoplethysmography
point-of-care testing
preanalytical error
precision
proficiency testing
quality control

Continued

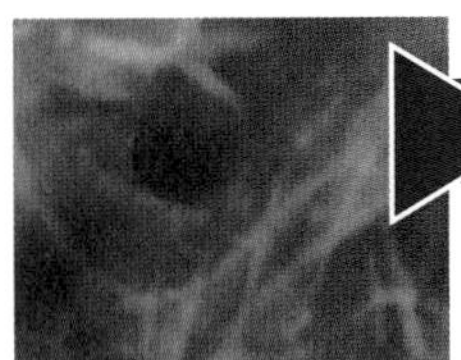

Key Terms—cont'd

spectrophotometry
systematic error
thrombolytic
thrombosis
undampened

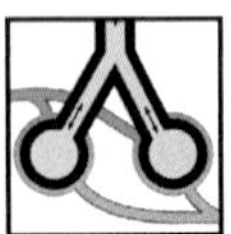

Ultimately, gas exchange takes place inside each of the body's cells, where complex metabolic pathways use oxygen to create energy while producing carbon dioxide as a waste product. Although it is possible to analyze gas exchange at the cellular level, clinical focus normally is on gas exchange between the lungs and blood or between the blood and tissues. Gas exchange between the lungs and blood is usually analyzed by measuring oxygen and carbon dioxide levels in the arterial blood. Clinicians also can measure carbon dioxide levels in the expired air to monitor ventilation. The most common approach to analyzing gas exchange between the blood and tissues is to measure oxygen levels in the mixed venous (pulmonary artery [PA]) blood. This chapter focuses on these important concepts and the parameters that reflect gas exchange.

▶ ANALYSIS VERSUS MONITORING

Although the term *analysis* is defined broadly as *study* or *interpretation*, analysis conducted in a clinical laboratory has a special meaning, as does the term *monitoring*. In clinical practice, laboratory analysis refers to discrete measurements of fluids or tissue that must be removed from the body. Such measurements are made by a laboratory **analyzer**. Conversely, monitoring is an ongoing process by which clinicians obtain and evaluate dynamic physiological processes in a timely manner, usually at the bedside. A **monitor** is a device that provides the appropriate data to the clinician in real time, usually without removal of samples from the body.

▶ INVASIVE VERSUS NONINVASIVE PROCEDURES

Invasive procedures require insertion of a sensor or collection device into the body, whereas **noninvasive** monitoring is a means of gathering data externally. Because laboratory analysis of gas exchange requires blood samples, it is usually considered invasive. On the other hand, monitoring can be either invasive or noninvasive. In general, invasive procedures tend to provide more accurate data than do noninvasive methods but carry greater risk.

When both approaches are available, the need for measurement accuracy should dictate which is chosen. However, clinicians can sometimes combine the two approaches, using the invasive approach to establish accurate baseline information, while applying the noninvasive method for ongoing monitoring.

▶ MEASURING F_{IO_2}

Analysis of gas exchange begins with knowledge of the system inputs—the inspired oxygen and carbon dioxide concentrations. Healthy individuals breathe air that contains a fixed oxygen concentration (21%) and negligible amounts of carbon dioxide. Patients who are ill often suffer from hypoxemia, and they are given supplemental oxygen. Oxygen analyzers are used to measure the inspired oxygen concentration (F_{IO_2}).

Instrumentation

Although many methods exist for measuring oxygen concentrations, most bedside systems apply **electrochemical** principles. There are two common types of electrochemical oxygen analyzers: (1) the polarographic (Clark) electrode and (2) the galvanic fuel cell. Under ideal conditions of temperature, pressure, and relative humidity, both types are accurate to within ±2% of the actual concentration.[1]

The Clark electrode is similar to those used in blood gas analyzers and transcutaneous monitors (see p. 372). This system typically consists of a platinum cathode and a silver-silver chloride anode (Figure 16-1). Oxygen molecules diffuse through the sensor membrane into the electrolyte, where a polarizing voltage causes electron flow between the anode and cathode. While silver is oxidized at the anode, the flow of electrons reduces oxygen (and water) to hydroxyl ions (OH^-) at the cathode. The more O_2 molecules that are reduced, the greater the electron flow is across the poles (current). The resulting change in current is proportional to the P_{O_2}, with its value displayed on a galvanometer, calibrated in percent oxygen. Response times for Clark electrode oxygen analyzers range between 10 and 30 seconds.

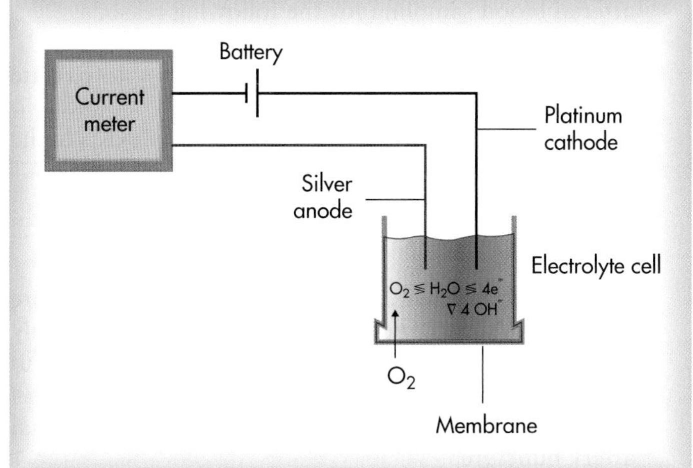

Figure 16-1
The basic principle underlying a Clark polarographic analyzer. *(From Kacmarek RM, Hess D, Stoller JK: Monitoring in respiratory care, St Louis, 1993, Mosby.)*

Most galvanic fuel cells use a gold anode and a lead cathode. Unlike the Clark electrode, current flow across these poles is generated by the chemical reaction itself. Thus, unless accessories such as alarms are included, a galvanic cell needs no external power. Unfortunately, this means that galvanic cells respond more slowly than do Clark electrodes, sometimes taking as long as 60 seconds.

The Clark electrode and galvanic cell are suitable for basic FIO_2 monitoring. When greater accuracy or faster response times are needed (such as when performing indirect calorimetry), either a paramagnetic, zirconium cell, Raman scattering, or mass spectroscopy analyzer should be selected.

Procedure

To obtain accurate results with an oxygen analyzer, the clinician first must calibrate it. Although procedures differ according to the manufacturer, the basic steps are similar, requiring exposure of the sensor to two gases with different oxygen concentrations, usually 100% O_2 and room air (21% O_2). In one common procedure, the sensor is first exposed to 100% O_2. If the analyzer fails to read 100%, the device's calibration, or balance control, must be adjusted until it reads 100%. Then the clinician exposes the sensor to room air and confirms a second reading of 21% (±2%). The clinician should use the analyzer to measure a patient's FIO_2 only after confirming both readings.

Problem-Solving and Troubleshooting

Because oxygen analyzers include replaceable components that deteriorate over time (batteries, electrodes, membranes, electrolyte), the best way to avoid problems is through preventive maintenance, which should include both scheduled parts replacement and routine operational testing by biomedical engineering personnel. As with any preventive maintenance program, it is essential that detailed records be kept on each piece of equipment.

Even with the best preventive maintenance, oxygen analyzers sometimes will malfunction. The clinician will know that an analyzer is not working if it fails to calibrate or gives an inconsistent reading during use. The most common causes of analyzer malfunction are low batteries (Clark electrode systems), sensor depletion, and electronic failure. Because a low battery condition is so common with Clark electrode systems, the first step in troubleshooting is to replace the batteries. If the analyzer still does not calibrate on fresh batteries, the problem is probably a depleted sensor. With most analyzers, a depleted sensor must be replaced (some Clark electrodes can be recharged). If an analyzer still fails to calibrate after battery and sensor replacement, the most likely problem is an internal failure of its electrical system. In this case, the device should be taken out of service and sent in for repair.

Inaccurate readings also can occur with electrochemical analyzers, resulting from either condensed water vapor or pressure fluctuations. Galvanic cells are particularly sensitive to condensation. To avoid this problem during continuous use in humidified circuits, the clinician should place the analyzer sensor *proximal* to any humidification device.

Fuel cell and Clark electrode readings also are affected by ambient pressure changes. Under conditions of low pressure (high altitude), these devices read lower than the actual oxygen concentration. Conversely, higher pressures, such as those that occur during positive pressure ventilation, cause these devices to read higher than the actual FIO_2. Of course, these observations are consistent with the fact that both devices actually measure the PO_2 but report a percent concentration scale.

▶ SAMPLING AND ANALYZING BLOOD GASES

In the clinical setting, it is common for the collection of blood specimens (sampling) to be performed separately from their analysis. Moreover, each procedure involves different knowledge and skill. For these reasons, these topics are covered separately.

Sampling

Clinicians have been using blood samples to assess gas exchange parameters for more than 30 years. In fact, the definition of respiratory failure still is based largely on blood gas measurements.

Depending on the need, blood gas samples can be obtained by percutaneous puncture of a peripheral artery, from an indwelling catheter (arterial, central venous, or PA), or by capillary sampling.

Arterial Puncture and Interpretation

Results obtained from sampling arterial blood gas (ABG) are the cornerstone in the diagnosis and management of oxygenation and acid-base disturbances. Indeed, ABGs are considered the gold standard of gas exchange analysis, against which all other methods are compared.

Arterial puncture involves drawing blood from a peripheral artery (radial, brachial, femoral, or dorsalis pedis) through a single percutaneous needle puncture (Figure 16-2). The radial artery is the preferred site for arterial blood sampling for the following reasons:

- It is near the surface and relatively easy to palpate and stabilize.
- Effective **collateral circulation** normally exists in the ulnar artery.
- The artery is not near any large veins.
- The procedure is relatively pain free.

Other sites (brachial, femoral, and dorsalis pedis) are riskier and should be used only by those specifically trained in their use. Likewise, arterial puncture in infants (through either the radial or the temporal artery) requires advanced training. The focus here is on radial artery puncture.

To guide practitioners in providing quality care, the American Association for Respiratory Care (AARC) has published *Clinical Practice Guideline: Sampling for Arterial Blood Gas Analysis*.[2] Complementary recommendations have been published by the National Committee for Clinical Laboratory Standards.[3] Modified excerpts from the AARC guideline appear on p. 359.

Equipment. Box 16-1 lists the equipment needed to perform an arterial puncture. Commercial vendors provide kits containing most of the equipment listed. If provided, the **needle capping device** serves two purposes. First, it isolates the sample from air exposure (to ensure accurate results). Second, it helps prevent inadvertent needlestick injuries. There are many different capping device designs; those that allow single-handed recapping are preferred. If a capping safety device is not provided, the clinician should use the

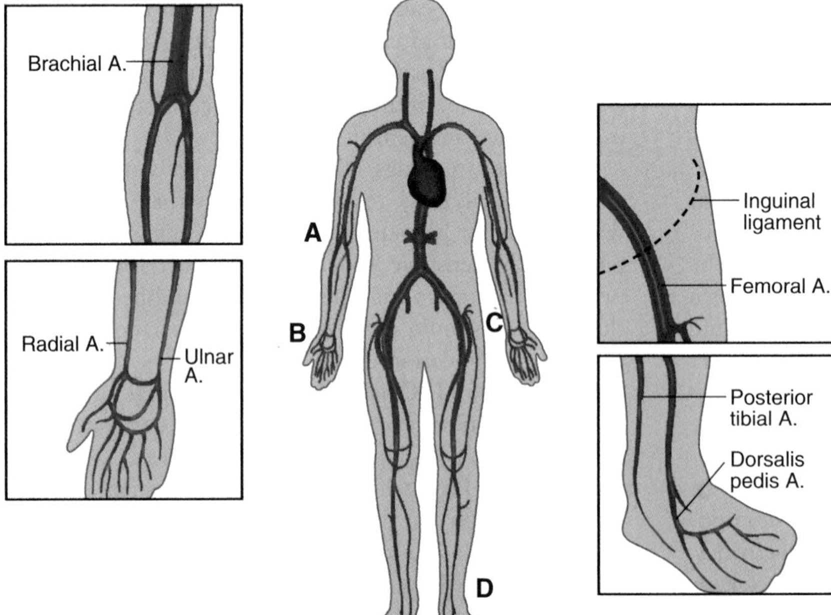

Figure 16-2
Arteries used for arterial puncture. **A**, Brachial artery. **B**, Radial artery (with collateral flow through the ulnar arteries). **C**, Femoral artery. **D**, Dorsalis pedis (with collateral flow through the posterior tibial artery). The radial artery is the preferred site.

SAMPLING FOR ARTERIAL BLOOD GAS ANALYSIS

AARC Clinical Practice Guideline (Excerpts)*

➤ INDICATIONS

- The need to evaluate ventilation ($PaCO_2$), acid-base (pH and $PaCO_2$), oxygenation (PaO_2 and SaO_2) status, and the oxygen-carrying capacity of blood (PaO_2, HbO_2, total Hb, and dyshemoglobins)
- The need to assess the patient's response to therapy and/or diagnostic tests (e.g., oxygen therapy or exercise testing)
- The need to monitor the severity and progression of a documented disease process

➤ CONTRAINDICATIONS

- Negative results of a **modified Allen test** (collateral circulation test) are indicative of inadequate blood supply to the hand and suggest the need to select another extremity for the puncture site.
- Arterial puncture should not be performed through a lesion or distal to a surgical shunt. For example, arterial puncture should not be performed on a patient undergoing dialysis. If there is evidence of infection or peripheral vascular disease involving the selected limb, an alternate site should be selected.
- Because of the need for monitoring the femoral puncture site for an extended period, femoral punctures should not be performed outside the hospital.
- A coagulopathy or medium- to high-dose anticoagulation therapy, such as heparin or warfarin (Coumadin), streptokinase, and tissue plasminogen activator (but not necessarily aspirin) may be a relative contraindication.

➤ PRECAUTIONS AND/OR POSSIBLE COMPLICATIONS

- Arteriospasm
- Air or clotted blood emboli
- Anaphylaxis from local anesthetic
- Patient or sampler contamination
- Hematoma
- Hemorrhage
- Trauma to the vessel
- Arterial occlusion
- Vasovagal response
- Pain

➤ ASSESSMENT OF NEED

The following findings may make it easier for the clinician to decide whether arterial blood sampling is needed:

- History and physical indicators, such as positive smoking history, recent onset of difficult breathing independent of activity level, or trauma
- Presence of other abnormal diagnostic tests or indexes, such as abnormal pulse oximetry reading or chest x-ray examination
- Initiation, change, or discontinuation of therapy (e.g., oxygen therapy or mechanical ventilation)
- Projected surgical interventions for patients at risk
- Projected enrollment in a pulmonary rehabilitation program

➤ FREQUENCY

The frequency with which sampling is repeated should depend on the clinical status of the patient and the indication for performing the procedure. Because repeated punctures at a single site can cause injury, clinicians should consider either finding alternate sites or using an indwelling catheter.

➤ MONITORING

The following should be monitored as part of arterial blood sampling:

- FIO_2 (analyzed) or prescribed flow
- Proper application of oxygen device
- Mode of ventilatory support and settings
- Pulsatile blood return
- Presence of air bubbles or clots in the syringe or sample
- Appearance of the puncture site (for hematoma) after application of pressure and before dressing
- Patient's respiratory rate
- Patient's temperature
- Patient's position and level of activity
- Patient's clinical appearance
- Ease or difficulty in obtaining a blood sample

*For the complete guideline, see Respir Care 37:913, 1992.

Box 16-1 • Recommended Equipment for Percutaneous Arterial Blood Sampling

- Standard precautions barrier protection (gloves, safety goggles)
- Anticoagulant (liquid sodium, lithium heparin, or dry lyophilized heparin)
- Sterile glass or low-diffusibility plastic syringe (1 to 5 mL)
- Short bevel 20- to 22-gauge needle with a clear hub (23- to 25-gauge for children and infants)
- Patient/sample label
- Isopropyl alcohol (70%) or povidone-iodine (Betadine) swabs (check patient for iodine sensitivity)
- Sterile gauze squares, tape, bandages
- Puncture-resistant container
- Ice chips (if specimen will not be analyzed within 15 minutes)
- Towels
- Sharps container
- Local anesthetic (0.5% lidocaine)*
- Hypodermic needle (25 or 26 gauge)
- Needle capping device

*Optional.

single-handed "scoop" method to cap the needle before removing it and plugging the syringe.[4]

Procedure. Box 16-2 outlines the basic procedure for radial artery puncture of adults.

Before any radial puncture is performed, a modified Allen test (Figure 16-3) should be performed. The test is positive (indicating adequate collateral circulation) if the palm, fingers, and thumb flush pink within 10 seconds after pressure on the ulnar artery is released. A positive test result is required to proceed with a radial puncture.

The Allen test cannot be performed on uncooperative or unconscious patients. In addition, prior radial artery cannulation, severe circulatory insufficiency, wrist or hand burns, or jaundice makes interpreting the results difficult. In such cases, a Doppler pulse transducer should be used to assess the pulsatile flow of the thumb, with and without ulnar occlusion. If quick release of pressure restores a good pulse, collateral flow is present, and the radial puncture can proceed. A similar procedure has been described using a pulse oximeter.[5]

In most cases, a sample volume of 2 to 4 mL of blood is adequate.The actual sample volume needed depends on the following: (1) the anticoagulant used, (2) the requirements of the specific analyzer used, and (3) whether other tests will be performed on the sample.

The following rules for careful handling of the needle will help avoid transmission of bloodborne diseases:

Box 16-2 • Procedure for Radial Artery Puncture

- Check the chart to (1) confirm the order and indications and (2) determine the patient's primary diagnosis, history (especially bleeding disorders or bloodborne infections), current status, respiratory care orders (especially oxygen therapy or mechanical ventilation), and anticoagulant or thrombolytic therapy.
- Confirm steady-state conditions (20 to 30 minutes after changes).
- Obtain and assemble the necessary equipment and supplies.
- Wash hands and don barrier protection (e.g., gloves, eyewear).
- Explain the procedure to the patient.
- Position the patient, extending his or her wrist to approximately 30 degrees.
- Perform a modified Allen test, and confirm collateral circulation.
- Thoroughly cleanse the site with 70% isopropyl alcohol or an equivalent antiseptic.
- Inject a local anesthetic subcutaneously and periarterially (wait 2 minutes for effect).*
- Heparinize the syringe and expel the excess (fill dead space only).
- Palpate and secure the artery with one hand.
- Slowly insert the needle, bevel up, through the skin at a 45-degree angle until blood pulsates into the syringe.
- Allow 2 to 4 mL of blood to fill the syringe (the need to aspirate indicates a venous puncture).
- Apply firm pressure to the puncture site with sterile gauze until the bleeding stops.
- Expel any air bubbles from the sample, and cap or plug the syringe.
- Mix the sample by rolling and inverting the syringe.
- Place the sample in a transport container (ice).
- Properly dispose of waste materials and sharps.
- Document the procedure and patient status in the chart and on the specimen label.
- Check the site after 20 minutes for hematoma and adequacy of distal circulation.

From Malley WJ: Clinical blood gases: application and noninvasive alternatives, Philadelphia, 1990, WB Saunders; Shapiro BA, Peruzzi WT, Kozelowski-Templin R: Clinical application of blood gases, ed 5, St Louis, 1994, Mosby; White GC: Basic clinical lab competencies for respiratory care: an integrated approach, ed 2, Albany, 1993, Delmar.
*Optional.

- Never recap a used needle without a safety device; never handle it using both hands, and never point it toward any part of the body.
- Never bend, break, or remove used needles from syringes by hand.
- Always dispose of used syringes, needles, and other sharp items in appropriate puncture-resistant sharps containers.[4]

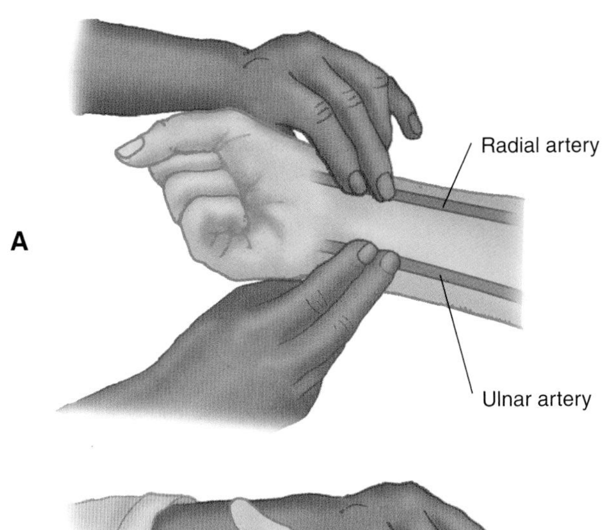

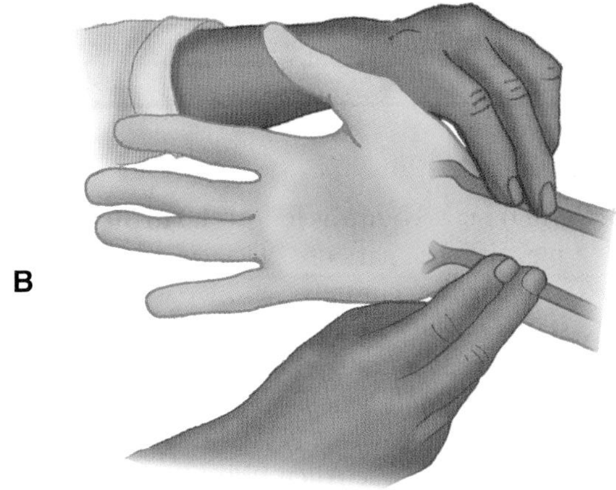

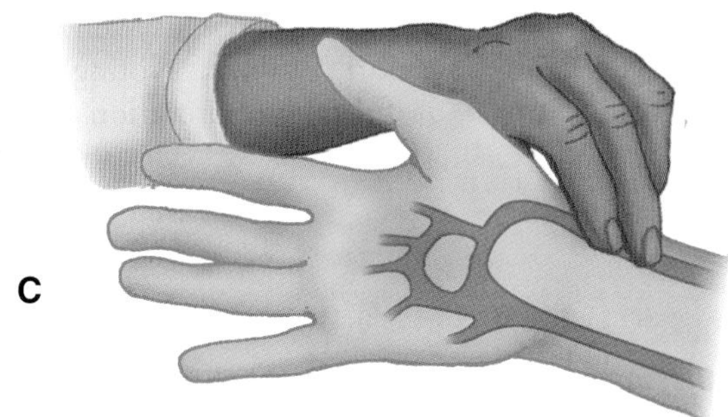

Figure 16-3
The modified Allen test. **A**, The hand is clenched into a tight fist and pressure is applied to the radial and ulnar arteries. **B**, The hand is opened (but not fully extended); the palm and fingers are blanched. **C**, Removal of pressure on the ulnar artery should result in flushing of the entire hand.

Indications for Blood Gas Sampling. Knowing when to obtain a blood gas sample is just as important as knowing how to perform the procedure. See the Clinical Practice Guideline on p. 359 for the general indications for ABG sampling. Box 16-3 lists the more common clinical situations associated with the need for ABG analysis.

Problem-Solving and Troubleshooting. There are two major problem areas associated with arterial puncture.

Box 16-3 • Clinical Indications for Arterial Blood Gas Analysis

- Sudden, unexplained dyspnea
- Cyanosis
- Abnormal breath sounds
- Severe, unexplained tachypnea
- Heavy use of accessory muscles
- Changes in ventilator settings
- Cardiopulmonary resuscitation
- Diffuse infiltrates in the chest radiograph

The first problem area involves difficulties in getting a good sample. The second problem area involves **preanalytical error.**

Getting a Good Sample. Problems with getting a good sample include an inaccessible artery, absent pulse, deficient sample return, and alteration of test results caused by the patient's response. If the selected artery cannot be located, another site should be considered. Likewise, if an adequate pulse cannot be palpated at the chosen site, another site should be selected or an acceptable noninvasive approach should be considered as an alternative.

If the clinician gets only a small spurt of blood, the needle has probably passed through the artery. In this situation, he or she should slowly withdraw the needle until a pulsatile flow fills the syringe. The clinician must never redirect the tip of the needle without first withdrawing it to the subcutaneous tissue. *If the needle must be withdrawn completely and the clinician does not have an adequate sample, he or she should repeat the procedure with a fresh ABG kit.*

Small sample volumes or the need to apply syringe suction also may indicate that venous blood has been obtained. However, when drawing arterial blood from hypotensive patients or when using small needles (smaller than 23 gauge), the clinician may need to pull gently on the syringe barrel. Excessive suction can alter the blood gas results.

If the clinician suspects that pain or anxiety during the procedure may have altered the results (most typically causing hyperventilation), he or she should consider using a local anesthetic for subsequent sampling attempts.

Preanalytical Error. Preanalytical errors are problems occurring *before* sample analysis, which can alter the accuracy of the blood gas results. Table 16-1 summarizes the most common errors associated with arterial blood sampling, including recommendations on how to recognize and avoid these problems.[6,7] Clinicians can avoid most preanalytical errors by ensuring that the sample is

Table 16-1 ▶ ▶ Preanalytical Errors Associated With Arterial Blood

Error	Effect on Parameters	How to Recognize	How to Avoid
Air in sample	Lowers P_{CO_2} Raises pH Raises low P_{O_2} Lowers high P_{O_2}	Visible bubbles or froth Low P_{CO_2} inconsistent with patient status	Discard frothy samples Fully expel bubbles Mix only after air is expelled Cap syringe quickly
Venous admixture	Raises P_{CO_2} Lowers pH Can greatly lower P_{O_2}	Failure of syringe to fill by pulsations Patient has no symptoms of hypoxemia	Avoid brachial/femoral sites Do not aspirate sample Use short-bevel needles Avoid artery "overshoot" Cross-check with Sp_{O_2}
Excess anticoagulant (dilution)	Lowers P_{CO_2} Raises pH Raises low P_{O_2} Lowers high P_{O_2}	Visible heparin remains in syringe before sampling	Fill dead space only Collect >2 mL (adults) and >0.6 mL (infants) Use dry heparin
Metabolic effects	Raises P_{CO_2} Lowers pH Lowers P_{O_2}	Excessive time lag since sample collection Values inconsistent with patient status	Analyze within 15 minutes Place sample in ice slush

obtained anaerobically, is properly anticoagulated (with immediate expulsion of air bubbles), and is analyzed within 15 minutes.

The traditional method used to avoid errors caused by blood cell metabolism is to quickly chill the sample by placing it in an ice slush. Recently, this practice has been called into question. Some dual-purpose electrolyte/blood gas analyzers require immediate analysis of unchilled blood to provide accurate potassium measurement. In addition, studies have shown that 30 minutes of chilling blood in plastic syringes can erroneously increase the P_{O_2} value.[8] Based on these findings, some authors recommend that blood gas samples collected with plastic syringes not be iced, but that they be kept at room temperature and analyzed within 30 minutes. If longer delays are expected, the blood should be collected in glass syringes and kept in ice. Even chilled samples should be discarded if they are not analyzed within 60 minutes.

Interpretation of ABGs. Given that gas exchange is a dynamic process, looking at results from a single blood sample is somewhat akin to looking at a single frame in a feature-length movie. If the scene is changing rapidly, the single frame can be misleading. Conversely, if the scene is relatively stable, a single frame can provide useful information. Thus blood gas results must be interpreted in light of the patient status at the time the sample was obtained.

Unfortunately, any major change in either patient condition or therapy disrupts the patient's steady state. However, over time, a steady state normally returns. The time needed to restore a steady state varies with the patient's pulmonary status. Patients with healthy lungs achieve a steady state in only 5 minutes after changes, whereas those with chronic obstructive pulmonary disease (COPD) may require as long as 20 to 30 minutes.[9] For example, if the patient's F_{IO_2} is changed, the measured Pa_{O_2} will accurately reflect the patient's gas exchange status within 5 minutes in healthy people but may require 20 to 30 minutes in patients with COPD.

To document the patient's status, clinicians must properly record the following: (1) date, time, and site of sampling; (2) results of the Allen test; (3) patient's body temperature, position, activity level, and respiratory rate; and (4) F_{IO_2} concentration or flow, as well as all applicable ventilatory support settings. Noting such information may prove useful in interpretation of the results.

RULE OF THUMB

To ensure a steady state, wait 20 to 30 minutes after any major change in support before sampling and analyzing the blood gases of a critically ill patient.

In the first step of interpretation of the results, the clinician must ensure that he or she is looking at the results of the correct patient. This is done by matching the name and patient identification number from the blood gas report with those of the patient. Interpretation of the results can be divided into two basic steps: (1) interpretation of the oxygenation status and (2) interpretation of the acid-base status.

The oxygenation status is determined by examination of the Pa_{O_2}, Sa_{O_2}, and Ca_{O_2}. The *Pa_{O_2}* represents the partial pressure of oxygen in the plasma of the arterial blood and is the result of gas exchange between the lung and blood. The Pa_{O_2} is reduced in a variety of settings but most often when lung disease is present. A $Pa{O_2}$ of less than 40 mm Hg is called *severe hypoxemia*, a $Pa{O_2}$ of 40 to 59 mm Hg is called *moderate hypoxemia*, and a $Pa{O_2}$ of 60 mm Hg to the predicted normal is called *mild hypoxemia*.

The *$Sa{O_2}$* represents the degree to which the hemoglobin is saturated with oxygen (see Chapter 10). Normally, the hemoglobin saturation with oxygen is 95% to 100% with healthy lungs. When the lungs cannot transfer oxygen into the blood at normal levels, in most cases the $Sa{O_2}$ drops in proportion to the degree of lung disease present.

The *$Ca{O_2}$* represents the content of oxygen in 100 mL of arterial blood and is a function of the amount of hemoglobin present and the degree to which it is saturated. A normal $Ca{O_2}$ is 18 to 20 mL of oxygen per 100 mL of arterial blood. A reduced $Ca{O_2}$ is often the result of low $Pa{O_2}$ and $Sa{O_2}$, reduced hemoglobin level, or both.

The acid-base status of the patient is determined by evaluating the pH, $Pa{CO_2}$, and plasma HCO_3^-. The steps to interpretation of the acid-base status of the ABG results are described in Chapter 12.

Indwelling Catheters (Arterial and Central Venous Pressure/Pulmonary Artery Lines)

Indwelling catheters provide ready access for blood sampling and allow continuous monitoring of vascular pressures, without the traumatic risks associated with repetitive percutaneous punctures.[10,11] However, infection and thrombosis are more likely with indwelling catheters than they are with intermittent punctures.[12]

The most common routes for indwelling vascular lines are a peripheral artery (usually radial or brachial), a central vein (usually the vena cava), and the PA. Table 16-2 summarizes the usefulness of these various sites in providing relevant clinical information. Chapter 43 provides details on the use of these systems for hemodynamic pressure and flow monitoring.

Equipment. Figure 16-4 shows the basic setup used for an indwelling vascular line, in this case a brachial artery catheter. The catheter connects to a disposable continuous-flush device (Intraflow). This device keeps the line open by providing a continuous low flow (2 to 4 mL/hr) of heparinized intravenous (IV) fluid through the system. Because arterial pressures are much higher than are venous pressures, the IV bag supplying these systems must be pressurized, usually by a hand bulb pump. A strain-gauge pressure transducer connected to the flush device provides an electrical signal to an amplifier or monitor, which displays the corresponding pressure waveform.

Procedure. Access for sampling blood from most intravascular lines is provided by a three-way stopcock (Figure 16-5). Equipment and supplies are the same as those specified for arterial puncture, with the addition of a second "waste" syringe. Box 16-4 outlines the proper procedure for taking an arterial blood sample from a three-way stopcock system.

The procedure is slightly different when obtaining mixed venous blood samples from PA catheters, because PA catheters have separate sampling and IV infusion ports and a balloon at the tip used to measure pulmonary capillary wedge pressure. First, the clinician draws the sample directly from the catheter's distal port (no three-way stopcock), ensuring that the balloon is deflated. Second, he or she slowly withdraws the sample. If the clinician fails to deflate the balloon or withdraws the sample too quickly, the venous blood may be contaminated with that from the pulmonary capillaries. The result is always a falsely high oxygen level. In addition, the clinician must pay close attention to the infusion rate through the catheter. Rapid flow of IV fluid can dilute the blood sample and affect oxygen content measures.

Table 16-2 ▶▶ Common Sites for Indwelling Vascular Catheters and the Information They Provide

	Blood Collection		Pressure Monitoring	
Location	**Sample**	**Reflects**	**Pressure**	**Reflects**
Peripheral artery	Arterial blood	Pulmonary gas exchange (O_2 uptake/CO_2 removal)	Systemic arterial pressure	LV afterload Vascular tone Blood volume
Central vein	Venous blood (unmixed)	Not useful for assessing gas exchange; can be used for some other laboratory tests	Central venous pressure (CVP)	Fluid volume Vascular tone RV preload
Pulmonary artery	Mixed venous blood (balloon deflated)	Gas exchange at the tissues (O_2 consumption/CO_2 production)	Pulmonary artery pressure (PAP) Pulmonary capillary wedge pressure (PCWP)	RV afterload Vascular tone Blood volume LV preload

LV, Left ventricular; *RV*, right ventricular.

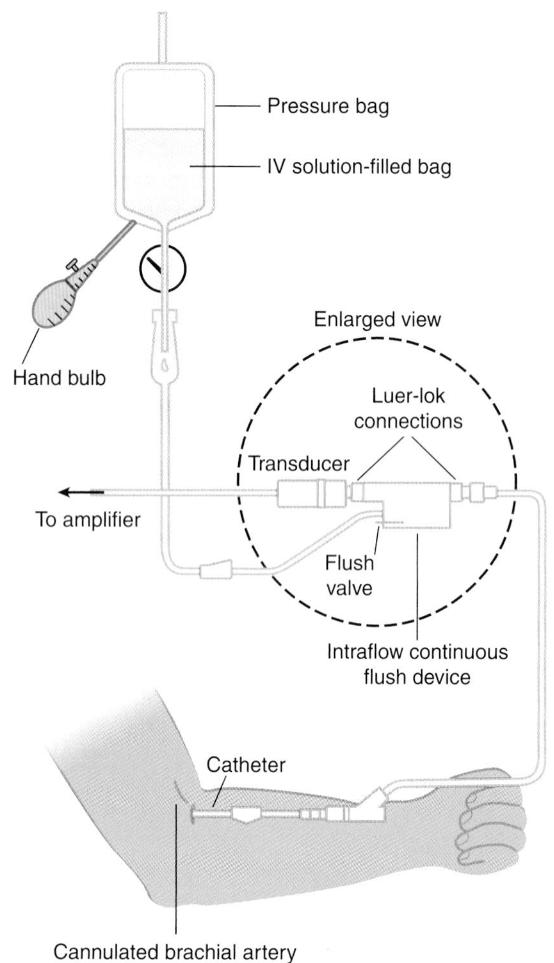

Figure 16-4
An indwelling vascular line (brachial artery catheter) used to monitor blood pressure and obtain a blood sample.

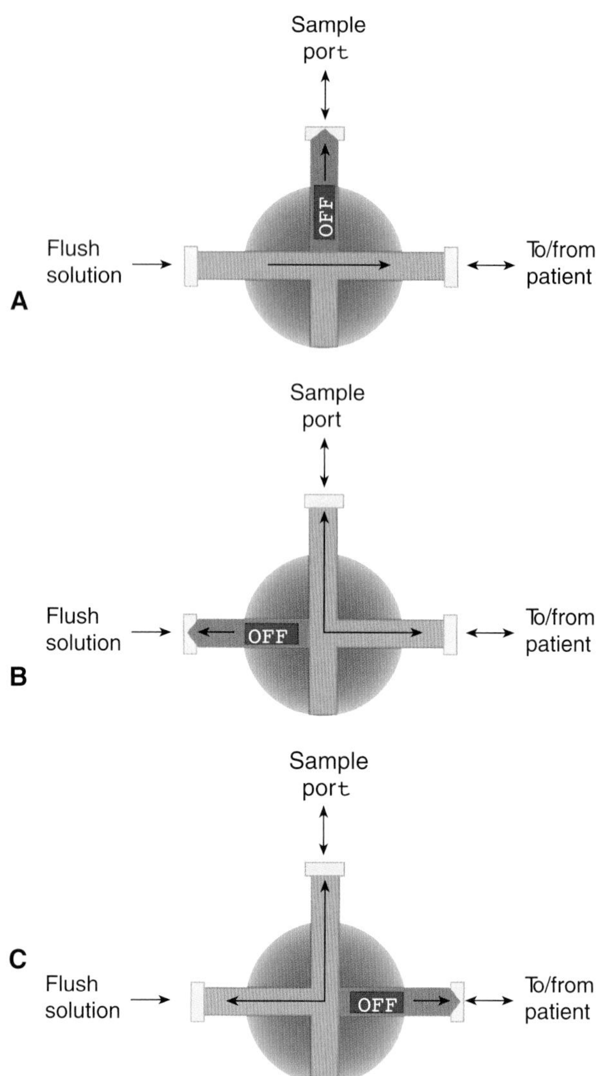

Figure 16-5
A three-way stopcock in a vascular line system showing the various positions used. **A**, Normal operating position, with flush solution going to the patient and the sample port closed. **B**, Position to draw a blood sample from the vascular line (closed to flush solution). **C**, Position to flush sample port (closed to patient). In any intermediary position, all ports are closed.

Problem-Solving and Troubleshooting. With the exception of venous admixture, the preanalytical errors that occur when sampling blood from a vascular line are the same as those occurring with intermittent puncture, as are the ways to avoid them. For clinicians, the challenge with vascular lines is properly maintaining their function and troubleshooting the many potential problems that can occur. Because these are key components of bedside monitoring skills, they are discussed in the section Hemodynamics in Chapter 43.

Capillary Blood Gases

Sometimes capillary blood gas sampling is used as an alternative to direct arterial access in infants and small children. Properly obtained capillary blood from a well-perfused patient can provide rough estimates of arterial pH and P_{CO_2} levels. However, the capillary P_{O_2} is of no value in estimating arterial oxygenation.[13] For this reason, direct arterial access is still the preferred approach for assessing gas exchange in infants and small children. The clinician must exercise extreme caution when using capillary blood gases to guide clinical decisions.

Capillary blood values are meaningful only if the sample site is properly warmed. Warming the skin (to approximately 42° C) causes dilation of the underlying blood vessels, which increases capillary flow well above tissue needs. Blood gas values resemble those in the arterial circulation. This is why a sample obtained from a warmed capillary site is often referred to as **arterialized blood.**

To guide practitioners in providing quality care, the AARC has published *Clinical Practice Guideline:*

Box 16-4 • Procedure for Sampling Arterial Blood From an Indwelling Catheter

- Check the chart (as per arterial puncture).
- Confirm steady-state conditions (20 to 30 minutes after changes).
- Obtain and assemble needed equipment and supplies.
- Wash hands and don barrier protection (e.g., gloves, eyewear).
- Explain the procedure to the patient.
- Attach the waste syringe to the stopcock port.
- Position the stopcock so that blood flows into the syringe and the IV bag port is closed.
- Aspirate at least 5 mL, or 5 to 6 times the tubing volume, of fluid or blood.
- Reposition the stopcock handle to close off all ports.
- Disconnect and properly discard the waste syringe.
- Attach a new heparinized syringe to the sampling port.
- Position the stopcock so that blood flows into the sample syringe and the IV bag port is closed.
- Allow 2 to 4 mL of blood to fill the syringe.
- Reposition the stopcock handle to close off the sampling port and open the IV bag port.
- Disconnect the syringe, expel air bubbles from the sample, and cap or plug the syringe.
- Flush the line and stopcock with the heparinized IV solution.
- Mix the sample by rolling and inverting the syringe.
- Confirm that the stopcock port is open to the IV bag solution and catheter.
- Confirm **undampened** pulse pressure waveform on the monitor graphic display.
- Place the sample in a transport container (ice).
- Properly dispose of waste materials.
- Document the procedure and patient status in the chart and on the specimen label.

Capillary Blood Gas Sampling for Neonatal and Pediatric Patients.[13] Modified excerpts from the AARC guideline appear on p. 366.

Equipment. Equipment needed for capillary blood sampling includes a lancet, preheparinized glass capillary tubes, metal "fleas," a magnet, clay or wax sealant or caps, gauze or cotton balls, bandages, ice, gloves, skin antiseptic, warming pads (42° C), sharps container, and labeling materials.

Procedure. Box 16-5 outlines the basic procedure for capillary blood sampling. The most common site for sampling is the heel, specifically the lateral aspect of the plantar surface.

Problem-Solving and Troubleshooting. Sampling of capillary blood is useful for patient management only if the procedure is carried out according to an established quality assurance program. The most common technical errors in capillary sampling are inadequate warming of the capillary bed and squeezing of the puncture site. Both errors will invalidate the test results. Other preanalytical errors are essentially the same as those described for arterial puncture. Because of the small sample and collection tube size, the clinician *must* ensure an adequate sample volume and avoid allowing it to clot.

Box 16-5 • Procedure for Capillary Blood Sampling

- Check the chart (as per arterial puncture).
- Confirm steady-state conditions (20 to 30 minutes after changes).
- Obtain and assemble the necessary equipment and supplies.
- Wash hands and don barrier protection (e.g., gloves, eyewear).
- Select site (e.g., heel, earlobe, great toe, finger).
- Warm the site to 42° C for 10 minutes using a compress, heat lamp, or commercial hot pack.
- Cleanse the skin with an antiseptic solution.
- Puncture the skin (<2.5 mm) with the lancet.
- Wipe away the first drop of blood and observe free flow (do not squeeze).
- Fill the sample tube from the middle of the blood drop until it is completely full (75 to 100 mL).
- Place the flea in the capillary tube and then seal the tube ends.
- Tape sterile cotton or a bandage over the puncture wound.
- Mix the sample by moving the magnet back and forth along the capillary tube.
- Place the sample in the transport container (ice).
- Properly dispose of waste materials.
- Document the procedure and patient status in the chart and on the specimen label.

Analyzing

The primary parameters of pH, P_{CO_2}, and P_{O_2} in a blood sample are measured with a blood gas analyzer. Typically, analyzers use these measures to compute several secondary values, such as plasma bicarbonate, base excess or deficit, and hemoglobin saturation. If actual measurement of hemoglobin (Hb) saturation (oxyhemoglobin [HbO_2], methemoglobin [metHb], and carboxyhemoglobin [HbCO]) is required, the sample usually must be analyzed separately using hemoximetry (see p. 377).

Blood gas analysis and hemoximetry are complex laboratory procedures. Clinicians performing these tests must have documented training and must demonstrate proficiency in performing the procedures, preventive

Capillary Blood Gas Sampling for Neonatal and Pediatric Patients

AARC Clinical Practice Guideline (Excerpts)*

INDICATIONS

Capillary blood gas sampling is indicated when:

- ABG analysis is indicated, but arterial access is not available
- Noninvasive monitor readings (e.g., $P_{tc}CO_2$:$P_{ET}CO_2$, SpO_2) are abnormal
- Assessment of initiation, administration, or change in therapy (e.g., mechanical ventilation) is indicated
- A change in patient status is detected by history or physical assessment
- Monitoring the severity and progression of a documented disease process is desirable

CONTRAINDICATIONS

Capillary punctures should not be performed at or through the following:

- The posterior curvature of the heel (because it can puncture the bone)
- The heel of a patient who has begun walking and has callous development
- The fingers of neonates (because it can cause nerve damage)
- Previous puncture sites
- Inflamed, swollen, or edematous tissues
- Cyanotic or poorly perfused tissues
- Localized areas of infection
- Peripheral arteries

Capillary punctures should not be performed:

- On patients younger than 24 hours old (because of poor peripheral perfusion)
- When there is a need for direct analysis of oxygenation
- When there is a need for direct analysis of arterial blood

Relative contraindications include:

- Peripheral vasoconstriction
- Polycythemia (caused by shorter clotting times)
- Hypotension

PRECAUTIONS AND/OR POSSIBLE COMPLICATIONS

- Contamination and infection of the patient, including calcaneus osteomyelitis and cellulitis
- Inadvertent puncture or incision and consequent infection in sample
- Burns
- Bone calcification
- Bruising
- Pain
- Inappropriate patient management may result from reliance on capillary PO_2 values
- Tibial artery laceration (puncture of posterior medial aspect of heel)
- Hematoma
- Nerve damage
- Scarring
- Bleeding

ASSESSMENT OF NEED

Capillary blood gas sampling is an intermittent procedure and should be performed only when a documented need exists and arterial access is unavailable or contraindicated. Documented need exists in response to initiation, administration, or change in therapy and is determined by history and physical assessment or the results of noninvasive respiratory monitoring.

MONITORING

The following should be monitored and documented in the medical record as part of the capillary sampling procedure:

- FIO_2 or prescribed oxygen flow
- Oxygen modality or ventilator settings
- Ease or difficulty of obtaining the sample
- Free flow of blood, without the necessity for "milking" the foot or finger to obtain a sample
- Presence or absence of air or clot in the sample
- Date, time, and sampling site
- Appearance of puncture site
- Complications or adverse reactions to the procedure
- Results of the blood gas analysis
- Patient's temperature, respiratory rate, position or level of activity, and clinical appearance
- Noninvasive monitoring values (e.g., SpO_2)

*For the complete guideline, see Respir Care 39:1180, 1994.

maintenance, troubleshooting, and instrument calibration. In addition, they must be skilled in validating test results using rigorous quality control methods.[14]

To guide practitioners in providing quality care, the AARC has published *Clinical Practice Guideline: In vitro pH and Blood Gas Analysis and Hemoximetry.*[15] Related recommendations have been published by the National Committee for Clinical Laboratory Standards.[16,17] Modified excerpts from the AARC guideline appear on p. 369.

Instrumentation

Many instrumentation companies manufacture laboratory blood gas analyzers. Although available in a range of designs, these devices typically share the following key components:

- An operator interface (e.g., operating controls, light-emitting diode [LED] or cathode ray tube [CRT] displays, keypads, software)
- A measuring chamber incorporating the typical three-electrode system
- Calibrating gas tanks
- Reagent containers (buffers used for calibration, rinse solutions)
- A waste container
- A results display, storage, and transmittal system (e.g., screen, printer, disk storage device, network interface)

Actual measurement of the three primary parameters —pH, P_{CO_2}, and P_{O_2}—is accomplished using three separate electrodes. To measure P_{O_2}, blood gas analyzers use the Clark polarographic electrode (see Figure 16-1).

The pH electrode actually consists of two electrodes or *half-cells* (Figure 16-6). The measuring half-cell contains a silver-silver chloride rod surrounded by a solution of constant pH and enclosed by a pH-sensitive glass membrane. As the sample passes this membrane, the difference in H^+ concentration on either side of the glass changes the potential of the measuring electrode. The reference half-cell (here mercury-mercurous chloride) produces a constant potential, regardless of sample pH. The difference in potential between the two electrodes is proportional to the H^+ concentration of the sample, which is displayed on a voltmeter calibrated in pH units.

To measure P_{CO_2}, blood gas analyzers use the Severinghaus electrode, which is essentially a pH electrode exposed to an electrolyte solution that is in equilibrium with the sample through a carbon dioxide–permeable membrane. As carbon dioxide diffuses through this membrane into the electrolyte solution, it undergoes the following hydration reaction:

$$CO_2 + H_2O \leftrightarrow H_2CO_3 \leftrightarrow H+ + HCO_3^-$$

The greater the partial pressure of CO_2, the more hydrogen ions are produced by this reaction, and the more pH of the electrolyte solution changes. The measuring electrode detects the pH change as a change in electrical potential, which is proportional to the P_{CO_2} of the sample.

Procedure

To provide accurate and clinically useful data, blood gas analysis must be performed as follows:

- On a sample free of preanalytical errors
- With a properly functioning analyzer (validated by quality control procedures)
- Using a procedure that follows the manufacturer's recommendations

Prior discussion addressed how to avoid preanalytical errors. Subsequent discussion focuses on blood gas quality control and key elements involved in the actual analysis procedure.

Box 16-6 outlines the steps commonly used in most established procedures for laboratory blood gas analysis.

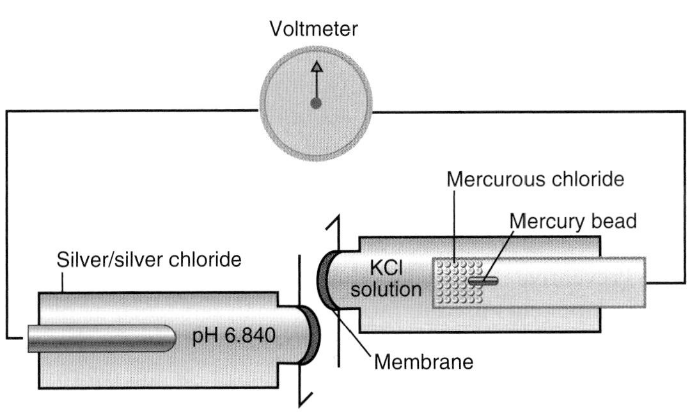

Figure 16-6
Blood gas analyzer pH electrode system, consisting of both a measurement and a reference electrode. *(From Shapiro BA, Peruzzi WT, Kozelowski-Templin R: Clinical application of blood gases, ed 5, St Louis, 1994, Mosby.)*

Box 16-6 • Basic Procedure for Analyzing a Blood Gas Sample

- Apply standard precautions.
- Confirm that the instrument and its electrodes are operating properly.
- Identify the specimen and confirm all relevant information provided on the request slip.
- Note the time at which the sample was obtained (discard the sample if >60 minutes has passed).
- Inspect the sample for obvious signs of preanalytical error (e.g., air bubbles, gross dilution, clotting, air exposure).
- Mix the sample (critical for hemoglobin and hematocrit measurements).
- Uncap the syringe and expel and discard a drop or two of blood from the syringe tip.
- Introduce the sample (manually or by automatic aspiration).
- Confirm the readings.
- Remove the syringe and clear the system.
- Properly dispose of waste materials.
- Transmit the results.
- Contact the responsible clinician if the results warrant it.

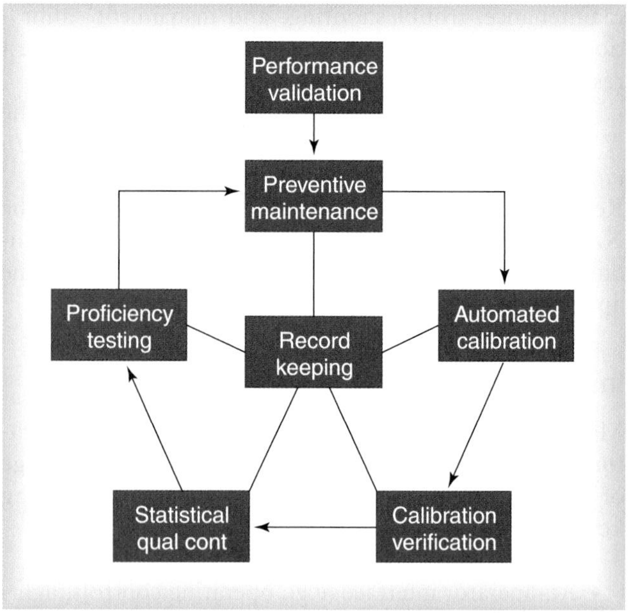

Figure 16-7
Blood gas analysis quality control program. *(Data from Kozelowski-Templin R: Respir Care Clin North Am 1:35, 1995.)*

Of course, the operator should always refer to the manufacturer's literature for the particular steps to use with a specific analyzer.

Rigorous application of Centers for Disease Control and Prevention (CDC) Standard Precautions is essential. In addition, the Occupational Safety and Health Administration (OSHA) requires personnel to wear gloves when handling all laboratory specimens. Although splashes are rare during analysis, some manufacturers provide extra protection by mounting splash shields on their instruments. If splashes are anticipated, the operator can wear a face shield.

Remember that waste fluids are potentially infectious and should be handled as if they were blood samples. In addition, the National Committee for Clinical Laboratory Standards recommends adding a strong disinfectant, such as 2% glutaraldehyde or a 1:4 solution of sodium hypochlorite, to the instrument's waste container either during use or before disposal.

Quality Assurance

Quality patient care depends on consistently accurate blood gas results. Modern laboratory analyzers are highly automated, computer-controlled, self-calibrating systems. Unfortunately, this sophistication has led to the false assumption that accurate results are "automatic," with clinicians needing only to properly input the sample and record the results. Nothing could be further from the truth. As with all diagnostic laboratory procedures, the accuracy of blood gas testing depends on rigorous quality control.

Although an in-depth review of laboratory quality control is beyond the scope of this text, all respiratory therapists (RTs) must understand the key elements. Figure 16-7 depicts the key components of laboratory quality control. Following is a brief description of each element.

Recordkeeping. Meticulous recordkeeping and clearly written and comprehensive policies and procedures are the hallmark of a comprehensive **quality control** program. Both statutory law and professional accreditation requirements emphasize this component as the basis for demonstrating and ensuring quality.

Performance Validation. Performance validation is the process of testing a *new instrument* to confirm a manufacturer's claims. Typically, this involves using samples with known values to assess both the accuracy (comparing the value from the tested instrument with a known value) and the **precision** (examining the repeatability of results) of the instrument.

Preventive Maintenance and Function Checks. Many components used in blood gas analyzers, such as filters, membranes, and electrolyte solution, have a limited life and can deteriorate, be consumed, or fail over time, resulting in faulty analysis. The best way to avoid these problems is by scheduling regular preventive maintenance.

BLOOD GAS ANALYSIS AND HEMOXIMETRY

AARC Clinical Practice Guideline (Excerpts)*

INDICATIONS

- The need to evaluate the adequacy of a patient's ventilation ($PaCO_2$), oxygenation (PaO_2 and HbO_2), and/or acid-base balance (pH, $PaCO_2$, HCO_3^-)
- The need to quantify the response to therapeutic intervention (e.g., oxygen therapy, mechanical ventilation) and/or diagnostic evaluation (e.g., exercise desaturation)
- The need to monitor the severity and progression of documented disease processes

CONTRAINDICATIONS

Contraindications to pH and blood gas analysis and hemoximetry include the following:

- An improperly functioning analyzer
- An analyzer for which the performance has not been validated by quality control or proficiency testing procedures
- Any specimen gathered with known or suspected preanalytical errors (e.g., air contamination, improper anticoagulation, improper storage or handling)
- An incomplete requisition that precludes adequate interpretation and documentation of results
- An inadequately labeled specimen lacking the patient's full name or other unique identifier, such as the medical record number, date, and time of sampling

PRECAUTIONS AND/OR POSSIBLE COMPLICATIONS

- Infection of specimen handler from blood (human immunodeficiency virus, hepatitis B, other bloodborne pathogens)
- Inappropriate patient medical treatment based on an improperly analyzed blood specimen, on analysis of an unacceptable specimen, or on incorrect reporting of results

ASSESSMENT OF NEED

Presence of the indications listed above in the patient to be tested supports the need for sampling and analysis.

FREQUENCY

The frequency with which pH-blood gas analysis is repeated (on different samples from the same patient) should depend on the clinical status of the patient and not on an arbitrarily designated time or frequency. The frequency of reanalysis of single specimens depends on laboratory protocol and technologist suspicion that preliminary results may not reflect the clinical status of the patient, because of preanalytical or instrument error, for example.

MONITORING

The following aspects of analysis should be monitored, and corrective action should be taken as indicated:

- Presence of air bubbles or clots in the specimen, with evacuation before mixing and sealing the syringe
- Assurance that a continuous sample is aspirated (or injected) into the analyzer and that all the electrodes are covered by the sample (confirmed by direct visualization if possible)
- Assurance that 8-hour quality control and calibration procedures have been completed and that instrumentation is functioning properly before patient sample analysis
- Assurance that the specimen was properly labeled, stored, and analyzed within an acceptable period
- Participation in an accredited (recognized) proficiency testing program
- As part of any quality assurance program, indicators must be developed to monitor potential sources of error:
  - There must be evidence of active review of quality control; proficiency testing; and physician alert, or "panic values" on a level commensurate with the number of tests performed
  - Personnel who do not meet acceptable performance thresholds should not be allowed to independently participate further, until they have received remedial instruction and have been reevaluated

*For the complete guideline, see Respir Care 46:498, 2001.

Preventive maintenance should include scheduled parts replacement and routine function tests, as recommended by the manufacturer.

Automated Calibration. Calibration is the only fully automated element of blood gas quality control. Blood gas analyzers regularly calibrate themselves by adjusting each electrode's output signal when exposed to media having known values. In most units, the media used to calibrate the gas electrodes are precision mixtures of oxygen and carbon dioxide. For the pH electrode, standard pH buffer solutions are used. **Calibration media** must meet the requirements set by nationally recognized standards organizations. Users are responsible for ensuring that calibration media are properly stored and that in-use life and expiration dates are strictly enforced.

Calibration is performed to ensure that the output of the analyzer is both accurate and linear across the range of measured values. Parameters must be measured with known input values representing at least two points, usually a low and a high value. Figure 16-8 shows a typical two-point calibration procedure. In this example, the instrument's initial precalibration response indicates that the output readings are consistently higher than the actual input, with this positive **bias** worsening at the higher levels. Calibration is performed first by adjusting the offset (or balance) of the instrument so that the low output equals the low input (in this case zero). Next, the gain (or slope) of the device is adjusted to ensure that the high output equals the high input. When both offset and gain are adjusted against known inputs, the instrument is properly calibrated and can undergo calibration verification with control samples.

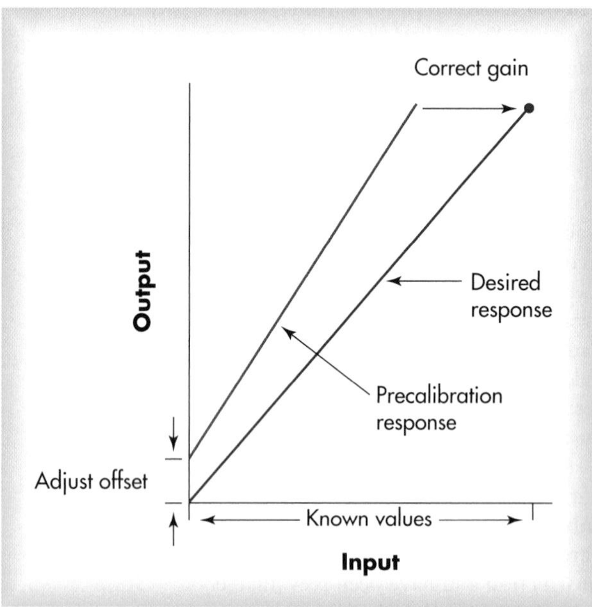

Figure 16-8

The two-point calibration procedure. *(From Chatburn RL: Fundamentals of metrology: evaluation of instrument error and method agreement. In Kacmarek RM, Hess D, Stoller JK, editors: Monitoring in respiratory care, St Louis, 1993, Mosby.)*

Calibration Verification by Control Media. Calibration verification establishes and periodically confirms the validity of blood gas analyzer results. Calibration verification requires analysis of at least three materials with known values spanning the *entire range* of values expected for clinical samples. Ideally, these materials, called *controls*, should mimic real blood samples chemically and physically. Because requirements for use of control media currently vary among the regulatory agencies, users should consult the applicable regulations directly. As a general recommendation, at least two levels of control media should be analyzed during every 8-hour shift. Rotation among the three levels should ensure that all three levels are analyzed at least once every 24 hours.

Internal Statistical Quality Control. Internal quality control takes calibration verification a step further by applying statistical and rule-based procedures to help detect, respond to, and correct instrument error. In one common approach, the results of control media analyses are plotted on a graph and compared with statistically derived limits, usually ±2 standard deviation (SD) ranges (Figure 16-9). Control results that fall outside these limits indicate analytical error.

There are two categories of analytical error: (1) random and (2) systematic. Random error is observed when sporadic, out-of-range data points occur (see Figure 16-9, *point A*). Random errors are errors of precision, or more precisely, **imprecision**. Conversely, either a trending or an abrupt shift in data points outside the statistical limits (see Figure 16-9, *point B*) will sometimes be observed. This phenomenon is called **systematic error** or sometimes *bias*. Bias plus imprecision equals total instrument error, or **inaccuracy**. Table 16-3 outlines the major factors causing these two types of error and suggests some common corrective actions.

External Quality Control (Proficiency Testing). The federal government mandated a rigorous program of external quality control for analytical laboratories in the late 1980s. To meet these standards, analytical laboratories must undergo regular proficiency testing designed to evaluate their operating procedures, as well as the competence of their personnel.

Proficiency testing requires analysis and reporting on externally provided control media with unknown values, usually three times per year, with five samples per test. These analyses must be performed along with

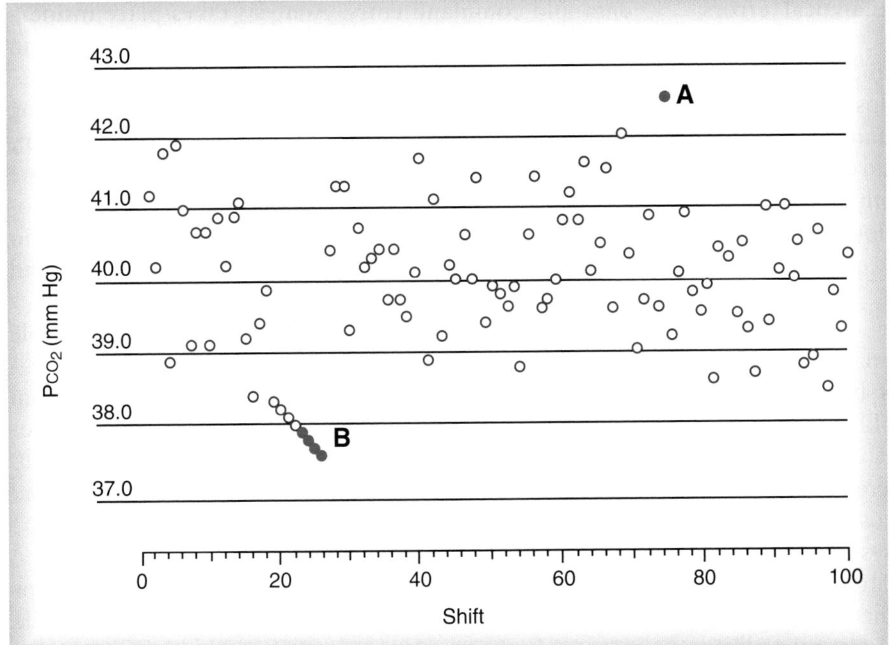

Figure 16-9

Schematic representation of a quality control plot for P_{CO_2}. The horizontal axis depicts 8-hour shifts. The blue circles represent values within two standard deviations of the mean; black circles represent values outside two standard deviations of the mean. *Point A* represents a random error; *point B* represents systematic errors. *(From Shapiro BA, Peruzzi WT, Kozelowski-Templin R: Clinical application of blood gases, ed 5, St Louis, 1994, Mosby.)*

Table 16-3 ▶▶ Correction of Analytical Errors

Error type	Common Contributing Factors	Common Corrective Actions
Imprecision (random) errors	Statistical probability Sample contamination Sample mishandling	Rerun the control Repeat analysis on a different instrument
Bias (systematic) errors	Contaminated buffers Incorrect gas concentrations Incorrect procedures Component failure	Perform function check of suspected problem area Repair/replace failed components

MINI CLINI

Blood Gas Quality Control

PROBLEM

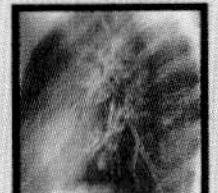

The RT is responsible for the quality control of a blood gas analyzer in the intensive care unit (ICU). Using control media for calibration verification, he notes that the readings on the "high P_{CO_2}" control have increased progressively over the last four quality control analyses from 60 mm Hg ±1 SD to 66 mm Hg ±1 SD. What is the likely problem, and what actions should he take?

SOLUTION

The observed problem indicates a trending, or systematic, error (bias). If the analyzer solutions and calibrating gases have not been changed during the error period, the likely problem is component failure—probably the P_{CO_2} electrode. The electrode should be checked, and any faulty components should be replaced.

the regular workload by the personnel routinely responsible for testing, following the laboratory's standard testing practices.

Criteria for acceptable performance specify a range around a target value, such as ±0.04 for pH. A single incidence of unsatisfactory performance requires documentation of remedial action. Multiple or recurring incidences of poor performance can result in severe sanctions, including suspension of Medicare and Medicaid reimbursement or even the loss of the laboratory's operating license.

Remedial Action. Remedial action is the ongoing process of applying appropriate measures to correct errors identified through the quality assurance cycle. Analytical errors include calibration and internal quality control failures, actual sample errors, and unsatisfactory proficiency test results. A comprehensive quality assurance program also will try to identify and correct both preanalytical and postanalytical errors, such as clerical misreporting.

Examples of remedial action include procedural changes, staff training and retraining, closer supervision, and more frequent preventive maintenance checks. Of course, the remedial action chosen should be appropriate for the identified problem. As with all other components of the process, meticulous documentation is necessary.

Point-of-Care Testing

Point-of-care testing takes blood gas analysis from the specialized laboratory to the patient's bedside.[18] This reduces turnaround time, which should improve care and lower costs. In theory, cost-savings can be accrued by eliminating delays in therapy, thereby decreasing patient length of stay. Additional cost-savings may occur if point-of-care testing decreases the need for specialized laboratory personnel. Current evidence supporting the cost-effectiveness of point-of-care testing over traditional laboratory methods is incomplete.[19]

Instrumentation. Figure 16-10 shows a typical point-of-care blood gas analyzer (SenDx 100 Blood Gas and Electrolyte Systems, SenDx Medical, Inc., Carlsbad, California). In addition to blood gas analysis, such devices can be used to measure several chemistry and hematology parameters, including serum electrolytes, blood glucose levels, blood urea nitrogen, hematocrit, and prothrombin and partial thromboplastin times.

These devices are portable and can perform up to 900 tests on a single set of batteries. They typically include a display screen for accessing menu functions and viewing results. Most also include a simple keypad for data and command entry. Analysis takes place inside a disposable cartridge, which is inserted into a chamber in the body of the unit.

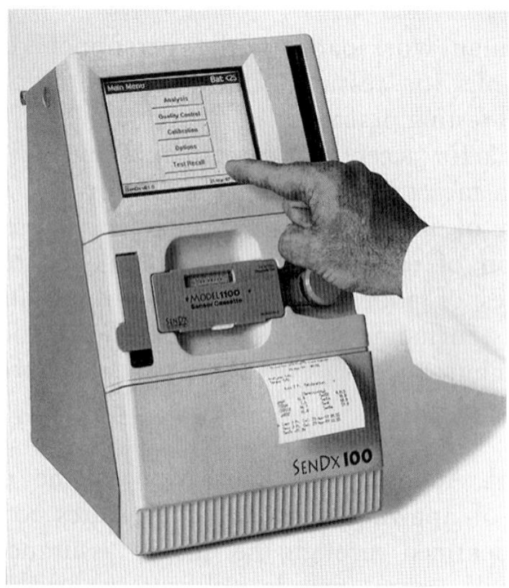

Figure 16-10
The SenDx 100 Blood Gas and Electrolyte System. *(Courtesy SenDx Medical, Inc., Carlsbad, Calif.)*

Sample cartridges differ according to the test being performed. Each cartridge contains the necessary calibration solution, a sample handling system, a waste chamber, and a miniaturized electrochemical or photochemical sensor.[20] The cartridge system requires no operator oversight because it is self-calibrating and disposable after a single use.

After self-calibration and introduction of the sample into the cartridge, the sensors measure the concentration of the analytes and conduct their output signal through conductive contact pads to the analyzer microprocessor. Test results usually are ready within 90 seconds. Waste management involves simple removal and proper disposal of the analysis cartridge.

Clinical Performance. Recent method comparisons indicate that portable point-of-care blood gas analyzers can achieve accuracy and precision levels comparable with laboratory-based analyzers.[14,21] Such findings are likely to result in more widespread use of these systems, especially if cost-effectiveness can be demonstrated. Guidelines for providers who are considering adoption of this new technology have been published in the clinical laboratory literature.[22]

▶ BLOOD GAS MONITORING

A blood gas monitor is a bedside tool (usually dedicated to a single patient) that can provide measurements either continuously or at appropriate intervals *without permanently removing blood from the patient.* Three such systems are in current clinical use: (1) the transcutaneous blood gas monitor, (2) the intraarterial (**in vivo**) blood gas monitor, and (3) the on-demand (**ex vivo**) blood gas monitor.

Transcutaneous

Transcutaneous blood gas monitoring provides continuous, noninvasive estimates of arterial PO_2 and PCO_2 through a surface skin sensor. As with capillary sampling, the device arterializes the underlying blood by heating the skin.[23] Warming also increases the permeability of the skin to oxygen and carbon dioxide, which allows them to diffuse more readily from the capillaries to the sensor, where they are measured as *transcutaneous* (tc) partial pressures ($P_{tc}O_2$ and $P_{tc}CO_2$).[24]

Numerous factors influence the agreement between arterial blood and transcutaneous gas measurements, with oxygen levels being affected most.[25] The two most important factors are age and perfusion status. Table

Table 16-4 ▶▶ Ratios Correlating $P_{tc}O_2$ With PaO_2

Age-Group	$P_{tc}O_2/PaO_2$ Ratio	Perfusion Status	$P_{tc}O_2/PaO_2$
Premature infants	1.14:1	Stable	0.79:1
Neonates	1.00:1	Moderate shock	0.48:1
Children	0.84:1	Severe shock	0.12:1
Adults	0.79:1		
Older adults	0.68:1		

From Tobin MJ: *JAMA* 264:244, 1990.

16-4 summarizes these relationships using the ratio of $P_{tc}O_2$ to PaO_2. A ratio of 1.0:1 indicates "perfect" agreement between $PtCO_2$ and PaO_2. As can be seen, this level of agreement occurs only in neonates.

In terms of age, the younger the patient, the better the agreement between the PaO_2 and $P_{tc}O_2$. This is mainly because of age-related differences in skin composition. With regard to perfusion status, the PaO_2 and $P_{tc}O_2$ are similar only in patients with normal cardiac output and fluid balance. This is because accurate transcutaneous measures require adequate skin perfusion. Low cardiac output, shock, and dehydration all cause peripheral vasoconstriction and impair capillary flow, which lowers the $PtCO_2$ level. In fact, some clinicians use the $PtCO_2$, not to monitor oxygenation, but to assess blood flow changes during procedures such as vascular surgery and resuscitation.[25]

Agreement between $PaCO_2$ and $P_{tc}CO_2$ is a little better, perhaps because CO_2 is more diffusible. In fact, $PaCO_2$ changes of as little as 5 mm Hg can be monitored or "trended" by transcutaneous blood gas analysis.

Based on these factors, transcutaneous monitoring is a reasonable choice when there is a need for continuous, noninvasive analysis of gas exchange in hemodynamically stable infants or children. In these patients, the PaO_2 can be "calibrated" against the $P_{tc}O_2$, thus decreasing the need for repeated arterial samples. Because pulse oximetry cannot provide accurate estimates of excessive blood oxygen, the transcutaneous monitor also is useful for monitoring hyperoxia in neonates.[24]

To guide practitioners in providing quality care, the AARC has published *Clinical Practice Guideline: Transcutaneous Blood Gas Monitoring for Neonatal and Pediatric Patients.*[23] Modified excerpts from the AARC guideline appear on p. 374.

Instrumentation

Figure 16-11 shows a simplified diagram of a transcutaneous blood gas monitor sensor. Included are a heating element and two electrodes, one for oxygen and one for carbon dioxide. These electrodes are similar in design to those found in bench-top analyzers. However, instead of measuring gas tensions in a blood sample, transcutaneous electrodes measure the PO_2 and PCO_2 in an electrolyte gel between the sensor and the skin. Once properly set up, the response time for these electrodes is between 20 and 30 seconds, a bit slower than the response time for pulse oximetry.

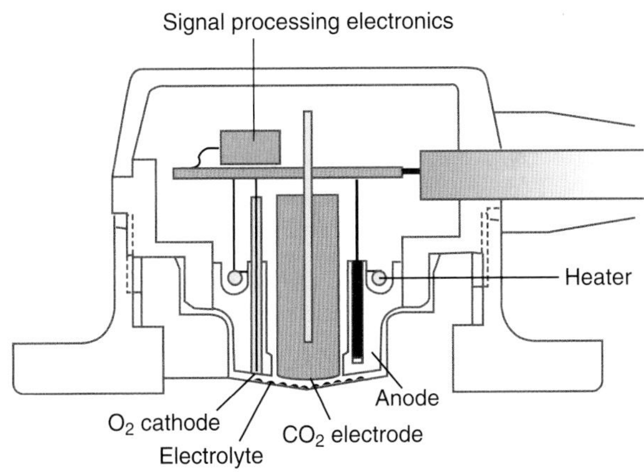

Figure 16-11
Schematic diagram of the oxygen–carbon dioxide sensor. *(Modified from Mahutte CK et al: Crit Care Med 12:1063, 1984.)*

MINI CLINI

Selecting a Monitoring System

PROBLEM

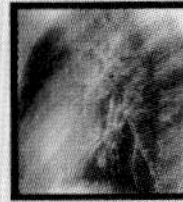

A neonatologist, concerned about retinopathy of prematurity, asks the RT to set up a noninvasive system to monitor a preterm infant for hyperoxia. What type of system should the RT choose and why?

SOLUTION

Because the neonatologist wants the infant *monitored* for hyperoxia, a system that provides continuous data would be the best choice. Because hyperoxia is best assessed using the PO_2 (as opposed to the hemoglobin saturation), the RT will need to use a PO_2 electrode system. A transcutaneous PO_2 electrode system will provide the needed measurement noninvasively.

Transcutaneous (TC) Blood Gas Monitoring for Neonatal and Pediatric Patients

AARC Clinical Practice Guideline (Excerpts)*

➤ INDICATIONS

- The need to continuously monitor the adequacy of arterial oxygenation and/or ventilation
- The need to quantify the real-time responses to diagnostic and therapeutic interventions, as evidenced by $P_{tc}O_2$ and/or $P_{tc}CO_2$ values

➤ CONTRAINDICATIONS

In patients with poor skin integrity or adhesive allergy, transcutaneous monitoring may be relatively contraindicated.

➤ PRECAUTIONS AND/OR POSSIBLE COMPLICATIONS

- False-negative or false-positive results may lead to inappropriate treatment
- Tissue injury (e.g., erythema, blisters, burns, skin tears) may occur at the measuring site

➤ ASSESSMENT OF NEED

- When direct measurement of arterial blood is not available or readily accessible, $P_{tc}O_2$ or $P_{tc}CO_2$ measurements may suffice temporarily if the limitations of the data are appreciated.
- Transcutaneous blood gas monitoring is appropriate for continuous and prolonged monitoring (e.g., during mechanical ventilation, continuous positive airway pressure [CPAP], and supplemental oxygen administration) of infants and children.
- $P_{tc}O_2$ values can be used for diagnostic purposes, such as in the assessment of functional shunts or in determining the response to oxygen challenge in the assessment of congenital heart disease.

➤ ASSESSMENT OF OUTCOME

- Results should reflect the patient's clinical condition (i.e., they should validate the basis for ordering the monitoring).
- Documentation of results, therapeutic intervention (or lack thereof), and clinical decisions based on the transcutaneous measurements should be noted in the medical record.

➤ MONITORING

The schedule of patient and equipment during transcutaneous monitoring should be integrated into assessment of the patient and determination of vital signs. Results should be documented in the patient's medical record and should detail the following conditions:

- Date and time of measurement, transcutaneous reading, patient's position, respiratory rate, and activity level
- Inspired oxygen concentration or supplemental oxygen flow, specifying the type of oxygen delivery device
- Mode of ventilatory support, ventilator, or CPAP settings
- Electrode placement site, electrode temperature, and time of placement
- Results of simultaneously obtained PaO_2, $PaCO_2$, and pH, when available
- Clinical appearance of the patient and subjective assessment of perfusion, pallor, and skin temperature

*For the complete guideline, see Respir Care 39:1176, 1994.

Procedure

Box 16-7 outlines the basic procedure for setting up a transcutaneous blood gas monitor. The most common sites for electrode placement are the abdomen, chest, and lower back. Once the electrodes are properly set up, the clinician should compare the monitor readings with those obtained with a concurrent ABG. Consistency between values validates monitor performance under the existing conditions. This validation should be repeated anytime the patient's status undergoes a major change. During validation studies of patients with anatomical shunts, the electrode site and arterial sampling site should be on the same "side" of the shunt.

Problem-Solving and Troubleshooting. Transcutaneous blood gas monitoring is a relatively complex and labor-intensive activity that requires ongoing training and

Box 16-7 • Procedure for Using a Transcutaneous Monitor

- Place the unit at bedside and provide manufacturer-specified warm-up time.
- Check the membrane to ensure that it is free of bubbles or scratches, and change it if necessary.
- Select the monitoring site by evaluating perfusion, skin thickness, and absence of bones.
- Prepare the sensor with an adhesive ring and electrolyte gel.
- Set the appropriate probe temperature (per the manufacturer's recommendations).
- Prepare the site by removing excess hair and cleansing the skin.
- Securely attach the probe to the patient.
- Allow for stabilization time (10 to 20 minutes).
- Schedule the site change time (2 to 6 hours, depending on patient).
- Set the high and low alarms.
- Monitor and document the results per institutional protocol.
- Change the site at appropriate intervals.
- Validate the reading against ABG values.

From Koff PB, Hess D: Transcutaneous oxygen and carbon dioxide measurements. In Kacmarek RM, Hess D, Stoller JK, editors: Monitoring in respiratory care, St Louis, 1993, Mosby.

Table 16-5 ▶▶ Factors Affecting Transcutaneous Blood Gas Monitors

Technical Factors	Clinical Factors
Labor-intensive, high-skill procedure	Poor perfusion
Lengthy stabilization time	Hyperoxemia
Improper calibration can be difficult to detect	Improper sensor application or placement
Heating required to obtain valid PO_2 results	Use of vasoactive drugs
Proper sensor-electrolyte contact is essential	Variation in skin characteristics

careful quality control. Table 16-5 lists the major factors that can affect the accuracy or limit the performance of a transcutaneous monitor.

In terms of technical limitations, the lengthy stabilization time needed by transcutaneous monitors precludes their use during short procedures or in emergencies. In such cases, the pulse oximeter is a better choice.

Sensors must be calibrated and maintained using methods similar to those described for bench-top analyzers. Improper calibration yields erroneous patient information. Unfortunately, improper calibration can be difficult to detect on some systems. Meticulous care of the sensor membranes is also essential for proper maintenance.

Because the sensor is heated, clinicians must take care to avoid thermal injury to the patient's skin. This is accomplished by (1) careful monitoring of sensor temperature (the safe upper limit is approximately 42° C) and (2) regularly rotating the sensor site.

Proper sensor-electrolyte contact is essential, as is proper application to the skin surface. A loosely applied sensor may have air leaks or may become dislodged. In either case, the resulting measurements will approach those in room air:

$$PO_2 = 159 \text{ mm Hg}$$
$$PCO_2 = 0 \text{ mm Hg}$$

Conversely, excessive pressure on the sensor compresses the underlying capillaries and produces a falsely low $P_{tc}O_2$. Even with proper application and placement, $P_{tc}O_2$ measures can vary by as much as 10% at different sites, with values from the extremities generally being lower than those obtained from the chest or abdomen.[22]

When arterial and transcutaneous blood gas values are inconsistent with each other or with the clinical status of the patient, the clinician should explore possible causes before reporting any results. Often, discrepancies can be reduced by switching the monitoring site or recalibrating the instrument. If these steps fail to resolve the inconsistencies, the clinician should recommend an alternative method for assessing gas exchange, such as pulse oximetry or more frequent ABG analysis.

Intraarterial (in vivo)

Over the last 20 years, the desire for continuous in vivo blood gas analysis has led to remarkable strides in technology. However, the clinical requirements for such systems (Box 16-8) are extremely demanding and have yet to be fully met.[26]

Early research focused on miniaturized versions of standard blood gas analyzer electrodes. However, problems with instrument drift, fouling of electrode surfaces, wire breakage, current leakage, and corrosion have limited clinical application of these systems.[27] Better success has been achieved using indwelling fiberoptic photochemical sensors, or *optodes*.

Instrumentation

Rather than using electrochemistry, optodes measure blood gas parameters by photochemical reactions, which alter light transmission through optical fibers. An **optode** contains a photosensitive dye at the distal end of an optical fiber. Light transmitted to this dye can be absorbed, reflected, or even re-emitted at a different wavelength (a phenomenon called **fluorescence**). The amount of light an optode dye absorbs, reflects, or re-emits changes when it is exposed to specific chemicals

Box 16-8 • Requirements for an Intraarterial Blood Gas Monitor

- Should accurately measure pH, P_{CO_2}, P_{O_2}, and temperature with a rapid response time
- Must operate within a 20-gauge catheter without affecting the following:
  - Continuous pressure measurement
  - Blood sampling procedures
  - Routine function of the arterial catheter system
- Must be biocompatible and nonthrombogenic
- Must be simple to operate and maintain
- Should withstand the abuse and rigors of clinical conditions common in the ICU and operating room
- Should remain stable and operate consistently for at least 72 hours
- Should not be adversely affected by a reduction in local blood flow or temperature
- Should not be adversely affected by hemodynamic changes
- Should be cost-effective

From Peruzzi WT, Shapiro BA: Respir Care Clin North Am 1:143, 1995.

or gases. By measuring the resulting changes in light transmission, the concentration of these substances can be measured.

Most photochemical blood gas systems use both absorbance- and fluorescence-based optodes. The absorbance-based pH and P_{CO_2} sensors use dye cells that absorb light in proportion to the concentration of the **analyte**. The intensity of light transmitted back to the instrument (after absorption) is measured and converted into the appropriate output signal (pH, P_{CO_2}). The fluorescence-based P_{O_2} sensor measures the amount of light re-emitted from the dye. Because oxygen "quenches" the dye's fluorescence, the intensity of this return signal is inversely proportional to the arterial P_{O_2}. Figure 16-12 shows how these three optodes are combined (with a thermocouple) at the tip of a flexible fiberoptic catheter.

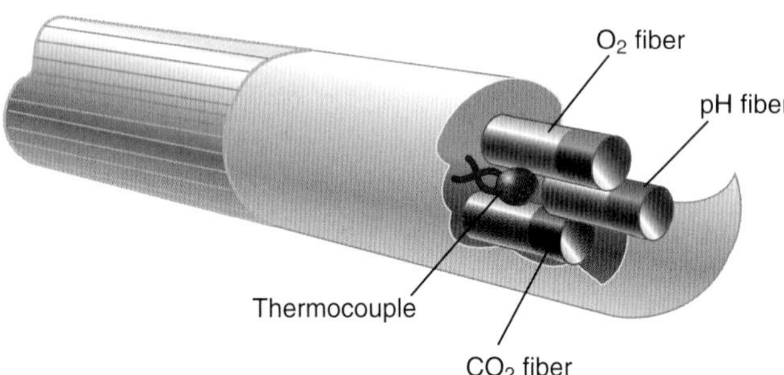

Figure 16-12
Simplified diagram of an indwelling optode-based arterial blood gas catheter showing the O_2, CO_2, pH, and thermocouple fibers.

Clinical Performance and Usefulness

Despite their potential, the actual performance of in vivo blood gas monitors still falls short of the clinical requirements previously specified. Accuracy and reliability are simply not as good as they are with standard blood gas analysis. Multicenter studies continue to reveal occasional, but large and unexplained, discrepancies between monitor readings and analyzer measurements, especially for P_{O_2}.[26] The frequency of these problems has led many to conclude that these devices are not yet reliable enough to replace traditional blood gas analysis.[28] However, current technology does provide clinically useful information at a level of accuracy and reliability sufficient for trend analysis.[28,29] Whether the use of these complex and expensive systems solely for trend monitoring makes sense is open to question.

On Demand (ex vivo)

On-demand (ex vivo) blood gas monitoring systems are a logical compromise between bench-top and in vivo blood gas analysis. Ex vivo systems eliminate all the problems associated with indwelling sensors, while still providing quick results. In concept, the only major shortcoming of ex vivo systems is their inability to provide real-time continuous data.

Instrumentation and Procedure

Figure 16-13 depicts an optode-based, ex vivo blood gas monitoring system in place on a patient. The optodes are located in a sensor cassette inserted in-line with the arterial catheter near the patient's wrist. To measure pH, P_{CO_2}, and P_{O_2}, the clinician first closes the system to the IV fluid source at *stopcock A*. Then he or she creates subatmospheric pressure in the syringe attached to *stopcock A*, which functions as an aspirating reservoir. This causes arterial blood to flow into the sensor cassette for analysis. During analysis, the clinician returns *stopcock A* to its original position (off to the aspirating syringe). This restores flow through the line and allows blood pressure monitoring to continue.

Blood gas parameter results are displayed in approximately 2 minutes. When analysis is complete, the clinician returns the blood sample to the patient by emptying the aspirating reservoir *(B)* and flushing the system through the flow valve at *D*.

Clinical Performance and Usefulness

In recent clinical trials of the U.S. Food and Drug Administration–approved ex vivo blood gas monitor CDI

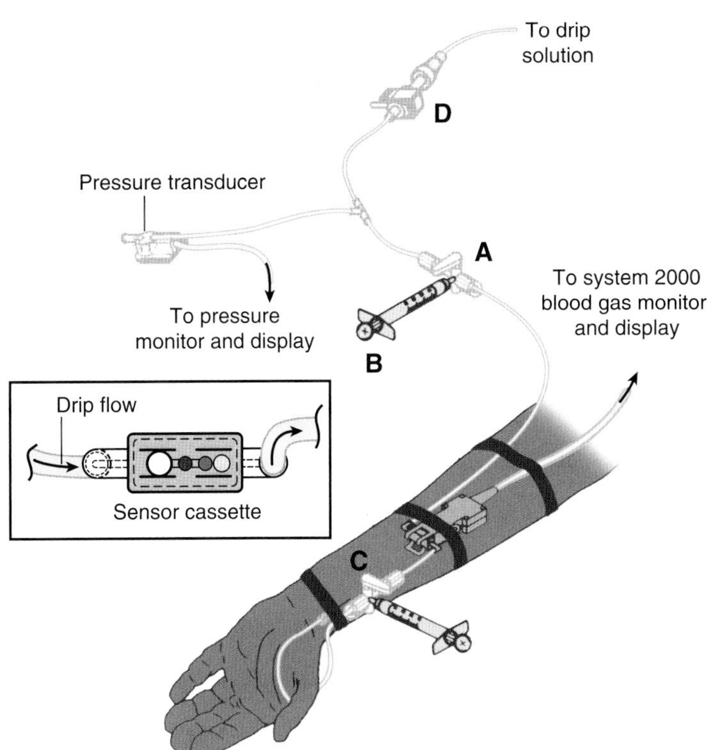

Figure 16-13

Schematic representation of an ex vivo blood gas monitoring system in place on a patient. The *inset* depicts a longitudinal section through the sensor cassette showing the three optodes (pH, Pco_2, Po_2) and the thermistor. **A**, "Upstream" stopcock, which permits function of the aspirating reservoir. **B**, A syringe used as an aspirating reservoir. **C**, A stopcock to permit blood sampling. **D**, A tubing flush valve connected to a pressure transducer. *(Modified from Shapiro BA et al: Crit Care Med 21:488, 1993.)*

2000, Gas-STAT (CDI, Irvine, California), the system tested performed as well as a laboratory blood gas analyzer in all patients, at all times.[26] Measurements could be obtained as often as every 3 minutes, and the intermittent errors commonly associated with in vivo systems were not observed.

▶ OXIMETRY

Oximetry is the measurement of blood hemoglobin saturations using **spectrophotometry**. According to the principles of spectrophotometry, every substance has a unique pattern of light absorption, much like a fingerprint. Moreover, a substance's pattern of light absorption varies predictably with the amount present. This is known as the *Lambert-Beer law*. Thus by measuring the light absorbed and transmitted by a substance, scientists can identify its presence and determine its concentration.

The particular pattern of light absorption exhibited by a substance at different wavelengths is called its *absorption spectrum*. As shown in Figure 16-14, each form of hemoglobin (e.g., Hb, HbO_2, HbCO) has its own unique pattern. By comparison of the amount of light transmitted through (or reflected from) a blood sample at two or more specific wavelengths, the relative concentrations of two or more forms of hemoglobin can be measured. For example, oxygenated hemoglobin absorbs less red light (600 to 750 nm) and more infrared light (850 to 1000 nm) than deoxygenated or reduced Hb does. Comparing a blood sample's light absorption with red and infrared light yields the $\%HbO_2$ and %Hb. For measurement of the concentration of additional forms of Hb, additional (more than two) wavelengths of light need to be used.

The following two types of oximetry are used in clinical practice: *hemoximetry* (also called *co-oximetry*) and *pulse oximetry*. Hemoximetry is a laboratory analytical procedure requiring invasive sampling of arterial blood. Pulse oximetry is a noninvasive monitoring technique performed at the bedside.

Hemoximetry

Hemoximetry is an analytical method of oximetry and is covered in the AARC *Clinical Practice Guideline: In vitro pH and Blood Gas Analysis and Hemoximetry*[15] (see p. 369). Related recommendations have been published by the National Committee for Clinical Laboratory Standards.[30]

Instrumentation

Figure 16-15 is a simplified diagram showing the key components of a laboratory hemoximeter. Light generated by a thallium cathode lamp passes through a series of lenses and filters, yielding the specific wavelengths needed for analysis. A beam splitter then divides the light into

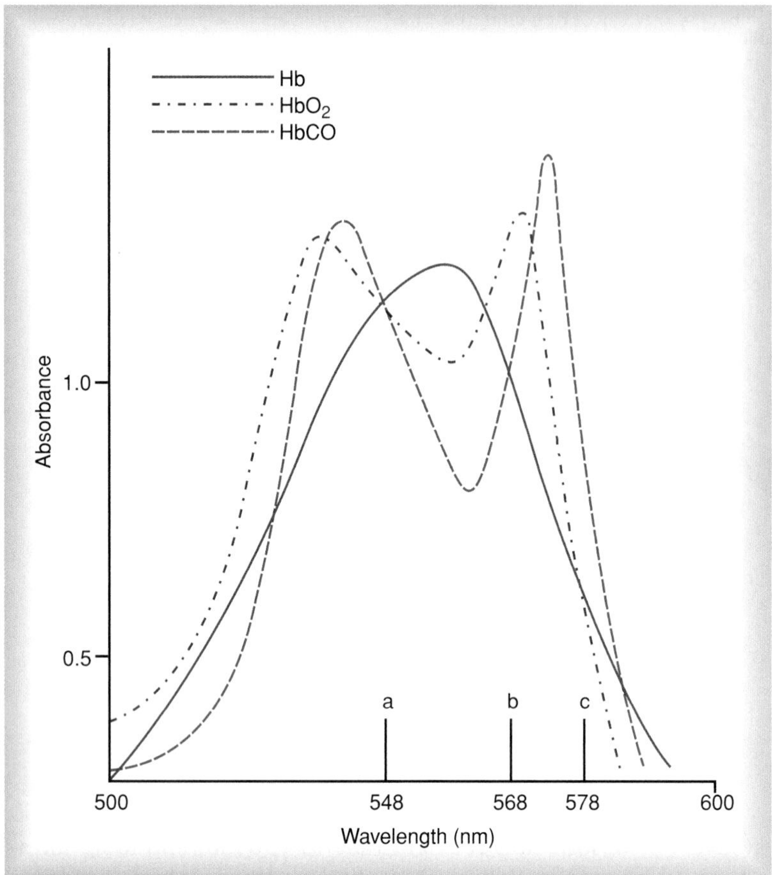

Figure 16-14
Principle of spectrophotometric oximetry. Different forms of hemoglobin (e.g., Hb, HbO_2, HbCO) absorb light differently at different wavelengths. By comparing points of equal absorbance (isobestic points) between pairs of Hb species (e.g., Hb versus HbO_2, Hb versus HbCO), the relative proportion of each can be measured.

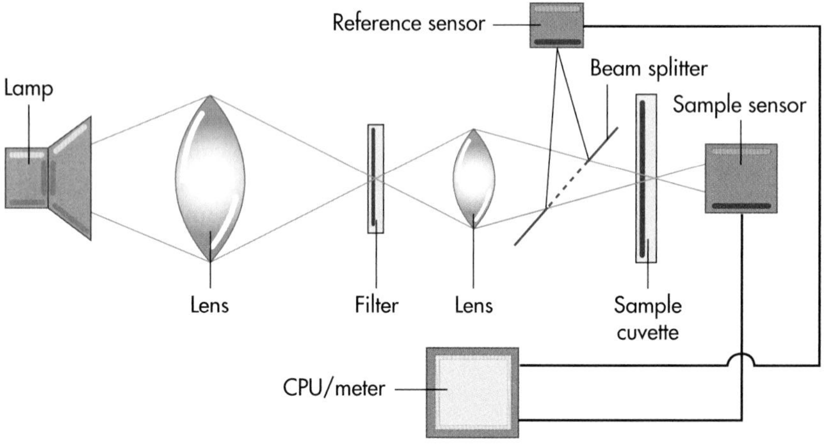

Figure 16-15
Simplified diagram showing the key components of a laboratory hemoximeter. *(From Lane EE: Clinical arterial blood gas analysis, St Louis, 1987, Mosby.)*

two portions, directing one through a reference solution and the other through a sample chamber, or **cuvette**. Photo detection sensors measure the amount of light transmitted through these two sources. By comparing the difference in light transmission through the reference and sample solutions, a microprocessor computes the relative amount of hemoglobin present, with its output sent to the calibrated device meter or display. Because a laboratory hemoximeter uses three different wavelengths of light, it can simultaneously compute the relative concentrations of multiple hemoglobin species, such as Hb, HbO_2, HbCO, and metHb.

Procedure and Quality Assurance

Like modern blood gas analyzers, laboratory hemoximeters are highly automated and simple to use. Indeed, some devices now combine both technologies into a single instrument. However, the caveats remain the same. Accurate and clinically useful hemoximetry results can be expected only if an error-free sample is assessed on a calibrated analyzer, using the manufacturer's protocol.

Although variations exist among devices, the basic procedure is similar. First, the blood is introduced into the sampling port of the analyzer, usually either by aspiration or injection. Required sample sizes vary from approximately 200 μL to as little as 40 μL (microanalysis). Once introduced, erythrocyte hemoglobin is released into the solution by hemolysis (incomplete hemolysis can cause erroneous results). After hemolysis, the sample is transported to the cuvette for analysis. On completion of the analysis, the sampling system (cuvette and tubing) is flushed and cleaned. As with blood gas analysis, operators must follow CDC Standard Precautions and ensure proper disposal of syringes and waste materials.

Quality assurance procedures for hemoximetry are essentially the same as those used for blood gas analysis, differing only with regard to the control materials used. In addition, careful cleaning and maintenance of the cuvette chamber is essential, because clouding of its walls decreases absorbance and can cause falsely high values.[31]

Problem-Solving and Troubleshooting

A major assumption underlying hemoximetry is that the measured changes in light absorbance result only from variations in the relative concentrations of various hemoglobins. In practice, this assumption does not always hold true. Table 16-6 outlines some of the potential problems and resulting errors that can occur with hemoximetry.

Table 16-6 ▶▶ Problems Causing Measurement Errors With Hemoximeters

Problem	Potential Error
Incomplete hemolysis	Falsely low total Hb, HbO_2
Sickle cell anemia (caused by incomplete hemolysis)	Falsely low HbO_2
Presence of vascular dyes (e.g., methylene blue)	Falsely low total Hb, HbO_2
High lipid levels (e.g., from parenteral nutrition)	Falsely low total Hb, HbO_2
Presence of high levels of fetal hemoglobin	Falsely high HbCO
Elevated bilirubin levels (>20 mg/dL)	Falsely high total Hb, HbO_2, metHb
Dirty cuvette chamber	Falsely high total Hb, HbO_2

Pulse Oximetry

A pulse oximeter is an inexpensive and portable noninvasive monitoring device that provides estimates of arterial blood oxyhemoglobin saturation levels. So as not to confuse these estimates with actual SaO_2 measures obtained by hemoximetry, the abbreviation SpO_2 is used to refer to pulse oximetry readings.

No other device in recent medical history has been so widely and quickly adopted into clinical practice.[20] Unfortunately, with this widespread use have come equally widespread misconceptions regarding the appropriate applications and limitations of this technology.[32]

To guide practitioners in providing quality care, the AARC has published *Clinical Practice Guideline: Pulse Oximetry*.[33] Modified excerpts from the AARC guideline appear on p. 380.

Instrumentation

The pulse oximeter combines the principle of spectrophotometry, as used by hemoximeters, with **photoplethysmography**. Photoplethysmography uses light to detect the tiny volume changes that occur in living tissue during pulsatile blood flow.

However, compared with a hemoximeter, the pulse oximeter uses only two wavelengths of light, one red (approximately 660 nm) and one infrared (approximately 940 nm). In addition, rather than measuring light transmission through a blood sample in a glass cuvette, the pulse oximeter actually measures transmission through living tissue, such as a finger or earlobe.

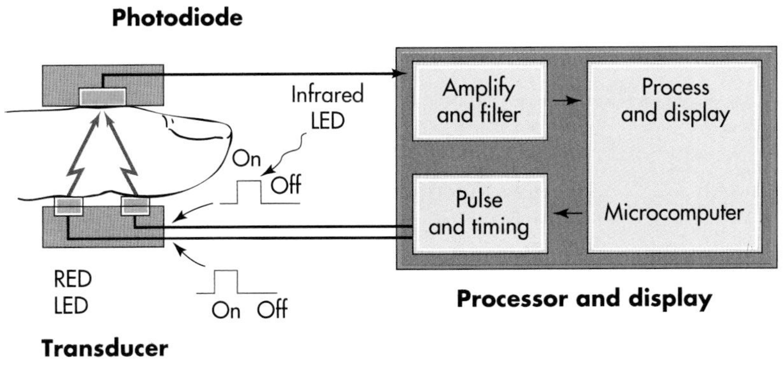

Figure 16-16
Schematic block diagram of a pulse oximeter. *(Modified from Gardner RM: J Cardiovasc Nurs; 1:79, 1987.)*

Pulse Oximetry

AARC Clinical Practice Guideline (Excerpts)*

➤ INDICATIONS

- To monitor the adequacy of arterial oxyhemoglobin saturation
- To quantify the response of arterial oxyhemoglobin saturation to therapeutic intervention or to diagnostic procedures, such as bronchoscopy
- To comply with mandated regulations or recommendations by authoritative groups

➤ CONTRAINDICATIONS

- The ongoing need for actual measurements of pH, $Pa{CO_2}$, total hemoglobin, and abnormal hemoglobins may be a relative contraindication to pulse oximetry.

➤ PRECAUTIONS AND/OR POSSIBLE COMPLICATIONS

- Device limitations causing false-negative results for hypoxemia or false-positive results for normoxemia or hyperoxemia may lead to inappropriate treatment of the patient
- Tissue injury may occur at the measuring site as a result of the following:
  - Pressure sores from prolonged application
  - Electrical shock and burns when using incompatible probes between instruments

➤ ASSESSMENT OF NEED

- When direct measurement of $Sa{O_2}$ is not available or accessible in a timely fashion, a pulse oximetry measurement may temporarily suffice if the limitations of the data are appreciated.
- $Sp{O_2}$ is appropriate for continuous and prolonged monitoring (e.g., during sleep, exercise, or bronchoscopy).
  - $Sp{O_2}$ may be adequate when assessment of acid-base status or $Pa{O_2}$ is not required.

➤ ASSESSMENT OF OUTCOME

The following should be used to evaluate the benefits of pulse oximetry:

- $Sp{O_2}$ results should reflect the patient's clinical condition (i.e., they should validate the basis for ordering the test)
- Documentation of results, therapeutic intervention (or lack thereof), and clinical decisions based on the $Sp{O_2}$ measurements should be noted in the medical record

➤ FREQUENCY

After agreement has been established initially between $Sa{O_2}$ and $Sp{O_2}$, the frequency of $Sp{O_2}$ monitoring (i.e., continuous versus spot check) depends on the clinical status of the patient, the indications for performing the procedure, and recommended guidelines. For example, continuous $Sp{O_2}$ monitoring may be indicated throughout a bronchoscopy to detect desaturation, whereas a spot check may suffice for evaluating the efficacy of oxygen therapy in a stable postoperative patient. Direct measurement of $Sa{O_2}$ is needed whenever the $Sp{O_2}$ does not confirm or verify suspicions about the patient's clinical state.

➤ MONITORING

During continuous pulse oximetry, the monitoring schedule for both the patient and the equipment should be correlated with the bedside assessment and determination of vital signs.

*For the complete guideline, see Respir Care 36:1406, 1991.

Figure 16-16 provides a schematic block diagram of a pulse oximeter, consisting of a sensor and a processor and display unit. The sensor has two sides. From one side, separate red and infrared LEDs alternately transmit their light through the tissue. The transmitted light intensity is measured by a photodetector on the other side. The resulting output signal is filtered and amplified by instrument electronics, with processing and display functions controlled by a microprocessor.

Figure 16-17 shows a typical output signal generated by the photodetector (the pulsatile component actually can be observed on instruments that have a plethysmographic display). A baseline component represents the stable absorbance of the tissue bed, which mainly is

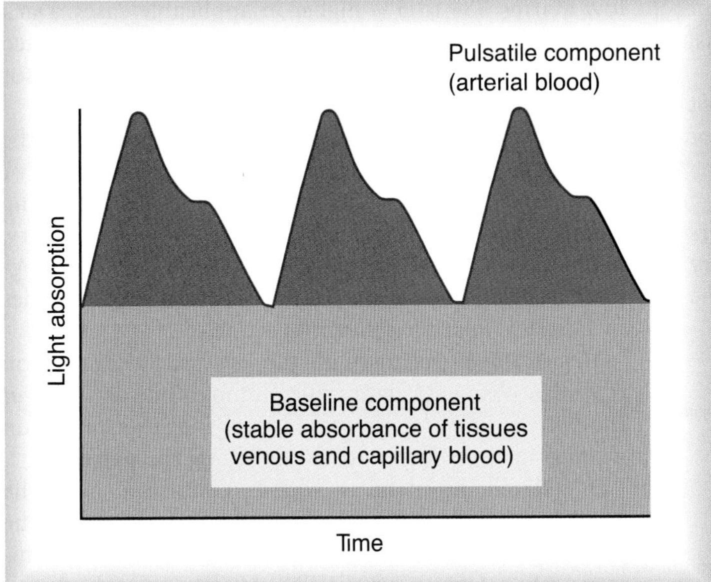

Figure 16-17

Output signal generated by pulse oximeter. Saturation is based on the ratio of light absorption during pulsatile and baseline phases.

the result of venous and capillary blood. At the top is the pulsatile component, caused by intermittent arterial flow through the tissues. By comparing light absorbance during the pulsatile phase with the baseline value at each wavelength, a pulse-added measure is obtained that is independent of incident light. Arterial oxyhemoglobin saturation ($Sa{O_2}$) is then computed as the ratio of the pulse-added absorbances at the two different wavelengths.

In terms of accuracy, the pulse oximetry readings of sick patients usually fall within ±3% to 5% of those obtained with invasive hemoximetry.[20] In general, the lower the actual $Sa{O_2}$, the less accurate and reliable the $Sp{O_2}$. Most clinicians consider pulse oximeter readings unreliable at saturations below 70%. Instrument response times vary by manufacturer, sensor location, and the patient's hemodynamic status from as few as 10 seconds to a full minute or longer.

Procedure

The actual procedure used to measure $Sp{O_2}$ varies according to the device used, sensor site selected, and whether a spot check or continuous monitoring is required. Box 16-9 lists key points to be considered when performing pulse oximetry.

Given the limits of this technology, meticulous documentation is a must. Specifically, all $Sp{O_2}$ results should be recorded in the patient's medical record. The following details should be documented:

1. Date, time of measurement, and reading
2. Patient's position, activity level, and location during monitoring
3. $F{I}{O_2}$ or oxygen flow and oxygen delivery device
4. Probe type and placement site
5. Model of device (if more than one device is available for use)
6. Results of simultaneously obtained ABGs and hemoximetry
7. Stability of readings (length of observation time and range of fluctuation)

Box 16-9 • Key Points for Performing Pulse Oximetry

- Always follow manufacturer's recommended protocol.
- Never mix sensors among different devices.
- Make sure the sensor is the correct size for the site chosen.
- Make sure the sensor is properly applied (not too tight or loose).
- Before taking or recording a reading, confirm the adequacy and accuracy of the pulse signal.
- When doing spot checks, be sure to allow sufficient response time before taking a reading, because response times vary greatly.
- For continuous monitoring of adults and children, set the low alarm in the 88% to 92% range.
- Whenever possible, validate the initial $Sp{O_2}$ reading against the actual $Sa{O_2}$.
- Clean multiuse sensors, and disinfect the instrument housing between patients.
- Inspect the sensor site frequently throughout the duration of continuous monitoring, and change it as needed.
- Never act on $Sp{O_2}$ readings alone.
- Avoid using pulse oximetry to monitor hyperoxia in neonates.

8. Patient's clinical appearance, including assessment of perfusion at the measuring site (e.g., cyanosis, skin temperature)
9. Agreement between oximeter and actual patient heart rate, as determined by palpation or electrocardiogram

If direct measurement of arterial blood parameters (Pa_{O_2}, Sa_{O_2}) cannot be performed when pulse oximetry is initiated, this limitation should be indicated in the patient's record.

> **RULE OF THUMB**
>
> When using a pulse oximeter to warn of hypoxemia in otherwise healthy adults, never set the low alarm below 92%. In general, this level will ensure that the alarm is activated before the real arterial saturation drops below the critical value of 90%.

Problem-Solving and Troubleshooting

Problems with pulse oximetry fall into the following two categories: (1) those inherent in the technology itself and (2) those associated with clinical interpretation and use of data.

Dozens of technical factors may affect the readings, limit the precision, or alter the performance of pulse oximeters. Table 16-7 summarizes the most important of these factors and the types of errors they cause.

Motion artifact probably is the most common source of error and false alarms. Although new technologies promise to reduce this, relocation of the sensor to the earlobe, toe, or external nares can minimize the problem. As a last resort, the patient may be restrained.

Because of the falsely high readings that can occur with dark skin pigmentation, most clinicians set oximeter low alarms 3% to 5% higher in applicable cases. Dark nail polish presents a similar error, but it is better corrected either by using a different site or by rotating the sensor so that the light path does not cross the fingernails.

If ambient light interference is creating problems, the sensor can be loosely covered with an opaque towel or cloth. Problems that occur during procedures producing electromagnetic interference (e.g., electrocautery, magnetic resonance imaging [MRI]) need only be recognized. Careful monitoring of the patient during episodes of false low alarms is essential.

Regarding problems with the use and interpretation of pulse oximetry data, rule number one is to *treat the patient, not the monitor*. Never interpret or act on monitoring data without first assessing the patient.

A related problem is simple confusion over the relationship between oxyhemoglobin saturation and the partial pressure of oxygen. Unfortunately, many clinicians rely solely on arterial P_{O_2} readings to assess oxygenation and do not really understand oxyhemoglobin saturation. To them, a Sp_{O_2} reading of 80% might be confused easily with a Pa_{O_2} of 80 mm Hg. Of course, the latter measure of partial pressure is normal, whereas a saturation of 80% indicates moderate to severe hypoxemia, equivalent to a Pa_{O_2} of approximately 50 mm Hg.

A similar interpretation error (Pa_{O_2} versus Sp_{O_2}) is because of the limited accuracy of most pulse oximeters. It is common practice to set a monitoring oximeter's low alarm to 90%. In theory this makes sense because a Sa_{O_2} reading of 90% normally corresponds to a P_{O_2} reading of approximately 60 mm Hg, which is the lower limit of clinically acceptable oxygenation. However, with the accuracy of some oximeters being only ±5%, an Sp_{O_2} reading of 90% could mean an actual Sa_{O_2} reading as low as 85%, corresponding to a P_{O_2} level of 55 mm Hg or less!

At the high end, oximetry data can be even less meaningful. Because of the characteristics of the oxy-

Table 16-7 ▶▶ Factors Affecting the Accuracy or Precision of Pulse Oximeters

Factor	Potential Error
Presence of HbCO	Falsely high %HbO_2
Presence of high levels of metHb	Falsely low %HbO_2 if Sa_{O_2} >85% Falsely high %HbO_2 if Sa_{O_2} <85%
Presence of fetal hemoglobin	No effect
Anemia (low hematocrit)	Falsely low %HbO_2
Vascular dyes (e.g., methylene blue)	Falsely low %HbO_2
Elevated bilirubin levels	No effect
Dark skin pigmentation	Falsely high %HbO_2 (3%-5%)
Nail polish (especially black)	Falsely high %HbO_2
Ambient light	Varies (e.g., falsely high %HbO_2 in sunlight); also may cause falsely high pulse reading
Poor perfusion (vasoconstriction)	Inadequate signal; unpredictable results
Motion artifact	Unpredictable, spurious readings
Electrocautery	Falsely low HbO_2
Magnetic resonance imaging	Falsely low HbO_2

hemoglobin dissociation curve (see Chapter 10), a patient with a Spo_2 reading of 100% could represent a Pao_2 level anywhere between 100 and 600 mm Hg. The lesson here is not to use the pulse oximeter for monitoring hyperoxia (as may be important for neonates).

It is also important to recognize that the pulse oximeter does not measure Pco_2. Thus a patient breathing an elevated Fio_2 can have normal Spo_2 readings despite severe hypercarbia. ABG analysis is needed when acute ventilatory failure may be present.

As with transcutaneous monitoring, if pulse oximetry and blood gas values are inconsistent with each other or the clinical status of the patient, the RT should explore possible causes before reporting, interpreting, or acting on results. Often, discrepancies can be reduced by switching sites or replacing the sensor probe. If these steps fail to resolve the inconsistencies, the RT should document the problem and recommend obtaining an ABG.

▶ CAPNOMETRY AND CAPNOGRAPHY

Capnometry is the measurement of CO_2 in respiratory gases. A capnometer is the device that measures the CO_2. **Capnography** is the graphic display of CO_2 levels as they change during breathing.

Although capnography can be applied to any patient, its primary clinical use is for monitoring during either general anesthesia (where it is a standard of care) or mechanical ventilation. The remainder of this section assumes application during mechanical ventilation.

To guide practitioners in providing quality care, the AARC has published *Clinical Practice Guideline: Capnography/Capnometry during Mechanical Ventilation.*[34] Modified excerpts from the AARC guideline appear on p. 384.

Instrumentation

The key component in a capnograph is a rapidly responding CO_2 analyzer. Rapid CO_2 analysis can be achieved using infrared absorption, Raman scattering, mass spectroscopy, or photoacoustic technology, with the infrared capnometer being the most common.

Figure 16-18 provides a simple schematic of a double-beam infrared capnometer. A filtered infrared light source passes through a sample chamber. (Because glass absorbs infrared radiation, the chamber "windows" usually are constructed of sodium chloride or sodium bromide). After the infrared light passes through the sample chamber, a lens focuses the remaining, unabsorbed radiation onto an electric photodetector. Because CO_2 absorbs infrared radiation, the greater the concentration of carbon dioxide in the sample, the less infrared light will arrive at the detector. Thus variations in the concentration of CO_2 alter the electrical output signal of the detector. This signal then is used either to display the CO_2 concentration with LEDs (capnometer) or to generate a real-time graphic display (capnogram).[35]

Capnometers use two different methods to sample the respiratory gases: mainstream sampling and sidestream sampling (Figure 16-19). The mainstream analyzer

MINI CLINI

Troubleshooting Pulse Oximetry

PROBLEM

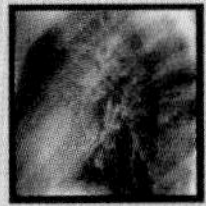

The RT draws an ABG sample from a conscious and alert patient in a postsurgical unit who also is being monitored with a pulse oximeter, which reads *80% saturation.* The patient is breathing 35% oxygen through an air-entrainment mask. The patient's extremities are pink and warm. After running the blood sample through a calibrated ABG analyzer with a hemoximeter, the RT obtains the following values:

Po_2 = 90 mm Hg
Hb = 12 g/dL
Sao_2 = 92%
metHb = 0.5%
HbCO = 1%

Explain the difference between the pulse oximeter and hemoximeter readings of this patient's blood oxygen levels and what action the RT should take.

SOLUTION

Given that a calibrated hemoximeter will provide more accurate results than will a pulse oximeter and that the patient exhibits no signs of hypoxemia, it is likely that the pulse oximeter reading is falsely low. Because the Hb and metHb levels are not grossly abnormal, potential problems include motion artifact, poor sensor placement, or device malfunction. The oximeter and sensor should be rechecked, and if found to be malfunctioning, they should be replaced.

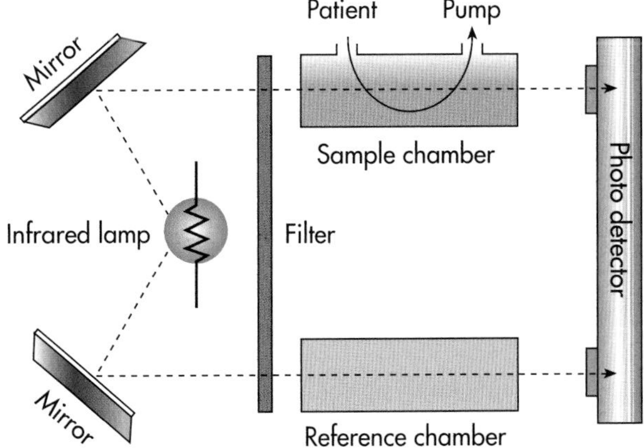

Figure 16-18
Schematic representation of an infrared capnometer.

Capnography/Capnometry during Mechanical Ventilation

AARC Clinical Practice Guideline (Excerpts)*

INDICATIONS

Based on available evidence, capnography may be indicated for the following:

- Evaluation of end-tidal CO_2 levels (P_{ETCO_2}) during mechanical ventilation
- Monitoring severity of pulmonary disease and evaluating the patient's response to therapy, especially that intended to do the following:
  - Improve the dead space to tidal volume ratio (V_D/V_T)
  - Improve the matching of ventilation to perfusion ($\dot{V}/\dot{Q}$)
  - Increase coronary blood flow
- Determining that tracheal, rather than esophageal, intubation has taken place
- Continued monitoring of the integrity of the ventilatory circuit, including the artificial airway
- Evaluation of the efficiency of mechanical ventilatory support (by the [Pa_{CO_2}-P_{ETCO_2}])
- Reflecting CO_2 elimination
- Monitoring adequacy of pulmonary and coronary blood flow
- Monitoring inspired CO_2 when CO_2 gas is being therapeutically administered
- Graphic evaluation of the ventilator-patient interface

CONTRAINDICATIONS

There are no absolute contraindications to capnography in mechanically ventilated adults, provided that the data obtained are evaluated with consideration given to the patient's clinical condition.

PRECAUTIONS AND/OR POSSIBLE COMPLICATIONS

- Misunderstanding of the data provided may lead to inappropriate treatment of the patient.
- With mainstream analyzers, too large a sampling window can excessively increase the mechanical dead space circuit.
- The sampling window or the sampling lines can place additional weight on the circuit and increase traction on the patient's artificial airway.

ASSESSMENT OF NEED

Capnography is a standard of care during anesthesia. The Society of Critical Care Medicine has suggested that capnography be available in every ICU. Assessment of the need to use capnography with a specific patient should be guided by the clinical situation. The patient's primary cause of respiratory failure and the acuteness of his or her condition should be considered. Patients with severe dynamic disease, such as adult respiratory distress syndrome (ARDS), should be considered candidates for capnography.

ASSESSMENT OF OUTCOME

Results should reflect the patient's condition and should validate the basis for ordering the monitoring. Documentation of results (along with all ventilatory and hemodynamic variables available), therapeutic interventions, and/or clinical decisions made based on the capnogram should be included in the patient's chart.

MONITORING

During capnography, the following should be considered and monitored:

- Ventilatory variables: tidal volume, respiratory rate, positive end-expiratory pressure (PEEP), inspiratory/expiratory time ratio (I:E), peak airway pressure, and concentrations of respiratory gas mixture
- Hemodynamic variables: systemic and pulmonary blood pressures, cardiac output, shunt, and ventilation-perfusion imbalances

*For the complete guideline, see Respir Care 40:1321, 1995.

places an in-line analysis chamber between the patient's airway and the ventilator circuit. The sidestream analyzer uses a sampling tube to continually pump a small volume of gas from the ventilator circuit into the analysis chamber within the device. Table 16-8 lists the advantages and disadvantages of these two approaches. Differences notwithstanding, clinicians should use the method best suited to the patient's needs and the device with which they are most experienced and familiar.

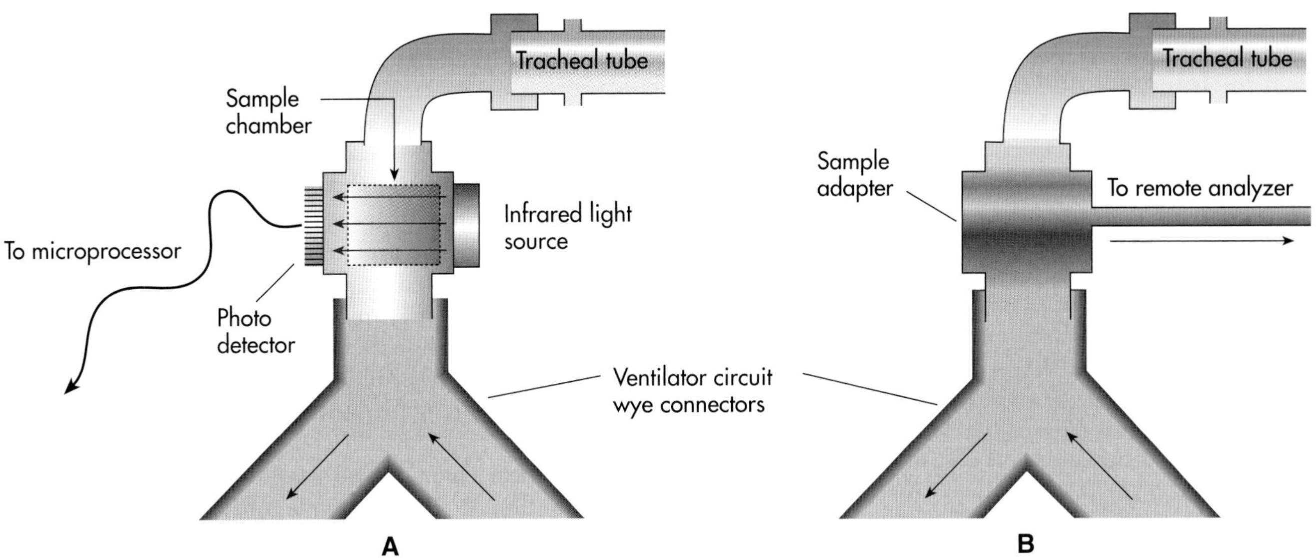

Figure 16-19
A, Mainstream CO_2 sampling. The sample chamber, light source, and photodetector are attached to the breathing circuit, with the output signal sent to a microprocessor for analysis and display. **B**, Sidestream CO_2 sampling through an in-line sampling adapter with a small-bore connector. A small sample of expired gas is drawn continuously through the tubing and analyzed inside a remote capnometer.

Table 16-8 ▶▶ Advantages and Disadvantages of Mainstream and Sidestream Capnometers

	Mainstream	Sidestream
Advantages	Sensor at patient airway	No bulky sensors or heaters at airway
	Fast response (crisp waveform)	Ability to measure N_2O
	Short lag time (real-time readings)	Disposable sample line
	No sample flow to reduce tidal volume	Ability to use with nonintubated patients
Disadvantages	Secretions and humidity can block sensor window	Secretions block sample tubing
	Sensor requires heating to prevent condensation	Trap required to remove water from the sample
	Requires frequent calibration	Frequent calibration required
	Bulky sensor at patient airway	Slow response to CO_2 changes
	Does not measure N_2O	Lag time between CO_2 change and measurement
	Difficult to use with nonintubated patients	Sample flow may decrease tidal volume
	Reusable adapters require cleaning and sterilization	

From Kacmarek RM, Hess D, Stoller J: Monitoring in respiratory care, St Louis, 1993, Mosby.

Interpretation

Interpretation of the capnogram can be useful in assessing trends in alveolar ventilation and detecting $\dot{V}/\dot{Q}$ imbalance caused by either pulmonary disease or cardiovascular disorders. Capnometry also has been used to estimate physiological dead space, to detect esophageal intubation, to assess blood flow during cardiac arrest, and to determine PEEP levels. To interpret abnormal events, clinicians first must understand the normal capnogram.

Normal Capnogram

Figure 16-20 shows a typical normal single-breath capnogram. Initially, the expired P_{CO_2} is 0 mm Hg, indicating exhalation of pure dead space gas. Soon after *(point A)*, alveolar gas begins mixing with dead space gas, causing a rapid rise in expired P_{CO_2}. Later in expiration *(point B)*, the CO_2 concentration begins leveling off. This plateau indicates exhalation of gas coming mainly from ventilated alveoli. Gas sampled at the end of exhalation *(point C)* is called *end-tidal gas*, with its partial pressure of carbon dioxide abbreviated as P_{ETCO_2}. In healthy individuals, the P_{ETCO_2} averages 1 to 5 mm Hg less than the Pa_{CO_2}, or between 35 and 43 mm Hg (approximately 5% to 6% CO_2). The sharp downstroke and return to baseline that normally occurs after the end-tidal point indicates inhalation of fresh gas with zero carbon dioxide.

Abnormal Capnogram

The first step in assessing the capnogram is to determine the actual P_{ETCO_2} and whether it has changed over time.

MINI CLINI

Interpreting Capnometry Data

PROBLEM

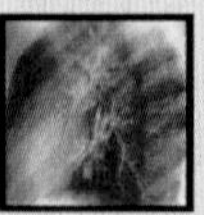

With a capnograph, the RT is monitoring an intubated, mechanically ventilated patient in the ICU. She notices the expired CO_2 level suddenly drop to near zero. On auscultation, the patient exhibits good bilateral breath sounds, and all connections between the airway and capnograph are tight. What is the likely problem?

SOLUTION

The most common causes of a zero P_{ETCO_2} are extubation and ventilator or monitoring system disconnection. However, a P_{ETCO_2} of zero also can occur with shock or cardiac arrest (no CO_2 returns to the lungs for exhalation). The RT should check this patient's cardiovascular status immediately. If the patient's cardiovascular system is functioning within normal limits, she should check the position of the endotracheal tube.

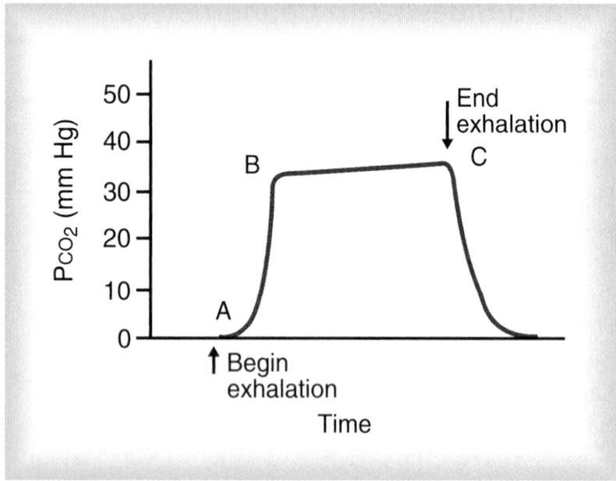

Figure 16-20
A normal single-breath capnograph tracing.

Table 16-9 differentiates between the causes of high and low P_{ETCO_2} readings by the suddenness of the change. Note that a P_{ETCO_2} of zero usually indicates a system leak, esophageal intubation, or cardiac arrest.

Once the capnogram has been assessed for changes in P_{ETCO_2}, the waveform and its pattern should be analyzed. A normal capnogram starts with a sharp upstroke, followed by a plateau, and then a rapid downstroke. As indicated in Figure 16-21, changes in this normal contour may indicate a ventilation-perfusion abnormality. Such patterns, although not diagnostic, can indicate the severity of the $\dot{V}/\dot{Q}$ disturbance and can warn of developing problems, such as acute pulmonary emboli.

Waveform changes also may occur with equipment malfunction.[36] For example, because the normal inspired CO_2 level is zero, the capnogram baseline also should be at zero. An elevated baseline (higher than 0 mm Hg) indicates rebreathing. However, an expired CO_2 level of zero might indicate patient disconnect. (For more information on the use of capnography during mechanical ventilation, see Chapter 43.)

Procedure

Bedside capnography procedures vary according to the type of equipment used and the manufacturer's recommended protocol. In general, a capnograph should be calibrated as recommended by its manufacturer, using precision CO_2 mixtures in the clinical range of measurement.

In terms of infection control, nondisposable components that contact the patient's airway or ventilator circuit should undergo high-level disinfection between patients. The monitor should be cleaned as needed, according to manufacturer's recommendations.

Table 16-9 ▶▶ Conditions Associated With Changes in P_{ETCO_2}

Change	High P_{ETCO_2}	Low P_{ETCO_2}
Sudden	Sudden increase in cardiac output Sudden release of a tourniquet Injection of sodium bicarbonate	Sudden hyperventilation Sudden decrease in cardiac output Massive pulmonary embolism Air embolism Disconnection of the ventilator Obstruction of the endotracheal tube Leakage in the circuit
Gradual	Hypoventilation Increase in CO_2 production	Hyperventilation Decrease in oxygen consumption Decreased pulmonary perfusion

An absent P_{ETCO_2} means that a system leak, esophageal intubation, or cardiac arrest has occurred.

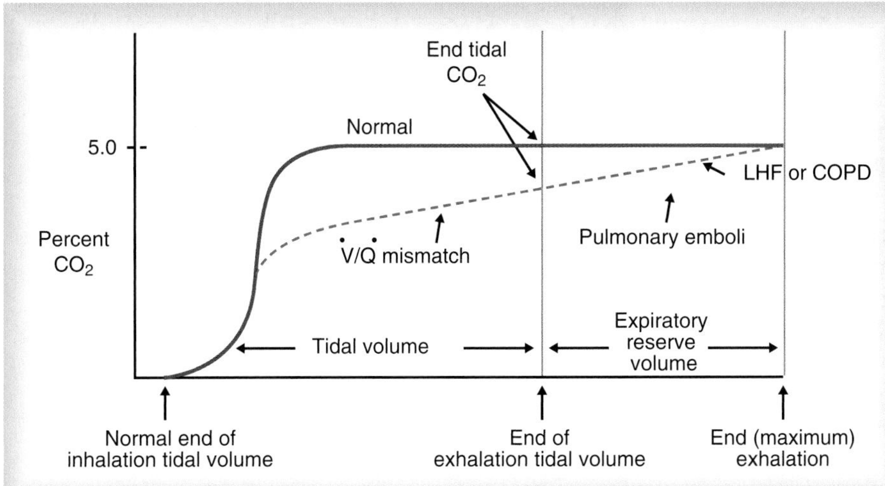

Figure 16-21 Normal and abnormal capnogram waveforms. For a healthy individual (*solid line*), the end-tidal CO_2 at the completion of normal tidal exhalation is equal to that at maximum exhalation. With shock caused by left ventricular heart failure (LHF) or chronic obstructive pulmonary disease (COPD), the CO_2 level rises more slowly and does not reach a true end-tidal plateau. Moreover, the end-tidal CO_2 is less than normal at the completion of a normal exhalation (but may rise slightly with a maximum exhalation). Similar findings can be noted with a pulmonary embolus, except that the low end-tidal CO_2 does not rise with a maximum exhalation. *(Modified from Pilbeam SP: Mechanical ventilation: physiological and clinical applications, ed 3, St Louis, 1998, Mosby.)*

Problem-Solving and Troubleshooting

Monitoring a patient with a capnograph that is properly calibrated and operating according to the manufacturer's specifications presents few major problems. The most significant error is assuming that the end-expired carbon dioxide levels can substitute for actual Pa_{CO_2} measurements. The most common problem is contamination or obstruction of the sampling system or monitor by secretions or condensate.[34] Proper use of water traps and regular changing of sample tubing or chambers can help prevent this problem. Other potential problems include the following:

- False reading caused by the presence of gases with infrared absorption spectra similar to CO_2 (e.g., nitrous oxide)
- Inaccurate readings with high frequencies of breathing (this is more of a problem with sidestream systems)
- Misinterpreting low or absent cardiac output as a disconnect or possible esophageal intubation (all three can result in a P_{ETCO_2} of zero)[36]

KEY POINTS

- To measure the inspired oxygen concentration, use a properly calibrated electrochemical oxygen analyzer.
- The most common causes of oxygen analyzer malfunction are low batteries, sensor depletion, and electronic failure.
- As the gold standard of gas exchange analysis, ABGs help assess ventilation, acid-

KEY POINTS—cont'd

base balance, oxygenation, and the oxygen-carrying capacity of blood.

- The radial artery is the preferred site for adult arterial blood sampling. Before radial puncture, perform a modified Allen test to confirm collateral circulation.
- For critically ill patients, wait 20 to 30 minutes after a change in treatment before sampling arterial blood.
- Most preanalytic blood gas errors can be avoided by ensuring that the sample was obtained anaerobically, is properly anticoagulated, and will be analyzed within 15 minutes.
- Indwelling peripheral artery, central venous, and pulmonary artery catheters give ready access for blood sampling and allow continuous pressure monitoring, but with increased risk of infection and thrombosis.
- Capillary blood pH and P_{CO_2} are sometimes used to assess acid-base status in infants and children. The capillary P_{O_2} is of no value in estimating arterial oxygenation.
- To perform blood gas analysis and hemoximetry, the clinician must be proficient in performing the procedures, preventive maintenance, troubleshooting, instrument calibration, and quality control.
- A blood gas analyzer measures pH, P_{CO_2}, and P_{O_2} using three separate electrodes.

Continued

KEY POINTS—cont'd

- To obtain accurate blood gas results, ensure that the sample is free of preanalytical error, and follow the manufacturer's recommended analysis protocol.
- Blood gas analysis quality control involves a cycle of performance validation for new instruments, preventive maintenance and function checks, automated calibration, calibration verification with control media, internal statistical quality control, external proficiency testing, and thorough recordkeeping of all processes.
- Portable point-of-care blood gas analyzers can achieve accuracy and precision levels comparable with those of laboratory-based analyzers.
- A blood gas monitor provides bedside measurements either continuously or at appropriate intervals, without permanently removing blood from the patient. This may be accomplished transcutaneously or with either in vivo or ex vivo blood analysis.
- Transcutaneous blood gas monitoring provides continuous noninvasive analysis of gas exchange, but it is useful only for hemodynamically stable infants or children.
- Current in vivo blood gas monitors are not yet reliable enough to replace traditional blood gas analysis, but they may provide information at a level of accuracy and reliability sufficient for trend analysis.
- Oximetry is the measurement of blood hemoglobin saturations using spectrophotometry. Hemoximetry is a laboratory procedure that requires an arterial blood sample. Pulse oximetry combines spectrophotometry with photoplethysmography to obtain a noninvasive measure of blood hemoglobin saturations.
- At best, pulse oximetry readings fall within ±3% to 5% of those obtained by hemoximetry.
- Dozens of technical factors affect the readings, limit the precision, or alter the performance of pulse oximeters. To interpret test results properly, clinicians must have in-depth knowledge of these factors.
- Capnometry is the measurement of CO_2 in respiratory gases. A capnometer is the device that actually measures the CO_2. Capnography is the graphic display of CO_2 levels as they change during breathing.
- A capnogram may be used to assess trends in alveolar ventilation, to identify $\dot{V}/\dot{Q}$ imbalance caused by cardiopulmonary disorders, to estimate physiological dead space, to detect esophageal intubation, and to determine the amount of blood flow during cardiac arrest.

References

1. Wahr JA, Tremper KK: Noninvasive oxygen monitoring techniques, Crit Care Clin 11:199, 1995.
2. American Association for Respiratory Care: Clinical practice guideline: sampling for arterial blood gas analysis, Respir Care 37:913, 1992.
3. Wiseman JD: Percutaneous collection of arterial blood for laboratory analysis, H11-A2, ed 2, Wayne, Penn, 1992, National Committee for Clinical Laboratory Standards.
4. Garner JS: Guideline for isolation precautions in hospitals, Infect Control Hosp Epidemiol 17:53, 1996.
5. Pillow K, Herrick IA: Pulse oximetry compared with Doppler ultrasound for assessment of collateral blood flow to the hand, Anesthesia 46:388, 1991.
6. Szaflarski NL: Preanalytic error associated with blood gas/pH measurement, Crit Care Nurse 16:89, 1996.
7. Ehrmeyer S: Blood gas preanalytical considerations: specimen collection, calibration, and controls, C27-A, Wayne, Penn, 1993, National Committee for Clinical Laboratory Standards.
8. Mahoney JJ, Harvey JA, Wong RI: Changes in oxygen measurements when whole blood is stored in iced plastic or glass syringes, Clin Chem 37:1244, 1991.
9. Hess D et al: The validity of assessing arterial blood gases 10 minutes after an F_{IO_2} change in mechanically ventilated patients without chronic pulmonary disease, Respir Care 30:1037, 1985.
10. Clark VL, Kruse JA: Arterial catheterization, Crit Care Clin 8:687, 1992.
11. Ermakov S, Hoyt JW: Pulmonary artery catheterization, Crit Care Clin 8:773, 1992.
12. Sladen A: Complications of invasive hemodynamic monitoring in the intensive care unit, Curr Probl Surg 25:69, 1988.
13. American Association for Respiratory Care: Clinical practice guideline: capillary blood gas sampling for neonatal and pediatric patients, Respir Care 39:1180, 1994.
14. MacIntyre NR et al: Accuracy and precision of a point-of-care blood gas analyzer incorporating optodes, Respir Care 41:800, 1996.
15. American Association for Respiratory Care: Clinical practice guideline: in vitro pH and blood gas analysis and hemoximetry, Respir Care 38:505, 1993.

16. Ehrmeyer S: Definitions of quantities and conventions related to blood pH and gas analysis, C12-A, Wayne, Penn, 1994, National Committee for Clinical Laboratory Standards.
17. Ehrmeyer S: Performance characteristics for devices measuring PO_2 and PCO_2 in blood samples, C21-A, Wayne, Penn, 1992, National Committee for Clinical Laboratory Standards.
18. Smith BL, Vender JS: Point-of-care testing, Respir Care Clin North Am 1:133, 1995.
19. Keffer JH: Economic considerations of point-of-care testing, Am J Clin Pathol 104:S107, 1995.
20. Wahr JA, Tremper KK, Diab M: Pulse oximetry, Respir Care Clin North Am 1:77, 1995.
21. Wahr JA et al: Accuracy and precision of a new, portable, handheld blood gas analyzer: the IRMA, J Clin Monit 12:317, 1996.
22. Goldsmith BM: Point-of-care in vitro diagnostic (IVD) testing: proposed guideline, AST2-P, Wayne, Penn, 1995, National Committee for Clinical Laboratory Standards.
23. American Association for Respiratory Care: Clinical practice guideline: transcutaneous blood gas monitoring for neonatal and pediatric patients, Respir Care 39:1176, 1994.
24. Wahr JA, Tremper KK: Noninvasive oxygen monitoring techniques, Crit Care Clin 11:199, 1995.
25. Frankin ML: Transcutaneous measurement of partial pressure of oxygen and carbon dioxide, Respir Care Clin North Am 1:119, 1995.
26. Peruzzi WT, Shapiro BA: Blood gas monitors, Respir Care Clin North Am 1:143, 1995.
27. Gilbert HC, Vender JS: Arterial blood gas monitoring, Crit Care Clin 11:233, 1995.
28. Uchida T et al: Clinical assessment of a continuous intra-arterial blood gas monitoring system, Can J Anaesth 41:64, 1994.
29. Hess D, Kacmarek RM: Techniques and devices for monitoring oxygenation, Respir Care 38:646, 1993.
30. Jones AR: Reference and selected procedures for the quantitative determination of hemoglobin in blood, H15-A2, ed 2, Wayne, Penn, 1994, National Committee for Clinical Laboratory Standards.
31. Mathews PJ: Co-oximetry, Respir Care Clin North Am 1:47, 1995.
32. Moyle JT: Uses and abuses of pulse oximetry, Arch Dis Child 74:77, 1996.
33. American Association for Respiratory Care: Clinical practice guideline: pulse oximetry, Respir Care 38:1406, 1991.
34. American Association for Respiratory Care: Clinical practice guideline: capnography/capnometry during mechanical ventilation, Respir Care 40:1321, 1995.
35. Stock MC: Capnography for adults, Crit Care Clin 11:219, 1995.
36. Schmitz BD, Shapiro BA: Capnography, Respir Care Clin North Am 1:107, 1995.

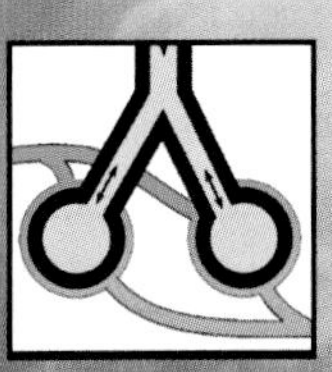

CHAPTER 17

Pulmonary Function Testing

F. Herbert Douce

In This Chapter You Will Learn:

- The principles used to perform spirometry and bronchial challenge testing and applied to measure lung volumes and diffusing capacity of the lung
- How to use pulmonary function data to evaluate patients and their respiratory care
- How to systematically review a pulmonary function report to identify patterns of pulmonary disease

Chapter Outline

Key Terms

diffusing capacity of the lung (DL)
diffusing capacity of the lung to alveolar volume ratio (DL_{CO}/V_A)
expiratory reserve volume (ERV)
forced expiratory flow at 25% ($FEF_{25\%}$) of FVC
forced expiratory flow at 50% ($FEF_{50\%}$) of FVC
forced expiratory flow at 75% ($FEF_{75\%}$) of FVC
forced expiratory flow between 25% and 75% of FVC ($FEF_{25\%-75\%}$)
forced expiratory flow between 75% and 85% of FVC ($FEF_{75\%-85\%}$)
forced expiratory flow between 200 mL and 1200 mL of FVC ($FEF_{200-1200}$)
forced expiratory volume in 1 second (FEV_1)
forced expiratory volume in 1 second to forced vital capacity ratio (FEV_1/FVC)
forced expiratory volume in half of a second ($FEV_{0.5}$)
forced inspiratory flow at 50% ($FIF_{50\%}$)
forced vital capacity (FVC)
functional residual capacity (FRC)
inspiratory capacity (IC)
inspiratory reserve volume (IRV)
maximal voluntary ventilation (MVV)
minute ventilation
obstructive pulmonary disease
peak expiratory flow rate (PEFR)
residual volume (RV)
restrictive pulmonary disease
tidal volume (V_T)

Continued

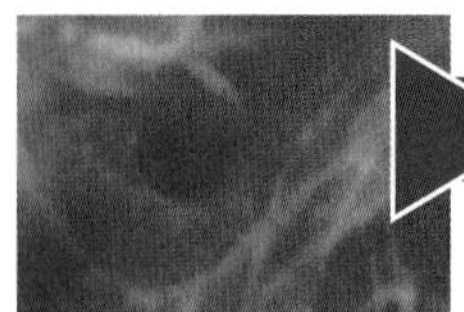

Key Terms—cont'd

total lung capacity (TLC)
vital capacity (VC)

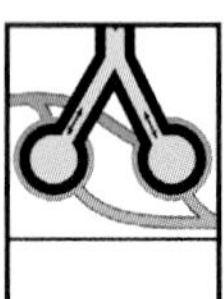

The primary function of the lungs is gas exchange. As mixed venous blood passes through the pulmonary circulation, the lungs add oxygen and remove excess carbon dioxide. Normal gas exchange results in normal arterial blood gases (ABGs). The ability of the lungs to perform gas exchange depends on the following four general physiological functions:

1. The diaphragm and thoracic muscles must be capable of expanding the thorax and lungs to produce a subatmospheric pressure.
2. The airways must be unobstructed to allow gas to flow into the lungs and reach the alveoli.
3. The cardiovascular system must circulate blood through the lungs.
4. Oxygen and carbon dioxide must be able to diffuse through the alveolar capillary membrane.

Pulmonary function tests can provide valuable information about these important components of gas exchange. A variety of measurements is available to aid in the diagnosis and assessment of pulmonary diseases, to determine the need for therapy, and to evaluate the effectiveness of respiratory care. For respiratory therapists (RTs), knowledge of these tests and the ability to interpret the measurements are essential for planning and implementing effective patient care.

▶ PULMONARY FUNCTION TESTING

A complete evaluation of the respiratory system includes pulmonary function testing and patient history, physical examination, chest x-ray examination, and ABG analysis. Pulmonary function test results become most meaningful when considered in the context of a complete evaluation. Diagnostic pulmonary function testing is performed in a laboratory setting and usually only on patients in a stable condition. There are three categories of pulmonary function tests, measuring (1) lung volumes and capacities, (2) flow rates of gases through the airways, and (3) the ability of the lungs to diffuse gases. A combination of these measurements provides a quantitative picture of lung function. Although pulmonary function tests do not diagnose specific pulmonary diseases, these tests identify the presence and degree of pulmonary impairments, as well as the type of pulmonary disease present. Some basic tests of pulmonary function can be performed at the bedside, and some tests also may provide immediate information about the effectiveness of therapy.

Purposes

The diagnostic and therapeutic roles of pulmonary function testing help clinicians answer some general questions about patients with lung disease (Box 17-1). In general, the purpose of pulmonary function testing is to identify and quantify pulmonary impairments.[1]

The specific purposes of pulmonary function assessment are as follows:

- *Identification and quantification of changes in pulmonary function.* The most common purpose of pulmonary function testing is to detect pulmonary disease, and over time pulmonary function tests help quantify the progress or the reversibility of the disease.[2]
- *Epidemiological surveillance for pulmonary disease.* Screening programs may detect pulmonary abnormalities caused by disease or environmental factors in general populations, occupational settings, smokers, or other high-risk groups. In addition, researchers

Box 17-1 • Basic Diagnostic and Therapeutic Questions for Clinical Pulmonary Function Testing

DIAGNOSTIC
- Is lung disease present?
- What type of lung impairment is present?
- What is the degree of lung impairment?
- Is more than one type of lung impairment present?
- Can multiple lung diseases be separated?

THERAPEUTIC
- Is therapy indicated?
- What treatments are most effective?
- To what degree is the disease reversible?
- Can treatments be evaluated?
- Is rehabilitation feasible?

have determined what normal pulmonary function is by measuring the pulmonary function of the average population.[3]

- *Assessment of postoperative pulmonary risk.* Preoperative testing can identify those patients who may have an increased risk of pulmonary complications after surgery.[4] Sometimes the risk for complications can be reduced by preoperative respiratory care.
- *Aid in the determination of pulmonary disability.*[5] Pulmonary function tests also can determine the degree of disability caused by lung diseases, including occupational diseases such as pneumoconiosis of coal workers. Some federal entitlement programs and insurance policies rely on pulmonary function tests to confirm claims for financial compensation.
- *Evaluation and quantification of therapeutic effectiveness.*[6] Pulmonary function tests may aid clinicians in selecting or modifying a specific therapeutic regimen or technique (e.g., bronchodilator medication, rehabilitation exercise protocol). Clinicians and researchers use pulmonary function tests to objectively measure changes in lung function before and after treatment.

Organization

In most pulmonary function laboratories, there are three components to pulmonary function testing: (1) measuring lung volumes and capacities, (2) measuring airway mechanics, and (3) measuring the diffusing capacity of the lung (DL). For each component, there are a variety of techniques and different types of equipment that make the measurements. When the purpose of the testing is to identify the presence and the degree of pulmonary impairment and the type of pulmonary disease, all three testing components are required. When the purpose of the testing is more limited, such as to assess postoperative pulmonary risk or to evaluate and quantify therapeutic effectiveness, the scope of measurement also is limited. Many pulmonary function laboratories also perform ABG analysis (see Chapter 16), and some laboratories provide more specialized and advanced tests, such as bronchial challenge tests and exercise stress tests (see Chapter 48).

Equipment

Measuring gas volumes and flow for pulmonary function testing can be accomplished using a variety of instruments and measurement principles. The types of instruments used for pulmonary function testing are outlined as follows:

I. Devices that measure gas volume
   A. Water-sealed spirometers
   B. Bellow spirometers
   C. Dry rolling seal spirometers
II. Devices that measure gas flow
   A. Pneumotachometers
   B. Thermistors
   C. Turbinometers
   D. Sonic devices
   E. Peak flow meters

Detailed descriptions and examples of each type of device are beyond the scope of this chapter and are available elsewhere.[7] Regardless of the type of device or the principle of measurement used, several important characteristics are common to all volume and flow measuring devices. Having an understanding of these common characteristics provides RTs the ability to select and use these devices properly. Every measuring instrument has capacity, accuracy, error, precision, linearity, and output.[8,9] The ideal instrument would have unlimited capacity to measure every pulmonary parameter, and it would have perfect accuracy and precision over its entire measurement range. Of course, there are no ideal instruments.

The *capacity* of an instrument refers to the range or limits of how much it can measure. Most instruments are designed with capacities to measure volumes and flow rates of all adults. The *accuracy* of a measuring instrument is how well it measures a known reference value. For volume measurements, standard reference values are provided by a graduated 3.0-L calibration syringe.[10,11] No measuring instrument is perfect, and there usually is an arithmetic difference between reference values and measured values. This difference is called the *error.* Accuracy and error are opposing terms; the greater the accuracy, the smaller the error. Accuracy and error are commonly expressed as percentages, with their sum always equaling 100%. To determine percent accuracy and percent error, several reference values are measured, and the mean of the measured values is computed and compared with the reference values according to the following equations:

$$\%\ \text{Accuracy} = \frac{\text{Mean measured value}}{\text{Reference value}} \times 100$$

or

$$\%\ \text{Error} = \frac{\text{Mean measured value - Reference value}}{\text{Reference value}} \times 100$$

Precision is synonymous with *reproducibility* and refers to the reliability of measurements. The *standard deviation* (SD) of the mean measured reference value is the statistic that indicates the precision of an instrument. *Linearity* refers to the accuracy of the instrument over its entire range of measurement, or its capacity. Some devices may accurately measure large volumes or high flow rates, but may be less accurate when measuring small volumes or low flow rates. To determine linearity, accuracy and precision are calculated at different points over the range (capacity) of the device.

Output includes the specific measurements made or computed by the instrument. Most volume and flow measuring devices measure the **forced vital capacity (FVC)** and **forced expiratory volume in 1 second (FEV_1)**. Others calculate a variety of forced expiratory flow (FEF) rates, and some measure **tidal volume (V_T)** and **minute ventilation.**

Diagnostic spirometers usually measure and calculate **vital capacity (VC)**, FVC, FEV_1, **peak expiratory flow rate (PEFR)**, and forced expiratory flow rates. Some measure and calculate **maximal voluntary ventilation (MVV)**. Some of these instruments may be a component of a laboratory system providing the volume or flow measuring capability for other diagnostic tests of pulmonary function. For example, they may be used with gas analyzers to measure **functional residual capacity (FRC)** and **total lung capacity** (TLC) or the inspiratory VC during the single breath diffusing capacity ($DL_{CO}SB$). Whether a spirometer is used in a diagnostic laboratory, a physician's office, or at the bedside in an intensive care unit, it should meet or exceed the national performance standards for volume and flow measuring devices.

In 1978, the American Thoracic Society (ATS) adopted the initial standards for diagnostic spirometers. These standards, which were updated in 1987 and 1994, have been adopted by other medical organizations and government agencies. Some spirometers have been independently evaluated against the ATS standards or compared with instruments that meet those standards. Regardless of the measuring principle used by the spirometer or the purpose of the patient testing, therapists should use only spirometers that meet or exceed the most current ATS performance standards. According to the ATS standards, when measuring a slow VC, the spirometer should be able to measure for up to 30 seconds, and for the FVC, the time capacity should be at least 15 seconds. When measuring the VC and forced expiratory volumes (FEV), a volume measuring spirometer should have a capacity of at least 8 L and should measure volumes with less than a 3% error or within 50 mL of a reference value, whichever is greater. These standards, even the 8-L standard for capacity, also apply to children. A diagnostic spirometer that measures flow should be at least 95% accurate (or within 0.2 L/sec, whichever is greater) over the entire 0 to 14 L/sec range of gas flow. A summary of the standards is provided in Table 17-1.

The spirometer standards also require spirometers to have a thermometer or to produce values corrected for body temperature, ambient pressure, and fully saturated with water vapor (BTPS); standards also require that a graphic recording be produced of sufficient size for diagnostic testing, validation, and hand measurements. For the diagnostic function, the scale of the volume axis must be 5 mm/L and the scale for the time axis must be 10 mm/sec. For validation and hand measurement functions, the scale of the volume axis must be 10 mm/L and the scale for the time axis must be 20 mm/sec. Most manufacturers have designed their spirometers to meet or exceed the validation and hand measurement standards. For quality control, the standards include verifying volume accuracy with a 3.0-L calibration syringe daily or every 4 hours, if the spirometer is in continuous use. Volume linearity should be verified quarterly over the entire volume range, and the recorder speed should be checked with a stopwatch quarterly.

Infection Control

Pulmonary function testing is safe, but a possibility of cross contamination exists, either from patients or from technologists. Standard precautions should be applied because of the potential exposure to saliva or mucus, which could possibly contain blood other potentially hazardous microorganisms. The use of proper low-resistance barrier filters and handwashing are important. RTs performing procedures on patients with potentially infectious airborne diseases should wear a personal respirator or a close-fitting surgical mask, especially if the testing itself induces coughing. The mouthpiece, tubing, and any parts of the spirometer that come into contact with any patient should be disposed, sterilized, or disinfected between patients. It is unnecessary to routinely clean the interior surface of the spirometer between patients.[12,13]

Table 17-1 ▶ ▶ 1994 Spirometer Performance Standards of the American Thoracic Society[10]

Test	Volume (L)	Flow (L/sec)	Accuracy	Time (sec)	Back Pressure (cm H_2O/L/sec)
VC	8 L	0-14	≤3% or 50 mL*	30	<1.5 at 14 L/sec
FVC	**	**	**	15	
FEV_1	**	**	**		
Flow	**	**	≤5% or 0.2 L/sec*		
MVV	250 L/min at 2 L/breath		2 L ±5%	12-15 ±1%	<10 at 14 L, 120 breaths/min

*Whichever is greater.
**Same as for VC.

▶ PRINCIPLES OF MEASUREMENT

For tests of pulmonary function, four important general principles must be considered. These are test specificity, sensitivity, validity, and reliability. Most tests of pulmonary function are not very specific, because several different diseases may cause the test result to be abnormal. This is a limitation of many pulmonary function tests, which explains why these tests identify a pattern of impairment rather than diagnose specific diseases. Some tests are extremely sensitive, and apparent healthy individuals may have an abnormal test result. However, some tests are not sensitive; individuals must be extremely sick to have an abnormal test result. To be meaningful, each test must be valid or the test is not measuring what it is intended to measure. When performing pulmonary function testing, strictly following testing procedures, ensuring patient effort and performance, and ensuring equipment accuracy and calibration will establish test validity. Test reliability is the consistency of the test results. A reliable test will produce consistent test results with some acceptable variability. To be reliable, each test must be performed more than once. Ensuring test validity and reliability is the most important role of the therapist. Test results that are not valid or not reliable can lead to misdiagnosis, mistreatment, and poor outcomes.

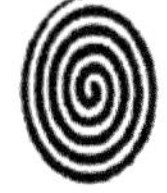

RULE OF THUMB

Never report test results that are not valid or not reliable!

Lung Volumes and Capacities

There are four lung volumes and four lung capacities.[14] A lung capacity consists of two or more lung volumes. The lung volumes are tidal volume, **inspiratory reserve volume (IRV)**, **expiratory reserve volume (ERV)**, and **residual volume (RV)**. The four lung capacities are TLC, **inspiratory capacity (IC)**, FRC, and the VC. These volumes and capacities are shown in Figure 17-1. The lung volumes that can be measured directly with a spirometer include tidal volume, IC, IRV, ERV, and VC. Because the RV cannot be exhaled, the RV, FRC, and TLC must be measured using indirect methods.

The tidal volume is measured directly from a spirogram (see Figure 17-1). For the purposes of ensuring test validity and standardization, the patient should be in a sitting position and wearing a nose clip. It sometimes takes the patient 2 to 3 minutes to become accustomed to the nose clip and mouthpiece. The patient breathes through a tight-fitting mouthpiece until a normal, rhythmic breathing pattern is established. Because the tidal volume will vary normally from breath to breath, an average tidal volume is a more reliable measurement. In the laboratory, an average tidal volume sometimes is measured during 3 minutes of quiet breathing while the spirometer records volumes and graphs volume and time. At the bedside, an average tidal volume usually is measured over 1 minute; the patient breathes normally into a spirometer that stores in a memory each volume exhaled for 1 minute and computes an average. An alternate approach is to measure the total volume of air exhaled for 1 minute ($\dot{V}_E$) and then divide by the breathing frequency (f) counted during the same period. The following formula can be used to calculate the tidal volume:

$$V_T = \frac{\dot{V}e}{f}$$

The IC is also measured directly from a spirogram. The patient is asked to inhale maximally at the end of a normal effortless exhalation. To ensure validity, a consistent resting expiratory level should be obvious on the spirogram before inhaling. To ensure reliability, the IC should be measured at least twice, and the two largest measurements should agree within 5%. Because the definition of IC is the maximal volume inhaled, the largest measurement is the patient's IC.

The ERV is measured directly from the spirogram (see Figure 17-1). The patient is asked to breathe normally for a few breaths and then exhale maximally. The ERV is that volume of air exhaled between the resting expiratory level and the maximal exhalation level on the spirogram. To ensure validity, a consistent resting expiratory level should be obvious on the spirogram before exhaling maximally. To ensure reliability, the ERV should be measured at least twice and the two largest measurements should agree within 5%. Because the definition of ERV is the maximal volume exhaled, the largest measurement is the patient's ERV.

The VC is the most commonly measured lung volume. There are several methods of measuring the VC. The VC can be measured during inspiration or during a slow prolonged expiration when air trapping is of concern. To measure the VC during inspiration, the patient exhales maximally and then inhales as deeply as possible. The volume of the maximal inspiration is the *inspiratory* VC. To measure the VC during expiration, the patient inhales maximally and then exhales maximally, taking all the time necessary to exhale completely. The exhaled volume is the *slow* VC. An alternate method is to measure the IC and the ERV and add these volumes together for a "combined" VC, but this method should be reserved only for patients who cannot otherwise execute the VC. The VC also is measured when it is exhaled forcefully and as rapidly as possible. This technique is called the *FVC*, and it is used to assess pulmonary mechanics.

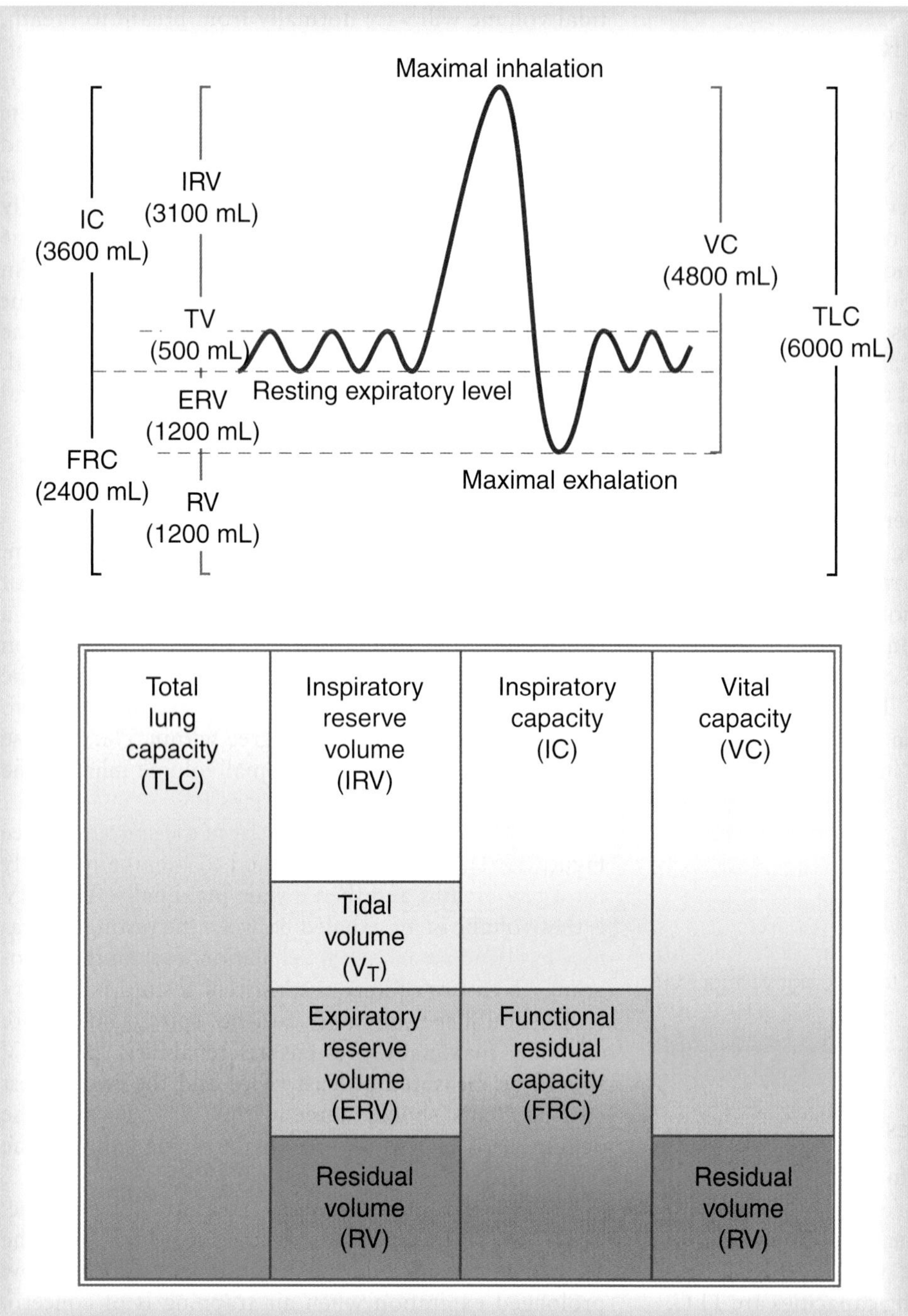

Figure 17-1
Lung volumes and capacities. Volumes listed are average normals for a young, healthy adult male.

Because the RV cannot be exhaled, neither it nor the FRC, or TLC, can be measured directly with a spirometer. There are three indirect techniques to measure these lung volumes: helium dilution, nitrogen washout, and body plethysmography. The helium dilution and nitrogen washout techniques measure whatever gas is in the lungs at the beginning of the test, if the gas is in communication with unobstructed airways. The body plethysmographic technique measures all the gas in the thorax at the resting expiratory volume. Because the plethysmographic technique measures all gas in the thorax, including gas that is trapped distal to obstructed airways or gas in the pleural space, the lung volume measured by this technique is called the *thoracic gas volume (TGV)*. In healthy individuals, the TGV is identical to the FRC measured by both the helium dilution and nitrogen washout techniques. Once the FRC is known, the RV can be calculated as the difference between the FRC and the ERV. The TLC also can be calculated by adding the RV to the VC.

The helium dilution technique for measuring lung volumes uses a closed, rebreathing circuit[15] (Figure 17-2). This technique is based on the assumptions that a known volume and concentration of helium in air begin

MINI CLINI

Why are FRC and RV Increased in Emphysema?

PROBLEM

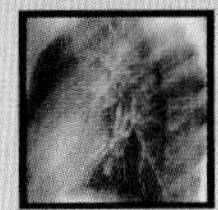

In the advanced stages of pulmonary emphysema, the FRC and the RV are increased; in addition, the VC is often decreased. Why do these changes occur?

SOLUTION

When the ventilatory muscles relax, the opposing forces of lung recoil and chest wall expansion determine the size of the FRC. Emphysema is characterized by a destruction of elastic tissue in the lung, which causes a lower lung recoil force. When lung recoil forces decrease, as in emphysema, chest wall expansion forces predominate, and the chest wall expands outward, pulling the lung with it. As the lung stretches to a larger volume, its recoil force increases, and eventually equilibrium is reestablished between the lung and chest wall. This new equilibrium occurs at an increased lung volume, so the FRC is increased. The RV is increased in emphysema because the VC is decreased because of small airway obstruction. When a person with emphysema tries to exhale completely, his or her bronchioles collapse, trapping air in the lungs and increasing the RV. An increased FRC is called *hyperinflation*, and an increased RV is called *air trapping*.

in the closed spirometer, that the patient has no helium in his or her lungs, and that an equilibration of helium can occur between the spirometer and the lungs. For the helium dilution procedure to be performed, a measurable volume of helium is added into the spirometer circuit, and the initial concentration of helium (F_iHe) is measured. Next, the valve is turned to connect the patient to the breathing circuit at a predetermined lung volume. The resting expiratory level of the FRC is a common point to begin the test. Starting the test at RV requires maximal expiratory effort by the patient and is not considered a reliable starting point. Although starting the test at the TLC level requires a maximal inspiration, TLC may be a reliable alternate beginning point.

The patient is connected to the helium-air mixture, and the concentration of helium is diluted slowly by the patient's lung volume. Wearing nose clips, the patient breathes normally in the closed circuit. Exhaled carbon dioxide is absorbed with soda lime, and oxygen is added at a rate equal to the patient's oxygen consumption. A constant volume is maintained to ensure accurate helium concentration measurements. The patient rebreathes the gas in the system until equilibrium of helium concentration is established. In healthy patients and those with a small FRC, equilibration occurs in 2 to 5 minutes. Patients with obstructive lung disease may require up to 20 minutes to equilibrate because of slow gas mixing in the lungs. The helium dilution time or the duration of the test is a gross index of the distribution of ventilation.

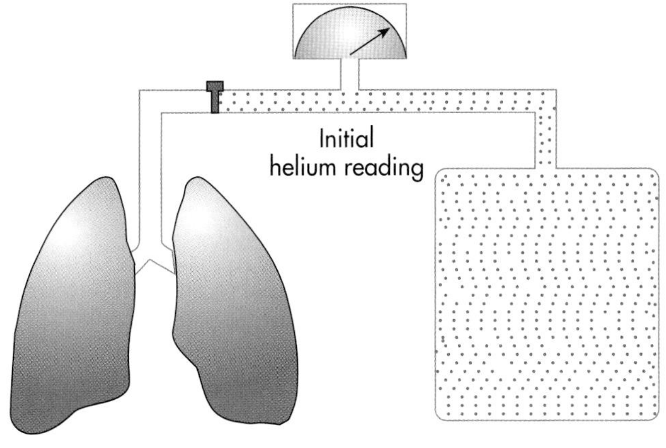

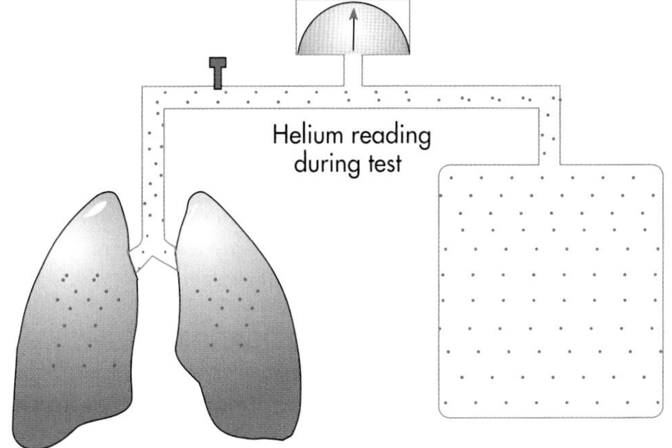

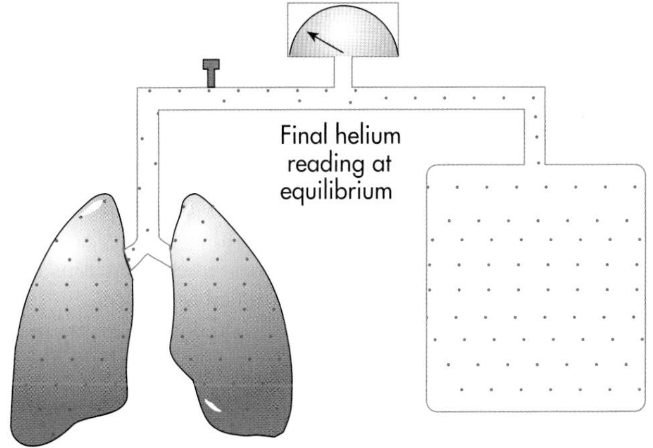

Figure 17-2
Helium dilution method for measuring the functional residual capacity, the residual volume, and the total lung capacity.

For the FRC to be calculated using the helium dilution technique, several observations must be made. These include the volume of helium added (vol He) to the closed spirometer, the initial helium concentration (F_iHe) before the patient is connected to the breathing

Static Lung Volumes

AARC Clinical Practice Guideline (Excerpts)*

INDICATIONS

Indications include the need to do the following:

- Diagnose restrictive disease patterns
- Differentiate between obstructive and restrictive disease patterns
- Assess response to therapeutic interventions (e.g., transplantation, radiation, chemotherapy, lobectomy)
- Aid in the interpretation of other lung function tests
- Make preoperative assessments in patients with impaired lung function that will be affected by surgery
- Evaluate pulmonary disability
- Quantify the amount of gas trapping by comparing results of different techniques

CONTRAINDICATIONS

- No apparent absolute contraindications exist; relative contraindications for spirometry include hemoptysis of unknown origin, untreated pneumothorax, unstable cardiovascular status, and thoracic and abdominal or cerebral aneurysms.
- With respect to whole-body plethysmography, factors such as claustrophobia, upper body paralysis, obtrusive body casts, or other conditions that immobilize or prevent the patient from fitting into or gaining access to the "body box" are a concern. In addition, the procedure may necessitate stopping intravenous therapy or supplemental oxygen.

HAZARDS AND COMPLICATIONS

- Nosocomial infection contracted from improperly cleaned tubing, mouthpieces, and pneumotachographs
- Hypoxemia from interruption of oxygen therapy with the body box
- Depressed ventilatory drive in susceptible subjects (i.e., CO_2 retainers) as a consequence of breathing 100% oxygen during the nitrogen washout; such patients should be carefully observed
- Hypercapnia and hypoxemia during helium-dilution FRC determinations as a consequence of failure to adequately remove CO_2 or add O_2

ASSESSMENT OF NEED

Determine that valid indications are present.

ASSESSMENT OF OUTCOME/TEST QUALITY

- Outcome and test quality are determined by ascertaining that the desired information has been generated for the specific indication and that validity and reproducibility have been ensured.
- Results are valid if the equipment functions acceptably and the subject is able to perform the maneuvers in an acceptable and reproducible fashion.
- Report of test results should contain a statement by the technician performing the test about test quality (including patient understanding of directions and effort expended) and, if appropriate, which recommendations were not met.
- Equipment calibration and quality control measures specific to measuring lung volumes should be applied and documented.

MONITORING

The following should be monitored during lung-volume determinations:

- Test data of repeated efforts (i.e., reproducibility of results) to ascertain the validity of results
- The patient for any adverse effects of testing (patients on supplemental oxygen may require periods of time to rest on oxygen between trials)

*For the complete guideline, see Respir Care 46:531, 2001.

circuit, the final helium concentration (F_fHe) after helium equilibrium between the spirometer and patient is established, the spirometer temperature, and the time necessary for helium equilibration to occur. The FRC can be calculated with the following equation:

$$FRC = (vol\ He \div F_iHe) \times [(F_iHe - F_fHe) \div F_fHe]$$

Corrections for temperature and helium absorption are normally applied.

All lung volumes and capacities must be reported under BTPS conditions. Volumes measured by spirometers are at ambient temperature, pressure, and saturated (ATPS) conditions and must be adjusted for the temperature difference between the spirometer and the patient's body temperature. This ATPS to BTPS adjustment can increase volumes 5% to 10%, and the difference is large enough to invalidate the test results, unless the correction is made.

Although helium is an inert gas with a negligible solubility in plasma, another correction is sometimes applied. A small amount of helium is thought to diffuse across the alveolar capillary membrane and is lost in the measurement of final helium concentration. To account for the loss, 30 mL of BTPS-corrected volume is subtracted for each minute of helium breathing, up to 200 mL for a 7-minute test.[16] Once these corrections are made, the RV can be calculated by subtracting the ERV from the FRC according to the following equation:

$$RV = FRC - ERV$$

The nitrogen washout technique uses a nonrebreathing or open circuit[17] (Figure 17-3). The technique is based on the assumptions that the nitrogen concentration in the lungs is 78% and in equilibrium with the atmosphere, that the patient inhales 100% oxygen, and that the oxygen replaces all of the nitrogen in the lungs. Similar to the helium dilution technique, the patient is connected to the system at either the resting expiratory level or the TLC. The lung volume when the patient begins breathing 100% oxygen and when exhaled gas is measured is the lung volume measured. The patient's exhaled gas is monitored, and its volume and nitrogen percentage are measured.

In general, two types of circuits are used to measure lung volumes with this technique. In one type of circuit, all of the exhaled gases are collected in a large container, where the volume and concentration of nitrogen are measured. In the second type of circuit, the volume and concentration of each exhaled breath are measured separately and stored in a memory; the sum of the volumes and the weighted average of the nitrogen concentration is calculated by a computer.

Wearing nose clips, the patient breathes 100% oxygen until nearly all of the nitrogen has been washed out of the lungs, leaving less than 2.5% nitrogen in the lungs. When the peak exhaled concentration of nitrogen is less than 2.5%, the patient exhales completely and the fractional concentration of alveolar nitrogen (F_AN_2) is noted. Similar to the helium technique, the time it

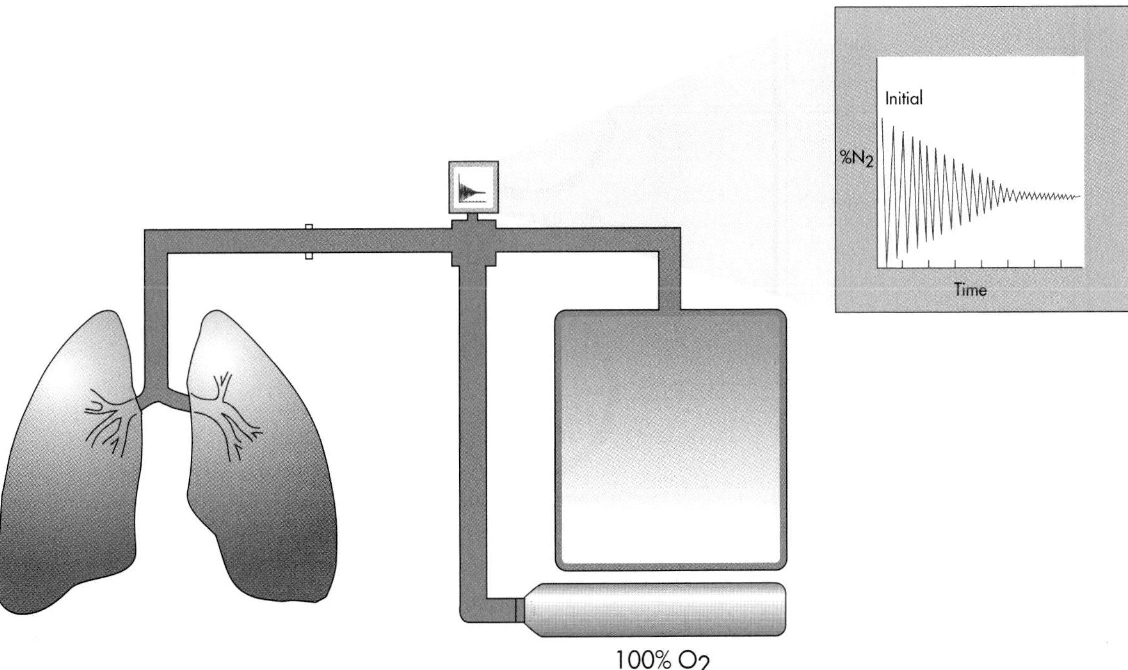

Figure 17-3
Nitrogen washout method for measuring the functional residual capacity, the residual volume, and the total lung capacity.

takes to wash out the nitrogen is approximately 2 to 5 minutes in healthy patients and longer in those with obstructive lung disease. The test must occur in a leak-proof circuit, because the presence of any air alters the measured nitrogen percentages.

For the FRC or TLC to be calculated by the nitrogen washout technique, several measurements must be made. These include the total volume of gas exhaled during the test (V_E), the fractional concentration of exhaled nitrogen in the total gas volume (F_EN_2), the fractional concentration of nitrogen in the alveoli at the end of the test (F_AN_2), and the spirometer temperature. The FRC (or TLC, if the test began at TLC) can be calculated with the following equation:

$$FRC = (V_E \times F_EN_2) \div (0.78 - F_AN_2)$$

The calculated FRC (or TLC) must be adjusted for the temperature difference between the spirometer and the patient's body temperature using the BTPS correction factor. During the test, some nitrogen from the plasma and body tissues is usually excreted and exhaled with lung nitrogen. For this reason, a correction is needed. The volume of tissue nitrogen excreted (V_{tis} in milliliters) is directly related to the time (t in minutes) of the test and weight (W in kilograms) of the patient. A correction for this extra nitrogen should be made according to the following formula:

$$V_{tis}\ (mL) = (0.1209\ \sqrt{t} - 0.0665) \times (W \div 70)$$

V_{tis} (mL) is subtracted from the BTPS-corrected lung volume. The RV is the difference between the ERV and the FRC.

The validity of the helium dilution and nitrogen washout techniques can be ensured by measuring known volumes accurately, such as a 3-L syringe, while recognizing that this method would not include oxygen consumption and oxygen titration for the helium method nor tissue nitrogen excretion for the nitrogen method. The reliability of these techniques can be established by repeated measurements of known volumes or healthy patients that agree within 5%.

When the FRC is measured by either He dilution or N_2 washout, any leak will increase the measured FRC and may be falsely interpreted as hyperinflation.

The whole-body plethysmography technique applies Boyle's law and uses volume and pressure changes to determine lung volume.[18] The plethysmograph consists of a sealed chamber in which the patient sits (Figure

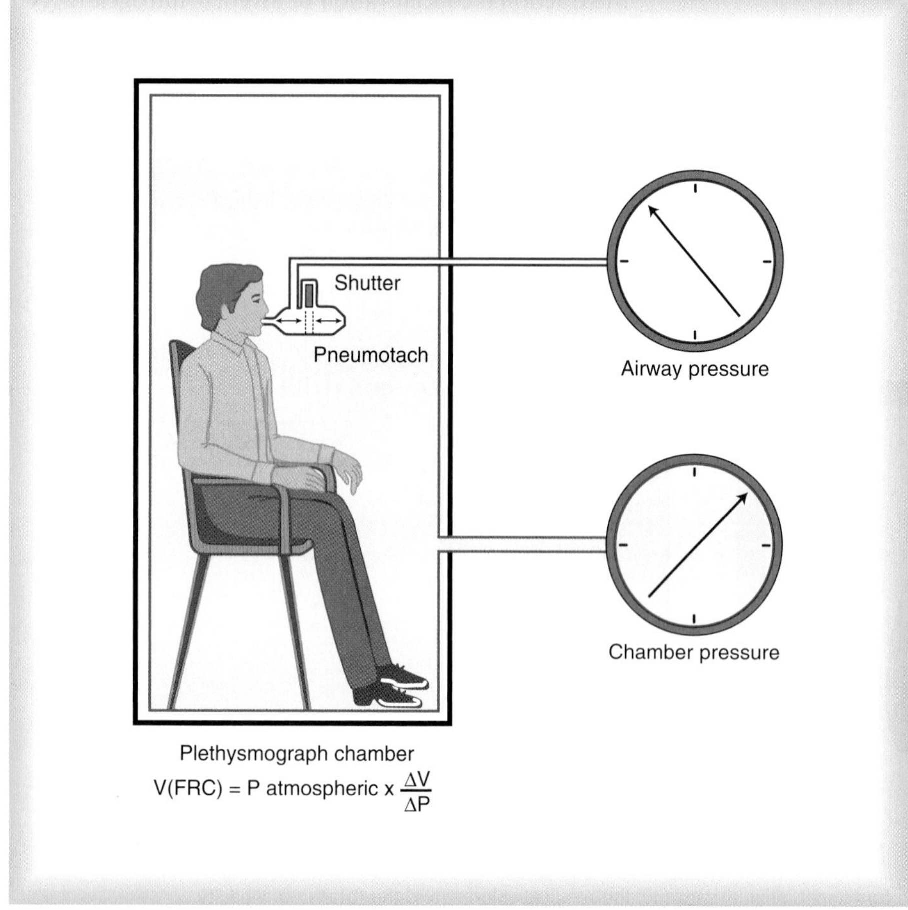

Figure 17-4 Body plethysmography method for measuring lung volumes. V is the change in gas volume in the lungs, as sensed by the chamber pressure manometer. P is the change in pressure produced by the respiratory efforts of breathing against the shutter, as sensed by the airway pressure manometer.

17-4). Pressure transducers (electronic manometers) measure pressure at the airway and in the chamber. An electronically controlled shutter allows the airway to be occluded periodically, thereby measuring airway pressure changes under conditions of no airflow. According to Boyle's law ($V \times P = k$), volume changes in the thorax create volume changes in the chamber, which in turn are reflected by pressure changes in the chamber. When the measurement of TGV is being conducted, the patient sits in the chamber, breathes normally through the mouth-

BODY PLETHYSMOGRAPHY

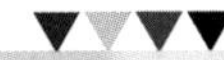

AARC Clinical Practice Guideline (Excerpts)*

INDICATIONS

Body plethysmographic determination of volume thoracic gas (VTG), airway resistance (Raw), and specific airway conductance (SGaw) may be indicated for the following:

- Measurement of lung volumes to distinguish between restrictive and obstructive processes
- Evaluation of obstructive lung diseases, such as bullous emphysema and cystic fibrosis, which may produce artifactually low results if measured by helium dilution or N_2 washout
- Measurement of lung volumes when multiple repeated trials are required or when the subject is unable to perform multibreath tests
- Evaluation of resistance to airflow
- Determination of the response to bronchodilators (Raw, SGaw, and VTG)
- Determination of bronchial hyperreactivity in response to methacholine, histamine, or isocapnic hyperventilation (VTG, Raw, and SGaw)
- After the course of disease and response to treatment

CONTRAINDICATIONS

The following are relative contraindications to body plethysmography:

- Mental confusion, muscular incoordination, body casts, or other conditions that prevent the subject from entering the plethysmograph cabinet or from adequately performing the required maneuvers (i.e., panting against a closed shutter)
- Claustrophobia that may be aggravated by entering the plethysmograph cabinet
- Presence of devices or other conditions, such as continuous intravenous infusions with pumps or other equipment that will not fit into the plethysmograph, that should not be discontinued, or that might interfere with pressure changes (e.g., chest tube, transtracheal O_2 catheter, ruptured eardrum)
- Continuous oxygen therapy that should not be temporarily discontinued

HAZARDS AND COMPLICATIONS

- VTG and Raw measurements require the subject to pant against a closed shutter; improper panting technique may result in excessive intrathoracic pressures
- Enclosure in the plethysmograph may cause symptoms of claustrophobia
- Prolonged confinement in the plethysmograph chamber could result in hypercapnia or hypoxia; however, because of the limited length of the test and the fact that the plethysmograph must be vented periodically, this is an uncommon occurrence
- Transmission of infection is possible through improperly cleaned equipment (i.e., mouthpieces) or as a consequence of the inadvertent spread of droplet nuclei or body fluids (patient-to-patient or patient-to-technologist)

ASSESSMENT OF NEED

The need for body plethysmography is based on the presence of the aforementioned test indications.

ASSESSMENT OF TEST QUALITY

- Each laboratory should standardize procedures and demonstrate intertechnician reliability. Test results can be considered valid only if they are derived according to and conform to established laboratory control and quality assurance protocols. These protocols should address test standardization and reproducibility criteria that include the methodology used to derive and report VTG and airway mechanics.
- Results are valid if the equipment functions acceptably and the subject is able to perform the maneuvers in an acceptable and reproducible fashion.

Continued

BODY PLETHYSMOGRAPHY—CONT'D

AARC Clinical Practice Guideline (Excerpts)*

- VTG maneuvers may be considered acceptable when the following occurs:
  - The displayed or recorded tracing indicates proper panting technique; the Pmouth/Pbox loop (closed shutter) should be closed or nearly so. The patient should support his or her cheeks with the hands to prevent pressure changes induced by the mouth.[20] This should be done without supporting the elbows or elevating the shoulders.
  - Recorded pressure changes should be within the calibrated pressure range of each transducer. The entire tracing should be visible. Pressure changes that are too large or too small may yield erroneous results.
  - There should be evidence of thermal equilibrium: tracings should not drift on the display or recording.
  - The panting frequency should be approximately 1 Hz. Nonpanting maneuvers may be acceptable if the plethysmograph system is specifically designed to perform such a maneuver.
- The following should be remembered about the reported VTG:
  - It should be averaged from a minimum of three to five separate, acceptable panting maneuvers.
  - It should be calculated using tangents or angles that agree within 10% of the mean; widely varying tangents or angles should be averaged and reported as variable.
  - It should indicate whether the thoracic volume was at FRC or at another level.
  - It should be compared with other lung volume determinations (He dilution, N_2 washout) if performed.
  - From some systems, it should be corrected for patient weight.
- A slow VC maneuver and its subdivisions, IC and ERV, should be performed during the same testing session. The ERV, IC, and IVC can be measured before disconnecting the patient from the measuring system. Alternatively, the patient can be disconnected and the ERC, IC, and IVC performed immediately afterward.
  - The largest VC obtained should be used for calculation of derived lung volumes (i.e., TLC, RV, and RV/TLC%).
  - The IC and ERV from the largest acceptable VC should be used to calculate derived volumes.
  - TLC may be calculated from the FRC: TLC = FRC + IC or TLC = RV + VC.
  - RV may be calculated from the plethysmograph FRC: RV = FRC - ERV or RV = TLC - VC.
- Raw and SGaw maneuvers may be considered acceptable if they meet criteria.
  - The open-shutter panting maneuver should show a relatively closed loop, particularly in the range of +0.5 to -0.5 L/sec.
  - The panting frequency during serial measurements in a given patient should be kept the same to aid in interpretation. Consensus of the group suggests a range of 1.5 to 3.0 Hz.
- The following should be remembered about the reported Raw and SGaw:
  - They should be calculated from the ratio of closed- and open-shutter tangents for each maneuver.[21] Airway resistance and lung volume are interdependent in a nonlinear fashion.
  - They should be averaged from three to five separate, acceptable maneuvers; reproducibility should be within 10%.
  - They should have the open-shutter tangent (V/Pbox) measured between flows of +0.5 and -0.5 L/sec. For loops that display hysteresis, the inspiratory limbs may be used.
  - The SGaw should be calculated using the VTG at which the shutter was closed for each individual maneuver.
- Report of test results should contain a statement by the technician performing the test about test quality and, if appropriate, which recommendations were not met.
- Equipment calibration and quality control measures specific to plethysmography should be applied and documented.

➤ MONITORING

- The final report should contain a statement regarding test quality.
- The final report should contain the VTG, Raw, and SGaw, if performed. If the VTG is measured at a lung volume other than FRC, both values should be reported.
- If the FRC is measured by more than one method, the report should indicate how lung volumes are reported.

*For complete guideline, see Respir Care 46:506, 2001.

piece, and then holds his cheeks and pants.[19] During the panting, the technologist closes the airway shutter and measures the airway pressure changes (ΔP) and the chamber volume changes (ΔV). As applied to whole-body plethysmography, the following equation is true:

$$TGV = P_B \times (\Delta V \div \Delta P)$$

where P_B is the barometric pressure in cm H_2O.

Because the body plethysmographic method of measuring FRC actually measures the TGV, the value obtained for some patients may be somewhat larger than those resulting from either the helium dilution or nitrogen washout techniques. Such a difference occurs whenever there is gas in the thorax that is not in communication with patent airways, as might be the case in pneumothorax, pneumomediastinum, or emphysema. The RV is the difference between the TGV and the ERV, and the TLC is the sum of the RV and the VC, or the sum of the TGV and the IC.

Pulmonary Mechanics: Spirometry

The tests of pulmonary mechanics include measurements of FEV, forced inspiratory flow rates (FIF), FEF, and the MVV. Measuring pulmonary mechanics is assessing the ability of the lungs to move large volumes of air quickly to identify airway obstruction. Some measurements are aimed at large intrathoracic airways, some are aimed at small airways, and some assess obstruction throughout the lungs.

The FVC is the most commonly performed test of pulmonary mechanics, and many measurements are made while the patient is performing the FVC maneuver, which is shown in Figure 17-5. Measuring FVC often occurs under baseline or untreated conditions. For baseline testing, patients should temporarily abstain from bronchodilator medications. When a patient's baseline results show airway obstruction, performing FVC following treatment, such as bronchodilator aerosol, can help determine if the treatment is effective. The FVC maneuver is also performed repeatedly during bronchial provocation testing. Although performing FVC is a safe procedure, some adverse reactions have occurred. These include pneumothorax,[22] syncope (fainting), chest pain, symptoms of paroxysmal coughing, and bronchospasm associated with exercise-induced asthma.[23] There are few contraindications to performing FVC maneuvers, and they are not considered absolute. These contra-

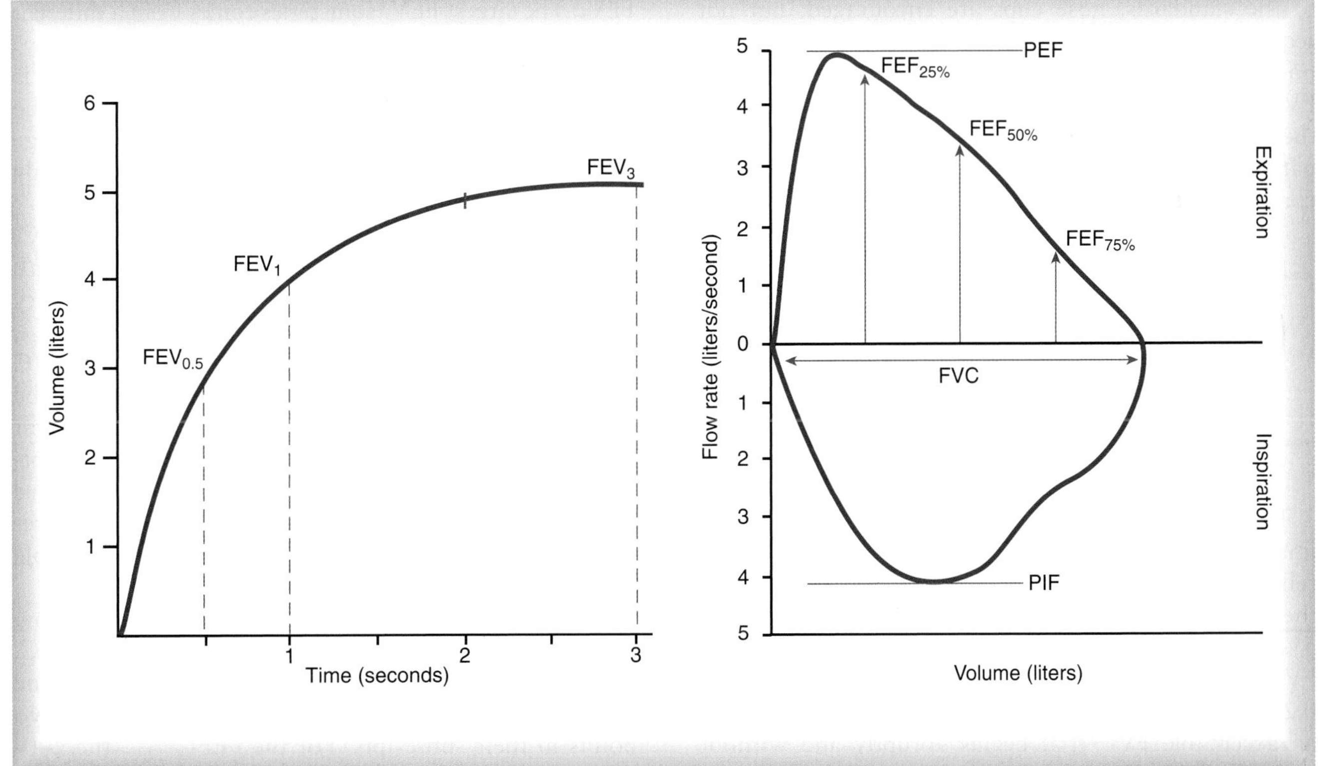

Figure 17-5
Forced vital capacity, forced expiratory volumes, and flow rates. **A**, The forced vital capacity on a volume-time graph. **B**, The forced vital capacity on a flow-volume graph.

indications include hemoptysis of unknown origin; untreated pneumothorax; and unstable cardiovascular status, which includes thoracic, abdominal, or cerebral aneurysms.[6] Patients who have recently had cataracts removed may be at risk because of an increase in cerebral pressure. Performing the FVC on patients who are acutely ill or who have recently smoked a cigarette may hinder test validity.

National professional standards for performing the FVC and for ensuring validity and reliability of the measurements and accuracy and precision of the measuring equipment have been adopted by the ATS, the American Association for Respiratory Care, and other professional and government agencies.[6,24-26] The FVC may be measured on a spirometer that measures volumes or flows, that presents a graph of volume and time or flow and volume, that is mechanical or electronic, and that has a calculator or computer. The forced expiratory VC sometimes is followed by a forced inspiratory VC to produce a complete loop of forced breathing.

The FVC is an effort-dependent maneuver that requires careful patient instruction, understanding, coordination, and cooperation. Spirometry standards for FVC specify that patients must be instructed in the FVC maneuver, that the appropriate technique be demonstrated, and that enthusiastic coaching occur. When measuring the FVC, the tester needs to coach the preceding IC as enthusiastically as the FVC. According to the standards, nose clips are encouraged, but not required. Patients may be tested in the sitting or standing position, although standing usually produces a larger FVC as compared with sitting. It is recommended that the position be consistent for repeat testing of the same patient. FVC should be converted to body temperature conditions and reported as liters under BTPS conditions.

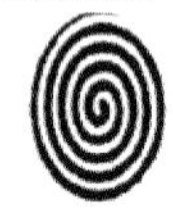

RULE OF THUMB

If you don't inhale it, you can't exhale it. So, coach the preceding IC as enthusiastically as the FVC.

To ensure validity, each patient must perform a minimum of three acceptable FVC maneuvers. To ensure reliability, the largest FVC and second largest FVC from the acceptable trials should not vary by more than 5% (expressed as a percentage of the largest observed FVC regardless of the trial on which it occurred) or 0.200 L, whichever is greater. The forced exhalation of an acceptable FVC trial begins abruptly and without hesitation. A satisfactory start of expiration is characterized by an extrapolated volume less than 5% of FVC or 0.150 L, whichever is greater (Figure 17-6). An acceptable FVC trial also is smooth, continuous, and complete. A cough, an inspiration, a Valsalva maneuver, a leak, or an obstructed mouthpiece while a FVC maneuver is being performed will disqualify the trial. The FVC must be completely exhaled, or an exhalation time of at least 6 seconds must occur (longer times are commonly needed for patients with airway obstruction). An end-expiratory plateau must be obvious in the volume-time curve; the former objective standard was less than 40 mL exhaled for at least 2 seconds of exhalation. Consistent with its definition, the largest acceptable FVC (BTPS) measured of the set of three acceptable trials is the patient's FVC.

During FVC testing several other measurements are also made. The FEV_1 is a measurement of the volume exhaled in the first second of the FVC (see Figure 17-2, *A*). To ensure validity of the FEV_1, the measurement must originate from a valid FVC trial. The first second of forced exhalation begins at the *zero time point* (see Figure 17-6). The volume exhaled before the zero time point is called the *extrapolated volume*. To be valid, no more than 5% of the VC, or 150 mL, is allowed to be exhaled before the zero time point. To ensure reliability of the FEV_1, the largest FEV_1 and second largest FEV_1 from the acceptable trials should not vary by more than 5% (expressed as a percentage of the largest observed FEV_1 regardless of the trial on which it occurred) or 0.100 L, whichever is greater. Consistent with its definition, the largest FEV_1 (BTPS) measured is the patient's FEV_1. The largest FEV_1 sometimes comes from a different trial than the largest FVC.

The $\%FEV_1/FVC$, also called the FEV_1/FVC ratio, is calculated by dividing the patient's largest FEV_1 by the patient's largest FVC and converting it to a percentage (by multiplying by 100). The two values do not necessarily have to come from the same trial.

All other measurements that originate from the FVC, such as PEFR, **forced expiratory flow between 200 mL and 1200 mL of FVC ($FEF_{200\text{-}1200}$)**, **forced expiratory flow between 25% and 75% of FVC ($FEF_{25\%\text{-}75\%}$)**, **forced expiratory flow between 75% and 85% of FVC ($FEF_{75\%\text{-}85\%}$)**, and/or the instantaneous FEF should be obtained from the single *best test*, or *best curve*. The best test curve is defined as the trial that meets the acceptability criteria and gives the largest sum of FVC plus FEV_1. The validity and reliability of these other measurements are based on their origin from a valid and reliable FVC.

The $FEF_{200\text{-}1200}$ and $FEF_{25\%\text{-}75\%}$ represent average flow rates that occur during specific intervals of the FVC. Both measurements can be made on a volume-time spirogram as the slope of a line connecting the two points in their subscripts. For the $FEF_{200\text{-}1200}$, the 200-mL point and the 1200-mL point are identified. A straight line is drawn connecting these points, and the line is extended to intersect two vertical time lines 1 second apart on the graph (Figure 17-7). The volume

SPIROMETRY

AARC Clinical Practice Guideline (Excerpts)*

➤ INDICATIONS

The indications for spirometry include the need to do the following:

- Detect the presence or absence of lung dysfunction suggested by history or physical signs and symptoms and/or the presence of other abnormal diagnostic tests (e.g., chest radiograph, ABGs)
- Quantify the severity of known lung disease
- Assess the change in lung function over time or following administration of or change in therapy
- Assess the potential effects or response to environmental or occupational exposure
- Assess the risk for surgical procedures known to affect lung function
- Assess impairment and/or disability (e.g., for rehabilitation, legal reasons, military)

➤ CONTRAINDICATIONS

Circumstances listed here could affect the reliability of spirometry measurements. In addition, forced expiratory maneuvers may aggravate these conditions, which may make test postponement necessary until the medical condition resolves. The following are some relative contraindications to performing spirometry:

- Hemoptysis of unknown origin (forced expiratory maneuver may aggravate the underlying condition)
- Pneumothorax
- Unstable cardiovascular status (forced expiratory maneuver may worsen angina or cause changes in blood pressure) or recent myocardial infarction or pulmonary embolus
- Thoracic, abdominal, or cerebral aneurysms (danger of rupture resulting from increased thoracic pressure)
- Recent eye surgery (e.g., cataract)
- Presence of an acute disease process that might interfere with test performance (e.g., nausea, vomiting)
- Recent surgery of thorax or abdomen

➤ HAZARDS AND COMPLICATIONS

Although spirometry is a safe procedure, untoward reactions may occur, and the value of the test data should be weighed against potential hazards. The following have been reported anecdotally:

- Pneumothorax
- Increased intracranial pressure
- Syncope, dizziness, light-headedness
- Chest pain
- Paroxysmal coughing
- Contraction of nosocomial infections
- Oxygen desaturation resulting from interruption of oxygen therapy
- Bronchospasm

➤ ASSESSMENT OF NEED

Need is assessed by determining that valid indications are present.

➤ ASSESSMENT OF TEST QUALITY

Spirometry performed for the listed indications is valid only if the spirometer functions acceptably and the subject is able to perform the maneuvers in an acceptable and reproducible fashion. All reports should contain a statement about the technician's assessment of test quality and specify which acceptability criteria were not met.

➤ *QUALITY CONTROL*

- Volume verification (i.e., calibration): At least daily before testing, use a calibrated known-volume syringe with a volume of at least 3 L to ascertain that the spirometer reads a known volume accurately. The known volume should be injected and/or withdrawn at least three times, at flows that vary between 2 and 12 L/sec (3-L injection times of approximately 1 second, 6 seconds, and somewhere between 1 and 6 seconds). The tolerance limits for an acceptable calibration are ±3% of the known volume. Thus for a 3-L calibration syringe, the acceptable recovered range is 2.91 to 3.09 L. The practitioner is encouraged to exceed this guideline whenever possible (i.e., reduce the tolerance limits to <±3%).
- Leak test: Volume-displacement spirometers must be evaluated for leaks daily. One recommendation is that any volume change of more than 10 mL/min while the spirometer is under at least 3 cm H_2O pressure be considered excessive.
- A spirometry procedure manual should be maintained.

Continued

SPIROMETRY—CONT'D

AARC Clinical Practice Guideline (Excerpts)*

- A log that documents daily instrument calibration, problems encountered, corrective action required, and system hardware and/or software changes should be maintained.
- Computer software for measurement and computer calculations should be checked against manual calculations if possible. In addition, biological laboratory standards (i.e., healthy, nonsmoking individuals) can be tested periodically to ensure historic reproducibility, to verify software upgrades, and to evaluate new or replacement spirometers.
- The known-volume syringe should be checked for accuracy at least quarterly using a second known-volume syringe, with the spirometer in the patient-test mode. This validates the calibration and ensures that the patient-test mode operates properly.
- For water-seal spirometers, water level and paper tracing speed should be checked daily. The entire range of volume displacement should be checked quarterly.

➤ *QUALITY ASSURANCE*

- Each laboratory or testing site should develop, establish, and implement quality assurance indicators for equipment calibration and maintenance and patient preparation.
- Methods should be devised and implemented to monitor technician performance (with appropriate feedback) while obtaining, recognizing, and documenting acceptability criteria.

➤ MONITORING

- The following should be evaluated during the performance of spirometric measurements to ascertain the validity of the results:
  - Acceptability of maneuver and reproducibility of FVC, FEV_1
  - Level of effort and cooperation by the subject
  - Equipment function or malfunction (e.g., calibration)
- The final report should contain a statement about test quality.
- Spirometry results should be subject to ongoing review by a supervisor, with feedback to the technologist.
- Quality assurance and/or quality improvement programs should be designed to monitor technician competency, both initially and ongoing.

*For the complete guideline, see Respir Care 41:629, 1996.

of air measured between the two time lines is the $FEF_{200\text{-}1200}$ in liters per second. The volume measured must be corrected to BTPS.

The $FEF_{25\%\text{-}75\%}$ is a measure of the flow during the middle portion of the FVC, or the time necessary to exhale the middle 50%. For the $FEF_{25\%\text{-}75\%}$, the VC of the best curve is multiplied by 25% and 75%, and the points are identified on the tracing. A straight line is drawn connecting these points, and the line is extended to intersect two vertical time lines 1 second apart on the graph. The volume of air measured between the two time lines is the $FEF_{25\%\text{-}75\%}$ in liters per second. The volume measured must be corrected to BTPS (Figure 17-8).

The PEFR is difficult to identify on a volume-time graph of the FVC. The peak flow is the slope of the tangent to the steepest portion of the FVC curve. The PEFR is easy to identify on a flow-volume graph as the highest point on the graph[27] (see Figure 17-2, *B*). The PEFR is sometimes measured independently of the FVC with a peak flow meter. These devices are designed to indicate only the greatest expiratory flow rate. The validity of PEFR is based on a preceding inspiration to TLC and a maximal effort. The FVC principles of ensuring reliability should apply to measurements of PEFR. The two largest repeated measurements should agree within 5%.

In addition to PEFR, the other instantaneous flow rates, such as **forced expiratory flow at 25% ($FEF_{25\%}$)**, **forced expiratory flow at 50% ($FEF_{50\%}$)**, and **forced expiratory flow at 75% ($FEF_{75\%}$)**, during a FVC are graphed on a flow-volume curve. When the FVC is followed by a forced inspiratory VC, a flow-volume loop is produced (see Figure 17-2, *B*). On the flow-volume loop, the maximal **forced inspiratory flow rate at 50% ($FIF_{50\%}$)** of the VC can be measured and compared with the $FEF_{50\%}$.

Methacholine Challenge Testing

AARC Clinical Practice Guideline (Excerpts)*

➤ INDICATIONS

Indications for testing include the need to do the following:

- Exclude the diagnosis of airway hyperreactivity
- Evaluate occupational asthma
- Assess the severity of hyperresponsiveness
- Determine the relative risk of developing asthma
- Assess the response to therapeutic interventions

➤ CONTRAINDICATIONS

The following are absolute contraindications to methacholine challenge testing:

- Presence of severe ventilatory impairment, defined as FEV_1 less than 50% predicted normal or less than 1.0 L
- Heart attack or stroke within the last 3 months
- Known aortic or cerebral aneurysm
- Uncontrolled hypertension, defined as systolic pressure greater than 200 mm Hg and/or diastolic pressure greater than 110 mm Hg

Relative contraindications include the following:

- Presence of moderate ventilatory impairment, defined as FEV_1 greater than 50% predicted normal or greater than 1.5 L, but less than 60% predicted
- Inability to perform spirometry
- Significant response to inhaling the diluent
- Recent respiratory tract infection, defined as within 2 to 6 weeks
- Current use of cholinesterase-inhibitor medication
- Pregnancy and lactation
- Recent ingestion of foods or medications that contain caffeine or other factors that may confound the test rest results

➤ HAZARDS AND COMPLICATIONS

Possible hazards or untoward reactions include the following:

- Bronchoconstriction
- Hyperinflation
- Severe coughing
- Dizziness, light-headedness
- Chest pain
- Nosocomial infection contracted from improperly cleaned tubing, mouthpieces, and pneumotachographs

➤ ASSESSMENT OF NEED

Need is assessed by determining that valid indications are present.

➤ ASSESSMENT OF OUTCOME/TEST QUALITY

- Outcome and test quality are determined by ascertaining that the desired information has been generated for the specific indication and that validity and reproducibility have been ensured.
- Results are valid if the equipment functions acceptably and the subject is able to perform the maneuvers in an acceptable and reproducible fashion.
- Report of test results should contain a statement by the technician performing the test about test quality (including patient understanding of directions and effort expended) and, if appropriate, which recommendations were not met.
- Equipment calibration and quality control measures specific to methacholine challenge should be applied and documented.

➤ MONITORING

- The FEV_1 is the primary variable to be monitored. Breath sounds, pulse rate, pulse oximetry, and/or blood pressure should be monitored. Patients should not be left unattended.
- Test data of repeated efforts (i.e., reproducibility of results) to ascertain the validity of results.
- Monitor the patient for a positive response to provocation, defined as a decrease in FEV_1 greater than 20% from baseline.

*For the complete guideline, see Respir Care 46:523, 2001.

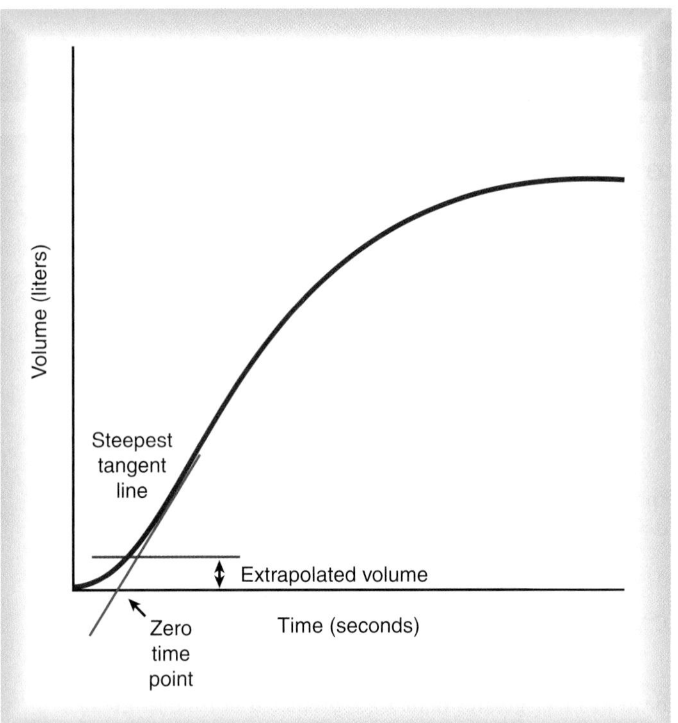

Figure 17-6
Extrapolated volume and zero time point determination.

MINI CLINI

Decreased FVC and FEV1: Is It Obstruction or Restriction?

PROBLEM

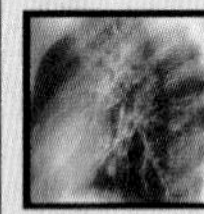

Both obstructive and restrictive diseases may exhibit decreased FVC and FEV_1. How can the two kinds of patterns be differentiated?

SOLUTION

FVC and FEV_1 are reduced in both obstructive and restrictive diseases for different reasons. With restrictive disease, lung expansion is reduced. If a person can inhale only a small volume, then he or she can exhale only a small volume. All lung volumes are smaller than normal, including the TLC, FVC, and FEV_1.

With obstructive disease, there is airway obstruction, which slows expiratory flow. FEV_1 is reduced because of the increased airway resistance, which decreases expiratory flow rates. FVC is reduced because airway obstruction in the bronchioles causes air trapping in the lung. If a person cannot exhale all of his or her air because some is trapped in the lungs, then the volume he or she does exhale is reduced.

To differentiate between obstructive and restrictive patterns of impairment, compare the FEV_1 with the FVC using the FEV_1/FVC ratio. Only those with airway obstruction will exhale less than 70% of their FVC in the first second. Those with restrictive disease and/or healthy lungs will be able to exhale more than 70% of their FVC during the first second.

Another measurement of pulmonary mechanics is the *MVV*. The MVV is another effort-dependent test for which the patient is asked to breathe as deeply and as rapidly as possible for at least 12 seconds. The MVV is a test that reflects patient cooperation and effort, the ability of the diaphragm and thoracic muscles to expand the thorax and lungs, and airway patency. The patient usually stands with a chair behind him or her and with nose clips in place. After a demonstration of the expected breathing pattern is performed, the patient should be instructed to breathe as rapidly and as deeply as possible for 12 or 15 seconds. The patient's breathing is measured on a spirogram (Figure 17-9) or electronically for the specific number of seconds (t) and the volume (V) breathed when the MVV is converted to liters per minute. As with all volumes measured on a spirometer, the recorded values should be in BTPS conditions.

Diffusing Capacity

The third major category of pulmonary function testing is measuring the ability of the lungs to transfer gases across the alveolar-capillary membrane. The **diffusing capacity of the lung** (DL) is sometimes called the *transfer factor*. Carbon monoxide (CO) is the gas normally used to measure the DL. The diffusing capacity of the lung for carbon monoxide (DL_{CO}) is expressed in mL/min/mm Hg under standard temperature and pressure and dry conditions (STPD). In general, DL_{CO} is the difference between the volume of CO inhaled (FICO) and the

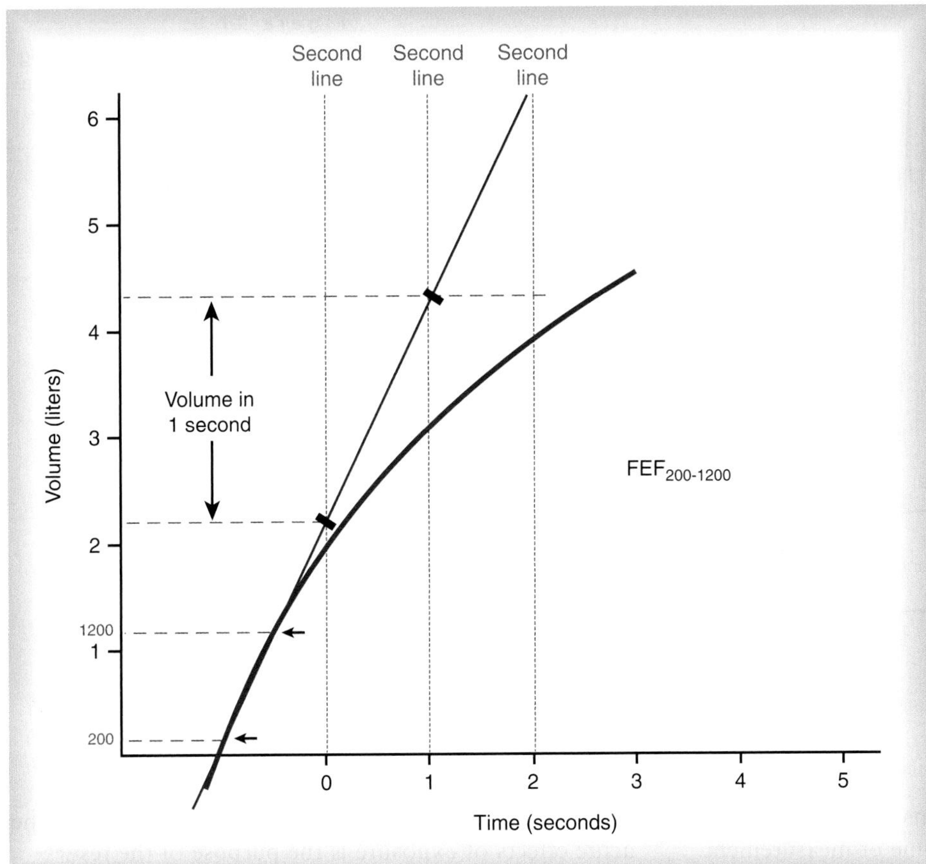

Figure 17-7
Forced expiratory flow rate 200 to 1200 mL.

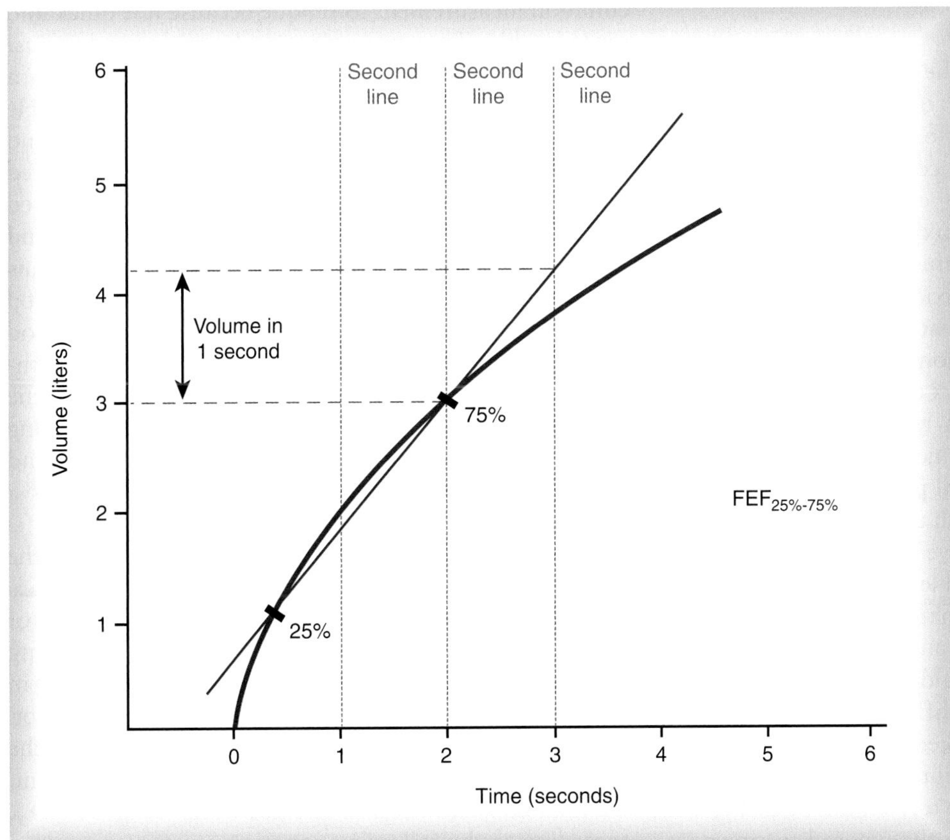

Figure 17-8
Forced expiratory flow rate 25% to 75% of the FVC.

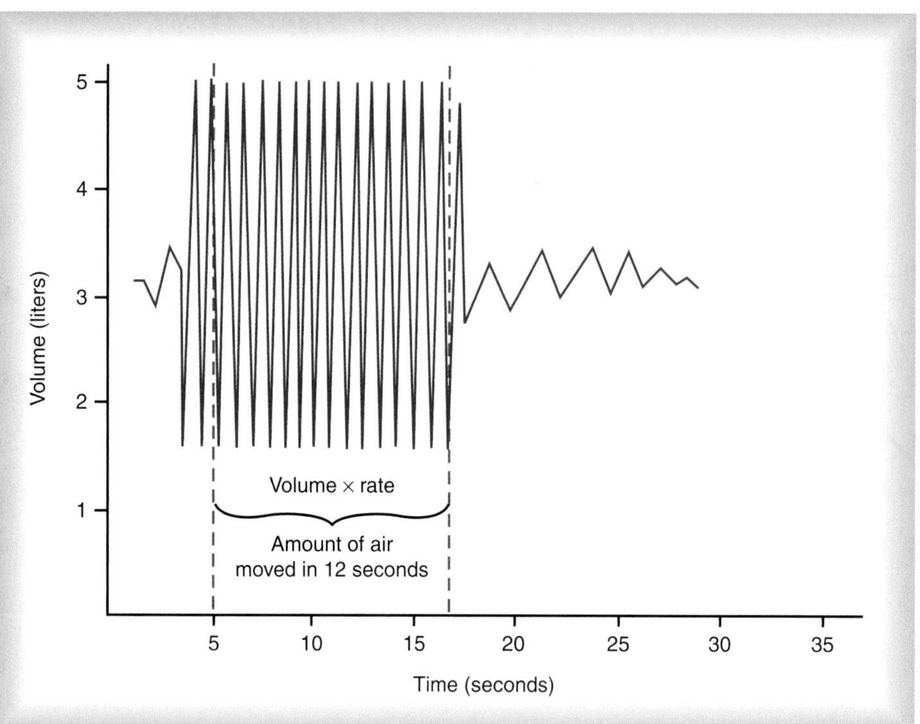

Figure 17-9

Maximal voluntary ventilation tracing. Actual ventilations recorded during a 12-second period.

volume of CO exhaled (FECO), considering the partial pressure of CO in the lung at the time of measurement. The equation format follows:

$$DL_{CO} = \frac{\dot{V}e\ (FICO - FECO)}{(PACO)}$$

Carbon monoxide is used as the transfer gas because carbon monoxide is similar to oxygen in important ways. Carbon monoxide and oxygen have similar molecular weights and solubility coefficients. Similar to oxygen, carbon monoxide also chemically combines with hemoglobin. Carbon monoxide has a very high affinity for hemoglobin and diffuses rapidly into the pulmonary blood. Carbon monoxide has an affinity for hemoglobin nearly 210 times greater than oxygen, and the high affinity keeps the pulmonary capillary partial pressure of carbon monoxide (PcCO) near zero. Consequently, the diffusion of carbon monoxide across the alveolar capillary membrane is membrane-limited and not limited as much by the partial pressure gradient. To focus the test on diffusion through the alveolar-capillary membrane, the patient should have a normal hematocrit and should not have an abnormal level of carboxyhemoglobin before the test. The hematocrit of all patients undergoing diffusing capacity should be measured, and a mathematical correction should be applied if it is abnormal.[20] Performing the diffusing capacity on patients who have recently smoked a cigarette or who have been exposed to environmental carbon monoxide may hinder test validity; thus the test should be delayed for patients who have been recently exposed to smoke or excessive auto emissions, unless determining the acute effects of exposure is the purpose of the test.[28]

The diffusing capacity of the lung for carbon monoxide using the single breath method ($DL_{CO}SB$) is the most common measurement technique because it is quick and reproducible. The entire test can be performed in just slightly longer than 10 seconds. The patient inspires a VC of a gas mixture containing 0.3% CO and 10% He in air, maintains breath-holding for 10 seconds, and then exhales rapidly at least 1 L. After a predesignated volume is exhaled, a sample of alveolar gas is collected and analyzed for expired carbon monoxide ($FECO_t$) and helium (FEHe). The breath-holding period (t) begins when inspiration of the gas mixture begins, and the period ends when the alveolar sample is collected; this period should not exceed 11 seconds. To regulate the breath-holding period, some measuring systems close the mouthpiece with a timed shutter. The suitable breathing pattern does require some patient cooperation and coordination; some patients benefit from a timer as a visual aid.[29]

The single breath method ($DL_{CO}SB$) is based on the diffusion decay curve described by Forster et al[30] (Figure 17-10). When a bolus of CO gas is inhaled, the rate of gas diffusion declines logarithmically. The diffusing capacity of the lung is a function of lung volume (V_A) in STPD conditions exposed to the test gas,[21] the duration (60 ÷ t) that the test gas is in contact with the lung, the initial concentration of test gas in the lung ($FACO_0$), and the final concentration of test gas in the lung ($FACO_t$), according to the following equation:

MINI CLINI

DL_{CO} in Chronic Obstructive Pulmonary Disease (COPD)

PROBLEM

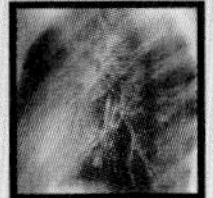

A patient has spirometry and lung volumes typical of the obstructive pattern. The FEV_1, FEV_1/FVC, and FEFs are significantly reduced, and the FRC and TLC are increased. Two common obstructive diseases are chronic bronchitis and pulmonary emphysema. How can pulmonary function data differentiate between these two diseases? The answer is the DL_{CO}.

SOLUTION

Chronic bronchitis involves mostly airways and is characterized by chronic inflammation of the mucosa, hypertrophy of mucous glands, excessive mucus, and possibly, bronchospasm, all of which narrow the airways. Pulmonary emphysema primarily involves alveolar structures and is characterized by destruction of alveolar architecture, elastic fibers, and alveolar-capillary membranes. Emphysema decreases gas exchange surface area. Chronic bronchitis does not involve alveoli and therefore does not change surface area for gas exchange. For these reasons, a decreased diffusion capacity is associated with emphysema rather than with chronic bronchitis. The test for diffusion capacity (DL_{CO}) is a useful way to find out the extent to which emphysema may be present in a patient with COPD.

$$DL_{CO}SB = [60(V_A) \div t(P_B - 47)] \times \ln (FACO_0 \div FACO_t)$$

where $(P_B - 47)$ is ambient barometric pressure corrected for water vapor pressure at 37° C.

Helium is in the gas mixture as a tracer gas for the dilution of the inspired carbon monoxide concentration by the RV and to measure the effective total lung capacity by a single breath helium dilution. The inspired carbon monoxide concentration of 0.3% is not the concentration of carbon monoxide received by the lungs, because the inspired volume is diluted by the RV of the patient. The dilution of carbon monoxide is reflected by the dilution of helium, and the $FACO_0$ can be calculated according to the following equation:

$$FaCO_0 = FICO \times (FEHe \div FIHe)$$

The $FACO_0$ is the concentration of carbon monoxide in the lung at "zero time" before any diffusion occurs. The single breath technique distributes the gas mixture through unobstructed airways to an alveolar volume that is also called the *effective total lung capacity*. The effective total lung capacity (V_A) can be calculated according to the following equation:

$$V_A = VC \times (FIHe \div FEHe)$$

The effective total lung capacity is necessary to calculate the DL_{CO}, and it also is used in the determination of the **diffusing capacity of the lung to alveolar volume ratio (DL_{CO}/V_A)**.

▶ INTERPRETATION OF TEST RESULTS

Pathophysiological Patterns

Pulmonary function testing provides the basis for classifying pulmonary diseases into two major categories: obstructive and restrictive. These two types of lung diseases sometimes occur together. Obstructive and restrictive types of lung diseases are different in several important ways. Figure 17-11 shows normal lungs with the pathophysiological aspects of obstructive lung diseases and restrictive lung diseases, and the differences are summarized in Table 17-2. The primary problem in obstructive pulmonary disease is an increased airway

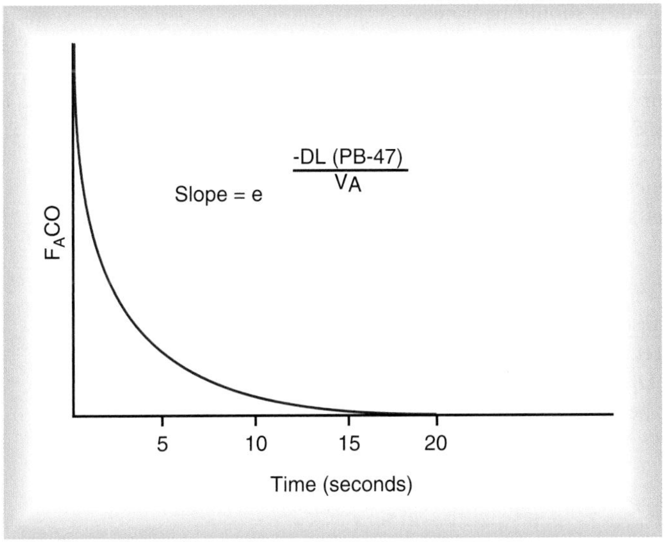

Figure 17-10

The concentration of alveolar carbon monoxide following a single breath to total lung capacity.

Single Breath Carbon Monoxide Diffusing Capacity

AARC Clinical Practice Guideline (Excerpts)*

➤ INDICATIONS

Tests of diffusing capacity may be indicated in the following situations:

- Evaluation and follow-up of parenchymal lung diseases associated with dusts (e.g., asbestos) or drug reactions (e.g., amiodarone) or related to sarcoidosis
- Evaluation and follow-up of emphysema and cystic fibrosis
- Differentiation among chronic bronchitis, emphysema, and asthma in patients with obstructive patterns
- Evaluation of pulmonary involvement in systemic diseases (e.g., rheumatoid arthritis, lupus erythematosus)
- Evaluation of cardiovascular diseases (e.g., pulmonary hypertension, pulmonary edema, thromboembolism)
- Prediction of arterial desaturation during exercise in chronic obstructive pulmonary disease
- Evaluation and quantification of disability associated with interstitial lung disease
- Evaluation of the effects of chemotherapy agents or other drugs known to induce pulmonary dysfunction
- Evaluation of hemorrhagic disorders

➤ CONTRAINDICATIONS

The following are relative contraindications to performing a diffusing capacity test:

- Mental confusion or incoordination preventing the subject from adequately performing the maneuver
- A large meal or vigorous exercise immediately before the test
- Smoking within 24 hours of test administration (may have effect on DL_{CO} independent of the carboxyhemoglobin [COHb])

➤ HAZARDS AND COMPLICATIONS

- $DL_{CO}SB$ requires breath-holding at TLC: some patients may perform either a Valsalva (high intrathoracic pressure) or Muller (low intrathoracic pressure) maneuver. Either of these can result in alteration of venous return to the heart.
- Transmission of infection is possible via improperly cleaned mouthpieces or from the inadvertent spread of droplet nuclei or body fluids (patient to patient or patient to technologist).

➤ ASSESSMENT OF NEED

The need for DL_{CO} testing exists when any of the aforementioned indications are present.

➤ ASSESSMENT OF TEST QUALITY

Individual test maneuvers and results should be evaluated according to the American Thoracic Society recommendations. In particular,

- The inspiratory volume should exceed 90% of the largest previously measured vital capacity (FVC or VC).
- Breath-hold time should be between 9 and 11 seconds, with a rapid inspiration.
- The washout volume (dead space) should be 0.75 to 1.00 L, or 0.50 L if the subject's VC is less than 2.0 L. If a washout volume other than 0.75 to 1.00 L is used, it should be noted.
- Two or more acceptable tests should be averaged: The maneuvers should be reproducible to within 10% or 3 mL CO/min/mm Hg, whichever is greater.
- The subject should have refrained from smoking for 24 hours before the test.
- Corrections for Hb and COHb should be included; correction for tests performed at high altitude is recommended.
- If Hb correction is made, both the corrected and uncorrected D_LCO values should be reported.
- Equipment calibration and quality control measures specific to measuring diffusing capacity should be applied and documented.

➤ MONITORING

- The final report should contain a statement about test quality.
- The final report should contain the D_LCO, the corrected D_LCO (Hb, COHb, altitude), and the Hb value used for correction. The alveolar volume (V_A) and D_L/V_A (i.e., the ratio of diffusing capacity to the lung volume at which the measurement was made) may be included in the report. These values are helpful for purposes of interpretation.

*For complete guideline, see Respir Care 44:91, 1999.

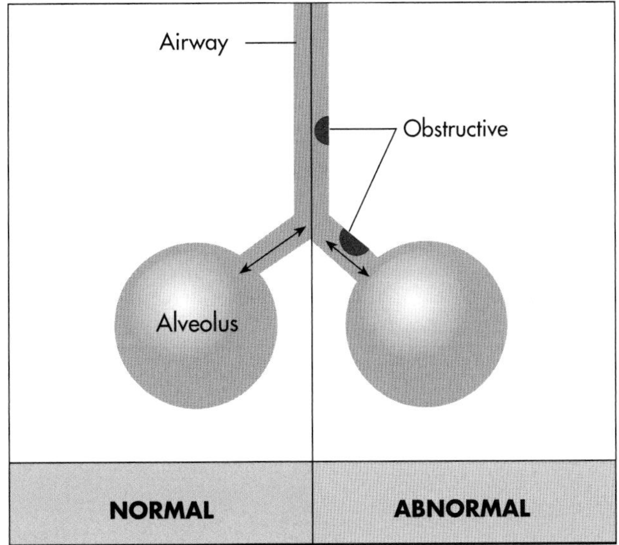

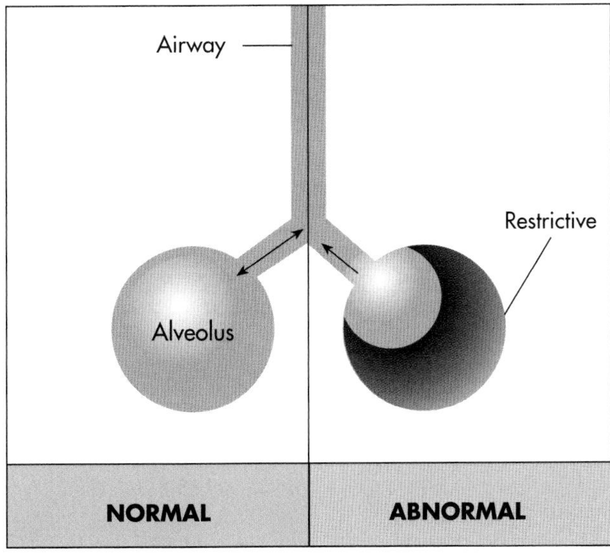

Figure 17-11
Pathophysiological aspects of lung disease.

resistance. Airway resistance (Raw) is the difference in pressure between the ends of the airways divided by the flow rate of gas moving through the airway, according to the following formula:

$$Raw = \frac{\Delta P}{\dot{V}}$$

There is an inverse relationship between airway resistance (Raw) and flow rates ($\dot{V}$). If the pressure difference is constant, a reduced flow rate indicates an increase in airway resistance. Because the radius of the airways normally lessens slightly during expiration, flow rates are usually measured during expiration. By rearranging the symbols in Poiseuille's law (see Chapter 5), airway resistance is inversely related to the radius of the airways according to the following formula:

$$Raw = \frac{\Delta P}{\dot{V} = \eta 8l \div r^4}$$

When airway radius (r) decreases, resistance (Raw) increases while the flow rate of gas through the airways ($\dot{V}$) decreases. Airway radius can be reduced by excessive contraction of the bronchial and bronchiolar muscles (bronchospasm), excessive secretions in the airways, swelling of the airway mucosa, airway tumors, collapse of the bronchioles, and other causes. By measuring flow rates, pulmonary function tests measure indirectly the size of the airways, airway resistance, and the presence of obstructive disease.

The primary problem in restrictive lung disease is reduced lung compliance, thoracic compliance, or both lung and thoracic compliances. Compliance is the volume of gas inspired per the amount of inspiratory effort; effort is measured as the amount of pressure created in the lung or in the pleural space when the inspiratory muscles contract. Compliance is calculated according to the following formula:

$$C = \frac{\Delta V}{\Delta P}$$

There is a direct relationship between compliance (C) and volume (V). If the pressure difference is constant, a reduced inspiratory volume indicates a reduction in compliance. A reduced lung compliance is usually the result of alveolar inflammation, pulmonary fibrosis, or neoplasms in the alveoli; a reduced thoracic compliance may be the result of thoracic wall abnormalities such as kyphoscoliosis. Neuromuscular diseases also can result in reduced lung volumes and restrictive type pulmonary impairments, mainly by affecting the function of the inspiratory muscles. In these circumstances, lung and thoracic compliances may be normal, but the patient is

Table 17-2 ▶▶ Comparisons of Obstructive and Restrictive Types of Pulmonary Diseases

Characteristic	Obstructive Disease	Restrictive Disease
Anatomy affected	Airways	Lung parenchyma/thoracic pump
Breathing phase difficulty	Expiration	Inspiration
Pathophysiology	Increased Raw	Decreased lung/thoracic compliance
Useful measurements	Flow rates	Volumes/capacities

MINI CLINI

Identifying Patterns of Pulmonary Impairment

PROBLEM

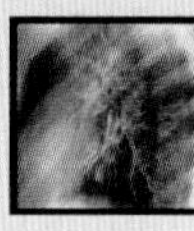

Following are three pulmonary function reports that show three distinct examples of pulmonary impairment. Using the algorithm in Figure 17-17 (p. 423), identify the patterns typical of asthma, pulmonary fibrosis, and chronic obstructive pulmonary disease (COPD).

PULMONARY FUNCTION REPORT #1

Pulmonary measurements	Predicted normal value	Measured baseline conditions	Percent predicted baseline	Measured after broncho-dilator treatment	Percent predicted after treatment
SVC (L)	5.00	3.00	60%		
FVC (L)	5.00	3.00	60%		
FEV_1 (L)	4.00	2.80	70%		
FEV_1/FVC	80%	94%	—		
$FEF_{25\%-75\%}$ (L/sec)	4.00	3.75	94%		
PEFR (L/sec)	8.00	8.25	103%		
TLC (L)	7.20	3.96	55%		
FRC (L)	4.10	2.00	49%		
RV (L)	2.20	1.40	60%		
DL_{CO} (mL/min/mm Hg)	34.0	15.9	47%		
DL_{CO}/V_A (mL/min/mm Hg/L)	7.20	3.50	49%		

SOLUTION: CASE #1

Although the FEV_1 is less than 80% of predicted, because the FEV_1/FVC is greater than 70%, there is no apparent airway obstruction. The FEV_1 is reduced because the FVC is reduced. The patient's measured FVC is less than the predicted FEV_1. Because the TLC is less than 80% predicted, the data suggest a restrictive impairment, and because the DlCO is less than 80% predicted, there is also a diffusion impairment. The low D_LCO/Va suggests that the diffusion impairment is out of proportion to the lung volume. This finding implies that the impairment to normal diffusion is the lung tissue. Overall, this report shows a moderate restrictive pattern consistent with pulmonary fibrosis.

PULMONARY FUNCTION REPORT #2

Pulmonary measurements	Predicted normal value	Measured baseline conditions	Percent predicted baseline	Measured after broncho-dilator treatment	Percent predicted after treatment
SVC (L)	5.00	3.50	70%	4.25	85%
FVC (L)	5.00	3.30	66%	4.00	80%
FEV_1 (L)	4.00	2.00	50%	2.50	62%
FEV_1/FVC	80%	57%	—	62%	—
$FEF_{25\%-75\%}$ (L/sec)	4.00	1.00	25%	2.00	50%
PEFR (L/sec)	8.00	6.00	7%	6.50	80%
TLC (L)	5.27	5.51	105%	5.36	102%
FRC (L)	3.11	4.55	146%	3.60	116%
RV (L)	1.67	2.60	156%	2.00	120%
DL_{CO} (mL/min/mm Hg)	28.7	25.25	88%	—	—
DL_{CO}/V_A (mL/min/mm Hg/L)	5.45	5.17	96%	—	—

SOLUTION: CASE #2

The FEV_1/FVC is less than 70%; therefore there is airway obstruction. The FEV_1 is 50% of predicted; therefore the obstruction is moderate. Because the $FEF_{25\%-75\%}$ is 25% of predicted, the major site of obstruction is in the bronchioles. Following bronchodilator inhalation, the FEV_1 improved by 24% (Remember to compute % change!), showing effective treatment and partial reversibility of the obstruction. The large FRC and RV show hyperinflation and air trapping, which also improved following bronchodilator therapy. Diffusing capacity is in the normal range, indicating no diffusion impairment and no alveolar problems. Overall, this report shows a moderate obstructive pattern with hyperinflation and air trapping responsive to bronchodilators and consistent with acute hyperreactive airways disease, such as asthma.

MINI CLINI—cont'd

PULMONARY FUNCTION REPORT #3

Pulmonary measurements	Predicted normal value	Measured baseline conditions	Percent predicted baseline	Measured after bronchodilator treatment	Percent predicted after treatment
SVC (L)	5.00	4.00	80%	4.25	85%
FVC (L)	5.00	3.50	70%	4.00	80%
FEV_1 (L)	4.00	2.00	50%	2.20	55%
FEV_1/FVC	80%	57%	—	55%	—
$FEF_{25\%-75\%}$ (L/sec)	4.00	1.75	50%	2.00	50%
PEFR (L/sec)	8.00	6.00	75%	6.50	80%
TLC (L)	5.27	5.51	105%	5.36	102%
FRC (L)	3.11	4.55	146%	3.79	122%
RV (L)	1.67	2.60	156%	2.24	134%
DlCO (mL/min/mm Hg)	28.7	14.25	56%	—	—
DlCO/Va (mL/min/ mm Hg/L)	5.45	3.17	58%	—	—

SOLUTION: CASE #3

This case is similar to case #2, but there are some important differences also. The FEV_1/FVC is less than 70%; therefore there is airway obstruction. The FEV_1 is 50% of predicted; therefore the obstruction is moderate. Following a single bronchodilator treatment, the FEV_1 improved by 10% (Remember to compute % change!)—not enough to show that the bronchodilator therapy was immediately effective. The large FRC and RV show hyperinflation and air trapping, which did improve following bronchodilator therapy. Diffusing capacity and the D_LCO/Va are reduced, suggesting alveolar involvement. This report shows a moderate obstructive pattern with hyperinflation and air trapping not responsive to bronchodilators. There is diffusion impairment and alveolar disease. Overall, this report is consistent with COPD, chronic bronchitis, and pulmonary emphysema.

unable to generate enough subatmospheric pressure to take a full, deep breath.

Some obstructive diseases and some restrictive diseases also may affect the ability of the lung to diffuse gases. In some diseases, there is damage to the alveolar capillary membrane or less alveolar surface area is accessible for diffusion. Measuring the DL_{CO} can identify the destruction of alveolar tissue or the loss of functioning alveolar surface area.

For each measurement of pulmonary function, there is a normal value and a range of normal limits. The severity of pulmonary impairment is based on a comparison of each patient's measurement with the predicted normal value for the patient. Several methods are used for comparison with the normal value. A common method of comparison is to compute a percentage of the predicted normal value according to the following equation:

$$\% \text{ Predicted} = \frac{\text{Measured value}}{\text{Predicted normal value}} \times 100$$

Determining if the patient's value is within one or two standard deviations of the predicted normal value is an alternate method used in some laboratories. The predicted percentage or the number of standard deviations from the predicted normal value can be used to quantify severity of impairment. Typical degrees of severity are listed in Table 17-3.

Table 17-3 Severity of Pulmonary Impairments Based on a Percentage of the Predicted Normal Value or Standard Deviations of the Mean Predicted Normal Value

Impairment	Percent (%) Predicted	Number of Standard Deviations (SD)
None, normal	80-120	±1
Mild	65-79 or 121-135	±1-2
Moderate	50-64 or 136-150	±2-3
Severe	35-49 or 151-165	>±3
Very severe	<35 or >165	

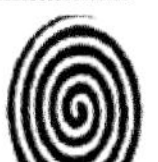

RULE OF THUMB

Normal pulmonary function values are predictably based on the subject's age, height, gender, ethnicity, and sometimes, weight. Normal pulmonary function predictably declines with age greater than 20 years.

Lung Volumes and Capacities

Some lung volumes provide valuable diagnostic information. For example, the TLC is always reduced in restrictive lung disease, unless obstruction and restriction occur together. Then the TLC may be a less sensitive measure of the restrictive impairment. Other volumes and capacities may remain normal with obstructive or restrictive disease. The pattern of lung volume changes also is important. Table 17-4 summarizes lung volume and capacity changes that may occur in obstructive and restrictive lung diseases.

The normal V_T is approximately 500 to 700 mL for the average healthy adult. In the normal population, great variation of tidal volumes and measurements beyond the normal range are not indicative of a disease process. Normal tidal volumes are often observed in both restrictive and obstructive lung diseases. Therefore the V_T alone is not a valid indicator of the type of lung disease.

The normal IC is approximately 3600 mL, with a significant variation in the normal population. The IC may be normal or reduced in restrictive and obstructive lung diseases. A reduction of IC occurs in restrictive lung diseases because the patient's inhaled volume is reduced, and there is a reduction in TLC. In mild obstructive lung diseases, the IC is usually normal. In moderate and severe obstructive diseases, the IC can be reduced because the resting expiratory level of the FRC has increased because of hyperinflation of the lungs. An increase in IC may occur when the patient inhales from below the resting expiratory level when the measurement is performed; athletes and musicians who play wind instruments may also have increased inspiratory capacities. Therapists use the measurement of IC in clinical protocols to decide between methods of lung inflation therapy (see Chapter 36).

The IRV is not commonly measured. Similar to the V_T and the IC, the IRV can be normal in both restrictive and obstructive diseases and is not a useful diagnostic measurement. The normal value for the IRV is 3.10 L.

The normal ERV is approximately 1.20 L and represents approximately 20% to 25% of the VC. It can be either normal or reduced in obstructive and restrictive lung diseases. The ERV is subtracted from the FRC to calculate the RV.

The normal value of the VC is 4.80 L and represents approximately 80% of the TLC. Normal values for VC can vary significantly depending on age, gender, height, and ethnicity. A reduction of VC occurs in restrictive lung diseases because the patient's inhaled volume is reduced and there is a reduction in TLC. In mild obstructive lung diseases, the slow VC is usually normal if the patient exhales leisurely and has had enough time to exhale completely, or if the VC is measured during inspiration. Measurements made from the FVC provide valuable data for pulmonary mechanics.

The RV, FRC, and TLC are the most important measurements of lung volumes. Age, height, gender, ethnicity, and sometimes, weight or body surface area (BSA) correlate with normal values for these lung volumes.[31] Table 17-5 provides common regression equations to predict the lung volumes for individuals of specific height (in centimeters), age (in years), gender, and BSA (in square meters). A positive correlation exists between lung volumes and height, and a negative correlation exists between lung volumes and age for patients older than 20 years. Male values are larger than female values when height and age are equal.

The typical normal TLC is 6.00 L. The normal RV is approximately 1.20 L and represents approximately 20% of the TLC. The FRC is approximately 2.40 L, which represents approximately 40% of the TLC. The RV and FRC are usually enlarged in acute and chronic obstructive lung diseases because of hyperinflation and air trapping (Figure 17-12).

In chronic obstructive pulmonary disease (COPD), the TLC may also be enlarged. The TLC is always reduced in restrictive lung diseases because of a loss of lung volume; the RV and FRC are often reduced proportionately. Certain acute disorders, such as pulmonary edema, atelectasis, and consolidation, also will cause a reduction of TLC and FRC.

Table 17-4 ▶▶ Pulmonary Function Changes in Advanced Lung Diseases

Measurement	Normal*	Obstructive	Restrictive
V_T	500 mL	N or ↑	N or ↓
IRV	3.10 L	N or ↓	↓
ERV	1.20 L	N or ↓	↓
RV	1.20 L	↑	↓
IC	3.60 L	N or ↓	↓
FRC	2.40 L	↑	↓
TLC	6.00 L	N or ↑	↓
FVC	4.80 L	↓	↓
FEV_1	4.20 L	↓	N or ↓
FEV_1/FVC	>70%	↓	N or ↑
$FEF_{200-1200}$	8.5 L/sec	↓	N
$FEF_{25\%-75\%}$	4.5 L/sec	↓	N
PEFR	9.5 L/sec	↓	N
$FEF_{25\%}$	9.0 L/sec	↓	N
$FEF_{50\%}$	6.5 L/sec	↓	N
$FEF_{75\%}$	3.5 L/sec	↓	N
MVV	160 L/min	↓	N or ↓
DL_{CO}	40 mL/min/mm Hg	N or ↓	N or ↓
DL_{CO}/VA	6.6 mL/min/mm Hg/L	N or ↓	N or ↓

N, No change.
*Values for 20-year-old, 70-kg male.

Pulmonary Mechanics: Spirometry

The normal values for the spirometric measurements of pulmonary mechanics are based on height, age, gender, and ethnicity. Table 17-6 provides common regression equations to predict normal values for the measurements of pulmonary mechanics for individuals of specific

Table 17-5 ▶▶ Examples of Equations for Predicting Normal Lung Volumes and Capacities in Adults

Lung Volumes	Gender	Equations	References
FRC (L)	♂	0.081 (Ht) - 1.792 (BSA) - 7.11	31
	♀	0.042 (Ht) - 0.00449 (A) - 3.825	31
RV (L)	♂	0.027 (Ht) - 0.017 (A) - 3.447	31
	♀	0.032 (Ht) - 0.009 (A) - 3.90	31
TLC (L)	♂	0.094 (Ht) - 0.015 (A) - 9.167	31
	♀	0.079 (Ht) - 0.008 (A) - 7.49	31
VC (L)	♂	0.0844 (Ht) - 0.0298 (A) - 8.7818	27
	♀	0.0427 (Ht) - 0.0174 (A) - 2.9001	27

A, Age (in years); *BSA*, body surface area; *Ht*, height (in centimeters).

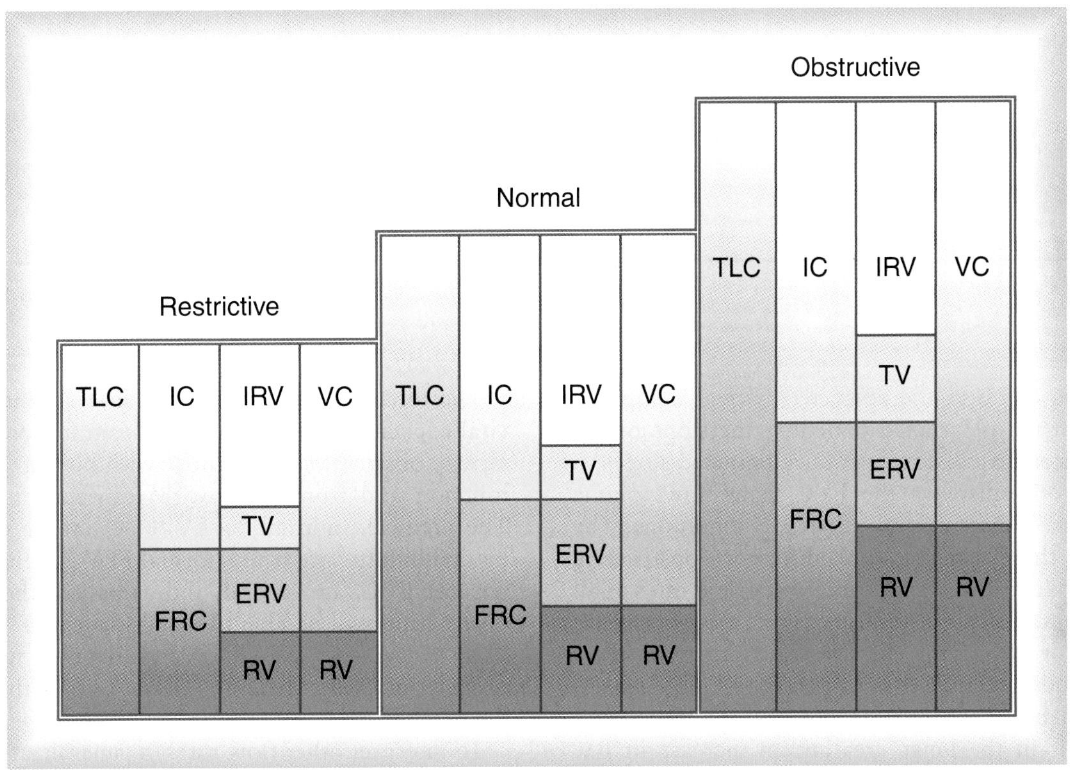

Figure 17-12
Changes in lung volumes and capacities with pulmonary disease.

height (in centimeters), age (in years), and gender.[32] A positive correlation exists between measurements of pulmonary mechanics and height, and a negative correlation exists between measurements of pulmonary mechanics and age for patients older than 20 years. Male values are larger than female values when height and age are equal. The populations that were studied to determine the normal values of pulmonary mechanics were predominately Caucasian. To account for ethnic differences of non-Caucasians, the predicted normal values for Caucasians commonly are reduced by 12% to 15% when applied to non-Caucasians. Figure 17-13 presents the nomogram produced by Morris in 1971 for predicting spirometric values of males and females. For patients of each gender, a line connecting the points of age and height is extended to identify the predicted normal values of FVC, FEV_1, $FEF_{200\text{-}1200}$, and $FEF_{25\%\text{-}75\%}$.

A typical normal FVC is 4.80 L. A reduced FVC may occur with obstructive or restrictive impairments. Figure 17-14 demonstrates FVC from volume-time spirometer tracings for the normal, obstructive, and restrictive conditions. The FVC in both the obstructed and restricted curves are shown as reduced volumes compared with the normal. The primary difference

Table 17-6 ▶▶ Examples of Regression Equations for Predicted Normal Pulmonary Mechanics in Adults

Lung Volumes	Gender	Equations	References
FVC (L)	♂	$(0.0580 \times Ht) - (0.025 \times A) - 4.24$	32
	♀	$(0.0453 \times Ht) - (0.024 \times A) - 2.852$	
FEV_1 (L)	♂	$(0.052 \times Ht) - (0.027 \times A) - 4.203$	32
	♀	$(0.027 \times Ht) - (0.021 \times A) - 0.794$	
%FEV_1/FVC	♂	$103.64 - (0.087 \times Ht) - (0.140 \times A)$	27
	♀	$107.38 - (0.111 \times Ht) - (0.109 \times A)$	
$FEF_{200-1200}$	♂	$(0.0429 \times Ht) - (0.047 \times A) + 2.010$	32
	♀	$(0.0570 \times Ht) - 0.036 \times A) - 2.532$	
$FEF_{25\%-75\%}$	♂	$(0.0185 \times Ht) - (0.045 \times A) - 2.513$	32
	♀	$(0.0236 \times Ht) - (0.030 \times A) - 0.551$	
$FEF_{75\%-85\%}$	♂	$(0.0051 \times Ht) - (0.023 \times A) + 1.21$	32
	♀	$(0.0098 \times Ht) - (0.021 \times A) + 0.321$	
PEFR	♂	$(0.0567 \times Ht) - (0.024 \times A) + 0.225$	27
	♀	$(0.0354 \times Ht) - (0.018 \times A) + 1.130$	
$FEF_{25\%}$	♂	$(0.088 \times Ht) - (0.035 \times A) - 5.618$	27
	♀	$(0.043 \times Ht) - (0.025 \times A) - 0.132$	
$FEF_{50\%}$	♂	$(0.069 \times Ht) - (0.015 \times A) - 5.4$	27
	♀	$(0.035 \times Ht) - (0.013 \times A) - 0.444$	
$FEF_{75\%}$	♂	$(0.44 \times Ht) - (0.012 \times A) - 4.143$	27
	♀	$3.042 - (0.014 \times A)$	
MVV	♂	$(1.19 \times Ht) - (0.816 \times A) - 37.9$	33
	♀	$(0.84 \times Ht) - (0.685 \times A) - 4.87$	

A, Age (in years); *Ht*, height (in centimeters).

between the curve in the restricted patient compared with that of the obstructed patient is the slope of the tracing; obstructive diseases produce flattened slopes.

Figure 17-15 displays the FVC from flow-volume tracings for obstructive and restrictive conditions. The shapes of these tracings are different; obstructive diseases produce lower peaks and lower flow rates at all lung volumes. Forced inspiratory flow rates sometimes are useful for identifying extrathoracic airway obstructions. In moderate and severe obstructive lung diseases, the FVC will be reduced if weakened bronchioles collapse and trap air in the lungs creating an increase in RV. Some laboratories compare the volumes of the SVC and the FVC to identify air trapping. VC is reduced in restrictive lung diseases because the patient's inhaled volume is reduced.

The **forced expiratory volume in half of a second ($FEV_{0.5}$)** is an indicator of patient effort during the initial phase of the FVC maneuver. With good effort, a patient should exhale at least 50% of his or her VC in the initial half of a second.

Although the FEV_1 is measured as a volume, the FEV_1 is considered a flow rate. A typical normal FEV_1 is 4.20 L. The FEV_1 may be reduced with obstructive or restrictive impairments. For patients with airway obstruction, the FEV_1 measures the general severity of airway obstruction. For patients with restrictive impairment, the FEV_1 may be reduced when the patient's VC is smaller than the predicted FEV_1.

The **forced expiratory volume in 1 second to forced vital capacity ratio (FEV_1/FVC)** separates patients with airway obstruction from those with normal pulmonary function and from those with restrictive impairment. The predicted normal %FEV_1/FVC can be determined by dividing the predicted normal FEV_1 by the predicted normal FVC. In general, individuals without airway obstruction will be able to exhale at least 70% of their FVC in the first second, and individuals with airway obstruction will exhale less than 70% of their FVC in the first second.

To interpret other flow rates, a generalization may be helpful. Gas exhaled during the early portion of the FVC reflects the resistance in the larger airways, and gas exhaled during the later portion of the FVC reflects the resistance in the smaller airways. As exhalation of the FVC proceeds, flow decreases, and the airways reflected in the measurements get smaller. Any flow measured in the first half of the FVC reflects on the bronchi; any flow measured beyond 50% of the VC reflects on the bronchioles.

The PEFR, $FEF_{200-1200}$, and $FEF_{25\%}$ occur near the onset of the FVC. Typical normal values are similar; PEFR is 9.5 L/sec; $FEF_{200-1200}$ is 8.5 L/sec; and $FEF_{25\%}$ is 9.0 L/sec. A reduced PEFR, $FEF_{200-1200}$, or $FEF_{25\%}$ may occur as a result of a large airway obstruction, as well as from lack of sufficient effort to inhale maximally and exhale forcibly. The $FEF_{25\%-75\%}$ and $FEF_{50\%}$ occur in the middle of the FVC. Because the $FEF_{25\%-75\%}$ is an average

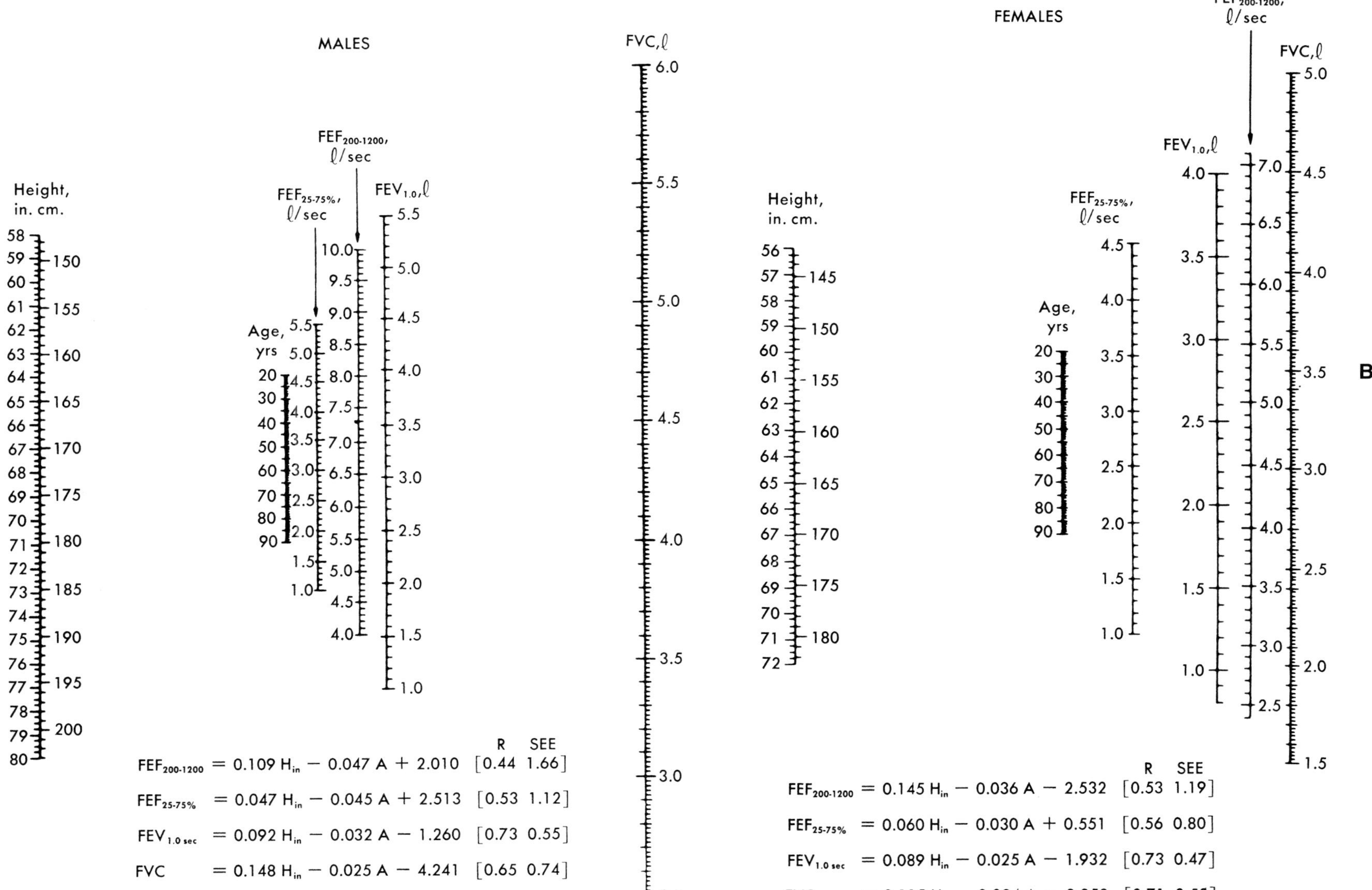

Figure 17-13
Spirometric standards for males (**A**) and females (**B**) (BTPS). *(From Morris JF, Koski A, Johnson LC: Am Rev Respir Dis 103:57, 1971.)*

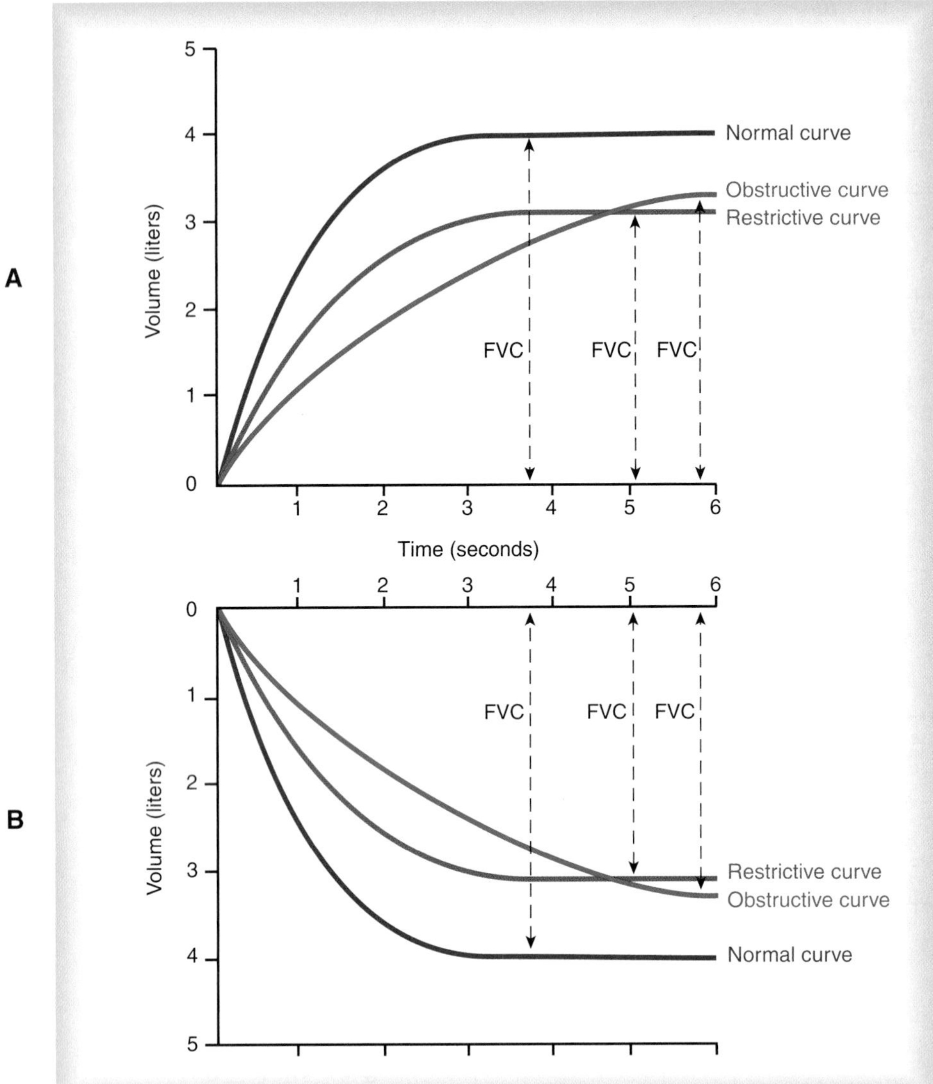

Figure 17-14
Forced vital capacity curves comparing normal, obstructive, and restrictive disorders. **A**, Curves as they appear on commonly available spirometers with tracings beginning at the bottom left corner. **B**, The same curves as they appear on some spirometers that begin tracings at upper left corner.

of half the VC and $FEF_{50\%}$ is an instantaneous flow, these typical normal values are less similar; $FEF_{25\%-75\%}$ is 4.5 L/sec; $FEF_{50\%}$ is 6.5 L/sec. A reduced $FEF_{25\%-75\%}$ or $FEF_{50\%}$ may occur because of small airway obstruction, as well as from lack of effort to sustain a maximal exhalation. The $FEF_{75\%}$ and $FEF_{75\%-85\%}$ occur late in the FVC and reflect on the smallest airways. Typical values are 3.5 L/sec for $FEF_{75\%}$ and 1.5 L/sec for $FEF_{75\%-85\%}$. Sometimes, patients who are asymptomatic for cough, sputum production, or dyspnea may have reduced flow in the small airways. A singular reduction in small airway flow may indicate nothing at all or may be an early indicator of obstruction.

The shape of the flow-volume loop and the $FEF_{50\%}/FIF_{50\%}$ ratio provide additional information about upper airway obstruction. Compared with the normal flow-volume loop, a fixed upper airway obstruction produces a curve that appears box-shaped. In Figure 17-16, both expiratory and inspiratory flows are decreased and limited by the solid obstruction; the $FEF_{50\%}/FIF_{50\%}$ ratio remains normal. Variable upper airway obstructions produce two different shapes depending on the site of the obstruction. Because the intraairway pressure during a forced inspiration is less than atmospheric outside the thorax, a variable extrathoracic upper airway obstruction limits inspiratory flow, and the $FEF_{50\%}/FIF_{50\%}$ ratio is greater than 1.0. Because the intraairway pressure during a forced inspiration is greater than atmospheric pressure inside the thorax, a variable intrathoracic upper airway obstruction limits expiratory flow, and the $FEF_{50\%}/FIF_{50\%}$ ratio is less than 1.0.

Similar to other spirometric measurements of pulmonary mechanics, normal values of the MVV are based on gender, age, and height. The MVV is reduced in patients with moderate and severe airway obstruction. A measured value less than 75% of the predicted is

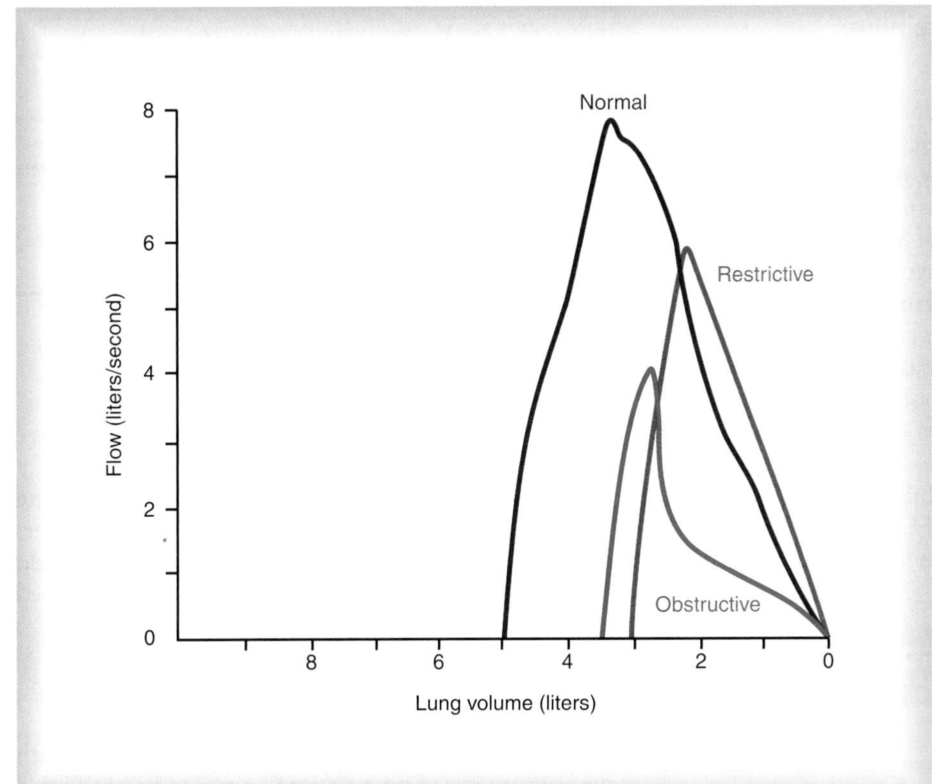

Figure 17-15
Maximal expiratory flow volume curves of normal, obstructive, and restrictive patterns.

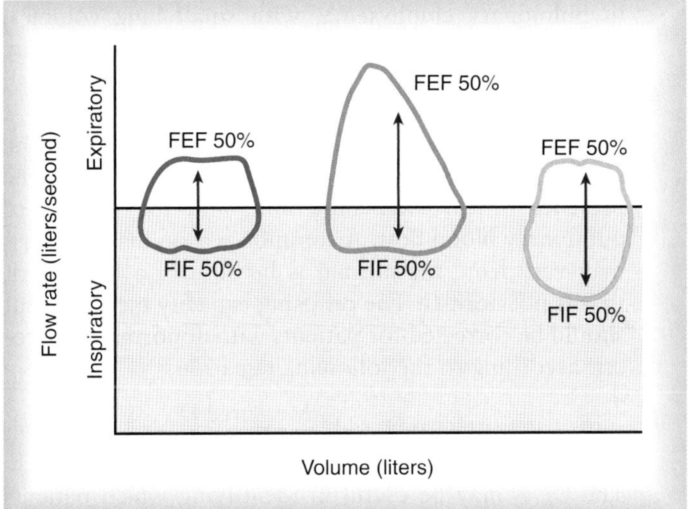

Figure 17-16
Flow-volume loops of fixed upper airway obstruction, variable extrathoracic upper airway obstruction, and variable intrathoracic upper airway obstruction.

significant. The normal for males is approximately 160 to 180 L/min; it is slightly lower in females. In restrictive lung disease, the MVV value may be normal or only slightly reduced. Respiratory muscle strength is a primary determinant of MVV in patients with interstitial lung disease and an important determinant in patients with COPD. Undernourished patients also may have a reduced MVV.[33]

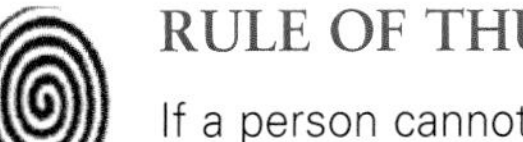

RULE OF THUMB

If a person cannot exhale at least 70% of his or her VC in 1 second, there must obstruction. A FEV_1/FVC of less than 70% indicates an obstructive impairment.

Pulmonary Mechanics: Reversibility and Bronchial Challenge

Based on the initial results of baseline spirometry, additional testing of pulmonary mechanics is often desirable. If the baseline test indicates airway obstruction, determining the reversibility of the obstruction is indicated. Therapists also use the concept of reversibility when evaluating routine therapy by performing spirometry before and after therapy. In the laboratory, the FVC maneuver is often repeated after the patient has received a bronchodilator administered by small-volume nebulizer or metered-dose inhaler. This laboratory protocol is commonly known as spirometry *before and after bronchodilator*. Reversibility of the airway obstruction indicates effective therapy; reversibility is defined as a 15% or greater improvement in FEV_1 and at least a 200-mL increase in FEV_1. Improvement is determined using the percent change formula:

$$\% \text{ Improvement} = \frac{\text{Post-FEV}_1 - \text{Pre-FEV}_1}{\text{Pre-FEV}_1} \times 100$$

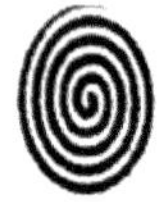

RULE OF THUMB

A *change in percent* (A% - B%) is not the same as a *percent change* $\frac{(B\% - A\%)}{A\%}$.

When the patient's history suggests episodic symptoms of hyperreactive airways and airway obstruction, such as seasonal or exercise-induced wheezing, and the results of baseline spirometry are normal, performing a bronchial provocation may be indicated. Bronchial provocation testing uses an agent to stimulate a hyperreactive airway response and to create airway obstruction. Although several types of provocations are possible, such as inhaling histamine or cold air or exercising, provoking a hyperreactive airway response by inhaling methacholine is likely the most popular and predicable technique. The procedure usually begins with the patient inhaling a normal saline aerosol and then repeating the FVC maneuver. Some very sensitive patients will demonstrate hyperreactive airways with saline alone; a positive response to saline is defined as a decrease in FEV_1 of 10% or greater. The methacholine provocation protocol systematically exposes the patient to increasing dosages of methacholine. Usually starting with a low dose of 0.03 mg/mL, patients inhale methacholine aerosol and then repeat the FVC maneuver. A positive response to methacholine is defined as a decrease in FEV_1 of 20% or greater (another example of percent change). If a positive response does not occur, the methacholine dosage is doubled to 0.06 mg/mL and then the FVC maneuver is repeated. The process of "double-dosing" and performing FVC maneuvers continues until there is either a positive response or until the full dose, 16 mg/mL, is given. If a positive response occurs, treatment with a fast-acting bronchodilator is indicated, and sometimes administering oxygen is helpful. The final test report should include the concentration of methacholine that caused the 20% decrease in FEV_1.

Table 17-7 ▶▶ Examples of Regression Equations for Predicted Normal Diffusion in Adults

Parameter	Regression Equations	References
$DL_{CO}SB$	(0.416 Ht) - (0.219 A) - 26.34	34
	(0.256 Ht) - (0.144 A) - 8.36	34
$DL_{CO}SB/\dot{V}_A$	6.61 - (0.034 A)*	34
	7.34 - (0.032 A)*	34

A, Age (in years); Ht, height (in centimeters).
*Hemoglobin corrected according to Dinakara.[35]

Diffusing Capacity

Normal values for the DL_{CO} using the single breath technique are based on a patient's age and height (Table 17-7); a typical normal value for a 20-year-old healthy male is 40 mL/min/mm Hg.[34] The DL_{CO} may be reduced from the predicted normal in patients with obstructive or restrictive lung diseases. With destruction of alveoli in pulmonary emphysema, with small lung volumes, and with fibrosis of alveoli in asbestosis, the DL_{CO} may be less than normal.

Pulmonary embolism also may decrease the DL_{CO}. Diffusion also can be influenced by hematological factors, such as hemoglobin type (Hgb) and concentration, the presence of carboxyhemoglobin, and the volume of pulmonary blood flow. A common reason that the DL_{CO} may vary from the normal is because of a hematocrit that is not normal. The diffusing capacity measurement should be corrected for patients with abnormal hematocrit according to the following equation[35]:

$$\text{Corrected } DL_{CO} = \frac{\text{Measured } DL_{CO}}{0.06965(\text{Hgb})}$$

The DL_{CO} may be useful in identifying which patients with obstructive impairment are likely to desaturate during exercise and which may benefit from oxygen therapy. The DL_{CO} may be increased in patients with polycythemia, congestive heart failure (resulting from an increase in pulmonary vascular blood volume), and elevated cardiac output. Factors that can alter the DL_{CO} above or below the normal value are summarized in Table 17-8.

The DL_{CO}/V_A ratio differentiates between diffusion abnormalities caused by having a small lung compared with diffusion abnormalities caused by alveolar-capillary

Table 17-8 ▶▶ Effect of Various Factors on the Diffusing Capacity of the Lung

Factors that Decrease DL_{CO}	Factors that Increase DL_{CO}
Anemia	Polycythemia
Carboxyhemoglobin	Exercise
Pulmonary embolism	Congestive heart failure
Diffuse pulmonary fibrosis	
Pulmonary emphysema	

membrane pathologies. Patients whose only problem is small lungs will have a decreased DL_{CO}, but their DL_{CO}/V_A ratio will be normal. Patients with pulmonary emphysema or fibrosis will have a decreased DL_{CO} and a decreased DL_{CO}/V_A ratio.

Interpretation of the Pulmonary Function Report

Many computer-based pulmonary function testing systems have an algorithm in their programs for computer-assisted interpretations of the pulmonary function report. Figure 17-17 presents a sample algorithm. The $\%FEV_1/FVC$ ratio is a good place to start, because it provides an initial focus as normal, restrictive, or obstructive impairment. If the $\%FEV_1/FVC$ ratio is greater than 70% and if the % predicted normal TLC is less than 80%, the patient has a restrictive impairment, according to this algorithm. The severity of the restriction is based on the % predicted or on the number of standard deviations from the mean predicted TLC according to Table 17-3.[36] If the $\%FEV_1/FVC$ ratio is less than 70%, the patient likely has an obstructive impairment; the severity of the obstruction is based on the % predicted normal FEV_1. If the % predicted normal DL_{CO} is less than 80%, the patient likely has a diffusion impairment, and if the DL_{CO}/V_A ratio is also less the 80% of the predicted normal value, the cause of the diffusion impairment is within the lung. The algorithm also can help identify patients with reversible airway obstruction, small airway disease, hyperinflation, and air trapping.

Most modern pulmonary function laboratories use computers for data acquisition and reduction. Computer-assisted testing can decrease the time necessary to

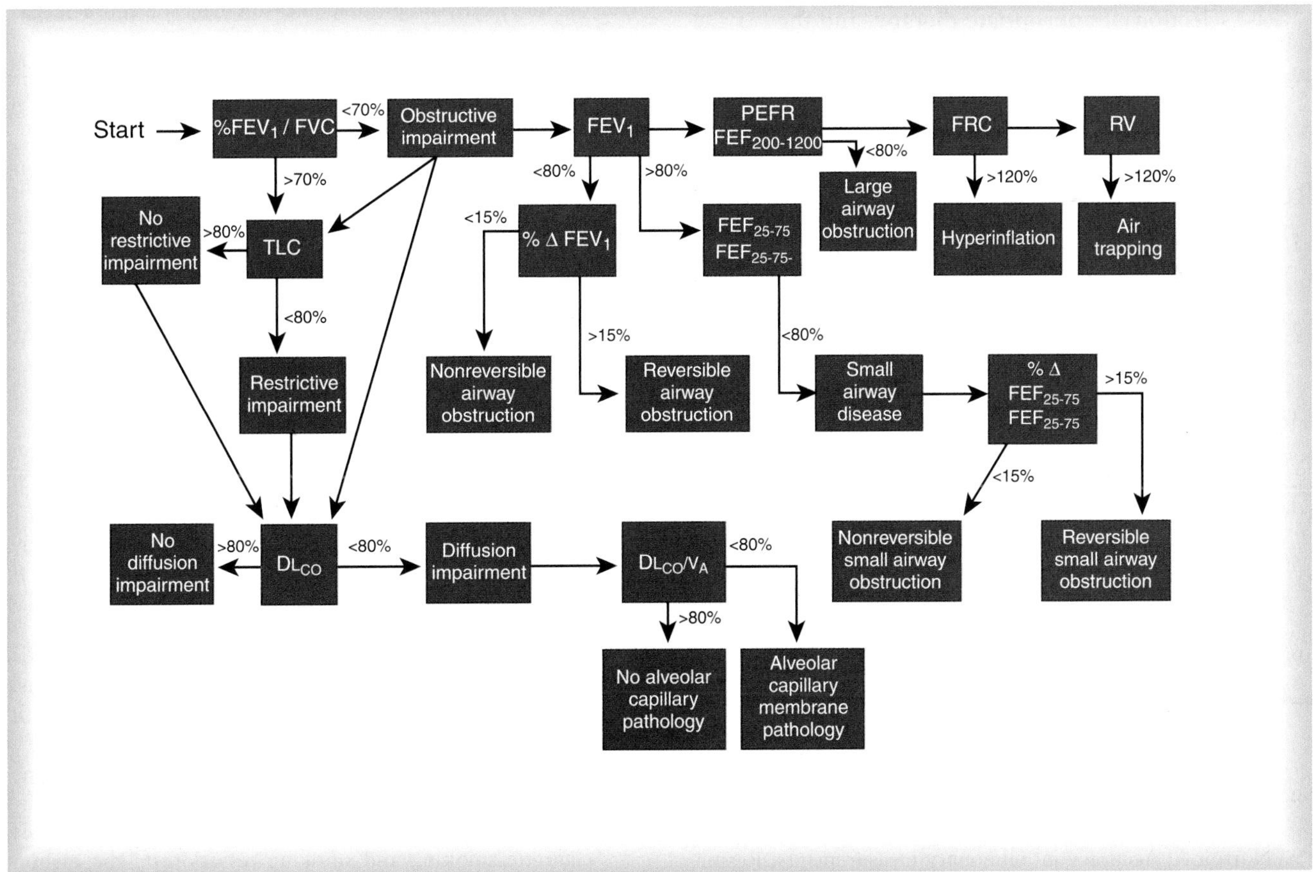

Figure 17-17
An algorithm for systematically assessing basic pulmonary function test results.

complete the test and its interpretation and enhance the effectiveness of pulmonary function testing by increasing accuracy, increasing patient acceptance, and enhancing patient performance.[37,38] Although ATS spirometry performance criteria are often applied by a computer, computer analysis should not replace human analysis.

KEY POINTS

- Pulmonary function testing provides valuable information on the components of gas exchange in health and disease.
- Pulmonary function testing includes measurements of lung volumes and capacities, airway mechanics, and the diffusing capacity of the lung.
- The results of pulmonary function testing can aid in the diagnosis of disease and include patterns of obstructive and restrictive impairments.
- Pulmonary function testing provides objective data on which decisions may be made regarding the status of the patient, the selection of appropriate therapy, and the evaluation of therapeutic outcomes.

References

1. Zibrak JD, O'Donnell CR, Marton K: Indications for pulmonary function testing, Ann Intern Med 112:793, 1990.
2. American Thoracic Society: Evaluation of impairment/disability secondary to respiratory disorders, Am Rev Respir Dis 133:1205, 1986.
3. Ferris BG: Epidemiology standardization project: recommended standardized procedures for pulmonary function testing, Am Rev Respir Dis 118:1, 1978.
4. Hodgkin JE: Preoperative assessment of respiratory function, Respir Care 29:496, 1984.
5. Renzetti AD Jr et al: Evaluation of impairment/disability secondary to respiratory disorders, Am Rev Respir Dis 133:1205, 1986.
6. American Association for Respiratory Care: Clinical practice guideline: spirometry, Respir Care 41:629, 1996.
7. Douce FH: Flow and volume measuring devices. In Branson R, Hess D, Chatburn R, editors: Respiratory care equipment, Philadelphia, 1995, JB Lippincott.
8. Shigeoka JW: Calibration and quality control of spirometer systems, Respir Care 28:747, 1983.
9. Norton A: Accuracy in pulmonary measurements, Respir Care 24:131, 1979.
10. American Thoracic Society: Standardization of spirometry, 1994 update, Am J Respir Crit Care Med 152:1107, 1995.
11. American Thoracic Society: Quality assurance in pulmonary function laboratories, Am Rev Respir Dis 134:6257, 1986.
12. Garner JS, Favero MS: CDC guidelines for the prevention and control of nosocomial infections: guideline for hand washing and hospital environmental control, Am J Infect Control 14:110, 1986.
13. Dooley SW et al: Guidelines for preventing the transmission of tuberculosis in health-care settings, with special focus on HIV-related issues, MMWR 39:1, 1990.
14. Pulmonary terms and symbols: a report of the ACCP-ATS Joint Committee on Pulmonary Nomenclature, Chest 67:583,1975.
15. Hathirat S, Renzetti AD, Mitchell M: Measurement of the total lung capacity by helium dilution in a constant volume system, Am Rev Respir Dis 102:760, 1970.
16. Birath G, Swenson EW: A correction factor for helium absorption in lung volume determination, Scand J Clin Lab Invest 8:155, 1956.
17. Boren HG, Kory RC, Snyder JC: The Veterans Administration–Army cooperative study of pulmonary function II: the lung volume and its subdivisions in normal men, Am J Med 41:96, 1966.
18. Dubois AB et al: A rapid plethysmographic method for measuring thoracic gas volume: a comparison with a nitrogen washout method for measuring FRC in normal patients, J Clin Invest 35:322, 1956.
19. Habib MP, Engel LA: Influence of the panting technique on the plethysmographic measurement of thoracic gas volume, Am Rev Respir Dis 117:265, 1978.
20. Knudson RJ et al: The single-breath carbon monoxide diffusing capacity: reference equations derived from a healthy nonsmoking population and effects of hematocrit, Am Rev Respir Dis 135:805, 1987.
21. Ogilvie CM et al: A standardized breath holding technique for the clinical measurement of the diffusing capacity of the lung for carbon monoxide, J Clin Invest 36:117, 1957.
22. Varkey B, Kory RC: Mediastinal and subcutaneous emphysema following pulmonary function tests, Am Rev Respir Dis 108:1393, 1973.
23. Stanescu DC, Teculescu DB: Exercise and cough induced asthma, Respiration 27:273, 1970.
24. Taussig LM et al: Conference Committee: standardization of lung function testing in children, J Pediatr 97:668, 1980.
25. Zamel N, Altose MD, Speir WA Jr: ACCP Scientific Section Recommendations: statement of spirometry: a report of the section on respiratory pathophysiology, Chest 83:547, 1983.
26. U.S. Department of Labor: Pulmonary function standards for cotton dust standard: 29 Code of Federal Regulations: 1910.1043 Appendix D. Occupational Safety and Health Administration 808832, 1980.
27. Knudson RJ et al: The maximal expiratory flow volume curve, Am Rev Respir Dis 113:587, 1976.
28. Knudson RJ, Kaltenborn WT, Burrows B: The effects of cigarette smoking and smoking cessation on the carbon monoxide diffusing capacity of the lung in asymptomatic patients, Am Rev Respir Dis 140:645, 1989.

29. American Thoracic Society: Single breath carbon monoxide diffusing capacity (transfer factor): recommendations for a standard technique, Am J Respir Crit Care Med 152:2185, 1995.
30. Forster RE et al: The absorption of carbon monoxide by the lungs during breathholding, J Clin Invest 33:1135, 1954.
31. Goldman HI, Becklake MR: Respiratory function tests: normal values at median altitudes and the prediction of normal values, Am Rev Tuberculosis 79:457, 1959.
32. Morris JF, Koski A, Johnson LC: Spirometric standards for healthy nonsmoking adults, Am Rev Respir Dis 116:209, 1971.
33. Aldrich TK, Arora NS, Rochester DF: The influence of airway obstruction and respiratory muscle strength on maximal voluntary ventilation in lung disease, Am Rev Respir Dis 126:1959, 1982.
34. Crapo RO, Morris AM: Standardized single breath normal values for carbon monoxide diffusing capacity, Am Rev Respir Dis 123:185, 1981.
35. Dinakara P et al: The effect of anemia on pulmonary diffusing capacity with derivation of a correction equation, Am Rev Respir Dis 102:965, 1970.
36. American Thoracic Society: Lung function testing: selection of reference values and interpretative strategies, Am Rev Respir Dis 144:1202, 1991.
37. Gardner RM et al: Computer guidelines for pulmonary laboratories, Am Rev Respir Dis 134:628, 1986.
38. Larson JK: Computer-assisted spirometry, Respir Care 27:839, 1982.

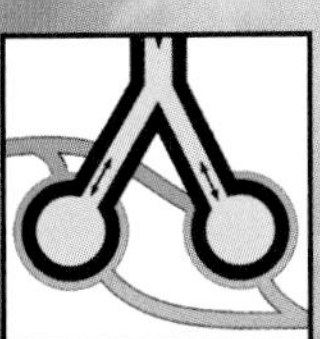

CHAPTER 18

A Synopsis of Thoracic Imaging

Peter B. O'Donovan and James K. Stoller

In This Chapter You Will Learn:

- How thoracic imaging assists in the diagnosis of pulmonary disease
- What steps are used to interpret thoracic imaging studies
- How to identify the more commonly encountered abnormalities seen on thoracic imaging studies
- How to apply some rules of thumb about thoracic imaging in the practice of respiratory care

Chapter Outline

Key Terms

Air bronchograms
Alveolar infiltrate
Chest radiograph
Computed tomography
Hydrothorax
Interstitial lung disease
Mediastinum
Plate atelectasis
Pneumothorax
Pulmonary infiltrates
Radiolucency
Radiopacity

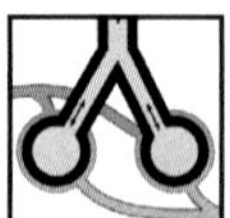

Because chest imaging is critically important in the practice of pulmonary and critical care medicine, it is essential that the respiratory therapist (RT) have a solid understanding of chest imaging. A variety of chest imaging modes exists, including the conventional chest x-ray (more accurately called a *radiograph* or *roentgenogram* after Wilhelm Conrad Roentgen who first discovered the x-ray beam), computed tomography (CT) scanning, ultrasound (which uses high-frequency sound rather than x-rays to image structures), and magnetic resonance imaging (MRI). An additional chest imaging technique is ventilation and perfusion scanning (also known as $\dot{V}/\dot{Q}$ *scanning*), which is often used in evaluating for pulmonary embolism.

This chapter summarizes important concepts in chest imaging for the RT, first addressing the basic elements of plain chest radiology and then describing the role of various imaging techniques used to evaluate the different components of the chest (e.g., the pleura, the mediastinum, the lung tissue [called the *parenchyma*]). Examples of abnormal findings are shown, including some obtained with the more sophisticated imaging techniques such as ultrasound, CT, and MRI.

By way of overview, ultrasound can be helpful in localizing pleural fluid collections, in characterizing them as simple or complex, and as a guidance tool in the drainage of such fluid collections.[1] Transesophageal ultrasound has become well established as a diagnostic tool in evaluation of cardiac and esophageal abnormalities. CT, which depicts the chest in cross-sectional slices like slices of bread in a loaf, has become indispensable in the staging of primary pulmonary cancers and lymphomas and in evaluating mediastinal masses. High-resolution CT uses thin slices to depict fine anatomical detail of the lung parenchyma. The applications of MRI to the pulmonary parenchyma are limited. The multiplanar display of MRI is useful in assessing the extent of disease involving the chest wall. More recently, it has been shown to have some value in assessing the lung vessels and in cases of suspected pulmonary embolism.[2]

▶ OVERVIEW OF THE PLAIN CHEST RADIOGRAPH

The plain **chest radiograph** is taken using one of two techniques: the posteroanterior (PA) view or the anteroposterior (AP) view. The standard chest film is obtained with the PA view, which indicates that the x-ray beam passes through the patient from back to front. This view minimizes magnification of the heart because it is closer to the film and is usually taken in the radiology department in a controlled setting. This allows for a high-quality film in most cases. The AP film is taken with a portable radiography machine with the film behind the patient, which causes slight magnification of the heart. It is usually taken in the intensive care setting because the patient is too ill to go to the radiology department, and it often results in a film of lesser quality as compared with the PA film.

A disciplined approach is required to get the maximal value out of any diagnostic imaging study. The plain chest x-ray perhaps best exemplifies this statement. An obvious abnormality such as a 6-cm mass is easily spotted, even by the untrained eye. The problem is that such an abnormality tends to immediately monopolize the observer's attention. This causes more subtle abnormalities, often with greater diagnostic importance, to go unnoticed. To avoid this pitfall, the observer must develop a step-by-step approach, which is applied in a disciplined fashion until it becomes second nature. The following suggestions are broad guidelines, and each observer must formulate an approach that he or she finds comfortable.

In broad terms, the steps in reviewing the chest film are as follows:

MINI CLINI

Evaluating the Heart Size on a Portable Chest Radiograph

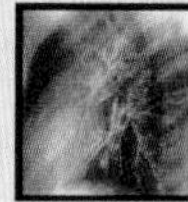

The standard chest film is obtained with the patient standing and facing the film cassette. The x-ray beam penetrates the patient's back first and then passes through the anterior chest and finally to the film. This standard technique is called the posteroanterior (PA) chest film. The heart is located very close to the film with the standard PA view, and magnification of the heart shadow is minimal.

PROBLEM

In the intensive care unit, the patient is too ill for a PA chest film to be obtained. Thus the chest film is obtained with the patient lying in bed and the film cassette placed behind the patient. The x-ray beam passes from anterior to posterior, producing an anteroposterior (AP) portable chest film. In examining the AP portable chest film, how will the appearance of the heart size be affected?

ANSWER

The AP portable radiograph is obtained with the patient's heart further from the film, thus producing a heart shadow artificially magnified as compared with the shadow produced with a PA chest film. This may give the appearance of an enlarged heart in some cases. The clinician interpreting the AP portable radiograph must keep this in mind to avoid misinterpreting the film. To illustrate this point, hold a flashlight 3 feet from a wall and turn it on. While holding the flashlight steady, place your hand in line with the beam. Note how the shadow created by your hand becomes smaller as you move your hand closer to the wall and further from the light source.

- Determine whether the radiograph is technically satisfactory and capable of being interpreted adequately.
- Systematically review the anatomical structures on the chest film to assess their normality or abnormality.

In the sections that follow, these steps are considered, first with an overview of the normal anatomical structures on the chest radiograph, and then with instruction on evaluating the technical quality and adequacy of the film. The remainder of the chapter considers each major anatomical component of the radiograph in order to discuss common abnormalities that the RT should recognize.

▶ OVERVIEW OF THE NORMAL ANATOMY SEEN ON THE CHEST RADIOGRAPH

As shown in Figure 18-1, the following are the main structures imaged on the routine chest radiograph:

1. Bones (e.g., ribs, clavicles, scapulae, vertebrae)
2. Soft tissues (e.g., tissues of the chest wall, upper abdomen, lymph nodes)
3. Lungs (including the trachea; bronchi; and tissue, or *parenchyma*)
4. Pleura (membranous coverings of lung, including the visceral pleura [the part attached to the lungs] and the parietal pleura [the part lining the inside of the chest wall]; although normally occupied by only a small amount of fluid, the space between the parietal and visceral pleura is called the *pleural space*)
5. Heart and mediastinum (i.e., the tissues between the two lungs in the center of the chest, bordered by the sternum and the vertebral column in the AP dimension and by the thoracic inlet [where the trachea enters the thorax] and the diaphragm in the cephalocaudal direction)
6. Upper abdomen
7. Lower neck

▶ TECHNICAL ADEQUACY OF A RADIOGRAPH

With these normal anatomical structures in mind, the RT's first step in evaluating the technical adequacy of the radiograph is to judge the patient's position when the chest x-ray was taken. The RT should ask himself or herself the following questions: Is the whole chest visible on the film? Is the patient well positioned?

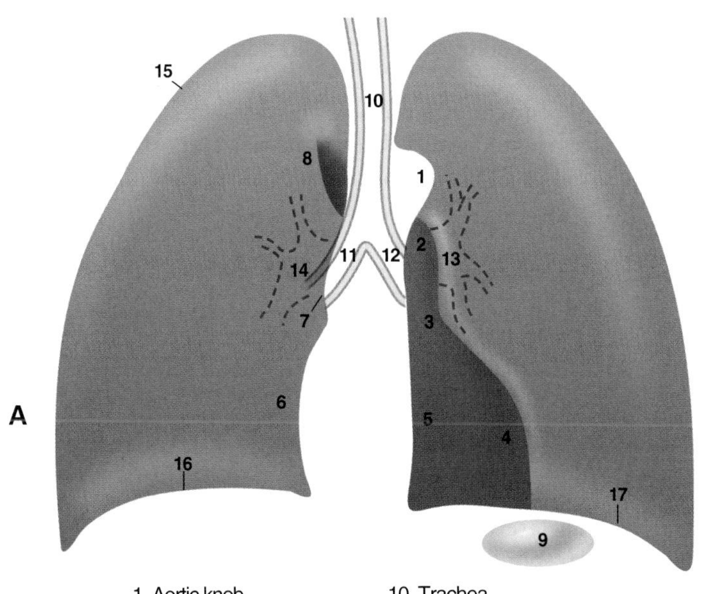

1. Aortic knob
2. Main pulmonary artery
3. Left atrium
4. Left ventricle
5. Descending aorta
6. Right atrium
7. Ascending aorta
8. Superior vena cava
9. Gastric bubble
10. Trachea
11. Right main bronchus
12. Left main bronchus
13. Left pulmonary artery
14. Right pulmonary artery
15. Pleural line
16. Right hemidiaphragm
17. Left hemidiaphragm

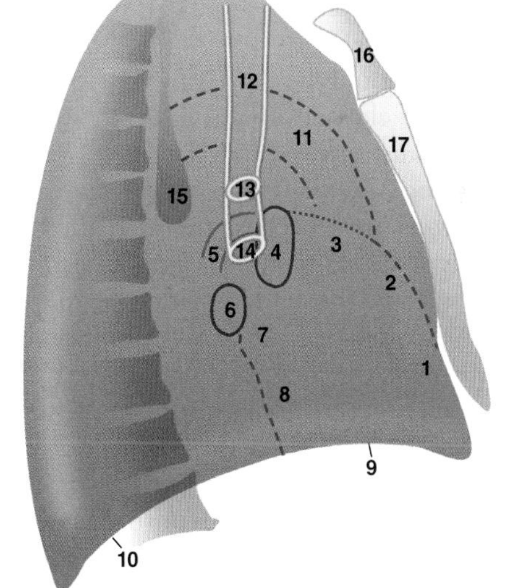

1. Right ventricle
2. Pulmonary outflow tract
3. Main pulmonary artery
4. Right pulmonary artery
5. Left pulmonary artery
6. Pulmonary veins
7. Left atrium
8. Left ventricle
9. Right hemidiaphragm
10. Left hemidiaphragm
11. Aortic arch
12. Trachea
13. Right upper lobe bronchus
14. Left upper lobe bronchus
15. Scapulae
16. Manubrium
17. Sternum

Figure 18-1
Schematic diagram of the normal structures seen on the chest x-ray. **A**, Posteroanterior view. **B**, Lateral view.

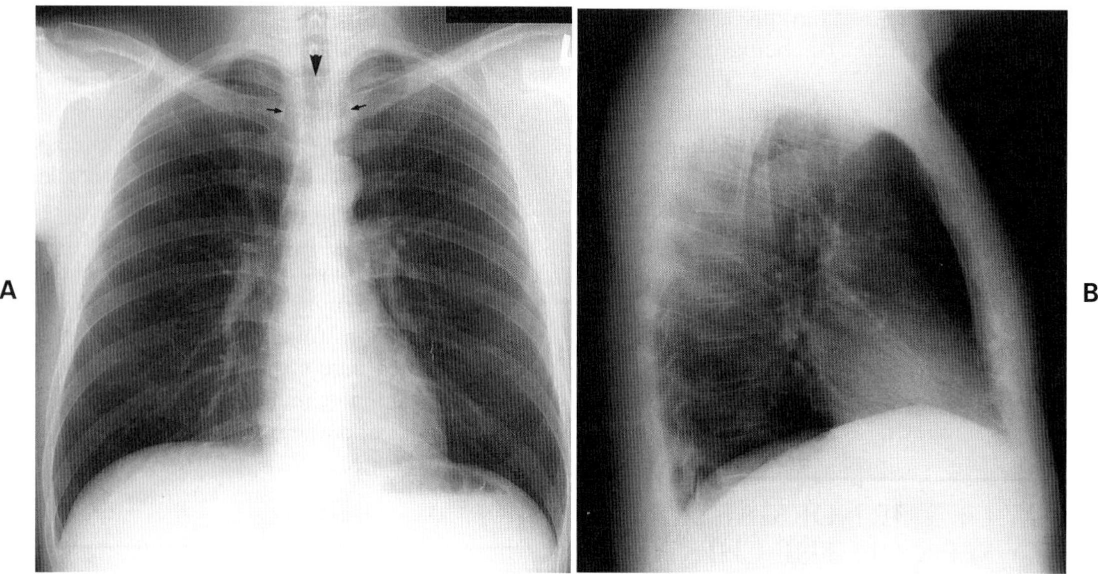

Figure 18-2
Normal frontal (**A**) and normal lateral (**B**) chest films. Note the medial ends of the clavicles (*arrows*) with the spinous process (*arrowhead*) framed between them (**A**).

Patient rotation can make interpretation more difficult by projecting midline structures (e.g., the trachea) to the right or left. The observer can assess for rotation by comparing anterior structures such as the medial (toward the middle) ends of the clavicles with a posterior structure such as the spinous process (midline structure of the spine). In a perfectly positioned chest film, the spinous process should be seen midway between the medial ends of the clavicles (Figure 18-2).

The RT also must ensure that the film is adequately penetrated, noting how the lungs appear relatively dark on the chest film. This is because they are filled with air, which is the least dense material in the chest. Most of the radiation passes through the lungs and produces exposure or blackening of the film (**radiolucency**). The bones are the densest material on the film, and they stop much of the radiation, thus appearing white on the chest film (**radiopacity**). The soft tissues (e.g., heart, blood vessels) are of intermediate density on the chest film. A chest x-ray with proper exposure should show the intervertebral disc spaces through the shadow of the **mediastinum** and should visualize the blood vessels in the lungs. A chest x-ray that is underexposed does not allow visualization of the intervertebral discs through the heart shadow. An over-penetrated x-ray overexposes the film, leaving the lung parenchyma black and no ability to visualize the peripheral blood vessels.

When satisfied that pertinent anatomy is included and that positioning and exposure are adequate, the observer should begin a systematic search for abnormality. This involves applying an individual approach to reviewing the chest x-ray. It may be helpful to divide the anatomy into the chest wall and pleura, the lung parenchyma, and the mediastinum. Assessment of the chest wall should include looking for symmetry, rib fractures or other bone changes, pleural abnormalities such as fluid in the pleural space (hydrothorax), and air in the pleural space (pneumothorax). Evaluation of the lungs is difficult because 80% to 90% of the parenchyma is overlaid with bone in the form of ribs, clavicles, and spine. The lateral film is most helpful in clarifying the presence or absence of lung abnormalities suspected on the frontal projections. The RT must pay specific attention to areas where subtle abnormalities may be hiding. These include the lung tissue behind the clavicles (especially medially), the area of lung that projects behind the heart, and part of the lung that lies deep in the posterior sulcus (the extreme bottom of the lung projecting below the diaphragm on the frontal view). Evaluation of the mediastinum should include assessment of heart size. In the PA projection, the diameter of the heart shadow should not exceed one half the diameter of the chest. The lateral contours of the mediastinum should correspond to normal anatomical structures as outlined in Figure 18-3.

Development and application of a reproducible, comprehensive approach to the assessment of the chest film is very important. The remainder of the chapter outlines commonly encountered abnormalities involving the pleura, the lung parenchyma, and the mediastinum. The reader is encouraged to finely tune his or her observational powers for assessment of imaging studies because, as noted by Pasteur, "In the field of observation, chance favors the prepared mind."

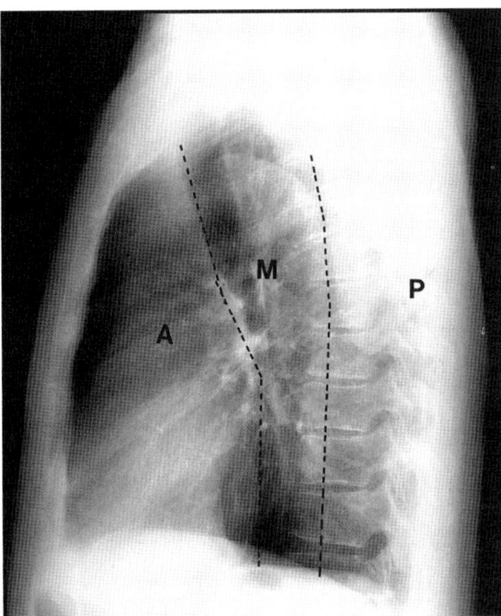

Figure 18-3

Lateral view of the chest, indicating the divisions of the mediastinum. *A*, Anterior; *M*, middle; *P*, posterior.

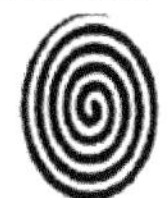

RULE OF THUMB

Three general steps to assessing the chest film:

1. Content assurance (Is the entire chest visible on the film?)
2. Quality assurance (Is the chest x-ray properly exposed and centered?)
3. Disciplined application of personalized search pattern

▶ THE PLEURA

The lungs are surrounded by two thin pleural membranes. The outer membrane, known as the *parietal pleura*, adheres to the inside of the chest wall, the upper surface of the diaphragm, and the lateral aspect of the mediastinal compartment. The inner pleural membrane, or *visceral pleura*, closely adheres to the surface of each lung. The visceral pleura extends into the lung along the fissures that separate the lobes. A small amount of fluid between the two pleural layers allows them to move freely over each other as the lung expands and contracts. The pleural membranes around the lung cannot be seen on the plain (or conventional) chest radiograph, because they blend into the water density of the chest wall, diaphragm, and mediastinum. However, the visceral pleura separating the lobes often can be seen. Although very thin, the visceral pleura is made more visible by the aerated lobes on either side of it, and to some extent, by the small amount of fluid necessary to keep it lubricated. Visibility of the interlobar fissures depends on their position with respect to the x-ray beam. For the fissure to be seen, the x-ray beam must be parallel to the fissure.

Hydrothorax

Hydrothorax refers to accumulation of an abnormal amount of fluid within the pleural space. Its presence is recognized on front and side (or lateral) views of the chest by the so-called pleural meniscus sign[3] (Figure 18-4). This sign is a shadow of uniform density that curves upward against the side of the chest on the front view. On the lateral film, this density also curves upward against the back wall of the chest. In the upright patient, abnormal amounts of pleural fluid accumulate first in a subpulmonic location[4] (i.e., between the pleural layers under the lung and above the diaphragm). The earliest sign of a left-sided pleural effusion on an upright chest x-ray is an increased distance between the inferior margin of the left lung and the stomach gas bubble. With a subpulmonic effusion, there may be an associated slight lateral shift of the point at which the diaphragm dips downward on the frontal chest x-ray (i.e., like a hockey stick with the blade toward the lateral chest wall).

A sharp costophrenic angle, the angle between the diaphragm and the lateral chest wall, is usually maintained on the frontal view, even if 175 to 200 mL of pleural fluid accumulates. With more fluid, the fluid usually spills laterally to blunt the costophrenic angle in the upright patient. Rarely, a sharp costophrenic angle is maintained with as much as 500 mL in the subpulmonic space.[5] The lateral film more sensitively indicates the presence of free fluid. The posterior costophrenic angle becomes blunted with as little as 75 to 100 mL of fluid. The most sensitive type of radiograph for detecting small amounts of pleural fluid is the so-called decubitus view, which is obtained with the patient lying on the side where the effusion is suspected. As little as 5 mL of pleural fluid can be detected on a decubitus radiograph.[6]

An air-fluid level in the pleural space indicates a hydropneumothorax (Figure 18-5). Occasionally, fluid occupies an unusual position such as within an interlobar fissure (which separates lobes of the lung). This is most commonly seen in the minor fissure, which is between the right middle lobe and right upper lobe. Fluid within a fissure can be diagnosed on the chest x-ray by a characteristic lenslike, elliptical shape on either the PA or the lateral projection (Figure 18-6).

In healthy individuals, it is estimated that 1 to 5 mL of pleural fluid is normally present.[7] In general, an increased volume of fluid is categorized as either a transudate or an exudate (see Chapter 22), but an exudate cannot be distinguished from a transudate on the chest x-ray. Rather, making this distinction requires analyzing a sample of the pleural fluid. Loculation of pleural fluid (or trapping so the fluid does not move

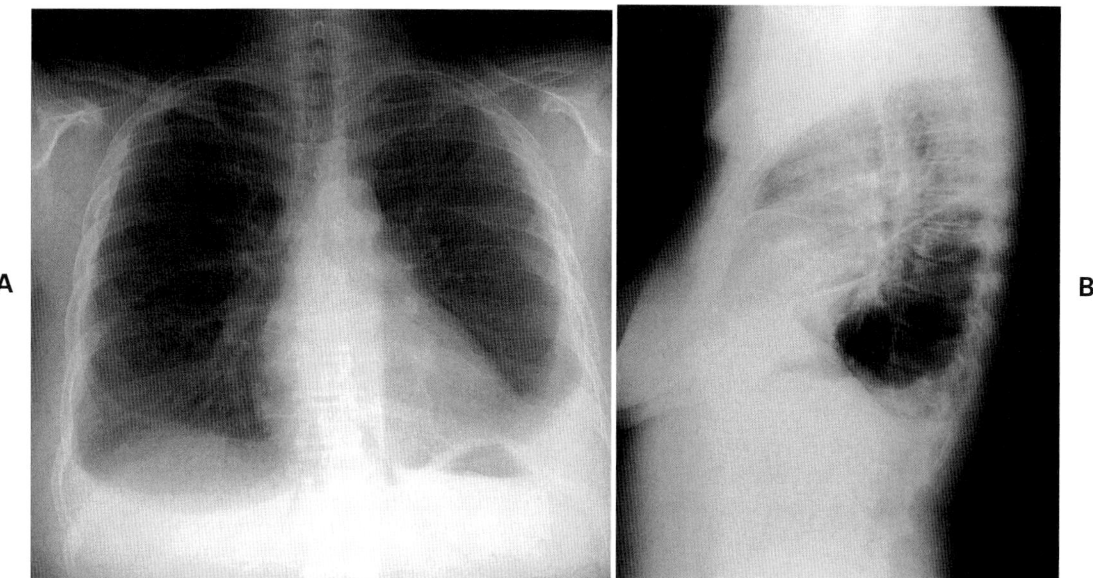

Figure 18-4 · Pleural Effusion
Posteroanterior (**A**) and lateral (**B**) chest films in a 43-year-old patient with longstanding bilateral pleural effusions resulting from rheumatoid arthritis. Note the bilateral meniscus sign is also visualized posteriorly on the lateral view.

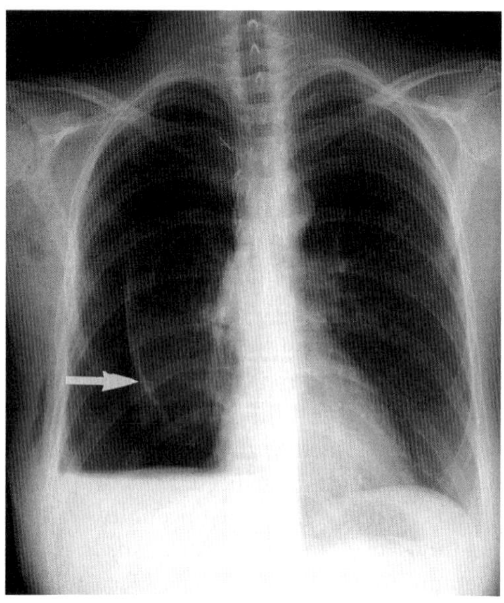

Figure 8-5 · Hydropneumothorax
A single posteroanterior view of the chest in a patient with a hydropneumothorax. Note the air-fluid level in the pleural space. The visceral pleura is slightly thickened (*arrow*) from prior surgery on the right.

freely with changing positions) is more commonly seen in exudative effusions, hemothorax (blood in the pleural space), and empyema (infection of the pleural fluid).

Ultrasound for Evaluating Pleural Fluid

Ultrasound is more sensitive than conventional chest x-rays for identifying exudative pleural effusions.[8,9] The presence of internal echoes, septations (e.g., strands or walls within the fluid), pleural thickening, or nodularity are ultrasound findings that strongly suggest an exudate. Pleural effusions with few echoes may be transudates or exudates (Figure 18-7). Ultrasound is reported to be 92% accurate in differentiating solid pleural lesions from pleural fluid and is a useful imaging way to characterize pleural abnormalities and to guide pleural drainage procedures.[10]

Computed Tomography

Pleural fluid can be identified easily on CT scans of the chest. In the supine patient, free fluid accumulates in the most dependent area of the pleura, which is posterior. CT is less accurate than ultrasound for differentiating exudates from transudates. Heterogeneity and septations within pleural fluid favor an exudate and are better demonstrated by ultrasound. Parietal pleural thickening, enhancement, and nodularity are well seen by CT. An elliptical pleural fluid collection with thickening and enhancement of the surrounding pleura (the split pleura sign) suggests an empyema, which is infected pleural fluid[11] (Figure 18-8). Contraction of the parietal pleura with movement away from the inner aspect of the chest wall and increased density in the extrapleural fat are additional strong signs of empyema. The presence of gas bubbles within the fluid without prior surgery or needle insertion (which can introduce air) establishes the diagnosis of empyema.

Clues to whether a pleural exudate results from inflammation or from cancer may be present on the chest x-ray. The surgical absence of a breast shadow

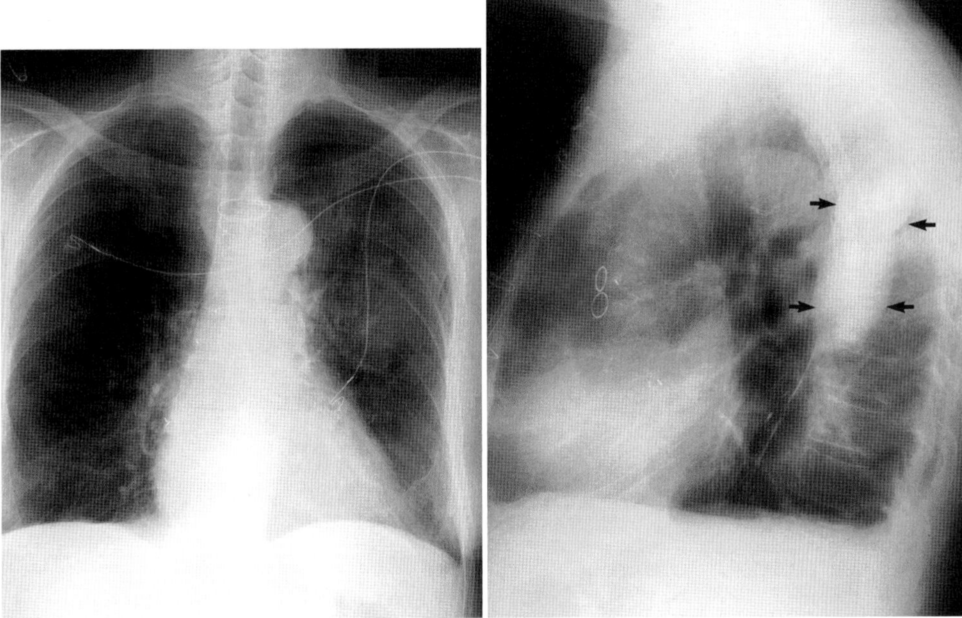

Figure 18-6 · Intrafissural Fluid
Two views of the chest showing fluid accumulating within the superior portion of the major fissure. In the posteroanterior view, the fluid is seen as vague increased density in the left upper lobe. Note the typical elliptical shape of the fluid on the lateral projection (*arrows*).

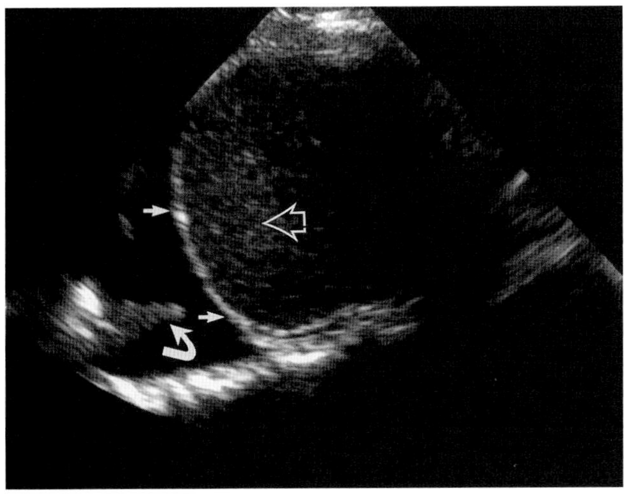

Figure 18-7 · Pleural Ultrasound
Sonographic image shows liver (*open arrow*) in the right upper abdomen with sharp demarcation of this from pleural fluid (anechoic area) by the diaphragm (*small arrows*). Note the tail of atelectatic lower lobe (*curved arrow*) surrounded by anechoic pleural fluid.

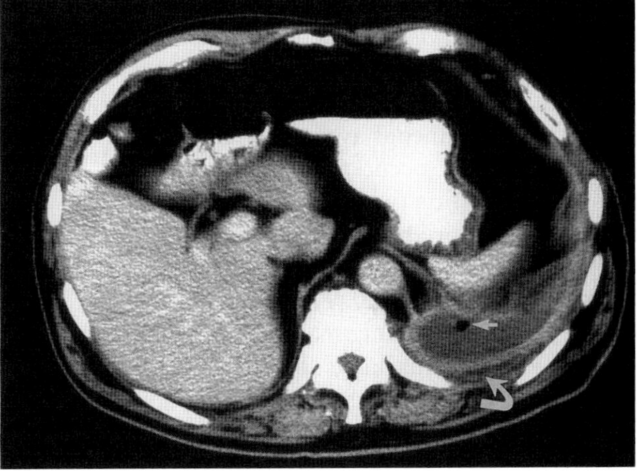

Figure 18-8 · Empyema
Cross-sectional computed tomographic image demonstrates an elliptical-shaped pleural fluid collection surrounded by thickened enhancing pleura (split pleural sign). The presence of the gas bubble (*arrow*) within the fluid and the thickened extrapleural subcostal tissues (*curved arrow*) is strongly suggestive of empyema.

or evidence of prior axillary (armpit) node dissection suggests breast cancer. The coexistence of an enlarging pulmonary parenchymal mass (lung cancer) or multiple lung masses (metastatic disease) suggests malignant pleural involvement. The presence of bone erosions involving the clavicles and shoulders suggests rheumatoid arthritis. Skin calcification may indicate dermatomyositis.

Although they are usefully imaged by chest CT, a discussion of specific focal pleural abnormalities is beyond the scope of this chapter.

Pneumothorax

The term **pneumothorax** refers to the abnormal collection of air within the pleural space. The visceral

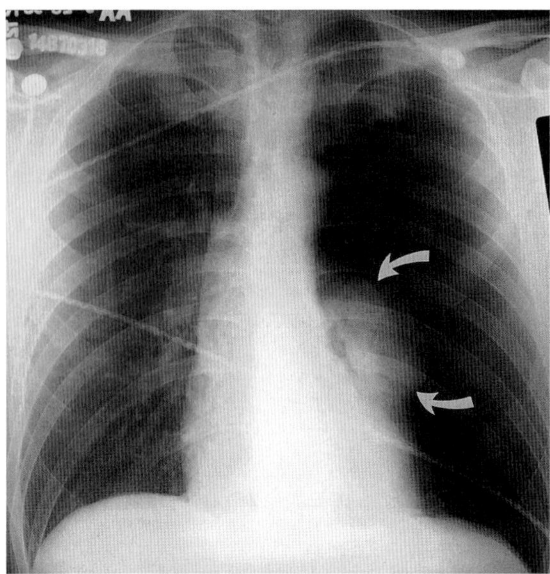

Figure 18-9 · Pneumothorax
Complete atelectasis of the left lung (*curved arrows*) resulting from a large left pneumothorax.

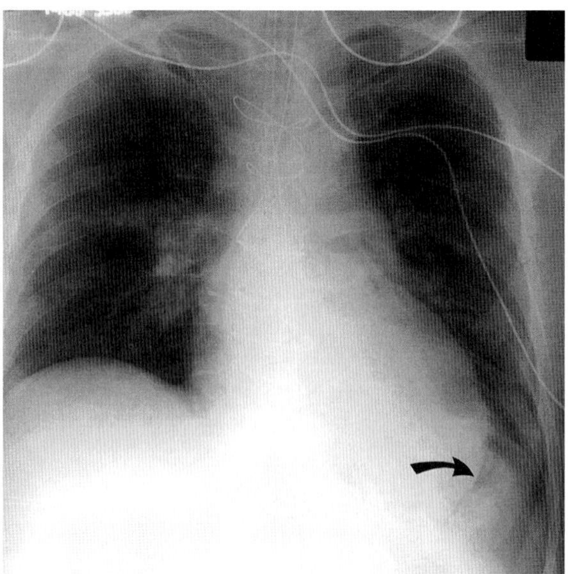

Figure 18-10 · Deep sulcus sign
Portable supine radiograph in a patient status-post median sternotomy. Note the increased lucency in the left upper quadrant. The highest portion of the thorax in the supine patient is the anterior cardiophrenic sulcus. This accounts for the well-defined low cardiac border (*arrow*) and the adjacent fat pad.

pleura surrounding the lung becomes visible when air accumulates in the pleural space. This may occur spontaneously because of rupture of a bleb (a gas-containing space within the visceral pleura of the lung—a form of pulmonary air cyst) or may result from an invasive procedure that punctures the pleura such as a transbronchial biopsy or percutaneous aspiration lung biopsy. Pneumothorax may also occur as a complication of positive pressure ventilation (which is called *barotrauma*). When the patient is upright, the intrapleural air accumulates over the top of the lung (apex) and pushes the lung away from the chest wall. The clinician can easily detect it here by seeing the lung margin and noting absence of bronchovascular markings between the lung margin and the inner aspect of the chest wall (Figure 18-9).

When the patient is supine, the free air in the pleural space moves to the highest point in the chest, which is the anterior cardiophrenic sulcus[12] (see Figure 18-1). Because air in this region does not create a visible edge between the pleura and the x-ray beam, radiographic clues to the presence of pneumothorax are more subtle in the supine patient.[13] If a diagnosis of pneumothorax is suspected, an upright chest radiograph should be taken. Visualizing a small pneumothorax may be assisted by taking the chest x-ray when the patient exhales. The supine patient with a pneumothorax may have a deep sulcus sign[14] (Figure 18-10), which refers to air accumulating anteriorly and outlining the heart border below the dome of the diaphragm. In addition, the upper abdomen on the same side often shows increased lucency. Sometimes, free air outlines fat at the cardiac apex (the "narrow" end of the heart). If the diagnosis remains in doubt, a decubitus radiograph or a cross-table lateral radiograph (in which the patient lies face up while the x-ray is directed across the body) can help make the diagnosis of pneumothorax.

Occasionally, air within the pleural space may be under pressure or tension (Figure 18-11); this is called a *tension pneumothorax*. It is a surgical emergency that occurs when the tear in the pleura (that allows air to leave the lung and enter the pleural space) opens on inspiration but closes on expiration. Air then continues to accumulate in the pleural space and can compress the heart and adjacent lung. A tension pneumothorax is suggested on chest films when the hemidiaphragm is pushed down inferiorly or when the mediastinum is shifted toward the opposite lung. A tension pneumothorax requires immediate decompression with a chest tube or Heimlich valve.

Abnormal Air Collections in the Thorax: Common Etiologies

Barotrauma

Mechanical ventilation may cause rupture of an alveolus, which is a type of barotrauma. Alveolar rupture allows air to leak into the interstitium of the lung, producing pulmonary interstitial emphysema. From this location, the air may migrate along the interstitium surrounding the bronchovascular bundles centrally to produce a pneumomediastinum or outwardly to the pleural surface, where the air may rupture into the pleural space, producing a pneumothorax.

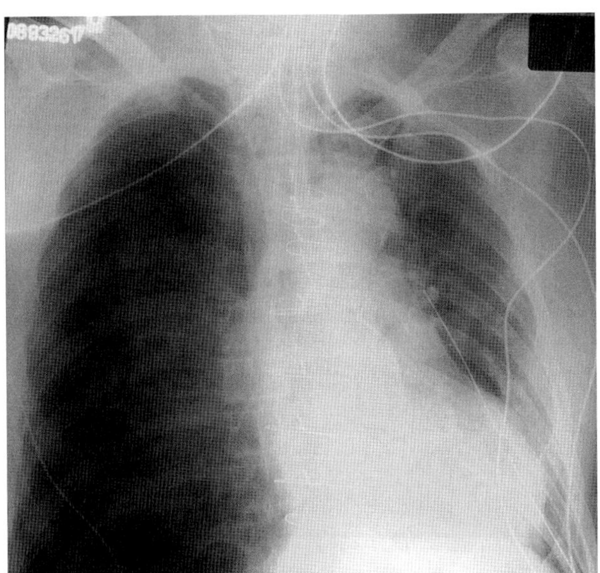

Figure 18-11 · Tension pneumothorax
Portable chest radiograph in a patient status-post median sternotomy and coronary artery bypass grafting. Note the large right pneumothorax displacing the mediastinum to the left and the right hemidiaphragm inferiorly. These findings indicate the presence of a tension pneumothorax on the right requiring immediate chest tube placement.

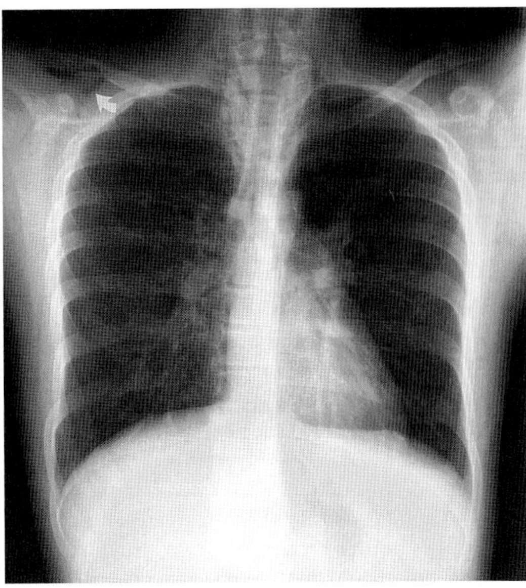

Figure 18-12 · Pneumomediastinum
Posteroanterior view of the chest of an 11-year-old asthmatic shows linear lucencies (free air) in the mediastinum and extending into the soft tissues of the neck bilaterally. Note the free air around the lateral aspect of the right clavicle (*arrow*).

Pneumothorax

As described previously, a pneumothorax may result from barotrauma, but also may result from spontaneous rupture of a paraseptal (subpleural) bleb or from unintended puncture of the lung while a central line is being placed (see Figures 18-9 and 18-10).

Pneumomediastinum

Pneumomediastinum, another sign of barotrauma, may result from movement of air into the mediastinum, as may also be seen in cases of esophageal rupture (Figure 18-12). This usually occurs in the distal portion of the esophagus in patients who undergo procedures to stretch or dilate the esophagus. Chest trauma may cause rupture of a main bronchus, also allowing movement of air into the mediastinum. Rarely, air dissects down from the soft tissues of the neck after thyroid, parathyroid, or tonsillar surgery. Gas associated with a retrotonsillar abscess may also move down to the mediastinum through the fascial planes of the neck. Air that accumulates in the retroperitoneum may enter the mediastinum via openings in the diaphragm for the aorta or esophagus.

▶ LUNG PARENCHYMA

The lung parenchyma is made up of two components, the air sacs (alveoli) and the interstitium (the supporting structures of the lung). Lung diseases that produce infiltrates usually involve both components, although one component is usually affected most. When filled, the alveoli have a characteristic radiographic appearance regardless of the material that fills them. The material that fills alveoli can be either water, pus, fat, or blood and varies depending on the cause of the infiltrate. In the case of a bacterial pneumonia, alveoli are filled with a watery inflammatory cellular exudate (pus), and in the case of pulmonary hemorrhage, they fill with blood. Both pneumonia and a bleeding lung may cause an identical-appearing shadow on the chest x-ray, which is referred to as an **alveolar infiltrate** and is characterized by patchy areas of increased density that tend to coalesce over time.

These shadows or opacities often have lucent tubular visible structures running through them that represent **air bronchograms** (Figure 18-13). Normally, patent airways are not visible in the outer two thirds of the lung on the chest x-ray. However, the increased contrast produced by filling of the surrounding alveoli makes the airways more visible and causes the *air bronchogram sign*. Air bronchograms are the hallmark of infiltrates that fill alveoli (so-called air space disease) (Figure 18-14) (Table 18-1).

RULE OF THUMB

Air bronchograms indicate that the opacification is located in the lung parenchyma and not in the pleural space. They suggest **pulmonary infiltrates** such as pneumonia.

MINI CLINI

Use of the Silhouette Sign

PROBLEM

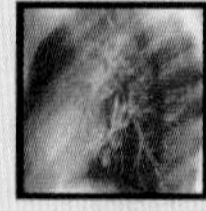

A patient has an infiltrate in the lower half of his right lung. It is not clear if this pneumonia is located in the right middle lobe or in the upper portion of the lower lobe. Is there a way to identify the location of this infiltrate?

ANSWER

If the right heart border is visible next to the infiltrate, the pneumonia is located in the lower lobe behind the heart. If the right heart border is not visible, the infiltrate must be located in the right middle lobe next to the right side of the heart.

Pneumonia is considered a water density, and when two structures of similar density are touching each other in the same plane, the border between the two structures will not be seen. Pneumonia in the upper segments of the lower lobe appears to be next to the heart on the PA chest film but does not obliterate the heart border in such cases. This is known as the *silhouette sign*.

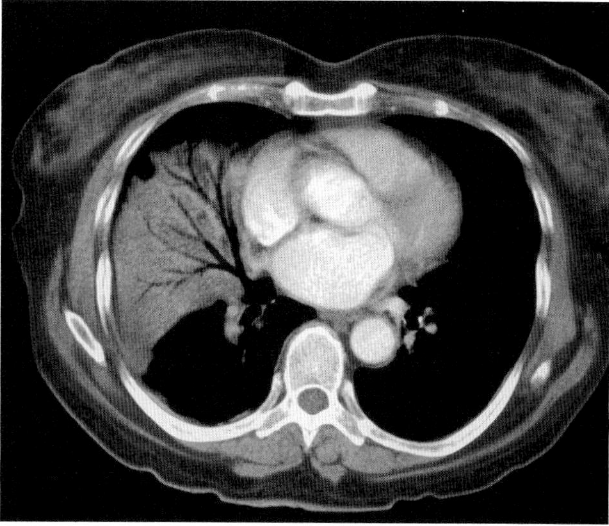

Figure 18-14 · Right Middle Lobe Pneumonia
Computed axial tomographic slice shows an alveolar filling process in the right middle lobe with tubular air bronchograms running through it. The patient is a 73-year-old female with right middle lobe pneumonia.

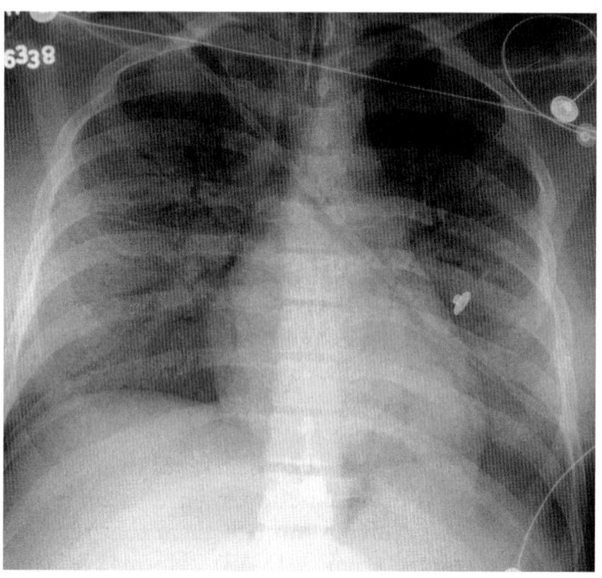

Figure 18-13 · Air Bronchograms
This portable radiograph shows diffuse increased density throughout both lungs highlighted by tubular lucencies. These are air bronchograms. They are visualized because of the alveolar filling that surrounds them. This typical alveolar-filling pattern (air space disease) suggests acute pneumonia, pulmonary hemorrhage, or pulmonary edema.

Table 18-1 ▶▶ Radiographic Features of Alveolar Versus Interstitial Processes

Alveolar (Air Space) Disease	Interstitial Disease
Air bronchograms	Nodules
Fluffy opacities	Linear/reticular opacities
Rapid coalescence	Septal lines
Acinar nodules	Cysts
Segmental/lobar distribution	Honeycombing

Diseases that mainly involve the interstitium have a different radiographic appearance (see Table 18-1). Such diseases involve that portion of the lung that frames the air spaces and supports the vessels and bronchi as they travel through the lung. The functional unit of the lung is the so-called secondary pulmonary lobule.[15] This structural unit is made up of the lung beyond the terminal bronchiole. The bronchovascular bundle runs in the center of the secondary pulmonary lobule, which is bounded by interlobular septa that contain the small veins and lymphatics (Figure 18-15). Thickening around the structures of the secondary pulmonary lobule and the interlobular septa produces the radiographic signs of **interstitial lung disease.** The secondary pulmonary lobules are arranged in an organized geometric fashion in the lung periphery; septal thickening there gives rise to so-called Kerley B lines. Kerley B lines are short, thin, faint linear shadows measuring 1 to 3 cm in length (Figure 18-16). They usually are best seen along the lower lateral lung margins, but wherever they occur, they are always perpendicular to the nearest pleural surface. Kerley A and C lines also represent thickened lymphatics but in different anatomical locations.[16] Kerley A lines are thin, nonbranching lines that radiate from the hila but are not arteries or veins. Kerley C lines are fine interlacing lines seen throughout the lung and

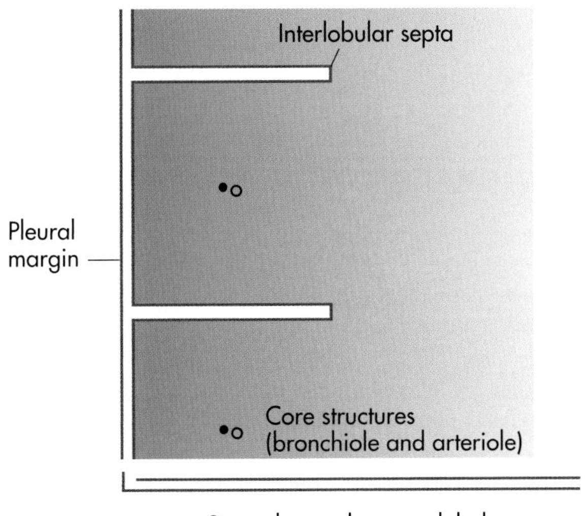

Figure 18-15
Diagramatic representation of the secondary pulmonary lobule.

Table 18-2 ▶▶ Clues on the Plain Chest Radiograph to the Specific Cause of Interstitial Lung Disease

Clue on Radiograph	Cause of Disease
Pneumothorax	Lymphangioleiomyomatosis Eosinophilic granuloma of lung
Pleural effusion	Rheumatoid arthritis Systemic lupus erythematosus
Dilated esophagus	Scleroderma CREST syndrome
Erosive arthropathy (shoulder joints, clavicles)	Rheumatoid arthritis
Mediastinal adenopathy	Sarcoidosis Scleroderma Metastatic disease
Soft tissue calcification	Dermatomyositis Scleroderma
Pleural plaques	Asbestosis

CREST, Calcinosis cutis, Raynaud's phenomenon, esophageal dysfunction, sclerodactyly, and telangiectasia.

represent septa of more haphazardly oriented secondary pulmonary lobules. Kerley lines may be seen for only a brief time (as in pulmonary edema) or persistently (as in some occupational inhalational diseases or lymphangitic metastases).

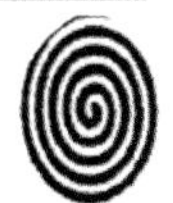

RULE OF THUMB

Radiographic signs of cardiac decompensation include the following:

- Cardiac enlargement
- Pleural effusion
- Redistribution of blood flow to the upper lobes
- Poor definition to central vessels (perihilar haze)
- Kerley B lines
- Alveolar filling

NOTE: These findings are seen in Figure 18-16.

In general, interstitial lung disease refers to inflammation of the interstitium characterized by accumulation of neutrophils, macrophages, or lymphocytes.[17] Through release of mediators, these inflammatory cells may cause pulmonary scarring or fibrosis. The radiographic signs of pulmonary fibrosis are volume loss and honeycombing, which is the development of cystic spaces with well-defined walls seen in the periphery of the lung and resembling a bee's honeycomb. Honeycombing is thought to represent irreversible scarring and indicates end-stage lung disease (Figure 18-17).

Many conditions may cause interstitial lung disease. These may be infectious (as in viral pneumonia) or occupational (e.g., asbestosis or silicosis) (see Chapter 21). The two most common interstitial lung diseases, sarcoidosis and fibrosing alveolitis, have no known cause.[18] Because many different types of interstitial lung diseases have the same appearance on the plain chest x-ray, the chest film rarely establishes the specific cause of interstitial disease. Clues to specific causes of interstitial lung disease on the plain chest x-ray are reviewed in Table 18-2.

Assessing Lung Volume

Volume loss, or atelectasis, is a common abnormality on chest x-rays, and the location and extent of volume loss produces characteristic chest x-ray patterns. Atelectasis may be localized to a subsegmental portion of the lung, where it has a classic radiographic appearance called **plate atelectasis**[19] (Figure 18-18). Plate atelectasis is associated with ventilatory disturbance, including restricted diaphragmatic motion, sometimes with resultant alveolar hypoventilation; retained secretions producing small airway obstruction; and diminished surfactant production.[20] Atelectasis commonly occurs after abdominal or thoracic surgery, with pleurisy, or following pleural irritation from rib fracture or pulmonary infarction.

Volume loss involving a whole lobe is usually caused by central airway obstruction.[21] The collapsed lobe assumes the shape of a wedge with the apex of the wedge at the hilum and the base of the wedge on the pleural surface. This wedge will be visible on the PA or lateral x-ray, depending on which lobe is collapsed (Figure 18-19). The central bronchial obstruction may be caused by a cancer, foreign body, or a mucous plug (Figure 18-20). As shown in Figure 18-21, a bulging convexity to the apex of the wedge indicates a central tumor.

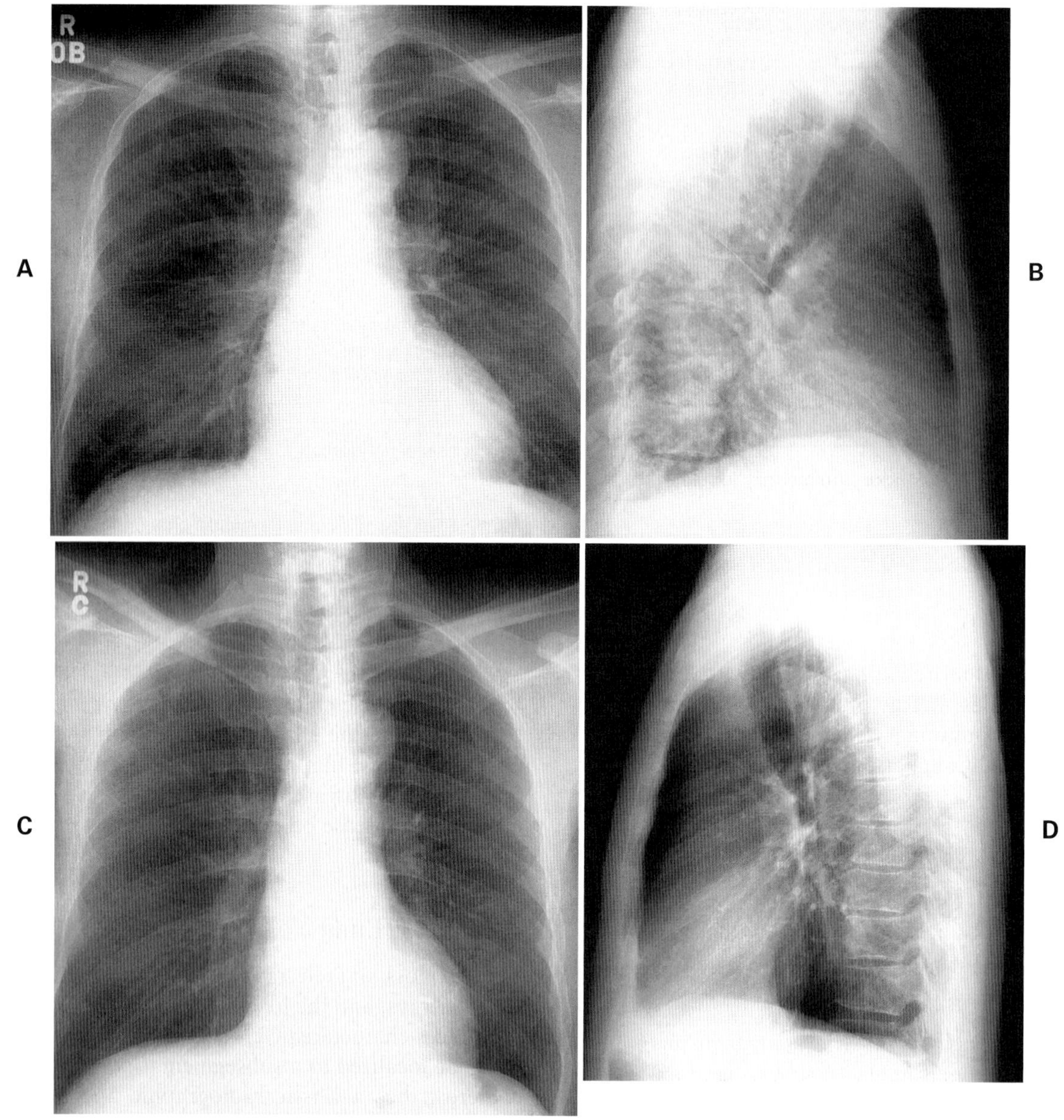

Figure 8-16

Posteroanterior (**A**) and lateral (**B**) chest films show an enlarged cardiac silhouette. The lateral lung margins are slightly displaced away from the inner chest wall in both costophrenic angles, which is consistent with bilateral effusions. There is thickening of the fissures on the lateral projection, indicating that the pleural fluid is extending into the interlobar fissures. Numerous Kerley B lines are seen as linear densities extending to the pleural surface in the right lower chest. The definition of the central vessels is suboptimal, indicating interstitial edema. **C** and **D**, Same patient following therapeutic diuresis. Note the decreased heart size, disappearance of Kerley B lines, and improved definition of central pulmonary vasculature.

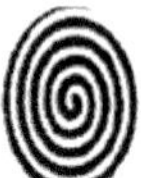

RULE OF THUMB

Radiographic signs of volume loss include the following:

1. Fissure displacement
2. Wedge of increased density (lobar collapse)
3. Unilateral diaphragmatic elevation
4. Mediastinal shift
5. Narrowing of rib cage
6. Compensatory hyperaeration
7. Hilar displacement

See Figures 18-19, 18-20, and 18-21.

Assessment of lung volumes on the chest x-ray requires several observations. Rib counting is a popular method to assess lung volume. With a good inspiration, the sixth and sometimes the seventh anterior rib should project above the diaphragm. If more than seven anterior ribs are visible above the diaphragm, hyperinflation is present. Obstructive pulmonary disease is classically associated with increased lung volumes (hyperinflation). In patients with chronic obstructive pulmonary disease, there may also be an increase in the AP diameter of the chest, with associated enlargement of the retrosternal

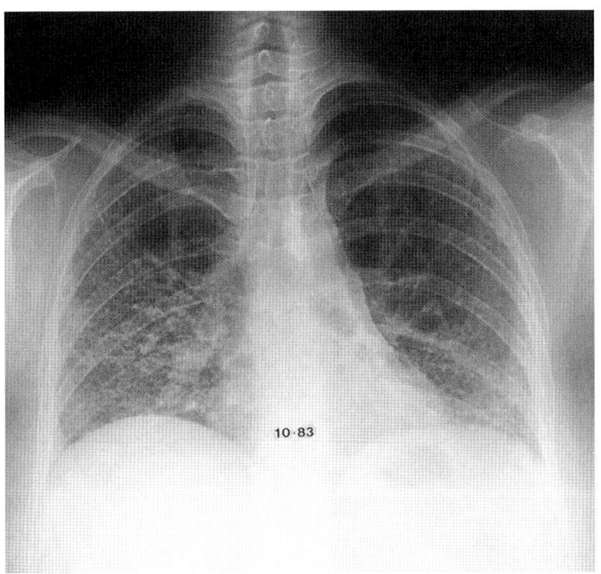

Figure 18-17

Posteroanterior view of the chest in a patient complaining of shortness of breath. The film demonstrates interstitial lung disease. The lung volumes are diminished. Several small cystic lucencies are visualized between the increased basilar interstitial markings representing honeycombing. The diagnosis is scleroderma lung. No esophageal abnormalities are evident on this film.

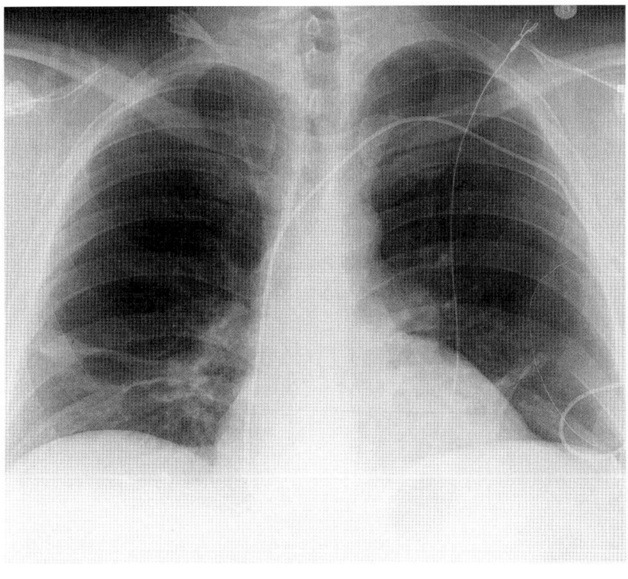

Figure 18-18 · Plate Atelectasis

Posteroanterior chest film shows linear areas of plate atelectasis in both lower lobes.

and retrocardiac air spaces and flattening of the hemidiaphragms. These are all secondary signs of pulmonary emphysema. The only primary signs of emphysema are loss and/or shifting of pulmonary vessel markings and the appearance of the walls of bullous air spaces (Figure 18-22).

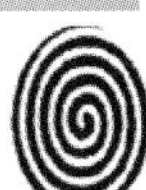

RULE OF THUMB

A good inspiratory effort by the patient is needed to obtain a quality chest film. Visualization of six anterior or ten posterior ribs above the level of the diaphragm indicates a good inspiratory effort by the patient.

Because radiographic signs of emphysema are apparent only with more advanced degrees of airflow obstruction, the chest x-ray is generally considered insensitive for detecting obstructive lung disease. However, CT is far more sensitive and may show evidence of emphysema even when pulmonary function test results are normal.[22] For example, Figure 18-23 demonstrates a case of upper lobe paraseptal emphysema, characterized by cysts on the pleural surface. Chest CT can also be used to assess the volume of lung destroyed by emphysema, using a computer program to identify all areas where the density falls below a value representing air rather than tissue.[23] These low-density areas have been shown to correspond to emphysema at autopsy. Chest CT may prove useful to define which patients may benefit from treatments such as lung volume reduction surgery.

Catheters, Lines, and Tubes

Endotracheal Tube

Endotracheal tubes are radiopaque or have an opaque marker indicating the end of the tube. Radiographs are routinely obtained at the bedside after intubation to assess correct tube position. The radiograph shows the distal tip of the endotracheal tube and the carina.[24] The position of the patient's neck is important. The neck position usually is neutral, but the position of the tip of the endotracheal tube can vary with neck position. Specifically, the difference between neck extension (high position) and neck flexion (low position) may be as much as 4 cm (which is one third the length of the average adult trachea). Goodman and Putman[25] suggest that when the head and neck are in the neutral position, the endotracheal tube should be midtrachea (5 to 7 cm from the carina). Placement below the thoracic inlet will ensure that the tube is beyond the vocal cords (usually at C5-6). Figure 18-24 shows a malpositioned endotracheal tube in the right mainstem bronchus.

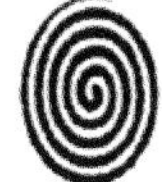

RULE OF THUMB

The distal tip of the endotracheal tube should be positioned approximately 5 cm above the level of the carina in the adult patient.

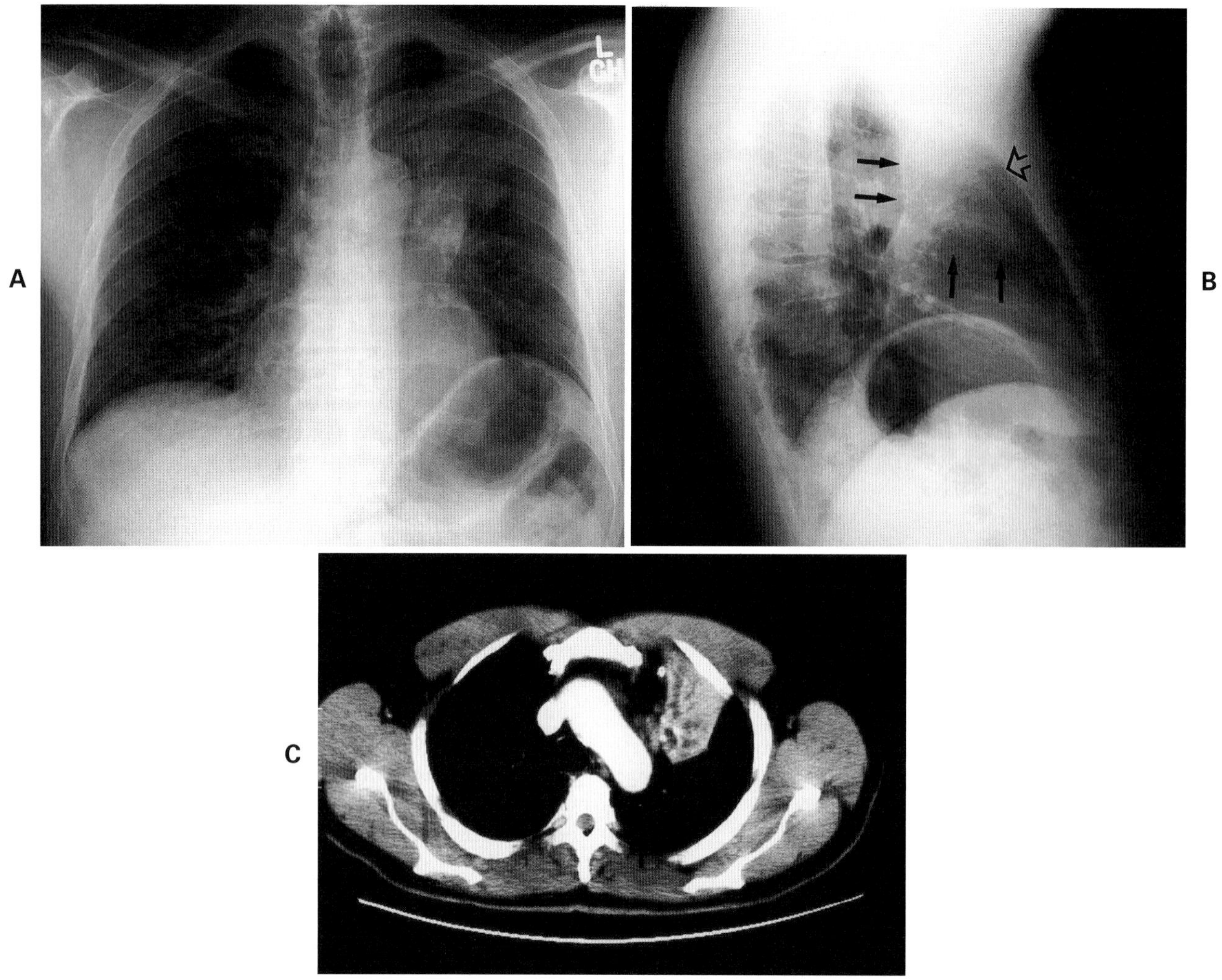

Figure 18-19

A, Posteroanterior view of the chest shows an elevated left hemidiaphragm, a left hilar mass, and increased density in the left upper chest. **B**, The lateral projection shows elevation of the left hemidiaphragm and a wedge of increased density (*arrows*), with its apex at the hilum and its base on the pleural surface. The lucency (*open arrow*) between the sternum and the wedge is herniated right upper lobe. **C**, The computed axial tomographic slice demonstrates the wedge of atelectatic left upper lobe. The tubular lucencies within it are mucous-filled bronchi.

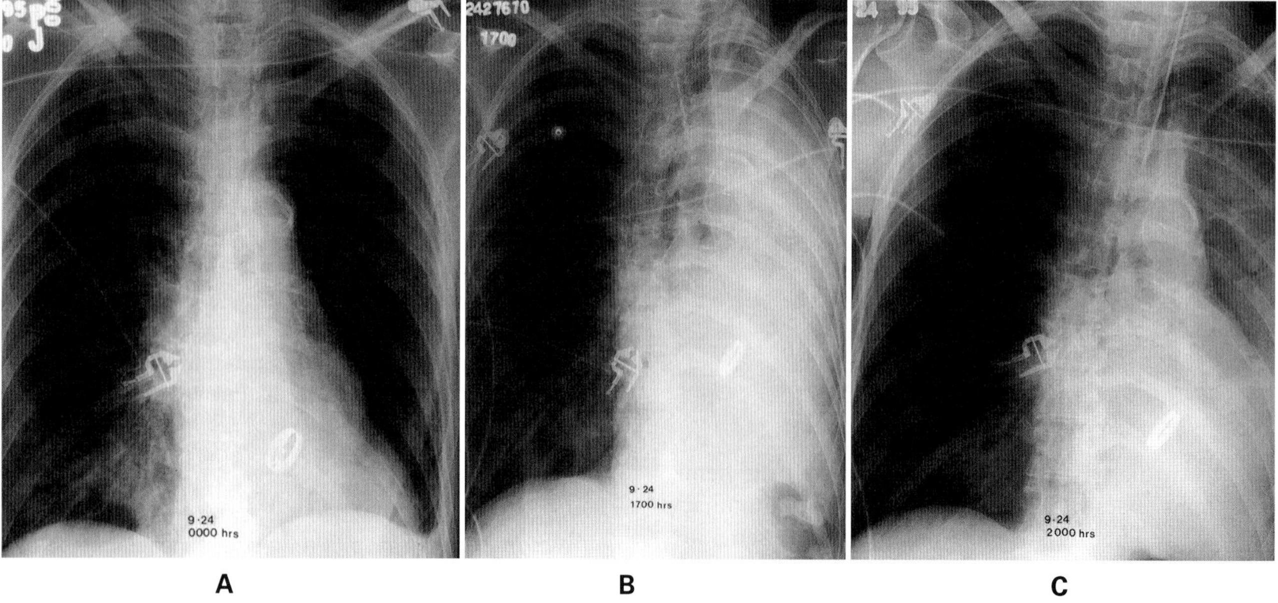

Figure 18-20

Three portable chest films obtained within a 20-hour time span. **A**, Good aeration of both lungs. **B**, Film obtained 17 hours later shows complete opacification of the left hemithorax. Bronchoscopy performed after this film revealed a mucous plug in the left main bronchus. It was removed at bronchoscopy. **C**, Partial reexpansion.

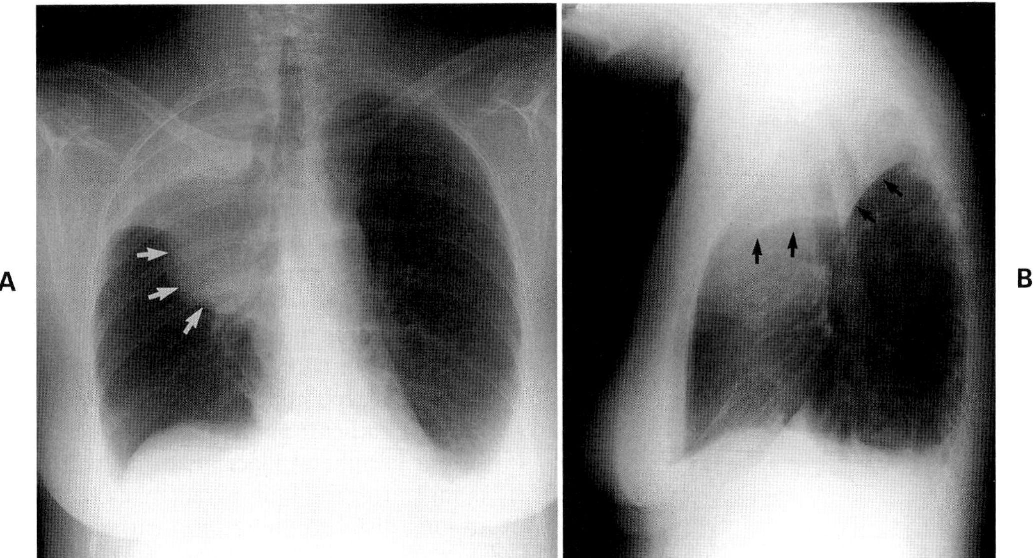

Figure 18-21
Posteroanterior (PA) (**A**) and lateral (**B**) views of the chest in a patient with right upper lobe collapse. **A**, Note the wedge opacity of the right upper lobe. Note the inferior bulge (*arrows*) of the minor fissure on the PA film. This indicates the presence of a central mass. **B**, The wedge shape of right upper lobe atelectasis (*arrows*) is well seen on the lateral film.

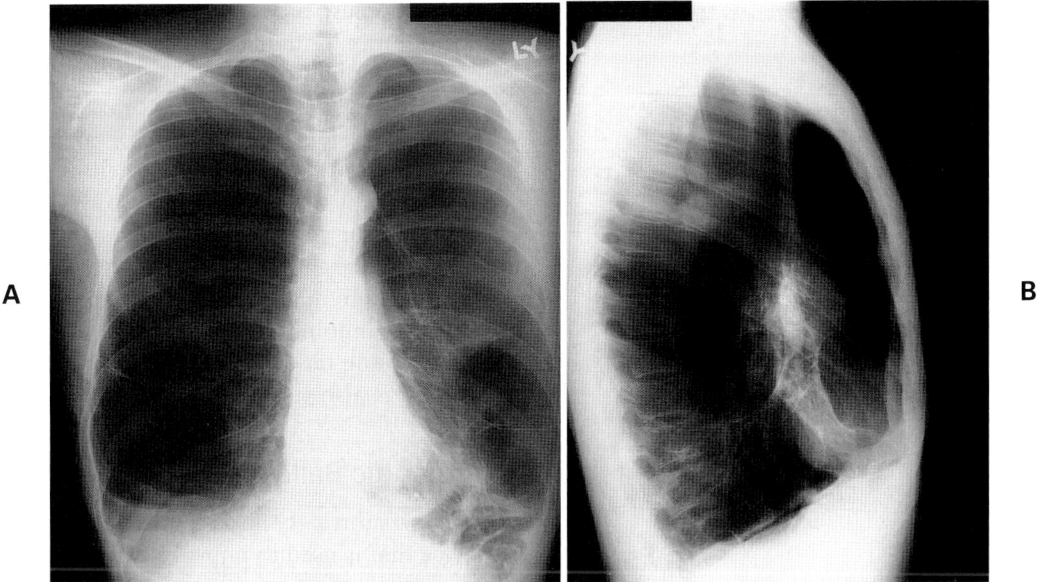

Figure 18-22
Posteroanterior and lateral views of the chest of a patient with bullous emphysema. Marked pulmonary hyperinflation is worse on the right. The asymmetrical hyperinflation is producing mediastinal shift to the left. There is flattening of the diaphragm, prominence of the clear spaces, and large areas in the upper lung zones that are devoid of any vascular markings. The walls of these bullous air spaces are well visualized.

Tracheostomy Tubes

Tracheostomy tubes should be two thirds the diameter of the trachea and should project within the borders of the trachea on the radiograph. The tip should extend beyond half the distance from the stoma to the carina.

Central Lines

The central venous pressure (CVP) catheter is often placed via the internal jugular veins or subclavian veins. A radiograph should be obtained after placement to assess position and to exclude procedural complications

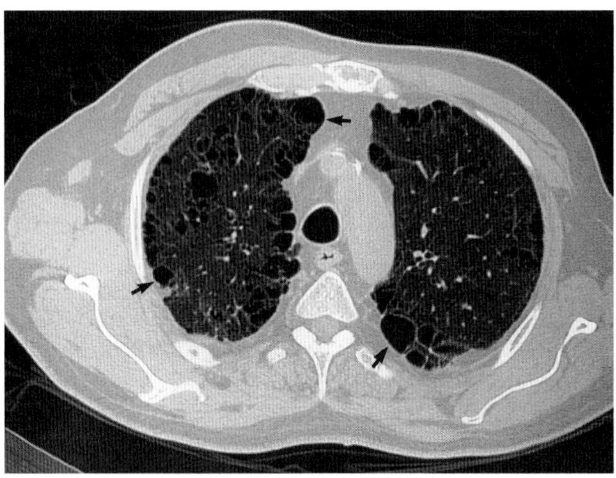

Figure 18-23
Computed tomographic slice through the upper lungs in a patient with pulmonary emphysema. Numerous cystic lucencies are present in both lungs. Note the absence of bronchovascular markings within the lucencies. Most of the emphysematous areas are located in a peripheral distribution (*arrows*) along the pleural surface (paraseptal).

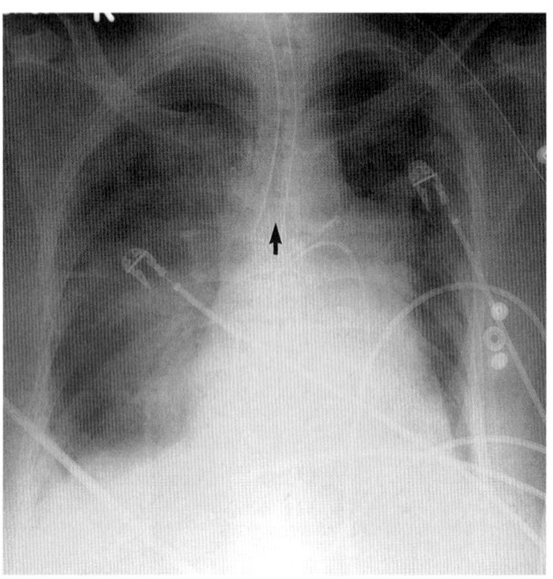

Figure 18-24
Portable supine chest film demonstrates malposition of an endotracheal tube in the right mainstem bronchus (*arrow*).

(e.g., pneumothorax, hemothorax). Ideally, the tip of the CVP catheter should be in the superior vena cava. This vessel usually forms at the level of the first anterior intercostal space where the brachiocephalic veins come together. The brachiocephalic veins contain valves and, ideally, these catheters should be placed central to any valves.

Pulmonary Artery (Swan-Ganz) Catheters

Swan-Ganz catheters are used to measure hemodynamic and central pressure variables such as pulmonary artery occlusion pressure. Pulmonary artery catheters are placed at the bedside and ideally should reside in the proximal right or left main pulmonary arteries. They are floated into position using an inflatable balloon on the catheter tip. Because of this floating, they are placed in the right pulmonary artery more than 90% of the time. When measuring the so-called wedge or pulmonary artery occlusion pressure, the balloon is inflated and the catheter moves out into a more peripheral vessel. As soon as the reading is accomplished, the balloon should be deflated and the catheter pulled back to a central location. Persistent peripheral placement (i.e., when the catheter tip is far out in the lung parenchyma) can cause infarction of lung distal to the wedged catheter (Figure 18-25).

Chest Tubes

Chest tubes are large-bore tubes placed into the pleural space from outside the chest wall. The most common indications for a chest tube are pneumothorax (air in the pleural space) and empyema (pus in the pleural space), although chest tubes may also be used to drain blood (hemothorax) or fluid (hydrothorax) or to install a sealant (e.g., the antibiotic doxycycline) to achieve closure of the pleural space when pneumothorax or hydrothorax are causing persistent dyspnea. Radiographically, chest tubes have radiopaque stripes along their axis so they can be seen on the plain chest radiograph. The chest tube should be within the pleural space; thus it usually follows the contour of the chest wall or diaphragm on one chest x-ray view. Clues to malposition of the chest tube may include persistent bubbling, which may indicate penetration into the lung tissue itself, especially if the radiographic position is also suspicious for parenchymal placement.

Intraaortic Balloon Pump

The intraaortic balloon pump is a counterpulsation device that is used to improve cardiac output and blood pressure in patients with cardiogenic shock. It is inserted through the femoral artery and advanced into the thoracic aorta. The device is approximately 26 cm long, and a radiopaque tip on the top allows radiographic verification of position. The pump inflates the balloon during diastole and it deflates during systole to enhance perfusion of the coronary arteries and cardiac output. The radiopaque tip should reside just beyond to the origin of the left subclavian artery.

Solitary Pulmonary Nodule

The solitary pulmonary nodule (SPN) is defined as parenchymal opacity smaller than 3 cm in diameter that

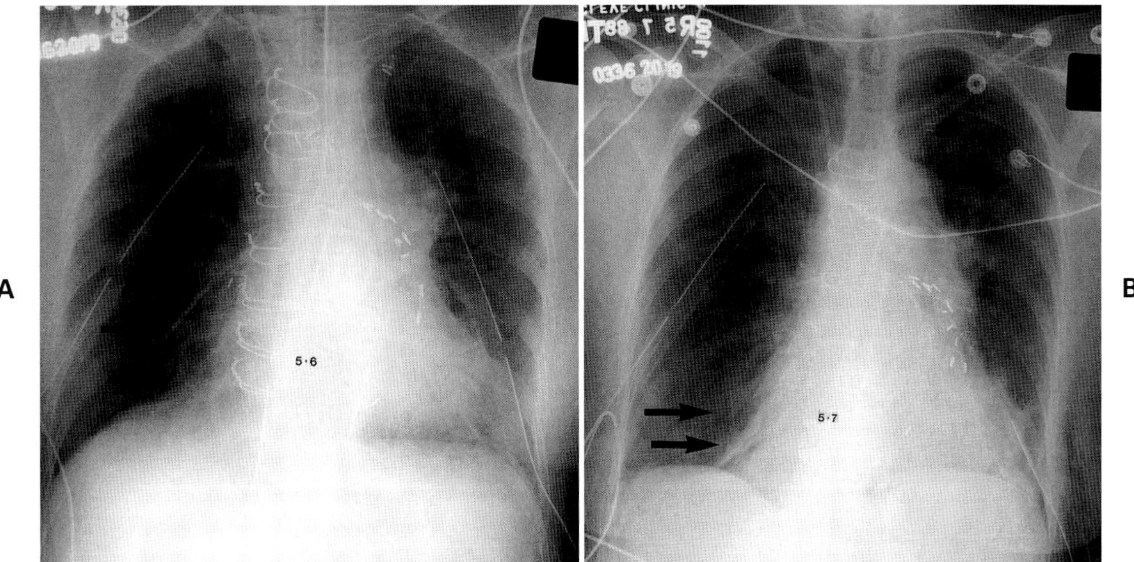

Figure 18-25

Two portable supine chest films obtained 30 hours apart. **A**, A wedged Swan-Ganz (pulmonary artery) catheter in the right lower lobe (*arrow*). **B**, Film obtained after retraction of the catheter shows increased density at the site, reflecting an area of infarction caused by prolonged inadvertent wedging of the catheter (*arrows*).

is totally surrounded by aerated lung. One or two SPNs are encountered in every 1000 chest radiographs. The reported prevalence of malignancy in an SPN varies from 3% to 6% in large surveys of the general population to 30% to 60% among resected nodules.[26]

When first encountered, an SPN should be assessed for features listed in Table 18-3 that may help establish a nonmalignant cause. The goal of imaging an SPN is to avoid resecting benign nodules while encouraging surgical removal of all potentially curable cancers. The axial anatomical display of CT coupled with the better density discriminating powers combine to make CT a favored tool for evaluating the SPN. CT provides a detailed evaluation of the shape and edges of pulmonary nodules in addition to helping identify whether calcification is present and, if so, the pattern of its calcification (Figure 18-26).

Table 18-3 ▶▶ Features Useful in Distinguishing Benign from Malignant Solitary Pulmonary Nodules

Feature	Favoring Malignant	Favoring Benign
Patient age	>40 years old	<40 years old
Smoking status	Current or former smoker	Never smoked
Size	>3 cm	<3 cm
Shape	Lobulated	Spherical
Margins	Spiculated	Well defined
If cavitary...	Thick wall	Thin wall
Doubling time*	7-465 days	<7 or >465 days
Calcification	Rare; usually eccentric	Central, lamellar, popcorn

*Time necessary for the nodule to double in volume.

Central or lamellar (swirls of concentric rings) calcification strongly suggests a benign cause of the SPN or a granuloma. Eccentric (off center), speckled, or amorphous calcification may be seen in cancers. A smooth-edged round nodule will more often be benign, whereas a lobulated or spiculated (having a spikelike appearance) edge is more likely to be a malignant nodule (see Figure 18-26).

▶ THE MEDIASTINUM

The mediastinum lies between the lungs and is divided into three compartments: anterior, middle, and posterior mediastinum. Once a mediastinal abnormality has been found, the precise anatomical placement will help determine possible causes. The mediastinal compartments are best defined on the lateral chest film (see Figure 18-3). A line extending from the diaphragm along the posterior margin of the heart and the anterior margin of the trachea to the neck divides the anterior mediastinum from the middle compartment. A second line traversing the vertebral bodies 1 cm behind their anterior margins and extending from the neck to the diaphragm divides the middle from the posterior compartment. Most mediastinal masses are visible on both front and lateral projections, and the specific location within the mediastinum offers the first clue to diagnosis.

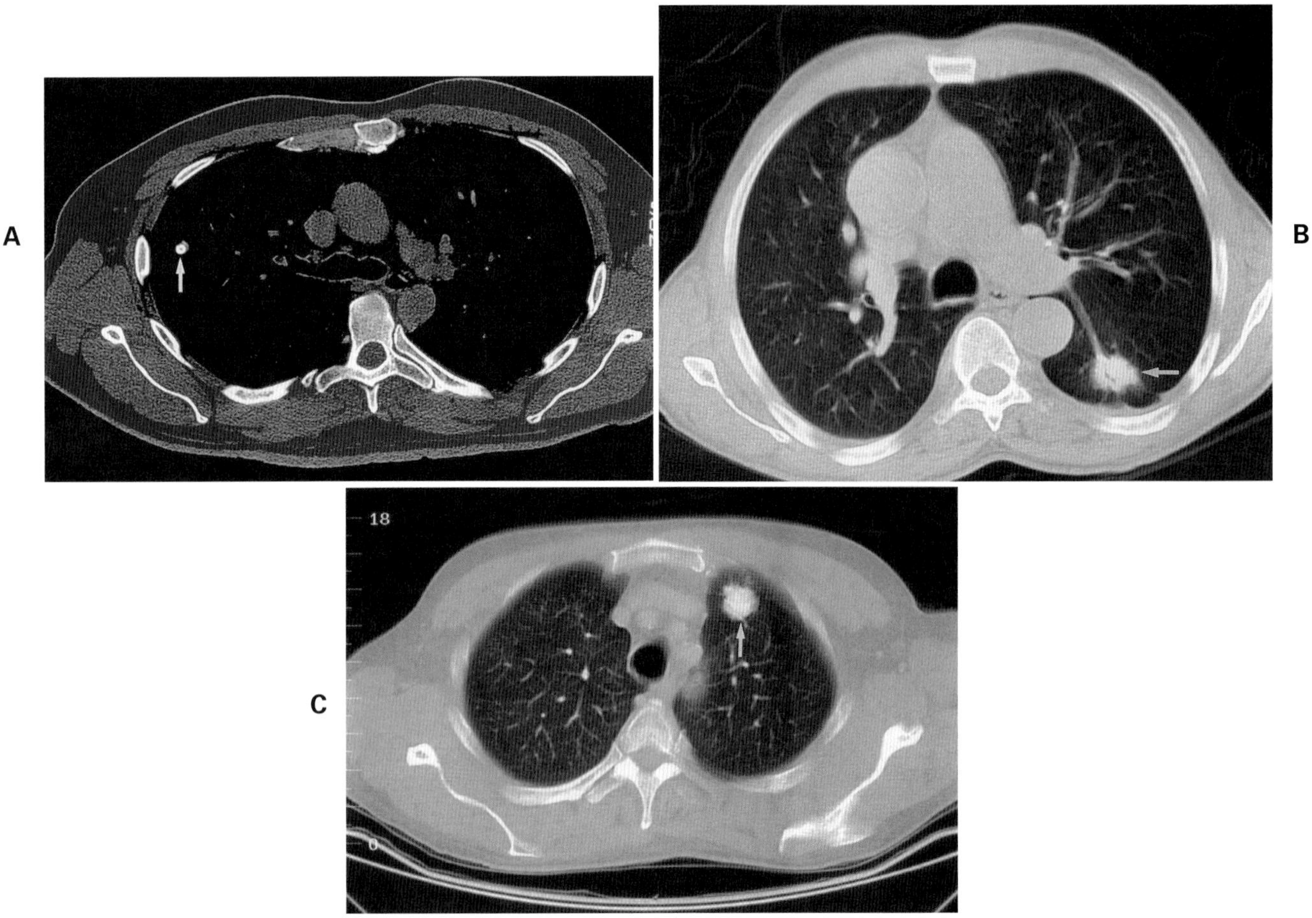

Figure 18-26

Computed tomography examples of solitary pulmonary nodules. **A**, Ringlike calcification in a right upper lobe solitary pulmonary nodule. This lamellar calcification indicates a granuloma (a benign nodule usually caused by an inhaled infectious agent, such as fungus) (*arrow*). **B**, Note the spiculated edge of this left lower lobe pulmonary nodule (*arrow*). This is a lung cancer. **C**, The lobulated edge of this nodule (*arrow*) indicates different growth rates within different areas of this bronchogenic carcinoma.

Table 18-4 ▶ ▶ Mediastinal Abnormalities By Compartment

Anterior Mediastinum	Middle	Posterior Mediastinum
Thyroid and parathyroid masses	Aortic aneurysm (ascending/arch)	Aortic aneurysm (descending)
Thymic lesions	Lymphadenopathy	Neurogenic tumors
Lymphoma	Bronchogenic cyst	Lymphoma
Pericardial cyst/fat pad	Tracheoesophageal masses	Neuroenteric cyst
Teratoma	Hiatal hernia	Bochdalek hernia*
Morgagni hernia*		
Ventricular aneurysm		

*Hernia in which the abdominal contents press through a gap in the diaphragm.

Table 18-4 lists the common causes of masses in the three mediastinal compartments. CT is the best type of imaging for assessing most mediastinal masses. Figure 18-27 demonstrates the normal axial anatomical display on contrast-enhanced CT at the levels of the great vessels, aortic arch, carina, and cardiac chambers. The CT appearance of an anterior mediastinal mass (thymoma) is demonstrated in Figure 18-28. Figure 18-29 shows a middle mediastinal mass (bronchogenic cyst) on both axial CT and MRI scans. The high signal intensity of the abnormality on the T_2-weighted image indicates its cystic nature. Figure 18-30 shows a large hiatal hernia in the posterior mediastinum containing stomach and omental fat.

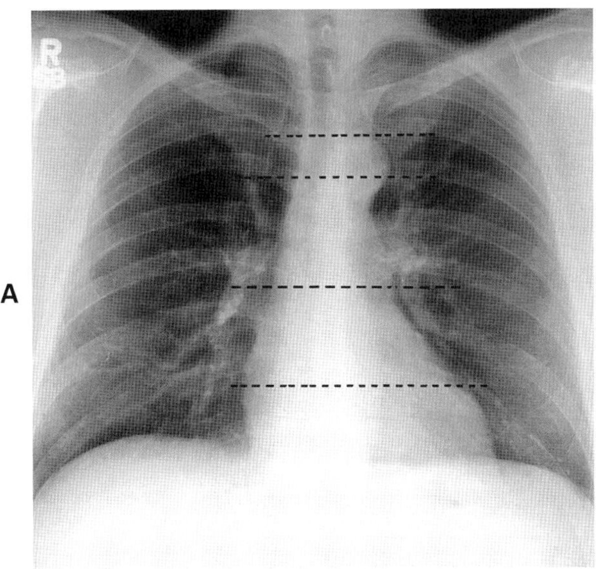

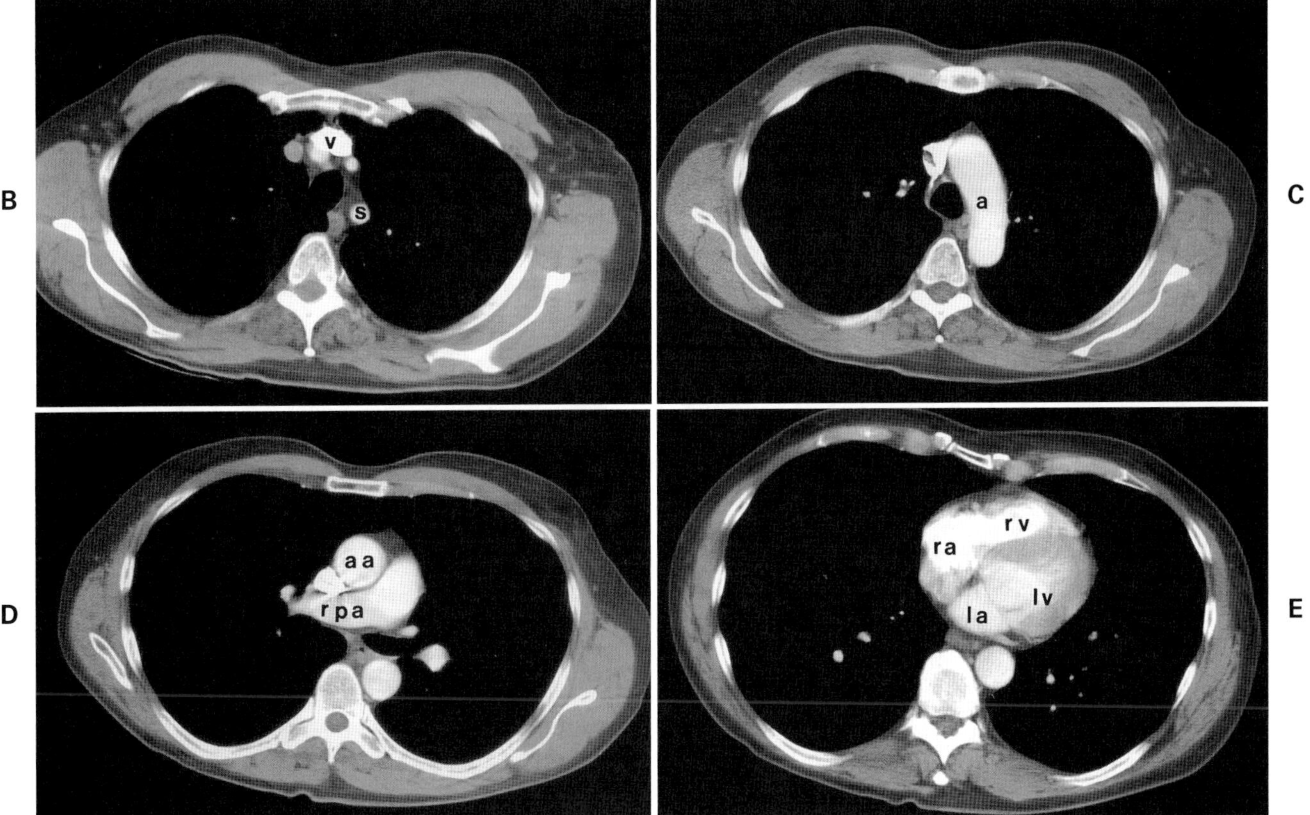

Figure 18-27

A, Posteroanterior chest film indicating the four levels at which computed tomographic scan slices B, C, D and E were obtained. **B**, The most superior image is at the level of the great vessels. Contrast fills the left brachiocephalic vein (*v*) as it courses across the anterior mediastinum to meet the right brachiocephalic vein and form the superior vena cava. The innominate artery and left common carotid are in front of the trachea behind the veins. The left subclavian artery (*s*) sits on the left of the airway next to the esophagus. **C**, At this level, the arch of the aorta (*a*) lies on the left side of the airway. The esophagus is seen in front of the vertebral body behind the airway. The opacified superior vena cava lies to the right of the arch anteriorly. **D**, At the carina, the airway bifurcates and the right pulmonary artery (*rpa*) crosses the mediastinum anterior to the right main bronchus. The vena cava lies to the right of the ascending aorta (*aa*). The lower lobe branch of the left pulmonary artery sits behind the left main bronchus. The descending aorta is seen next to the vertebral body. **E**, At the level of the heart, contrast is seen filling the right atrium (*ra*) and crossing the atrioventricular valve into the right ventricle (*rv*). The thick, muscular left ventricular (*lv*) wall is visualized as it contracts. The left atrium (*la*) is seen anterior to the esophagus.

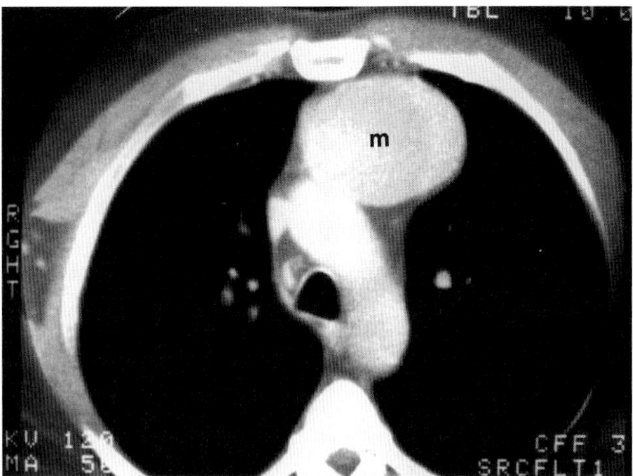

Figure 18-28 · Anterior Mediastinal Mass

Computed axial tomographic slice at the level of the aortic arch showing a homogenous encapsulated anterior mediastinal mass (*m*). Diagnosis: Thymoma.

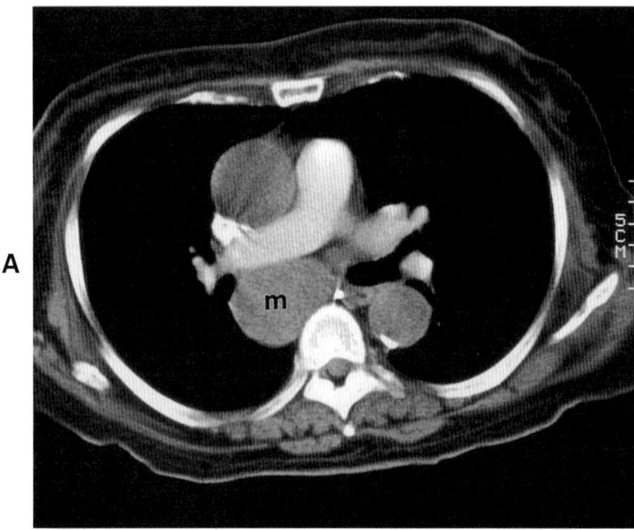

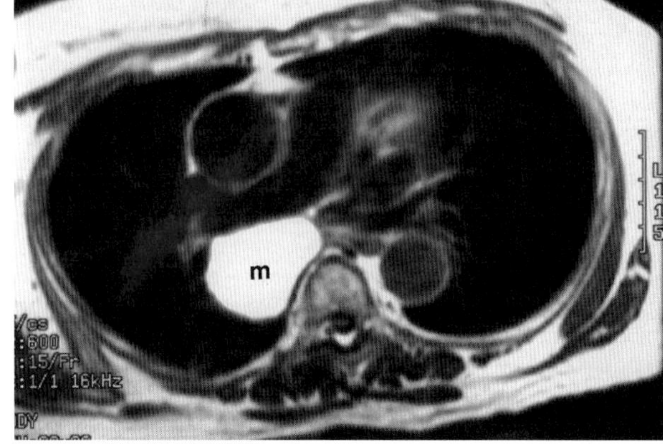

Figure 18-29

Middle mediastinal mass. Computed axial tomographic (**A**) and magnetic resonance image (**B**) scans at the subcarinal level show a large cystic mass (*m*) in the middle mediastinum. Diagnosis: Bronchogenic cyst.

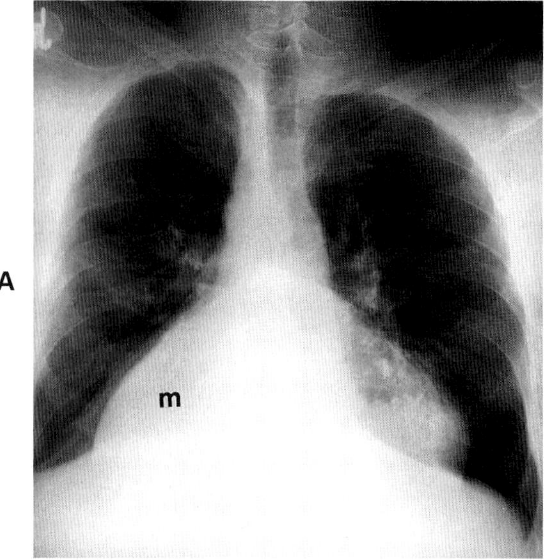

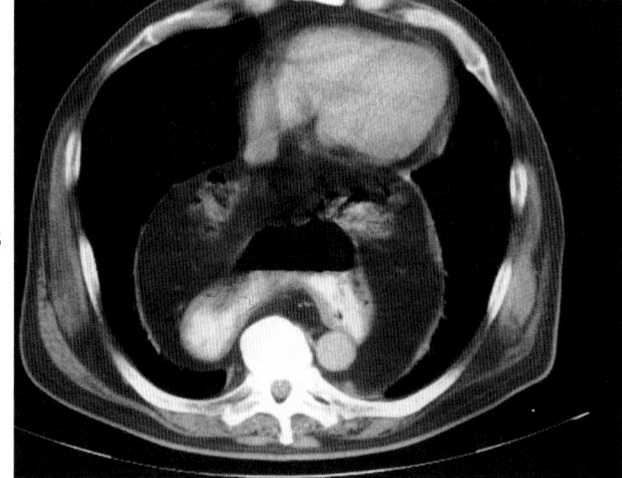

Figure 18-30 · Posterior Mediastinal Mass

A, Posteroanterior chest film shows a large soft tissue density (*m*) obscuring the right heart border and the right hemidiaphragm. **B**, Computed axial tomographic image at this level shows a large retrocardiac diaphragmatic hernia containing omentum and stomach.

KEY POINTS

- Thoracic imaging is an important tool for evaluating the cause and degree of various pulmonary diseases. A variety of imaging modalities is available for pulmonary diagnosis.
- The three general steps to interpretation of the chest film include (1) making sure the entire chest is visible on the film; (2) making sure the quality of the film is acceptable; and (3) taking a disciplined approach to review of all anatomy seen on the chest film.

KEY POINTS—cont'd

- The lungs are considered radiolucent and the bones are radiopaque.
- The chest x-ray is useful for detecting abnormalities in the pleural space such as hydrothorax and pneumothorax.
- Alveolar infiltrates will be seen as areas of white in the involved lung tissue and may represent pus, blood, or water in the lung.
- Air bronchograms are seen when alveolar infiltrates are surrounded by air-filled airways.
- Radiographic signs of cardiac failure include (1) cardiac enlargement, (2) pleural effusion, (3) redistribution of blood flow to the upper lobes, (4) Kerley B lines, and (5) alveolar filling.
- Signs of volume loss in the lungs include (1) fissure displacement, (2) lobar collapse, (3) unilateral diaphragmatic elevation, (4) mediastinal shift, (5) narrowing of the space between the ribs, (6) compensatory hyperaeration, and (7) hilar displacement.
- The chest film is useful in identifying the position of catheters and tubes. The tip of the endotracheal tube should be 5 to 7 cm from the carina.

References

1. McLoud TC, Flower CD: Imaging the pleura: sonography, CT and MR imaging, AJR Am J Roentgenol 156:1145, 1991.
2. Gefter WB, Hatabu H: Evaluation of pulmonary vascular anatomy and blood flow by magnetic resonance, J Thorac Imaging 8:122, 1993.
3. Raasch BN et al: Pleural effusion: explanation of some typical appearances, AJR Am J Roentgenol 139:899, 1982.
4. Hessen I: Roentgen examination of pleural fluid: a study of the localization of free effusions, the potentialities of diagnosing minimal quantities of fluid and its existence under physiological conditions, Acta Radiol 86:1, 1951.
5. Collins JD et al: Minimum detectable pleural effusions: a roentgen pathology model, Radiology 105:51, 1972.
6. Moskowitz H et al: Roentgen visualization of minute pleural effusions: an experimental study to determine the minimum amount of pleural fluid visible on a radiograph, Radiology 109:33, 1973.
7. Black LF: The pleural space and pleural fluid, Mayo Clin Proc 47:493, 1972.
8. Hirsch JH, Rogers JV, Mack LA: Real time sonography of the pleural opacities, AJR Am J Roentgenol 136:297, 1981.
9. Yang PC et al: Value of sonography in determining the nature of pleural effusions: analysis of 300 cases, AJR Am J Roentgenol 159:29, 1992.
10. Lipscomb DJ, Flower CDR, Hadfield JW: Ultrasound of the pleura: an assessment of its clinical value, Clin Radiol 32:289, 1981.
11. Stark DD et al: Differentiating lung abscess and empyema: radiography and computed tomography, AJR Am J Roentgenol 141:163, 1983.
12. Chiles C, Ravin C: Radiographic recognition of pneumothorax in the intensive care unit, Crit Care Med 14:677, 1986.
13. Tocino IM: Pneumothorax in the supine patient: radiographic anatomy, Radiographics 5:557, 1985.
14. Gordon R: The deep sulcus sign, Radiology 136:25, 1980.
15. Bergin C et al: The secondary pulmonary lobule: normal and abnormal CT appearances, AJR Am J Roentgenol 151:21, 1988.
16. Felson B: The lymphatic vessels. In Chest roentgenology, Philadelphia, 1973, WB Saunders.
17. Crystal R et al: Interstitial lung diseases of unknown cause: disorders characterized by chronic inflammation of the lower respiratory tract, N Engl J Med 310:154, 1984.
18. Lynch DA: Radiology of interstitial lung disease. In Newell JD Jr, Tarver RD, editors: Thoracic radiology, New York, 1993, Raven Press.
19. Wescott JL, Cole S: Plate atelectasis, Radiology 155:1, 1985.
20. Fraser RG, Pare JA: Diagnosis of diseases of the chest, Philadelphia, 1977, WB Saunders.
21. Woodring JH, Reed JC: Types and mechanisms of pulmonary atelectasis, J Thorac Imaging 11:92, 1996.
22. Gurney JW et al: Regional distribution of emphysema: correlation of high-resolution CT with pulmonary function tests in unselected smokers, Radiology 183:457, 1992.
23. Muller NL et al: "Density mask": an objective method to quantitate emphysema using computed tomography, Chest 94:782, 1988.
24. Studer SM, Meade A, Combs AH: Management of airway difficulties in the intensive care unit, Hosp Physician 31:15, 1995.
25. Goodman LR, Putman CE: Radiological evaluation of patients receiving assisted ventilation, JAMA 245:858, 1981.
26. Steele JD: The solitary pulmonary nodule, J Thorac Cardiovasc Surg 46:21, 1963.

SECTION IV

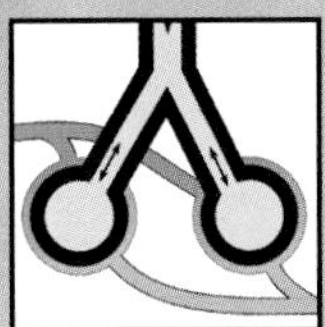

Synopsis of Cardiopulmonary Disease

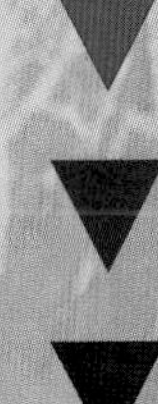

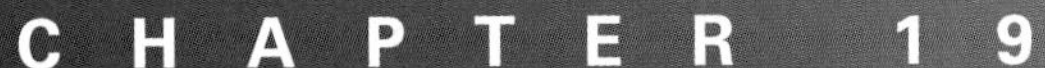

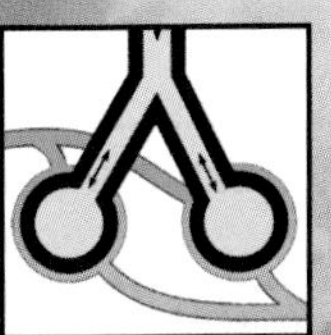

CHAPTER 19

Pulmonary Infections

David L. Longworth and Steven K. Schmitt

In This Chapter You Will Learn:

- The pathogenesis of and current classification scheme for pneumonia
- How to recognize the common causes of lower respiratory tract infection in specific clinical settings
- How the respiratory therapist aides in diagnosis and management of patients with suspected pneumonia
- The latest recommendations regarding what antibiotic regimens are used to treat various types of pneumonia, both empirical and pathogen specific
- What strategies can be used to prevent pneumonia

Chapter Outline

Key Terms

antibiotic therapy
atypical pathogens
community-acquired pneumonia
criteria for hospitalization
lower respiratory tract infection
nosocomial pneumonia
pneumonia
prevention
tuberculosis
ventilator-associated pneumonia

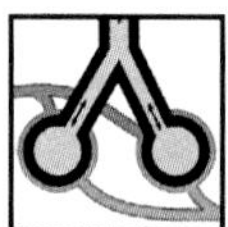

Infection involving the lungs is called **pneumonia** or **lower respiratory tract infection** and is a common clinical problem in the practice of respiratory care. In the late 1800s, Sir William Osler remarked that pneumonia is "captain of the men of death" because of its poor prognosis in the pre-antibiotic era. More than a century later, pneumonia remains a major cause of morbidity and mortality in the United States and around the world. Five million people die from pneumonia worldwide each year. In the United States, it is estimated that 4 million cases of pneumonia occur annually, of which approximately 600,000 require hospitalization, at a projected yearly cost of 20 billion dollars.[1] Pneumonia is the sixth leading cause of death in the United States and the most common cause of infection-related mortality.[2]

▶ CLASSIFICATION

Pneumonia can be classified based on the clinical setting in which it occurs (Table 19-1). This classification is useful because it predicts the likely microbial causes and determines empirical antimicrobial chemotherapy while a definitive microbiological diagnosis is awaited. (The term *empirical therapy* refers to treatment that is initiated based on the most likely cause of infection when the specific causative organism is still unknown.)

Community-acquired pneumonia can be divided into two types—*acute* and *chronic*—based on its clinical presentation. Acute pneumonia generally appears as an illness of relatively sudden onset over a few hours to several days. The clinical presentation may be *typical* or *atypical*, depending on the pathogen. The onset of chronic pneumonia is more insidious than that of acute pneumonia, often with gradually escalating symptoms over days, weeks, or even months. Nursing home–acquired pneumonia is defined as lower respiratory tract infections occurring in residents of chronic care facilities.

Nosocomial pneumonia, also known as *hospital-acquired pneumonia*, is defined as lower respiratory tract infection that develops in hospitalized patients more than 48 hours after admission and excludes community-acquired infections that are incubating at the time of admission. Nosocomial pneumonia can occur in non-intubated or mechanically ventilated patients. Hospital-acquired pneumonia is a common clinical problem and represents the second most common nosocomial infection in the United States, accounting for 15% to 18% of all such infections.[3,4] Current estimates suggest that more than 250,000 individuals develop this complication each year. In selected patient populations, such as patients in the intensive care unit (ICU) and bone marrow transplant recipients, the crude mortality rate from hospital-acquired pneumonia may approach 70%, especially with certain organisms such as *Pseudomonas aeruginosa*.[5]

Table 19-1 ▶▶ Classifications and Possible Causes of Pneumonia

Classification	Likely Organisms
Community-Acquired: Acute	
Typical	*Streptococcus pneumoniae* *Haemophilus influenzae* *Moraxella catarrhalis*
Atypical	*Legionella pneumophila* *Chlamydia pneumoniae* *Mycoplasma pneumoniae* Viruses *Coxiella burnetii*
Community-Acquired: Chronic	*Mycobacterium tuberculosis* *Histoplasma capsulatum* *Blastomyces dermatitidis* *Coccidioides immitis*
Nursing Home–Acquired	Mixed aerobic and anaerobic mouth flora *Staphylococcus aureus* Enteric gram-negative bacilli Influenza *M. tuberculosis*
Immunocompromised Host	*Pneumocystis carinii* Cytomegalovirus *Aspergillus* sp. *Cryptococcus neoformans* Reactivation tuberculosis or histoplasmosis
Nosocomial	
Aspiration	Mixed aerobes and anaerobes Gram-negative bacilli *S. aureus*
Ventilator associated	*Pseudomonas aeruginosa* *Acinetobacter* sp. *Enterobacter* sp. *Klebsiella* sp. *Stenotrophomonas maltophilia* *S. aureus*

▶ PATHOGENESIS

Six pathogenetic mechanisms may contribute to the development of pneumonia (Table 19-2). To minimize nosocomial spread, knowledge of these mechanisms is important to the understanding of the various disease processes, as well as to the formulation of effective infection control strategies within the hospital. For example, the fact that **tuberculosis** is acquired by *inhalation* of infectious particles is the basis for a policy whereby patients with suspected or proven tuberculosis who are coughing are placed in respiratory isolation, thereby minimizing the risk of disease transmission within the hospital setting.

Aspiration of oropharyngeal secretions is the second mechanism that may contribute to the development of lower respiratory tract infection. Healthy individuals may aspirate periodically, especially at night during sleep, and a small volume of oropharyngeal secretions, which are colonized with potential pathogens such as *Streptococcus pneumoniae* and *Haemophilus influenzae*, may contribute to the development of community-acquired pneumonia. Certain patient populations are at risk of large-volume aspiration, such as those with impaired gag reflexes from narcotic use, alcohol intoxication, or prior stroke. Aspiration also may occur as a result of seizure disorder, cardiac arrest, or syncope.

Aspiration appears to be the major mechanism responsible for the development of some types of hospital-acquired mixed aerobic and anaerobic, gram-negative, and staphylococcal pneumonias. In intubated patients, chronic aspiration of colonized secretions through a tracheal cuff has been linked to the subsequent occurrence of pneumonia,[3] which has led to the development of novel strategies to prevent hospital-acquired pneumonia, such as continuous suctioning of subglottic secretions in mechanically ventilated patients and elevation of the head of the bed.[6,7]

Direct inoculation of microorganisms into the lower airway is a less common cause of lower respiratory tract infection, which may contribute to the development of nosocomial pneumonia in mechanically ventilated patients who undergo frequent suctioning of lower airway secretions. In this instance, passage of a suction catheter through the oropharynx may result in inoculation of colonizing organisms into the trachea.

Contiguous spread of microorganisms to the lungs or pleural space from adjacent areas of infection, such as subdiaphragmatic or liver abscesses, is an infrequent cause of pneumonia. This pathogenetic mechanism may occur in patients with pyogenic or amebic liver abscesses involving the dome of the liver in whom rupture of the abscess through the diaphragm leads to the development of pulmonary infection or empyema.

The spread of infection through the bloodstream from a remote site is called *hematogenous dissemination*. This is an uncommon cause of pneumonia, which may occur in patients with right-sided bacterial endocarditis in whom fragments of an infected heart valve break off, embolize through the pulmonary arteries to the lungs, and produce either pneumonia or septic pulmonary infarcts. Certain parasitic pneumonias, including strongyloidiasis, ascariasis, and hookworm, arise through hematogenous dissemination. In such cases, migrating parasite larvae travel to the lungs through the bloodstream from remote sites of infection, such as the skin or the gastrointestinal tract.

Pneumonia also may develop when a latent infection, acquired earlier in life, is *reactivated*. This may occur for no apparent reason, as in the case of reactivation pulmonary tuberculosis, but most often it is attributable to the development of cellular immunodeficiency. *Pneumocystis carinii* pneumonia is a prime example of lower respiratory tract infection arising as a result of this mechanism. In developed countries, most healthy individuals have acquired *P. carinii* by the age of 3 years and demonstrate serological evidence of prior infection. The organism remains dormant in the lung but may reactivate later in life and produce pneumonia in individuals with compromised cell-mediated immunity, such as those with human immunodeficiency virus (HIV) or recipients of chronic immunosuppressive therapy. Cytomegalovirus pneumonia is another example of a latent infection that can reactivate during chronic immunosuppression, especially in solid organ and bone marrow transplant recipients. Cellular immunodeficiency also may reactivate pulmonary and extrapulmonary tuberculosis.

Table 19-2 ▶ ▶ Pathogenetic Mechanisms Responsible for the Development of Pneumonia

Mechanism of Disease	Examples of Specific Infections
Inhalation of aerosolized infectious particles	Tuberculosis Histoplasmosis Cryptococcosis Blastomycosis Coccidioidomycosis Q fever Legionellosis
Aspiration of organisms colonizing the oropharynx	Community-acquired bacterial pneumonia Aspiration pneumonia Nosocomial pneumonia
Direct inoculation of organisms into the lower airway	Nosocomial pneumonia
Spread of infection to the lungs from adjacent structures	Mixed anaerobic and aerobic pneumonia from subdiaphragmatic abscess Amebic pneumonia from rupture of amebic liver abscess into the lung
Spread of infection to the lung through the blood	*Staphylococcus aureus* pneumonia arising from right-sided bacterial endocarditis Parasitic pneumonia: strongyloidiasis, ascariasis, hookworm
Reactivation of latent infection, usually resulting from immunosuppression	*Pneumocystis carinii* pneumonia Reactivation tuberculosis Cytomegalovirus

▶ MICROBIOLOGY

The microbiology of community-acquired and nosocomial pneumonia has been studied extensively. A knowledge of which organisms are most commonly associated with pneumonia in different settings is essential, because the microbial differential diagnosis guides the diagnostic evaluation and the selection of empirical antimicrobial therapy.

In most studies, *S. pneumoniae*, also called *pneumococcus*, has been the most commonly identified cause of community-acquired pneumonia, accounting for 20% to 75% of cases (Table 19-3). A variety of other organisms has been implicated with varying frequencies. *H. influenzae*, *Staphylococcus aureus*, and gram-negative bacilli each account for 3% to 10% of isolates in many reports.[8] *Legionella* species, *Chlamydia pneumoniae*, and *Mycoplasma pneumoniae* together account for 10% to 20% of cases. These latter organisms, called **atypical pathogens**, vary in frequency in recent reports, depending on the age of the patient population, the season of the year, and geographical locale. Legionellosis and *C. pneumoniae*, in particular, seem to exhibit significant geographical variation in incidence.

Many studies examining the epidemiology and microbiology of community-acquired pneumonia are potentially biased because they focus on patients requiring hospitalization. In patients with less severe illnesses not requiring hospitalization, recent studies suggest that organisms such as *M. pneumoniae* and *C. pneumoniae* account for up to 38% of cases and may be more common than typical bacterial pathogens such as pneumococcus and *H. influenzae*.[9] In patients who are ill enough to require admission to the ICU, *Legionella* species, gram-negative bacilli, and pneumococcus are disproportionately more common.[1] In urban settings that have a high incidence of endemic HIV infection, *P. carinii* may be a more common cause of community-acquired pneumonia and, according to one recent report, may account for up to 13% of cases.[10] Viruses such as influenza, respiratory syncytial virus (RSV), and adenovirus are occasional causes of community-acquired pneumonia, especially in patients with milder illnesses not requiring hospitalization encountered in the late fall and winter months. Mixed aerobic and anaerobic aspiration pneumonia accounts for up to 10% of cases and is an important consideration for nursing home residents and for those with impaired gag reflexes or recent loss of consciousness.

Table 19-3 ▶▶ Frequency of Pathogens in Community-Acquired Pneumonia

Cause	Percentage of Cases (%)
Streptococcus pneumoniae	20–75
Aspiration	6–10
Chlamydia pneumoniae	4–11
Haemophilus influenzae	3–10
Gram-negative bacilli	3–10
Staphylococcus aureus	3–5
Legionella sp.	2–8
Viruses	2–16
Moraxella catarrhalis	1–3
Mycoplasma pneumoniae	1–24
Pneumocystis carinii	0–13
Mycobacterium tuberculosis	0–5
No diagnosis	25–50

The recent outbreak of inhalation anthrax in the United States adds another microbial differential diagnostic consideration in patients with suspected community-acquired lower respiratory tract infection.[11] Fortunately, to date inhalation anthrax remains a rare disease. However, it must be considered in selected clinical and epidemiological settings as discussed later in this chapter.

In most published series, no microbiological diagnosis is established in up to 50% of patients. This is attributable to many factors, including the following:

- Inability of many patients to produce sputum
- Failure to routinely perform numerous serological studies in all patients
- The fact that many organisms (such as viruses and anaerobic bacteria) were not routinely sought
- Failure, until recently, to recognize "new" pneumonia pathogens such as *C. pneumoniae*

The common microbial agents producing nosocomial pneumonia are summarized in Table 19-1 and include gram-negative bacilli, *S. aureus*, *Legionella* species, and rarely, viruses such as influenza or RSV. The latter viruses are considerations only during the winter months, when they are endemic in the community and may be brought into the hospital by healthcare workers or patients with incubating or active infections.

The relative frequencies and antimicrobial susceptibilities of these respective bacteria may vary considerably from one institution to another. Knowledge of which nosocomial isolates are most common within one's own institution, along with their drug-sensitivity profiles, has important implications with regard to selection of **antibiotic therapy**, formulation of infection control policies, investigation of potential outbreaks, and selection of antimicrobial agents for the hospital formulary. For example, nosocomial legionellosis is so uncommon in some institutions that empirical therapy in critically ill patients with nosocomial lower respiratory tract infection does not require coverage of this pathogen. However, in other institutions nosocomial legionellosis occurs more frequently, and patients with hospital-acquired pneumonia may require empirical treatment for this organism.

Nosocomial pathogens capable of producing hospital-acquired pneumonia can be transmitted directly from one patient to another, as in the case of tuberculosis. However, transmission from healthcare workers (including respiratory therapists [RTs]), contaminated equipment, or fomites (objects capable of transmitting infection through physical contact with them) is more common, especially for gram-negative bacilli and *S. aureus*. The RT has an important role to play in preventing the transmission and development of nosocomial pneumonia (see further discussion later in the chapter).

▶ CLINICAL MANIFESTATIONS

Patients with community-acquired pneumonia typically have fever and respiratory symptoms, such as cough, sputum production, pleuritic chest pain, and dyspnea. Not all of these symptoms are invariably present, especially in elderly individuals in whom the presentation may be subtle. Other problems, such as hoarseness, sore throat, headache, and diarrhea, may accompany certain pathogens. Fever, cough, and sputum production may occur in other illnesses such as acute bronchitis or flare-ups of chronic bronchitis.

In the past, clinicians often distinguished between typical and atypical clinical syndromes as a means of predicting the most likely microbial causes. A *typical presentation* consisted of the sudden onset of high fever, shaking, chills, and cough with purulent sputum. Such a presentation was considered more common with bacterial pathogens such as pneumococcus and *H. influenzae*. An *atypical presentation* was an illness characterized by the gradual onset of fever, headache, constitutional symptoms, diarrhea, and cough, often with minimal sputum production. Coughing was often a relatively minor symptom at the outset, and the illness was initially dominated by nonrespiratory symptoms. Such a presentation was thought to be more common with pathogens such as *M. pneumoniae*, *C. pneumoniae*, *Legionella* species, and viruses. More recent studies have demonstrated that these distinctions are not ironclad and that considerable overlap exists in the clinical presentations of pneumonia with typical and atypical pathogens.[12] The occurrence of concomitant diarrhea, once considered indicative of legionellosis, is now known to be common in pneumococcal and mycoplasma pneumonia.

Despite the limitations in predicting with absolute certainty the microbial diagnosis based on the clinical presentation, clinicians use certain historical clues and physical findings at the bedside to determine the likely cause of pneumonia in patients presenting from the community. In patients presenting with high fever, teeth-chattering chills, pleuritic pain, and a cough producing rust-colored sputum, pneumococcal pneumonia is the most likely diagnosis. Patients with pneumonia accompanied by foul-smelling breath, an absent gag reflex, or recent loss of consciousness are most likely to have a mixed aerobic and anaerobic infection as a consequence of aspiration. Community-acquired pneumonia accompanied by hoarseness suggests that the culprit is *C. pneumoniae*. Pneumonia in a patient with a history of splenectomy suggests infection with an encapsulated pathogen such as pneumococcus or *H. influenzae*. Epidemics of pneumonia occurring within households or closed communities, such as dormitories or barracks, suggest pathogens such as *M. pneumoniae* or *C. pneumoniae*. Pneumonia accompanied by splenomegaly prompts consideration of psittacosis or Q fever. Bullous myringitis and erythema multiforme are associated with *Mycoplasma* infection. Relative bradycardia, defined as a heart rate of less than 100 beats/min, in the presence of fever and the absence of preexisting cardiac conduction system disease or β-blocker therapy, may suggest infection with one of the atypical pathogens. Pneumonia accompanied by conjunctivitis suggests adenovirus infection.

The clinical presentation of community-acquired pneumonia in elderly patients deserves special mention because it may be subtle. Older individuals with pneumonia may not have a fever or cough and may simply present with shortness of breath, confusion, worsening congestive heart failure (CHF), or failure to thrive.

As previously mentioned, inhalation anthrax is a rare disease, but it deserves consideration because of the small epidemic believed to be an act of bioterrorism.[11] This outbreak affected mainly postal workers who were exposed to mail containing anthrax spores. Most patients presented with a febrile flulike illness of several days' duration accompanied by dry cough and shortness of breath. Some patients in whom the diagnosis was not quickly considered went on to develop septic shock, meningitis, and disseminated intravascular coagulation over several days, culminating in death.

Nosocomial pneumonia usually presents with a new onset of fever in hospitalized patients. Nonintubated patients may have a recent history of vomiting, seizure, or syncope, during which aspiration of oropharyngeal or gastric secretions may have occurred. In intubated patients, nosocomial pneumonia traditionally presents with a new onset of fever, purulent endotracheal secretions, and a new pulmonary infiltrate. The diagnosis of nosocomial pneumonia can be extremely difficult to make in patients with preexisting abnormalities on the chest radiograph, such as CHF or adult respiratory distress syndrome (ARDS). In mechanically ventilated patients, purulent tracheobronchitis may be accompanied by fever, and in patients with preexisting abnormalities on the chest x-ray film, the distinction between bronchitis and pneumonia can be especially difficult.

▶ CHEST RADIOGRAPH

In patients with a compatible clinical syndrome, the diagnosis of community-acquired pneumonia is established by the presence of a new pulmonary infiltrate on the chest radiograph. Not all healthy outpatients with suspected pneumonia require a chest radiograph, and physicians may elect to forego radiography and treat empirically for community-acquired pneumonia in individuals with mild illnesses who are at low risk for morbidity or mortality.

A normal chest x-ray film does not exclude the diagnosis of pneumonia. The chest radiograph may be normal in patients with early infection, dehydration, or *P. carinii* infection. The pattern of radiographic abnormality is not diagnostic of the causative agent, although specific radiographic findings should suggest specific microbial differential diagnoses (Table 19-4).

Consolidation involving an entire lobe is called *lobar consolidation*, whereas *bronchopneumonia* refers to the presence of a patchy infiltrate surrounding one or more bronchus, without opacification of an entire lobe. Both radiographic patterns suggest the presence of a bacterial pathogen. Pleural effusions are common in patients with bacterial pneumonia and uncommon in those with viral, *P. carinii*, *C. pneumoniae*, or fungal pneumonias. Pleural effusions are seen in approximately 10% of patients with *M. pneumoniae* and *Legionella pneumophila* pneumonia, and they occur occasionally in patients with reactivation pulmonary tuberculosis. Interstitial infiltrates, especially if diffuse, suggest viral disease, *P. carinii*, or miliary tuberculosis in patients with community-acquired pneumonia. Cavitary infiltrates are seen in reactivation pulmonary tuberculosis; fungal pneumonias, such as histoplasmosis and blastomycosis; nocardiosis; pyogenic lung abscess; and rarely, *P. carinii* pneumonia. Patients with severe staphylococcal or gram-negative pneumonias may develop small cavities called *pneumatoceles*. Legionellosis should be seriously considered in sicker patients with pneumonia of a single lobe, which quickly spreads to involve multiple lobes over 24 to 48 hours. Inhalation anthrax presents with widening of the mediastinal silhouette resulting from mediastinal lymphadenopathy. Parenchymal pulmonary infiltrates are typically absent and pleural effusions are common.

Table 19-4 ▶▶ Radiographic Patterns Produced by Pathogens in Community-Acquired Pneumonia

Pattern	Pathogens
Lobar consolidation	Bacterial
Bronchopneumonia	Bacterial
Pleural effusion	Bacterial Inhalation anthrax
Interstitial infiltrates	Viruses *Pneumocystis carinii*
Cavities	Mycobacteria Fungi *Nocardia* sp. *Staphylococcus aureus* Gram-negative bacilli Polymicrobial aerobic and anaerobic lung abscess *P. carinii* (rare)
Mediastinal widening without infiltrates	Inhalation anthrax
Rapidly progressive multilobar	*Legionella* sp. *Streptococcus pneumoniae* Endobronchial tuberculosis

The chest radiograph may be helpful in diagnosing nosocomial pneumonia in nonintubated patients with a suspected aspiration event and a previously normal chest film. In such cases, the development of a new infiltrate may confirm the clinical suspicion of aspiration pneumonia. The chest radiograph is often less helpful in the diagnosis of nosocomial pneumonia in mechanically ventilated patients in the ICU because these individuals often have other reasons for radiographic abnormalities, such as ARDS, CHF, pulmonary thromboembolism, alveolar hemorrhage, or atelectasis. In these patients, the accurate diagnosis of a new nosocomial lower respiratory tract infection can be difficult. Clinical diagnosis, defined as the presence of fever, purulent respiratory secretions, new leucocytosis, and a new pulmonary infiltrate, is sensitive but not specific for the diagnosis of nosocomial pneumonia. This has led to the investigation of other strategies to diagnose nosocomial lower respiratory tract infection in intubated patients more accurately.

▶ RISK FACTORS FOR MORTALITY AND ASSESSING THE NEED FOR HOSPITALIZATION

Many cases of community-acquired pneumonia can be managed successfully on an outpatient basis. The challenge for the clinician is to identify those individuals at higher risk of morbidity and mortality for whom hospitalization is indicated.

Over the past decade, a number of studies have analyzed risk factors for mortality in patients with community-acquired pneumonia.[13-15] Risk factors predictive of a high risk of death are summarized in Box 19-1.

Fine et al[14] performed a meta-analysis of 127 cohorts of patients with community-acquired pneumonia. The study examined risk factors for fatal outcome. The overall mortality for the 33,148 patients in these cohorts was 13.7%. Eleven prognostic variables were significantly associated with mortality, including male sex, the absence of pleuritic chest pain, hypothermia, systolic hypotension, tachypnea, diabetes mellitus, cancer, neurological disease, bacteremia, leukopenia, and multilobar infiltrates on chest radiograph. Mortality varied according to the infecting agent and was highest for *P. aeruginosa* (61.1%), *Klebsiella* species (35.7%), *Escherichia coli* (35.3%), and *S. aureus* (31.8%). Mortality rates for more common pathogens were lower but still substantial and included *Legionella* species (14.7%), *S. pneumoniae* (12.3%), *C. pneumoniae* (9.8%), and *M. pneumoniae* (1.4%).

Box 19-1 • Risk Factors for Mortality in Community-Acquired Pneumonia From Multiple Studies[14]

I. Patient variables
  A. Age greater than 50 years
  B. Male sex
  C. Comorbid illnesses
    1. Cerebrovascular disease
    2. Cancer
    3. Congestive heart failure
    4. Renal disease
    5. Liver disease
    6. Immunosuppression
    7. Alcoholism
    8. Diabetes mellitus
    9. Chronic lung disease
II. Clinical parameters at presentation
  A. Altered mentation
  B. Systolic hypotension <90 mm Hg
  C. Tachypnea >30 breaths/min
  D. Hypothermia (temperature <35° C)
  E. Fever >40° C
  F. Pulse rate >125 beats/min
  G. Extrapulmonary site of infection
III. Laboratory and radiographic findings at presentation
  A. Arterial pH <7.35
  B. Blood urea nitrogen >30 mg/dL
  C. Serum sodium <130 mmol/L
  D. Glucose >250 mg/dL
  E. Hematocrit <30%
  F. Hypoxia (Pao_2 <60 mm Hg) or hypercarbia (Pco_2 >50 mm Hg) on room air
  G. White blood cell count <4 × 10^9/L or >30 × 10^9/L or an absolute neutrophil count <1 × 10^9
  H. Multilobar infiltrate
  I. Bacteremia
  J. Pleural effusion
  K. High-risk cause
    1. Gram-negative bacilli
    2. *Staphylococcus aureus*
    3. Postobstructive pneumonia
    4. Aspiration

Because some variables are unknown at the time a patient seeks treatment for pneumonia, such as the causative agent and whether bacteremia is present, more recent studies have sought to assess the risk of fatal outcome by using clinical and laboratory data that are readily available at the time of the initial evaluation. Based on an analysis of more than 40,000 patients regarding 30-day mortality, Fine et al[15] have proposed a prediction rule to identify both low-risk and high-risk patients with community-acquired pneumonia. Their algorithm uses the demographic, clinical, and laboratory data available at presentation to stratify the risk of fatal outcome and the **criteria for hospitalization** in outpatient groups. Points are assigned for the presence of a number of variables, and cumulative point scores are used to stratify patients into one of five different risk groups with predictable mortality rates (Tables 19-5 and 19-6). In this model, which has been validated in large prospective cohorts of patients, those at the lowest risk of death fall into groups I and II. In most instances, these patients may be treated successfully as outpatients, unless they are hypoxic, vomiting and unable to take oral antibiotics, noncompliant, or immunocompromised. Patients in group I are those younger than 50 years of age who lack comorbid illnesses and abnormal physical findings at presentation (see Box 19-1 and Table 19-5). This group of patients has a risk of fatal outcome of 0.1%.

Patients with nosocomial pneumonia are, by definition, already hospitalized at the time pneumonia develops, and a decision regarding the need for hospitalization is unnecessary. Many studies have examined risk factors for the development of nosocomial pneumonia, which in broad terms can be divided into (1) factors that interfere with host defense and (2) factors that facilitate exposure to large numbers of bacteria.[5] Examples of the former include the following:

- Underlying illnesses such as diabetes mellitus, malignancy, chronic heart and lung disease, and renal failure
- Critical illnesses such as sepsis syndrome and ARDS
- Certain therapeutic interventions such as endotracheal intubation, tracheostomy, and the administration of medications such as sedatives and corticosteroids

Factors that promote exposure of the lung to large numbers of microorganisms or smaller numbers of virulent pathogens include the following:

Table 19-5 ▶ ▶ Scoring System for Stratifying Risk of 30-Day Mortality in Adults With Community-Acquired Pneumonia

Variable	Points Assigned
Age	
Men	Age (years)
Women	Age (years) - 10
Nursing Home Resident	+10
Comorbid Illnesses	
Cancer	+30
Liver disease	+20
Kidney disease	+10
Cerebrovascular disease	+10
Congestive heart failure	+10
Physical Findings	
Altered mentation	+20
Tachypnea >30 breaths/min	+20
Systolic hypotension <90 mm Hg	+20
Temperature <35° C or >40° C	+15
Heart rate >125 beats/min	+10
Laboratory and Radiographic Findings	
Acidemia (arterial pH <7.35)	+30
Azotemia (BUN >30 mg/dL)	+20
Hyponatremia (sodium <130 mmol/L)	+20
Hypoxia (Pa_{O_2} <60 mm Hg)	+10
Hyperglycemia (glucose >250 mg/dL)	+10
Anemia (Hct <30%)	+10
Pleural effusion	+10

Modified from Fine MJ et al: N Engl J Med 336:243, 1997.
BUN, Blood urea nitrogen; Hct, hematocrit.
Plus sign (+) denotes adding points; minus sign (–) denotes subtracting points (e.g., for women, points assigned equal age in years –10).

Table 19-6 ▶ ▶ Risk Class Mortality Rates Using Prediction Model Cumulative Point Scores in Patients with Community-Acquired Pneumonia

Risk Class (Cumulative Point Score)	Mortality Rate (%)
I	0.1
II (≤70)	0.6
III (71-90)	2.8
IV (91-130)	8.2
V (>130)	29.2

Modified from Fine MJ et al: N Engl J Med 336:243, 1997.
Note: Patients in risk class I are younger than age 50 years and lack existing illness or physical findings listed in Table 19-5. Points are assigned to patients in risk classes II or higher.

- Use of endotracheal or nasogastric tubes
- Contaminated ventilator equipment or water supplies
- Prior antibiotic therapy
- Neutralization of gastric pH

Although numerous studies have highlighted the substantial mortality rate (20% to 50%) for patients

MINI CLINI

Estimating Risk From Pneumonia

PROBLEM

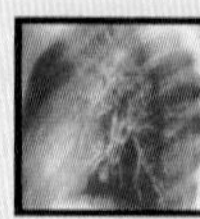

The RT is called to the emergency department (ED) to perform an arterial blood gas analysis on a 70-year-old woman who has been sent from a nursing home with confusion and shortness of breath. Her history is notable for end-stage renal disease caused by hypertension and a recent stroke, which has resulted in a left-sided hemiplegia. The ED physician ordered a chest x-ray examination, which revealed a right lower lobe infiltrate and a right pleural effusion.

On physical examination, the patient is somnolent. Her vital signs are as follows: temperature, 35° C; blood pressure, 85/50 mm Hg; and heart rate, 130 beats/min. Additional findings are as follows:

- Absent gag reflex
- Right basilar rales and a left hemiplegia
- Peripheral white blood cell count, 3000 cells/mm^3
- Blood urea nitrogen, 100 mg/dL
- Hematocrit, 31%
- Blood glucose, 110 mg/dL
- Serum sodium, 144 mmol/L

The RT collects the arterial blood gas on room air, which discloses a pH level of 7.30, a Pa_{O_2} reading of 58 mm Hg, and a P_{CO_2} level of 25 mm Hg. Should the patient be admitted to the hospital, or should she be sent back to the nursing home? What is her risk of 30-day mortality?

DISCUSSION

This patient is at substantial risk of dying from pneumonia and should be admitted to the hospital. The Fine prediction rule[15] may be used as follows to estimate the risk of 30-day mortality (see Tables 19-5 and 19-6):

Variable	Points
Age: 70 years	+70
Sex: female	-10
Nursing home resident	+10
Cerebrovascular disease	+10
Renal disease	+10
Altered mentation	+20
Systolic hypotension	+20
Hypothermia	+15
Tachycardia	+10
Acidemia	+30
Renal failure	+20
Hypoxemia, with Pa_{O_2} <60 mm Hg	+10
Pleural effusion	+10
Total	225

Her cumulative point score is 225, she belongs to risk class V, and her estimated risk of mortality is 29.2% (see Table 19-6). She should be admitted to the hospital for treatment.

who develop nosocomial pneumonia, few studies have examined the specific risk factors associated with mortality in hospital-acquired lower respiratory tract infection. For nonventilated patients, risk factors for mortality include bilateral infiltrates, respiratory failure, and infection with high-risk organisms.[16,17] In mechanically ventilated patients, factors associated with fatal outcome include the following[17,18]:

- Infection with high-risk organisms such as *P. aeruginosa*, *Acinetobacter* species, and *Stenotrophomonas maltophilia*
- Multisystem organ failure
- Nonsurgical diagnosis
- Therapy with antacids or H_2-receptor antagonists
- Transfer from another hospital or ward
- Renal failure
- Prolonged mechanical ventilation
- Coma or shock
- Inappropriate antibiotic therapy
- Hospitalization in a noncardiac ICU

▶ DIAGNOSTIC STUDIES

Community-Acquired Pneumonia

Many patients with community-acquired pneumonia who are treated as outpatients never have an established microbiological diagnosis. Many are treated based on the history and on compatible findings on physical examination, with or without a chest radiograph to confirm the presence of an infiltrate. Patients who are sick enough to warrant hospitalization or its consideration should receive a number of studies to stratify risk of mortality and to establish a microbiological diagnosis (Box 19-2). The complete blood count, blood glucose, serum sodium, and blood urea nitrogen are all necessary to derive a point score for estimating the risk of mortality. An arterial blood gas analysis is used to detect the presence of hypoxemia and acidemia, which indicate a more serious illness.

The value of the Gram stain and culture of expectorated sputum has been debated for years.[19] Many patients lack a productive cough, making collection of an adequate specimen difficult. Prior antibiotic therapy reduces the yield from both of these tests. Only approximately 50% of patients with bacteremic pneumococcal pneumonia have a positive sputum culture.[20] Nevertheless, the finding of a predominant organism on Gram stain in an appropriately collected specimen has a high predictive value for the selection of appropriate antibiotic therapy.[21] In addition, isolation of penicillin-resistant pneumococci from sputum has important implications for therapy. It is important to emphasize that a routine sputum culture can be interpreted only within the context of the sputum Gram stain. Specimens contaminated with oropharyngeal epithelial cells are unsatisfactory for analysis.

Box 19-2 • Recommended Tests for Adults With Community-Acquired Pneumonia Warranting Consideration of Hospitalization

- Chest radiograph
- Complete blood count
- Blood chemistries
  - Glucose
  - Serum sodium
  - Blood urea nitrogen
- Arterial blood gas
- Sputum Gram stain and culture
- Additional sputum studies as clinically indicated
  - Acid-fast stains and culture for mycobacteria
  - Potassium hydroxide examination and fungal culture
  - Stain for *Pneumocystis carinii*
  - Direct fluorescent antibody stain for *Legionella* sp.
- Blood cultures
- Pleural fluid analysis if sizable effusion is present
  - Cell count with differential
  - Glucose, protein, and lactate dehydrogenase
  - pH
  - Gram stain and routine aerobic and anaerobic culture
  - Acid-fast stain and culture for mycobacteria
- Additional other studies as clinically indicated
  - *Legionella* urinary antigen
  - Acute and convalescent sera for *M. pneumoniae*, *Legionella* sp., and *C. pneumoniae*
  - Fungal serologies
  - HIV test for individuals ages 15 to 54 years or for those engaging in high-risk behavior

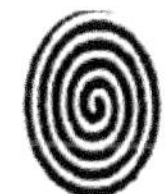

RULE OF THUMB

A routine sputum culture can be interpreted only within the context of the sputum Gram stain.

The RT has an important role in the collection of an appropriate specimen of expectorated sputum. Patients should be advised to rid the mouth of contaminating saliva, either by rinsing with water or by spitting, and then to expectorate a specimen from deep within the tracheobronchial tree into a collection container. Prompt transportation to the laboratory is essential and improves the diagnostic yield from culture.[8] Most microbiology laboratories screen the adequacy of the specimen by cytological examination. A satisfactory specimen contains more than 25 leucocytes and less than 10 squamous epithelial cells per high-power field.[22] In routine sputum culture, the isolation of bacteria, such as *S. pneumoniae* and *H. influenzae*, must be interpreted within the context of the Gram stain because these organisms can colonize the oropharynx, and their presence in culture may not signify true lower respiratory tract infection. The culture isolation of other organisms such as *Mycobacterium tuberculosis*, *Histoplasma capsulatum*, *Blastomyces dermatitidis*, *Coccidioides immitis*, and *Legionella* species is diagnostic of disease because these organisms almost never colonize just the respiratory tract.

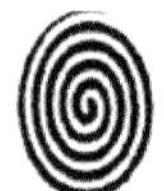

RULE OF THUMB

The presence of *Candida* species on sputum smear or culture is almost never clinically significant.

Other stains and cultures of expectorated sputum should be obtained as dictated by the clinical circumstance. In patients with suspected tuberculosis, the finding of acid-fact bacilli in stained specimens of sputum often prompts initiation of antituberculous therapy, because culture isolation of *M. tuberculosis* may take up to 6 weeks. A direct fluorescent antibody stain of sputum for *Legionella* species may reveal the organism in 25% to 80% of individuals with Legionnaires' disease, and cultures are positive in 50% to 70% of these individuals.[23] Toluidine blue O stains of sputum may disclose the organism in up to 80% of patients with *P. carinii* pneumonia. Potassium hydroxide preparations of sputum disclose fungi in a minority of patients with histoplasmosis, blastomycosis, or coccidioidomycosis but are very helpful if positive. In inhalation anthrax, patients typically do not produce sputum, and the organism is usually absent if they do.

Blood cultures should be obtained in hospitalized patients with community-acquired pneumonia and may be helpful in establishing the diagnosis in patients with typical bacterial pathogens. Blood cultures are positive in approximately 30% of patients with pneumococcal pneumonia and in up to 70% of those with *H. influenzae* pneumonia.[24] Blood cultures are often positive in patients with inhalation anthrax and should be collected if the diagnosis is suspected. They are not helpful in patients with legionellosis, *M. pneumoniae*, *C. pneumoniae*, *P. carinii*, or most viral infections. Collection of blood cultures within 24 hours of hospitalization in elderly patients with pneumonia has been associated with improved survival.[25]

Parapneumonic pleural effusions are common and occur in 30% to 50% of cases of community-acquired pneumonia.[8] Hemorrhagic pleural effusions are typically present in patients with inhalation anthrax. Thoracentesis is indicated for patients with large pleural effusions and for those with smaller effusions who fail to respond to therapy or for whom the microbiological diagnosis is not established. Pleural fluid should also be sampled in patients with suspected inhalation anthrax. Pleural fluid should be tested for cell count, glucose, protein, pH, lactate dehydrogenase, Gram and acid-fast bacilli stains, and routine (aerobic and anaerobic) and mycobacterial cultures. Patients having effusions with a pH less than 7.30 or a high white blood cell count require tube thoracostomy for drainage.[26]

Other studies may be helpful in establishing a microbiological diagnosis in the appropriate clinical setting. *L. pneumophila* serogroup 1 accounts for 80% of cases of Legionnaires' disease.[27] The urinary antigen test for *L. pneumophila* serogroup 1 is a sensitive and rapid test and usually becomes positive within 3 days of onset of illness. The test has several limitations. First is its inability to detect the non–serogroup 1 *L. pneumophila* and nonpneumophila species that account for 20% of cases of Legionnaire's disease. Second, the test may remain positive for up to 1 year, obviating the ability to distinguish new from remote infection in those with a recent history of pneumonia.

Serological tests for IgM and IgG antibodies to *M. pneumoniae*, *Legionella* species, or *C. pneumoniae* are rarely helpful during the initial stages of pneumonia, but convalescent titers 3 to 4 weeks later may permit a retrospective microbiological diagnosis by demonstrating a fourfold rise in IgG titer or the development of IgM antibody against a specific pathogen. Acute sera should be analyzed in patients who are critically ill with pneumonia and for whom microbiological diagnosis is enigmatic. Fungal serologies are occasionally helpful in supporting the diagnosis of blastomycosis, histoplasmosis, or coccidioidomycosis, pending culture isolation of the organism.

Because pneumococcal and *H. influenzae* pneumonia occur with higher frequency in patients with HIV than they do in the average population, an HIV test is recommended for patients with community-acquired pneumonia who are between the ages of 15 and 54 years. HIV testing also is recommended for other individuals who engage in behaviors that put them at risk for HIV.

Molecular techniques, such as DNA probes and polymerase chain reaction, used for detecting specific organisms, such as *M. pneumoniae or M. tuberculosis*, for confirming identity in culture isolates are being developed but are not yet widely available.

Fiberoptic bronchoscopy is usually reserved for severe cases of community-acquired pneumonia, for immunocompromised individuals in whom opportunistic pathogens must be excluded, or if HIV or *P. carinii* infection is suspected. The yield from fiberoptic bronchoscopy is higher if performed before the initiation of antibiotic therapy in patients with bacterial pneumonia. Open lung

MINI CLINI

The Importance of Clinical Setting for Determining the Cause of Pneumonia

PROBLEM

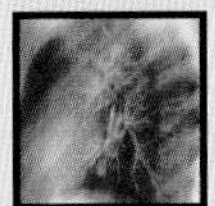

The RT is caring for a 32-year-old man admitted to the hospital 24 hours earlier with fever, shaking chills, and a new left lower lobe infiltrate. His white blood cell count on admission was 3500 cells/mm^3, with 96% neutrophils and 4% lymphocytes. A sputum Gram stain disclosed many polymorphonuclear leucocytes and lancet-shaped, gram-positive diplococci. Blood cultures have grown *S. pneumoniae* at 24 hours. He remains febrile 24 hours into therapy with penicillin G. While checking pulse oximetry, the RT notes that the patient is emaciated and that multiple needle tracks are present in each antecubital fossa. He tells the RT that he uses intravenous (IV) heroin. What other tests are indicated?

DISCUSSION

This patient, who is an IV drug user, has bacteremic pneumococcal pneumonia. These findings, along with the presence of cachexia and leukopenia with lymphopenia, should suggest the possibility of underlying HIV infection. An HIV test is indicated and should be performed after the patient's consent is obtained.

Both pneumococcal and *H. influenzae* pneumonia occur with higher frequency in HIV-infected individuals than they do in the general population. Occasionally, the development of one of these infections results in an HIV-infected patient's first contact with the healthcare system. Adults with these infections between the ages of 15 and 54 years should be offered HIV testing.

The RT would also want to know the antibiotic susceptibility profile of this patient's pneumococcus. Although fever 24 hours into therapy for pneumococcal pneumonia is not unusual, penicillin resistance to *S. pneumoniae* is becoming increasingly common. If this patient's isolate were penicillin resistant, he would likely require therapy with vancomycin.

biopsy is rarely indicated for patients with community-acquired pneumonia.

Nosocomial Pneumonia

The accurate diagnosis of nosocomial pneumonia is fraught with difficulty and has been the subject of intense investigation over the past decade. A number of techniques have been extensively reviewed (Box 19-3).[28-30] None is absolutely sensitive and specific. Clinical diagnosis has been defined as the development of a new infiltrate on chest radiograph, in the setting of fever, purulent tracheal secretions, and leucocytosis, in hospitalized patients. Clinical diagnosis lacks specificity because many other causes of pulmonary infiltrates exist in hospitalized patients, especially those on mechanical ventilation.[31] In addition, the upper airway commonly is colonized with nosocomial gram-negative bacilli and staphylococci, even in the absence of pneumonia. The qualitative culture isolation of these organisms from tracheal secretions correlates poorly with the presence or absence of pneumonia.

Box 19-3 • Techniques for Diagnosing Nosocomial Pneumonia

- Clinical diagnosis
- Direct visualization of the airway by bronchoscopy
- Quantitative cultures of endotracheal aspirates
- Quantitative cultures of protected brush-bronchoscopy specimens
- Quantitative cultures of nonbronchoscopic distally protected specimens
- Quantitative cultures of conventional or protected bronchoalveolar lavage (BAL) specimens, plus microscopic examination of recovered cells
- Quantitative cultures of protected specimen brush and BAL specimens, plus microscopic examination of BAL fluid cells
- Therapist-directed mini-BAL
- Transthoracic fine-needle aspiration

Direct visualization by bronchoscopy of the lower airway in ventilated patients is sometimes helpful in supporting the diagnosis of nosocomial pneumonia. In one recent study, the presence of distal, purulent secretions; persistence of secretions surging from distal bronchi during exhalation; and a decrease in the PaO_2/FIO_2 ratio of less than 50 mm Hg were independently associated with the presence of pneumonia. The presence of two of three of these factors had a sensitivity of 78% in the diagnosis of nosocomial pneumonia, and these factors were absent when there was no pneumonia 89% of the time (89% specific).[32]

Because the specificity of qualitative sputum cultures has been unreliable, several studies have examined the role of quantitative cultures of endotracheal aspirates using various break points ranging from 10^3 to 10^7 colony-forming units (CFU) per milliliter of respiratory secretions. Results with this techniques have been best using a break point of 10^6 CFU/mL, but sensitivities have been only 68% to 82%, with specificities of 84% to 96% with this modality.[33,34]

Protected specimen brush (PSB) was developed in the 1970s and uses a special double-catheter brush system to minimize contamination by upper airway flora. Specimens obtained with this technique are cultured quantitatively. A number of studies have validated the sensitivity of this technique in the diagnosis of nosocomial pneumonia.[35,36] However, its usefulness may be suboptimal for cases in which antibiotic therapy has already been initiated, cases of early infection, and cases in which the wrong lobe is sampled.[29]

Nonbronchoscopic techniques using telescoping protected catheters have been developed to obtain specimens for quantitative culture from the lower airway. In most studies, sensitivity has been comparable with that of bronchoscopic techniques, but discordant results, compared with those of bronchoscopy, have been noted in up to 20% of cases.[29]

Bronchoalveolar lavage (BAL), in which a lung segment is lavaged with sterile saline through the bronchoscope and recovered fluid is quantitatively cultured, has been studied extensively as a tool for diagnosing nosocomial pneumonia. Some studies have supported the usefulness of this technique, whereas others have questioned its specificity because of upper airway contamination.[35,36] BAL has been proven useful for obtaining alveolar cells for microscopic analysis, and several studies have suggested that the presence of intracellular bacteria in 3% to 5% of BAL cells distinguishes those patients with nosocomial pneumonia from those without it.[35,36] In one study, the combination of PSB cultures and microscopic examination of BAL cells for intracellular bacteria was 100% sensitive and 96% specific in identifying patients with nosocomial pneumonia.[35]

Recently, mini-BAL performed by RTs has been advocated for diagnosing ventilator-associated pneumonia. In one study, results obtained using this technique were comparable with those obtained by bronchoscopy using PSB.[37] Transthoracic ultrathin needle aspiration of the lung in nonventilated patients with nosocomial pneumonia also has been studied recently, and in one report was found to have a sensitivity of 60%, a specificity of 100%, and a positive predictive value of 100%.[38]

In summary, the accurate diagnosis of nosocomial pneumonia remains a challenge for the physician and the RT. None of the available diagnostic techniques is 100% sensitive or specific, and all of them are limited in the populations at the greatest risk for contracting nosocomial pneumonia, namely mechanically-ventilated patients and those receiving prior antibiotic therapy.

▶ THERAPY

The selection of antibiotic therapy for patients with community-acquired pneumonia should be guided by several considerations. These include the age of the patient, the severity of the illness, the presence of risk factors for specific organisms, and results of initial diagnostic studies. Pathogen-specific therapy should be used when clinical circumstances and initial evaluation strongly suggest the microbiological diagnosis or when cultures or other studies confirm the cause. In many instances, initial studies fail to establish a diagnosis, and empirical therapy must be initiated. Major classes of antibiotics used to treat pneumonia are listed in Table 19-7. Guidelines for therapy have been published recently by the American Thoracic Society (ATS)[39] and the Infectious Disease Society of America (IDSA).[40] These are summarized in Table 19-8. Therapy initiated within 8 hours of hospital admission has been associated with improved survival.[25]

For hospitalized patients who are not critically ill and are admitted to the ward, an empirical regimen of erythromycin plus a second- or third-generation cephalosporin or a β-lactam/β-lactamase inhibitor combination is recommended by the IDSA. Another acceptable alternative is a fluoroquinolone alone (see Table 19-8). The ATS stratifies empirical therapy in this setting based on the presence or absence of underlying cardiopulmonary

Table 19-7 ▶ ▶ Major Classes of Antibiotics Used in the Treatment of Pneumonia

Antibiotic Class	Representative Drugs
Penicillins	Penicillin G, ampicillin
Ureidopenicillins	Ticarcillin, piperacillin, mezlocillin
Semisynthetic penicillins	Oxacillin, nafcillin
First-generation cephalosporins	Cefazolin
Second-generation cephalosporins	Cefuroxime
Third-generation cephalosporins	Cefotaxime, ceftriaxone, ceftizoxime
Antipseudomonal cephalosporins	Ceftazidime, cefepime
Carbapenems	Imipenem, meropenem
Monobactams	Aztreonam
β-Lactam/β-lactamase inhibitor combinations	Ticarcillin/clavulanate, piperacillin/tazobactam, ampicillin/sulbactam
Quinolones	Ciprofloxacin, levofloxacin, gatifloxacin
Macrolides	Erythromycin, clarithromycin, azithromycin
Tetracyclines	Doxycycline
Glycopeptides	Vancomycin

Table 19-8 ▶ ▶ Empirical Regimens for Treatment of Hospitalized Adults With Community-Acquired Pneumonia: American Thoracic Society (ATS) and Infectious Disease Society of America (IDSA) Guidelines

Patient Group	Likely Pathogens	ATS Regimens	IDSA Regimens
Hospitalized on ward	*S. pneumoniae* *H. influenzae* *C. pneumoniae* *S. aureus* *M. pneumoniae* Anaerobes Viruses	No cardiopulmonary disease or risk factors: IV azithromycin or a fluoroquinolone Cardiopulmonary disease or risk factors: IV β-lactam plus IV/PO macrolide or doxycycline *or* IV fluoroquinolone alone	Extended-spectrum cephalosporin or β-lactam/β-lactamase inhibitor plus macrolide or a fluoroquinolone alone
Critically ill, ICU	*S. pneumoniae* *Legionella* sp. *S. aureus* Gram-negative bacilli *M. pneumoniae* *C. pneumoniae*	*P. aeruginosa* unlikely: IV β-lactam plus either IV macrolide or fluoroquinolone *P. aeruginosa* possible: IV antipseudomonal β-lactam plus fluoroquinolone or IV antipseudomonal β-lactam plus aminoglycoside plus either IV macrolide or fluoroquinolone	Extended-spectrum cephalosporin or β-lactam/β-lactamase plus either macrolide or fluoroquinolone

From American Thoracic Society: Am J Respir Crit Care Med 163:1730, 2001 and Bartlett JG et al: Clin Infect Dis 31:347, 2001.
IV, Intravenous; *PO*, by mouth.

disease or risk factors for mortality. For individuals without these, intravenous (IV) azithromycin or a fluoroquinolone is recommended. For higher-risk patients with these comorbidities, acceptable alternatives include an IV β-lactam plus an IV or oral macrolide or doxycycline; alternatively, a parenteral fluoroquinolone may be used alone.

In certain geographical areas, *S. pneumoniae* resistant to penicillin is common. Some strains are multidrug resistant and not covered by doxycycline, macrolides, or trimethoprim-sulfamethoxazole (TMP-SMX). When such isolates are suspected, empirical therapy with a fluoroquinolone or ceftriaxone is indicated. Vancomycin is another alternative, although the ATS guidelines suggest avoiding vancomycin unless methicillin-resistant *S. aureus* is a concern.

For critically ill patients requiring admission to the ICU, the IDSA guidelines recommend as empirical therapy an extended-spectrum cephalosporin or β-lactam/β-lactamase inhibitor combination together with either a macrolide or fluoroquinolone (see Table 19-8). The ATS recommendations for such patients are stratified based on whether *P. aeruginosa* is a likely pathogen. If it is not a likely pathogen, the ATS recommends a parenteral β-lactam along with either a macrolide or a fluoroquinolone. If *P. aeruginosa* is a possibility, empirical therapy should include an IV antipseudomonal β-lactam plus a fluoroquinolone or, alternatively, an antipseudomonal β-lactam plus an aminoglycoside plus either a fluoroquinolone or a macrolide.

Once a microbiological diagnosis is established, the antimicrobial regimen should be tailored to the isolated pathogen. Pathogen-specific treatment recommendations from the IDSA are summarized in Table 19-9; these are not provided by the ATS. For isolates of *S. pneumoniae* susceptible to penicillin, penicillin remains the preferred agent. Many strains of *H. influenzae* produce β-lactamase, rendering them resistant to penicillin. Second- or third-generation cephalosporins, azithromycin, or TMP-SMX are the agents of choice. Legionellosis should be treated with a macrolide with or without rifampin or, alternatively, with a fluoroquinolone alone. Mycoplasma and *C. pneumoniae* pneumonia should be treated with a macrolide or doxycycline. TMP-SMX is the drug of choice for *P. carinii* pneumonia. However, up to 50% of HIV-infected patients will develop fever or a rash while taking this medication. Therefore pentamidine is an acceptable alternative. Treatment for staphylococcal or gram-negative pneumonias is dictated by the antibiotic susceptibility profiles of the offending organism. For patients with staphylococcal pneumonia, vancomycin is preferred, pending antibiotic susceptibility results. If the isolate is methicillin susceptible, a semisynthetic penicillin such as oxacillin or nafcillin should be used; in seriously ill patients, rifampin or an aminoglycoside may be added. In patients with suspected or proven inhalation anthrax, either doxycycline or ciprofloxacin should be administered along with one or two of the following antibiotics: penicillin, ampicillin, vancomycin, rifampin, chloramphenicol, imipenem, clindamycin, or clarithromycin. A detailed discussion of antibiotic therapy for the treatment of pulmonary tuberculosis is beyond the scope of this chapter. In general, however, three drugs are initiated in patients with suspected or confirmed tuberculosis, unless a multidrug-resistant strain is suspected. In this case, four or five drugs usually are administered.

The duration of therapy of community-acquired pneumonia is guided by the specific pathogen and the patient's clinical course. In general, 10 to 14 days of

Table 19-9 ▶▶ Pathogen-Specific Treatment Recommendations for Adults With Community-Acquired Pneumonia: IDSA Guidelines[40]

Pathogen	Recommended Regimen
S. pneumoniae	
Penicillin susceptible	Penicillin G or amoxicillin
Penicillin resistant	Ceftriaxone, cefotaxime, fluoroquinolone or vancomycin
H. influenzae	Second- or third-generation cephalosporin, azithromycin, or TMP-SMX
Legionella species	Macrolide ± rifampin or fluoroquinolone alone
M. pneumoniae	Macrolide or doxycycline
C. pneumoniae	Macrolide or doxycycline
S. aureus	
Methicillin susceptible	Semisynthetic penicillin ± rifampin or gentamicin
Methicillin resistant	Vancomycin ± rifampin or gentamicin
Enterobacteriaceae	Third generation cephalosporin ± aminoglycoside or carbapenem
P. aeruginosa	Aminoglycoside + antipseudomonal β-lactam or carbapenem

therapy will suffice, except in cases of Legionnaires' disease, where a minimum of 2 weeks of therapy is recommended. Older individuals and those with comorbidities may require longer courses of treatment. Once fever has resolved and patients begin to improve clinically, oral therapy may be used to complete the treatment program. Failure of the patient's temperature to normalize within 4 or 5 days suggests the following possibilities: a missed pathogen, a metastatic or closed-space infection (e.g., empyema), drug fever, or the presence of an obstructing endobronchial lesion. Empyema should be treated with tube thoracostomy. Abnormal findings on physical examination may persist beyond 1 week in 20% to 40% of patients, despite clinical improvement. By 1 month, radiographic resolution occurs in 90% of individuals younger than the age of 50 years.[41] After 1 month, radiographic abnormalities may persist in up to 70% of cases involving older individuals or in those with significant underlying illnesses.[41]

MINI CLINI

Recognizing Unusual Exposures in Patients With Suspected Pneumonia

PROBLEM

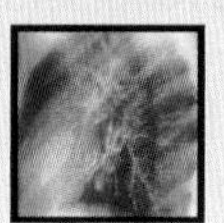

It is October 2001 and the RT is called to the ED to see a 50-year-old male postal worker in Washington, DC. He presents with a 3-day history of fever, dry cough, muscle and joint pain, and slight shortness of breath. Several of his colleagues who work in the mail sorting room with him have developed similar illnesses in the past few days. His history is notable for mild chronic obstructive pulmonary disease, obesity, and hypertension. He has smoked two packs of cigarettes per day for the past 30 years. He takes enalapril for his hypertension and denies recent travel.

On physical examination, his temperature is 38.5° C, blood pressure is 100/60 mm Hg, heart rate is 100 beats/min, and respiratory rate is 18 breaths/min. His examination is notable for slight dullness to percussion at both lung bases but is otherwise unremarkable. His white blood cell count is 15,000 cells/mm^3. Pulse oximetry discloses an oxygen saturation of 90%. A chest radiograph demonstrates widening of the mediastinal silhouette, clear lung fields, and bilateral pleural effusions of moderate size. What is the most likely diagnosis? Can this patient be safely discharged home? What antibiotics, if any, should be administered?

DISCUSSION

The most likely diagnosis is inhalation pulmonary anthrax. Clues to the diagnosis are the patient's occupation as a postal worker in Washington DC during the bioterrorist outbreak of inhalation anthrax during October 2001, along with the typical radiographic findings of mediastinal widening caused by suppurative lymphadenitis and bilateral pleural effusions, which are typically hemorrhagic in anthrax. The lack of pulmonary parenchymal infiltrates in the setting of these other radiographic findings also suggests the diagnosis.

The recognition of important epidemiological exposures and aspects of a patient's history is crucial for the RT, because these historical clues may provide the key to the diagnosis. Certain occupations and epidemiological exposures predispose to specific unusual infections. For example, healthcare workers may be more likely to encounter patients with unrecognized tuberculosis. Abattoir workers and sheep farmers are at higher risk of Q fever. Recent travel to the southwestern United States may expose patients to unusual pathogens such as *Coccidioides immitis* or hantavirus. Exposure to streams or rivers with beaver dams in the upper midwestern United States may lead to the development of pulmonary blastomycosis.

The fatality rate of inhalation anthrax is high and exceeds 40% even with aggressive therapy. This patient should be admitted to hospital and treated aggressively with intravenous antibiotics. Current Centers for Disease Control and Prevention recommendations for the treatment of pulmonary anthrax call for a regimen of either ciprofloxacin or doxycycline, along with one or two other agents, which may include penicillin, ampicillin, vancomycin, rifampin, chloramphenicol, imipenem, clindamycin, or clarithromycin. Sputum samples are rarely helpful in identifying the organism. Cultures of blood and pleural fluid should be obtained. Serology may be helpful in establishing a retrospective diagnosis.

RULE OF THUMB

Empyema should be ruled out in patients with community-acquired pneumonia and a large pleural effusion who fail to respond to therapy.

Empirical and definitive therapy of nosocomial pneumonia is dictated by institution-specific data regarding the most common organisms and their antibiotic-susceptibility profiles, as well as by patient-specific risk factors. Although general guidelines have been published,[28] the importance of local data cannot be overemphasized, because considerable geographical and institutional variability exists regarding the prevalence and susceptibility profiles of specific pathogens.

In general, in-hospital aspiration should be treated with a regimen that provides coverage against anaerobes and gram-negative bacilli, such as a β-lactam/β-lactamase inhibitor combination or clindamycin along with a third-generation cephalosporin. Vancomycin should be added if methicillin-resistant *S. aureus* is suspected. For **ventilator-associated pneumonia**, empirical coverage may be targeted at organisms known to colonize the patient's oropharynx or pathogens endemic to the ICU. Patients with *P. aeruginosa* pneumonia usually are treated with two agents, such as a ureidopenicillin or antipseudomonal cephalosporin together with an aminoglycoside or fluoroquinolone. In general, other gram-negative pneumonias are treated with a single agent, except in cases involving critically ill patients for whom a second drug is sometimes added. If legionellosis is endemic as a nosocomial infection within an institution, a macrolide may be added to the empirical regimen.

MINI CLINI

Evaluating Persisting Fever in Pneumonia

PROBLEM

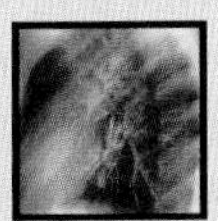

The RT is caring for a 68-year-old man admitted 1 week ago with bacteremic *H. influenzae* pneumonia. His admitting chest radiograph disclosed right lower lobe consolidation and a large right pleural effusion. He has a history of chronic obstructive pulmonary disease (COPD) and reports a 100 pack/year smoking history. He was treated initially with erythromycin and ceftizoxime until his blood cultures became positive. The organism was susceptible to ceftizoxime, which was continued as monotherapy. Despite this, he has remained persistently febrile (39° C), and his chest x-ray film has not improved. Why is he not responding to therapy?

DISCUSSION

Patients with community-acquired pneumonia who have comorbid illnesses such as alcoholism or COPD may recover more slowly than healthy individuals, despite appropriate therapy. Nevertheless, persistent fever 7 days into optimal treatment should prompt several considerations.

The two most likely concerns for this patient are (1) an undrained empyema and (2) an obstructing endobronchial malignancy, given his substantial smoking history. Other less likely considerations are as follows: drug fever; a new nosocomial infection; a missed pathogen, which is not responsive to ceftizoxime, contributing to his pneumonia; or a deep venous thrombosis resulting from bed rest.

The next step should be to repeat the history and physical examination. If these do not reveal a cause of the persistent fever, a thoracentesis should be performed to exclude empyema. If this is negative, further investigation in search of an occult endobronchial-obstructing lesion should be considered.

As with community-acquired pneumonia, the duration of therapy for cases of nosocomial pneumonia is dictated by the clinical course. Usually, a minimum of 2 weeks is required. Failure of the patient to improve should prompt the following considerations: the presence of an occult empyema; an unrecognized pathogen; a new and unrelated nosocomial infection; or other noninfectious causes of fever common in the ICU, such as deep venous thrombosis, drug fever, occult pancreatitis, or acalculous cholecystitis (gallbladder inflammation without gallstones).

Some organisms, such as *P. aeruginosa* and *Acinetobacter* species, are associated with a poor prognosis in ventilator-associated pneumonia, despite optimal therapy.[42] The mortality rate for these organisms may approach 90%, despite appropriate treatment.

The RT has an important role in the diagnosis and management of patients with community-acquired and nosocomial pneumonia. Ensuring mobilization of infected secretions facilitates clinical improvement, and maintenance of adequate oxygenation is essential. The usefulness of chest physiotherapy in the treatment of pneumonia is still unproved, but some patients seem to benefit from it.

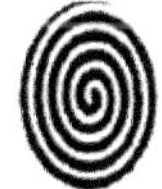

RULE OF THUMB

In cases of community-acquired pneumonia, patients often get better before their x-ray examinations show any improvement.

▶ PREVENTION

Preventive strategies for community-acquired pneumonia have focused on immunization of high-risk individuals against influenza and *S. pneumoniae*. Influenza is a risk factor for the subsequent development of community-acquired pneumonia during the fall and winter months. Immunization is indicated for individuals older than the age of 60 years, because it reduces the incidence of illness for their age-group by half.[43] Immunization also is indicated for individuals with chronic lung or heart disease or for whom the morbidity of influenza may be substantial. Recent studies have suggested that widespread immunization of healthy working adults may be cost-effective, because the number of sick days taken and the number of visits to a physician are reduced.[44] Healthcare workers, including RTs, should be immunized annually to prevent transmission of influenza to patients.

Currently available pneumococcal vaccines provide protection against the 23 serotypes of *S. pneumoniae*, which cause 85% to 90% of invasive pneumococcal infections in the United States. Vaccination is indicated for all individuals older than the age of 65 years and for those older than the age of 2 years who have functional or anatomical asplenia. Vaccination is also indicated in patients with chronic illnesses such as CHF, chronic lung disease, chronic liver disease, alcoholism, cerebrospinal fluid leaks, or conditions characterized by impaired immunity.[45] Routine pneumococcal vaccination of all healthcare workers is not currently recommended, unless they possess one of the specific indications for vaccination outlined previously.

The **prevention** of nosocomial pneumonia has been an area of intense investigation over the past 20 years. Table 19-10 summarizes currently available strategies and their relative efficacy. None are uniformly effective.

Handwashing is an important but frequently neglected measure that can reduce transmission of nosocomial bacteria from one patient to another. It is especially important for RTs who may be caring for several ventilated patients in the ICU. Failure to wash the hands between patient contact may result in transmission of respiratory pathogens from one patient to another. Handwashing is important even if gloves are worn. Gloves should be changed between patient contact, because they too can become contaminated with and transmit bacteria.

Table 19-10 ▶ ▶ Strategies for the Prevention of Nosocomial Pneumonia

Strategy	Efficacy
Handwashing	Probably effective
Isolation of patients with resistant organisms	Probably effective
Infection control and surveillance	Probably effective
Enteral feeding, rather than TPN	Possibly effective
Semierect position	Possibly effective
Sucralfate for bleeding prophylaxis	Possibly effective
Careful handling of respiratory therapy equipment	Possibly effective
Subglottic secretion aspiration	Possibly effective
Selective digestive decontamination	Unproved efficacy
Topical tracheobronchial antibiotics	Unproved efficacy

TPN, Total parenteral nutrition.

Infection control surveillance to detect outbreaks of nosocomial pneumonia with specific pathogens and to monitor antibiotic resistance patterns is an important strategy, because isolation and cohorting of infected patients can limit the scope and duration of outbreaks, especially in ICUs.

In patients requiring nutritional support, the use of enteral feeding by means of jejunostomy has been associated with a lower risk of nosocomial pneumonia than that associated with the use of total parenteral nutrition.[46] In addition, patients who are fed enterally have a lower incidence of pneumonia if kept semierect rather than recumbent.[6]

Two studies have suggested that gastrointestinal bleeding prophylaxis with sucralfate is associated with a lower risk of pneumonia, compared with antacid or H_2-blockers.[47,48] Careful handling of respiratory therapy equipment may reduce the risk of lower respiratory tract infection in ventilated patients. Condensate within the tubing may be colonized with bacteria and should be drained away from the patient, because passage of this material into the airway may facilitate colonization with nosocomial pathogens. One study found that continuous subglottic aspiration of secretions was effective in reducing the incidence of nosocomial pneumonia in intubated patients.[49] A number of studies have failed to demonstrate the efficacy of selective digestive decontamination in the prevention of nosocomial pneumonia, a strategy that uses topical antibiotics in the oropharynx and gastrointestinal tract, along with a brief course of systemic therapy.

In summary, prevention of nosocomial pneumonia remains a challenge to the RT. Even so, careful attention to basic infection control practices, such as frequent handwashing, using new gloves with each patient contact, and careful handling of respiratory care equipment, are important practices in the prevention of nosocomial pneumonia.

KEY POINTS

- ➤ Community-acquired and nosocomial pneumonia are common and important clinical problems with significant morbidity and mortality.
- ➤ Most studies find that *S. pneumoniae* remains the most common cause of community-acquired pneumonia.

KEY POINTS—cont'd

- Gram-negative bacilli and *S. aureus* are the most common pathogens producing nosocomial pneumonia, but their relative incidence and antimicrobial susceptibility profiles may vary from one institution to another.
- The risk of mortality can be quantified at presentation for most patients with community-acquired pneumonia, which may help in determining the need for hospitalization.
- Routine sputum cultures for patients with community-acquired pneumonia must be interpreted within the context of the sputum Gram stain, which provides valuable information regarding the adequacy of the specimen and the predominance of potential pathogens.
- The accurate diagnosis of nosocomial pneumonia remains a challenge, and none of the diagnostic modalities currently available is completely reliable.
- Guidelines exist for the treatment of community-acquired and nosocomial pneumonia. To whatever extent possible, pathogen-specific antibiotic therapy should be used.
- Immunization of high-risk individuals against influenza and *S. pneumoniae*, although imperfect, is the major strategy in the prevention of community-acquired pneumonia.
- Strategies for preventing nosocomial pneumonia are not uniformly effective.
- The RT can help prevent nosocomial pneumonia by careful attention to basic infection control procedures such as handwashing.

References

1. Meeker DP, Longworth DL: Community-acquired pneumonia: an update, Cleve Clin J Med 63:16, 1996.
2. American Thoracic Society: Guidelines for the initial management of adults with community-acquired pneumonia: diagnosis, assessment of severity, and initial antimicrobial therapy, Am J Respir Crit Care Med 163:1730, 2001.
3. Craven DE, Steger KA, Barber TW: Preventing nosocomial pneumonia: state of the art and perspectives for the 1990s, Am J Med 91:44S, 1991.
4. Wiblin RT, Wenzel RP: Hospital-acquired pneumonia, Curr Clin Top Infect Dis 16:194, 1996.
5. Bassin A, Niederman MS: New approaches to prevention and treatment of nosocomial pneumonia, Semin Thorac Cardiovasc Surg 7:70, 1995.
6. Torres A et al: Pulmonary aspiration of gastric contents in patients receiving mechanical ventilation: the effect of body position, Ann Intern Med 116:540, 1992.
7. Valles J et al: Continuous aspiration of subglottic secretions in preventing ventilator-associated pneumonia, Ann Intern Med 122:179, 1995.
8. Bartlett JG, Mundy LM: Community-acquired pneumonia, N Engl J Med 333:1618, 1995.
9. Marrie TJ et al: Ambulatory patients with community-acquired pneumonia: the frequency of atypical agents and clinical course, Am J Med 101:508, 1996.
10. Mundy LM et al: Community-acquired pneumonia: impact of immune status, Am J Respir Crit Care Med 152:1309, 1995.
11. Bush LM et al: Index case of fatal inhalational anthrax due to bioterrorism in the United States, New Engl J Med 345:1607, 2001.
12. Fang GD et al: New and emerging etiologies for community-acquired pneumonia with implications for therapy: a prospective multicenter study of 359 cases, Medicine 69:307, 1990.
13. Fine MJ, Smith DN, Singer DE: Hospitalization decision in patients with community-acquired pneumonia: a prospective cohort study, Am J Med 89:713, 1990.
14. Fine MJ et al: Prognosis and outcomes of patients with community-acquired pneumonia: A metaanalysis, JAMA 274:134, 1995.
15. Fine MJ et al: A prediction rule to identify low-risk patients with community-acquired pneumonia, N Engl J Med 336:243, 1997.
16. Torres A et al: Incidence, risk, and prognosis factors of nosocomial pneumonia in mechanically ventilated patients, Am Rev Respir Dis 142:523, 1990.
17. Craven DE, Steger KA: Epidemiology of nosocomial pneumonia: new perspectives on an old disease, Chest 108:1S, 1995.
18. Kollef MH et al: The effect of late-onset ventilator-associated pneumonia in determining patient mortality, Chest 108:1655, 1995.
19. Rein MF et al: Accuracy of Gram's stain in identifying pneumococci in sputum, JAMA 239:2671, 1978.
20. Barrett-Connor E: The nonvalue of sputum culture in the diagnosis of pneumococcal pneumonia, Am Rev Respir Dis 103:845, 1970.
21. Gleckman R et al: Sputum Gram's stain assessment in community-acquired bacteremic pneumonia, J Clin Microbiol 26:846, 1988.
22. Murray PR, Washington JA: Microscopic and bacteriologic analysis of expectorated sputum, Mayo Clin Proc 50:339, 1975.
23. Nguyen MLT, Yu VL: Legionella infection, Clin Chest Med 12:257,1991.
24. Farley MM et al: Invasive *Haemophilus influenzae* disease in adults, Ann Intern Med 116:806, 1992.
25. Meehan TP et al: Quality of care, process, and outcomes in elderly patients with pneumonia, JAMA 278:2080, 1997.

26. Heffner JE et al: Pleural fluid chemical analysis in parapneumonic effusions: a meta-analysis, Am J Respir Crit Care Med 151:1700, 1995.
27. Kohler RB: Antigen detection for the rapid diagnosis of mycoplasma and Legionella pneumonia, Diagn Microbiol Infect Dis 4:47S, 1986.
28. American Thoracic Society: Hospital-acquired pneumonia in adults: diagnosis, assessment of severity, initial antimicrobial therapy, and preventative strategies, Am J Respir Crit Care Med 153:1711, 1995.
29. Chastre J, Fagon JV, Trouillet JL: Diagnosis and treatment of nosocomial pneumonia in patients in intensive care units, Clin Infect Dis 21(Suppl 3):S226, 1995.
30. Garrard CS, A'Court CD: The diagnosis of pneumonia in the critically ill, Chest 108 (Suppl 2):17S, 1995.
31. Fagon JY et al: Evaluation of clinical judgment in the identification and treatment of nosocomial pneumonia in ventilated patients, Chest 103:547, 1993.
32. Timsit JF et al: Usefulness of airway visualization in the diagnosis of nosocomial pneumonia in ventilated patients, Chest 110:172, 1996.
33. Marquette C et al: Diagnostic efficacy of endotracheal aspirates with quantitative bacterial cultures in intubated patients with suspected pneumonia, Am Rev Respir Dis 148:138, 1993.
34. Jourdain B et al: Role of quantitative cultures of endotracheal aspirates in the diagnosis of nosocomial pneumonia, Am J Respir Crit Care Med 152:241, 1995.
35. Chastre J et al: Quantification of BAL cells containing intracellular bacteria rapidly identifies ventilated patients with nosocomial pneumonia, Chest 95:190, 1989.
36. Chastre J et al: Diagnosis of nosocomial bacterial pneumonia in intubated patients undergoing ventilation: comparison of the usefulness of bronchoalveolar lavage and the protected specimen brush, Am J Med 85:499, 1988.
37. Kollef MH et al: The safety and diagnostic accuracy of minibronchoalveolar lavage in patients with suspected ventilator-associated pneumonia, Ann Intern Med 122:743, 1995.
38. Dorca J et al: Efficacy, safety, and therapeutic relevance of transthoracic aspiration with ultrathin needle in nonventilated nosocomial pneumonia, Am J Respir Crit Care Med 151:1491, 1995.
39. American Thoracic Society: Guidelines for the management of adults with community-acquired pneumonia, Am J Respir Crit Care Med 163:1730, 2001.
40. Bartlett JG et al: Guidelines from the IDSA for the management of community-acquired pneumonia, Clin Infect Dis 31:347, 2001.
41. Mittl RL et al: Radiographic resolution of community-acquired pneumonia, Am J Respir Crit Care Med 149:630, 1994.
42. Fagon JY et al: Nosocomial pneumonia in patients receiving continuous mechanical ventilation, Am Rev Respir Dis 139:877, 1989.
43. Govaert TM et al: The efficacy of influenza vaccination in elderly individuals: a randomized double-blind placebo-controlled trial, JAMA 272:1661, 1994.
44. Nichol KL et al: The effectiveness of vaccination against influenza in healthy, working adults, N Engl J Med 333:889, 1995.
45. Centers for Disease Control and Prevention: Prevention of pneumococcal disease: recommendations of the Advisory Committee on Immunization Practices (ACIP), MMWR CDC Surveill Summ 46(RR-8):1, 1997.
46. Moore FA et al: TEN versus TPN following major abdominal trauma: reduced septic mortality, J Trauma 29:916, 1989.
47. Tryba M: Sucralfate versus antacids or H_2-antagonists for stress ulcer prophylaxis: a meta-analysis on efficacy and pneumonia rate, Crit Care Med 19:942, 1991.
48. Cook DJ et al: Nosocomial pneumonia and the role of gastric pH: a meta-analysis, Chest 100:7, 1991.
49. Valles J et al: Continuous aspiration of subglottic secretions in preventing ventilator-associated pneumonia, Ann Intern Med 122:179, 1995.

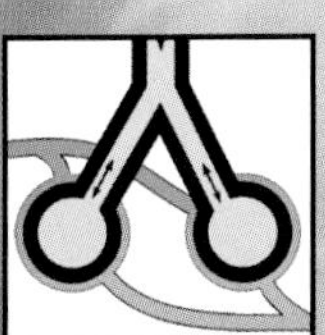

CHAPTER 20

Obstructive Lung Disease: COPD, Asthma, and Related Diseases

Raed Dweik and James K. Stoller

In This Chapter You Will Learn:

- How many Americans are diagnosed with chronic obstructive pulmonary disease (COPD) and how many deaths from COPD occur each year
- What two major risk factors are associated with the onset of COPD
- What common signs and symptoms are associated with COPD
- How to develop a treatment plan for the patient with stable COPD and for the patient with an acute exacerbation
- What factors are associated with the onset of asthma
- What clinical presentation is typical for the patient with asthma
- What treatment is currently available for the patient with acute asthma
- What treatment is currently available for patients with bronchiectasis

Chapter Outline

Key Terms

acute exacerbations of COPD
airway hyperresponsiveness
airway inflammation
airway obstruction
α_1-antitrypsin deficiency
asthma
bronchiectasis
bronchodilator
bronchospasm
chronic bronchitis
emphysema
noninvasive ventilation
supplemental oxygen

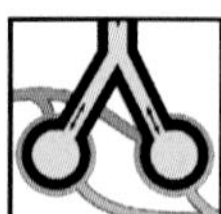

The spectrum of obstructive lung diseases is broad and includes chronic obstructive pulmonary disease (COPD) and **asthma** as the most common components, as well as less common entities such as **bronchiectasis** and cystic fibrosis. This chapter reviews the major diseases that comprise obstructive lung disease, emphasizing their defining features, epidemiology, pathophysiology, clinical signs and symptoms, prognosis, and management. Cystic fibrosis is discussed in Chapter 28.

▶ CHRONIC OBSTRUCTIVE PULMONARY DISEASE

Overview and Definitions

The term *chronic obstructive pulmonary disease,* abbreviated COPD or sometimes COLD ("L" for lung), refers to a disease state characterized by the presence of airflow obstruction resulting from **chronic bronchitis** or **emphysema.** As defined by the American Thoracic Society (ATS),[1] airflow obstruction in COPD is usually progressive, may be accompanied by airway hyperreactivity, and may be partially reversible. The spectrum of COPD is usefully represented by Figure 20-1, which presents a nonproportional Venn diagram representing the major components of COPD: chronic bronchitis and emphysema. Although asthma is no longer conventionally considered to be part of the spectrum of COPD, the overlap of asthma with COPD represents individuals with asthma but incompletely reversible airflow obstruction who are indistinguishable from patients with COPD. Whereas the ATS definition of COPD emphasizes chronic bronchitis and emphysema,[1] the Global Initiative for Chronic Obstructive Lung Disease (GOLD) proposes a definition that focuses on the progressive nature of airflow limitation and its association with abnormal inflammatory response of the lungs to various noxious particles or gases.[2] According to the GOLD document, COPD is "a disease state characterized by airflow limitation that is not fully reversible. The airflow limitation is usually both progressive and associated with an abnormal inflammatory response of the lungs to noxious particles or gases."[2]

The two major entities composing COPD—emphysema and chronic bronchitis—are defined in different ways. Emphysema is defined in anatomical terms as a condition characterized by abnormal, permanent enlargement of the airspaces beyond the terminal bronchiole, accompanied by destruction of the walls of the airspaces without fibrosis. In contrast, chronic bronchitis is defined in clinical terms as a condition in which chronic productive cough is present for at least 3 months per year for at least 2 consecutive years. The definition specifies further that other causes of chronic cough (e.g., gastroesophageal reflux, asthma, and postnasal drip) have been excluded. Figure 20-1 shows considerable overlap between chronic bronchitis and emphysema and some overlap with asthma (i.e., when airflow obstruction is incompletely reversible). Figure 20-1 also shows that chronic bronchitis and emphysema can occur without airflow obstruction, although the clinical significance of these entities usually stems from obstruction to airflow.

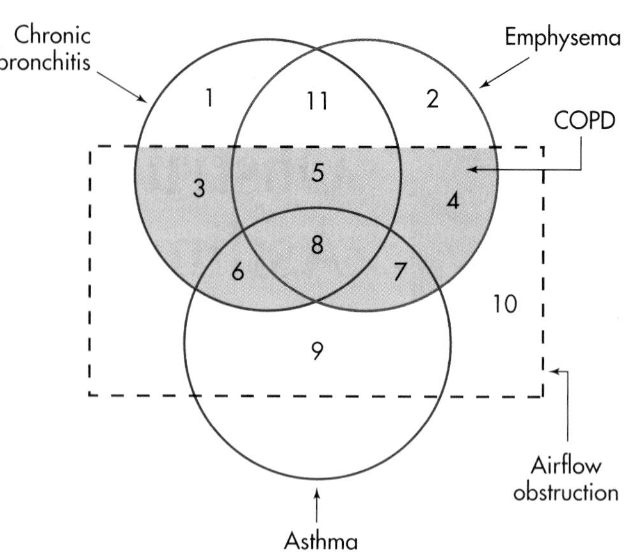

Figure 20-1 · Schema of Chronic Obstructive Pulmonary Disease (COPD)

This nonproportional Venn diagram shows subsets of patients with chronic bronchitis, emphysema, and asthma. The subsets composing COPD are shaded. Subset areas are not proportional to actual relative subset sizes. Asthma is by definition associated with reversible airflow obstruction, although in variant asthma special maneuvers may be necessary to make the obstruction evident. Patients with asthma whose airflow obstruction is completely reversible *(subset 9)* are not considered to have COPD. In many cases, it is virtually impossible to differentiate patients with asthma whose airflow obstruction does not remit completely from patients with chronic bronchitis and emphysema who have partially reversible airflow obstruction with airway hyperreactivity; therefore patients with unremitting asthma are classified as having COPD *(subsets 6, 7, and 8)*. Chronic bronchitis and emphysema with airflow obstruction usually occur together *(subset 5)*, and some patients may have asthma associated with these two disorders *(subset 8)*. Individuals with asthma who are exposed to chronic irritation (e.g., from cigarette smoke) may develop a chronic, productive cough, a feature of chronic bronchitis *(subset 6)*. Such patients are often referred to as having asthmatic bronchitis or the asthmatic form of COPD. Persons with chronic bronchitis and/or emphysema without airflow obstruction *(subsets 1, 2, and 11)* are not classified as having COPD. Patients with airway obstruction caused by diseases with known etiology or specific pathology, such as cystic fibrosis or obliterative bronchiolitis *(subset 10)*, are not included in this definition.

Epidemiology

COPD is common, with recent estimates suggesting that 16 million Americans are affected—approximately 14 million with chronic bronchitis and another 2 million with emphysema.[1] COPD is now the fourth leading cause of death in the United States, accounting for an estimated 105,000 deaths (approximately 4% of all deaths) annually. Unlike the rates for more common causes of death (e.g., stroke, cardiovascular disease), the rate of deaths from COPD has risen steadily between 1966 and 1986, likely paralleling (with a lag time) prior smoking trends. The health burden caused by COPD is great; in 1993, COPD caused 505,000 hospitalizations, 14,258,000 office visits to physicians, and a health expenditure of almost $24 billion. In this regard, COPD is a problem that is a frequent challenge for the respiratory therapist (RT).

Risk Factors and Pathophysiology

Although many risk factors exist for COPD (Box 20-1), the two most common are cigarette smoking (which has been estimated to account for 80% to 90% of all COPD-related deaths) and **α_1-antitrypsin deficiency.**[3,4] Evidence linking cigarette smoking to the development of COPD is strong and includes several different lines of evidence:

1. The symptoms of COPD (e.g., chronic cough and phlegm production) are more common in smokers than in nonsmokers.
2. Impaired lung function with evidence of an obstructive pattern of lung dysfunction is more common in smokers than in nonsmokers.
3. Pathological changes of airflow obstruction and chronic bronchitis are evident in smokers' lungs.
4. Susceptible smokers (representing approximately 15% of all cigarette smokers) experience more rapid rates of decline of lung function than do nonsmokers.

Indeed, recent information from the Lung Health Study (Figure 20-2) highlights the accelerated rate of decrease of the forced expiratory volume in one second (FEV_1) in smokers compared with former smokers who have achieved sustained cessation.[5] Overall, the strength of evidence implicating cigarette smoking as a cause of COPD has allowed the Surgeon General to conclude: "Cigarette smoking is the major cause of chronic obstructive lung disease in the United States for both men and women. The contribution of cigarette smoking to chronic obstructive lung disease morbidity and mortality far outweighs all other factors."[6]

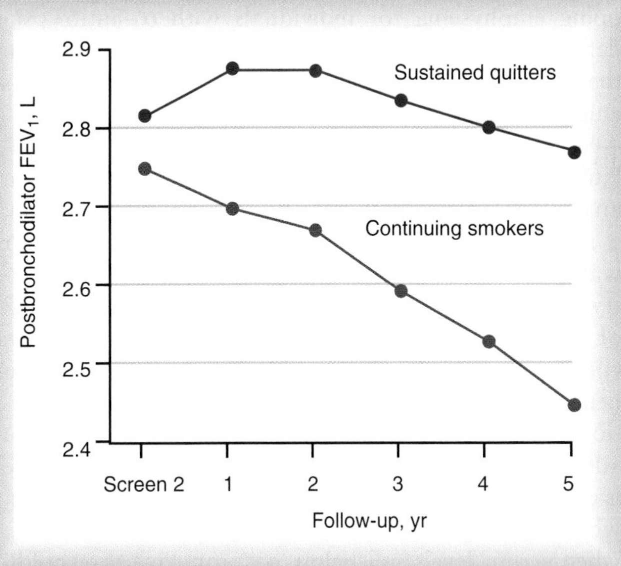

Figure 20-2
Mean postbronchodilator FEV_1 for participants in the smoking intervention and placebo groups who were sustained quitters *(red circles)* and continuous smokers *(purple circles)*. The two curves diverge sharply after baseline. *(Modified from Anthonisen SR et al: JAMA 272:1497, 1994.)*

Box 20-1 • Causes of COPD*

Cigarette smoking
α_1-Antitrypsin deficiency†
Hypocomplementemic urticarial vasculitis
Intravenous Ritalin abuse
Ehlers-Danlos syndrome; Marfan syndrome
Salla disease†
α_1-Antichymotrypsin deficiency†
HIV (emphysema-like illness)

*Multiple causes (e.g., cigarette smoking and α_1-antitrypsin deficiency may coexist in a single patient).
†Putative cause; firm evidence unavailable.

The second well-recognized cause of emphysema, α_1-antitrypsin deficiency, sometimes called *genetic emphysema,* is a condition characterized by a deficient amount of a protein called *α_1-antitrypsin* that may result in the early onset of emphysema and that is inherited as a so-called autosomal-codominant condition. Accounting for 2% to 3% of all cases of COPD, α_1-antitrypsin deficiency is severely underrecognized by healthcare providers, but affects an estimated 100,000 Americans.[3,4] For example, in one survey, the mean interval between the first onset of pulmonary symptoms and initial diagnosis of α_1-antitrypsin deficiency was 7.2 years, and 43% of individuals with severe α_1-antitrypsin deficiency reported seeing at least three physicians before the diagnosis of α_1-antitrypsin deficiency was first made.[3] The importance of early identification is emphasized by the need to test (by simply sending a serum level for α_1-antitrypsin testing) first-degree relatives (e.g., siblings, parents, children), by the favorable effect of primary prevention of smoking among individuals identified early, and by the availability of a specific therapy called *intravenous (IV) augmentation therapy.* The risk of developing emphysema for individuals with α_1-antitrypsin deficiency increases as the level of α_1-antitrypsin in the serum falls below 11 μmol/L, or 80 mg/dL, and is enhanced greatly by cigarette smoking.

Study of α_1-antitrypsin deficiency has helped formulate the protease-antiprotease hypothesis of emphysema, an explanatory model (Figure 20-3) in which lung elastin, a major structural protein that supports the alveolar walls of the lung, is normally protected by α_1-antitrypsin, a protein that opposes the degradative threat of neutrophil elastase.[7] Neutrophil elastase is a protein contained within neutrophils that is disgorged when neutrophils are attracted to the lung during inflammation or infection. Under normal circumstances of an adequate amount of α_1-antitrypsin, neutrophil elastase is counteracted so as not to digest lung elastin. However, when severe α_1-antitrypsin deficiency is present (i.e., when serum levels fall below a "protective threshold" value of 11 mmol/L or 80 mg/dL), neutrophil elastase may go unchecked, causing breakdown of elastin and resulting dissolution of alveolar walls. This protease-antiprotease model is believed to explain, at least partially, the pathogenesis of emphysema in α_1-antitrypsin deficiency, but evidence suggesting its role in COPD in individuals with normal amounts of α_1-antitrypsin is conflicting.

The mechanisms of airflow obstruction in COPD include inflammation and obstruction of small airways (less than 2-mm diameter), loss of the elasticity that keeps small airways open when elastin is destroyed in emphysema, and active **bronchospasm.** Although traditionally considered to be characteristic of asthma, some reversibility of airflow obstruction has been observed in up to two thirds of patients with COPD when tested serially with inhaled bronchodilators.[8]

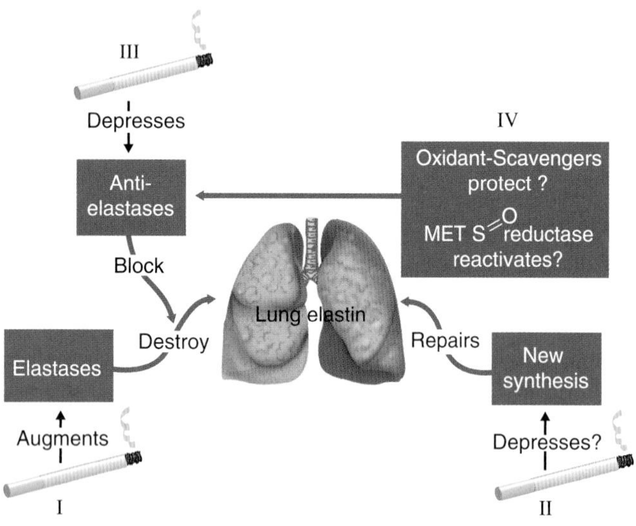

Figure 20-3

Proposed biochemical links between cigarette smoking and the pathogenesis of emphysema. *(I)* Smoking recruits monocytes, macrophages, and (through macrophage chemotactic factors) polymorphonuclear neutrophils to the lung, elevating the connective tissue "burden" of elastolytic serine and metalloproteases. *(III)* At the same time, oxidants in smoke plus those produced by smoke-stimulated lung phagocytes (as well as oxidizing products of chemical interactions between these two) inactivate bronchial mucus proteinase inhibitor and α_1-antitrypsin, the latter representing the major antielastase "shield" of the respiratory units. *(II)* Other unidentified, water-soluble, gas-phase components of cigarette smoke (cyanide? copper-chelators?) inhibit lysyl oxidase–catalyzed oxidative deamination of epsilon-amino groups in tropoelastin and block formation of desmosine and presumably other cross-links during elastin synthesis, thus decreasing connective tissue repair. *(IV)* Antioxidants (ceruloplasmin? methionine-sulfoxide-reductase) may protect or reactivate elastase inhibitors, and other unidentified factors may modulate the chemical lesions induced in the lung by smoking to influence the risk of developing COPD. *(Modified from Janoff A et al: Am Rev Respir Dis 127[Suppl]:S31, 1983.)*

Clinical Signs and Symptoms

Common symptoms of COPD include cough, phlegm production, wheezing, and shortness of breath, typically on exertion. Dyspnea is often slow but progressive in onset and occurs later in the course of the disease, characteristically in the late sixth or seventh decade of life. One notable exception is α_1-antitrypsin deficiency, in which dyspnea begins sooner (mean age, approximately 45). Table 20-1 reviews the characteristic features of both emphysema and chronic bronchitis and emphasizes traits that should suggest the possibility of α_1-antitrypsin deficiency, including early onset of emphysema, emphysema in a nonsmoker, or a family history of emphysema. Suspicion of α_1-antitrypsin deficiency should lead to a simple blood test by which the serum level can be established; serum levels of α_1-antitrypsin below 11 μmol/L or 80 mg/dL suggest severe deficiency.

Physical examination of the chest in a patient with COPD may show wheezing or diminished breath sounds early. Later, signs of hyperinflation may be evident (i.e., increased anteroposterior diameter, diaphragm flattening, and dimpling inward of the chest wall at the level of the diaphragm on inspiration [called *Hoover's sign*]). Other late signs of COPD include the use of accessory muscles of respiration, edema resulting from cor pulmonale, mental status changes caused by hypercapnia (especially if acute, as in acute exacerbations of chronic, severe disease), or asterixis (i.e., involuntary flapping of the hands when held in an extended position, as in "stopping traffic").

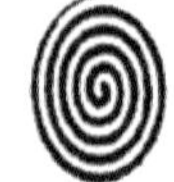

RULE OF THUMB

In patients with COPD, the $Paco_2$ is usually preserved until airflow obstruction is severe (i.e., FEV_1 <1 L), when $Paco_2$ may rise.

Table 20-1 ▶▶ Clinical Features of COPD: Distinctions Between Chronic Bronchitis and Emphysema, With Emphasis on Distinguishing Features of α_1-Antitrypsin Deficiency

Features	Chronic Bronchitis*	Emphysema[†]	Severe α_1-Antitrypsin Deficiency
Symptoms and Signs			
Chronic cough, phlegm	Common	Less common	Less common, but may be present
Dyspnea on exertion	Less common	Common	Common
Cor pulmonale	Present (often with multiple exacerbations)	Present (but often in end-stage emphysema)	Present (but often in end-stage emphysema)
Age of patient at symptom onset	Sixth to seventh decade	Sixth to seventh decade	Fourth to fifth decade (although late onset is possible)
Family history of COPD	Possible but not characteristic	Possible but not characteristic	Common in parents, children, and siblings
History of cigarette smoking	Present, often heavy	Present, often heavy	May be present, but COPD can occur in the absence of smoking
Physiological Function			
Airflow (FEV_1, FEV_1/FVC)	Decreased	Decreased	Decreased
Lung volumes, residual volume	Normal	Increased, suggesting air trapping	Increased
Gas exchange, diffusion			
Pao_2	Often decreased	Often preserved until advanced stage	Often preserved until advanced stage
$Paco_2$	May be increased	Often preserved until advanced disease, then elevated	Often preserved until advanced disease, then elevated
Diffusion capacity	Often normal	Decreased	Decreased
Static lung compliance	Normal	Increased	Increased
Chest radiograph	"Dirty lungs" with peribronchial cuffing, suggesting thickened bronchial walls	Hyperinflation, with evidence of emphysema; greater at the lung apex than at the lung base	Hyperinflation, with evidence of emphysema; greater at the lung base than at the lung apex (basilar hyperlucency)

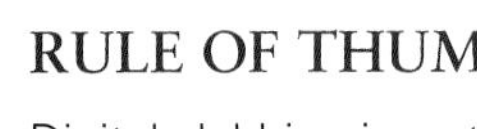

RULE OF THUMB

Digital clubbing is *not* caused by COPD alone, even if hypoxemia is present. Rather, clubbing in a patient with COPD should invite consideration of another cause (e.g., bronchogenic cancer, bronchiectasis).

Management

In managing patients with chronic stable COPD, several goals must guide the clinician. These goals are as follows:

1. Establish the diagnosis of COPD.
2. Optimize lung function.
3. Maximize the patient's functional status.
4. Simplify the medical regimen as much as possible.
5. Whenever possible, prolong survival.

In managing patients with **acute exacerbations of COPD,** additional considerations are to reestablish the patient to the baseline status as quickly and with as little morbidity and mortality as possible. Each of the treatments discussed in this section is considered in the context of these goals, recognizing differences in management between patients with chronic stable versus acute exacerbations of COPD. Figures 20-4 and 20-5 present algorithms that guide general management.

Establishing the Diagnosis of COPD

Although a spectrum of diseases can give rise to obstructive lung disease (e.g., including some unusual entities such as chronic eosinophilic pneumonia, bronchiectasis, and allergic bronchopulmonary aspergillosis), the major challenge facing the clinician who encounters a patient with airflow obstruction is to distinguish COPD (i.e., emphysema and/or chronic bronchitis) from asthma (see Figure 20-4 and Table 20-1). Features that favor COPD include chronic daily phlegm (which establishes the diagnosis of chronic bronchitis), diminished vascularity on the chest radiograph, and a decreased diffusing capacity, whereas the diagnosis of asthma is favored if the diminished FEV_1 obtained on spirometry can be normalized after an inhaled bronchodilator. Once the diagnosis of COPD is established, a secondary issue is for the clinician to consider whether the patient has an unusual cause for COPD, such as α_1-antitrypsin deficiency or another etiology listed in Box 20-1. Such underlying etiologies will be present in fewer than 5% of patients with COPD, with α_1-antitrypsin deficiency the most common (2% to 3% of all patients with COPD).

MINI CLINI

Determining the Severity of COPD

PROBLEM

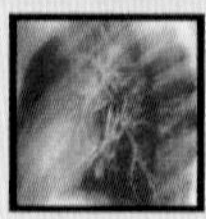

The RT is called to see a patient with COPD and is asked to describe the severity of the patient's illness to a colleague. How is the severity of COPD characterized?

DISCUSSION

The severity of COPD is described by the degree of airflow obstruction. Certainly, developments such as hypoxemia and hypercapnia are useful to characterize patients with COPD and have been traditional descriptors. The American Thoracic Society (ATS) has proposed a staging system for COPD,[1] as have other societies.[2,9,10] According to the ATS staging system, patients are categorized into one of three stages as follows: Stage I is assigned to patients with FEV_1 >50% predicted, stage II is assigned to patients with FEV_1 35%–49% predicted, and stage III is assigned to patients with FEV_1 <35% predicted. In general, stages correspond to other physiological features of COPD. For example, patients with stage I COPD usually do not have severe hypoxemia. In addition, hypercapnia from airflow obstruction is not expected in patients with stage I COPD, and an arterial blood gas (ABG) is not usually recommended. Patients with stages II or III COPD may require supplemental oxygen, so an ABG may be helpful in their assessment.

Optimizing Lung Function

Stable COPD. Although the airflow obstruction resulting from emphysema itself is irreversible, most (up to two thirds) patients with stable COPD will demonstrate a reversible component of airflow obstruction, defined as a 12% and 200-mL rise in the postbronchodilator FEV_1 or functional vital capacity (FVC). For this reason, **bronchodilator** therapy is recommended for patients with COPD. Both anticholinergic and sympathomimetic bronchodilators can improve airflow in patients with COPD, although many clinicians favor an inhaled anticholinergic medication (e.g., ipratropium bromide) as first-line therapy[11] (see Figure 20-5). The addition of a sympathomimetic bronchodilator (e.g., a β_2-agonist) may offer additive bronchodilation. Importantly, results of the Lung Health Study,[5] which compared the effects of inhaled ipratropium bromide (2 puffs four times daily) with placebo in patients with mild stable COPD, showed that regular, long-term use of ipratropium did not change the rate of decline of lung function, but offered a one-time, small rise in FEV_1. The lack of a demonstrable survival benefit of inhaled bronchodilators in COPD suggests that patients with symptoms or functional limitation from COPD should be treated, but that bronchodilator therapy can be deferred in patients with minimal or no symptoms.

Other treatment options to optimize lung function include administering corticosteroids and methyl-

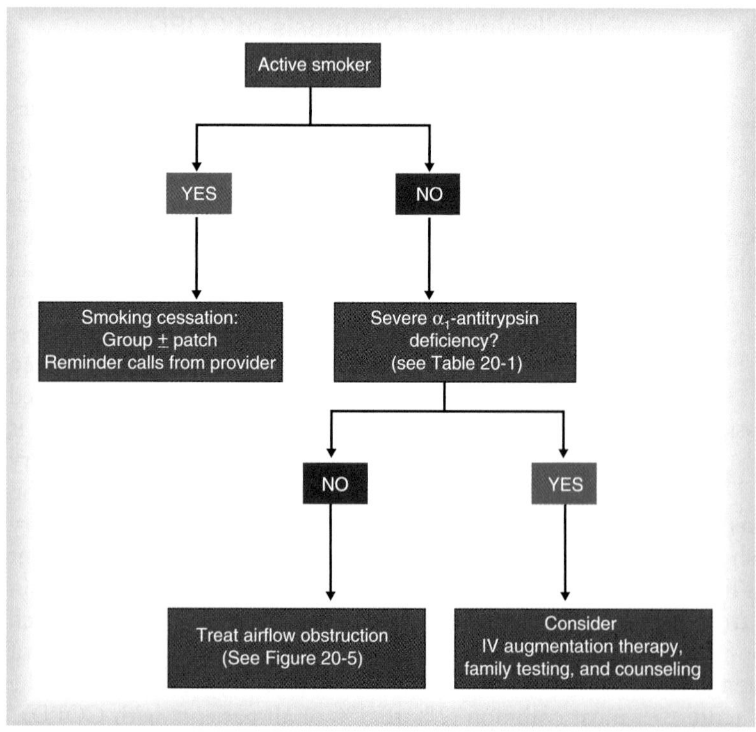

Figure 20-4
General management of COPD.

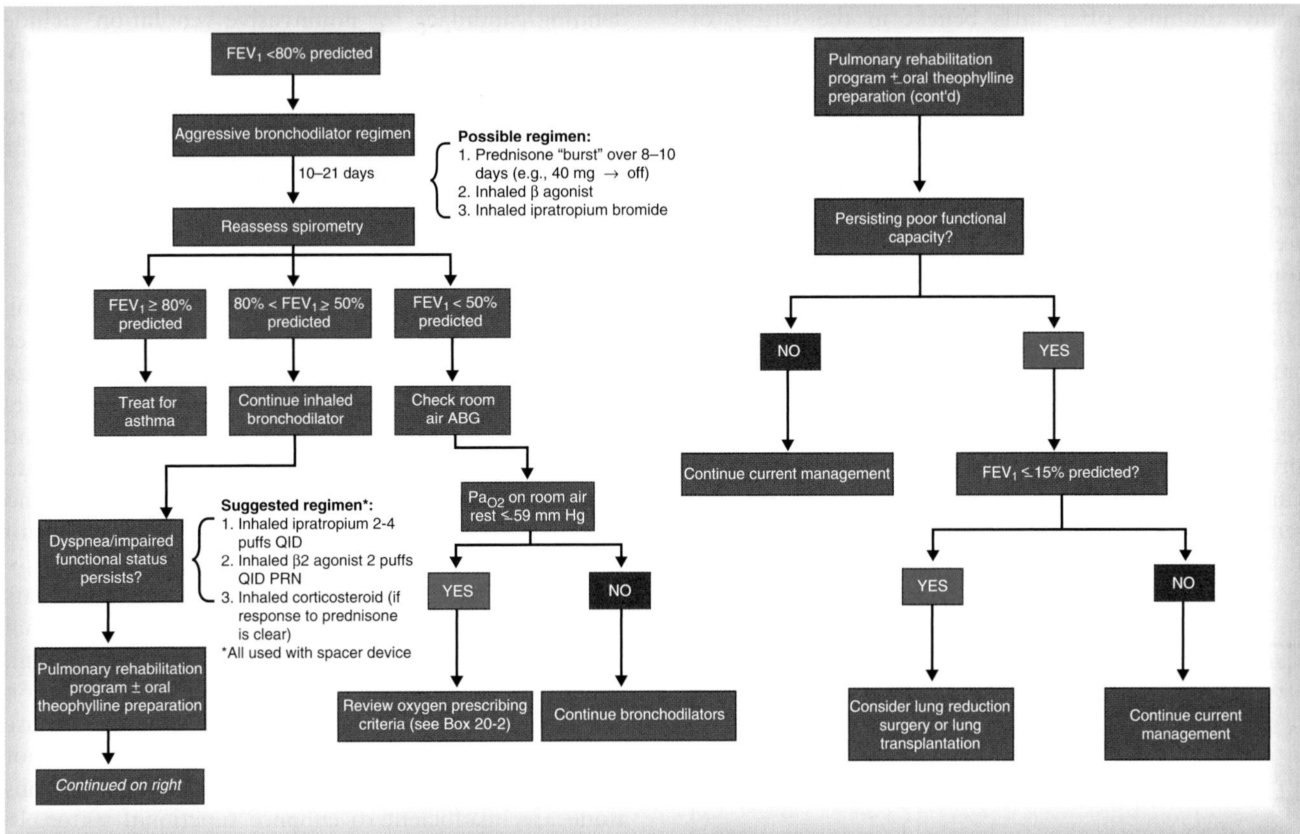

Figure 20-5
COPD management algorithm. *ABG*, Arterial blood gas; *PRN*, as needed; *QID*, four times daily.

xanthines. Systemic corticosteroids can produce significant improvements in airflow in a minority (6% to 29%) of patients with stable COPD.[12] Both to assess whether airflow obstruction is completely reversible (i.e., the patient has asthma) and whether the patient with COPD is steroid responsive, a brief course of corticosteroids (i.e., 20 to 40 mg/day of prednisone or equivalent for 10 to 14 days) is often recommended as part of the initial assessment of the patient with stable COPD.[2,9,10] Patients with a significant clinical response are often managed with chronic inhaled corticosteroids or the least necessary dose of systemic corticosteroids, while recognizing that long-term systemic steroid therapy poses risk.[13] Recently, several randomized, placebo-controlled trials of inhaled corticosteroids in patients with COPD have shown no effect on the rate of FEV_1 decline.[14-17] However, one of those studies suggested that patients with COPD who received inhaled steroids experienced fewer COPD exacerbations than patients who did not receive them.[15]

Methylxanthine therapy offers little additional bronchodilation in patients on inhaled bronchodilators and generally is reserved for patients with debilitating symptoms from stable COPD despite optimal inhaled bronchodilator therapy. Controlled trials do show lessened dyspnea in methylxanthine recipients despite lack of measurable increases in airflow.[18] Side effects of methylxanthines include anxiety, tremulousness, nausea, cardiac arrhythmias, and seizures. To minimize the chance of toxicity, current recommendations suggest maintaining serum theophylline levels at 8 to 10 μg/mL.

Acute exacerbations of COPD. Strategies to improve lung function in acute exacerbations of COPD generally include inhaled bronchodilators (especially β_2-agonists) and systemic corticosteroids.[19] An early randomized, controlled trial of IV methylprednisolone for patients with acute exacerbations has shown accelerated improvement in FEV_1 within 72 hours.[20]

Recent randomized clinical trials support the use of systemic corticosteroids to enhance airflow and to lessen treatment failure in acute exacerbations of COPD, but show no benefits of prolonged therapy beyond 2 weeks.[21-23]

For patients with purulent phlegm as an underlying feature of their acute exacerbation, oral antibiotics (e.g., trimethoprim-sulfamethoxazole, amoxicillin, doxycycline) administered for 7 to 10 days have produced accelerated improvement of peak flow rates compared with the rates of placebo recipients.[24,25] Finally, IV methylxanthines offer little benefit in the setting of acute exacerbations of COPD and have fallen into disfavor in this setting.[19,26]

For patients presenting with hypercapnia and acute respiratory acidemia, the clinician must determine whether to institute ventilatory assistance. Although intubation and mechanical ventilation have historically been the preferred approach, more recent studies suggest that noninvasive positive pressure ventilation can be an appealing alternative for selected patients with acute exacerbations of COPD. Specifically, based on available randomized, controlled clinical trials showing that noninvasive positive pressure ventilation can shorten intensive care unit (ICU) stay and avert the need for intubation, the American Association for Respiratory Care (AARC) Consensus Conference on noninvasive ventilation has endorsed this approach.[27] Criteria defining candidacy for **noninvasive ventilation** include acute respiratory acidosis (without frank respiratory arrest); hemodynamic stability; ability to tolerate the interface needed for noninvasive ventilation; ability to protect the airway; and lack of craniofacial trauma or burns, copious secretions, or massive obesity.[19,27]

MINI CLINI

Recognizing and Managing an Acute Exacerbation of COPD

PROBLEM

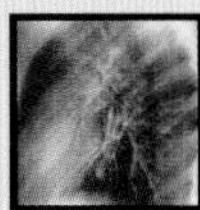

A 70-year-old patient with longstanding COPD is admitted to the hospital with an acute exacerbation. On physical examination, he is not dehydrated, and his chest examination shows diminished breath sounds bilaterally without wheezing. Pertinent laboratory values show a hematocrit of 54% (normal, 41% to 47%) and an arterial blood gas on room air as follows: PaO_2 47 mm Hg, PCO_2 67 mm Hg, pH 7.33, HCO_3^- 34 mEq/L. How could his current status be described, what do his current laboratory values suggest about his chronic gas exchange status, and what treatment should be considered?

DISCUSSION

The patient presents with an acute exacerbation of his COPD. His arterial blood gases indicate an acute rise in his PCO_2 superimposed on chronic hypercapnia, the latter suggested by the elevated serum bicarbonate (HCO_3^-) that represents renal compensation for chronic respiratory acidosis. Although his current hypoxemia may be a result of worsened gas exchange accompanying the current flare of his COPD, his elevated hematocrit in the absence of dehydration suggests chronic hypoxemia and compensatory erythrocytosis. The goal of therapy is to restore his gas exchange to baseline and to avoid invasive and/or high-risk interventions while optimizing survival. For these goals to be achieved, current treatment would consist of aggressive bronchodilators, IV corticosteroids, an antibiotic (if there is evidence of acute lung infection, either as a bronchitis or a pneumonia), and supplemental oxygen.[20] Ventilatory support should be considered in view of his acute chronic respiratory acidemia and, as shown in several recent randomized controlled trials, noninvasive positive pressure ventilation represents an effective alternative to intubation.

Maximizing Functional Status

In symptomatic patients with stable COPD, maximizing the ability to perform daily activities is a priority (see Figure 20-5). Pharmacological treatments to maximize functional status include administering bronchodilators to enhance lung function as much as possible and considering methylxanthine therapy, based on data indicating that such drugs can lessen dyspnea and improve functional status ratings even in the absence of improved airflow.[19]

Comprehensive pulmonary rehabilitation represents an additional important strategy to improve functional status. Recent randomized, controlled trials show that a pulmonary rehabilitation program including education and a progressive exercise program can enhance exercise capacity, although lung function and survival are not improved.[28,29] Although important, educational sessions alone are insufficient to enhance functional status. In addition, based on data showing that upper extremity training can enhance ventilatory function, exercise training in pulmonary rehabilitation should also include a program to strengthen the muscles of the shoulder girdle.[29]

Preventing Progression of COPD and Enhancing Survival

Cigarette smoking is widely recognized as the major risk factor for accelerating airflow obstruction in the 15% of smokers who are "susceptible." For these individuals, smoking cessation can slow the rate of decline of FEV_1 and restore the rate of lung decline to that seen in a normal, age-matched nonsmoker. Data from the Lung Health Study[5] confirm that with a comprehensive smoking cessation program (including instruction, group counseling, and nicotine replacement therapy), 22% of participants can achieve sustained smoking cessation and that the rate of annual FEV_1 decline in these sustained nonsmokers was significantly less than in continuing smokers. Critical success elements in achieving abstinence from smoking include identifying "teachable moments" (i.e., during episodes of illness where smoking can be identified as a contributing factor), identifying the role of smoking in adverse health outcomes in the subject, negotiating a "quit date," and providing frequent follow-up reminders from healthcare providers.[30] In this regard, the RT who frequently sees the patient has a special responsibility to provide

Box 20-2 • Indications for Long-Term Oxygen Therapy

I. Continuous oxygen
  A. Resting Pa_{O_2} of ≤55 mm Hg
  B. Resting Pa_{O_2} of 56–59 mm Hg or Sa_{O_2} of 89% in the presence of any of the following:
    1. Dependent edema, suggesting congestive heart failure
    2. P pulmonale on the electrocardiogram (P wave >3 mm in standard lead II, III, or aV_F)
    3. Erythrocythemia (hematocrit >56%)
      (a) Reimbursable only with additional documentation justifying the oxygen prescription and a summary of more conservative therapy that has failed

II. Noncontinuous oxygen
  A. Oxygen flow rate and number of hours per day must be specified
    1. During exercise: Pa_{O_2} of ≤55 mm Hg or Sa_{O_2} of ≤88% with a low level of exertion
    2. During sleep: Pa_{O_2} of ≤55 mm Hg or Sa_{O_2} of ≤88% with associated complications, such as pulmonary hypertension, daytime somnolence, or cardiac arrhythmias

From Tarpy SP, Celli BR: N Engl J Med 333:710, 1995.

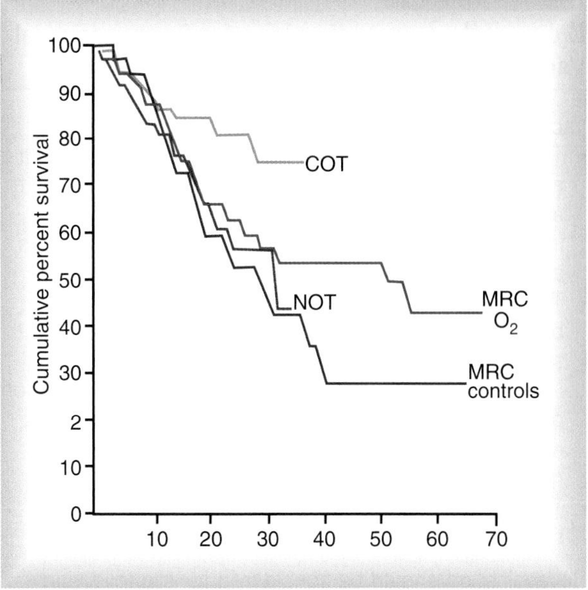

Figure 20-6

Cumulative percentage survival of patients in the Nocturnal Oxygen Therapy Trial (NOTT) and Medical Research Council (MRC) controlled trials of long-term domiciliary oxygen therapy for men older than 70 years of age. The MRC control subjects (-·-·-·-) received no oxygen. NOTT subjects (···) received oxygen for 12 hours in the 24-hour day, including the sleeping hours. MRC 0_2 subjects (—) received oxygen for 15 hours in the 24-hour day, including the sleep hours. Continuous oxygen therapy (COT) subjects (—) received oxygen for 24 hours in the 24-hour day (on average, 19 hours). *(Modified from Flenley DC: Chest 87:99, 1985.)*

frequent constructive reminders about the advisability of smoking cessation.

Among the available treatments for COPD, only **supplemental oxygen** has been shown to prolong survival. Box 20-2 reviews the indications for supplemental oxygen, and Figure 20-6 shows the results of the American Nocturnal Oxygen Therapy Trial[31] and the British Medical Research Council trial of domiciliary oxygen in 1980 to 1981.[32,33] As shown, survival was improved when eligible patients used supplemental oxygen for as close to 24 hours as possible and that survival improved less for those using oxygen only 15 hours per day. No survival advantage was observed when oxygen use was confined to sleeping hours. It is important to remember that patients should be assessed for supplemental oxygen use only after receiving optimal bronchodilator therapy, because up to one third of potential oxygen candidates can experience enough improvement with aggressive bronchodilation to obviate the need for supplemental oxygen.

Finally, preventive strategies such as an annual influenza vaccination and a pneumococcal vaccination, when indicated, are recommended for all patients with chronic debilitating conditions such as COPD.[34] Specific indications for pneumococcal vaccination are presented in Box 20-3.

Miscellaneous Therapies for Patients with COPD

Additional therapies for individuals with end-stage COPD include lung transplantation[35] and lung-volume reduction surgery (LVRS),[36-40] in which small portions of emphysematous lung are removed to reduce hyperinflation and to improve lung mechanics of the remaining tissue.

Lung transplantation is a consideration for patients with severe airflow obstruction (i.e., FEV_1 less than 20% predicted) who are less than 65 years old, who lack major dysfunction of other organs, and who are psychologically and motivationally suitable. Given the scarcity of available lungs to transplant, single lung transplantation is usually performed for individuals with COPD, and COPD represents the most common current indication for lung transplantation. Although lung transplantation may be associated with significantly improved quality of life and functional status, major risks include rejection (manifested as bronchiolitis obliterans and progressive, debilitating airflow obstruction), infection with unusual opportunistic organisms, and death from these and other complications. Five-year actuarial survival rates following single lung transplantation are approximately 40% (Figure 20-7).

Box 20-3 • Indications for Pneumococcal Vaccine Administration

Vaccination is recommended for the following adults:

- Those age 65 years and older, as well as adults of all ages with long-term illnesses that are associated with a high risk of contracting pneumococcal disease, including those with heart or lung diseases, diabetes, alcoholism, cirrhosis, or cerebrospinal fluid leaks
- Those with diseases or conditions that lower the body's resistance to infections or those who are taking drugs that lower the body's resistance to infections, including individuals with abnormal function of the spleen or removed spleen, Hodgkin's disease, lymphoma, multiple myeloma, kidney failure, nephrotic syndrome, or organ transplantation
- Those with HIV/AIDS infection, with or without symptoms

Revaccination should be considered for the following groups:

- Individuals at the highest risk of fatal pneumococcal infection, such as those with abnormal function or removal of the spleen, who received the original pneumococcal vaccination (between 1979 and 1983) or who received the current vaccine (1983 to present) 6 or more years ago.
- Individuals shown to lose protection rapidly (e.g., those with nephrotic syndrome, kidney failure, or transplants), who received the current vaccine 6 or more years ago.
- Children age 10 years or younger with nephrotic syndrome, abnormal function or removal of the spleen, or sickle cell anemia, who received the vaccine 3 to 5 years ago.

LVRS has been repopularized recently after initial experience was reported in 1957.[36] Initial studies suggested that LVRS can improve FEV_1, walking endurance, and oxygenation, although response to LVRS remains heterogeneous and current understanding of predictors of ideal response remains imperfect. Currently, the efficacy of LVRS is being evaluated in a National Institutes of Health multicenter study initiated in 1997, which is expected to clarify the role of LVRS. Available reports to date show that LVRS is contraindicated in individuals with severely impaired lung function (i.e., FEV_1 less than 20% predicted, homogeneous emphysema, and/or lung diffusing capacity for carbon monoxide less than 20% predicted),[39] but that LVRS recipients with moderate degrees of airflow obstruction may experience an improved FEV_1, walking distance, and quality of life.[40]

In addition, for patients with α_1-antitrypsin deficiency and established COPD, so-called IV augmentation with a purified preparation of α_1-antitrypsin from human blood donors is recommended.[41,42] Although no confirmatory randomized, controlled trial is available,[42,43] observational studies suggest that for individuals with severe α_1-antitrypsin deficiency and moderate degrees of airflow obstruction (e.g., FEV_1 35% to 49% predicted), weekly augmentation therapy may be associated with a slowed rate of decline of lung function and improved survival.[42,44] Difficulties with IV augmentation therapy include great expense (approximately $25,000 to $50,000 per year); the inconvenience of frequent IV infusions for life; and the infusion itself, which confers a theoretical risk of transmitting a bloodborne infection.

▶ ASTHMA

Definition

Asthma is a clinical syndrome characterized by **airway obstruction** (which is partially or completely reversible either spontaneously or with treatment), **airway inflammation,** and **airway hyperresponsiveness** to a variety of stimuli.[45-47] Although past definitions of asthma emphasized airway hyperresponsiveness and reversible obstruction, newer and more accurate definitions of asthma focus on asthma as a primary inflammatory disease of the airways with clinical manifestations of increased bronchial hyperreactivity and airflow obstruction secondary to this inflammation.

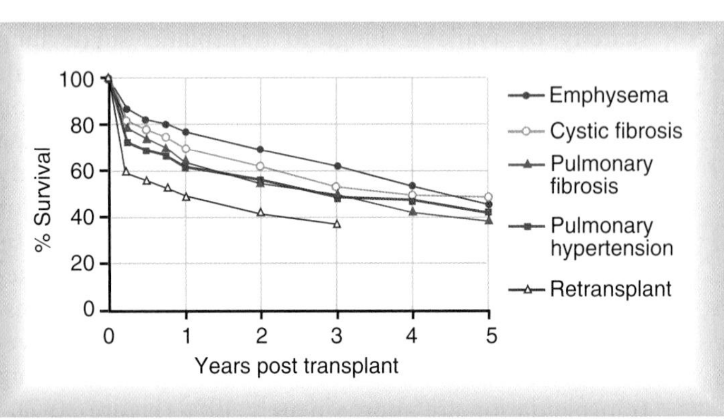

Figure 20-7
Actuarial survival curves according to pretransplant diagnosis. The overall survival rate of patients with emphysema (including α_1-antitrypsin deficiency) is significantly higher than that of patients with cystic fibrosis, pulmonary fibrosis, or primary pulmonary hypertension. *(Modified from Williams TJ, Snell GI: Clin Chest Med 18:245, 1997.)*

Epidemiology

Asthma affects more than 5% of the population in industrialized countries but is underdiagnosed and undertreated. In the United States from 1980 to 1987, the prevalence of asthma increased by 29%, and in 1988 alone, asthma-related healthcare expenditures exceeded $4 billion. Asthma mortality is also on the rise contrary to the trend for other common treatable conditions. From 1980 to 1987, death rates for asthma as the first listed diagnosis increased by 31% in the United States.[47,48]

Etiology and Pathogenesis

In the genetically susceptible host, allergens, respiratory infections, certain occupational and environmental exposures, and many unknown host or environmental stimuli can produce the full spectrum of asthma with persistent airway inflammation, bronchial hyperreactivity, and subsequent airflow obstruction. Once the inflammation and bronchial hyperreactivity are present, asthma can be triggered by additional factors including exercise; inhalation of cold, dry air; hyperventilation; cigarette smoke; physical or emotional stress; inhalation of irritants; and pharmacological agents such as methacholine and histamine.[45-48]

When a patient with asthma inhales an allergen to which he or she is sensitized, the antigen crosslinks to specific immunoglobulin E (IgE) molecules attached to the surface of mast cells in the bronchial mucosa and submucosa. The mast cells degranulate rapidly (within 30 minutes), releasing multiple mediators including leukotrienes (previously known as *slow-reacting substance of anaphylaxis [SRS-A]*), histamine, prostaglandins, platelet-activating factor, and other mediators. These mediators lead to smooth muscle contraction and vascular congestion and leakage, resulting in airflow obstruction that can be assessed clinically as a drop in the FEV_1 or peak expiratory flow rate (PEFR) (Figure 20-8). This is the early (acute) asthmatic response (EAR), which is an immediate hypersensitivity reaction that usually subsides in approximately 30 to 60 minutes. However, in approximately half of patients with asthma, airflow obstruction recurs in 3 to 8 hours. This late asthmatic response (LAR) is usually more severe and lasts longer than the EAR (Figure 20-9). The LAR is characterized by increasing influx and activation of inflammatory cells such as mast cells, eosinophils, and lymphocytes.[47,48]

Clinical Presentation and Diagnosis

The diagnosis of asthma requires clinical assessment supported by laboratory evaluation. Because no single measurement can establish the diagnosis with certainty and the physical examination can be entirely normal between episodes, the history plays a key role in suggesting and later establishing the diagnosis of asthma. Classic symptoms suggestive of asthma are episodic wheezing, shortness of breath, chest tightness, or cough. The absence of wheezing does not exclude asthma and sometimes cough can be the only manifestation (cough-variant asthma). Conversely, it is important to recognize

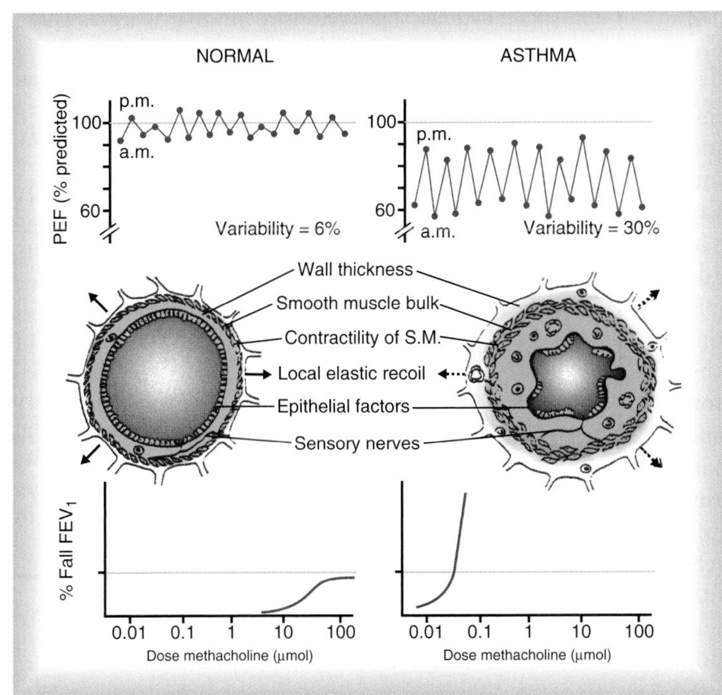

Figure 20-8 · Inflammation in Asthma
Cross sections of an airway from a healthy individual and a patient with asthma. Multiple cells and multiple mediators are involved in asthma. Inflammatory cells, such as mast cells, eosinophils, lymphocytes, and macrophages, release a variety of chemical mediators, such as histamine, prostaglandins, and leukotrienes. These mediators result in increased wall thickness, airway smooth muscle hypertrophy and constriction, epithelial sloughing, mucus hypersecretion, mucosal edema, and stimulation of nerve endings. The upper panel shows the daily variability in peak airflow measurements. The normal increase in smooth muscle tone in the early morning, which causes airway narrowing in healthy individuals, is more exaggerated in asthmatics. The lower panel shows the dose response curves to methacholine. *PEF*, Peak expiratory flow; *SM*, smooth muscle. *(Modified from Woolcock AJ: Asthma. In Murray JF, Nadel JA, editors: Textbook of respiratory medicine, Philadelphia, 1994, WB Saunders.)*

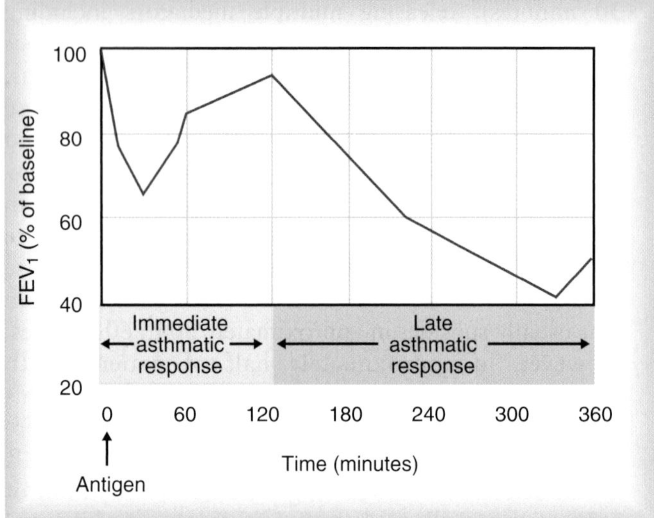

Figure 20-9

The early and late asthmatic responses. When a person with asthma is exposed to an allergen to which he or she is sensitized, the challenge results in a biphasic decline in respiratory function. An early asthmatic response (EAR) occurs within minutes and usually subsides within 2 hours. In approximately half of asthmatic patients, a late asthmatic response (LAR) occurs within 3 to 8 hours and may last for 24 hours or longer. *(Modified from Wiedemann HP, Kavuru MS: Diagnosis and management of asthma, Caddo, Okla., 1994, Professional Communications.)*

that not all wheezing is a result of asthma. Obstruction of the upper airway by tumors, laryngospasm, aspirated foreign objects, tracheal stenosis, or even functional laryngospasm (vocal cord dysfunction) can mimic the wheezing of asthma.[49]

Confirmation of the diagnosis of asthma requires demonstration of reversible airflow obstruction. Pulmonary function tests may be normal in asymptomatic patients with asthma, but more commonly reveal airway obstruction of some degree, manifested by decreased FEV_1 and FEV_1 to FVC ratio. By convention, improvement in the FEV_1 by at least 12% and 200 mL following administration of a bronchodilator is considered evidence of reversibility. Spontaneous variation in self-recorded PEFR by 15% or more can also provide evidence of reversibility of airway obstruction (see Figure 20-8).

Patients with asthma who are evaluated in a symptom-free period may have a normal chest examination and normal pulmonary function tests. Under these circumstances, provocative testing can be used to induce airway obstruction. The most commonly used bronchoprovocative stimulus is methacholine. Other stimuli include histamine, exercise, and inhaled hypotonic or hypertonic saline. The generally accepted criterion for hyperresponsiveness is the demonstration of a decrease in FEV_1 by 20% or more below the baseline value after inhalation of methacholine (see Figure 20-8). The methacholine provocation test has few false-negative results (less than 5%), but a false-positive result may be found in as many as 7% to 8% of the normal population and in patients with other obstructive lung diseases. Elevated IgE levels and eosinophilia may be present in patients with asthma, but their presence is not specific and their absence does not exclude asthma, rendering them not useful for the diagnosis.[45-47]

MINI CLINI

Diagnosis of Wheezing

PROBLEM

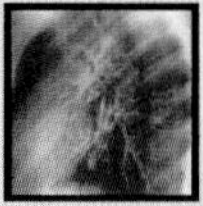

The RT is asked to see a patient with a history of wheezing. The patient notes that the wheezing has been continuous; present for several months; and absolutely unresponsive to bronchodilator medications, including systemic corticosteroids and various inhaled bronchodilators. How does the RT explain this and what management is suggested?

DISCUSSION

The patient has either refractory asthma or a condition mimicking asthma. The aphorism "all that wheezes is not asthma" applies very well here, and the clinician should suspect alternative diagnoses. Features that are somewhat atypical for asthma in this patient are the continuous nature of the wheezing and its complete refractoriness to medication. With this in mind, consideration of other "wheezy" disorders should include abnormalities of the upper airway. Specifically, tracheal stenosis or fixed upper airway obstruction (e.g., resulting from tracheal tumors) could well account for the patient's symptoms. Another asthma mimic is vocal cord dysfunction. Most characteristically, vocal cord dysfunction causes stridor with convergence of the vocal cords on inspiration (a paradoxic response). However, vocal cord dysfunction can also cause expiratory wheezing with closure of the vocal cords on expiration. Further assessment of this patient might include a flow-volume loop or a fiberoptic examination of the upper airway, observing both the vocal cords and the trachea to the level of the mainstem bronchi.

Management

The goals of asthma management are to maintain a high quality of life for the patient, uninterrupted by asthma symptoms, by side effects from medications, or by limitations on the job or during exercise. These goals can be accomplished by preventing acute exacerbations with potential mortality and morbidity or by returning the patient to a stable baseline when exacerbations occur. To achieve these goals effectively, asthma management relies on four integral components as recommended by the National Asthma Education Program (NAEP) expert panel.[45-47] These components are objective measurements and monitoring of lung function, pharmacological therapy, environmental control, and patient education.[38]

Table 20-2 outlines the step approach currently recommended for the long-term management of asthma. This approach provides a framework for an individually tailored dose of medication based on the severity of asthma present in any patient at a particular time. This approach acknowledges that asthma is a chronic and dynamic disease that needs optimal control. Control of asthma is defined as minimal to no chronic daytime or nocturnal symptoms, infrequent exacerbations, minimal to no need for β_2-agonists, no limitation to exercise activity, PEFR or FEV_1 greater than 80% predicted with less than 20% diurnal variation, and minimal to no adverse effects of medication.[45-47,50]

Objective Measurement and Monitoring

Objective measurement of lung function is particularly important in asthma, because subjective measures, such as patient reports, and physical examination findings often do not correlate with the variability and severity

Table 20-2 ▶▶▶ The Stepwise Approach to Long-Term Management of Asthma Based on Severity

Severity*	Clinical Features Before Treatment†	PEFR or FEV_1	Long-term Preventive Medications	Quick-relief Medications
Step 4 Severe persistent *Red zone*	Continuous symptoms Frequent exacerbations Nocturnal symptoms Symptoms limit activity	≤60% predicted >30% variability	Inhaled corticosteroids 800–2000 μg/day or more Long-acting bronchodilator‡ Oral corticosteroids	Inhaled β_2-agonist as needed for symptoms
Step 3 Moderate persistent *Yellow zone*	Daily symptoms Exacerbations affect activity and sleep Nocturnal symptoms more than once per week Daily use of short-acting β_2-agonist	>60%-<80% predicted >30% variability	Inhaled corticosteroids 800–2000 μg/day or more Long-acting bronchodilator,‡ especially for nocturnal symptoms	Inhaled β_2-agonist as needed for symptoms, not to exceed three to four times per day
Step 2 Mild persistent *Yellow zone*	Symptoms at least once per week but less than one time per day Exacerbations may affect activity or sleep Nocturnal symptoms more than twice per month	≥80% predicted 20%-30% variability	Either inhaled corticosteroid, 200–500 mg/day, cromolyn, or nedocromil Long-acting bronchodilator‡ for nocturnal symptoms	Inhaled β_2-agonist as needed for symptoms, not to exceed three to four times per day
Step 1 Intermittent *Green zone*	Intermittent symptoms less than once per week Nocturnal symptoms not more than twice per month Asymptomatic with normal lung function between exacerbations	≥80% predicted <20% variability	None needed	Inhaled β_2-agonist needed for symptoms, but less than once per week Inhaled β_2-agonist or cromolyn before exercise or exposure to allergen

Modified from Global Initiative for Asthma: Asthma management and prevention: a practical guide for public health officials and health care professionals, Bethesda, Md, 1995, National Institutes of Health, National Heart, Lung, and Blood Institute, and World Health Organization, NIH publication no. 96-3659A.

FEV_1, Forced expiratory volume in 1 second; PEFR, peak expiratory flow rate.

*Step-down: Review treatment every 3 to 6 months. If control is sustained for at least 3 months, consider a gradual stepwise reduction in treatment. Step-up: If control is not achieved, consider step-up, but first review patient medication technique, compliance, and environmental control.

†The presence of one of the features of severity is sufficient to place a patient in that category.

‡Long-acting β_2-agonist or sustained-release theophylline

of airflow obstruction. It is recommended that spirometry be performed as part of the initial assessment of all patients being evaluated for asthma and periodically thereafter as needed. Either spirometry or PEFR measurement can be used to assess response to therapy in the outpatient setting, emergency department, or hospital. It is also recommended that home PEFR measurement be used in patients with moderate to severe asthma. Once patients learn how to take PEFR measurements at home, the clinician's ability to provide effective treatment is improved. Daily monitoring of PEFR helps in detecting early stages of airway obstruction. All PEFR measurements are compared with the patient's personal best value, which can be established during a 2- to 3-week asymptomatic period when the patient is optimally treated.[45-47,51,52] To help patients understand home PEFR monitoring, a zonal system adapted to the traffic light system may be helpful (see Table 20-2). A PEFR measurement of 80% to 100% of personal best is considered to fall in the green zone. No asthma symptoms are present and maintenance medications can be continued or tapered. A PEFR in the 60%-to-80% range of personal best is in the yellow zone, may indicate an acute exacerbation, and requires a temporary step up in treatment. A PEFR lower than 60% is in the red zone and signals a medical alert and requires immediate medical attention if it does not return to the yellow or green zone with bronchodilator treatment.[45-47]

Pharmacotherapy

Pharmacotherapy for asthma reflects the basic understanding that asthma is a chronic inflammatory airway disease that requires long-term antiinflammatory therapy for adequate control.[51-54] Antiinflammatory agents such as corticosteroids and cromolyn suppress the primary disease process and its resultant airway hyperreactivity. Bronchodilators, such as β_2-adrenergic agonists, anticholinergics, and theophylline, relieve the symptoms of asthma. Because asthma is a disease of the airways, inhalation therapy is preferred over oral or other systemic therapy. Inhaled therapy using metered-dose inhalers (MDIs) or powders allows a high concentration of the medication to be delivered directly to the airways, resulting in fewer systemic side effects. Spacer devices can be used to improve delivery of inhaled medication, but training and coordination are still required of patients using MDIs. Table 20-3 lists some of the commonly used medications in the treatment of asthma.

Corticosteroids

Corticosteroids are clearly the most effective currently available medication for the treatment of asthma. Although their mode of action is still uncertain, corticosteroids probably act on various components of the inflammatory response in asthma.[52-54] Inhaled corticosteroids are very effective locally, and their regular use suppresses inflammation in the airways, decreases bronchial hyperreactivity and airflow obstruction, and reduces symptoms and mortality in asthma. Long-term, high-dose inhaled corticosteroids have far fewer side effects than do oral corticosteroids. Oropharyngeal candidiasis and dysphonia are controllable with spacer usage and with mouth washing after each treatment. Oral corticosteroids are very effective in asthma, but the potential for devastating side effects during chronic use restricts their use to patients not responding to other forms of asthma therapy. On the other hand, short-term, high-dose (0.5 to 1.0 mg/kg/day) oral corticosteroid therapy in exacerbations reduces the severity and duration of the exacerbation, decreases the need for emergency department visits and hospitalization, and reduces mortality.[53]

Cromolyn

Cromolyn sodium is a noncorticosteroid antiinflammatory medication. Its mechanism of action is not completely understood. It has a protective effect against provocative stimuli such as allergens, cold air, and exercise. The drug is most effective when administered prophylactically. Cromolyn does not dilate smooth muscle, and hence is not useful to treat the symptoms of an acute asthma attack. Cromolyn is useful in cough-variant asthma and exercise-induced asthma (EIA), but has otherwise gained only limited utility in the treatment of adults with asthma. However, many believe that cromolyn is the drug of choice for atopic children with asthma.[54]

Nedocromil

Nedocromil was approved for use in MDIs in the United States in 1993. It is structurally different from cromolyn but has similar pharmacological activity and is 4 to 10 times more potent in preventing acute allergic bronchospasm. It can be used as an alternative to cromolyn, but neither of these medications has a clear advantage over inhaled corticosteroids.

Leukotriene Inhibitors

Leukotrienes are mediators of inflammation and bronchoconstriction and are thought to play a role in the pathogenesis of asthma.[55,56] Leukotriene activity can be inhibited by synthesis inhibition, as can be achieved by zileuton (Zyflo) (Abbott Laboratories, North Chicago, Illinois), or by receptor blocking, as can be achieved by the leukotriene receptor antagonists zafirlukast (Accolate) (Astra Zeneca Pharmaceuticals, Wilmington, Delaware)

Table 20-3 ▶▶ Medications Commonly Used in the Treatment of Asthma and COPD

Medication	Trade Names	Available Preparations	Usual Dosage
Inhaled Corticosteroids			
Beclomethasone	Beclovent, Vanceril	MDI 42 μg/puff, 200 puffs/canister	2 puffs tid-qid, max 20 puffs/day
Triamcinolone	Azmacort	MDI 100 μg/puff, 240 puffs/canister	2-4 puffs qid, max 16 puffs/day
Flunisolide	Aerobid	MDI 250 mg/puff, 100 puffs/canister	2 puffs bid, max 8 puffs/day
Fluticasone	Flovent	MDI 44, 110, 220 μg/puff	88-880 μg/day
Systemic Corticosteroids			
Prednisone	Many	Tablets 1, 5, 20, 50 mg	5-50 mg/day
Methylprednisolone	Medrol	Tablets 2, 4, 8, 16, 24, 32 mg	4-48 mg/day
	Solu-Medrol	IV 40, 125, 500, 1000 mg	1-2 mg/kg q4-6h
Hydrocortisone	Solu-Cortef	IV 100, 250, 500, 1000 mg	4 mg/kg q4-6h
β_2-Agonists			
Albuterol	Proventil	MDI 90 μg/puff, 200 puffs/canister	2–4 puffs q4-6h, max 20 puffs/day
	Ventolin	Solution for nebulizer 0.083% and 0.5%	2.5-10 mg q6-8h
		Tablets 2, 4 mg	2-4 mg q6-8h
	Volmax	Sustained-release tablets 4, 8 mg	4-8 mg q12h
Metaproterenol	Alupent	MDI 650 μg/puff, 200 puffs/canister	2-3 puffs q3-4h, max 12 puffs/day
	Metaprel	Solution 0.5%	2.5-10 mg q4-6h
		Tablets 10, 20 mg	10 mg q6-8h
Pirbuterol	Maxair 300 puffs/canister	MDI 200 μg/puff,	1-2 puffs q4-6h, max 12 puffs/day
Terbutaline	Breathaire	MDI 200 μg/puff, 300 puffs/canister 1-2 puffs q4-6h	
	Bricanyl	Tablets 2.5, 5 mg	2.5-5 mg tid, max 15 mg/day
		Solution 1 mg/mL	0.25 mg SC q15-30min
Salmeterol	Serevent	MDI 50 μg/puff	2 puffs q12h
Anticholinergics			
Ipratropinum bromide	Atrovent	MDI 18 μg/puff, 200 puffs/canister Solution for nebulizer 0.02% 0.5 mg/2.5 mL vial 0.5 mg qid	2-4 puffs q6h
Methylxanthines			
Aminophylline	Amoline	IV Tablets or capsules	Load 5-6 mg/kg, maintenance 0.5-0.9 mg/kg/hr
Theophylline	Theodur Slo-Bid Theovent Uniphyl (Immediate or sustained release)		300-1200 mg/day divided q6-8h for immediate and q12-24h for sustained
Leukotriene Inhibitors			
Zafirlukast	Accolate	Tablets 20 mg	20 mg bid
Zileuton	Zyflo	Tablets 600 mg	600 mg qid
Montelukast	Singulair	Tablets 10 mg	10 mg qd
Other			
Cromolyn	Intal	MDI 800 μg/puff, 112 puffs/canister	2 puffs qid
		Spinhaler 20 mg/capsule	20 mg qid
Nedocromil	Tilade	MDI 1.75 mg/puff, 112 puffs/canister	2 puffs bid-qid

IV, Intravenous; *MDI*, metered-dose inhaler; *SC*, subcutaneous.

and montelukast sodium (Singulair) (Merck & Co., Inc., Whitehouse Station, New Jersey). Leukotriene inhibitors are modestly effective for maintenance treatment of mild to moderate asthma. They may allow the dose of corticosteroids to be reduced in moderate to severe asthma. They are particularly useful for patients with aspirin-sensitive asthma, who tend to produce large amounts of leukotrienes, although the exact role of leukotriene inhibitors in asthma therapy is yet to be fully determined.[55,56] Inhaled steroids remain the antiinflammatory drugs of choice for the treatment of asthma.

β_2-Adrenergic Agonists

Inhaled β_2 agents are the most rapid and effective bronchodilators for the treatment of asthma. They are the drugs of choice for all types of acute bronchospasm, and, when given prophylactically, they protect from all bronchoconstrictor challenges, but they do not prevent the LAR. β_2-Agonists are the drugs of choice for EIA. They exert their action by attaching to β_2-receptors on the cell to produce smooth muscle relaxation and by blocking mediator release from mast cells.

The effectiveness of β-agonists as bronchodilators is not disputed, and they remain the drugs of choice for acute emergency management of asthma. However, there is a concern that they may worsen asthma control if used regularly and that excessive use may increase the risk of death from asthma, which makes their role in long-term maintenance therapy less clear. Although there is sufficient concern regarding fenoterol to justify avoiding its use, it remains unclear whether the association between excessive β-agonist use and death from asthma is a causal or spurious association.[48,51] However, it is clear that excessive β-agonist use by people with asthma indicates an increased risk of death from asthma and indicates the need for more effective antiinflammatory therapy. There is currently little evidence to suggest that treatment with conventional doses of β_2-agonists available in the United States is harmful to patients with asthma.[48,51] The NAEP guidelines recommend that inhaled β_2-agonists be used as needed. If a patient needs more than 3 or 4 puffs/day of a β-agonist, additional antiinflammatory therapy should be considered.[45]

Newer, longer-acting (12 to 24 hours) β_2-agonists are now available. Salmeterol is a long-acting β_2-agonist that is available in the United States. Salmeterol's mechanism of action is clearly different from the shorter-acting β_2-agonists discussed previously. The utility of salmeterol in nocturnal asthma is obvious, but understanding of its utility in the chronic management of asthma is currently evolving.[45-47,54]

Methylxanthines

The role of theophylline and similar drugs in the treatment of acute asthma remains controversial. Sustained-release theophyllines added to chronic asthma management may be helpful in controlling nocturnal asthma symptoms (because they maintain therapeutic plasma concentrations overnight) and in soothing the symptoms of the labile asthmatic. However, the utility of theophylline is limited by its side effects of nausea, vomiting, headache, insomnia, seizures, and cardiac arrhythmias. Toxicity increases with blood levels above 15 μg/mL, but levels of 8 to 10 mg/mL are adequate for chronic therapy and are associated with fewer side effects. Several factors affect the plasma levels of theophylline by increasing or decreasing hepatic metabolism of the drug. Conditions that tend to increase plasma concentrations include acute viral infections, cardiac failure, hepatic disease, and the concomitant use of certain medications such as erythromycin or cimetidine. In these cases, the maintenance dose should be halved and the theophylline blood levels should be monitored. Conditions that tend to decrease plasma levels of theophylline include cigarette smoking and the administration of medications that increase hepatic clearance, such as phenobarbital.[54]

Anticholinergics

Inhaled anticholinergic agents, such as ipratropium bromide, are effective dilators of airway smooth muscles. Although the regular use of these agents appears to be effective in patients with COPD, their benefit in the day-to-day management of asthma has not been established. Ipratropium produces bronchodilation by reducing intrinsic vagal tone and by blocking vagal reflex bronchospasm, but this drug does not stabilize mast cells or prevent mediator release and is a less potent bronchodilator than are β_2-agonists. Ipratropium has few side effects, is safe because it is poorly absorbed, has an additive bronchodilator effect to the β_2-agonists, and is useful in cough-variant asthma.[37-39]

Newer Therapies

Omalizumab. Omalizumab (Xolair) (Genentech, Inc., South San Francisco, California and Novartis Pharmaceuticals Corporation, East Hanover, New Jersey) is a recombinant humanized antibody that binds IgE with high affinity.[57-59] It has recently been developed for the treatment of allergic diseases and is currently under review by the U.S. Food and Drug Administration for the treatment of allergic asthma. IgE plays a central role in the pathogenesis of allergic diseases (including asthma) and IgE-mediated immunological pathways have long represented an attractive target for therapeutic agents in asthma. An important property of this newly developed antibody is that it binds to the circulating IgE without activating mast cells or basophils. The antibody is specific to IgE and does not bind to IgG or IgA. Omalizumab is not yet licensed for clinical use in the United States, but pilot studies suggest that it is effective when administered by subcutaneous injection every 2 to 4 weeks in a dose that is determined by the levels of serum IgE. Results of initial studies suggest that omalizumab may have a role as an additional treatment in patients with steroid-dependent asthma.[57-59]

Levalbuterol. Levalbuterol (Xopenex) (Sepracor, Inc., Marlborough, Massachusetts) is the therapeutically active (R)-isomer of the standard albuterol, which is a racemic mixture of equal amounts of the R and S isomers.[60] Levalbuterol is currently available for clinical use only as a solution for nebulization. A small dose of 0.63 mg provides bronchodilation similar to 2.5 mg of the standard (mixed) albuterol. Although the newer preparation is reported to have fewer side effects, the exact role of levalbuterol in asthma therapy remains to be determined.[54,60]

Emergency Department and Hospital Management

Emergency management of acute asthma should include early and frequent administration of aerosolized β_2-agonists and therapy with systemic corticosteroids. Frequent assessment for response with PEFR should be performed. Which subset of patients may benefit from continuous aerosolized β_2-agonists is not clear.

Hospital and ICU care for patients with asthma should be very aggressive. The aim is to decrease mortality and morbidity and to return the patient to preadmission stability and function as quickly as possible. Management includes oxygen supplementation, frequent administration of high doses of aerosolized β_2-agonists (limited only by tachycardia or tremor), high-dose parenteral corticosteroids (more than 0.5 to 1.0 mg/kg/day), and antibiotics if there is evidence of infection. Sedatives and hypnotics should be avoided. Symptoms, PEFR, and arterial blood gases should be monitored.

Patients who need ventilatory support present special challenges. Mortality rates in these patients can be as high as 22% and complications are common, especially barotrauma. These complications can be minimized by limiting peak inspiratory pressure to less than 50 cm H_2O and by using small tidal volumes, allowing "permissive hypercapnia" if necessary.

RULE OF THUMB

In a patient presenting with an acute asthma attack, the Pa_{CO_2} is usually low because of hyperventilation. A normal Pa_{CO_2} in this situation indicates a severe attack and impending respiratory failure.

When asthma control is achieved, hospital discharge criteria include being free from supplemental oxygen with a Pa_{O_2} of more than 60 mm Hg, stable PEFR or FEV_1 with values close to the patient's best or greater than 70% of predicted, asthma symptoms that have returned to preadmission levels, freedom from nocturnal symptoms, and 12 to 24 hours of stability on discharge medications.[45-47]

MINI CLINI

Assessing the Severity of an Acute Asthma Attack

PROBLEM

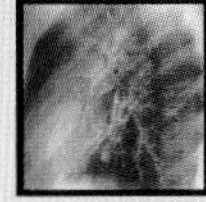

The RT has just obtained an arterial blood gas (ABG) analysis on a patient who presented to the emergency department with an acute attack of asthma. How does the ABG analysis help the RT assess the severity of the attack?

DISCUSSION

In the early stages of an asthma attack, the ABG analysis shows a low Pa_{CO_2} caused by hyperventilation. As the asthma attack progresses and FEV_1 drops below 25% of predicted, the Pa_{CO_2} returns to normal. When FEV1 drops to below 15% of predicted, CO_2 retention begins to occur. Changes in the pH reflect changes in Pa_{CO_2}. The accompanying table summarizes the ABG abnormalities based on the severity of an asthma attack.

Asthma Severity	Stage	Pa_{O_2}	Pa_{CO_2}	pH
Mild	I	Normal	Decreased	Increased
Moderate	II	Decreased	Decreased	Increased
Severe	III	Decreased	Normal	Normal
Very severe (respiratory failure)	IV	Decreased	Increased	Decreased

Immunotherapy

Although immunotherapy is accepted in the treatment of allergic rhinitis, its use in asthma is not standardized and remains controversial. The role of immunotherapy in asthma is currently limited to patients with allergic asthma who are unable to achieve substantial relief of symptoms with avoidance measures and pharmacotherapy. It is hoped that future studies will define the role and efficacy of immunotherapy more clearly.[56]

Environmental Control

The association between asthma and allergy has long been recognized. Between 75% and 85% of patients with asthma are reported to have positive immediate skin test reaction to common inhalant allergens. For the clinician to diagnose whether a patient's asthma has an allergic component, a thorough history is essential to determine the relationship between exposure to an allergen and occurrence of symptoms. Skin tests are more helpful in excluding an allergen as a cause of asthma symptoms, because clinical sensitivity to an aeroallergen is rare in the absence of a positive skin test, whereas many positive skin tests do not have clinical relevance. To prevent allergic reactions in asthma patients, environmental control measures to reduce exposure to indoor and outdoor allergens and irritants are essential.

Patients should be advised to avoid outdoor antigens, primarily ragweed, grass, pollens, and molds. Exposure to outdoor allergens is best reduced by staying indoors with the windows closed in an air-conditioned environment, particularly during the midday and afternoon when pollen and some mold counts are highest. Patients who are allergic to indoor allergens, primarily house-dust components and indoor molds, should implement strategies for eliminating these allergens from the home environment. All warm-blooded pets, including small rodents and birds, should be removed from the house because they can produce dander, urine, and saliva that can cause allergic reactions. House-dust mites depend on atmospheric moisture and human dander for survival. Essential house-dust mite control measures include encasing mattresses and pillows in airtight covers, washing the bedding weekly in water that is 130° F, avoiding sleeping on upholstered furniture, and removing carpets that are laid on concrete. Additional helpful control measures include reducing the indoor humidity to less than 50%, removing carpets from the bedroom, and using chemical agents to kill mites. Indoor air cleaning devices, especially the high-efficiency, particulate-air (HEPA) filters, may be useful but cannot substitute for controlling the source of allergen. Conversely, humidifiers are potentially harmful because they can harbor and aerosolize mold spores, and the increased humidity they generate may encourage production of both mold and house-dust mites.[45-47]

Patient Education

Much of the day-to-day responsibility for managing asthma falls on the patient and the patient's family. Patient education is a powerful tool for helping the patient gain motivation, skill, and confidence to control his or her asthma. Patient education involves helping patients understand asthma and learn and practice the skills necessary to manage it. This includes providing information, developing a partnership with the patient, involving the patient in decision making, and demonstrating and observing asthma management practices such as the proper use of inhalers, nebulizers, and peak flow meters.[61]

Special Considerations in Asthma Management

Exercise-Induced Asthma

EIA is common in asthmatics, especially after outdoor activities in cold weather. Swimming is less likely to cause EIA. Although the etiology of EIA is not fully understood, heat loss from the airways appears to be one of the causes. Treatment consists of prophylactic inhalation of a β_2-agonist or cromolyn before exercise. Leukotriene inhibitors may also have a role in treatment of EIA.[55,56]

Occupational Asthma

An estimated 2% to 5% of all asthma may be caused by exposure to a specific sensitizing agent in the workplace. Occupational asthma is now the most common form of occupational lung disease in many industrialized countries. In an attempt to distinguish occupational from preexisting asthma, occupational asthma is defined as a disease characterized by a variable airflow limitation and/or airway hyperresponsiveness resulting from causes and conditions attributable to a particular working environment and not to stimuli encountered outside the workplace. Toluene diisocyanate is the most common and best studied cause of occupational asthma. Other selected causes of occupational asthma are listed in Table 20-4.

In general, the treatment of occupational asthma is identical to that of other types of asthma. However, early diagnosis is important and emphasis is placed on environmental control, particularly cessation of exposure. Complete cessation of exposure is usually necessary, because once sensitization has occurred, bronchoconstriction can be triggered by minimal subsequent exposure.[62]

Cough-Variant Asthma

Cough may be the sole complaint of patients with asthma. In such patients, the cough may be relieved by

Table 20-4 ▶▶▶ Selected Occupational Causes of Asthma

Occupation/Industry	Agent
Laboratory animal workers, veterinarians	Animals (dander, urine protein)
Food processing	Shellfish, egg proteins, pancreatic enzymes
Dairy farming	Storage mites
Poultry farming	Poultry mites, droppings, feathers
Detergent manufacturing	*Bacillus subtilis* enzymes
Baking	Flour
Sawmill workers, carpentry	Wood dust (western red cedar, oak, mahogany, zebrawood, redwood)
Nursing	Psyllium
Refining	Platinum salts
Plating	Nickel salts
Stainless steel welding	Chromium salts
Cosmetology	Persulfate
Refinery workers	Vanadium
Rubber processing	Formaldehyde, ethylenediamine
Plastics industry	Toluene diisocyanate, trimellitic anhydride

a bronchodilator or the avoidance of inhaled allergens. If bronchospasm is not present at the time of examination and spirometry is normal (which is often the case), the diagnosis can be confirmed by demonstrating reversible airway obstruction by provocative testing (e.g., a methacholine challenge test). Ipratropium bromide may be particularly helpful in the treatment of cough-variant asthma. Otherwise, the treatment of cough-variant asthma is the same as with other types of asthma.

Nocturnal Asthma

Nocturnal asthma is a characteristic problem in poorly controlled asthma and is reported by more than two thirds of suboptimally treated patients. This is probably caused by the known physiological decrease in the airway tone during sleep that has been attributed to variation in catecholamine and cortisol secretion. After ensuring adequate antiinflammatory therapy, medications for nocturnal asthma should be focused toward the night and especially the early morning hours when the airway tone is lowest. Sustained-release theophylline and long-acting β_2-agonists such as salmeterol are particularly helpful for controlling nocturnal asthma symptoms.[45-47]

Aspirin Sensitivity

At least 5% of adults with asthma will experience severe and even fatal exacerbation of asthma after taking aspirin or other nonsteroidal antiinflammatory drugs (NSAIDs). Many of these aspirin-sensitive patients have nasal polyps, although the relationship is not causal. The presumed mechanism of aspirin sensitivity is the inhibition of the cyclooxygenase pathway by aspirin and NSAIDs, with subsequent shunting of all arachidonic acid into the 5-lipoxygenase pathway, causing overproduction of bronchoconstrictor leukotrienes. It is prudent to avoid these medications in patients with asthma and instead use alternatives such as acetaminophen. Patients should also be informed that many over-the-counter medications contain aspirin and should be avoided.[61] As discussed previously in this chapter, leukotriene inhibitors are particularly useful in treating patients with aspirin-sensitive asthma, because they tend to produce large amounts of leukotrienes.[55]

Gastroesophageal Reflux

The relationship between asthma and gastroesophageal reflux (GER) remains controversial, although GER is nearly three times more prevalent in patients with asthma than in others. Presumably, acid reflux into the esophagus causes vagal stimulation, resulting in a reflex increase in bronchial tone in patients with asthma. Medical management includes antireflux measures, H_2 blockers, or proton-pump inhibitors.

Asthma in Pregnancy

During pregnancy, one third of patients have worse asthma, one third have better control of their asthma, and one third experience no change in their asthma. The potential threat of adverse effects from asthma medications is far outweighed by the danger of uncontrolled asthma to the fetus and mother. Poorly controlled asthma during pregnancy can cause increased perinatal mortality, increased prematurity, and low birth weight. Theophylline, β_2-agonists, inhaled or oral corticosteroids, or cromolyn can be used during pregnancy without significant threat of increasing fetal abnormalities.[63]

Sinusitis

Acute and chronic sinusitis has been related to exacerbations and poor control of asthma. A limited computed tomographic (CT) scan of the sinuses should be obtained in patients with uncontrolled asthma. If sinusitis is present, therapy with antibiotics for 2 to 3 weeks, nasal decongestants, and nasal corticosteroid inhalers may help improve asthma control.

Surgery

Patients with asthma are predisposed to respiratory complications following surgery, including respiratory arrest during induction, hypoxemia and possible hypercapnia, impaired effectiveness of cough, atelectasis, and respiratory infection. The likelihood of these complications depends on the severity of the patient's airway hyperresponsiveness, the degree of airflow obstruction, and the amount of excess airway secretions at the time of surgery. Optimizing the patient's lung function before surgery, including the administration of perioperative corticosteroids, is an important strategy to minimize perioperative complications.[45-47]

▶ BRONCHIECTASIS

Clinical Presentation

Bronchiectasis refers to the abnormal irreversible dilation of the bronchi resulting from destructive and inflammatory changes in the airway walls. Three major anatomical patterns are described. In cylindrical bronchiectasis, the airway wall is regularly and uniformly dilated. Varicose bronchiectasis refers to an irregular pattern, with alternating areas of constriction and dilation. Cystic bronchiectasis is characterized by progressive, distal enlargement of the airways resulting

Box 20-4 • Causes of Bronchiectasis

LOCAL BRONCHIECTASIS

- Foreign body
- Benign airway tumor (e.g., adenoma)
- Bronchial compression by surrounding lymph nodes (e.g., middle lobe syndrome)

DIFFUSE BRONCHIECTASIS

- Cystic fibrosis
- Ciliary dyskinesia disorders (e.g., Kartagener's syndrome, Young's syndrome)
- Hypogammaglobulinemia
- α_1-Antitrypsin deficiency
- Allergic bronchopulmonary aspergillosis
- Rheumatoid arthritis
- Serious lung infection (e.g., from whooping cough, measles, or influenza)

in saclike dilations.[64] Bronchiectasis is thought to result from damage to the bronchial wall by chronic inflammation. Predisposing conditions are listed in Box 20-4.

Evaluation

The hallmark of bronchiectasis is the chronic production of large quantities of purulent and often foul-smelling sputum. Dyspnea is variable and depends on the extent of involvement and the underlying disease. Hemoptysis occurs frequently and is usually mild, but severe hemoptysis can occur. Radiographic studies confirm the diagnosis by demonstrating airway dilation. A chest radiograph may show cystic spaces and tram tracks (thin parallel lines representing the airway walls). So-called fine-cut (or high-resolution) CT scanning has replaced bronchography as the definitive diagnostic test for bronchiectasis.[65] Because reversible airway changes consistent with bronchiectasis can follow pneumonia, CT should be deferred for 2 to 4 weeks after pneumonia resolves before a diagnosis of bronchiectasis can be made.

Management

Antibiotics and bronchopulmonary hygiene are the mainstays of managing patients with bronchiectasis. Antibiotics can be given as needed or following a regularly scheduled regimen. Sputum cultures may be helpful in guiding antibiotic choice. Inhaled aminoglycosides may be a useful option in patients with chronic colonization by *Pseudomonas aeruginosa*. Secretions can be cleared by chest physiotherapy with postural drainage, cough maneuvers, and humidification. Inhaled bronchodilators may be helpful in some patients, because accompanying airflow obstruction is common. In cases that are complicated by massive hemoptysis, embolization of the bleeding bronchial artery may be helpful. Surgical resection should be reserved for patients with localized disease who develop massive hemoptysis or who are severely symptomatic despite appropriate medical therapy.[66-68]

KEY POINTS

- COPD is common, affecting 16 million people. It is now the fourth leading cause of death in the United States, accounting for an estimated 105,000 (or approximately 4% of all) deaths annually.
- The two most common risk factors for COPD are cigarette smoking (which accounts for 80% to 90% of all COPD-related deaths) and α_1-antitrypsin deficiency.
- Common symptoms of COPD include cough, phlegm production, wheezing, and shortness of breath, typically on exertion.
- The goals of managing patients with chronic stable COPD are to establish the diagnosis; optimize lung function; maximize the patient's functional status; simplify the medical regimen; and, whenever possible, prolong survival.
- The goals of managing patients with acute exacerbations of COPD are to reestablish the patient to the baseline status as quickly and with as little morbidity and mortality as possible.
- Asthma is a clinical syndrome characterized by airway obstruction (which is partially or completely reversible, either spontaneously or with treatment), airway inflammation, and airway hyperresponsiveness to a variety of stimuli.
- Asthma affects more than 5% of the population in industrialized countries, and asthma mortality is increasing.
- Allergens, respiratory infections, certain occupational and environmental exposures, and many unknown host or environmental stimuli can produce the full spectrum of asthma.
- Classic symptoms of asthma are episodic wheezing, shortness of breath, chest tightness, and cough.
- The goals of stable asthma management are to maintain a high quality of life for the patient, uninterrupted by asthma symptoms,

KEY POINTS—cont'd

side effects from medications, or limitations on the job or during exercise. This can be accomplished by objective measurements, monitoring lung function, pharmacological therapy, environmental control, and patient education.

- The goal of emergency management of acute asthma is to decrease mortality and morbidity and to return the patient to preadmission stability and function as quickly as possible. This is accomplished by oxygen supplementation, frequent administration of high doses of aerosolized β_2-agonists, high-dose parenteral corticosteroids, and antibiotics if there is evidence of infection.
- The hallmark of bronchiectasis is the chronic production of large quantities of purulent sputum. Dyspnea is variable and depends on the extent of involvement and the underlying disease. Antibiotics and bronchopulmonary hygiene are the mainstays of management.

References

1. American Thoracic Society: Standards for the diagnosis and care of patients with chronic obstructive pulmonary disease, Am J Respir Crit Care Med 152:S77, 1995.
2. Pauwels RA et al: Global strategy for the diagnosis, management, and prevention of chronic obstructive pulmonary disease: NHLBI/WHO Global Initiative for Chronic Obstructive Lung Disease (GOLD) Workshop summary, Am J Respir Crit Care Med 163:1256, 2001.
3. Stoller JK: Clinical features of alpha 1-antitrypsin deficiency: Roger S. Mitchell Lecture, Chest 111:123S, 1997.
4. Alpha 1-antitrypsin deficiency: memorandum from a WHO meeting, Bull World Health Organ 75:397, 1997.
5. Anthonisen NR et al: Effects of smoking intervention and the use of an inhaled anticholinergic bronchodilator on the rate of decline of FEV_1: The Lung Health Study, JAMA 272:1497, 1994.
6. U.S. Department of Health and Human Services: The health consequences of smoking: chronic obstructive lung disease—a report of the Surgeon General, Rockville, Md, 1984, U.S. Department of Health and Human Services, Public Health Service, Office on Smoking and Health, DHHS publication no. (PHS) 84-50205.
7. Gadek JE et al: Antielastase of the human alveolar structures: implications for the protease-antiprotease therapy of emphysema, J Clin Invest 68:889, 1981.
8. Anthonisen NR, Wright EC: Response to inhaled bronchodilators in COPD, Chest 91:36S, 1987.
9. Siafakas NM et al: Optimal assessment and management of chronic obstructive pulmonary disease (COPD): the European Respiratory Society Task Force, Eur Respir J 8:1398, 1995.
10. BTS guidelines for the management of chronic obstructive pulmonary disease: the COPD Guidelines Group of the Standards of Care Committee of the BTS, Thorax 52(Suppl 5):S1, 1997.
11. Ferguson GT, Cherniack RM: Management of chronic obstructive pulmonary disease, N Engl J Med 328:1017, 1993.
12. Callahan D, Dittus R, Katz B: Oral corticosteroid therapy for patients with stable chronic obstructive pulmonary disease: a meta-analysis, Ann Intern Med 114:216, 1991.
13. McEvoy CE, Niewoehner DE: Adverse effects of corticosteroid therapy for COPD: a critical review, Chest 111:732, 1997.
14. Pauwels RA et al: Long-term treatment with inhaled budesonide in persons with mild chronic obstructive pulmonary disease who continue smoking: European Respiratory Society Study on Chronic Obstructive Pulmonary Disease, N Engl J Med 340:1948, 1999.
15. Burge PS et al: Randomised, double blind, placebo controlled study of fluticasone propionate in patients with moderate to severe chronic obstructive pulmonary disease: the ISOLDE trial, BMJ 320:1297, 2000.
16. Vestbo J et al: Long-term effect of inhaled budesonide in mild and moderate chronic obstructive pulmonary disease: a randomised controlled trial, Lancet 353:1819, 1999.
17. Effect of inhaled triamcinolone on the decline in pulmonary function in chronic obstructive pulmonary disease: the Lung Health Study Research Group, N Engl J Med 343:1902, 2000.
18. Mahler D et al: Sustained-release theophylline reduces dyspnea in nonreversible obstructive airway disease, Am Rev Respir Dis 131:22, 1985.
19. Stoller JK: Management of acute exacerbations in the patient with chronic obstructive pulmonary disease, N Engl J Med 346:988-994, 2002.
20. Albert R, Martin T, Lewis S: Controlled clinical trial of methylprednisolone in patients with chronic bronchitis and acute respiratory insufficiency, Ann Intern Med 92:753, 1980.
21. Niewoehner DE et al: Effect of systemic glucocorticoids on exacerbations of chronic obstructive pulmonary disease: Department of Veterans Affairs Cooperative Study Group, N Engl J Med 340:1941, 1999.
22. Davies L, Angus RM, Calverley PM: Oral corticosteroids in patients admitted to hospital with exacerbations of chronic obstructive pulmonary disease: a prospective randomised controlled trial, Lancet 354:456, 1999.
23. Thompson WH et al: Controlled trial of oral prednisone in outpatients with acute COPD exacerbation, Am J Respir Crit Care Med 154:407, 1996.
24. Saint S et al: Antibiotics in chronic obstructive pulmonary disease exacerbations: a meta-analysis, JAMA 273:957, 1995.
25. Anthonisen NR et al: Antibiotic therapy in exacerbations of chronic obstructive pulmonary disease, Ann Intern Med 106:196, 1987.
26. Rice KL et al: Aminophylline for acute exacerbations of chronic obstructive pulmonary disease: a controlled trial, Ann Intern Med 107:305, 1987.
27. Bach JR et al: Consensus statement: non-invasive positive pressure ventilation, Respir Care 42:365, 1997.

28. Ries AL et al: Effects of pulmonary rehabilitation on physiologic and psychosocial outcomes in patients with chronic obstructive pulmonary disease, Ann Intern Med 122:823, 1995.
29. Celli BR: Is pulmonary rehabilitation an effective treatment for chronic obstructive pulmonary disease? Am J Respir Crit Care Med 155:781, 1997.
30. Kottke TE et al: Attributes of successful cessation interventions in medical practice: a meta-analysis of 39 controlled trials, JAMA 259:2882, 1988.
31. Continuous or nocturnal oxygen therapy in hypoxemic chronic obstructive lung disease: a clinical trial—Nocturnal Oxygen Therapy Trial Group, Ann Intern Med 93:391, 1980.
32. Long-term domiciliary oxygen therapy in chronic hypoxic cor pulmonale complicating chronic bronchitis and emphysema: Report of the Medical Research Council Working Party, Lancet 1:681, 1981.
33. Flenley DC: Long-term oxygen therapy, Chest 87:99, 1985.
34. Gardner P, Schaffner W: Immunization of adults, N Engl J Med 328:1252, 1993.
35. Williams TJ, Snell GI: Early and long-term functional outcomes in unilateral, bilateral, and living-related transplant recipients, Clin Chest Med 18:245, 1997.
36. Brantigan OC, Mueller E: Surgical treatment of pulmonary emphysema, Am Surg 23:789, 1957.
37. Sciurba FC: Early and long-term functional outcomes following lung volume reduction surgery, Clin Chest Med 18:259, 1997.
38. Gelb AF, McKenna RJ Jr, Brenner M: Expanding knowledge of lung volume reduction, Chest 119:1300, 2001.
39. Patients at high risk of death after lung-volume-reduction surgery: National Emphysema Treatment Trial Research Group, N Engl J Med 345:1075, 2001.
40. Geddes D et al: Effect of lung-volume-reduction surgery in patients with severe emphysema, N Engl J Med 343:239, 2000.
41. Abboud RT, Ford GT, Chapman KR: Alpha 1-antitrypsin deficiency: a position statement of the Canadian Thoracic Society, Can Respir J 8:81, 2001.
42. Survival and FEV1 decline in individuals with severe deficiency of alpha 1-antitrypsin: the Alpha-1-Antitrypsin Deficiency Registry Study Group, Am J Respir Crit Care Med 158:49, 1998.
43. Dirksen A et al: A randomized clinical trial of alpha 1-antitrypsin augmentation therapy, Am J Respir Crit Care Med 160:1468, 1999.
44. Wencker M et al: Longitudinal follow-up of patients with alpha(1)-protease inhibitor deficiency before and during therapy with IV alpha(1)-protease inhibitor, Chest 119:737, 2001.
45. National Asthma Education and Prevention Program: Expert Panel Report 2: guidelines for the diagnosis and management of asthma, Bethesda, Md, 1997, National Heart, Lung, and Blood Institute, National Institutes of Health, NIH publication no. 97-4051.
46. U.S. Department of Health and Human Services: International Consensus report on diagnosis and treatment of asthma, Bethesda, Md, 1992, National Heart, Lung, and Blood Institute, NIH publication no. 92-3091.
47. Global Initiative for Asthma: Asthma management and prevention: a practical guide for public health officials and health care professionals, Bethesda, Md, 1995, National Institutes of Health, National Heart, Lung, and Blood Institute, and World Health Organization, NIH publication no. 96-3659A.
48. McFadden ER Jr, Gilbert IA: Asthma, N Engl J Med 327:1928, 1992.
49. Aboussouan LS, Stoller JK: Diagnosis and management of upper airway obstruction, Clin Chest Med 15:35, 1994.
50. Barnes PJ: A new approach to the treatment of asthma, N Engl J Med 321:1517, 1989.
51. Martin RJ, editor: Asthma, Clin Chest Med 16:557, 1995.
52. Barnes PJ: Inhaled corticosteroids for asthma, N Engl J Med 332:868, 1995.
53. Dweik RA, Ahmad M: Diagnosis and treatment of asthma, Resident and Staff Physician 44:36, 1998.
54. Drugs for asthma, The Medical Letter on Drugs and Therapeutics 42:19, 2000.
55. Drazen JM, Israel E, O'Byrne PM: Treatment of asthma with drugs modifying the leukotriene pathway, N Engl J Med 340:197, 1999.
56. Kavuru MS et al: Asthma: current controversies and emerging therapies, Cleve Clin J Med 62:293, 1995.
57. Barnes PJ: Anti-IgE antibody therapy for asthma, N Engl J Med 341:2006, 1999.
58. Milgrom H et al: Treatment of allergic asthma with monoclonal anti-IgE antibody: rhuMAb-E25 Study Group, N Engl J Med 341:1966, 1999.
59. Busse W et al: Omalizumab, anti-IgE recombinant humanized monoclonal antibody, for the treatment of severe allergic asthma, J Allergy Clin Immunol 108:184, 2001.
60. Levalbuterol for asthma, The Medical Letter on Drugs and Therapeutics 41:51, 1999.
61. Teach your patient about asthma: a clinician's guide, Bethesda, Md, 1992, United States Department of Health and Human Services, NIH publication no. 92-2737.
62. Chan-Yeung M, Malo JL: Occupational asthma, N Engl J Med 333:107, 1995.
63. National Asthma Education Program: Report of the Working Group on Asthma and Pregnancy: executive summary—management of asthma during pregnancy, Bethesda, Md, 1993, National Institutes of Health, National Heart, Lung, and Blood Institute, NIH publication no. 93-3279A.
64. Reid LM: Reduction in bronchial subdivision in bronchiectasis, Thorax 5:233, 1950.
65. Stanford W, Galvin JR: The diagnosis of bronchiectasis, Clin Chest Med 9:691, 1988.
66. Barker AF, Bardana EJ Jr: Bronchiectasis: update of an orphan disease, Am Rev Respir Dis 137:969, 1988.
67. Swigris J, Stoller JK: Review of bronchiectasis, Clin Pulm Med 7:223, 2000.
68. Luce JM: Bronchiectasis. In Murray JF, Nadel JA, editors: Textbook of respiratory medicine, Philadelphia, 1994, WB Saunders.

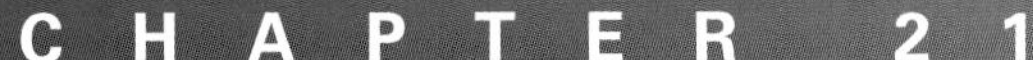

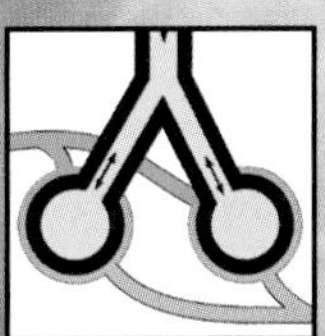

CHAPTER 21

Interstitial Lung Disease

Kevin K. Brown and Eugene J. Sullivan

In This Chapter You Will Learn:

- How to classify the wide variety of pulmonary disorders grouped under the term *interstitial lung disease* (ILD)
- How to interpret the common clinical signs and symptoms of ILD
- How to interpret common pulmonary function testing abnormalities in patients with ILD
- What specific characteristics are associated with some of the more common types of ILD
- How some specific ILDs can be managed

Chapter Outline

Key Terms

asbestosis
chronic hypersensitivity pneumonitis
connective tissue disease
corticosteroids
cytotoxic agents
drug-related lung disease
eosinophilic granuloma
idiopathic pulmonary fibrosis
interstitial lung disease
lymphangioleiomyomatosis
occupational ILD
pulmonary vasculitis
respiratory bronchiolitis
sarcoidosis
silicosis

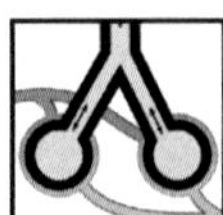

The term **interstitial lung disease** (ILD) refers to a broad category of lung diseases rather than to a specific disease entity.[1] These diseases are grouped together because of general similarities in their clinical presentations, plain chest radiographic appearance, and physiological features. However, the category includes a variety of illnesses with diverse causes, treatments, and prognoses.

▶ CLASSIFICATION OF ILD

Because of the diverse nature of these diseases, it is helpful to subclassify them according to certain characteristics. A simple classification scheme based on etiologic factor is presented in Box 21-1. The diseases are broken down into those associated with occupational exposures, drug exposures (Box 21-2), hypersensitivity (allergic) reactions (Table 21-1), underlying connective tissue (rheumatologic) diseases, and conditions that remain idiopathic or unclassified. It is evident from this classification scheme that a critical component for evaluating a patient with ILD is a careful and complete history with a review of any and all exposures in the home, in the workplace, and with avocations and travel that could result in pulmonary inflammation and scarring.

▶ PATHOPHYSIOLOGY

As the name implies, the histologic abnormalities that characterize ILD generally involve the pulmonary interstitium to a greater extent than they do the alveolar spaces or airways, although exceptions exist. Figure 21-1 illustrates the components of the normal pulmonary parenchyma. The interstitium is generally considered the area between the capillaries and the alveolar space. As Figure 21-1 shows, in the normal state this space contains connective tissue matrix, a few fibroblasts, and occasional inflammatory cells such as macrophages. As a general concept, many of the ILDs are caused by an injury to the lung that results in chronic inflammation with accumulation of inflammatory cells, frequently lymphocytes and occasionally macrophages, within the interstitial space. This injury could be from occupational exposure (e.g., asbestos), drug exposure (e.g., nitrofurantoin macrocrystals [Macrodantin]), an inhaled antigen to which a patient is allergic (e.g., farmer's lung), a connective tissue disease (e.g., rheumatoid arthritis), or an unknown cause (e.g., sarcoidosis). The resulting chronic inflammation, in some cases, can lead to scarring or fibrosis. In other cases, it appears the scarring or fibrosis of the interstitium is primary, without significant inflammation (e.g., idiopathic pulmonary fibrosis).

Box 21-1 • Interstitial Lung Diseases

Occupation related
- Asbestosis
- Silicosis
- Coal worker's pneumoconiosis
- Berylliosis
- Talc pneumoconiosis
- Hard metal fibrosis

Drug induced*

Hypersensitivity (allergic) reactions†

Connective tissue disease
- Rheumatoid arthritis
- Scleroderma
- Polymyositis/dermatomyositis
- Systemic lupus erythematosus
- Mixed connective tissue disease
- Sjögren's syndrome
- Behçet's syndrome
- Ankylosing spondylitis

Idiopathic and unclassified diseases
- Idiopathic pulmonary fibrosis (IPF)
- Nonspecific interstitial pneumonia (NSIP)
- Desquamative interstitial pneumonia (DIP)
- Respiratory bronchiolitis–interstitial lung disease (RB-ILD)
- Acute interstitial pneumonitis (AIP)
- Bronchiolitis obliterans organizing pneumonia (BOOP)
- Sarcoidosis
- Lymphocytic interstitial pneumonitis (LIP)
- Eosinophilic granuloma (EG)
- Lymphangioleiomyomatosis
- Tuberous sclerosis
- Acute and chronic eosinophilic pneumonia
- Pulmonary alveolar proteinosis (PAP)
- Pulmonary vasculitis and capillaritis
- Inflammatory bowel disease
- Hepatic cirrhosis
- Neurofibromatosis
- Amyloidosis
- Cryoglobulinemia

Modified from Schwarz MI: Clinical overview of interstitial lung disease. In Schwarz MI, King TE, editors: *Interstitial lung disease*, ed 2, St Louis, 1993, Mosby.
*See Box 21-2.
†See Table 21-1.

Therefore the term *interstitial lung disease* is a clinically relevant and useful designation, but it can be somewhat confusing because of the diverse nature of these diseases.

▶ CLINICAL SIGNS AND SYMPTOMS OF ILD

Many of the ILDs have similar clinical features. Symptoms are generally limited to the respiratory tract. Exertional breathlessness (dyspnea), often slowly pro-

Box 21-2 • Medications Associated With the Development of ILD

ANTIBIOTICS
Nitrofurantoin*
Sulfasalazine

ANTIINFLAMMATORY AGENTS
Aspirin
Gold
Penicillamine
Methotrexate

CARDIOVASCULAR AGENTS
Amiodarone
Tocainide

CHEMOTHERAPEUTIC AGENTS

ANTIBIOTICS
Bleomycin
Mitomycin-C

ALKYLATING AGENTS
Busulfan
Cyclophosphamide
Chlorambucil
Melphalan

ANTIMETABOLITES
Azathioprine
Cytosine arabinoside
Methotrexate

NITROSOUREAS
Carmustine
Lomustine
Methyl-CCNU

OTHER AGENTS
Procarbazine
Zinostatin
Etoposide
Vinblastine

DRUG-INDUCED SYSTEMIC LUPUS ERYTHEMATOSUS
Procainamide
Isoniazid
Hydralazine
Hydantoins
Penicillamine

ILLICIT DRUGS
Heroin
Methadone
Propoxyphene
Talc

MISCELLANEOUS AGENTS
Oxygen
Drugs inducing pulmonary infiltrate and eosinophilia
L-tryptophan
Hydrochlorothiazide

From Rosenow EC, Martin WJ: Drug-induced interstitial lung disease. In Schwarz MI, King TE, eds: *Interstitial lung disease*, ed 2, St Louis, 1993, Mosby.
*Associated with both acute and chronic ILD.

gressive, and a nonproductive cough are the most common reasons patients seek medical attention. However, sputum production, hemoptysis, or wheezing can occur and is helpful in classifying the disease. If the patient also has prominent nonrespiratory symptoms, such as pain, erythema, and swelling of the joints of the hands, ILD resulting from a systemic illness such as rheumatoid arthritis or other underlying **connective tissue disease** may be present.

Physical Examination

At examination, most patients with ILD have bilateral inspiratory, fine crackles, which usually are most prominent at the lung bases. Expiratory wheezing is relatively uncommon in uncomplicated ILD, and its presence would suggest concomitant airways disease. In rare instances, wheezing may be a clue to a particular diagnosis. For example, in diseases such as **sarcoidosis**, which may involve the airways as well as the interstitium, localized wheezing may indicate focal airway narrowing caused by inflammation or scarring.

Clubbing of the digits and signs of pulmonary hypertension with right ventricular dysfunction, such as lower-extremity edema or jugular venous distension, may occur late in the course of any of the ILDs.

Examination also may disclose features of underlying connective tissue disease, including active joint inflammation (synovitis), joint deformities, or skin rash.

Radiographic Features

For most ILDs, a plain chest radiograph reveals reduced lung volumes with bilateral reticular or reticulonodular opacities. However, there is variability among the specific diseases in the character and distribution of parenchymal abnormalities. The ready availability of high-resolution computed tomography (HRCT) has highlighted significant radiographic differences between diseases that have otherwise very similar plain chest radiographic patterns.

Table 21-1 ▶▶ Etiologies of Hypersensitivity Pneumonitis

Antigen	Exposure	Syndrome
Bacteria		
Thermophilic Bacteria		
Micropolyspora faeni	Moldy hay	Farmer's lung
Thermoactinomyces vulgaris	Moldy sugarcane	Bagassosis
T. sacchari	Mushroom compost	Mushroom worker's lung
T. candidus	Heated water reservoirs	Humidifier lung
		Air conditioner lung
Nonthermophilic Bacteria		
Bacillus subtilis, B. cereus	Water, detergent	Humidifier lung
		Washing powder lung
Fungi		
Aspergillus sp.	Moldy hay	Farmer's lung
	Water	Ventilation pneumonitis
A. clavatus	Barley	Malt worker's lung
Penicillium casei, P. roqueforti	Cheese	Cheese washer's lung
Alternaria sp.	Wood pulp	Wood pulp worker's lung
Cryptostroma corticale	Wood bark	Maple bark stripper's lung
Graphium, Aureobasidium pullulans	Wood dust	Sequoiosis
Merulius lacrymans	Rotten wood	Dry rot lung
Penicillium frequentans	Cork dust	Suberosis
A. pullulans	Water	Humidifier lung
Cladosporium sp.	Hot-tub mists	Hot tub HSP
Trichosporon cutaneum	Damp wood and mats	Japanese summer-type HSP
Amoebae		
Naegleria gruberi	Contaminated water	Humidifier lung
Acanthamoeba polyphaga	Contaminated water	Humidifier lung
A. castellani	Contaminated water	Humidifier lung
Animal Proteins		
Avian proteins	Bird droppings, feathers	Bird-breeder's lung
Urine, serum, pelts	Rats, gerbils	Animal handler's lung
Wheat weevil (*Sitophilus granarius*)	Infested flour	Wheat weevil lung
Chemicals		
Toluene diisocyanate	Paints, resins, isocyanate	HSP
Diphenylmethane diisocyanate		
Polyurethane foams		
Hexamethylene diisocyanate		
Trimellitic anhydride (TMA)	Plastics, resins, paints	TMA-HSP
Copper sulfate	Bordeaux mixture	Vineyard sprayer's lung
Sodium diazobenzene sulfate	Chromatography reagent	Pauli's reagent alveolitis
Pyrethrum	Pesticide, pyrethrum	HSP

From Rose CS, Newman LS: Hypersensitivity pneumonitis and chronic beryllium disease. In Schwarz MI, King TE, eds: *Interstitial lung disease*, ed 2, St Louis, 1993, Mosby.
HSP, Hypersensitivity pneumonitis.

HRCT has the ability to better define the specific characteristics of parenchymal abnormalities. The increased sensitivity of HRCT for these features significantly increases the chance of making a confident diagnosis of the underlying lung disease. HRCT is considered a standard technique in the evaluation of ILD.

The radiographic features of **idiopathic pulmonary fibrosis** (IPF) often are considered the classic ILD pattern, primarily because IPF is one of the most common ILDs and because several other ILDs have a similar appearance. As shown in Figure 21-2, the x-ray film and CT scan in IPF usually reveal bilateral reticulonodular infiltrates with a peripheral and basilar predominance. Disease involvement and volume loss tend to be greatest in the lung bases. Therefore the hilar structures appear closer than normal to the diaphragm. Pleural disease and significant lymphadenopathy are not seen. In later stages of the disease, the chest x-ray examination may reveal multiple, tiny cysts in the most markedly involved regions. This cystic pattern, called *honeycombing*, reflects end-stage fibrosis in these areas and is a feature of many end-stage ILDs.

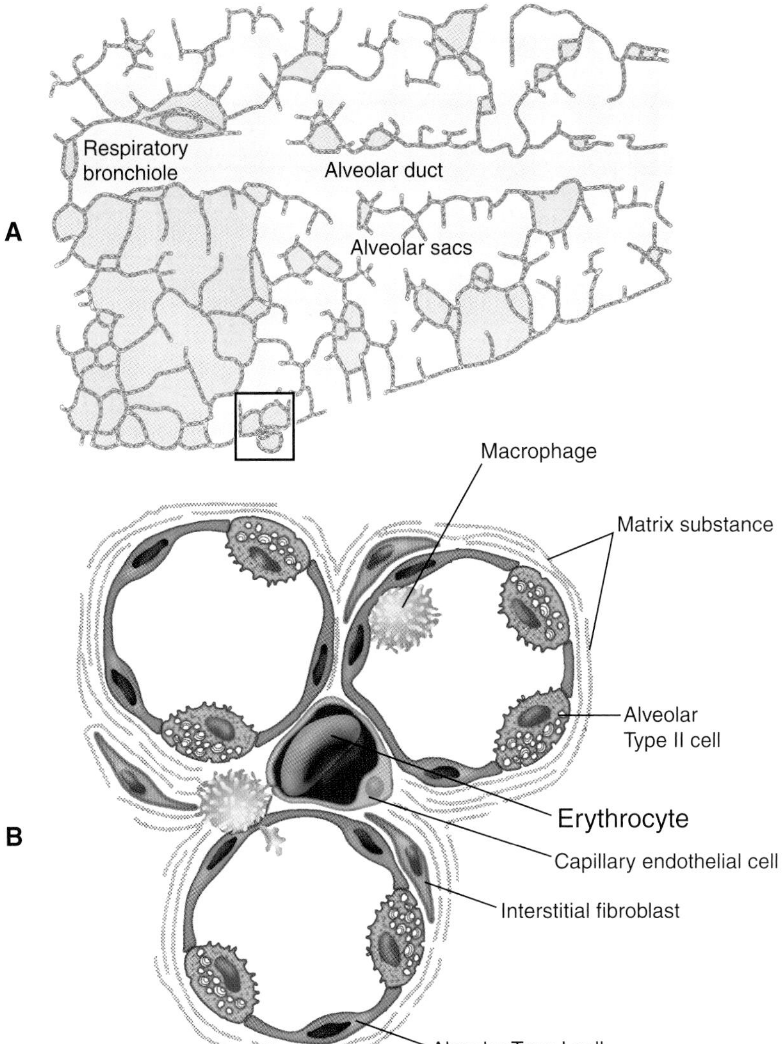

Figure 21-1

A, Diagram of the pulmonary parenchyma shows the respiratory bronchiole, alveolar duct, and alveolar sacs. **B**, The constituents of the interstitial space, including type I and type II alveolar epithelial cells, a capillary with vascular endothelial cells and erythrocytes in transit, resident macrophages, interstitial fibroblasts, and matrix substance.

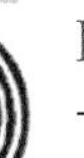

RULE OF THUMB

In the diagnosis of pneumothorax and interstitial infiltrates confirmed by chest x-ray examination, lymphangioleiomyomatosis (in women) and histiocytosis X (eosinophilic granuloma [EG]) should be considered.

RULE OF THUMB

The presence of calcification along the pleura on a chest x-ray film suggests previous exposure to asbestos. Although such plaques do not cause symptoms or physiological abnormality by themselves, they can provide a clue to the cause of ILD.

Physiological Features

The ILDs in general result in restrictive physiological impairment.[2] Thus both forced expiratory volume in 1 second (FEV_1) and forced vital capacity (FVC) are diminished, and the FEV_1/FVC ratio is preserved or often even supranormal. Lung volumes are reduced, as is the diffusing capacity of the lung for carbon monoxide (D_{LCO}). When corrected for alveolar volume, the D_{LCO} usually improves toward normal. This reduction in diffusing capacity reflects a pathological disturbance of the alveolus-capillary interface.

Although not commonly pursued, the compliance characteristics of the lungs can be evaluated with an esophageal balloon to measure intrathoracic pressure at various lung volumes. The pulmonary parenchymal inflammation and scarring characteristic of ILD cause the lungs to be stiff and poorly compliant. This lack of compliance results in small lung volumes, and abnormally high transthoracic pressures are necessary to achieve any particular lung volume (Figure 21-3).

As ILD becomes more severe, hypoxemia develops. In early stages, hypoxemia may be evident only with exertion, but as the disease progresses, patients begin to experience hypoxemia even at rest. It has been suggested

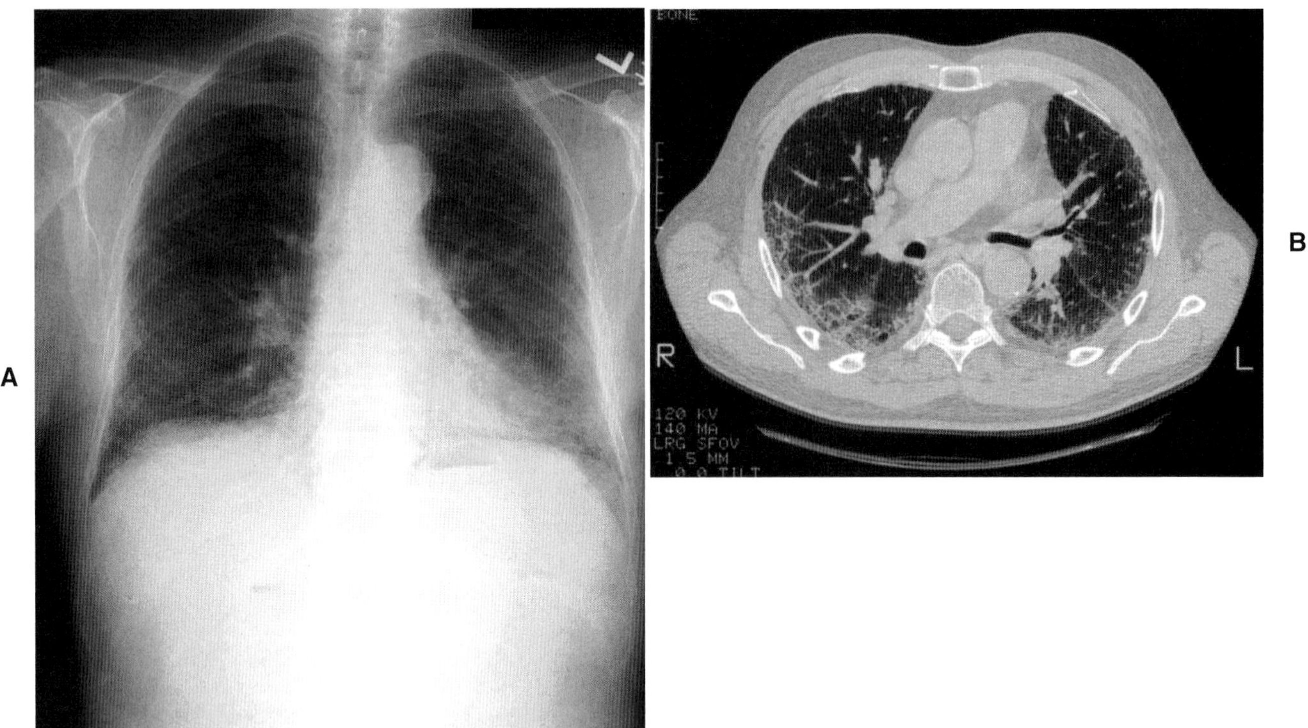

Figure 21-2

A, Posteroanterior chest radiograph shows the characteristic features of IPF, a common ILD. Notice the bilateral lower zone reticulonodular infiltrates and the loss of lung volume in the lower lobes. **B**, Chest CT scan shows the peripheral nature of the infiltrates.

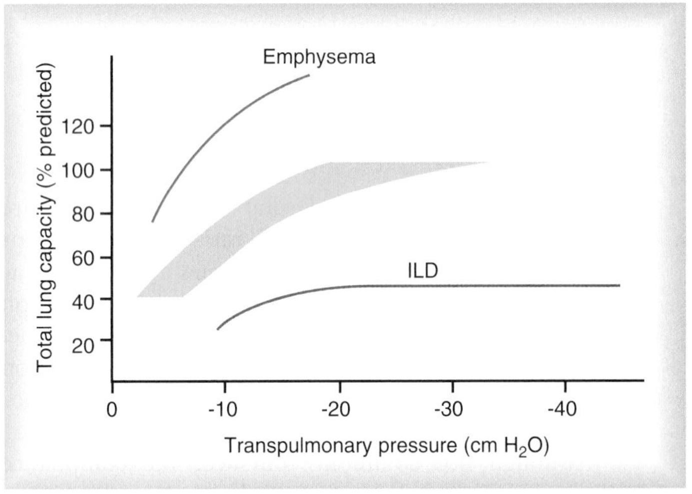

Figure 21-3

The static pressure-volume curve. The compliance characteristics of the lung are illustrated with a plot of lung volume against the corresponding transthoracic pressure measured during static (i.e., no flow) conditions. The shaded area represents the range of values expected with a normally compliant lung. The line labeled *ILD* represents an example of a patient with ILD. At any particular lung volume, the transthoracic pressure is greater than expected. For comparison, the line labeled *Emphysema* shows the compliance characteristics of patients with emphysema.

that the exercise limitation among patients with ILD is related more to pulmonary vascular compromise and impaired gas exchange through ventilation/perfusion mismatching than to the restrictive ventilatory impairment.[3]

The physiological characteristics of ILD may be altered by concomitant obstructive lung disease.[4,5] The loss of pulmonary parenchymal tissue that occurs in emphysema makes the lungs excessively compliant. Thus if ILD develops in a patient with significant emphysema, the opposing physiological effects of the two diseases may result in apparently normally compliant lungs. In this circumstance, spirometry and lung volume measurements may be deceptively normal. However, because both emphysema and ILD result in impaired gas exchange, the D_{LCO} is significantly decreased. In smokers with IPF, normal results at spirometry and lung volumes with a reduced D_{LCO} suggest coexisting emphysema.

MINI CLINI

ILD With Normal Lung Volumes

PROBLEM

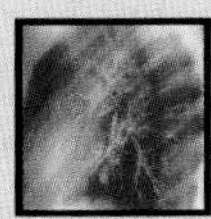

A 50-year-old woman has symptoms and physical examination findings suggestive of ILD. However, pulmonary physiologic testing reveals normal lung volumes. How is it possible to have marked ILD yet have normal lung volumes?

SOLUTION

Because of inflammation and scarring in the lung tissue, patients with ILD have stiff, noncompliant lungs. The result is restrictive physiology and reduced lung volumes at chest x-ray examination. However, several entities can result in normal lung volumes despite significant ILD. Examples are as follows:

- *Sarcoidosis and chronic hypersensitivity pneumonitis (CHP).* In both of these disorders, the inflammation in the lung tends to be centered in the airways. In CHP, this condition likely is due to the route of exposure to the antigen (i.e., inhalation). It is not known why the inflammation in sarcoidosis tends to follow the bronchovascular structures of the lung. If significant airway involvement results in compromise of the lumens of the bronchioles and bronchi, there may be a component of obstructive physiology. Airway obstruction may lead to increased lung volumes and balance the restrictive effect of the ILD.
- *Eosinophilic granuloma* (also known as *histiocytosis X*) and *lymphangioleiomyomatosis.* These two rare ILDs are characterized by extensive cystic changes in addition to interstitial thickening. These cysts result in air-trapping, which often results in preservation or even an increase of lung volumes.
- *Emphysema.* Normal or even increased lung volumes may be present when any ILD occurs in a patient with emphysema. The loss of lung parenchyma seen that occurs in emphysema results in the loss of normal elastic recoil and thus pulmonary hyperinflation. If the remaining parenchyma becomes involved with inflammation and scarring, the elastic properties (and thus lung volumes) may normalize. In a patient with both ILD and emphysema, the measured lung volumes reflect the relative proportions of each disease.

RULE OF THUMB

Among smokers with IPF, normal spirometric results and lung volumes with a reduced D_{LCO} suggest the presence of coexisting emphysema.

▶ SPECIFIC TYPES OF ILD

Occupational

The three most common types of **occupational ILD** are **asbestosis**, chronic **silicosis**, and coal worker's pneumoconiosis (CWP).

Numerous clinical and radiographic abnormalities occur in patients who have been exposed to asbestos.[6] These abnormalities include pleural plaques, pleural fibrosis, pleural effusions, rounded atelectasis, parenchymal scarring, lung cancer, and mesothelioma. The term *asbestos-related pulmonary disease* may be used to encompass all of these entities. The term *asbestosis* is reserved for patients who have evidence of parenchymal scarring or fibrosis. Most patients with asbestosis have had considerable asbestos exposure many years before manifestation of the lung disease. Exposure frequently is associated with occupations such as ship building or insulation work. Patients report dyspnea on exertion and have crackles at lung examination. Physiological testing shows restrictive impairment with reduced D_{LCO}. The chest x-ray examination reveals bilateral lower-zone reticulonodular infiltrates.[7] In the correct clinical setting, the presence of radiographic pleural plaques or pleural effusion may indicate that asbestos is the cause, although neither of these findings is necessary or sufficient for establishing the diagnosis. Management of asbestosis frequently is similar to that of IPF. However, the rates of response to currently available therapy are dismal.

Chronic silicosis occurs in patients with chronic exposure to silica over many years.[8] In addition to the chronic form, *acute* and *accelerated* forms of silicosis occur, and in these forms exposure is more intense. Occupations that commonly entail exposure to silica include mining, tunneling, sandblasting, and foundry work. The chest x-ray examination commonly shows an upper-lung-zone predominant abnormality characterized by multiple small nodular opacities.[9] These nodules may slowly coalesce into large masses known as *progressive massive fibrosis* (PMF). Enlargement and often calcification of the hilar lymph nodes are common. Functional and physiological impairment in chronic silicosis is quite variable. Some patients may report few, if any, symptoms and may have no abnormal examination findings and only mild physiological impairment, despite significant chest x-ray abnormalities. Any physiological impairment may remain stable or, if PMF occurs, may progress even in the absence of continued exposure.

Coal worker's pneumoconiosis develops as the result of chronic inhalation of coal mine dust. In the past, it was assumed that silica dust was responsible for the pulmonary disease seen among coal miners because the clinical and radiographic features are quite similar.

MINI CLINI

Chest X-ray Clues to Specific ILD Diagnoses

PROBLEM

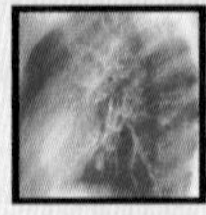

In the care of patients with ILD, arriving at a specific diagnosis often requires histological confirmation in addition to careful clinical evaluation. Clues to the diagnosis may be found with close questioning regarding previous illnesses or exposures, physical examination, physiological testing, or radiographic studies. Although they generally are nonspecific, the chest radiographic findings occasionally suggest the possibility of certain diagnoses. What chest x-ray patterns are helpful in differential diagnosis?

SOLUTION

The distribution of changes on the chest x-ray film may help narrow the differential diagnosis. Diseases such as IPF, connective tissue disease, and asbestosis tend to have a lower-zone predominance. The presence of predominantly upper-zone disease indicates the possibility of silicosis, CHP, sarcoidosis, EG, or ankylosing spondylitis. The presence of infiltrates within and respecting the borders of previous radiation treatment ports suggests radiation pneumonitis. Chronic eosinophilic pneumonia may have a distinctly peripheral distribution or the so-called radiographic negative of the central changes often seen in cardiogenic pulmonary edema.

In addition to the distribution of radiographic changes, the character of the opacities may be helpful. Reticulonodular opacities are common. Primarily nodular opacities may be seen in sarcoidosis, silicosis, CWP, and bronchiolitis obliterans. Cystic changes (called *honeycomb lung*) are characteristic of EG and lymphangioleiomyomatosis. They often are present in the late stages of many ILDs.

Certain other chest x-ray findings may be helpful. For example, the presence of pleural plaques raises the possibility of asbestosis. Pleural effusions may be seen in asbestosis, connective tissue disease, and lymphangioleiomyomatosis. Enlarged lymph nodes in the hila are seen in sarcoidosis and silicosis. Pneumothorax may occur in EG or lymphangioleiomyomatosis.

Although a specific diagnosis cannot be made solely on the basis of chest x-ray findings, certain radiographic findings may be helpful in narrowing the differential diagnosis. For example, sarcoidosis, silicosis, or CWP should be considered in this case.

However, it is now recognized that CWP and silicosis are the result of distinct exposures.[10] Simple CWP, characterized by multiple small nodular opacities on the chest x-ray film, is asymptomatic. Cough and shortness of breath do not develop unless the disease progresses to PMF similar to that seen in silicosis. It is not clear that any therapeutic approach is useful in either CWP or silicosis, although corticosteroids often are tried.

Drug Related

Many drugs have been associated with pulmonary complications of various types, including interstitial inflammation and fibrosis, bronchospasm, pulmonary edema, and pleural effusions.[11] Numerous drugs have been associated with ILD. Coming from many different therapeutic classes, these drugs include chemotherapeutic agents, antibiotics, antiarrhythmic drugs, and anti-inflammatory agents (see Box 21-2). In addition, therapeutic exposure to radiation in the management of cancer may result in ILD. Given the variety of pulmonary pathologic responses possible, it is not surprising that the clinical presentations also vary. Dyspnea and cough are common presentations with rales at examination. Physiology may be restricted with a decreased D_{LCO}. The results of radiographic studies vary; examples include airspace disease, lung fibrosis, and pleural changes. In a few cases, simply discontinuing the offending agent may lead to improvement, but in many instances systemic **corticosteroids** may be needed.

Connective Tissue Disease

ILD is a well-known complication of various connective tissue (rheumatologic) disorders. The most commonly implicated disorders are rheumatoid arthritis, scleroderma, Sjögren's syndrome, polymyositis/dermatomyositis, and systemic lupus erythematosus.

In any of these disorders, pulmonary involvement may remain undetected until significant impairment is present, because patients with these disorders may be inactive because of the underlying rheumatologic disease. For example, a patient whose activity is severely limited by joint pain and deformity related to rheumatoid arthritis may not detect dyspnea until lung function is severely impaired. However, there is generally poor correlation between the severity of the pulmonary and nonpulmonary manifestations of these diseases. In some instances the lung disease may overshadow or even predate the other symptoms of the underlying disease. When symptoms develop, dyspnea and cough are common. At chest examination, rales (crackles), wheezing, or even a pleural rub may be heard because of the varied patterns of lung involvement in these disorders. Physiology may be restricted with a decreased D_{LCO} or even may be obstructive depending on the type of involvement. The results of radiographic studies vary; examples include airspace disease, lung fibrosis, and pleural changes.

The interstitial inflammation associated with these diseases can occur in a variety of patterns. Some patterns of inflammation are associated with a disease that may be responsive to aggressive treatment with antiinflammatory agents, such as corticosteroids or cytotoxic agents; others may be much less responsive and therefore tend to have a poorer prognosis.

Allergic, or Hypersensitivity, Responses

Acute hypersensitivity pneumonitis results from intermittent, acute exposure to modest or high levels of organic antigens (e.g., animal proteins or microorganisms). These exposures may be associated with acute pulmonary reactions that may mimic pneumonia. Patients who have been exposed to high levels of organic antigens may come to medical attention with acute shortness of breath, chest pain, fever, chills, and a cough that may be productive of purulent sputum.[12] The symptoms associated with such a reaction usually are dramatic enough that the patient will seek medical attention promptly.

In comparison, some patients who are chronically exposed to low levels of inhaled organic antigens may have subtle interstitial inflammatory reactions in the lung that do not result in noticeable symptoms for months to years. Such chronic inflammation may lead to slowly progressive scarring in the lung that is known as **chronic hypersensitivity pneumonitis** (CHP).[12,13] Common sources of the types of organic antigens known to cause this type of disease include bacteria and fungi, which may be found in moldy hay (farmer's lung) or in the home environment, particularly in association with central humidification systems (humidifier lung), animal proteins (e.g., bird breeder's lung), and various chemicals. Numerous established antigens are listed in Table 21-1 along with the typical source of exposure to each and the associated syndrome.

Chronic hypersensitivity pneumonitis is more common among nonsmokers than it is among smokers.[14] Patients experience progressive shortness of breath. They usually do not describe the episodic symptomatic worsening with exposures that patients with acute disease report.[12] For this reason, the clinical presentation may be quite similar to that of IPF. Examination abnormalities are restricted to the chest, inspiratory rales or crackles being detected. The plain chest x-ray examination reveals bilateral reticulonodular infiltrates, which may have an upper lobe distribution. Because the symptoms may not betray the association and because the source of antigenic exposure often is unknown to the patient, a careful environmental history is critical in evaluating patients with ILD of unknown causation.

Blood samples may be obtained to determine whether there has been an antibody response to certain antigens associated with CHP. Unfortunately, the presence of such antibodies is not sufficient to establish the diagnosis of CHP because many persons develop antibodies in the absence of disease. Likewise, the absence of detectable antibodies does not rule out the diagnosis of CHP because the culprit may be an antigen that is not included in the blood analysis.[13]

In general, patients with CHP must practice strict antigen avoidance and may respond to corticosteroids. However, the course of the disease is quite variable. Variability in response to steroids and disease progression may be related to the characteristics of the antigen or to those of the host.[13]

Idiopathic and Unclassified Disease

In addition to the entities just described in which there is an identifiable cause, there are many ILDs that are of unknown causation (i.e., they are idiopathic).

Idiopathic Pulmonary Fibrosis

Idiopathic pulmonary fibrosis is one of the most common ILDs and is the most common of a group of disorders referred to as the *idiopathic interstitial pneumonias*[15] (IPF, nonspecific interstitial pneumonia, desquamative interstitial pneumonia [DIP], respiratory bronchiolitis ILD [RB-ILD], and acute interstitial pneumonia). Idiopathic pulmonary fibrosis develops in persons of all ages, but it occurs most commonly during the fifth to seventh decades of life. A small number of patients have a family history of IPF, but most cases occur sporadically.[16] Although one report suggests that persons with a history of tobacco abuse may be at increased risk of development of IPF,[17] the disease commonly occurs among nonsmokers.

Patients with IPF commonly have progressive dyspnea on exertion and have a nonproductive cough. Results of chest examination are abnormal, mid to late inspiratory rales (crackles) being found in the lower half of the chest. The chest x-ray findings, described previously, may have been present and progressing slowly for years before the diagnosis is actually rendered.

Prednisone and **cytotoxic agents** are the standard management of IPF.[18] Unfortunately, fewer than 30% of patients have clear physiological or subjective improvement with treatment. Although currently available treatments may slow the progression of IPF, this disease is almost uniformly fatal. The median survival time is approximately 3 to 5 years from the time of diagnosis. New approaches to treatment are focused on antifibrotic therapies.

Sarcoidosis

Sarcoidosis is an idiopathic multisystem inflammatory disorder that commonly involves the lung.[19] The tissue inflammation that occurs in sarcoidosis has a characteristic pattern in which the inflammatory cells collect in microscopic nodules called *granulomas*. Unlike IPF, sarcoidosis is more common among young adults than it is among older persons. Sarcoidosis often follows a quite benign course; spontaneous remission occurs frequently.

The most common clinical manifestation of sarcoidosis is an asymptomatic chest x-ray abnormality. When symptoms do occur, they include cough, chest pain, dyspnea, and wheezing. The most common radiographic finding is bilateral hilar lymphadenopathy without parenchymal opacities. When they do occur, parenchymal opacities may be nodular, reticulonodular, or, occasionally, alveolar. Results of pulmonary function tests may be normal or may demonstrate restrictive physiology with reduced D_{LCO}. Coexisting obstructive impairment may be related to endobronchial granulomatous inflammation or scarring.

Corticosteroids are commonly used in the management of sarcoidosis, but treatment usually is reserved for patients with marked symptoms or physiological impairment attributable to the disease.

Pulmonary Vasculitis

Pulmonary vasculitis is a rare group of respiratory illnesses often classified with the ILDs, mainly because they can present radiographically in a pattern similar to that of other ILDs. The diseases are characterized by acute and chronic inflammation of the blood vessels (occasionally with associated granulomas, known as a *granulomatous vasculitis*)[20] in more than one organ system. Pulmonary vasculitis often occurs with a variety of seemingly unrelated symptoms in several organ systems, and diagnosis often becomes confused.

The cause of pulmonary vasculitis is obscure. Although an abnormal response to infection or an antigen has been identified, the primary cause is a matter of speculation for almost all forms of vasculitis. Fundamentally, disease occurs when the body's immune system attacks the blood vessels in the lung and other organs. Symptoms and signs often indicate a systemic disease rather than a particular lung disease, although hemoptysis occasionally occurs. Examination findings are nonspecific.

The main differential diagnostic concern usually is infection. The diagnosis of pulmonary vasculitis often is considered when the result of an antinuclear cytoplasmic antibody blood test is positive. The diagnosis usually requires surgical biopsy of the involved organ, and therapy consists of an aggressive antiinflammatory approach with a combination of corticosteroids and cytotoxic agents.

▶ TREATMENT ISSUES

Specific comments about the management of specific ILDs are presented earlier. The following comments are general guides.

Medical Treatment

Corticosteroids

Corticosteroids are a primary therapy for many types of ILD. Because an uncontrolled inflammatory reaction may be the cause of many of these diseases, it makes sense to use these antiinflammatory drugs. For some types of the ILD, the course of therapy can be limited to a few weeks or months. For others, therapy may well be continued for years.

Unfortunately, not all patients with an ILD respond to corticosteroid therapy, and additional therapies may be needed. One limitation of corticosteroid therapy is the frequency of side effects, some of which can be confused with progression of the underlying lung disease. For this reason, patients undergoing steroid therapy need regular assessments of the underlying lung disease, response to therapy, and tolerance of the medication.

Cytotoxic Agents

A number of medicines used in the management of ILD fall into the category of *cytotoxic medications*.[21] Examples include cyclophosphamide (Cytoxan), azathioprine (Imuran), and cyclosporine (Neoral, Sandimmune). Many of these drugs have been used in cancer chemotherapy, as have corticosteroids, for preventing transplant rejection, and for managing connective tissue diseases. All of these medications have antiinflammatory actions and are considered more potent than steroids. Because of this property, cytotoxic agents often have been added to a therapeutic regimen when steroids alone are unhelpful. Cyclophosphamide has proved particularly helpful in the management of one type of pulmonary vasculitis, Wegener's granulomatosis. The side effects of cytotoxic medicines include depression of the immune system. As with steroids, monitoring of side effects becomes an important part of disease management.

Oxygen Therapy

The use of oxygen therapy in the management of ILDs and vasculitis has not been studied as extensively as it has in the management of chronic obstructive pulmonary disease (COPD). Use of oxygen therapy is important to patients with hypoxemia. Evaluation for hypoxemia should include measurement of oxygen saturation at rest, during exercise, and, if clinically indicated, during sleep. Maintenance of normal oxygen tension is necessary to prevent secondary hypertension and subsequent right-sided heart failure, complications of ILD that amplify a patient's sense of breathlessness.

Avoiding Exposure

For a number of the ILDs, such as hypersensitivity pneumonitis (e.g., bird breeder's lung), drug-induced ILD, and occupational ILDs (e.g., silicosis), exposure to an antigen, fume, or potentially toxic substance leads to lung injury. In these cases, removal from or avoidance of the offending agent is critical because continued

MINI CLINI

Clinical Deterioration in a Patient Being Treated for ILD

PROBLEM

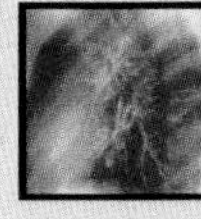

A 50-year-old man with IPF is being treated with high-dose corticosteroids and cyclophosphamide. After 6 months of therapy, he begins to report progressive breathlessness. Why is this occurring?

SOLUTION

Many ILDs follow a gradually progressive course to end-stage disease and death. The available treatments may result in temporary improvement or retarded progression of the disease. Unfortunately, these treatments seldom are curative. Decline in the condition of a patient being treated for ILD often, although not always, is indicative of disease progression.[22]

The following possibilities must be considered and separated from progression of the disease.

- *Superimposed infection.* The antiinflammatory agents used in the management of ILD increase the risk of infection in the lung and elsewhere. Common bacteria or uncommon opportunistic infections may be responsible. Pneumonia may be difficult to detect radiographically because of preexisting radiographic abnormalities, and bronchoscopy with bronchoalveolar lavage may be needed.
- *Steroid-related muscle weakness* is a less common complication of therapy, which can provoke breathlessness indistinguishable from that of progression of the underlying disease. Steroid-related muscle weakness is difficult to diagnose because the weakness results in worsening of the established restrictive physiology. The development of proximal muscle weakness concurrent with worsening respiratory status should raise the possibility of complication of steroid treatment.
- *Pulmonary embolism.* Inactivity as a result of disease-related physiological impairment and right ventricular dysfunction may be risk factors for thromboembolic disease. A sudden decline in respiratory status, sometimes associated with pleuritic chest pain, should raise the possibility of the presence of pulmonary embolism. These symptoms also suggest the development of pneumothorax. An increased incidence of pneumothorax has been associated with certain ILDs.
- *Bronchogenic carcinoma* may develop in patients with pulmonary fibrosis and may contribute to clinical decline.
- *Atherosclerotic vascular disease.* Many patients with ILD have independent risk factors for atherosclerotic vascular disease. Therefore they may have unrelated cardiac disease, such as coronary artery disease, left ventricular dysfunction, or valvular disease, which can be mistaken for a worsening of the pulmonary process.

Each of the possible explanations for the patient's breathlessness should be considered before ascribing it to disease progression.

MINI CLINI

Tobacco Use and ILD

PROBLEM

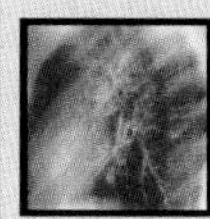

A 30-year-old woman has ILD and is addicted to cigarettes. She is concerned that quitting on her own is too difficult and comments that tobacco use is associated with emphysema not with scarring. Should she be encouraged to quit smoking? Why or why not?

SOLUTION

Yes! Although the association between tobacco use and emphysema and COPD is clear, in general, the association is not thought to play a large role in the development of most types of ILD. However, the following three types of ILD have a strong association with cigarette smoking: (1) DIP, (2) RB-ILD, and (3) EG, also known as pulmonary histiocytosis X.

Approximately 90% of patients with DIP are current or former smokers. More than 90% of patients with identified EG smoke, often quite heavily, and can have considerable difficulty quitting. Essentially all patients with RB smoke. As with other toxic exposures, complete smoking cessation and probably avoidance of all secondhand smoke is important for all patients with RB and EG.

In both RB and EG, physiological stabilization and even improvement can occur after abstinence from tobacco. Abstinence alone is more beneficial than any currently available drug therapy. In DIP, the benefits of smoking cessation are unclear.

In all these illnesses, use of one of the numerous smoking cessation techniques often is necessary, even after the patient has been informed of the severity of the problem. The underlying mechanism by which these three diseases are related to cigarette smoking is unclear. In addition to having concerns about these specific disease considerations, patients with ILD of any type cannot afford to risk the development of additional, smoking-related respiratory impairment. Thus the patient should be encouraged to stop smoking.

The diseases considered under the category of ILD are a diverse group of illnesses of varied causation, treatment, and prognosis. In general, these diseases manifest as chronic, progressive dyspnea on exertion and as cough. Abnormalities at examination generally are limited to the chest in the form of fine, inspiratory crackles. The most common chest x-ray finding is diffuse reticular or reticulonodular infiltrates with reduced lung volumes. Pulmonary function testing usually reveals restrictive physiology. Therapy often includes the use of antiinflammatory drugs (corticosteroids and cytotoxic agents) and the avoidance of disease-inducing exposures.

exposure often leads to progressive loss of lung function.

Identification of the exposure requires a complete medical history, including medications and previous occupational and environmental exposures. In many instances, the source of the exposure is obvious, such as birds in the home or previous work with asbestos insulation. Sometimes, however, the source is less clear, and additional measures such as the use of the services of an industrial hygienist to review a home or workplace environment may be necessary. Once the exposure is identified, every effort must be made to avoid it, a measure often not trivial and possibly necessitating removal of pets, changing jobs, or even moving to a new home.

Pulmonary Rehabilitation and Exercise Therapy

Like oxygen therapy, the use of pulmonary rehabilitation in the management of ILD has not been as well studied as its use in COPD has. Pulmonary rehabilitation is important in building aerobic fitness, maintaining physical activity, and preventing the musculoskeletal side effects of corticosteroids.

Vaccinations

As do most patients with chronic illnesses, particularly those with chronic lung illnesses, patients with ILD should receive a pneumococcal vaccine and a yearly influenza virus vaccine, unless there are contraindications.

Transplantation

The therapy of last resort for end-stage ILD is lung transplantation. Transplantation has been performed successfully in the management of most ILDs. However, in ILDs related to systemic diseases, such as connective tissue disease, there is some concern that the outcome is not as good as when transplantation is performed in the setting of an illness affecting only the lung (e.g., emphysema).

KEY POINTS

- The ILDs are a diverse group of illnesses of varied causes, treatments, and prognoses.
- In general, these diseases manifest as chronic, progressive dyspnea on exertion and as cough.
- The most common chest x-ray finding is diffuse reticular or reticulonodular infiltrates with reduced lung volumes.
- Pulmonary function testing usually reveals restrictive physiology.
- Therapy often includes the use of antiinflammatory drugs (corticosteroids and cytotoxic agents) and the avoidance of disease-inducing exposures.

References

1. Schwarz MI: Clinical overview of interstitial lung disease. In Schwarz MI, King TE, editors: *Interstitial lung disease*, ed 2, St Louis, 1993, Mosby.
2. Keogh BA, Crystal RG: Pulmonary function testing in interstitial pulmonary disease: what does it tell us? Chest 78:856, 1980.
3. Hansen JE, Wasserman K: Pathophysiology of activity limitation in patients with interstitial lung disease, Chest 109:1566, 1996.
4. Wiggins J, Strickland B, Turner-Warwick M: Combined cryptogenic fibrosing alveolitis and emphysema: the value of high resolution computed tomography in assessment, *Respir Med* 84:365, 1990.
5. Hanley ME, and others: The impact of smoking on mechanical properties of the lungs in idiopathic pulmonary fibrosis and sarcoidosis, *Am Rev Respir Dis* 144:1102, 1991.
6. Mossman BT, Gee JB: Asbestos-related diseases, *N Engl J Med* 320:1721, 1989.
7. McLoud TC: Conventional radiography in the diagnosis of asbestos-related disease, *Radiol Clin North Am* 30:1177, 1992.
8. Graham WGB: Silicosis, *Clin Chest Med* 13:253, 1992.
9. Stark P, Jacobson F, Shaffer K: Standard imaging in silicosis and coal worker's pneumoconiosis, *Radiol Clin North Am* 30:1147, 1992.
10. Lapp NL, Parker JE: Coal workers' pneumoconiosis, *Clin Chest Med* 13:243, 1992.
11. Rosenow III EC, and others: Drug-induced pulmonary disease: an update, Chest 102:239, 1992.
12. Kaltreider HB: Hypersensitivity pneumonitis, *West J Med* 159:570, 1993.
13. Rose C, King TE: Controversies in hypersensitivity pneumonitis, *Am Rev Respir Dis* 145:1, 1992.
14. Schuyler M: Lessons from hypersensitivity pneumonitis, *West J Med* 159:620, 1993.
15. Katzenstein AL, Myers JL: Idiopathic pulmonary fibrosis: clinical relevance of pathologic classification, *Am J Respir Crit Care Med* 157:1301, 1998.
16. Meier-Sydow J, and others: Idiopathic pulmonary fibrosis: current clinical concepts and challenges in management, *Semin Respir Crit Care Med* 15:77, 1994.
17. Baumgartner KB, and others: Cigarette smoking: a risk factor for idiopathic pulmonary fibrosis, *Am J Respir Crit Care Med* 155:242, 1997.
18. American Thoracic Society. Idiopathic pulmonary fibrosis: diagnosis and treatment. International consensus statement. American Thoracic Society (ATS), and the European Respiratory Society (ERS). *Am J Respir Crit Care Med* 161:646-64, 2000.
19. Sharma OP: Sarcoidosis, *Dis Mon* 36:469, 1990.
20. King TE, Mortenson R, Brown K: Granulomatous vasculitides. In Kelley W, editor: *Textbook of internal medicine*, ed 3, Philadelphia, 1996, JB Lippincott.
21. Lynch JP, McCure WJ: Immunosuppressive and cytotoxic pharmacotherapy for pulmonary disorders, *Am J Respir Crit Care Med* 155:395, 1997.
22. Panos RJ, and others: Clinical deterioration in patients with idiopathic pulmonary fibrosis: causes and assessment, *Am J Med* 88:396, 1990.

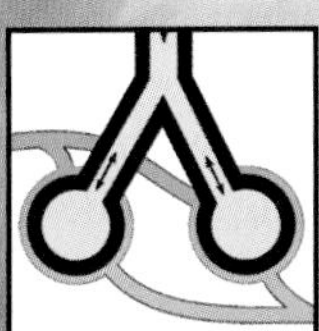

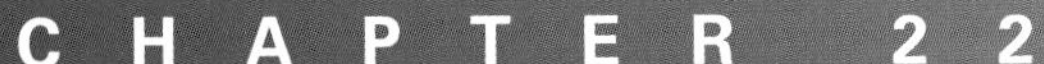

CHAPTER 22

Pleural Diseases

Charlie Strange

In This Chapter You Will Learn:

- Why diagnostic thoracentesis is an important tool for the assessment of pleural effusion
- Why spirometric improvements after thoracentesis usually are modest
- Why it is important to know the physiology of ventilation and oxygenation when treating patients with pleural effusion or pneumothorax
- How to properly manage chest tubes and water-seal chambers
- How to manage ventilators for patients with bronchopleural fistulas

Chapter Outline

The Pleural Space
 Overview and definitions
Pleural Effusions
 Transudative
 Exudative
 Physiological importance
 Diagnostic tests
Pneumothorax
 Traumatic
 Spontaneous
 Complications
 Diagnosis
 Therapy
 Bronchopleural fistula
 Pleurodesis

Key Terms

bronchopleural fistula
chylothorax
empyema
exudative pleural effusion
hemothorax
parietal pleura
pleural effusion
pleural space
pleurisy
pleurodesis
pneumothorax
primary spontaneous pneumothorax
reexpansion pulmonary edema
secondary spontaneous pneumothorax
tension pneumothorax
thoracentesis
transudative pleural effusion
visceral pleura

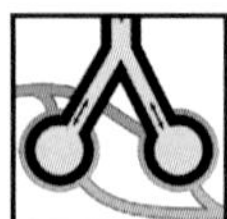

A spectrum of pleural diseases affects respiratory function. An understanding of pleural anatomy, physiology, and pathology is essential to delivering effective respiratory care. This chapter focuses on the two major disease processes that occur in the **pleural space: pleural effusion** and **pneumothorax**.

▶ THE PLEURAL SPACE

Overview and Definitions

Each lung is covered by a thin membrane called the **visceral pleura**, which adheres closely to the subjacent alveoli of the lung. The visceral pleura dips into the fissures of the lung, allowing the surgeon easy access between the lung lobes and allowing pleural fluid to travel freely between the lobes while remaining in the pleural space.

The ribs and connective tissue of the chest wall are covered on the inner surface by a similar membrane called the **parietal pleura**. The parietal pleura can be thought of as a sac that covers not only the rib surface (costal pleura) but also the diaphragm (diaphragmatic pleura) and the mediastinum (mediastinal pleura).

The blood vessels and airways that enter the lung connect to the mediastinum at the lung hilum. It is at this juncture that the visceral pleura meets the mediastinal parietal pleura to form a single, continuous pleural membrane (Figure 22-1).

Because the lung usually is completely inflated, one would think that the pleural membranes always touch. However, freeze-fracturing has demonstrated that there is a space between the visceral and parietal pleura that averages 10 to 20 mm in width and is filled with pleural fluid. This thin film of fluid allows the lung to slide over the ribs and allows for a gliding movement that takes little energy and produces little friction.

The average person has approximately 8 mL of pleural fluid per hemithorax.[1] It is estimated that this pleural fluid has a total protein concentration similar to that of interstitial fluid elsewhere in the body: between 1.3 and 1.4 g/dL.[2]

In human beings, the pleural spaces surrounding each lung are completely independent, being separated by the mediastinum. This is not the case in all other mammals. The slaughter of the American buffalo could occur with a single spear or rifle shot because the pleural spaces of the buffalo lung are connected. Consequently, air in the pleural space collapses both lungs. An analogous situation can occur in any patient who has undergone median sternotomy, during which both pleural spaces were entered. Common operations resulting in this condition are lung volume reduction surgery and bilateral lung transplantation.

The pleural space is under negative pressure except during forced expiration. The intact thoracic rib cage provides elastic recoil pressure outward, whereas the intrinsic recoil pressure of the lung is inward toward the lung hilum. The diaphragm further decreases the intrapleural pressure below the atmospheric pressure to allow inspiration to occur. In an upright person, the pressure is more negative at the lung apex than at the lung base because of the weight of the lung and the effects of gravity. The net effect of the negatively pressurized pleural space is that fluid moves into the pleural space from adjacent sites when a communication is present. A patient with ascitic fluid and a diaphragmatic defect preferentially pulls fluid into the chest.

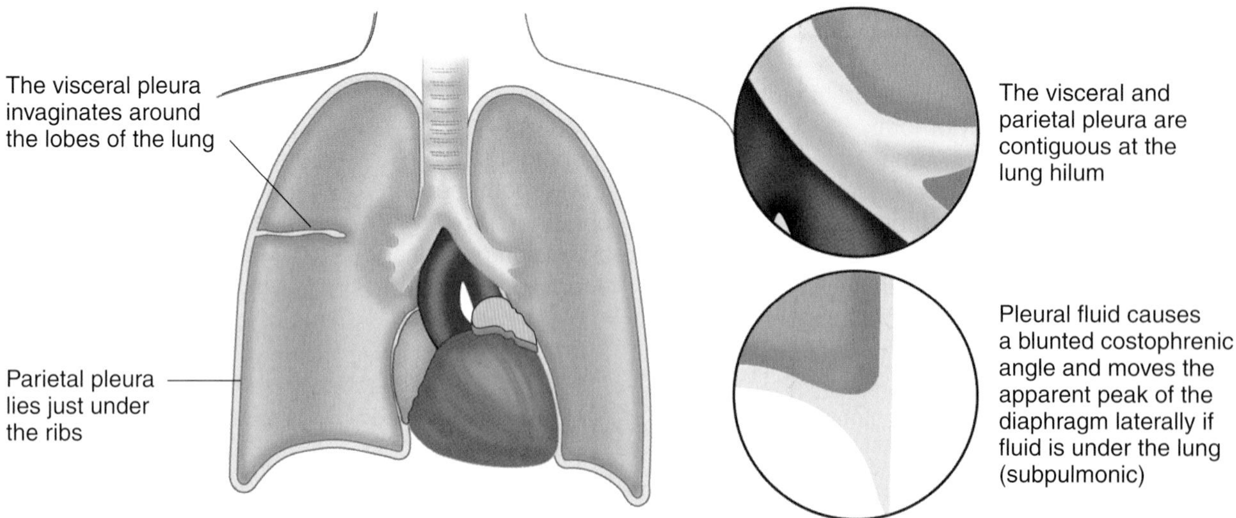

Figure 22-1
Anatomy of the pleura.

▶ PLEURAL EFFUSIONS

Any abnormal amount of pleural fluid in the pleural space is called *pleural effusion*. The many causes of pleural effusion are categorized according to etiologic factor and the content of the fluid.[3]

Pleural fluid enters the pleural space across both the visceral and the parietal pleurae, particularly when the interstitial pressure within either the lung or the chest wall is increased. The main route for pleural fluid removal is small holes within the parietal pleura called *stomata*, which are large enough to allow a red blood cell to enter and be cleared from the pleural space. The parietal pleural stomata connect with intercostal lymphatic vessels under the ribs that drain posteriorly into the mediastinum. In the mediastinum, these lymphatic vessels enter lymph nodes before draining into the thoracic duct, a large lymphatic channel within the chest, which empties into the left subclavian vein. Abnormalities of increased pleural fluid production or blockade of drainage can cause pleural fluid to accumulate.

Transudative

Any pleural effusion that forms when the integrity of the pleural space is undamaged is called a **transudative pleural effusion**. A pleural fluid total protein concentration less than 50% of the serum total protein level and lactate dehydrogenase (LDH) values in the pleural fluid less than 60% of the serum value indicate the presence of a transudative pleural effusion. In the absence of serum values, an absolute pleural fluid LDH level less than two-thirds normal for serum suggests the presence of a transudate. These numbers were derived from large patient series in which pleural fluid and serum protein concentrations were measured while the cause of the effusion was being determined and corrected.[4]

Box 22-1 • Causes of Pleural Effusion

TRANSUDATIVE PLEURAL EFFUSION
- Congestive heart failure
- Cirrhosis
- Nephrotic syndrome
- Hypoalbuminemia
- Lymphatic obstruction
- Peritoneal dialysis
- Atelectasis
- Central venous catheter in pleural space
- Urinothorax

EXUDATIVE PLEURAL EFFUSION

NEOPLASTIC DISEASE
- Carcinoma
- Lymphoma
- Mesothelioma

INFECTIOUS DISEASE
- Bacterial infection
- Tuberculosis
- Fungal infection
- Paragonimiasis
- Viral pleurisy

PULMONARY EMBOLISM

GASTROINTESTINAL DISEASE
- Pancreatic disease
- Intraabdominal abscess
- Splenic infarction
- Esophageal perforation
- Abdominal surgery
- Endoscopic variceal sclerotherapy

COLLAGEN VASCULAR DISEASE
- Rheumatoid pleurisy
- Systemic lupus erythematosus
- Drug-induced lupus
- Immunoblastic lymphadenopathy
- Sjögren's syndrome
- Familial Mediterranean fever
- Churg-Strauss syndrome
- Wegener's granulomatosis

DRUG-INDUCED PLEURAL DISEASE
- Nitrofurantoin
- Minoxidil
- Dantrolene
- Methysergide
- Bromocriptine
- Amiodarone
- Procarbazine, bleomycin, mitomycin
- Methotrexate
- Practolol

MISCELLANEOUS DISEASES AND CONDITIONS
- Benign asbestos pleural effusion
- Postcardiac injury syndrome
- Meigs' syndrome
- Yellow nail syndrome
- Sarcoidosis
- Pericardial disease
- Fetal pleural effusion
- Uremic pleural effusion
- Trapped lung
- Radiation pleurisy
- Amyloidosis
- Electrical burns

HEMOTHORAX

CHYLOTHORAX

The classification system listed in Box 22-1 is not perfect, and refinements continue to be proposed. For practical purposes, these numbers help narrow the possible causes of pleural fluid formation.

Transudative pleural effusions form when hydrostatic and oncotic pressure is abnormal (Figure 22-2).[5] The list of diseases that cause transudative pleural effusions is short. Therefore these diseases remain relatively easy to diagnose.

Congestive Heart Failure

Elevation of pressure in the left atrium and pulmonary veins is the hallmark of congestive heart failure (CHF). Elevation of pulmonary venous pressure increases the amount of interstitial fluid in the lung. In severe cases, flooding of the alveoli causes pulmonary edema, but in less severe cases, interstitial lung water increases and decompresses into the pleural space. Because systemic venous pressure also is elevated, there is limited capability to remove pleural fluid through the intercostal veins. Therefore all pleural fluid must enter the lymphatic vessels. Pleural effusions result when the capacity of pleural lymphatic drainage is overcome.[6]

Congestive heart failure is the most common cause of clinical pleural effusions. The effusions can be massive, filling the entire hemithorax and compressing the lung. More commonly, they are small and bilateral. The effusions are rarely drained because outcome is heavily influenced by successful management of the underlying CHF, which also clears the effusions.[7]

Nephrotic Syndrome

In nephrotic syndrome (also known as *nephrosis*), the kidneys leak more than 3 g of protein per day into the urine. Because they become protein depleted, patients have insufficient oncotic pressure within the blood to hold appropriate amounts of fluid within the blood vessels. These patients become very edematous, and fluid leaks into the lung interstitium and pleural space. Pleural effusions are common but usually are small.

Patients with nephrosis are at increased risk of deep venous thrombosis and pulmonary emboli. In nephrosis, protein S, which keeps blood from clotting, becomes deficient from leaking into the urine. Therefore the presence of large or asymmetrical pleural effusions should raise the possibility of the presence of pulmonary emboli. Pleural effusions associated with pulmonary emboli usually are exudates and contain large numbers of red blood cells.

Hypoalbuminemia

Hypoalbuminemia is caused by a variety of debilitating diseases, such as acquired immunodeficiency syndrome and chronic liver disease. Pleural effusions rarely form until the serum albumin level is less than 1.8 g/dL. The mechanism of formation of pleural fluid is identical to that of nephrotic syndrome. Low protein levels in the blood allow fluid to leak into interstitial tissues and the pleural space. The effusions usually are small.

Liver Disease

End-stage liver disease causes transudative fluid to accumulate in the abdomen. This is called *ascites*. Because the pleural space is under negative pressure during inspiration and because ascitic fluid often is under positive pressure, any small hole in the diaphragm can result in movement of ascitic fluid into the pleural space to form *hepatic hydrothorax*.

All ascitic fluid can end up in the chest because of the pressure gradient, and true ascites can be absent. This condition often is quite difficult to manage except with methods that limit ascites formation, such as sodium restriction and diuretics. Excessive pleural fluid is present in approximately 6% of patients with ascites, and 70% of these fluid collections are on the right side.[8]

Atelectasis

When segments of the lung collapse, intrapleural pressure becomes more negative and can produce small effusions. With relief of bronchial obstruction and postoperative pain, these effusions regress.

Lymphatic Obstruction

Lymphatic obstruction within the mediastinum causes poor pleural fluid egress from the pleural space, although the pleural space is otherwise normal. The most common condition that causes this abnormality is cancer that metastasizes to the mediastinum. This condition should be differentiated from a true malignant pleural effusion, defined as cancer cells within the pleural space.

Rare Causes

There are other rare causes of transudative pleural effusions. Urinothorax occurs after rupture of the ureter when urine leaks into the retroperitoneal space and refluxes into the chest. The pleural fluid has a low pH. A central venous line that is inappropriately placed into the pleural space can put large amounts of transudative fluid into the pleural space before this abnormality is recognized. The level of glucose in the pleural fluid can be very elevated, depending on the infusion. Peritoneal dialysate can migrate into the pleural cavity in patients undergoing continuous ambulatory peritoneal dialysis.

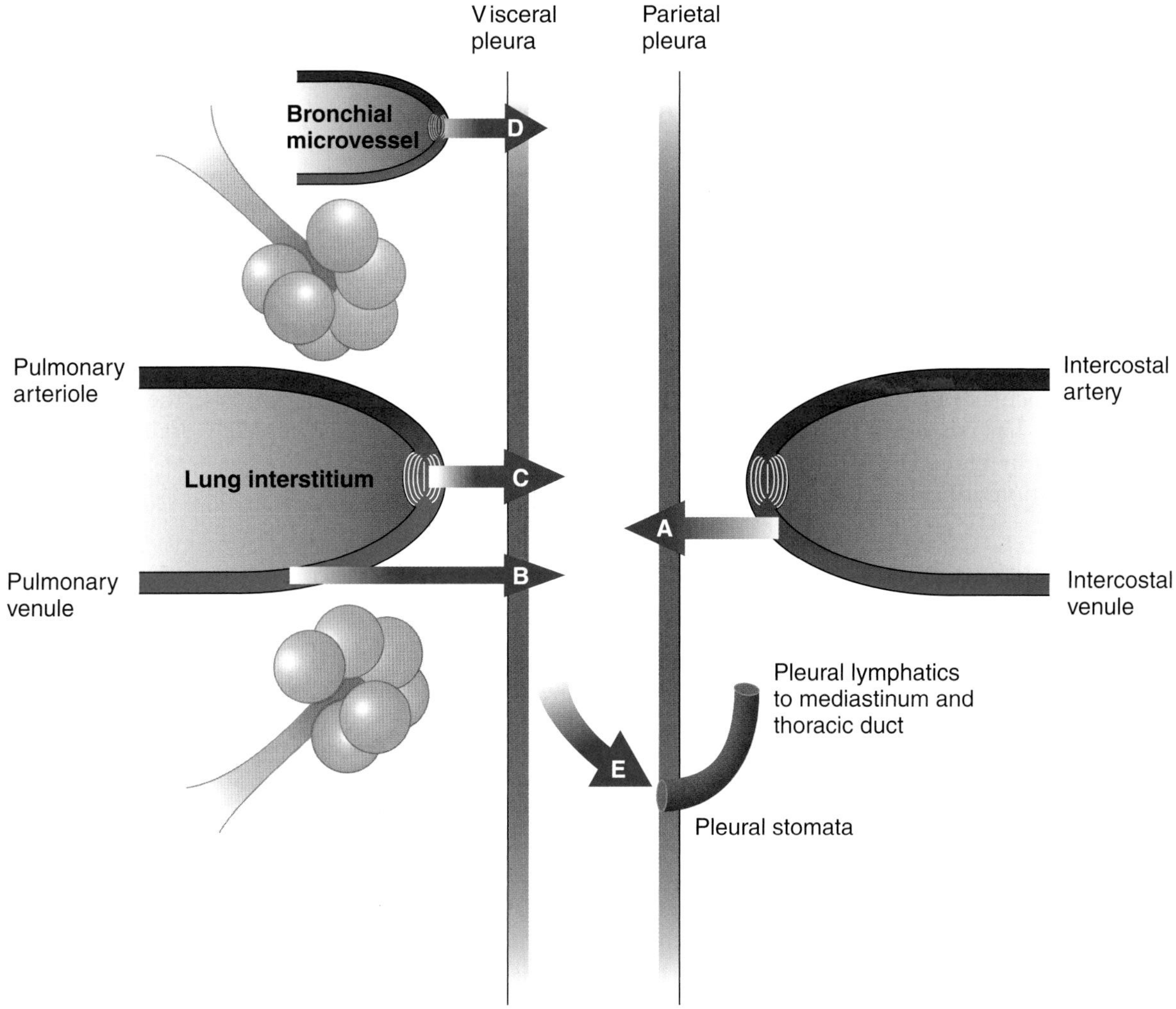

Figure 22-2

Pleural fluid formation requires both excess fluid formation and decreased elimination. In diseases such as pulmonary hypertension, in which right-sided heart pressure is increased and systemic veins, such as the intercostal veins (A), are pressurized, pleural fluid does not form because pleural drainage is rapid. However, when left ventricular failure causes pulmonary venule pressure (B) to increase, the addition of interstitial lung water overwhelms the drainage and produces a transudative pleural effusion. Injury to the capillaries (C), as in pneumonia or ARDS, causes fluid to leak into the lung interstitium and pleural space at increased rates. Under these conditions, fibrin can occlude the pleural lymphatic vessels (E) and cause fluid to accumulate. The bronchial microvessels (D) supply the pleura with blood and likely participate to some extent in production of pleural fluid.

Exudative

An **exudative pleural effusion** is caused by inflammation in the lung or pleura. This type of pleural effusion has more protein and inflammatory cells present than does a transudative effusion. Because therapy for pleural effusion depends on the cause, **thoracentesis** often is performed to determine the specific biochemical and cellular characteristics of the pleural effusion. Box 22-1 lists the common causes of exudative pleural effusion. They account for approximately 70% of all pleural effusions.

Parapneumonic

Pleural effusions form in pneumonia because inflammation in the lung increases interstitial lung water and pleural fluid production. Most effusions are small and resolve with resolution of the bacterial pneumonia.[9] Complicated parapneumonic pleural effusion develops when the pleural fluid has a high enough protein content to clot. The clotting causes fibrin strands to span the visceral and parietal pleurae. The net result is collection of pleural fluid into different loculi within the pleural cavity. These cannot be drained by a single chest tube.

Progression to **empyema** is marked by the presence of bacteria within the pleural space, seen as pus or bacteria with Gram stain. Empyema necessitates drainage. Whether complicated parapneumonic effusions necessitate drainage remains controversial, although most physicians perform drainage because some of these effusions can progress to empyema.[10]

Parapneumonic effusions are common causes of persistent fever among intensive care unit (ICU) patients with pneumonia. Sampling by thoracentesis is commonly performed to exclude empyema. Pleural fluid drainage can improve ventilation if the fluid volume is large.

Viral Pleurisy

Viral lung infections can cause pleural inflammation, small pleural effusions, and pain. The effusions may be so small they may be overlooked on a routine chest radiograph, and even when they can be seen, the effusions often are too small to sample. Pleural pain, which is called *pleurodynia*, and which can be the result of many other pleural processes, often is difficult to manage. The typical patient with pleurodynia has shallow respirations; deeper breaths are limited by pain. The subsequent atelectasis can cause oxygenation difficulty caused by shunting.

Tuberculous Pleurisy

In many parts of the world, any lymphocyte-predominant exudative effusion is considered tuberculosis until proved otherwise. Tuberculous pleural effusions occur when a caseous granuloma in the lung ruptures through the visceral pleural surface causing an exudative inflammatory effusion. Experiments in which purified protein derivative (PPD) is placed into the pleural space of animals have shown that such effusions result from the body's immune reaction to tuberculin proteins.

Although these patients need respiratory isolation, only 25% of them have sputum that subsequently grows *Mycobacterium tuberculosis*. The PPD skin test result is negative in 30% of patients when they come to medical attention but turns positive in 6 to 8 weeks in almost everyone.[11]

Malignant

Malignant disease is the most common cause of large unilateral pleural effusions among persons older than 60 years. Common cancers that form malignant pleural effusions include lung cancer and breast cancer, although any cancer can metastasize to the pleural surface. The effusions usually are lymphocyte predominant; malignant cells are found during cytologic examination of the pleural fluid.

Some malignant pleural effusions, such as those from lymphoma, respond to therapy for the malignant disease. However, patients with symptoms who have the common pleural fluid malignancies need primary therapy with **pleurodesis**, which is fusion of the pleural membranes to obliterate the pleural space.

Postoperative

A variety of operations involving the chest or upper abdomen produce pleural fluid.[12] Effusions following cardiac surgery usually are predominant on the left side and tend to be bloody. These effusions are particularly prevalent after a cutdown of the internal mammary artery for coronary artery bypass.

Small transudative pleural effusions are common when there is any atelectasis in the lung. Upper abdominal operations cause inflammation of the diaphragm and effusion that has been termed *sympathetic*. Lung surgery in which the lung is unable to fill the thoracic cavity leaves a space under negative pressure, which fills with inflammatory pleural fluid. When the lung is unable to fill the space because of small postoperative size or visceral pleural fibrosis, the resulting pleural effusion can never be completely drained because of the "trapped lung."

Chylothorax

The thoracic duct is a lymphatic channel that runs from the abdomen through the mediastinum to enter the left subclavian vein. Disruption of the thoracic duct anywhere along its course can cause leakage of chyle into the mediastinum, which then may rupture into the pleural space. The most common causes of rupture are as follows: malignancy (50%), surgery (20%), and trauma (5%).[13] The thoracic duct courses through the right side of the mediastinum in the lower thoracic cavity before crossing to the left side of the mediastinum at T4 to T6. Rupture below this level causes right-sided pleural effusion, whereas rupture above this level causes left-sided pleural effusion.

In a patient who has eaten recently, the effusions are milky white as a result of the presence of chylomicrons (microscopic fat particles) absorbed by abdominal lymphatic vessels. In a fasting patient, these effusions usually are yellow and may be bloody. A pleural fluid triglyceride concentration greater than 110 mg/dL confirms the diagnosis.[14] Computed tomography (CT) should be performed to evaluate the cause of the chylothorax.

Hemothorax

Hemothorax is the presence of blood in the pleural space. Hemothorax is arbitrarily defined as a pleural fluid hematocrit more than 50% greater than the serum value. It must be understood that small amounts of blood in otherwise clear fluid can turn the fluid red.

Although hemothorax is seen most commonly after blunt or penetrating chest trauma, a number of medical conditions can give rise to blood in the pleural space. These should be considered in the absence of trauma. Any vein or artery in the thorax can bleed into the pleural space. A chest tube usually is inserted to monitor the rate of bleeding and determine whether the source is arterial or venous.[15]

Connective Tissue Diseases

Pleural effusions are found in a variety of connective diseases, although the effusions usually are small. Effusions caused by inflammation of small blood vessels are the most common chest manifestation of systemic lupus erythematosus (SLE). Pleural effusions often accompany pericardial effusions in SLE and disappear with corticosteroid therapy.

Rheumatoid arthritis produces a characteristic effusion with a very low glucose content and low pH. These effusions can cause visceral pleural fibrosis and a trapped lung.

Uremic

Uremic pleurisy occurs under the same conditions as uremic pericarditis. The typical patient is undergoing dialysis, and the dialysis is inadequate. Although the cause of pleural and pericardial inflammation in kidney failure remains unknown, the inflammatory process can take weeks to resolve.

Miscellaneous Causes

Discussion of the other causes of exudative effusions is beyond the scope of this chapter. Nevertheless, thoracentesis that yields findings compatible with any of the systemic diseases listed in Box 22-1 can narrow the differential diagnosis.

Physiological Importance

Mechanics of Ventilation

Pleural effusions cause lung atelectasis because the capacity of the thorax is limited, and fluid collapses the lung. Spirometry shows restriction. Studies correlating the volume of pleural fluid removed with improvement in forced vital capacity (FVC) show much variability from patient to patient.

> **RULE OF THUMB**
>
> The patient's vital capacity improves by one third of the pleural fluid volume removed.[16] The remainder of the pleural fluid volume causes diaphragmatic compression and chest wall expansion. Some patients have a delay of 24 to 48 hours before the improvement can be seen as atelectasis resolves. Lack of any improvement suggests that lung consolidation or endobronchial obstruction is present.

Dyspnea is common with small pleural effusions, even when lung mechanics are relatively preserved. The mechanisms remain unknown but likely involve activation of stretch receptors, irritant receptors within the airways, or nonadrenergic, noncholinergic C fibers in the chest wall or diaphragm. The net result is that dyspnea relief is variable after pleural fluid removal. Some patients have symptomatic relief after removal of small pleural fluid volumes. Others can actually have more dyspnea if the fluid is removed in situations such as trapped lung, in which neural activation may increase with fluid withdrawal.

In rare instances, the pleura thickens with a disease process sufficient to cause fibrothorax. Technically, fibrothorax is any process that causes fibrosis of the thoracic cage that affects pulmonary function. Fibrothorax can be caused by skin (such as fibrothorax that occurs rarely in scleroderma), soft tissue, bone (e.g., myositis ossificans, a disease in which muscles calcify), or pleura. The causes of pleural thickening significant enough to produce restriction include severe asbestos pleurisy, rheumatoid pleurisy, complicated trauma, cancer, and empyema.

Hypoxemia

Most patients with a pleural effusion have an increased alveolar-arterial (A-a) gradient resulting from the pathologic changes in the lung that are causing the effusion. Oxygenation can worsen after thoracentesis because changes in ventilation-perfusion matching are not instantaneous. Recovery to baseline PO_2 and subsequent small improvement usually occur within 90 minutes.[16]

Diagnostic Tests

Chest Radiography

The chest radiograph is the most common method of detecting a pleural effusion. It is important that, if possible, the chest radiograph be obtained with the patient in an upright position to show a pleural fluid meniscus at the costophrenic angles. When the same patient undergoes radiography in the supine position, the effusion is distributed throughout the posterior part of the chest. The chest radiograph shows a generalized haze, which interferes with the detection of pulmonary infiltrates and quantification of pleural effusion.

A lateral decubitus chest radiograph helps delineate the presence or absence of pleural effusion. Although pleural fluid volumes of as little as 5 mL may be seen on a lateral decubitus chest radiograph, the presence of a 1-cm meniscus from the lung to the rib margin suggests that the effusion is large enough for safe sampling by means of thoracentesis. Bilateral decubitus chest radiographs can ensure that any pleural thickening is differentiated from a free-flowing effusion. These radiographs also can show underlying parenchymal lung abnormalities when the effusion is moved toward the mediastinum.

Ultrasonography and Computed Tomography

Pleural fluid and loculi can be detected easily with ultrasonography of the chest. The sensitivity of ultrasonography for pleural effusions is high, although ultrasonography is an operator-dependent study.

Computed tomography of the chest is the most sensitive study for identification of pleural effusion. A contrast-enhanced scan is essential to delineate the pleural membrane and differentiate peripheral lung consolidation from pleural fluid formation. In addition to showing the size and location of a pleural effusion, the chest CT scan often gives information about the underlying lung parenchyma and the primary process causing the effusion.

Thoracentesis

In thoracentesis, pleural fluid is sampled percutaneously by means of insertion of a needle into the pleural space (Figure 22-3). Administration of adequate local anesthetic ensures a painless procedure if care is taken to place lidocaine at the skin insertion site, along the periosteum of the involved rib, and at the parietal pleura, which is richly innervated with sensory nerve fibers. Diagnostic sampling of pleural fluid for cell counts, cultures, chemistries, and cytologic examination usually can be performed with a single syringe and a small needle. Samples for pleural pH should be kept from contact with room air. Pleural fluid drainage with lung reexpansion involves more extensive placement of the catheter into the pleural space.

Thoracentesis involves the following three major risks: (1) intercostal artery laceration, (2) infection, and (3) pneumothorax.[17] Both an artery and a vein course under every rib, and the vessels become increasingly serpiginous with aging. Ensuring needle passage just superior to the rib margin makes bleeding during thoracentesis rare.

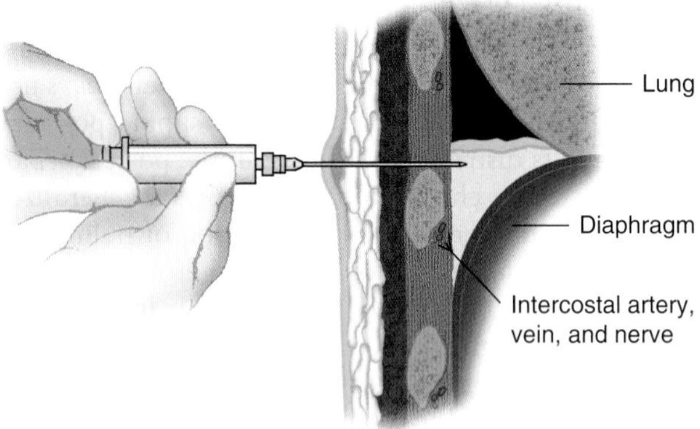

Figure 22-3
The technique of thoracentesis involves passage of a needle just superior to the rib. If the needle is placed too high on the chest, the lung can be punctured, and air is withdrawn. If the needle is placed too low on the chest, the diaphragm or organs below the diaphragm can be punctured. Diagnostic thoracentesis can be performed with small amounts of pleural fluid.

Because infection can be introduced into the pleural space, a totally sterile procedure is necessary. In some situations the risk of infection is so high that thoracentesis rarely should be performed. When a lung is surgically removed, the space fills with sterile fluid. An infection introduced into this space usually necessitates open surgical drainage. Any trapped lung also carries a high risk of empyema because of the inability of the visceral and parietal pleurae to meet and contain any infectious process. Needle puncture remains one of the most common causes of pneumothorax (see later, Pneumothorax).

Chest Thoracotomy Tubes

Chest tubes currently are manufactured in a variety of sizes and shapes, from 7F to 40F catheters. Catheter choice is frequently a matter of physician preference. Larger tubes are less likely to become obstructed and are capable of high airflow rates.

Intercostal placement is designed for the skin and soft tissue to approximate the tube and prevent air from entering the pleural space from the outside. The chest tube is then connected to a water-sealed chamber, which usually is contained within a commercially marketed three-bottle system that also regulates pleural pressure and is used to measure pleural fluid volume (Figure 22-4).

Thoracoscopy

The video-assisted thoracoscope is ideally designed for diagnostic and therapeutic work in the pleural space. Diagnostic thoracoscopy often is performed in a medical procedure room with the use of local anesthesia and conscious sedation. The procedure involves placing the thoracoscope through an intercostal incision for visualization of the lung surfaces, drainage of pleural fluid, biopsy under direct visualization, and pleurodesis if needed.

Pleurodesis

Pleurodesis is the process of fusing the parietal and visceral pleurae with a fibrotic reaction that prevents further pleural fluid formation. Methods to produce pleural symphysis include surgical abrasion and the application of intrapleural chemicals such as doxycycline, minocycline, and talc. Talc has been applied as a powder suspended in sterile saline solution and injected through the chest tube (talc slurry) or dusted through a thoracoscope (talc insufflation). The success of talc pleurodesis, approximately 90%, is higher than

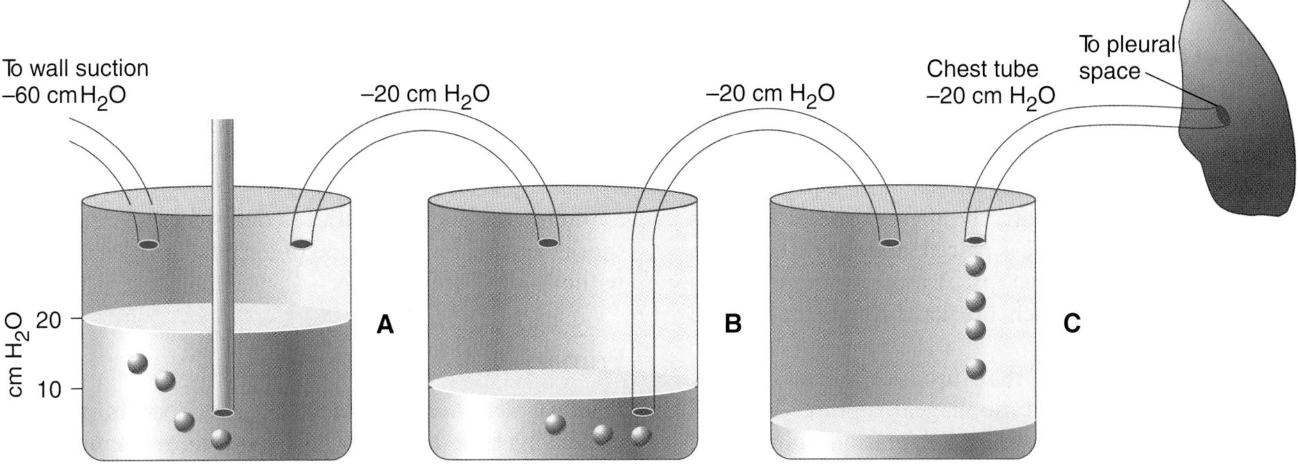

Figure 22-4

The standard three-bottle system is the basis for all commercial chest tube drainage systems. Pleural fluid and pleural air enter compartment **C**, which serves as a fluid collection trap so that the water-seal fluid volume will not rise (compartment B) and create resistance to air escaping the chest. Air cannot be inspired into the chest because of the water in compartment **B**. Open entrainment of room air through a submerged tube in compartment **A** buffers the amount of wall suction applied (–60 cm H_20) to the height of the water column to standardize the pressure (–20 cm H_20) transmitted to the chest.

that of all alternatives except surgical abrasion.[18,19] Pleurodesis is used most commonly in the management of symptomatic pleural effusions caused by cancer.

Although pleurodesis of benign effusions, such as those occurring with CHF, nephrotic syndrome, and idiopathic chylothorax, have been performed successfully, the procedure is discouraged for pleural effusions that are not malignant. Most pleural effusions are best managed by control of the underlying condition.[20]

Pleuroperitoneal Shunt and Pleurex Catheter

In refractory pleural effusions that cannot be treated adequately with pleurodesis, a small pump can be placed subcutaneously, and tubes are placed in the pleural and peritoneal spaces. The pleuroperitoneal connection must have a one-way valve and a pumping mechanism to allow the patient to expel pleural fluid from the negatively pressurized chest to the positively pressurized peritoneum. The pleuroperitoneal shunt is placed as a last resort for refractory pleural effusions for which there is no other treatment. A Pleurex catheter has an adapter for connection to vacuum bottles. It is inserted into the pleural space so that pleural fluid can be removed at home for recurrent effusions.

▶ PNEUMOTHORAX

Pneumothorax is air in the pleural space. Although air can enter the pleural space from outside the body, as occurs in sucking chest wounds, most cases of pneumothorax occur when disruption of the visceral pleura allows air from the lung to enter the pleural space. Pneumothorax is discussed according to etiologic factor because traumatic pneumothorax is managed differently from spontaneous pneumothorax.

Spontaneous pneumothoraces are of two types: (1) **primary spontaneous pneumothorax**, in which there is no underlying lung disease, and (2) **secondary spontaneous pneumothorax**, in which lung disease is present.

Chest pain, which is typically sharp and abrupt, occurs in nearly every patient with pneumothorax. Palpation of the chest wall does not worsen the pain, although respiratory efforts may be difficult. Dyspnea occurs in approximately two thirds of patients when decreases in vital capacity and PO_2, probably due to airway closure at low lung volumes, cause ventilation-perfusion defects and shunting. When spontaneous pneumothorax is evacuated, hypoxemia may persist in some patients.

The following sections describe the diseases that cause pneumothorax and the important treatment differences between them.

Traumatic

Blunt and Penetrating Chest Trauma

Traumatic pneumothorax can be caused by either blunt or penetrating wounds of the thorax. The common causes of penetrating wounds include gunshots and knife punctures. In many cases, penetrating trauma to the chest can be managed conservatively with a chest tube. The clear indications for entering the chest surgically are uncontrolled bleeding from intercostal or pulmonary arteries and injury to the heart or great vessels. In these situations, the pneumothorax becomes secondary. The chest tube is multifunctional to allow measurement of the rate of bleeding, to allow the lung to be pulled to the parietal pleural surface to tamponade bleeding, and to allow maximum ventilation.

In blunt trauma to the chest, pneumothorax can be the result of a rib fracture that enters the lung parenchyma and allows air to leak into the pleural space. For this type of injury, a chest tube is placed, and the rib fractures necessitate no specific therapy. A more common injury is alveolar rupture, which breaks through the pleural membrane.

Two special injuries that produce pneumothorax are tracheal fracture and esophageal rupture. Tracheal fracture results from severe deceleration injury and often occurs in concert with fractures of the anterior aspect of the first through third ribs. In this case, urgent bronchoscopy is appropriate because tracheal fracture must be corrected surgically. Esophageal rupture produces an air fluid level in the pleural space. Pleural fluid amylase level is elevated from a salivary source.

Large-caliber chest tubes are placed for trauma-related pneumothoraces to allow exit of blood and blood clots, which can be difficult to remove through small-bore catheters. Air leaks from an injured lung can be large. When bleeding is a major component of pleural injury, two chest tubes are used: a posterior chest tube to drain blood that is gravity dependent and an anterior and apical chest tube to drain air that moves to the lung apex in the absence of pleural disease.

Iatrogenic

Iatrogenic pneumothorax is the most common type of traumatic pneumothorax. Common causes are punctures of the lung from needle aspiration lung biopsy, thoracentesis, and central venous catheter placement. Unusual causes, such as Dobbhoff tube placement into the pleural space, also have been recorded. Because the pleural rupture is typically small in the absence of parenchymal lung disease, these lung punctures usually resolve within 24 hours and can be observed without chest tubes as long as serial radiographs are obtained.

Neonatal

In radiographic series, spontaneous pneumothorax occurs in 1% to 2% of all infants soon after birth.[21] The cause of pneumothorax is likely high transpulmonary pressure during birth coupled with transient bronchial blockade caused by meconium, mucus, or aspiration of blood that can produce transpulmonary pressure gradients as high as 100 cm H_2O.

Recognizing pneumothorax is difficult because breath sounds are transmitted widely through the chest of the neonate. A shift of the heart sounds away from the side of the pneumothorax may provide a clue. Transillumination of the chest with a high-intensity light is used in some centers. Almost all neonates with pneumothorax need a chest tube.

Spontaneous

Spontaneous pneumothorax is defined as any pneumothorax caused by the escape of air into the pleural space without an obvious cause.

Primary

Primary spontaneous pneumothorax occurs without underlying lung disease. In a way, this term is a misnomer because high-resolution CT scans have shown the presence of small subpleural blebs in more than 80% of patients.[22]

Primary spontaneous pneumothorax usually occurs in patients in their late teenage years or early twenties. Patients often are tall and slender, and the lungs and pleural membrane may not have grown at the same pace; the result is airspace enlargement and a thin pleural membrane.

Results of some studies suggest that cigarette smoking is a risk factor in more than 90% of cases of primary spontaneous pneumothorax.[23] The smoking history is typically short, and smoking cessation is recommended.

Secondary

Secondary spontaneous pneumothorax occurs in patients with underlying lung disease. In most cases, the underlying lung disease is chronic obstructive pulmonary disease with some component of emphysema. Pneumothorax also can occur with asthma and cystic fibrosis, usually during an exacerbation of disease.

Interstitial lung diseases in which lung volumes are spared, such as sarcoidosis, bronchiolitis obliterans with organizing pneumonia, histiocytosis X, and lymphangioleiomyomatosis, have a higher incidence than do diseases without any component of obstruction, such as idiopathic pulmonary fibrosis.

Depending on the extent of parenchymal lung disease, pneumothorax in this population can be devastating. A Veterans Affairs cooperative study included 185 patients with secondary spontaneous pneumothorax and monitored them for 5 years.[24] Although only three patients died of pneumothorax, the mortality rate was 43%.[1] Severe underlying lung disease caused most of these deaths. This finding suggested that most pneumothoraces occur in patients with severe lung dysfunction. The degree of dyspnea is disproportionate to the size of pneumothorax in this group of patients because pulmonary reserve is already diminished. Pneumothorax usually should be evacuated and not observed in this patient cohort.

Catamenial

Catamenial pneumothorax occurs in conjunction with menstruation and usually is recurrent and right-sided. The reason for the right-sided predominance is unclear. Many patients have endometriosis on the pleural surface, although it may be impossible to see because of hormonal involution during menses. Once the diagnosis is considered, catamenial pneumothorax is not difficult to manage in that most patients do not have a recurrence when ovulation is suppressed.

Complications

Tension Pneumothorax

Tension pneumothorax occurs when air in the pleural space exceeds atmospheric pressure. The radiographic appearance includes mediastinal shift to the contralateral side, diaphragmatic depression, and expansion of the ribs. The lung does not necessarily collapse completely if it is involved with a disease process such as acute respiratory distress syndrome (ARDS).

Not all patients with radiographic tension have the physiological changes commonly associated with tension pneumothorax. However, almost all pneumothoraces that occur during mechanical ventilation enlarge if not drained.

As pressure in the thorax increases and mediastinal shift places torsion on the inferior vena cava, venous return to the right side of the heart decreases. Cardiac output decreases, and hypotension with tachycardia results. Hypoxemia occurs as the lung continues to compress because of intrapulmonary shunting through the collapsed lung.

The respiratory therapist can make the diagnosis of tension pneumothorax. Treatment is emergency decompression of the chest. This procedure usually is done with an 18-gauge Jelco catheter inserted just over the second rib on the anterior aspect of the chest in the midclavicular line. Catheter placement should elicit a rush of air through the catheter, and this sign confirms the diagnosis. Blood pressure recovery should be rapid, although resolution of hypoxemia depends on complete lung reexpansion and can be delayed. The soft Jelco catheter can be left in place while a more conventional chest tube is inserted.

MINI CLINI

Subcutaneous Emphysema

PROBLEM

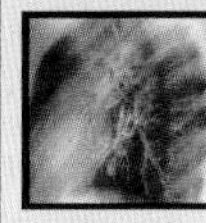

A patient with ARDS experiences subcutaneous emphysema. How do you determine where the air leak is occurring? Is a pneumothorax always present?

SOLUTION

Subcutaneous emphysema occurs when air enters the soft tissues. Although physical examination reveals subcutaneous bubbles, the patient's family needs to be reassured that the condition is rarely, if ever, physiologically significant. What is important to recognize, however, is that alveolar disruption has occurred, most commonly as the result of barotrauma.

Barotrauma disrupts alveoli and allows air to enter the interstitium of the lung. Rupture of the visceral pleura allows air to produce pneumothorax, or the air can travel along the low-resistance tissue planes of the bronchovascular bundles and through the hilum of the lung to enter the mediastinum. From the mediastinum, air has easy access to the retroperitoneal space, including the scrotum and the neck. The presence of subcutaneous air does not necessarily mean that pneumothorax has occurred, although the risk factors for its development are present. Air under pressure in the pleural space can enter the subcutaneous tissues through the intercostal incision made for chest tube placement. Subcutaneous air often is seen on a chest radiograph after chest tube placement, but the air rarely spreads unless the chest tube is occluded.

In the absence of pneumothorax, there is no way to determine which lung is causing subcutaneous emphysema. For any deterioration in gas exchange, radiographs should be repeated. Because air in the mediastinum can displace the mediastinal parietal pleura, it can be difficult to tell without chest CT whether a small pneumothorax is present. Because patients often are in too unstable condition to be moved, a chest tube sometimes is placed because the potential benefits are greater than the risks.

RULE OF THUMB

Tension pneumothorax is a clinical diagnosis made at the bedside in more than 50% of cases. The clinical signs are diminished breath sounds, hyperresonance to percussion, tachycardia, and hypotension.

In one case series of 74 patients with tension pneumothorax, a clinical diagnosis was made for 45 patients; the associated mortality rate was 7%. In the other cases, the diagnosis was delayed from the onset of clinical signs by 30 minutes to 8 hours, resulting in a 31% mortality rate.[25]

Respiratory therapists are in the perfect position to make a timely diagnosis because ventilator alarms give early warnings.

Reexpansion Pulmonary Edema

Reexpansion pulmonary edema occurs in a lung that has been rapidly reinflated from low lung volumes, particularly when the pneumothorax has been longstanding or when the pressure gradient across the lung has become high, as might occur when there is endobronchial obstruction from cancer, mucus, or blood.

For many years, it was believed that alveolar edema occurs because intraalveolar pressure becomes negative and pulls fluid from the vasculature. However, the lung fluid has a high protein content, a finding that suggests blood vessels have been injured as well.

One of the proposed mechanisms of vascular injury is a phenomenon of reperfusion injury caused by reactive oxygen species. Support for this hypothesis has come from experimental studies that have shown administration of antioxidants before reexpansion decreases the amount of reexpansion pulmonary edema.

Regardless of the cause, lung reexpansion in nonemergency situations should proceed slowly, and transpulmonary pressure should not become excessive. Most physicians who insert a chest tube for a large pneumothorax first place it to water seal without suction. If the lung is not completely inflated on the subsequent chest radiograph, the chest tube is placed to suction. Reexpansion pulmonary edema also occurs after drainage of pleural effusions. As a rule, thoracentesis should be limited to 1000 mL, unless pleural pressures are monitored and not allowed to fall below –20 cm H_2O.

Diagnosis

The diagnosis of pneumothorax is established with chest radiography. The diagnosis requires a high-quality film for visualization of a visceral pleural line. In the ICU, as many as 30% of cases of pneumothorax may be missed in retrospect on a chest radiograph. Impediments to diagnosis include a low-quality radiograph, supine position of the patient, concomitant presence of mediastinal air, and subpulmonic or mediastinal position of the pneumothorax. Diagnosis is enhanced with additional upright radiographs or decubitus views.

The size of a pneumothorax is difficult to assess with a chest radiograph because a two-dimensional picture is being taken of a three-dimensional thorax. Size can be confirmed with CT if needed.

RULE OF THUMB

The size of a pneumothorax on a chest radiograph can be estimated with the knowledge that the volume of the lung and thorax is proportional to the cube of their diameters.

For example, on a chest radiograph, the chest measures 8 cm from the spine to the lateral chest wall. A pneumothorax is measured 2 cm from the chest wall.

Volume of the lung ≈ $(6\ \text{cm})^3 = 216\ \text{cm}^3$
Volume of the hemithorax ≈ $(8\ \text{cm})^3 = 512\ \text{cm}^3$
Lung size = 216/512 = 42%
Pneumothorax size ≈ 58%

The equation shows the large volume of lung that a pneumothorax can displace despite a "small" distance from the lung to the chest wall. Use of the equation is not as accurate as chest CT because many pneumothoraces collapse asymmetrically.

Therapy

Oxygen

Oxygen should be administered to all patients who have a pneumothorax. Most of the air in a pneumothorax is nitrogen because oxygen is readily absorbed. If an air leak is continuing, supplemental oxygen rather than nitrogen leaks into the pleural space. After an air leak has been stopped, administration of oxygen decreases the blood and tissue partial pressure of nitrogen surrounding the pleural space. Pneumothorax resolution is normally 1.25% of the air per day. Oxygen speeds recovery by increasing the gradient of nitrogen from the pleural space to the pleural tissues.

Observation

A 2001 consensus conference recommended observation of patients in stable condition with primary spontaneous pneumothorax and of some patients with small secondary spontaneous pneumothorax before recurrence prevention is administered.[26] Small iatrogenic pneumothorax also should be managed with observation. Primary spontaneous pneumothorax often is observed for 4 hours in the emergency department before discharge to home follow-up care as long as no pneumothorax enlargement is found on chest radiographs. Discharged patients should have ready access to emergency care facilities.

Patients with secondary spontaneous pneumothorax should be admitted to the hospital. During observation, it is important to record the respiratory rate and any signs of deteriorating respiratory function. An oximetry decrease can be an early warning of pneumothorax enlargement. Any deterioration indicates that the pneumothorax must be drained.

Simple Aspiration

Simple aspiration can be used in the emergency department when pneumothorax is first identified. A small catheter is placed into the pleural space, and air is sequentially evacuated with a three-way stopcock until no more air can be removed. If more than 4 L of air is aspirated and no resistance to further aspiration is felt, a chest tube is needed for continuing pleural air leak.

The goal of aspiration is to reexpand the lung. Many patients have a pneumothorax from air leak that subsequently heals between the time of onset and the time treatment is sought in the emergency department. Patients with primary spontaneous pneumothorax who undergo simple aspiration for lung reexpansion and who have a stable chest radiograph 4 hours after aspiration can go home without hospital admission.

Chest Tubes

Chest thoracostomy tubes (chest tubes) come in a variety of sizes, from 7F to 40F, and can be connected to a variety of one-way devices (e.g., Heimlich valves) that prevent entry of air into the pleural space from the outside environment. Regardless of chest tube size and the presence of a Heimlich valve or water seal, the effectiveness of chest tube placement for pneumothorax resolution depends more on lung surface healing than on the device used.

Small-Bore. One simple device is a small-bore 7F catheter with a one-way valve apparatus (Heimlich valve) that prevents air movement back into the chest. Small-bore catheters can be placed with a small skin incision, although they do require a trocar for transthoracic placement, and the trocar can injure the lung.

All chest tubes used to drain pneumothorax should be directed to the apex of the lung. Small-bore catheters can be placed in the second intercostal space anteriorly in the midclavicular line or laterally in the chest from the fifth through the seventh intercostal space.

It is difficult to determine whether a Heimlich valve has an ongoing leak unless it is placed to underwater seal. This procedure can be done in the emergency department by placing the Heimlich valve into a cup of water or by placing it in line with a water-seal chamber to see whether an air leak is continuing after lung expansion.

Large-Bore. Large-bore chest tubes usually are connected to a commercial equivalent of a three-bottle system to collect any pleural fluid present, to determine whether an air leak is ongoing, and to measure intrapleural pressure (Figure 22-5). Insertion of large-bore catheters is accomplished with local anesthetic and blunt dissection of soft tissue down to the parietal pleura.

Dissection should be wide enough to allow insertion of a finger into the pleural space to ensure that no adhesions are holding the lung close to the insertion site and to allow unobstructed entrance of the tube into the pleural space, where it can be directed to the position of choice.

Chest tubes are secured with sutures. The insertion distance should be recorded and be checked on subsequent days to ensure that the chest tube does not migrate outward. Should the most proximal hole in the tube emerge from the skin, air will enter the tube, and it will appear as if the lung is persistently leaking.

Another problem of apparent chest tube leak can occur when the insertion wound is large enough to allow air entry into the pleural space. This usually is accompanied by a sucking sound at the entrance, which can be occluded with petroleum gauze.

A chest radiograph is routinely obtained, although unless a lateral radiograph also is obtained, confirmation of precise placement often is difficult. In addition, many chest tubes end up in the major fissure, where their function may be suboptimal.

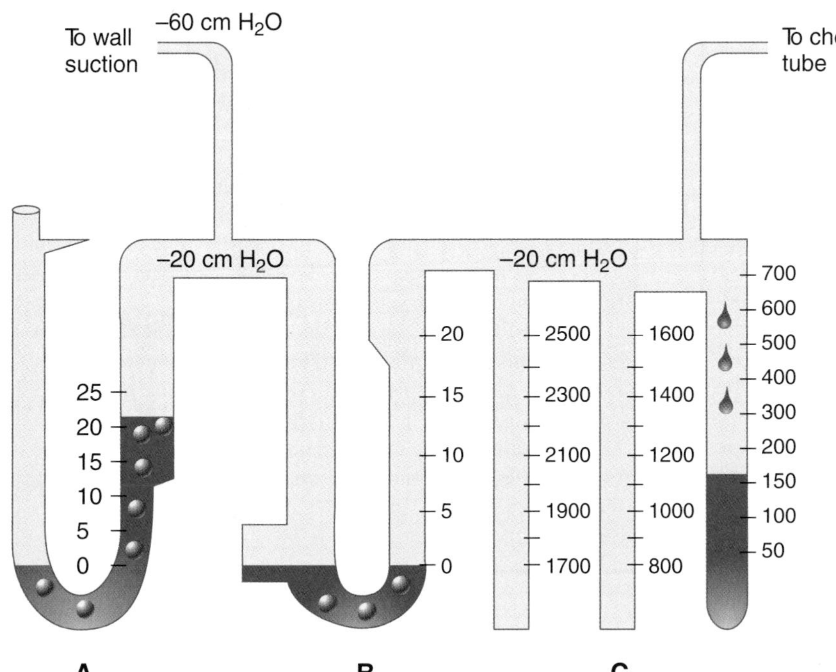

Figure 22-5 The Pleur-evac chest tube collection system collects fluid in compartment **C** so that it will not spill into the water-seal compartment (**B**). A patent chest tube should cause respiratory variation to be seen on the scale adjacent to compartment **B**, which measures intrapleural pressure. Compartment **B** also is the place to see bubbles if an air leak is present. The water level in compartment **A** controls intrapleural pressure and should be adjusted daily.

Chest tube removal remains a highly variable practice. Removal of a chest tube as soon as an air leak visually ceases is associated with a 25% rate of recurrence of pneumothorax. The recurrence rate is near zero when chest tubes are removed 48 hours after the air leak no longer is seen in the water-seal chamber.[27] A common practice of clamping the chest tube, with chest radiographs before and after a 4-hour observation period, can be accompanied by the return of pneumothorax. If symptoms develop during chest tube clamping, the clamp should be removed immediately, and the presence of air leak assessed.

Bronchopleural Fistula

Although any air leak from the lung through a chest tube is technically considered a *bronchopleural fistula* (BPF), the term often is reserved for large air leaks that

MINI CLINI

Bronchopleural Fistula

PROBLEM

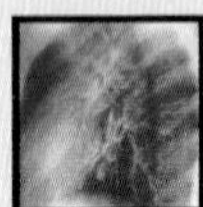

Pneumothorax develops in a patient undergoing ventilation for pneumonia. A 20F chest tube is placed, and the lung fails to reexpand, although a large amount of air is passing through the water-seal chamber. The patient's minute ventilation is 20 L/min to keep gas exchange stable. What is the problem?

SOLUTION

The problem is a BPF caused by a large hole in the pleura, which is difficult to manage. The lung surface of patients with underlying emphysema can contain large bullae that do not heal readily once ruptured. Large pleural holes also can develop in patients with necrotizing pneumonia and those who have undergone surgery on the lung.

The Fanning equation tells us that humidified airflow through a chest tube is proportional to the chest tube radius to the fifth power. Therefore the chest tube radius is the most important determinant of maximal airflow. Airflow through large BPFs has been measured as high as 16 L/min, a volume impossible to remove through a chest tube smaller than 24F, regardless of the amount of pressure applied.

This patient should receive a second, larger chest tube. The seal of the chest tube at the skin surface should be inspected to ensure that no air is entering the body from the outside. The position of both chest tubes should be confirmed either radiographically or manually to ensure the tubes are in the pleural space. Once the lung is expanded, the minute ventilation should decrease because effective alveolar ventilation will be improved.

Flow through stopcocks and chest tube collection devices is governed by the same considerations as chest tube size. The manufacturer of the chest tube collection device in your hospital will have the resistance figures necessary to ensure that 16 L/min of airflow can be accommodated.

MINI CLINI

Measuring a BPF

PROBLEM

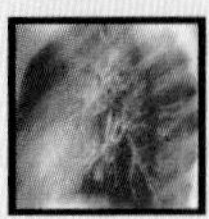

Pneumothorax develops in a patient with ARDS, and a chest tube is placed to reexpand the lung. Before the pneumothorax developed, the patient was ventilated easily at a rate of 16 breaths/min, which delivered a tidal volume (V_T) of 700 mL, and was exhaling 650 mL (a small difference caused by endotracheal cuff leak and tubing compliance). Since the pneumothorax developed, the patient needs a rate of 30 breaths at the same V_T to keep the $Pa{CO_2}$ level the same. Exhaled V_T is 500 mL. What is the approximate size of this patient's BPF? What ventilation options are appropriate?

SOLUTION

Although research laboratories can measure bronchopleural airflow through a chest tube with a pneumotachometer, clinical care can be provided by estimating the pleural air leak.

The following simple calculations suggest that the excess difference in returned V_T (650–500 mL) is due to air passing through the BPF:

30 breaths/min × 150 mL differential = 4.5 L of pleural ventilation

The problem is that large amounts of CO_2 (up to 20%) may be removed through the chest tube.[29] Removal of CO_2 is beneficial because it allows lower V_T and respiratory rates for any given $P{CO_2}$. However, as the BPF closes, CO_2 will have to be eliminated from the endotracheal tube, necessitating higher minute ventilation. The higher respiratory rates and V_T indicate a BPF size that is not improving when the true air leak is decreased.

Nevertheless, when the air leak is measured with every ventilatory change, the mode of ventilation that minimizes air leak is the one most likely to allow pleural healing. Breath-by-breath analysis shows the difference between delivered V_T and exhaled V_T and approximates the volume of the pleural leak.

PEEP can be a major cause of large BPF and should be turned off. Because there is no such thing as a true plateau pressure when air is exiting a BPF, V_T should be adjusted to produce the lowest peak airway pressure that can sustain ventilation and oxygenation. Position the patient so that the lung with the air leak is in the bed.[30]

Auto-PEEP can be impossible to measure if the fistula is large and decompressing the airways. Therefore, long expiratory times are preferred. Trials of pressure-controlled and high-frequency jet ventilation are appropriate. In a practical sense, these adjustments are the same ones made to prevent barotrauma in the first place and are limited by the severity of lung injury, which requires more support than would optimally close the BPF.

MINI CLINI

Management of BPF

PROBLEM

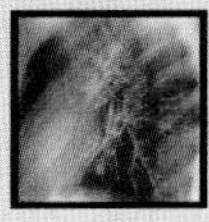

A 40-year-old trauma patient with ARDS cannot be ventilated because of a large (16 L/min) BPF located entirely in the left lung. If surgery is not possible, what ventilatory options would be appropriate?

SOLUTION

Two ventilatory interventions have been attempted for large BPFs. The first is placement of a double-lumen endotracheal tube, which can carry most ventilation and PEEP on the right lung while underventilating the lung with the fistula to aid in its closure.[31] Long-term double-lumen ventilation is difficult for the following reasons: tenuous tube position, the need for continuous paralysis, difficulty with secretion clearance, and high airway resistance through the small endotracheal tube lumens.

The second intervention is application of positive pressure to the chest tube. This back pressure increases resistance across the BPF and allows the remainder of the lung to better ventilate. One simple way to add chest tube resistance is to connect a PEEP valve to the expiratory port of the water-seal chamber.[32] PEEP usually is placed at the same level as the ventilator. Inspiratory pressures exceed PEEP, and air flows through the chest tube. However, as expiratory pressures equilibrate, PEEP can be held within the lung, allowing the beneficial effects on oxygenation.

Pressurizing the chest tube entails synchronous closure of the chest tube during inspiration[33] and requires specialized equipment, which must be set up under controlled conditions. When used in combination with an in-line PEEP valve, BPF flow can be slowed during both inspiration and expiration.

These techniques usually increase the volume of intrapleural air. The net effect on oxygenation necessitates careful bedside observation because hypoxemia can worsen with any degree of lung collapse. Tension pneumothorax can occur and should be managed expectantly.

do not heal rapidly. Many patients with a BPF are receiving mechanical ventilation, and positive airway pressures contribute to the perpetuation of pleural air.

Because a BPF can leak large quantities of air, more than one chest tube may be used to approximate the lung to the chest wall. This maneuver results in tamponade of the site of the air leak and allows pleural healing to occur.

Therapy for BPF involves meticulous monitoring of tidal volume, airway pressures, and positive end-expiratory pressure (PEEP); avoidance of auto-PEEP; and consideration of bronchoscopic closure or thoracoscopic surgery.[28]

Pleurodesis

Patients who have had one pneumothorax are more likely than is the general population to have a second. The recurrence rate is greater than 30% among patients with primary spontaneous pneumothorax and approximately 40% among patients with secondary spontaneous pneumothorax. These high recurrence rates indicate that prevention of recurrence of pneumothorax should be undertaken, particularly for patients in whom pneumothorax may be life threatening. Preventing recurrence involves production of adhesions between the parietal and the visceral pleura in the involved area and is termed **pleurodesis**.

The most noninvasive approaches to pleurodesis entail chemical sclerosis of the pleural space through the chest tube once the pleural air leak has ceased. The two most common preparations used currently in the United States include 500 mg of doxycycline or 5 g of talc mixed into a 50-mL syringe of sterile saline solution. The agent is injected through the chest tube into the pleural space. Then the chest tube is clamped for 2 hours before drainage is allowed.

More invasive methods have included thoracoscopy with pleural poudrage (blowing talc onto the pleural surface under direct visualization), pleural abrasion through a thoracoscope, and thoracotomy with pleurectomy (removing the pleural surface to ensure lung adhesion). Recent recommendations are pleurodesis after the first secondary spontaneous pneumothorax with thoracoscopic bullae stapling and talc poudrage.[26]

Because the diseases that produce pneumothorax often involve both lungs, patients may experience sequential events in opposite lungs. In this situation, median sternotomy with bilateral abrasion or pleurectomy can be performed, particularly for patients at considerable risk of development of pneumothorax, such as divers and aviators.

KEY POINTS

- Pleural effusions form when excess pleural fluid is produced by the lung or chest wall in sufficient quantities to overcome the resorptive capacity of the pleural lymphatic vessels.
- Pleural fluid analysis is the key to understanding the specific cause of any pleural effusion.
- Transudates have a pleural fluid total protein level less than 0.5 and an LDH level less than 0.6 of the respective serum values. Common diagnoses include CHF, nephrosis, and cirrhosis.

Continued

KEY POINTS—cont'd

- Pleural fluid drainage returns approximately one third of the volume in FVC. The other two thirds allows the diaphragm to rise and the chest wall to normalize.
- Pneumothorax size is underestimated with a one-dimensional view of the chest. Measurement accuracy requires a three-dimensional perspective.
- The risk factors for pneumothorax and pneumomediastinum are the same. Air ruptures a pleural membrane in pneumothorax, and air passes through the lung hilum in pneumomediastinum.
- Oxygen therapy speeds resolution of all pneumothoraces by improving nitrogen absorption.
- Chest tube flow depends on tube size, stopcock size, and collection system resistance.
- Breath-by-breath measurement of a BPF can be approximated by the difference between inspired and expired volumes in the absence of endotracheal cuff leaks.
- The type of ventilator that produces the least fistula airflow is the most likely to effect healing.
- Methods to decrease BPF airflow include lowering V_T, lowering respiratory rate, lowering PEEP, and avoiding auto-PEEP. In more severe cases, positioning the affected lung down, double-lumen tube ventilation, adding PEEP valves to the chest tube, inspiratory chest tube occlusion, or thoracic surgery should be considered.

References

1. Noppen M, and others: Volume and cellular content of normal pleural fluid in humans examined by pleural lavage, Am J Respir Crit Care Med 162:1023, 2000.
2. Light RW: Pleural diseases, ed 2, Philadelphia, 1990, Lea & Febiger.
3. Sahn SA: The diagnostic value of pleural fluid analysis, Semin Respir Crit Care Med 16:269, 1995.
4. Light RW, and others: Pleural effusions: the diagnostic separation of transudates and exudates, Ann Intern Med 77:507, 1972.
5. Staub NC, Wiener-Kronish JP, Albertine KH: Transport through the pleura: physiology of normal liquid and solute exchange in the pleural space. In Chretien J, Bignon J, Hirsch A, editors: The pleura in health and disease, New York, 1985, Marcel Dekker.
6. Wiener-Kronish JP, and others: Relationship of pleural effusions to pulmonary hemodynamics in patients with congestive heart failure, Am Rev Respir Dis 132:1253, 1985.
7. Peterman TA, Brothers SK: Pleural effusions in congestive heart failure and in pericardial disease, N Engl J Med 309:313, 1983.
8. Lieberman FL, and others: Pathogenesis and treatment of hydrothorax complicating cirrhosis with ascites, Ann Intern Med 64:341, 1966.
9. Light RW, and others: Parapneumonic effusions, Am J Med 69:507, 1980.
10. Colice GL, and others: Medical and surgical treatment of parapneumonic effusions: an evidence-based guideline, Chest 118:1158, 2000.
11. Berger HW, Mejia E: Tuberculous pleurisy, Chest 63:88, 1973.
12. Light RW, George RB: Incidence and significance of pleural effusion after abdominal surgery, Chest 69:621, 1976.
13. Sahn SA: State of the art: the pleura, Am Rev Respir Dis 138:184, 1988.
14. Seriff NS, and others: Chylothorax: diagnosis by lipoprotein electrophoresis of serum and pleural fluid, Thorax 32:98, 1977.
15. Strange C: Hemothorax, Semin Respir Crit Care Med 16:324, 1995.
16. Judson MA, Sahn SA: Pulmonary physiological abnormalities caused by pleural disease, Semin Respir Crit Care Med 16:346, 1995.
17. Collins TR, Sahn SA: Thoracentesis: complications, patient experience and diagnostic value, Chest 91:817, 1987.
18. Walker-Renard PB, Vaughan LM, Sahn SA: Chemical pleurodesis for malignant pleural effusions, Ann Intern Med 120:56, 1994.
19. Kennedy L, Sahn SA: Talc pleurodesis for the treatment of pneumothorax and pleural effusion, Chest 106:1215, 1994.
20. Sudduth CD, Sahn SA: Pleurodesis for nonmalignant pleural effusions: recommendations, Chest 102:1855, 1992.
21. Chernick V, Reed MH: Pneumothorax and chylothorax in the neonatal period, J Pediatr 76:624, 1970.
22. Bense L, and others: Nonsmoking, non-alpha 1-antitrypsin deficiency-induced emphysema in nonsmokers with healed spontaneous pneumothorax, identified by computed tomography of the lungs, Chest 103:433, 1993.
23. Bense L, Ecklund G, Wiman LG: Smoking and the increased risk of contracting spontaneous pneumothorax, Chest 92:1009, 1987.
24. Light RW, and others: Intrapleural tetracycline for the prevention of recurrent spontaneous pneumothorax: results of a Department of Veterans Affairs cooperative study, JAMA 264:2224, 1990.
25. Steier M, Ching N, Roberts EB: Pneumothorax complicating continuous ventilatory support, J Thorac Cardiovasc Surg 67:17, 1979.
26. Baumann MH, and others: Management of spontaneous pneumothorax: an American College of Chest Physicians Delphi consensus statement, Chest 119:590, 2001.

27. Sharma TN, Agnihotri SP, Jain NK: Intercostal tube thoracostomy in pneumothorax, Indian J Chest Dis Allied Sci 30:32, 1988.
28. Baumann MH, Sahn SA: Medical management and therapy of bronchopleural fistulas in the mechanically ventilated patient, Chest 97:721, 1990.
29. Bishop MJ, Benson MS, Pierson DJ: Carbon dioxide excretion via bronchopleural fistulas in adult respiratory distress syndrome, Chest 91:400, 1987.
30. Lau KY: Postural management of bronchopleural fistula, Chest 94:1122, 1988.
31. Dodds CP, Hillman KM: Management of massive air leak with asynchronous independent lung ventilation, Intensive Care Med 8:287, 1982.
32. Weksler N, Ovadia L: The challenge of bilateral bronchopleural fistula, Chest 95:938, 1989.
33. Gallagher TJ, and others: Intermittent inspiratory chest tube occlusion to limit bronchopleural cutaneous airleaks, Crit Care Med 4:328, 1976.

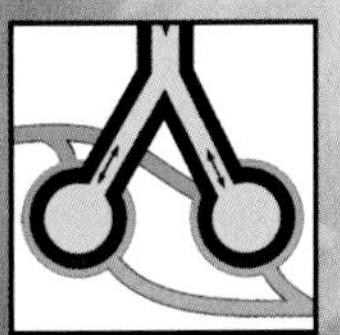

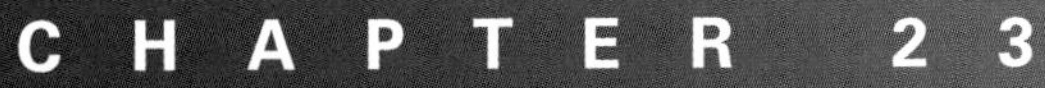

CHAPTER 23

Pulmonary Vascular Disease

Alejandro C. Arroliga

In This Chapter You Will Learn:

- How many patients will develop venous thromboembolism each year
- How and where thromboemboli originate
- How pulmonary emboli alter lung and cardiac function
- What clinical features, electrocardiographic, chest x-ray, and arterial blood gas findings are associated with pulmonary embolism
- How pulmonary embolism is diagnosed and managed
- What characteristics are associated with primary pulmonary hypertension (PPH)
- What possible mechanisms are believed to be responsible for the onset of PPH
- Who is at risk of development of PPH
- What clinical features are associated with PPH
- What treatment is used to care for patients with PPH
- What are the pathogenesis and management of pulmonary hypertension associated with COPD

Chapter Outline

Venous Thromboembolic Disease
- Pathogenesis
- Pathology
- Pathophysiology
- Clinical features
- Diagnostic modalities
- Treatment

Primary Pulmonary Hypertension
- Pathogenesis
- Epidemiology and clinical findings
- Diagnosis
- Management of pulmonary hypertension

Key Terms

deep venous thrombosis
pulmonary embolism
pulmonary hypertension
venous thromboembolism

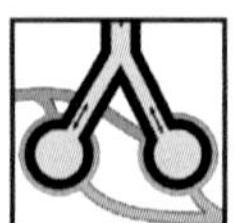

The pulmonary vasculature is affected by a variety of diseases, ranging from obstructive airway disease to parenchymal disease such as interstitial fibrosis. In general, the presence of pulmonary hypertension is dictated by the severity of the underlying lung disease. Pulmonary hypertension is present in other entities such as heart disease (congenital and acquired) and in systemic disorders, the most common of which are connective tissue diseases such as systemic sclerosis and systemic lupus erythematosus. Another systemic problem that affects the pulmonary vasculature is venous thromboembolic disease (deep venous thrombosis [DVT] and pulmonary embolism). This chapter reviews disorders associated with the pulmonary vasculature. It focuses on venous thromboembolic disease and primary pulmonary hypertension (PPH), a rare but lethal disease affecting young people, and briefly reviews pulmonary heart disease (cor pulmonale).

▶ VENOUS THROMBOEMBOLIC DISEASE

Venous thromboembolism is a major national health problem. The prevalence of venous thromboembolism has been calculated to be 117 cases per 100,000 persons (the prevalence of deep venous thrombosis is 48 cases per 100,000 and of pulmonary embolism is 69 cases per 100,000). It is estimated that 200,000 to 300,000 new cases a year occur in the United States.[1]

One third of deaths of pulmonary embolism occur within 1 hour of the onset of symptoms. More than 70% of patients who die of pulmonary embolism are not suspected of having it before death.[2] The mortality rate for the first episode of pulmonary embolism among hospitalized patients may be as high as 12%.[3] The diagnosis is not even suspected in approximately two thirds of patients who die, and the frequency of recognizable emboli in routine autopsies of adult patients varies from 1.5% to almost 30%.[4-6] In a population-based study of pulmonary embolism as a cause of death in New Mexico, only 34% of 812 postmortem documented cases of pulmonary embolism were diagnosed before death.[5] Morpurgo and Schmid[7] reported their experience with 92 postmortem cases of massive or submassive pulmonary embolism found from 1986 to 1989. Only 28% of the cases were diagnosed before death, a finding that emphasizes the underdiagnosis of venous thromboembolic disease.

Two thirds of cases of initial embolus from which patients survive remain undiagnosed. The mortality among this group of patients with undiagnosed embolism is approximately 30%.[8] Recognition of pulmonary embolism therefore is essential. If venous thromboembolism is recognized and treated, the mortality falls below 8%.[9] The reported long-term survival rates after venous thromboembolism in an inception cohort of 2218 patients were 72% and 63% at 1 month and 1 year, respectively.[10]

Objective tests therefore are needed to confirm or exclude the diagnosis of venous thromboembolism, because the accuracy of clinical diagnosis is less than 50%.[11] Patients with multiple injuries, immobilization, bed rest, or intravascular catheters and elderly patients are at high risk of venous thromboembolic disease (Table 23-1).

Pathogenesis

The point of origin of pulmonary emboli is found in only one half of patients.[7] Pulmonary emboli arise from detached portions of venous thrombi that form, in most cases, in deep veins of the lower extremities or pelvis (86%). A small percentage of pulmonary emboli arise from the right heart chambers (3.15%) or the superior vena cava (3%).[7]

Thrombus formation occurs by blood stasis, the presence of hypercoagulable states, or vessel wall abnormalities. The causes of stasis include local pressure, venous obstruction, and immobilization. Other causes of stasis include congestive heart failure, shock and dehydration, varicose veins, and enlargement of the right heart chambers.

Several conditions enhance the intravascular coagulability of the blood and predispose the patient to venous thromboembolic disease. Such conditions include acquired diseases, such as cancer, and primary diseases, such as hyperhomocysteinemia, a mutation in the gene coding for factor V (factor V Leiden), mutation of the prothrombin gene, antithrombin deficiency, antiphospholipid antibody, deficiency of proteins C and S, elevated factor VIII level, abnormalities of fibrinogen,

Table 23-1 ▶▶ Frequency of Venous Thrombosis in Various Hospitalized Patient Groups

Group	Frequency (%)
Orthopedic (e.g., fractured hip)	54-67
Urologic (e.g., prostatectomy)	25
Surgical patients older than 40 y	28
Gynecologic surgery	18
Cardiovascular surgery (e.g., acute myocardial infarction)	39
Obstetrics	3

From Arroliga AC, Matthay MA, Matthay RA: Pulmonary thromboembolism and other pulmonary vascular diseases. In George RB et al, eds: Chest medicine: essentials of pulmonary and critical care medicine, ed 3, Baltimore, 1995, Williams & Wilkins.

Box 23-1 • Conditions Predisposing to Venous Thrombosis and Pulmonary Thromboembolism

- Advanced age
- Postoperative status
- Previous venous thrombosis
- Trauma
- Cerebrovascular accidents
- Thrombocytosis
- Erythrocytosis
- Hyperhomocysteinemia
- Antithrombin deficiency
- Proteins C and S deficiency
- Sickle cell anemia
- Oral contraceptive use
- Pregnancy
- Prolonged bed rest
- Long periods of travel
- Carcinoma
- Obesity
- Antiphospholipid syndrome
- Myeloproliferative disorder
- Paroxysmal nocturia hemoglobinuria
- Heparin-induced thrombocytopenia

From Arroliga AC, Matthay MA, Matthay RA: Pulmonary thromboembolism and other pulmonary vascular diseases. In George RB et al, eds: Chest medicine: essentials of pulmonary and critical care medicine, ed 3, Baltimore, 1995, Williams & Wilkins.

and deficiency of plasminogen[12] (Box 23-1). Vessel wall abnormalities are found most often in patients who have sustained trauma or have undergone major surgery.

Pathology

Stasis, an important factor for the formation of DVT, is rarely the only risk factor.[13] Deposition of platelets and fibrin in the venous valve cups of the lower extremities occurs as a result of stasis. The combination of diminished blood flow and the presence of trauma and toxins can exacerbate endothelial damage and promote the release of mediators that encourage adhesion, aggregation, and degranulation of platelets. The result is activation of the coagulation cascade and production of thrombi and fibrin. Pulmonary embolism occurs when a fragment of the thrombus in the venous system travels to the pulmonary circulation. Pulmonary emboli occur more frequently in the lower lobes and are more often found in the right than in the left lung, a phenomenon probably related to the flow distribution that favors the right lung and the lower lobes.[4] Embolism to the pulmonary circulation produces pulmonary hemorrhage in the ischemic area and infarction in fewer than 10% of cases of pulmonary embolism. Infarction is less common than thromboembolism because the lung has two blood supplies: the pulmonary arterial circulation and the bronchial circulation. At a capillary level, extensive connections exist within the pulmonary and bronchial circulation and prevent serious damage to lung tissue deprived of its pulmonary artery supply.[4] Patients with underlying cardiovascular disease may have compromise with the remaining bronchial circulation; the result is necrosis of lung tissue when emboli occur. Pulmonary infarction is associated with thromboembolic obstruction of a medium-sized pulmonary artery. In general, infarcts occur at the lung bases, are pleural-based, and may be accompanied by pleural effusion. Microscopic examination shows a pulmonary infarct comprises necrosis of alveolar walls, alveoli filled with erythrocytes, and a mild inflammatory response in the periphery.[4]

RULE OF THUMB

Pulmonary embolism is a complication of venous thrombosis. Patients with venous thrombosis in the proximal venous system of the lower extremities and in the upper extremities are at high risk of development of pulmonary embolism.

Pathophysiology

The sudden obstruction of a pulmonary arterial branch causes a decrease in or total cessation of blood flow to the distal zone that leads to respiratory and hemodynamic alterations.[14] Death of massive pulmonary embolism is the result of cardiovascular collapse rather than of respiratory failure.

Embolic obstruction of the pulmonary artery increases the alveolar dead space, causes bronchoconstriction, and decreases the production of alveolar surfactant. Wasted or dead space areas occur because of the presence of ventilated but nonperfused lung parenchyma. The response is to increase total ventilation ($\dot{V}$). The increased $\dot{V}$ contributes to the sensation of dyspnea that accompanies pulmonary embolism. Bronchoconstriction from diminished carbon dioxide concentration, regional hypoxia, and the production of serotonin and histamine cause further ventilation/perfusion ($\dot{V}/\dot{Q}$) mismatching.[15]

The depletion of surfactant material as a result of embolic occlusion leads to atelectasis and intrapulmonary shunt.[14] Not all patients with pulmonary embolism have arterial hypoxemia, but the presence of a wide alveolar-arterial oxygen tension gradient and a reduced arterial oxygen tension (Pa_{O_2}) are common. Hypoxemia develops because of high and low $\dot{V}/\dot{Q}$ mismatch, intrapulmonary shunt, or cardiogenic shock. Shock is caused by obstruction of the pulmonary vasculature by massive emboli or by numerous small emboli in the presence of cardiopulmonary disease. Cardiac output decreases, and oxygen delivery falls. With the decrease in oxygen delivery, the peripheral tissues increase oxygen extraction. The result is venous oxygen desaturation. In patients with significantly increased right heart pressure, intracardiac shunt may develop because of the presence of a patent foramen ovale.[14,15]

The main hemodynamic consequence of pulmonary embolism is increased resistance to blood flow caused by obstruction of the pulmonary arterial bed. The hemodynamic consequences are determined by the extent of the cross-sectional area of the pulmonary circulation involved, the underlying cardiopulmonary reserve, and the neurohumoral response to the embolism. Pulmonary hypertension occurs when 50% of the pulmonary vascular bed has been occluded.[14,15] To maintain the same flow at a higher pressure, the right ventricle must work harder. The result is an increase in right ventricular work that causes the right ventricle to become dilated and ischemic. The thin-walled right ventricle is not designed to work with acute heavy pressure loads. When the mean pulmonary arterial pressure increases to greater than 40 mm Hg, the right ventricle fails, and hemodynamic collapse occurs. The role of vasoconstriction in the pathogenesis of pulmonary hypertension is uncertain, but vasoconstrictors such as serotonin and thromboxane A_2 may play a role in the development of pulmonary hypertension after acute pulmonary embolism.

The course of pulmonary embolism is to resolve rapidly. Permanent residual emboli[16] do occur, although fewer than 10% of patients have perfusion defects after 6 weeks. Even massive emboli are likely to resolve within weeks, particularly in young persons. Emboli are lysed by fibrinolytic factors. Vascular patency is restored by organization of the emboli.

Clinical Features

A high index of suspicion for DVT and pulmonary thromboembolism is important to make the diagnosis for patients at risk. Unfortunately, no specific signs or symptoms indicate the presence of venous thromboembolic disease, although most patients with DVT have pain or swelling, or both, of the extremity.[2] In patients who have swelling above and below the knee, fever, and a history of immobility and cancer, the likelihood of finding DVT on a venogram is only 42%.[17] Fewer than 35% of patients in whom pulmonary embolism is suspected actually have it.[2] The physical findings of DVT in the lower extremities include erythema and warm skin in one third of patients and swelling and tenderness in three fourths. Prolonged empiric therapy should not be based on the symptoms, even if the clinical suspicion is high; therefore confirming or excluding the diagnosis with further testing is necessary.

The most frequent symptom in patients with angiographically confirmed pulmonary embolism is dyspnea, followed by pleuritic chest pain, cough, apprehension, leg swelling, and pain. Hemoptysis occurs in 13% to 20% of patients. The combination of dyspnea of sudden onset, fainting, and chest pain should raise suspicion of pulmonary embolism. In one study, this combination of symptoms was present in 96% of patients with confirmed pulmonary embolism compared with 59% of patients in whom pulmonary embolism was suspected but not confirmed.[18] In some patients, dyspnea lasts only a few minutes, and this episode may be considered trivial[14,18-20] (Table 23-2). There are no characteristic physical findings of pulmonary embolism. The most frequent physical findings include tachypnea, crackles, and tachycardia. These signs, like dyspnea, may be transient. Other common physical findings include an accentuated pulmonary component of the second heart sound (loud P_2) consistent with pulmonary hypertension. Fever may be present in as many as 54% of cases.[18-20]

Chest Radiograph

The chest radiograph by itself is helpful to rule out other potentially life-threatening conditions, such as pneumothorax. In dyspneic patients, a normal chest radiograph may be a clue to the presence of pulmonary embolism. The chest radiograph is abnormal in more than 80% of cases. Some of the abnormalities include enlargement of the right descending pulmonary artery (66%), elevation of diaphragm (61%), enlargement of the heart shadow (55%), and small pleural effusion (50%). Parenchymal densities are present in patients who have infarction or atelectasis. The densities may be present as patchy infiltrates or round nodular lesions. Abutment against a pleural surface is the only unique feature. Other less common findings include the Westermark sign, in which pulmonary hyperlucency caused by a marked reduction in blood flow is present. The so-called Hampton hump, an opacity in the costophrenic angle, is present in 25% to 30% of patients.[18]

Table 23-2 ▶▶ Symptoms in Patients With Pulmonary Embolism and No Cardiac or Pulmonary Disease

Symptom	Frequency (%)
Dyspnea	73
Pleuritic pain	66
Cough	37
Leg swelling	28
Leg pain	26
Hemoptysis	13
Palpitation	10
Wheezing	9
Angina-like pain	4

From Stein PD et al: Chest 100:598, 1991.

Electrocardiogram

The electrocardiogram is helpful to rule out other diagnoses, such as acute myocardial infarction and pericarditis. Most abnormalities are nonspecific in 70% to 75% of cases; tachycardia and ST-segment depression are the most common findings.[18] Abnormalities such as T-wave inversion in right precordial leads, depression of the ST segment, and T-wave inversion in V_1 and V_2 may be present. A so-called $S_1Q_3T_3$ pattern is associated with massive pulmonary embolism and is present in 19% of patients.[17] Only 13% of patients with pulmonary embolism have a normal electrocardiogram.

Arterial Blood Gases

Most patients with acute pulmonary embolism have hypoxemia and hypocapnia,[18] but a significant percentage of patients (15% to 25%) with or without previous cardiopulmonary disease have a PaO_2 exceeding 80 mm Hg. A normal alveolar-arterial oxygen gradient may be present in approximately 20% of patients with angiographically documented pulmonary embolism.[18,20] In an intubated patient or in patients with chronic obstructive lung disease (COPD), a decrease in PaO_2 and an increase in arterial carbon dioxide content should raise the suspicion of pulmonary embolism. Measurement of arterial blood gases (ABGs) is not helpful to confirm or exclude the diagnosis of venous thromboembolic disease. The utility of measuring ABGs is to document hypoxemia and direct oxygen supplementation. In the care of patients with limited cardiopulmonary reserve, ABG levels are used to document the level of carbon dioxide.

Byproducts of Thrombin and Plasmin

Clot formation is invariably associated with thrombin generation. Measurement of fibrin split products (D-dimers), products of cross-linked fibrin, has been found sensitive for acute venous thromboembolism. The specificity D-dimer enzyme-linked immunosorbent assay has excluded all but 5% to 10% of patients with acute pulmonary embolism.[21] The specificity of the test is only 39%, but a value less than 500 mg/L has been shown to rule out venous thromboembolic disease in 98% of patients.[22-24] In patients in whom DVT is suspected clinically, negative results of the D-dimer assay combined with negative findings at impedance plethysmography have a negative predictive value of 98% for DVT.[22] D-dimer results have been useful in the emergency department and outpatient area for the evaluation of patients with suspected DVT[22] and pulmonary embolism.[24] In patients with a low pretest probability of DVT or pulmonary embolism and a negative result (whole-blood agglutination D-dimer test), the negative predictive value for the strategy has been greater than 99%.[23,24]

Diagnostic Modalities

The diagnosis of venous thromboembolic disease relies on the diagnosis of DVT or pulmonary embolism. The absence of one condition does not exclude the other.

Testing for Lower-Extremity DVT

The most widely used modalities for diagnosing DVT in the extremities are compression ultrasonography, impedance plethysmography, and venography.

Venography is the standard for the diagnosis of DVT. However, many problems may be encountered, including inability to cannulate the vein, reaction to contrast material, and, in a small percentage of patients, formation of deep venous thrombi. When results of noninvasive studies are negative, venography is recommended for the evaluation of patients at high risk in whom iliac or pelvic vein thrombus is suspected.

Impedance plethysmography, a noninvasive modality, measures electrical impedance to blood flow, which changes with inflation and deflation of a lower-extremity cuff. The test is operator dependent and requires that the patient be supine and still for at least 2 minutes. The test has a sensitivity and specificity of 91% and 96%, respectively, for symptomatic proximal venous thrombi. A lower sensitivity of 65% has been reported.[25,26]

Compression ultrasonography has proved sensitive and specific for the diagnosis of symptomatic proximal DVT. Compression ultrasonography is noninvasive, portable, and accurate and is the test of choice for the diagnosis of venous thromboembolic disease. Compression ultrasonography combines B-mode scanning with a tightly focused pulse Doppler beam directed at the vessels of interest. Deep venous thrombosis is diagnosed with the findings of venous noncompressibility, an echogenic filling defect, free-floating thrombus in the vein, and venous distension.[27] The most reliable sign of DVT is lack of compressibility of the vein, although a free-floating thrombus has the highest embolic potential. The sensitivity and specificity of compression ultrasound in symptomatic patients vary between 95% and 100% for the detection of a proximal lower-extremity thrombus.[27,28] Areas not well visualized with compression ultrasonography include the iliac veins, superficial femoral veins in the adductor canal, and the calf veins. However, the accuracy of compression ultrasound, even with the addition of color Doppler ultrasonography, is moderate to low for the detection of DVT in patients at high risk who do not have symptoms.[29] These results suggest that ultrasonography, although sensitive and specific for the diagnosis of DVT, is not a good screening test for patients at high risk who do not have symptoms.

The increased incidence of upper extremity DVT poses diagnostic problems. Ultrasonography still may be the initial diagnostic test of choice, although venography is more commonly used for detection of thrombi in hidden areas that cannot be assessed with ultrasonography and in the evaluation of patients without symptoms who have negative findings with noninvasive modalities but have a high risk of DVT.

Testing for Pulmonary Embolism

Noninvasive leg tests for the diagnosis of DVT are complemented with a $\dot{V}/\dot{Q}$ scan for the diagnosis of pulmonary embolism. Either of these tests, depending on the resources available, may be the initial diagnostic examination if the presence of acute venous thromboembolism is suspected on the basis of the clinical findings.[30] Only $\dot{V}/\dot{Q}$ lung scanning and pulmonary angiography are reasonably sensitive and reliable tests in the diagnosis of pulmonary embolism. Ventilation/perfusion scanning involves the inhalation of a radiolabeled gas (usually xenon-133, xenon-127, krypton-181m, or technetium-99m) and the intravenous injection of macroaggregated albumin tagged with a gamma-emitting radioisotope. The distribution of lung $\dot{V}$ and lung $\dot{Q}$ is studied, and areas of mismatch where $\dot{Q}$ is less than $\dot{V}$ are sought. The presence of mismatches most often indicates embolic occlusion of the blood vessel, although other rare causes of mismatches exist, such as extrinsic compression of the vessel by a mass, intraluminal obstruction by angiosarcoma, or obliteration of a vessel by vasculitis. The $\dot{V}$ scan increases the specificity of the $\dot{Q}$ scan.[31] In general, with the presence of a parenchymal abnormality, the $\dot{V}$ defect coincides with the $\dot{Q}$ defect, and matched abnormalities are found. Normal results of a $\dot{Q}$ scan exclude the presence of a clinically significant pulmonary embolism in the presence of low clinical probability of pulmonary embolism. In these cases, long-term anticoagulant therapy can be safely withheld.[32] Abnormal $\dot{V}/\dot{Q}$ scan results can be classified as high probability, intermediate (or indeterminate) probability, and low probability for pulmonary embolism, according to the size of the defect and the degree of mismatch between the $\dot{V}/\dot{Q}$ scan and chest radiographic abnormalities[31] (Table 23-3). The presence of concomitant cardiopulmonary disease even if severe (e.g., hypoxemia with or without ventilatory support, a condition that necessitates intensive care), or COPD does not diminish the diagnostic usefulness of $\dot{V}/\dot{Q}$ scans in the diagnosis of acute pulmonary embolism.[33-35]

For the one third of patients who do not receive a definitive diagnosis on the basis of the results of noninvasive studies, pulmonary angiography is the test of choice. The mortality for pulmonary angiography is 0.5%, and the prevalence of major nonfatal complications is 1%. However, patients in a medical intensive care unit are at higher risk of morbidity and mortality (approximately 4%), including respiratory failure, renal failure, and hematoma necessitating transfusion, than are other patients.[36] Pulmonary angiographic signs of acute pulmonary embolism include filling defects and cutoff of the pulmonary artery. Other angiographic signs include absent, decreased, or delayed filling of pulmonary arteries, delayed venous emptying, pruning, and abnormal tapering. None of these findings is as specific as filling defects, particularly in the presence of

Table 23-3 ▶▶▶ Revised PIOPED $\dot{V}/\dot{Q}$ Scan Interpretation Criteria

High probability	Two or more large (>75% of a segment) segmental $\dot{Q}$ defects without corresponding $\dot{V}$ or abnormalities on chest radiograph
	One large segmental $\dot{Q}$ defect and two or more moderate (25%-75% of a segment) segmental $\dot{Q}$ defects without corresponding $\dot{V}$ or abnormalities on chest radiograph
	Four or more moderate segmental $\dot{Q}$ defects without corresponding $\dot{V}$ or abnormalities on chest radiograph
Intermediate probability	One moderate or up to two large segmental $\dot{Q}$ defects without corresponding $\dot{V}$ defect or abnormalities on chest radiograph
	Corresponding $\dot{V}/\dot{Q}$ defects and parenchymal opacity in lower lung zone on chest radiograph
	Corresponding $\dot{V}/\dot{Q}$ defects and small pleural effusion
	Single moderate matched $\dot{V}/\dot{Q}$ defects with normal findings on chest radiograph
	Findings difficult to categorize as normal, low, or high probability
Low probability	Multiple matched $\dot{V}/\dot{Q}$ defects, regardless of size, with normal findings on chest radiograph
	Corresponding $\dot{V}/\dot{Q}$ defects and parenchymal opacity in upper or middle lung zone on chest radiograph
	Corresponding $\dot{V}/\dot{Q}$ defects and large pleural effusion
	Any $\dot{Q}$ defects with substantially larger abnormality on chest radiograph
	Defects surrounded by normally perfused lung (stripe sign)
	Single or multiple small (<25% of a segment) segmental $\dot{Q}$ defects with a normal chest radiograph
	Nonsegmental $\dot{Q}$ defects (cardiomegaly, aortic impression, enlarged hila)
Normal	No $\dot{Q}$ defects; $\dot{Q}$ outlines the shape of the lung on chest radiograph

Modified from Worsley DF, Alavi A, Palevsky JH: Radiol Clin North Am 31:849, 1993.
PIOPED, Prospective Investigation of Pulmonary Embolism Diagnosis.

Table 23-4 ▶▶ Likelihood of Identifying Pulmonary Embolism on Pulmonary Angiogram on the Basis of Results of $\dot{V}/\dot{Q}$ Lung Scan and Clinical Probability

Scan Interpretation	High Clinical Probability	Intermediate Clinical Probability	Low Clinical Probability
High probability	96%	88%	56%
Intermediate probability	66%	28%	16%
Low probability	40%	16%	4%
Near normal/normal	0%	6%	2%

From Arroliga AC, Matthay MA, Matthay RA: Pulmonary thromboembolism and other pulmonary vascular diseases. In George RB et al, eds: *Chest medicine: essentials of pulmonary and critical care medicine*, ed 3, Baltimore, 1995, Williams & Wilkins.

other cardiopulmonary diseases. The probability of finding pulmonary embolism with angiography on the basis of results of $\dot{V}/\dot{Q}$ scan and clinical probability is shown in Table 23-4.[36]

A definite diagnosis can be established with noninvasive diagnostic tools in two thirds of cases.[37] In one study, if the pretest clinical probability was low or moderate for pulmonary embolism and the $\dot{V}/\dot{Q}$ scan result was not high probability, 0.5% of the patients had pulmonary embolism or DVT diagnosed during a 90-day follow-up period.[38] Figure 23-1 summarizes the diagnostic approach to pulmonary embolus.

Other diagnostic modalities have been used to make the diagnosis of pulmonary embolism. Helical computed tomography has been used extensively.[39] The reported sensitivity of helical computed tomography ranges from 53% to 100%, and the specificity ranges from 81% to 100%. However, the safety of withholding therapy for pulmonary embolism in the presence of negative study results is unclear.[40] Magnetic resonance imaging has been suggested as an alternative noninvasive means for confirming the presence or absence of DVT. The sensitivity, specificity, and accuracy of magnetic resonance imaging are approximately 97%.[41] Magnetic resonance imaging with radial pulse acquisition appears accurate in the diagnosis of acute DVT. Because of its limited availability, magnetic resonance imaging may not be useful in the acute setting.

Treatment

Prophylaxis

Prophylactic therapy reduces the risk of venous thromboembolism in patients at risk. The frequency of proximal DVT varies from 2% to 4% among general surgical patients undergoing minor surgery to 40% to 80% among patients at the highest risk, such as those who have undergone hip or knee surgery.[42] Patients at

MINI CLINI

Respiratory Distress After Hip Replacement

PROBLEM

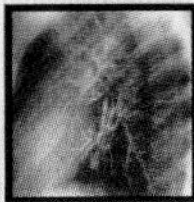

You are told to evaluate a 65-year-old man who has undergone right hip replacement. On the third day after surgery, the patient experienced dyspnea and pleuritic chest pain in the right hemithorax. On physical examination, his heart rate is 120 beats/min; respiratory rate, 25 breaths/min; and blood pressure, 120/85 mm Hg. The lungs are clear, and the heart examination does not show any gallops or murmurs. Arterial blood gas measurements on room air yield a pH of 7.49; Pa_{CO_2}, 30 mm Hg; and P_{O_2}, 85 mm Hg. The chest radiograph is unremarkable. What is your differential diagnosis, and how do you treat this patient?

DISCUSSION

The differential diagnosis is extensive and should include an ischemic cardiac event such as myocardial infarction as well as bacterial pneumonia. The type of chest pain is not typical of myocardial infarction. An electrocardiogram may be of value because in patients with myocardial infarction, elevation of the ST segments is prominent in the acute phase. Other laboratory data include elevation of the creatinine kinase and troponin levels. The normal chest radiograph decreases the likelihood of the presence of pneumonia.

Because of the history of surgery on the right hip, DVT and pulmonary embolism are the most likely diagnoses. The next examinations are duplex ultrasonography of the lower extremities and a $\dot{V}/\dot{Q}$ radionuclide study. The presence of a thrombus in the proximal venous system of the lower extremities or high-probability results of a $\dot{V}/\dot{Q}$ scan establish the diagnosis. The patient needs to be treated with heparin, continuous intravenous drip, followed by warfarin. The presence of a "normal" Pa_{O_2} of 85 mm Hg in this patient may be misleading. The wide alveolar-arterial gradient probably is caused by the presence of a pulmonary embolus.

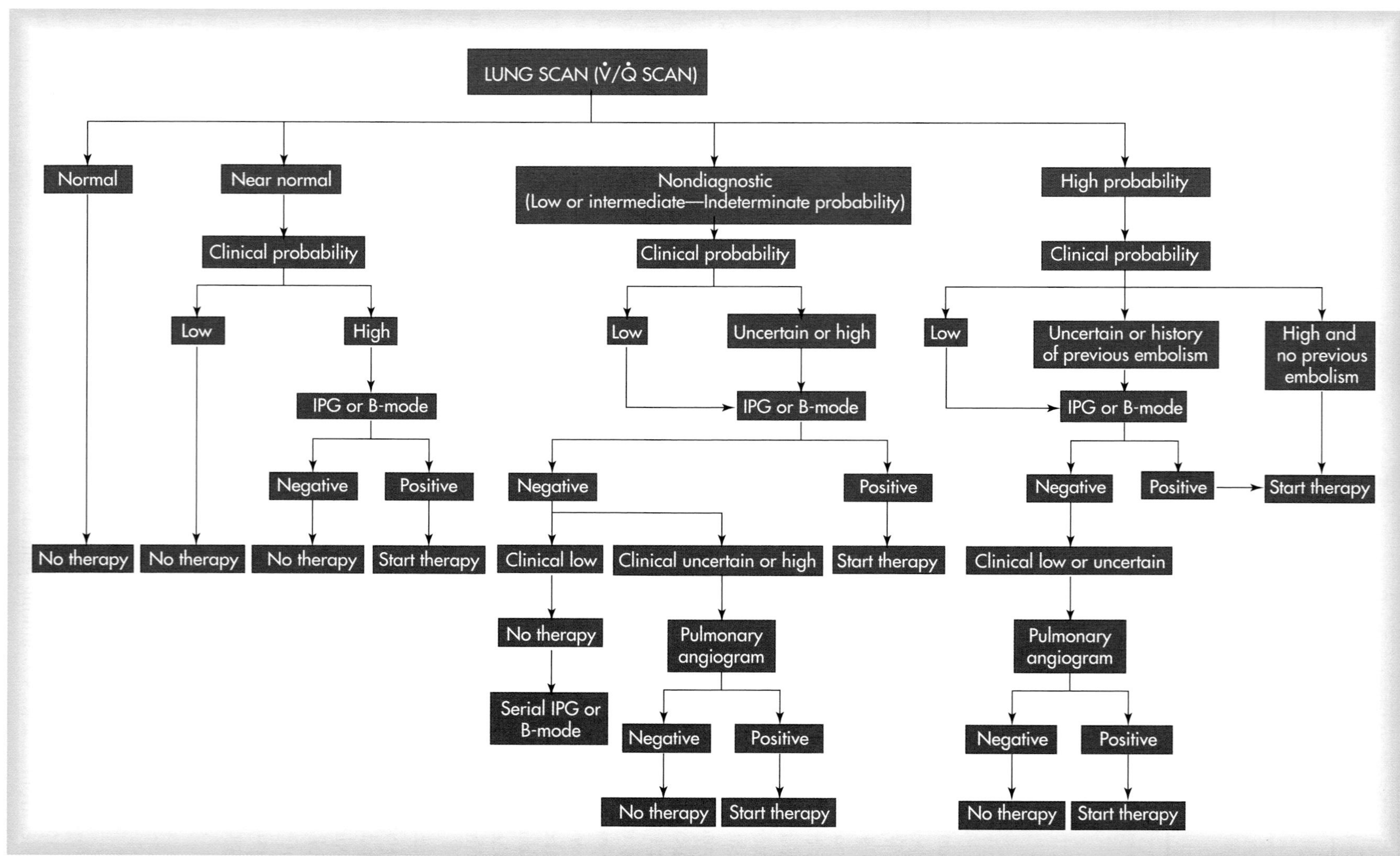

Figure 23-1 · Therapist-Driven Protocol

Strategy for diagnosis of pulmonary embolism for patients in stable condition. Diagnosis is based on clinical suspicion and the results of lung scan, pulmonary angiography, and noninvasive tests for DVT. *IPG*, Impedance plethysmography; *B-mode*, duplex, compression ultrasonography. *(Modified from Stein PD et al: Chest 103:1553-1559, 1993.)*

moderate to high risk include those with acute spinal cord injury, myocardial infarction, ischemic stroke, or other medical conditions, such as heart failure and pneumonia.[42] Another group at risk of DVT is patients admitted to medical intensive care units; DVT has been detected in 33% of these patients.[43] Unfortunately, compliance in the use of prophylaxis varies between 28% and 100%.[42]

Pharmacological choices for prophylaxis include low-dose subcutaneous heparin, warfarin, low-molecular-weight heparin, heparinoids, and dextran. Mechanical measures to reduce venous stasis include early ambulation, wearing elastic stockings, pneumatic calf compression, and electrical stimulation of calf muscles. Current prophylactic strategies for DVT and pulmonary embolism are summarized in Table 23-5. Most hospitalized patients who are immobile need prophylaxis for venous thromboembolism.

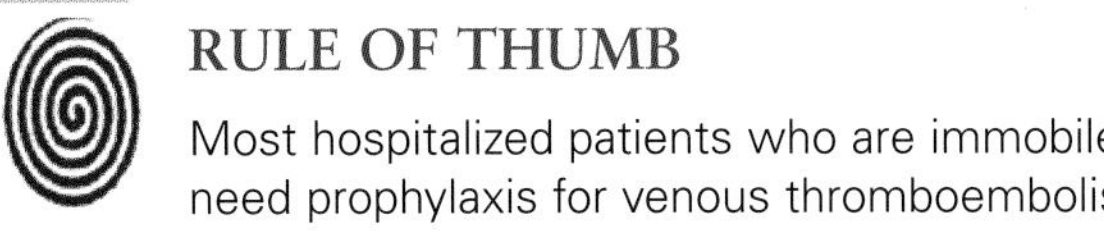

RULE OF THUMB

Most hospitalized patients who are immobile need prophylaxis for venous thromboembolism.

Management of Acute DVT and Pulmonary Embolism

The therapies for DVT and pulmonary embolism are similar. Heparin is the standard therapy for venous thromboembolic disease; it has an immediate action and is relatively safe. Heparin is an acidic glycosaminoglycan that inhibits the coagulation system. It potentiates the action of antithrombin and heparin cofactor 2 and in this way inactivates thrombin, factor IXa, and factor Xa. Heparin does not lyse existing clots but prevents formation and propagation of new clots. Unfractionated

Table 23-5 ▶▶ Prophylaxis of DVT and Pulmonary Embolism

Type of Operation or Condition	Patient at Usual Risk	Patient at High Risk (e.g., Previous DVT or Pulmonary Embolism)
General abdominothoracic surgery	<40 y of age: surgery lasting <30 min; no risk factors; no prophylaxis, early ambulation All other patients: low-dose heparin,* SC, q12h starting 2 h preoperatively plus ES *or* IPC	Very high risk with multiple risk factors: low-dose heparin or LMW or dextran plus IPC
Orthopedic surgery		
Hip replacement	Low-dose warfarin (2 mg per day) or warfarin (INR 2-3) *or* LMW or adjusted-dose heparin (aPTT 31-36 sec)	Combination of methods *or* Selected patients: IVCF?
Hip fractures	Warfarin or LMW	Selected patients: IVCF?
Knee operations	IPC or LMW or warfarin	Selected patients: IVCF?
Eye surgery or neurosurgery	IPC with or without ES	
Acute spinal cord injury with paralysis	Adjusted-dose heparin (aPTT 31-36 s) *or* LMW, warfarin? IPC?	Adjusted-dose heparin (aPTT 31-36 sec) *or* LMW, warfarin? IPC?
Multiple trauma	IPC? or warfarin? or LMW?	IPC? or warfarin? or LMW?
General medical patient		
Myocardial infarction	Low-dose heparin or warfarin (INR 2-3) LMW? IPC? ES?	Low-dose heparin or warfarin (INR 2-3) LMW? IPC? ES?
Ischemic stroke and lower-extremity paralysis	LMW or low-dose heparin Warfarin? IPC? ES?	LMW or low-dose heparin Warfarin? IPC? ES?
Other medical condition (e.g., heart failure, pneumonia, malignancy)	Low-dose heparin?	Low-dose heparin?
Long-term indwelling catheter and malignant disease	Warfarin 1 mg per day	Warfarin 1 mg per day

Data from Clagett GP, Anderson FA Jr, Levine MN: Chest 102:391S-407S, 1992. In Arroliga AC, Matthay MA, Matthay RA: Pulmonary thromboembolism and other pulmonary vascular diseases. In Chest medicine: essentials of pulmonary and critical care medicine, ed 3, Baltimore, 1995, Williams & Wilkins.

aPTT, Activated partial thromboplastin time; *ES*, graduated compression elastic stockings; *INR*, international normalized ratio; *IPC*, intermittent pneumatic compression; *IVCF*, inferior vena caval filter; *LMW*, low-molecular-weight heparin; *PE*, pulmonary embolism; *SC*, subcutaneously; ?, probably indicated but insufficient data.

*Low-dose heparin is 5000 units per dose.

heparin should be administered as a bolus followed by a continuous infusion.[42] Continuous infusion therapy may be superior to intermittent intravenous bolus infusion and subcutaneous administration of large doses.[44]

The heparin regimen should be selected to maximize its antithrombotic effect without increasing the risk of bleeding. It is very important to achieve a therapeutic effect in the first 24 to 48 hours of starting therapy. The goal of heparin therapy is to maintain an activated partial thromboplastin time (aPTT) greater than 1.5 times the control value.[45] Clinical recurrence of DVT and pulmonary embolism is rare when heparin is infused at doses of at least 1250 units per hour.[45] The fastest way to achieve a therapeutic heparin effect is to follow an established nomogram. Several nomograms are currently available, and one is shown in Table 23-6.[45-47] These nomograms have been well accepted by clinicians and have led to aggressive heparin dosing and improvement in intermediate outcome. The use of nomograms has been associated with decreasing time to achieve therapeutic aPTT (85%-90% of patients achieve a therapeutic level within 24 hours) and a decrease in the variance of these parameters without any changes in bleeding rate.[47] The complications of intravenous heparin administration include major bleeding (3.8%), thrombocytopenia caused by immunoglobulin G antiheparin antibodies (2.5%-3% of patients to whom heparin is given therapeutically, <0.5% of patients to whom it is given prophylactically). If thrombocytopenia or bleedings occurs, heparin should be discontinued promptly. Long-term administration of heparin can cause hypoaldosteronism and osteoporosis.

Heparin should be given for a minimum of 5 to 7 days.[45] During the first or second day, oral anticoagulation should be started. Coumarin derivatives are drugs that inhibit the formation of factors II, VII, IX, and X. The coumarin derivative racemic warfarin sodium is the most commonly used oral anticoagulant. It must be given for 6 to 7 consecutive days to achieve a full antithrombotic effect. Warfarin should not be used solely for the initial management of venous thromboembolism because the peak effect is delayed for at least 72 to 96 hours. Because warfarin decreases production of proteins C and S, a relative hypercoagulable state may occur in the first 24 hours as a result of the depletion of these proteins. The loading dose of coumarin varies between 5 and 10 mg/d. The 5-mg/d dose produces a lesser degree of anticoagulation and avoids the development of a potential hypercoagulable state caused by the decrease in the level of protein C during the first 36 hours of therapy.[48] Patients generally need treatment with oral anticoagulants for 6 months, although in patients with transient risk of DVT (postoperative period), a 4- to 6-week course of anticoagulation may be adequate.[45,49] Patients who need therapy for more than 6 months include those with idiopathic venous thromboembolism. Patients who need therapy for more than 1 year or for life are those with a history of cancer, anticardiolipin antibody, or antithrombin deficiency.[45]

Table 23-6 ▶▶ Weight-Based Nomogram for Administration of Heparin

Initial dose	80 U/kg bolus, then 18 U/kg per hour
aPTT <35 s (<1.2 × control value)	80U/kg bolus, then 4 U/kg per hour
aPTT 35-45 s (1.2-1.5 × control value)	40 U/kg bolus, then 2 U/kg per hour
aPTT 46-70 s (1.5-2.3 × control value)	No change
aPTT 71-90 s (2.3-3 × control value)	Decrease infusion rate by 2 U/kg per hour
aPTT >90 s (>3 × control value)	Hold infusion 1 h, then decrease infusion rate by 3 U/kg per hour

Modified from Raschke RA, Gollihake B, Pierce JC. *Arch Intern Med* 156:1645, 1996.
Doses are calculated on actual body weight.

Low-molecular-weight heparin, as a single dose or twice a day by the subcutaneous route, is a new modality of therapy for proximal DVT. This agent has been shown to be as effective and as safe as, and less expensive than, intravenous heparin therapy. At the same time, in selected patients low molecular-weight heparin can be administered at home in an efficacious and safe way that can potentially decrease the number of days of hospital admission for acute DVT.[45] It has been suggested that as much as $250 million could be saved annually in the United States if patients were treated in the outpatient setting. The patients chosen for outpatient therapy should be in stable condition, should have a low risk of bleeding, and should not have renal insufficiency. Home administration of low molecular-weight heparin should be closely supervised.

The role of thrombolytic therapy with streptokinase, urokinase, or tissue plasminogen activator is not well defined in the management of acute DVT. The administration of early thrombolytic therapy decreases the pain and the incidence of postphlebitic syndrome, but the risks and benefits of this particular therapy are not well established.[45] A systematic review of the efficacy and the safety of the use of recombinant tissue plasminogen activator in the management of lower extremity DVT did not support the routine use of this medication. Knowledge of the patient's values and preferences must be used to guide the best decision.[50]

Management of Pulmonary Embolism

The management of pulmonary embolism depends on the extent and status of the cardiopulmonary system. Therapy with heparin followed by oral coumarin in a regimen similar to that for acute DVT is the modality of choice. Patients with an acute pulmonary embolism need additional supportive measures. Supplemental oxygen should be administered to patients who have hypoxemia, and adequate analgesia should be prescribed for patients who have pain and anxiety. Resuscitation with fluids and vasopressor agents is necessary for patients who are hypotensive and in shock. The vasopressors of choice include agents that may reduce pulmonary vascular resistance and increase cardiac output, such as norepinephrine and dopamine.[51,52] In the care of patients with severe hypoxemia, acute right heart failure, or shock, thrombolytic therapy may be administered for lysis of the emboli. However, for patients with no evidence of hypotension, thrombolytic administration has to be individualized. When thrombolytic therapy with streptokinase and urokinase is used, heparin should not be infused concurrently. However, the use of heparin is optional in the treatment of patients receiving tissue plasminogen activator or reteplase.[45]

Other options in the care of a patient with massive pulmonary embolism include pulmonary embolectomy, catheter tip embolectomy, and catheter tip fragmentation. These techniques can be used in centers with appropriate experience.[30] Patients who have undergone attempts at embolectomy and catheter extraction have had massive embolism, shock, unsuccessful thrombolytic therapy, or contraindications to thrombolytic therapy.[45]

The main indications for the insertion of an inferior vena caval filter are the presence of contraindications to the administration of anticoagulant or the presence of complications of anticoagulation. Other indications for filter insertion include recurrent embolism despite adequate anticoagulation and the presence of chronic thromboembolic disease. Filter placement reduces the incidence of pulmonary embolism in the period immediately after insertion but is associated with a higher incidence of recurrent DVT.[45,53]

▶ PRIMARY PULMONARY HYPERTENSION

Primary pulmonary hypertension is characterized by an elevation in mean pulmonary arterial pressure greater than 25 mm Hg at rest and 30 mm Hg during exercise, increased pulmonary vascular resistance, and normal left heart ventricular function in the absence of other secondary causes of pulmonary hypertension.[54] Pulmonary arterial hypertension is an elevation in pulmonary arterial pressure and may be associated with other conditions, including congenital heart disease, collagen vascular disease, cirrhosis of the liver, viral infections (human immunodeficiency virus), and drug effects (anorexigenics), to name a few.[55]

Pathogenesis

The initial event of PPH is probably an insult to the pulmonary endothelium. A genetic predisposition is probably necessary. The damage to the endothelium alters the balance between vasoconstrictive mediators such as thromboxane and endothelin I and vasodilators such as endothelium-derived relaxing factor and prostacyclin; the result is vasoconstriction. Vasoconstriction may not be the primary event, but it is an important component in the pathophysiology of PPH.[56-59] Other abnormalities that have been observed in patients with PPH include the presence of thrombi in situ, elevation of the level of serotonin, monoclonal proliferation of endothelial cells, vascular remodeling, and alteration in the regulation of the potassium channel in the smooth-muscle cells of the pulmonary artery. Down-regulation of the potassium channel is associated with reduction of the potassium current and results in membrane depolarization and subsequent elevation of the cellular calcium level. The current thinking is that these abnormalities in potassium and calcium transport may cause pulmonary vasoconstriction.[55]

Epidemiology and Clinical Findings

Primary pulmonary hypertension is more common among women than among men, with a ratio of 3 to 1. Approximately 7% of all cases are familial disease. Primary pulmonary hypertension is rare and can occur at any age, although it is more common in the third and fourth decades. On average, the diagnosis is delayed 2 years. The condition frequently is misdiagnosed as hyperventilation and depression. Primary pulmonary hypertension is characterized by onset of vague symptoms. The most common initial symptom is dyspnea (60% of patients). Angina, probably due to underperfusion of the right ventricle or stretching of the large pulmonary arteries, is present in approximately 50% of patients. Syncope is present in 8% of patients as an early symptom. Other symptoms include cough, hemoptysis, hoarseness, and Raynaud's phenomenon (blanching of the fingers on exposure to cold) in approximately 10% of patients. Physical findings associated with PPH include a loud second heart sound and a right-sided third or fourth heart sound. Other common signs are a palpable right ventricular heave and impulse of the pulmonary artery and both pulmonary ejection and pulmonary tricuspid regurgitation murmurs. Signs of right ventricular failure are common. Cyanosis often is present as a result of low cardiac output or the presence of an intracardiac right-to-left shunt that occurs as cor pulmonale develops. Clubbing does not occur in PPH. The chest radiographic findings include enlargement of the main and hilar pulmonary arteries, "pruning" (or narrowing) of the peripheral arteries, and enlargement of the right ventricle and atrium. The chest radiograph may be normal in 6% of patients. Pleural effusions are not present. In pulmonary venoocclusive disease, a histopathological type of PPH, there is an increase in vascular markings, and Kerley's B lines may be present.[56]

Diagnosis

Entities that can cause secondary pulmonary hypertension need to be ruled out. Electrocardiographic findings usually include right axis deviation, right ventricular hypertrophy, and strain. The echocardiogram shows dilatation of the right ventricle and right atrium but no other abnormalities. The most important noninvasive test for PPH is the $\dot{V}/\dot{Q}$ scan lung scan. The $\dot{V}/\dot{Q}$ scan helps to rule out the possibility of chronic thromboembolic pulmonary hypertension (a mimic of PPH). In patients with PPH, the $\dot{Q}$ scan is normal or shows only patchy subsegmental defects. In patients with chronic thromboembolic pulmonary hypertension, the $\dot{V}/\dot{Q}$ scan shows segmental defects, and in these cases pulmonary angiography is necessary.

High-resolution computed tomography is necessary to rule out secondary causes and may be useful in evaluation of the small group of patients with chronic interstitial disease and normal chest radiographs. Pulmonary function tests are useful to rule out the presence of significant restrictive or obstructive airway disease. The most common abnormality at pulmonary function testing of patients with PPH is low carbon monoxide diffusing capacity (D_{LCO}).

In patients with shortness of breath with unremarkable results at physical examination, the presence of a low D_{LCO} and normal pulmonary mechanics suggests a pulmonary vascular cause (e.g., pulmonary hypertension) of the symptoms.

Systemic lupus erythematosus, systemic sclerosis, and mixed connective tissue disease are some of the entities that may be ruled out by the appropriate clinical examinations and laboratory tests. Schistosomiasis, a parasitic disease and the most common cause of pulmonary hypertension worldwide, must be ruled out in the appropriate setting.

Invasive studies such as pulmonary angiography and open lung biopsy are occasionally needed in the diagnosis of PPH. Right heart catheterization is useful to determine the degree of hemodynamic impairment and the prognosis of patients with PPH. Patients with severe degrees of pulmonary hypertension, high right atrial pressure, and low cardiac output have a very poor prognosis.[56]

Management of Pulmonary Hypertension

Primary pulmonary hypertension often is a fatal disease. Without therapy, only 33% of patients are alive 5 years after the onset of the disorder. During the last decade, treatment has improved considerably. Medical treatment consists of supplemental oxygen, anticoagulation with coumarin, and vasodilators. Lung transplantation is an option for patients with severe PPH.[54,56]

Oxygen is administered to patients who are hypoxemic at rest or during exercise. Arterial oxygen saturation should be maintained above 90%. Long-term coumarin therapy has been shown to improve the survival of patients with PPH. Prothrombin time is monitored to maintain the INR around 2 when warfarin is used. Adjusted doses of heparin may be an alternative to warfarin therapy.[54] Digoxin may be used to counteract the negative inotropic effect of calcium channel blockers. Diuretics may be used carefully to control hepatic congestion and pedal edema.

Treatment with vasodilators has been advocated for the last few decades. The goal of vasodilator therapy is to reduce the mean pulmonary arterial pressure and pulmonary vascular resistance by at least 20% with an increase in cardiac output while not inducing systemic hypotension.[60] Only 26% of patients have a therapeutic response to oral vasodilators. Calcium channel blockers have been the oral vasodilators used most commonly; nifedipine and diltiazem are preferred because they have less negative inotropic effect. Calcium channel blockers are given through titration with hourly doses under close hemodynamic monitoring (pulmonary arterial catheter) until a maximal effect or adverse effects occur. Patients who respond to vasodilator therapy have a better survival than do patients who do not respond. The average daily dose of sustained-released nifedipine is 120 to 140 mg/d. Diltiazem in doses up to 900 mg/d is used as an alternative if the patient has marked tachycardia.

Intravenous prostacyclin was initially used as a screening agent for pulmonary vasoreactivity. Prostacyclin has been used in continuous infusion with improvement in hemodynamic values, exercise tolerance, and, most important, survival.[61] Even if a patient does not respond immediately to prostacyclin administration, benefit can be achieved with long-term administration.[62-64] Patients who receive prostacyclin need close monitoring because tachyphylaxis (resistance to further drug effect) occurs with long-term use, and adjustment of the dosage is necessary. Another medication that improves outcome among patients with PPH is the endothelin receptor antagonist bosentan.

Single or double lung transplantation has been used successfully in the treatment of patients with PPH. Patients who undergo lung transplantation have an immediate decrease in pulmonary artery pressure at the time of surgery and rapid improvement in right heart function despite severe preoperative cor pulmonale. Lung transplantation is indicated in the care of patients who do not respond to vasodilators and have significant cardiac impairment. Transplantation is generally reserved for patients who are in New York Heart Association functional class III or IV. Although lung transplantation is an alternative in the treatment of patients with PPH, the disadvantages of transplantation are the need for lifelong immunosuppression and the morbidity and mortality of lung transplantation, which increase as a function of time. The survival rate 3 years after lung transplantation is approximately 60%.

RULE OF THUMB

In patients with shortness of breath who have unremarkable results at physical examination, the presence of a low D_Lco and normal pulmonary mechanics suggests a pulmonary vascular cause (e.g., pulmonary hypertension) of the symptoms.

MINI CLINI

Dyspnea and Near-Syncope

PROBLEM

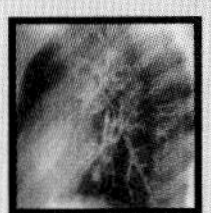

A 35-year-old woman has shortness of breath. She had an episode of near-syncope approximately 6 months ago; a diagnostic evaluation was done, and the results were negative. The physical examination shows a loud second heart sound. A chest radiograph shows questionable cardiomegaly. The forced vital capacity and forced expiratory volume in 1 second are normal, but the D_{LCO} is only 40% of the predicted value. What is the cause of the dyspnea and the low D_{LCO}?

DISCUSSION

This patient could have pulmonary hypertension of unknown cause, that is, PPH. She has physical findings consistent with high pressure in the right side of the heart (a loud second heart sound), and she has symptoms that are common in this disorder, such as dyspnea and near-syncope or syncope. The diagnosis is difficult, but a low D_{LCO} in the presence of normal lung mechanics could indicate an abnormality of the pulmonary vasculature.

Venous thromboembolism (DVT and pulmonary embolism) is an important cause of morbidity and mortality among hospitalized patients. One third of deaths caused by pulmonary embolism occur within 1 hour of the symptoms. The mortality in the group of patients with pulmonary embolism that remains undiagnosed is 30%; if the venous thrombosis is recognized and managed, the mortality is less than 8%. The point of origin of pulmonary embolism is DVT of the lower extremities or pelvis in 86% of cases. Most of the time, the clinical presentation of pulmonary embolism and DVT is nonspecific. A high index of suspicion is important to make the diagnosis in patients at risk.

Pulmonary Hypertension in Chronic Lung Disease

Pulmonary hypertension is a frequent complication of chronic pulmonary disease (see Chapter 20). Approximately 50% of elderly patients with chronic COPD have pulmonary hypertension with significant reduction of survival and quality of life.[65]

The pulmonary hypertension associated with COPD is multifactorial. Loss of vascular surface caused by destruction of lung parenchyma, compression of the vascular bed as a result of hyperinflation, hyperviscosity of the blood as a result of polycythemia, and left ventricular dysfunction are important contributory factors. Alveolar hypoxia, because of its potent pulmonary vasoconstrictive effect, is probably the most important factor contributing to pulmonary hypertension in patients with COPD. Sustained alveolar hypoxia causes pulmonary vasoconstriction and eventually medial hypertrophy, fibrosis of the intima, and narrowing of the lumen of the pulmonary blood vessels.[65,66] The increases in pulmonary arterial pressure and vascular resistance cause an increase in the afterload of the right ventricle with dilation and hypertrophy in an effort to maintain the cardiac output.[66] Patients with COPD may have worsening of dyspnea and a decrease in exercise tolerance without a change in the degree of airway obstruction.

At examination, patients may have right ventricular lift in the subxiphoid area, an accentuated pulmonic component of the second heart sound,[65] and a fourth heart sound in the right parasternal or subxiphoid area that indicates right ventricular overload. The presence of jugular venous distension and hepatojugular reflex may be caused by right ventricular failure or by hyperinflation of the lung with decreased venous return to the thorax.[66,67]

The presence of pulmonary hypertension in patients with COPD correlates with the severity of the disease. Patients with severe hypoxemia (PaO_2 <55 mm Hg) in general have severe pulmonary hypertension.[65] The chest radiograph shows an increase in the diameter of the right descending pulmonary artery to more than 20 mm and an increased ratio of hilar width to the transverse diameter of the thorax.[68] The electrocardiogram is useful for confirming the presence of right ventricular hypertrophy, dilatation of the ventricle, and the degree of pulmonary hypertension.

Management of pulmonary hypertension associated with severe lung disease must include optimization of therapy for the underlying lung disease. In patients with COPD, β_2 agonists and aminophylline improve right ventricular function but may have side effects such as tachyarrhythmia.[65,66] Digitalis therapy is of little help to these patients because it does not improve right ventricular function. Digitalis should be used only in the presence of left ventricular failure.

Oral vasodilators such as β-adrenergic agonists, α-adrenergic antagonists, calcium channel blockers, nitrates, inhibitors of angiotensin-converting enzyme, and direct vasodilators such as hydralazine have not proved of benefit to patients with pulmonary hypertension and COPD. Furthermore, these drugs may be associated with systemic hypotension and worsening of gas exchange.[65-67] At present, there is no role for oral vasodilators in the treatment of patients with COPD and pulmonary hypertension.

Other potentially useful vasodilator agents include inhaled nitric oxide and intravenous prostacyclin, although results of large clinical trials are not yet available.[69]

Oxygen therapy is the only treatment that improves survival among patients with COPD and pulmonary hypertension. Current criteria for recommending long-term oxygen therapy in the care of patients with COPD whose condition is stable include PaO_2 less than 55 mm Hg or oxygen saturation less than 88%. Other indications for supplemental oxygen use include a PaO_2 between 55 and 59 mm Hg or oxygen saturation less than 89% in the presence of findings suggestive of cor pulmonale, such as "P pulmonale" on the electrocardiogram, hematocrit greater than 55%, or the presence of congestive heart failure.[70] Oxygen administration may be adjusted for rest, exertion, and sleep to maintain an oxygen saturation of 90% or greater. At least 20 minutes of administration of oxygen may be needed for full equilibration. Other situations in which oxygen is sometimes prescribed include desaturation with exercise or with sleep to a partial pressure of oxygen less than 55 mm Hg, although evidence that supplemental oxygen enhances survival in these specific settings is lacking. In case of desaturation during sleep, continuous positive airway pressure may be considered as well.[70]

KEY POINTS

- Venous thromboembolism (DVT and pulmonary embolism) is an important cause of morbidity and mortality among hospitalized patients.
- One third of the deaths caused by pulmonary embolism occur within 1 hour of the symptoms. The mortality in the group of patients with pulmonary embolism that remains undiagnosed is 30%; if the venous thrombosis is recognized and managed, the mortality is less than 8%.
- The point of origin of pulmonary embolism is DVT of the lower extremities or pelvis in 86% of cases.

KEY POINTS—cont'd

- Most of the time, the clinical presentation of pulmonary embolism and DVT is nonspecific. A high index of suspicion is important to make the diagnosis in patients at risk.
- Prophylactic therapy reduces the risk of venous thromboembolism in patients at risk. Unfortunately, prophylactic therapy is underutilized.
- Pharmacological choices for prophylaxis include low-dose subcutaneous heparin, warfarin, low molecular-weight heparin, and dextran. Mechanical measures include early ambulation, wearing elastic stockings, pneumatic calf compression, and electric stimulation of calf muscles.
- Management of venous thromboembolism includes anticoagulation therapy (heparin and warfarin).
- PPH is a rare disease that mainly affects young adults. In PPH, damage to the endothelium of the pulmonary artery alters the balance between vasoconstrictors and vasodilators, favoring vasoconstriction.
- Management of PPH includes warfarin and vasodilators (calcium channel blockers and epoprostenol). Lung transplantation is an option.

References

1. Silverstein M et al: Trends in the incidence of deep vein thrombosis and pulmonary embolism: a 25-year population-based study, Arch Intern Med 158:585, 1998.
2. Rosenow EC: Venous and pulmonary thromboembolism: an algorithmic approach to diagnosis and management, Mayo Clin Proc 70:45, 1995.
3. Anderson FA Jr et al: A population based perspective of the hospital incidence and case fatality rates of deep vein thrombosis and pulmonary embolus: the Worcester DVT Study, Arch Intern Med 151:933, 1991.
4. Wagenvoort CA: Pathology of pulmonary thromboembolism, Chest 107:10S, 1995.
5. Sperry KL, Key CR, Anderson RE: Toward a population-based assessment of death due to pulmonary embolism in New Mexico, Hum Pathol 21:159, 1990.
6. Sandler DA, Martin JF: Autopsy proven pulmonary embolism in hospital patients: are we detecting enough deep vein thrombosis? J R Soc Med 82:203, 1989.
7. Morpurgo M, Schmid C: The spectrum of pulmonary embolism: clinicopathologic correlations, Chest 107:18S, 1995.
8. Dalen JE, Alpert JS: Natural history of pulmonary embolism, Prog Cardiovasc Dis 17:257, 1975.

9. Carson JL et al: The clinical course of pulmonary embolism, N Engl J Med 326:1240, 1992.
10. Heit JA, Silverstein M, Mohr D, et al: Predictors of survival after deep vein thrombosis and pulmonary embolism: a population-based cohort study, Arch Intern Med 159:445, 1999.
11. Dalen JE: When can treatment be withheld in patients with suspected pulmonary embolism? Arch Intern Med 153:1415, 1993.
12. Arroliga AC, Matthay MA, Matthay RA: Pulmonary thromboembolism and other pulmonary vascular diseases. In George RB et al, editors: Chest medicine: essentials of pulmonary and critical care medicine, ed 4, Philadelphia, 2000, Lippincott Williams & Wilkins.
13. Walker ID, Greaves M, Preston FE: Investigation and management of heritable thrombophilia, Br J Haematol 114:512, 2001.
14. Riedel M: Acute pulmonary embolism, 1: pathophysiology, clinical presentation, and diagnosis, Heart 85:229, 2001.
15. Elliott CG: Pulmonary physiology during pulmonary embolism, Chest 101:163S, 1992.
16. Thomas D et al: Mechanisms of bronchoconstrictions produced by thromboemboli in dogs, Am J Physiol 206:1207, 1964.
17. Landefeld CS, McGuire E, Cohen AM: Clinical findings associated with acute proximal deep vein thrombosis: a basis of quantifying clinical judgment, Am J Med 88:382, 1990.
18. Miniati M et al: Accuracy of clinical assessment in the diagnosis of pulmonary embolism, Am J Respir Crit Care Med 159:864, 1999.
19. Manganelli D et al: Clinical features of pulmonary embolism: doubts and certainties, Chest 107:25S, 1995.
20. Stein PD et al: Clinical, laboratory, roentgenographic, and electrocardiographic findings in patients with acute pulmonary embolism and no pre-existing cardiac or pulmonary disease, Chest 100:598, 1991.
21. Goldhaber SZ et al: Quantitative plasma D-dimer levels among patients undergoing pulmonary angiography for suspected pulmonary embolism, JAMA 270:2819, 1993.
22. Ginsberg JS et al: The use of D-dimer testing and impedance plethysmographic examination in patients with clinical indications of deep vein thrombosis, Arch Intern Med 157:1077, 1997.
23. Kearon C et al: Management of suspected deep venous thrombosis in outpatients by using clinical assessment and D-dimer testing, Ann Intern Med 135:108, 2001.
24. Wells P et al: Excluding pulmonary embolism at the bedside without diagnostic imaging: management of patients with suspected pulmonary embolism presenting to the emergency department by using a simple clinical model and D-dimer, Ann Intern Med 135:98, 2001.
25. Hull RD et al: Impedance plethysmography: the relationship between venous filling and sensitivity and specificity for proximal vein thrombosis, Circulation 58:898, 1978.
26. Ginsberg JS et al: Reevaluation of the sensitivity of impedance plethysmography for the detection of proximal deep vein thrombosis, Arch Intern Med 154:1930, 1994.
27. Cronan JJ: Venous thromboembolic disease: the role of ultrasound, Radiology 186:619, 1993.
28. Lensing AWA et al: Detection of deep vein thrombosis by real-time B-mode ultrasonography, N Engl J Med 320:342, 1989.
29. Lensing AWA et al: A comparison of compression ultrasound with color Doppler ultrasound for the diagnosis of symptomless postoperative deep vein thrombosis, Arch Intern Med 157:765, 1997.
30. ACCP Consensus Committee on Pulmonary Embolism: Opinions regarding the diagnosis and management of venous thromboembolic disease, Chest 109:233, 1996.
31. Worsley DF, Alavi A, Palevsky JH: Role of radionuclide imaging in patients with suspected pulmonary embolism, Radiol Clin North Am 31:849, 1993.
32. Van Beek EJR et al: A normal perfusion lung scan in patients with clinically suspected pulmonary embolism: frequency and clinical validity, Chest 108:170, 1995.
33. Stein PD et al: Diagnostic utility of ventilation/perfusion lung scans in acute pulmonary embolism is not diminished by pre-existing cardiac or pulmonary disease, Chest 100:604, 1991.
34. Henry JW et al: Scintigraphic lung scans and clinical assessment in critically ill patients with suspected acute pulmonary embolism, Chest 109:462, 1996.
35. Hartmann IJ et al: Diagnosing acute pulmonary embolism: effect of chronic obstruction pulmonary disease on the performance of D-dimer testing, ventilation/perfusion scintigraphy, spiral computed tomographic angiography, and conventional angiography, Am J Respir Crit Care Med 162:2232, 2000.
36. The PIOPED Investigators: Value of the ventilation/perfusion scan in acute pulmonary embolism: results of the prospective investigation of pulmonary embolism diagnosis (PIOPED), JAMA 263:2753, 1990.
37. Perrier A et al: Diagnosis of pulmonary embolism by a decision analysis-based strategy including clinical probability, D-dimer levels, and ultrasonography: a management study, Arch Intern Med 156:531, 1996.
38. Wells PS et al: Use of a clinical model for safe management of patients with suspected pulmonary embolism, Ann Intern Med 129:997, 1998.
39. Remy-Jardin M et al: Diagnosis of pulmonary embolism with spiral CT: comparison with pulmonary angiography and scintigraphy, Radiology 200:699, 1996.
40. Rathbun S, Raskob GE, Whitsett TL: Sensitivity and specificity of helical computed tomography in the diagnosis of pulmonary embolism: a systematic review, Ann Intern Med 132:227, 2000.
41. Spritzer CE et al: Detection of deep venous thrombosis by magnetic resonance imaging, Chest 104:54, 1993.
42. Geerts WH et al: Prevention of venous thromboembolism, Chest 119:132S, 2001.
43. Hirsch DR, Ingenito EP, Goldhaber SZ: Prevalence of deep venous thrombosis among patients in medical intensive care, JAMA 274:335, 1995.
44. Hull RD et al: Continuous intravenous heparin compared with intermittent subacute heparin in the initial treatment of proximal vein thrombosis, N Engl J Med 315:1109, 1986.
45. Hyers TM et al: Antithrombotic therapy for venous thromboembolic disease, Chest 2001:119:176S.

46. Raschke RA et al: The weight-based heparin dosing nomogram compared with a "standard care" nomogram, Ann Intern Med 119:874, 1993.
47. Raschke RA, Gollihare B, Pierce JC: The effectiveness of implementing the weight-based heparin nomogram as a practice guideline, Arch Intern Med 156:1645, 1996.
48. Harrison L et al: Comparison of 5 mg and 10 mg loading doses in initiation of warfarin therapy, Ann Intern Med 126:133, 1997.
49. Pinede L et al: Comparison of 3 and 6 months of oral anticoagulant therapy after a first episode of proximal deep vein thrombosis or pulmonary embolism and comparison of 6 and 12 weeks of therapy after isolated calf deep vein thrombosis, Circulation 103:2453, 2001.
50. O'Heara JJ et al: A decision analysis of streptokinase plus heparin as compared with heparin alone for deep-vein thrombosis, N Engl J Med 330:1864, 1994.
51. Tapson VF, Witty LA: Massive pulmonary embolism, Clin Chest Med 16:329, 1995.
52. Goldhaber SZ: Contemporary pulmonary embolism thrombolysis, Chest 107:50S, 1995.
53. Decousus H et al: A clinical trial of vena caval filters in the prevention of pulmonary embolism in patients with proximal deep-vein thrombosis, N Engl J Med 338:409, 1998.
54. Rubin LJ: Primary pulmonary hypertension, Chest 104:236, 1993.
55. Archer S, Rich S: Primary pulmonary hypertension: a vascular biology and translational research "work in progress," Circulation 102:2781, 2000.
56. Arroliga AC et al: Primary pulmonary hypertension: update on pathogenesis and novel therapies, Cleve Clin J Med 67:175, 2000.
57. Giaid A et al: Expression of endothelin-1 in the lung of patients with pulmonary hypertension, N Engl J Med 328:1732, 1993.
58. Christman BW et al: Imbalance between the excretion of thromboxane and prostacyclin metabolites in pulmonary hypertension, N Engl J Med 327:70, 1992.
59. Rich S, Brundage BH: Pulmonary hypertension: a cellular basis for understanding the pathophysiology and treatment, J Am Coll Cardiol 14:545, 1991.
60. Rich S, Kaufmann G, Levy PS: The effect of high doses of calcium channel blockers on survival in primary pulmonary hypertension, N Engl J Med 327:76, 1992.
61. Barst RJ et al: Survival in primary pulmonary hypertension with long-term continuous intravenous prostacyclin, Ann Intern Med 121:409, 1994.
62. Barst RJ et al: A comparison of continuous intravenous epoprostenol (prostacyclin) with conventional therapy for primary pulmonary hypertension, N Engl J Med 334:296, 1996.
63. Shapiro SM et al: Primary pulmonary hypertension: improved long-term effect and survival with continuous intravenous epoprostenol infusion, J Am Coll Cardiol 30:343, 1997.
64. Mc Laughlin VV et al: Reduction in pulmonary vascular resistance with long-term epoprostenol (prostacyclin) therapy in primary pulmonary hypertension, N Engl J Med 338:273, 1998.
65. Salvaterra CG, Rubin LJ: Investigation and management of pulmonary hypertension in chronic obstructive pulmonary disease, Am Rev Respir Dis 148:1414, 1993.
66. Matthay RA et al: Right ventricular function at rest and during exercise in chronic obstructive pulmonary disease, Chest 101:255S, 1992.
67. Weitzenblum E et al: Medical treatment of pulmonary hypertension in chronic lung disease, Eur Respir J 7:148, 1994.
68. Matthay RA et al: Pulmonary artery hypertension in chronic obstructive pulmonary disease: chest radiographic assessment, Invest Radiol 16:95, 1981.
69. Yoshida M et al: Combined inhalation of nitric oxide and oxygen in chronic obstructive pulmonary disease, Am J Respir Crit Care Med 155:526, 1997.
70. Celli BR et al: Standards for the diagnosis and care for patients with chronic obstructive pulmonary disease, Am J Respir Crit Care Med 152:77S, 1995.

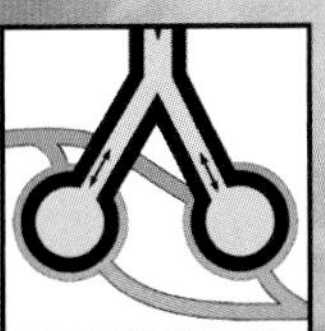

CHAPTER 24

Acute Lung Injury, Pulmonary Edema, and Multiple System Organ Failure

Elliott D. Crouser and Ruairi J. Fahy

In This Chapter You Will Learn:

- What clinical conditions lead to hydrostatic pulmonary edema (congestive heart failure [CHF]) and nonhydrostatic pulmonary edema (acute respiratory distress syndrome [ARDS])
- What criteria are considered for the diagnosis of CHF, ARDS, and multiple organ dysfunction syndrome (MODS)
- What pathophysiology is associated with hydrostatic and nonhydrostatic pulmonary edema
- How hydrostatic and nonhydrostatic pulmonary edema are differentiated from one another in the clinical setting
- What principles of supportive care are followed for patients with ARDS
- How ventilator settings (e.g., tidal volume, positive end-expiratory pressure) are adjusted for patients with ARDS and MODS
- How mechanical ventilation can cause lung injury and how ventilator-induced lung injury can be avoided
- What approaches to the management of ARDS and MODS are being implemented

Chapter Outline

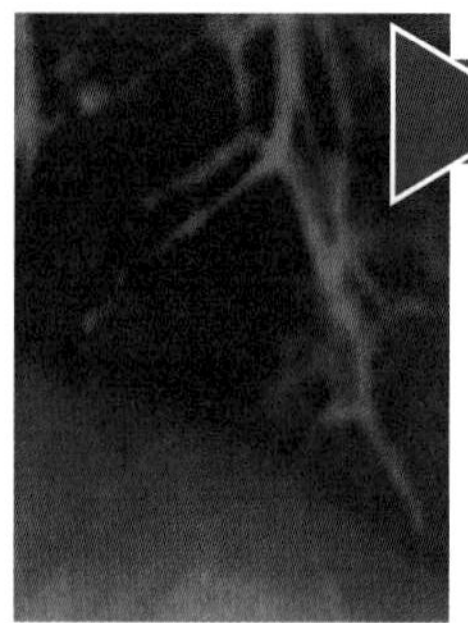

Key Terms

acute lung injury (ALI)
airway pressure release ventilation (APRV)
acute respiratory distress syndrome (ARDS)
congestive heart failure (CHF)
compliance
extracorporeal carbon dioxide removal ($ECCO_2R$)
extracorporeal membrane oxygenation (ECMO)
high-frequency ventilation
hydrostatic
multiple organ dysfunction syndrome (MODS)
positive end-expiratory pressure (PEEP)
surfactant

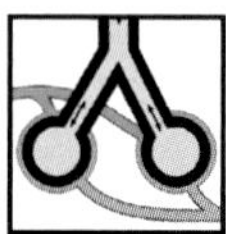

Acute hypoxemic respiratory failure may develop in many clinical settings and is a common reason for admission to intensive care units. Most causes of acute hypoxemic respiratory failure develop as a result of abnormal accumulations of fluid within the lung parenchyma and alveoli. These accumulations are collectively referred to as *pulmonary edema*. Pulmonary edema may arise from acute illnesses associated with increased pulmonary venous pressure (hydrostatic pulmonary edema or **congestive heart failure** [CHF]) or may result from conditions associated with **acute lung injury** (ALI), in which the normal barriers to fluid movement within the lungs are disrupted (nonhydrostatic pulmonary edema). Acute lung injury of sufficient severity to cause acute hypoxemic respiratory failure is commonly referred to as **acute respiratory distress syndrome** (ARDS). Thus ALI and ARDS represent a spectrum of lung injury, the term *ARDS* being reserved for more severe gas exchange abnormalities[1] (Table 24-1).

The arbitrary dividing line between ALI and ARDS may have clinical relevance, because patients with more severe lung injury often have simultaneous injury to other systemic organs. Acute illnesses associated with widespread systemic organ injury are referred to as **multiple organ dysfunction syndrome** (MODS), which is the most common cause of death in intensive care units.

Congestive heart failure and ARDS are manifestations of unique diseases demanding different management strategies. Failure to differentiate these two forms of pulmonary edema may delay appropriate therapy for the underlying disease, and the result is prolonged hospitalization and worse outcome. Unfortunately, because of similarities in clinical presentations, differentiating **hydrostatic** and nonhydrostatic pulmonary edema often is often difficult for even the most skilled clinician.

This chapter initially focuses on the mechanisms responsible for acute respiratory failure due to hydrostatic and to nonhydrostatic pulmonary edema. Emphasis is on identifying key clinical features that differentiate these two forms of respiratory failure. This discussion sets the stage for a better understanding of the established principles of supportive care and of the rationale behind innovative treatments of patients with ARDS and MODS.

▶ EPIDEMIOLOGY

Acute respiratory distress syndrome is a common cause of respiratory failure. It can occur as a consequence of critical illnesses of diverse causes. The incidence of ARDS is unknown but was initially estimated to be approximately 150,000 cases per year in the United States. This figure has been questioned, but precise figures remain unavailable. However, the incidence is probably substantially lower and more closely approximates 20,000 to 30,000 cases per year.

Table 24-1 ▶▶ Recommended Criteria for Acute Lung Injury (ALI) and Acute Respiratory Distress Syndrome (ARDS)

Criteria Pressure	Timing	Oxygenation	Chest Radiograph	Pulmonary Artery Wedge
ALI	Acute onset	$PaO_2/FIO_2 \leq 300$ mm Hg (regardless of PEEP level)	Bilateral infiltrates seen on frontal chest radiograph	≤18 mm Hg when measured or no clinical evidence of left atrial hypertension
ARDS	Acute onset	$PaO_2/FIO_2 \leq 200$ mm Hg (regardless of PEEP level)	Bilateral infiltrates seen on frontal chest radiograph	≤18 mm Hg when measured or no clinical evidence of left atrial hypertension

Modified from Bernard GR et al: Am J Respir Crit Care 149:819, 1994.

Despite uncertainties regarding the incidence of ARDS, it appears that the mortality associated with ARDS has declined over the past two decades from more than 90% to its present level of 40%.[2] The explanation for this favorable trend is likely multifactorial and includes advances in supportive care, early detection, and effective management of comorbid diseases, such as nosocomial infection, and the broad application of innovative mechanical ventilation techniques. However, the cumulative cost of ARDS and MODS in terms of both human lives and medical resource utilization remains unacceptably high. The medical community awaits the results of ongoing investigations that may provide insight into the pathogenesis and management of ARDS.

▶ ARDS RISK FACTORS

It has been proposed that ARDS can develop by different mechanisms and that the risk factors for ARDS should therefore be categorized as either direct or indirect[1] (Box 24-1). However, all of these risk factors share the common ability to initiate a systemic inflammatory reaction, which if sufficiently vigorous, may lead to diffuse lung injury (ARDS). In this regard, the probability of development of ARDS may depend in part on the severity and characteristics of the initial injury. For example, gastric aspiration and septic shock (sepsis with hypotension) are associated with a greater than 25% risk of development of ARDS, whereas use of multiple blood transfusions carries a risk of ARDS of less than 5%.[3] The risk of development of ARDS also appears to be additive when multiple risk factors are present.[4]

Box 24-1 • Risk Factors for ALI and ARDS

PRIMARY

- Pneumonia (viral, bacterial, fungal)
- Gastric aspiration
- Toxic inhalation (phosgene, cocaine, smoke, high concentration of oxygen)
- Near-drowning
- Lung contusion

SECONDARY

- Sepsis
- Burn injury (chemical or heat induced)
- Prolonged systemic hypotension and shock
- Multiple trauma
- Pancreatitis
- Gynecologic (abruptio placentae, amniotic embolism, eclampsia)
- Drug effect (salicylates, thiazides)
- Fulminant hepatic failure
- Sickle cell crisis
- Multiple drug transfusions

▶ PATHOPHYSIOLOGY

Normal Physiology

The lung structure is optimally designed to fulfill its physiologic functions. These are as follows:

1. To deliver inhaled oxygen to the site of gas exchange, namely the alveoli
2. To diffuse gases, mainly oxygen and carbon dioxide, between the alveolar capillary membrane and the lumen of the alveolus
3. To match alveolar ventilation with pulmonary capillary blood flow such that gas exchange is optimized
4. To maintain a net flux of fluid through the lung parenchyma without inducing lung edema or alveolar consolidation.

For optimization of gas exchange, the entire cardiac output passes through the vascular system of the lungs. Gas exchange primarily occurs through the extensive capillary network surrounding the alveolar air spaces. The entire surface of alveolar walls is in approximation to pulmonary capillaries. As such, the diffusion distances between inspired gases and capillary blood are very small (less than 0.5 μm). Diffusion of gases at the alveolar-capillary interface depends on the relative concentrations of gases in the inspired air and in the blood. Thus there is net diffusion of oxygen from the alveolus into the blood, whereas carbon dioxide diffuses from the blood to the alveolus. These diffusion gradients are constantly renewed by provision of deoxygenated and carbon dioxide-rich blood from the systemic circulation to the lungs and by ventilation of the lungs with oxygenated, carbon dioxide-depleted air. Thus the heart and lungs are vitally linked.

Pulmonary Blood Flow

The intricate design of the pulmonary circulation provides for the efficient transfer of gases between the alveoli and the blood. On average, the entire blood volume of the body circulates through the lungs in 1 minute or less. This incredible feat is achieved through an ingenious design. Starting at the outflow tract of the right ventricle (pulmonary valve), the relatively thick-walled, smooth muscle-lined pulmonary artery branches successively and follows the divisions of the bronchi as far as the terminal bronchioles. Beyond the terminal bronchioles, the pulmonary vasculature further divides to form a fine capillary meshwork surrounding the alveoli. The large surface area of the capillary network provides for a low-pressure (5-12 mm Hg), high-volume system wherein large volumes of blood come into immediate contact with alveolar gases. At a capillary level, the vessel walls are composed solely of endothelial cells bound to a basal lamina. Because of the delicate nature of the alveolar-capillary interface, it is not surprising that injury to the alveolar-capillary interface and high capillary blood pressure result in disruption of pulmonary gas exchange (see later "Pulmonary Edema").

The Lung Interstitium

The interstitial space of the lung is the space between the alveolar epithelium and the capillaries. The interstitium is composed of several structural proteins (type I, III, and IV collagen and elastin) and proteoglycans. The proteoglycans make up the ground substance of the interstitium and are composed of 20% protein and 80% glycosaminoglycans. The alveolar-capillary interstitial space is composed of endothelial and epithelial cell membranes bound to a common basement membrane with a very thin (<0.5 μm) interstitial space. In contrast, the interstitium on the nonalveolar side of the capillaries contains separate basement membranes for both epithelial cells and endothelial cells, as well as fibroblasts, structural collagen, elastin proteins, and mucopolysaccharides in a hyaluronic acid gel (Figure 24-1).

The physical properties of the matrix allow absorption of water into the interstitial space without an increase in hydrostatic pressure and without an effect on pulmonary gas exchange. The interstitium is highly compliant under normal circumstances (large increases in fluid volume produce little change in interstitial pressure). However, the compliance of the interstitium dramatically decreases when the interstitial space becomes saturated. This phenomenon has important implications in protecting against pulmonary edema.

Liquid and Solute Transport in the Lungs

The alveolar capillaries are selectively permeable to protein and are consequently "leaky." This capillary porosity allows movement of solutes between the intravascular space and the interstitium of the lungs. The net exchange of fluids between the intravascular space and the interstitium of the lungs is determined by the combined influences of hydrostatic and osmotic forces. The relation between these two forces is described by the Starling equation:

$$Q_f = K_{fc}[(P_{mv} - P_i) - (s_d)(TT_{mv} - TT_i)]$$

where Q_f is net fluid filtration; K_{fc}, the capillary filtration coefficient (permeability constant) of the microvascular endothelium; P_{mv}, microvascular hydrostatic pressure; P_i, interstitial hydrostatic pressure; (s_d), the average osmotic reflection coefficient; TT_{mv}, microvascular osmotic pressure; and TT_i, interstitial osmotic pressure.

Under normal conditions, forces influencing the movement of fluid from the bloodstream to the interstitium of the lungs [microvascular hydrostatic pressure (P_{mv}) + interstitial osmotic pressure (TT_i)] are slightly greater than forces opposing this movement [microvascular osmotic pressure (TT_{mv}) + interstitial hydrostatic pressure (P_i)]. Thus as fluid and proteins move from the vascular space into the interstitium, a small fraction of the cardiac output (approximately 0.01%) normally filters through the interstitium of the lungs. This filtration process plays a role in the immune defenses of the lung and is a major determinant of total lung fluid content.

The lung protects itself from the devastating consequences of excessive fluid accumulation by several mechanisms. The lung **lymphatic drainage system** is the primary operant system under nonpathological conditions. The lymphatic drainage system is the main conduit for the removal of filtered fluid and protein from the lungs.

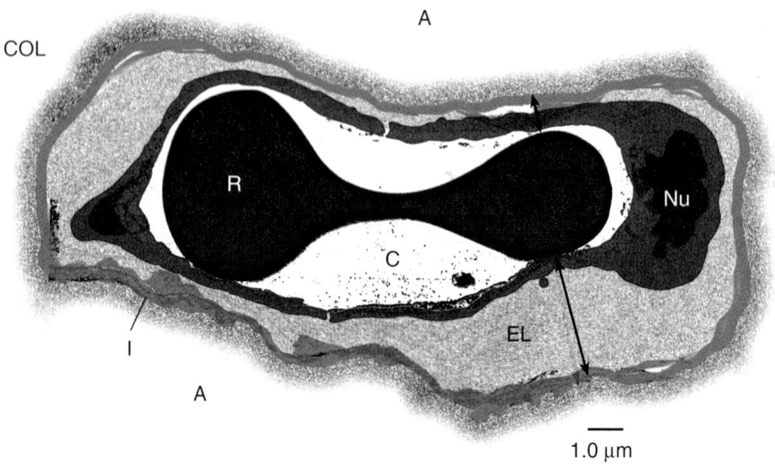

Figure 24-1
Cross-section of an alveolar wall shows the path for oxygen and carbon dioxide diffusion. The thin side of the alveolar wall barrier (short double arrow) consists of type I epithelium (*I*), interstitium (*) formed by the fused basal laminae of the epithelial and endothelial cells, capillary endothelium (*E*), plasma in the alveolar capillary (*C*), and finally the cytoplasm of the red blood cell (R). The thick side of the gas exchange barrier (long double arrow) has an accumulation of elastin (*EL*), collagen (*COL*), and matrix that separates the alveolar epithelium from the alveolar capillary endothelium. As long as the red blood cells are flowing, oxygen and carbon dioxide diffusion probably occur across both sides of the air-blood barrier. *A*, alveolus; *Nu*, nucleus of the capillary endothelial cell. (Human lung surgical specimen, transmission electron photomicrograph.)

From small lymphatic capillaries located around the respiratory bronchioles, fluid and solutes enter the lymphatic drainage channels. This process is assisted by the presence of a modest pressure gradient within the lungs. That is, pressure is greatest within the dense alveolar interstitium and gradually decreases in the nonalveolar interstitium and terminal lymphatic vessels (Figure 24-2). Drainage is further enhanced by intrathoracic pressure alterations that occur with respiration, and retrograde flow is prevented by the presence of one-way lymphatic valves. Ultimately, lymphatic fluid drains into the superior vena cava through the thoracic duct.[5]

When fluid filtration exceeds the capacity for drainage through pulmonary lymphatic vessels, several "backup" systems exist for storing additional fluid and for protection against alveolar flooding. **Loose connective tissue** located along the peribronchovascular space and extending to the level of the bronchiole is capable of storing twice the normal fluid content of the lungs.[5] Filling of these spaces or cuffs manifests radiographically as increased interstitial infiltrates (Figure 24-3), or Kerley's lines, which are caused by increased fluid in interlobular septal spaces. The peribronchovascular spaces drain into the local blood vessels or follow the intrinsic pressure gradient in the lung and empty into pulmonary lymphatic vessels. As total lung fluid accumulation increases further, the gel-like **matrix** of the lung is capable of absorbing additional fluid without affecting interstitial pressure. The latter property is important because fluid is allowed to accumulate in the lungs without transmitting additional hydrostatic pressure to the alveolar barrier. Additional fluid movement into the lungs thereby is avoided. The dense connective tissue making up the **alveolar matrix** resists edema formation in response to elevated hydrostatic or oncotic pressure.

Pulmonary Edema

Despite these protective mechanisms, during certain disease states, fluid flux into the lungs exceeds the capacity of the lung to remove or store the fluid. Under such circumstances, small increases in lung fluid content produce large increases in interstitial hydrostatic pressure. The result is alveolar flooding (pulmonary edema). Impaired gas exchange in the setting of pulmonary edema is further complicated by an increase in the work of breathing caused by dramatic reductions in lung compliance resulting from alveolar collapse and interstitial fluid accumulation. Thus patients with pulmonary edema experience impaired gas exchange with increases in metabolic demand, a situation that often leads to acute respiratory failure.

Hydrostatic Pulmonary Edema

The alveolar barrier is made up of the dense alveolar matrix (described earlier), the epithelial basement membrane, and the lining epithelial cells. The alveolar basement membrane is selectively permeable to only very small solutes such that osmotic forces favor the retention of fluid in the intravascular space. Moreover, alveolar pressure generally is slightly higher than

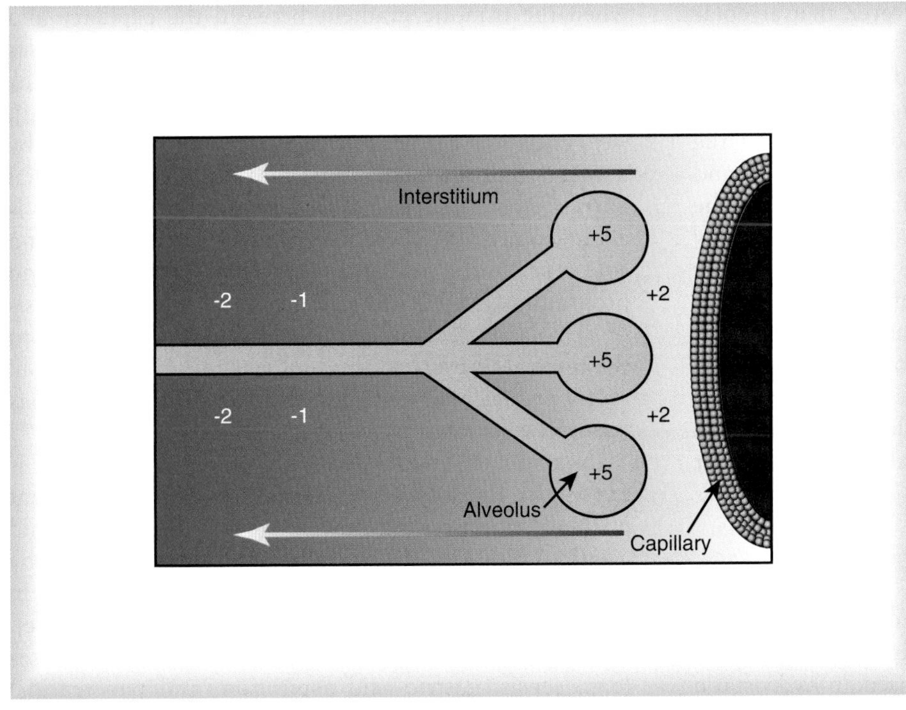

Figure 24-2
The relative hydrostatic pressures (in cm H_2O) that typically exist within the various compartments of the lung. Hydrostatic forces favor the movement of fluid along the pressure gradient (arrows) between the alveolar and pericapillary spaces and pulmonary lymphatic vessels. This hydrostatic pressure gradient favors the movement of fluid away from the alveolar capillary interface and protects against alveolar and interstitial edema formation.

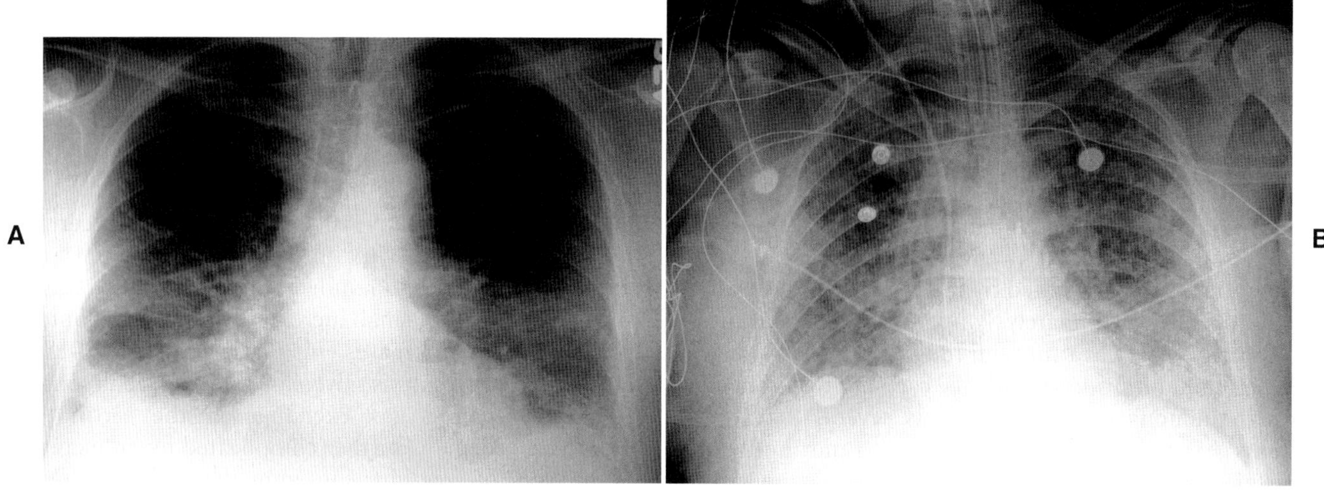

Figure 24-3

Chest radiographs show the typical radiographic features of CHF and ARDS. **A**, CHF is characterized by cardiomegaly, interstitial infiltrates, bilateral perihilar and basilar alveolar infiltrates, and bilateral pleural effusions, which cause blunting of the costophrenic angles. **B**, ARDS is commonly associated with normal cardiac size, diffuse peripheral alveolar infiltrates, and minimal or absent pleural effusions.

interstitial pressure, and this difference provides further protection against alveolar fluid accumulation (see Figure 24-2). Thus under normal circumstances there is little fluid movement into the alveoli across the alveolar barrier. Fluid that does form is composed of low-molecular-weight proteins and is actively transported back into the interstitium by type II pneumocytes.[6] In contrast, when the defense mechanisms against fluid accumulation in the lung are overwhelmed, hydrostatic pressure increases sharply within the interstitium of the lung, and alveolar flooding ensues. The precise mechanism of alveolar flooding during hydrostatic pulmonary edema is unknown. It has been shown, however, that alveolar flooding tends to occur in an "all or none" manner. Moreover, the alveolar fluid formed in the setting of increased hydrostatic pressure has characteristics identical to those of interstitial fluid even though the alveolar epithelium is impermeable to large proteins and molecules.[7] This observation lends support to the findings of Conhaim,[8] who demonstrated experimentally that high interstitial fluid pressure leads to alveolar flooding through leakage of fluid from the epithelium of respiratory bronchioles, alveolar ducts, and their associated alveoli. The epithelium of the respiratory bronchioles and alveolar ducts may be particularly prone to hydrostatic injury, because these locations represent the transition zone between respiratory and alveolar epithelium.

Nonhydrostatic Pulmonary Edema

Unlike hydrostatic pulmonary edema, nonhydrostatic pulmonary edema is associated with increased total lung water despite normal microvascular hydrostatic pressure. The mechanisms of nonhydrostatic pulmonary edema that ultimately lead to ARDS are more complex than those responsible for hydrostatic pulmonary edema. Although many seemingly unrelated risk factors for ARDS have been identified, all causes of ARDS evoke disruption of endothelial and epithelial barriers and typically occur under conditions associated with widespread microvascular injury to the lungs. Vascular endothelial injury in the lungs in turn results in increased microvascular permeability and fluid filtration, such that there is uninhibited entry of protein-rich fluid into the pulmonary interstitium. Alveolar flooding develops when the osmotic gradient between the capillary and the lung becomes essentially zero and no longer opposes the hydrostatic forces favoring fluid movement from the capillary into the lung $[K_{fc}(Pmv - Pi) >> (s_d)(TT_{mv} - T_{ti})]$, (see Equation 1). This process may be facilitated by damage to the normally impermeable alveolar epithelial barrier. Acute injury to alveolar epithelial lining cells is a key feature of ARDS.[9] Recent investigations support a role for both necrotic epithelial cell death and programmed cell death (apoptosis) in the pathogenesis of alveolar wall damage.[10,11] In addition to damage to the normal barriers to fluid movement into the alveoli, recent evidence for impaired alveolar fluid clearance has been demonstrated in ALI and ARDS.[12]

In summary, nonhydrostatic pulmonary edema is caused by the loss of the normal osmotic forces that normally oppose fluid movement into the lungs. Fluid accumulation in the lung is further promoted by impaired pulmonary fluid clearance and by increases in hydrostatic pressure (i.e., pulmonary capillary pressure).

A mechanism to explain how different acute illnesses (e.g., sepsis, gastric acid aspiration, and pancreatitis) can lead to the development of ARDS has been proposed by Weiland et al.[13] These investigators demonstrated that ARDS, regardless of the cause, is associated with an influx of neutrophils (PMNs) and PMN-derived inflammatory byproducts (such as neutrophil elastase and myeloperoxidase) into the lung. The PMN-activating cytokine interleukin-8 (IL-8) has been shown to be increased in the lungs of patients with ARDS, whereas a reduction in IL-8 and PMNs has been shown to correlate with recovery from ARDS.[14] Taken together, the results of these studies suggest that the common mechanism for the development of ARDS is activation of inflammation, which can occur as a result of events that are largely localized to the lungs or that originate systemically.

Although PMNs play a central role in the development of ARDS, ARDS has been reported to occur in neutropenic patients. In this regard, other chemical (e.g., gastric aspiration) and immunological pathways participate in the initiation and development of the systemic inflammatory response to critical illnesses associated with ARDS. For example, sepsis is associated with intense activation of systemic inflammatory pathways such that cytokines (e.g., tumor necrosis factor α [TNF-α], IL-1, IL-6, and IL-8), arachidonic acid metabolites (e.g., platelet-activating factor, leukotrienes), and nitric oxide (NO) all contribute to the hemodynamic and inflammatory events characteristic of this syndrome.[15] The relative contributions and exact roles of these proinflammatory mediators in the pathogenesis of ARDS and MODS remain a topic of intense investigation and controversy.[16,17] Attempts to control the inflammatory response during sepsis by blocking specific mediators, such as anti-TNF antibodies, have not proved beneficial and may worsen outcome.

Gas Exchange and Lung Mechanics During ARDS

ARDS is associated with restrictive physiology and refractory hypoxemia, which are largely a result of pulmonary microvascular injury. Specifically, increased pulmonary capillary permeability facilitates the influx of inflammatory fluid into the lung interstitium and alveolar spaces and causes decreased lung **compliance** and alveolar consolidation. The presence of intraalveolar inflammatory fluid impairs surfactant synthesis and function such that pulmonary gas exchange (i.e., related to atelectasis) and compliance are further impaired. The negative effects of alveolar consolidation and atelectasis on pulmonary gas exchange are exacerbated by a loss of the normal vascular response to alveolar hypoxemia. Unaerated alveoli receive excessive blood flow, which contributes to severe ventilation/perfusion mismatching and intrapulmonary shunt during ARDS.

Box 24-2 • Clinical Features of CHF and ARDS

FEATURES COMMON TO CHF AND ARDS

- Symptoms of anxiety, dyspnea, tachypnea
- Reduced lung volumes and decreased compliance
- Arterial blood gases initially show respiratory alkalosis and arterial hypoxemia
- Chest radiograph shows diffuse alveolar and interstitial infiltrates

FEATURES FAVORING CHF

- Clinical history suggestive of CHF (see Box 24-1)
- Cardiomegaly or pleural effusions on chest radiograph (see Figure 24-3)
- PCWP >18 mm Hg
- Bronchoalveolar lavage fluid (BALF) nonproteinaceous and noninflammatory

FEATURES FAVORING ARDS

- Clinical history of risk factors for ARDS (see Table 24-1)
- Peripheral infiltrates on chest radiograph (see Figure 24-3)
- PCWP <18 mm Hg
- BALF is proteinaceous and inflammatory
- Pathological examination shows diffuse alveolar damage, type II pneumocyte hyperplasia with or without fibrosis

The pulmonary manifestations of ARDS and CHF are summarized in Box 24-2.

The Role of Organ-Organ Interactions in the Pathogenesis of ARDS and MODS

The notion that factors operating outside the lungs may participate in the initiation and progression of ARDS has generated interest in the role of organ system interactions in the pathogenesis of ARDS and MODS. For example, injury to remote systemic organs is known to occur after ALI,[18] apparently along PMN-mediated pathways.[19] In this way, ALI may perpetuate the systemic inflammatory response and lead to further lung and systemic organ injury. The gut-liver-lung axis may be most influential in causing the systemic inflammatory response associated with ARDS and MODS. The gastrointestinal (GI) tract contains large quantities of potentially pathogenic bacteria and endotoxin against which the host is normally protected by intact mucosal barriers and the reticuloendothelial (RE) system. However, during critical illness, the function of the GI tract and the liver often is compromised. The widespread use of broad-spectrum antibiotics in the care of critically ill patients often leads to overgrowth of bacterial populations within the GI tract. These populations are characterized by antibiotic resistance and a greater chance for spread within the host. The bacteria and their toxic byproducts (such as endotoxin) escape from the GI tract and are taken up by the RE cells of the liver, spleen, and regional lymph nodes. The resultant activation of the RE system may initiate and perpetuate a systemic inflammatory response that leads to systemic organ injury (i.e., ARDS and MODS).[20] This sequence of events forms the basis for strategies designed to reduce the release of proinflammatory mediators from the GI tract, including selective decontamination, early enteral feeding, and other approaches designed to moderate the systemic inflammatory response during ARDS and MODS (see later, Therapeutic Approach to ARDS).

Why ARDS/MODS develops in some patients with ALI and not others is unknown. The determinants of ARDS may relate to the balance between proinflammatory and antiinflammatory factors within the body. In this regard, the liver plays a major role in both induction and *modulation* of the systemic inflammatory response to all kinds of initiating events and is primarily responsible for the breakdown of endogenous proinflammatory mediators, including TNF-α, leukotrienes, and others.[21] It is not surprising that patients with liver disease have higher levels of circulating proinflammatory mediators and are more prone to bacteremia than are patients without liver disease.

The liver is not the sole determinant of ARDS and MODS in critically ill patients. Other factors, such as the severity of the primary illness and comorbid diseases (e.g., cardiac disease, advanced age, renal failure, malignant disease), also appear to predispose patients to ARDS and MODS.[20,21]

▶ HISTOPATHOLOGY AND CLINICAL CORRELATES OF ARDS

Exudative Phase (1 to 3 days)

The exudative phase is characterized by diffuse alveolar damage, diffuse microvascular injury, and the influx of inflammatory cells into the interstitium. Many of the alveolar spaces are filled with a proteinaceous, eosinophilic (on hematoxylin and eosin stain) material called *hyaline membranes,* which are composed of cellular debris and condensed plasma proteins. Pathologically there is destruction of type I pneumocytes, which are normally the predominant cells lining the alveoli, whereas type II pneumocytes are relatively resistant to injury.[22] Patients with ARDS have profound dyspnea, tachypnea, and refractory hypoxemia. This phase of ARDS often is difficult to differentiate from respiratory failure related to hydrostatic pulmonary edema (CHF). The clinical presentations of these two forms of acute respiratory failure are discussed later (see Differentiating Hydrostatic from Nonhydrostatic Pulmonary Edema in the Clinical Setting). The exudative phase may be self-limited or may progress to a fibroproliferative phase.

> **RULE OF THUMB**
>
> A careful history and physical examination often are the most useful means by which CHF and ARDS can be initially differentiated in a patient who has refractory hypoxemia and bilateral infiltrates on chest radiographs. A history consistent with one of the common causes of CHF (Box 24-3) together with physical examination findings of jugular venous distension, cardiac murmurs or gallops, bibasilar crackles, or peripheral edema suggests a diagnosis of CHF. Acute respiratory distress syndrome is more likely when the history is positive for one of the established risk factors (see Box 24-1) and there is no clinical evidence in support of CHF.

Fibroproliferative Phase (3 to 7 days)

After inflammatory injury to the lung is established and the initiating events are controlled, a process of lung repair begins. Pathologically, there are hyperplasia of alveolar type II pneumocytes and proliferation of fibroblasts within the alveolar basement membrane and intraalveolar spaces. Fibroblasts mediate the formation of intraalveolar and interstitial fibrosis.[22] The extent of fibrosis determines the degree of pulmonary disability in patients who survive ARDS.

The exact mechanisms controlling lung remodeling during ALI are not well established but very likely involve byproducts of inflammatory cells (e.g., proteases, antiproteases, IL-6) and various growth factors (TGF-α, TGF-β).[23] However, the remodeling process following ARDS is quite variable. In some cases, the architecture of the lung never returns to normal, and patients

Box 24-3 • Common Causes of Hydrostatic Pulmonary Edema

CARDIAC
- Left ventricular failure (e.g., myocardial infarction, myocarditis)
- Cardiac valvular disease (aortic, mitral)

VASCULAR
- Systemic hypertension
- Pulmonary embolism

VOLUME OVERLOAD
- Excessive fluid administration
- Renal failure

of the lung never returns to normal, and patients experience severe respiratory disability related to extensive pulmonary fibrosis and obliteration of the pulmonary vasculature. In other cases, patients have nearly complete normalization of lung compliance and oxygenation over a period of 6 to 12 months after the illness. The pattern of fibrosis following ALI suggests that, as in repair of the skin, an intact basement membrane is necessary for normal repair of the epithelium of the alveoli. It follows that disruption of the alveolar basement membrane is a prerequisite to the development of fibrosis after ALI. This line of reasoning is supported by the observation that the extent of recovery depends on the severity of the initial lung injury and on the influence of secondary forms of injury. Secondary forms of lung injury include nosocomial infection, oxygen toxicity, and barotrauma (see later, Therapeutic Approach to ARDS).

Differentiating Hydrostatic From Nonhydrostatic Pulmonary Edema in the Clinical Setting

The diagnostic criteria for ARDS are shown in Table 24-1. However, despite the existence of distinct pathophysiological mechanisms of hydrostatic and nonhydrostatic pulmonary edema, differentiating these two forms of acute respiratory failure may be difficult because of similarities in their early clinical presentations. Congestive heart failure is more common than ARDS and should be considered when any patient has pulmonary edema, particularly when the history and physical examination findings suggest one of the causes of CHF listed in Box 24-3. Alveolar flooding by either hydrostatic or nonhydrostatic mechanisms results in diffuse radiographic infiltrates, altered gas exchange, and abnormal mechanical properties of the lung (see Box 24-2). A clinical history of infection, recent trauma, or risk factors for aspiration may be present in either patient group. Likewise, many patients with ARDS are older and have preexisting illnesses that place them at risk of CHF. In patients with acute hypoxemic respiratory failure, CHF must always be considered, even when the patient has obvious risk factors for ARDS.

The ability to discern CHF and ARDS solely on the basis of radiographic findings is difficult or impossible and is complicated by technical limitations associated with obtaining chest radiographs in the intensive care unit. Both CHF and ARDS are characterized by diffuse alveolar infiltrates prevalent in dependent lung zones. Congestive heart failure is more often associated with cardiomegaly and the presence of perihilar infiltrates and pleural effusions. Acute respiratory distress syndrome is more often associated with the presence of peripheral alveolar infiltrates, air bronchograms, sparing of the costophrenic angles, and normal cardiac size. However, cardiac size may be difficult to interpret on an anteroposterior radiograph, and when images are obtained with the patient in the supine position, pleural effusions may be obscured. The hallmark radiographic features of CHF and ARDS consequently often are invisible to the clinician, a situation further complicated by the occasional coexistence of both hydrostatic and nonhydrostatic pulmonary edema.

Alveolar flooding of any cause (i.e., hydrostatic or nonhydrostatic) is associated with impaired gas exchange and abnormal lung mechanics. Both CHF and early ARDS (the exudative phase) are associated with interstitial and alveolar accumulation of fluid. As a result of ventilation/perfusion mismatching and shunt attendant to this fluid accumulation, arterial hypoxemia develops. Patients with interstitial and alveolar edema of any cause use a higher fraction (up to 25%-50%) of their total metabolic output to support the increased work of breathing attendant to reduced lung compliance and higher ventilatory rates. However, on the basis of gas exchange and lung mechanics alone, alveolar flooding related to hydrostatic causes may be indistinguishable from that related to nonhydrostatic causes.

In many cases, measurement of hemodynamic variables is necessary to determine whether hydrostatic or nonhydrostatic forces underlie the development of acute hypoxemic respiratory failure. To this end, a pulmonary artery (Swan-Ganz) catheter is a useful clinical tool because it allows estimation of clinically relevant data, such as cardiac output and pulmonary capillary wedge pressure (PCWP). Under ideal circumstances, PCWP closely corresponds to left ventricular end-diastolic pressure and is a reflection of the hydrostatic forces applied to the pulmonary capillary system. In this regard, a PCWP in excess of 18 mm Hg is necessary for the development of hydrostatic pulmonary edema. Conversely, alveolar flooding resulting from nonhydrostatic pulmonary edema can occur at any PCWP and is the exclusive cause of pulmonary edema at PCWP less than 18 mm Hg. Unfortunately, invasive hemodynamic monitoring may be unreliable in patients with high airway pressure. In particular, high levels of **positive end-expiratory pressure** (**PEEP**) lead to expansion of non-zone 3 lung areas in which alveolar pressure exceeds venous pressure. A PCWP in non-zone 3 lung actually reflects alveolar pressure and not left ventricular pressure.[24] During ARDS, hydrostatic forces may be overestimated or misdiagnosed as hydrostatic pulmonary edema.

Another useful means of separating nonhydrostatic from hydrostatic pulmonary edema is based on differences in the characteristics of the edema fluid. As previously discussed (see Pathophysiology), ARDS is associated with inflammatory injury to the pulmonary microvasculature, which allows the influx of inflammatory cells and proteinaceous fluid into the interstitium and alveolar spaces. The inflammatory nature of this quantities of inflammatory cells (predominantly neutrophils) in bronchoalveolar lavage fluid (BALF). Moreover, the BALF findings may be enough for establishing a diagnosis if infection or signs of aspiration (e.g., food particles) are present. In contrast, although hydrostatic pulmonary edema is associated with alveolar flooding, the edema fluid typically is noninflammatory, and the protein content is much lower than the protein content of BALF.[25] Thus BALF often provides useful insight into the underlying cause of hypoxemic respiratory failure.

The clinical characteristics that differentiate acute hypoxemic failure due to hydrostatic pulmonary edema from that caused by nonhydrostatic pulmonary edema are summarized in Box 24-2.

▶ THERAPEUTIC APPROACH TO ARDS

The management of critical illness associated with ARDS once was confined to supportive therapy (Box 24-4) designed to preserve systemic organ function and allow recovery from the underlying illness. Strategies have evolved for controlling the systemic inflammatory response that leads to lung and organ injury. The following section presents an overview of the current approach to supportive care and new potential therapies for ARDS and MODS.

Supportive Care of Patients With ARDS and MODS

General Principles

An outline of the fundamental principles of supportive care of patients with ARDS and MODS is presented in Box 24-4.

Hemodynamics and Fluid Management During ARDS

Preservation of systemic organ integrity is one of the principal goals of supportive management of all causes of respiratory failure. Ventilator strategies designed to improve arterial oxygenation must be weighed against any potential changes in hemodynamic values incurred as a result of these strategies. Because of the deleterious cardiopulmonary effects of high-pressure mechanical ventilation during ARDS, invasive monitoring of both cardiac output and systemic oxygen delivery (DO_2) may be necessary. This topic is controversial.

Gas exchange is highly dependent on total lung fluid during the exudative phase of ARDS, and small increases in hydrostatic forces (PCWP) lead to significant decreases in oxygenation as a result of alveolar flooding and associated right-to-left shunting. Measures that restrict intravascular volume are associated with improved oxygenation. However, as with increasing PEEP, im-

Box 24-4 • Supportive Care of Patients With ARDS

1. Identify and manage underlying cause of ARDS.
2. Avoid secondary (iatrogenic or nosocomial) lung injury:
   a. O_2 toxicity
   b. Aspiration
   c. Barotrauma, volume trauma
   d. Identify and manage nosocomial infection and pneumonia.
   e. Extubate as soon as is feasible.
3. Maintain adequate DO_2 to systemic organs.
   a. Minimize demand by reducing metabolic rate:
      (1) Control fever.
      (2) Control anxiety and pain.
   b. Support cardiovascular system with intravenous fluids and vasopressor agents, as necessary, to
      (1) Prevent hypotension (systolic blood pressure >90 mm Hg and mean arterial pressure >70 mm Hg).
      (2) Reverse lactic acidosis.
      (3) Maintain adequate urine output.
4. Provide nutritional support.

MINI CLINI

Determination of "Optimal" PEEP

PROBLEM

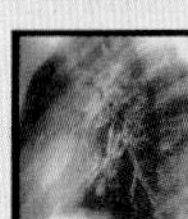

Although it is capable of recruiting collapsed alveolar units in patients with ARDS, PEEP adversely affects cardiac output and increases ventilatory pressure. The clinician must approach PEEP as a therapy that has risks and benefits.

DISCUSSION

In patients with ARDS, increasing levels of PEEP are associated with improved oxygenation and a reduction in the measured shunt fraction (FIO_2/PaO_2 ratio) (Figure 24-4). Despite progressive increases in oxygenation above the level of PEEP designated the "optimal level" in Figure 24-4, there is a net decrease in systemic DO_2. Lung compliance may begin to decline at higher levels of PEEP, and the risk of volume trauma increases. The pressure-volume relations of the lungs may be used to adjust PEEP such that end-expiratory alveolar collapse and end-inspiratory overinflation are minimized (Figure 24-5).

Although the optimal PEEP must be determined for each patient, optimal levels of PEEP usually fall in the range of 8 to 15 cm H_2O. The tidal volume may have to be decreased whenever PEEP is increased to avoid alveolar overdistension.

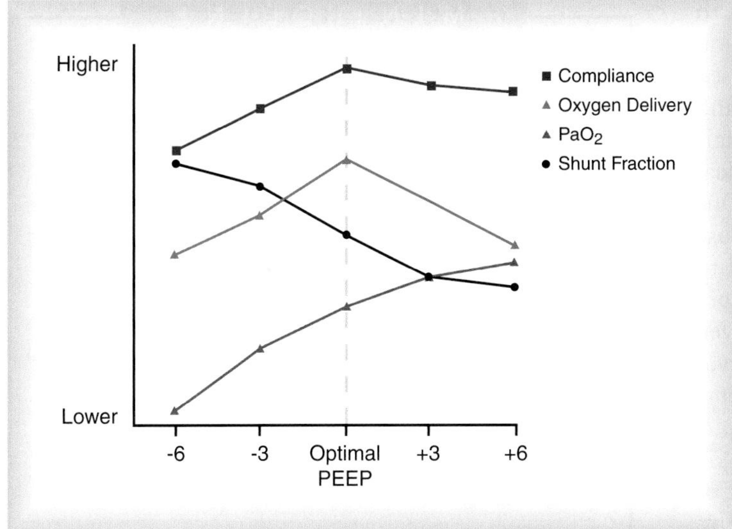

Figure 24-4

Determination of "optimal PEEP" from simultaneous measurements of hemodynamic (Do_2), gas exchange (shunt fraction and arterial oxygenation [Pao_2]), and physiological values. Optimal PEEP does not necessarily correspond to the PEEP associated with optimal pulmonary gas exchange. When adjusting PEEP, the clinician should consider its effects on systemic Do_2 and lung compliance such that systemic organ injury and lung injury are minimized.

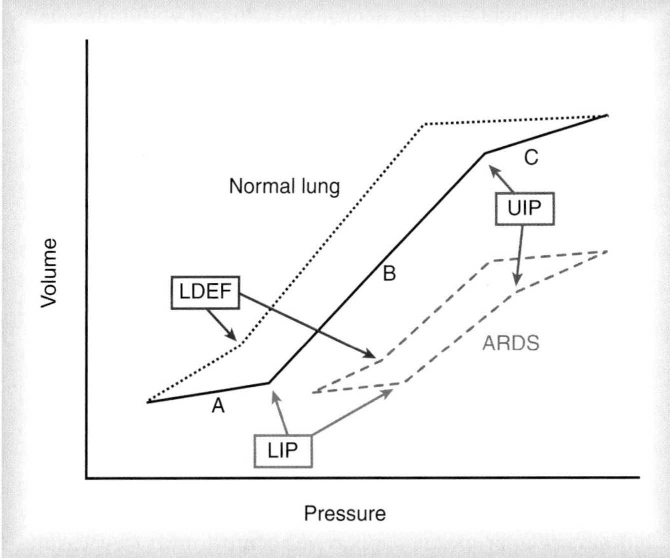

Figure 24-5

Typical pressure-volume (P-V) relations during normal conditions and during ARDS. At low lung volume, inspiratory pressure increases faster than does lung volume (line A) owing to high alveolar surface tension. As alveoli open, surface tension decreases and the pressure required to further increase lung volume decreases (line B). The lower inflection point (*LIP*) occurs between lines A and B and represents the volume above which most alveolar units are open. The upper inflection point (*UIP*) occurs at near-maximal lung volume and corresponds to the point at which further increases in pressure result in minimal increases in lung volume (line C). Pressure applied above the UIP are associated with alveolar distension. During the expiratory phase of the respiratory cycle (dotted line), the lower deflection point (*LDEF*) is the point below which lung volumes slowly decrease (alveolar units collapse). During ARDS (gray dashed curve), pressure-volume relations change such that higher pressure is needed to maintain alveolar patency, and alveolar distension occurs at lower tidal volumes. Near-maximal lung volumes are typically achieved at an inspiratory pressure of approximately 35 cm H_2O in normal conditions and during ARDS. Attempts to increase inspiratory pressure to more than 35 cm H_2O provide little additional ventilation and substantially increase the risk of volume trauma to the lungs. The LIP corresponds to pressure below which alveolar collapse occurs (line A). Under normal conditions the LIP may not be evident (i.e., minimal alveolar collapse occurs at end-inspiration under normal conditions). In contrast, during ARDS, the LIP often is evident during measurements of P-V relations and frequently occurs at a pressure of 5 to 15 cm H_2O. Positive end-expiratory pressure at levels greater than LIP may prevent end-expiratory alveolar collapse and thereby reduce lung injury due to alveolar shear stress.

provements in arterial oxygenation related to reduced PCWP must be balanced against the resultant reduction in cardiac output, as reflected by the measured Do_2 or other measures of systemic tissue oxygenation.

RULE OF THUMB

The beneficial effects of PEEP are optimal at a pressure of 15 cm H_20 or less in most patients with ARDS. Therefore, levels of PEEP greater than 15 cm H_2O should not be routinely used unless the benefits of higher levels of PEEP are supported by objective endpoints, such as improved lung compliance (see Figure 24-4) or optimal alveolar recruitment (see Figure 24-5).

With regard to tissue oxygenation during critical illness, various investigations have shown that an abnormal dependence of oxygen consumption (Vo_2) on Do_2 exists throughout the physiologic range of oxygen deliveries in many critically ill patients.[26] This abnormal dependence of Vo_2 on Do_2 is associated with impaired oxygen extraction. These observations have been interpreted to imply that tissue hypoxia may exist and contributes to organ failure (MODS) in these patients. This notion formed the basis for studies in which Do_2 was increased to "supranormal" levels in patients *at risk* of sepsis and ARDS. However, the encouraging results of early trials of this strategy[27,28] were not supported in larger clinical trials with patients with *established* sepsis.[29,30] One study showed a higher mortality associated with the use of this strategy.[30] Because of these findings, efforts to increase Do_2 beyond normal values (3.5 L/min per kilogram) are not currently recommended. Moreover, the "optimal Do_2" for critically ill patients may never be established, because the needs of individual patients must be factored into the decision to augment Do_2. It follows that new techniques for detecting tissue hypoxia are needed for guiding the hemodynamic treatment of these patients. Until such tools become available, it seems prudent to prevent hypotension (systolic blood pressure >90 mm Hg, mean blood pressure >60 mm Hg) and lactic acidosis and to ensure adequate urine output.

Mechanical Ventilation During ARDS

Despite the presence of widespread pulmonary injury and altered gas exchange during ARDS, recent investigation has shown that aerated portions of the lung have near-normal mechanical characteristics. Gattinoni and Pesenti[31] have suggested that three distinct zones exist in the lungs of patients with ARDS. The most dependent lung zones are characterized by dense pulmonary infiltrates corresponding to nonventilated lung units. A second lung zone also has dense pulmonary infiltrates and nonventilated alveolar units but is distinct from the more dependent lung zones in that these areas may be made available for gas exchange through changes in the mode of mechanical ventilation. Finally, nondependent lung zones appear to be overinflated and receive most of the ventilation. Moreover, the aerated lung zones have been shown to retain normal mechanical characteristics as reflected by the measured specific compliance (static compliance adjusted for the volume of ventilated lung). Thus in ARDS, the lungs are effectively diminished in size to 20% to 30% of normal, but the aerated portions of the lungs retain near-normal physiological properties.

Setting Tidal Volume

Because of the heterogeneous properties of the lungs during ARDS, conventional mechanical ventilation may not be appropriate for these patients. For example, conventional tidal volumes of 10 to 15 mL/kg are distributed primarily to the aerated lung zones, which then become hyperinflated. In animal models, alveolar hyperinflation has been shown to result in altered alveolar capillary permeability identical to that associated with ARDS. Moreover, the excessive volume, not high pressure, is responsible for lung injury.[32] Lung tissue injury induced by alveolar hyperinflation has been termed *volume trauma* ("volu-trauma") and can be avoided with the use of lower tidal volumes.

Tidal volume ideally would be selected on the basis of each patient's own pressure-volume relation. Pressure volume relations can be established for each patient by

MINI CLINI

Managing Hydrostatic Pressure in Patients With ARDS

PROBLEM

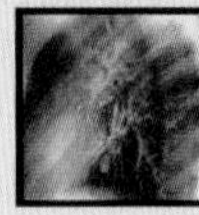

Critically ill patients who need mechanical ventilation for acute respiratory failure often receive large volumes of fluid in the form of intravenous medications, maintenance fluids, and enteral or parenteral feedings. These patients consequently are at risk of iatrogenic pulmonary edema due to increased pulmonary vascular hydrostatic pressure (increased intravascular volume). Excessive fluid administration is of particular concern in patients with ARDS who have "leaky capillaries" and are remarkably sensitive to changes in pulmonary vascular hydrostatic pressure. How can iatrogenic pulmonary edema be avoided in these patients?

DISCUSSION

Patients with respiratory insufficiency of any cause may not tolerate additional demands on the cardiorespiratory system, including the demands associated with pulmonary edema due to intravascular volume overload. Therefore the patient's volume status must be monitored closely by noninvasive and, in the care of more severely ill patients, invasive means. Noninvasive estimates of total body water, such as daily weights and total fluid intake/total fluid output measurements, are prone to error related to confounding variables. For example, limited patient mobility interferes with the ability to obtain exact measurements of the patient's weight. Likewise, total fluid intake and total fluid output measurements are limited by the loss of information related to insensible fluid losses (e.g., perspiration and respiration-related fluid loss).

Inaccuracies related to noninvasive estimates of total body fluid content are tolerable as long as the patient's clinical status is improving and the patient's condition remains hemodynamically stable. In situations in which pulmonary gas exchange or systemic Do_2 is unsatisfactory despite appropriate supportive therapy, invasive measurement of intravascular volume status (e.g., pulmonary artery catheterization) often is necessary to optimize pulmonary and systemic gas exchange. *In this regard*, the goals of invasive monitoring should be to guide therapy such that the minimum intravascular volume associated with safe levels of inspired oxygen ($Fio_2 \leq 0.6$) and adequate systemic Do_2 are attained. Invasive monitoring is particularly useful in the care of patients with ARDS, who have increased pulmonary capillary permeability and are consequently very sensitive to increases in pulmonary hydrostatic pressure.

means of measurement of airway pressure changes over a wide range of tidal volumes. These measurements are used to describe lower inflection point (P_{FLEX}) and upper P_{FLEX} (Figure 24-5). The upper P_{FLEX} (UIP) corresponds to the development of regional lung overdistension. Ventilatory pressure exceeding that associated with the UIP is likely to cause lung injury. In contrast, the lower P_{FLEX} (LIP) represents the point in the pressure-volume relation where dynamic collapse of alveolar units begins to occur. At ventilator pressure associated with lung volumes below the LIP, alveoli begin to collapse, and oxygenation is impaired. As airway pressure falls below the LIP at end-expiration and increases above the LIP, the alveoli undergo cyclical collapse and reexpansion. The shear stress induced by this cyclical opening and closing represents another possible mechanism of ventilator-associated lung injury.

Ventilator strategies designed to optimize pressure-volume relations and minimize ventilator-associated lung injury were initially described by Amato et al.[33] and are under investigation by the ARDS Network sponsored by the National Institutes of Health (NIH). These strategies have been termed *volume-controlled* ventilation strategies (see later, Innovative Ventilation Strategies for ARDS).

Adjusting PEEP

The rationale behind the use of PEEP in the care of patients with ARDS is not directly related to its effect on lung injury. Positive end-expiratory pressure may contribute to further pulmonary injury (volume trauma) in these patients. The benefits of PEEP relate to recruitment of additional alveoli, which results in an increase in functional residual capacity (FRC) and improved oxygenation. By improving arterial oxygenation, PEEP may enable reduction of the fraction of inspired oxygen (FIO_2) and thus diminish the risk of oxygen toxicity to the lungs. When patency of alveolar units is maintained throughout the ventilatory cycle, the damaging effects of opening and closing alveoli with each ventilatory cycle can be avoided. The form of lung injury occurring at lower lung volumes has been termed *airway shear trauma*, and the point at which it occurs is reflected by the LIP of the pressure-volume curve (see Figure 24-5).

The beneficial effects of PEEP must be balanced against the negative effects. Because the primary goal of mechanical ventilation is to provide adequate oxygenation at safe levels of FIO_2 while maintaining adequate DO_2 to the body, the inverse relation between PEEP and cardiac output must be considered. For example, one common clinical scenario (see Mini Clini on p. 546) involves increasing PEEP to improve arterial oxygenation at the expense of a reduction in the overall DO_2 to the body. For this reason, patients with ARDS necessitating PEEP may need invasive hemodynamic monitoring.

As with tidal volume adjustments, the optimal level of PEEP is different for each patient. On the basis of the previous discussion, the goals of PEEP therapy are as follows:

1. Provide adequate oxygenation (PaO_2 >60 mm Hg) at a safe FIO_2 (<0.6).
2. Ensure adequate tissue oxygenation.

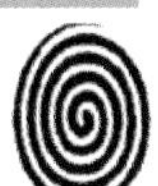

RULE OF THUMB

Administration of high levels of supplemental oxygen (FIO_2 >0.6) for more than 24 hours can cause lung injury as a result of oxygen toxicity (oxidative stress), which advances ARDS and lung fibrosis. Moreover, as the FIO_2 increases above 0.6, the time required to cause lung injury decreases. Thus the FIO_2 should be lowered to 0.6 as soon as possible by means of supportive therapy, such as positive-pressure ventilation, PEEP, manipulations of pulmonary vascular pressure, or another recommended therapy (Tables 24-2 and 24-3).

3. Maintain the patency of alveolar units throughout the ventilatory cycle (see Figure 24-5).
4. Avoid barotrauma by maintaining mean airway pressure less than 35 cm H_2O or below the pressure that corresponds to the UIP of the pressure-volume curve (see Figure 24-5).

Table 24-2 ▶▶ Criteria for Evidence-Based Recommendations for Management of ARDS

	Criteria
Quality of Evidence	
Level 1	Randomized, prospective, controlled investigations of ARDS
Level 2	Nonrandomized, concurrent cohort investigations, historical cohort investigations, and case series of patients with ARDS
Level 3	Randomized, prospective, controlled investigations of sepsis or other relevant conditions that have potential application to ARDS
Level 4	Case reports of ARDS
Grading of Recommendations	
A	Supported by at least two level 1 investigations
B	Supported by only one level 1 investigation
C	Supported by level 2 investigations only
D	Supported by at least one level 3 investigation
Ungraded	No available clinical investigations

Modified from Kollef MH, Schuster D: Dis Mon 42:302, 1996.

Table 24-3 ▶▶ Recommendations for the Nonpharmacologic Management of ARDS

Treatment	Recommendation	Grade
Mechanical ventilation		Ungraded
Initial settings: assist control mode; FIO_2 1.0; PEEP ≤5 cm H_2O; inspiratory flow, 60 L/min	Yes	
Tidal volume, 6-10 mL/kg	Yes	C
Prophylactic PEEP (≤5 cm H_2O)	No	B
Least PEEP with SaO_2 ≥0.9 and FIO_2 ≤0.6	Yes	Ungraded
Permissive hypercapnia to maintain peak airway pressure <40-45 cm H_2O and plateau pressure <35 cm H_2O	Yes	C
Routine use of IRV	No	C
IRV for persistent hypoxemia or elevated airway pressure	Yes	C
APRV	No*	
HFV	No	B
Tracheal gas insufflation	—*	
Partial liquid ventilation	—*	
ECMO	No	B
$ECCO_2R$	No	B
Patient repositioning (including prone position)	Yes	C
Early fluid restriction or diuresis	Yes	B
Supranormal DO_2 goals	No	D

Modified from Kolief MH, Schuster D: Dis Mon 42:303, 1996.
*Pending results of ongoing clinical trials.
APRV, airway pressure release ventilation; *$ECCO_2R$*, extracorporeal carbon dioxide removal; *ECMO*, extracorporeal membrane oxygenation; *HFV*, high-frequency ventilation; IRV, inverse-ratio ventilation.

Adjusting the Ventilatory Rate

Acute respiratory distress syndrome is associated with alveolar consolidation and ventilation/perfusion mismatching, which results in a decrease in the number of normally functioning alveoli. Moreover, critically ill patients often have elevated metabolic rates such that carbon dioxide (CO_2) production is increased. Relative to persons with normal lungs, patients with ARDS need much higher minute ventilation to maintain a normal $PaCO_2$. In patients with ARDS, it is desirable to maintain lower tidal volumes and thus avoid volume trauma. The goal of reducing tidal volume and controlling ventilatory rate is achieved at the expense of considerable CO_2 retention in patients with ARDS. In most cases, the $PaCO_2$ increases to 60 to 80 mm Hg and the pH decreases to approximately 7.25. Subsequent metabolic compensation tends to correct the acidosis over several days.[34] In some cases the acidosis is more severe but appears to be well tolerated as long as tissue oxygenation is maintained. This ventilatory strategy has been designated permissive hypercapnia or controlled hypoventilation and often requires sedation and paralysis.[34]

Animal models and human studies have confirmed the safety of controlled hypoventilation. Several studies have shown a survival benefit of low-volume ventilation and permissive hypercapnia in patients with ARDS. This strategy is contraindicated in the care of patients with elevated intracranial pressure or unstable hemodynamic status, because these conditions may be negatively affected by elevated $PaCO_2$ and reductions in tissue pH, respectively.

Innovative Ventilation Strategies for ARDS

Patients with ARDS who need high levels of inspired oxygen (FIO_2 >0.6) despite conventional supportive therapy may benefit from alternative ventilatory strategies.

Volume-Controlled Mechanical Ventilation

Volume-controlled mechanical ventilation represents an exciting new area of ARDS research. A large, well-designed clinical trial sponsored by the NIH ARDS Network showed a significant reduction in mortality (approximately 20%) when lower tidal volumes were used in patients with ALI and ARDS.[35] Volume-controlled ventilation is now considered a preferred ventilation strategy for patients with ARDS. This ventilation technique is typically adjusted to the specific pressure-volume relations of each patient; however, a range of optimal initial ventilator settings can be derived from recent experimental observations. A tidal volume of 10 mL/kg exceeds the volume at which the UIP is reached in more than 80% of patients with ARDS, and most patients need only 5 to 7 mL/kg tidal volume to reach this inflection point.[36] On the basis of these observations, it is now recommended that the tidal volume for patients with ARDS be initiated at 5 to 7 mL/kg. Subsequent tidal volume adjustments should then be made on the basis of each patient's pressure-volume relations (see Figure 24-5). Ideal PEEP should be determined as previously described (see Figure 24-4 and Mini Clini on page 546).

High-Frequency Ventilation

High-frequency ventilation (HFV) was designed to simultaneously maintain adequate ventilation and reduce alveolar collapse through ventilation with high expiratory lung volumes and rapid (up to 300 breaths/min), small tidal volumes (3-5 mL/kg). This technique has been successfully applied to the ventilation of neonates with respiratory distress related to insufficient surfactant production.[37] However, despite preliminary evidence suggesting that HFV may be beneficial to adults with ARDS,[38,39] no randomized controlled trials have verified these findings.

Inverse-Ratio Ventilation

Inverse-ratio ventilation (IRV) is designed to recruit alveolar units through prolongation of the inspiratory phase of the ventilatory cycle and thereby improve oxygenation. In conventional modes of mechanical ventilation, the respiratory cycle is characterized by inspiratory to expiratory ratios exceeding 1:2. During IRV, the inspiratory time on the ventilator is prolonged such that the inspiratory to expiratory (I:E) ratio is reversed and may exceed 4:1. Initial reports of the use of this strategy showed significant improvement in oxygenation in patients with ARDS.[40] However, these studies did not take into account other variables, such as the level of PEEP. More recent studies have not substantiated the claims of earlier studies regarding improved oxygenation in patients with ARDS,[41] and no study has shown a significant survival benefit of IRV. Because of the discomfort associated with this mode of ventilation and the risk of asynchronous spontaneous ventilatory efforts, patients often need heavy sedation or paralysis during IRV. The routine use of IRV during ARDS cannot be advocated at this time.

Pressure Control Ventilation

Pressure control ventilation (PCV) is designed to prevent ventilator-associated lung injury. The clinician sets the maximal inspiratory airway pressure. A maximal inspiratory pressure (30-35 cm H_2O) is chosen that is likely to avert alveolar overdistension and prevent volume-associated lung injury. Ventilation is maintained by setting the ventilator rate. Tidal volume becomes a dynamic variable during PCV. That is, tidal volume is primarily dependent on the driving pressure (maximum inspiratory pressure, PEEP), airway resistance, and the lung compliance. Changes in intrathoracic pressure (e.g., due to spontaneous inspiratory efforts) or airway resistance or changes in lung compliance influence tidal volume. Large swings in ventilation (increases or decreases in Pa_{CO_2}) may be observed during PCV. Therefore close monitoring of the ventilatory status of the patient must be maintained while the PC mode is in use.

Despite its theoretical benefits, PCV has not been shown superior to volume-controlled ventilation in clinical trials.[42,43]

Airway Pressure Release Ventilation

Airway pressure release ventilation (APRV) was designed to optimize ventilation by recruiting collapsed alveolar units while minimizing ventilator-induced barotrauma in patients with ARDS. Like IRV, APRV prolongs the inspiratory phase of the ventilatory cycle. However, when fixed inspiratory volume is used, APRV supports the patency of alveolar units by maintaining a constant inspiratory pressure. During APRV, tidal volumes are delivered during transient decreases in intrathoracic pressure, which may be triggered by the patient. As a result, patients appear to tolerate this form of mechanical ventilation better than they do IRV. Nonetheless, because of prolonged inspiratory times, APRV is associated with an increase in mean airway pressure and a tendency to stack breaths (increased intrinsic PEEP [PEEPi]). Increased PEEPi may explain how APRV improves arterial oxygenation.

Comparisons of APRV with other forms of mechanical ventilation, including pressure support and synchronized intermittent mandatory ventilation, have shown APRV to be an effective and well-tolerated mode of mechanical ventilation that is associated with lower peak airway pressure. In a study by Sydow et al.,[44] in which APRV was compared with IRV in ARDS patients, APRV was better tolerated and was associated with lower peak airway pressure. Moreover, alveolar recruitment improved over time with APRV but not with IRV. Despite these potential advantages, APRV has not proved superior to conventional mechanical ventilation in large clinical trials.

Positioning of the Patient

In view of the heterogeneous distribution of lung injury in patients with ARDS, it has been proposed that changing the position of the patient could result in improved ventilation/perfusion matching within the lungs. It is known that alveolar consolidation tends to be most pronounced in the dependent lung zones in patients with ARDS.[45] These observations led investigators to experiment with positioning the patient such that aerated lung fields (nondependent lung zones) become dependent (by positioning of the patient in the prone position). Douglas et al.[46] were the first to describe improved oxygenation with prone positioning of patients with ARDS. For unclear reasons this ventilation strategy was not popularized until more recently when other investigators demonstrated similar beneficial effects in patients with ARDS.[47] The mechanisms by which prone positioning improves oxygenation are the subject of ongoing debate. Some of the possible mechanisms include improved matching of ventilation with perfusion, increased FRC, increased cardiac output, more thorough drainage of secretions, and improved diaphragmatic excursion. Investigations with an animal model of ALI have shown that ventilation in the supine position results in compressive forces on the dorsal airspaces that causes derecruitment of lung units. This phenomenon is reversed by prone-position ventilation.[48]

Despite the demonstrated improvement in oxygenation during prone positioning, some patients do not tolerate prone positioning because of hemodynamic instability or worsening gas exchange. All patients need specialized

MINI CLINI

Avoiding Ventilator-Induced Lung Injury

PROBLEM

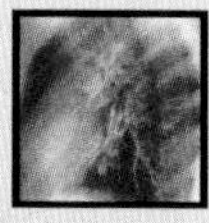

How can ventilator-induced lung injury be minimized in patients with ARDS through adjustments of PEEP and tidal volume?

DISCUSSION

Alveolar shear stress occurs when alveoli collapse during expiration and are reopened as the next tidal volume is delivered. Patients with ARDS are prone to development of this form of lung injury, because surface tension increases as a result of impaired surfactant synthesis and function and decreased lung compliance. Alveolar collapse at end-expiration (the LIP of the pressure-volume curve) can be avoided with PEEP, which reduces alveolar shear stress by preventing the cyclical opening and closing of the alveoli during each ventilatory cycle. Because partially patent alveoli require less pressure to inflate than do collapsed alveoli, PEEP also improves lung compliance. Improved compliance is reflected by an increase in the slope of the pressure-volume curve (see Figure 24-5).

Many of the newer ventilators can provide pressure-volume relations. The information allows the clinician to estimate the PEEP needed to maintain alveolar patency (see Figure 24-5). Alternatively, the clinician can gauge the effects of PEEP on the basis of calculated changes in lung compliance (see Figure 24-4). In the clinical setting, changes in lung compliance are estimated from the compliance of the entire respiratory system, which includes the combined influences of lung compliance, chest wall compliance, and abdominal pressure:

Compliance of the respiratory system = Tidal volume ÷ (Plateau pressure − Total PEEP)

Unfortunately, as PEEP increases, so do airway pressure and the risk of lung injury due to volume trauma. Volume trauma occurs when alveoli are exposed to pressure in excess of that necessary to provide optimal ventilation. Volume trauma is particularly problematic in the care of patients with ARDS, because the tidal volume necessary for complete inflation of the lungs is reduced. Thus during ARDS, tidal volumes must be adjusted to avoid lung injury related to alveolar overinflation.

Just as alveolar collapse during end-expiration is associated with decreased lung compliance, alveolar overinflation during end-inspiration is reflected by decreasing compliance and corresponds to the UIP of the pressure-volume curve (Figure 24-5). Tidal volumes should be adjusted such that maximal inspiratory pressure does not exceed the pressure corresponding to the UIP of the pressure-volume curve. In most patients, the UIP is attained at tidal volumes less than 10 mL/kg and plateau pressure less than 35 cm H_2O.[34]

nursing care. The improvements in gas exchange related to repositioning the patient tend to be transient such that subsequent repositioning is needed. This ventilation strategy requires experienced nursing staff and special equipment (e.g., special beds to facilitate prone positioning and to minimize complications). Implementation of this technique should be restricted to facilities experienced in its use.

The risk-benefit analysis of prone-position ventilation for patients with ARDS must be based on results of clinical evaluation of the effect on ARDS-related mortality. A large multicenter, randomized trial demonstrated a lack of survival benefit when prone-position ventilation was used (152 patients) instead of conventional ventilation (152 patients) for at least 6 hours a day in the care of patients with ALI or ARDS[49] (see Table 24-1).

Extracorporeal Membrane Oxygenation and Extracorporeal Carbon Dioxide Removal

Extracorporeal membrane oxygenation (ECMO) was first introduced in 1972 as a form of respiratory support for patients with severe, acute hypoxemic respiratory failure. This modality involves the establishment of an arteriovenous circuit for diverting a large proportion of the cardiac output through an artificial lung to facilitate the exchange of CO_2 and O_2. After an initial flurry of interest during the 1970s, a trial comparing ECMO plus conventional mechanical ventilation with conventional mechanical ventilation alone demonstrated no survival benefit with ECMO.[50]

Like ECMO, **extracorporeal carbon dioxide removal** ($ECCO_2R$) entails the use of artificial membrane lungs. Unlike ECMO, $ECCO_2R$ has a venovenous circuit that diverts a fraction of the cardiac output (approximately 20%) through the membrane lung, is primarily designed to remove CO_2, and does not directly influence oxygenation. Oxygenation is indirectly facilitated through the removal of CO_2, which would otherwise compete with O_2 exchange within the alveoli. By this mechanism, $ECCO_2R$ allows the clinician to maintain the same level of oxygenation at lower ventilatory rates and thereby reduce the risk of lung injury related to mechanical ventilation.

Clinical trials comparing $ECCO_2R$ with conventional mechanical ventilation in the care of adults with ARDS have demonstrated improved gas exchange, lower peak airway pressure, lower ventilatory rate, and reduced thoracic volume (less overinflation of the lungs) in patients treated with $ECCO_2R$ ventilation.[51] Technological advances in $ECCO_2R$ renewed interest in extracorporeal technology in the care of patients with ARDS. Results of several recent uncontrolled clinical trials have suggested a survival benefit among ARDS patients treated with ECMO. However, the only controlled clinical trial performed with adults with ARDS did not show a survival benefit with $ECCO_2R$ at 30 days in a relatively small group of patients (n = 40).[52] The authors of the study concluded that "extracorporeal support for ARDS patients should be restricted to controlled clinical trials" and cannot be recommended for routine management of ARDS at this time.

Exogenous Surfactant Administration

The assumed role of **surfactant** deficiency in the pathogenesis of infant respiratory distress is well established. Exogenous surfactant administration is one of the cornerstones of therapy for infant respiratory distress syndrome. However, the pathogenesis of ARDS is more complex (see earlier, Pathophysiology). Although surfactant is known to be qualitatively and quantitatively altered during ARDS, other factors, such as the severity of pulmonary microvascular injury, contribute to the gas exchange abnormalities associated with this condition. Nonetheless, surfactant has been shown to have immunomodulating properties that may reduce microvascular injury in the lungs. Thus surfactant dysfunction may contribute to the development of ARDS by promoting instability of the alveolar units (airway shear trauma, atelectasis, and right-to-left shunt) and by allowing inflammatory injury to alveoli to continue unchecked. This rationale explains the observed correlation between the degree of surfactant dysfunction and the severity of gas exchange abnormalities during adult ARDS and forms the basis for clinical trials of exogenous surfactant administration during ARDS.

Exogenous surfactant replacement is of greatest benefit in models of pure surfactant deficiency, such as infant respiratory distress or the aftermath of saline lavage. However, in adult ARDS, in which deactivation of surfactant relates to the influx of inflammatory cells and mediators into the alveolar space, the effects of exogenous surfactant are less apparent. In initial studies, a surfactant preparation composed of phosphatidylcholine (Exosurf) and administered by nebulization was ineffective. However, the preliminary results of a trial of a preparation that contains apoproteins and lipids similar to those of human surfactant (Alveofact) and administered by means of direct instillation have been promising.[53] Similar results were reported with the use of modified bovine lung surfactant[54] (Survanta). Recommendations regarding the use of surfactant in the management of ARDS await the results of larger clinical trials.

Liquid (Perfluorocarbon) Mechanical Ventilation

Perfluorocarbon-associated gas exchange, or liquid mechanical ventilation, is a promising new alternative to conventional mechanical ventilation in the care of patients with ARDS. Perfluorocarbons are carbon-based molecules in which hydrogen ions are replaced by fluoride ions. They are nontoxic substances that are both hydrophobic and lipophobic. Unlike saline solution, perfluorocarbons do not eliminate surfactant after instillation into the lungs. Perfluorocarbons dissolve large quantities of oxygen (2.5 times as much as the same volume of air) and carbon dioxide such that gas exchange within the lungs is facilitated in their presence. The unique physical properties of perfluorocarbons allow adequate gas exchange when the lungs are partially filled with the liquid and ventilation is provided from gases delivered with conventional ventilators. This mode of ventilation has been referred to as "partial liquid ventilation" and is more easily used and better tolerated than total liquid ventilation. Perfluorocarbons have very low surface tension, which facilitates their delivery to the terminal airways and their effects on lung compliance in surfactant-deficient lungs.[55]

Because of its unique properties, liquid mechanical ventilation with perfluorocarbons may be of benefit in the management of ARDS. In animal models of ARDS, ventilation with perfluorocarbons has been shown to improve oxygenation, lung mechanics, and survival.[56] In other studies, liquid mechanical ventilation has been shown to locally reduce the inflammatory response in the lungs during ARDS,[57] and it has been shown to be safe and feasible in humans.[58] Partial liquid mechanical ventilation appears to be a promising alternative to conventional mechanical ventilation for patients with ARDS. However, as with other innovative therapies, recommendations regarding the use of liquid mechanical ventilation must await the results of ongoing, multicenter clinical trials.

Pharmacologic Therapies for ARDS

Inhaled Nitric Oxide

Nitric oxide (NO) is a potent vasodilator that plays a critical role in the regulation of blood flow within the lungs. Nitric oxide is soluble in liquids and gases and diffuses readily through various tissues. In vitro, the vasodilatory effects of NO are short-lived, because NO is quickly bound and neutralized by hemoglobin and competes with oxygen for mitochondrial oxidization. Consequently, the effects of NO are localized and temporally self-limited.

The potential role of inhaled NO during ARDS is based on the notion that NO will be preferentially distributed to well-ventilated portions of the lung, where it will cause local vasodilation. In this way, well-ventilated areas of the lung would receive a greater portion of the total pulmonary blood flow, which would result in improved oxygenation by reducing ventilation/perfusion mismatch. In practice, the effects of inhaled NO in patients with ARDS have been variable. In general, patients with high pulmonary vascular resistance, who presumably have more severe alterations in pulmonary vascular regulation, appear to benefit the most. The beneficial effects of NO can be achieved at relatively low concentrations of inhaled NO; thus the incidence of systemic hypotension associated with its use is low. However, sudden discontinuation of inhaled NO may be associated with severe pulmonary vasoconstriction; slow weaning is necessary.

Despite encouraging results of animal studies demonstrating tolerance of low doses of inhaled NO for up to 6 months, the safety and effectiveness of inhaled NO therapy for ARDS have not been established. The breakdown products of NO are potentially toxic and include highly reactive free radicals (e.g., peroxynitrite) and methemoglobin. Thus NO may contribute to further lung injury in patients with ARDS. The use of inhaled NO during mechanical ventilation involves close monitoring and special exhaust systems to prevent exposure of healthcare personnel to NO and its potentially toxic byproducts. Many phase II and phase III studies have been completed with NO. Unfortunately, none has shown that NO improves outcome or mortality.[59,60] Because of these uncertainties, inhaled NO remains a promising but experimental therapy for ARDS.

A comprehensive discussion of investigational therapies for ARDS is beyond the scope of this chapter. Several excellent reviews have been published.[1,61,62]

Corticosteroids for Late, Uncomplicated ARDS

Although most patients who survive ARDS have minimal residual pulmonary impairment, a small but significant number of patients cannot be weaned from mechanical ventilatory support because of abundant fibroproliferation during recovery from ARDS. The high mortality among these patients appears to be related to the extent and severity of pulmonary fibrosis.[63] High-dose corticosteroids have been used to manage uncomplicated pulmonary fibrosis following ARDS.[64-66] In a well-publicized but uncontrolled study by Meduri et al.,[65] patients treated with corticosteroids for ARDS-related pulmonary fibrosis had improved gas exchange and a low mortality (24%). Subsequently, the same investigators performed a randomized double-blind placebo-controlled trial to determine the effect of prolonged methylprednisolone therapy for unresolving ARDS. The results were encouraging, demonstrating improvement in lung injury scores and reduced mortality.[66] The NIH ARDS Network is conducting a large multicenter trial of corticosteroids in the treatment of patients with late ARDS and the timing of steroid therapy for established ARDS. These investigations should clarify the role of corticosteroids for ARDS that progress to the fibroproliferative phase.

KEY POINTS

- CHF and ARDS are common causes of acute respiratory failure that often are difficult to differentiate on the basis of the results of the initial clinical evaluation.

KEY POINTS—cont'd

- Although CHF and ARDS both cause pulmonary edema, CHF-associated pulmonary edema is caused by elevated hydrostatic pressure in the pulmonary vasculature. Pulmonary edema associated with ARDS results from inflammatory injury to the lungs and occurs at normal hydrostatic pressure.
- ARDS is the likely diagnosis in a patient who has an established risk factor for ARDS (see Box 24-1) and whose history is not suggestive of one of the causes of CHF (see Box 24-3).
- When the clinical history, physical examination, and chest radiograph do not provide enough information for a diagnosis, alternative diagnostic techniques, such as bronchoscopy or pulmonary artery catheterization, may be necessary to differentiate CHF and ARDS.
- No therapy has proved effective against the systemic inflammatory reaction responsible for ARDS and MODS. Recommendations regarding the management of ARDS have focused on supporting gas exchange and systemic organ function until the patient recovers from the underlying illness.
- There is no consensus regarding supportive care of patients with ARDS. However, currently recommended ventilatory strategies for patients with ARDS are designed to minimize ventilator-induced lung injury by use of PEEP, low tidal volumes, and nontoxic levels of inspired oxygen.
- Innovative ventilatory strategies and therapies for ARDS that does not resolve with conventional supportive therapy are under investigation.
- Ambiguity surrounds the treatment of patients with ARDS because of the heterogeneous nature of the patient population, the complex pathophysiological determinants of ARDS and MODS, and the limitations of the studies designed to evaluate each form of therapy.
- An evidence-based approach to the development of a rational therapeutic plan for the treatment of patients with ARDS is needed to standardize the care of these patients (see Tables 24-2 and 24-3).

References

1. Bernard GR et al: The American-European consensus conference on ARDS: definitions, mechanisms, relevant outcomes, and clinical trial coordination, Am J Respir Crit Care Med 149:818, 1994.
2. Milberg JA et al: Improved survival of patients with acute respiratory distress syndrome (ARDS): 1983-1993, JAMA 273:306, 1995.
3. Fowler AA et al: Adult respiratory distress syndrome: risk with common predispositions, Ann Intern Med 98:593, 1983.
4. Sloane PJ et al: A multicenter registry of patients with acute respiratory distress syndrome: physiology and outcome, Am Rev Respir Dis 146:419, 1992.
5. Flick MR: Pulmonary edema and acute lung injury. In Murray JF, Nadel JA, editors: Textbook of respiratory medicine, Philadelphia, 1994, WB Saunders.
6. Matthay MA, Berthiaume Y, Staub NC: Long-term clearance of liquid and protein from the lungs of unanesthetized sheep, J Appl Physiol 59:928, 1985.
7. Egan EA, Nelson RM, Gessner IH: Solute permeability of the alveolar epithelium in acute hemodynamic pulmonary edema in dogs, Am J Physiol 233:H80, 1977.
8. Conhaim RL: Airway level at which edema liquid enters the air space of isolated dog lungs, J Appl Physiol 67:2234, 1989.
9. Pugin J et al: The alveolar space is the site of intense inflammatory and profibrotic reactions in the early phase of acute respiratory distress syndrome, Crit Care Med 27:304, 1999.
10. Matute-Bello G et al: Soluble Fas ligand induces epithelial cell apoptosis in humans with acute lung injury (ARDS), J Immunol 163:2217, 1999.
11. Katzenstein AA, Bloor CM, Leibow AA: Diffuse alveolar damage: the role of oxygen, shock and related factors, Am J Pathol 85:210, 1976.
12. Ware LB, Matthay MA: Alveolar fluid clearance is impaired in the majority of patients with acute lung injury and the acute respiratory distress syndrome, Am J Respir Crit Care Med 163:1376, 2001.
13. Weiland JE et al: Lung neutrophils in the adult respiratory distress syndrome, Am Rev Respir Dis 133:218, 1986.
14. Baughman RP et al: Changes in the inflammatory response of the lung during acute respiratory distress syndrome: prognostic indicators, Am J Respir Crit Care Med 154:76, 1996.
15. Marsh CB, Wewers MD: The pathogenesis of sepsis: factors that modulate the response of gram-negative bacterial infection, Clin Chest Med 17:183, 1996.
16. Parsons PE. Mediators and mechanisms of acute lung injury, Clin Chest Med, 3:467, 2000.
17. Ware LB, Matthay MA: The acute respiratory distress syndrome, N Engl J Med 342:1334, 2000.
18. Crouser ED et al: Acid aspiration results in ileal injury without altering ileal VO2-DO2 relationships, Am J Respir Crit Care Med 153:1965, 1996.
19. St John RC et al: Acid aspiration-induced acute lung injury causes leukocyte-dependent systemic organ injury, J Appl Physiol 74:1994, 1993.
20. Crouser ED, Dorinsky PM: Gastrointestinal tract dysfunction in critical illness: pathophysiology and interaction with acute lung injury in adult respiratory distress syndrome/multiple organ dysfunction syndrome, New Horizons 2:476, 1994.
21. Matuschak GM: Liver-lung interactions in critical illness, New Horizons 2:488, 1994.
22. Tomashefski JF: Pulmonary pathology of the adult respiratory distress syndrome, Clin Chest Med 11:593, 1990.
23. Marinelli WA et al: Mechanisms of alveolar fibrosis after acute lung injury, Clin Chest Med 11:657, 1990.
24. O'Quin R, Marini JJ: Pulmonary artery occlusion pressure: clinical physiology, measurement, and interpretation, Am Rev Respir Dis 128:319, 1983.
25. Idell S, Cohen AB: Bronchoalveolar lavage in patients with the adult respiratory distress syndrome, Clin Chest Med 6:459, 1985.
26. Schumacker PT, Samsel RW: Oxygen supply and consumption in the adult respiratory distress syndrome, Clin Chest Med 11:715, 1990.
27. Tuchschmidt J et al: Elevation of cardiac output and oxygen delivery improves outcome in septic shock, Chest 102:216, 1992.
28. Shoemaker WC et al: Prospective trial of supranormal values as therapeutic goals in high risk surgical patients, Chest 94: 1176, 1988.
29. Hayes TM et al: Elevation of systemic oxygen delivery in the treatment of critically ill patients, N Engl J Med 330:1717, 1994.
30. Gattinoni L et al: A trial of goal-directed hemodynamic therapy in critically ill patients, N Engl J Med 333:1025, 1995.
31. Gattinoni L, Pesenti A: Computerized tomography scanning in acute respiratory failure. In Zapol WM, Lemaire F, editors: Adult respiratory distress syndrome, New York, 1991, Marcel Dekker.
32. Dreyfuss D et al: High inflation pressure pulmonary edema: respective effects of high airway pressure, high tidal volume, and positive end-expiratory pressure, Am J Respir Dis 137:1159, 1988.
33. Amato MB et al: Beneficial effects of the "open lung approach" with low distending pressures in acute respiratory distress syndrome: a prospective randomized study on mechanical ventilation, Am J Respir Crit Care Med, 152:1835, 1995.
34. Lessard MR: New concepts in mechanical ventilation for ARDS, Can J Anaesth 43:R50, 1996.
35. Adult Respiratory Distress Syndrome Network: Ventilation with lower tidal volumes as compared with traditional tidal volumes for acute lung injury and the acute respiratory distress syndrome, N Engl J Med 342:1301, 2000.
36. Roupie E et al: Titration of tidal volume and induced hypercapnia in acute respiratory distress syndrome, Am J Respir Crit Care Med 152:121, 1995.
37. Paulson TE et al: High-frequency pressure-control ventilation with high positive end-expiratory pressure in children with acute respiratory distress syndrome, J Pediatr 129:566, 1996.

38. Gluck E et al: Use of ultrahigh frequency ventilation in patients with ARDS: a preliminary report, Chest 103:1413, 1993.
39. Fort P et al: High frequency oscillatory ventilation for adult respiratory distress syndrome: a pilot study, Crit Care Med 25:937, 1997.
40. Tharratt RS, Allen RP, Albertson TE: Pressure controlled inverse ratio ventilation in severe adult respiratory failure, Chest 94:755, 1988.
41. Mercat A et al: Cardiorespiratory effects of pressure-controlled ventilation with and without inverse ratio in the adult respiratory distress syndrome, Chest 104:871, 1993.
42. Lessard MR et al: Effects of pressure-controlled with different I/E ratios versus volume controlled ventilation on respiratory mechanics, gas exchange, and hemodynamics in patients with adult respiratory distress syndrome, Anesthesiology 80:983, 1994.
43. Esteban A et al: Prospective randomized clinical trial comparing pressure-controlled ventilation and volume-controlled ventilation in ARDS, Chest 117:1690, 2000.
44. Sydow M et al: Long-term effects of two different ventilatory modes on oxygenation in acute lung injury: comparison of airway pressure release ventilation and volume-controlled inverse ratio ventilation, Am J Respir Crit Care Med 149:1550, 1994.
45. Gattinoni L et al: Body position changes redistribute lung computed tomographic density in patients with acute respiratory failure, Anesthesiology 74:15, 1991.
46. Douglas WW et al: Improved oxygenation in patients with acute respiratory failure: the prone position, Am Rev Respir Dis 1977;115:559, 1977.
47. Chatte G et al: Prone position in mechanically ventilated patients with severe acute respiratory failure, Am J Respir Crit Care Med 155:473, 1997.
48. Mutoh T et al: Prone position alters the effects of volume overload on regional pleural pressures and improves hypoxemia in pigs in-vivo, Am Rev Respir Dis 146:300, 1992.
49. Gattinoni L et al: Effects of prone positioning on the survival of patients with acute respiratory failure, N Engl J Med 345:568, 2001.
50. Zapol WM et al: Extracorporeal membrane oxygenation in severe acute respiratory failure, JAMA 242:2193, 1979.
51. Brunet F et al: Extracorporeal carbon dioxide removal technique improves oxygenation without causing overinflation, Am J Respir Crit Care Med 149:1557, 1994.
52. Morris AH et al: Randomized clinical trial of pressure-controlled inverse ratio ventilation and extracorporeal CO_2 removal for adult respiratory distress syndrome, Am J Respir Crit Care Med 149:295, 1994.
53. Walmrath D et al: Bronchoscopic surfactant administration in patients with severe adult respiratory distress syndrome and sepsis, Am J Respir Crit Care Med 154:57, 1996.
54. Gregory TJ et al: Bovine surfactant therapy for patients with acute respiratory distress, Am J Respir Crit Care Med 155:1309, 1997
55. Leach CL et al: Perfluorocarbon-associated gas exchange (partial liquid ventilation) in respiratory distress syndrome: a prospective, randomized, controlled study, Crit Care Med 21:1270, 1993.
56. Papo MC et al: Perfluorocarbon-associated gas exchange improves oxygenation, lung mechanics, and survival in a model of adult respiratory distress syndrome, Crit Care Med 24:466, 1996.
57. Smith TM et al: A liquid perfluorochemical decreases in vitro production of reactive oxygen species by nuclear macrophages, Crit Care Med 23:1533, 1995.
58. Hirschl RB et al: Initial experience with partial liquid ventilation in adult patients with the acute respiratory distress syndrome, JAMA 275:383, 1996.
59. Dellinger RP et al: Effects of inhaled nitric oxide on patients with acute respiratory distress syndrome: results of a randomized phase II trial, Crit Care Med 26:15, 1998.
60. Payen D et al: Results of the French prospective multicenter randomized double-blind placebo controlled trial on inhaled nitric oxide in ARDS, Intensive Care Med 25(suppl):S166, 1999.
61. Kollef MH, Schuster D: Acute respiratory distress syndrome, Dis Mon 42:266, 1996.
62. Hudson LD: New therapies for ARDS, Chest 108:79S, 1995.
63. Martin C et al: Pulmonary fibrosis correlates with outcome in adult respiratory distress syndrome, Chest 107:196, 1995.
64. Hooper RG, Kearl RA: Treatment of established ARDS: steroids, antibiotics, and fungal therapy, Chest 100:137S, 1991.
65. Meduri GU et al: Corticosteroid rescue treatment of progressive fibroproliferation in late ARDS, Chest 105:1516, 1994.
66. Meduri GU et al: Effect of prolonged methylprednisolone therapy in unresolving acute respiratory distress syndrome: a randomized controlled trial, JAMA 280:159, 1998.

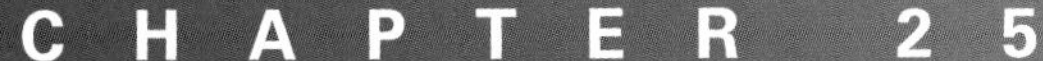

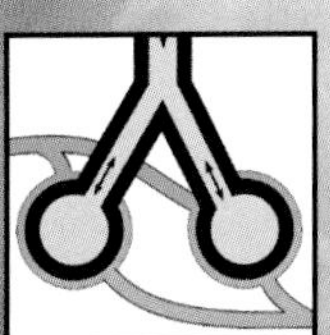

CHAPTER 25

Lung Neoplasms

Raed Dweik and Alejandro C. Arroliga

In This Chapter You Will Learn:

- What is the incidence of lung cancer in the United States
- What relationship exists between smoking and lung cancer
- How to describe the major histopathologic types of lung cancer
- What clinical manifestations are signs of lung cancer
- How lung cancer is staged
- What current approaches are being implemented in lung cancer treatment
- How lung cancer can be prevented

Chapter Outline

Key Terms

chemotherapy
lung cancer
metastasis
neoplasms
non–small cell bronchogenic carcinoma
radiation therapy
small cell cancer
staging

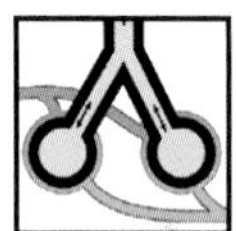

It is estimated that in 2001, 169,500 cases of bronchogenic carcinoma were newly diagnosed in the United States, making bronchogenic carcinoma a major health hazard and the leading cause of cancer deaths in the United States.[1] Bronchogenic carcinoma is responsible for 23% of all deaths related to cancer in the United States and is currently the most frequently diagnosed major cancer in the world. The World Health Organization estimates that there will be 2 million cases of bronchogenic carcinoma worldwide each year.

The total number of deaths peaked in the late 1990s and will remain high over the next 2 or 3 decades. The incidence of bronchogenic carcinoma has risen dramatically in the last decades, but in the 1980s, it was apparent that the increase among men had begun to taper. Current data indicate that the peak incidence of **lung cancer** among white and black men occurred in the mid 1980s. The incidence of bronchogenic carcinoma has been stable since the early 1990s among women, and a decline among women 40 to 59 years of age has been noticed. The effect of these different trends among men and women has resulted in a slight decline in the incidence of bronchogenic carcinoma among all persons.[1,2]

▶ ETIOLOGY

Approximately 85% of all cases of bronchogenic carcinoma are linked to smoking. The most important cause of the increase in the incidence of bronchogenic carcinoma is tobacco smoking. The carcinogenic substances in cigarette smoke are only partially understood, but the association between chemicals in tobacco smoke and bronchogenic carcinoma has been known for more than 50 years.[3] More than 40 carcinogens have been identified in cigarette smoke; some of these include polycyclic aromatic hydrocarbons, vinyl chloride, nickel, aldehydes, peroxide, nitrosamines, and benzo[a]pyrene. A direct link has been made between benzo[a]pyrene, one of the most potent mitogens and carcinogens known, and molecular changes that result in gene mutation in the cell. This sequence provides a direct etiological link between bronchogenic carcinoma and a chemical carcinogen present in tobacco smoke.[4]

It is estimated that 78% of cases of bronchogenic carcinoma among women and 90% among men are directly related to tobacco smoking.[5] The incidence of lung cancer among smokers is 10- to 25-fold higher than that among nonsmokers, and smoking increases the risk of all four major histologic types of bronchogenic carcinoma. When smoking is discontinued, there is a progressive decline in lung cancer risk. After a long period of abstinence (15 to 30 years), the risk of development of lung cancer among smokers is near that of lifelong nonsmokers. Factors related to the high risk of development of bronchogenic carcinoma include number of cigarettes smoked, duration in years of smoking, early age at initiation of smoking, depth of inhalation, and tar and nicotine content in the cigarette.[6] Cigar smoking has increased markedly over the last few years. Persons who smoke cigars are at higher risk of development of carcinoma of the lung. The relative risk of bronchogenic carcinoma among cigar smokers is 2.14.

Approximately 46 million adults in the United States (26% of the population) are smokers. The number of smokers who reported they were heavy smokers (defined as consumption of 20 or more cigarettes per day) changed little from 26% in 1974 to 27% in 1985. In the decades from 1970 to 1990, the percentage of women who smoked declined from 33% to 25%, and the rate of smoking among men decreased from 43% to 28%. Unfortunately, the annual decline that had occurred since the early 1970s was unchanged from 1990 to 1991: 25.7% for the combined groups despite mounting evidence associating smoking with disease and death (Figure 25-1).[7]

No decrease in smoking has been observed among adults 18 to 24 years of age, and cigarette smoking among young persons remains a major public health concern. Among college students, smoking has increased during the last decade. In a survey, 33% of young adults

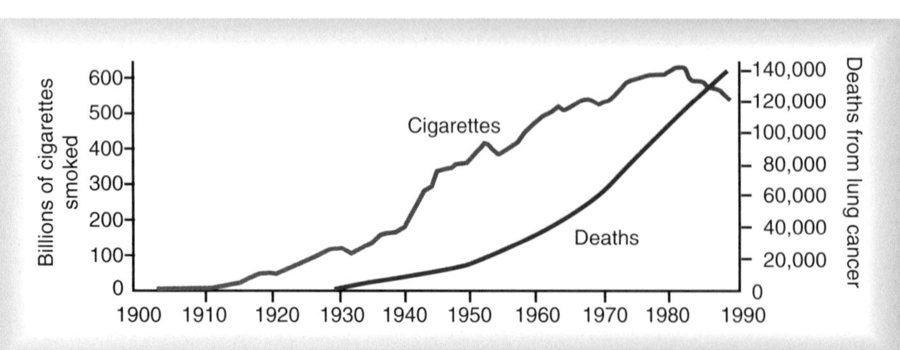

Figure 25-1 · Smoking Trends
Cigarette consumption and total deaths from lung cancer in the United States from 1900 to 1989. (From US Dept of Health and Human Services: Smoking, tobacco and cancer program: 1985–1989 status report, NIH publication no. 90–3107, Bethesda, Md, 1990.)

(18 to 24 years of age) were current users of tobacco.[8] Each day approximately 3000 teenagers begin smoking, and almost all begin using tobacco before high school graduation.[9] A person who has not started smoking as a teenager is unlikely to ever become a smoker. It is clear that the tobacco industry has focused on young people as the primary source of new customers, replacing adults who have either quit smoking or have died. Nicotine, the drug in tobacco, has been shown to cause addiction and dependence.[10]

The carcinogenic effect of passive exposure or second-hand smoke has been determined. Second-hand smoke increases the risk of bronchogenic carcinoma. In 1993, the Environmental Protection Agency concluded that environmental tobacco is a human lung carcinogen responsible for approximately 3000 lung cancer deaths a year among nonsmokers in the United States. It is estimated that second-hand smoking from spouses of heavy smokers may explain 3000 to 5000 bronchogenic carcinoma deaths in the United States every year. The inhalation of tobacco by spouses of nonsmokers is associated with a 30% excess risk of bronchogenic carcinoma. An increase in relative risk is observed with an increase in pack-years of spousal environmental tobacco exposure. Subjects with 80 or greater pack-year exposure from their spouses have an 80% excess risk of bronchogenic carcinoma. This excess risk of bronchogenic carcinoma among women exposed to environmental tobacco is present when they are exposed in the household, workplace, and social settings.[11]

Many other potential carcinogens have been linked with an increased incidence of bronchogenic carcinoma. These carcinogens include atmospheric pollution,[12,13] occupational factors (Box 25-1), and dietary and genetic factors. Asbestos and radon are the two substances encountered in the workplace that have received the most attention. Inhalation of asbestos fibers causes malignant tumors of the lung (bronchogenic carcinoma) and pleura (pleural mesothelioma). Asbestos exposure increases the incidence of bronchogenic cancer 3- to 5-fold among nonsmokers, but among smokers, this risk may increase to 70- to 90-fold. A dose-response relation exists between cumulative asbestos exposure and the development of lung cancer.[14] All four major types of lung cancer occur with asbestos exposure. Tumors related to asbestos exposure appear to have a predilection for the lower lobe and the lung periphery. Radon gas is the decayed product of uranium in the earth and has been recognized as a carcinogen for many years. Nonsmoking miners exposed to radioactive substances derived from radon have a 10- to 15-fold increased risk of lung cancer.[15,16] The interaction between exposure to radon and smoking is synergistic.

Box 25-1 • Causative Substances for Bronchogenic Carcinoma

- Arsenic
- Asbestos
- Bis(chloromethyl)ether and chloromethyl ether
- Chromium
- Ionizing radiation, γ-rays, x-rays
- Synthetic mineral fibers (certain kinds only)
- Mustard gas
- Nickel
- Radon (decay products)
- Soot, tars, mineral oils (polycyclic aromatic hydrocarbons)
- Vinyl chloride

▶ PATHOGENESIS AND PATHOLOGY

Bronchogenic carcinoma, like other malignant lesions, is the result of stimuli that damage the genetic material (DNA) of cells and of spontaneous mutations of stem cell lines of the lungs.[4] The damage to DNA occurs after exposure to carcinogens such as tobacco smoke.[17] These changes result in growth independence of cells. Genetic changes in the respiratory cells include expression of oncogenes, deletion of tumor suppressor gene, deletion of chromosomes, and secretion of growth factors.

The major histopathologic types of bronchogenic carcinoma include adenocarcinoma, squamous cell carcinoma, small cell carcinoma, and large cell carcinoma. Other malignant epithelial lung tumors include adenosquamous carcinoma, carcinoma with pleomorphic, sarcomatoid, or sarcomatous elements, carcinoid tumors, carcinoma of salivary gland type, and unclassified carcinoma.[18] Only the first four major histopathologic types are reviewed.

Adenocarcinoma represents 30% to 35% of all lung cancers and is currently the most common category, surpassing squamous cell carcinoma in the mid 1980s. The increasing prevalence of adenocarcinoma is probably related to more frequent occurrence among women, changes in environmental exposure, and changes in the histopathologic criteria of bronchogenic carcinoma. Adenocarcinoma forms glandular structures and may arise from lung scars (Figure 25-2, *A*). Adenocarcinoma is divided into acinar, papillary, solid adenocarcinoma with mucin formation, mixed type, and other rare variants. Bronchoalveolar cell carcinoma, a type of adenocarcinoma, has a unique histologic and clinical presentation. Bronchoalveolar carcinoma may manifest as an isolated nodule or as multiple shadows (multicentric). Most localized bronchoalveolar carcinomas are resectable, and the prognosis of the localized type is better than that of the diffuse or multicentric type.[19] Approximately 15% of all adenocarcinomas are bronchoalveolar cell carcinoma.

Squamous cell carcinoma accounts for 30% to 32% of cases of bronchogenic carcinoma. Squamous cell carcinoma is composed of flattened or polygonal, stratified epithelial cells that form intercellular bridges (intercellular desmosomes) and elaborate keratin (Figure 25-2, *B*). Squamous cell carcinoma arises from areas of damaged epithelium. Squamous cell carcinoma is the cell type more prone to cavitation, although in recent years, a higher incidence of cavitating adenocarcinoma has been reported.

Large cell carcinoma constitutes 15% to 20% of adult cases of bronchogenic carcinoma. Large cell carcinoma is composed of pleomorphic cells with variably enlarged nuclei and prominent nucleoli with abundant cytoplasm (Figure 25-2, *C*). Large cell carcinoma lacks glandular and squamous differentiation. The diagnosis of large cell carcinoma sometimes is inaccurate because tumors without clear differentiation frequently are classified as large cell tumors. Large cell carcinoma usually is a large, peripheral lesion and may have aggressive behavior. When the patient comes to medical attention, the tumor most commonly is in an advanced stage. Large cell carcinoma tends to metastasize widely.[12]

Small cell bronchogenic carcinoma accounts for 20% to 25% of primary lung cancers. **Small cell lung cancer** develops from a common pulmonary stem cell with secondary differentiation into a cell type with neural characteristics (Figure 25-2, *D*).[12] The cells in small cell bronchogenic carcinoma are pleomorphic, no larger than a lymphocyte nucleus. The cells may be round, angulated, or oval, and the cytoplasmic size is variable. Approximately 80% of small cell tumors are centrally located in the lungs (i.e., in the central bronchi). The tumor usually infiltrates the submucosal tissue. The tumor tends to spread into the mediastinal lymph nodes very early in the course of the disease and usually is extensive when discovered. The most common sites of metastatic lesions include bone, liver, bone marrow, and brain.

Clinical Manifestations

Early recognition of bronchogenic carcinoma is important. The clinical manifestations of bronchogenic carcinoma result from local growth of the tumor, metastasis

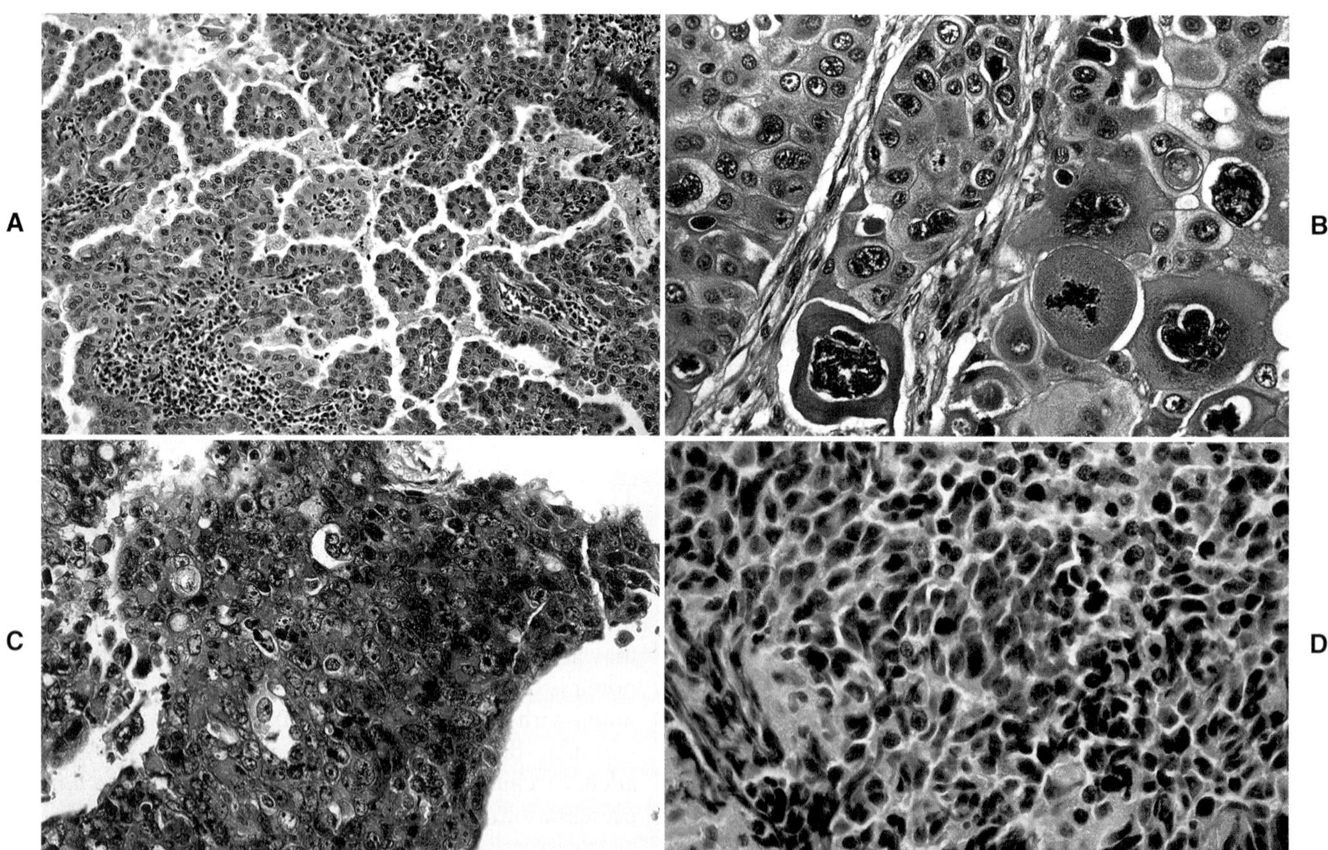

Figure 25-2 · Major Histopathologic Types of Bronchogenic Carcinoma

A, Adenocarcinoma. The well-differentiated glandular structures are evident. **B**, Squamous cell carcinoma with flattened polygonal epithelial cells and elaborate formation of keratin. **C**, Large cell carcinoma with pleomorphic cells and variably enlarged nuclei and prominent nucleoli with abundant cytoplasm. There is no tendency to form glands and no formation of keratin. **D**, Small cell undifferentiated carcinoma composed of sheets of small malignant cells with little cytoplasm. *(Courtesy Carol Farver, MD.)*

to extrathoracic and intrathoracic organs, and paraneoplastic syndrome.[20] Some of the clinical manifestations of bronchogenic carcinoma depend on the cell type. Small cell lung cancer has very aggressive behavior with marked mediastinal and early extrathoracic spread. Squamous cell carcinoma, however, usually causes local symptoms because these tumors invade locally before spreading systemically. Patients with adenocarcinoma and large cell carcinoma tend to have systemic manifestations relatively early in the course of disease.

A large percentage of patients (15%) with bronchogenic carcinoma, usually with peripheral lesions, have no symptoms. Local tumor growth in the central airways or in the mediastinal structure causes cough, hemoptysis, wheezing, dyspnea, dysphagia, postobstructive pneumonitis, hoarseness due to involvement of the recurrent laryngeal nerve, superior vena cava syndrome due to obstruction of the superior vena cava, chylothorax due to compression and obstruction of the thoracic duct, vague chest pain, palpitation, and syncope due to pericardial and cardiac involvement. Cavitation of the tumor in cases of squamous cell carcinoma and adenocarcinoma can cause fever, chills, and cough. Bronchorrhea, characterized by excessive production of bronchial secretions, occurs in 20% of patients with bronchoalveolar cell carcinoma and may be an initial manifestation. Bronchorrhea usually indicates extensive lung involvement. Patients with pleural or chest wall involvement may have chest pain, dyspnea, and cough. The pleura is involved in approximately 10% to 15% of patients with bronchogenic carcinoma.[20] In the case of superior sulcus tumor (Pancoast's syndrome), involvement of the cervical sympathetic chain causes C7-T2 neuropathy and Horner's syndrome (ptosis or droopy eyelid, miosis [small pupil], and hemifacial anhidrosis [lack of sweating]). Most patients with Pancoast's syndrome have squamous cell carcinoma.

The extrathoracic manifestation of bronchogenic carcinoma may be caused by tumor infiltration (metastasis) or nonmetastatic complications known as *paraneoplastic syndromes*. Lung metastasis results from hematogenous, lymphatic, or intraalveolar dissemination (Table 25-1).[20] Some of the extrathoracic, nonmetastatic manifestations of bronchogenic carcinoma are caused by paraneoplastic syndromes and occur in approximately 10% of patients with bronchogenic carcinoma. The clinical manifestations of paraneoplastic syndromes are not related to tumor invasion, metastasis, or side effects of therapy. Rather, these syndromes are caused by production of peptides, growth factors, and cytokines by the tumor or by the host in response to the tumor or by production of antibodies against a tumor antigen that cross-reacts with normal structures in the host and causes anatomical and functional abnormalities. For the diagnosis of paraneoplastic syndrome, primary electrolyte and metabolic, infectious, and nutritional abnormalities must be ruled out. The paraneoplastic syndromes more commonly associated with bronchogenic carcinoma are hypercalcemia of malignancy, syndrome of inappropriate antidiuresis, ectopic Cushing's syndrome, and less commonly, paraneoplastic neurologic syndromes, which affect approximately 3% of patients with small cell lung carcinoma. Other paraneoplastic syndromes include skeletal abnormalities, such as clubbing and hypertrophic osteoarthropathy, and systemic symptoms, such as weight loss, fever, and general malaise.

Table 25-1 ▶▶ Frequency of Metastatic Involvement of Organ Systems by Lung Cancer

Site or Type of Involvement	Frequency (%)
Central nervous system	20-50
Cervical lymph nodes	15-60
Bone	25
Heart and pericardium	20
Pleural effusion	8-15
Superior vena cava syndrome	4
Liver	1-35
Bone marrow in small cell carcinoma*	50

Modified from Patel AM, Peters SG: Mayo Clin Proc 68:273, 1993.
*Small cell carcinoma, with or without hematologic abnormalities.

Hypercalcemia of malignancy affects patients with non–small cell lung cancer (most commonly with squamous cell carcinoma and occasionally with adenocarcinoma and large cell carcinoma). It may be present in approximately 15% of patients with advanced bronchogenic carcinoma. In approximately 85% of cases, the syndrome is caused by secretion by the tumor of a peptide called *parathyroid hormone–related peptide* (PTH-rP). This peptide has structural characteristics and functions similar to those of parathyroid hormone. The PTH-rP increases the osteoclast activity, and the result is resorption of the bone. The final abnormality in these patients is elevation of ionized serum calcium, which causes lethargy, confusion, fatigue, nausea, anorexia, and weakness. Therapy for hypercalcemia of malignancy associated with bronchogenic carcinoma includes hydration, calcitonin, mithramycin, biphosphonates, and gallium nitrite.

The other two common paraendocrine syndromes are inappropriate antidiuresis and ectopic Cushing's syndrome. These two paraneoplastic disorders are associated with small cell lung cancer. Inappropriate antidiuresis occurs when the tumor secretes the hormone arginine vasopressin. Some tumors produce atrial natriuretic factor. Patients with a syndrome of inappropriate antidiuresis usually have inappropriate thirst, which plays an important role in the pathogenesis of this disorder. The final biochemical manifestation of inappropriate antidiuresis is the presence of hyponatremia (serum sodium level less than 135 mmol/L with associated plasma hypoosmolality; that is, <280 mOsm/kg).

Arginine vasopressin makes the epithelium of the distal and collective tubules of the kidney permeable to water. Management of this syndrome includes therapy for the underlying tumor, water restriction, demeclocycline, and fludrocortisone.

Ectopic Cushing's syndrome is caused by secretion of the prohormone propiomelanocortin, a precursor of the hormone adrenocorticotropin. Adrenocorticotropin causes hyperfunction of the adrenal cortex; the result is a high cortisol level. Patients with ectopic Cushing's syndrome usually have peripheral edema, hypertension, muscle weakness, and moon facies. Metabolic abnormalities such as hypokalemic metabolic alkalosis and hyperglycemia are frequent. The diagnosis is based on the clinical presentation (most of these patients have obvious bronchogenic carcinoma) and the presence of elevated levels of cortisol and corticotropin. Other forms of biochemical diagnosis include use of metyrapone and the dexamethasone suppression test. Management of the syndrome includes therapy for the underlying malignant disease and administration of adrenal enzyme inhibitors such as ketoconazole (an antifungal agent), metyrapone, aminoglutethimide, mifepristone, and octreotide.

Paraneoplastic neurologic syndromes are more commonly associated with small cell lung cancer. They are present in 1% to 3% of patients with small cell lung cancer. The most common of these disorders is *Eaton-Lambert syndrome.* Eaton-Lambert syndrome is a disorder of neuromuscular transmission characterized by a deficit in the release of acetylcholine at the motor nerve terminals. The syndrome is caused by production of immunoglobulin G antibody against the tumor that cross-reacts with the calcium channel complex, inhibiting calcium flux and the liberation of acetylcholine. These patients have fatigability and muscle weakness, although strength may improve after a sustained maximal effort. The syndrome is characterized by a very-low-amplitude compound muscle action potential with normal conduction velocity in the electromyogram. These muscle action potentials increase in size after exercise or fast stimulation. Management of this syndrome includes therapy for the malignant tumor, use of corticosteroids, use of azathioprine, plasma exchange, and intravenous administration of γ-globulin. Other paraneoplastic neurologic disorders include subacute cerebellar degeneration, subacute sensory neuronopathy, limbic encephalitis, and polyneuropathy.

Radiographic Manifestations

For most patients with asymptomatic lung cancer, the tumor is diagnosed with plain chest radiography. Lesions smaller than 5 to 6 mm are difficult to see on a chest radiograph. Although the radiographic appearance of a lesion cannot be used to differentiate benign and malignant processes, some radiographic characteristics

MINI CLINI

Hilar Adenopathy

PROBLEM

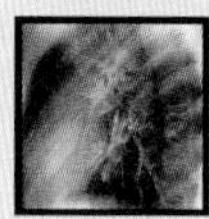

A 60-year-old man has been found to have small cell lung cancer on the basis of results of bronchoscopic biopsy. A CT scan of the chest shows extensive hilar adenopathy. The patient has been admitted to the oncology floor for **chemotherapy**. You are called to assess him because he cannot lie down owing to shortness of breath (orthopnea). When you arrive, the patient is sitting on the edge of the bed. You notice that his face and neck are swollen. He also has dilated veins over the face, neck, chest, and arms. How do you explain these findings?

DISCUSSION

This patient has superior vena caval (SVC) obstruction due to compression by the mediastinal tumor. The swelling of the face, neck, and arms is caused by impairment of the venous drainage from the upper body (the SVC distribution). The dilated chest and arm veins are collateral vessels (or alternative pathway vessels) that compensate for the SVC obstruction. Superior vena caval obstruction can be caused by a variety of benign or malignant conditions that involve the mediastinum or the right upper lung. Treatment usually is therapy for the underlying problem. For this patient, the preferred treatment is chemotherapy because small cell lung cancer is highly responsive to this modality. Other cancers usually are more responsive to radiation. Good responses occur in 75% of patients within 2 weeks of initiation of therapy. Surgical resection rarely is needed.

MINI CLINI

Pancoast's Tumor

PROBLEM

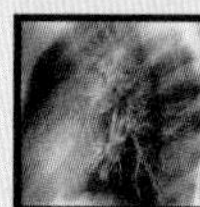

A 65-year-old man who has smoked two packs of cigarettes per day for the past 40 years has had drooping of the left eyelid for the past 3 weeks. A chest radiograph reveals a mass in the apex of the left lung. Is there a link between the drooping of the eyelid and the lung mass?

DISCUSSION

Lung tumors involving the apex of the lung (superior sulcus tumors) also are known as *Pancoast's tumors.* If they involve the cervical sympathetic nerves in the neck, these tumors result in Horner's syndrome. This syndrome is characterized by ptosis (drooping of the eyelid), anhidrosis (absence of sweating), and miosis (constricted pupil) on the same side as the tumor. Most cases of Pancoast's tumors are caused by squamous cell carcinoma. Other manifestations of Pancoast's tumors include pain and weakness in the upper extremity (due to involvement of the brachial plexus), rib destruction, and destruction of vertebral bodies. This condition usually reflects the presence of advanced disease that may not be amenable to surgical resection.

MINI CLINI

Paraneoplastic Syndrome

PROBLEM

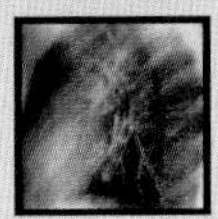

A 55-year-old man is brought to the emergency department by family members because of confusion and progressive generalized weakness. Examination in the emergency department shows the patient is dehydrated, lethargic, and confused. A chest radiograph reveals a cavitary lesion in the right upper lobe. Results of arterial blood gas analysis are normal. Results of chemical analysis urgently performed with the blood gas analysis reveal a sodium level of 150 mEq/L (normal, 135-145 mEq/L) and a calcium level of 17 mg/dL (normal, 9-10.5 mg/dL). How is the lung mass related to this patient's presentation and biochemical abnormalities?

DISCUSSION

This patient's confusion and weakness are due to hypercalcemia, which is a paraneoplastic presentation of lung cancer, especially squamous cell carcinoma (the cavitating mass on the chest radiograph). Paraneoplastic syndromes are systemic manifestations of lung cancer that are not caused by metastasis. Most paraneoplastic syndromes are associated with small cell lung cancer. Hypercalcemia, however, is more common with squamous cell carcinoma and is caused by secretion by the tumor of PTH-rP. Treatment consists of hydration, diuresis, and the use of medications that can reduce the levels of calcium.

MINI CLINI

No Response to Antibiotics

PROBLEM

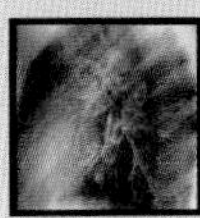

A 55-year-old woman who does not smoke has a 3-month history of dyspnea on exertion, weight loss, and cough productive of copious amounts of clear, frothy sputum. She has no fever or chills. She has been treated for 2 weeks for "double pneumonia" without relief of the symptoms. Examination reveals finger clubbing and decreased air entry in both lung bases with dullness to percussion. A chest radiograph shows bilateral alveolar infiltrates. What should be done next?

DISCUSSION

The patient has bronchoalveolar cell carcinoma. Cough productive of copious amounts of clear, frothy sputum is characteristic of this type of lung cancer. The radiographic appearance may be indistinguishable from that of pneumonia, especially when sputum production occurs. The absence of fever, the chronic presence of infiltrates, and the lack of response to antibiotic therapy should raise the suspicion of bronchoalveolar cell carcinoma. Bronchoscopy with transbronchial biopsy would be a reasonable next step to confirm the diagnosis.

that suggest the presence of malignant growth include margins that are shaggy and poorly defined and lobulation of the mass. Adenocarcinoma manifests in 40% of cases as a peripheral mass and in another 40% as a central lesion. Bronchoalveolar cell carcinoma, a type of adenocarcinoma, may manifest as a solitary nodule, as numerous small unilateral or bilateral nodules, or as lobular or segmental unilateral or bilateral consolidation mimicking a pneumonic process.

Squamous cell carcinoma usually manifests as a central lesion and may obstruct the airways and cause atelectasis, postobstructive pneumonia, or lung abscess. Peripheral squamous cell carcinoma may cavitate. Large cell carcinoma is more frequently a peripheral lesion and usually manifests as a lobulated, well-defined mass that may cavitate occasionally. Small cell lung cancer occurs centrally and may manifest as a hilar mass. Small cell lung cancer almost never cavitates. Mediastinal adenopathy may cause external compression of the airways with atelectasis and postobstructive pneumonia. Small cell lung cancer occurs peripherally in approximately 5% of instances.

Solitary Pulmonary Nodule

A solitary nodule is defined as a single lesion up to 3 cm in diameter surrounded by lung parenchyma. A solitary pulmonary nodule represents a diagnostic dilemma.[21] The two most common causes of solitary nodules are bronchogenic carcinoma and granulomatous disease. Approximately 30% of all cases of bronchogenic carcinoma manifest as a solitary nodule, and in medical practice, approximately 50% of solitary nodules are malignant. Most of the malignant lesions are bronchogenic carcinoma, although a small number (10%) are metastatic lesions, and approximately 2% are carcinoid tumors.

Solitary nodules often do not produce symptoms. Most of the time a solitary nodule is an incidental finding on a chest radiograph. Establishing the cause of a nodule is the main clinical challenge. The final goal in the treatment of these patients is identifying who has a malignant nodule that necessitates surgery while avoiding thoracotomy on patients with benign nodules. The most reliable finding that suggests a benign cause is the absence of growth of a nodule for more than 24 months. Growth is evaluated by review of old radiographs. Another important characteristic is the presence and pattern of calcification in the nodule. A nodule that is homogeneous, popcorn-like, laminated, and concentric is likely benign (Figure 25-3). If a nodule is noncalcified and the pattern of growth for the last 24 months cannot be determined, the probability of cancer must be assessed on the basis of the clinical features. Clinical features suggestive of the presence of malignant disease include a high incidence of expected malignant disease in the population, a nodule more than 2 cm in diameter, history of smoking, history of previous malignant disease, and the radiographic characteristics of the edge of the nodule. The nodular margins are better assessed with computed tomography (CT) of the chest. Spiculated (irregular) borders suggest a malignant cause, whereas smooth borders favor a benign cause.

The most important step in evaluating a patient with a solitary pulmonary nodule is to obtain previous radiographs to determine the stability of the size of the nodule over the previous 2 years. Other imaging techniques include magnetic resonance imaging and positron emission tomography (PET). The combined sensitivity and specificity of PET are 91.2%. If the patient is at high risk of bronchogenic carcinoma, the false-negative rate remains unacceptable, and the patient needs either biopsy or surgical removal of the nodule.[22]

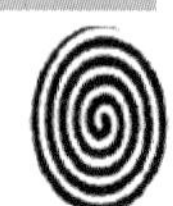

RULE OF THUMB

A solitary pulmonary nodule that has not grown in 24 months is unlikely to be malignant.

If a nodule is not calcified, the cause is undetermined after radiologic studies, and the probability of cancer is moderate, biopsy is indicated and is performed by means of transthoracic needle aspiration (TTNA) or thoracotomy. If the probability of cancer is high, immediate thoracotomy has the highest expected utility. For patients with a low probability of cancer, a wait and watch strategy is favored.[21]

▶ DIAGNOSIS

Current methods of tissue diagnosis of bronchogenic carcinoma include sputum cytologic examination, flexible fiberoptic bronchoscopy (FFB), TTNA, in which a needle is passed into the nodule from outside the chest wall under radiologic guidance, and thoracotomy. Other techniques that are useful in selected cases include thoracentesis with percutaneous pleural biopsy, pleuroscopy, and mediastinoscopy. Cytologic examination of a sputum specimen is helpful in the diagnosis of central, proximal tumors (more frequently squamous cell carcinoma and small cell carcinoma). The results of sputum cytologic examination are variable, and interpretation may be difficult owing to poor sample preparation and lack of an experienced cytologist. A negative result does not rule out bronchogenic carcinoma in the appropriate setting. Fiberoptic bronchoscopy is helpful in the diagnosis of central airway bronchogenic carcinoma. The diagnostic yield of FFB of a centrally located lesion is approximately 90%.[23] The diagnostic yield of transbronchial biopsy, brushing, and lavage in cases of peripheral lesions (tumors not visible at FFB) is 48% to 80%, with an average of 69%. The size of the lesion is the most important determinant of the diagnostic yield of peripheral lesions. The yield is less than 30% in lesions less than 2 cm in diameter and approximately 65% in lesions greater than 2 cm in diameter. In some lesions 4 cm or larger, the diagnostic yield is approximately 80%. Complications of bronchoscopy occur in fewer than 5% of procedures. They include laryngospasm, transient hypoxemia in patients with severe lung disease, airway bleeding, and pneumothorax.

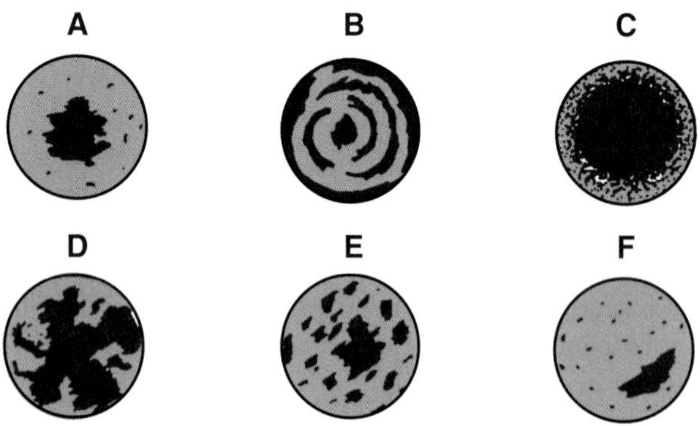

Figure 25-3 · Patterns of Calcification in a Solitary Pulmonary Nodule

A, Central. **B**, Laminated. **C**, Diffuse. **D**, Popcorn. **E**, Stippled. **F**, Eccentric. **A** through **D** show benign patterns of calcification. **E** and **F** show patterns of calcification that may be seen in either benign or malignant nodules. *(Modified from Lillington GA: Systematic diagnostic approach to pulmonary nodules. In Fishman AP, editor: Pulmonary disease and disorders, ed 2, New York, 1988, McGraw-Hill.)*

Transthoracic needle aspiration is useful in the diagnosis of lung masses and of mediastinal abnormalities. It complements bronchoscopy in the diagnosis of peripheral pulmonary lesions.[23-25] Transthoracic needle aspiration should be considered in the evaluation of peripheral, small (<2 to 3 cm) nodules. The diagnostic yield of TTNA is greater than 90% for lesions >1.5 cm in diameter, but the frequency of complications is between 25% and 30%. Only 15% of patients with complications need treatment (i.e., insertion of a chest tube after pneumothorax). Unless a negative TTNA result for bronchogenic carcinoma indicates a specific benign diagnosis, such as teratoma, the result cannot be used to exclude bronchogenic carcinoma. If TTNA does not yield a diagnosis, the clinician should proceed to thoracotomy.

The combination of thoracentesis and pleural biopsy has a diagnostic yield of 80% to 90% in evaluation for bronchogenic carcinoma and pleural involvement. Other diagnostic techniques, such as thoracoscopy (a procedure that allows biopsy under direct vision), increase the diagnostic yield in the evaluation of pleural involvement.

Staging

After the histopathologic diagnosis is made, tumor staging is the most important prognostic variable in bronchogenic carcinoma.[26] Staging is important for

Table 25-2 ▶▶ New International System for Staging Lung Cancer

Stage	TNM	Survival at 5 Years by Stage Pathologically Confirmed (%)
0	In situ	?
IA	$T_1N_0M_0$	67
IB*	$T_2N_0M_0$	57
IIA*	$T_1N_1M_0$	55
IIB*	$T_2N_1M_0$	39
	$T_3N_0\ M_0$*	38
IIIA	$T_3N_1M_0$	25
	$T_{1,2,3}N_2M_0$	23
IIIB	$T_4N_{0,1,2}M_0$	7
	$T_{1,2,3}N_3M_0$	3
IV	M_1	1

From Mountain CG: Chest 111:1710, 1997.
The survival is given for pathologically confirmed cases, except stages IIIB and IV, which are clinical stages.
*Changes in the staging system.

assessing the extent of the disease, selection of therapy, and prognosis. The staging system most commonly used for **non–small cell bronchogenic carcinoma** is based on the status of the primary tumor (T), local and regional lymph node involvement (N), and the presence of metastasis (M). The TNM classification groups patients in stages or categories (Table 25-2, Figure 25-4).[26] The stage has prognostic importance because non–small cell lung cancer in stages I and II and selected cases in stage IIIA are considered surgically resectable. Lesions in stages IIIB and IV are considered unresectable. Stage of disease also correlates with survival (see Table 25-2 and Figures 25-4 and 25-5).

Staging of small cell lung cancer is different from that of non–small cell lung cancer. Small cell lung cancer has only two stages: limited and extensive. Limited disease implies that the tumor is confined to the ipsilateral hemithorax and that the tumor is confined within a radiation port. Extensive disease is defined as spread beyond the hemithorax and adjacent lymph nodes, recurrent disease after radiation of the primary tumor, or cytologically positive pleural effusion.

Complete evaluation of the hilar and mediastinal areas is essential for accurate staging. Computed tomography of the chest is useful because it offers significant advantage over chest radiography. The sensitivity for detecting malignant mediastinal disease at chest CT is approximately 90%, although the specificity is low. Histologic examination of the lymph nodes therefore is required because the enlargement may be the result of an inflammatory nonneoplastic process. Transbronchial needle aspiration by FFB and mediastinoscopy has been used for sampling of mediastinal lymph nodes. Mediastinoscopy remains the standard procedure for mediastinal staging of non–small cell bronchogenic carcinoma. Any lymph node enlargement detected with CT should be subjected to biopsy with the previously mentioned techniques to confirm or exclude the presence of metastasis.

Another radiologic technique used in staging bronchogenic carcinoma is magnetic resonance imaging for evaluation of the chest wall and pleura. Magnetic resonance imaging may be particularly useful in the evaluation of patients with a contraindication to the use of the intravenous contrast materials used in CT. Positron emission tomography with [^{18}F]fluorodeoxyglucose has been used for identification of malignant pulmonary lesions in the mediastinum.[27] The test characteristics of PET appear better than the characteristics of CT; the overall sensitivity and specificity of PET are 96% and 93%, respectively.[27]

Detection of extrapulmonary metastasis begins with an adequate history and physical examination. Bronchogenic carcinoma tends to metastasize to the liver, central nervous system, adrenal glands, bone, and supraclavicular lymph nodes. The presence of symptoms such as weight loss, anorexia, neurologic symptoms, and localized bone pain is highly suggestive of the presence of metastasis. Laboratory evaluation includes liver function tests and measurement of alkaline phosphatase and calcium. The presence of abnormalities indicates the need for further evaluation. Imaging techniques used for detection of extrapulmonary metastasis include CT of the chest (which should include the liver and adrenal glands) and bone and liver-spleen scans if the clinical history suggests involvement of these organs. Computed tomography of the central nervous system is indicated in the evaluation of patients who have clinical neurologic involvement and patients who have adenocarcinoma. Patients with squamous cell carcinoma or large cell carcinoma do not need routine CT of the head. Positron emission tomography has a sensitivity and specificity of 95% and 83%, respectively, for the detection of mediastinal and distant metastasis.[28]

For patients with small cell lung cancer, accurate extrathoracic staging is important. Routine nuclear scans of the bone, liver, and spleen in addition to a CT of the head are necessary for detection of tumor metastasis. Bone marrow aspiration and biopsy often are used for detection of tumors in this area if results of the noninvasive evaluation for metastasis have been negative.

Screening

Mass screening of patients at high risk of bronchogenic carcinoma with chest radiography and sputum cytologic examination does not confer any significant improvement in overall survival of bronchogenic carcinoma.[29] There is no current consensus that patients at high risk should undergo yearly chest radiography or sputum cytologic examination. Low-dose spiral CT has shown some promise as a screening test for lung cancer because

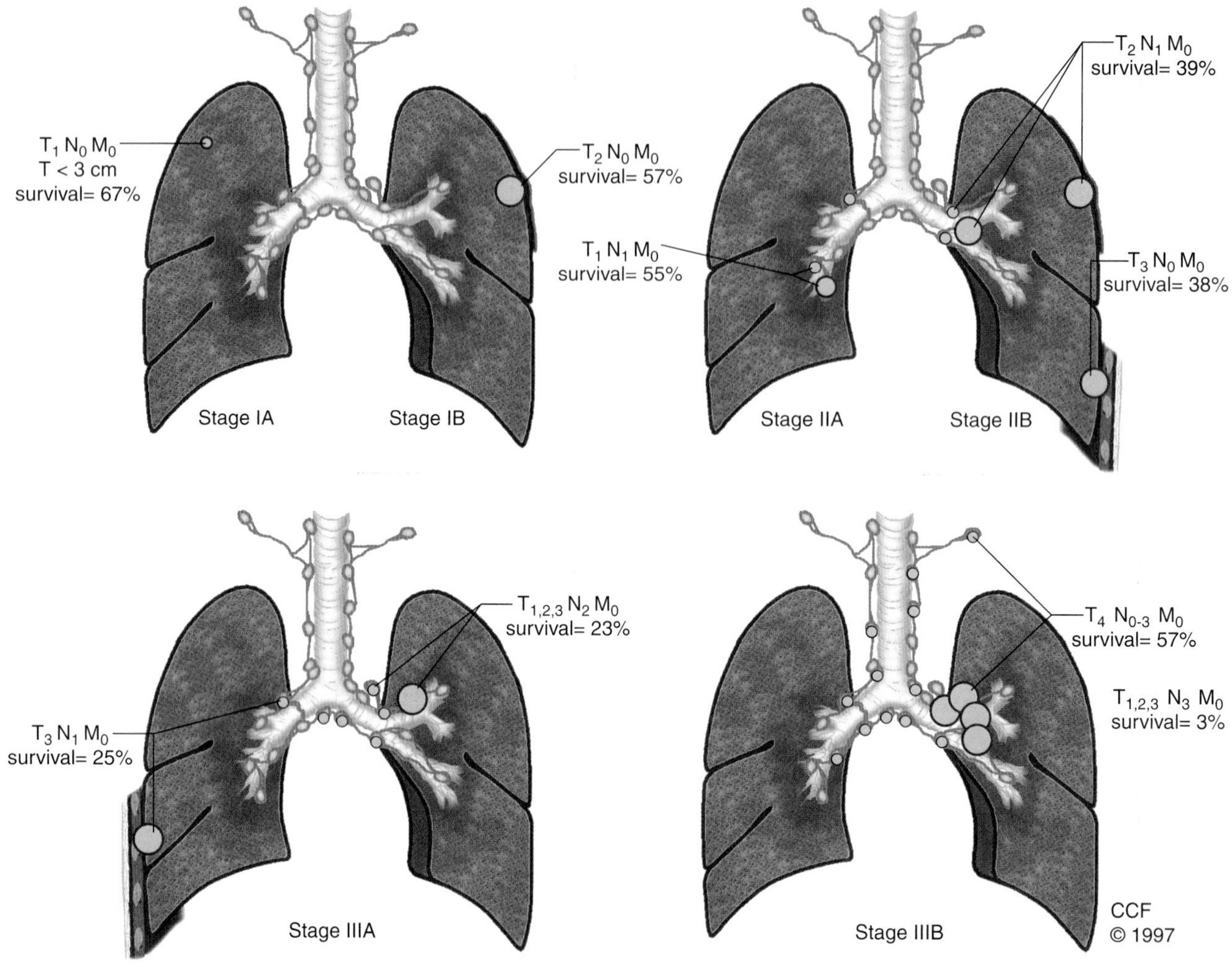

Figure 25-4 · **Lung Cancer Stages**

The stages are summarized in Table 25-2. The survival rate is based on results of clinical staging (see Figure 25-5).

this technique can depict more nodules than can chest radiography. Although there is growing enthusiasm for such low-dose CT screening, no guidelines or definitive data support screening of patients with low-dose spiral CT. Additional data are needed before this technique can be recommended for routine office practice.[29]

▶ TREATMENT

Non–Small Cell Lung Cancer

The most commonly used modalities of treatment of patients with non–small cell lung cancer are surgical resection, radiation therapy, and chemotherapy.[30] Modalities used for palliative therapy include endobronchial laser therapy and endobronchial radiation (brachytherapy).[31] Surgical resection should be considered the initial modality in the treatment of all patients with non–small cell lung cancer because it offers the best prospect of long-term survival. The survival rate among patients who have undergone surgery varies from 70% among patients with small tumors and stage I disease (T_1,N_0,M_0) to 25% among patients with stage IIIA disease, in which the ipsilateral mediastinal nodes are involved (see Table 25-2).[32] Although surgical resection is the treatment of choice because it offers the best prospect of long-term survival, only one third of patients have disease that may be resectable at the time of the diagnosis. Most patients with non–small cell lung cancer come to medical attention with locally advanced stage IIIB or metastatic stage IV disease and are not candidates for surgery.

Lung reserve must be evaluated with pulmonary function testing in the care of patients who are candidates for lung resection. The preoperative forced expiratory volume in 1 second (FEV_1) is probably the value most commonly used for predicting postoperative lung function. A preoperative FEV_1 of more than 2 L or more than 70% of predicted value indicates good lung reserve, and the patient may even tolerate pneumonectomy. Patients who have an FEV_1 of less than 70% of

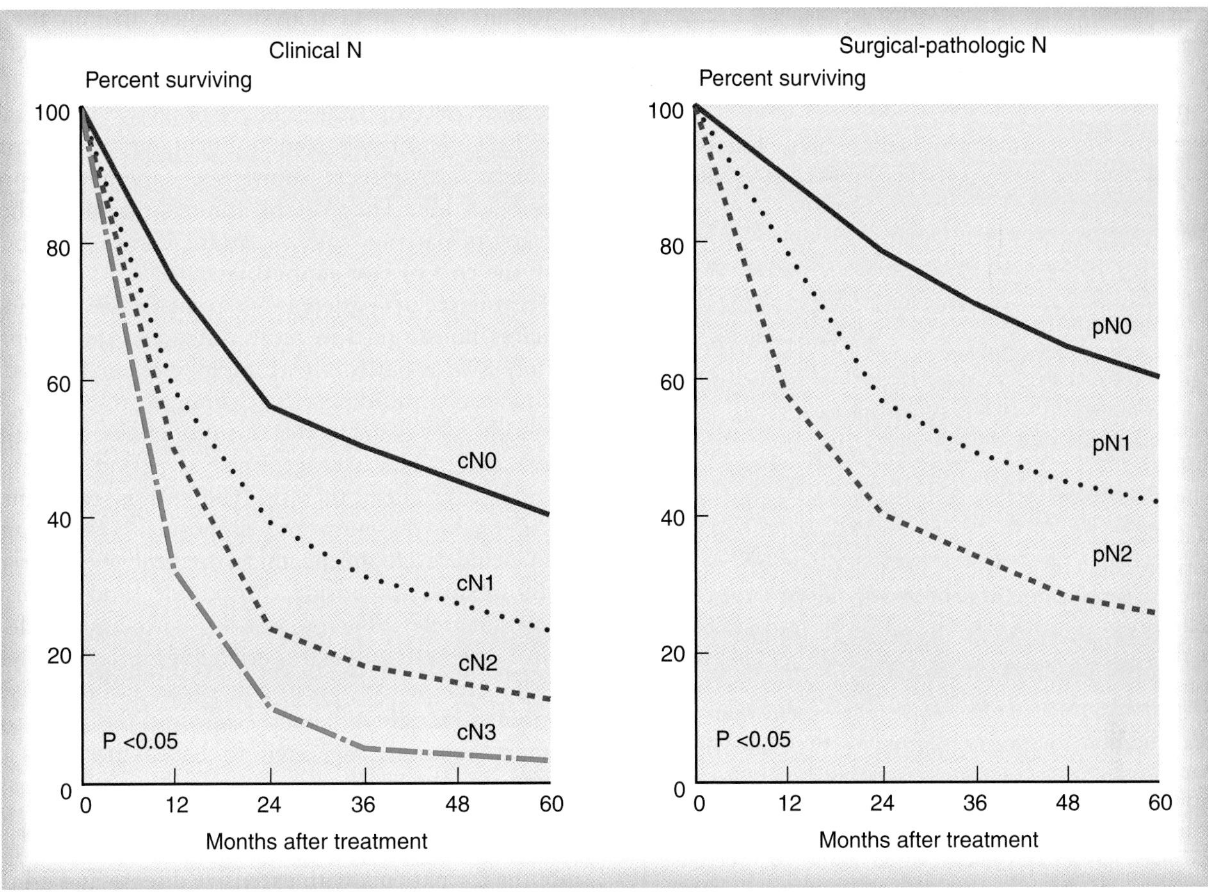

Figure 25-5 · Lung Cancer Survival

Cumulative percentage of patients surviving 5 years or longer after treatment according to the status of lymph nodes. Left, survival based on clinical stage. Right, survival based on pathological stage. *(Modified from Mountain CF: Chest 111:1710, 1997.)*

predicted value need a quantitative ventilation-perfusion scan for prediction of postoperative lung function. A postoperative predicted FEV_1 of less than 40% of predicted value, postoperative predicted diffusing capacity of the lung for carbon monoxide of less than 40%, and the presence of marked dyspnea before surgery suggest a high morbidity and mortality among patients scheduled to undergo lung resection.

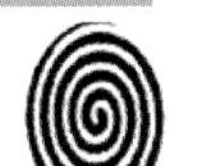

RULE OF THUMB

Patients with an FEV1 of more than 70% predicted value or 2 L can safely undergo resectional surgery for lung cancer, even if pneumonectomy is needed.

Cardiopulmonary exercise testing is a noninvasive procedure used for evaluation of candidates with borderline lung function. Patients able to achieve a maximal measured oxygen consumption ($\dot{V}O_{2max}$) of 20 mL/kg per minute are likely to tolerate surgical resection without major complications. However, among patients who achieve only 10 mL/kg per minute, a high mortality is expected. For patients who achieve a $\dot{V}O_{2max}$ between these values, the surgical approach has to be individualized.

Lobectomy and pneumonectomy are the procedures of choice in the care of patients with stage I and stage II bronchogenic carcinoma. Because of the frequent coexistence of significant chronic obstructive lung disease in patients with lung cancer, other procedures designed to spare pulmonary parenchyma, such as segmentectomy, wedge resection, and bronchial sleeve resection, have been used frequently in operations on patients with limited lung function. Local recurrence remains a problem after such limited resection. In addition, limited pulmonary resection does not improve perioperative morbidity or mortality or late postoperative pulmonary function.[32-34]

The value of surgery in the management of extensive local disease (stage IIIA and IIIB) is controversial.[30] Although patients with stage IIIB non–small cell bronchogenic carcinoma have not been considered surgical candidates in the past and have been treated only with

MINI CLINI

Evaluating Surgical Risk

PROBLEM

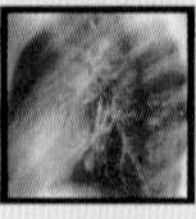

A 62-year-old man with a long history of smoking has a chronic, productive cough. A chest radiograph obtained because of a recent episode of hemoptysis reveals a right lung mass. Results of transbronchial biopsy suggest the presence of large cell carcinoma. There is no evidence of metastasis. As part of the patient's evaluation for surgery, he has the following spirometry results:

Forced vital capacity (FVC), 4.2 L (80% of predicted value)
FEV_1, 1.6 L (60% of predicted value)
FEV_1/FVC, 0.4
Can he undergo surgery?

DISCUSSION

Assessment of lung reserve is an important step in the preoperative evaluation of patients with lung cancer being considered for surgical resection. A preoperative FEV_1 of more than 2 L (or >70% of predicted value) indicates good lung reserve with low surgical risk even if pneumonectomy is needed. An FEV_1 less than 35% of predicted value is a contraindication to surgery because of the high risk of postoperative mortality and morbidity. Other options, such as radiation therapy or chemotherapy, must be considered for these patients. This patient, like most patients with lung cancer, has an FEV_1 between 35% and 70% because of underlying chronic obstructive pulmonary disease (COPD). He needs reevaluation after appropriate management of the underlying COPD. If the patient's lung function does not improve to the low-risk level with treatment, a quantitative lung perfusion scan may be necessary for assessment of the percentage of functional contribution by each lung and for prediction of residual lung function after surgical resection.

radiation and chemotherapy, recent experience suggests that these patients may be candidates for treatment under strict study protocols incorporating neoadjuvant therapy (radiation and chemotherapy before surgery).[35]

Radiation therapy is useful in decreasing the size of local tumors and is helpful as a palliative measure, especially in the treatment of patients who have obstruction of the airways, compression of vital chest structures, pain, or hemoptysis. The addition of chemotherapy to radiation therapy may improve survival for a small group of patients with non–small cell lung cancer with locally advanced, unresectable disease. The benefit of this combination therapy is relatively small and should be balanced against the toxicity associated with the addition of chemotherapy.[36] Radiation therapy may be curative in a small percentage (approximately 15%) of patients with stage I non–small cell lung cancer. Chemotherapy is ineffective as the sole therapy for non–small cell lung cancer.

Results of a meta-analysis suggest that in the care of patients with advanced, non–surgically resectable, non–small cell lung cancer, chemotherapy with vinca alkaloids or etoposide, and, especially, *cis*-platinum–based regimens offers a small but significant advantage in survival over best supportive care and improves quality of life. The cost of administration of chemotherapy to patients with metastatic disease may be less than the cost of best supportive care.[30,37]

Treatment of patients with small cell carcinoma remains nonsurgical in most instances. Only approximately 8% of patients with peripheral small cell carcinoma are candidates for surgical resection, and chemotherapy is the management of choice of small cell lung cancer. The average survival period is 7 to 10 months after chemotherapy. The current regimens are based on *cis*-platinum and etoposide.[30] Other agents used include cyclophosphamide, doxorubicin, vincristine, methotrexate, teniposide, ifosfamide, and lomustine. Approximately 20% of patients with limited disease have a disease-free survival period of more than 3 years. In the treatment of patients with limited disease, combined-modality chemotherapy and radiation to the primary tumor are suggested. Radiation therapy is given to decrease the likelihood of local relapse. Patients with extensive disease have very poor response and long-term survival. The median survival period is 7 to 10 months for patients with extensive disease and 14 to 20 months for patients with limited disease.[30]

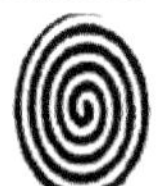

RULE OF THUMB

Chemotherapy is the modality of choice for small cell lung cancer. Management of all other forms of lung cancer is surgery if feasible.

Prevention

The most effective way to prevent lung cancer is to prevent smoking. Healthcare professionals, especially respiratory therapists, have the duty of advising patients about stopping smoking. Indeed, Frequent reminders by healthcare providers have been shown to be an important factor in achieving smoking cessation. The most common pharmacologic measures to assist smoking cessation include nicotine preparations and bupropion. Use of bupropion alone or in combination with a nicotine patch has been associated with an abstinence rate of 30% to 35% and with a 1-year continuous abstinence rate of 20% versus 6% in a group of patients using placebo.[38] Secondary prevention with the administration of vitamin E and β-carotene to decrease the incidence of bronchogenic carcinoma has shown no benefit in decreasing the incidence of these **neoplasms**.[39-41]

KEY POINTS

- It is estimated that in 2001, 169,500 cases of bronchogenic carcinoma were newly diagnosed in the United States, making bronchogenic carcinoma a major health hazard and the leading cause of cancer deaths in the United States.
- Approximately 85% of all cases of bronchogenic carcinoma are linked to smoking. The most important cause of the increased incidence of bronchogenic carcinoma is tobacco smoking.
- The major histopathologic types of bronchogenic carcinoma include adenocarcinoma, squamous cell carcinoma, small cell carcinoma, and large cell carcinoma. Adenocarcinoma represents 30% to 35% of all cases of lung cancer and is currently the most common type of cancer.
- The clinical manifestations of bronchogenic carcinoma result from local growth of the tumor, metastasis to extrathoracic and intrathoracic organs, and paraneoplastic syndromes.
- The staging system most commonly used for non–small cell bronchogenic carcinoma is based on status of the primary tumor (T), local and regional lymph node involvement (N), and the presence of metastasis (M). The TNM classification groups patients in stages or categories that correlate with survival. Small cell lung cancer is classified in two stages: limited and extensive.
- The most commonly used modalities of treatment of patients with non–small cell lung cancer are surgical resection, radiation therapy, and chemotherapy. Treatment of most patients with small cell carcinoma remains nonsurgical in the form of chemotherapy.
- The most effective way to prevent lung cancer is to prevent smoking.

References

1. Greenlee RT et al: Cancer statistics, 2001, CA Cancer J Clin 51:15, 2001.
2. Travis WD et al: United States lung carcinoma incidence trends: declining for most histologic types among males, increasing among females, Cancer 77:464, 1996.
3. Davila DG, Williams DE: The etiology of lung cancer, Mayo Clin Proc 68:170, 1993.
4. Denissenko MF et al: Preferential formation of benzo(a)pyrene adducts at lung cancer mutational hot spots, Science 274:430, 1996.
5. Shopland DR, Eyre HJ, Pechacek TF: Smoking-attributable cancer mortality in 1991: is lung cancer now the leading cause of death among smokers in the United States? J Natl Cancer Inst 83:1142, 1991.
6. Loeb LA et al: Smoking and lung cancer: an overview, Cancer Res 44:5940, 1984.
7. Bartecchi CE, MacKenzie TD, Schrien RW: The human cost of tobacco use, N Engl J Med 330:907, 1994.
8. Rigotti NA, Lee JE, Wechsler H: US college students use of tobacco products: results of a national survey, JAMA 284:699, 2000.
9. Kessler DA: Nicotine addiction in young people, N Engl J Med 333:186, 1995.
10. Fontham ETH et al: Environmental tobacco smoke and lung cancer in nonsmoking women: a multi-center study, JAMA 271:1752, 1994.
11. Office of Health and Environmental Assessment, Office of Research and Development: Respiratory health effect of passive smoking: lung cancer and other disorders, Washington, DC, 1992, US Environmental Protection Agency.
12. Filderman AE, Matthay RA: Bronchogenic carcinoma. In Bone RC et al, editors: Pulmonary and critical care medicine, St. Louis, 1995, Mosby.
13. Craighead JE, Mossman BT: The pathogenesis of asbestos-related diseases, N Engl J Med 306:1446, 1982.
14. Roscoe RJ et al: Lung cancer mortality among non-smoking uranium miners exposed to radon daughters, JAMA 262:629, 1989.
15. Pershagen G et al: Residential exposure and lung cancer in Sweden, N Engl J Med 330:159, 1994.
16. Nuorva K et al: 53 protein accumulation in lung carcinomas of patients exposed to asbestos and tobacco smoke, Am J Respir Crit Care Med 150:528, 1994.
17. Christiani DC: Smoking and the molecular epidemiology of lung cancer, Clin Chest Med 21:87, 2000.
18. Travis WD et al: The World Health Organization histological type of lungs and pleural tumors, ed 3, Berlin, 1999, Springer-Verlag.
19. Hsu C, Chen C, Hsu N: Bronchioloalveolar carcinoma, J Thorac Cardiovasc Surg 110:374, 1995.
20. Patel AM, Peters SG: Clinical manifestations of lung cancer, Mayo Clin Proc 68:273, 1993
21. Jain P, Kathawalla SA, Arroliga AC: Managing solitary pulmonary nodules, Cleve Clin J Med 65:316, 1998.
22. Gould MK et al: Accuracy of positron emission tomography for diagnosis of pulmonary nodules and mass lesions: a meta-analysis, JAMA 285:914, 2001.
23. Mazzone P et al: Bronchoscopy and needle biopsy techniques for diagnosis and staging of lung cancer, Clin Chest Med 23:137, 2002.
24. Harrow EM et al: The utility of transbronchial needle aspiration in the staging of bronchogenic carcinoma, Am J Respir Crit Care Med 161:601, 2000.
25. Gasparini S et al: Integration of transbronchial and percutaneous approach in the diagnosis of peripheral pulmonary nodules or masses, Chest 108:131, 1995.

26. Mountain CF: Revisions in the International System for staging lung cancer, Chest 111:1710, 1997.
27. Gupta NC, Graeber GM, Bishop HA: Comparative efficacy of positron emission tomography with fluorodeoxyglucose in evaluation of small (<1cm), intermediate (1 to 3 cm), and large (>3 cm) lymph node lesions, Chest 117:773, 2000.
28. Pieterman RM et al: Preoperative staging of non-small cell lung cancer with positron emission tomography, N Engl J Med 343:254, 2000.
29. Jain P, Arroliga AC: Spiral CT for lung cancer screening: Is it ready for prime time? Cleve Clin J Med 68:74, 2001.
30. Hoffman PC, Mauer AM, Vokes EE: Lung cancer, Lancet 355:479, 2000.
31. Dweik RA, Mehta AC: Bronchoscopic management of malignant airway disease, Clin Pulm Med 3:43, 1996.
32. Shields TW: Surgical therapy for carcinomas of the lung, Clin Chest Med 14:121, 1993.
33. Warren WH, Faber LP: Segmentectomy versus lobectomy in patients with stage I pulmonary carcinoma, J Thorac Cardiovasc Surg 107:1087, 1994.
34. Ginsberg RJ, Rubinstein LV: Randomized trial of lobectomy versus limited resection for T1N0 non-small cell lung cancer, Lung Cancer Study Group, Ann Thorac Surg 60:615, 1995.
35. Rusch VW et al: Neoadjuvant therapy: a novel and effective treatment for stage III non-small cell lung cancer, Ann Thorac Surg 58:290, 1994.
36. Pritchard RS, Anthony SP: Chemotherapy plus radiotherapy compared with radiotherapy alone in the treatment of locally advanced unresectable, non-small cell lung cancer: a meta-analysis, Ann Intern Med 125:723, 1996.
37. LeChevalier T: Chemotherapy for advanced non-small cell lung cancer: will meta-analysis provide the answer? Chest 109:107S, 1996.
38. Jorenby DE et al: A controlled trial of sustained release bupropion, a nicotine patch, or both for smoking cessation, N Engl J Med 340:685, 1999.
39. The effect of vitamin E and beta carotene on the incidence of lung cancer and other cancers in male smokers, The Alpha-Tocopherol, Beta Carotene Cancer Prevention Study Group, N Engl J Med 330:1029, 1994.
40. Hennekens CH et al: Lack of effect of long-term supplementation with beta carotene on the incidence of malignant neoplasm and cardiovascular disease, N Engl J Med 334:1145, 1996.
41. Omenn GS et al: Effect of a combination of beta carotene and vitamin A on lung cancer and cardiovascular disease, N Engl J Med 334:1150, 1996.

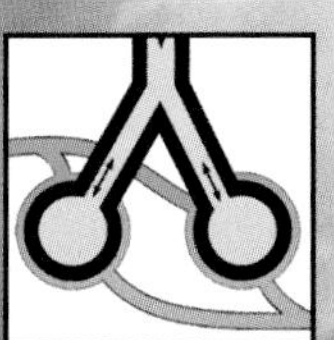

CHAPTER 26

Neuromuscular and Other Diseases of the Chest Wall

Robert Schilz

In This Chapter You Will Learn:

- What major components make up the respiratory neuromuscular system and how their dysfunction can affect ventilation
- What major effects neuromuscular disease has on the respiratory system
- How to assess patients for signs and symptoms of neuromuscular weakness of the ventilatory muscles
- What common pulmonary function abnormalities appear in patients with neuromuscular weakness of the respiratory muscles
- Which neuromuscular diseases affect respiration
- How to describe abnormalities of respiration that appear in patients with spinal cord injury
- How to describe thoracic cage deformities such as flail chest and scoliosis and their effects on the respiratory system

Chapter Outline

Key Terms

amyotrophic lateral sclerosis (ALS)
ankylosing spondylitis
Cheyne-Stokes respiration
demyelination
flail chest
Guillain-Barré syndrome (GBS)
Lambert-Eaton syndrome (LES)
myasthenia gravis (MG)
myopathy
myositis
myotonic dystrophy
neuromuscular
neuropathy
paradoxical breathing
polymyositis
scoliosis
traumatic brain injury

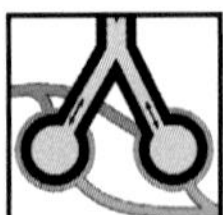

The respiratory system is composed of the lungs, which mediate gas exchange; the thoracic cage, which forms the structure of the ventilatory pump; and the muscles of respiration, which are linked to respiratory centers in the brainstem by nerves exiting the spinal column. The **neuromuscular** organization of the components of the respiratory system is shown in Figure 26-1.

Maintenance of normal ventilation is critically dependent on intact, functional components of the neuromuscular system. Diseases that affect the brain, nerves, muscles, or thoracic cage can lead to respiratory failure or hypoxemia even if the lungs are normal. The pulmonary consequences of neuromuscular disease can include the following:

1. Hyperventilation or hypoventilation
2. Sleep apnea
3. Aspiration
4. Atelectasis with resulting hypoxemia
5. Pulmonary hypertension
6. Cor pulmonale

Figure 26-1

The neuromuscular components of the respiratory system include elements of the cortex (which allow conscious alteration of breathing) and motor centers (which maintain upper airway tone). Brainstem structures receive input from peripheral oxygen, pH, and stretch receptors and generate automatic respiration. Efferent nerves carry central nervous impulses to the muscles of respiration through the phrenic and spinal nerves, which drive the muscles of respiration.

Some systemic diseases that affect the neuromuscular system also cause interstitial lung disease, which can lead to considerable dysfunction (see Chapter 21). Finally, respiratory failure, often accompanied by pulmonary infection, is a frequent cause of death among patients with neuromuscular disorders.

A thorough understanding of the physiology of ventilation and chest wall mechanics (Chapter 9) will help the reader understand how abnormalities of the upper airway, chest wall, diaphragm, and abdominal muscles cause disease. This chapter reviews major disorders of the neuromuscular and skeletal systems of the chest. The chapter is organized anatomically, focusing on pulmonary manifestations of these disease processes (Table 26-1).

▶ GENERAL PRINCIPLES RELATING TO NEUROMUSCULAR WEAKNESS OF THE VENTILATORY MUSCLES

Among the many neuromuscular problems causing pulmonary dysfunction, respiratory muscle weakness that leads to atelectasis, hypoxemia, and ventilatory insufficiency is among the best recognized. The following general considerations describe the evaluation and testing of patients with suspected neuromuscular weakness of the respiratory muscles regardless of the disease that produced the weakness.

Table 26-1 ▶ ▶ Locations at Which Several Neuromuscular Diseases Affect the Respiratory System

Location	Disease
Cortex and upper motor neurons	Stroke, traumatic brain injury
Spinal cord	Trauma, transverse myelitis, multiple sclerosis
Anterior horn cells (lower motor neurons)	Amyotrophic lateral sclerosis, spinal muscular atrophy, poliomyelitis and postpoliomyelitis
Peripheral nerves	Guillain-Barré syndrome, critical illness polyneuropathy, Lyme disease
Neuromuscular junction	Myasthenia gravis, Lambert-Eaton syndrome, botulism
Muscle	Duchenne's muscular dystrophy, polymyositis, acid maltase deficiency
Interstitial lung disease*	Polymyositis, dermatomyositis, tuberous sclerosis, neurofibromatosis

*A category of systemic diseases that can affect the neuromuscular

Clinical Signs and Symptoms

Patients with respiratory muscle weakness due to neuromuscular disease may initially report exertional dyspnea, fatigue, orthopnea, or symptoms of cor pulmonale. These symptoms occur because the muscles involved with respiration can no longer generate or maintain normal ventilation. Continued progression of respiratory muscle weakness or reduction in lung and chest wall compliance can lead to a rapid, shallow breathing pattern. Patients with poor inspiratory muscle function may have marked orthopnea and prefer to sleep in a seated position. A decline in the volume and power of voice occasionally is reported. Progressive muscle weakness can reach the point at which adequate ventilation is no longer maintained, and hypercapnia occurs. The hypoventilation that occurs with progressive neuromuscular disease may be a protective mechanism that avoids acute respiratory muscle fatigue.[1] Some recent evidence, however, suggests that purely mechanical factors, such as elastic load and respiratory muscle strength alone, lead to rapid, shallow breathing and hypercarbia.[2] Accompanying expiratory muscle weakness is characterized by poor cough and secretion clearance.

Pathophysiology and Pulmonary Function Testing

Neuromuscular weakness of the respiratory muscles is characterized by the inability to generate or maintain normal respiratory pressures. Pulmonary function testing in patients with neuromuscular weakness and otherwise normal pulmonary parenchyma typically reveals a restrictive ventilatory defect. Vital capacity (VC), forced expiratory volume in 1 second (FEV_1), and total lung capacity (TLC) are decreased. Residual volume (RV) is normal or increased, and diffusing capacity corrected for alveolar volume is normal or near normal but has been reported to be decreased.[3] Comparison of spirometric results obtained with the patient in the seated position can be useful in showing orthopnea is caused by neuromuscular weakness. A decrease in FEV_1 and VC of greater than 20% when a patient moves from the seated to the supine position suggests diaphragmatic weakness. The inability to generate normal respiratory pressures is reflected in a decreased maximal inspiratory pressure (PI_{max}). Expiratory muscle weakness is characterized by a decreased maximal expiratory pressure (PE_{max}). Arterial blood gases in the setting of a rapid, shallow breathing pattern may show a decreased arterial partial pressure of carbon dioxide ($Pa{CO_2}$), although progressive inspiratory muscle weakness leads to hypoventilation and hypercapnia. Hypoxemia can occur in patients unable to take deep breaths and may be caused by microatelectasis, which leads to ventilation/perfusion mismatching within the lung and a resulting decrease in arterial partial pressure of oxygen ($Pa{O_2}$) (Figure 26-2).

MINI CLINI

Assessment of a Patient With Neuromuscular Weakness

PROBLEM

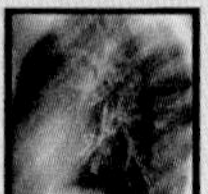

A 50-year-old man with amyotrophic lateral sclerosis (ALS) is admitted to the hospital because of right lower lobe pneumonia. The patient is moderately hypoxemic, with a partial pressure of oxygen ($P{O_2}$) of 68 mm Hg on room air. He has carried a diagnosis of ALS for 3 years, during which time he has had progressive worsening of dyspnea. These symptoms first occurred with mild exertion and then with supine position, which the patient has noticed in the last month or two. A recent measurement of vital capacity at the physician's office was 35 mL/kg. The patient has noticed recent difficulty with swallowing and frequent coughing at meals. What features in the patient's history may be relevant with regard to management?

DISCUSSION

It is important to identify this patient as having a disease that is associated with respiratory compromise. All patients with ALS ultimately have respiratory insufficiency. The earliest symptom of neuromuscular weakness in the respiratory muscles is exertional dyspnea, which this patient has had for some time. A more significant finding is orthopnea, which is highly suggestive of diaphragmatic weakness. Patients with significant diaphragmatic weakness prefer the upright seated position, which allows the abdominal contents to shift toward the feet and allows unimpeded diaphragmatic descent. Although the patient may not have had a critically low vital capacity recently, this value is low. Additional loading of already compromised ventilatory machinery can lead to fatigue and frank respiratory failure. It is therefore important to recognize that the underlying neuromuscular weakness coupled with pneumonia may predispose this patient to respiratory fatigue and subsequent failure. The historical element of difficulty with feeding may suggest the pneumonia is related to aspiration. The location of pneumonia in the lower lobe also favors the diagnosis if the aspiration occurs when the patient is seated.

PROBLEM

What physical findings may suggest respiratory distress in a patient with diaphragmatic weakness?

DISCUSSION

Patients whose diaphragmatic strength is inadequate to meet their ventilatory needs may use "accessory" muscles of inspiration. The sternocleidomastoid, intercostal, and scalene muscles all may be found active in the setting of respiratory distress. Activation of these muscles in the setting of a weak or paralyzed diaphragm can lead to cephalic movement of the diaphragm during inspiration that is accompanied by paradoxical inward movement of the abdomen during inspiration (paradoxical breathing). The presence of these signs in this patient should prompt evaluation of ventilatory adequacy and the need for ventilatory support.

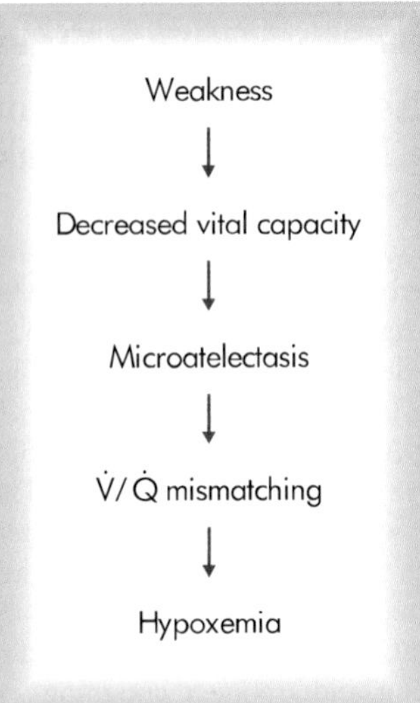

Figure 26-2
Atelectasis as a mechanism of hypoxemia in patients with respiratory muscle weakness. $\dot{V}/\dot{Q}$, Ventilation/perfusion.

> **RULE OF THUMB**
>
> Expiratory muscle strength measured with a PI_{max} maneuver is necessary for the production of adequate cough. Pressures of 40 cm H_2O or more are generally needed to produce cough adequate to clear pulmonary secretions.

> **RULE OF THUMB**
>
> Neuromuscular weakness of the respiratory muscles may be present before any substantial decrease in VC or FEV_1 is noticed. Values of PI_{max} and PE_{max} may be decreased 50% or more before any decrement in VC or FEV_1 is noticed.

Monitoring and Assessing Patients for Respiratory Insufficiency

The result of progressive neuromuscular weakness of the inspiratory muscles is respiratory failure. The onset of respiratory failure is acute or chronic depending on the disease process and the circumstances of the patient. Careful follow-up and monitoring of symptoms and pulmonary function are necessary for assessment of the need for mechanical ventilation.

Monitoring the ventilatory function of a patient with neuromuscular weakness can involve repeated measurement of inspiratory pressure, VC, and arterial blood gas values for assessment of the need for ventilatory assistance. At least two caveats to this general approach should be mentioned. First, patients with myasthenia gravis having an acute myasthenic crisis may have normal test results even within minutes of acute ventilatory failure, because of the nature of the disorder.[4] Second, the need to protect the upper airway from secretions and aspiration may not be clearly reflected in results of pulmonary function tests. Neuromuscular weakness may not manifest uniformly in all muscle groups. Thus ventilation may be only moderately reduced in patients with gross oropharyngeal dysfunction leading to aspiration. In general, patients with ventilatory weakness can face high risk of acute respiratory failure if acute upper respiratory tract infection or pneumonia develops. In these patients, inability to clear secretions can increase the work of breathing; the results are muscle fatigue, hypoventilation, and acute respiratory failure.

Patients with significant weakness of the respiratory muscles can be at high risk of respiratory failure when pulmonary processes increase the work of breathing. Pulmonary edema, pneumonia, and mucous plugging are examples of clinical conditions that can precipitate respiratory failure rapidly in patients with significant neuromuscular weakness. Such patients may need observation of their respiratory status when they are in the hospital with these conditions.

Nocturnal oximetry or formal sleep testing with polysomnography may be suggested in some clinical settings when patients have cor pulmonale, sleep disturbance, or excessive daytime somnolence that is otherwise unexplained.

Management of Respiratory Muscle Weakness

Respiratory insufficiency and failure to clear secretions are the major consequences of inspiratory and expiratory muscle weakness, respectively. Treatment of these patients involves consideration of mechanical ventilation by means of face mask or other noninvasive interfaces or by means of tracheostomy. Although often overlooked, therapies to augment secretion clearance and cough are important in this patient population (see Chapter 37). Used together, these interventions can decrease hospitalizations due to respiratory complications in patients with neuromuscular disease.[5]

Noninvasive ventilation is being used increasingly to manage acute deterioration of the condition of patients with neuromuscular disease[6] (during a pneumonia, for example) and for temporary support for surgical procedures such as gastrostomy tube insertion.[7] Institution of mechanical ventilation in some patients with neuromuscular weakness may be subject to significant variability between physicians.[8] Although uniform recommendations cannot be made, long-term mechanical ventilation is best instituted with adequate planning and management of a variety of issues related to respiratory care in alternative settings. These issues are summarized in consensus statements[9] and are discussed in Chapter 49.

MINI CLINI

Care of a Patient With Neuromuscular Weakness

PROBLEM

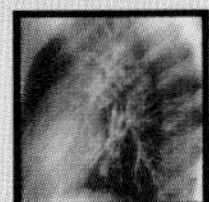

A 45-year-old man has been found to have myotonic dystrophy. He has progressive dyspnea that has increased particularly in the last year. The partial pressure of carbon dioxide (P_{CO_2}) determined from arterial blood gas analysis is 55 mm Hg. The VC is 45% of the predicted value. The patient has no underlying pulmonary disease. Cough is decreased, but the patient maintains adequate control of secretions. The patient sleeps in a seated to semirecumbent position. What interventions are indicated for this patient?

DISCUSSION

The patient has a disease that can result in respiratory insufficiency. The VC is decreased, and arterial carbon dioxide levels are increased. These factors are consistent with hypoventilation due to neuromuscular weakness. The patient has dyspnea on exertion and orthopnea. All these factors suggest that mechanical ventilation should be considered.

Noninvasive positive pressure ventilation (NIPPV) may be a reasonable first choice in the care of this patient. The patient's mental status and bulbar function are intact. He has no significant problems with secretions. (Important factors for successful application of NIPPV are discussed in Chapter 42). Use of a nasal mask with a biphasic positive airway pressure (BiPAP) unit may be instituted and titrated to patient tolerance. (However, most pressure or volume-cycled ventilators can be used to deliver NIPPV.) Patients with neuromuscular weakness in general prefer a relative low expiratory pressure (2-3 cm H_2O) with a significantly higher inspiratory pressure (7-15 cm H_2O). A time-cycled backup rate can be set on some ventilators to facilitate ventilation of patients who may inadequately trigger the ventilator. If the ability to clear secretions becomes compromised, cough augmentation strategies should be implemented.

▶ SPECIFIC NEUROMUSCULAR DISEASES

Disorders of the Muscle (Myopathic Disease)

Primary muscle disease can decrease the ability of a normal depolarizing impulse to generate effective muscle contraction. Some commonly recognized **myopathies** include Duchenne's muscular dystrophy, myotonic dystrophy, and polymyositis. Box 26-1 contains a more complete list of myopathic diseases associated with ventilatory dysfunction.

Box 26-1 • Myopathic Diseases With Associated Respiratory Dysfunction

MUSCULAR DYSTROPHIES
- Duchenne's muscular dystrophy
- Myotonic dystrophy
- Facioscapulohumeral muscular dystrophy
- Limb-girdle dystrophy
- Oculopharyngeal dystrophy

MYOPATHIES
- Congenital myopathies
  - Nemaline rod myopathy
  - Centronuclear myopathy
- Metabolic myopathies
  - Acid maltase deficiency
  - Mitochondrial myopathies (Kearns-Sayre syndrome)
- Inflammatory myopathies
  - Polymyositis
  - Dermatomyositis
- Endocrine myopathies
  - Hypothyroid- and hyperthyroid-related myopathies
  - Steroid-induced myopathies
- Miscellaneous myopathies
  - Electrolyte disorders (e.g., hypophosphatemia, hypokalemia)
  - Rhabdomyolysis
  - Periodic paralysis
  - Post–neuromuscular blockade myopathy

Duchenne's (and Becker's) Muscular Dystrophy

Duchenne's (and Becker's) muscular dystrophy (DMD), an inherited form, is an X-linked recessive muscle-wasting disorder caused by mutations in the dystrophin gene.[10] A conclusive diagnosis is made when these genetic alterations are found in DNA samples from peripheral white blood cells or when abnormal dystrophin or the absence of the dystrophin protein is identified in muscle biopsy specimens.

Duchenne's muscular dystrophy manifests early in life with proximal muscle weakness that leads to a waddling gait, exaggerated lumbar curvature (lordosis), and frequent falls. Most of these children need a wheelchair by 12 years of age. Death generally occurs by 20 years of age, as a result of complications of declining respiratory muscle strength and subsequent infection. Becker's muscular dystrophy, a milder form of DMD, also is associated with dysregulation of the dystrophin gene and manifests later in life. Other systemic effects of DMD include scarring of the left ventricle and decreased bowel motility (intestinal pseudoobstruction).

The progressive decline in respiratory function in patients with DMD parallels limb weakness and typically occurs at the point of wheelchair dependence. Respiratory weakness is primarily due to loss of muscle strength and leads to a lower PI_{max} at all lung volumes than is present in healthy persons. The response to hypoxia and respiratory drive, measured with airway occlusion pressure ($P_{0.1}$), is preserved in patients with DMD.[11] This is frequently the case in neuromuscular weakness. Patients with DMD increase minute ventilation by increasing respiratory rate and adopting a rapid, shallow breathing pattern.

Progressive scoliosis is associated with DMD and can further contribute to respiratory insufficiency. Although spinal fusion with correction of the scoliosis improves comfort and ability to maintain a seated posture, several studies have failed to demonstrate improvement or stabilization of pulmonary function after such a procedure.[12] Institution of positive pressure ventilation (PPV) is a decision most patients face at some point in the disease. The need for mechanical ventilation correlates with the degree of disability and with FVC less than 30%.[13] Nocturnal PPV can be instituted in response to oxygen desaturation during sleep, which is common in patients with increased disability and scoliosis. Nocturnal ventilation appears to improve daytime ventilatory function in patients with DMD,[14] presumably through the prevention of fatigue of the affected respiratory muscles. Despite this improvement, results of studies of early "prophylactic" institution of PPV in the care of patients with DMD have failed to delay the need for formal ventilatory support.[15]

Myotonic Dystrophy

Myotonic dystrophy is the most common form of muscular dystrophy in adults, with an estimated frequency of 1 case in 8000 persons.[16] Myotonia, or delayed muscle relaxation, is the hallmark of this neuromuscular disorder but does not clearly occur in respiratory muscles or lead to respiratory insufficiency.[17] This autosomal-dominant disorder has the clinical features of progressive muscle weakness, abnormalities of the cardiac conduction system, endocrine dysfunction, and cataracts. The genetic defect in myotonic dystrophy is located on chromosome 19 and involves a specific cytosine-thymine-guanine (CTG) sequence of DNA.[18]

Respiratory dysfunction in myotonic dystrophy is common and can include respiratory muscle weakness, obstructive sleep apnea, central sleep apnea, and bulbar muscle dysfunction leading to aspiration. Sleep-related disorders are particularly common, even at an early age. Patients with myotonic dystrophy can be very sensitive to anesthesia and respiratory depressants. Both respiratory failure and prolonged neuromuscular blockade have been reported in myotonic dystrophy patients given usual doses of these agents. For this reason, prolonged perioperative monitoring after surgery is important.

Nocturnal ventilation by nasal mask often is effective for these patients and should be considered if the patient has declining oxygen saturation or hypercapnia.[19] If present, central hypoventilation may necessitate tracheostomy and mechanical ventilation.

Polymyositis

Polymyositis, dermatomyositis, and inclusion body **myositis** are examples of inflammatory myopathies of unknown causation. Respiratory compromise is rare in inclusion body myositis but can be seen in both polymyositis and dermatomyositis. Clinical respiratory muscle weakness is not common but can lead to respiratory weakness or failure within weeks to months in the setting of rapidly progressing disease. Diagnosis of these diseases is based on clinical findings of myalgia, elevated muscle enzymes (creatine phosphokinase or aldolase), and compatible electromyographic or muscle biopsy results.

Ventilatory insufficiency and failure caused by this myopathy are unusual but tend to parallel the development of limb muscle weakness when they occur. In rare instances, diaphragmatic function is decreased disproportionately to the degree of limb weakness.[20]

Corticosteroids are typically the mainstay of management of polymyositis and dermatomyositis, although other immunosuppressive regimens have been used. Ten percent to 30% of patients with inflammatory myopathy have interstitial lung disease.[21] This lung disease appears as diffuse interstitial infiltrates that usually involve the lung bases. Antibodies to a specific protein called Jo-1 antigen, a histidyl-transfer RNA synthetase, are found in more than 50% of patients with inflammatory myopathy and interstitial lung disease.[22] The role of these antibodies in the pathogenesis of this process is unclear. Pulmonary vasculitis can occur with polymyositis and dermatomyositis and can lead to oxygen exchange abnormalities and pulmonary hypertension.

Disorders of the Neuromuscular Junction

Although they arise from different molecular defects, disorders of the neuromuscular junction decrease conduction of central nervous system impulses to the peripheral muscles. The result is syndromes characterized by muscle weakness. The neuromuscular junction is represented schematically in Figure 26-3. Disorders of the neuromuscular junction include the following:

1. Myasthenia gravis
2. Lambert-Eaton syndrome
3. Poisoning (organophosphate, tetanus, botulism)

Myasthenia Gravis

Myasthenia gravis (MG) is characterized by intermittent muscular weakness, which worsens on repetitive stim-

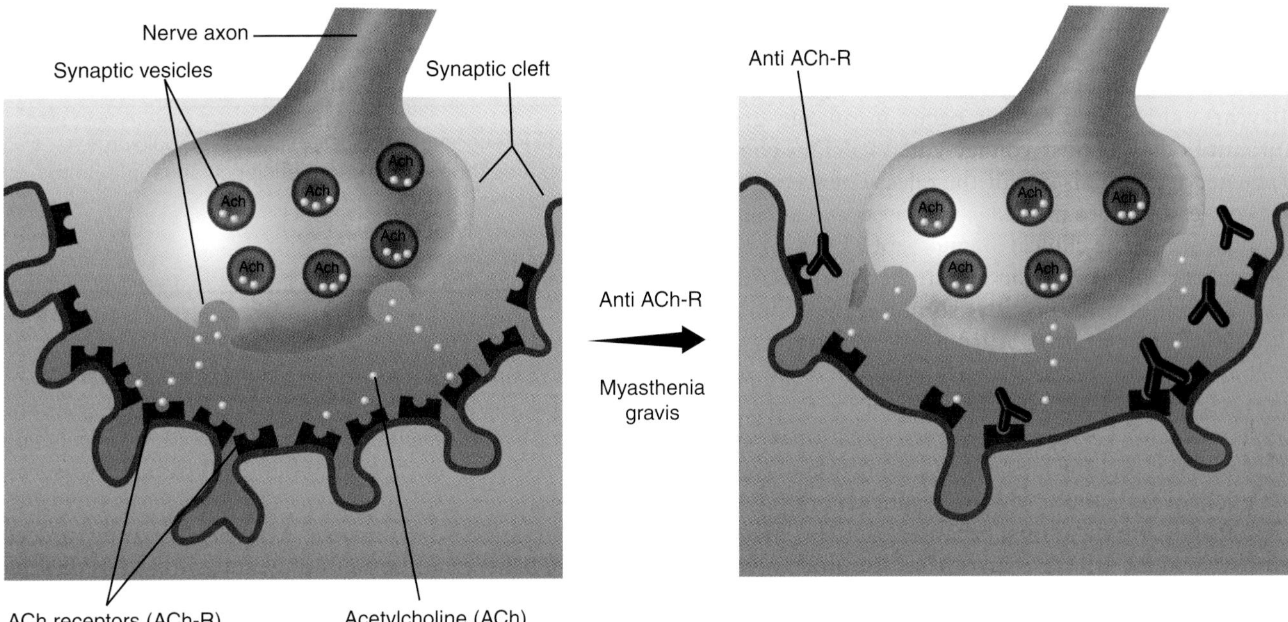

Figure 26-3
The neuromuscular junction with acetylcholine (ACh) stored in presynaptic vesicles. The ACh is released by exocytosis into the synaptic cleft in response to a presynaptic nerve impulse. The ACh binds to its cognate acetylcholine receptor (ACh-R) on the postsynaptic membrane. This process depolarizes the nerve, propagates the impulse, and causes muscle contraction. Binding of anti-ACh-R antibodies to ACh-R mediates autoimmune destruction of the receptors. This process leads to abnormal muscle activation and the weakness that occurs in patients with myasthenia gravis.

ulation and improves with the administration of anticholinesterase medications, such as edrophonium (Tensilon) or neostigmine. Most cases of MG arise from production of antibodies directed against the acetylcholine receptor (ACh-R). The antibodies inactivate the ACh-R and block transmission of electrical impulses from the nerve to the muscle. Abnormalities of the thymus gland are common in MG. Approximately 10% of myasthenic patients have an abnormal growth called *thymoma*. Patients without thymoma typically have some degree of thymic hyperplasia. Congenital or fetal myasthenic syndromes are caused by either autoantibodies or inherited defects in the ACh-R.

Myasthenia gravis typically occurs in younger patients with a female predominance (female-to-male ratios typically are 3:1 to 4.5:1).[23] The disease is characterized by progressive loss of muscular function, which may affect only the eye muscles (ocular myasthenia) or may be more widespread. The patient typically reports weakness of the affected muscles that may progress during the day or with repetitive use. The diagnosis of MG is supported by the detection of anti-ACh-R antibodies in the blood, a characteristic fading of nerve impulses with repeated nerve stimulation testing during electromyography, and improvement of strength or symptoms in response to an anticholinesterase inhibitor drug (edrophonium). Management of MG includes thymectomy and administration of anticholinesterases with or without corticosteroids or other immunosuppressants, such as azathioprine or cyclosporine. Circulating antibodies in this disease can be removed by **plasmapheresis,** which results in clinical improvement[24,25] and has been used to facilitate weaning from mechanical ventilation in the care of patients with myasthenic crisis.[26]

The pulmonary complications of MG depend on the magnitude and location of the affected muscle groups and tend to occur in patients most severely disabled with the disease. Upper airway obstruction, exertional dyspnea, and overt ventilatory failure all have been reported in MG. Pulmonary function testing of MG patients who have respiratory muscle weakness shows decreased TLC, VC, PI_{max}, and PE_{max} similar to that in other neuromuscular disorders, PI_{max} and PE_{max} being more sensitive markers of early respiratory muscle weakness.[27] "Myasthenic crisis" is an acute event in MG and is characterized either by respiratory failure or by inability to maintain a patent airway. Myasthenic crisis can occur acutely in response to worsening of disease, intercurrent infection, or surgery or when excess anticholinesterase inhibitors have been given. Endotracheal intubation and mechanical ventilation are required immediately and may be prolonged.[28]

Lambert-Eaton Syndrome

Another syndrome of neuromuscular weakness arising from a disorder at the neuromuscular junction is **Lambert-Eaton syndrome** (LES). More than 66% of cases of LES are associated with cancer. Of these cancer-related cases, 50% are associated with small cell carcinoma of the lung.[29] The mean age at presentation is approximately 60 years, although LES can occur in all age groups. Autoantibodies against voltage-gated calcium channels at the nerve terminals impair the release of acetylcholine and can lead to both muscular weakness and autonomic insufficiency.[30] The clinical diagnosis of LES is supported by results of nerve conduction studies. Potentiation of muscle strength with repetitive stimuli is the hallmark of LES, which differentiates it from MG. In contrast, MG is characterized by progressive fatigue of muscular contraction with repetitive stimulation.

Symptoms of LES usually are tiredness or weakness of proximal muscle groups out of proportion to findings at clinical examination. Although patients are subject to respiratory complications because of their increased sensitivity to the effects of anesthesia, respiratory failure is rare. The clinical course of LES tends to be one of relative stability with less fluctuation than MG. Management of LES includes therapy for the underlying malignant disease when present, use of anticholinesterase medications such as pyridostigmine (Mestinon), and immunosuppressive therapy with prednisone or azathioprine.

Disorders of the Nerves

The peripheral nerves may be affected by toxic agents, inflammatory processes, vascular disorders, malignant diseases, and metabolic or nutritional imbalances. Hundreds of conditions have been associated with neuropathies leading to respiratory muscle dysfunction. Representative conditions are listed in Box 26-2.

Guillain-Barré Syndrome

Guillain-Barré syndrome (GBS) is the most common peripheral **neuropathy** causing respiratory insufficiency. Guillain-Barré syndrome is characterized by paralysis and hyporeflexia with or without sensory symptoms. Guillain-Barré syndrome is typically a self-limited disease, but overall mortality ranges from 3% to 6%.[31]

Box 26-2 • Causes of Phrenic Nerve Dysfunction Leading to Respiratory Dysfunction

- Cardiac surgery (cold cardioplegia to arrest the heart can cause "frostbitten" phrenic nerves)
- Diabetes
- Trauma
- Thoracic aneurysm

Box 26-3 • Factors Predisposing to Guillain-Barré Syndrome

- Viral infection (mononucleosis, cytomegalovirus, hepatitis, human immunodeficiency virus infection)
- Pregnancy
- Hodgkin's lymphoma
- General surgery

The proportion of patients with significant disability 1 year after the onset of the disease can be 20%.[32] Autonomic nervous system problems, such as hypotension, flushing, bronchorrhea, dermatographia, and bradycardia, are common.

Guillain-Barré syndrome is a demyelinating process widely believed to be caused by autoantibodies directed against the myelin constituting the nerve sheath. Patients with GBS often have a history of upper respiratory infections or a flu-like illness that precedes the onset of symptoms and is thought to be related. A number of other entities have been associated with the subsequent development of this syndrome (Box 26-3).

The diagnosis of GBS is based on a combination of clinical, laboratory, and electrophysiological data. Cerebrospinal fluid protein levels are elevated with minimal cellularity after approximately 1 week of illness. Nerve conduction studies show slowing of conduction with preserved amplitude, which is typical of **demyelination.** Treatment strategies that have improved outcome in GBS include intravenous immunoglobulin infusions[33] and plasmapheresis.[34]

Approximately one third of all patients with GBS have respiratory muscle compromise. Although the diaphragm is typically affected later in the course of GBS, cases of respiratory failure in the absence of substantial peripheral weakness have been reported. Patients with dyspnea, orthopnea, or impaired ability to maintain a patent airway should receive spirometry every 4 to 6 hours for documentation of function and assessment of the need for endotracheal intubation. Figure 26-4 shows a typical relation between symptoms of respiratory compromise and declining VC.[35] Some authors have suggested that comparison of seated and supine VC measurements may be more helpful in assessing imminent respiratory decompensation.[36] Patients with poor upper airway control, weak cough, or large amounts of secretions should be considered for endotracheal intubation even though their VC is greater than 20 mL/kg. The increased work of breathing imposed by mucous plugging or atelectasis can hasten decompensation. As many as two thirds of patients with GBS need mechanical ventilation for more than 2 weeks, after which tracheostomy should be considered.[37] A small subgroup may need mechanical ventilation for a

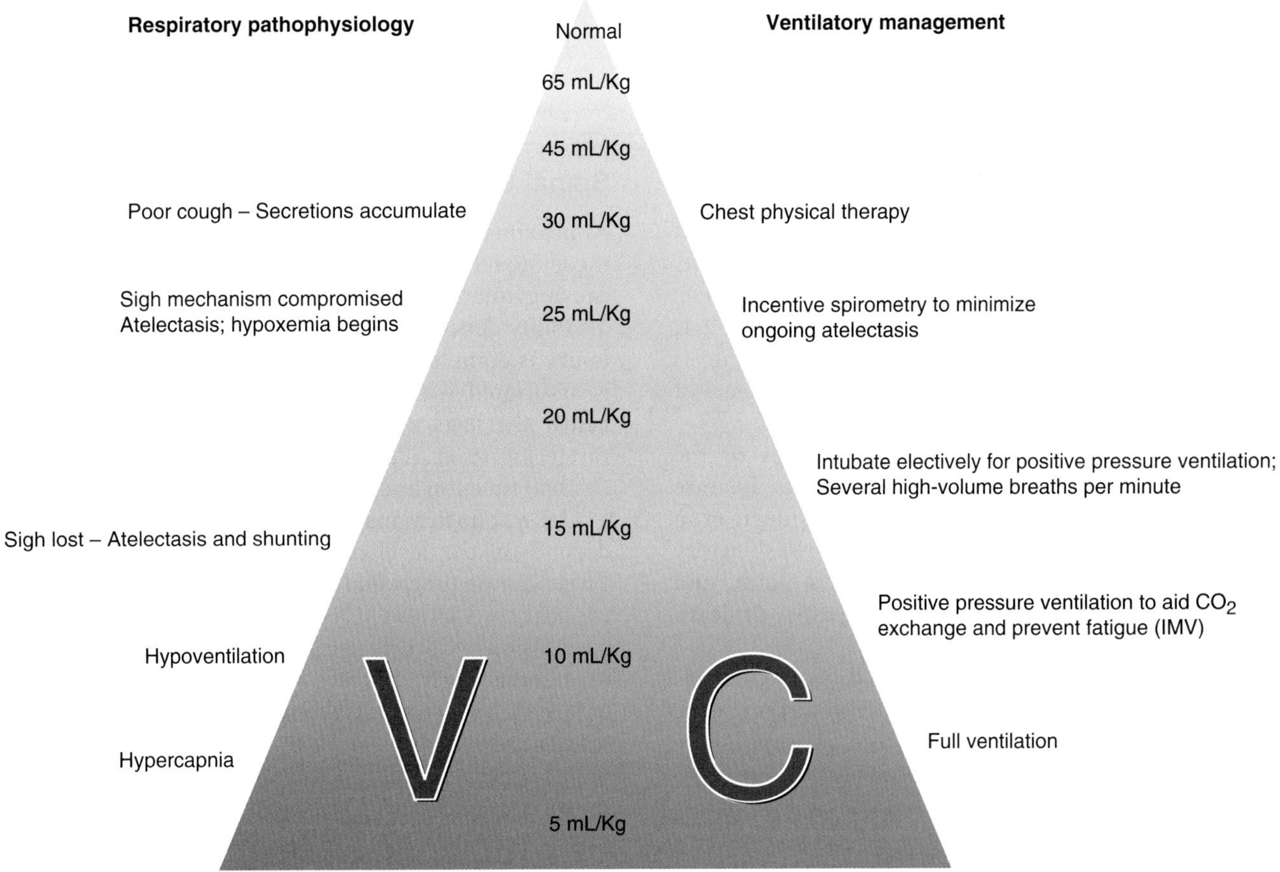

Figure 26-4

Approximate VC levels correspond to each event during deterioration. At a VC of 12 to 15 mL/kg, most patients need intubation and mechanical ventilation. *(From Ropper AH: Critical care of Guillain-Barré syndrome. In Ropper AH, ed: Neurological and neurosurgical intensive care, New York, 1993, Raven Press.)*

year or more. Weaning of patients with GBS from mechanical ventilation is predicted by VC greater than 18 mL/kg,[38] transdiaphragmatic pressure greater than 31 cm H_2O, or a PI_{max} greater than 30 cm H_2O.[39]

Phrenic Nerve Damage and Diaphragmatic Paralysis

Each hemidiaphragm is supplied by its own phrenic nerve. The phrenic nerve emerges from the spinal cord at level C3 through C5 and descends in proximity to the great vessels of the chest and pericardium. Damage to or interruption of this nerve leads to the paralysis of the ipsilateral hemidiaphragm. Bilateral interruption is seen in high cervical cord injury and causes complete diaphragmatic paralysis. Unilateral diaphragmatic paralysis can be seen in a variety of disease processes. Reversible unilateral diaphragmatic paralysis is a rare complication of acute pneumonia but occurs frequently after cardiac surgery.

Patients with unilateral diaphragmatic paralysis may have a 15% to 20% reduction in VC and TLC in the upright position and a further reduction while supine. If they have no other diseases, patients with unilateral diaphragmatic paralysis continue to have no symptoms. Diaphragmatic paralysis is diagnosed most often with chest radiography. The paralyzed side retains its contour but is displaced upward. At fluoroscopy, the paralyzed hemidiaphragm paradoxically rises into the thorax during a sudden forceful inspiration (sniff test). There is no effective therapy for permanent unilateral diaphragmatic paralysis.

Disorders of the Spinal Cord

Upper motor neurons arise from cell bodies in the motor areas of the brain and terminate at the anterior horn cells, which constitute the lower motor neurons. Disorders in this group (e.g., amyotrophic lateral sclerosis) can affect specific parts of this chain or nonspecifically disrupt these tracts (e.g., spinal cord injury). Other examples of lesions in this anatomical location include transverse myelitis, syringomyelia, poliomyelitis, and spinal cord tumors.

Amyotrophic Lateral Sclerosis

Amyotrophic lateral sclerosis (ALS), or Lou Gehrig's disease, is a neuromuscular disease characterized by progressive degeneration of both upper and lower motor neurons, although either may predominate early in the disease. Approximately 8% to 10% of cases are familial; the others are sporadic. The typical patient with ALS experiences the onset in middle to late life, and the occurrence of ALS increases linearly with age. The male-to-female ratio for ALS is approximately 2:1, and the mean age at onset is 56 years. The prognosis of ALS is poor, 80% of patients dying within 5 years of the onset of the disease.

Although weakness of large muscle groups or the bulbar muscles is common, ALS manifests in rare instances as isolated respiratory muscle dysfunction in an otherwise relatively intact patient.[40] Respiratory involvement occurs in all patients at some point, and pulmonary complications are a frequent cause of death among these patients.

Inspiratory muscle decline, measured by FVC, tends to be linear with time in any one patient, although the rate of decline may be different between patients. Acute respiratory decompensation may occur in the setting of respiratory infection or aspiration. Nocturnal hypoxemia and hypoventilation can lead to disrupted sleep, frequent arousal, daytime headaches, and somnolence.

Monitoring of FVC, PI_{max}, and PE_{max} is helpful in this group of patients and can provide important information regarding the ability to clear secretions and maintain gas exchange. Effective cough typically requires a PE_{max} greater than 40 cm H_2O to compress airways and generate high flow velocities within the tracheobronchial tree. Ineffective cough can lead to atelectasis and pneumonia as well as worsening gas exchange and hypoxemia.

The prevention of respiratory complications and assessment of the need for ventilatory assistance remain the central themes in caring for patients with advancing ALS. Helpful therapeutic interventions include (1) modification of food consistency or placement of feeding tubes in patients with marked bulbar dysfunction, (2) clearing of secretions with assisted cough techniques or postural drainage, and (3) ventilatory assistance with positive- or negative-pressure devices.

The timing and type of ventilatory intervention in the care of patients with ALS are the subject of much discussion. General guidelines for considering ventilatory assistance[41] include the following:

1. PI_{max}, 30 cm H_2O
2. $PaCO_2$ greater than 45 mm Hg
3. Vital capacity less than 20 mL/kg

Although many patients decide not to accept ventilation, 90% of those who do accept it report satisfaction with their decision and would choose tracheostomy and ventilation again in the same situation.[42] Although overall survival with ALS is poor, prolonged survival of ventilated patients has been reported.

Spinal Cord Trauma

Approximately 10,000 new spinal cord injuries occur in the United States each year, 5% to 10% of these injuries causing quadriplegia. The degree and distribution of disability depend on the level of injury and whether the injury is complete or incomplete. Complete cord injury is associated with absent motor and sensory function below the level of injury, and the patient's condition rarely improves. Patients with incomplete injury have residual function and tend to improve to varying degrees.

The respiratory manifestations of spinal cord injury depend on the level of injury and extent of damage. These can be functionally divided into two classes: high cervical cord lesions (C1-2) and middle to low cervical cord lesions (C3 through C8). The diaphragm receives its innervation from nerve roots exiting the spinal cord at levels C3 through C5. Complete injury above this level results in total respiratory muscle paralysis and death, unless urgent intubation and ventilation are performed. Injury to the cord at C3 through C5 can severely reduce respiratory strength as manifested by reductions in PE_{max}, PI_{max}, FVC, and FEV_1 consistent with a restrictive ventilatory defect. Patients adopt a rapid, shallow breathing pattern and use accessory inspiratory muscles (scalene and sternocleidomastoid muscles). Abdominal paradox (inward movement of the abdomen while the thorax expands) is the hallmark of significant bilateral diaphragmatic weakness. Despite the serious nature of injury between C3 and C5, as many as 80% of intubated patients with this lesion can ultimately become liberated from mechanical ventilation. The muscles of expiration receive neural input from spinal levels T1 through L1 and are predominantly affected by middle to low cervical cord lesions. This condition manifests as a marked reduction in PE_{max} compared with PI_{max} and a diminished or absent effective cough.

The differential weakness of respective muscle groups in patients with neuromuscular weakness affects ventilatory capacity in the supine and seated positions. Patients with predominantly diaphragmatic weakness have orthopnea and are most comfortable in the upright seated position. This position favors gravity-assisted descent of the diaphragm, which is relatively unencumbered by abdominal contents that shift caudad in the seated patient. Recumbent patients with bilateral diaphragmatic weakness accompanying spinal cord injury may display **paradoxical breathing** or "abdominal paradox." Observation of the chest and abdomen of these patients reveals paradoxical inward movement of the abdomen during inspiration. Conversely, patients with expiratory muscle weakness similar to that produced by low cervical cord injury prefer the supine position, in which the tendency of the abdominal contents to move toward the head assists expiration in the absence of marked expiratory muscle tone. These physiological principles form the basis for the use of "rocking beds" and pneumatic belt devices as ventilatory adjuncts in the care of patients with considerable respiratory muscle weakness (see Chapter 39).

Disorders of the Brain

Traumatic brain injury, stroke, hemorrhage, and infection can lead to derangements of respiration through a variety of mechanisms. The motor cortex contains voluntary centers for control of the upper airway and pharynx (see Chapter 13). The pons and medulla, located in the brainstem, contain (1) chemoreceptors for the automatic control of ventilation in response to increasing pH and hypercapnia, and (2) centers that generate and modify patterns of automatic ventilation in response to visceral and chemical afferent information (see Figure 26-1). Both stroke and traumatic brain injury can lead to disordered patterns of breathing, such as apnea, hyperpnea, or **Cheyne-Stokes respirations** as well as abnormalities in the lungs themselves. The following sections discuss the clinical entities of stroke and traumatic brain injury and their effects on the respiratory system.

MINI CLINI

Respiratory Dysfunction in Spinal Cord Injury

PROBLEM

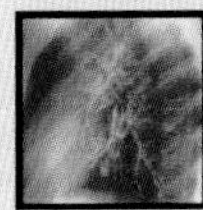

A young person who is otherwise healthy falls from a ladder and transects the spinal cord at the level of C6. Which muscles of the respiratory system will be affected, and what will be the effect?

DISCUSSION

Transection of the spinal cord at the level of the sixth cervical vertebra paralyzes any muscle group that receives its innervation from nerve roots that exit the spinal vertebral canal below C6. A review of the innervation of the major muscles of inspiration and expiration is important:

Upper airway, tongue, palate: cranial nerves IX, X, XI, and XII
C3 through C5: diaphragm
C4 through C8: shoulder girdle muscle (scalenes)
T1 through T12: intercostal muscles
T7 through L1: abdominal muscles

The upper airway, tongue, shoulder girdle muscles, and diaphragm should be intact in this patient's injury. Maintenance of intrathoracic volume depends in part on continuous activation of intercostal muscles, which stabilize and expand the thoracic cage. With these muscles paralyzed, expiratory reserve volume decreases, and normal activation of the diaphragm results in a tendency toward inward excursion of the chest wall and loss of effective volume. Forceful exhalation and the development of cough depend on activation of abdominal and intercostal muscle groups, both of which are paralyzed in this injury. Although he has an intact diaphragm, this patient has an increased reserve and poor cough, both of which are predisposing factors for atelectasis, pooling of secretions, and pneumonia. Successful management of spinal cord injury at this level includes aggressive postural drainage and percussion (once the injury has been stabilized) and possibly assisted cough in the respiratory care regimen.

Stroke

Stroke is a clinical syndrome produced by acute interruption of the normal blood flow to an area of the brain. The result is persistent dysfunction related to the affected structures. Stroke can be thrombotic (related to local formation of a clot), embolic (related to a clot traveling from a remote place in the body), or hemorrhagic. The effect of a stroke on respiration depends on which of the control elements of ventilation are damaged.

A common location for stroke is the cerebral cortex. Although decreased chest wall movement and diaphragmatic movement have been reported in patients with hemispheric stroke in the cerebral cortex, infarction in this area usually does not lead to significant alteration of ventilation. The patient may, however, have significant impairment of speech and movement, including impairment of muscles that affect upper airway tone and control secretions. Stroke in these regions of the motor cortex can lead to obstructive sleep apnea or aspiration pneumonia as a result of the loss of bulbar muscle function. There have been reports of localized stroke leading to profound alterations of the respiratory system. These relatively unusual events are summarized in Table 26-2, according to their location and the effect on respiration.

Therapy for stroke has evolved considerably. Previous therapy for thrombotic stroke was largely supportive. Now early use of **thrombolytic** therapy to dissolve the clot and restore circulation and function has been shown to improve function and survival, particularly if the thrombolytic agent is given less than 3 to 6 hours after the onset of symptoms.[43,44] Physical therapy and occupational therapy continue to be important components for optimizing function in the setting of residual deficit after stroke. Patients with substantial impairment of speech and swallowing may be at risk of aspiration pneumonia.

Traumatic Brain Injury

Traumatic brain injury is a general term referring to any of a number of focal or diffuse lesions of the brain

Table 26-2 ▶ ▶ Effect of Stroke Syndromes on the Respiratory System

Location	Effect on Respiration
Cerebral cortex—hemispheric infarct	Mild hyperventilation Contralateral decreased chest wall movement Decreased diaphragm excursion Sleep apnea
Bilateral hemispheric infarct	Cheyne-Stokes respiration
Lateral medulla and tegmentum (rare)	Loss of automatic rhythmically effective breathing (apnea)
Midpons (rare)	Loss of conscious control of respiration with preserved automatic ventilation

Data from Vingerhoets F, Bogousslavsky J: Respiratory dysfunction in stroke. In: Fanburg B, Sicilian L, editors: Clinics in chest medicine, Philadelphia, 1994, WB Saunders.

resulting from blunt or penetrating force. Although direct trauma to the respiratory centers in the brain also can cause the derangements of ventilation listed in Table 26-2, traumatic brain injury can cause neurogenic pulmonary edema and hypersecretion of mucus, which lead to hypoxemia and respiratory insufficiency through mechanisms other than muscular weakness. Head injury sufficient to produce loss of consciousness often causes apnea.

▶ DISORDERS OF THE THORACIC CAGE

The thoracic cage contains the lungs and supports the muscles of respiration. Normal ventilatory mechanics depend on a compliant thoracic cage with free excursion throughout the respiratory cycle.

Kyphoscoliosis

Kyphosis is posterior angulation of the thoracic cage. **Scoliosis** is lateral curvature of the spine. These two deformities typically occur together (called kyphoscoliosis) as a result of the compensatory effects of the spine in response to the primary lateral curve in scoliosis. Scoliosis is typically noticed during childhood and progresses during adolescence, although idiopathic adult kyphoscoliosis has been reported. The degree of scoliosis is measured by the Cobb angle, which is determined by the intersection of lines drawn between the upper and lower limbs of the primary curve in scoliosis (Figure 26-5).

Long-standing, severe kyphoscoliosis (Cobb angle greater than 90 to 100 degrees) can lead to hypoventilation, hypercapnia, and, if untreated, complications of pulmonary hypertension. However, the degree of pulmonary dysfunction cannot be predicted with the angle of curvature alone.[45,46] This respiratory dysfunction is probably multifactorial in most patients. Compliance of the chest wall and lung is decreased in patients with significant kyphoscoliosis. The result is decreased TLC and VC and detection of a restrictive ventilatory defect at pulmonary function testing. Maximal transdiaphragmatic pressure also is decreased, a sign of impaired diaphragmatic function in the pathogenesis of respiratory dysfunction in severe kyphoscoliosis. However, patients with even mild curvature can have reductions in measured VC.

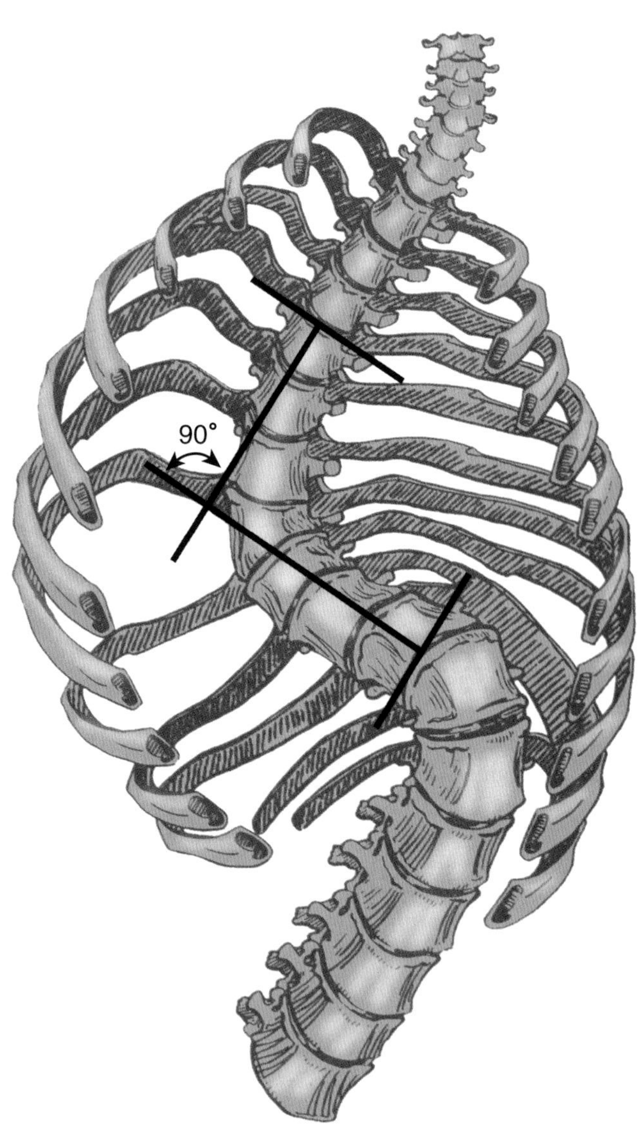

Figure 26-5
Scoliosis is lateral curvature of the spine. The degree of scoliosis is measured by the Cobb angle, which is determined by the intersection of lines drawn between the upper and lower limbs of the primary curve in scoliosis. Respiratory insufficiency rarely occurs until the Cobb angle exceeds 90 to 100 degrees. *(From Fishman AP: Acute respiratory failure. In Fishman AP, ed: Pulmonary disease, New York, 1992, McGraw-Hill, p 2300.)*

Anterior or posterior spinal fixation can stabilize kyphoscoliosis and restore the thoracic curvature to a condition close to normal. Fixation prevents complications due to progressive curvature, loss of compliance, and subsequent ventilatory dysfunction. Unfortunately, little is available to restore pulmonary function to older patients with established kyphoscoliosis. Surgery to correct the deformity can be undertaken, but this treatment generally does not improve pulmonary function.[47]

Nocturnal ventilation can assist patients with marked nocturnal desaturation and hypoventilation. Both negative pressure[48] and positive pressure[49] ventilation have been reported to stabilize respiratory function in patients with severe kyphoscoliosis.

Flail Chest

Flail chest is defined in different ways but occurs as a result of multiple rib fractures that cause a portion of the chest wall to become free-floating. The destabilized segment of the thoracic cage exhibits paradoxical motion during the respiratory cycle, bowing out with expiration and collapsing inward during a spontaneous breath. The movement is associated with a negative intrathoracic pressure gradient. Flail chest frequently is accompanied by other pulmonary injuries as a result of the mechanism of injury and the force required to fracture multiple ribs. Pulmonary contusion, hemothorax, and pneumothorax are frequently associated with flail chest and often necessitate urgent or emergency treatment of the trauma patient.[50]

There has been a great deal of debate about the mechanism of respiratory dysfunction in patients with flail chest. The movement of the flail segment has been postulated to lead to dysfunction of the remaining unaffected segments and to cause "exhalation" of the alveoli immediately adjacent to the injury. This leads to collapse, atelectasis, ventilation/perfusion mismatch, decreased compliance, and hypoxemia. Accompanying injuries, especially pulmonary contusion, are thought to lead to hypoxemia and decreased compliance in this patient population. Some studies of animal models of flail chest support the latter view and have led some authors to favor this explanation. In either case, PPV, with or without surgical stabilization of the rib cage, and adequate analgesia are the mainstays of management of flail chest.

Ankylosing Spondylitis

Ankylosing spondylitis is a rheumatologic disease that affects the spine and thoracic cage. Chronic joint inflammation ultimately leads to fusion of the vertebral bodies and the costovertebral joints and causes a dramatic decrease in thoracic cage compliance. Because diaphragmatic movement is retained, TLC and VC are only slightly reduced. Parenchymal lung disease in the form of apical fibrocystic changes occurs in some patients with ankylosing spondylitis.

KEY POINTS

- The components of the neuromuscular system that affect respiration include the brain (especially respiratory centers in the brainstem), the nerves (which lead to peripheral muscles, such as the diaphragm), the neuromuscular junction, and the muscles of inspiration, expiration, and upper airway control.
- Weakness or ventilatory failure is probably the most important dysfunction of the respiratory system in many neuromuscular diseases.
- Other effects of neuromuscular disease on the respiratory system can be hyperventilation or hypoventilation, sleep apnea, aspiration, atelectasis, pulmonary hypertension, and cor pulmonale.
- Signs and symptoms that may indicate weakness of the respiratory muscles include exertional dyspnea, orthopnea, decreased volume of voice, weak or ineffective cough, accessory muscle use, and a paradoxical breathing pattern (abdominal paradox).
- Pulmonary function abnormalities in patients with inspiratory muscle weakness typically include decreases in Pi_{max}, TLC, VC, and FEV_1. Residual volume can be increased. There often is an abnormally large decrease in FVC and FEV_1 (30% to 50%) when patients undergo testing in the seated and supine positions. Diffusing capacity corrected for alveolar volume typically is normal.
- Some common neuromuscular disorders that cause respiratory compromise include amyotrophic lateral sclerosis, myotonic dystrophy, spinal cord injury, Guillain-Barré syndrome, Duchenne's muscular dystrophy, and myasthenia gravis.
- Cervical spinal injury above the C3 level results in complete paralysis of the respiratory muscles and necessitates emergency mechanical entilation. Cervical spinal injury below C5 leads to weakness of the expiratory muscles with decreased ability to cough and clear secretions.

Continued

KEY POINTS—cont'd

- Unilateral diaphragmatic paralysis due to phrenic nerve damage usually is asymptomatic and is associated with minor reductions in respiratory function in an otherwise healthy patient.
- Scoliosis is abnormal lateral curvature of the spine. Respiratory insufficiency can occur if the curve is severe.
- Flail chest typically results from trauma to the chest. Multiple fractures of adjacent ribs produce a "free-floating" segment of the thoracic cage, which displays paradoxical excursion during the respiratory cycle. Flail chest often is associated with serious damage to the lungs, heart, or great vessels. Respiratory insufficiency in patients with flail chest can occur through a number of mechanisms.

References

1. Moxham J: Respiratory muscle fatigue: mechanisms, evaluation and therapy, Br J Anaesth 65:43, 1990.
2. Misuri G et al: Mechanism of CO_2 retention in patients with neuromuscular disease, Chest 117:447, 2000.
3. Rochester D, Aldrich T: The lungs and neuromuscular disease. In Murray J, Nadel J, editors: Textbook of respiratory medicine, ed 2, Philadelphia, 1994, WB Saunders.
4. Bennett D, Bleck T: Recognizing impending respiratory failure from neuromuscular causes, J Crit Illn 3:46, 1988.
5. Tzeng AC, Bach JR: Prevention of pulmonary morbidity for patients with neuromuscular disease, Chest 118:1390, 2000.
6. Vianello A et al: Non-invasive ventilatory approach to treatment of acute respiratory failure in neuromuscular disorders: a comparison with endotracheal intubation, Intensive Care Med 26:384, 2000.
7. Boitano LJ, Jordan T, Benditt JO: Noninvasive ventilation allows gastrostomy tube placement in patients with advanced ALS, Neurology 56:413, 2001.
8. Melo J et al: Pulmonary evaluation and prevalence of non-invasive ventilation in patients with amyotrophic lateral sclerosis: a multicenter survey and proposal of a pulmonary protocol, J Neurol Sci 169:114, 1999.
9. Make BJ et al: Mechanical ventilation beyond the intensive care unit: report of a consensus conference of the American College of Chest Physicians, Chest 113(suppl):289S, 1998.
10. Hoffman E, Brown R, Kunkel L: Dystrophin: the product of the Duchenne muscular dystrophy locus, Cell 51:919, 1987.
11. Begin R et al: Control of breathing in Duchenne's muscular dystrophy, Am J Med 69:227, 1980.
12. Miller R et al: The effect of spine fusion on respiratory function in Duchenne's muscular dystrophy, Neurology 41:38, 1991.
13. Lyager S, Steffensen B, Juhl B: Indicators of the need for mechanical ventilation in Duchenne muscular dystrophy and spinal muscular atrophy, Chest 108:779, 1995.
14. Mohr C, Hill N: Long-term follow-up of nocturnal ventilatory assistance in patients with respiratory failure due to Duchenne-type muscular dystrophy, Chest 97:91, 1990.
15. Raphael JC et al: Randomized trial of preventive nasal ventilation in Duchenne muscular dystrophy: French Multicentre Cooperative Group on Home Mechanical Ventilation Assistance in Duchenne de Boulogne Muscular Dystrophy, Lancet 343:1600, 1994.
16. Harper P: Myotonic dystrophy: major problems in neurology, vol 21, Philadelphia, 1989, WB Saunders.
17. Rimmer K et al: Myotonia of the respiratory muscles in myotonic dystrophy, Am Rev Respir Dis 148:1018, 1993.
18. Pizzuti A, Friedman D, Caskey C: The myotonic dystrophy gene, Arch Neurol 50:1173, 1993.
19. Moxley RI: Myotonic muscular dystrophy. In Rowland L, DiMauro S, editors: Handbook of clinical neurology, Amsterdam, 1992, Elsevier Science.
20. Blumbergs P, Byrne E, Kakulas B: Polymyositis presenting with respiratory failure, J Neurol Sci 65:221, 1984.
21. Dickey B, Myers A: Pulmonary disease in polymyositis/dermatomyositis, Semin Arthritis Rheum 14:60, 1984.
22. Arnett F et al: The Jo-1 antibody system in myositis: relationships to clinical features and HLA, J Rheumatol 8:925, 1981.
23. Simpson J: Myasthenia gravis and myasthenic syndromes. In Walton J, editor. Disorders of the voluntary muscle, Edinburgh, 1981, Churchill Livingstone.
24. Norris FH Jr, Denys EH, Mielke CH Jr: Plasmapheresis (plasma exchange) in neurologic disorders, Clin Neuropharmacol 5:93, 1982.
25. Batocchi AP et al: Therapeutic apheresis in myasthenia gravis, Ther Apher 4:275, 2000.
26. Gracey DR, Howard FM Jr., Divertie MB: Plasmapheresis in the treatment of ventilator-dependent myasthenia gravis patients: report of four cases, Chest 85:739, 1984.
27. Mier-Jedzejowicz A, Brophy C, Green M: Respiratory muscle function in myasthenia gravis, Am Rev Respir Dis 138:867, 1988.
28. Gracey D, Divertie M, Howard FJ: Mechanical ventilation for respiratory failure in myasthenia gravis: two year experience with 22 patients, Mayo Clin Proc 58:597, 1983.
29. McEvoy K: Diagnosis and treatment of Lambert-Eaton myasthenic syndrome, Neurol Clin 12:387, 1994.
30. Lennon VA, Lambert EH: Autoantibodies bind solubilized calcium channel-omega-conotoxin complexes from small cell carcinoma: a diagnostic aid for Lambert-Eaton myasthenic syndrome, Mayo Clin Proc 64:1498, 1989.
31. Ropper AH, Kehne S: Guillain-Barré syndrome: management of respiratory failure, Neurology 35:1662, 1985.
32. Winer J, Hughes R, Osmond C: A prospective study of acute idiopathic neuropathy, I: clinical features and their prognostic value, J Neurol Neurosurg Psychiatry 51:605, 1988.

33. Van der Meché FG, Schmitz P: A randomized trial comparing intravenous immune globulin and plasma exchange in Guillain-Barré syndrome, Dutch Guillain-Barré Study Group, N Engl J Med 326:1123, 1992.
34. French Cooperative Group on Plasma Exchange in Guillain Barré Syndrome: Efficacy of plasma exchange in Guillain Barré Syndrome: role of replacement fluids, Ann Neurol 22:753, 1987.
35. Ropper AH: Critical care of Guillain-Barré syndrome. In Ropper AH, editor: Neurological and neurosurgical intensive care, New York, 1993, Raven Press.
36. Mier-Jedzejowicz A et al: Assessment of diaphragm weakness, Am Rev Respir Dis 134:877, 1998.
37. Marsh M, Gillespie D, Baumgartner A: Timing of tracheostomy in critically ill patients, Chest 96:190, 1989.
38. Chevrolet JC, Deleamont P: Repeated vital capacity measurements as predictive parameters for mechanical ventilation need and weaning success in Guillain-Barré syndrome, Am Rev Respir Dis 144:814, 1991.
39. Borel CO, Teitelbaum J, Hanley D: Ventilatory drive and CO_2-response in ventilatory failure due to myasthenia gravis and Guillain-Barré, Crit Care Med 21:1717, 1993.
40. Hill R, Martin J, Hakim A: Acute respiratory failure in motor neuron disease, Arch Neurol 40:32, 1983.
41. Braun S: Respiratory system in amyotrophic lateral sclerosis, Neurol Clin 5:9, 1987.
42. Moss AH, Casey P: Home ventilation for amyotrophic lateral sclerosis patients: outcomes, costs and patient, family and physician attitudes, Neurology 43:438, 1993.
43. Adams HP Jr et al: Guidelines for thrombolytic therapy for acute stroke: a supplement to the guidelines for the management of patients with acute ischemic stroke: a statement for healthcare professionals from a Special Writing Group of the Stroke Council, American Heart Association, Circulation 94:1167, 1996.
44. Pereira AC, Martin PJ, Warburton EA: Thrombolysis in acute ischaemic stroke, Postgrad Med J 77:166, 2001.
45. Upadhyay S et al: Evaluation of deformities and pulmonary function in adolescent idiopathic thoracic scoliosis, Eur Spine J 4:274, 1995.
46. Kearon C et al: Factors determining pulmonary function in adolescent idiopathic thoracic scoliosis, Am Rev Respir Dis 148:288, 1993.
47. Wong C et al: Pulmonary function before and after anterior spinal surgery in adult idiopathic scoliosis, Thorax 51:534, 1996.
48. Jackson M et al: The effects of five years of nocturnal cuirass-assisted ventilation in chest wall disease, Eur Respir J 6:630, 1993.
49. Hoeppner V et al: Nighttime ventilation improves respiratory failure in secondary kyphoscoliosis, Am Rev Respir Dis 129:240, 1984.
50. Ciraulo D et al: Flail chest as a marker for significant injuries, J Am Coll Surg 178:466, 1994.

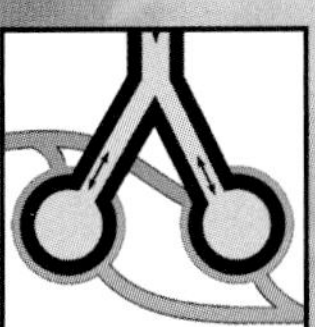

CHAPTER 27

Disorders of Sleep

Laurie A. Kilkenny, Karl S. Fernandes, and Patrick J. Strollo, Jr.

In This Chapter You Will Learn:

- How to define obstructive sleep apnea (OSA)
- Why airway closure occurs only during sleep
- What are the long-term consequences of uncontrolled OSA
- How a diagnosis of OSA is made
- What groups of patients are at particular risk of OSA
- What treatments are available for patients with OSA
- How continuous positive airway pressure (CPAP) works
- What problems are associated with CPAP
- When bilevel pressure is useful
- What "auto-titrating" CPAP means
- What are the surgical alternatives

Chapter Outline

Key Terms

bilevel positive airway pressure (BiPAP)
central sleep apnea (CSA)
continuous positive airway pressure (CPAP)
obesity hypoventilation
obstructive sleep apnea (OSA)
sleep-disordered breathing
uvulopalatopharyngoplasty (UVPPP)

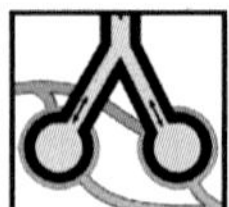

Obstructive sleep apnea (OSA) syndrome is a clinical common problem that continues to be underdiagnosed.[1] It is estimated that approximately 2% to 4% of the adult population has OSA.[2-4] This prevalence is equivalent to that of asthma and diabetes in the general population. The spectrum of disease ranges from sleep disruption related to increased airway resistance to profound daytime sleepiness in conjunction with severe oxyhemoglobin desaturation, pulmonary hypertension, and right heart failure. The common feature in all the variants of OSA syndrome is sleep disruption secondary to increased ventilatory effort that results in daytime hypersomnolence (Figure 27-1).[5] Effective treatment that decreases morbidity and mortality is available.

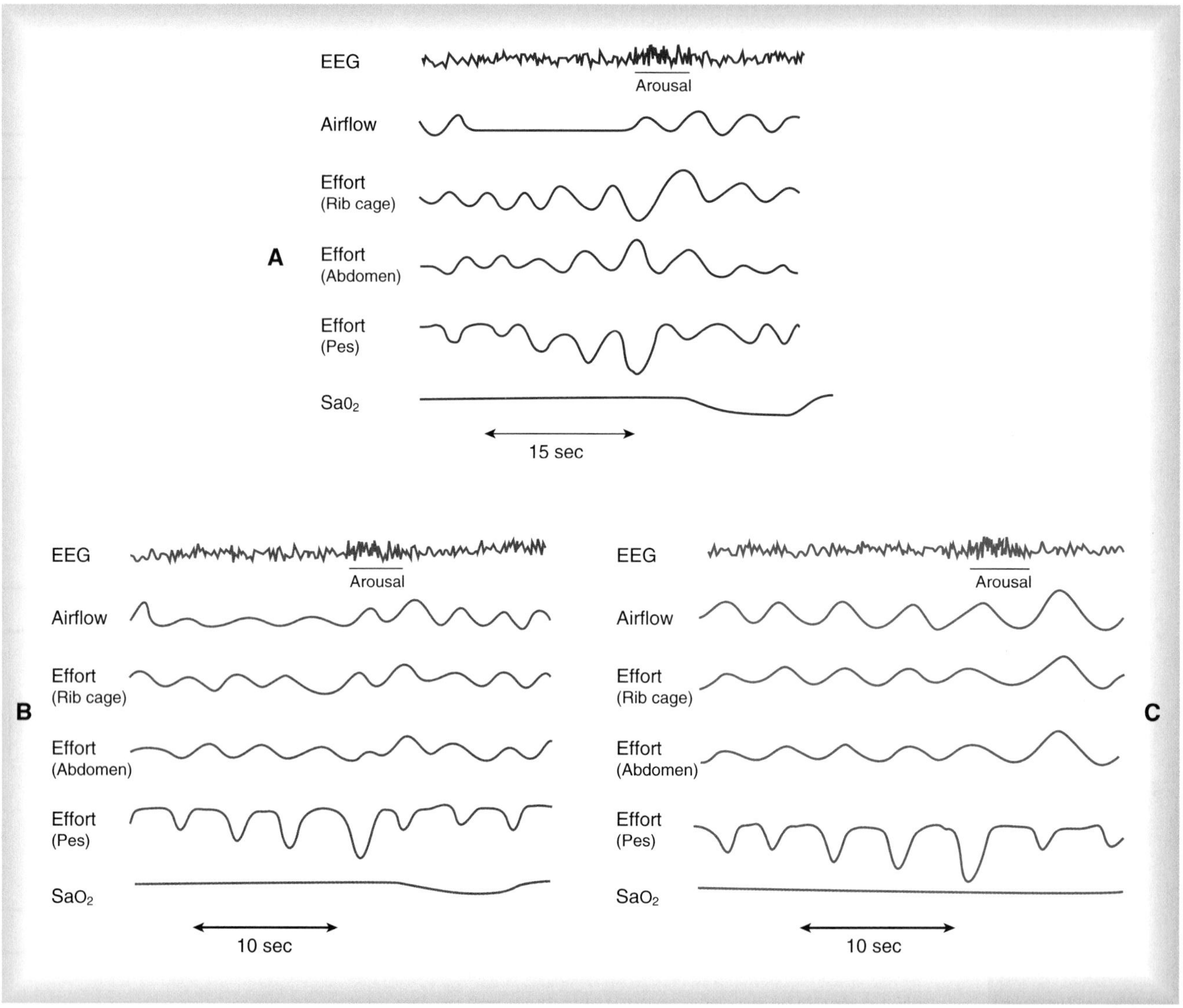

Figure 27-1 · Spectrum of Sleep-Related Upper Airway Obstruction

A, Obstructive apnea. These events are defined as cessation of airflow for 10 seconds or longer. Paradoxical movement of the rib cage and abdomen in response to the closed airway occurs. Ventilatory effort, measured with an esophageal balloon (Pes), usually increases until a threshold is reached that triggers a brief arousal seen on the EEG, and airway opening occurs. Oxyhemoglobin desaturation usually accompanies the event. **B,** Obstructive hypopnea. These events have been defined as a reduction of airflow by 30% to 50% for 10 seconds or longer. Paradoxical movement of the rib cage and abdomen in response to the narrowed airway occurs. Ventilatory effort, measured with an esophageal balloon (Pes), usually increases until a threshold is reached that triggers a brief arousal seen on an EEG, and complete airway opening occurs. Oxyhemoglobin desaturation usually accompanies the event and usually is of a lesser degree than that which occurs with apnea. **C,** Respiratory effort–related arousals. These events are characterized by no discernible reduction in airflow. Subtle paradoxical movement of the rib cage and abdomen in response to narrowing of the airway may occur. As in apnea and hypopnea, ventilatory effort, measured with an esophageal balloon (Pes), usually increases until a threshold is reached that triggers a brief arousal seen on an EEG, and complete airway opening occurs. By definition, no oxyhemoglobin desaturation is associated with the event.

▶ DEFINITIONS

Sleep apnea can be defined as repeated episodes of complete cessation of airflow for 10 seconds or longer. The events can be obstructive (due to upper airway closure) or central (due to lack of ventilatory effort).

Primary central nervous system lesions, stroke, congestive heart failure, and high-altitude hypoxemia can diminish respiratory control and cause central apnea events.[6] **Central sleep apnea** (CSA) is not as common as OSA. Only 10% to 15% of patients with sleep disordered breathing are classified as having CSA.[7] Mixed apnea has both a central component and an obstructive component (Figure 27-2).

Hypopnea is a significant decrease in without complete cessation of airflow.[4] Hypopnea is defined as a 30% decrease in airflow in conjunction with 4% oxygen desaturation.[8] Most investigators agree that physiologically significant hypopnea is associated with a decrease in oxygen saturation or arousal from sleep.[9]

The respiratory therapist is likely to encounter both OSA and CSA when treating patients. Because OSA is the most commonly encountered type of sleep apnea and is underdiagnosed by health professionals, the focus of this chapter is the pathophysiology and management of the variants of OSA.

▶ PATHOPHYSIOLOGY

Obstructive Sleep Apnea

The primary cause of OSA is a small or unstable pharyngeal airway. This condition can be caused by soft-tissue factors, such as upper body obesity or

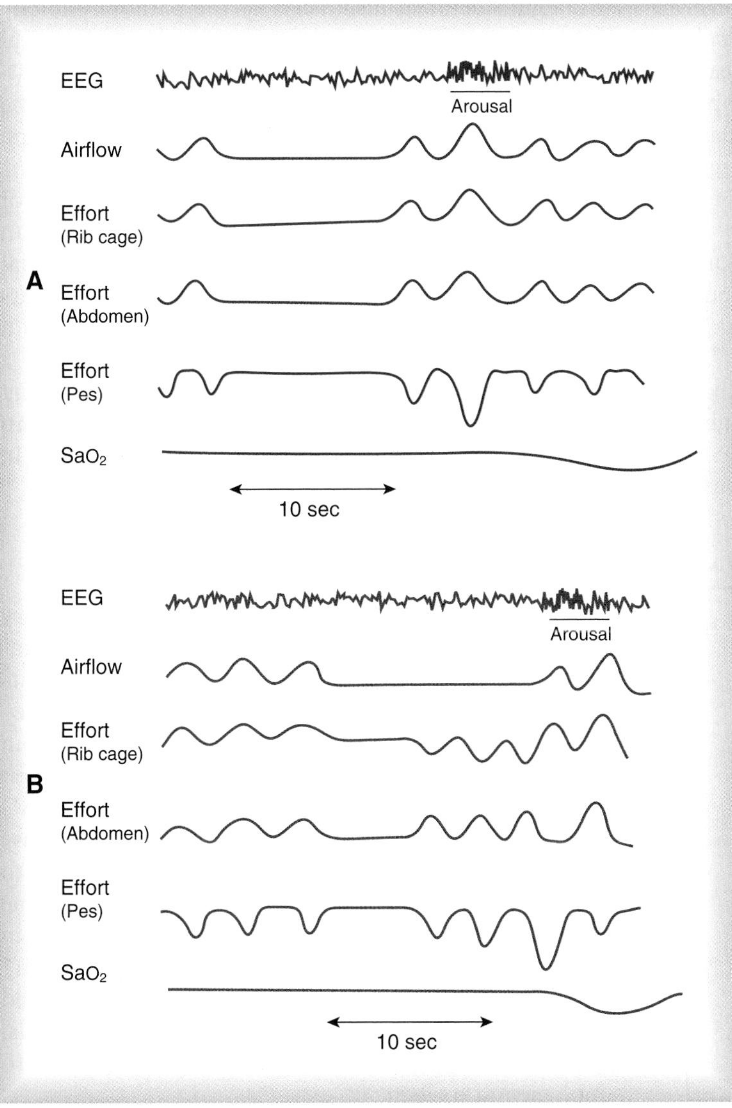

Figure 27-2 · Central and Mixed Apnea

A, Central apnea. These events are defined as cessation of airflow for 10 seconds or longer. Compared with the events of obstructive apnea, no movement of the rib cage or abdomen is present and the airway remains open. During an apneic event, there is a lack of ventilatory effort, measured with an esophageal balloon (Pes). A brief arousal on the EEG is associated with a maximal ventilatory effort that usually follows the episode of apnea. Oxyhemoglobin desaturation may be associated with the event. **B,** Mixed apnea. These events have characteristics of both central and obstructive apnea. They are 10 seconds or longer in duration, and the central portion precedes the obstructive component. As with other sleep-related upper airway obstructive events, termination of the event is characterized by a maximal ventilatory effort and is associated with brief arousal on the EEG. Mixed apnea usually is associated with oxyhemoglobin desaturation.

tonsillar hypertrophy (rare in adults), as well as skeletal factors, such as a small or recessed chin.[10] During the waking state, pharyngeal patency is maintained by increased activity of the upper airway dilator muscles. Sleep onset is associated with a decrease in the activity of these muscles. The result is airway narrowing or closure of airways that are at risk.[11,12] In the unstable upper airway, narrowing and closure during sleep involve multiple sites.[13]

Partial or complete closure of the upper airway during sleep has many serious neurobehavioral and cardiopulmonary consequences (Box 27-1). Patients with untreated OSA, compared with the general population, have an increased risk of systemic and pulmonary hypertension, stroke, nocturnal arrhythmia, heart failure, and myocardial infarction.[14-17] The repetitive cycle of upper airway closure and opening during sleep is believed to have effects on the autonomic nervous system, specifically an increase in sympathetic tone.[16] These effects are caused in part by episodes of hypoxemia and hypercapnia due to airway closure and hypoventilation that can occur throughout the night in patients with OSA. The arousals and microarousals during sleep also play an important role in the increase in sympathetic tone.[18-20] Over time, increased sympathetic tone may result in systemic and pulmonary hypertension.[21,22] Patients with OSA may have right ventricular hypertrophy and failure if they are not treated.[23]

Obesity, especially of the upper body, has been found to correlate positively with the presence of OSA. Patients with OSA frequently are obese with a large amount of peripharyngeal tissue and adipose tissue in the neck.[24] A body mass index (BMI) greater than 28 (more than 120% of ideal body weight normalized for height) should alert the practitioner to the possibility of OSA, particularly if the patient has excessive daytime sleepiness (EDS).[25]

Box 27-1 • Adverse Consequences of OSA

CARDIOPULMONARY
- Nocturnal arrhythmia
- Diurnal hypertension
- Pulmonary hypertension
- Right or left ventricular failure
- Myocardial infarction
- Stroke

NEUROBEHAVIORAL
- Excessive daytime sleepiness
- Diminished quality of life
- Adverse personality change
- Motor vehicle accidents

Patients who are of normal body weight can be predisposed to OSA if they have an abnormal craniofacial configuration. Men often grow a beard to disguise such a craniofacial abnormality. If the chin is recessed (retrognathic) or small (micrognathic), the upper airway space may be narrow, and the risk of airway closure during sleep increases.[2,10,11,21,25] Patients with a deviated nasal septum or trauma to the nasal passages may be predisposed to upper airway closure during sleep as a result of the increased resistive load to the upper airway. An isolated nasal abnormality is an unusual cause of OSA.

Obstructive sleep apnea may have a genetic predisposition. There have been reports of families in which obesity alone does not explain the increased prevalence of OSA.[26] It has been postulated that craniofacial abnormalities and defects in ventilatory control explain the increased frequency of OSA in these families.

Central Sleep Apnea

Although a detailed discussion of the pathophysiology of CSA is beyond the scope of this chapter, several concepts are important to the respiratory therapist. Unlike OSA, which represents a spectrum of the same disease, CSA is a heterogeneous group of disorders. Patients have a ventilatory pattern known as *periodic breathing*, in which there is a waxing and waning of respiratory drive, which is reflected clinically as an increase and then a decrease in respiratory rate and tidal volume. Cheyne-Stokes respiration, which often occurs in patients with congestive heart failure or stroke, is a severe type of periodic breathing characterized by a crescendo-decrescendo pattern of hyperpnea alternating with apnea. After apnea occurs, there may be an increase in central ventilatory drive and an increase in tidal volume.[6,7]

Overlap Syndrome

Some patients with chronic obstructive pulmonary disease (COPD) also have coexisting OSA. This combination is referred to as *overlap syndrome*. Patients usually are obese and have a history of smoking. They have moderate to severe nocturnal oxyhemoglobin desaturation due to both OSA and COPD. The worst desaturations occur during rapid eye movement (REM) sleep and are related to the loss of accessory muscle use encountered in this physiological state. Patients tend to have a worse prognosis than do patients with the same degree of OSA but without COPD. They may arrive in the intensive care unit with a "COPD exacerbation" and decompensated right heart failure. Undiagnosed OSA complicates the course at night with arousals, increased dyspnea, and desaturations resistant to supplemental oxygen.[27]

▶ CLINICAL FEATURES

Patients with sleep apnea usually are men (three times greater frequency than among women), are older than 40 years, and have hypertension (Box 27-2). Most patients with sleep apnea report habitual snoring that may date to early adulthood but has become progressively worse.[2,3,5,24] Sensations of nocturnal choking, gasping, or resuscitative snorting are commonly reported. A bed partner may observe periods of apnea, which is almost enough to confirm the diagnosis of OSA.

The presence of EDS may be underestimated because OSA manifests in a subacute manner. As a result, patients with OSA may report symptoms of fatigue alone. These patients also frequently report nocturnal reflux, nocturia, chronic nasal obstruction, morning headaches, and depression.

Patients with OSA have arousals from sleep and sleep fragmentation, which can lead to fatigue, EDS, and irritability.[28,29] Patients who have an increased frequency of awakenings and microarousals have more daytime sleepiness and greater difficulty with daytime functioning than does the general population.[30] Patients with OSA may have neuropsychological deficits and impairment in vigilance.[31] Compared with the general population, untreated OSA patients are at increased risk of motor vehicle accidents because of EDS.[31-34]

The physical examination of most patients reveal evidence of obesity, particularly in the upper body. Upper body obesity can be quantitated with neck size. A neck circumference of 42 cm (16.5 in) increases the likelihood of the diagnosis of sleep apnea at diagnostic testing.[21] Examination of the oropharynx frequently reveals a long soft palate. Although tonsillar hypertrophy is common in children with sleep apnea, it is seldom found in adults. Large palatine tonsils may increase the risk of airway closure during sleep. The retrognathic or micrognathic mandible can narrow the pharyngeal airway, placing a patient of normal weight at risk of airway closure during sleep.[10,11]

The cardiovascular examination may reveal evidence of pulmonary hypertension or right heart failure (lower-extremity edema).[35] These findings are determined primarily by the hypoxic burden experienced by the patient.[22] Pulmonary hypertension or right heart failure is more commonly encountered in patients with concomitant daytime hypoxemia. Patients with OSA and COPD or severe obesity (BMI ≥40) appear to be at particular risk of these complications.[36]

Box 27-2 • Obstructive Sleep Apnea: Common Clinical Features

- Male
- Age older than 40 years
- Upper body obesity (neck >16.5 in)
- Habitual snoring
- Fatigue or daytime sleepiness
- Diurnal hypertension

RULE OF THUMB

Uncontrolled OSA can cause daytime hypoxemia. The diagnosis of OSA should be considered when the degree of hypoxemia is out of proportion to the pulmonary spirometric defect. When the arterial partial pressure of oxygen is less than 60 mm Hg and the forced expiratory volume in 1 second is greater than 30% of that predicted, COPD in itself is inadequate to explain the hypoxemia, and coexisting OSA should be considered.[37] Obstructive sleep apnea in this setting is frequently associated with pulmonary hypertension and evidence of right heart failure at physical examination. Hypoxemia, pulmonary hypertension, and right heart failure can be substantially improved with management of OSA. If the patient adheres to therapy, the need for supplemental oxygen may be reduced or eliminated.

Recurrent moderate to severe oxyhemoglobin desaturation and resaturation due to OSA can be associated with an increased incidence of cardiac arrhythmia. Repeated nocturnal desaturation can be a cause of secondary polycythemia.[15,21]

▶ LABORATORY TESTING

When sleep apnea is suspected, an overnight polysomnogram (PSG) should be obtained for confirmation of the clinical diagnosis. A full-night PSG in the sleep laboratory monitored by a sleep technologist is considered the standard or reference.

In a laboratory sleep study, the technologist records several physiological signals to determine whether airway closure occurs during sleep and to what extent the closure disturbs sleep continuity and cardiopulmonary function. An electroencephalogram (EEG), electrooculogram (EOG), and chin electromyogram (EMG) are obtained for assessment of sleep stage and documentation of sleep disruption due to sleep-related breathing disturbance. Airflow (measured at nose and mouth), ventilatory effort (assessed with inductance PSG monitoring of rib cage and abdominal movement), cardiac rhythm (monitored with a continuous electrocardiogram [ECG] for evaluation of the effect of apnea), and oxygen saturation (measured with pulse oximetry) also are assessed.

POLYSOMNOGRAPHY

AARC Clinical Practice Guideline (Excerpts)*

➤ INDICATIONS

Polysomnography may be indicated in patients with:

- COPD whose awake PaO_2 is >55 mm Hg but whose illness is complicated by pulmonary hypertension, right heart failure, polycythemia, or excessive daytime sleepiness
- Restrictive ventilatory impairment secondary to chest-wall and neuromuscular disturbances whose illness is complicated by chronic hypoventilation, polycythemia, pulmonary hypertension, disturbed sleep, morning headaches, or daytime somnolence/fatigue
- Disturbances in respiratory control whose awake $PaCO_2$ is >45 mm Hg or whose illness is complicated by pulmonary hypertension, polycythemia, disturbed sleep, morning headaches, or daytime somnolence/fatigue
- Nocturnal cyclic bradyarrhythmias or tachyarrhythmias, nocturnal abnormalities of atrioventricular conduction, or ventricular ectopy that appear to increase in frequency during sleep
- Excessive daytime sleepiness or insomnia
- Snoring associated with observed apneas and/or excessive daytime sleepiness
- Other symptoms of sleep-disordered breathing as described in the International Classification of Sleep Disorders

➤ CONTRAINDICATIONS

There are no absolute contraindications to polysomnography when indications are clearly established. However, risk-benefit ratios should be assessed if transferring medically unstable inpatients.

➤ PRECAUTIONS AND COMPLICATIONS

- Skin irritation may occur as a result of the adhesive used to attach electrodes to the patient.
- At the conclusion of the study, adhesive remover is used to dissolve adhesive on the patient's skin. Adhesive removers (e.g., acetone) should be used only in well-ventilated areas.
- The integrity of the electrical isolation of polysomnographic equipment must be certified by engineering or biomedical personnel qualified to make such assessment.
- The adhesive used to attach EEG electrodes should not be used to attach electrodes near the patient's eyes and should always be used in well-ventilated areas.
- Because of the high flammability of adhesives and acetone, these substances should be used with caution, especially in patients who require supplemental oxygen.
- Adhesives should be used with caution in patients with reactive airways disease and in small infants.
- Patients with parasomnias or seizures may be at risk of injury related to movements during sleep.
- Institution-specific policies and guidelines describing personnel responsibilities and appropriate responses should be developed.

➤ ASSESSMENT OF NEED

Polysomnography is indicated for patients suspected of having sleep-related respiratory disturbances described in *The International Classification of Sleep Disorders, Diagnostic and Coding Manual.*

➤ ASSESSMENT OF TEST QUALITY

- Polysomnography should either confirm or eliminate a sleep-related diagnosis.
- Documentation of findings, suggested therapeutic intervention, and/or other clinical decisions resulting from polysomnography should be noted in the patient's chart.
- Each laboratory should implement a quality assurance program that addresses equipment calibration and maintenance, patient preparation/monitoring, scoring methodology, and intertechnician scoring variances.

➤ MONITORING

- Patient variables to be monitored include EEG, EOG, EMG, EGG, respiratory effort, nasal or oral airflow, SpO_2, body position, limb movement: intervention should occur if the physiological signals are lost.
- Infrared or low-light video cameras and recording equipment should permit visualization of the patient by the technician throughout the procedure.
- The technician should intervene if an acute change in physiologic status occurs and communicate that change to appropriate medical personnel.

---

*For complete guidelines see Respir Care 40:1336, 1995.

In obstructive apnea or hypopnea, airflow is absent or decreased in the presence of ventilatory effort. Asynchronous (paradoxical) movement of the abdomen and rib cage often occurs. Oxygen desaturation may or may not occur, depending on factors including the length of the apneic event and the patient's baseline saturation (see Figure 27-1). Respiratory effort–related arousals (RERA) are characterized by increased respiratory effort, leading to arousal from sleep that does not meet the criteria of an apneic or a hypopneic event (see Figure 27-1).[38]

Measuring devices that are adequate for assessing hypopnea also are adequate for assessing apnea; however, devices used for measuring apnea cannot always detect hypopnea. The diagnosis of hypopnea may be affected by the measurement technique used. In 1999, an American Academy of Sleep Medicine task force conducted an evidence-based review of measurement techniques for the detection of hypopnea.[39] The scoring system was as follows: A, good to excellent agreement with a reference standard (face mask pneumotachygraph); B, limited data but good theoretical framework and clinical experience suggest the method is valid; C, no data, weak theoretical framework or clinical experience; and D, research or clinical experience suggests that method is not valid.

The measuring techniques were scored as follows: nasal pressure, B; respiratory inductance plethysmography (RIP) with sum of chest and abdominal signals, B; dual-channel RIP, C; single-channel RIP, C; piezo sensors, strain gauges, and thoracic impedence, D; breathing measurement signal with a desaturation or arousal, B; expired CO_2, D; and thermal sensors, D. The face mask pneumotachygraph was graded A and became the reference standard. Unfortunately, a face mask pneumotachygraph is poorly tolerated. Nasal pressure is a reliable way to detect hypopnea and is well tolerated by patients undergoing diagnostic PSG.[39]

Once the sleep study is completed, the sleep technologist scores it. The number of events of apnea and of hypopnea per hour of sleep are reported as an apnea-hypopnea index (AHI) or respiratory disturbance index. Although there is incomplete agreement on the exact number that defines the severity of **sleep-disordered breathing**, an AHI greater than 30 is compatible with moderate to severe sleep apnea. An AHI less than 5 is considered within the normal range. The number of arousals per hour (arousal index), the percentage of each sleep stage, the frequency of oxygen desaturations, mean oxygen saturation, and the nadir of oxygen saturation also are reported (Box 27-3).

Box 27-3 • Obstructive Sleep Apnea: Key Features of Sleep Studies to Be Analyzed and Reported

- Apnea-hypopnea index
- Arousal index
- Sleep stage distribution
- Frequency of oxyhemoglobin desaturations
- Mean oxyhemoglobin saturation
- Nadir of oxyhemoglobin saturation

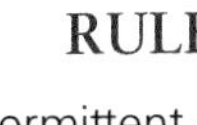

RULE OF THUMB

Intermittent checks of oxygen saturation cannot reliably exclude sleep-related desaturation due to OSA. Placing the oximetry probe on the patient frequently awakens the patient. In addition, isolated readings may not allow sampling of all sleep stages, especially REM sleep, during which sleep-disordered breathing and nocturnal desaturation tend to be prominent. Continuous overnight oximetry is a better assessment of the degree of oxyhemoglobin desaturation with sleep.

Abbreviated (portable) cardiopulmonary testing has been used to confirm a diagnosis of OSA. These studies do not record the electrophysiological signals (EEG, EOG, EMG) required to stage and score sleep. The portable studies vary in the type and number of cardiopulmonary values recorded. Controversy exists whether portable systems can show sleep apnea as well as traditional full-night PSG does. Many variables, such as airflow, ventilatory effort, sleep stage, and oxygen saturation values, may be less precise or may not be measured at all with these systems.[40,41]

▶ TREATMENT

Management of OSA should be individualized but generally can be divided into three options: behavioral, medical, and surgical interventions. Behavioral therapy should be pursued in the care of all patients. Medical therapy and surgical therapy must be tailored to the patient. The likelihood of acceptance of and adherence to the prescribed therapeutic intervention must be considered. The goals of treatment are to normalize oxygen saturation and ventilation; eliminate apnea, hypopnea, and snoring; and improve sleep architecture and continuity (Box 27-4).

Behavioral Interventions and Risk Counseling

Patients need to be informed of the risks of uncontrolled sleep apnea. Several behavioral interventions can be beneficial, including weight loss by obese patients;

MINI CLINI

Nocturnal Angina in an Obese Middle-Aged Man

HISTORY

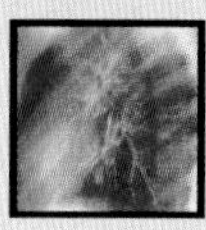

A 45-year-old morbidly obese nonsmoker is admitted to the coronary care unit after awakening at 4 am with chest pain typical of angina pectoris. The pain has resolved by the time he reaches the emergency department. The patient is unsure of the duration of the pain before he called for his wife, who sleeps in a separate bedroom because of his very loud habitual snoring. The patient reports exertional shortness of breath but no chest pain before this event. He states that he frequently gets "indigestion" that at times is worse at night but that this pain was different.

MEDICATIONS

- Captopril 25 mg by mouth twice a day
- Furosemide (Lasix) 20 mg by mouth every day
- Cimetidine (Tagamet) 300 mg by mouth at bedtime

MEDICAL HISTORY

Hypertension and gastroesophageal reflux. No significant cardiac disease. Cardiac catheterization 1 year ago showed normal left ventricular function and minimal coronary artery occlusion.

PHYSICAL EXAMINATION

- Vital signs: blood pressure, 160/98 mm Hg; heart rate, 100 beats/min; temperature, 98.6° F (37° C); respiration, 18 breaths/min
- General: mildly diaphoretic obese white man
- Neck: 52 cm (20.5 in) in circumference
- Lungs: clear breath sounds bilaterally
- Heart: regular rate and rhythm
- Abdomen: obese, soft, normal bowel sounds
- Extremities: 4 mm pretibial pitting edema

LABORATORY DATA

- Room air arterial blood gases: pH, 7.36; P_{CO_2}, 37 mm Hg; P_{O_2}, 62 mm Hg; Sa_{O_2}, 92%
- Chest radiograph: pulmonary congestion; otherwise normal
- ECG: sinus tachycardia without acute changes

Why did the patient experience angina during sleep?

DISCUSSION

Serial cardiac enzyme values show no myocardial infarction. A stress test result is negative, but a submaximal effort is obtained. The patient's weight precludes an adenosine thallium stress test. Repeated cardiac catheterization shows no change in the minimal coronary artery occlusion reported previously. The pulmonary consultant called to evaluate the patient's shortness of breath recommends nocturnal PSG to rule out sleep apnea. The sleep study result is positive for severe sleep apnea (AHI, 110; lowest Sa_{O_2}, 7% on the oximeter during REM sleep). A continuous positive airway pressure (CPAP) titration test is performed. The patient is discharged home on CPAP 17.5 cm H_2O through a nasal mask. He returns to the pulmonary clinic 1 month after discharge. He reported no further episodes of nocturnal angina. Reflux and shortness of breath have been relieved. The patient has lost 10 pounds (4.5 kg) without dieting. The lower extremity edema is markedly relieved.

Box 27-4 • Obstructive Sleep Apnea: Goals of Treatment

- Eliminate apnea, hypopnea, and snoring
- Normalize oxygen saturation and ventilation
- Improve sleep architecture and continuity

avoidance of alcohol, sedatives, and hypnotics; and avoidance of sleep deprivation. Weight loss by obese patients can decrease the severity of sleep apnea; however, weight reduction is one of the more difficult behavioral strategies to implement. Involvement of the patient with a dietitian or nutritionist can be helpful.[25] Alcohol decreases the arousal threshold and thus can cause each apnea episode to last longer. Alcohol also reduces upper airway muscle tone, causing the airway to be more compliant and prone to complete or partial closure and thus apnea.[42,43] For these reasons, alcohol is to be avoided by patients believed to have sleep apnea. Sedatives and hypnotics can decrease the stability of the upper airway and suppress certain stages of sleep. Most notably, REM sleep is suppressed when benzodiazepines are used.[44]

Positional Therapy

When a sleep study indicates that apnea and snoring occur only in the supine position, instruction on sleeping in the lateral position can be beneficial. Use of the "tennis ball" technique, in which a ball is sewn onto the back of the patient's sleeping garment, discourages the patient from rolling into the supine position. The long-term effects of positional therapy are unknown. Positional therapy is generally recommended for milder cases of positional OSA.

Medical Interventions

Positive Pressure Therapy: Continuous Positive Airway Pressure Therapy

Continuous positive airway pressure (CPAP) therapy was introduced for management of OSA in 1981.[45] It has become the first-line medical therapy for OSA. Numerous studies have documented the effectiveness of CPAP in decreasing the morbidity and mortality associated with OSA.[14,30,46-50] For most patients, obstruction

MINI CLINI

Young Man Hospitalized for Observation After a Single-Vehicle Accident in the Mid Afternoon

HISTORY

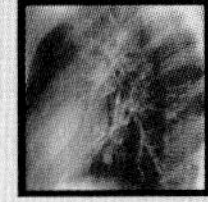

A 27-year-old nonsmoker is admitted to the coronary care unit for monitoring so that the diagnosis of cardiac contusion can be ruled out. The patient has been involved in a single-vehicle automobile accident. The accident occurred at 3:30 pm on a clear day. The patient felt drowsy immediately before the event. He became conscious after hitting the guardrail. The patient's chest hit the steering wheel. The patient reports anterior chest wall pain and denies having angina or presyncope.

MEDICATIONS

None

MEDICAL HISTORY

Negative

PHYSICAL EXAMINATION

- Vital signs: blood pressure, 140/88 mm Hg; heart rate, 100 beats/min; temperature, 98.6° F (37° C); respirations, 16 breaths/min
- General: well-developed, well-nourished white man
- Head, eyes, ears, nose throat: elongated soft palate, mild crowding of the tonsillar pillars, retrognathic chin
- Neck: 40 cm (16 in) in circumference
- Chest: contusion on the anterior portion of the chest
- Lungs: clear breath sounds bilaterally
- Heart: regular rate and rhythm
- Abdomen: soft with normal bowel sounds
- Extremities: no clubbing, cyanosis, or edema
- Skin: multiple small lacerations

LABORATORY DATA

- Chest radiograph: no cardiomegaly, mass, infiltrate, or effusion
- ECG: sinus tachycardia
- Creatine kinase: 350 IU/L (no MB fraction)

What caused the patient to fall asleep at the wheel?

DISCUSSION

The patient is found to be bradycardiac during sleep on the night of admission. This sign is associated with snoring and oxyhemoglobin desaturation on oxygen at 2 L/min through a nasal cannula. The cardiology consultant recommends diagnostic nocturnal PSG to rule out sleep apnea. The study shows severe sleep apnea (AHI 85 with a low SaO_2 of 60%). A CPAP titration study shows the patient needs 10 cm H_2O of CPAP through nasal pillows. One month later the patient states he no longer experiences the fatigue he had previously. In retrospect, the patient believes that before treatment with CPAP, he was quite sleepy during the day. Despite this improvement, he wants to explore other treatment options. A surgical consultation is obtained.

of the upper airway is abolished by CPAP pressures between 7.5 and 12.5 cm H_2O.[51-53] The level of CPAP required for optimal management of OSA is patient based and is best determined with a titration performed in the sleep laboratory.[54] Attempts to use an algorithm or a prediction equation as a replacement for in-laboratory titration have not been uniformly successful.[55]

Continuous positive airway pressure therapy has been shown to decrease daytime sleepiness, improve neurocognitive testing and vigilance scores, decrease the incidence of pulmonary hypertension and right heart failure, and decrease the number of ventilation-related arousals and nocturnal cardiac events. Reductions in daytime hypoxemia and hypercapnia also have been attributed to CPAP therapy.[31,46,49-51,56]

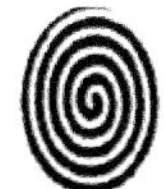

RULE OF THUMB

Retrognathia can be the cause of OSA in young patients who are at or close to ideal body weight. Continuous positive airway pressure is highly effective for these patients, but upper airway reconstruction (phases I and II surgery) can be curative.

Continuous positive airway pressure therapy is believed to work by splinting the upper airway open, thus raising the intraluminal pressure of the upper airway above a critical transmural pressure of the pharynx and hypopharynx that is associated with airway closure. The soft palate is effectively moved anteriorly up against the tongue, which pressurizes the upper airway (Figure 27-3).[57] Continuous positive airway pressure allows the upper airway to be splinted open whether there is a single site (uncommon) or there are multiple sites (more common) of airway narrowing or closure. Investigators have found that when nasal CPAP is applied, EMG activity of the upper airway dilator muscles is depressed.[58]

To be successful, CPAP titration should obliterate all apneic episodes and reduce the number of hypopneic episodes for prevention of arterial oxygen desaturation. Paradoxical thoracoabdominal movement and snoring should be eliminated.[59] For improvement of sleep continuity, respiration-related EEG arousals and microarousals must be abolished. There is no evidence to support the misconception that a higher level of CPAP always is necessary in patients with severe sleep apnea. There is a great degree of variability in CPAP across the spectrum of OSA. Some patients with relatively mild elevations of the AHI need higher levels of CPAP pressures than do those with substantially higher AHIs.[60]

Patients who report EDS without an increase in AHI may have repetitive 2- to 3-second transient EEG arousals during episodes of snoring. These short arousals occur

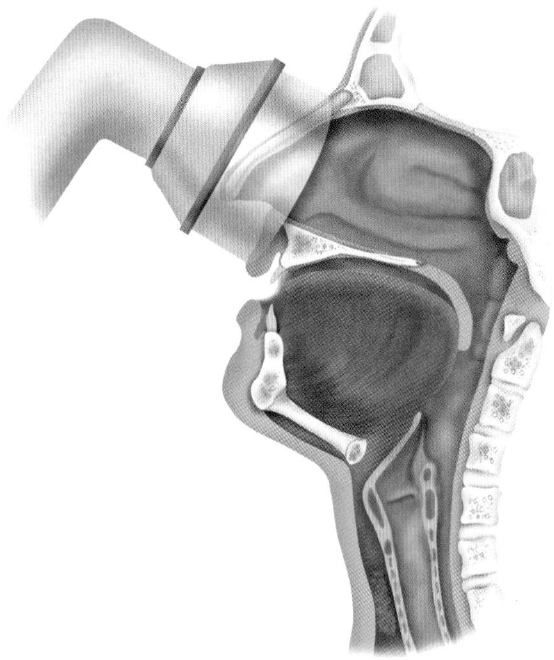

Figure 27-3 · Nasal Continuous Positive Airway Pressure (CPAP)

Positive airway pressure is applied with a nasal mask. The soft palate falls against the base of the tongue so that the upper airway is pneumatically splinted open.

during episodes of increased upper airway resistance, and although not associated with any significant arterial oxygen desaturation, they may cause EDS and fatigue.[5,29] This pattern generally occurs in younger patients, is known as *upper airway resistance syndrome* (UARS), and is characterized by RERA (see Figure 27-1). With the emergence of UARS as a clinical entity, some researchers have suggested that CPAP titrations may be suboptimal without measurement of esophageal pressure.[60-62] Many sleep laboratories, however, do not have the technical capability to measure esophageal pressure. In addition, many patients refuse this type of monitoring because of discomfort.

Results of analysis have shown the contour of the inspiratory flow signal correlates with ventilatory effort as reflected by esophageal pressure swings.[38] These results suggest that this value best predicts the optimum CPAP titration when esophageal balloons are not used.[62] Condos et al.[38] have hypothesized that during CPAP titration, there is a period during the transition to deeper stages of sleep when there is flow limitation and increased intrathoracic pressure without EEG arousals. These investigators surmised that if this condition is not corrected, patients may have incomplete and suboptimal titrations. However, the authors have admitted that evidence is lacking regarding the clinical significance of flow limitation without EEG arousals.

Despite numerous studies documenting the efficacy of CPAP in the treatment of patients in the sleep laboratory, clinicians have encountered difficulty with patients' adherence to CPAP therapy. Approximately 80% of patients accept CPAP, although long-term objective compliance is less than optimal. Objective compliance, defined as use of the machine for more than 4 hours per night for more than 70% of observed nights, has been measured to be as low as 46%.[63] Severity of the AHI does not always correlate with compliance, but the benefit perceived by the patient is a better predictor.[51,59,63,64] Data reported by Douglas et al. indicate that patients who are subjectively sleepy and have an AHI >30 are likely to accept and comply with CPAP therapy.[65] Follow-up study with objective compliance monitoring is essential. Compliance 1 month after the initiation of therapy is reported to be a good predictor of CPAP use at 3 months.[63]

It is unclear whether higher levels of CPAP cause a decrease in compliance. Some patients believe that increased pressure, particularly during expiration, is uncomfortable. Discomfort with the interface and the device may reduce acceptance and compliance.[53,63,66] Since the introduction of CPAP, a variety of interfaces have been designed to improve compliance by increasing the patient's comfort. Nasal pillows or prongs, nasal masks with comfort flaps or bubbles, oral-nasal masks, and full-face masks are available.[12,67-70] No studies have been conducted for direct comparison of efficacy, subjective patient comfort, or objective patient compliance with these interfaces.[12] In clinical practice, some patients tolerate one interface better than another. Sleep laboratories may prefer to use a certain interface primarily on the basis of technician bias rather than objective data.

Positive Pressure Therapy: Bilevel Pressure Therapy

Another form of positive-pressure therapy is **bilevel positive airway pressure** (BiPAP). Bilevel positive airway pressure therapy was developed to take advantage of the fact that some patients may have different pressure requirements between inspiration and expiration.[67] It was hypothesized that because a patient may have a lower expiratory pressure requirement to splint the airway open, patient acceptance and compliance would be favorably affected. Bilevel units operate on household electricity and are similar in size and appearance to conventional CPAP units. There is a substantial difference in cost, a bilevel unit being almost twice the price of a CPAP unit.

Although patient acceptance may be slightly better with bilevel pressure, the published data have shown no difference in compliance between conventional CPAP and BiPAP.[70,71] Nonetheless, BiPAP may be better tolerated by the subgroup of patients who need higher CPAP pressures.

MINI CLINI

Middle-Aged Woman With Primary Pulmonary Hypertension

HISTORY

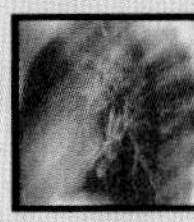

A 59-year-old former smoker is admitted to the hospital for right and left heart catheterization. A previous echocardiographic examination showed pulmonary hypertension. The patient denies having angina or exertional chest discomfort. She admits to dyspnea on exertion that has been increasing over the past few months and to a chronic nonproductive cough. She denies taking "diet pills."

MEDICATIONS

- Nifedipine 10 mg by mouth three times a day
- Furosemide (Lasix) 20 mg by mouth daily
- Potassium chloride 20 mEq by mouth twice a day

MEDICAL HISTORY

Hypertension and allergic rhinitis, no cardiac disease

PHYSICAL EXAMINATION

- Vital signs: blood pressure, 140/88 mm Hg; heart rate, 90 beats/min; temperature, 98.6° F (37° C); respirations, 12 breaths/min
- General: obese white woman in no acute distress
- Neck: 40 cm (16 in) in circumference
- Lungs: clear breath sounds bilaterally
- Heart: regular rate and rhythm, increased second heart sound (P_2)
- Abdomen: obese, soft, normal bowel sounds
- Extremities: 2-mm pretibial pitting edema

LABORATORY DATA

- Chest radiograph: mildly enlarged heart, no mass, infiltrate, or effusion
- ECG: normal sinus rhythm with P pulmonale
- Left heart catheterization: no significant coronary artery disease, normal left ventricular function
- Right heart catheterization: pulmonary hypertension (75/25 mm Hg); pulmonary artery wedge pressure, 23 mm Hg
- Room air arterial blood gases: pH, 7.45; Pco_2, 41 mm Hg; Po_2, 54 mm Hg; Sao_2, 84%
- Spirometry: forced vital capacity (FVC), 1.69 L (55% of predicted value); FEV_1, 1.27 L (55% of predicted value); FEV_1/FVC, 75; forced expiratory flow, midexpiratory phase ($FEF_{25\%-75\%}$), 0.96 L/s (37% of predicted value); no significant improvement with a single-dose bronchodilator

What is the cause of the pulmonary hypertension?

DISCUSSION

The pulmonary service is consulted for evaluation for pulmonary hypertension in association with abnormal spirometric results. Results of bilateral lower extremity Doppler examinations and a ventilation/perfusion scan are normal. Because of a history of snoring, an overnight portable cardiopulmonary sleep study is performed. The study reveals evidence of snoring, nonpositional apnea and hypopnea, and desaturation to less than 60% on the oximeter for most of the monitoring period. Results of an "in-lab" PSG verify the presence of moderate to severe OSA, which responds well to the application of CPAP. Follow-up examinations show the dyspnea is relieved and arterial blood gas values have improved. The patient no longer needs portable liquid oxygen to maintain oxygen saturation greater than 90% at rest or with exercise.

It is unlikely this patient has primary pulmonary hypertension, which generally affects younger women. Chronic thromboembolic disease should be excluded, as it was in this case. Chronic right heart failure due to sleep apnea will be relieved with proper treatment.

Unlike conventional CPAP, BiPAP is titrated by increasing inspiratory positive airway pressure (IPAP) and expiratory positive airway pressure (EPAP) separately in response to apnea, hypopnea, and desaturation. Although the specific algorithm may vary from laboratory to laboratory, in general, IPAP is increased above the level of EPAP (usually in increments of 2.5 cm H_2O) in response to apnea or hypopnea that occur when both pressures are equal. If apnea or hypopnea occurs after IPAP has been increased over EPAP, the EPAP is increased. For snoring, arousals, and nonapneic oxygen desaturation, IPAP is increased.

Positive-Pressure Therapy: Autotitrating Devices

A new generation of self-titrating CPAP devices have been developed to address the issues of patient compliance, patient comfort, and the requirements for changes in upper airway pressure throughout the night.[72-74] These devices are referred to as "auto-CPAP," "intelligent CPAP," or "smart CPAP." Use of these devices entails a computer algorithm for adjusting CPAP pressure in real time when abnormal upper airway functioning is detected. Abnormal function manifests as snoring, hypopnea, and apnea. These devices may reduce the average overnight pressure required to treat patients and may minimize interface-related leaks because of the lower overall pressures required. It remains to be seen whether these devices are capable of eliminating the need for standard CPAP titration in a sleep laboratory. Self-titrating devices may be useful in facilitating therapeutic CPAP titrations by technologists in the sleep laboratory. Further studies are needed to determine whether self-titrating CPAP devices provide any improvement over conventional CPAP units in the areas of compliance and EDS .

Positive-Pressure Therapy: Side Effects and Troubleshooting Strategies

Side effects of positive-pressure therapy are related to the interface and to the pressure prescribed. These effects

MINI CLINI

Worsening Right-Sided Heart Failure in a Patient With COPD Who Is Using Oxygen

HISTORY

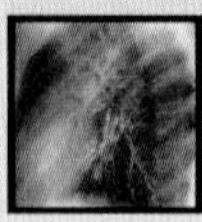

A 50-year-old former smoker previously found to have severe COPD, FEV_1 0.9 L (30% of predicted value), is admitted to the hospital for evaluation and management of worsening shortness of breath and persistent bilateral leg swelling. He has been using oxygen at 2 L/min 24 hours per day for the last 3 months. A chronic productive cough of clear sputum has been unchanged. He denies having chest pain.

MEDICATIONS

- Ipratropium bromide by metered dose inhaler 4 puffs 4 times a day
- Oxygen 2 L/min 24 hours per day
- Hydrochlorothiazide 50 mg by mouth daily
- Theophylline 300 mg by mouth twice a day

MEDICAL HISTORY

Hypertension and chronic bronchitis. No cardiac disease.

PHYSICAL EXAMINATION

- Vital signs: blood pressure, 150/90 mm Hg; heart rate, 100 beats/min; temperature, 98.6° F (37° C); respirations, 18 breaths/min
- General: obese white man who appears short of breath
- Neck: 46 cm (18 in) in circumference
- Lungs: decreased breath sounds bilaterally
- Heart: faint sounds but regular rate and rhythm
- Abdomen: obese, soft, normal bowel sounds
- Extremities: "dusky" lower extremities with 4-mm pitting edema to the knees

LABORATORY DATA

- Theophylline level, 12 μg/mL
- Arterial blood gases: pH, 7.36; Pco_2 44 mm Hg; Po_2 56 mm Hg; Sao_2, 89% (on 2 L/min oxygen)
- Chest radiograph: "pulmonary congestion"; otherwise normal
- ECG: sinus tachycardia without acute changes
- Echocardiogram: "technically limited" but reported to be without segmental wall abnormalities or to demonstrate normal left ventricular function
- Bilateral lower extremity Doppler examination: negative for deep venous thrombosis

What could be the cause of this patient's continued signs of right heart failure?

DISCUSSION

The patient has overlap syndrome (COPD and OSA). He has been appropriately treated for COPD (bronchodilators and oxygen) but has not been treated for sleep apnea. His physician never asked and the patient never volunteered a history of nightly loud snoring with observed apnea and daytime fatigue. Subsequent evaluation with nocturnal PSG reveals severe nocturnal desaturation to 40% on the oximeter despite treatment with oxygen at 2 L/min. A CPAP titration study is performed. The patient is discharged with CPAP set at 15 cm H_2O through a nasal mask. Three months later, he returns to the outpatient clinic "feeling great." He reports that the shortness of breath has decreased and that he has much more energy during the day. Physical examination shows trace pedal edema. Arterial blood gas studies on 2 L/min of oxygen reveal pH, 7.40; Pco_2, 40 mm Hg; Po_2, 75 mm Hg; Sao_2, 93%.

include feelings of claustrophobia, nasal congestion, rhinorrhea, skin irritation, and nasal dryness (Figure 27-4). Claustrophobia and skin irritation can be managed by changing the interface to one that is more easily tolerated by the patient. Nasal congestion, rhinorrhea, skin irritation, and nasal dryness can be managed by use of combinations of topical nasal steroids, antihistamines, nasal saline sprays, and lotions. A humidifier can be used in-line with the machine. Heated humidification can assist with compliance.[75] If the patient has a sensation of too much pressure in the nose, adding a system equipped with a ramp may prove beneficial.[55] The ramp allows a gradual increase in pressure over 5 to 45 minutes. The ramp time is empirically determined by the prescribing physician. There is no objective evidence that ramps improve patient acceptance or compliance.[76]

Another problem respiratory therapists encounter is pressure leaks. Most interfaces are of the nasal variety. Some patients tend to breathe partially or mainly through the mouth. The addition of a chin strap may not resolve the problem. Changing the interface to an oral-nasal mask may be required for effective "pressurization" of the upper airway in these patients.[12]

Oral Appliances

Oral appliances are devices that enlarge the airway by moving the mandible forward or by keeping the tongue in an anterior position (Figure 27-5). Patients who have mild sleep apnea and are unwilling to use CPAP may benefit from these devices. Oral appliances are worn only during sleep and come in a variety of forms. The appliances are custom fitted by dentists and are generally well tolerated by patients. They are overall less effective than CPAP therapy and therefore are regarded as a second-line intervention.[77]

Medications

Medications have proved ineffective for most patients with sleep apnea. Benzodiazepines and other sedative hypnotics should be avoided, because they can potentiate upper airway collapse. The antidepressants pro-

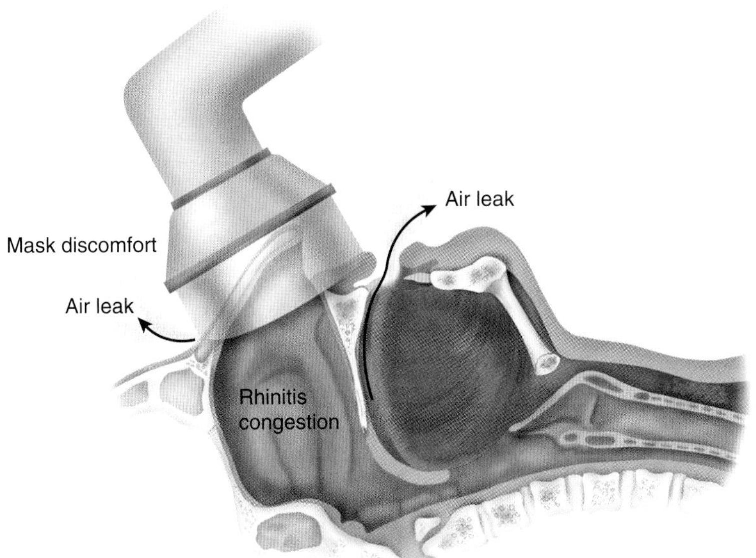

Figure 27-4 · Positive Airway Pressure Problems
A variety of problems encountered with CPAP.

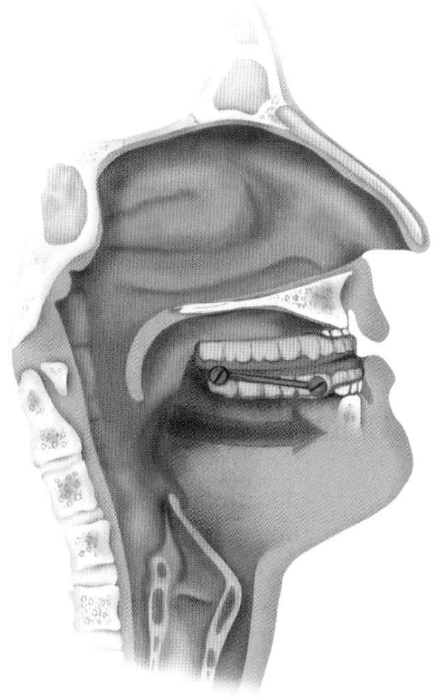

Figure 27-5 · Oral Appliance
The oral appliance covers the teeth of the upper and lower jaws and is adjusted to mechanically move the mandible (lower jaw) forward to open the airway.

triptyline and fluoxetine have been used to manage mild sleep apnea but are ineffective in most patients.[21] Oxygen therapy is useful for patients with oxyhemoglobin desaturation who refuse positive-pressure therapy. Oxygen therapy can improve nocturnal desaturation but has no significant effect on ventilatory arousals and daytime sleepiness.[78] Oxygen therapy should be used with caution by patients with concomitant COPD, who may retain carbon dioxide.

Box 27-5 • Obstructive Sleep Apnea: Surgical Alternatives

- Bypass of the upper airway
- Tracheostomy
- Reconstruction of the upper airway
- Nasal surgery
- Palatal surgery
- Maxillofacial surgery

Surgical Interventions

Surgical alternatives can be divided into two broad categories: procedures that bypass the upper airway and procedures that reconstruct the upper airway (Box 27-5). Before the advent of CPAP therapy, tracheostomy was the primary therapy for severe OSA. Because of the psychosocial and medical morbidity associated with the procedure, use of tracheostomy today is limited to management of severe OSA when all other therapy has been exhausted.[79, 80]

Palatal Surgery

Uvulopalatopharyngoplasty (UPPP) is palatal surgery performed with a standard "cold knife" technique and a laser. In these procedures, portions of the soft palate, the uvula, and additional redundant tissue are removed. The success rate of UPPP is less than 50% overall, less among obese patients.[81] The site of the physiological obstruction cannot be predicted correctly with preoperative imaging. Laser-assisted UPPP has been marketed as an outpatient procedure; however, substantial efficacy in the management of OSA has not been documented.

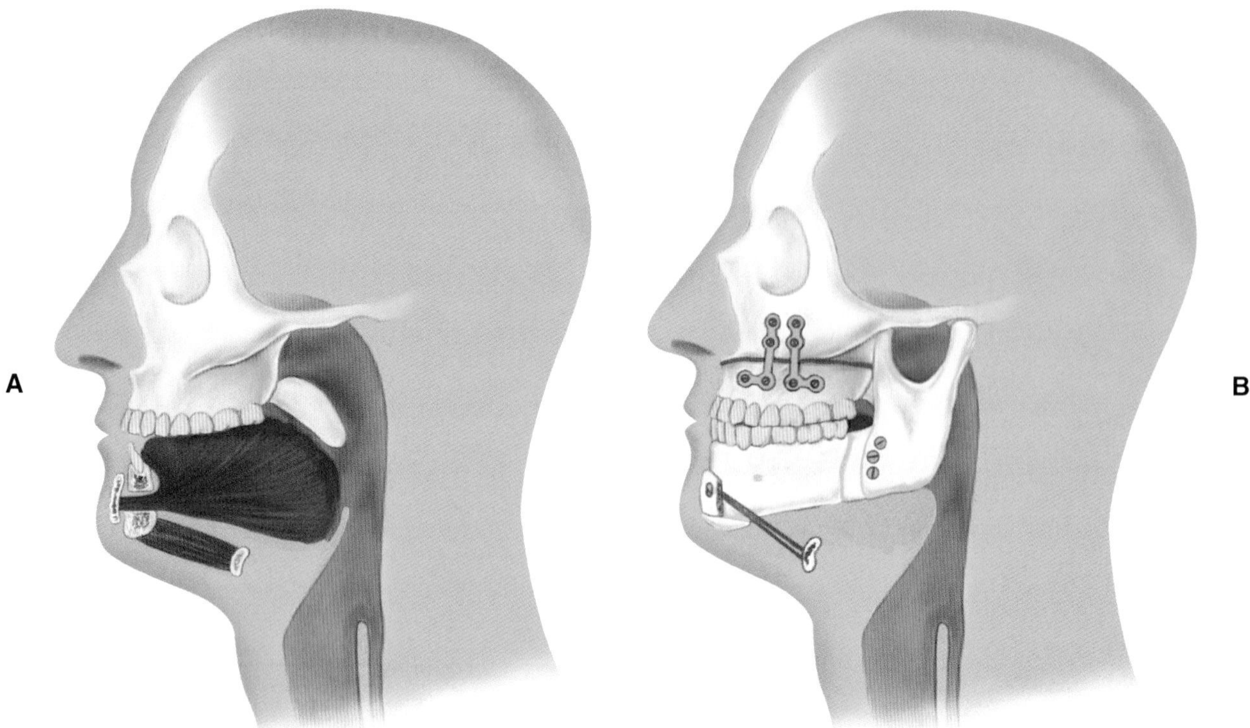

Figure 27-6 · Phase I and Phase II Upper Airway Reconstruction

A, Phase I surgery. Lateral cutaway view of the skull shows tongue (genioglossal) and hyoid bone advancement in conjunction with UPPP. **B,** Phase II surgery. Lateral cutaway view of the skull shows advancement of the maxilla (upper jaw) and mandible (lower jaw) in a patient who has undergone a phase I procedure.

This surgery cannot currently be recommended for the management of OSA.[82,83]

Maxillofacial Surgery

Maxillofacial surgery shows more promise for patients with OSA (Figure 27-6). Phase I surgical procedures combine UPPP with genioglossal advancement and resuspension of the hyoid bone. These patients are identified preoperatively with a combination of radiologic imaging and direct visualization of the upper airway during sleep. It is beneficial to have these patients use CPAP therapy perioperatively to reduce the chronic upper airway swelling and edema present before surgery and to reduce postoperative airway edema.[84] When phase I surgery is unsuccessful, phase II surgery involves advancement of the maxilla and the mandible.[83,85] These surgical procedures are performed at only a few specialized centers. A coordinated effort by a dedicated team of otolaryngologists, oral surgeons, and sleep specialists is essential. Regardless of the surgical option chosen, a formal PSG should be obtained before surgery and several weeks after for assessment of the effectiveness of the procedure.[83]

▶ CONCLUSIONS

Assessment, patient education, initiation of therapy, continued monitoring, and reassessment are critical. These needs are best met by a core of dedicated professionals. Respiratory therapists can play an invaluable role as members of the sleep medicine team.

KEY POINTS

- There are three types of sleep apnea: obstructive, central, and mixed, of which OSA is the most common.
- Obstructive sleep apnea is common, underdiagnosed, and controllable.
- The predominant risk factor for airway narrowing or closure during sleep is a small or unstable upper airway.

KEY POINTS—cont'd

- The shift in physiological state from wakefulness to sleep results in partial or complete airway closure at several sites in the upper airway of patients at risk of OSA.
- The long-term adverse consequences of OSA include poor daytime functioning and increased risk of cardiovascular morbidity and mortality.
- Risk factors for OSA include male sex, age older than 40 years, upper body obesity (neck size >16.5 in), habitual snoring, and diurnal hypertension.
- A formal PSG is the best way to make the diagnosis of OSA. This test measures several physiological variables and allows for the staging of sleep and measurement of airflow, ventilatory effort, ECG, and oxygen saturation.
- First-line medical therapy for OSA is CPAP. This modality is almost always effective in the laboratory, although long-term compliance with therapy may be less than optimal.
- Bilevel positive airway pressure therapy may be useful in salvaging selected patients who have difficulty accepting or complying with CPAP.
- The role of "auto-titrating" CPAP devices in the management of OSA remains to be defined.
- Surgical therapy may be an option for a select group of patients who have undergone an extensive preoperative analysis of the upper airway and do not accept or comply poorly with medical therapy. Optimal management of OSA, regardless of the modality, requires patient education, continued monitoring, and reassessment.

References

1. Haponik EF et al: Challenges for primary care physicians, J Gen Intern Med 11:759, 1996.
2. Young T et al: The occurrence of sleep-disordered breathing among middle-aged adults, N Engl J Med 328:1230, 1993.
3. Lavie P: Incidence of sleep apnea in a presumably healthy working population: a significant relationship with excessive daytime sleepiness, Sleep 6:312, 1983.
4. American Thoracic Society: Indications and standards for use of nasal continuous positive airway pressure (CPAP) in sleep apnea syndromes, Am J Respir Crit Care Med 150:1738, 1994.
5. Guilleminault C et al: From obstructive sleep apnea syndrome to upper airway resistance syndrome: consistency of daytime sleepiness, Sleep 15:S13, 1992.
6. Martin TJ, Sanders MH: Chronic alveolar hypoventilation: a review for the clinician, Sleep 18:617, 1995.
7. Bradley TD, Phillipson EA: Breathing disorders in sleep: central sleep apnea, Clin Chest Med 13:493, 1992.
8. Meoli A: Hypopnea in sleep-disordered breathing in adults, Sleep 24:469, 2001.
9. Moser NJ et al: What is hypopnea anyway? Chest 105:426, 1994.
10. Lowe A: The tongue and airway, Otolaryngol Clin North Am 23:677, 1990.
11. Rivlin J et al: Upper airway morphology in patients with idiopathic obstructive sleep apnea, Am Rev Respir Dis 129:355, 1984.
12. Sanders MH et al: CPAP therapy via oronasal mask for obstructive sleep apnea, Chest 106:774, 1994.
13. Launois SH et al: Pharyngeal narrowing and closing pressures in patients with obstructive sleep apnea, Am Rev Respir Dis 148:606,1993.
14. He J et al: Mortality and apnea index in obstructive sleep apnea: experience in 385 male patients, Chest 94:9, 1988.
15. Yamashiro Y, Kryger MH: Why should sleep apnea be diagnosed and treated? Clin Pulm Med 1:250, 1994.
16. Dimsdale JE et al: Sympathetic nervous system alterations in sleep apnea: the relative importance of respiratory disturbance, hypoxia, and sleep quality, Chest 111:639, 1997.
17. Shahar E, et al: Sleep- disordered breathing and cardiovascular disease: cross sectional results of the Sleep Heart Health Study, Am J Respir Crit Care Med 163:19, 2001.
18. Weiss JW et al: Hemodynamic consequences of obstructive sleep apnea, Sleep 19:388, 1996.
19. Ringler J et al: Hypoxemia alone does not explain blood pressure elevations after obstructive sleep apneas, J Appl Physiol 69:2143, 1990.
20. Suzuki M et al: Blood pressure "dipping" and "non-dipping" in obstructive sleep apnea syndrome patients, Sleep 19:382, 1996.
21. Strollo PJ, Rogers RM: Obstructive sleep apnea, N Engl J Med 334:99, 1996.
22. Laks L et al: Pulmonary hypertension in obstructive sleep apnea, Eur Respir J 8:537, 1995.
23. Ursula C: Echocardiographic features of the right heart in sleep-disordered breathing, Am J Respir Crit Care Med 164:933, 2001.
24. Block AJ et al: Sleep apnea, hypopnea and oxygen desaturation in normal subjects: a strong male predominance, N Engl J Med 300:513, 1979.
25. Wittels EH, Thompson S: Obstructive sleep apnea and obesity, Otolaryngol Clin North Am 23:751, 1990.
26. Mathur R, Douglas NJ: Family studies in patients with the sleep apnea-hypopnea syndrome, Ann Intern Med 122:174, 1995.
27. Fletcher EC, Schaaf JW, Miller J: Long-term cardiopulmonary sequelae in patients with sleep apnea and chronic lung disease, Am Rev Respir Dis 135:525, 1987.
28. Cheshire K et al: Factors impairing daytime performance in patients with sleep apnea/hypopnea syndrome, Arch Intern Med 152:538, 1992.

29. Guilleminault C et al: A cause of excessive daytime sleepiness: the upper airway resistance syndrome, Chest 104:781, 1993.
30. Roehrs T et al: Predictors of objective level of daytime sleepiness in patients with sleep-related breathing disorders, Chest 95:1202, 1989.
31. Engleman HM et al: Effect of continuous positive airway pressure treatment on daytime function in sleep apnea/hypopnea syndrome, Lancet 343:572, 1994.
32. Findley LJ, Unverzagt ME, Suratt PM: Automobile accidents involving patients with obstructive sleep apnea, Am Rev Respir Dis 138:337, 1998.
33. George CFP: Sleep apnea and automobile crashes, Sleep 22:790, 1999.
34. Teran Santos J: The association between sleep apnea and the risk of traffic accidents, N Engl J Med 340:847, 1999.
35. Blankfield RP: Bilateral leg edema, obesity, pulmonary hypertension and obstructive sleep apnea, Arch Intern Med 160:2357, 2000.
36. Weitzenblum E et al: The obesity in hypoventilation syndrome revisited: a prospective study of 34 consecutive cases, Chest 120:369, 2001.
37. McNicholas W: Impact of sleep in chronic obstructive pulmonary disease, Chest 117 (suppl 2):48S, 2000.
38. Condos R et al: Flow limitation as a noninvasive assessment of residual upper-airway resistance during continuous positive airway pressure therapy of obstructive sleep apnea, Am J Respir Crit Care Med 150:475, 1994.
39. American Academy of Sleep Medicine Task Force: Sleep-related breathing disorders in adults: recommendations for syndrome definition and measurement techniques in clinical research, Sleep 22:667,1999.
40. Stiller RA, Strollo PJ, Sanders MH: Unattended recording in the diagnosis and treatment of sleep-disordered breathing: unproven accuracy, untested assumptions, and unready for routine use, Chest 105:1306, 1994.
41. Ferber R et al: Portable recording in the assessment of obstructive sleep apnea: ASDA standards and practice, Sleep 17:378, 1994.
42. Krol RC, Knuth SL, Bartlett D: Selective reduction of genioglossal muscle activity by alcohol in normal human subjects, Am Rev Respir Dis 129:247, 1984.
43. Scrima L et al: Increased severity of obstructive sleep apnea after bedtime alcohol ingestion: diagnostic potential and proposed mechanism of action, Sleep 5:318, 1982.
44. Dolly FR, Block AJ: Effect of flurazepam on sleep-disordered breathing and nocturnal oxygen desaturation in asymptomatic subjects, Am J Med 73:239, 1982.
45. Sullivan CE et al: Reversal of obstructive sleep apnea by continuous positive pressure applied through the nares, Lancet 1:862, 1981.
46. Sforza E, Lugaresi E: Daytime sleepiness and nasal continuous positive airway pressure therapy in obstructive sleep apnea syndrome patients: effect of chronic treatment and 1-night therapy withdrawal, Sleep 18:195, 1995.
47. Sanders MH: Nasal CPAP effect on patterns of sleep apnea, Chest 86:839, 1984.
48. Rajagopal KR et al: Overnight nasal CPAP improves hypersomnolence in sleep apnea, Chest 90:172, 1986.
49. Montplaisir J et al: Neurobehavioral manifestations in obstructive sleep apnea syndrome before and after treatment with continuous positive airway pressure, Sleep 15:S17, 1992.
50. Lamphere J et al: Recovery of alertness after CPAP in apnea, Chest 96:1364, 1989.
51. Hoffstein V et al: Treatment of obstructive sleep apnea with nasal CPAP: Patients' compliance, perception of benefits, and side effects, Am Rev Respir Dis 145:841, 1992.
52. Nino-Murcia G et al: Compliance and side effects in sleep apnea patients treated with nasal continuous positive airway pressure, West J Med 150:165, 1989.
53. Sanders MH, Gruendl CA, Rogers RM: Patient compliance with nasal CPAP therapy for sleep apnea, Chest 90:330, 1986.
54. Strollo PJ et al: Predicting the positive pressure prescription in sleep apnea/hypopnea, Am J Respir Crit Care Med 151:A155, 1995.
55. Miljetig H, Hoffstein V: Determinants of continuous positive airway pressure level for treatment of obstructive sleep apnea, Am Rev Respir Dis 147:1526, 1993.
56. Leech JA, Onal E, Lopata M: Nasal CPAP continues to improve sleep-disordered breathing and daytime oxygenation over long-term follow-up of occlusive sleep apnea syndrome, Chest 102:1651, 1992.
57. Strollo PJ, Sanders MH, Stiller RA: Continuous and bilevel positive airway pressure therapy in sleep disordered breathing, Oral Maxillofac Surg Clin North Am 7:221, 1995.
58. Strohl KP, Redline S: Nasal CPAP therapy, upper airway activation and obstructive sleep apnea, Am Rev Respir Dis 134:555, 1986.
59. Grunstein RR: Sleep-related breathing disorders, 5: nasal continuous positive airway pressure treatment for obstructive sleep apnoea, Thorax 50:1106, 1995.
60. Sforza E et al: Determinants of effective continuous positive airway pressure in obstructive sleep apnea, Am J Respir Crit Care Med 151:1852, 1995.
61. Guilleminault C, Stoohs R, Duncan S: Snoring: daytime sleepiness in regular heavy snorers, Chest 99:40, 1991.
62. Montserrat JM et al: Time-course of stepwise CPAP titration, Am J Respir Crit Care Med 152:1854, 1995.
63. Kribbs NB et al: Objective measurement of patterns of nasal CPAP use by patients with obstructive sleep apnea, Am Rev Respir Dis 147:887, 1993.
64. Kribbs NB, Getsy JE: Patient compliance with CPAP therapy, Clin Pulm Med 2:180, 1995.
65. McCardle N: Long term use of CPAP therapy for sleep apnea/hypopnea syndrome, Am J Respir Crit Care Med 159:1108, 1999.
66. Sanders MH, Kern N: Obstructive sleep apnea treated by independently adjusted inspiratory and expiratory positive airway pressure via nasal mask: physiological and clinical implications, Chest 98:317, 1990.
67. Prosise GL, Berry RB: Oral-nasal continuous positive airway pressure as a treatment for obstructive sleep apnea, Chest 106:180, 1994.
68. Criner GJ et al: Efficacy of a new full face mask for non-invasive positive pressure ventilation, Chest 106:1109, 1994.

69. Mayer LS, Kerby GR, Whitman RA: Evaluation of a new nasal device for administration of continuous positive airway pressure for obstructive sleep apnea, Am Rev Respir Dis 139:A114, 1989.
70. Harris C et al: Comparison of cannula and mask systems for administration of nasal continuous positive airway pressure for treatment of obstructive sleep apnea, Sleep Res 19:233, 1990 (abstract).
71. Reeves-Hoche MK, Meck R, Zwillich CW : Nasal CPAP: an objective evaluation of patient compliance, Am J Respir Crit Care Med 149:149, 1994.
72. Scharf MB, et al: Evaluation of automatic adjustable nasal positive airway pressure versus standard nasal continuous positive airway pressure. Presented at the Ninth Annual Meeting of the Association of Professional Sleep Societies, May 31-June 4, 1995, Nashville.
73. Sharma S et al: Evaluation of a self-titrating continuous positive airway pressure (CPAP) system. Presented at the Ninth Annual Meeting of the Association of Professional Sleep Societies, May 31-June 4, 1995, Nashville.
74. Meurice JC, Marc I, Series F: Efficacy of auto-CPAP in the treatment of obstructive sleep apnea/hypopnea syndrome, Am J Respir Crit Care Med 153:794, 1996.
75. Fleury B et al. Predictive factors for the need for additional humidification during nasal continuous positive airway pressure therapy, Chest 199:460, 2001.
76. Rosen R et al: Compliance with continuous positive airway pressure therapy: assessing and improving treatment outcomes, Curr Opin Pulm Med 7:391, 2001.
77. Schmidt-Nowara W et al: Oral appliances for the treatment of snoring and obstructive sleep apnea: a review, Sleep 18:501, 1995.
78. Fletcher EC, Munafo DA: Role of nocturnal oxygen therapy in obstructive sleep apnea: when should it be used? Chest 98:1497, 1990.
79. Guilleminault C et al: Obstructive sleep apnea syndrome and tracheostomy: long-term follow up experience, Arch Intern Med 141:985, 1981.
80. Conway WA et al: Adverse effect of tracheostomy for sleep apnea, JAMA 246:347, 1981.
81. Sher AE: The efficacy of surgical modifications of the upper airway in adults with obstructive sleep apnoea syndrome, Sleep 19:156, 1996.
82. Sher AE: Uvulopalatopharyngoplasty, Oral Maxillofac Surg Clin North Am 7:293, 1995.
83. Sher AE: When is upper airway surgery appropriate for obstructive sleep apnea? Clin Pulm Med 3:78, 1996.
84. Johnson NT, Chinn J: Uvolopalatopharyngoplasty and inferior sagittal mandibular osteotomy with genioglossus advancement for treatment of obstructive sleep apnea, Chest 105:278, 1994.
85. Riley RW, Powell NB, Guilleminault C: Obstructive sleep apnea syndrome: a review of 306 consecutively treated surgical patients, Otolaryngol Head Neck Surg 108:117, 1993.

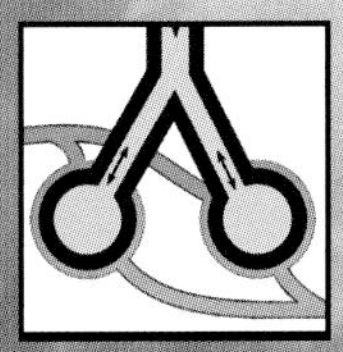

CHAPTER 28

Neonatal and Pediatric Respiratory Disorders

Douglas Deming and N. Lennard Specht

In This Chapter You Will Learn:

- How many infants are found to have respiratory distress syndrome (RDS) each year in the United States
- How RDS alters gas exchange in the lung
- What clinical findings and radiographic abnormalities are seen in RDS
- How to treat the patient with RDS
- What clinical manifestations are seen in transient tachypnea of the newborn (TTN)
- How to treat an infant with TTN
- How meconium aspiration syndrome occurs
- How meconium aspiration syndrome alters lung function and pulmonary hemodynamic values
- What clinical findings are typical of meconium aspiration syndrome (MAS)
- What treatment modalities are used to manage MAS
- How bronchopulmonary dysplasia (BPD) develops in the preterm infant
- What clinical signs and symptoms are seen in BPD
- How to treat an infant with BPD
- What etiologic factors are associated with apnea of prematurity
- How to treat infants with apnea of prematurity
- How persistent pulmonary hypertension of the newborn (PPHN) occurs and the three fundamental types
- How to diagnose PPHN and the treatment to apply
- What pathological changes are seen with congenital diaphragmatic hernia
- What anatomic defects are associated with tetralogy of Fallot
- How ventricular septal defect manifests clinically
- How many infants die of sudden infant death syndrome (SIDS) each year in the United States
- What epidemiologic factors are associated with increased risk of SIDS
- What respiratory problems are associated with gastroesophageal reflux disease
- What clinical findings are common in cases of bronchiolitis
- How to care for an infant with bronchiolitis
- What clinical features are seen in children with croup
- How to treat a child with croup
- What clinical manifestations are commonly seen with epiglottitis
- How to treat a patient with epiglottitis
- How many people in the United States have cystic fibrosis
- What clinical manifestations are common in patients with cystic fibrosis
- How to treat a patient with cystic fibrosis

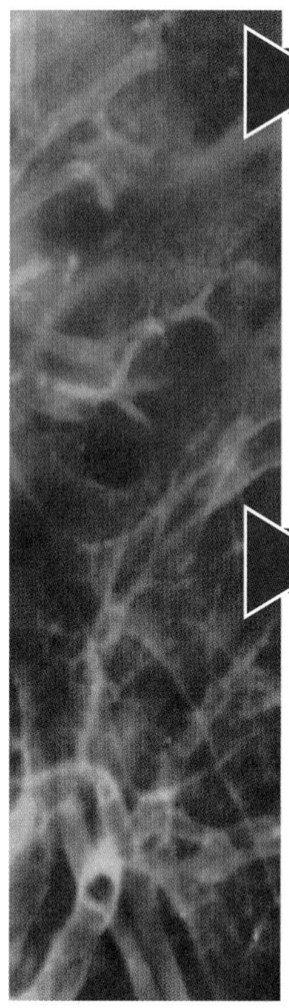

Chapter Outline

Neonatal Respiratory Disorders
- Lung parenchymal disease
- Control of breathing
- Pulmonary vascular disease
- Congenital abnormalities affecting respiration
- Congenital heart disease

Pediatric Respiratory Disorders
- Sudden infant death syndrome
- Gastroesophageal reflux disease
- Bronchiolitis
- Croup
- Epiglottitis
- Cystic fibrosis

Key Terms

apnea of prematurity
bronchiolitis
bronchopulmonary dysplasia
croup
cystic fibrosis
ductus arteriosus
epiglottitis
foramen ovale
meconium aspiration syndrome (MAS)
nasal flaring
neutral thermal environment
persistent pulmonary hypertension of the newborn (PPHN)
respiratory distress syndrome (RDS)
retractions
sudden infant death syndrome (SIDS)
tetralogy of Fallot
transient tachypnea of the newborn (TTN)
transposition of the great arteries

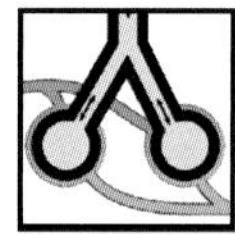

Many perinatal disorders affect the respiratory system. Some disorders are developmental abnormalities of the heart, lungs, or airways; some are caused by prematurity, some by problems during labor and delivery, and some by treatment. Common disorders in the neonatal period are meconium aspiration syndrome, respiratory distress syndrome, transient tachypnea of the newborn, apnea of prematurity, bronchopulmonary dysplasia, persistent pulmonary hypertension, and congenital cardiopulmonary abnormalities.

▶ NEONATAL RESPIRATORY DISORDERS

Lung Parenchymal Disease

Respiratory Distress Syndrome

Background. Neonatal respiratory distress syndrome (RDS) affects 60,000 to 70,000 infants each year in the United States. Although the death rate has decreased dramatically over the last three decades, many infants still die or have chronic effects of the syndrome. Respiratory distress syndrome, or hyaline membrane disease, is a disease of prematurity. The incidence increases with decreasing gestational age. The major factors in the pathophysiology of RDS are qualitative surfactant deficiency, decreased alveolar surface area, increased small airways compliance, and the presence of the ductus arteriosus.

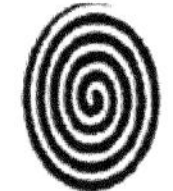

RULE OF THUMB

The incidence of RDS increases with decreasing gestational age.

Surfactant production depends on both the relative maturity of the lung and the adequacy of fetal perfusion. Maternal factors that impair fetal blood flow, such as abruptio placentae and maternal diabetes, also may lead to RDS.

Pathophysiology. In preterm infants adequate amounts of surfactant are present in the lung; however, the surfactant is trapped inside type II cells. In infants with RDS, type II cells do not release adequate amounts of surfactant. The surfactant that is released is incomplete in formation, so it does not make tubular myelin and thus does not cause a decrease in alveolar surface tension.

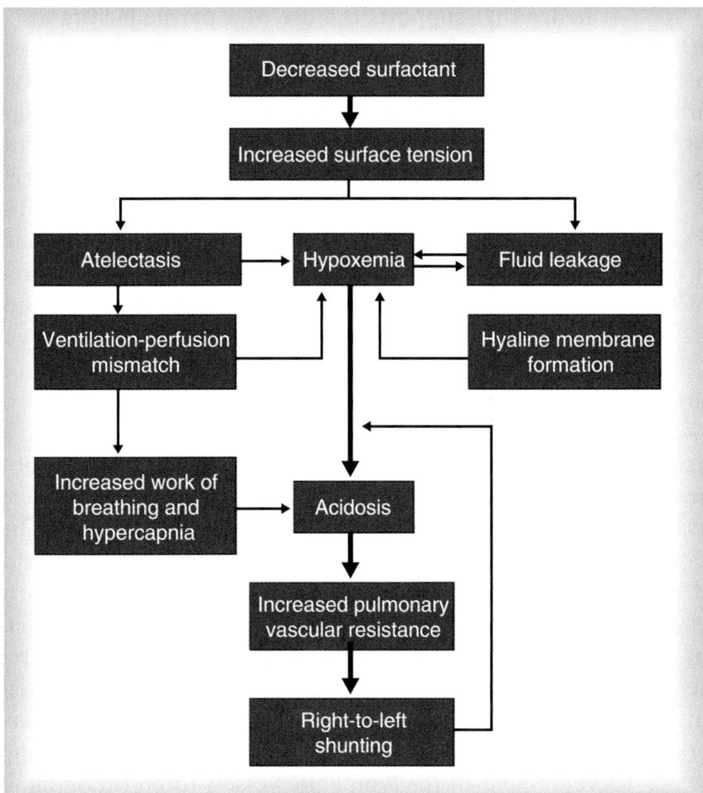

Figure 28-1
Clinical progression of hyaline membrane disease.

Because the surfactant molecule in the alveolus is structurally not normal, the type II cells and alveolar macrophages have more rapid uptake for recycling. Thus there is a qualitative deficiency of alveolar surfactant.

Figure 28-1 outlines the pathophysiologic events associated with RDS. A qualitative decrease in surfactant increases alveolar surface tension forces. This process causes alveoli to become unstable and collapse and leads to atelectasis and increased work of breathing. At the same time, the increased surface tension draws fluid from the pulmonary capillaries into the alveoli. In combination these factors impair oxygen exchange and cause severe hypoxemia. The severe hypoxemia and acidosis increase pulmonary vascular resistance (PVR). As pulmonary arterial pressure increases, extrapulmonary right-to-left shunting increases, and hypoxemia worsens. Hypoxia and acidosis also impair further surfactant production.

Clinical Manifestations. The first signs of respiratory distress in infants with RDS usually occur soon after birth. Tachypnea usually occurs first. After tachypnea, worsening retractions, paradoxical breathing, and audible grunting are observed. Nasal flaring also may be seen. Chest auscultation often reveals fine inspiratory crackles. Cyanosis may or may not be present. If central cyanosis is observed, it is likely that the infant has severe hypoxemia. Certain other conditions, such as systemic

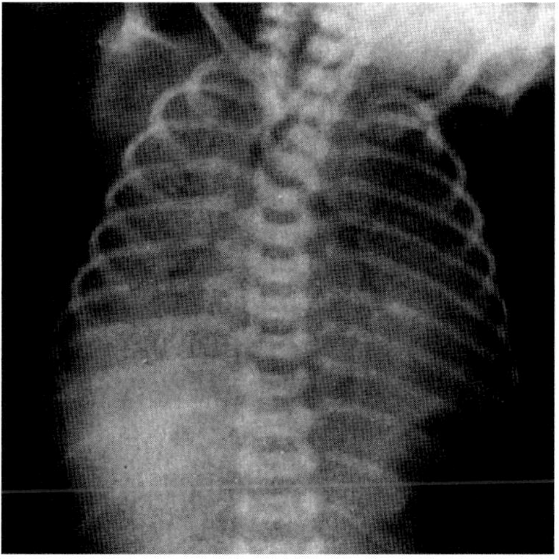

Figure 28-2
Radiopaque appearance of severe hyaline membrane disease. The lungs are dense. The cardiac shadow is barely discernible in the left side of the chest. Prominent black streaks emanating from both hilar areas are air bronchograms. *(From Korones SB: High-risk newborn infants: the basis for intensive nursing care, ed 4, St Louis, 1986, Mosby.)*

hypotension, hypothermia, and poor perfusion, can mimic this aspect of RDS.

Definitive diagnosis of RDS usually is made with chest radiography (Figure 28-2). Diffuse, hazy, reticulogranular densities with the presence of air bronchograms with low lung volumes are typical of RDS. The reticulogranular pattern is caused by aeration of respiratory bronchioles and collapse of the alveoli. Air bronchograms appear as aerated, dark, major bronchi surrounded by the collapsed or consolidated lung tissue.

Treatment. Continuous positive airway pressure (CPAP) and positive end-expiratory pressure (PEEP) are the traditional support modes used to manage RDS. Surfactant replacement therapy and high-frequency ventilation (HFV) have been added to these traditional approaches.[1] Unless the infant's condition is severe, a trial of nasal CPAP is indicated. Because of the hazards of endotracheal (ET) tubes, nasal prongs are preferred. If signs of respiratory distress persist after CPAP is started, the airway pressure should be raised in small increments (1-2 cm H_2O). If the infant's clinical condition deteriorates rapidly, a more aggressive approach is required. Endotracheal intubation should be performed under controlled conditions as an elective procedure. A trial of endotracheal CPAP with the same settings used for the nasal route may be tried before mechanical ventilation is considered. Endotracheal CPAP might provide better oxygenation than the nasal route, because there is less pressure leakage. If oxygenation does not improve with CPAP and a given fractional inspired oxygen concentration (F_{IO_2}), or if the patient is apneic or acidotic, mechanical ventilation with PEEP should be initiated.

The aim of mechanical ventilation for RDS is to prevent lung collapse and maintain alveolar inflation. In severe RDS, collapse of alveoli with every breath necessitates very high reinflation pressure. To prevent the need for this high reinflation pressure, use of end-tidal pressure is desirable.

Because of the relation between arterial partial pressure of carbon dioxide (Pa_{CO_2}) and functional residual capacity (FRC), Pa_{CO_2} is lowest when PEEP is used to optimize FRC. The time constant of the lungs in RDS is short, so the lung empties very quickly with each ventilator cycle. If alveolar ventilation is inadequate, either peak inspiratory pressure (PIP) or rate should be increased. For minimization of the potential for volutrauma, the PIP should be kept less than 30 cm H_2O for larger premature infants and even lower PIP for more immature infants.

Three surfactant preparations are being used in the United States for management of neonatal RDS: beractant (Survanta), calfactant (Infasurf), and poractant alfa (Curosurf).[2,3] Survanta and Infasurf are natural bovine surfactant extracts. Curosurf is a natural porcine surfactant extract. All of these preparations are liquid suspensions that are instilled directly into the trachea. The current standard of care is to deliver replacement surfactant to all infants with RDS. There is currently no evidence that supports the use of a particular brand of surfactant. Surfactant replacement therapy also is used as both a rescue treatment (of infants who already have RDS) and a prophylactic therapy (in the care of infants delivered prematurely).[4-6] Some centers use prophylactic surfactant replacement therapy in the care of all very small infants (<1500 g). Therapies aimed at decreasing pulmonary edema, improving cardiac output, and weaning from oxygen and high ventilator pressures are essential in the successful treatment of infants undergoing surfactant therapy.[6]

Transient Tachypnea of the Newborn

Background. Transient tachypnea of the newborn (TTN), often called type II RDS, is probably the most common respiratory disorder of the newborn. The cause of TTN is unclear, but it is most likely related to delayed clearance of fetal lung liquid.[7] During most births, approximately two thirds of this fluid is expelled by thoracic squeeze in the birth canal; the rest is reabsorbed through the lymphatic vessels during initial breathing. These mechanisms are impaired in infants born by cesarean section or infants with incomplete development of the lymphatic vessels (preterm or small for gestational age infants).[7] The residual lung fluid causes an increase in airway resistance and an overall decrease in lung compliance. Because compliance is low, the infant must generate more negative pleural pressure to breathe. This process can result in hyperinflation of some areas and air-trapping in others. Most infants with TTN are born at term without any specific predisposing factors in common. Mothers of neonates who have TTN tend to have longer labor intervals and a higher incidence of failure to progress in labor, which leads to cesarean delivery.[7] In many cases, however, maternal history and labor and delivery are normal.

Clinical Manifestations. During the first few hours of life, infants with TTN breathe rapidly. Alveolar ventilation, as measured by arterial pH and partial pressure of carbon dioxide, usually is normal. The chest radiographic findings, which may initially be indistinguishable from those of pneumonia, are hyperinflation, which is secondary to air-trapping, and perihilar streaking. The perihilar streaking probably represents lymphatic engorgement. Pleural effusions may be evident in the costophrenic angles and interlobar fissures.

Treatment. Infants with TTN usually respond readily to a low F_{IO_2} by infant oxygen hood (Oxyhood) or nasal cannula. Infants requiring a higher F_{IO_2} may benefit from CPAP. Because the retention of lung fluid may be gravity dependent, frequent changes in the infant's position may help speed lung fluid clearance. Because

TTN and neonatal pneumonia have similar clinical signs, intravenous administration of antibiotics should be considered for at least 3 days after appropriate culture samples are obtained. The need for mechanical ventilation is rare and probably indicates a complication. Clearing of the lungs evident on both a chest radiograph and with clinical improvement usually occurs within 24 to 48 hours. A small number of infants with TTN eventually have persistent pulmonary hypertension.

Meconium Aspiration Syndrome

Background. Meconium aspiration syndrome (MAS) is a disease of term and near-term infants. It involves aspiration of meconium into the central airways of the lung. It usually is associated with perinatal depression and asphyxia.

Pathophysiology. Amniotic fluid consists mainly of fetal lung fluid, fetal urine, and transudate from the uterine wall. Meconium, the contents of the fetal intestine, occasionally is expelled from the fetus into the surrounding amniotic fluid. Meconium consists of mucopolysaccharides, cholesterol, bile acids and salts, intestinal enzymes, and other substances. Meconium normally is not passed until after delivery.[8] Infants who have marked perinatal depression or perinatal asphyxia may pass meconium in utero. Understanding of the pathophysiologic control mechanisms for the passage of meconium in utero is incomplete. It is widely accepted that infants can have meconium aspiration in utero. Amniotic fluid stained with meconium is found in approximately 12% of all births.[8] Meconium-stained amniotic fluid is rare among infants of less than 37 weeks' gestational age. The clinical syndrome develops in only 2 of every 1000 infants. Ninety-five percent of infants with inhaled meconium clear their lungs spontaneously.[8]

For many years, the aspirated meconium itself was considered the primary cause of the syndrome. Recent evidence suggests that the real causative agent is the fetal asphyxia that precedes aspiration.[8] Fetal asphyxia causes pulmonary vasospasm and hyperreactivity of the vasculature, which lead to persistent pulmonary hypertension.

Meconium aspiration syndrome involves three primary problems: pulmonary obstruction, lung tissue damage, and pulmonary hypertension.[9] Obstruction occurs because of plugging of the airways with particulate meconium. This obstruction often is of the ball-valve type, which allows gas entry but prevents gas exit. Ball-valve obstruction causes air-trapping and can lead to volutrauma (Figure 28-3). The lung tissue injury caused by MAS is chemical pneumonitis. Persistent pulmonary hypertension with intracardiac and extracardiac right-to-left shunting frequently complicates MAS.[8]

Clinical Manifestations. Before birth, thick meconium, fetal tachycardia, and absent fetal cardiac accelerations during labor are evidence that the fetus is at high risk of MAS.[10] If after delivery the infant has a low umbilical artery pH, an Apgar score less than 5, and meconium aspirated from the trachea, intensive care and close observation for MAS are warranted. Infants with MAS typically have gasping respirations, tachypnea, grunting, and retractions. The chest radiograph usually shows irregular pulmonary densities, which represent areas of atelectasis, and hyperlucent areas, which represent hyperinflation due to air-trapping. Arterial blood gases typically show hypoxemia with mixed respiratory and metabolic acidosis.[9] In the most severe cases there is right-to-left shunting and persistent pulmonary hypertension.[8]

Treatment. In the presence of meconium-stained amniotic fluid, the oropharynx should be suctioned as the

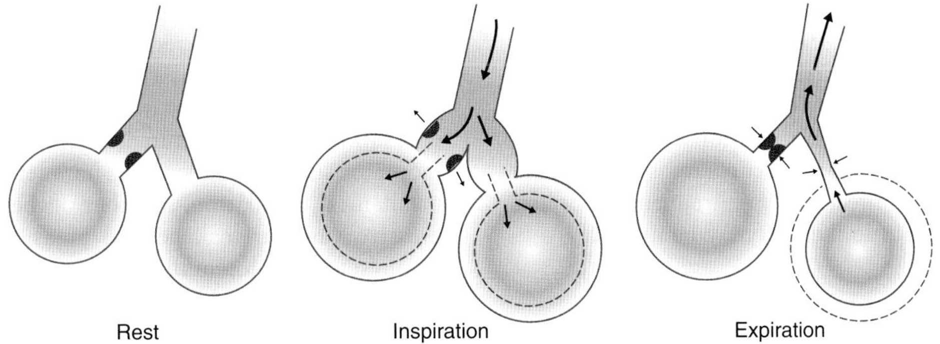

Figure 28-3 · Ball-Valve Effect

At rest the airway lumen is partially obstructed. With inspiration negative intrathoracic pressure opens the airway and relieves obstruction. Gas enters and expands the alveoli. With expiration, intrathoracic pressure changes to positive force, which narrows the airway and causes total occlusion. Gas cannot be expelled and is trapped within the alveoli. *(Modified from Koff PB, Eitzman DV, Neu J: Neonatal and pediatric care, ed 2, St. Louis, 1993, Mosby.)*

head presents during delivery, before the first breath is taken. Once delivery is complete and if the infant is depressed, an ET tube should be inserted immediately, and suction should be applied directly to the ET tube. The ET tube is removed and inspected for meconium. If meconium is present, the procedure is repeated with a new ET tube until no further meconium is aspirated or until two to four aspirations have been performed. The ET tube should be left in place, and mechanical ventilation should be started. For prevention of hypoxia, a flow of warmed 100% oxygen should be blown across the infant's face during the aspiration efforts. There is no evidence that suggests an improved outcome due to ET suctioning in the care of infants who have meconium and are vigorous.[11]

Should the infant's condition worsen, CPAP or mechanical ventilation may be indicated. Continuous positive airway pressure is indicated if the primary problem is hypoxemia. By distending the small airways, CPAP can sometimes overcome the ball-valve obstruction and improve both oxygenation and ventilation. On the other hand, if respiratory acidosis is severe or clinical assessment indicates excessive work in breathing, mechanical ventilation should be started. Figure 28-3 shows the ball-valve effect. At rest, the airway lumen is partially obstructed. With inspiration, negative intrathoracic pressure opens the airway and relieves the obstruction. Gas enters and expands the alveoli. With expiration, intrathoracic pressure changes to a positive force, which narrows the airway and causes total occlusion. Gas cannot be expelled and is trapped within the alveoli. It is difficult to provide ventilation to infants with severe MAS. These infants often retain carbon dioxide and need increased ventilator support. Because of high airways resistance, the lungs have a long time constant. High ventilator rates and pressures increase the risk of volutrauma, especially in the presence of trapping. Evidence suggests that both HFV and synchronous intermittent mechanical ventilation decrease the risk of air leak.[12] Various studies have shown improvement in MAS with the use of HFV and surfactant.[13] Nitric oxide has become a major adjunct in the management of persistent pulmonary hypertension.[14] High mean airway pressures may worsen pulmonary hypertension and aggravate right-to-left cardiac shunting.[10,15] Because pulmonary infections are frequent complications of MAS, antibiotic therapy may be needed.

Bronchopulmonary Dysplasia

Infants, especially preterm infants, with severe respiratory failure in the first few weeks of life may develop a chronic pulmonary condition called *bronchopulmonary dysplasia* (BPD). Immaturity, malnutrition, oxygen toxicity, and mechanical ventilation all have been implicated in the origin of BPD.[16-20]

Pathophysiology. The development of BPD is complex and involves many pathways. The initiating factors are related to atelectrauma (lung collapse) and volutrauma (large tidal volumes). *Atelectrauma* is the term coined to describe loss of alveolar volume that is both a consequence and a cause of lung injury. *Volutrauma* is the term used to describe local overinflation (and thus stretch) of airways and alveoli. Atelectrauma leads to derecuitment of the lung. Volutrauma leads to damage to airways, pulmonary capillary endothelium, alveolar and airway epithelium, and basement membranes. The combination of atelectrauma and volutrauma synergistically increases lung injury.

Both atelectrauma and volutrauma cause a need for increased supplemental oxygen concentrations. This use of supplemental oxygen leads to overproduction of superoxide, hydrogen peroxide, and perhydroxyl radicals. Preterm infants are particularly susceptible to oxygen radicals because the antioxidant systems are developed in the last trimester of pregnancy. Prolonged hyperoxia begins a sequence of lung injury that leads to inflammation, diffuse alveolar damage, pulmonary dysfunction, and death.

The response of the lungs to the combination of trauma and oxygen toxicity is the production and release of soluble mediators. These mediators probably are released from granulocytes resident in the lung. The release of these mediators can injure the alveolar-capillary barrier and induce an inflammatory response.[16]

A "new" BPD is being described that shows decreased alveolarization rather than the prominent airway damage of the "old" BPD. This change in the pathological characteristics of BPD is thought related to improvements in ventilator management, the use of surfactant, and processes that interrupt alveolar development (e.g., postnatal steroid therapy).

Clinical Manifestations. There are a variety of clinical manifestations of BPD. Some very immature infants may start with little or no oxygen requirement and little or no mechanical ventilation requirement. Progressive respiratory distress develops at approximately 2 to 3 weeks of life, and then the infant needs oxygen and mechanical ventilation. Other immature infants may begin with pneumonia or sepsis and need very high levels of oxygen and mechanical ventilation. In either of these scenarios, progressive vascular leakage and areas of atelectasis and emphysema develop in the lungs, and progressive pulmonary damage occurs. Arterial blood gas measurements reveal varying degrees of hypoxemia and hypercapnia secondary to airway obstruction, air trapping, pulmonary fibrosis, and atelectasis. There is a marked increase in airway resistance with an overall decrease in lung compliance.

Treatment. The best management of BPD is prevention. Prevention of atelectrauma and volutrauma begins in the delivery room. Establishment of an optimal FRC without overstretching the lung requires careful attention to detail in providing end-tidal pressure and avoiding large tidal volumes. Surfactant should be delivered early in the course of treatment.

Treatment of infants with BPD involves steps to minimize additional lung damage and prevent pulmonary hypertension and cor pulmonale. Infants with severe disease may be dependent on supplemental oxygen or mechanical ventilation for months and have symptoms of airway obstruction for years. Therapy usually is supportive throughout the course of the disease. An infant with BPD is given respiratory support as needed. Supplemental oxygen can help decrease the pulmonary hypertension that is common with this disorder. Diuretics are given as needed to decrease pulmonary edema; antibiotics are given to manage existing pulmonary infection.[21] Chest physical therapy may help mobilize secretions and prevent further atelectasis. Bronchodilator therapy may be useful in decreasing airway resistance.[22] Steroid therapy with dexamethasone can produce substantial short-term improvement in lung function, often allowing rapid weaning from ventilatory support. Steroid therapy, however, apparently has little effect on long-term outcome such as mortality and duration of oxygen therapy.[23,24] Steroid therapy also has been implicated in decreasing alveolarization and increased developmental delay. Although steroids are still given in clinical practice, they should be used cautiously and only after the risks have been thoroughly explored.

Control of Breathing

Apnea of Prematurity

Apnea is a common, controllable disorder among premature infants. It usually resolves over time.[25] Premature infants frequently have periodic respiration, which is sequential short apneic episodes of 5 to 10 seconds followed by 10 to 15 seconds of rapid respiration. Apneic spells are abnormal if (1) they last more than 15 seconds or (2) they are associated with cyanosis, pallor, hypotonia, or bradycardia.

If no effort to breathe occurs during a spell, the apnea is called *central apnea*. If breathing efforts occur but obstruction prevents air flow, the apnea is termed *obstructive*. Mixed apnea is a combination of the central and obstructive types that starts as obstructive apnea and then develops into central apnea.[26]

Etiology. Premature infants have an immature chemocontrol of respiratory drive. In mature animals an increase in alveolar partial pressure of carbon dioxide (P_{ACO_2}) elicits an increase in tidal volume and respiratory rate. A decrease in F_{IO_2} below room air also triggers an increase in tidal volume. Conversely, in premature animals, an increase in P_{ACO_2} temporarily increases tidal volume but does not increase respiratory rate. A decrease in F_{IO_2} below room air decreases tidal volume and respiratory rate. This effect can lead to apnea in a premature infant. Several factors in addition to prematurity can cause apnea in infants. Table 28-1 describes the potential causes, associated signs, and diagnostic indicators.[27]

Treatment. Infants with apnea need continuous monitoring of heart and respiratory rates. Continuous noninvasive monitoring of oxygenation by transcutaneous electrode or pulse oximetry is recommended. Most apneic incidents can be quickly terminated with gentle mechanical stimulation, such as picking the infant up, flicking the sole of the foot, or rubbing the skin.[26] If the cause of apnea is not prematurity, treatment must be directed at resolving the underlying condition. Table 28-2 outlines current treatment strategies for infants with apnea.[27]

Apnea secondary to prematurity responds well to the methylxanthines, especially theophylline and caffeine.[28] These agents stimulate the central nervous system and

Table 28-1 ▶▶▶ Evaluation of an Infant With Apnea

Possible Cause	Associated Signs	Investigation
Infection	Lethargy, respiratory distress, temperature instability	Complete blood count, sepsis evaluation
Metabolic disorder	Poor feeding, lethargy, jitteriness	Glucose, calcium, electrolyte levels
Impaired oxygenation	Respiratory distress, tachypnea, cyanosis	Oxygen monitoring, arterial blood gases, chest radiograph
Maternal drugs	Maternal history, hypotonia, central nervous system depression	Magnesium level, urine drug screen
Intracranial lesion	Abnormal neurologic findings, seizures	Cranial ultrasonography
Environmental	Lethargy	Monitor temperature (infant and environment)
Gastroesophageal reflux	Feeding difficulty	Specific observation, radiographic barium swallow examination

From Stark AR: Respir Care 36:673, 1991.

Table 28-2 ▶▶ Treatment Strategies for Infants With Apnea

Treatment	Rationale
Manage underlying cause if identified	Removes precipitating factor
Tactile stimulation	Increases respiratory drive by sensory stimulation
CPAP	Reduces mixed and obstructive apnea by splinting the upper airway
Theophylline or caffeine	Increases respiratory center output and CO_2 response, enhances diaphragm strength; adenosine antagonist
Doxapram	Stimulates respiratory center and peripheral chemoreceptors
Transfusion	Decreases hypoxic depression by increasing oxygen-carrying capacity
Mechanical ventilation	Provides support when respiratory effort is inadequate

From Stark AR: Respir Care 36:673, 1991.

increase the infant's responsiveness to carbon dioxide. For infants with apnea that is refractory to treatment with theophylline, doxapram can be used.[29] Continuous positive airway pressure also is used to manage infant apnea. Although its mechanism of action is not clearly established, CPAP probably increases FRC and thus improves arterial partial pressure of oxygen ($Pa{O_2}$) and $Pa{CO_2}$. It is possible that CPAP also stimulates vagal receptors in the lung, thereby increasing the output of the brainstem respiratory centers. Severe or recurrent apnea that is not responsive to these interventions may necessitate mechanical ventilatory support.

As the respiratory control mechanisms mature, apnea of prematurity normally resolves itself. Apneic spells begin to disappear by the 37th to 44th week of postmenstrual age with no apparent long-term effects. Infants who have apnea of prematurity are not at higher risk of SIDS than are other infants.[26]

Pulmonary Vascular Disease

Persistent Pulmonary Hypertension of the Newborn

Background. Persistent pulmonary hypertension of the newborn (PPHN) is a complex syndrome with many causes. The common denominator in PPHN is a return to fetal circulatory pathways, usually because of high PVR. This condition results in further right-to-left shunting, severe hypoxemia, and metabolic and respiratory acidosis.

Pathophysiology. In the uterus the fetus does not use the lungs as a gas exchange organ. The PVR is high and the systemic vascular resistance (SVR) is low. This condition produces a PVR/SVR ratio greater than 1. A fetus has two anatomic shunts that are not present in older infants, children, or adults: the foramen ovale and the ductus arteriosus. With a PVR/SVR ratio greater than 1 and the anatomic shunts, blood flow bypasses the lung either at the atrial level (foramen ovale) or the pulmonary artery (ductus arteriosus). Thus intrauterine total pulmonary blood flow is low.

In the transition to extrauterine life, PVR decreases owing to gas filling of the lung and increasing $Pa{O_2}$ in the pulmonary venous circulation. Systemic vascular resistance increases with the removal of the placenta from the circulation. This makes the PVR/SVR ratio less than 1. Should PVR not decrease to allow the PVR/SVR ratio to become less than 1, the infant has PPHN.

There are three fundamental types of PPHN: vascular spasm, increased muscle wall thickness, and decreased cross-sectional area of pulmonary vessels. Vascular spasm is an acute event that can be triggered by many different conditions, including hypoxemia, hypoglycemia, hypotension, and pain. Increased muscle wall thickness is a chronic condition that develops in utero in response to several different etiologic factors, including chronic fetal hypoxia, increased pulmonary blood flow (e.g., intrauterine closure of the ductus arteriosus), pulmonary venous obstruction (e.g., total anomalous pulmonary venous return with obstructed below-diaphragm return). Decreased cross-sectional area is related to hypoplasia of the lungs and occurs with congenital diaphragmatic hernia, Potter's sequence (absent kidneys), and oligohydramnios syndromes (decreased amniotic fluid).

Clinical Manifestations. Persistent pulmonary hypertension should be suspected when an infant has rapidly changing oxygen saturation without changes in $F{IO_2}$ or has hypoxemia out of proportion to the lung disease detected with chest radiography or $Pa{CO_2}$ measurement. In infants with a significant shunt through the ductus arteriosus, there usually is a substantial gradient (>5%) between preductal and postductal oxygen saturation. This gradient can be easily found if two pulse oximeters are placed on the infant, one on the right arm and the other on either leg.

Treatment. Initial therapy for PPHN is removal of the underlying cause, such as administration of oxygen for hypoxemia, surfactant for RDS, glucose for hypoglycemia, and inotropic agents for low cardiac output and systemic hypotension. If correction of the underlying problem does not correct the hypoxemia, the infant needs intubation and mechanical ventilation. Because pain and anxiety may contribute to PPHN, the infant may need sedation and, frequently, paralysis. If these measures do not improve oxygenation, the next step is HFV. This mode of ventilation allows a higher FRC without a large tidal volume. Inhaled nitric oxide is now considered the next intervention.[30-32] Should all of these modalities fail to improve oxygenation, the infant may be a candidate for extracorporeal membrane oxygenation (ECMO).[30,33,34] Even with all these therapeutic modalities, PPHN remains a complex disease with high morbidity.

Congenital Abnormalities Affecting Respiration

Congenital abnormalities that affect respiration can be divided into several groups: airway diseases, lung malformations, chest wall abnormalities, abdominal wall abnormalities, and diseases of neuromuscular control.

Airway Diseases

Airway abnormalities have three fundamental mechanisms: internal obstruction, external obstruction, and disruption. Internal obstruction includes common problems, such as laryngomalacia, that cause obstructive apnea. Less common problems caused by internal obstruction are tracheomalacia, laryngeal webs, tracheal stenosis, and hemangiomas. All of these diseases usually manifest as a combination of inspiratory stridor, gas trapping, expiratory wheezing, and accessory respiratory muscle activity.

External compression can be caused by hemangiomas, neck or thoracic masses, and vascular rings. These lesions are far less common than diseases caused by internal obstruction, but they are by no means rare. The symptoms are similar to those of internal obstruction. Neck masses usually are obvious at visual inspection. Intrathoracic masses and vascular rings must be suspected on the basis of the clinical manifestations: noise during the respiratory cycle that worsens with exertion. The infant may have difficulty with swallowing.

Airway disruptions usually are related to tracheoesophageal fistula (TEF) in a newborn. This malformation usually is associated with esophageal atresia. There are five types of TEF: esophageal atresia with a proximal fistula, esophageal atresia with a distal fistula, esophageal atresia with both a proximal and a distal fistula, esophageal atresia without either fistula, and an intact esophagus with an H fistula. The most common of these malformations is esophageal atresia with a distal fistula, which comprises 85% to 90% of all TEFs. The least common is the H fistula. All of these malformations manifest as difficulty swallowing, bubbling and frothing at the mouth, and choking, particularly during attempts at feeding. These anomalies can occur in isolation or as part of an association of defects. The most common is the VATER or VACTERL association of *v*ertebral anomalies, imperforate *a*nus, *t*racheo*e*sophageal fistula, and *r*enal or *r*adial anomalies. In VACTERL, *c*ardiac anomalies are added, and *r*enal and *l*imb anomalies replace renal or radial anomalies in the initialism. These associated anomalies must be sought in any infant with TEF. Tracheoesophageal fistula is managed with surgical ligation of the fistula and reconnection of the interrupted esophagus. Most infants with TEF have a good outcome; however, some have severe malformations that can cause chronic problems. Infants with TEF usually need only supportive respiratory care. They usually do not have lung disease. Some infants, however, need HFV because the air leak through the fistula can become larger than the airflow to the alveoli.

Lung Malformations

Several lung malformations occur in the newborn period. The most common is congenital cyst adenomatoid malformation of the lung (C-CAM). This disease is classified into three types on the basis of the type and size of the cyst. The disease usually affects entire lobes of the lung. The affected parts of the lung do not exchange gas and can become infected. The usual treatment is surgical removal of the affected lobe. Most infants with C-CAM have symptoms of lung volume loss. As the mass expands, the normal surrounding lung is compressed. A few of these infants have severe cardiorespiratory compromise and need respiratory support and emergency surgery.

Other less common lung malformations include pulmonary sequestration and lobar emphysema. Both of these diseases involve maldevelopment of lobes of the lung. These malformations manifest as space-occupying masses within the thorax. They usually are managed with surgical resection.

Congenital Diaphragmatic Hernia

Congenital diaphragmatic hernia is a severe disease that usually manifests in newborns as severe respiratory distress. The pathophysiologic mechanism is a complex combination of lung hypoplasia, including decreased alveolar count and decreased pulmonary vasculature, pulmonary hypertension, and unusual anatomy of the inferior vena cava.[35] This disorder varies between asymptomatic (rare) to severe life-threatening disease (frequent). There are two types of hernia: Bochdalek's hernia (lateral and posterior defect, usually on the left) and Morgagni's hernia (medial and anterior). Hernias that occur in the right hemidiaphragm usually are less severe because the liver blocks the defect and decreases the volume of abdominal contents that can enter the thorax.

Most cases of congenital diaphragmatic hernia can be diagnosed in utero with ultrasonography. Physical examination may yield the following findings: scaphoid abdomen (because the abdominal contents are in the thorax), decreased breath sounds, displaced heart sounds (because the heart is pushed away from the hernia), and severe cyanosis (from lung hypoplasia and pulmonary hypertension). The diagnosis is established with chest radiography.

The general treatment of infants with congenital diaphragmatic hernia involves both neonatologists and pediatric surgeons. Initial treatment is insertion of an ET tube, paralysis, and mechanical ventilation. A large sump tube is placed into the stomach and connected to continuous suction. These therapies allow adequate ventilation and oxygenation and prevent gas insufflation of the intestine. Most centers delay surgical repair for several days to allow the natural decrease in PVR. On the seventh to tenth day of life, a surgeon closes the defect. This scenario occurs only for infants with easily correctable pulmonary hypertension. Infants with severe pulmonary hypertension need HFV and ECMO.[36-38] At some centers the diaphragm is repaired during ECMO. Most centers try to wean the infant from ECMO and then perform the repair. In spite of all these advanced therapies, the mortality for this disease is high.

Abdominal Wall Abnormalities

Because all newborns are primarily abdominal breathers, the abdominal wall is an intrinsic part of the respiratory system. Large defects in the abdominal wall can cause severe respiratory compromise. The most common of these defects is omphalocele. Usually only large omphaloceles cause respiratory distress. When they are greater than 10 cm in diameter, these defects can cause severe respiratory distress and frequently necessitate prolonged mechanical ventilation.

Neuromuscular Control

Many diseases of poor neuromuscular control affect newborns. These include spinal muscular atrophy, congenital myasthenia gravis, myotonic dystrophy, and many others. These diseases frequently necessitate respiratory support in the newborn period. The morbidity and mortality of these diseases are extremely variable. Some diseases can be quite severe in the newborn period and be relieved with age. It is important to make an accurate diagnosis both to be able to estimate prognosis and to provide genetic counseling. Many of these diseases are inherited with known inheritance patterns.

Congenital Heart Disease

A full discussion of congenital heart disease is beyond the scope of this chapter. Basic knowledge of the common defects, however, is essential to good practice in pediatric and neonatal respiratory care. Congenital heart diseases usually are divided into two large categories: cyanotic and acyanotic heart disease. Cyanotic heart diseases are diseases in which blood shunts from right to left, bypassing the lungs, and is thus deoxygenated. Acyanotic heart diseases are diseases in which blood shunts from left to right and thus cause congestive heart failure. Figure 28-4 compares normal cardiac anatomy with the features of the five most common congenital defects.

Cyanotic

The two most common cyanotic heart diseases are tetralogy of Fallot and transposition of the great arteries.

Tetralogy of Fallot. Tetralogy of Fallot is a defect that includes (1) obstruction of right ventricular outflow (pulmonary stenosis), (2) ventricular septal defect (a hole between the right and left ventricles), (3) dextroposition of the aorta, and (4) right ventricular hypertrophy. Tetralogy of Fallot varies between mild disease, which is initially diagnosed in early childhood, and severe disease, which is diagnosed in the newborn period. The mild form of the disease manifests as a heart murmur, intermittent severe cyanotic spells, a history of the infant squatting or entering a knee chest position, or a combination of these features. The severe form of the disease manifests as a heart murmur and severe continuous cyanosis. Most types of tetralogy of Fallot can be managed surgically. The type and timing of the surgery depend on the anatomy of the defects. Children with this defect are at increased risk of sudden death of arrhythmia later in life.

Transposition of the Great Arteries. Transposition of the great arteries is the heart disease that most frequently causes severe cyanosis. It usually manifests as moderate to severe cyanosis immediately after birth. A murmur may be present. Infants with this abnormality frequently need emergency atrial septostomy (cutting a hole in the wall between the two atria). This procedure historically has been performed in heart catheterization laboratories. Many pediatric cardiologists who perform invasive procedures have begun performing this procedure with ultrasound guidance in the neonatal intensive care unit. The condition of infants who need atrial septostomy usually stabilizes. The goal is to allow PVR to decrease and then to perform the arterial switch operation in the second or third week of life.

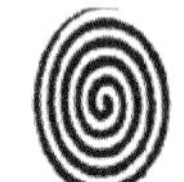

RULE OF THUMB

An infant with profound cyanosis at birth most likely has cyanotic heart disease or persistent pulmonary hypertension.

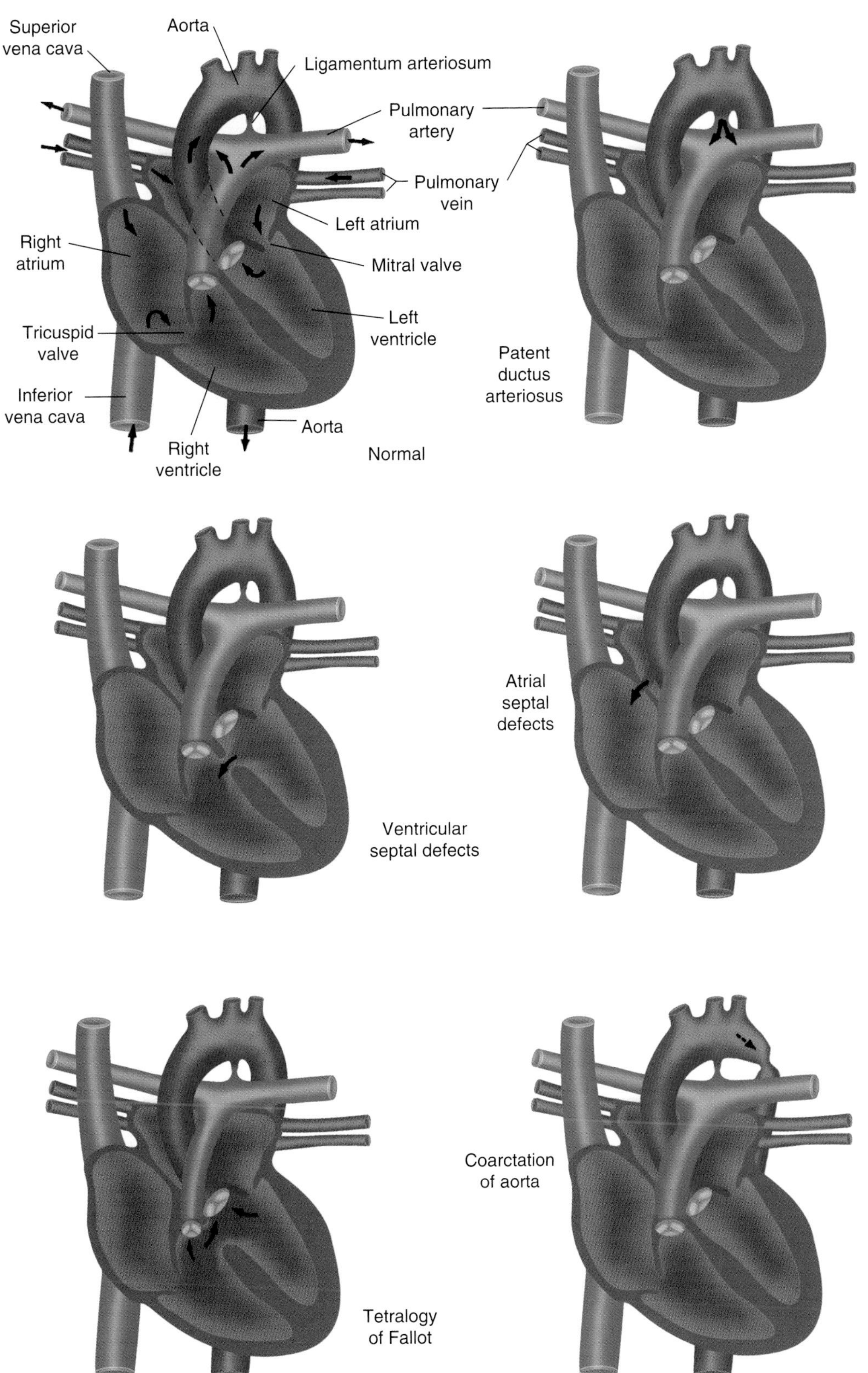

Figure 28-4

Normal flow of blood through the heart and some congenital defects that cause abnormal flow. *(Modified from Jacob S, Francone C, Lossow WJ: Structure and function in man, ed 5, Philadelphia, 1982, WB Saunders.)*

Acyanotic

Some of the most common and most severe congenital heart diseases are acyanotic. Ventricular septal defect is probably the most common congenital heart disease. Hypoplastic left heart syndrome is among the most severe of congenital heart diseases.

Ventricular Septal Defect. Defects along the septum separating the right and left ventricles are quite common. Ventricular septal defect can occur alone or in combination with other anomalies. A simple ventricular septal defect usually causes left-to-right shunting and congestive heart failure. This defect usually does not appear immediately after birth. It appears at 6 to 8 weeks of age, when the PVR has decreased enough that the shunt becomes large.

Atrial Septal Defect. The most common type of atrial septal defect is a small, slit-like opening that persists after closure of the foramen ovale. An isolated atrial septal defect is of little clinical importance.

Patent Ductus Arteriosus. In a fetus most of the pulmonary blood flow is shunted through the ductus arteriosus to the aorta. Closure of the ductus normally occurs 5 to 7 days after the birth of term infants.[39,40] Patent ductus arteriosus usually is a disease of immature, preterm infants. Factors altering pressure gradients or affecting smooth muscle contraction can cause the ductus to not close or to reopen after it has closed. Depending on the pressure gradients established, shunting through an open ductus may be either right to left (pulmonary pressure greater than aortic) or left to right (aortic pressure greater than pulmonary). Treatment is either pharmacologic (indomethacin) or surgical (ligation).

Hypoplastic Left Heart Syndrome, Interrupted Aortic Arch, and Coarctation of the Aorta. Hypoplastic left heart syndrome (Figure 28-5), interrupted aortic arch, and coarctation of the aorta have in common obstruction of left ventricular outflow. They all manifest in the newborn period with symptoms of acute heart failure. Systemic blood flow depends on patency of the ductus arteriosus. When the ductus spontaneously closes (usually at 5-7 days of age), severe congestive heart failure develops. The symptoms range from moderate respiratory distress to complete cardiovascular collapse. Initial treatment is the intravenous administration of prostaglandin E_1. Most infants with these defects need support with mechanical ventilation. These infants do not have lung disease. The pressures and rates used should be set appropriately.

There are standard surgical repairs for both interrupted aortic arch and coarctation of the aorta.

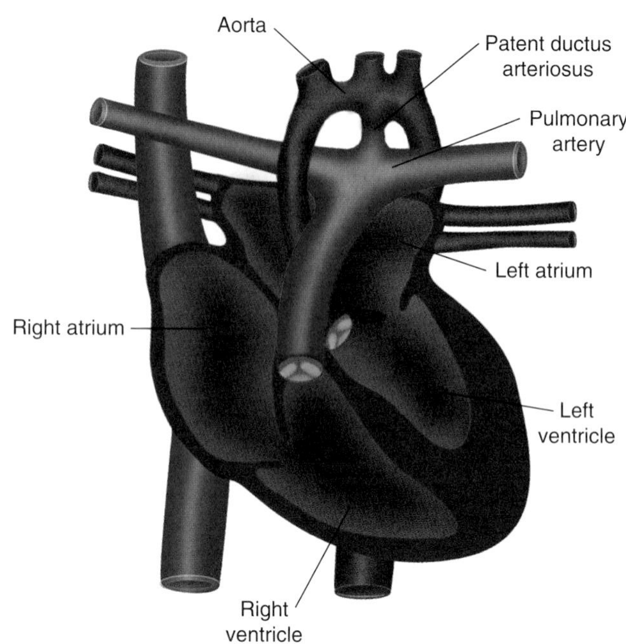

Figure 28-5
Hypoplastic left heart syndrome.

Hypoplastic left heart syndrome has three accepted treatments: comfort care (allowing the infant to die), a palliative surgical procedure (Norwood), and transplantation.[41-44] None of these options is ideal. Each has significant associated problems. The decision must be made with the family.

▶ PEDIATRIC RESPIRATORY DISORDERS

Compared with the common cardiopulmonary diseases in the neonatal period, the pulmonary conditions that occur among older infants and children commonly result from airway obstruction caused by bacterial or viral infections. Other entities discussed in this section include asthma, sudden infant death syndrome, gastroesophageal reflux, and cystic fibrosis.

Sudden Infant Death Syndrome

Sudden infant death syndrome (SIDS) is the leading cause of death (40%) among infants younger than 1 year in the United States. Approximately 7000 infants die of SIDS each year in the United States.[45] A presumptive diagnosis is based on the conditions of death in which a previously healthy baby dies unexpectedly, usually during sleep. Autopsy shows that many infants who die of SIDS have evidence of repeated episodes of hypoxia or ischemia. Factors associated with increased frequency of SIDS are presented in Box 28-1.

Box 28-1 • Factors Associated With Increased Frequency of SIDS

MATERNAL CHARACTERISTICS
- Younger than 20 years
- Poor
- Black, Native American, or Alaskan native
- Previous fetal loss
- Cigarette smoking
- Narcotic abuse
- Illness during pregnancy
- Inadequate prenatal care

INFANT CHARACTERISTICS AT BIRTH
- Male gender
- Premature birth
- Small for gestational age
- Low Apgar score
- Resuscitation with oxygen and ventilation at birth
- Second or third in birth order or of a multiple birth
- Sibling death of SIDS

From Koff PB, Eitzman DV, Neu J: Neonatal and pediatric respiratory care, ed 2 St Louis, 1993, Mosby.

Etiology

The cause of SIDS remains unknown. Apnea of prematurity is not a predisposing factor, and there is no evidence that immaturity of the respiratory centers is a cause. Although infants in families in which two or more SIDS deaths have occurred are at slightly higher risk, there is no evidence of a genetic link. The best knowledge of SIDS comes from population or epidemiological studies and is summarized in Box 28-2. An infant who dies of SIDS typically is a preterm black boy born to a poor mother younger than 20 years of age who received inadequate prenatal care. Infants 1 to 3 months of age are most susceptible, and death is most likely to occur at night during the winter months. The risk of SIDS also is high among infants who previously experienced an apparent life-threatening event. Such an event occurs when a baby becomes apneic, cyanotic, or limp enough to frighten the parent or caregiver. The prone sleeping position has been strongly associated with increased risk of SIDS. It is difficult to differentiate death of SIDS from death of intentional suffocation. The possibility of intentional suffocation must be investigated, but with great sensitivity.[46]

Prevention

Because of the unknown causation and unexpected occurrence, there is no current therapy for SIDS. Prevention is the goal. Successful prevention requires that infants at high risk be identified through a history of risk factors and documented monitoring or event recording. After identification that an infant is at risk, the family is trained in apnea monitoring and cardiopulmonary resuscitation (CPR). The American Academy of Pediatrics recommends that infants be placed in either the supine or the side-lying position for the first 6 months of life.[45] To define the need and appropriate approach for home monitoring of infants, the National Institutes of Health (NIH) developed a consensus statement on infantile apnea and home monitoring. The eight specific NIH recommendations regarding the need for and use of home monitoring are summarized in Box 28-3.

Box 28-2 • Infant Characteristics Near Time of SIDS Death

- Age <6 months (peak between 1 and 3 months)
- Winter season
- Asleep at night
- Mild illness in week before death
- History of apparent life-threatening event
- Prone sleep position

Gastroesophageal Reflux Disease

Gastroesophageal reflux disease (GERD) is the regurgitation of stomach contents into the esophagus and is common in childhood. Some causes of GERD are physiological. There is general agreement that there are important interactions between GERD and a variety of disorders of the respiratory system.[47] Respiratory problems caused by gastroesophageal reflux include reactive airways disease, aspiration pneumonia, laryngospasm, stridor, chronic cough, choking spells, and apnea. Gastroesophageal reflux disease should be considered when an infant has faced a sudden life-threatening event and when an older child has unexplained chronic head and neck problems. Gastroesophageal reflux disease can be diagnosed with esophageal pH testing, upper gastrointestinal contrast studies, and gastric scintiscanning. Once GERD has been diagnosed, medical therapy can begin. Occasional cases that do not respond to medical management may require surgical intervention.

Bronchiolitis

Bronchiolitis is an acute infection of the lower respiratory tract, usually caused by the respiratory syncytial virus (RSV). Nearly 1 in 10 infants younger than 2 years acquires a bronchiolitis infection. The outcome is generally good, although approximately 1% of infants hospitalized for bronchiolitis die of respiratory failure. Those most prone to respiratory failure as a consequence

Box 28-3 • NIH Consensus Statement on Infantile Apnea and Home Monitoring

1. Home cardiorespiratory monitoring is medically indicated in certain groups of infants at high risk for sudden death including the following:
   a. Infants with one or more severe ALTEs [apparent life-threatening events] requiring vigorous stimulation, mouth-to-mouth resuscitation, or CPR.
   b. Siblings of two or more victims of SIDS.
   c. Preterm infants with apnea of prematurity who are otherwise ready for discharge.
   d. Infants with conditions such as central hypoventilation or tracheostomy.
2. It is not clear from existing evidence whether the potential benefits of monitoring outweigh the risk for other groups of infants in whom the risk of sudden death is elevated. These groups include the following:
   a. Siblings of one SIDS victim.
   b. Infants with less severe ALTEs.
   c. Infants of opiate-abusing or cocaine-abusing mothers.
3. Cardiorespiratory monitoring is not medically indicated for normal infants or asymptomatic preterm infants.
4. Caregivers must be trained and demonstrate proficiency in infant CPR and must understand that cardiorespiratory monitoring does not guarantee survival.
5. Pneumocardiograms are not useful in screening infants in an attempt to predict SIDS victims or victims of infantile apnea.
6. Decisions for stopping home monitoring should be based on clinical criteria. It is reasonable to discontinue the monitor when the infant has had 2 or 3 months free of events requiring vigorous stimulation, mouth-to-mouth resuscitation, or CPR.
7. Effective home monitoring requires a coordinated, interdisciplinary effort from physicians, nursing and social work services, healthcare agencies, and medical equipment vendors.
8. In the rare infant with recurrent severe apnea of infancy requiring resuscitation, prolonged hospitalization may be necessary. The vast majority of infants with an ALTE and apnea of infancy have an excellent prognosis without after effects.

of bronchiolitis are very young and immunodeficient and have comorbidity, such as congenital heart disease, bronchopulmonary dysplasia, cystic fibrosis, or childhood asthma.

Clinical Manifestations

The clinical manifestations of bronchiolitis are inflammation and obstruction of the small bronchi and bronchioles. Bronchiolitis commonly occurs soon after a viral upper respiratory infection. The infant may have a slight fever with an intermittent cough. After a few days, signs of respiratory distress develop, particularly dyspnea and tachypnea. Progressive inflammation and narrowing of the airways cause inspiratory and expiratory wheezing and increase airway resistance. The chest radiograph shows signs of hyperinflation with areas of consolidation. The diagnosis of RSV infection can be established by immunofluorescent assay the same day and assists in the implementation of a treatment plan.

Box 28-4 • American Academy of Pediatrics Recommendations for the Use of Ribavirin to Manage RSV Pneumonia

1. Presence of underlying congenital heart disease
2. Presence of underlying chronic lung conditions (BPD)
3. Immunosuppression (human immunodeficiency virus infection, organ transplantation)
4. Infant younger than 6 weeks
5. Severe pneumonitis caused by RSV with Pa_{O_2} <65 mm Hg and increasing Pa_{CO_2}

Treatment

Treatment of a patient with bronchiolitis varies with the severity of the infection and the clinical signs and symptoms. Many patients can be treated at home with humidification and oral decongestants. Patients with more severe symptoms (apnea) and comorbidity usually are hospitalized, and treatment is directed at relieving the airway obstruction and associated hypoxemia. Hospitalized children frequently are treated with systemic hydration and oxygen by Oxyhood, croup tent, or nasal cannula and assisted with airway clearance. Because bronchiolitis and childhood asthma have similar symptoms, a trial course of bronchodilator therapy with a β-agonist may be useful if airway obstruction is relieved after administration.[48] This practice is controversial, and practitioners should assess the efficacy of all bronchodilator therapy before continuing. Antibiotics may be administered to control secondary bacterial infections. Severe cases may be managed with ribavirin[49] (Box 28-4). Ribavirin is a broad-spectrum virustatic agent active against a wide range of viruses. However, clinical efficacy outside children with complex comorbidity is questionable, and use of ribavirin is highly controversial. Should bronchiolitis progress to acute respiratory failure, mechanical ventilation is required. Because of the obstructive nature of this disorder, low respiratory rates and long expiratory times may be needed to prevent air trapping. Vigorous bronchial hygiene, occasionally including tracheobronchial aspiration, usually is needed to maintain a patent airway.

Croup

Croup is a viral disorder of the upper airway that normally results in subglottic swelling and obstruction. Termed *laryngotracheobronchitis*, viral croup is caused by the parainfluenza virus and is the most common form of airway obstruction in children between 6 months and 6 years of age. Less common as causative agents are RSV and influenza virus. Bacterial superinfection with *Staphylococcus aureus*, group A *Streptococcus pyogenes*, or *Haemophilus influenzae* may worsen croup.

Clinical Manifestations

Symptoms become evident after 2 or 3 days of nasal congestion, fever, and coughing. The child typically has slow, progressive inspiratory and expiratory stridor and a barking cough. As the disease progresses, dyspnea, cyanosis, exhaustion, and agitation occur. Upper airway radiographic examination is helpful in confirming the diagnosis and ruling out epiglottitis but is usually not needed in most cases of croup.[50] Classic croup manifests on an anteroposterior radiograph as characteristic subglottic narrowing of the trachea, called the *steeple sign* (Figure 28-6).

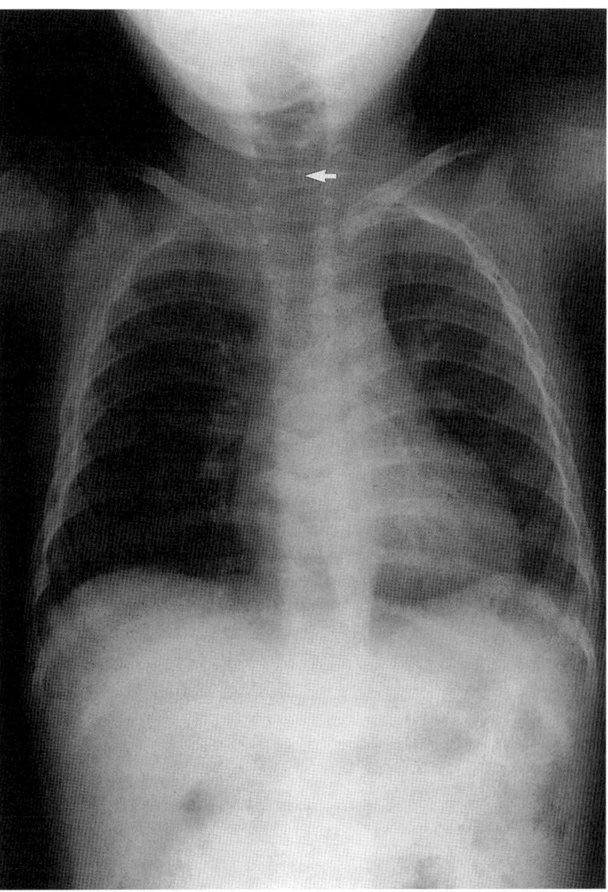

Figure 28-6
Anteroposterior chest radiograph of a patient with croup. The subglottic narrowing typical of croup is evident (*arrow*).

Treatment

The evaluation and treatment of a child with croup must focus on the degree of respiratory distress and associated clinical findings. If stridor is mild or occurs only on exertion and cyanosis is not present, hospitalization is generally not required, and the child is treated at home. If there is stridor at rest (accompanied by harsh breath sounds, suprasternal retractions, and cyanosis with breathing of room air), hospitalization is indicated. Although there is little research to support the practice,[51] treatment of a child with mild to moderate croup traditionally involves cool mist therapy with or without supplemental oxygen. Aerosolized racemic epinephrine and dexamethasone (0.3 mg/kg) are effective in decreasing the length and severity of respiratory symptoms associated with viral croup.[51] The addition of budesonide has been shown to reduce the severity of symptoms in mild to moderate cases of croup.[52] Progressive worsening of the clinical signs despite treatment indicates the need for intubation and mechanical ventilation.

Epiglottitis

Epiglottitis is an acute and often life-threatening infection of the upper airway that causes severe obstruction secondary to supraglottic swelling. Evidence suggests that the incidence of epiglottitis is decreasing among children, probably because of the use of vaccines.[53-55] The most common cause is *H. influenzae* type B infection.

Clinical Manifestations

A child with epiglottitis usually has a high fever, sore throat, stridor, and labored breathing.[56] The patient does not have a croupy bark but instead has a muffled voice. Older children may report a sore throat and difficulty in swallowing. Difficulty swallowing may cause drooling. Lateral neck radiographic results (Figure 28-7) indicate the epiglottis is markedly thickened and flattened (thumb sign) and the aryepiglottic folds are swollen; the vallecula may not be visualized. Visual examination of the upper airway is dangerous in these children and always should be performed in a controlled setting by personnel expert in emergency intubation. Inadvertent traction of the tongue can cause further and immediate swelling of the epiglottis and abrupt and total upper airway obstruction. Children with suspected epiglottitis should be accompanied by personnel expert in emergency intubation during any transport for diagnostic procedures.

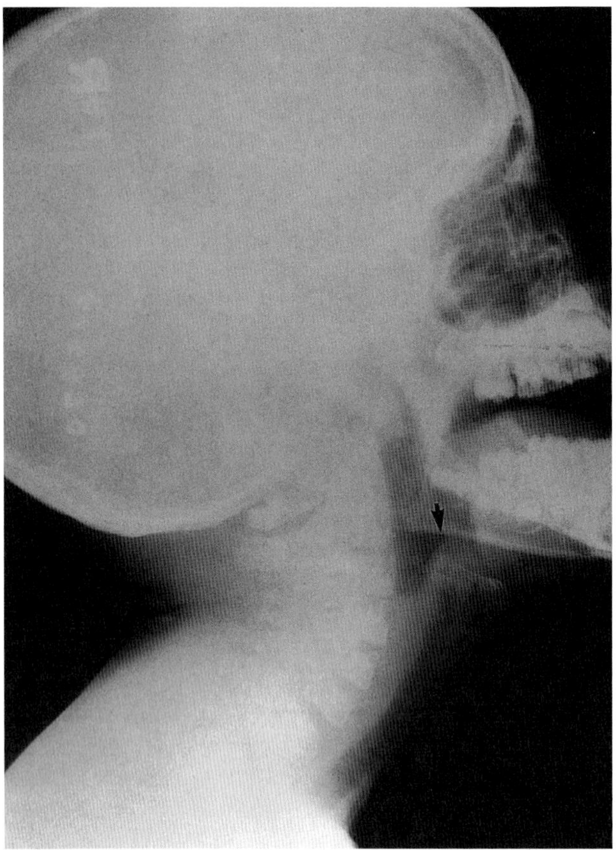

Figure 28-7

Lateral radiograph of the neck of a patient with epiglottitis. The thumb sign is prominent *(arrow)*.

MINI CLINI

Extubation

PROBLEM

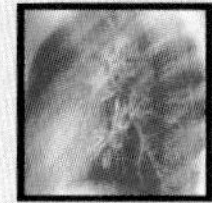

A 3-year-old child underwent emergency intubation 5 days ago for epiglottitis. The physician asks you to evaluate the patient for extubation. What would you evaluate before making the decision for extubation? What equipment would you want to have at the bedside during extubation?

DISCUSSION

Clinical examination of vital signs (e.g., body temperature), breath sounds, sensorium, and degree of airway leak should be considered. Equipment for rapid reintubation must be at the bedside, including racemic epinephrine for aerosolization.

Extubation of any patient should take into consideration the pathophysiologic condition that led to intubation. In this case, the respiratory therapist should look for evidence that the infection is resolving and that the upper airway is no longer inflamed. A lack of fever for at least 12 hours and visual inspection of the throat that reveals minimal inflammation would be most helpful. After extubation, close monitoring must be performed for evidence of airway compromise. Cool mist may be helpful to minimize inflammation after extubation.

Treatment

Children with epiglottitis need elective intubation under general anesthesia in the operating room. Tracheostomy may be needed if the patient's condition warrants it; however, this practice is rarely used. There should be no attempt to lie the child down or attempts to intubate until the patient is sedated. Premature attempts at intubation can precipitate acute airway obstruction and respiratory arrest. Once an airway is secured, a sample for bacterial culture should be obtained and antibiotic therapy started. Children with an ET tube should be sedated and restrained to prevent inadvertent extubation. Pressure support ventilation with 3 cm H_2O CPAP should be used; FIO_2 greater than 0.40 is rarely required unless there is associated pneumonia. Children should be assessed daily for the presence of an airway leak. Extubation should not be attempted until an upper airway leak is readily detected.

Cystic Fibrosis

Cystic fibrosis is the most common lethal genetic disorder among white persons. It is inherited as an autosomal recessive trait that affects approximately 30,000 persons in the United States alone. The disease is caused by a genetic mutation of a large protein that controls the movement of chloride ions through the cell membrane.[57] Movement of chloride ions is vital to the proper regulation of secretions. In cystic fibrosis, abnormalities of chloride movement cause markedly abnormal exocrine secretions.

RULE OF THUMB

Both parents must be carriers of the CF gene for any child to be born with cystic fibrosis. If both parents carry the CF gene, the odds that cystic fibrosis will develop in offspring are 1:4.

Clinical Manifestations

Patients with cystic fibrosis experience many clinical syndromes caused by the abnormal secretions. All organs with exocrine function are affected in one way or another; however, the most severely affected organs are the sweat glands, pancreas, and lungs. Sweat glands of patients with cystic fibrosis are unable to properly remove salt from sweat.[58] As a result the skin develops a salty taste, and patients are prone to dehydration during hot weather.[59] The sweat chloride test used for diagnosis of the disease is based on the high salt concentration in the sweat of patients with cystic fibrosis.[60] Most patients with cystic fibrosis have exocrine pancreatic insufficiency, usually in infancy. Exocrine pancreatic insufficiency dramatically reduces the number digestive enzymes. Patients who lack digestive enzymes experience malnutrition and diarrhea. Digestion of fats is severely compromised in patients with cystic fibrosis. These patients often have deficiencies of the fat-soluble vitamins A, D, E, and K and have large amounts of undigested fat in the stool (steatorrhea).

Complications of lung disease are the leading cause of death among patients with cystic fibrosis. Patients have recurring pulmonary infections. On occasion the infections begin during the first few days of life. The organisms associated with these infections include *S. aureus*, *H. influnzae*, and *Pseudomonas aeruginosa*. Patients with cystic fibrosis have bronchiolitis and bronchiectasis and produce copious amounts of thick mucinous secretions. At times, mucus obstructs the airways and causes atelectasis, pneumonia, or lung abscesses. As the disease progresses, the lungs become hyperinflated, and the frequency of bronchiectatic exacerbations increases. Patients at the end stage of cystic fibrosis have severe debility with marked hypoxemia, pulmonary hypertension, and cor pulmonale.

Diagnosis

The diagnosis of cystic fibrosis is suspected when a patient has multiple clinical manifestations of the disease. The diagnosis usually is confirmed with the sweat chloride test. In evaluation of a child, a sweat chloride level greater than 60 mEq/L confirms the diagnosis of cystic fibrosis.[61]

Treatment

The deficiency of pancreatic enzymes that occurs among patients with cystic fibrosis is managed with pancreatic enzyme supplementation. Several important steps are taken to help patients with cystic fibrosis maintain lung function. Regular chest physical therapy improves lung function and clearance of secretions.[62] Many patients with cystic fibrosis have no partner to assist with chest physiotherapy. For these patients, strenuous exercise, PEEP devices, or autogenic drainage may substitute for regular chest physiotherapy. Another mucous clearance adjunct is inhaled recombinant deoxyribonuclease (DNase). The routine daily use of inhaled DNase reduces the frequency of respiratory infections.[63]

Antibiotics directed against the usual infectious organisms are required with each bronchiectatic exacerbation. A nebulized form of the antibiotic tobramycin is used to prevent infection. When inhaled tobramycin is used twice daily every other month, there is a marked reduction in the number of bronchiectatic exacerbations.[64]

Patients younger than 13 years have a marked reduction in loss of lung function when they use high doses of the antiinflammatory drug ibuprofen.[65] Many cystic fibrosis patients have asthma symptoms. These patients benefit from bronchodilators.

Lung transplantation is commonly used in the care of patients with advanced cystic fibrosis lung disease. Sequential double-lung transplantation is the most commonly used form of lung transplantation in the treatment of patients with cystic fibrosis.

Prognosis

When cystic fibrosis was first described more than 60 years ago, children with the disease rarely lived more than a few years. Today more than half of all patients with cystic fibrosis live beyond 30 years of age.

KEY POINTS

- Neonatal RDS affects 60,000 to 70,000 infants each year in the United States.
- The incidence of RDS increases with decreasing gestational age.
- A qualitative decrease in surfactant increases alveolar surface tension forces in RDS patients. This process causes alveoli to become unstable and collapse and leads to atelectasis and increased work of breathing.
- The definitive diagnosis of RDS usually is made with chest radiography. Diffuse, hazy, reticulogranular densities with the presence of air bronchograms and low lung volumes are typical of RDS.
- Continuous positive airway pressure and PEEP are the traditional support modes used to manage RDS. Surfactant replacement therapy and HFV have been added to these traditional approaches.
- Transient tachypnea of the newborn, often referred to as type II RDS, is probably the most common respiratory disorder of the newborn. The cause of TTN is unclear but is most likely related to delayed clearance of fetal lung liquid.
- Infants with TTN usually respond readily to low FIO_2 by Oxyhood or nasal cannula. Infants who need higher FIO_2 levels may benefit from CPAP.

Continued

KEY POINTS—cont'd

- Meconium aspiration syndrome is a disease of term and near-term infants. It involves aspiration of meconium into the central airways of the lung. This disorder usually is associated with perinatal depression and asphyxia.
- Meconium aspiration syndrome involves three primary problems: pulmonary obstruction, lung tissue damage, and pulmonary hypertension.
- Infants with MAS typically have gasping respirations, tachypnea, grunting, and retractions. The chest radiograph usually shows irregular pulmonary densities, which represent areas of atelectasis, combined with hyperlucent areas, which represent hyperinflation due to air-trapping.
- Management of MAS is complex and involves a variety of modalities, including airway intubation, suctioning, oxygen, CPAP, and sometimes mechanical ventilation.
- Infants, especially preterm infants, with severe respiratory failure in the first few weeks of life may develop a chronic pulmonary condition called *bronchopulmonary dysplasia*. Immaturity, malnutrition, oxygen toxicity, and mechanical ventilation all have been implicated in the origin of BPD.
- The best management of BPD is prevention. Prevention of atelectrauma and volutrauma begins in the delivery room.
- Infants with severe BPD may be dependent on supplemental oxygen or mechanical ventilation for months and have symptoms of airway obstruction for years. Therapy usually is supportive throughout the course of the disease.
- Persistent pulmonary hypertension of the newborn is a complex syndrome with many causes. The common denominator in PPHN is a return to fetal circulatory pathways, usually because of high PVR.
- Persistent pulmonary hypertension should be suspected when an infant has rapidly changing oxygen saturation without changes in FIO_2 or has hypoxemia out of proportion to the lung disease detected with a chest radiograph or on the basis of $PaCO_2$.

KEY POINTS—cont'd

- Congenital diaphragmatic hernia is severe disease that usually manifests as severe respiratory distress in the newborn period. The pathophysiologic mechanism is a complex combination of lung hypoplasia, including decreased alveolar count and decreased pulmonary vasculature, pulmonary hypertension, and unusual anatomy of the inferior vena cava.
- The general treatment of infants with congenital diaphragmatic hernia involves both neonatology and pediatric surgery. Initially, an ET tube is inserted, paralysis is induced, and mechanical ventilation is begun.
- Tetralogy of Fallot is a defect that includes (1) obstruction of right ventricular outflow (pulmonary stenosis), (2) ventricular septal defect (a hole between the right and left ventricles), (3) dextroposition of the aorta, and (4) right ventricular hypertrophy. Most patients are treated with surgery.
- Sudden infant death syndrome is the leading cause of death (40%) among infants younger than 1 year old in the United States. Approximately 7000 infants die of SIDS each year in the United States.
- The cause of SIDS remains unknown. Apnea of prematurity is not a predisposing factor, and there is no evidence that immaturity of the respiratory centers is a cause.
- Bronchiolitis is an acute infection of the lower respiratory tract usually caused by RSV.
- Bronchiolitis commonly occurs soon after a viral upper respiratory infection. The infant may have a slight fever with an intermittent cough. After a few days, signs of respiratory distress develop, particularly dyspnea and tachypnea. Progressive inflammation and narrowing of the airways causes inspiratory and expiratory wheezing and increases airway resistance. The chest radiographic examination shows signs of hyperinflation with areas of consolidation.
- Croup is a viral disorder of the upper airway that normally results in subglottic swelling and obstruction. Termed *laryngotracheobronchitis*, viral croup is caused by the parainfluenza virus and is the most common form of airway obstruction in children 6 months to 6 years of age.

KEY POINTS—cont'd

- Although little research supports the practice, treatment of a child with mild to moderate croup traditionally involves cool mist therapy with or without supplemental oxygen. Aerosolized racemic epinephrine and dexamethasone (0.3 mg/kg) are effective in decreasing the length and severity of respiratory symptoms associated with viral croup.
- Epiglottitis is an acute and often life-threatening infection of the upper airway that causes severe obstruction secondary to supraglottic swelling. Evidence suggests that the incidence of epiglottitis is decreasing among children, probably because of the use of vaccines.
- A child with epiglottitis usually has a high fever, sore throat, stridor, and labored breathing.
- A child with epiglottitis usually undergoes intubation for airway maintenance, and antibiotics are used for control of infection.
- Cystic fibrosis is the most common lethal genetic disorder among white persons. It is inherited as an autosomal recessive trait that affects approximately 30,000 people in the United States alone.
- Management of cystic fibrosis is complex. A respiratory therapist often provides postural drainage and aerosol therapy to maintain bronchial hygiene.

References

1. Wiswell TE, Mendiola J Jr: Respiratory distress syndrome in the newborn: innovative therapies. Am Fam Physician 47:407, 1993.
2. Phibbs RH et al: Initial clinical trial of EXOSURF, a protein-free synthetic surfactant, for the prophylaxis and early treatment of hyaline membrane disease, Pediatrics 88:1, 1991.
3. Hoekstra RE et al: Improved neonatal survival following multiple doses of bovine surfactant in very premature neonates at risk for respiratory distress syndrome, Pediatrics 88:10, 1991.
4. Jobe AH: Pulmonary surfactant therapy. N Engl J Med 328:861, 1993.
5. Yee WF, Scarpelli EM: Surfactant replacement therapy, Pediatr Pulmonol 11:65, 1991.
6. Hallman M et al: Factors affecting surfactant responsiveness, Ann Med 1991;23:693, 1991.
7. Rawlings JS, Smith FR: Transient tachypnea of the newborn: an analysis of neonatal and obstetric risk factors, Am J Dis Child 138:869, 1984.
8. Katz VL, Bowes WA Jr: Meconium aspiration syndrome: reflections on a murky subject, Am J Obstet Gynecol 166:171, 1992.
9. Burchfield DJ. Neonatal parenchymal diseases. In Koff PB, Eitzman DV, Neu J, editors: Neonatal and pediatric respiratory care, St Louis, 1988, Mosby.
10. Rossi EM et al: Meconium aspiration syndrome: intrapartum and neonatal attributes, Am J Obstet Gynecol 1989;161:1106, 1989.
11. Halliday HL: Endotracheal intubation at birth for preventing morbidity and mortality in vigorous, meconium-stained infants born at term, Cochrane Database Syst Rev CD000500, 2001.
12. Greenough A, Milner AD, Dimitriou G: Synchronized mechanical ventilation for respiratory support in newborn infants, Cochrane Database Syst Rev CD000456, 2001.
13. Soll RF, Dargaville P: Surfactant for meconium aspiration syndrome in full term infants, Cochrane Database Syst Rev CD002054, 2000.
14. Finer NN, Barrington KJ: Nitric oxide for respiratory failure in infants born at or near term, Cochrane Database Syst Rev CD000399, 2001.
15. Keszler M et al: Combined high-frequency jet ventilation in a meconium aspiration model, Crit Care Med 1986;14:34, 1986.
16. Clark RH et al: Lung injury in neonates: causes, strategies for prevention, and long- term consequences, J Pediatr 139:478, 2001.
17. Nickerson BG: Bronchopulmonary dysplasia: chronic pulmonary disease following neonatal respiratory failure, Chest 87:528, 1985.
18. Bancalari E, Gerhardt T: Bronchopulmonary dysplasia, Pediatr Clin North Am 33:1, 1986.
19. Chambers HM, van Velzen D: Ventilator-related pathology in the extremely immature lung, Pathology 21:79, 1989.
20. Frank L, Sosenko IR: Undernutrition as a major contributing factor in the pathogenesis of bronchopulmonary dysplasia, Am Rev Respir Dis 138:725, 1988.
21. Blanchard PW, Brown TM, Coates AL: Pharmacotherapy in bronchopulmonary dysplasia, Clin Perinatol 14:881, 1987.
22. Wilkie RA, Bryan MH: Effect of bronchodilators on airway resistance in ventilator-dependent neonates with chronic lung disease, J Pediatr 111:278-82, 1987.
23. Benini F et al: Dexamethasone in the treatment of bronchopulmonary dysplasia, Acta Paediatr Scand Suppl 360:108, 1989.
24. Harkavy KL et al: Dexamethasone therapy for chronic lung disease in ventilator- and oxygen-dependent infants: a controlled trial, J Pediatr 115:979, 1989.
25. Miller MJ, Martin RJ: Apnea of prematurity, Clin Perinatol 19:789, 1992.
26. Chesrown SE: Sudden infant death syndrome and apnea disorders. In Koff PB, Eitzman DV, Neu J, editors: Neonatal and pediatric respiratory care, ed 2, St. Louis, 1993, Mosby.

27. Stark AR: Disorders of respiratory control in infants, Respir Care 36:673, 1991.
28. Kriter KE, Blanchard J: Management of apnea in infants, Clin Pharm 8:577, 1989.
29. Barrington KJ et al: Physiologic effects of doxapram in idiopathic apnea of prematurity, J Pediatr 108:124, 1986.
30. Walsh MC, Stork EK: Persistent pulmonary hypertension of the newborn: rational therapy based on pathophysiology, Clin Perinatol 28:609, 2001.
31. Weinberger B et al: Pharmacologic therapy of persistent pulmonary hypertension of the newborn, Pharmacol Ther 89:67, 2001.
32. Golombek SG: The use of inhaled nitric oxide in newborn medicine, Heart Dis 2:342, 2000.
33. Somme S, Liu DC: New trends in extracorporeal membrane oxygenation in newborn pulmonary diseases, Artif Organs 25:633, 2001.
34. Kinsella JP, Abman SH: Inhaled nitric oxide: current and future uses in neonates, Semin Perinatol 24:387, 2000.
35. Cullen ML, Klein MD, Philippart AI: Congenital diaphragmatic hernia, Surg Clin North Am 65:1115, 1985.
36. Sawyer SF et al: Improving survival in the treatment of congenital diaphragmatic hernia, Ann Thorac Surg 41:75, 1986.
37. Bloom BT et al: Respiratory distress syndrome and tracheoesophageal fistula: management with high-frequency ventilation, Crit Care Med 18:447, 1990.
38. Goldberg LA, Marmon LM, Keszler M: High-frequency jet ventilation decreases air flow through a tracheoesophageal fistula, Crit Care Med 20:547, 1992.
39. Hiraishi S et al: Two-dimensional Doppler echocardiographic assessment of closure of the ductus arteriosus in normal newborn infants, J Pediatr 111:755, 1987.
40. Gentile R et al: Pulsed Doppler echocardiographic determination of time of ductal closure in normal newborn infants, J Pediatr 98:443, 1981.
41. Bailey LL, Gundry SR: Hypoplastic left heart syndrome, Pediatr Clin North Am 37:137, 1990.
42. Bardo DM et al: Hypoplastic left heart syndrome, Radiographics 21:705, 2001.
43. Cohen DM, Allen HD: New developments in the treatment of hypoplastic left heart syndrome, Curr Opin Cardiol 12:44, 1997.
44. Ungerleider RM: Pediatric cardiac surgery, Curr Opin Cardiol 7:73, 1992.
45. American Academy of Pediatrics AAP Task Force on Infant Positioning and SIDS: Positioning and SIDS, Pediatrics 89:1120, 1992.
46. Hunt CE: Sudden infant death syndrome and other causes of infant mortality: diagnosis, mechanisms, and risk for recurrence in siblings, Am J Respir Crit Care Med 164:346, 2001.
47. Bernard F, Dupont C, Viala P: Gastroesophageal reflux and upper airway diseases, Clin Rev Allergy 8:403, 1990.
48. Schuh S et al: Nebulized albuterol in acute bronchiolitis, J Pediatr 117:633, 1990.
49. Englund JA et al: High-dose, short-duration ribavirin aerosol therapy in children with suspected respiratory syncytial virus infection, J Pediatr 117:313, 1990.
50. Dawson KP, Steinberg A, Capaldi N: The lateral radiograph of neck in laryngo-tracheo-bronchitis (croup), J Qual Clin Pract 14:39, 1994.
51. Skolnik NS: Treatment of croup: a critical review, Am J Dis Child 143:1045, 1989.
52. Klassen TP et al: The efficacy of nebulized budesonide in dexamethasone-treated outpatients with croup, Pediatrics 97:463, 1996.
53. Kucera CM et al: Epiglottitis in adults and children in Olmsted County, Minnesota, 1976 through 1990, Mayo Clin Proc 71:1155, 1996.
54. Mayo-Smith MF et al: Acute epiglottitis: an 18-year experience in Rhode Island, Chest 108:1640, 1995.
55. Gonzalez Valdepena H et al: Epiglottitis and Haemophilus influenzae immunization: the Pittsburgh experience—a five-year review, Pediatrics 96:424, 1995.
56. Benjamin B: Acute epiglottitis, Ann Acad Med Singapore 20:696, 1991.
57. Anderson MP et al: Demonstration that CFTR is a chloride channel by alteration of its anion selectivity, Science 253:202, 1991.
58. Quinton PM Bijman J: Higher bioelectiric potentials due to decreased chloride absorption in the sweat glands of patient with cystic fibrosis, N Engl J Med 308:1185, 1983.
59. Di Sant'Agnese PA et al: Abnormal electrolyte composition of sweat in cystic fibrosis of the pancreas, Pediatrics 12:549, 1953.
60. Gibson LE, Cooke TR: A test for concentration of electrolytes in sweat in cystic fibrosis of the pancreas utilizing pilocarpine by iontophoresis, Pediatrics 23:545, 1959.
61. Stern RC: The diagnosis of cystic fibrosis, N Engl J Med 336:487, 1997.
62. Thomas J, Cook DJ, Brooks D: Chest physical therapy management of patients with cystic fibrosis: a meta-analysis, J Respir Crit Care Med 151:846, 1995.
63. Fuchs HJ et al: Effect of aerosolized recombinant DNase on exacerbations of respiratory symptoms and on pulmonary function in patients with cystic fibrosis. The Pulmozyme Study Group, N Engl J Med 331:637, 1994.
64. Ramsey BW et al: Intermittent administration of inhaled tobramycin in patients with cystic fibrosis. The Cystic Fibrosis Inhaled Tobramycin Study Group, N Engl J Med 340:23, 1999.
65. Konstan MW et al: Effect of high dose ibuprofen in patients with cystic fibrosis, N Engl J Med 332:848, 1995.

SECTION V

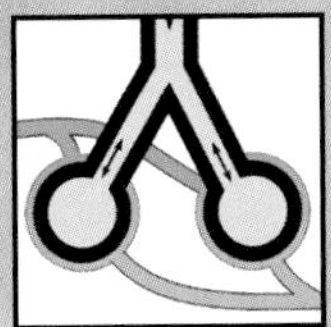

Basic Therapeutics

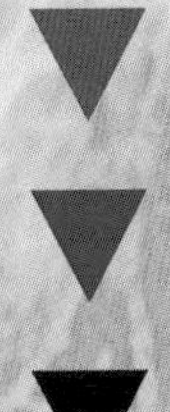

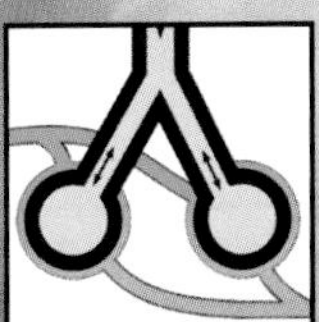

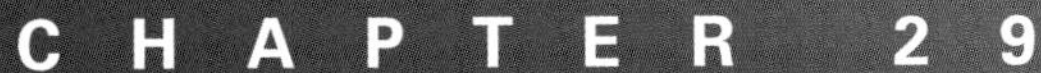
CHAPTER 29

Airway Pharmacology

Joseph L. Rau

In This Chapter You Will Learn:

- What three phases constitute the course of drug action from dose to effect
- What classes of drugs are delivered via the aerosol route
- What mode of action, indications, and adverse effects characterize each major class of aerosolized drug
- What the available aerosol formulations, brand names, and dosages are for specific drugs in each class
- How to select the appropriate drug class for a given patient or clinical situation
- How to assess the outcomes for each class of aerosol drug therapy

Chapter Outline

Key Terms

adrenergic
agonists
antagonists
antiadrenergic
anticholinergic
catecholamine
cholinergic
COMT
degranulation

Continued

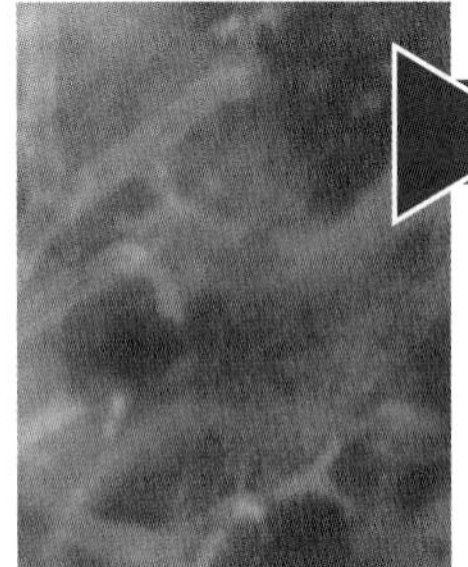

Key Terms—cont'd

drug signaling
L/T ratio
leukotriene
muscarinic
mydriasis
neutropenia
pancreatitis
pharmacodynamic phase
pharmacokinetic phase
prodrug
stomatitis
tachyphylaxis
transcription
vasopressor

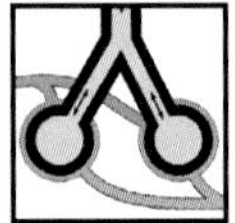

The primary focus of respiratory care pharmacology is the delivery of bronchoactive inhaled aerosols to the respiratory tract for the diagnosis and treatment of pulmonary diseases. Although other drug classes are used in respiratory care, this chapter will limit discussion to bronchoactive inhaled aerosols. Reviews of other drug classes can be found in pharmacology texts.[1-3]

▶ PRINCIPLES OF PHARMACOLOGY

Three phases constitute the course of drug action from dose to effect: the drug administration, pharmacokinetic, and pharmacodynamic phases. These three phases of drug action can be applied to drug treatment of the respiratory tract with bronchoactive inhaled agents.

The Drug Administration Phase

The drug administration phase describes the method by which a drug dose is made available to the body. Administering drugs directly to the respiratory tract uses the *inhalation route*, and the dose form is an *aerosol* of liquid solutions, suspensions, or dry powders. The most commonly used devices to administer orally or nasally inhaled aerosols are the metered-dose inhaler (MDI), the small-volume nebulizer (SVN), and the dry-powder inhaler (DPI). Reservoir devices, including both holding chambers with one-way inspiratory valves and simple, nonvalved spacer devices, are often added to an MDI to reduce the need for complex hand-breathing coordination and to reduce oropharyngeal impaction of the aerosol drug (see Chapter 33).

The advantages for treatment of the respiratory tract with inhaled aerosols are as follows:

- Aerosol doses are usually smaller than doses for systemic administration.
- Onset of drug action is rapid.
- Delivery is targeted to the organ requiring treatment.
- Systemic side effects are often fewer and less severe.

There are also disadvantages to the delivery of inhaled aerosols in treating respiratory disease, and these include the number of variables affecting the delivered dose and lack of adequate knowledge on device performance and use among patients and caregivers.[4]

The Pharmacokinetic Phase

The pharmacokinetic phase of drug action describes the time course and disposition of a drug in the body based on its absorption, distribution, metabolism, and elimination. Inhaled bronchoactive aerosols are intended for local effects in the airway. Undesired systemic effects result from absorption and distribution throughout the body. One method of limiting distribution of inhaled aerosols is use of a fully ionized drug rather than a nonionized agent. A fully ionized drug is not absorbed across lipid membranes, while a nonionized drug is lipid-soluble and diffuses across cell membranes and into the bloodstream. An example of this is ipratropium, in comparison with atropine sulfate. Ipratropium is a fully ionized quaternary ammonium compound that diffuses poorly across lipid membranes. Atropine is poorly ionized and diffuses well, distributing throughout the body. As a result, atropine produces systemic side effects such as mydriasis and blurring of vision. The effects of ipratropium are largely local to the airway, and systemic effects are nonexistent or minimal.

An inhaled aerosol distributes to the lung and stomach through swallowing of a drug that deposits in the oropharynx. The therapeutic effect of the aerosol drug is caused by the portion in the airway. Systemic effects are due to absorption of the drug from the airway and gastrointestinal (GI) tract. The ideal aerosol would distribute only to the airway with none reaching the stomach. The lung availability/total systemic availability ratio (L/T ratio) quantifies the efficiency of aerosol delivery to the lung.

L/T ratio = Lung availability/(Lung + GI Availability)

This concept, proposed by Borgström and elaborated by Thorsson, is illustrated in Figure 29-1, showing delivery of albuterol by inhalation using an MDI and a DPI.[5-6]

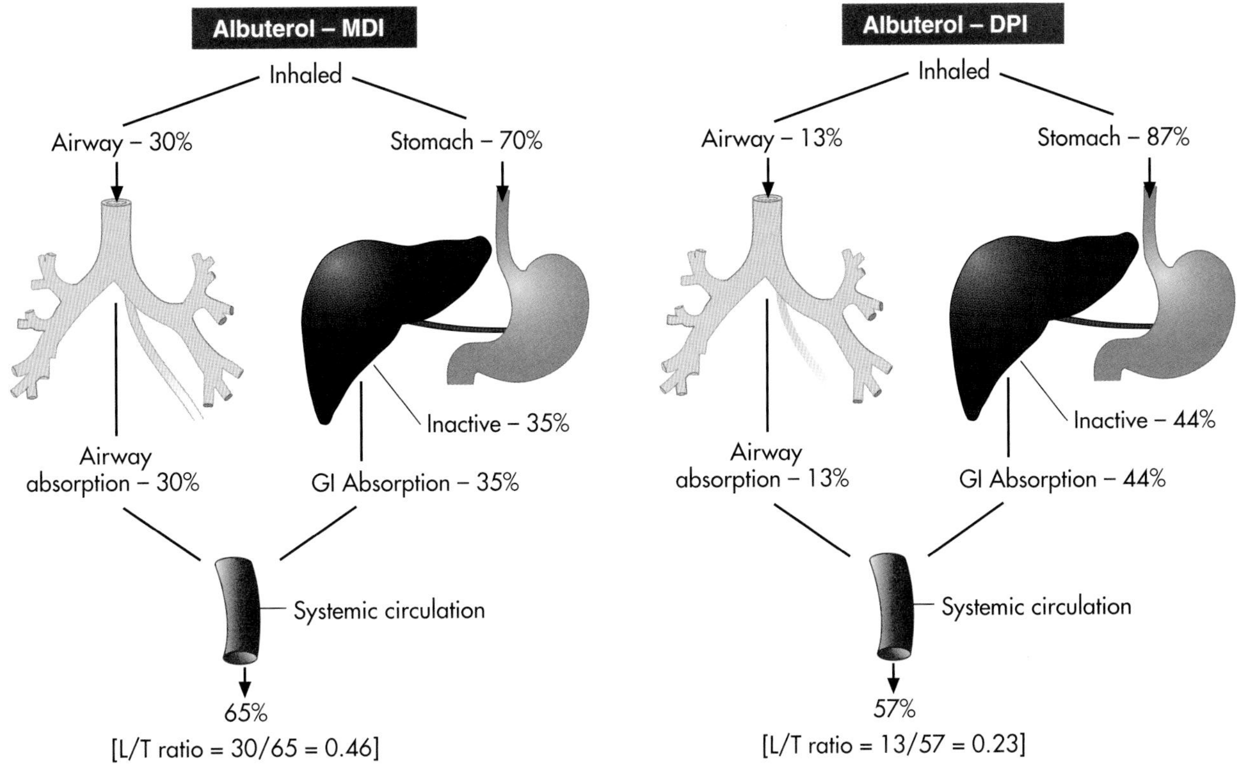

Figure 29-1 • **Comparison of Efficiency of Aerosol Delivery With Two Devices, Using the L/T Availability Ratio**
MDI, metered dose inhaler; *DPI*, dry powder inhaler. *(From Rau JL: Respiratory care pharmacology, ed 6, St. Louis, 2002, Mosby.)*

The Pharmacodynamic Phase

The pharmacodynamic phase describes the mechanisms of drug action by which a drug molecule causes its effects in the body. Drug effects are caused by the combination of a drug with a matching receptor. Drug signaling mechanisms include the following:

Signaling Mechanism	Example
Mediation by G protein (guanine nucleotide)-linked receptors	β-adrenergic agonists, antimuscarinic agents
Attachment to intracellular receptors by lipid-soluble drugs	Corticosteroids

The mechanisms of drug action will be briefly described for each class of bronchoactive drug.

Airway Receptors and Neural Control of the Lung

Pharmacological control of the airway is mediated by receptors found on airway smooth muscle, secretory cells, bronchial epithelium, and pulmonary and bronchial blood vessels. There are both sympathetic (adrenergic) and parasympathetic (cholinergic) receptors in the lung. The terminology for drugs acting on these receptors is based on the usual neurotransmitter that acts on the receptor. The usual neurotransmitter in the sympathetic system is norepinephrine, which is similar to epinephrine, also known as *adrenalin*. The usual neurotransmitter in the parasympathetic system is acetylcholine. The receptors responding to these neurotransmitters are termed *adrenergic* and *cholinergic* respectively. Agonists (stimulating agents) and antagonists (blocking agents) that act on these receptors are given the following classifications:

- **Adrenergic (adrenomimetic):** A drug that stimulates a receptor responding to norepinephrine or epinephrine
- **Antiadrenergic:** A drug that blocks a receptor for norepinephrine or epinephrine
- **Cholinergic (cholinomimetic):** A drug that stimulates a receptor for acetylcholine
- **Anticholinergic:** A drug that blocks a receptor for acetylcholine
- **Muscarinic:** A drug that stimulates acetylcholine receptors specifically at parasympathetic nerve-ending sites

Because cholinergic receptors exist at autonomic ganglia as well as at the myoneural junction in skeletal muscle, the terms *muscarinic* and *antimuscarinic* distinguish cholinergic agents whose action is limited to parasympathetic sites. For example, neostigmine is a *cholinergic* (indirect acting) drug that increases receptor

Table 29-1 ▶▶ Airway Receptors and Their Effects in the Cardiopulmonary System*

Location	Receptor	Effect
Heart	β_1-adrenergic	Increased rate, force
	M_2-cholinergic	Decreased rate
Bronchiolar smooth muscle	β_2-adrenergic	Bronchodilation
	M_3-cholinergic	Bronchoconstriction
Pulmonary blood vessels	α_1-adrenergic	Vasoconstriction
	β_2-adrenergic	Vasodilation
	M_3-cholinergic	Vasodilation
Bronchial blood vessels	α_1-adrenergic	Vasoconstriction
	β_2-adrenergic	Vasodilation
Submucosal glands	α_1-adrenergic	Increased fluid, mucin
	β_2-adrenergic	Increased fluid, mucin
	M_3-cholinergic	Exocytosis, secretion

*Adrenergic and muscarinic cholinergic receptor subtypes are indicated. M_2, M_3, subtypes of muscarinic (*M*) cholinergic receptors.

stimulation at both the myoneural junction and the parasympathetic sites. By contrast, atropine is an *antimuscarinic* agent, which only blocks the action of acetylcholine at the parasympathetic sites. Table 29-1 summarizes receptors and their effects for the cardiopulmonary system. A more detailed description of the autonomic nervous system and receptor subtypes can be found in Katzung's[3] text of general pharmacology.

▶ ADRENERGIC BRONCHODILATORS

The adrenergic bronchodilators represent the largest single group of drugs among the aerosolized agents used for oral inhalation. Some of the drugs in this group are now considered clinically obsolete, although all agents are included for completeness. Table 29-2 lists bronchodilators in this group, with their aerosol formulations, selected brand names, and dosages. A more detailed review of this class is offered by Jenne, Aranson and Rau, and Rau.[7-9]

Indications for Use

The general indication for use of an adrenergic bronchodilator is the presence of reversible airflow obstruction. The most common use of these agents clinically is to improve flowrates in asthma (including exercise-induced asthma), acute and chronic bronchitis, emphysema, bronchiectasis, cystic fibrosis, and other obstructive airway states.

Indication for Short-Acting Agents

Short-acting β_2-agonists such as albuterol, levalbuterol, or pirbuterol, are indicated for relief of *acute* reversible airflow obstruction in asthma or other obstructive airway diseases.

Short-acting agents are termed "rescue" agents in the 1997 National Asthma Education and Prevention Program Expert Panel II (NAEPP EPR II) guidelines.[10]

Indication for Long-Acting Agents

Long-acting agents, such as salmeterol or formoterol, are indicated for maintenance bronchodilation and control of bronchospasm and nocturnal symptoms in asthma or other obstructive diseases.

NAEPP EPR II guidelines consider salmeterol a "controller"; its slow time-to-peak effect makes it a poor rescue drug. In asthma, a long-acting bronchodilator is usually combined with antiinflammatory medication for control of airway inflammation and bronchospasm. Even though formoterol has a rapid onset and peak effect similar to albuterol, its prolonged activity makes it a better maintenance drug rather than an acute reliever or rescue agent.

Indication for Racemic Epinephrine

Racemic epinephrine is often used either by inhaled aerosol or by direct lung instillation for its strong α-adrenergic vasoconstricting effect; to reduce airway swelling after extubation, during epiglottitis, croup, or bronchiolitis; or to control airway bleeding during endoscopy.

Mode of Action and Effects

Adrenergic bronchodilators can stimulate one or more of the following receptors, with the effects described:

Table 29-2 ▶▶ Inhaled Adrenergic Brochodilator Agents Currently Available in the United States

Drug	Brand Name	Receptor Preference	Adult Dosage	Time Course (Onset, Peak, Duration)
Epinephrine	Adrenalin Cl	(α, β)	SVN: 1% solution (1:100), 0.25-0.5 mL (2.5-5.0 mg) qid MDI: 0.2 mg/puff, 2 puffs as ordered or needed	3-5 min 5-20 min 1-3 hr
Racemic epinephrine	MicroNefrin, AsthmaNefrin, various	(α, β)	SVN: 2.25% solution, 0.25-0.5 mL (5.63-11.25 mg) qid	3-5 min 5-20 min 0.5-2 hr
Isoproterenol	Isuprel, Isuprel Mistometer	(β)	SVN: 0.5% solution (1:200), 0.25-0.5 mL (1.25-2.5 mg) qid MDI: 103 μg/puff, 2 puffs qid	2-5 min 5-30 min 0.5-2 hr
Isoetharine	Isoetharine HCl	(β_2)	SVN: 1% solution, 0.25-0.5 mL (2.5-5.0 mg) qid	1-6 min 15-60 min
Terbutaline	Brethaire	(β_2)	MDI: 200 μg/puff, 2 puffs q 4-6 hr TABS: 2.5 or 5 mg, 5 mg q 6 hr INJ: 1 mg/mL, 0.25 mg sc	1-3 hr 5-30 min 30-60 min 3-6 hr
Metaproterenol	Alupent	(β_2)	SVN: 5% solution, 0.3 mL (15 mg), tid, qid MDI: 650 μg/puff, 2-3 puffs tid, qid TABS: 10 or 20 mg, 20 mg tid, qid SYRUP: 10 mg/5 mL, 2 tsp tid, qid	1-5 min 60 min 2-6 hr
Albuterol	Proventil, Proventil HFA, Ventolin	(β_2)	SVN: 0.5% solution, 0.5 mL (2.5 mg) tid, qid MDI: 90 μg/puff, 2 puffs tid, qid TABS: 2 mg, 4 mg tid, qid SYRUP: 2 mg/5 mL, 1-2 tsp tid, qid	15 min 30-60 min
Bitolterol	Tornalate	(β_2)	SVN: 0.31 mg and 0.2% solution, 1.25 mL (2.5 mg) bid-qid MDI: 370 μg/puff, 2 puffs q 8 hr	3-4 min 30-60 min 5-8 hr
Pirbuterol	Maxair	(β_2)	MDI: 200 μg/puff, 2 puffs q 4-6 hr	5 min 30 min 5 hr
Levalbuterol	Xopenex	(β_2)	SVN: 0.31 mg and 0.63 mg/3 mL tid or 1.25 mg/3 mL tid	15 min 30-60 min 5-8 hr
Salmeterol	Serevent	(β_2)	MDI: 25 μg/puff, 2 puffs bid DPI: 50 μg/blister bid	20 min 3-5 hr 12 hr
Formoterol	Foradil	(β_2)	DPI: 12 μg/inhalation bid	5 min 30-60 min 12 hr

- α-receptor stimulation: Causes vasoconstriction and a vasopressor effect (increased blood pressure).
- β_1-receptor stimulation: Causes increased heart rate and myocardial contractility.
- β_2-receptor stimulation: Relaxes bronchial smooth muscle, stimulates mucociliary activity, and has some inhibitory action on inflammatory mediator release.

Bronchodilation, through stimulation of β_2-receptors, is the desired therapeutic effect. Both α- and β-adrenergic receptors are G protein-linked receptors. Figure 29-2 illustrates the mode of action for relaxation of airway smooth muscle when a β_2-receptor is stimulated. The nature of the β-receptor and its activity is presented in detail in a 1995 review by Barnes.[11]

Adrenergic Bronchodilator Agents

The group of adrenergic bronchodilator agents represents the evolution of a drug class. Although all of these agents are adrenergic agonists, the differences among individual agents are due to their receptor preference (α-, β_1-, β_2-adrenergic) and their different pharmacokinetics as listed in Table 29-2. These differences determine the optimal clinical application of individual agents, as discussed subsequently. The adrenergic bronchodilators actually form three subgroups.

Ultra-Short-Acting Catecholamines

The older agents, such as *epinephrine*, *isoproterenol*, and *isoetharine*, were all catecholamines. These agents

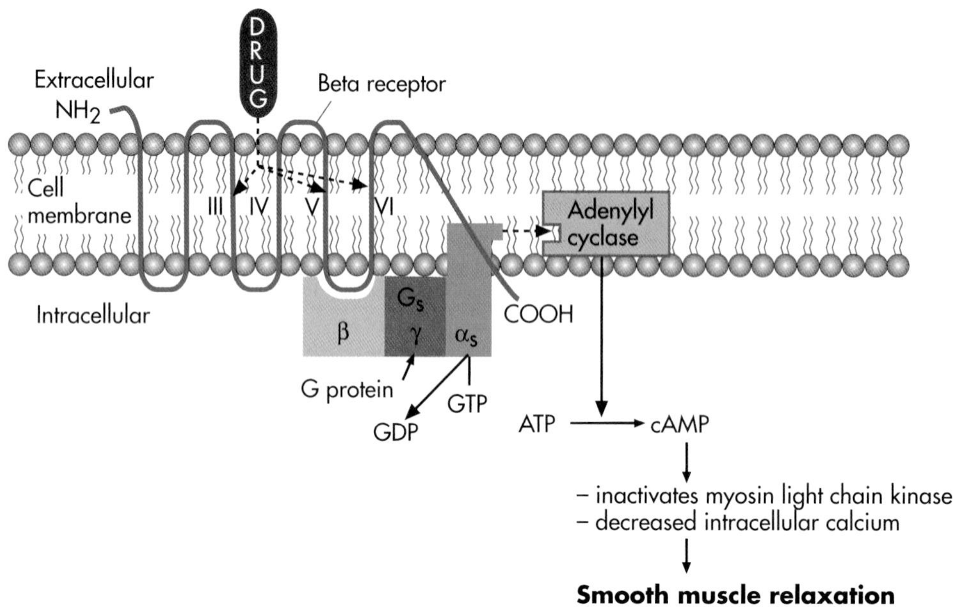

Figure 29-2 · Illustration of Mode of Action by Which a β-Agonist Stimulates the G Protein-Linked β-Receptor to Cause Smooth Muscle Relaxation

Adrenergic agonists such as albuterol or epinephrine attach to β-receptors, which are polypeptide chains traversing the cell membrane seven times. This causes activation of the stimulatory G protein, designated G_S, linked to the receptor. When stimulated, the receptor undergoes a conformational change, and the α subunit of the G protein attaches to adenylyl cyclase. Activation of adenylyl cyclase by the G_S protein causes an increased synthesis of the second messenger, cyclic adenosine monophosphate (cAMP). This ultimately causes smooth muscle relaxation and bronchodilation. *(From Rau JL: Respiratory care pharmacology, ed 6, St. Louis, 2002, Mosby.)*

lacked β_2-specificity. As a result, cardiac effects, especially tachycardia and increased blood pressure, were common. As catecholamines, they were metabolized rapidly by the enzyme catechol O-methyltransferase (COMT) and had a short duration of action. Because of their strong α_1-activity and vasoconstricting effect, epinephrine and the synthetic racemic epinephrine are used to reduce swelling in the nose (nasal decongestant), larynx (croup, epiglottitis), and to control bleeding during bronchoscopic biopsy.

Short-Acting Noncatecholamine Agents

Because of their short duration of action and lack of β_2-specificity, the catecholamines were replaced with longer-acting, β_2-specific agents. These have included *metaproterenol*, *terbutaline*, *albuterol*, and *pirbuterol*. Because their duration of action is approximately 4 to 6 hours, these drugs were more suited to maintenance therapy than the catecholamines and could be taken on a qid schedule. However, their modest duration of action results in the loss of bronchodilating effect overnight.

Bitolterol is a prodrug, which is metabolized by ester enzymes to the active form, colterol. Colterol is a catecholamine and its duration of action is due to the gradual hydrolysis of the prodrug, giving a sustained-release effect.

Single-Isomer β Agonists. In March, 1999, *levalbuterol* was approved as a single-isomer β_2-selective agonist. Previous inhaled formulations of adrenergic bronchodilators were all synthetic racemic mixtures, containing both the R-isomer and S-isomer in equal amounts. Levalbuterol is the pure R-isomer of racemic albuterol. Both stereoisomers of albuterol are shown in Figure 29-3 with the single-isomer (R-isomer) form of levalbuterol. Although the S-isomer is physiologically inactive on adrenergic receptors, there is accumulating evidence that the S-isomer is *not* inactive completely. Box 29-1 lists some of the physiological effects of S-albuterol noted in the literature.[12-18] The effects noted would antagonize the bronchodilating effects of the R-isomer and promote bronchoconstriction. In addition, the S-isomer is more slowly metabolized than the R-isomer. Levalbuterol was released as a nebulization solution in two strengths: 0.63-mg and 1.25-mg, with a later 0.31-mg dose. In a study by Nelson et al,[19] the 0.63-mg dose has been found comparable to the 2.5-mg racemic albuterol dose in onset and duration. Side effects of tremor and heart rate changes were less with the single-isomer formulation. The 1.25-mg dose showed a higher peak effect on FEV_1 with an 8-hour duration compared to racemic albuterol. Side effects with this dose were equivalent to those seen with racemic albuterol. It is significant that an equivalent clinical response was seen with one fourth of the racemic dose (0.63 mg) using the pure isomer,

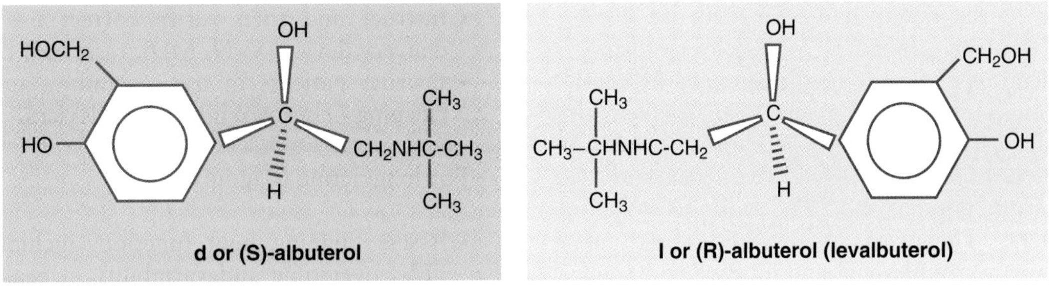

d or (S)-albuterol

l or (R)-albuterol (levalbuterol)

Figure 29-3 · R- and S-Isomers of Racemic Albuterol
Levalbuterol is the single, R-isomer form of racemic albuterol and contains no S-isomer.

Box 29-1 • Effects and Characteristics of the S-Isomer of Albuterol

- Increases intracellular calcium concentration in vitro.[12]
- Activity is blocked by the anticholinergic atropine.[12]
- Does not produce pulmonary or extrapulmonary β_2-mediated effects.[13]
- Enhances experimental airway responsiveness in vitro.[14]
- Increases contractile response of bronchial tissue to histamine or leukotriene C_4 (LTC_4) in vitro.[15]
- Enhances eosinophil superoxide production with interleukin-5 (IL-5) stimulation.[16]
- Slower metabolism than R-albuterol in vivo.[17]
- Preferential retention in the lung when inhaled by MDI (in vivo).[18]

although the racemic mixture contains 1.25 mg of the R-isomer (half of the total 2.5 mg dose). A detailed review of levalbuterol and differences between the R- and S-isomers of albuterol is available.[20]

Long-Acting Adrenergic Bronchodilators

The release of *salmeterol* offered the first long-acting adrenergic bronchodilator in the United States. In contrast to previous agents, salmeterol's duration of action is about 12 hours. The pharmacokinetics of salmeterol make it suitable for maintenance therapy, particularly with nocturnal asthma. However, it is not well suited for relief of acute airflow obstruction or bronchospasm because its onset is longer than 20 minutes, with a peak effect occurring by 3 to 5 hours. Although this agent is a β_2-agonist, its exact mode of action differs from previous β_2-agonists, allowing persistent receptor stimulation over a prolonged period of hours. A more detailed discussion of the action of salmeterol can be found in a review by Johnson.[21]

In 2001, *formoterol* was approved for general clinical use in the United States and represents a second long-acting, β_2-specific agent. The duration of effect is approximately 12 hours, but in contrast with salmeterol, the onset of action and peak effect of formoterol are rapid and similar to that of albuterol.[22] Nonetheless, patients should be cautioned about the risk of accumulation and toxicity if formoterol is used as a rescue agent in the same way that shorter-acting β-agonists, such as albuterol, are. As with salmeterol, the extensive side chain or tail makes formoterol more lipophilic than the shorter-acting bronchodilators and is the basis for its longer duration of effect. The approved formulation of formoterol is a racemic mixture (RR-, SS-formoterol), and the single-isomer of RR-formoterol is under investigation.

Adverse Effects

The older adrenergic agents such as isoproterenol commonly caused tachycardia, palpitations, and an "adrenalin effect" of shakiness and nervousness. The newer, more β_2-selective agents are safe and typically cause tremor as the main side effect. Other common side effects with the inhaled agents include headache, insomnia, and nervousness. Patients should be reassured that some tolerance to these effects will occur. Potential adverse effects with use of adrenergic bronchodilators include the following:

- Chlorofluorocarbon (CFC) propellant-induced bronchospasm
- Dizziness
- Hypokalemia
- Loss of bronchoprotection
- Nausea
- Tolerance (tachyphylaxis)
- Worsening ventilation-perfusion ratio (decrease in Pa_{O_2})

Inhalation gives fewer and less severe side effects than oral administration. Although tolerance develops to the bronchodilating effect, this is not a contraindication to use of the drugs, and relaxation of airway smooth muscle still occurs. Desaturation due to mismatching of ventilation and perfusion with inhalation of the aerosol is not clinically significant and reverses quickly. Bronchospasm due to CFC propellants can be prevented by changing to the newer hydrofluoroalkane (HFA)-propelled MDIs or a different aerosol delivery form.

The implication of β_2-adrenergic agonists in deaths due to asthma, termed the *asthma paradox* or the *β-agonist controversy*, remains debated.[23] There is evidence of loss of a bronchoprotective effect with use of β-agonists, and patients should be cautioned to avoid asthma triggers.[24] The increased prevalence of asthma in general remains a troublesome and unresolved issue.

Assessment of Bronchodilator Therapy

Assessment of therapy with adrenergic bronchodilators should be based on the indication(s) for the aerosol agent (presence of reversible airflow due to primary bronchospasm or other obstruction secondary to an inflammatory response and/or secretions, either acute or chronic). With all aerosol drug therapy, basic vital signs (respiratory rate and pattern, pulse, breath sounds) should be assessed before and after treatment, especially for initial drug use, as well as the patient's subjective reaction (complaints of breathing difficulty). Patients should be instructed in the correct use of the aerosol device used, with verification of correct use. Finally, the patient's subjective reaction to the treatment should be monitored for any change in breathing effort. The previous assessment applies to all subsequent drug groups by aerosol and is not repeated for each class. The following specific actions are suggested to evaluate patient response to this class of drugs:

- Monitor flow rates using bedside peak flow meters, portable spirometry, or laboratory reports of pulmonary function before and after bronchodilator studies to assess reversibility of airflow obstruction.
- Assess arterial blood gases (ABGs) or pulse oximeter saturation, as needed, for acute states with asthma or chronic obstructive pulmonary disease (COPD) to monitor changes in ventilation and gas exchange (oxygenation).
- Note effect of β-agonists on blood glucose (increase) and K^+ (decrease) laboratory values, if high doses, such as with continuous nebulization or emergency department treatment, are used.
- Long-term: Monitor pulmonary function studies of lung volumes, capacities, and flows.
- Instruct asthmatic patients in use and interpretation of disposable peak flow meters to assess severity of asthmatic episodes and provide an action plan for treatment modification.
- Patient education should emphasize that β-agonists do not treat underlying inflammation nor prevent progression of asthma, and additional antiinflammatory treatment or more aggressive medical therapy may be needed if there is a poor response to the rescue β-agonist.
- Instruct and then verify correct use of aerosol delivery device (SVN, MDI, reservoir, DPI).
- Instruct patients in use, assembly, and especially cleaning of aerosol inhalation devices.

For long-acting β-agonists:

- Assess ongoing lung function, including predose FEV_1 over time and variability in peak expiratory flows.
- Assess amount of rescue β-agonist use and nocturnal symptoms.
- Assess number of exacerbations, unscheduled clinic visits, and hospitalizations.
- Assess days of absence due to symptoms.
- Assess ability to reduce the dose of concomitant inhaled corticosteroids.

NOTE: Death has been associated with excessive use of inhaled adrenergic agents in severe acute asthma crises. Individuals using such drugs should be instructed to contact a physician or an emergency room if there is no response to the usual dose of the inhaled agent.

RULE OF THUMB

Choosing an Aerosol Agent

Choose an aerosol agent to treat the respiratory tract based on the indication for the agent or class of drugs and a corresponding presence of the indication in the patient.

Example: Adrenergic bronchodilator. The indication is presence of reversible airflow obstruction. The patient demonstrates a 20% improvement in FEV_1 on spirometry with use of inhaled albuterol. Choose an adrenergic bronchodilator.

Example: Inhaled corticosteroid. The indication is mild-to-moderate, persistent asthma. The patient with asthma reports a need to use a β-agonist inhaler more than 5 days each week and complains of waking up at night with shortness of breath. Choose an inhaled corticosteroid.

▶ ANTICHOLINERGIC BRONCHODILATORS

A second method of producing airway relaxation is through blockade of cholinergic-induced bronchoconstriction. An important difference between the β-agonists and the anticholinergic bronchodilators is the active stimulatory action of the former versus the passive blockade of the latter. A cholinergic blocking agent is only effective if bronchoconstriction exists due to cholinergic activity.

MINI CLINI

Assessing β-Agonist's Side Effects

PROBLEM

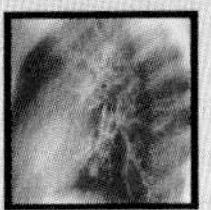

You have administered an aerosol treatment of albuterol using an MDI with a holding chamber to a 67-year-old patient with newly diagnosed COPD who was admitted for an acute exacerbation and shortness of breath. When you return for the second treatment that day, he informs you that he began to feel very shaky and nervous, beginning about 30 minutes after the previous treatment. He also noticed a tremor when he held his water cup and took a drink. His pulse during the earlier treatment was 84 beats per minute. Your clinical assessment shows that he is coherent, has good color, is not diaphoretic, and is in no respiratory distress. His respiratory rate is 16 breaths per minute and regular and his pulse is now 82 beats per minute and regular. Auscultation reveals mild wheezing and scattered rhonchi, with little change from earlier breath sounds. You observe a mild tremor when he holds his hand out. On questioning, he states that he is now feeling better and the "shakiness" has subsided a bit.

DISCUSSION

This patient's situation exemplifies a common reaction to inhaled adrenergic bronchodilators. Although albuterol is β_2-preferential, it is still an epinephrine-like drug and can produce side effects due to sympathetic stimulation. The description of the symptoms is suggestive of common adrenergic side effects (tremor, shakiness). The timing of the symptoms coincides with the pharmacokinetics of albuterol (peak effect in 30 to 60 minutes). As presented in the case description, it is important to rule out other complications. Your physical examination shows no changes from the earlier treatment in his vital signs.

It is important to caution patients about "normal" expected side effects and to reassure them that the side effects will decrease with tolerance to the medication. In addition, be alert to the possibility that patients may have deteriorated or changed in their respiratory status.

Indications for Use

Ipratropium bromide is the only agent approved as an inhaled aerosol bronchodilator at this time, although approval of the long-acting agent, tiotropium bromide, is anticipated. Table 29-3 lists the dosage forms and pharmacokinetics of ipratropium and several other anticholinergic (antimuscarinic) agents used as bronchodilators. Generally, anticholinergic agents have been found to be as effective as the β-agonists in airflow improvement in COPD but less so in asthma. A nasal formulation of ipratropium is also available for relief of allergic and nonallergic perennial rhinitis, including the common cold.[25]

Indication for anticholinergic bronchodilator: Ipratropium or other anticholinergic agents are indicated as bronchodilators for maintenance treatment in COPD, including chronic bronchitis and emphysema.

Indication for combined anticholinergic and β-agonist bronchodilators: A combination anticholinergic and β-agonist, such as ipratropium bromide and albuterol (Combivent), is indicated for use in patients with COPD on regular treatment who require additional bronchodilation for relief of airflow obstruction. Ipratropium bromide is also commonly used in severe asthma in addition to β-agonists, especially in acute bronchoconstriction that does not respond well to β-agonist therapy.

Mode of Action

As antimuscarinic agents, ipratropium and tiotropium act as competitive antagonists for acetylcholine at muscarinic receptors on airway smooth muscle. Part of the airflow obstruction in COPD may be due to vagally-mediated, reflex cholinergic stimulation. Airway irritation and inflammation stimulate afferent sensory C-fibers in the airway, which synapse with efferent vagal (cholinergic) fibers to the airway and mucus glands. The muscarinic receptor subtype on smooth muscle and submucosal mucus glands is the M_3 receptor, which is a G protein-linked receptor. The effect of acetylcholine, the usual neurotransmitter, on the muscarinic (M_3) receptors on airway smooth muscle is bronchoconstriction. The M_1 receptor at the ganglionic junction enhances cholinergic nerve transmission. The M_2 receptor is an auto-receptor inhibiting further release of acetylcholine, so that blockade can increase acetylcholine release and may offset the bronchodilating effect of ipratropium.[26]

Ipratropium bromide and tiotropium bromide block the action of acetylcholine at the M_3 receptor in the airway, reversing bronchoconstriction due to cholinergic activity. Ipratropium is a nonselective muscarinic receptor blocker and has affinity for M_1, M_2, and M_3 receptors. Blockade of the M_2 receptor can theoretically reverse the bronchodilating effect of ipratropium or other nonselective muscarinic receptor antagonists, because the autoinhibitory action of the M_2 receptor is blocked. Both ipratropium and tiotropium are quaternary ammonium compounds and are poorly absorbed following inhalation.

Tiotropium exhibits receptor subtype selectivity for M_1 and M_3 receptors. The drug binds to all three muscarinic receptors (M_1, M_2, and M_3) but dissociates much more slowly than ipratropium from the M_1 and M_3 receptors. This results in a selectivity of action on M_1 and M_3 receptors. In patients with COPD, tiotropium gives a bronchodilating effect for up to 24 hours, with an adequate dose. Inhalation of a single dose gives a peak plasma level within 5 minutes, with a rapid decline to very low levels within 1 hour.[26]

Table 29-3 ▶▶ Inhaled Anticholinergic Brochodilator Agents*

Drug	Brand Name	Adult Dosage	Time Course (Onset, Peak, Duration)
Ipratropium bromide	Atrovent	MDI: 18 μg/puff, 2 puffs qid SVN: 0.02% solution (0.2 mg/mL), 500 μg tid, qid Nasal spray: 0.03%, 0.06%; 2 sprays per nostril 2 to 4 times daily (dosage varies)	15 min 1-2 hr 4-6 hr
Ipratropium bromide and albuterol	Combivent DuoNeb	MDI: Ipratropium 18 μg/puff and albuterol 90 μg/puff, 2 puffs qid SVN: Ipratropium 0.5 mg and albuterol sulfate 3.0 mg (equal to albuterol base 2.5 mg)	15 min 1-2 hr 4-6 hr
Oxitropium bromide†	Oxivent	MDI: 100 mg/puff, 2 puffs bid, tid	15 min 1-2 hr 8 hr
Tiotropium bromide‡	Spiriva	DPI: 18 μg/inhalation, 1 inhalation daily	30 min 3 hr 24 hr

*A holding chamber is recommended with MDI administration to prevent accidental eye exposure.
† Available outside the United States.
‡ Investigational.

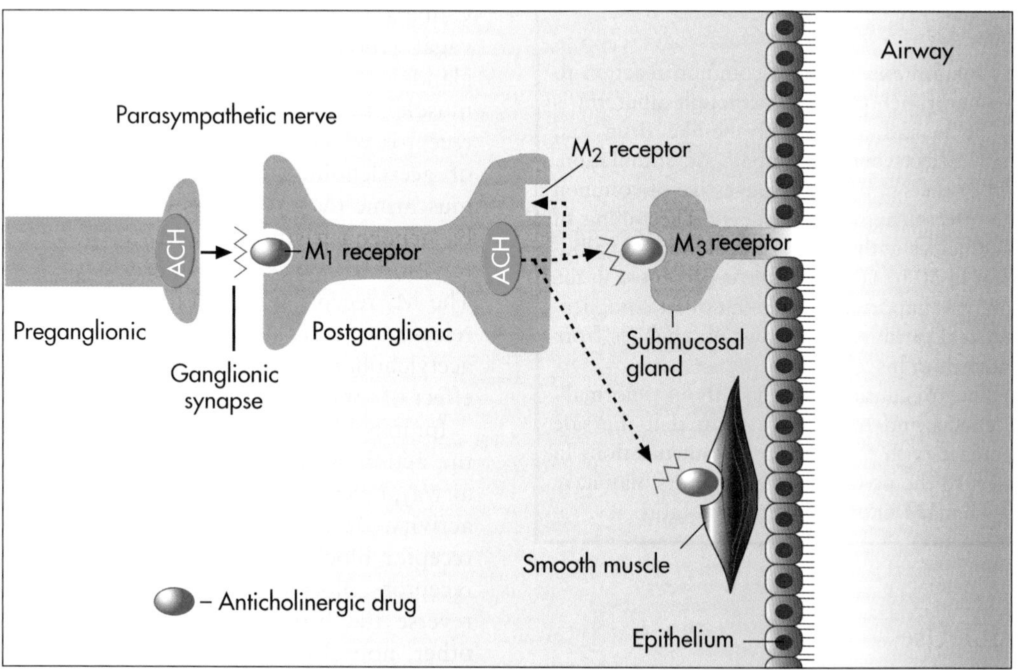

Figure 29-4 · Illustration of Mode of Action of Anticholinergic Agents in Blocking Muscarinic Receptors in the Airway to Inhibit Cholinergic-Induced Bronchoconstriction

(From Rau JL: Respiratory care pharmacology, ed 6, St. Louis, 2002, Mosby.)

The site of action of ipratropium and anticholinergic agents in reversing cholinergic-induced airflow obstruction is shown in Figure 29-4.

Adverse Effects

Ipratropium bromide and tiotropium bromide are fully ionized compounds that are not well absorbed and distributed throughout the body, whereas atropine sulfate is a tertiary ammonium compound that is easily absorbed into the bloodstream. As a result, atropine produces many systemic side effects when inhaled, even though it is delivered locally to the lung. Side effects include the local topical effect of dry mouth, as well as pupillary dilation, lens paralysis, increased intraocular pressure, increased heart rate, urinary retention, and altered mental state. Because of its many side effects and the availability of ionized compounds such as ipratro-

Box 29-2 • Side Effects Seen With Anticholinergic Aerosol Ipratropium Bromide*

MDI and SVN (Common):
- Cough, dry mouth

MDI (Occasional):
- Nervousness, irritation, dizziness, headache, palpitation, rash

SVN:
- Pharyngitis, dyspnea, flu-like symptoms, bronchitis, upper respiratory infections, nausea, occasional bronchoconstriction, eye pain, urinary retention

*Side effects were reported in a small percentage (1% to 5%) of patients.
Precautions: Use with caution in patients with narrow-angle glaucoma, prostatic hypertrophy, bladder neck obstruction, constipation, bowel obstruction, or tachycardia.

pium, the use of atropine sulfate by nebulization is not recommended. In contrast, the side effects of ipratropium are largely limited to its local site of action (Box 29-2).

It should be noted that the amount of drug in the nebulizer dose of ipratropium is more than 10 times greater than the MDI dose (500 µg versus 40 µg). If the patient receives approximately 10% of an inhaled aerosol to the lung, a much larger dose is given with an SVN. Although ipratropium is not contraindicated in subjects with prostatic hypertrophy, urinary retention, or glaucoma, the drug should be used with precaution and adequate evaluation for possible systemic side effects in these subjects. *The eye must be protected from drug exposure with aerosol use* due to accidental spraying from an MDI or with nebulizer-mask delivery. There is a lesser chance of eye exposure with the MDI formulation than the SVN solution; a holding chamber is recommended with MDI use. Cugell[27] gives a clear review of the clinical pharmacology and toxicology of ipratropium.

MINI CLINI

Calculating Drug Doses

PROBLEM

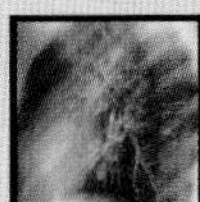

The dose of ipratropium bromide (Atrovent) released from the valve of the MDI is 20 µg, with approximately 18 µg released from the mouthpiece itself. With a usual dose of two actuations, this would release 40 µg total. The SVN solution is a vial of 2.5 mL of a 0.02% strength concentration, all of which is placed in the nebulizer. Does the nebulizer dose contain the same amount of drug as the two actuations from the MDI?

DISCUSSION

The amount of drug in mg or µg can be calculated for the nebulizer solution, using the formula for percentage strength:

$$\%\ (\text{as decimal}) = \frac{\text{drug solute (in g)}}{\text{total solution (in mL)}}$$

$$0.0002 = \frac{X\ g}{2.5\ mL}$$

$$X\ \text{grams} = 0.0002 \times 2.5\ mL = 0.0005\ \text{grams}$$

Converting 0.0005 g to mg gives 0.5 mg, or 500 µg. Therefore two actuations of the MDI releases 40 µg, whereas the dose contained in the SVN is 500 µg, or over 10 times more. The lower dose MDI is the reason that additional actuations of 4 or even 6 are needed if a patient does not obtain relief. The SVN solution may also provide relief by giving a higher dose of the drug.

Assessment

The assessment of bronchodilator therapy with an anticholinergic agent such as ipratropium is the same as that for adrenergic agents. In addition, preexisting conditions of narrow-angle glaucoma, prostatic hypertrophy, or urinary retention warrant caution with continued evaluation.

▶ MUCUS-CONTROLLING AGENTS

The two agents currently approved in the United States for oral inhalation with an effect on mucus are acetylcysteine and dornase alfa. Both agents are mucolytic, although their modes of action differ. Table 29-4 lists both agents, their formulations, and dosages, along with bland aqueous aerosols. A recent review with additional detail can be found in King and Rubin.[28]

Acetylcysteine

Acetylcysteine is the N-acetyl derivative of the amino acid L-cysteine and is given either by nebulization or by direct tracheal instillation.

Indications for Use

Acetylcysteine is indicated for treatment to reduce accumulation of airway secretions, with concomitant improvement in pulmonary function and gas exchange, and prevention of recurrent respiratory infection and airway damage. Diseases of excessive viscous mucus secretions and poor airway clearance include COPD, acute tracheobronchitis, and bronchiectasis. Acetylcysteine also is used to treat or prevent the liver damage that can occur when a patient takes an overdose of acetaminophen. Despite excellent in vitro mucolytic activity and a long history of use, there are no data to clearly demonstrate that oral or aerosolized acetylcysteine is effective therapy for any lung disease.

Table 29-4 ▶▶ Mucoactive Agents Available for Aerosol Administration

Drug	Brand Name	Adult Dosage	Use
Acetylcysteine 10%	Mucomyst Mucosil-10	SVN: 3-5 mL	Bronchitis, efficacy not proven
Acetylcysteine 20%	Mucomyst Mycosil-20	SVN: 3-5 mL	Bronchitis, efficacy not proven
Dornase alfa	Pulmozyme	SVN: 2.5 mg/ampule, 1 ampule daily*	CF
Aqueous aerosols: water, saline (0.45%, 0.9%, 5%-10%)	NA	SVN: 3-5 mL, as ordered USN: 3-5 mL, as ordered	Sputum induction, secretion mobilization

NA, Not applicable.
*Use recommended nebulizer system (see package insert); approved nebulizers: Hudson T Updraft II, Marquest II with Pulmo-Aide compressor, or the PARI LC Jet Plus with the PARI Inhaler Boy compressor.

This may be partially due to acetylcysteine selectively depolymerizing the essential mucin polymer structure and leaving the pathological polymers of DNA and F-actin intact in respiratory secretions.

Mode of Action

The mucus macromolecule consists of a polypeptide (protein) chain of amino acids, to which carbohydrate side chains are attached. There is internal cross-linking between strands with disulfide (–S–S–) bonds and hydrogen bonds.[28]

Acetylcysteine acts as a classic mucolytic to reduce the viscosity of mucus by substituting its own sulfhydryl group for the disulfide group in mucus, thereby breaking a portion of the bond forming the gel structure. The drug is effective in lowering viscosity and can be helpful by direct bronchial instillation during bronchoscopy to remove mucus plugs.

Side Effects

Several side effects to acetylcysteine have led to less use in patients with hypersecretory states. The drug is irritating to the airway and can produce bronchospasm, especially in subjects with asthma and hyperreactive airways. The general effect of airway irritation is counterproductive to reduction of mucus hypersecretion. To reduce the occurrence of bronchospasm, use of the 10% solution, which is less hypertonic than the 20%, is recommended. Pretreatment with an adrenergic bronchodilator, allowing adequate time for a bronchodilatory effect to be produced, can prevent or reduce airway resistance with acetylcysteine.

Other side effects that can occur include the following:

- Airway obstruction due to rapid liquefaction of secretions
- Disagreeable odor due to hydrogen sulfide
- Incompatibility with certain antibiotics (ampicillin, amphotericin B, erythromycin, and tetracyclines) if mixed in solution
- Increased concentration and tonicity of nebulizer solution toward end of treatment
- Nausea and rhinorrhea
- Stomatitis
- Reactivity of acetylcysteine with rubber, copper, iron, and cork

If acetylcysteine is administered by direct tracheal instillation, tracheobronchial suction should be immediately available to maintain the airway. To prevent concentration of solution in the nebulizer during treatment, it is suggested that the last fourth of the solution in the nebulizer be diluted with an equal volume of sterile water.

Dornase Alfa

Dornase alfa is a genetically engineered clone of the natural human pancreatic DNase enzyme, which can digest extracellular DNA material. It is a peptide mucolytic and can reduce extracellular DNA and F-actin polymers. It was originally referred to as *rhDNase*, for "recombinant human DNase." It is designated as an orphan drug. Administration and dosage are given in Table 29-4.

Indications for Use

Dornase alfa is indicated in the management of cystic fibrosis (CF), to treat purulent mucoid secretions, and to reduce the frequency of exacerbations due to respiratory infections, with attendant use of antibiotics or hospitalizations.[29]

Mode of Action

Dornase alfa is a proteolytic enzyme that can break down the DNA material from neutrophils found in

Reduction in Viscosity: (Pourability)	0 min.	15 min.	30 min.
Saline	0	+1	+1
rhDNase, 50 μg/ml	0	+3	+4
Bovine DNase, 50 μg/ml	0	+2	+4

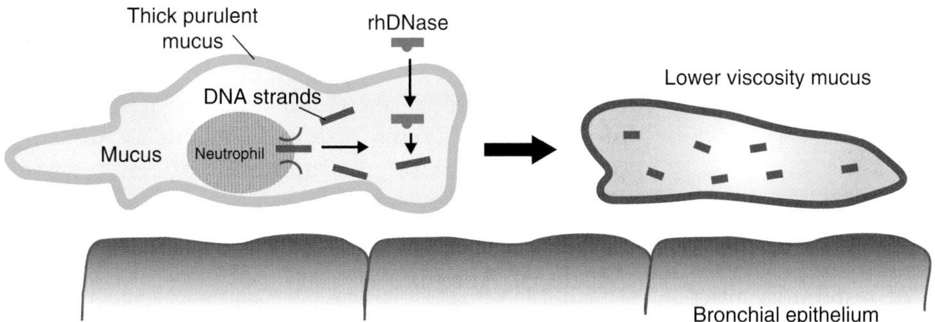

Figure 29-5
Mode of Action of Dornase Alfa (rhDNase) in Reducing Viscosity of Infected Sputum, Based on Data of Shak et al[30] *(From Rau JL: Respiratory care pharmacology, ed 5, St. Louis, 1998, Mosby.)*

purulent secretions (Figure 29-5). This agent has been shown to be more effective than acetylcysteine in reducing the viscosity of infected sputum in CF.[30]

Side Effects

Unlike its predecessor pancreatic dornase (Dornavac), a natural enzyme obtained from animal preparations, dornase alfa has not been shown to produce antibodies that might cause allergic reactions, including bronchospasm. Common side effects with the drug have included pharyngitis and voice alteration, laryngitis, rash, chest pain, and conjunctivitis. Other effects are less common but are reported as a variety of respiratory symptoms (cough, dyspnea, pneumothorax, hemoptysis, rhinitis, sinusitis), flu syndrome, GI obstruction, hypoxia, and weight loss. Contraindications to the drug include hypersensitivity to dornase, Chinese Hamster Ovary cell products, or other components of the drug preparation.

Other Mucoactive Agents

Bland aerosols of water, including distilled water and normo-, hyper-, and hypotonic saline, have traditionally been nebulized to improve mobilization of secretions in respiratory disease states. The mucus gel layer is relatively resistant to the addition or removal of water once it is formed. Bland aerosols have been found to increase secretion clearance and sputum production and cause productive coughing.[31] The effect is probably a vagally-mediated reflex production of cough and mucus secretion. Bland aerosols are therefore more properly considered expectorants rather than mucolytic agents. Clinicians must be alert to the possibility of bronchospasm with nonisotonic solutions, particularly in patients with hyperreactive airways.

Sodium bicarbonate has been aerosolized as well as directly instilled into the airway in intubated subjects to reduce the viscosity of airway secretions. This agent is not approved for such use. The reduction in secretion viscosity is thought to be caused by the increase in topical airway pH, with degradation of bonding in the mucin polysaccharide.

Expectorants are mucoactive but stimulate the production and clearance of airway secretions rather than cause mucolysis. Examples of such agents include guaifenesin, also known as glyceryl guaiacolate, iodinated glycerol, and saturated solution of potassium iodide (SSKI). Guaifenesin is found over the counter in many cough and cold products.

Assessment of Mucoactive Drug Therapy

Assessment of drug therapy for respiratory secretions is difficult: FEV_1 is relatively insensitive to changes in mucociliary clearance. The rate of change in lung function over time is a better marker. In addition, during maintenance therapy the volume of sputum expectorated is variable from day to day and does not reflect effective therapy. Therefore the following assessments should be performed.

Prior to treatment:

- Assess patient's adequacy of cough and level of consciousness to determine need for mechanical suctioning or adjunct bronchial hygiene (postural drainage or percussion, positive expiratory pressure [PEP] therapy) to clear airway with treatment, or if treatment is contraindicated.

During treatment and short-term:

- Instruct and then verify correct use of aerosol nebulization system, including cleaning.
- Assess therapy based on indication for drug: mucolysis and improved clearance of secretions.
- Monitor airflow changes or adverse effects such as a decrease in FEV_1.
- Assess breathing pattern and rate.
- Assess patient's subjective reaction to treatment (changes in breathing effort or pattern).
- Discontinue therapy if patient experiences adverse reactions.

Long term:

- Discontinue therapy if patient experiences adverse reactions.
- Monitor number and severity of respiratory tract infections, need for antibiotic therapy, emergency visits, and hospitalizations.
- Monitor pulmonary function for improvement or slowing in the rate of deterioration.

General contraindications:[28]

- Use mucoactive therapy with caution in patients with severely compromised vital capacity and expiratory flow, such as in the presence of end-stage pulmonary disease or neuromuscular disorders. Generally, if the FEV_1 is less than 25% of predicted, it becomes difficult to mobilize and expectorate secretions. Theoretically, with profound airflow compromise, secretion clearance could decline.

Gastroesophageal reflux and/or inability of the patient to protect the airway are risk factors for postural drainage, if that is necessary with mucoactive therapy. Mucoactive agents should be discontinued if there is evidence of clinical deterioration.

Patients with acute bronchitis or exacerbation of chronic disease (CF, COPD) may be less responsive to mucoactive therapy, possibly due to infection and muscular weakness, which can further reduce airflow dependent mechanisms.

▶ INHALED CORTICOSTEROIDS

Corticosteroids are endogenous hormones produced in the adrenal cortex, which regulate basic metabolic functions in the body, as well as exert an antiinflammatory effect. The use of aerosolized corticosteroids will be reviewed in this section. Corticosteroids used to treat asthma are all glucocorticoids. The term "steroid" in this section will be used to refer to glucocorticoid agents.

Indications and Purposes

The two general formulations of aerosolized glucocorticoids are orally inhaled and intranasal aerosol preparations. Orally inhaled preparations are listed in Table 29-5. The primary use of orally inhaled corticosteroids is for antiinflammatory maintenance therapy of mild-to-moderate persistent asthma, as defined by the 1997 NAEPP guidelines.[10] The use of intranasal steroids is for control of seasonal allergic or nonallergic rhinitis. All of the agents in Table 29-5 are available as intranasal preparations, with the addition of mometasone (Nasonex).

Mode of Action

Glucocorticoids are examples of lipid-soluble drugs that act on intracellular receptors. The complex action of steroids is illustrated in Figure 29-6.[32-34] Because steroid action involves modification of cell transcription, full antiinflammatory effects require hours to days. It is important for patients to understand that inhalation of a steroid aerosol will not provide immediate relief as with an adrenergic bronchodilator. However, daily compliance with the inhaled medication is essential to controlling the inflammation of asthma. Oral corticosteroids may be needed to initially clear the airway or as "burst" therapy to control asthma exacerbations.

Adverse Effects

The type and severity of side effects seen with inhaled aerosolized corticosteroids are much less than with systemic use, as with other classes of aerosolized drugs. Box 29-3 lists both systemic and local effects that are possible with inhaled steroids. The systemic effect of adrenal suppression is not usually seen with inhaled doses less than 800 μg per day in adults or less than 400 μg per day in children. Use of a reservoir device should be routine with inhaled steroids to prevent a swallowed portion adding to the systemic effect and to prevent the local effects of oral candidiasis and dysphonia. Growth retardation with inhaled steroids in asthma is debated. Some investigators found no growth suppression even with high-dose inhaled steroids. Kamada et al[35] provide a comprehensive review of possible side effects with inhaled steroids.

Assessment of Drug Therapy

The basic actions to evaluate an aerosol drug treatment should be followed (see Assessment of Bronchodilator Therapy). As with other drug therapy, the indications

Table 29-5 ▶▶▶ Corticosteroids Available by Aerosol for Oral Inhalation

Drug	Brand Name	Formulation and Dosage
Beclomethasone dipropionate	QVAR	MDI: 40 μg/puff and 80 μg/puff Adults ≥ 12 yr: 40 to 80 μg twice daily* or 40 to 160 μg twice daily† Children 5-11 yr: 40 μg twice daily*†
Triamcinolone acetonide	Azmacort	MDI: 100 μg/puff Adults: 2 puffs tid or qid Children: 1-2 puffs tid or qid
Flunisolide	AeroBid, AeroBid-M	MDI: 250 mg/puff Adults: 2 puffs bid Children: 2 puffs bid
Fluticasone propionate	Flovent	MDI: 44 μg/puff, 110 μg/puff, 220 μg/puff Adults ≥ 12 yr: 88 μg bid*, 88-220 μg bid†, or 880 μg bid‡
	Flovent Rotadisk	DPI: 50 μg, 100 μg, 250 μg Adults: 100 μg bid*, 100-250 μg bid†, 1000 μg bid‡ Children 4-11 yr: 50 μg bid
Budesonide	Pulmicort Turbuhaler	DPI: 200 μg/actuation Adults: 200-400 μg bid*, 200-400 μg bid†, 400-800 μg bid‡ Children ≥ 6 yr: 200 μg bid
	Pulmicort Respules	SVN: 0.25 mg/2 mL, 0.5 mg/2 mL Children 1-8 yr: 0.5 mg total dose given qd or bid in divided doses*†; 1 mg given as 0.5 mg bid, or qd‡
Fluticasone propionate/salmeterol	Advair Diskus	DPI: 100 μg fluticasone/50 μg salmeterol, 250 μg fluticasone/50 μg salmeterol, or 500 μg fluticasone/50 μg salmeterol Adults and children ≥ 12 yr: 100 μg fluticasone/50 μg salmeterol, 1 inhalation bid about 12 hr apart (starting dose if not currently on inhaled corticosteroids); maximum recommended dose is 500 μg fluticasone/50 μg salmeterol bid

Note: Individual agents are discussed in a separate section. Detailed information on each agent should be obtained from the manufacturer's drug insert.
*Recommended starting dose if on bronchodilators alone.
†Recommended starting dose if on inhaled corticosteroids previously.
‡Recommended starting dose if on oral corticosteroids previously.

for this class of drug should be present. The NAEPP guidelines released in 1997 are recommended for guidance.[10] In addition, with inhaled corticosteroid use the following are suggested:

- Verify that the patient understands that a corticosteroid is a controller agent and its difference from a rescue bronchodilator (relieving agent); assess patient's understanding of the need for consistent use of an inhaled corticosteroid (compliance with therapy).
- Instruct subject in use of a peak flow meter, to monitor baseline peak expiratory flow (PEF) and changes. Verify that there is a specific action plan, based on symptoms and peak flow results. Subject should be clear on when to contact a physician with deterioration in PEFs or exacerbation of symptoms.

Long-term:

- Assess severity of symptoms (coughing, wheezing, nocturnal awakenings, symptoms during exertion; use of rescue bronchodilator; number of exacerbations, missed work/school days; and pulmonary function) and modify level of asthma therapy (up or down, as described in NAEPP EPR-II guidelines for step therapy).
- Assess for presence of side effects with inhaled steroid therapy (oral thrush, hoarseness or voice changes, cough/wheezing with MDI use); use a reservoir (preferably a holding chamber) with MDI use and verify correct use.

▶ NONSTEROIDAL ANTIASTHMA DRUGS

Nonsteroidal antiinflammatory agents constitute a growing class of drugs in the treatment of asthma. These include the cromolyn-like agents (cromolyn sodium, nedocromil sodium) and the antileukotrienes, also termed *leukotriene modifiers* (zafirlukast, zileuton,

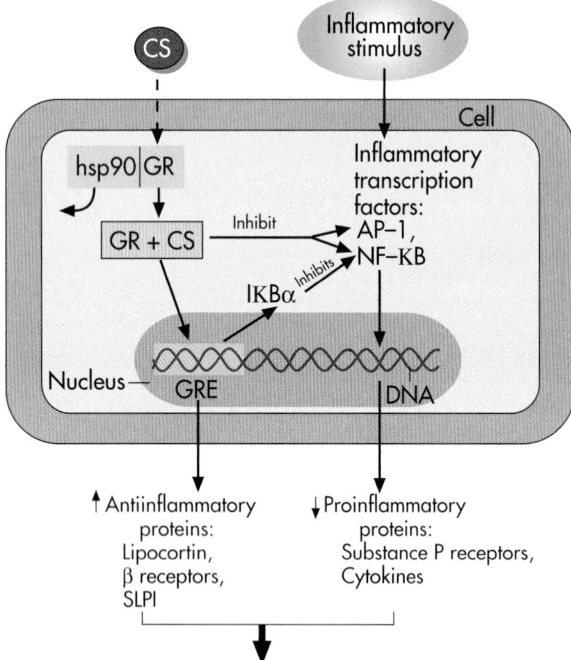

Figure 29-6 · Illustration of Mode of Action by Which Corticosteroids Modify Cell Response to Inhibit Inflammatory Response in the Airway

Corticosteroids (CS) diffuse into the cell and bind to a glucocorticoid receptor (GR). When the steroid binds to the GR, a protein, hsp 90, dissociates from the GR, and the steroid-GR complex moves into the cell nucleus. The drug-receptor complex binds to glucocorticoid response elements (GRE) of the nuclear DNA to up regulate transcription of antiinflammatory substances such as lipocortin, a protein which inhibits the generation of the arachidonic acid cascade by phospholipase A_2. There is evidence that steroids also up regulate inhibitors of factors in the cell, such as Nuclear Factor-kappa B (NF-kB), which can cause transcription of inflammatory substances. There may be direct inhibition of factors such as NF-kB, to further limit the inflammatory process. *(From Rau JL: Respiratory care pharmacology, ed 6, St. Louis, 2002, Mosby.)*

Box 29-3 • Potential Hazards and Side Effects of Aerosolized Corticosteroids

SYSTEMIC
- Adrenal insufficiency*
- Extrapulmonary allergy*
- Acute asthma*
- HPA suppression (minimal, dose-dependent)
- Growth retardation?
- Osteoporosis?

LOCAL (TOPICAL)
- Oropharyngeal fungal infections
- Dysphonia
- Cough, bronchoconstriction
- Incorrect use of MDI

*Following substitution for systemic corticosteroid therapy.
?Effect with inhaled corticosteroids alone is unclear.
HPA, Hypothalamic, pituitary, adrenal.

MINI CLINI

Patient Education

PROBLEM

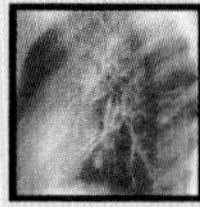

A 24-year-old patient with asthma has complained of waking up at night and being short of breath. She also reports feeling tight in her chest and needs to use her albuterol inhaler 5 to 6 days a week to get relief. She is not currently on other inhaled medications. Her allergist prescribes an inhaled MDI corticosteroid and salmeterol to be taken on a daily basis. What instructions should she be given in using these agents by inhalation?

DISCUSSION

Review the key points with corticosteroid inhalation. These are small doses and safe to take. However, it is important to take the prescribed corticosteroid dose regularly every day if the drug is to have an antiinflammatory effect in the lung. She should also use a reservoir device with the MDI. Rinsing her mouth with water after a treatment can further reduce the chance of oral candidiasis or dysphonia. With the salmeterol, she should also be instructed to follow her prescribed dose, which is usually two inhalations, twice daily. Salmeterol is considered a long-term controller and not a quick-reliever due to its pharmacokinetics. It is not helpful in relieving bronchospasm if she experiences acute difficulty in breathing. For acute respiratory problems, she should have a shorter- and quicker-acting adrenergic agent such as albuterol, pirbuterol, or terbutaline. If she experiences wheezing or chest tightness, one to two actuations of one of these agents will help. The salmeterol should then be taken at the regularly prescribed time.

and montelukast). The antileukotrienes are administered orally but are included as bronchoactive drugs. Table 29-6 lists pharmaceutical details on each agent.

Indications for Use

The general indication for clinical use of nonsteroidal antiasthma agents is *prophylactic* management (control) of mild persistent asthma (Step 2 or greater asthma, using the classification in the 1997 NAEPP guidelines). Step 2 Asthma is defined as: more than 2 days/week of symptoms, more than 2 nights/month with symptoms, FEV_1 or PEF ≥80%, but PEF variability is 20% to 30%.[10]

The following are qualifications to the general indication for use of these agents:

- Cromolyn-like drugs and the antileukotrienes are typically recommended as alternatives to introducing inhaled corticosteroids in Step 2 asthma.
- Cromolyn and nedocromil in particular are often used with infants and young children as alternatives to inhaled corticosteroids in Step 2 asthma because of their safety profiles.

Table 29-6 ▶▶ Nonsteroidal Antiasthma Medications*

Drug	Brand Name	Formulation and Dosage
Cromolyn-like (mast cell stabilizers)		
Cromolyn sodium†	Intal	MDI: 800 μg/actuation Adults and children ≥ 5 yr: 2 inhalations qid SVN: 20 mg/amp or 20 mg/vial Adults and children ≥ 2 yr: 20 mg inhaled qid
	Nasalcrom	Spray: 40 mg/mL (4%) Adults and children ≥ 6 yr: 1 spray each nostril 3-6 times daily every 4-6 hr
Nedocromil sodium	Tilade	MDI: 1.75 mg/actuation Adults and children ≥12 yr: 2 inhalations qid
Antileukotrienes		
Zafirlukast	Accolate	Tablets: 10 mg, 20 mg Adults and children ≥ 12 yr: 20 mg (1 tablet) bid, without food Children 5-11 yr: 10 mg twice daily
Montelukast	Singulair	Tablets: 10 mg, 5 mg, and 4 mg (cherry-flavored chewable) Adults and children ≥ 15 yr: 1 10-mg tablet each evening Children 6-14 yr: 1 5-mg chewable tablet each evening Children 2-5 yr: 1 4-mg chewable tablet each evening Children 12-23 mo: 4 mg oral granules each evening
Zileuton	Zyflo	Tablets: 600 mg Adults and children ≥ 12 yr: 1 600-mg tablet qid

*Detailed prescribing information should be obtained from the manufacturer's package insert.
†Cromolyn sodium is also available in an oral concentrate giving 100 mg in 5 mL (Gastrocrom), for treatment of systemic mastocytosis, and as an ophthalmic 4% solution (Opticrom, 40 mg/mL) for treatment of vernal keratoconjunctivitis.

- The antileukotriene agents can be useful in combination with inhaled steroids to reduce the dose of the steroid.

All of the nonsteroidal antiasthma drugs described in this chapter are controllers, not relievers, and are used in asthma requiring antiinflammatory drug therapy (Box 29-4).

Box 29-4 • Bronchoactive Agents Distinguished as Controllers or Relievers in Treating Asthma[10]

LONG-TERM CONTROL
- Inhaled corticosteroids
- Cromolyn sodium
- Nedocromil
- Long-acting β_2-agonists
  - Inhaled: salmeterol, formoterol
  - Oral: sustained-release albuterol
- Leukotriene modifiers
- Corticosteroids
- Methylxanthines (theophylline)

QUICK-RELIEF
- Short-acting inhaled β_2 agonists: albuterol, bitolterol, pirbuterol, terbutaline
- Anticholinergic (antimuscarinic): ipratropium
- Systemic corticosteroids (oral burst therapy, intravenous)

Mode of Action

Cromolyn sodium acts by inhibiting the degranulation of mast cells in response to allergic and nonallergic stimuli. This prevents release of histamine and other mediators of inflammation. These mediators cause bronchospasm and trigger an increasing cascade of further mediator release and inflammatory cell activity in the airway.[36]

Nedocromil sodium acts by inhibiting the activity of a variety of cells, including mast cells, eosinophils, airway epithelial cells, and sensory neurons called *C-fibers* (Figure 29-7). These cells can release a wide range of mediators, inflammatory cytokines, and enzymes that produce airway inflammation.[37]

Zafirlukast and montelukast act as leukotriene receptor antagonists and are selective competitive antagonists of leukotriene receptors LTD_4 and LTE_4. Leukotrienes such as LTC_4, LTD_4, and LTE_4 (previously known as *SRS-A*) stimulate leukotriene receptors termed $CysLT_1$ to cause bronchoconstriction, mucus secretion, vascular permeability, and plasma exudation into the airway. The mode of action is shown in Figure 29-8. The drug inhibits asthma reactions induced by exercise, cold air, allergens, and aspirin.[38-39]

Zileuton inhibits the 5-lipoxygenase enzyme that catalyzes the formation of leukotrienes from arachidonic acid, as also shown in Figure 29-8.[39]

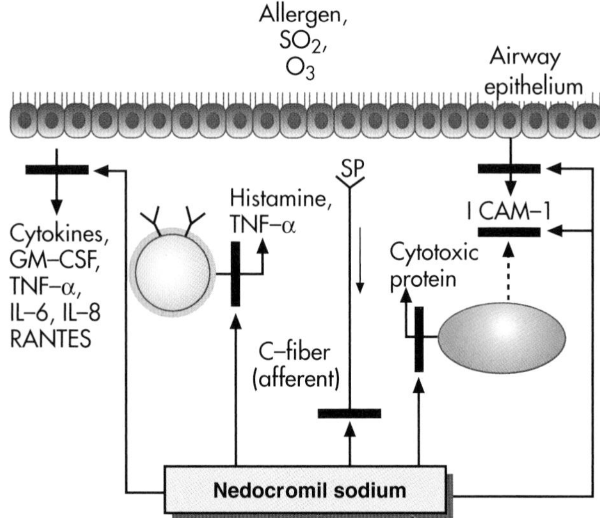

Figure 29-7 · Multiple Sites of Action by Which Nedocromil Sodium Inhibits Mediator Release and Airway Inflammation

(From Rau JL: Respiratory care pharmacology, ed 6, St. Louis, 2002, Mosby.)

Adverse Effects

A potential adverse effect with any of the nonsteroidal antiasthma drugs is inappropriate use. *None of these agents is a bronchodilator and offers no benefit for acute airway obstruction in asthma.* All of these agents are controllers rather than relievers, using the NAEPP terminology.[10] Cromolyn and nedocromil sodium are considered extremely safe agents. Because of their safety profile, the NAEPP guidelines recommend a trial of cromolyn or nedocromil sodium in children. Common side effects noted for cromolyn include cough, nasal congestion, throat irritation, dry mouth, and hoarseness. Nedocromil sodium has an unpleasant taste by aerosol and caused headache, nausea, and vomiting in a small percentage of patients.

Table 29-7 summarizes information and comparative features of the three antileukotriene agents, including drug interactions, common side effects, and contraindications.

Assessment of Drug Therapy

The basic actions to evaluate an aerosol drug treatment should be followed (see Assessment of Bronchodilator Therapy). As with other drug therapy, the indication for this class of drug should be present.

- Verify that the patient understands that nonsteroidal antiasthma agents are controller drugs and their difference from rescue bronchodilators (relieving agents); assess the patient's understanding of the need for consistent use of these agents (compliance with therapy).
- Instruct subject in use of a peak flow meter, to monitor baseline PEF and changes. Verify that there is a specific action plan, based on symptoms and peak flow results. Subject should be clear on when to contact a physician with deterioration in PEF or exacerbation of symptoms.

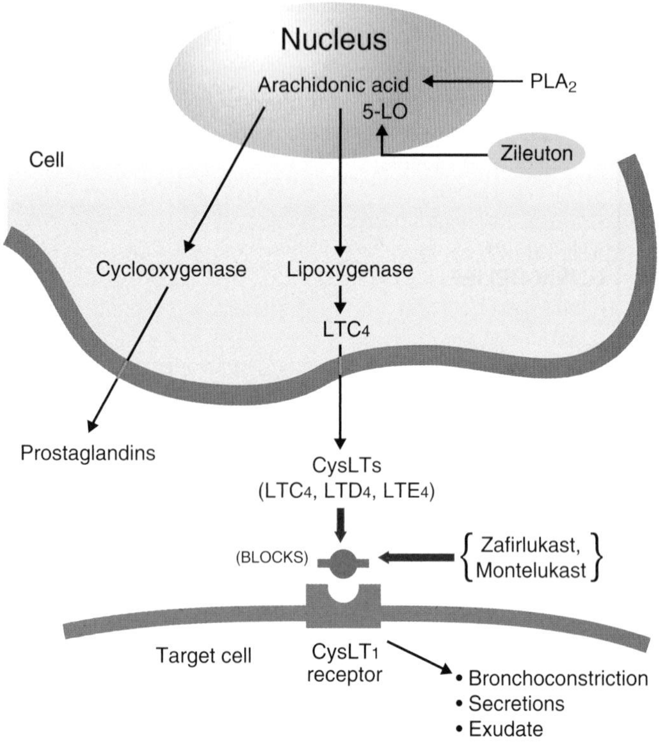

Figure 29-8 · Illustration of Modes and Sites of Action for Leukotriene Modifiers, Zileuton, Zafirlukast, and Montelukast

Zileuton inhibits the 5-LO enzyme, while zafirlukast and montelukast block the leukotriene receptor ($CysLT_1$).

Table 29-7 ▶▶ Summary of Comparative Features of the Three Currently Available Antileukotriene Agents

	Zileuton	Zafirlukast	Montelukast
Brand name	Zyflo	Accolate	Singulair
Action	5-LO inhibitor	$CysLT_1$ receptor block	$CysLT_1$ receptor block
Age range	≥12 years	≥12 years	≥2 years
Dose	600-mg tab, qid	Adult: 20-mg tab, bid Children 5-11 yr: 10-mg tab, bid	Adult: 10-mg tab, q evening 6-14 years: 5-mg tab, q evening 2-5 years: 4-mg tab, q evening 12-23 mo: 4 mg oral granules q evening
Administration	Can be taken with food	1 hr before or 2 hr after meal	Taken with or without food
Drug interaction	Yes (theophyllilne, warfarin, propranolol)	Yes (warfarin, theophylline, aspirin)	No
Side effects (common)	Headache, dyspepsia, unspecified pain, liver enzyme elevations	Headache, infection, nausea, possible liver enzyme changes	Headache, influenza, abdominal pain
Contraindications	Active liver disease or elevated liver enzyme levels, hypersensitivity to components	Hypersensitivity to components	Hypersensitivity to components

Table 29-8 ▶▶ Currently Available Inhaled Antiinfective Agents*

Drug	Brand Name	Formulation and Dosage	Clinical Use
Pentamidine isethionate	Nebupent	300 mg powder in 6 mL sterile water; 300 mg once every 4 wks	*P. carinii* pneumonia prophylaxis
Ribavirin	Virazole	6 g powder in 300 mL sterile water (20-mg/mL solution); given every 12-18 hrs/ day for 3-7 days by SPAG nebulizer	Respiratory syncytial virus
Tobramycin	TOBI	300-mg/5-mL ampule; adults and children ≥6 years: 300 mg bid, 28 days on/28 days off the drug	*P. aeruginosa* infection in CF
Zanamivir	Relenza	DPI: 5 mg/inhalation; adults ≥12 years: 2 inhalations (one 5-mg blister per inhalation) bid, 12 hrs apart for 5 days	Influenza

*Details on use and administration should be obtained from manufacturer's drug insert material prior to use.

Long-term:

- Assess severity of symptoms (coughing, wheezing, nocturnal awakenings, symptoms during exertion); use of rescue medication; number of exacerbations, missed work/school days; pulmonary function; and modify level of asthma therapy (up or down, as described in NAEPP EPR-II guidelines for step therapy).
- Assess for presence of side effects with nonsteroidal antiasthma agents; refer to particular agent and its side effects listed previously.

▶ AEROSOLIZED ANTIINFECTIVE AGENTS

In addition to the older aerosolized antiinfective agents pentamidine and ribavirin, an inhaled formulation of tobramycin is now available for use in CF, and zanamivir is available as a dry powder aerosol for treatment of influenza A and B. These antiinfective agents will be briefly outlined. Drug formulations and dosages are given in Table 29-8.

Pentamidine Isethionate

Pentamidine isethionate is an antiprotozoal agent that has been used in the treatment of opportunistic pneumonia caused by *Pneumocystis carinii* (PCP), which is seen in immunocompromised subjects, especially acquired immunodeficiency syndrome (AIDS).

Indication for Use

Pentamidine by inhalation is indicated as second-line therapy for the *prevention* of PCP in high-risk HIV-infected subjects who have a history of one or more episodes of PCP or a peripheral CD4+ (T4 helper cell) lymphocyte count ≤200/mm^3.[40]

Adverse Effects

Possible side effects with aerosolized pentamidine include cough, bronchial irritation, bronchospasm and wheezing, shortness of breath, fatigue, bad or metallic taste, pharyngitis, conjunctivitis, rash, and chest pain. Systemic effects have also been noted with inhaled pentamidine, including decreased appetite, dizziness, rash, nausea, night sweats, chills, spontaneous pneumothoraces, neutropenia, pancreatitis, renal insufficiency, and hypoglycemia. It is difficult to distinguish systemic effects caused by the drug versus the disease. Extrapulmonary infection with *P. carinii* can occur with prophylactic inhaled pentamidine.

Assessment

When administering aerosolized pentamidine, isolation, an environmental containment system (e.g., a booth or negative pressure room), and personnel barrier protection should be provided. Subjects should be screened for tuberculosis. The drug is given using a nebulizer system with one-way valves and scavenging expiratory filters (e.g., the Respirgard). This reduces environmental contamination. Nebulizer systems capable of producing a mass median astrodynamic diameter (MMAD) of 1 to 2 μm for peripheral lung deposition may reduce coughing. Monitor the patient for onset of any of the previously described adverse reactions. In addition, the following actions are recommended:

- Monitor for coughing and bronchospasm and provide a short-acting β-agonist or an anticholinergic bronchodilator such as ipratropium if present with inhaled pentamidine.
- Monitor for occurrence rate of PCP and rate of hospitalizations long-term.
- Monitor for presence of side effects (shortness of breath, possible pneumothorax, conjunctivitis, rash, neutropenia, dysglycemia) or appearance of extrapulmonary *P. carinii* infection.
- Evaluate need for prior use of a bronchodilator if symptoms of bronchospasm or coughing occur after inhalation of pentamidine.

Long-term:

- Monitor efficacy of pentamidine prophylaxis in preventing episodes of PCP.

Ribavirin

Ribavirin is an antiviral agent used in the treatment of severe respiratory syncytial virus (RSV) infection or in patients at risk for severe infection. RSV is a common seasonal respiratory infection in infants and young children, which is usually self-limiting. The cost-effectiveness of ribavirin continues to be debated. Recommendations for use of the drug can be found in a statement by the American Academy of Pediatrics.[41] Administration of the aerosol requires use of a special large-reservoir nebulizer called the *small particle aerosol generator* (SPAG). The mode of action of ribavirin is ascribed to the drug's similarity to guanosine, a natural nucleoside. Substitution of ribavirin for the natural nucleoside interrupts the viral replication process in the host cell.

Adverse Effects

Skin rash, eyelid erythema, and conjunctivitis have been noted with aerosol administration. Important equipment-related effects during mechanical ventilation include endotracheal tube occlusion and occlusion of ventilator expiratory valves or sensors. Deterioration of pulmonary function can occur.

Assessment

- Monitor signs of improvement in RSV infection severity, including vital signs, respiratory pattern and work of breathing (clinically), level of FIO_2 needed, level of ventilatory support, ABGs, body temperature, and other indicators of pulmonary gas exchange.
- Monitor patient for evidence of side effects such as deterioration in lung function, bronchospasm, occlusion of endotracheal tube (if present), cardiovascular instability, skin irritation from the aerosol drug, and equipment malfunction related to drug residue.

Inhaled Tobramycin

Patients with CF have chronic respiratory infection with *Pseudomonas aeruginosa*, as well as other microorganisms. Such chronic infection causes recurrent acute respiratory infections and deterioration of lung function. With the exception of the quinoline derivatives such as ciprofloxacin, antibiotics such as the aminoglycosides (e.g., tobramycin), which are effective against *Pseudomonas* organisms, have poor lung bioavailability when taken orally. Consequently, such antibiotics must be given either intravenously or by inhalation. The aminoglycoside, tobramycin, has been approved for inhaled administration and is intended to manage chronic infection with *P. aeruginosa* in CF. Goals of therapy are to treat or prevent early colonization with *P. aeruginosa* and maintain present lung function or reduce the rate of deterioration. The emergence of bacterial resistance was not seen in clinical trials with inhaled tobramycin.[42]

Adverse Effects

Side effects with parenteral aminoglycosides include possible auditory and vestibular damage with potential for deafness and nephrotoxicity. Other possible effects are listed in Box 29-5. Side effects observed since the introduction of inhaled tobramycin have been minimal and include voice alteration and tinnitus in a small percentage of patients. The risk for more serious side effects with tobramycin, whether by inhaled or parenteral routes, increases with the use of other aminoglycosides, in the presence of poor renal function and dehydration, with preexisting neuromuscular impairment, or with use of other ototoxic drugs.

The following precautions are suggested with use of inhaled tobramycin:

- Use with caution in patients with preexisting renal, auditory, vestibular, or neuromuscular dysfunction.
- Tobramycin solution should not be mixed with β-lactam antibiotics (penicillins, cephalosporins) due to admixture incompatibility, and in general mixing with other drugs is discouraged.
- Nebulization of antibiotics during hospitalization should be performed under conditions of containment, as previously described for pentamidine and ribavirin, to prevent environmental saturation and development of resistant organisms in the hospital.
- Aminoglycosides can cause fetal harm if administered to pregnant women; exposure to ambient aerosol drug should be avoided by women who are pregnant or trying to become pregnant.
- Local airway irritation resulting in cough and bronchospasm with decreased ventilatory flowrates is a possibility with inhaled antibiotics and seems to be related to the osmolality of the solution.[43-44] Peak flowrates and chest auscultation should be used before and after treatments to evaluate airway changes. Pretreatment with a β-agonist may be needed.
- Allergies in the patient, staff, or family should be considered, if exposure to the aerosolized drug is not controlled. The use of a nebulizing system with scavenging filter, one-way valves, and thumb control could reduce ambient contamination with the drug, as previously described.

Box 29-5 • Side Effects With Aminoglycosides and Tobramycin

PARENTERAL ADMINISTRATION

- Ototoxicity (auditory and vestibular)
- Nephrotoxicity
- Neuromuscular blockade
- Hypomagnesemia
- Cross-allergenicity
- Fetal harm (deafness)

INHALED NEBULIZED TOBRAMCYIN

- Voice alteration
- Tinnitus
- Nonsignificant increase in bacterial resistance

In clinical trials, inhaled tobramycin was administered using the PARI LC Plus nebulizer with a DeVilbiss Pulmo-Aide compressor. Other nebulizer systems must be tested to ensure adequate drug output and particle size, because antibiotic solutions differ in viscosity from the aqueous bronchodilator solutions used in common disposable nebulizers. Studies have reported that not all nebulizer-compressor systems perform adequately with antibiotic solutions, and higher flowrates of 10-12 LPM may be needed with nebulizers.[45-46]

Assessment

- Verify the patient understands that nebulized tobramycin should be given after other CF therapies, including other inhaled drugs.
- Check whether the patient has renal, auditory, vestibular, or neuromuscular problems or is taking other aminoglycosides or ototoxic drugs. Consider whether tobramycin should be used in the patient based on severity of preexisting or concomitant risk factors.
- Monitor lung function to note improvement in FEV_1.
- Assess rate of hospitalization before and after institution of inhaled tobramycin.
- Assess need for intravenous antipseudomonal therapy.
- Assess improvement in weight.
- Monitor for occurrence of side effects such as tinnitus or voice alteration; have patient rinse and expectorate after aerosol treatments.
- Evaluate for changes in hearing or renal function during use of inhaled tobramycin.

Inhaled Zanamivir

Zanamivir was approved for use in the treatment of uncomplicated influenza illness in adults in 1999, as an inhaled powder aerosol. Despite the availability of zanamivir, as well as the oral antiinfluenza agent, oseltamivir (Tamiflu), prophylactic vaccination against influenza is still recommended, especially in high-risk subjects with cardiovascular or pulmonary disease. Previous agents for treatment of influenza included amantadine (Symmetrel) and rimantadine (Flumadine). Zanamivir and oseltamivir represent a new class of antiviral agents termed *neuraminidase inhibitors*.

Indication for Use

Inhaled zanamivir is indicated for the treatment of uncomplicated acute illness due to influenza virus in adults and adolescents 12 years of age or older, who have been symptomatic for no more than two days.

Mode of Action

The influenza virus attaches to respiratory tract cells by binding of viral surface hemagglutinin to the cell's surface molecule of sialic acid (Figure 29-9). The viral particle also has an enzyme, neuraminidase, on its surface. When replicated viral particles are released from the host cell following infection, the viral neuraminidase cleaves the sialic acid on both the host cell surface and on other viral particle surfaces, so that mature virus can be released and spread. Without neuraminidase, influenza virus would clump together and to the host cell, preventing spread. Zanamivir, and also oseltamivir, combine with the surface neuraminidase, preventing its action and the spread of viral particles.

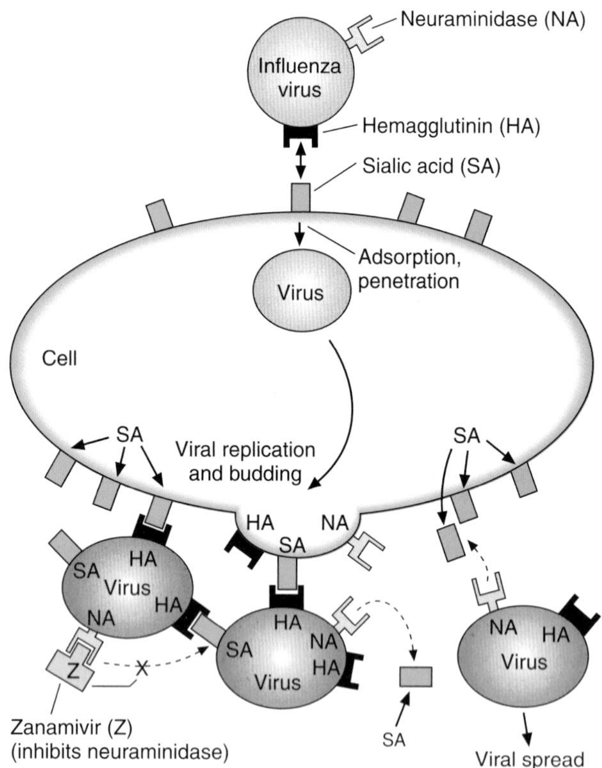

Figure 29-9 · Mode of Action by Which Inhaled Zanamivir Exerts Antiviral Effect on Influenza Virus

Zanamivir is a sialic acid analogue and binds to neuraminidase, the enzyme responsible for cleaving sialic acid and preventing viral binding to sialic acid. This causes viral aggregation, with binding of viral particles to each other and to the host cell, preventing viral spread. *(From Rau JL: Respiratory care pharmacology, ed 6, St. Louis, 2002, Mosby.)*

Adverse Effects

Several adverse effects can occur with inhaled zanamivir:

- Bronchospasm and deterioration in lung function, especially in patients with COPD or asthma
- Possible undertreatment of bacterial infection masquerading as a viral infection or a secondary bacterial infection in the presence of influenza
- Allergic reactions, as may occur with any drug
- Adverse reactions such as diarrhea, nausea, vomiting, bronchitis, cough, sinusitis, dizziness, and headaches

Because of the effect on lung function in respiratory disease patients and reports of adverse reactions, revised labeling for the drug carries a warning that zanamivir is not generally recommended for patients with underlying airways disease.[47]

Clinical Efficacy

In studies of clinical efficacy, use of zanamivir resulted in shortening of the median time to alleviation of symptoms by one day. In subjects who began treatment within 30 hours of illness, the median time to alleviation of symptoms was reduced by approximately 3 days.[48] Zanamivir is not approved for prophylaxis of influenza although there are data to suggest a preventative effect in those exposed to influenza virus.[49] Cost versus efficacy issues revolve around the modest reduction in symptoms as well as inability to confirm presence of influenza quickly, easily, and inexpensively as the basis for the drug treatment.

Assessment

- Assess improvement in influenza symptoms: fever reduction, less myalgia and headache, reduced coughing and sore throat, and less systemic fatigue.
- Monitor for airway irritation and symptoms of bronchospasm, especially during initial use of the dry powder aerosol. Provide a short-acting β-agonist if needed, or if patient is at risk for airway reactivity (COPD, asthma).

Inhaled Antifungal Therapy

No FDA-approved antifungal drugs are available for inhalation at this time. However, invasive pulmonary fungal infections such as aspergillosis are complications often seen in immunocompromised patients, such as those on anticancer chemotherapy or receiving lung, heart, or heart-lung transplants. Intravenous amphotericin B is an effective antifungal therapy, and amphotericin B is most often cited in the literature as an antifungal agent given by inhalation. Two recent reviews of inhaled antimicrobial therapy have included sections on inhaled antifungal therapy.[50,51]

Use of Aerosolized Amphotericin B

In lung transplantation, infections at the site of the bronchial anastomosis remain a serious airway complication. Such infection is due to poor blood flow, the use of corticosteroids for immunosuppression, which impairs healing, and airway colonization with infecting agents. A common anastomotic infection is caused by *Aspergillus* organisms.[52,53] *Candida* organisms are seen less frequently, as reported in two series of patients.[52, 54]

The rationale for inhaled antifungal therapy remains the same as with other inhaled agents: direct, targeted, local airway delivery with minimal systemic blood levels and exposure to a potentially toxic drug. Although effective, intravenous amphotericin B has a risk of nephrotoxicity.[55] Amphotericin B given intravenously in combination with other nephrotoxic drugs such as cyclosporine (used as an immunosuppressant in transplantation) can significantly increase the risk of renal damage.[52, 55]

Efficacy of Aerosolized Amphotericin B

A study published in 1997 reported a significant reduction in the incidence of fungal airway infections with prophylactic use of aerosolized amphotericin B after lung, heart, and heart-lung transplantation.[56] Birsan and colleagues[57] reported that prophylactic antifungal therapy with aerosolized amphotericin B 10 mg tid for 6 to 8 weeks after lung transplantation postponed but did not prevent aspergillus-related tracheobronchitis. Subsequent infection required further treatment with aerosolized amphotericin B and an oral antifungal agent. The authors suggested that longer prophylactic treatment is needed until complete healing of the anastomosis occurs. Palmer and colleagues[52] reported successful treatment of invasive candidal anastomotic infection with a sequential combination of intravenous amphotericin B followed by inhaled amphotericin B and oral fluconazole. In another study aimed primarily at assessing adverse events with inhaled antifungal therapy, Palmer and colleagues[55] found that anastomotic fungal infection occurred early after lung transplantation in only 4% (2 of 51) of patients studied, with no pneumonia in any patients.

Aerosol Dose

One of the major issues facing the use of aerosolized antifungal agents such as amphotericin B is the lack of standardized dosing based on studies of dose-response and pharmacokinetics with aerosol administration. Two formulations of amphotericin B have been aerosolized by nebulizer: an aqueous and a liposomal formulation.[50] In the studies cited in this summary, aerosol dosages ranged from 10 mg tid for 6 to 8 weeks postoperatively,[57] to 50 to 100 mg of the lipid complex given once daily for 4 days, and then once a week.[55]

Adverse Events

There have been reports of toxicity with inhaled amphotericin B, including nausea, vomiting and significant worsening of peak flow values reflecting bronchoconstriction.[58,59] In their study of 381 treatments with aerosolized amphotericin B lipid complex given to 51 lung transplant patients, Palmer and associates[55] reported that only one patient was withdrawn for drug intolerance. Nausea or vomiting occurred with less than 2% of treatments. No clinically significant bronchospasm was noted, and only 5% of all treatments in extubated patients exhibited a 20% or greater decline in the FEV_1/FVC ratio. Wheezing, as assessed by a respiratory therapist, was not documented on any posttreatment pulmonary examination. These results may indicate that the liposomal formulation of amphotericin B used will be better tolerated than the aqueous formulation. In their study of the safety of aerosolized amphotericin B lipid complex, Palmer and associates[55] were unable to detect blood levels after aerosol dosing, indicating minimal or no systemic drug exposure.

Issues

Although the published reports of aerosolized amphotericin B have been favorable, a scientific basis for a standardized clinical aerosol dose has not been established in humans. Aerosol administration results in much higher amphotericin B levels in pulmonary tissues than is possible with systemic administration.[60] It should be noted that with undetectable plasma levels of drug, extrapulmonary fungal infections are not prevented using inhalation only.[55] Other issues include the following:

- What is the optimal dose and duration of treatment with aerosol use, in either prophylactic maintenance, or acute treatment of pulmonary aspergillosis?
- Is combined systemic and inhaled treatment mandatory or efficient in all cases of local aspergillosis infection?
- What is the optimal aerosol formulation and which nebulizing systems produce adequate particle size and output levels for the formulation?

These questions require the same types of studies used to establish the standardized dosing regimen of inhaled tobramycin in CF.

KEY POINTS

- Orally-inhaled aerosol drug classes include the β-agonist bronchodilators, the anticholinergic (antimuscarinic) bronchodilators, the mucolytics, the corticosteroids, nonsteroidal antiasthma drugs, and antiinfective agents.
- The β-agonist and anticholinergic bronchodilators are used to reverse or improve airflow obstruction; the mucolytics are used to reduce mucus viscosity and improve mucociliary clearance; the corticosteroids and nonsteroidal antiasthma agents are used to reduce or prevent airway inflammation in asthma; the antiinfective agent pentamidine is used to treat PCP, especially in patients with AIDS; ribavirin is used for RSV infection in at-risk infants and children; inhaled tobramycin is used in CF to prevent or manage gram-negative *Pseudomonas* infections; and inhaled zanamivir is used to treat acute influenza.
- Selection of an appropriate aerosol class of drug is based on matching the indications for the drug class to the presence of the indications in the patient. For example, the presence of repeated respiratory infections requiring intravenous antibiotics, hospitalizations, and causing declining lung function in a patient with CF matches the indication for the use of dornase alfa and/or inhaled tobramycin.
- All aerosol treatments are assessed immediately by monitoring respiratory "vital signs," which include respiratory rate and pattern, pulse, breath sounds on auscultation, general patient appearance (e.g., color, diaphoresis), and patient report of subjective reaction (e.g., "chest tightness"). Additional assessment should be related to the indication for the drug: monitoring of peak flowrates or bedside spirometry with bronchodilator use; frequency of exacerbation or β-agonist use with inhaled corticosteroids in asthma.
- Each class of aerosol drug has its own mode of action: The β-agonists stimulate G protein-linked β-receptors to increase cyclic AMP and relax smooth muscle; the anticholinergic agents block cholinergic (muscarinic) receptors in the airway to prevent bronchoconstriction; the mucolytics lyse mucus; the corticosteroids modify cell nuclear

KEY POINTS—cont'd

transcription to cause an antiinflammatory effect; the cromolyn-like agents inhibit inflammatory mediator release or action; leukotriene modifiers competitively block leukotriene receptors (montelukast, zafirlukast) or 5-LO enzyme (zileuton); the antiinfectives inhibit particular infecting organisms (*P. carinii*, RSV, *Pseudomonas*, influenza).

- Common side effects with each class of drug include: tremor and shakiness with β-agonists; dry mouth with anticholinergic agents; bronchial irritation with acetylcysteine; dysphonia and voice changes with dornase alfa; oral fungal infections with corticosteroids; and miscellaneous reactions such as cough, unpleasant taste, headache, and liver enzyme changes (zileuton) with nonsteroidal antiasthma agents, depending on the specific agent; bronchial irritation and bronchospasm (pentamidine), skin rash, conjunctivitis, bronchial irritation, and equipment/endotracheal tube occlusion by drug precipitate (ribavirin); nebulized antibiotics and zanamivir may cause bronchospasm and require higher-than-normal power gas flowrates (10 to 12 L/min).
- Quick-relief agents used in asthma include: short-acting β-agonists (including albuterol, terbutaline, pirbuterol) and anticholinergic bronchodilators. Long-term control agents include: long-acting β-agonists (salmeterol), inhaled corticosteroids, and nonsteroidal antiasthma drugs (cromolyn, nedocromil, montelukast, and other leukotriene antagonists). Systemic corticosteroids are used for both quick relief (intravenously) and long-term control (orally).

References

1. Rau JL: Respiratory care pharmacology, ed 6, St. Louis, 2002, Mosby.
2. Leff AR, editor: Pulmonary and critical care pharmacology and therapeutics, New York, 1996, McGraw-Hill.
3. Katzung BG, editor: Basic & clinical pharmacology, ed 7, Norwalk, Conn, 1998, Appleton & Lange.
4. Hanania NA et al: Medical personnel's knowledge of and ability to use inhaling devices: metered-dose inhalers, spacing chambers, and breath-actuated dry powder inhalers, Chest 105:111, 1994.

5. Borgström L: A possible new approach of comparing different inhalers and inhaled substances, J Aerosol Med 4:A13, 1991.
6. Thorsson L: Influence of inhaler systems on systemic availability, with focus on inhaled corticosteroids, J Aerosol Med 8(suppl 3):S29, 1995.
7. Aranson R, Rau JL: The evolution of ?-agonists, Respir Care Clin N Am 5:479, 1999.
8. Rau JL: Inhaled adrenergic bronchodilators: historical development and clinical application, Respir Care 45:854, 2000.
9. Jenne JW: β-adrenergic pharmaceuticals. In Leff AR, editor: Pulmonary and critical care pharmacology and therapeutics, New York, 1996, McGraw-Hill.
10. National Asthma Education and Prevention Program. Expert Panel Report II: Guidelines for the diagnosis and management of asthma, National Institutes of Health, 1997.
11. Barnes PJ: ?-adrenergic receptors and their regulation, Am J Respir Crit Care Med 152:838, 1995.
12. Mitra S et al: (S)-albuterol increases intracellular free calcium by muscarinic receptor activation and a phospholipase C-dependent mechanism in airway smooth muscle, Mol Pharmacol 53:347, 1998.
13. Lipworth BJ et al: Pharmacokinetics and extrapulmonary β_2 adrenoceptor activity of nebulised racemic salbutamol and its R- and S-isomers in healthy volunteers, Thorax 52:849, 1997.
14. Johansson FJ et al: Effects of albuterol enantiomers on in vitro bronchial reactivity, Clin Rev Allergy Immunol 14:57, 1996.
15. Templeton AGB et al: Effects of S-salbutamol on human isolated bronchus, Pulm Pharmacol Ther 11:1, 1998.
16. Volcheck GW, Gleich GJ, Kita H: Pro- and anti-inflammatory effects of β-adrenergic agonists on eosinophil response to IL-5, J Allergy Clin Immunol 101:S35, 1998.
17.Schmekel B et al: Stereoselective pharmacokinetics of S-salbutamol after administration of the racemate in healthy volunteers, Eur Respir J 13:1230,1999.
18. Dhand R et al: Preferential pulmonary retention of (S)-albuterol after inhalation of racemic albuterol, Am J Respir Crit Care Med 160:1136,1999.
19. Nelson HS et al: Improved bronchodilation with levalbuterol compared with racemic albuterol in patients with asthma, J Allergy Clin Immunol 102:943, 1998.
20. Rau JL: Introduction of a single isomer β-agonist, Respir Care 45:962, 2000.
21. Johnson M et al: The pharmacology of salmeterol, Life Sci 52:2131, 1993.
22. Bartow RA, Brogden RN: Formoterol: an update of its pharmacological properties and therapeutic efficacy in the management of asthma, Drugs 56:303, 1998.
23. McFadden ER, Jr: The β_2-agonist controversy revisited, Ann Allergy Asthma Immunol 75:173, 1995.
24. Jenne JW: Adverse effects of β-adrenergic agonists. In Leff AR, editor: Pulmonary and critical care pharmacology and therapeutics, New York, 1996, McGraw-Hill.
25. Meltzer EO: Intranasal anticholinergic therapy of rhinorrhea, J Allergy Clin Immunol 90:1055, 1992.
26. Barnes PJ: The pharmacological properties of tiotropium, Chest 117:63S, 2000.
27. Cugell DW: Clinical pharmacology and toxicology of ipratropium bromide, Am J Med 81(suppl 5A):27, 1986.
28. King M, Rubin BK: Mucus-controlling agents: past and present, Respir Care Clin N Am 5:575, 1999.
29. Consensus Conference: Practical applications of Pulmozyme, Pediatr Pulmonol 17:404, 1994.
30. Shak S et al: Recombinant human DNase I reduces the viscosity of cystic fibrosis sputum, Proc Natl Acad Sci USA 87:9188, 1990.
31. Robinson M et al: Effect of hypertonic saline, amiloride, and cough on mucociliary clearance in patients with cystic fibrosis, Am J Respir Crit Care Med 153:1503, 1996.
32. Baraniuk JN: Molecular actions of glucocorticoids: an introduction, J Allergy Clin Immunol 97:141, 1996.
33. Barnes PJ: Molecular mechanisms of steroid action in asthma, J Allergy Clin Immunol 97:159, 1996.
34. Barnes PJ: Inhaled glucocorticoids for asthma, N Engl J Med 332:868, 1995.
35. Kamada AK et al: Issues in the use of inhaled glucocorticoids, Am J Respir Crit Care Med 153:1739, 1996.
36. Holgate ST: Inhaled sodium cromoglycate, Respir Med 90:387, 1996.
37. Devalia JL et al: Nedocromil sodium and airway inflammation in vivo and in vitro, J Allergy Clin Immunol 98:S51, 1996.
38. Bisgaard H: Role of leukotrienes in asthma pathophysiology, Pediatr Pulmonol 30:166, 2000.
39. Drazen JM, Israel E, O'Byrne PM: Treatment of asthma with drugs modifying the leukotriene pathway, N Engl J Med 340:197, 1999.
40. Centers for Disease Control: Recommendations for prophylaxis against Pneumocystic carinii pneumonia for adults and adolescents infected with human immunodeficiency virus, MMWR 41:1, 1992.
41. American Academy of Pediatrics Committee on Infectious Diseases: Use of ribavirin in the treatment of respiratory syncytial virus infection, Pediatrics 92:501, 1993.
42. Ramsey BW et al: Intermittent administration of inhaled tobramycin in patients with cystic fibrosis, N Engl J Med 340:23, 1999.
43. Littlewood JM, Smye SW, Cunliffe H: Aerosol antibiotic treatment in cystic fibrosis, Arch Dis Child 68:788, 1993.
44. Dally MB, Kurrle S, Breslin ABX: Ventilatory effects of aerosol gentamicin, Thorax 33:54, 1978.
45. Hurley PK, Smye SW, Cunliffe H: Assessment of antibiotic aerosol generation using commercial jet nebulizers, J Aerosol Med 7:217, 1994.
46. Newman SP et al: Evaluation of jet nebulizers for use with gentamicin solution, Thorax 40:671, 1985.
47. Federal Drug Administration: Revised labeling for zanamivir, JAMA 284:1234, 2000.
48. Hayden FG et al: Efficacy and safety of the neuraminidase inhibitor zanamivir in the treatment of influenza virus infections, N Engl J Med 337:874, 1997.
49. Hayden FG et al: Inhaled zanamivir for the prevention of influenza in families, N Engl J Med 343:1282, 2000.
50. O'Riordan T, Faris M: Inhaled antimicrobial therapy, Respir Care Clinics N Amer 5:617, 1999.

51. O'Riordan TG: Inhaled antimicrobial therapy: from cystic fibrosis to the flu, Respir Care 45:836, 2000.
52. Palmer SM et al: Candidal anastomotic infection in lung transplant recipients: successful treatment with a combination of systemic and inhaled antifungal agents, J Heart Lung Transplant 17:1029, 1998.
53. Kraemer MR et al: Ulcerative tracheobronchitis after lung transplantation: a new form of invasive aspergillosis, Am Rev Respir Dis 144:552, 1991.
54. Husain AN et al: Post-lung transplant biopsies: an 8-year Loyola experience, Mod Pathol 9:126, 1996.
55. Palmer SM et al: Safety of aerosolized amphotericin B lipid complex in lung transplant recipients, Transplantation 72:545, 2001.
56. Reichenspurner H et al: Significant reduction in the number of fungal infections after lung-, heart-lung, and heart transplantation using aerosolized amphotericin B prophylaxis, Transplant Proc 29:627, 1997.
57. Birsan T, Taghavi S, Klepetko W: Treatment of aspergillus-related ulcerative tracheobronchitis in lung transplant recipients, J Heart Lung Transplant 17:437, 1998.
58. Gryn J et al: The toxicity of daily inhaled amphotericin B, Am J Clin Oncol 16:43, 1993.
59. DuBois J et al: The physiologic effects of inhaled amphotericin B, Chest 108:750, 1995.
60. Niki Y et al: Pharmacokinetics of aerosol amphotericin B in rats, Antimicrob Agents Chemother 34:29, 1990.

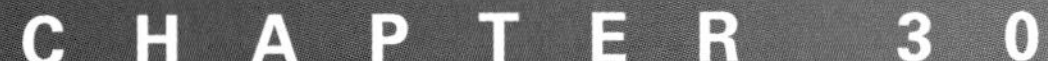

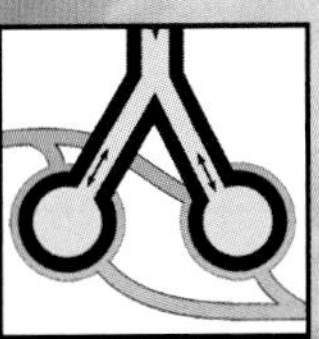

CHAPTER 30

Airway Management

Kim F. Simmons and Craig L. Scanlan

In This Chapter You Will Learn:

- How to safely perform endotracheal and nasotracheal suctioning
- How to properly obtain sputum samples
- How to assess the need for and select an artificial airway
- What complications and hazards are associated with insertion of artificial airways
- How to perform orotracheal and nasotracheal intubation of an adult
- How to assess and confirm proper endotracheal tube placement
- How and why tracheotomy is performed
- What types of damage artificial airways can cause
- How to properly maintain and troubleshoot artificial airways
- How to measure and adjust tracheal tube cuff pressures
- When and how to extubate or decannulate a patient
- How to use alternative airway devices
- How to assist a physician in setting up and performing bronchoscopy

Chapter Outline

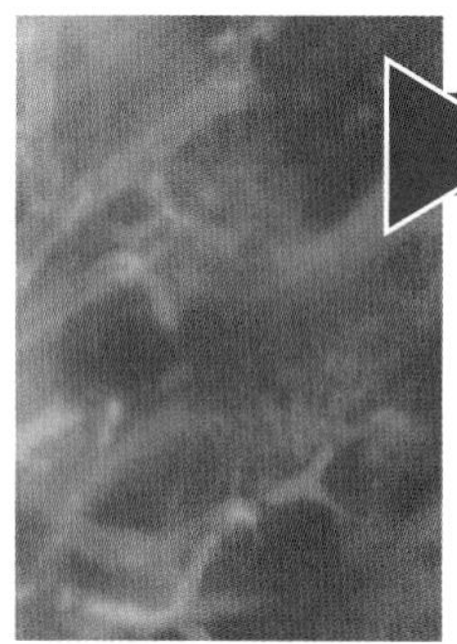

Key Terms

angioedema
American Society for Testing and Materials (ASTM)
bacteremia
colorimetry
fenestrated
fiberoptic
fistula
granuloma
obturator
peritubular
polyp
radiopaque
tracheomalacia
trismus

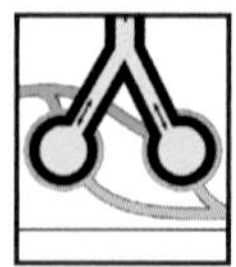

Respiratory therapists work with patients who have diseased lungs and impaired gas exchange. Because adequate gas exchange is not possible without a patent airway, respiratory therapists often assume key responsibility for airway management of patients in both the acute and postacute care settings.

Respiratory therapists must develop skills in three broad areas of airway care. First, the respiratory therapist must be proficient in airway clearance techniques, including those methods designed to ensure the patency of the patient's airway, natural or artificial. Second, the respiratory therapist must be able to insert and maintain artificial airways designed to support patients whose own natural airways are inadequate. Last, the respiratory therapist must be able to assist physicians in performing special procedures related to airway management. This chapter will explore each of these areas.

▶ SUCTIONING

Airway obstruction can be caused by retained secretions, foreign bodies, and structural changes such as edema, tumors, or trauma. Retained secretions increase airway resistance and the work of breathing and can cause hypoxemia, hypercapnia, atelectasis, and infection. Difficulty in clearing secretions may be due to their thickness or amount, or to the patient's inability to generate an effective cough.

Respiratory therapists can remove retained secretions or other semiliquid fluids from the airways by using mechanical aspiration, or suctioning. Suctioning involves application of negative pressure (vacuum) to the airways through a collecting tube (flexible catheter or suction tip). Removal of foreign bodies, secretions, or tissue masses beyond the mainstem bronchi requires bronchoscopy, which is performed by a physician. Respiratory therapists often assist physicians in performing bronchoscopy, which will be discussed at the end of the chapter.

Suction can be performed in either the upper airway (oropharynx) or the lower airway (trachea and bronchi). Secretions or fluids can also be removed from the oropharynx by using a rigid tonsillar, or Yankauer, suction tip (Figure 30-1). Access to the lower airway is via introduction of a flexible suction catheter (Figure 30-2) through the nose (nasotracheal suctioning) or artificial airway (endotracheal suctioning). Tracheal

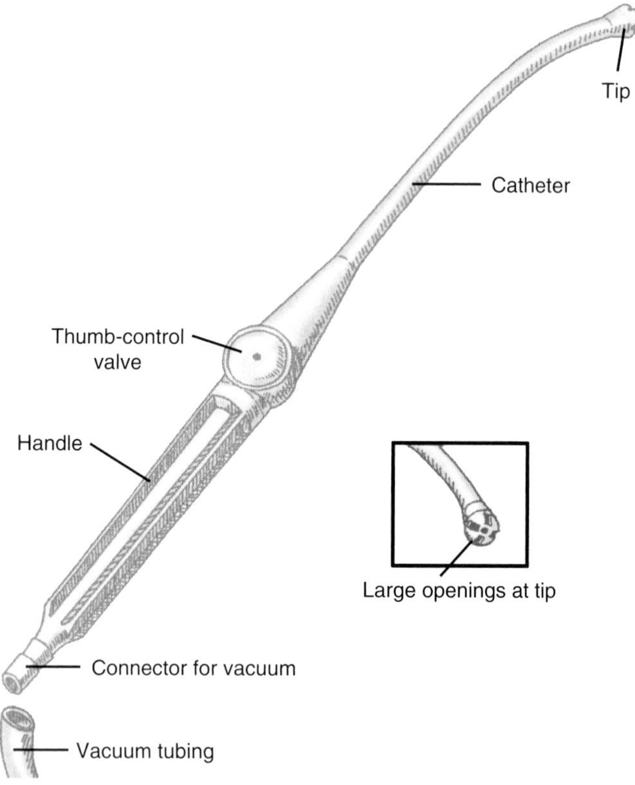

Figure 30-1
Rigid tonsillar, or Yankauer, suction tip. *(Modified from Sills JR: Entry Level Respiratory Therapist Exam Guide, St. Louis, 2000, Mosby.)*

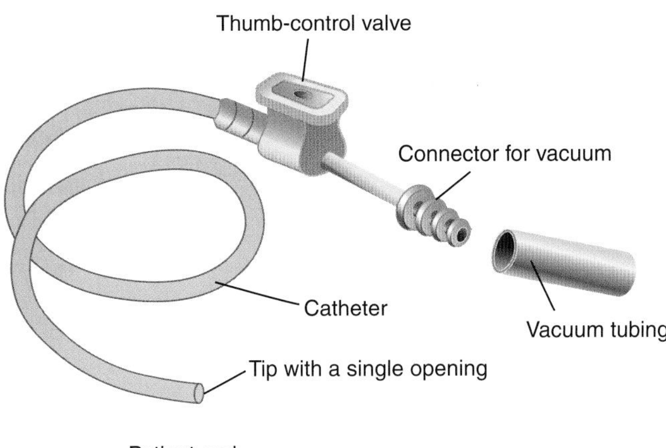

Figure 30-2
Flexible suction catheter for lower airway suctioning.

suctioning through the mouth should be avoided, as it causes gagging. Because endotracheal suctioning is the more common procedure, we discuss it first.

Endotracheal Suctioning

Clinical Practice Guideline

To guide practitioners in safe and effective application of this procedure, the American Association for Respiratory Care (AARC) has developed and published a clinical practice guideline on endotracheal suctioning of mechanically ventilated adults and children with artificial airways. Excerpts from the AARC guideline, including indications, contraindications, hazards and complications, assessment of need, assessment of outcome, and monitoring, appear on p. 656.[1]

Equipment and Procedure

The procedure described below is for endotracheal suctioning of adults or children. Nasotracheal suctioning is covered separately.

Step 1: Assess the Patient for Indications (Refer to Practice Guideline). A patient should never be suctioned by a preset schedule. However, although breath sounds are clear, you still should pass a suction catheter occasionally to ensure that the tip of the tube is not plugged. In addition, very thick secretions may not move with airflow and thus may not create any adventitious sounds.

Step 2: Assemble and Check Equipment. The equipment needed for endotracheal suctioning is listed in Box 30-1. Commonly, the suction catheter, glove(s), and basin are prepackaged together in disposable sterile kits.

Set the suction pressure as low as possible, yet high enough to effectively clear secretions. For adults, a pressure of –100 to –120 mm Hg is usually adequate. For children, limit the suction pressure to –80 to –100 mm Hg. With infants, –60 to –80 mm Hg is the limit.[2]

Suction catheters come in various designs, with most including side port s to minimize mucosal damage. Most general-purpose suction catheters are 22 inches long (sufficient to reach the mainstem bronchi) and sized in French units (external circumference). A curved-tip or coude-tip, catheter is available to increase the likelihood of left mainstem bronchial access. Perhaps more important than the catheter design is its size. Too large a catheter can obstruct the tracheal airway. During application of negative pressure, this quickly evacuates lung volume and causes atelectasis and hypoxemia. To avoid this problem, never suction a patient with a catheter whose outer diameter is greater than one half the internal diameter of the tracheal tube.[3]

RULE OF THUMB

To quickly estimate the proper size of suction catheter to use with a given tracheal tube, first multiply the tube's inner diameter by 2. Then use the *next smallest* size catheter.
Example: 6.0 mm endotracheal tube: 2 × 6 = 12; next smallest catheter is 10 French
Example: 8.0 mm endotracheal tube: 2 × 8 = 16; next smallest catheter is 14 French

For patients receiving ventilatory support, a closed-system multiuse suction catheter can be used (Figure 30-3). These systems are incorporated directly into the ventilator circuit and used repeatedly over 24 to 48 hours. Because you can perform suctioning without disconnecting the patient from the ventilator, high F_{IO_2} and positive end-expiratory pressure (PEEP) can be maintained, resulting in less likelihood of hypoxemia (preoxygenation with 100% O_2 is still required)[4]. In addition, cross-contamination is less likely and cost is lower than with single-use catheters.[5] However, the

Box 30-1 • Equipment Needed for Suctioning

- Adjustable suction source/collection system
- Sterile suction catheter with thumb port
- Sterile glove(s)
- Goggles, mask, and gown (standard precautions)
- Sterile basin
- Sterile bulk water or saline
- Sterile saline for instillation
- Oxygen delivery system (BVM or ventilator)

Endotracheal Suctioning of Mechanically Ventilated Adults and Children With Artificial Airways

AARC Clinical Practice Guideline (Excerpts)*

➤ INDICATIONS

The need to remove accumulated pulmonary secretions as evidenced by one of the following:

- Coarse breath sounds or "noisy" breathing
- Patient's inability to generate an effective spontaneous cough
- Radiograph changes consistent with retained secretions
- Changes in monitored flow/pressure graphics
- Increased peak inspiratory pressure (PIP) on volume-control ventilation (VCV); decreased V_T on pressure control ventilation (PCV)
- Visible secretions in the airway
- Suspected aspiration of gastric or upper airway secretions
- Clinically apparent increased work of breathing
- Deterioration of arterial blood gas values
- The need to obtain a sputum specimen for microbiological or cytological examination
- The need to maintain the patency and integrity of the artificial airway
- The need to stimulate a cough in patients unable to cough effectively secondary to changes in mental status or the influence of medication
- Presence of pulmonary atelectasis or consolidation, presumed to be associated with secretion retention

➤ CONTRAINDICATIONS

Endotracheal suctioning is a necessary procedure for patients with artificial airways. Most contraindications are relative to the patient's risk of developing adverse reactions or worsening clinical condition as a result of the procedure. When indicated, there is no absolute contraindication to endotracheal suctioning because abstaining from suctioning in order to avoid possible adverse reaction may, in fact, be lethal.

➤ HAZARDS AND COMPLICATIONS

- Hypoxia/hypoxemia
- Tracheal and/or bronchial mucosal trauma
- Cardiac or respiratory arrest
- Cardiac arrhythmias
- Pulmonary atelectasis
- Bronchoconstriction/bronchospasm
- Infection (patient and/or caregiver)
- Pulmonary hemorrhage/bleeding
- Elevated intracranial pressure
- Interruption of mechanical ventilation
- Hypertension
- Hypotension

➤ ASSESSMENT OF NEED

Qualified personnel should assess the need for endotracheal suctioning as a routine part of a patient/ventilator system check.

➤ ASSESSMENT OF OUTCOME

- Improvement in breath sounds
- Decreased PIP with narrowing of PIP-plateau; decreased airway resistance or increased dynamic compliance; increased tidal volume delivery during pressure-limited ventilation
- Improvement in arterial blood gas values or saturation as reflected by pulse oximetry (Spo_2)
- Removal of pulmonary secretions

➤ MONITORING

The following should be monitored prior to, during, and after the procedure:

- Breath sounds
- Oxygen saturation (Spo_2)

ENDOTRACHEAL SUCTIONING OF MECHANICALLY VENTILATED ADULTS AND CHILDREN WITH ARTIFICIAL AIRWAYS—CONT'D

AARC Clinical Practice Guideline (Excerpts)*

- Respiratory rate and pattern
- Pulse rate, blood pressure, ECG (if indicated and available)
- Sputum (color, volume, consistency, odor)
- Ventilator parameters
- Arterial blood gases
- Cough effort and ICP (if indicated and available)

*For complete guidelines see Respir Care 38:500, 1993.

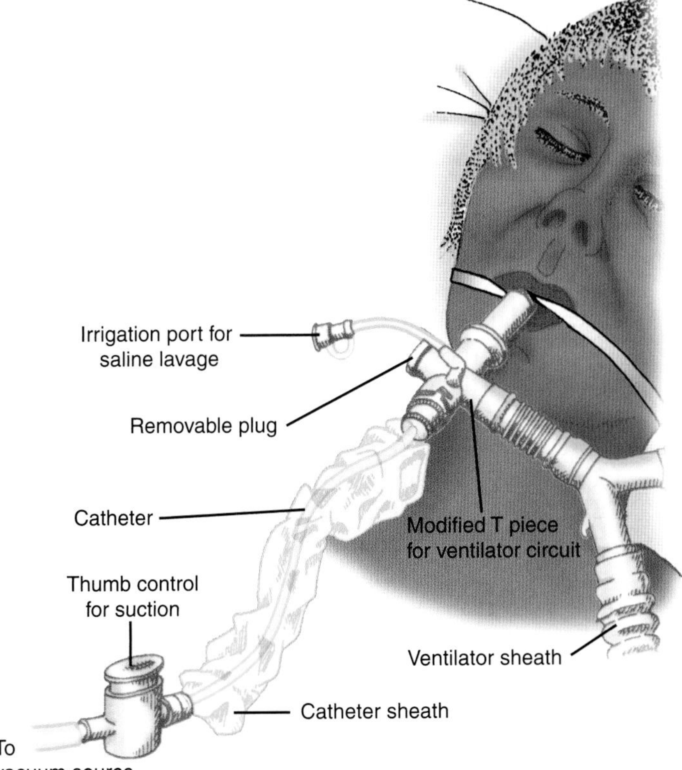

Figure 30-3
Closed-system multiuse suction catheter. *(Modified from Sills JR: Entry level respiratory therapist exam guide, St. Louis, 2000, Mosby.)*

extra weight an in-line catheter adds to a ventilator circuit may increase tension on the tracheal tube. Also, the presence of the catheter in the airway increases resistance and can alter the volumes delivered by the ventilator. Last, the reduced airway pressure during suctioning can cause the ventilator to inadvertently trigger on.[6] Basic indications for the use of closed suction catheters can be found in Box 30-2.[4]

Although many clinicians use 5 to 10 mL of sterile saline for instillation prior to suctioning an adult's airway, whether this practice actually aids secretion removal remains unclear. Moreover, saline irrigation may actually increase the incidence of nosocomial pneumonia by displacing bacteria from the wall of the airways.[7] For these reasons, we recommend against standard use of saline irrigation before endotracheal suctioning.[4] If the secretions are extremely tenacious, instillation of acetylcysteine or sodium bicarbonate (2%) tends to be more effective than normal saline. This may require a physician's order.

Box 30-2 • Indications for Use of Closed Suctioning Techniques

- High ventilator requirements:
  - Positive end-expiratory pressure ≥ 10 cm H_2O
  - Mean airway pressure ≥ 20 cm H_2O
  - Inspiratory time ≥ 1.5 seconds
  - Fraction of inspired oxygen ≥ 0.60
- Mechanically ventilated patients receiving frequent suctioning (≥ 6/day)
- Hemodynamic instability associated with ventilator disconnection
- Mechanically ventilated patients with active tuberculosis
- Patients receiving inhaled agents that cannot be interrupted by ventilator disconnection (e.g., nitric oxide, helium/oxygen mixture)

After connecting the catheter to the suction source, check the level of suction pressure by closing the catheter thumb port and aspirating some sterile water or saline from the basin. If no vacuum is generated, check for leaks in the tubing, at the collection container or at the suction regulator. In addition, if the collecting bottle is full, the float-valve will close and prevent vacuum transmission.

Step 3: Preoxygenate and Hyperinflate the Patient. You can easily hyperinflate the patient with a BVM unit (bag-valve-mask or manual resuscitator). If the patient is on a ventilator, you can hyperinflate the patient by using a machine breath; however, be sure to avoid breath stacking or insufficient expiratory time. To preoxygenate the patient, give 100% oxygen for at least 30 seconds. You can deliver the oxygen via either the BVM or the ventilator. If you use the ventilator to provide extra oxygen, be sure to allow adequate "washout time."[8] This will ensure the delivery of 100% oxygen prior to suctioning. When working with patients with chronic obstructive pulmonary disease (COPD), you may need to hyperinflate them without increasing the F_{IO_2}.

Step 4: Insert the Catheter. Insert the catheter carefully, until it can go no farther. Then withdraw the catheter a few centimeters before applying suction.

Step 5: Apply Suction/Clear Catheter. Apply suction, while withdrawing the catheter using a rotating motion. Keep total suction time less than 10 to 15 seconds.[9] After removing the catheter, clear it using the sterile basin and bulk water/saline. The closed suction catheter has an adapter for saline vials to be placed in line with the device. The catheter is cleared by squeezing the saline vial and applying suction at the same time. Caution must be used to ensure the saline is being drawn into the catheter and not down the airway. If any untoward response occurs during suctioning, immediately remove the catheter and oxygenate the patient.

Step 6: Reoxygenate and Hyperinflate the Patient. Reapply oxygen and repeat Step 3. Maintain the increased F_{IO_2} for at least 1 minute.

Step 7: Monitor the Patient and Assess Outcomes. Repeat Steps 3 through 7 as needed until you see improvement or observe an adverse response. Take any corrective steps necessary.

Minimizing Complications and Adverse Responses

Careful adherence to procedure is the best way to avoid or minimize the complications of endotracheal suctioning. First, preoxygenation helps minimize the incidence of hypoxemia during suctioning. Preoxygenation combined with hyperinflation provides even more protection and helps prevent atelectasis.[10] However, hyperinflation may agitate some patients. Preoxygenation and hyperinflation are more effective when done through the ventilator, as opposed to a manual resuscitator.[11] This appears especially true for patients on high levels of support, such as PEEP. Moreover, manual resuscitators cannot always provide 100% oxygen or deliver a consistent tidal volume, and maintaining sterile technique and PEEP levels is difficult with some of these devices. Insertion of the catheter through an adapter that does not require ventilator disconnection may also be helpful in preventing hypoxemia. You should use this technique for patients receiving high levels of support, especially PEEP levels greater than 10 cm H_2O.

As previously described, use of a closed-system catheter on ventilator patients can decrease the likelihood of hypoxemia. A second design, the double-lumen catheter, can provide both suction and oxygen delivery. When the valve on this catheter is closed, suction is applied to the airway; when the valve is opened, oxygen is delivered. This also appears to reduce the incidence of hypoxemia.[12]

Cardiac arrhythmias occur mainly as a result of hypoxemia.[9] Mechanical stimulation of the airway also can cause arrhythmias. If the patient is connected to a cardiac monitor, check it often for gross arrhythmias. Vagal stimulation can cause bradycardia or asystole. Tachycardia may result from patient agitation and hypoxemia. If any major change is seen in the heart rate or rhythm, immediately stop suctioning and administer oxygen to the patient, providing manual ventilation as needed.

Hypotension during suctioning may be due to cardiac arrhythmias or severe coughing episodes that decrease venous return. As with arrhythmias, if the patient becomes hypotensive, stop the procedure and restore oxygenation and ventilation. Hypertension may be caused by hypoxemia or increased sympathetic tone due to stress, anxiety, pain, or changes in hemodynamics resulting from manual hyperventilation.[13]

Atelectasis is due to removal of too much air from the lungs. You can avoid this complication by (1) limiting the amount of negative pressure used, (2) keeping the duration of suctioning as short as possible, and (3) providing hyperinflation before and after the procedure.

Mucosal trauma also occurs when the catheter adheres to the wall of the airway during suctioning. To avoid this problem, limit the amount of negative pressure used and always rotate the catheter while withdrawing. Once the depth of insertion is approximated on the first pass, it is not necessary to touch the carina on subsequent passes.

Increased intracranial pressure (ICP) has been reported during suctioning. These changes are only transient, with values normally returning to baseline within 1 minute. However, in patients who already have an elevated ICP, these changes could be significant. Should this problem occur, an aerosolized topical anesthetic given 15 minutes prior to suctioning may help reduce the rise in ICP.[14]

Nasotracheal Suctioning

Nasotracheal suctioning is indicated for patients who retain secretions but do not have an artificial tracheal airway.

Clinical Practice Guideline

To guide practitioners in safe and effective application of this procedure, the AARC has developed and published a clinical practice guideline on nasotracheal suctioning. Excerpts from the AARC guideline, including indications, contraindications, hazards and complications, assessment of need, assessment of outcome, and monitoring, appear on p. 660.[15]

Equipment and Procedure

The equipment and procedure for nasotracheal suctioning are similar to those for endotracheal suctioning. Here we highlight only the key differences.

In addition to the equipment and supplies used for endotracheal suctioning (see Box 30-1), you will need sterile water-soluble lubricating jelly to aid catheter passage through the nose. You should also consider using a nasopharyngeal airway to help reduce mucosal trauma in the nose of patients who require long-term nasotracheal suctioning.

The key aspect of the nasotracheal suctioning procedure is catheter insertion. After you lubricate the catheter, insert it gently through the nostril, directing it toward the septum and floor of the nasal cavity, without applying negative pressure. If you feel any resistance in the nose, gently twist the catheter. If this does not help, withdraw the catheter and try inserting it through the other nostril.

As you move the catheter into the lower pharynx, have the patient assume a "sniffing" position (Figure 30-4). This position helps align the opening of the larynx with the lower pharynx, making catheter passage through the larynx more likely. You should continue to advance the catheter until the patient coughs, or a resistance is felt much lower in the airway.

Minimizing Complications and Adverse Responses

Pushing the catheter into the oropharynx or esophagus may cause gagging or regurgitation. Always be ready to reposition the patient and suction the oropharynx if this occurs. The risk of regurgitation can also be minimized by avoiding suctioning too soon after a meal or tube feeding. This can be done by close coordination with nursing personnel.

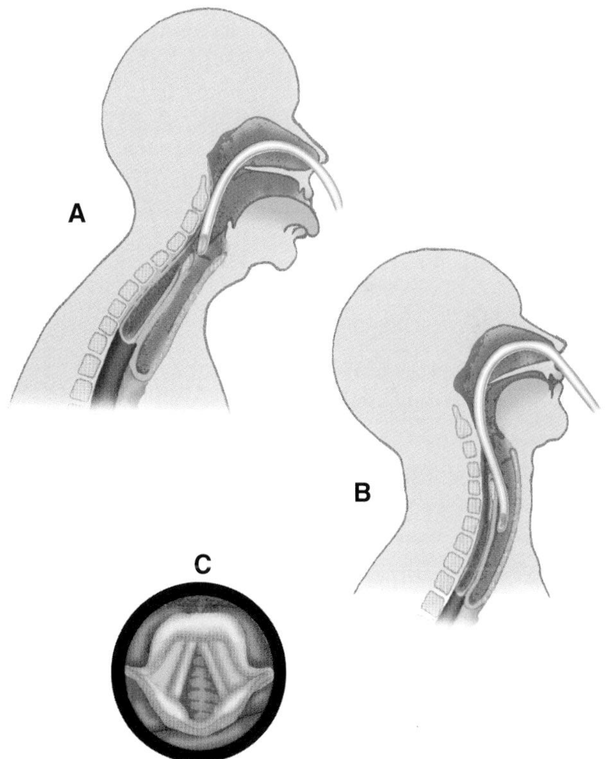

Figure 30-4 · Nasotracheal Suctioning Technique
A, Optimal position of head to insert catheter into the trachea. The neck is flexed and the head is extended. The tongue is protruded (and held by a 4 x 4 gauze pad). **B,** After catheter has advanced into the trachea, the tongue is released and the patient's head allowed to assume a comfortable position. **C,** View of vocal cords from above. The cords are most widely separated during inspiration. *(Modified from Sanderson RG: The cardiac patient: a comprehensive approach, Philadelphia, 1972, WB Saunders.)*

Nasotracheal Suctioning

AARC Clinical Practice Guideline (Excerpts)*

➤ INDICATIONS

The need to maintain a patent airway and remove secretions or foreign material from the trachea in the presence of:

- Inability to clear secretions
- Audible evidence of secretions in the large airways that persist in spite of patient's best cough effort

➤ CONTRAINDICATIONS

The only absolute contraindications to nasotracheal suctioning are epiglottitis and croup. Relative contraindications include:

- Occluded nasal passages
- Nasal bleeding
- Acute head, facial, or neck injury
- Coagulopathy or bleeding disorder
- Laryngospasm
- Irritable airway
- Upper respiratory tract infection

➤ HAZARDS AND COMPLICATIONS

- Hypoxia/hypoxemia
- Nasal, pharyngeal, tracheal trauma/pain
- Cardiac or respiratory arrest
- Cardiac arrhythmias/bradycardia
- Pulmonary atelectasis
- Bronchoconstriction/bronchospasm
- Infection (patient and/or caregiver)
- Mucosal hemorrhage
- Elevated ICP
- Uncontrolled coughing/laryngospasm
- Hyper/hypotension
- Gagging/vomiting

➤ ASSESSMENT OF NEED

- Personnel should auscultate chest for indications for nasotracheal suctioning.
- Personnel should assess effectiveness of cough.

➤ ASSESSMENT OF OUTCOME

- Effectiveness of nasotracheal suctioning should be reflected by improved breath sounds.
- Effectiveness of nasotracheal suctioning should be reflected by removal of secretions.

➤ MONITORING

The following should be monitored prior to, during, and after the procedure:

- Breath sounds
- Skin color/Spo_2
- Respiratory rate and pattern
- Pulse rate, arrhythmia, ECG (if available)
- Sputum (color, volume, consistency, odor)
- Presence of bleeding/evidence of trauma
- Subjective response, including pain
- Cough effort and ICP (if indicated/available)

---

*For complete guidelines see Respir Care 37:898-901, 1992.

Airway trauma can occur as you pass the catheter through the upper airway. The presence of blood in the catheter or patient's nose or mouth suggests tissue damage. Trauma can range from simple mucosal bleeding to laceration of nasal turbinates and pharyngeal perforation. To minimize airway trauma, you should avoid using excessive force when advancing the catheter. Lubrication of the catheter also eases its passage. As previously indicated, placement of a nasopharyngeal airway can help minimize nasal trauma when repeated access is needed.

Contamination of the lungs with bacteria from the upper airway is another complication of nasotracheal suctioning. Immunosuppressed patients are likely to develop more serious complications. Sterile technique and gentle insertion help minimize this complication.

The presence of the catheter in the lower airway may stimulate normal protective mechanisms, resulting in coughing, laryngospasm, or bronchospasm. The bronchospastic response may be particularly strong in patients with hyperactive airway disease. These patients should be assessed for the development of wheezes associated with suctioning.

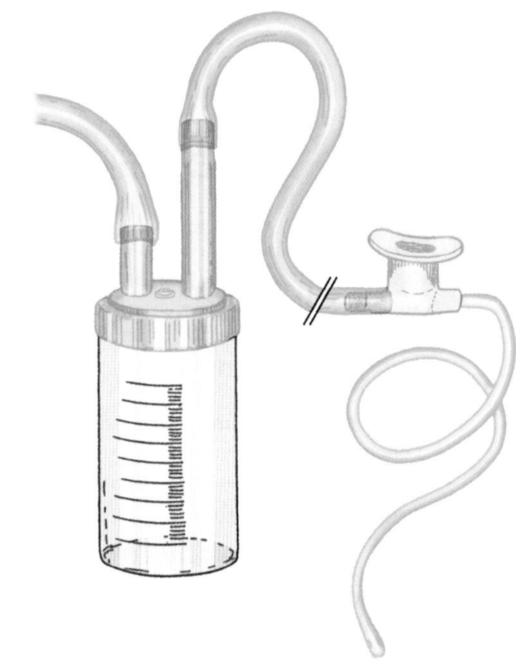

Figure 30-5
Specimen container placement between the suction catheter and wall suction source.

Sputum Sampling

Sputum samples are often collected to identify organisms infecting the airway. To obtain the samples, the suctioning procedures described previously are followed. In addition to the usual equipment, a specimen container is needed. This device consists of a plastic tube or cup with a flexible hose on one end to attach to the suction catheter. The other outlet is a stiff plastic nozzle that connects to the suction tubing from the wall vacuum unit (Figure 30-5).

It is very important to maintain sterile techniques when touching the connection points on the trap. If a closed suction system is in use, a new catheter should be placed just prior to suctioning the patient for the sample. Once an adequate sample is obtained, the container is removed from the suction catheter and suction tubing. The flexible tubing on the container is attached to the open nozzle. This will make a closed container. The container should be labeled and processed according to hospital policy. The suctioning procedure can be completed as previously described.

▶ ESTABLISHING AN ARTIFICIAL AIRWAY

Clinical Practice Guideline

An artificial airway is required when the patient's natural airway can no longer perform its proper functions. To guide practitioners in the identification, assessment, and treatment of patients requiring artificial airways, the AARC has developed and published a clinical practice guideline on management of airway emergencies. Excerpts from the AARC guideline, including indications; contraindications; precautions, hazards, and/or possible complications; assessment of need and outcome; and monitoring, appear on p. 662.[16]

Routes

In general, artificial airways are inserted by one of two routes, either through the pharynx or directly into the trachea.

Pharyngeal Airways

Pharyngeal airways prevent airway obstruction by keeping the tongue pulled forward and away from the posterior pharynx. This type of obstruction is common in the unconscious patient, as a result of a loss of muscle tone.

A nasal pharyngeal airway is most often placed in a patient who requires frequent nasotracheal suctioning. Although it does not ensure entry into the trachea, it does minimize damage to the nasal mucosa that can be caused by the suction catheter. The nasopharyngeal airway may also be placed in a patient who was recently extubated following facial surgery. This will help to maintain the patency of the upper airway.

Management of Airway Emergencies

AARC Clinical Practice Guideline (Excerpts)*

➤ INDICATIONS

- General conditions requiring airway management are impending or actual (1) airway compromise, (2) respiratory failure, and (3) need to protect the airway. Specific conditions include but are not limited to:
  - Airway emergency prior to endotracheal intubation
  - Artificial airway obstruction
  - Apnea
  - Acute traumatic coma
  - Penetrating neck trauma
  - Cardiopulmonary arrest and unstable arrhythmias
  - Severe bronchospasm
  - Self-extubation
  - Pulmonary edema
  - Sedative/narcotic drug effect
  - Severe allergic reactions with cardiopulmonary compromise
  - Foreign body obstruction
  - Choanal atresia in neonates
  - Aspiration/risk of aspiration
  - Severe laryngospasm
- Conditions requiring emergency tracheal intubation include, but are not limited to:
  - Accidental extubation of mechanically ventilated patient
  - Traumatic upper airway obstruction
  - Obstructive angioedema
  - Massive hemoptysis
  - Infection-related upper airway obstruction
  - Massive upper airway bleeding
  - Coma with increased ICP
  - Persistent apnea
  - Neonatal- or pediatric-specific (e.g., meconium aspiration)
  - Upper airway or laryngeal edema
  - Loss of protective reflexes
  - Cardiopulmonary arrest
- The patient in whom airway control is not possible by other methods may require surgical placement of an airway (needle or surgical cricothyrotomy).
- Conditions in which endotracheal intubation may not be possible and in which alternative techniques may be used include but are not limited to (1) restriction of endotracheal intubation by policy or statute; (2) difficult or failed intubation in the presence of risk factors associated with difficult tracheal intubations; and (3) when endotracheal intubation is not immediately possible.

➤ CONTRAINDICATIONS

Aggressive airway management (intubation or establishment of a surgical airway) may be contraindicated when the patient's desire not to be resuscitated has been clearly expressed and documented in the patient's medical record or other valid legal document.

➤ PRECAUTIONS, HAZARDS, AND/OR COMPLICATIONS

- Possible hazards or complications related to emergency airway management itself:
  - Failure to establish a patient airway, to intubate the trachea, or recognize esophageal intubation
  - Trauma to nose, mouth, tongue, pharynx, larynx, vocal cords, trachea, esophagus, spine, eyes, teeth
  - Aspiration and/or infection (pneumonia, sinusitis, otitis media)
  - Endotracheal tube problems (cuffs, pilot tubes, kinking, occlusion, extubation)
  - Autonomic or protective neural responses (hypo/hypertension, brady/tachycardia, arrhythmias, laryngospasm, bronchospasm)
  - Bleeding, hematoma formation, stomal stenosis, innominate artery erosion

MANAGEMENT OF AIRWAY EMERGENCIES—CONT'D

AARC Clinical Practice Guideline (Excerpts)*

- Possible hazards/complications related to emergency ventilation:
  - Inadequate O_2 delivery
  - Hypo/hyperventilation
  - Gastric insufflation and/or rupture
  - Barotrauma
  - Reduced venous return
  - Aspiration, vomiting,
  - Prolonged interruption of ventilation for intubation
  - Failure to establish adequate functional residual capacity (FRC) (neonates)
  - Movement of unstable cervical spine
  - Failure to exhale due to upper airway obstruction during percutaneous transtracheal ventilation

➤ ASSESSMENT OF NEED

The need for airway management is dictated by the patient's clinical condition. Careful observation, the implementation of basic airway management techniques, and laboratory and clinical data should help determine the need for more aggressive measures. Specific conditions requiring intervention include:

- Inability to adequately protect airway (e.g., coma, lack of gag reflex, inability to cough)
- Partially obstructed airway. Signs of a particularly obstructed upper airway include ineffective efforts to ventilate, paradoxical respiration, stridor, use of accessory muscles, patient's pointing to neck, choking motions, cyanosis, and distress. Signs of lower airway obstruction may include the above and wheezing.
- Complete airway obstruction. Respiratory efforts with no breath sounds or suggestion of air movement are indicative of complete obstruction.
- Apnea. No respiratory efforts are seen. May be associated with cardiac arrest.
- Hypoxemia, hypercarbia, and/or acidemia seen on ABG analysis, oximetry, or exhaled gas analysis.
- Respiratory distress. Elevated respiratory rate, high or low ventilatory volumes, and signs of sympathetic nervous system hyperacitivity may be associated with respiratory distress.

➤ ASSESSMENT OF OUTCOME

Timely intervention to maintain the patient's airway can improve outcomes. Under rare circumstances, maintenance of an airway by nonsurgical means may not be possible. Despite optimal airway maintenance, outcomes are affected by patient-specific factors. Lack of appropriate equipment and personnel may adversely affect outcomes. Monitoring and recording can help improve emergency airway management. Some aspects (e.g., intubation complication rates, time to establishment of a definitive airway) are easy to quantify and can help improve hospital-wide systems.

➤ MONITORING

- **Clinical signs:** Continuous patient observation and repeated clinical assessment by a trained observer provide optimal monitoring of the airway. Special consideration should be given to the following:
  - Level of consciousness
  - Ease of ventilation
  - Symmetry/amount of chest movement
  - Presence and character of breath sounds
  - Skin color and character (temperature, presence or absence of diaphoresis)
  - Presence of retractions
  - Presence of nasal flaring
  - Presence of upper airway sounds (e.g., stridor)
  - Presence of epigastric sounds
  - Presence of excessive secretions, blood, vomitus, or foreign objects in the airway
- **Physiological variables:** repeated assessment of physiological data supplements clinical assessment in managing patients with airway difficulties. Monitoring devices should be available, accessible, functional, and periodically evaluated for function. These data include but are not limited to:
  - Ventilatory rate, VT, airway pressure
  - Presence of CO_2 in exhaled gas

Continued

MANAGEMENT OF AIRWAY EMERGENCIES—CONT'D

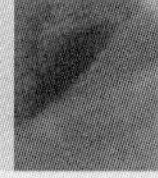

AARC Clinical Practice Guideline (Excerpts)*

- Heart rate and rhythm
- Pulse oximetry
- ABG values
- Chest radiograph
- **Endotracheal tube position:** regardless of the method of ventilation used, the most important consideration is detection of esophageal intubation.
- Tracheal intubation is suggested but may not be confirmed by bilateral breath sounds over the chest; symmetrical chest movement; and absence of ventilation sounds over the epigastrium; presence of condensation inside the tube, corresponding with exhalation; visualization of the tip of the tube passing through the vocal cords; esophageal detector devices may be useful in differentiating esophageal from tracheal intubation.
- Tracheal intubation is confirmed by detection of CO_2 in the exhaled gas, although cases of transient CO_2 excretion from the stomach have been reported.
- Tracheal intubation is confirmed by endoscopic visualization of the carina or tracheal rings through the tube.
- The position of the endotracheal tube (i.e., depth of insertion) should be appropriate on chest radiograph.
- **Airway management process:** a properly managed airway may improve patient outcome. Continuous evaluation of the process will identify components needing improvement. These include response time, equipment function, equipment availability, practitioner performance, complication rate, and patient survival and functional status.

*For complete guidelines see Respir Care 40:749, 1995.

Oral pharyngeal airways are inserted into the mouth and over the tongue. Their use should be restricted to the unconscious patient to avoid gagging and regurgitation. These airways maintain a patent airway when the tongue obstructs the oropharynx or the nasal passages are blocked. The airway can also be used as a bite block for patients with oral tubes.

Since pharyngeal airways are used mainly in emergency life support, further details on their use, insertion techniques, and size selection are found in Chapter 31.

Tracheal Airways

Tracheal airways extend beyond the pharynx, into the trachea. The two basic types of tracheal airways are endotracheal (translaryngeal) tubes and tracheostomy tubes. Endotracheal tubes are inserted through either the mouth or nose (orotracheal or nasotracheal), through the larynx, and into the trachea. Tracheostomy tubes are inserted through a surgically created opening directly into the trachea. A summary of the advantages and disadvantages of each of these three approaches appears in Table 30-1.

Airway Tubes

Endotracheal Tubes

Endotracheal tubes are semirigid tubes, most often made from polyvinyl chloride or related plastic polymers.[17] Specifications covering the sizing, labeling, performance requirements, and test methods for endotracheal tubes are established by the American Society for Testing and Materials (ASTM).[18] Figure 30-6 portrays a typical endotracheal tube and its key components. The proximal end of the tube is attached to a standard adapter with a 15-mm external diameter. The curved body of the tube usually has length marking, indicating the distance (in cm) from the beveled tube tip. In addition to the beveled opening at the tip, there should be an additional side port or "Murphy eye," which ensures gas flow if the main port should become obstructed. The angle of the bevel minimizes mucosal trauma during insertion. The tube cuff is permanently bonded to the tube body. Inflation of the cuff seals off the lower airway, either for protection from aspiration or to provide positive pressure ventilation. A small filling-tube leads from the cuff to a pilot balloon, used to monitor cuff status and

Table 30-1 ▶ ▶ Advantages and Disadvantages of Tracheal Airway Routes

Route	Advantages	Disadvantages
Oral intubation	Insertion is faster, easier, less traumatic, and more comfortable Larger tube is tolerated Easier suctioning Less airflow resistance Decreased work of breathing Easier passage of bronchoscope Reduced risk of the tube kinking Avoidance of nasal and paranasal complications, including epistaxis and sinusitis	Aesthetically displeasing, especially long-term Greater risk of self-extubation or inadvertent extubation Greater risk of mainstem intubation Risk of tube occlusion by biting/trismus Risk of injury to lips, teeth, tongue, palate, and oral soft tissues May require additional use of oral airway Great risk of retching, vomiting, and aspiration
Nasal intubation	Less retching and gagging Greater comfort in long-term use Less salivation Improved ability to swallow oral secretions Improved communication Improved mouth care/oral hygiene Avoidance of occlusion by biting/trismus Easier nursing care Avoidance of oral route complications Less posterior laryngeal ulceration Better tube anchoring; less chance of inadvertent extubation Reduced risk of mainstem intubation Some patients can swallow liquids, providing a means of nutritional support Blind nasal intubation does not require muscle relaxants or sedatives May avert "crash" oral intubation	Pain and discomfort, especially with inadequate preparation Nasal and paranasal complications, including epistaxis, sinusitis, otitis More difficult to perform Spontaneous breathing is required for blind nasal intubation Smaller tube is necessary Greater suctioning difficulty Increased airflow resistance Increased work of breathing Difficulty passing bronchoscope Smaller risk of transient bacteremia
Tracheotomy	Avoidance of laryngeal and upper airway complications of translaryngeal intubation Greater comfort Aids feeding, oral care, suctioning, speech Psychological benefit (improved motivation) Easier passage of fiberoptic bronchoscope Easier reinsertion Aesthetically less objectionable Facilitation of weaning from ventilator Elimination of risk of mainstem intubation Reduced work of breathing Better anchoring (reduced risk of decannulation) Improved ability to place a curve-tipped suction catheter in the left bronchus Improved mobility (transfer out of ICU to ward or extended-care facility)	Greater expense Requirement for use of operating room in most cases Need for general anesthesia in most cases Permanent scar More severe complications Greater mortality rate Delayed decannulation Increased frequency of aspiration Greater bacterial colonization rate Persistent open stoma after decannulation, reducing cough efficiency

From Stauffer JL, Silvestri RC: Respir Care 27:417, 1982.

pressure once the tube is in place. Finally, a spring-loaded valve with a standard connector for a syringe allows inflation and deflation of the cuff. Not shown, but included with most modern endotracheal tubes, is a radiopaque indicator that is embedded in the distal end of the tube body. This indicator allows for easy identification of tube position on radiograph.

Specialized Endtotracheal Tubes

The standard endotracheal tube has been modified for specific uses, including special ventilation methods, lung pathology, or surgical procedures. A detailed description of the variety of tubes is beyond the scope of this chapter but is provided elsewhere.[14] Two of the more common tubes, double lumen and jet ventilation, will be discussed.

Special mechanical ventilation techniques may require unique types of endotracheal tubes. When unilateral lung disease occurs, independent lung ventilation may be needed. This requires the use of a double lumen endotracheal tube (Figure 30-7).[14] This tube has two proximal ventilator connectors (15-mm adapter), two inner lumens for gas flow, two cuffs, and two distal

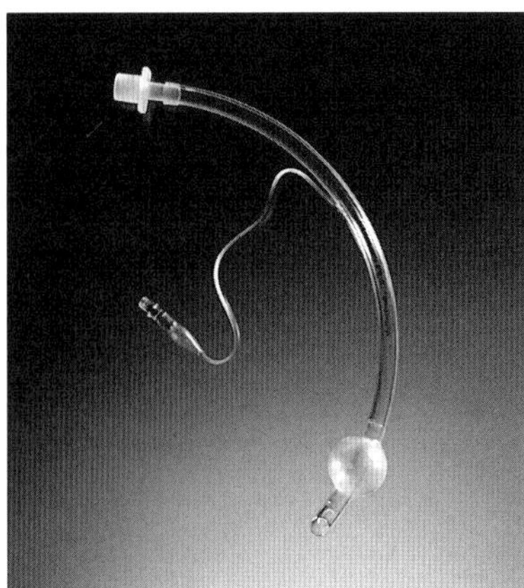

Figure 30-6
Typical endotracheal tube. *(Courtesy of Nellcor Puritan Bennett, Pleasanton, California.)*

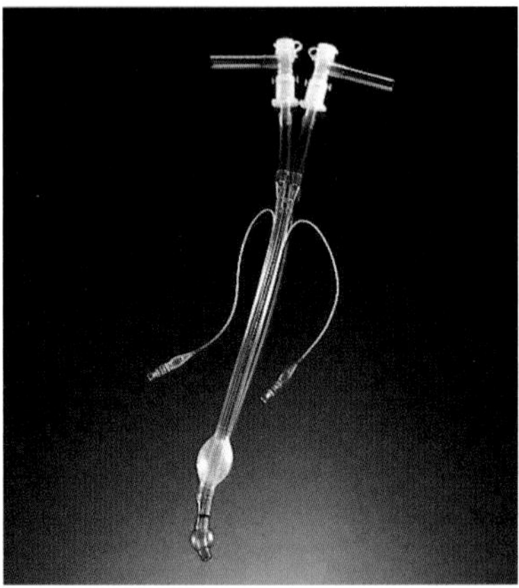

Figure 30-7
Double lumen endotracheal tube for independent lung ventilation *(Courtesy of Nellcor Puritan Bennett, Pleasanton, California.)*

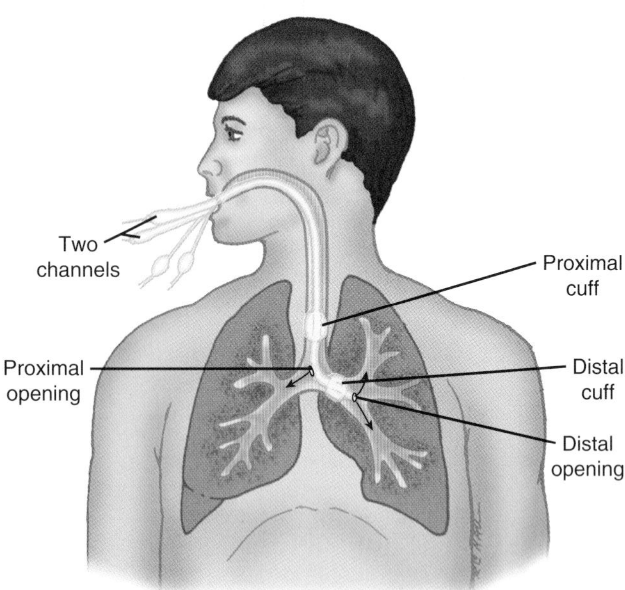

Figure 30-8
Correct positioning of double lumen endotracheal tube.

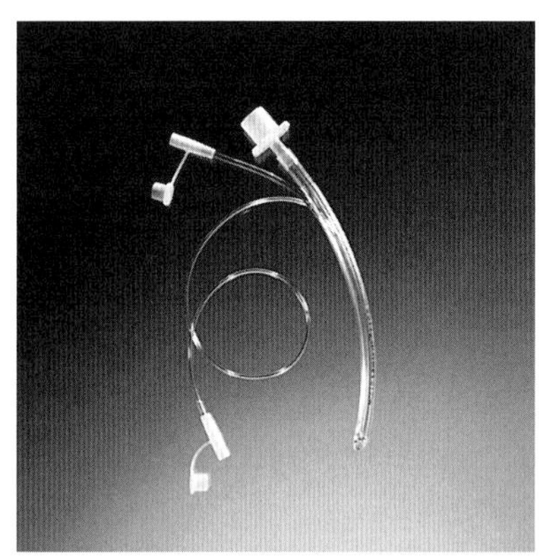

Figure 30-9 · Endotracheal tube modified for jet ventilation.
(Courtesy of Nellcor Puritan Bennett, Pleasanton, California.)

openings. The larger cuff seals the tracheal lumen and allows gas to flow into one bronchus. The smaller cuff seals the opposite bronchial lumen (Figure 30-8).

There are important points to consider when using double lumen endotracheal tubes. They are stiffer and bulkier to insert than standard tubes and must be rotated during insertion to align with the proper bronchus. Fiberoptic bronchsocopy should be performed to ensure the proper placement. The resistance to flow through each tube will be increased since each lumen is smaller than the same size single lumen tubes. A longer suction catheter will be needed to access the bronchial tube.

High frequency jet ventilation also may use a specially designed tube (Figure 30-9). The main body of the tube permits conventional ventilation. The insufflation port allows for the injection of high flow from the jet ventilator. A monitoring line is also available for monitoring pressures or instilling fluids.

Tracheostomy Tubes

As with endotracheal tubes, tracheostomy tubes are generally made from plastic polymers, although some are still made from silver. Specifications covering the sizing, labeling, performance requirements, and test methods for endotracheal tubes are established by the ASTM.[19]

Figure 30-10 portrays a typical plastic tracheostomy tube and its key components. The outer cannula forms the primary structural unit of the tube, to which is attached the cuff and a flange. The flange prevents tube slippage into the trachea and provides the means to secure the tube to the neck. A removable inner cannula with a standard 15-mm adapter is normally kept in

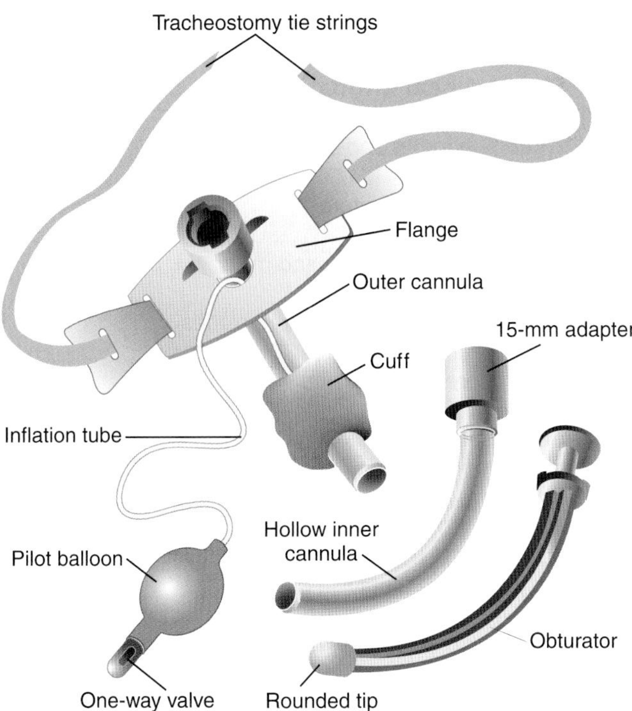

Figure 30-10
Parts of a tracheostomy tube.

place within the outer cannula but can be removed for routine cleaning or if it becomes obstructed. To prevent accidental removal, the inner cannula can be locked in place at the proximal end of the outer cannula. As with the endotracheal tube, an inflation tube leads from the cuff to a pilot balloon and spring-loaded valve. The tube is stabilized at the stoma site with cotton tape, which attaches to the flange and is tied around the neck. An obturator with a rounded tip is used for tube insertion. Prior to insertion, the obturator is placed within the outer cannula, with its tip extending just beyond the far end of the tube. This minimizes mucosal trauma during insertion, particularly the "snowplowing" effect that a rough tube edge can exert on the tracheal wall. Last, as with endotracheal tubes, a radiopaque indicator in the distal end of the tube helps confirm tube position on radiograph.

As with the endotracheal tubes, there are a variety of modified tracheostomy tubes. The Jackson tracheostomy tube is made of silver with an inner and outer cannula (Figure 30-11). It is important to realize there is no cuff at the distal end or 15-mm adapter at the proximal end. These tracheostomy tubes are generally found in patients with a long-term need for an airway but who do not require a seal to protect the airway from aspiration or to facilitate positive pressure ventilation. If the patient requires manual ventilation, a 15-mm adapter should be inserted into the proximal opening. If the patient requires a sealed airway, a cuff can be placed on the Jackson tracheostomy tube or it can be replaced by the standard tube described above.

Procedures

Orotracheal Intubation

Orotracheal intubation is the preferred route for establishing an emergency tracheal airway.[20] This is because oral passage is the quickest and easiest route in most cases. Orotracheal intubation can be safely performed by any appropriately trained physician, respiratory therapist, nurse, or paramedic.[21] Typically, this training involves manikin practice and application on anesthetized patients under the guidance of an anesthesiologist or other appropriately skilled individual. A description of the basic steps in orotracheal intubation is provided below.[22] Proficiency in this technique can be developed only with extensive training.

Step 1: Assemble and Check Equipment. Box 30-3 lists the equipment necessary for intubation. An easy way to remember all the necessary equipment is the mnemonic SOAPME.[22] *S*uction equipment, *o*xygen, *a*irway equipment, *p*osition the patient, *m*onitors, and *e*sophageal dectors describe both the equipment and basic steps of the process. Assemble all suction equipment and check the vacuum pressure prior to intubation, since vomitus

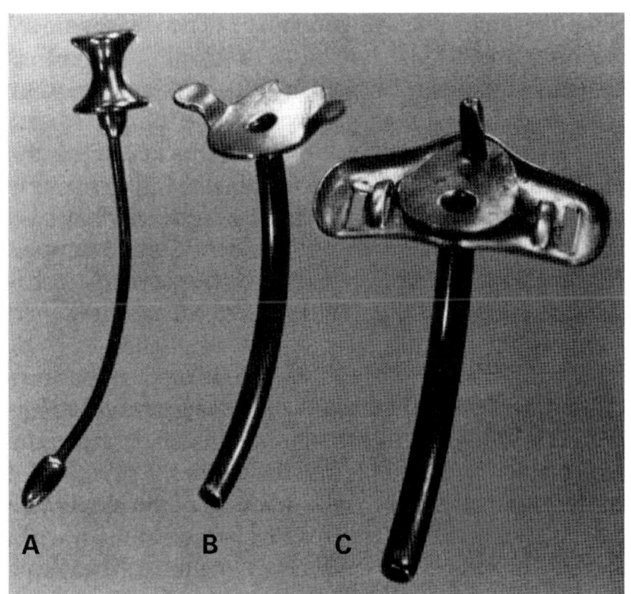

Figure 30-11
Jackson tracheostomy tube made from silver. It has no cuff and no 15-mm adapter. **A,** Obturator. **B,** Inner cannula. **C,** Outer cannula. *(Modified from Eubanks DH, Bones RC: Principles and applications for cardiorespiratory care equipment, St. Louis, 1994, Mosby.)*

MINI CLINI

Indications for Artificial Airway Management

PROBLEM

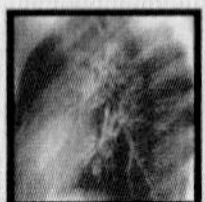

A patient is admitted to the emergency department after suffering chest trauma during a motor vehicle accident. The patient is unconscious, cyanotic, and tachypneic and has blood in her mouth and pharynx. Breath sounds are diminished on both sides. The physician requests that you immediately perform orotracheal intubation. Why?

DISCUSSION

This patient exhibits several indications for insertion of an artificial airway. First, being unconscious, the patient is probably not able to adequately protect her lower airway. With blood in the mouth and pharynx, we should be doubly concerned about protecting her lungs from aspiration. The blood also may indicate partial airway obstruction, with the breath sounds, cyanosis, and respiratory distress contributing to that conclusion. Finally, the cyanosis and chest trauma indicate a potential hypoxemic respiratory failure, which may require positive-pressure ventilatory support via a cuffed endotracheal tube.

Box 30-3 • Equipment Needed for Endotracheal Intubation

- Oxygen flowmeter and tubing
- Suction apparatus
- Flexible suction catheters
- Yankauer (tonsillar) tip
- Manual resuscitation bag and mask
- Oropharyngeal airway(s)
- Laryngoscope (2) with assorted blades
- Endotracheal tubes (3 sizes)
- Tongue depressor
- Stylet
- Stethoscope
- Tape
- Syringe
- Lubricating jelly
- Magill forceps
- Local anesthetic (spray)
- Towels (for positioning)
- CDC barrier precautions (gloves, gowns, masks, eyewear)

or secretions may obscure the pharynx or glottis. Also attach the laryngoscope blade to its handle, and check the light source for secure attachment and brightness. If the light does not function, first check that the bulb is tight. If the scope still does not light, check the batteries or replace the bulb.

Select a tube that is the right size for the patient, but be sure to have available at least one size larger tube and one size smaller tube. Table 30-2 lists recommended orotracheal tube sizes according to patient weight or age. Note that endotracheal tubes are sized by their internal diameter, in millimeters. Tube lengths in Table 30-2 are averages after insertion, confirmed placement, and fixation (teeth to tube tip).

After selecting the correct size of tube, you should inflate the tube cuff and check it for leaks. This can be done either with a pressure manometer or by submerging the inflated cuff in a cup of sterile water. A leak exists if either the pressure does not hold or bubbles escape underwater. Of course, you must be sure to deflate the cuff prior to insertion. To ease insertion, the outer surface of the tube should be lubricated with a water-soluble gel. Last, some clinicians insert a stylet into the tube to add rigidity and maintain shape during insertion. *The tip of the stylet must never extend beyond the endotracheal tube tip.*

Table 30-2 ▶▶ Pediatric to Adult Oral Endotracheal Tube Sizes

Age	Tube Size (mm Internal Diameter)	Tube Length, cm (Incisors to Tip)
Infant, <1000 g	2.5	9-11
Infant, 1000-2000 g	3.0	9-11
Infant, 2000-3000 g	3.5	10-12
Infant, >3000 g	4.0	11-12
6 months	3.0-4.0	11-12
18 months	3.5-4.5	11-13
3 years	4.5-5.0	12-14
5 years	4.5-5.0	13-15
6 years	5.5-6.0	14-16
8 years	6.0-6.5	15-17
12 years	6.0-7.0	17-19
16 years/small adult female	6.5-7.5	18-20
Adult females (average)	8.0	19-21
Adult males	9.0	21-23

Step 2: Position the Patient. To visualize the glottis and insert the tube, you must align the mouth, pharynx, and larynx. You achieve this alignment by combining moderate cervical flexion with extension of the atlanto-occipital joint. Placement of one or more rolled towels under the patient's head helps. You then flex the neck and tilt the head backward with your hand (Figure 30-12).

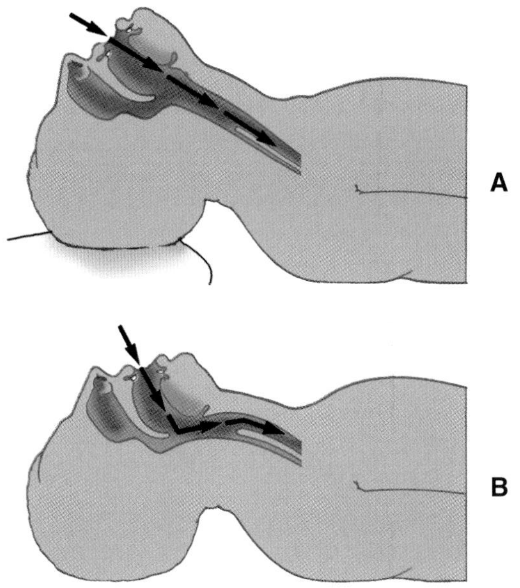

Figure 30-12
A, Correct preintubation head position. **B,** Incorrect preintubation head position.

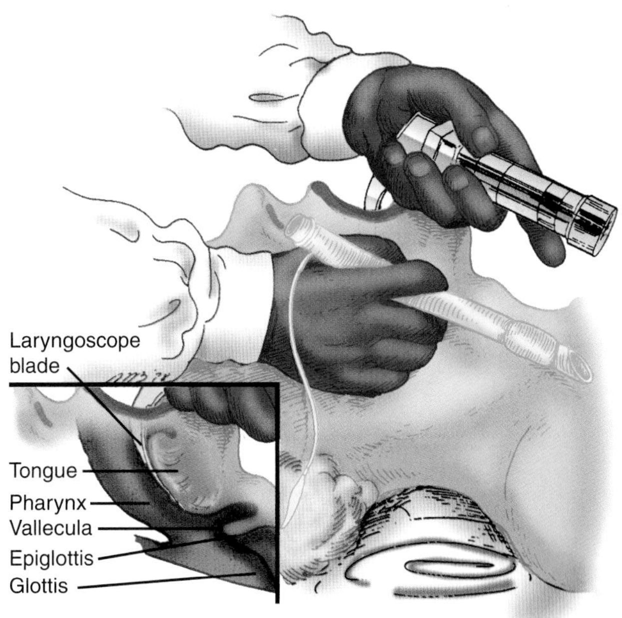

Figure 30-13
To achieve orotracheal intubation, hold laryngoscope in left hand, introduce the blade into right side of mouth, and displace the tongue to the left. *(Modified from Ellis PD, Billings DM: Cardiopulmonary resuscitation: procedures for basic and advanced life support, St Louis, 1980, Mosby.)*

Step 3: Preoxygenate the Patient. A patient in need of intubation is often apneic or in respiratory distress. You therefore must provide adequate ventilation and oxygenation by bag and mask prior to intubation. 100% oxygen provides the patient with a reserve during the intubation procedure. Do not devote more than 30 seconds to any intubation attempt. If intubation fails, you should immediately ventilate and oxygenate the patient for 3 to 5 minutes before a repeat attempt.

Step 4: Insert the Laryngoscope. Use your left hand to hold the laryngoscope, with the right hand used to open the mouth (Figure 30-13). Insert the laryngoscope into the right side of the mouth and move it toward the center, displacing the tongue to the left. Advance the tip of the blade along the curve of the tongue until you visualize the epiglottis.

Step 5: Visualize the Glottis. As the laryngoscope blade reaches the base of the tongue, you will begin to see the arytenoid cartilage and epiglottis (Figure 30-14). If you cannot see these structures, you have probably advanced the blade too far and may be in the esophagus. If this is the case, you should maintain upward force on the laryngoscope and slowly withdraw it until you see the larynx.

Step 6: Displace the Epiglottis. Which technique you use to displace the epiglottis depends on the type of blade chosen (Figure 30-15). With the curved or MacIntosh blade, you displace the epiglottis indirectly by advancing the tip of the blade into the vallecula (at the base of the tongue) and lifting the laryngoscope up and forward (Figure 30-15, *A*). With the straight or Miller blade, you displace the epiglottis directly by advancing the tip of the blade over its posterior surface and lifting the laryngoscope up and forward (Figure 30-15, *B*).

In lifting the tip of the blade, you should avoid levering the laryngoscope against the teeth, as this can damage the teeth and gums. You can avoid this problem by keeping the wrist fixed and moving the handle of the laryngoscope in the direction it is pointing when you visualize the epiglottis.

Step 7: Insert the Tube. Once you displace the epiglottis and can visualize the glottis, insert the tube from the right side of the mouth and advance it without obscuring the glottic opening (Figure 30-16). Once you see the tube tip pass through the glottis, advance it until the cuff has passed the vocal cords.

Once the tube is in place, stabilize it with the right hand, and use the left hand to remove the laryngoscope and stylet. Then inflate the cuff to seal the airway and immediately provide ventilation and oxygenation.

Step 8: Assess Tube Position. Ideally, the tip of an endotracheal tube should be positioned in the trachea about 5 cm above the carina.[4] You can use one or more of several bedside methods to assess positioning of the endotracheal tube before stabilization (Box 30-4).

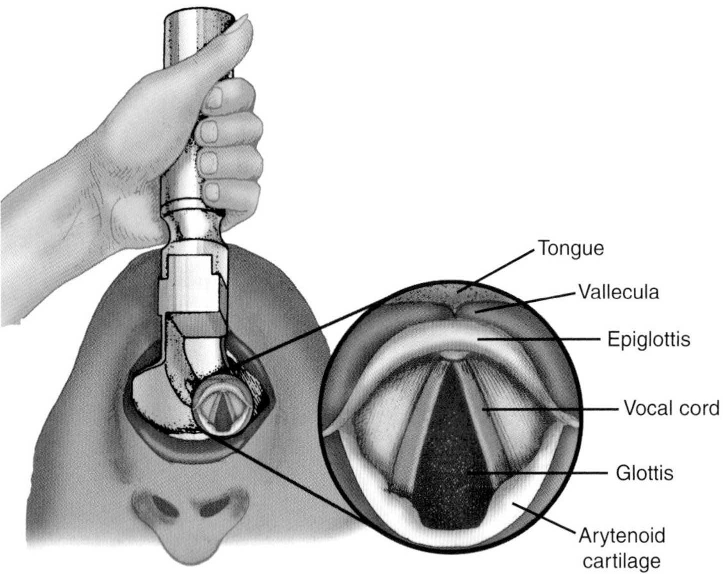

Figure 30-14
Visualization of vocal cords is achieved with laryngoscope. *(Modified from Ellis PD, Billings DM: Cardiopulmonary resuscitation: procedures for basic and advanced life support, St Louis, 1980, Mosby.)*

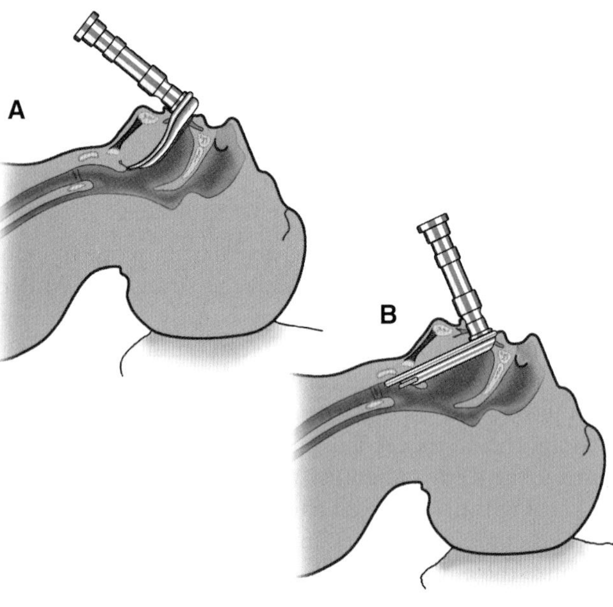

Figure 30-15
Placement of, **A,** curved versus, **B,** straight laryngoscope blade.

With the exception of fiberoptic laryngoscopy, none of these methods can absolutely confirm proper tube placement.

After tube passage and cuff inflation, first listen for equal and bilateral breath sounds as the patient is being ventilated. Air movement or gurgling sounds over the epigastrium indicate possible esophageal intubation. In addition, you should observe the chest wall for adequate and equal chest expansion. These movements, combined with auscultation, are reinforcing. For example, the combination of decreased breath sounds *and* decreased chest wall movement on the left side indicates right mainstem bronchial intubation. Correct right mainstem intubation by slowly withdrawing the tube, while listening for the return of left-side breath sounds. Remember other things will cause decreased breath sounds in the left lung (e.g., atelectasis, pleural effusion). Observe how far you retract the tube so as not to extubate the patient.

You can also use the depth of tube insertion (length from teeth to tip) to help determine tube position. As indicated in Table 30-2, the average length from the teeth (incisors) to the tip of a properly positioned oral endotracheal tube in males is between 21 and 23 cm. For females, this distance is about 2 cm less. Obviously, tube length alone cannot confirm proper placement; a tube with the 23-cm mark positioned at the teeth could just as well be in the esophagus as in the trachea.

You can quickly and easily detect whether the tube is in the esophagus or trachea by using a simple esophageal detection device.[23] The original device consists of a squeeze-bulb aspirator attached to a standard 15-mm adapter. After you create a negative pressure (-80 to -90 mm Hg) by squeezing the bulb, you attach it to the positioned endotracheal tube. If the tube is placed correctly, the bulb quickly reexpands upon release. This is because the trachea is held open by cartilaginous rings. On the other hand, if the tube is in the esophagus, it will not reinflate because the esophagus collapses around the endotracheal tube. Instead of a squeeze-bulb, you can use a large syringe with a 15-mm adapter. If the endotracheal tube is in the esophagus, you will feel strong resistance when you try to aspirate air (the barrel will actually tend to recoil if released); if the tube is in the trachea, you can freely aspirate air into the syringe. In patients with copious secretions, the esophageal detection device may become occluded and

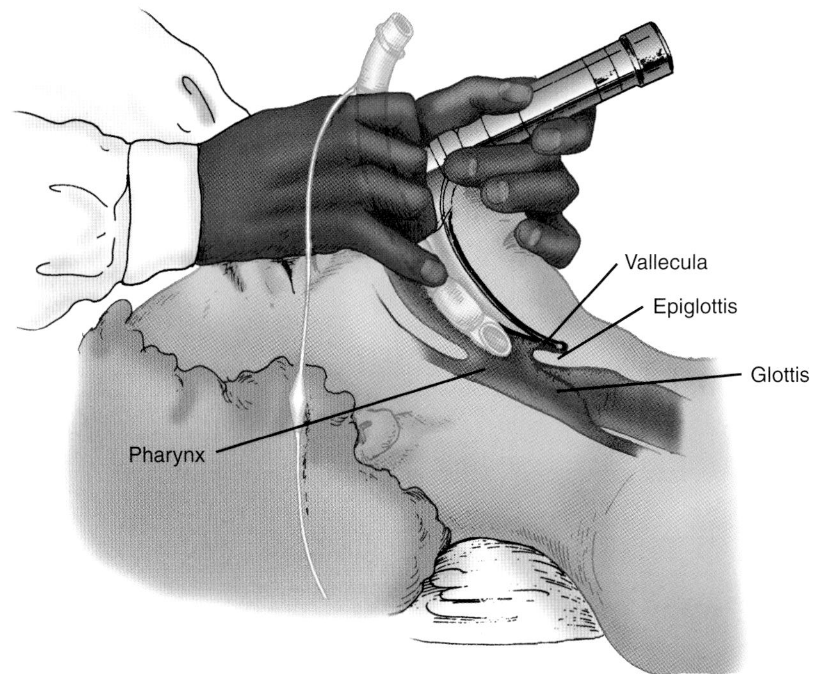

Figure 30-16

Insertion of endotracheal tube. *(Modified from Ellis PD, Billings DM: Cardiopulmonary resuscitation: procedures for basic and advanced life support, St Louis, 1980, Mosby.)*

Box 30-4 • Bedside Methods to Assess Endotracheal Tube Position

- Auscultation of chest and abdomen
- Observation of chest movement
- Tube length (cm to teeth)
- Esophageal detection device
- Light wand
- Capnometry
- Colorimetry
- Fiberoptic laryngoscopy

Table 30-3 ▶▶ Approximate Tracheostomy Tube Sizes

Jackson Size	Internal Diameter (mm)	External Diameter (mm)	French Size
00	2.5	4.5	13.0
0	3.0	5.0	15.0
1	3.5	5.5	16.5
2	4.0	6.0	18.0
3	4.5-5.0	7.0	21.0
4	5.5	8.0	24.0
5	6.0-6.5	9.0	27.0
6	7.0	10.0	11.0
7	7.5-8.0	11.0	33.0
8	8.5	12.0	36.0
9	9.0-11.0	13.0	39.0
10	10.0	14.0	42.0
11	10.5-11.0	15.0	45.0
12	11.5	16.0	48.0

not reexpand.[24] The esophageal detection device is *not* recommended for detecting esophageal intubation in children younger than 1 year of age.[25]

A light wand is a flexible stylet with a lighted bulb at the tip. If a light wand is used during intubation, as you pass the stylet and endotracheal tube into the larynx, you can observe a characteristic glow (described as a "jack-o'-lantern" effect) under the skin, just above the thyroid cartilage.[26] This glow is not as bright or focused if the tube is in the esophagus. When a light wand is used after intubation to confirm placement, you can observe the same glow in the trachea itself.

You also can detect esophageal intubation using exhaled CO_2 analysis (capnometry).[24] Since inspired air contains only about 0.04% CO_2 and end-tidal gas about 6% CO_2, placement of an endotracheal tube in the respiratory tract will cause CO_2 levels to abruptly rise during expiration. This will be evident on a capnographic display (Figure 30-17). On the other hand, if the tube is in the esophagus, CO_2 levels remain near zero.[27]

Colorimetric CO_2 analysis is an inexpensive alternative to capnometry. Functioning much like pH paper, a colorimetric system has an indicator that changes color when exposed to different CO_2 levels.[28] Figure 30-18 shows a disposable colorimetric system designed specifically to confirm tube placement during intubation. Colorimetric devices have the advantage of being portable and disposable.

Both devices are effective in detecting most esophageal intubations. In cardiac arrest victims, however,

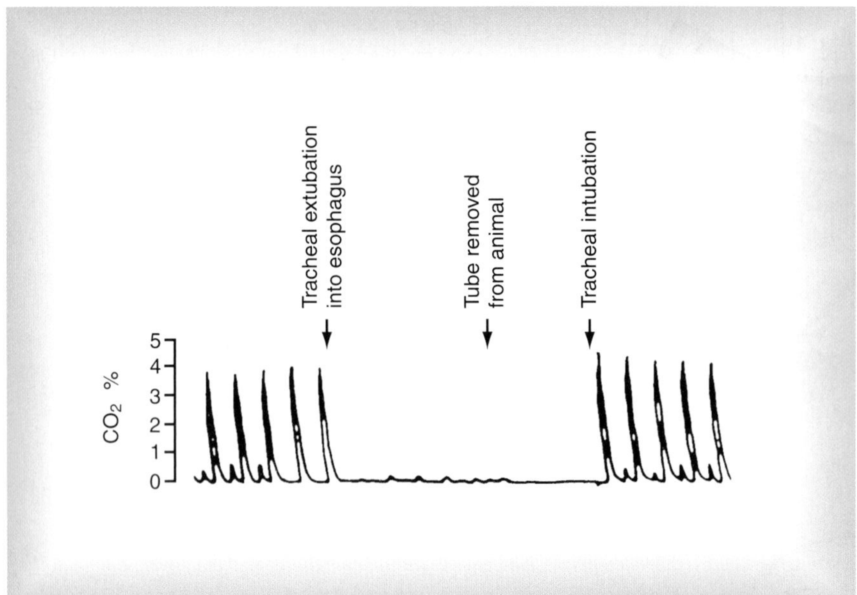

Figure 30-17
Capnogram tracing showing changes in expired percent CO_2 with proper and improper placement of endotracheal tube in test animals.

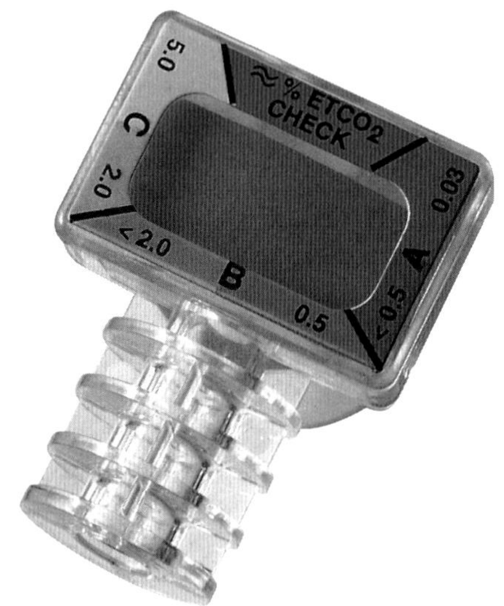

Figure 30-18
A disposable colorimetric CO_2 detector for confirming tracheal intubation. *(Courtesy Nellcor Puritan Bennett, Pleasanton, California.)*

MINI CLINI

Capnometry and Endotracheal Tube Placement

PROBLEM

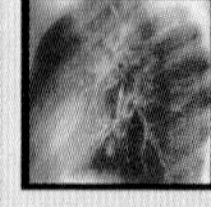

At a Code Blue in the emergency room a patient is intubated by a respiratory therapist. A capnometer is attached to the endotracheal tube to confirm placement in the trachea. The end-expired CO_2 reads 0% as the patient is ventilated with a manual resuscitator. At this time, no one is performing cardiac compressions. Should the therapist conclude that the endotracheal tube is not in the trachea?

DISCUSSION

Not necessarily. If the patient is in cardiac arrest, no blood is perfusing the alveoli, and therefore no CO_2 is entering the alveoli. The result is an end-tidal CO_2 of 0%. Once cardiac compressions begin (and they should begin immediately in confirmed cardiac arrest) and if compressions are effective, one should see an increase in end-tidal CO_2 as blood begins to perfuse the alveoli and CO_2 diffuses the blood.

Of course, there are other simple ways to assess endotracheal tube placement in the trachea, such as bilateral breath sounds upon auscultation and chest excursions. A rise in end-tidal CO_2, however, is a sure indication that the endotracheal tube is in the lungs, since the only source of CO_2 is in the alveoli.

expired CO_2 levels may be near zero because of poor pulmonary blood flow, yielding a false-negative result.[29] Generally, expired CO_2 levels increase with the return of spontaneous circulation. If bag-mask ventilation has occurred for some time, some CO_2 maybe present in the stomach.[30] Four to five additional breaths may be needed before the color of the detectors returns to the esophageal color.[24,30] Unfortunately, CO_2 analysis is not a reliable indicator of mainstem bronchial intubation.

Proper tube placement in the trachea can be confirmed without a chest radiograph by using a fiberoptic laryngoscope.[31] After ensuring patient reoxygenation, the clinician inserts a fiberoptic laryngoscope directly into the endotracheal tube (Figure 30-19). Visualization of the carina distal to the tip of the endotracheal tube ensures proper placement in the trachea. More precise placement is possible by moving the laryngoscope from the tube tip to the carina, while measuring this distance.

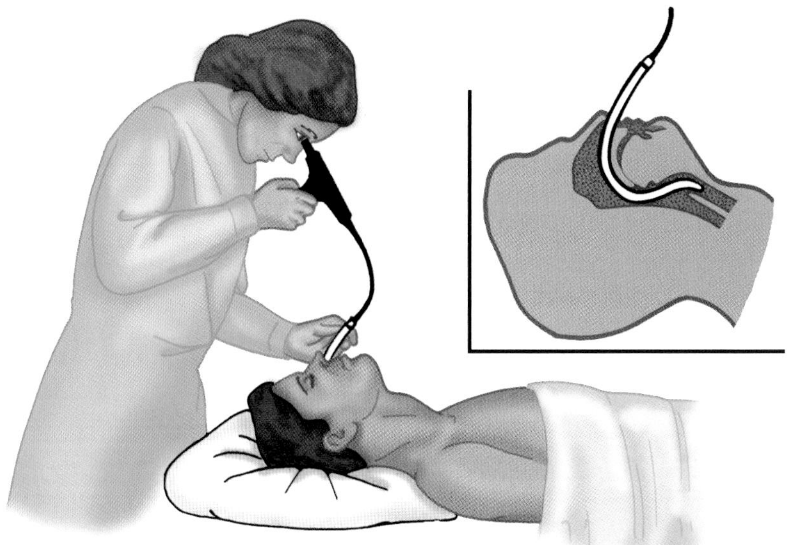

Figure 30-19
Fiberoptic laryngoscopy used to confirm endotracheal tube placement.

Step 9: Stabilize the Tube/Confirm Placement. Do not secure the tube until you have assessed placement by using one or more of the above methods. After assessing placement and while holding the tube in position, secure the tube to the skin above the lip and on the cheeks using tape. Normally you will need a bite block, oropharyngeal airway, or similar device to prevent the patient from biting down on the tube (Figure 30-20). After you stabilize the tube, you should make sure that a chest radiograph is taken to confirm its position.

The most common complication of emergency airway management is tissue trauma. The most serious complications are acute hypoxemia, hypercapnia, bradycardia, and cardiac arrest.[32] You can minimize or avoid these problems by using proper technique, providing the patient with adequate ventilation and oxygenation (before, during, and after), and strictly adhering to intubation time limits. In addition, sedation and anesthesia can reduce complications and facilitate intubation in the semicomatose or combative patient.[20,24] Paralysis can be used in the combative patient who cannot be controlled by sedation. It is important to remember the paralyzed patient has no ability to compensate for hypoxemia or hypercapnea. It is imperative the patient can be adequately ventilated by bag and mask. Rapid sequence induction is used to describe the administration of a sedative, hypnotic medication, and a paralyzing agent.

Difficult intubations occur because of the inability to open the mouth, position the patient, or unusual airway anatomy. Special intubation equipment (laryngoscope blades or stylets) or alternative techniques can be performed. Details of these techniques are beyond the scope of this chapter.[33]

Nasotracheal Intubation

Although nasotracheal intubation is more difficult than orotracheal intubation, it is the route of choice in certain clinical situations. Examples include intubation of patients when the oral route is unavailable, such as maxillofacial injuries or oral surgery.

Nasotracheal intubation is performed either blindly or by direct visualization.[37] The direct visualization approach requires either a standard or fiberoptic laryngoscope. For the blind technique to work, the patient must be breathing spontaneously. Equipment assembly, patient positioning, and preoxygenation are essentially the same as with oral intubation. Sprays of 0.25% racemic epinephrine and 2% lidocaine may also be needed to provide local anesthesia and vasoconstriction of the nasal passage.

Direct Visualization. The equipment needed for nasal intubation by direct visualization is the same as for oral intubation, with the addition of Magill forceps. A smaller radius endotracheal tube may also be needed. Prelubricate the tube to aid passage. To insert the tube, position the bevel toward the septum and advance it along the floor of the inferior meatus (inferiorly). When the tip of the tube is in the oropharynx, open the mouth, insert the laryngoscope (with your left hand), and visualize the glottis. With your right hand, use the Magill forceps to grasp the tube just above the cuff and direct it between the vocal cords (Figure 30-21). To help advance the tube past the vocal cords, you may need to flex the neck. The average depth of tube insertion from the external naris is 28 cm for adult males and 26 cm

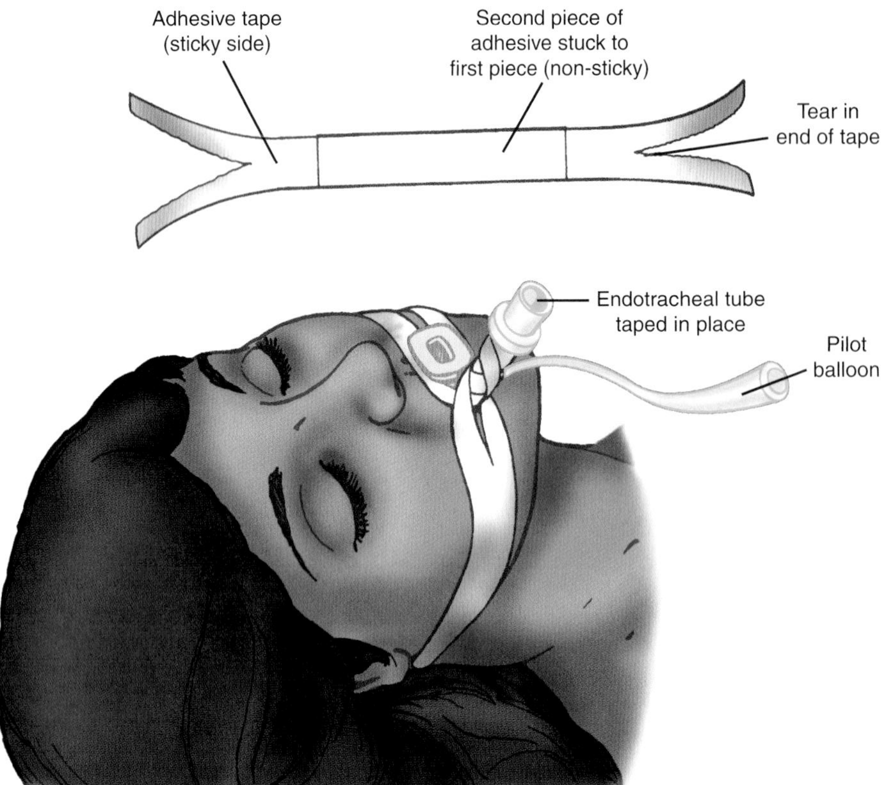

Figure 30-20
Securing the endotracheal tube.

for females.[8] Confirmation of position and stabilization follows, as with the oral route.

Alternatively, you can use a fiberoptic bronchoscope or laryngoscope to guide tube passage.[33] With the bronchoscopic method, pass the distal end of the scope through the endotracheal tube and directed into the trachea. Once placement is ensured, slide the endotracheal tube down over the scope into proper position. The procedure is similar with a fiberoptic laryngoscope. However, since directional control of the scope is limited, you may have to reposition the patient's head and neck to help guide the tube.

Blind Passage. For blind nasal intubation, place the patient in either the supine or sitting position.[34] As with direct visualization, insert the tube through the nose. As the tube approaches the larynx, listen through the tube for air movement. The breath sounds become louder and more tubular when the tube passes through the larynx. Successful passage of the tube through the larynx usually is indicated by a harsh cough, followed by vocal silence. If the sounds disappear, the tube is moving toward the esophagus. You can correct a malpositioned tube by manipulating the tube and reposition-

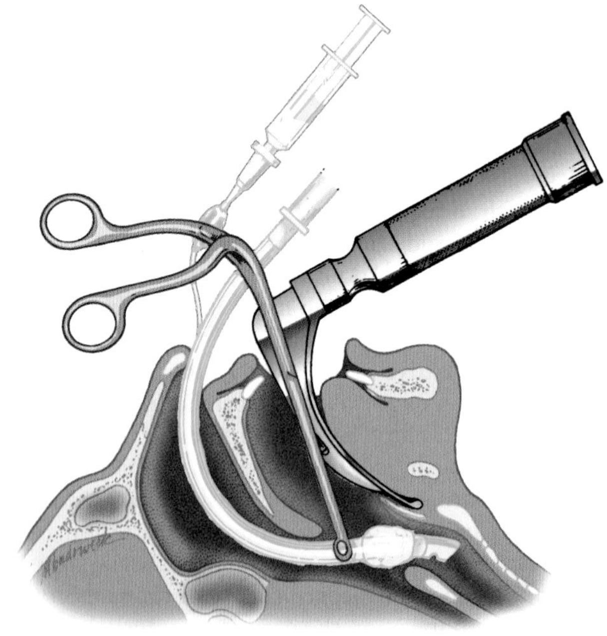

Figure 30-21
Nasal intubation using Magill forceps. *(Modified from Finucane BT, Santora AH: Principles of airway management, Philadelphia, 1988, FA Davis.)*

ing the patient's head and neck. Confirmation of tube placement and stabilization should follow. As previously indicated, a light wand can help ensure proper tracheal placement during blind nasotracheal intubation.

Tracheotomy

Tracheotomy is the procedure of establishing access to the trachea via neck incision. The opening created via this procedure is called a *tracheostomy*. Tracheotomy may be performed as a regular surgical procedure, or by using a special dilator kit (percutaneous dilatational tracheotomy).

Tracheotomy is the preferred, primary route for overcoming upper airway obstruction or trauma and for long-term care of patients with neuromuscular disease. Another indication for tracheotomy is the continuing need for an artificial airway after a prolonged period of oral or nasal intubation.[35] As with most other interventions, the decision as to when to switch from endotracheal tube to tracheostomy tube should be individualized.[36] Pertinent factors that should be considered in making this decision are summarized in Box 30-5. A decision-making algorithm useful in timing tracheotomy in critically ill patients is found in Figure 30-22.

Procedure. Tracheotomy should be performed as an elective procedure by a skilled physician or surgeon after the patient's airway is stabilized. Mortality and morbidity are higher when the procedure is performed

Box 30-5 • Factors to Consider in Switching From Endotracheal Tube to Tracheostomy

- The projected time the patient will need an artificial airway
- The patient's tolerance of the endotracheal tube
- The patient's overall condition (including nutritional, cardiovascular, and infection status)
- The patient's ability to tolerate a surgical procedure
- The relative risks of continued endotracheal intubation versus tracheostomy

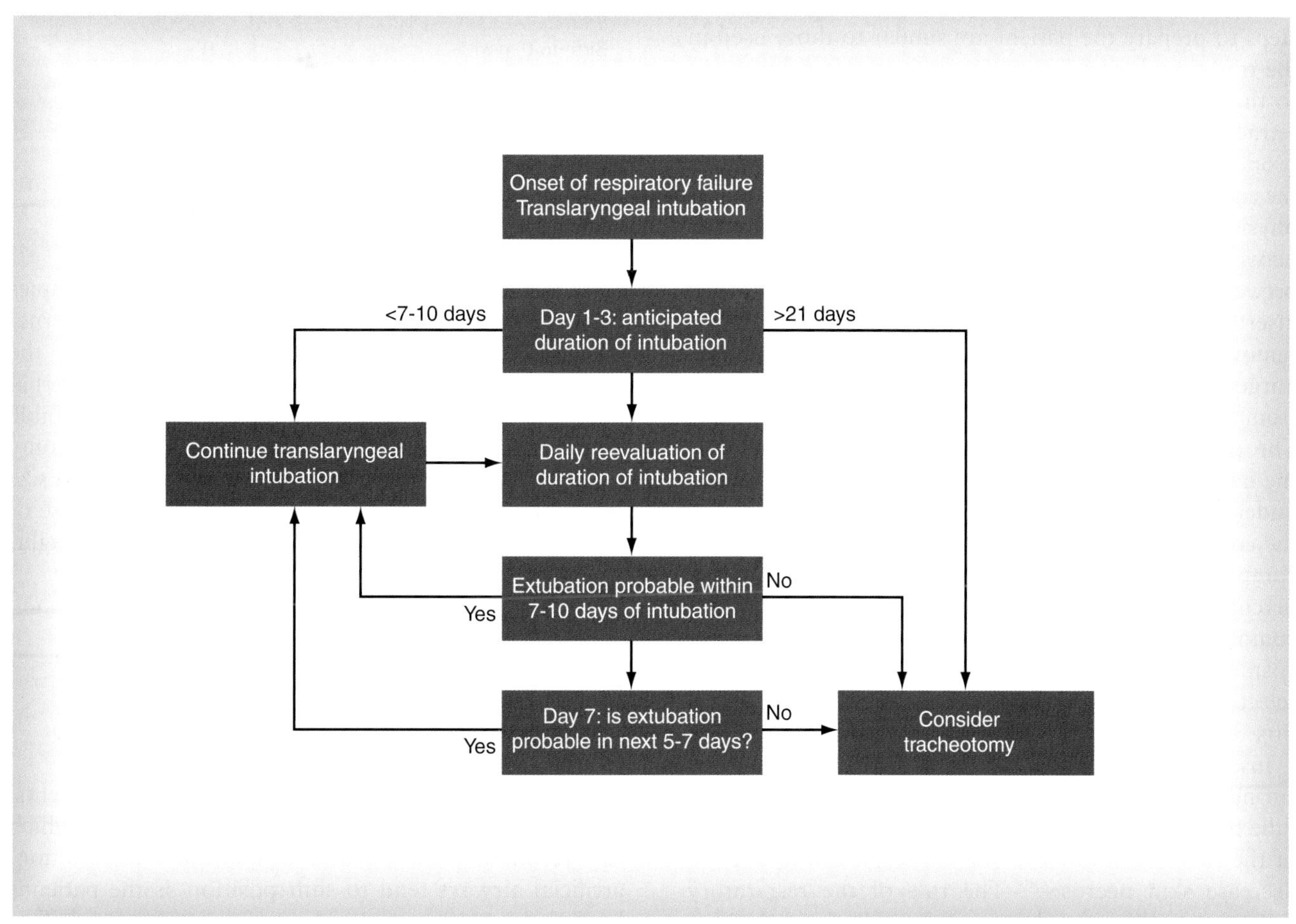

Figure 30-22
An approach to timing tracheotomy in patients intubated and mechanically ventilated for respiratory failure. *(From Heffner JE: Clin Chest Med 12:611, 1991.)*

on an emergency basis. The respiratory therapist may be asked to assist in tracheotomy, especially if performed at the bedside. For this reason we will briefly describe both the traditional surgical procedure and the new dilatational method.[37,38]

A local anesthetic is used and the patient mildly sedated, conditions permitting. If an endotracheal tube is in place, it should not be removed until just prior to the insertion of the tracheostomy tube. This ensures a patent airway and provides additional stability to the trachea during the procedure.

In the traditional surgical tracheotomy, the surgeon makes an incision in the neck over the second or third tracheal ring. Once the skin and subcutaneous tissue have been incised, the surgeon divides the platysma muscles and locates the underlying thyroid gland. The surgeon then divides and ligates the thyroid isthmus, which overlies the second and third tracheal rings. The surgeon then enters the trachea through either a horizontal incision between rings or a vertical one through the second and third rings. As little cartilage as possible should be removed, in order to promote better closure after extubation.

In percutaneous dilatational tracheotomy, the initial steps to prepare the patient are similar to those used in the traditional tracheotomy procedure. After dissection to the anterior tracheal wall, the endotracheal tube is retracted to keep the cuff just below the vocal cords. A bronchoscope can be used to reassess the placement for the endotracheal tube for duration of the procedure. The physician inserts a needle and sheath into the trachea between either the cricoid and first tracheal ring, or between the first and second rings. The physician then inserts a guidewire through the sheath, the sheath is removed, and a dilator is passed over the guidewire. Larger and larger dilators are introduced, until the stoma is large enough for a standard tracheostomy tube. The physician then slips the tracheostomy tube over the last dilator used. The procedure may be performed under direct vision with a bronchoscope passed through the endotracheal tube or a laryngeal mask airway.[39] As compared with the traditional surgical procedure, percutaneous dilatational tracheotomy is rapid with less complications from the surgical site and has a better cosmetic appearance after decannulation. Patient selection factors for percutaneous tracheotomy are in Box 30-6.

Insertion of the tube, inflation of the cuff, and securing of the tube follow both methods. Tracheostomy tube ties should be secure enough to prevent movement of the tube but allow for one finger's width of play to decrease skin necrosis.[40] The role of the respiratory therapist in the procedure may include managing the endotracheal tube, making ventilator changes as needed, assisting with the bronchoscope, and monitoring the patient.

Box 30-6 • Patient Selection Factors for Percutaneous Tracheostomy

PRO

- Easy reintubation (A)
- No coagulopathy (R)
- Adult (R)
- Favorable neck anatomy (R)
- Good extension
- No goiter
- No prior anterior surgery

CON

- Difficult reintubation (A)
- Coagulopathy (A)
- Unfavorable anatomy (R)

A, Absolute indication; *R*, relative indication.

Table 30-4 ▶ ▶ Pediatric to Adult Tracheostomy Tube Sizes

Age	Jackson Reference
Premature	000-00
Birth to 6 months	0
6-18 months	1
18 months to 4-5 years	1-2
4-5 years to 10 years	2-3
10 to 14 years	3-5
14 years to adult	5-9+

In general, the tube size is correct if it occupies between two thirds to three quarters of the internal tracheal diameter. Table 30-3 (on p. 671) lists the various tracheostomy tube sizes, using Jackson, internal diameter, external diameter, and French scales. Table 30-4 provides guidelines for selecting a tracheostomy tube according to a patient's age, using the Jackson size for reference. Within an age category, the exact size of tube chosen depends on the patient's height and weight.

▶ AIRWAY TRAUMA ASSOCIATED WITH TRACHEAL TUBES

Artificial airways do not exactly conform to patients' anatomies. The result is pressure on soft tissues, which can result in ischemia and ulceration.[32] In addition, artificial airways tend to shift position as the patient's head and neck move or as the tube is manipulated. This can result in friction-like injuries. Occasional reaction to the materials composing the tube may also cause problems.

Depending on the type of tube, damage to the patient's airway can occur anywhere from the nose down into the lower trachea. Since tracheostomy tubes do not pass through the larynx, structural injury due to these airways is limited to tracheal sites. Laryngeal dysfunction may occur secondary to a lack of stimulation from airflow or restricted movement secondary to equipment.[36]

Because injury often cannot be assessed while an artificial airway is in place, the patient's airway should always be evaluated carefully after extubation. Techniques commonly used to diagnose airway damage include physical examination, air tomography, fluoroscopy, laryngoscopy, bronchoscopy, magnetic resonance imaging, and pulmonary function studies.[41]

Laryngeal Lesions

The most common laryngeal injuries associated with endotracheal intubation are glottic edema, vocal cord inflammation, laryngeal/vocal cord ulcerations, and vocal cord polyps or granulomas. Less common and more serious are vocal cord paralysis and laryngeal stenosis.[32,41]

Glottic edema and vocal cord inflammation are transient changes that occur as a result of pressure from the endotracheal tube, or trauma during intubation.[32] The primary concern with glottic edema and vocal cord inflammation occurs *after* extubation. Since swelling can worsen over 24 hours after extubation, patients should be evaluated periodically for the delayed development of glottic edema.

The primary symptoms of glottic edema and vocal cord inflammation are hoarseness and stridor. Hoarseness occurs in most extubated patients and usually resolves quickly. Stridor is a more serious symptom than hoarseness, indicating a significant decrease in diameter of the airway. Stridor is often treated with racemic epinephrine (2.25% Vaponephrin) via aerosol.[32] The goal of the treatment is to reduce glottic or airway edema by mucosal vasoconstriction. A steroid may also be added to the aerosol to further reduce inflammation. Both of these techniques are more commonly used in children rather than adults.

To reduce laryngeal edema in patients who have had prolonged intubation or those who have failed prior extubation because of glottic edema, intravenous steroids may be given 24 hours prior to extubation.[32] If stridor continues and is unresponsive to treatment, structural changes that narrow the airway should be suspected.

Laryngeal and vocal cord ulcerations may also cause hoarseness soon after extubation. Symptoms usually resolve spontaneously, and no treatment is indicated. Vocal cord polyps and granulomas develop more slowly, taking weeks or months to form.[41] Symptoms include difficulty in swallowing, hoarseness, and stridor. If symptoms are severe or persistent, the polyps or granulomas may have to be removed surgically.

Vocal cord paralysis is likely in extubated patients with hoarseness and stridor that does not resolve with treatment or time. In some patients, symptoms may resolve within 24 hours, and full movement of the vocal cords can return over several days. If the obstructive symptoms continue, tracheotomy may be indicated.

Laryngeal stenosis occurs when the normal tissue of the larynx is replaced by scar tissue, which causes stricture and decreased mobility. The symptoms of laryngeal stenosis are similar to those of vocal cord paralysis, namely, stridor and hoarseness. The onset of dyspnea occurring within one year of intubation may be the result of larygneal injury.[41] Since laryngeal stenosis does not resolve spontaneously, surgical correction is usually required. Some patients will need a permanent tracheostomy.

Tracheal Lesions

Whereas laryngeal lesions occur only with oral or nasal endotracheal tubes, tracheal lesions can occur with any tracheal airway. The most common tracheal lesions are granulomas, tracheomalacia, and tracheal stenosis.[32,41] Less common, but more serious, complications are tracheoesophageal and tracheoinnominate fistulas.

Tracheomalacia and tracheal stenosis can occur either separately or together. Tracheomalacia is the softening of the cartilaginous rings, which causes collapse of the trachea during inspiration. Tracheal stenosis is a narrowing of the lumen of the trachea, which can occur as fibrous scarring causes the airway to narrow. In patients with endotracheal tubes, this type of damage most often occurs at the cuff site. In patients with tracheostomy tubes, stenosis may occur at the cuff, tube tip, or stoma sites, with the stoma site being the most common. Stenosis at the stoma site is associated with too large a stoma, infection of the stoma, movement of the tube, or frequent tube changes.[42]

Signs of possible tracheal damage prior to extubation include difficulty in sealing the trachea with the cuff and evidence of tracheal dilation on chest radiograph.[32] Postextubation signs and symptoms include difficulty with expectoration, dyspnea, and stridor. Although these findings may appear acutely, they more commonly develop over several months and may not be symptomatic until the radius is reduced by as much as 50%. Symptoms are often attributed to the development of asthma or chronic lung disease.[41]

Tomography, fluoroscopy, and pulmonary function studies (especially flow-volume loops) may be helpful in quantifying the severity of the damage. Flow-volume loops are also helpful in distinguishing between tracheomalacia and tracheal stenosis.[43] Tracheomalacia will appear as a variable obstruction with different inspira-

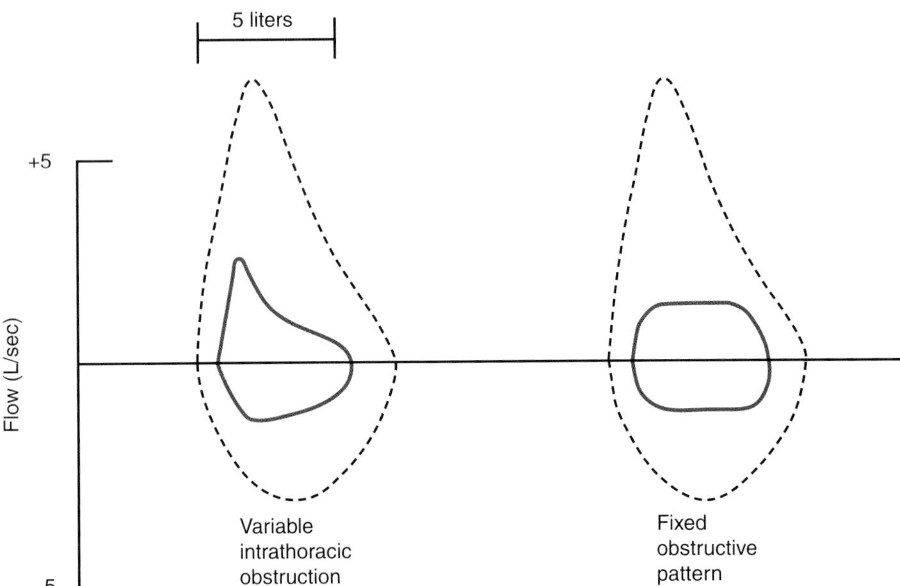

Figure 30-23
Variable intrathoracic *(left)* versus fixed obstructive pattern *(right)* flow-volume loops. Dotted lines are normals for comparison. Tracheomalacia is typically seen as a variable obstruction, while tracheal stenosis most often presents with a fixed pattern.

tory and expiratory patterns. Tracheal stenosis will appear as a fixed obstructive pattern, with flattening of both the inspiratory and expiratory limbs of the flow-volume loop (Figure 30-23).

Treatment depends on the severity, especially the length and circumference of the damage.[32,43] Laser therapy may be useful if the lesion is small. Resection and end-to-end anastomosis may be indicated when the damage involves less than three tracheal rings. More involved damage may require staged repair.

A tracheoesophageal fistula is a direct communication between the trachea and esophagus. Tracheoesophageal fistula is a relatively rare complication of both tracheotomy and endotracheal intubation. If it occurs soon after tracheotomy, incorrect surgical technique may be the cause. Later development is related to sepsis, malnutrition, tracheal erosion from the cuff and tube, and esophageal erosion from nasogastric tubes. [32,44] Diagnosis can be made by a history of recurrent aspiration and abdominal distention as air is forced into the esophagus during positive pressure ventilation. Diagnosis is made by direct endoscopic examination of the trachea and esophagus. Treatment involves surgical closure of the defect.

A tracheoinnominate fistula can occur when a tracheostomy tube causes tissue erosion through the innominate artery. The result is massive hemorrhage and, in most cases, death. Luckily, tracheoinnominate fistula is a rare complication, probably caused by improper low positioning of the stoma. Pulsation of the tracheostomy tube may be the only clue prior to actual hemorrhage. Once hemorrhage begins, hyperinflation of the cuff may slow the bleeding, but the patient will still need surgical intervention.[42] Even with proper corrective action, only 25% of patients who develop this serious complication survive.

Prevention

Several actions can minimize the trauma caused by tracheal airways. Many studies suggest that tube movement is a primary cause of injury.[34] Several methods can be used to limit tube movement. Sedation can help keep patients comfortable and decrease the likelihood of self-extubation. Nasotracheal tubes are easier to stabilize and may move less than orotracheal tubes. Swivel adapters can be used to minimize tube traction whenever respiratory therapy equipment is attached to patients with tracheostomies.[43] If the tracheostomy patient requires oxygen therapy, tracheostomy collars are preferred to T-tubes or Briggs adapters.

Selection of the correct size of airway is also important. Once in place, endotracheal and tracheostomy tubes should not be changed unless necessary. To minimize vocal cord closure around endotracheal tubes, patients should be discouraged from unnecessary coughing or efforts to talk. Pressure necrosis from the endotracheal or tracheostomy tube cuff can be reduced by limiting cuff pressures to those needed to minimize aspiration or provide ventilation.[4,41] If the airway is in place solely for suctioning or to bypass an obstruction, a cuff may not be needed at all.

Infected secretions have been implicated in the development of tracheitis and mucosal destruction, and infection of the tracheotomy stoma has been linked to tracheal stenosis.[45] Therefore sterile techniques should be used in working with these tubes. Good tracheostomy care, including aseptic cleaning of the stoma with hydrogen peroxide, should be carried out routinely. Soiled tracheostomy dressings should also be changed as needed.

▶ AIRWAY MAINTENANCE

Once a tracheal airway is in place, the respiratory therapist must attend to several aspects of airway maintenance. Among the critical responsibilities in this area are (1) securing the tube and maintaining its proper placement, (2) providing for patient communication, (3) ensuring adequate humidification, (4) minimizing the possibility of infection, (5) aiding secretions clearance, (6) providing appropriate cuff care, and (7) trouble-shooting airway-related problems.

Securing the Airway and Confirming Placement

The most common way to secure endotracheal tubes is with tape. The tape is secured to one side of the face, then wound around the tube and airway once or twice before the end is secured to the skin again (refer to Figure 30-19). Silk tape is adequate if the period of intubation is short, such as during surgery, however, silk tape is easily loosened by oral secretions. Cloth tape seems to be better for longer use and may adhere better if the skin is prepared with tincture of benzoin. Instead of using tape to secure the tube, practitioners can choose among several endotracheal tube harnesses. Case reports indicate that use of these harnesses can result in less skin damage, tube movement, and self-extubations than with traditional taping. However, of and by themselves, these stabilizing devices cannot prevent airway trauma.

You normally secure a tracheostomy tube by threading cloth ties through the tube flange and tying them together on the side of the patient's neck. Alternatively, you can use a special strip of foam rubber with Velcro attachments threaded through the tube flange. This system is easier to change and does not cause skin necrosis as often as cloth ties. Whichever system is used, you can minimize skin damage by keeping the ties loose enough to easily slip one finger underneath. Proper placement of an endotracheal or tracheostomy tube normally is confirmed by radiograph. The tube tip should be about 4 to 6 cm above the carina, or between the second and fourth tracheal rings.[32,34,46] Keeping the tube position in this range will minimize the chance of the tube moving down into the mainstem bronchi or up into the larynx. Even so, the endotracheal tube position will change with movement of the head and neck (Figure 30-24).[47] Flexion of the neck moves the tube toward the carina, while extension pulls the tube toward the larynx. Therefore when reviewing a radiograph for tube placement, you should also check the position of the head and neck. If the tube is malpositioned, you should remove the old tape and reposition the tube, using the centimeter markings as a guide. This often requires two people to prevent extubation.

As an alternative to using chest films to confirm tube placement, a practitioner trained in fiberoptic laryngoscopy or bronchoscopy may confirm the position of the tube visually.[48] With this method, the fiberoptic scope is inserted into the tube, and the carina directly visualized. By moving the scope from the tube tip to the carina, and measuring the distance of laryngoscope displacement, the exact distance of insertion can be determined.

Providing for Patient Communication

One of the most frustrating aspects of caring for a patient with a tracheal tube is his or her inability to talk. Phonation requires moving vocal cords, resulting in airflow between them. Endotracheal tubes prevent vocal cord movement and airflow through the cords.

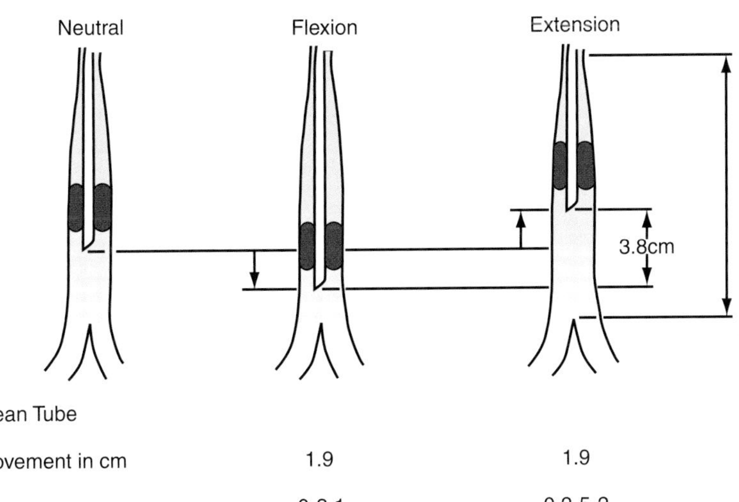

Figure 30-24
Effect of neck flexion and extension on endotracheal tube position. *(Modified from Conrardy PA et al: Crit Care Med 4:8, 1976.)*

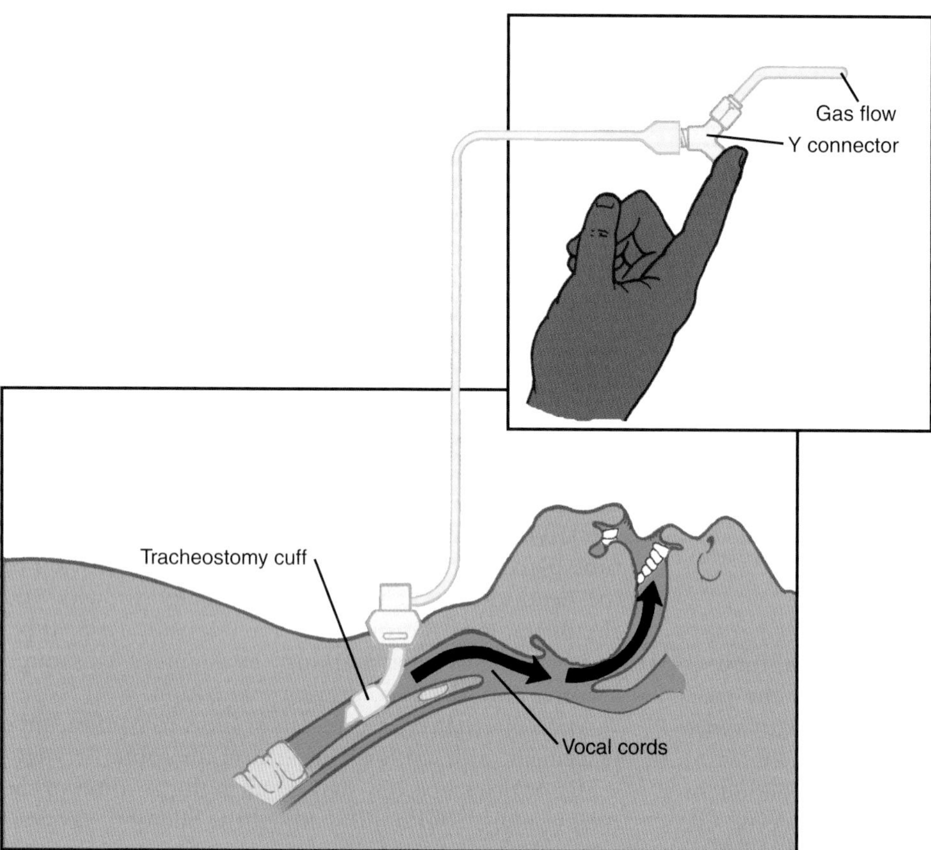

Figure 30-25
"Talking" tracheostomy tube.

Standard tracheostomy tubes allow vocal cord movement but prevent airflow.

The experienced practitioner may use lipreading, but this technique is very difficult in patients with orotracheal tubes. As an alternative, the alert patient may write messages on paper or some other writing surface. For many patients, however, restricted hand movement due to restraints or vascular lines makes writing impossible. Moreover, some critically ill patients simply cannot hold up their heads. A better solution is a letter, phrase, or picture board.[49] These devices allow patients to communicate by simple pointing. Large and simple drawings are particularly important for patients who cannot clearly see print.

In conscious patients with a long-term tracheostomy, communication can be enhanced with a "talking" tracheostomy tube (Figure 30-25).[50] These special airways provide a separate inlet for compressed gas, which escapes above the tube, thereby allowing phonation. There are, however, some problems associated with these tubes. The continuous gas flow through a new tracheostomy may cause air leaks. High flowrates may cause mucosal drying and irritation. Last, secretions may occlude the speaking gas outlets. Although not life-threatening, these problems can be frustrating for both patient and practitioner.

An alternative to the speaking tracheostomy tube is to place a one-way valve on the external opening of the tracheostomy tube.[51] With this device, the patient inhales through the tube and exhales through the larynx. Speech is coordinated with exhalation through the larynx. The Passy-Muir Valve is an example of this type of valve (Fig. 30-26). It can be used with spontaneously breathing or ventilator-dependent patients. When using the speaking valve, the cuff on the tube must be deflated to allow airflow around the tube. This will cause a leak

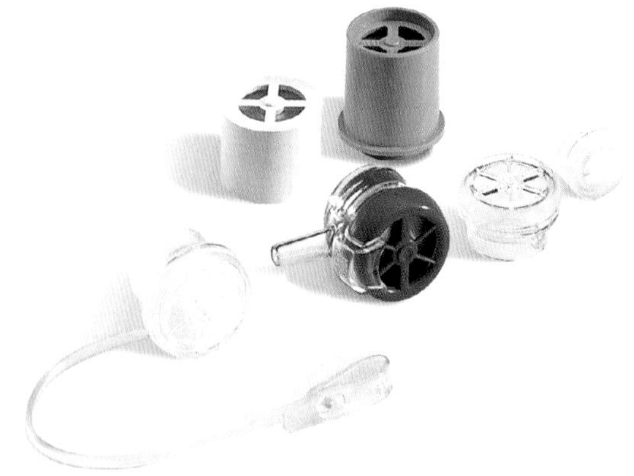

Figure 30-26
Passy Muir family of valves including one that can be used to deliver oxygen to the tracheostomy patient. *(Courtesy of Passy Muir, Inc., Irvine, California.)*

on inspiration and a decrease in tidal volume delivery. However, an increase in the set tidal volume on the ventilator during initial trials of the valve should compensate for this.

Assessment of heart rate, respiratory rate, and saturation should follow initial placement of the valve for all patients.[51,52] Expiratory effort should also be assessed. Since the expiratory flow now has to travel a longer distance through the upper airway, resistance to exhalation will be slightly increased. Air trapping may be detected by a rush of air when the valve is removed after the patient exhales. The most common cause of this problem is the size of the tracheostomy tube relative to the size of the trachea, or an upper airway abnormality. Once those issues have been addressed, the patient can again be tried on a speaking valve. Assessment of the patient for a speaking valve includes a respiratory therapist, speech pathologist, and otolaryngologist.[51]

In addition to facilitating communication, other benefits of airflow over the upper airway include better function of the vocal cords, sense of smell, and fewer secretion problems. Improved swallowing function and less aspiration have been reported with the Passy Muir Valve.[53,54]

Ensuring Adequate Humidification

Although tracheal tubes provide an airway to conduct gas to and from the lungs, they do not function as well as our natural airways. Specifically, artificial tracheal airways bypass the normal humidification, filtration, and heating functions of the upper airway. It has been shown that decreased humidity in the inspired air will cause secretions to thicken.[9] Cool air also can decrease ciliary function. These conditions may impair mucociliary clearance and cause retention of secretions. If a patient is intubated to help clear secretions, failure to provide adequate humidification will worsen the problem. In the worst case, thick secretions can plug a tracheal tube and cause asphyxiation.

To deliver humidity, we normally use either a heated humidifier or a large-volume jet nebulizer or heat and moisture exchangers (HME). These devices can provide saturated gas to the airway at temperatures between 32° and 35° C.[55] Ultimately, the selection of a humidification device should be based on patient needs and assessment of the airway, to include the volume and thickness of secretions and the history of mucus plugging or tube occlusions. More details can be found in the AARC Clinical Practice Guideline for humidification during mechanical ventilation, which is included in the chapter on humidity and aerosol therapy.[56]

Minimizing Nosocomial Infections

Patients with tracheal airways are very susceptible to bacterial colonization and infection of the lower respiratory tract. The presence of infection is suggested by changes in the patient's sputum (color, consistency, or amount), breath sounds (wheezes, crackles, or rhonchi), and/or chest radiograph (infiltrates or atelectasis).[57] Additional changes associated with bacterial infection include fever, increased heart rate, and leukocytosis.

As indicated in Box 30-7, there are several reasons why tracheal tubes increase the incidence of pulmonary infection.[57,58] To guard against infection, you should first avoid introducing organisms into the airway. This is done by (1) adhering to sterile technique during suctioning, (2) ensuring that only aseptically clean or sterile respiratory equipment is used for each patient, and (3) consistently washing hands between patient contacts (refer to Chapter 3).[57]

In addition, efforts should be made to prevent retention of secretions. Suctioning, chest physiotherapy, and adequate humidification are useful to this end. Routinely changing the inner cannula on tracheostomy tubes may also help minimize bacterial contamination and infection. Techniques to decrease the consequences of pharyngeal aspiration include (1) use of ulcer medications, such as sucralfate, that maintain normal gastric pH, (2) positioning of patients to decrease reflux, (3) using an oropharyngeal antibiotic paste, and (4) continuous aspiration of subglottic secretions.[57-60]

Facilitating Secretion Clearance

The most common cause of airway obstruction in critically ill patients is retained secretions. To remove retained secretions, blood, or other semiliquid fluids from the large airways, suction the patient as described previously in this chapter. Suctioning involves application of negative pressure to the large airways through a catheter. This method may be used alone or in combination with noninvasive techniques described in Chapter 37.

Providing Cuff Care

Tracheal tube cuffs are used to seal the airway for mechanical ventilation or to prevent or minimize aspira-

Box 30-7 • Why Tracheal Airways Increase the Incidence of Pulmonary Infection

- Bypassed upper airway filtration
- Increased aspiration of pharyngeal material
- Contaminated equipment or solutions
- Impaired mucociliary clearance in trachea
- Increased mucosal damage due to tube or suctioning
- Ineffective clearance via cough

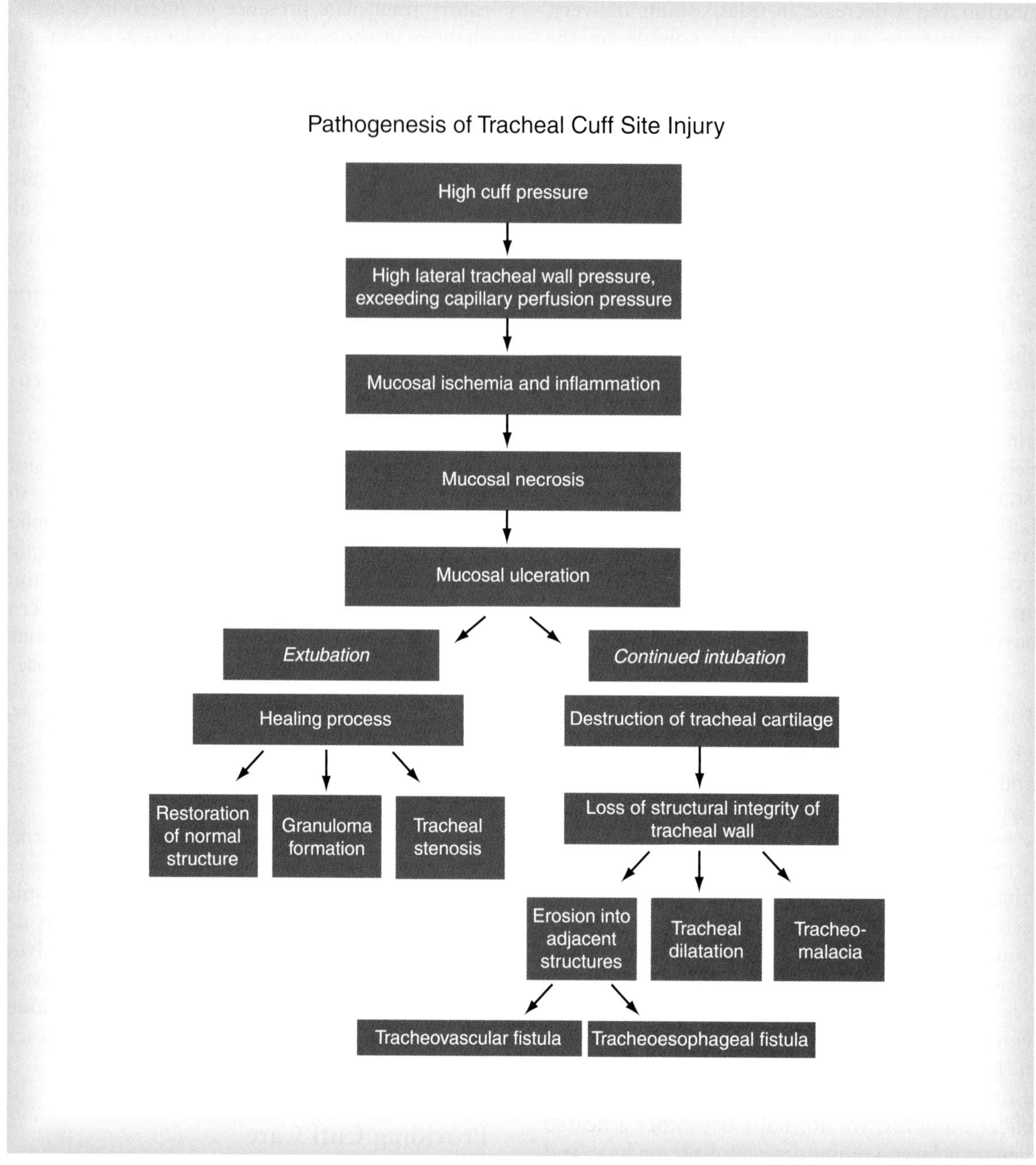

Figure 30-27
Tracheal injury may occur secondary to trauma from the cuff. *(Modified from Stauffer JL: Respir Care 44:828, 1999.)*

tion. As previously mentioned, tracheal stenosis and tracheomalacia are associated with cuff use. The pathogenesis of these problems is related to the amount of cuff pressure transmitted to the tracheal wall. If cuff pressure exceeds the mucosal perfusion pressure, ischemia, ulceration, necrosis, and exposure of the cartilage may result (Figure 30-27).

The Importance of Cuff Pressure

In the past, high-pressure tracheal tube cuffs were a major cause of airway damage. Since the 1970s, high-residual-volume, low-pressure cuffs have become the norm (Figure 30-28). The fully inflated diameter of these cuffs is greater than the diameter of the trachea. This means that the cuff does not have to be fully inflated to seal the airway, and less internal cuff pressure is needed. Thus, when properly used, these cuffs transmit less pressure to the tracheal wall than the old high-pressure designs. Although low-pressure cuffs have lessened the incidence of tracheal damage, they have not eliminated the problem.

A 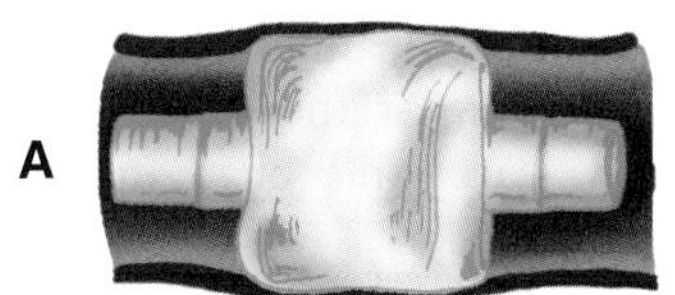

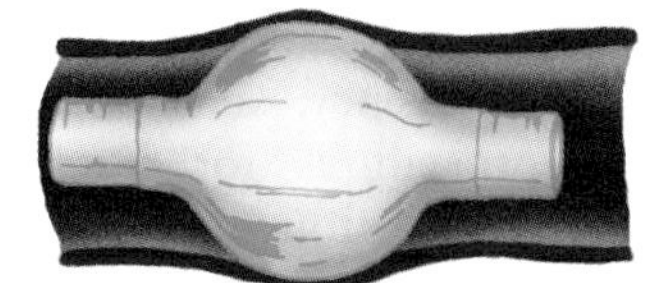 B

Figure 30-28
Comparison of shapes of high-residual-volume, low-pressure cuff, **A,** and low-residual-volume, high-pressure cuff, **B.** *(Modified from McPherson SP: Respiratory therapy equipment, ed 4, St Louis, 1989, Mosby.)*

Measuring and Adjusting Cuff Pressure

A key aspect of airway care is cuff pressure measurement and adjustment. The goal is to keep cuff pressures below the tracheal mucosal capillary perfusion pressure, estimated to range between 20 and 25 mm Hg.[32] Higher pressure will cut off mucosal blood flow and cause tissue damage.

You can measure and adjust cuff pressure with a device designed for this purpose. These devices have the ability to measure the pressure and allow for air to be added or withdrawn from the cuff. There are two key considerations when making these adjustments. First, most manometers are calibrated in cm H_2O and not mm Hg. Thus the "acceptable range" of 20 to 25 mm Hg equates to between 25 and 30 cm H_2O.[41] Second, attaching the measurement system to the pilot tube evacuates some volume from the cuff (and lowers its pressure). For this reason, you should always adjust the pressure to the desired level, never just measure it.

Do not inflate the cuff to the "acceptable range" if the trachea can be sealed with less pressure. Overinflation of a high-volume, low-pressure cuff is equivalent to using a high-pressure cuff.[32,43] This problem is common if the tube chosen is too small for the patient's trachea or positioned too high in the trachea. Another cause of high cuff pressures is high airway pressures generated by mechanical ventilation. Distention of the lumen of the tube occurs when pressure is the highest and will push on the trachea. Over time, this may cause tracheal dilation.

Always use the *lowest* inflation pressure needed to obtain a satisfactory seal with a tracheal tube cuff. Note, however, that the nature of a "satisfactory seal" may vary according to the patient, tube size, and conditions of treatment (e.g., positive-pressure ventilation, enteral feeding, aspiration risk).

Cuff Inflation

Two alternative inflation techniques are commonly used: (1) the minimal occluding volume technique and (2) the minimal leak technique.[4] Both techniques require that adjustments be made during positive-pressure breaths, and both require readjustment as airway pressures change. For patients with cuffed tracheal airways who are not on ventilators, cuff inflation pressures should be adjusted to the lowest pressure needed to prevent aspiration of pharyngeal secretions (see below).

When utilizing the minimal occluding volume technique, slowly inflate the cuff until the airflow heard escaping around the cuff during a positive-pressure breath ceases. Because the airways expand during the application of positive pressure, pressure on the trachea during inspiration is less than during expiration. The amount of ischemia that may result from using this technique depends on both the cuff pressure used and the rate of the positive-pressure breaths.

The minimal leak technique is similar to the minimal occluding volume technique in that air is slowly injected into the cuff until the leak stops. However, once a seal is obtained, you remove a small amount of air, allowing a slight leak at peak inflation pressure. Because this leak occurs during the positive-pressure breath, pharyngeal secretions tend to be blown up at peak inflation, minimizing the likelihood of aspiration.

It is important to realize that achieving a minimal leak in some patients may require cuff pressures exceeding 20 to 25 mm Hg. This is common at high ventilator pressures or if the tube is too small for the patient's airway. For this reason, cuff pressure measurements should still be conducted, regardless of the inflation method used.[4]

Alternative Cuff Designs

Several different types of cuffs have been designed to minimize mucosal trauma.[14] The Lanz tube incorporates an external pressure regulating valve and control reservoir designed to limit the cuff pressure between 16 and 18 mm Hg. The foam cuff is another alternative, which is designed to seal the trachea with atmospheric pressure in the cuff (Figure 30-29). Prior to insertion, the foam cuff must be deflated. Once in position, the pilot tube is opened to the atmosphere, and the foam is allowed to expand against the tracheal wall. Expansion of the cuff stops when the tracheal wall is encountered. If this results in too much air leak and volume loss around the tube, the pilot tube can be placed in line with the endotracheal tube.

Minimizing the Likelihood of Aspiration

When judging the adequacy of a tracheal seal, you must also take into account the potential for aspiration. The use of minimal leak technique and high-volume cuffs does not absolutely prevent aspiration, especially with cuff pressures less than 20 cm H_2O.[59] Also, aspiration is

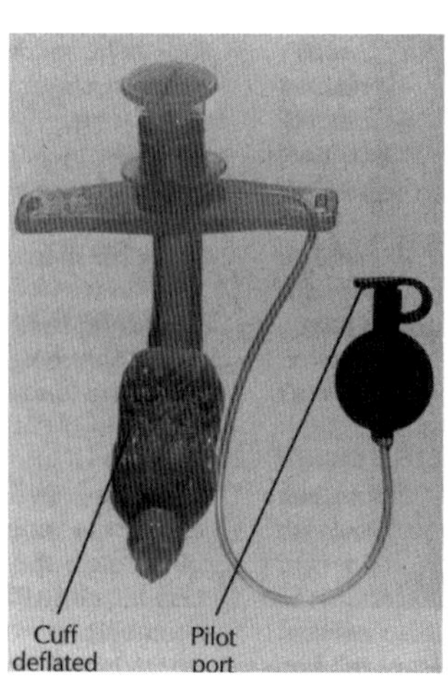

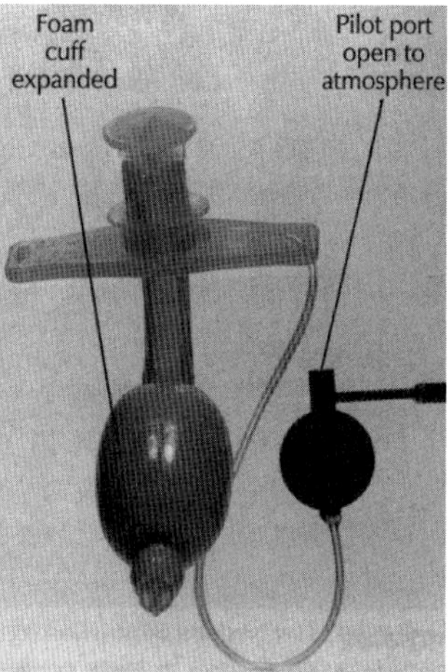

Figure 30-29
Foam cuff is deflated on insertion. The pilot tube is opened after the tube is in place. *(From Eubanks DH, Bones RC: Principles and applications of cardiorespiratory care equipment, St. Louis, 1994, Mosby.)*

reported to be more common in spontaneously breathing patients than in those receiving positive pressure ventilation. This may be due to the movement of pharyngeal secretions around the cuff during the negative-pressure phase of a spontaneous inspiration. Aspiration has also been reported to be more common with tracheostomy tubes than with endotracheal tubes.[51]

The methylene blue test can help determine whether this "leakage" type of aspiration is occurring.[51] To perform this test, add methylene blue to the patient's feedings or have the patient swallow a small amount in water. You then suction the patient's trachea through the artificial airway. If you obtain blue-tinged secretions when performing suctioning, you know that aspiration is occurring.

If leakage aspiration is confirmed, efforts must be made to minimize it. Ideally, the patient should be switched to a system that continually aspirates subglottic secretions. If this is not possible, oropharyngeal suctioning (above the tube cuff) should be performed as needed. To decrease the possibility of aspiration with feedings, the head of the bed should be elevated (where possible). Also, the feeding tube can be inserted into the duodenum, with its position confirmed by radiograph. The use of slightly higher cuff pressure during and after feedings may also minimize aspiration.

Care of the Tracheostomy and Tube

Tracheostomy tubes require daily care to clean the site and change the ties securing the tube. They may also be removed and replaced for routine cleaning or in an emergency, such as an obstruction of the tube. The procedures for tracheostomy care and changing a tracheostomy are describe below.[40]

Tracheostomy Care

Step 1: Assemble and Check Equipment. Box 30-8 lists the equipment needed for routine tracheostomy care. The equipment you will need is for cleaning through the tube, around the tube, and the tube itself. Protective equipment will be needed since the stimulation of the trachea may result in coughing. Suction equipment to clean through the tube prior to the procedure will decrease the possibility of secretion mobilization. Oxygen and a manual resuscitator will be needed for the suctioning procedure and in case any problems such as desaturation occurs. To clean around the tube, you will need peroxide, sterile water, cotton-tipped applicators, tracheostomy sponges, and new ties to secure the tube. A tracheostomy tube kit will include a basin and brushes to clean the inner cannula of the tube. Be sure to check the function of the manual resuscitator, oxygen flow, and suction control before starting.

Step 2: Explain the Procedure to the Patient.

Step 3: Suction the Patient. The procedures previously describe for endotracheal suctioning are appropriate for this situation. Remember, you will not have to insert the catheter very far. This is a short tube.

Step 4: Clean the Inner Cannula. Remove the inner cannula and place in the basin. Insert the disposable inner cannula if the patient requires mechanical ventilation. If not, reapply the oxygen therapy device as necessary. Add sterile water and peroxide to the basin

Box 30-8 • Equipment for Tracheostomy Care

- Gloves and goggles
- Suction equipment
- Resuscitation bag
- Oxygen
- Tracheostomy care kit (basin and brushes)
- Spare inner cannula
- Peroxide/sterile water
- Cotton-tipped applicators
- Precut gauze or 4 x 4 pad
- New tracheostomy tube ties/Velcro strap
- Additional equipment for changing tracheostomy tube
- New tracheostomy tube and component parts
- Water-soluble lubricant
- Syringe

and allow the cannula to soak. Use the brush to remove any dried secretions from the inner lumen or the outside of the cannula. Rinse with sterile water and allow to air dry on sterile gauze.

Step 5: Clean the Stoma Site. Remove the gauze dressing and dispose in a biohazard container. Using the applicators dipped in the peroxide/water solution, clean around the stoma site. Place clean gauze under the flange of the tube. Do not cut gauze for this purpose as fibers may become loose and caught in the stoma. Use either precut gauze or fold two 4 x 4 gauze pads.

Step 6: Change the Ties. Cut the old ties or loosen the Velcro holder. Keep one hand on the flange of the tracheostomy tube to keep it secure. Remove the old ties and discard. Replace the ties and keep one finger's width of space between the neck and ties.

Step 7: Replace the Clean Inner Cannula.

Step 8: Reassess the Patient. Listen to breath sounds and check vital signs and saturations.

Changing a Tracheostomy Tube

A tracheostomy tube may need to be replaced if the current tube becomes plugged or if a different size is needed. A single cannula tube has no inner cannula to remove for cleaning and may be replaced periodically.

Step 1: Assemble and Prepare Equipment. In addition to the equipment described above, you will need the new tube, an extra tube one size smaller, and water-soluable lubricant.

Step 2: Explain the Procedure to the Patient.

Step 3: Prepare the Equipment. Always maintain sterile technique for the distal portion of the cannula, which goes into the trachea. Remove the inner cannula and place on a sterile surface. Insert the obturator. Attach the ties to the flange of the tube. Inflate the cuff, check for leaks, and deflate the cuff. Apply lubricant to the distal portion of the cannula.

Step 4: Prepare the Patient. The patient should be placed with the neck extended so the trachea is accessible. Suction the patient and hyperoxygenate.

Step 5: Remove the Old Tube. Cut the ties or open the Velcro straps. Deflate the cuff. Remove the tube by following the curve of the tube. Grasp the outer portion of the tracheostomy tube with one hand and rotate your wrist toward the chest. Inspect the stoma for any bleeding or other problems.

Step 6: Insert the New Tube. Pick up the new tube by the proximal portion. Do not touch the surface that enters the trachea. Insert the tip of the obturator into the stoma and advance the tube following the curve of the tube. While holding the flange of the tube against the neck, immediately remove the obturator. Assess for airflow through the tube. Coughing may reflect pressure on the outside of the trachea.

Step 7: Secure the Tube. While still holding onto the flange, secure the tracheostomy tube ties and do not over tighten. Insert the inner cannula. Reassess for airflow and reapply the oxygen therapy device or ventilator.

Step 8: Reassess the Patient. Suctioning may be required again. Check vital signs and saturation.

Troubleshooting Airway Emergencies

The areas discussed so far are routine aspects of airway care. Three emergency situations that may occur are tube obstruction, cuff leaks, and accidental extubation. Clinical signs frequently encountered under these circumstances include various degrees of respiratory distress, changes in breath sounds, air movement through the mouth, or if mechanically ventilated, changes in pressures.

Decreased breath sounds are a common finding in airway emergencies. The respiratory therapist must try to identify specific indicators for each of these problems, such as the inability to pass a suction catheter (obstruction), the ability to fully pass a catheter (extubation), or airflow around the tube (leaky cuff). Replacement airways should be kept at the bedside, as well as a manual resuscitator, mask, and gauze pads (for patients with tracheostomies).

Tube Obstruction

Obstruction of the tube is one of the most common causes of airway emergencies. Tube obstruction can be caused by (1) kinking of or biting on the tube, (2) herniation of the cuff over the tube tip,[61] (3) jamming of the tube orifice against the tracheal wall, and (4) mucus plugging (Figure 30-30).

Depending on whether the tube obstruction is partial or complete, different clinical signs will be present.[32] A spontaneously breathing patient with partial airway obstruction will exhibit decreased breath sounds and decreased airflow through the tube. If the patient is receiving volume-controlled ventilation, peak inspiratory pressures will rise, often causing the high pressure alarm to sound; during pressure-controlled ventilation, delivered tidal volumes will fall. With complete tube obstruction, the patient will exhibit severe distress, no breath sounds will be heard, and there will be no gas flow through the tube.

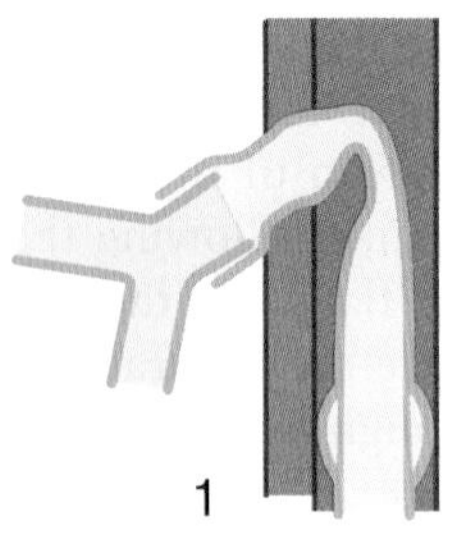

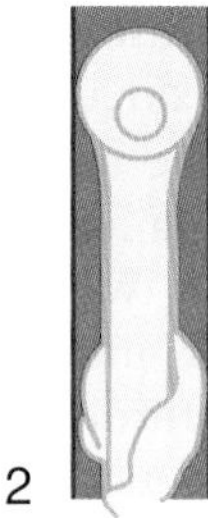

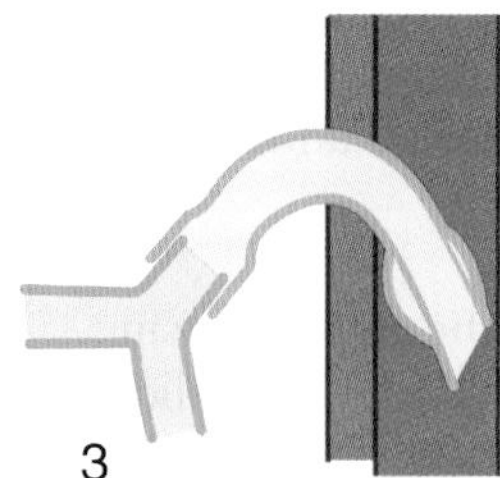

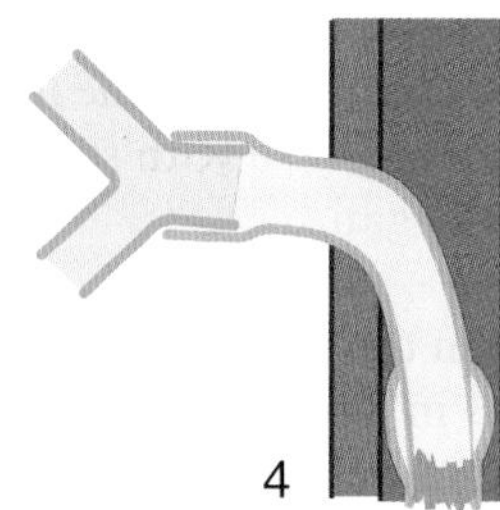

Figure 30-30
Causes of tube obstruction. (See text for details.) *(Modified from Sykes MK, McNichol MW, Campbell EJM: Respiratory failure, Philadelphia, 1969, FA Davis.)*

If the tube is kinked or jammed against the tracheal wall, you can sometimes relieve the obstruction by moving the patient's head and neck.[9, 32] If this does not relieve the obstruction, a herniated cuff may be blocking the airway, and you should deflate the tube cuff. If these steps fail to overcome the obstruction, you should try to pass a suction catheter through the tube.[9] How far you can insert the catheter helps determine the site of obstruction. If you cannot insert the catheter much beyond the tube tip and insertion does not cause coughing, the likely problem is a herniated cuff or a mucus plug. In the case of mucus plugging, you should attempt to suction the plug before considering more drastic action.

When the patient has a tracheostomy tube with an inner cannula, you should remove the inner cannula and check to see if the plug is lodged in the tube. You can provide oxygen to the patient through the outer cannula, or you can replace the inner cannula with a spare one to facilitate manual ventilation.

If you cannot clear the obstruction by using the above techniques, you must remove the airway and replace it. In patients having undergone recent tracheotomy (4 or 5 days previously), the stoma may not be well established and may close when you remove the tube. If suture ties were left in place by the surgeon, you can use these to pull open the stoma.

Once you remove an obstructed airway, you must immediately try to restore adequate ventilation and oxygenation. For a patient with a tracheotomy stoma, this may require sealing the wound with a gauze pad such as that used to temporarily close chest wounds in the field. Only after you restore adequate ventilation and oxygenation should airway reinsertion be undertaken.

Cuff Leaks

A leak in the cuff, pilot tube, or one-way valve is a problem mostly for patients receiving mechanical ventilation. This will cause a system leak, with a resultant loss of delivered volume and/or decreased inspiratory pressure.

You can detect a small cuff leak by noting decreasing cuff pressures over time. A large leak, such as occurs with a blown cuff, has a more rapid onset. Breath sounds will be decreased, but the spontaneously breathing patient will have air movement through the tube. With

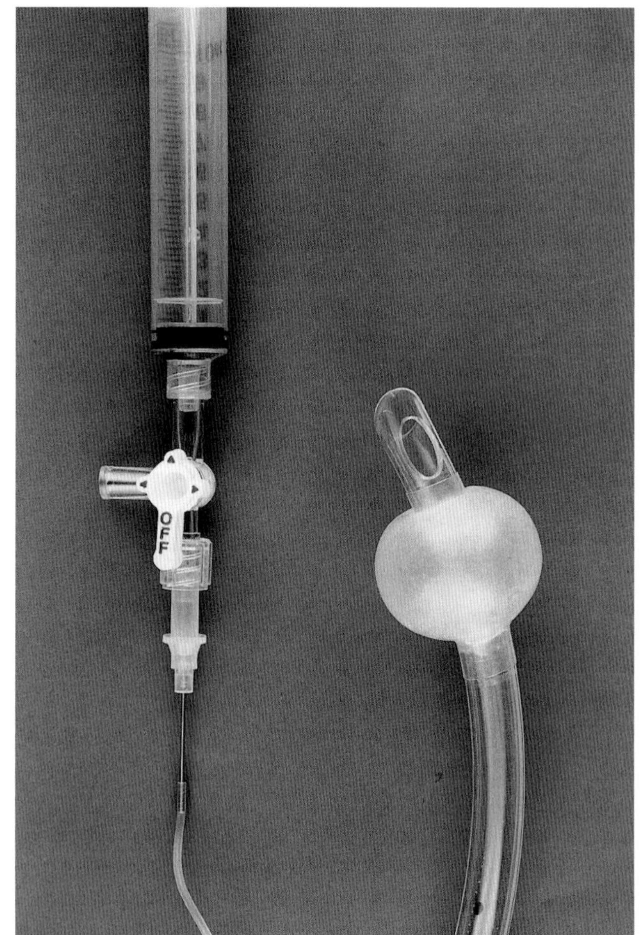

Figure 30-31
The pilot valve may be removed and a blunt needle and stopcock may be placed in the pilot tube. *(From Cairo JM, Pilbeam SP: Mosby's respiratory care equipment, ed 6, St Louis, 1999, Mosby.)*

positive-pressure breaths, you will often be able to feel airflow at the mouth. Under such circumstances, you should try to reinflate the cuff, while checking the pilot tube and valve for leaks.[4]

Leaks at the valve or in the pilot tube can be bypassed by placing a needle and stopcock in the pilot tube distal to the leak (Figure 30-31).[62] Using this method, you can reinflate the cuff and avoid emergency reintubation. A ruptured cuff requires extubation and reintubation.

Similar findings can occur when an endotracheal tube is positioned too high in the trachea, either near the glottic opening or in the esophagus.[20] Before presuming a cuff leak, attempt to advance the tube slightly and reassess the leak and equality of breath sounds in both lung fields.

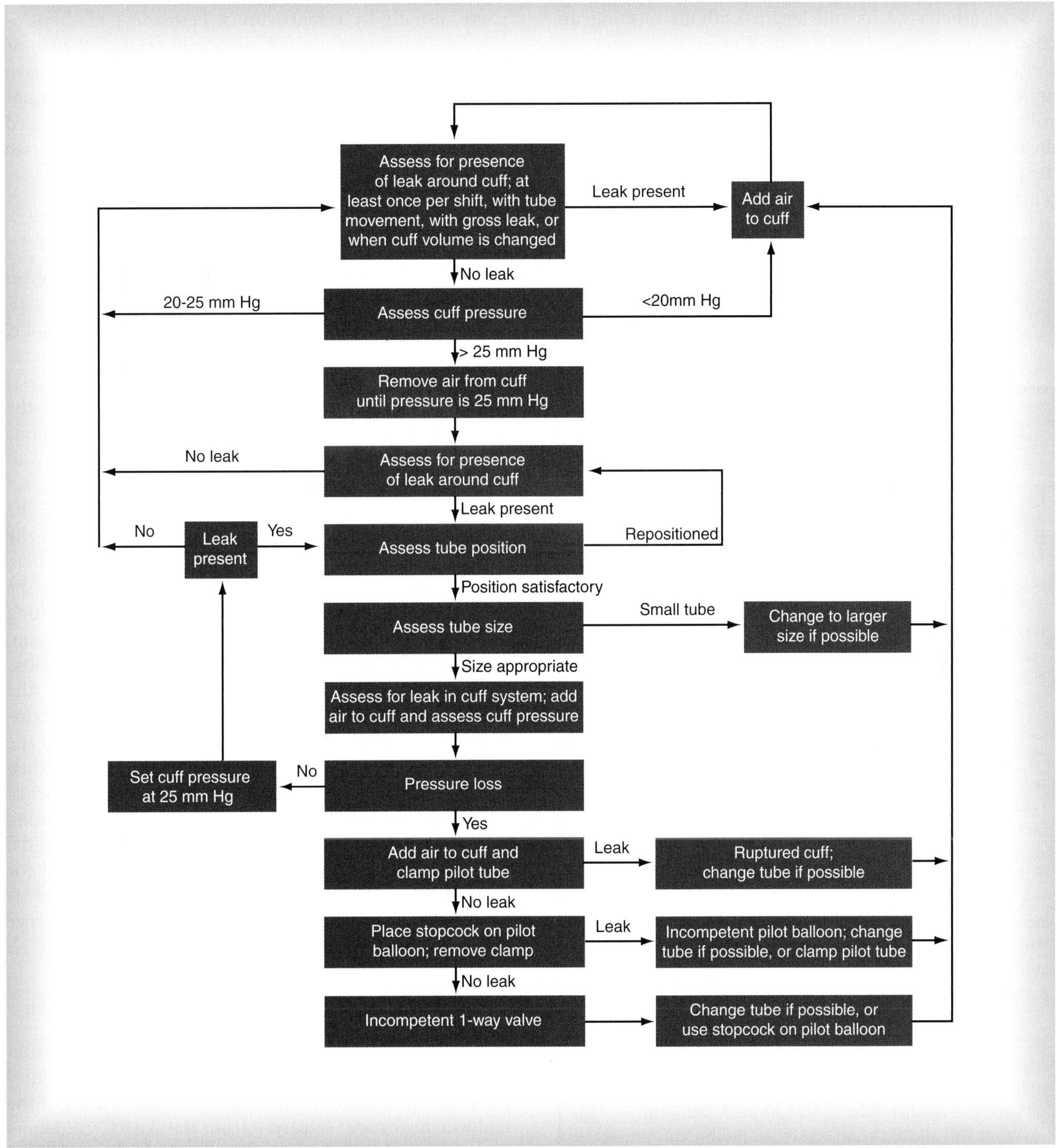

Figure 30-32
Algorithm for solving leaking cuff problems. *(From Hess D, Respir Care 44: 759, 1999.)*

A leak around a tracheal tube can occur from a tube or cuff problem. Figure 30-32 is a diagram of the process to investigate the source of a leak around a tube.[4]

Accidental Extubation

You can detect partial displacement of an airway out of the trachea by noting decreased breath sounds, decreased airflow through the tube, and the ability to pass a catheter to its full length without meeting an obstruction or eliciting a cough. With positive pressure ventilation, you may hear airflow through the mouth or into the stomach and note a decrease in delivered volumes or pressures. In these cases, completely remove the tube and provide ventilatory support as needed until the patient can be reintubated or the tracheostomy tube reinserted.

MINI CLINI

Airway/Cuff Problems

PROBLEM

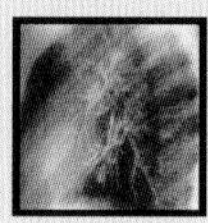

You are called for assistance on a 220-pound, 6′2″ male patient who is intubated with a 7.0-mm endotracheal tube and receiving positive pressure ventilation. The patient's nurse reports to you that over the last week it has been increasingly difficult to get a good seal with the tube cuff and that she has had to use "more and more air" to prevent gross leakage. When asked if she has been monitoring cuff pressures, she says "no." What are the likely problem and solution?

DISCUSSION

"Low-pressure" cuffs can exert high pressure at high inflation volumes. The need for high volumes to get a good seal usually indicates that the endotracheal or tracheostomy tube is too small for the patient. This large adult male should probably have been intubated with at least a 9.9 mm tube. In addition, because cuff pressures were not monitored, it is possible that tracheal damage has already occurred. The fact that the nurse reports having to use "more and more air" to get a seal suggests tracheomalacia, which could be confirmed by radiographic or bronchoscopic examination.

Tracheomalacia can cause a vicious cycle in which high pressure causes more tracheal dilation, which requires higher pressures to seal the cuff, and so on. If tracheomalacia is confirmed and the patient still needs an artificial airway, the smaller tube should be replaced with a larger one that will allow a good seal at acceptable cuff pressures. It may also be necessary to reposition the tube so that the cuff is not proximal to the original site of damage.

▶ EXTUBATION/DECANNULATION

For most patients, tracheal intubation is a temporary measure. Once the artificial airway is no longer needed, it should be removed. The process of removing an artificial tracheal airway is called *extubation.* Although most patients eventually undergo extubation, a small number will need to maintain a permanent artificial route, usually by tracheostomy. Permanent tracheostomies are common among surgically treated throat or laryngeal cancer patients and those requiring long-term positive pressure ventilation. Recent advances in noninvasive mechanical ventilation have lessened the need for permanent tracheostomies in the latter group (see Chapter 42).

Assessing Patient Readiness for Extubation

A patient is ready to extubate when the original need for the artificial airway no longer exists. Given that artificial airways are inserted for many different reasons, several different criteria to establish readiness for extubation need to be considered.[62] Some of the basic assessments include the ability to protect the airway by the presence of a gag reflex, the ability to manage secretions based on cough strength, the quantity and thickness of secretions, and the patency of the upper airway.

The decision to remove the airway may not be the same as the decision to remove the ventilator.[62] In the case of patients intubated for surgery and immediate postoperative care, the ventilator and airway may be removed simultaneously. However, if a patient's lung disease has improved, but the airway problems remain, the ventilator may be removed but the airway remains.

The cuff-leak test is designed to help predict the occurrence of glottic edema and/or stridor after extubation.[64] There are two ways to perform the test. In the first method, you totally deflate the tube cuff and then completely occlude the endotracheal tube. The presence of a peritubular leak during spontaneous breathing indicates no encroachment of airway (a positive test). A negative test (no leak) indicates a high potential for postextubation obstruction. The second method is similar, but the leak is assessed during positive pressure ventilation.

Clinical Practice Guideline

To guide practitioners in safe and effective application of this procedure, the AARC has developed and published a clinical practice guideline on removal of the endotracheal tube. Excerpts from the AARC guideline, including indications, contraindications, hazards and complications, assessment of need, assessment of outcome, and monitoring, appear on p. 689.[64]

Removal of the Endotracheal Tube

AARC Clinical Practice Guideline (Excerpts)*

➤ INDICATIONS

- When the airway control afforded by the endotracheal tube is no longer necessary.
- Patient should be capable of maintaining a patent airway and adequate spontaneous ventilation and should not require high levels of positive airway pressure.
- The endotracheal tube should be removed if acute severe obstruction of the tube is present and it cannot be cleared rapidly.
- The endotracheal tube should be removed in an environment in which the patient can be monitored and in which the equipment and personnel trained in airway management are immediately available.

➤ CONTRAINDICATIONS

There are no absolute contraindications to extubation.

➤ HAZARDS/COMPLICATIONS

- Hypoxemia
- Hypercapnia

➤ ASSESSMENT OF NEED

Patients receiving an artificial airway to facilitate treatment of respiratory failure should be considered for extubation when they have met traditional weaning criteria. Examples of weaning criteria include:

- The capacity to maintain adequate arterial oxygenation on inspired oxygen fractions provided with simple oxygen devices and with low levels of positive airway pressure
- The capacity to maintain appropriate pH and pCO_2 during spontaneous ventilation
- Adequate respiratory muscle strength
- Maximum negative inspiratory pressure >30 cm H_2O
- Vital capacity >10 mL/kg ideal body weight
- Pressure measured across the diaphragm during spontaneous ventilation less than 15% of maximum
- In adults, respiratory rate <35/min during spontaneous breathing
- In adults, a rapid shallow breathing index of <98-130
- Thoracic compliance >25 mL/cm
- Work of breathing <0.8 J/L
- Oxygen cost of breathing <15% total
- Dead space-to-tidal-volume ratio <0.6
- Absolute tracheal pressure in the first 0.1 second of occlusion <6 cm H_2O
- Maximum voluntary ventilation > twice the resting minute ventilation
- In addition to treatment of respiratory failure, artificial airways are sometimes placed for airway protection. Resolution of the need for airway protection may be assessed by but is not limited to:
- Normal consciousness
- Adequate airway protective reflexes
- Easily managed secretions

➤ ASSESSMENT OF OUTCOME

Clinical outcome may be assessed by physical examination, measurements of gas exchange, and chest radiography.

*For complete guidelines see Respir Care 44:749, 1995.

Procedures

Because respiratory therapists play a key role in extubation and the techniques differ somewhat, we will review the procedures for removing orotracheal or nasotracheal and tracheostomy tubes separately.

Orotracheal or Nasotracheal Tubes

The following procedure is recommended for orotracheal or nasotracheal extubation.[9,32]

Step 1: Assemble Needed Equipment. Needed equipment includes suctioning apparatus, two suction kits, oxygen and aerosol therapy equipment, manual resuscitator and mask, aerosol nebulizer with racemic epinephrine and normal saline (if ordered), and an intubation tray.

Step 2: Suction the Endotracheal Tube and Pharynx to Above the Cuff. Suctioning prior to extubation helps prevent aspiration of secretions after cuff deflation. After use, dispose of the first suction kit and prepare another for use, or prepare a rigid tonsillar (Yankauer) suction tip. Because patients will often cough after the tube is pulled, you may need to help them clear secretions.

Step 3: Oxygenate the Patient Well After Suctioning. Extubation is a stressful procedure that can cause hypoxemia and unwanted cardiovascular side effects. Give 100% oxygen for 1 to 2 minutes to help avoid these problems.

Step 4: Deflate the Cuff. Slowly remove all the air possible. Some practitioners then cut the valve off the pilot tube to ensure that any remaining air is easily displaced during removal.

Step 5: Remove the Tube. The technique used to remove the tube should help avoid aspiration of pharyngeal secretions and maximally abduct the vocal cords. Clinicians use one of two different techniques to accomplish these goals. In the first method, you give a large breath with the manual resuscitator and remove the tube at peak inspiration (when the vocal cords are maximally abducted).[34] In the second method, you have the patient cough, then pull the tube during the expulsive expiratory phase. This also results in maximal abduction of the vocal cords.

Step 6: Apply Appropriate Oxygen and Humidity Therapy. Patients who have been receiving mechanical ventilation may still require some oxygen therapy, usually at a higher F_{IO_2}. Other patients may require some oxygen, since this is a stressful procedure. If humidity therapy is indicated, most clinicians suggest a cool mist after extubation. A heated mist may only increase the swelling that normally occurs after extubation, thereby worsening airway obstruction.

Step 7: Assess/Reassess the Patient. After extubation, check for good air movement by auscultation. Stridor or decreased air movement after extubation indicates upper airway problems. Next assess the patient's respiratory rate, heart rate, color, and blood pressure. Mild hypertension and tachycardia immediately after extubation are common and resolve spontaneously in most cases. Also, watch for nosebleeding following nasotracheal extubation. Encourage the patient to cough, with assistance as needed. Because laryngeal edema may worsen with time and stridor may develop, be sure that racemic epinephrine is available. Sample and analyze ABG values as needed.

The most common problems that occur after extubation are hoarseness, sore throat, and cough.[41] These are benign and will improve with time. A rare, but serious, complication associated with extubation is laryngospasm. Postextubation laryngospasm is usually a transient event, lasting a matter of seconds. Should this occur, oxygenation can be maintained with a high F_{IO_2} and the application of positive pressure. If laryngospasm persists, a neuromuscular blocking agent may have to be given, which will necessitate manual ventilation or reintubation.

Since the vocal cords have had limited function during the intubation period, they may not fully close as needed once the airway has been removed. To avoid aspiration, oral feedings, especially liquids, should be withheld for 24 hours after extubation. Patients may aspirate liquids even with an intact gag reflex.[51]

Extubation failure, defined as reinsertion of the airway, due to airway problems often occurs within eight hours of extubation. Aspiration and edema are the most common problems. If the patient was also mechanically ventilated, reintubation may be required for work of breathing issues unrelated to the airway. [62]

MINI CLINI

Extubation Assessment

PROBLEM

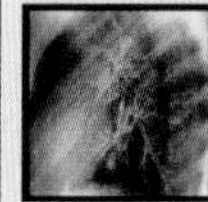

A physician indicates to you that a patient recently removed from a ventilator is maintaining adequate oxygenation and ventilation via spontaneous breathing through an oral endotracheal tube. She requests that you evaluate the patient for extubation. What would you assess and why?

DISCUSSION

Since the patient is maintaining adequate oxygenation and ventilation off the ventilator, two key criteria for extubation have already been met. Further assessment is needed to determine (1) the risk for upper airway obstruction after extubation, (2) the level of protection against aspiration, and (3) the ability of the patient to clear secretions, once extubated. First, you should perform a leak test to assess for upper airway edema. Second, you should determine the patient's level of consciousness and neuromuscular function by assessing the gag reflex or having the patient try to raise and hold his head off the bed. Last, you should determine the patient's ability to cough, using either subjective assessment (on suctioning) or measurement of maximum expiratory pressure or peak cough flow. Only if all three areas yield positive results should you recommend extubation.

Tracheostomy Tube Removal

There are several approaches to removing tracheostomy tubes.[66] Since patients with tracheostomies often have problems with aspiration or secretions, a weaning process is used rather than abrupt removal of the tube. Weaning is accomplished by using either fenestrated tubes, progressively smaller tubes, or tracheostomy buttons.

Prior to decannulation, a comprehensive patient assessment is required. The patient should have sufficient muscle strength to generate an effective cough. Ideally, there should be no active pulmonary infection and the volume and thickness of secretions should be acceptable. Patency of the upper airway should be assessed via bronchoscopy. Since dead space will be increased when the tube is removed, adequate nutrition and muscle strength must be present.[66] After removal of the tube, the stoma will close on its own in a matter of days. The particular decannulation technique used will depend on the patient's needs and the experience and preferences of the attending physician.

Fenestrated Tracheostomy Tubes

A fenestrated tracheotomy tube is a double cannulated tube that has an opening in the posterior wall of the outer cannula above the cuff (Figure 30-33). Removal of the inner cannula opens the fenestration. Plugging of the proximal opening of the tube's outer cannula, accompanied by deflation of the cuff, allows for assessment of upper airway function. Removal of the plug allows access for suctioning. If the need for mechanical ventilation occurs, the inner cannula can be reinserted.

One problem associated with this type of tracheostomy tube is malposition of the fenestration, such as between the skin and stoma, or against the posterior wall of the larynx.[67] Customizing the fenestration can help avoid this problem.[68] Proper placement can be confirmed by using fiberoptic bronchoscopy.

Case reports have demonstrated granular tissue formation in some patients using a fenestrated tracheostomy tube. This tends to occur on the anterior tracheal wall, above the tube fenestration. This granular tissue may occlude the fenestration, cause bleeding (especially with tube changes), or result in airway obstruction upon decannulation. Given the location of this granular tissue, these problems may be due to poor positioning of the fenestration within the airway.

Progressively Smaller Tubes

A second airway weaning technique is to use smaller and smaller tracheostomy tubes. As with fenestrated tubes, this approach maintains the airway, but allows for increasing use of the upper airway. This technique is also indicated in patients whose airway is too small for the fenestrated tubes that are currently available. The use of progressively smaller tubes may also allow for better healing of the stoma.

The problem with these techniques is the continued presence of a tube within the lumen of the airway.[66] The presence of the tube (cuffed or uncuffed) increases airway resistance. In patients with preexisting obstructive disorders, this added airway resistance may be too much to bear, resulting in failed decannulation. These tubes can also impair coughing by preventing full compression of the inspired thoracic volume.

Tracheal Buttons

The tracheal button also may be used to maintain a tracheal stoma.[65] Unlike the fenestrated tube, the

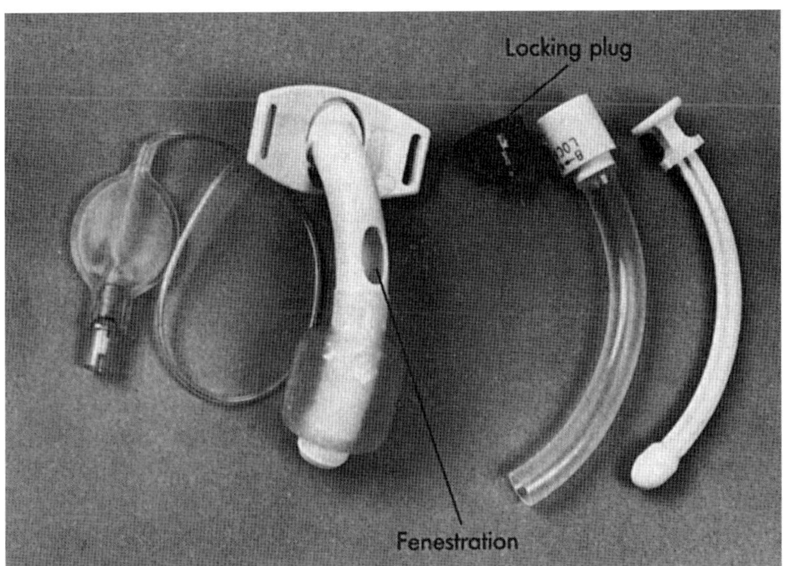

Figure 30-33
Fenestrated tracheostomy tube.

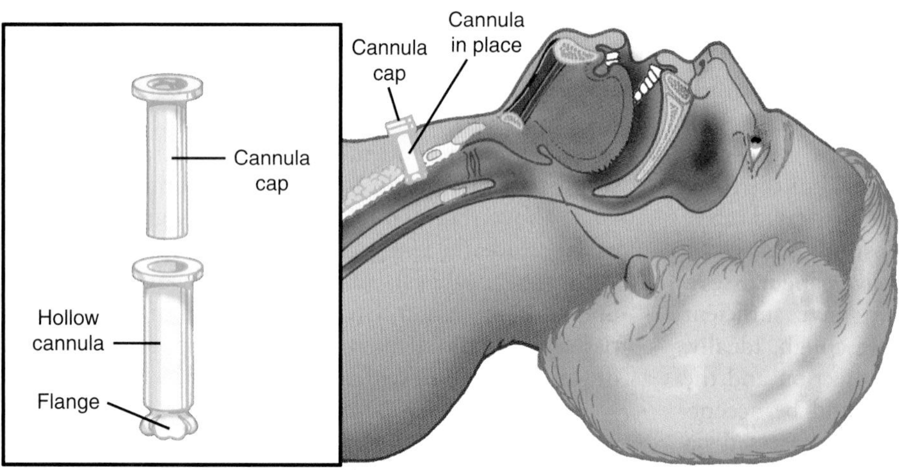

Figure 30-34
Tracheostomy button.

tracheal button fits from the skin just inside the anterior wall of the trachea (Figure 30-34). This avoids the problem of added resistance. Since the tracheal button has no cuff, its use is limited to relieving airway obstruction and aiding the removal of secretions. Adapters can be used that allow suctioning through the button. An optional one-way valve on the external end of the button allows for inspiration with less dead space and expiration with speech.

After tracheostomy decannulation, the patient should be assessed for vocal cord responses.[66] The problems seen with vocal cords may be related to laryngeal injury during intubation. Alternatively, decreased vocal cord responsiveness may occur as a result of the loss of laryngeal stimulation when the upper airway was bypassed. Vocal cord abnormalities can result in either aspiration or acute airway obstruction. A replacement tracheostomy tube and suctioning equipment should be available. If no complications develop, the stoma will close spontaneously over a few days. Surgery may be needed if there is any infection at the stoma site.

▶ ALTERNATIVE AIRWAY DEVICES

Placement of an endotracheal tube is a complex skill and is not always accomplished easily, even in experienced hands. Emergency medical service personnel are not always in the best situation to intubate. A patient's particular anatomy may make intubation difficult. Several alternative devices and techniques can be used in such circumstances. The American Society of Anesthesiology has an algorithm for difficult intubations, which provides extensive options.[69] Two devices, the laryngeal mask airway and the Combitube or double lumen airway, are referred to as nonintermediate airways. You can ventilate with them, but an endotracheal tube or tracheostomy tube will be needed eventually.[20] These two devices may be inserted by respiratory care practitioners and will be discussed below. The advantages and disadvantages of each device are described in Table 30-5.

Laryngeal Mask Airway

The algorithm for the management of a difficult airway has been modified to show the various uses of the laryngeal mask airway (LMA). The LMA consists of a short tube and a small mask that is inserted deep into the oropharynx[33, 70] (Figure 30-35). The open surface of the mask faces the laryngeal opening and the tip of the mask is just above the esophageal sphincter. The short tube has a 15-mm adapter that can be connected to a manual resuscitator bag. A small tube is used to inflate a cuff once the device is in place.

When compared to bag and mask ventilation, a greater amount of ventilation is directed to the lungs by the LMA. The ease and speed of insertion offer an advantage over intubation when the intubator is inexperienced, the patient cannot be positioned for intubation, or when the intubation is difficult.

The insertion of the LMA does not require any equipment[70] (Figure 30-36). The posterior surface of the mask must be lubricated and the cuff fully deflated prior to insertion. The index finger is used to guide insertion of the mask along the palate and down into the oropharynx. Once in place, the cuff is inflated to maximum of 60 cm H_2O. This causes the mask to rise slightly out of the mouth.

There are two major limitations to its use.[70] First, it cannot be used in the conscious or semicomatose patient due to stimulation of the gag reflex. Second, if ventilating pressures greater than 20 cm H_2O are needed, gastric distention may occur. It is important to remember this device does not protect against aspiration should regurgitation occur.

The classic LMA can be used to facilitate intubation since the opening faces the glottis. However, due to the

Table 30-5 ▶ ▶ Advantages and Disadvantages of Alternatives to Endotracheal Intubation for Maintaining Upper Airway Patency

	Advantages	Disadvantages
Oral and nasal airways	Little training required No special equipment necessary Inexpensive Can be quickly placed	Does not guarantee airway patency May worsen obstruction Poorly tolerated by awake patient Does not prevent aspiration Short-term use Does not facilitate positive pressure ventilation
Combitube placement	Less skill than bag-valve-mask or intubation No special equipment necessary Protection against aspiration Facilitates positive pressure ventilation	Difficulty distinguishing tracheal versus esophageal Short-term use Aspiration during removal Cannot suction in esophageal position Only one size (adult) Potential for esophageal injury
Laryngeal mask airway	Easy to insert No special equipment necessary Can intubate without removing laryngeal mask airway Avoids laryngeal and tracheal trauma	Short-term use Aspiration not absolutely avoided Cannot provide high ventilation pressures if needed

small size of the ventilating tube on the mask, a small endotracheal tube will be needed. A specially designed LMA with a small handle has been designed to facilitate intubation (Figure 30-37).

Double Lumen Airway

The double lumen airway (Combitube) is designed to be inserted blindly through the oropharynx and into the trachea or the esophagus[70] (Figure 30-38). Its external design is similar to the double lumen endotracheal tube with two external openings, two 15-mm adapters, two lumens, and two cuffs. One cuff seals the oropharynx. The second seals the trachea or the esophagus.

If the tube is placed into the esophagus and the cuffs are inflated, ventilation is accomplished by air passing through a series of holes in the area of the hypopharnyx and into the trachea. The pharyngeal cuff prevents air from leaving through the mouth. The distal cuff in the esophagus helps to decrease reguritation. If the tube is placed in the trachea, it will function like an endotracheal tube. To assess placement, manually ventilate through the external adapters and determine which gives you the best breath sounds.

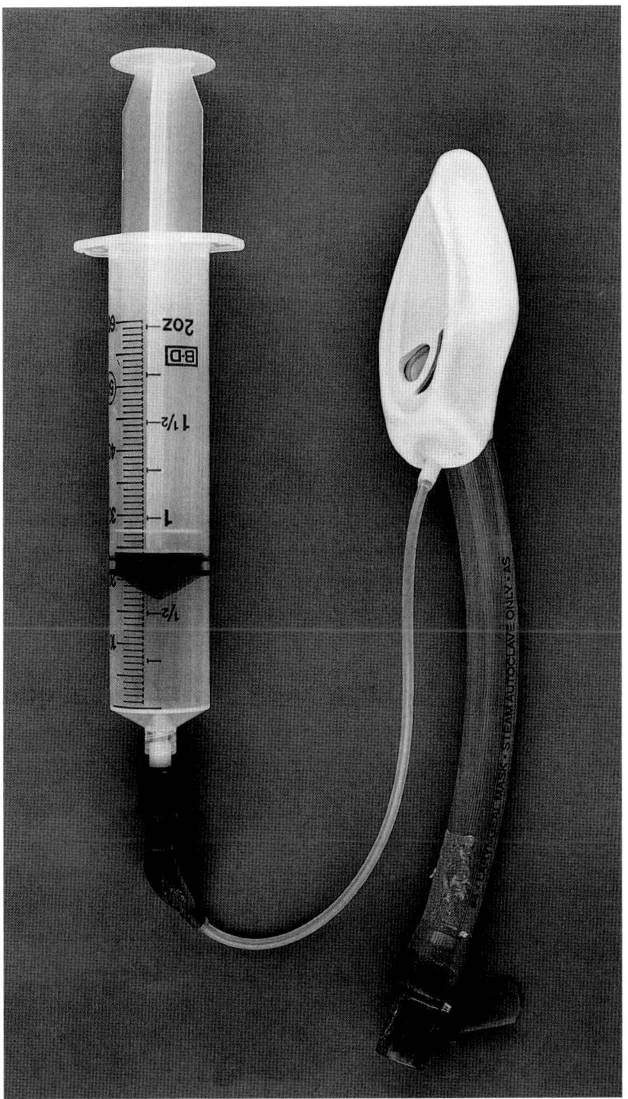

Figure 30-35
Laryngeal mask airway. *(From Cairo JM, Pilbeam SP: Mosby's respiratory care equipment, ed 6, St Louis, 1999, Mosby.)*

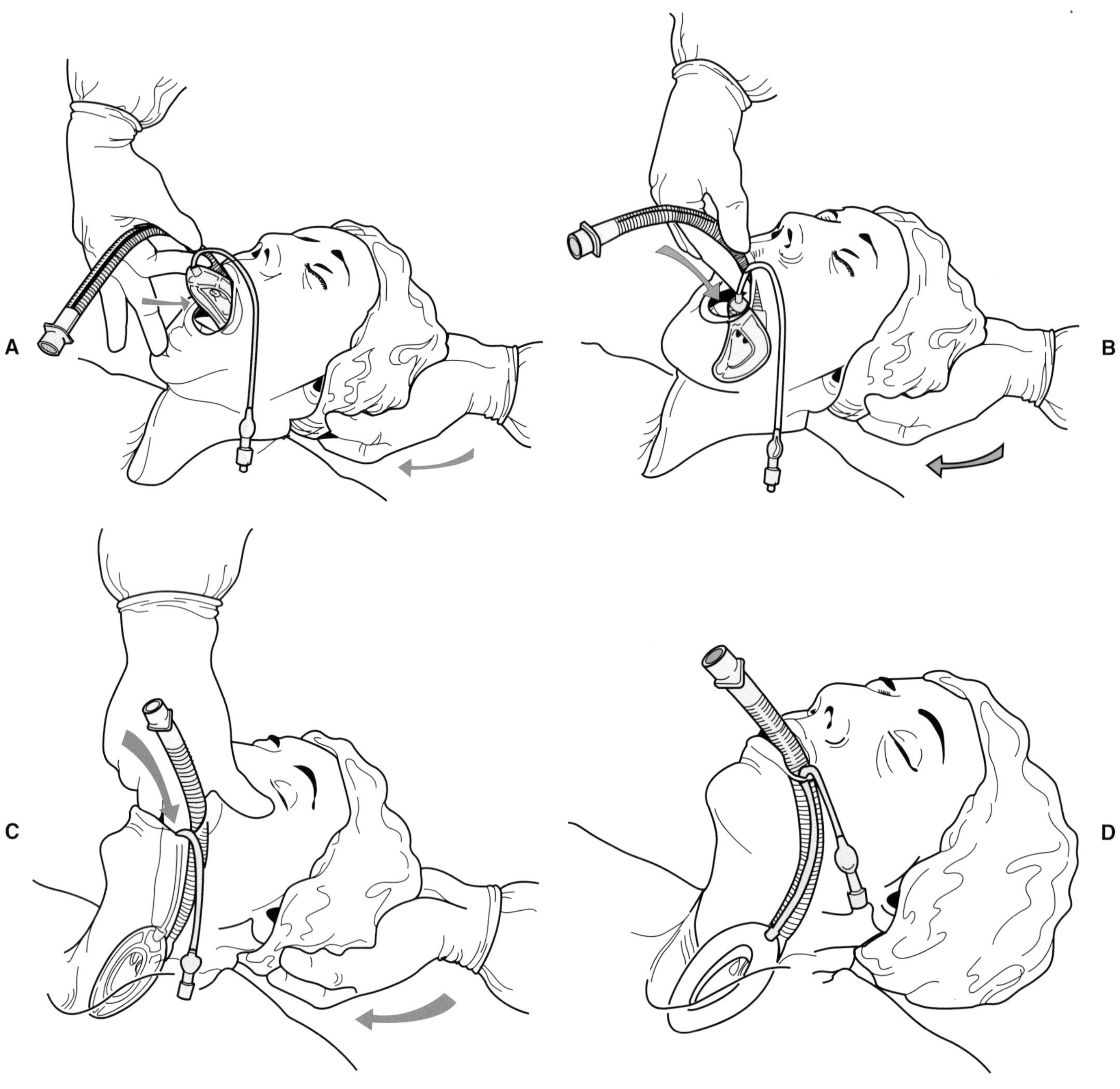

Figure 30-36
Insertion of laryngeal mask airway. *(Modified from Cairo JM, Pilbeam SP: Mosby's respiratory care equipment, 6 ed, St. Louis, 1999, Mosby.)*

Surgical Emergency Airways

In spite of the various alternatives to establish ventilation, occasionally the problem of "cannot intubate/cannot ventilate" occurs.[33] In these situations a surgical transtracheal airway must be established. Cricothyroidotomy and percutaneous transtracheal ventilation are options. Commercial kits are available or a series of available supplies can be used[20] (Figures 30-39 and 30-40).

Complications include bleeding, subcutaneous emphysema secondary to inspiratory airway resistance through a small lumen, and air trapping secondary to expiratory flow resistance. Nevertheless, cricothyroidotomy and percutaneous transtracheal ventilation are the preferred routes over emergent tracheotomy until a more definitive airway can be placed once the emergency has passed.

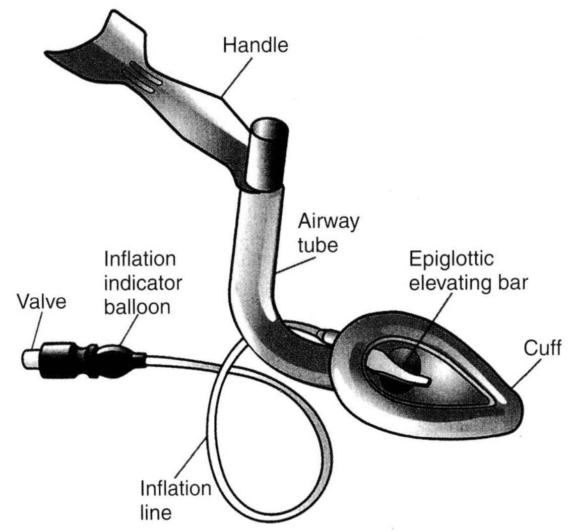

Figure 30-37
Intubating laryngeal mask airway. *(Courtesy of LMA North America, San Diego, California.)*

▶ BRONCHOSCOPY

Bronchoscopy is the general term used to describe the insertion of a visualization instrument (endoscope) into the bronchi. The purposes of bronchoscopy are to inspect the airway, remove objects from the airway, collect samples from the airway, and place devices into the airway. [31]

There are two different bronchoscopic techniques in current use: rigid tube bronchoscopy and flexible bronchoscopy. Although respiratory therapists most often assist in flexible fiberoptic bronchoscopy, they should understand the differences between these two approaches.

Rigid Tube Bronchoscopy

The rigid bronchoscope is an open metal tube with a distal light source and a port for attaching oxygen or ventilating equipment. The rigid bronchoscope is used most often by otorhinolaryngologists or thoracic surgeons. The tube is passed through the mouth, down into the trachea, and as far as the bronchi. A telescoping tube with mirrors is used to advance to and view segmental bronchi. Suctioning is via a metal tube passed through the bronchoscope. The large internal diameter of this suction tube allows for aspiration of thick inspissated secretions and large mucus plugs. Grasping forceps passed through the device allow removal of foreign bodies and biopsies of airway tumors.

Rigid bronchoscopy has several disadvantages. First, it is very uncomfortable for conscious patients. Moreover, it usually requires the assistance of an anesthesiologist and the use of an operating room. Last, and most important, rigid bronchoscopy cannot access the smaller airways.

Flexible Fiberoptic Bronchoscopy

In contrast, flexible fiberoptic bronchoscopy has gained popularity over the years as a result of both its versatility and ability to access very small airways.

The typical fiberoptic bronchoscope has a light transmission channel, a visualizing channel, and a multipurpose open channel (Figure 30-41). The open channel can be used for aspiration, tissue sampling, or oxygen administration. After insertion, the physician can direct the tip of the scope via the control section to the location desired. This type of bronchoscope is most often used by the pulmonologist, often with the assistance of a respiratory therapist.[71]

To guide practitioners in assisting physicians performing this procedure, the AARC has developed and published a clinical practice guideline on fiberoptic bronchoscopy assisting. Excerpts from the AARC guideline, including indications, contraindications, precautions and/or possible complications, assessment of need, assessment of outcome, and monitoring, appear on p. 698.[72]

Fiberoptic Bronchoscopy Procedure[73,74]

Key points to consider in planning and conducting fiberoptic bronchoscopy include premedication, equipment preparation, airway preparation, and monitoring. Also, to reduce the risk of aspiration due to gagging and loss of airway reflexes, the patient should refrain from food or drink for at least 8 hours prior to the start of the procedure. In addition, if the intravenous route is not already available, vascular access should be obtained prior to the start of the procedure.

Premedication

Bronchoscopy is an uncomfortable procedure. To decrease anxiety, the patient should be premedicated 1 to 2 hours in advance. The patient should be calm but alert enough to follow commands, such as taking a deep breath. Tranquilizers, such as the benzodiazepines (Valium, Versed), are frequently used for this purpose.

Another goal of premedication is to dry the patient's airway. This promotes anesthetic deposition, aids visibility, and can reduce procedure time. Atropine, given 1 to 2 hours prior to the procedure, is used for this purpose. Atropine may also help decrease vagal responses (such as bradycardia and hypotension) that can occur during bronchoscopy.

Narcotic analgesics such as morphine or fentanyl may also be given. In addition to reducing pain, these agents help diminish laryngeal reflexes. However, narcotics

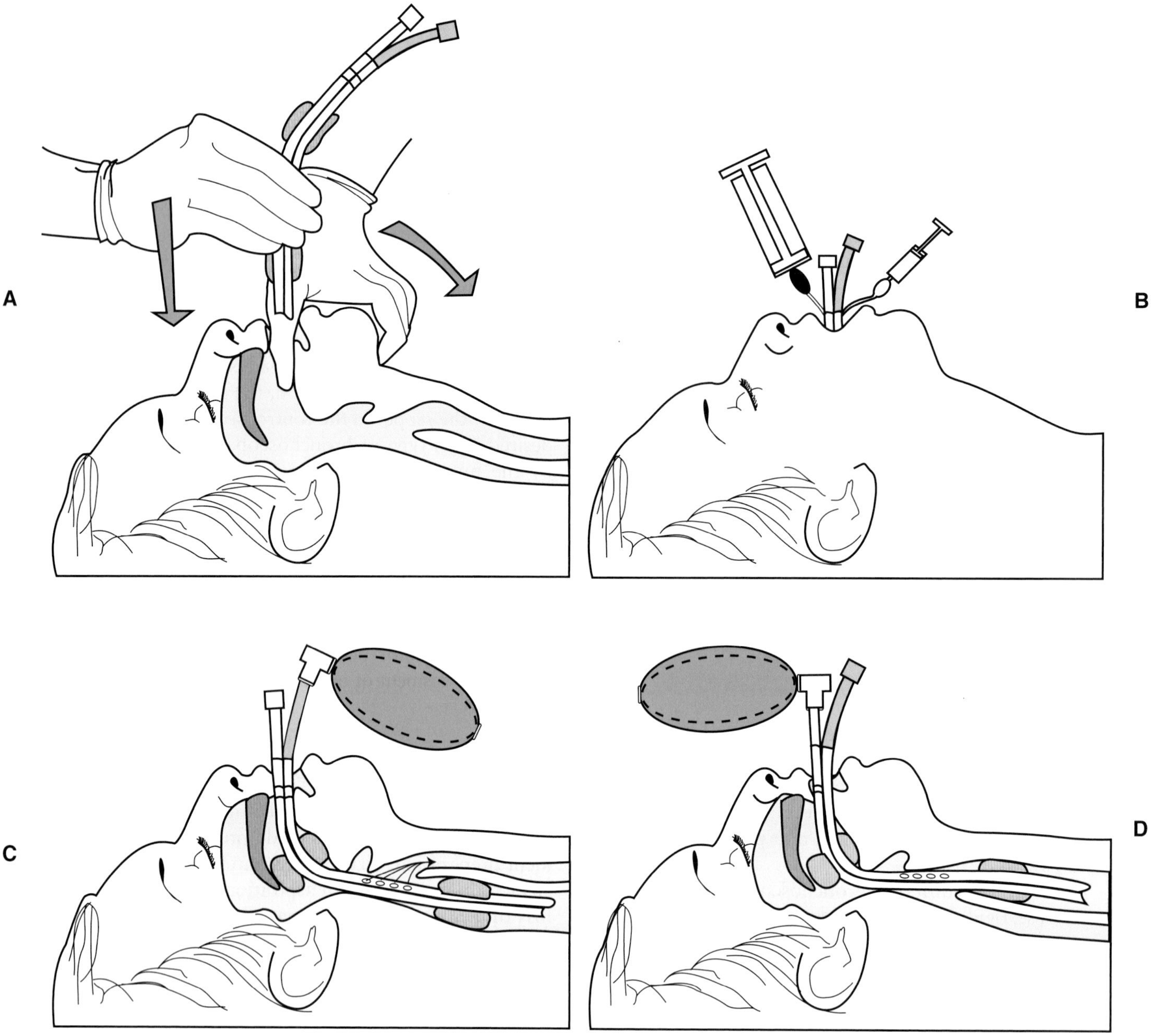

A

B

C

D

Figure 30-38

Insertion of the Combitube. *(Modified from Cairo JM, Pilbeam SP: Mosby's respiratory care equipment, 6 ed, St Louis, 1999, Mosby.)*

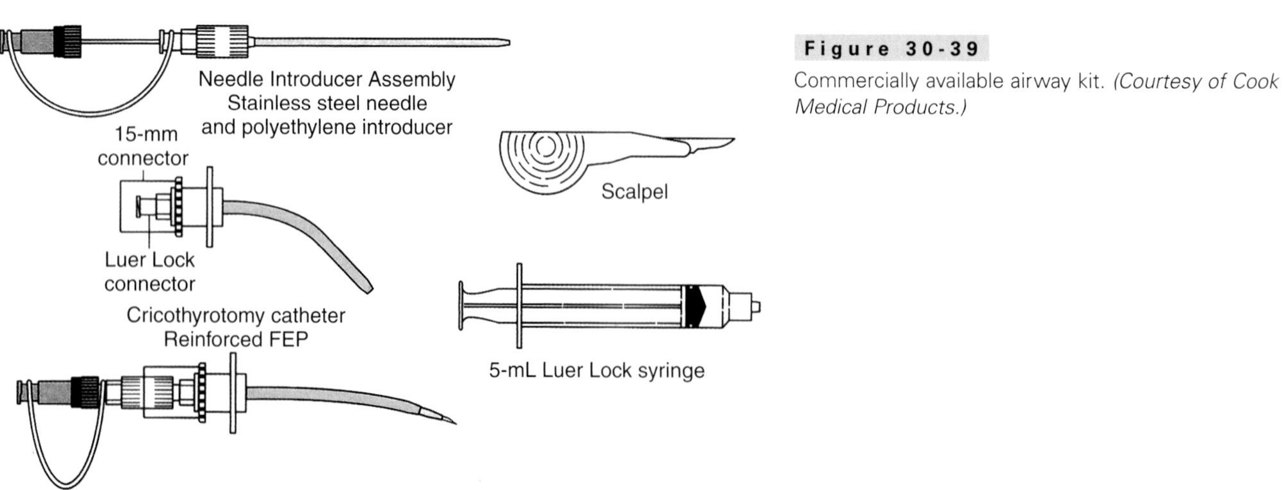

Figure 30-39

Commercially available airway kit. *(Courtesy of Cook Medical Products.)*

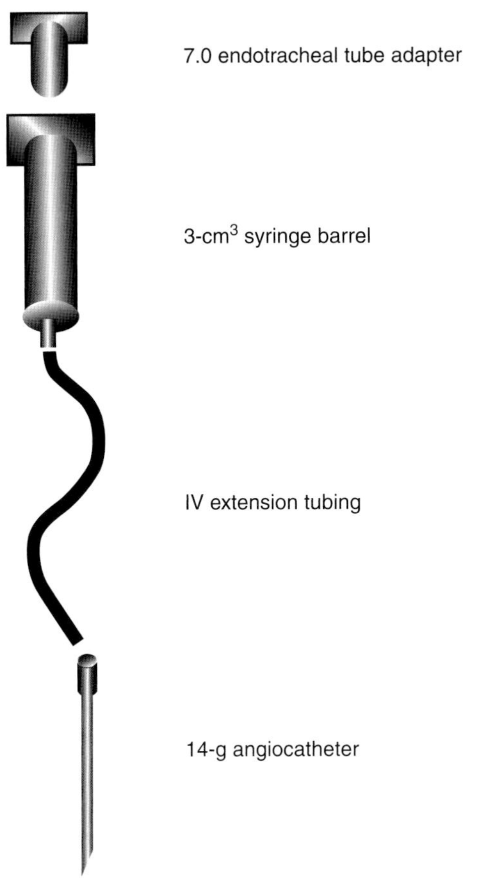

Figure 30-40
Percutaneous tracheal ventilation supplies. *(Modified from Rodricks MB, Deutschman CS: Crit Care Clinics 16(3): 396, 2000.)*

should be withheld until those procedures requiring patient cooperation are completed. Of course, caution must be taken to avoid respiratory depression. Should it occur, naloxone (Narcan) must be available.

Additional narcotics and sedatives may be needed for patient comfort and should be available. The need for antiarrhythmics, resuscitative drugs, narcotic antagonists, and intravenous fluids is harder to predict. Therefore advance preparation will result in a more efficient and rapid response.

Equipment Preparation

The respiratory therapist is often responsible for preparing equipment. Box 30-9 provides a list of needed equipment. Special procedure rooms are often used for bronchoscopy and usually have most of the ancillary equipment already in place. All equipment must be thoroughly checked for function, tight connections, and integrity. This is especially true for small parts and connectors, which can be aspirated if they loosen and disconnect.

Airway Preparation

The goals of airway preparation are to prevent bleeding, decrease cough and gagging, and decrease pain. Topical vasoconstrictors such as phenylephrine and cocaine are frequently used to prevent bleeding. Cocaine has the added advantage of increased sedation. Soaked cotton pledgets are introduced into the nostrils and advanced into the nasopharynx.

Airway anesthesia is achieved by topical anesthetics or nerve block. Topical anesthetics are more common. The particular anesthetic and route of administration vary depending on experience and locale. Lidocaine, viscous lidocaine, lignocaine, and cocaine are often used. Eutectic mixture of local anesthetics (EMLA) cream and lignocaine gel have been reported for use in the nasopharynx. However, they may affect visibility through the bronchoscope.

Lidocaine is commonly delivered by an atomizer to the nose, by mouthwash to the oropharynx, and by nebulizer and bronchoscope (instillation) to the lower airways. Cocaine has also been given by intratracheal injection through the cricoid membrane and through

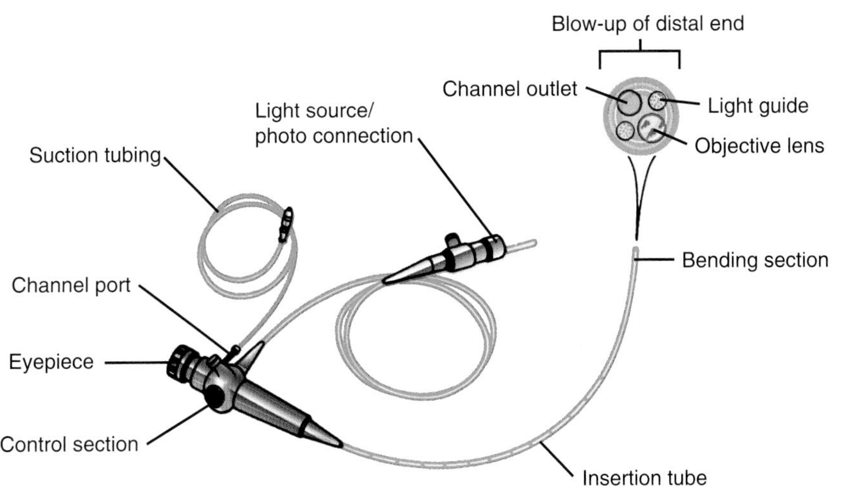

Figure 30-41
Flexible fiberoptic bronchoscope.

Fiberoptic Bronchoscopy Assisting

AARC Clinical Practice Guideline (Excerpts)*

➤ INDICATIONS

- The presence of lesions of unknown etiology on the chest radiograph or the need to evaluate atelectasis or infiltrates
- The need to assess upper airway patency or mechanical properties
- Suspicious or positive sputum cytology results
- The suspicion that secretions or mucus plugs are causing atelectasis
- The need to obtain lower respiratory tract secretions, cell washings, or biopsy samples for evaluation
- The need to investigate hemoptysis, unexplained cough, wheeze, or stridor
- The need to evaluate endotracheal or tracheostomy tube problems
- The need in performing difficult intubations
- The need to determine the location/extent of inhalation or aspiration injuries
- The need to remove abnormal tissue or foreign material
- The need to retrieve a foreign body

➤ CONTRAINDICATIONS

- **Absolute (do not perform):**
    - Absence of patient informed consent, unless a medical emergency exists and patient is not competent
    - Absence of an experienced bronchoscopist to perform or supervise the procedure
    - Lack of adequate facilities and personnel to care for such emergencies
    - Inability to adequately oxygenate the patient during the procedure
- **Perform only if benefit outweighs risk:**
    - Coagulopathy or bleeding diathesis that cannot be corrected
    - Severe obstructive airways disease
    - Refractory hypoxemia
    - Unstable hemodynamic status including arrhythmias
- **Relative (recognize increased risk):**
    - Lack of patient cooperation
    - Recent myocardial infarction/unstable angina
    - Partial tracheal obstruction
    - Moderate-to-severe hypoxemia
    - Any hypercapnia
    - Uremia/pulmonary hypertension
    - Lung abscess
    - Obstruction of the superior vena cava
    - Debility, advanced age, and malnutrition
    - Respiratory failure requiring laser therapy, large airway, or multiple transbronchial lung biopsies
    - Known or suspected pregnancy (radiation exposure)

➤ PRECAUTIONS AND/OR POSSIBLE COMPLICATIONS

- Adverse effects of medication used before and during the bronchoscopic procedure
- Hypoxemia
- Hypotension
- Caregiver/patient infection
- Laryngospasm, bradycardia, or other vagally-mediated phenomena
- Hypercapnia
- Increased airway resistance
- Cross-contamination of specimens or bronchoscopes
- Mechanical complications (e.g., epistaxis, pneumothorax, and hemoptysis)
- Wheezing
- Death

FIBEROPTIC BRONCHOSCOPY ASSISTING—CONT'D

AARC Clinical Practice Guideline (Excerpts)*

➤ **ASSESSMENT OF NEED**
Need is determined by the presence of clinical indications and the absence of contraindications, as described above.

➤ **ASSESSMENT OF OUTCOME**
Patient outcome is determined by clinical, physiological, and pathological assessment. Procedural outcome is determined by the accomplishment of the procedural goals as indicated above and by appropriate quality assessment indicators.

➤ **MONITORING**
The following should be monitored continuously before, during, and/or after bronchoscopy, until the patient returns to his or her presedation level of consciousness.

- Patient:
  - Level of consciousness
  - Blood pressure, heart rate, rhythm, and changes in cardiac status
  - Lavage volumes (delivered and retrieved)
  - Medications administered, dosage, route, and time of delivery
  - Documentation of site of biopsies/washings and tests requested on each sample
  - SpO_2 and FIO_2
  - Subjective response to procedure (e.g., pain, discomfort, dyspena)
  - Ventilation parameters if subject is mechanically ventilated
  - Periodic postprocedure follow-up of patient for 24 to 48 hours
- Technical devices:
  - Bronchoscope integrity (fiberoptic or channel damage, passage of leak test)
  - Strict adherence to the recommended procedures for cleaning, disinfection, and sterilization of the devices and the integrity of disinfection or sterilization packaging
  - Smooth, unhampered operation of biopsy devices (forceps, needles)
- Recordkeeping:
  - Quality assessment indicators are determined appropriate by the institution's quality assessment committee
  - Documentation of patient/device monitoring
  - Identification of bronchoscope used for each patient
  - Annual assessment of the institutional or departmental bronchoscopy procedure, including an evaluation of (a) the adequacy of bronchoscopic specimens; (b) infection control procedures and compliance with the current guidelines for semicritical patient-care objects; (c) synopsis of complications; (d) control washings to ensure that infection control and disinfection/sterilization procedures are adequate, and that cross-contamination of specimens does not occur; and (e) all of the above listed records with the physician bronchoscopists

*For complete guidelines see Respir Care 38:1173, 1993.

the bronchoscope. If lidocaine is nebulized, it is usually the respiratory therapist who performs this function. The use of nebulized lidocaine prior to bronchoscopy may limit the need for lidocaine instillations into the lower airways and can make the procedure less unpleasant for the patient.

Superior laryngeal nerve block will provide anesthesia in the upper larynx, but it does not affect the vocal cords. Transtracheal block through the cricoid membrane will anesthetize both the vocal cords and the trachea.

Monitoring

The respiratory therapist has an active role in monitoring the patient and should communicate any changes to the physician. Oxygenation should be monitored continuously via pulse oximetry. If desaturation occurs, the FIO_2 should be increased with an oxygen therapy device. Alternatively, the procedure can be temporarily halted, and oxygen can be given through the scope's open channel. The latter technique has the advantage of defogging the scope and diffusing any secretions.

Box 30-9 • Bronchoscopy Equipment

FOR OPERATOR AND ASSISTANT
- Masks
- Gloves
- Gown

FOR AIRWAY MANAGEMENT
- Endotracheal tubes
- Bronchoscope adapter for endotracheal tube
- Yankauer-type suction catheters
- Suction pump
- Suction tubing
- Bite block
- Adhesive tape
- Water-soluble lubricant

SYRINGES, NEEDLES, AND SOLUTION
- 10- and 20-mL syringes, Luer-Lok
- 10- and 20-mL syringes, nonLuer-Lok
- Needles, sharp tip
- Needles, blunt tip
- Saline
- Nonbacteriostatic saline

FOR OBTAINING SPECIMENS
- Bronchoscope accessories
- Specimen cups
- Sputum traps

FOR HANDLING SPECIMENS
- Microscope slides
- Viral and anaerobic transport media
- Carbowax
- Formalin

MISCELLANEOUS ITEMS
- Bronchoscope light source
- Denture cups
- Emesis basins
- Medicine cups
- Cotton 4 × 4 and 2 × 2 pads

FOR PATIENT SUPPORT AND MONITORING
- Pulse oximeter
- Oxygen cannulae
- ECG leads
- Cardiac monitor

FOR ANESTHESIA AND SEDATION
- Jackson forceps
- Cotton balls
- Heparin locks or caps
- Intravenous catheters or "butterflies"
- Alcohol wipes
- Band-Aids
- Sterile swabs
- Atomizer and accessories

MEDICATIONS
- Epinephrine 1:1000
- Heparin lock flush solution
- Sedatives (e.g., meperidine, codeine, morphine, diazepam, midazolam)
- Topical anesthetics (e.g., lidocaine [1%, 2%, and 4%], cocaine [4% or 10%], Cetacaine)

PAPERWORK
- Consent forms
- Specimen labels
- Laboratory specimen forms
- Radiology requisitions
- Bronchoscopy charge slips
- Physician's order forms

From Johnsom NT, Pierson DJ: Pulmonary diagnostic procedures. In Pierson DJ, Kacmarek RM, eds: Foundations of respiratory care, New York, 1992, Churchill Livingstone.

Suctioning for brief periods will help reduce the incidence or severity of hypoxemia.

Respiratory rate and depth should also be observed. Decreases in rate or depth may indicate over-sedation. Continuous electrocardiogram (ECG) and periodic blood pressure monitoring should also be routine. Arrhythmias and changes in blood pressure that occur are usually due to hypoxemia, vagal stimulation, pain, or anxiety. Prompt recognition of a problem and appropriate response will aid recovery.

Assisting With the Procedure

The physician inserts the bronchoscope into the airway and guides it by directing the tip by the thumb lever. While monitoring the patient, respiratory therapists may also assist the physician by supplying syringes filled with anesthetic, vasoconstrictor, mucolytic agents, or lavage solutions. Forceps or brushes are often inserted into the bronchoscope by the respiratory therapist. The physician then guides these devices to the desired area. In addition, sputum or tissue samples obtained by the physician may be collected by the respiratory therapist and prepared for laboratory analysis. Once the goals of the procedure have been achieved, the bronchoscope is removed, and the patient's recovery period begins.

Recovery

Hypoxemia that occurs during the procedure may persist after completion. Oxygen therapy should be maintained for up to 4 hours. Adequate oxygenation via pulse oximetry should be confirmed before therapy is discontinued.

The risk of aspiration persists as long as the airway is anesthetized. Therefore patients should remain in a sitting position and refrain from eating or drinking until sensation returns.

Patients should also be assessed for the development of stridor or wheezes. The physician should be notified, and appropriate aerosol therapy with racemic epinephrine or bronchodilators should be instituted.

Complications

The complications of bronchoscopy are similar to those for suctioning (Table 30-6). However, the greater patient discomfort, longer duration, and the extent of airway penetration make this a more hazardous and complex procedure.

Hypoxemia is most severe in patients with underlying lung disease. To minimize this problem, all patients should receive oxygen before and during the procedure. When the nasal route is used to insert the bronchoscope, oxygen can be administered by a nasal catheter (in the opposite naris) or by a mask adapted to allow passage of the scope.

Hemodynamic changes (heart rate, blood pressure, and cardiac output) vary and may be related to differences in techniques or medications.

Bronchospasm also has been reported and is most severe in patients with asthma. Premedication with albuterol and ipratropium bromide may help relieve this problem, as will the use of sedatives or narcotic analgesics, which do not release histamine. Demerol and fentanyl are better for the patient with asthma.[31]

In patients with artificial airways, placing a scope through an endotracheal tube or tracheostomy tube may decrease the radius by 50%. If the patient is on a ventilator, peak inspiratory pressure may increase or tidal volumes decrease. Inadvertent PEEP may increase as well. Respiratory therapists are needed to adjust the ventilator and monitor saturations and exhaled volumes.[31]

Table 30-6 ▶▶ Complications of Fiberoptic Bronchoscopy

Complication	Incidence (%)
Vasovagal reaction	2.4
Fever	1.2
Cardiac dysrhythmia	0.9
Bleeding	0.7
Pneumonia	0.6
Pneumothorax	0.4
Airway obstruction	0.4
Respiratory arrest	0.2
Nausea and vomiting	0.2
ECG abnormality	0.2
Death	0.1
Psychotic reaction	0.1
Aphonia	0.1

KEY POINTS

- Remove retained secretions, or other semiliquid fluids, from the large airways via suctioning. Removal of foreign bodies or tissue masses beyond the mainstem bronchi requires bronchoscopy.
- To avoid or minimize the complications of suctioning, (1) preoxygenate (2) limit negative pressure and suction time, and (3) use sterile technique.
- The primary indications for an artificial tracheal airway are (1) to relieve airway obstruction, (2) to facilitate secretion removal, (3) to protect against aspiration, and (4) to provide positive pressure ventilation.
- There are two basic types of tracheal airways: endotracheal (translaryngeal) tubes and tracheostomy tubes.
- Orotracheal intubation is the preferred route for establishing an emergency tracheal airway.
- Provide adequate ventilation and 100% oxygen by bag and mask prior to intubation.
- Do not devote any more than 30 seconds to any intubation attempt.
- There are many ways to assess endotracheal tube position; only laryngoscopy can confirm correct position.
- The serious complications of emergency airway management are acute hypoxemia, hypercapnia, bradycardia, and cardiac arrest.
- Nasotracheal intubation is the route of choice for intubation of patients with maxillofacial injuries.
- The primary indication for tracheotomy is the continuing need for an artificial airway after a prolonged period of oral or nasal intubation; the decision as to when to switch from endotracheal tube to tracheostomy tube should be individualized.
- The most common laryngeal injuries associated with endotracheal intubation are glottic edema, vocal cord inflammation, laryngeal/vocal cord ulcerations, and vocal cord polyps or granulomas.
- Whereas laryngeal lesions occur only with oral or nasal endotracheal tubes, tracheal lesions can occur with any tracheal airway. The most common tracheal lesions are granulomas, tracheomalacia, and tracheal stenosis.

Continued

KEY POINTS—cont'd

- To minimize or prevent trauma due to tracheal airways, (1) select the correct size of airway, (2) avoid tube movement or traction, (3) limit cuff pressures, and (4) use sterile techniques.
- Endotracheal tube obstruction can be caused by (1) kinking of or biting on the tube, (2) herniation of the cuff over the tube tip, (3) jamming of the tube orifice against the tracheal wall, and (4) mucus plugging.
- If a tracheal airway appears completely obstructed, proceed through these steps in order until the obstruction is relieved: (1) reposition the patient's head and neck; (2) deflate the tube cuff; (3) try passing a suction catheter; (4) try removing a tracheostomy tube's inner cannula; (5) remove the airway and provide bag-valve-mask ventilation/oxygenation.
- A patient is ready to extubate if he or she (1) can maintain adequate spontaneous oxygenation and ventilation, (2) is at minimal risk for upper airway obstruction, (3) has adequate airway protective reflexes, and (4) can adequately clear secretions.
- Tracheostomy decannulation can be accomplished by using fenestrated tubes, progressively smaller tubes, or tracheostomy buttons.
- A laryngeal mask airway or a Combitube can be used in a difficult intubation.
- Cricothyroidotomy is performed when you cannot intubate/cannot ventilate.
- Key points in planning and conducting fiberoptic bronchoscopy include premedication, equipment preparation, airway preparation, and monitoring.

References

1. American Association for Respiratory Care: Clinical practice guideline. Endotracheal suctioning of mechanically ventilated adults and children with artificial airways, Respir Care 38:500, 1993.
2. Birdstal C: What suction pressures should I use? Am J Nurs 866, 1985.
3. Tiffin NH, Keim MR, Trewen TC: The effects of variations in flow through an insufflating catheter and endotracheal tube and suction catheter size on test lung pressures, Respir Care 35:889, 1990.
4. Hess DR: Managing the artificial airway, Respir Care 44:759, 1999.
5. Johnson KL et al: Closed versus open endotracheal suctioning: costs and physiologic consequences, Crit Care Med 22:658, 1994.
6. Craig KC, Benson MS, Pierson DJ: Prevention of arterial oxygen desaturation during closed-airway endotracheal suction: effect of ventilator mode, Respir Care 29:1013, 1984.
7. Hagler DA, Traver GA: Endotracheal saline and suction catheters: sources of lower airway contamination, Am J Crit Care 3:444, 1994.
8. Campbell RS, Branson RD: How ventilators provide temporary O_2 enrichment: what happens when you press the 100% suction button, Respir Care 37:933, 1992.
9. Shapiro B et al: Clinical applications of respiratory care, ed 4, St Louis, 1991, Mosby.
10. Goodnough SK: The effects of oxygen and hyperinflation on arterial oxygen tension after endotracheal suctioning, Heart Lung 14:11, 1985.
11. Chulay M: Arterial blood gas changes with a hyperinflation and hyperoxygenation suctioning intervention in critically ill patients, Heart Lung 17:654, 1988.
12. Taft AA et al: A comparison of two methods of preoxygenation during endotracheal suctioning, Respir Care 36:1195, 1991.
13. Stone KS, Bell SP, Preusser BA: The effect of repeated suctioning on arterial blood pressure, Appl Nurs Res 4:152, 1991.
14. Jaeger JM, Durbin CG: Special purpose endotracheal tubes, Respir Care 44:661, 1999.
15. American Association for Respiratory Care: Clinical practice guideline. Nasotracheal suctioning, Respir Care 37:898, 1992.
16. American Association for Respiratory Care: Clinical practice guideline. Management of airway emergencies, Respir Care 40:749, 1995.
17. Colice GL: Technical standards for tracheal tubes, Clin Chest Med 12: 433, 1991.
18. American Society for Testing and Materials: Standard specification for cuffed and uncuffed tracheal tubes (F1242-96), Conshohocken, Pa, 1996, ASTM.
19. American Society for Testing and Materials: Standard specification for adult tracheostomy tubes (F1666-95), Conshohocken, Pa, 1996, ASTM.
20. Rodrick MB, Duetschman CS: Emergent airway management: indications and methods in the face of confounding conditions, Crit Care Med 16:389, 2000.
21. Thalman JJ, Rinaldo-Gallo S, MacIntyre, NR: Analysis of an endotracheal intubation service provided by respiratory care practitioners, Respir Care 38: 469, 1993.
22. Levitan R, Ochroch EA: Airway management and direct laryngoscopy: a review and update, Crit Care Clin 16:373, 2000.
23. Donahue PL: The oesophageal detector device: an assessment of accuracy and ease of use by paramedics, Anaesthesia 49:863, 1994.
24. Hurford WE: Orotracheal intubation outside the OR: anatomic considerations and techniques. Respir Care 44:651, 1999.

25. Haynes SR, Morton NS: Use of the oesophageal detector device in children under one year of age, Anaesthesia 45:1067, 1990.
26. Blosser SA, Stauffer JL: Intubation of critically ill patients, Clin Chest Med 17:355, 1996.
27. Murray IP, Modell JH: Early detection of endotracheal tube accidents by monitoring carbon dioxide concentrations in respiratory gas, Anesthesiology 59:344, 1983.
28. Goldberg JS et al: Colorimetric end-tidal carbon dioxide monitoring for tracheal intubation, Anesth Analg 70:191, 1990.
29. Varon AJ, Morrina J, Civetta JM: Clinical utility of colometric end-tidal CO_2 detector in cardiopulmonary resuscitation and emergency intubation, J Clin Monit 7: 289, 1991.
30. Sum-Ping ST, Mehk MD, Anderson JM: A comparative study of methods of detection of esophageal intubation, Anesth Analg 69:627, 1989.
31. Leibler JM, Markin CJ: Fiberoptic bronchoscopy for diagnosis and treatment, Crit Care Clin 16:83, 2000.
32. Mcculloch TM, Bishop MJ: Complications of translaryngeal intubation, Clin Chest Med 12:507, 1991.
33. Watson CB: Prediction of a difficult intubation: methods for successful intubation, Respir Care 44:777.
34. Stauffer JL: Medical management of the airway, Clin Chest Med 12: 449, 1991.
35. Goldman RK: Minimally invasive surgery, Crit Care Clin 16:113, 2000.
36. Heffner JE: Tracheostomy: indications and timing, Respir Care 44:807, 1999.
37. Finucane BT, Santora AH: Principles of Airway Management, ed 2, St Louis, 1996, Mosby.
38. Riebel JF: Trachotomy/tracheostomy, Respir Care 44:820, 1999.
39. Durbin CG, Seay W: Use of laryngeal mask airway during performance of percutaneous bedside tracheostomy, Respir Care 43:838, 1998 (abstract).
40. Butler TJ, Close JR, Close RJ: Laboratory exercises for competency in respiratory care, Philadelphia, 1998, FA Davis.
41. Stauffer JL: Complications of endotracheal intubation and tracheostomy, Respir Care 44:828, 1999.
42. Wood DE, Mathesen DJ: Late complications of tracheostomy, Clin Chest Med 12:597, 1991.
43. Streitz JM, Shaphay SM: Airway injury after tracheostomy and endotracheal intubation, Surg Clin North Am 71:1211, 1991.
44. Wissing DR, Romero MR, Payne K: An unusual complication of prolonged intubation, Respir Care 32:359, 1987.
45. Weber AL, Grillo HC: Tracheal stenosis: an analysis of 151 cases, Radiol Clin North Am 16:291, 1978.
46. Goodman LR et al: Radiographic evaluation of endotracheal tube position, Am J Roentgenol 127:433, 1976.
47. Conrardy PA et al: Alteration of endotracheal tube position: flexion and extension of the neck, Crit Care Med 4:8, 1976.
48. Reyes G et al: Use of an optical fiber scope to confirm endotracheal tube placement in pediatric patients, Crit Care Med 24:175, 2001.
49. Appel-Hardin SJ: Communicating with intubated patients, Crit Care Nurs 4:26, 1984.
50. Goodwin JE, Heffner JE: Special critical care considerations in tracheostomy management, Clin Chest Med 12:573, 1991.
51. Orringer MK: Tracheostomy: communication and swallowing, Respir Care 44:845, 1999.
52. Passy Muir Valve Clinical Inservice Outline, Passy Muir Inc, Irvine, Ca, November 1999.
53. Lichtman SW, Birnbaum IL, Sanfilippo MR: Effect of a tracheostomy speaking valve on secretions, arterial oxygenation, and olfaction: a quantitative evaluation, J Speech Lang Hear Res 38:549, 1995.
54. Dettelbach MS et al: Effect of the PMV on aspiration in patients with tracheostomy, Head and Neck 17:297, 1995.
55. Branson RD: Humdification for patients with artificial airways, Respir Care 44:630, 1999.
56. American Association for Respiratory Care: Clinical practice guideline. Humidification during mechanical ventilation. Respir Care 37:887, 1992.
57. Levine SA, Neederman MS: The impact of tracheal intubation on host defenses and risks for nosocomial pneumonia, Clin Chest Med 12:523, 1991.
58. Craven DE, Steiger KA: Nosocomial pneumonia in the intubated patient. New concepts on pathogenesis and prevention, Infect Dis Clin North Am 3:843, 1989.
59. Rello J et al: Pneumonia in intubated patients: role of respiratory airway care, Am J Respir Crit Care Med 154:111, 1996.
60. Rodriguez-Roldan JM et al: Prevention of nosocomial lung infection in ventilated patients: use of an antimicrobial pharyngeal nonabsorbable paste, Crit Care Med 18:1239, 1990.
61. OtolaryngolHead Neck Surg 122:768, 2000.
62. Sills J: An emergency cuff inflation technique, Respir Care 31:199, 1986.
63. Campbell RS: Extubation and the consequences of reintubation, Respir Care 44:799, 1999.
64. Marik PE: The cuff-leak test as a predictor of postextubation stridor: a prospective study, Respir Care 41:509, 1996.
65. American Association for Respiratory Care: Clinical practice guideline: removal of the endotracheal tube, Respir Care 44:85, 1999.
66. Godwin JE, Heffner JE: Special critical care considerations in tracheostomy management, Clin Chest Med 12:573, 1991.
67. Siddharth P, Mazzarella L: Granuloma associated with fenestrated tracheostomy tubes, Am J Surg 150:279, 1985.
68. Synder GM: Individualized placement of tracheostomy tube fenestration and in-situ examinations with the fiberoptic laryngoscope, Respir Care 28:1294, 1983.
69. American Society of Anesthesiologists: Practice guidelines for management of the difficult airway, Anesthesiology 78:597, 1993.
70. Foley LJ, Ochroch EA: Bridges to establish an emergency airway and alternate intubating techniques, Crit Care Clinics 16:429, 2000.
71. Treanor S, Benitez WD, Raffin TA: Respiratory therapists as fiberoptic bronchoscopy assistants, Respir Care 30:321, 1985.

72. American Association for Respiratory Care: Clinical practice guideline: fiberoptic bronchoscopy assisting, Respir Care 38:1173, 1993.
73. Johnson NT, Pierson DJ: Pulmonary diagnostic procedures. In Pierson DJ, Kacmarek RM, eds: Foundations of Respiratory Care, New York, 1992, Churchill Livingstone.
74. Reed AP: Preparation of the patient for awake flexible fiberoptic bronchoscopy, Chest 101:244, 1992.

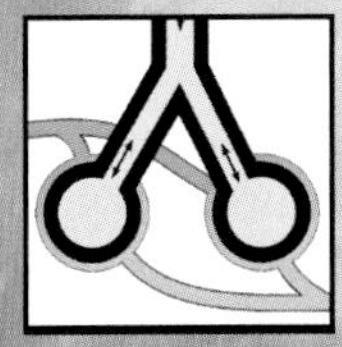

CHAPTER 31

Emergency Life Support

Arthur B. Marshak

In This Chapter You Will Learn:

- What causes sudden death
- How to assess a victim's need for emergency life support
- How to perform basic life support procedures on adults, children, and infants
- How to assess the effectiveness of basic life support procedures
- What complications can occur as a result of resuscitation efforts
- When not to initiate cardiopulmonary resuscitation (CPR)
- How to apply key adjunct equipment during advanced life support
- What common drugs and drug routes are used during advanced life support
- How patients who survive resuscitation are managed

Chapter Outline

Key Terms

advanced cardiac life support (ACLS)
automatic external defibrillators (AEDs)
basic life support (BLS)
cardiopulmonary resuscitation (CPR)
gastric distension
Heimlich maneuver

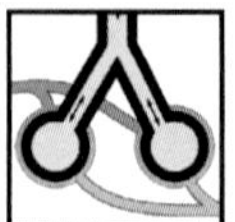

Emergency life support involves a variety of procedures designed to deal with sudden, life-threatening events caused by cardiac or respiratory failure. Respiratory therapists (RTs) play a vital role in emergency life support.[1] In the hospital setting, RTs normally serve as key members of the resuscitation team. In addition to managing the airway, RTs often participate in circulatory support, drug and electrical therapy, and postresuscitative care.

In the community, RTs may also be certified as **cardiopulmonary resuscitation (CPR)** instructors, extending their knowledge to lay personnel through organizations such as the American Heart Association (AHA) or the American Red Cross (ARC). Those who serve as CPR instructors need to be aware of the misconceptions the public may have about the success rate that is depicted on television shows. A recent survey found that approximately 75% of the CPR situations on television were successful in recovering the victim.[2] This percentage is far higher than what has been found in scientific surveys of CPR cases.[3,4] Thus the public may have an unrealistic expectation of outcome in cases of sudden death if CPR is given.

Both teaching and performing CPR require mastery of an extensive knowledge base and the development of a variety of sometimes difficult manual skills. Although this chapter is no substitute for the official AHA or ARC life support manuals or supervised practice under simulated conditions, it does provide a summary of the information needed to apply both basic and advanced life support techniques. The practitioner is encouraged to obtain further competencies by completion of formal courses in CPR, **advanced cardiac life support (ACLS)**, pediatric advanced life support (PALS), and neonatal resuscitation.

▶ CAUSES AND PREVENTION OF SUDDEN DEATH

Sudden death is a common event both inside and outside the hospital. Cardiovascular disease is the primary cause of sudden death among adults, for both men and women, accounting for approximately 950,000 fatalities in the United States in 1997.[5] Each year in the United States, approximately 2 million people are diagnosed with acute coronary syndrome. Of these, more than 500,000 will be hospitalized with the diagnosis of unstable angina, and approximately 1.5 million will experience an acute myocardial infarction (MI). Approximately 500,000 of the 1.5 million patients diagnosed with acute MI will die, and approximately 50% of these deaths will be sudden, occurring within 60 minutes of onset of symptoms.[6]

Accidents are the leading cause of sudden death among individuals ages 1 to 37 years in the United States and the fourth leading cause of death overall. In accidental death among adults, motor vehicle accidents, drowning, electrocution, burns, suffocation, and drug intoxication are the major causes of trauma.[6]

Among children, accidents are the leading cause of sudden death, accounting for approximately 44% of the fatalities in the 1- to 14-year-old age-group.[7] A particularly serious cause of sudden death in children is obstruction of the airway by foreign bodies. Foreign body obstruction accounts for more than 3000 deaths annually, most of which occur in children younger than 5 years of age.[5]

Although not all of these deaths are preventable, early use of life support methods can reduce this alarming toll of sudden death. CPR performed by bystanders can at least double the survival rate of victims of cardiac or respiratory arrest.[3,8,9] In addition, early intervention can decrease the subsequent likelihood of neurological impairment by as much as tenfold.[6] It is estimated that comprehensive implementation of emergency life support on a community-wide basis throughout the nation could save between 100,000 and 200,000 lives per year.[5]

Emergency life support involves a variety of methods and procedures designed to deal with sudden, life-threatening events caused by cardiac or respiratory failure. Emergency life support traditionally consists of two related phases: (1) **basic life support (BLS)** and (2) ACLS.[6]

▶ BASIC LIFE SUPPORT

The goal of BLS is to restore ventilation and circulation to victims of airway obstruction and respiratory or cardiac arrest. These skills can be used by a single practitioner to restore ventilation and circulation until the victim is revived or until ACLS equipment and personnel are available.

The steps for administering BLS are as follows:

1. Initial assessment to determine unresponsiveness
2. Activation of the emergency medical system
3. Airway restoration
4. Ventilation
5. Restoration of circulation
6. Automated external defibrillation

The last four steps are referred to as the *ABCDs of resuscitation*—Airway, Breathing, Circulation, and Defibrillation. Each of the ABCDs starts with a victim evaluation phase. The first phase determines unresponsiveness, the second determines breathlessness, and the third determines pulselessness. Box 31-1 and Table 31-1 summarize the ABCDs of CPR for adults, children, and infants.

Box 31-1 • The ABCDs of CPR

FIRST STEP
- Check for responsiveness (shake and shout).

ACT
- For adults: If no response, contact emergency medical services (EMS) immediately.
- For children and infants: Go through the ABCDs.

AIRWAY

ACT
- Open airway (tilt head, lift chin).

BREATHING

ASSESS
- Check for breathing (look, listen, touch).

ACT
- Give two breaths (reposition head if necessary).

CIRCULATION

ASSESS
- Check pulse
- For adults and children: Check the carotid artery.
- For infants: Check the brachial artery.

ACT
- For children and infants: If there is no pulse, initiate CPR for 1 minute; after 1 minute of CPR, contact EMS.
- For adults: The EMS should be on the way. If there is no pulse, begin CPR for 1 minute. If the pulse does not return spontaneously, resume CPR. Check pulse every few minutes thereafter, or until the automatic external defibrillator (AED) arrives.

DEFIBRILLATION

ASSESS
- Hook up the AED and determine if shockable rhythm is present.

ACT
- If shockable rhythm is present, charge and shock.

RESCUE BREATHING
- If the victim has a pulse and is not breathing, give ventilations at a normal respiratory rate.
- For adults: Give one breath every 5 seconds.
- For children and infants: Give one breath every 3 seconds.

OBSTRUCTED AIRWAY

CONSCIOUS
- For adults and children: Repeat the Heimlich maneuver.
- For infants: Give five back blows, five chest compressions.

UNCONSCIOUS
- Check mouth (sweep for adults only).
- Give ventilations.
- Attempt to relieve obstructions.

Modified from BLS Pre-course Material, Loma Linda, Calif, Loma Linda University, Life Support Education, 2001.
RULE: Always move forward through the ABCDs. If at some point a positive result is achieved (e.g., victim regains a pulse), go back to the beginning, and go through the ABCDs again.

Determining Unresponsiveness

Basic life support begins when a victim is found in an unresponsive or collapsed state. Because many hospitalized patients exhibit decreased levels of consciousness, healthcare personnel should avoid needless intervention by being fully aware of the patient's mental status.

When a person comes upon a collapsed victim outside the hospital setting who appears to be unconscious, he or she should first look for any obvious head or neck injuries. If such injuries are apparent, great care should be taken in subsequent manipulation of the neck and in any effort to move the individual.

Whatever the location, the victim's level of consciousness should be assessed quickly by tapping or gently shaking his or her shoulder and shouting, "Are you OK?" If this fails to stir the victim, the rescuer should call for help and activate the emergency medical service (EMS). Outside the hospital, this may mean having someone call 911 or the local EMS. Within the hospital, specific protocols exist for "calling a code." All RTs must be familiar with their institution's protocols for handling these emergency situations.

Restoring the Airway

After calling for help and activating the EMS, the rescuer should try to open the victim's airway. First, the victim should be quickly inspected for any neck or facial trauma. If spinal cord trauma is suspected, the neck must be carefully positioned in a neutral in-line position, and procedures requiring hyperextension must be modified. In addition, when a victim is found lying on his or her side or stomach, he or she should be moved to a supine position before airway procedures are begun. The "logroll" technique* is useful in doing this. The rescuer must ensure that the victim is positioned on a hard, flat surface.

*Rolling the patient as a unit so that the head, shoulders, and body move simultaneously without twisting.

Table 31-1 ▶▶▶ Steps for CPR in the Adult, Child, and Infant

Procedure	Adult	Child	Infant
Breathing			
Obstructive procedure	Conscious: Repeat Heimlich maneuver until the foreign body is expelled or the victim becomes unconscious Unconscious: Perform finger sweep of mouth, ventilate; perform abdominal thrusts five times; repeat sequence until successful	Conscious: Repeat Heimlich maneuver until the foreign body is expelled or the victim becomes unconscious Unconscious: Look into mouth, remove foreign body if found, ventilate; perform abdominal thrusts five times; repeat sequence until successful	Conscious: Perform five back blows and five chest compressions; repeat until foreign body is expelled or the infant becomes unconscious Unconscious: Look into mouth, remove foreign body if found, ventilate; perform five back flows, five chest compressions; repeat sequence until successful
Rescue Breathing	12 breaths/min, 1 breath every 5 seconds; count "One 1000, two 1000..."	20 breaths/min, 1 breath every 3 seconds; count "One 1000, two 1000..."	20 breaths/min, 1 breath every 3 seconds; count "One 1000, two 1000..."
Compressions			
Where to check pulse	Carotid artery	Carotid artery	Brachial artery, above elbow
Pulse check time	5-10 sec	5-10 sec	5-10 sec
Hand placement	One finger width above the xiphoid process with heel of both hands on the lower half of the sternum	One finger width above the xiphoid process with heel of one hand on the lower half of the sternum	One finger width below the nipple line with two fingers on the lower half of the sternum
Compressions to ventilation ratio	One rescuer: 15:2 Two rescuer: 15:2	One rescuer: 5:1	One rescuer: 5:1
Cycles	4 at 15:2	20 at 5:1	20 at 5:1
Approximate depth of compressions	1½-2 in	1-1½ in	½-1 in
Compression rate	100 beats/min	100 beats/min	120 beats/min

Modified from BLS Pre-course Material, Loma Linda, Calif, Loma Linda University, Life Support Education.

The most common cause of airway obstruction is loss of muscle tone, which causes the tongue to fall back into the pharynx, thereby blocking airflow. Movement of the lower jaw and extension of the neck pulls the tongue from the posterior pharyngeal wall and opens the airway. One of the two following procedures can be used to do this: (1) The *head-tilt/chin-lift* method is the primary procedure recommended for the layperson when spinal trauma is not suspected (Figure 31-1); (2) the *jaw thrust* is used mainly by trained clinicians when spinal neck injuries are suspected (Figure 31-2). One of these maneuvers will usually open the airway and may be the only lifesaving measure required. Once the airway is cleared and opened, immediately assess the victim's ventilation.

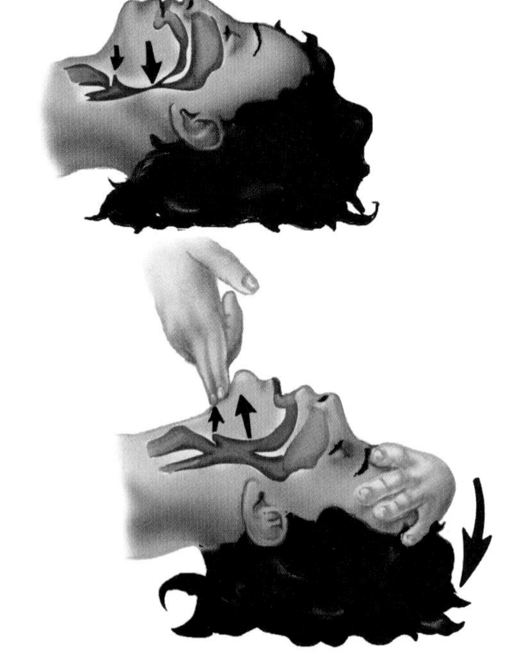

Figure 31-1 · Opening the Airway
Top, Airway obstruction produced by tongue and epiglottis. *Bottom,* Relief by head-tilt/chin-lift method.

Restoring Ventilation

Before attempting to provide artificial ventilation, the rescuer should assess for the presence of breathing. To determine breathlessness, he or she should place his or her ear over the victim's mouth and nose while simultaneously observing for spontaneous chest movement (Figure 31-3). Breathlessness exists if no chest movement

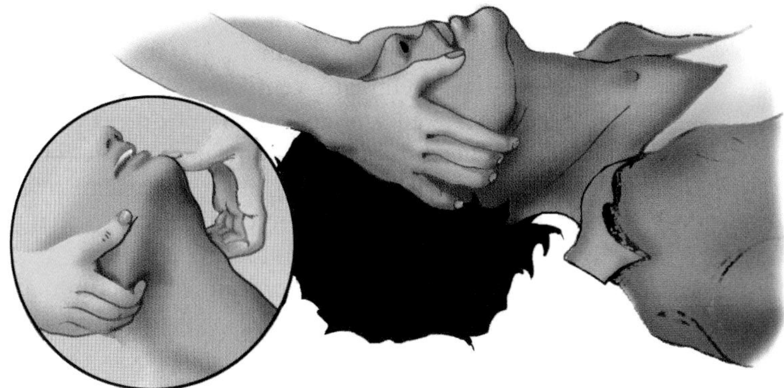

Figure 31-2
Jaw thrust maneuver.

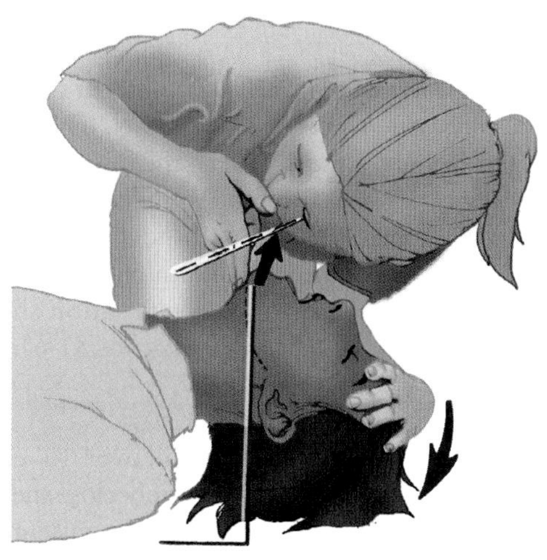

Figure 31-3
Determining breathlessness.

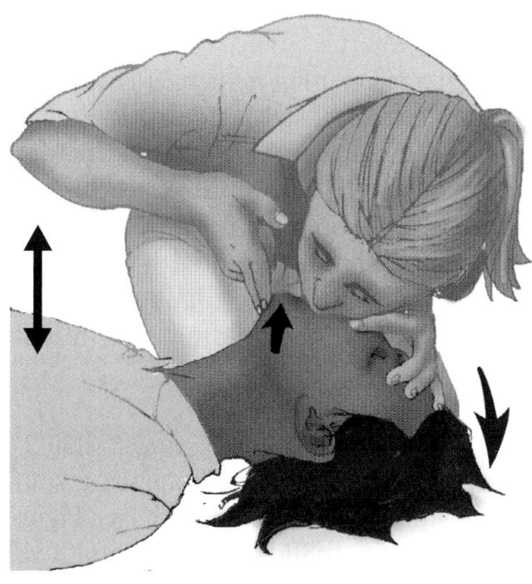

Figure 31-4
Adult mouth-to-mouth ventilation.

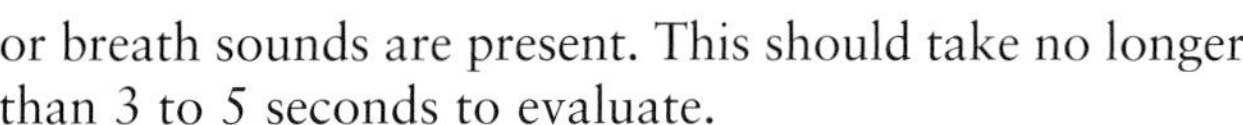

or breath sounds are present. This should take no longer than 3 to 5 seconds to evaluate.

Providing Artificial Ventilation

During respiratory arrest, the victim must be provided with oxygen within 4 to 6 minutes, or biological death will follow. The rescuer can restore an oxygen supply to the victim's lungs by exhaling into the victim's mouth, nose, or tracheal stoma. These procedures can be used for any victim, with appropriate modification for the patient's age.

Mouth-to-Mouth Ventilation. Adequate oxygenation can be restored through mouth-to-mouth ventilation. To do this, the rescuer must take a deep breath and exhale directly into the victim's mouth. Exhaled air provides approximately 16% oxygen, which is sufficient to achieve an arterial oxygen tension (PaO_2) of between 50 and 60 mm Hg. A tidal volume (V_T) between 800 and 1200 mL is ideal for most adults. Children require proportionally smaller volumes.

Initially, two slow, deep breaths should be given over a period of 1 to 2 seconds each. Excessive volumes or an inspiratory rate that is too fast must be avoided, because this can push air into the stomach and cause **gastric distension.** An amount sufficient to cause a rise and fall of the chest should be used to gauge the volume needed in both children and adults.

The procedure for adults is as follows (Figure 31-4):

1. Place the victim on his or her back, on a hard, flat surface.
2. Kneel at the patient's side, and open and clear the airway as previously described. Pinch the victim's nose with your thumb and index finger close to the nares to prevent air from escaping during ventilation.
3. Take a deep breath and, while making a seal over the victim's mouth, exhale slowly but forcibly for 2 seconds for each breath. A good seal over the patient's mouth is essential. If you cannot get a good seal using this method, you should attempt mouth-to-nose ventilation.

4. Remove your mouth from the patient's mouth and allow him or her to exhale passively. Provide a second breath after exhalation is complete.
5. After successfully delivering two slow breaths, immediately assess the circulatory status.
6. Should the initial attempt to ventilate fail, reposition the victim's head and repeat the effort. If a second attempt at ventilation fails, the victim may have a foreign body airway obstruction, so proceed with methods described on p. 720.
7. Assuming mouth-to-mouth ventilation is successful and the patient remains apneic, continue the effort at a rate of one breath every 5 seconds to maintain the minimal adult rate of 12 breaths/min.

Although airway opening maneuvers for children and infants are similar to those for adults, there are several key differences. Anatomical differences in the infant's airway make it especially susceptible to occlusion by the tongue. Therefore the infant's head should be extended only slightly, or it should be tilted back gently into a neutral position when the head-tilt/chin-lift maneuver is used. The procedure for children and infants is as follows (Figure 31-5):

1. If the patient is an infant (younger than 1 year of age), create an airtight seal by placing your mouth over the infant's nose and mouth (see Figure 31-5).
2. If the patient is a child between 1 and 8 years old, ventilate his or her lungs using the same technique you would use for an adult (see Figure 31-4).
3. Provide an initial slow breath (1 to 1.5 seconds per breath) sufficient to cause a rise in the chest. In infants, small puffs of air from the rescuer's cheeks are usually sufficient to achieve adequate ventilation.
4. Remove your mouth and allow the victim to exhale passively. Provide a second breath after this deflation pause.

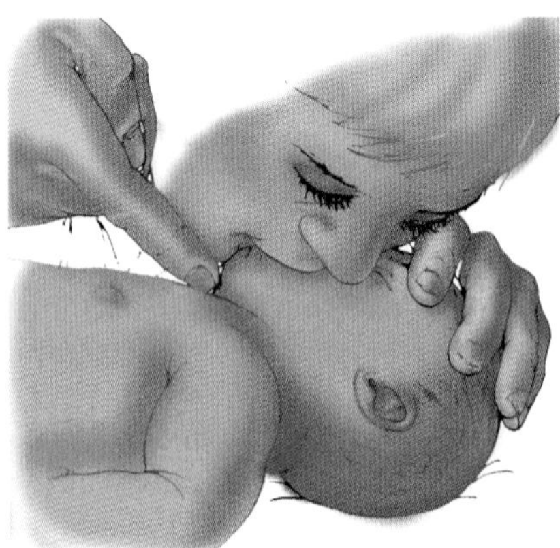

Figure 31-5
Mouth-to-mouth and nose seal for infants.

5. After successfully delivering two slow breaths, immediately assess the circulatory status.
6. If the initial attempt to ventilate fails, reposition the victim's head and repeat the effort. A child's head may need to be moved through a wide range of positions to secure an open airway. Remember that hyperextension of a child's neck can actually cause obstruction and should be avoided. If a second attempt at ventilation fails, the victim may have a foreign body airway obstruction, so proceed with the methods described on p. 720.
7. Assuming mouth-to-mouth ventilation is successful and the patient remains apneic, continue to provide one breath every 3 seconds to maintain a rate of 20 breaths/min.

Mouth-to-Nose Ventilation. Mouth-to-mouth ventilation cannot be performed in some situations. These include trismus (involuntary contraction of the jaw muscles; also known as *lockjaw*) and traumatic jaw or mouth injury. There are also times when it is difficult to maintain a tight seal with the lips using the mouth-to-mouth method. In these situations, mouth-to-nose ventilation should be used. The procedure is as follows (Figure 31-6):

1. Place the victim on his or her back.
2. Use the head-tilt/chin-lift maneuver to establish the airway, being sure to completely close the mouth.
3. Inhale deeply, and exhale into the patient's nose. Greater force may need to be applied than would be used with mouth-to-mouth ventilation, because the nasal passageways are smaller.

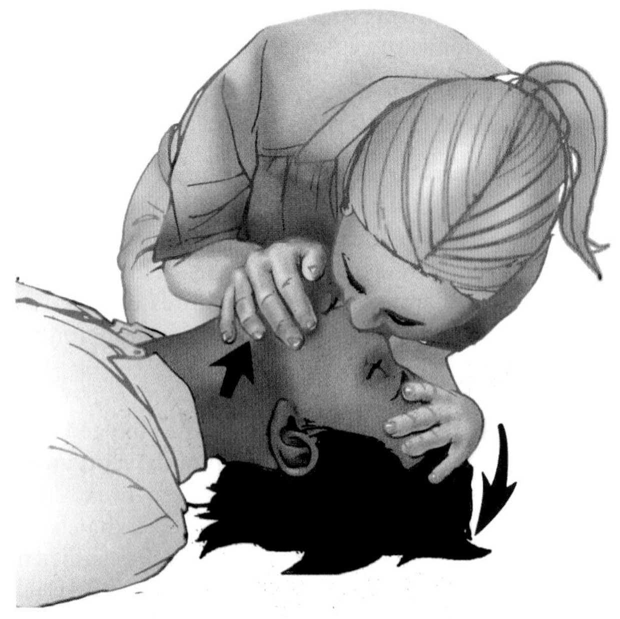

Figure 31-6
Mouth-to-nose ventilation.

4. Remove your mouth from the victim's nose to allow the patient to exhale passively. If the patient does not exhale through the nose (because of nasopharyngeal obstruction from the soft palate), open the victim's mouth or separate his or her lips to facilitate exhalation.
5. After successfully delivering two slow breaths, immediately assess the circulatory status.
6. If the victim remains apneic, maintain ventilation at the rate appropriate for his or her age.

Mouth-to-Stoma Ventilation. Patients with tracheostomies or laryngectomies can be ventilated directly through the stoma or tube. These patients can be identified by an obvious stoma or a tracheostomy or laryngectomy tube in place. Some patients wear a medical alert tag or bracelet indicating that a stoma is present. The procedure for mouth-to-stoma ventilation is as follows:

1. Place the victim on his or her back with the neck in vertical alignment. Usually, the neck does not need to be extended nor the nose or mouth sealed, because oropharyngeal structures are bypassed by the stoma.
2. Ensure that the stoma is clear of any obstructing matter and breathe directly into the stoma (or tube). If the victim has a cuffed tracheostomy tube in place, inflate the cuff to prevent air from escaping around the tube. If the tube is uncuffed, the mouth and nose may need to be sealed off with your hand or a tight-fitting face mask, if available.
3. After delivering two slow breaths, immediately assess the circulatory status.
4. If the victim remains apneic, maintain ventilation at the rate appropriate for his or her age.

Restoring Circulation

Determining Pulselessness

After giving two slow breaths, the rescuer should immediately determine whether a pulse is present. The rescuer must not attempt to restore circulation until pulselessness has been confirmed.

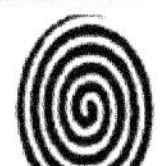

RULE OF THUMB

Careful assessment of the pulse for 5 to 10 seconds may help avoid unnecessary cardiac compressions.

Pulselessness is evaluated by palpating a major artery. In adults and children older than 1 year of age, the carotid artery in the neck should be palpated. To locate the carotid artery, the rescuer should maintain the head-tilt with one hand while sliding the fingers of the other hand into the groove created by the trachea and the large neck muscles (Figure 31-7). The carotid artery area must be palpated gently to avoid compressing the artery or pushing on the carotid sinus. Because the pulse may be slow, weak, or irregular, the artery must be assessed for approximately 8 to 10 seconds for the presence or absence of a pulse to be confirmed.

For infants, the brachial artery is preferred for assessing pulselessness. To palpate the brachial artery, the rescuer must grasp the infant's arm with his or her thumb outward, slide his or her fingers down toward the antecubital fossa, and press gently to feel for a pulse. The femoral artery also can be palpated, which may be done for an adult, a child, or an infant.

In hospital critical care settings, bedside monitoring equipment may provide supporting or confirming information regarding the respiratory or circulatory status of a patient. However, information obtained from these devices should never be a substitute for careful clinical assessment.

If the patient has a pulse but is not breathing, ventilation must be started immediately, at the appropriate rate. If no pulse is palpable, external chest compressions must be interposed with ventilatory support.

Providing Chest Compressions

Adequate circulation can be restored in the pulseless victim, using external chest compressions. To accomplish this, the rescuer manually compresses the lower half of the sternum (for the adult patient) in a serial fashion. Cardiac output produced by external chest compressions

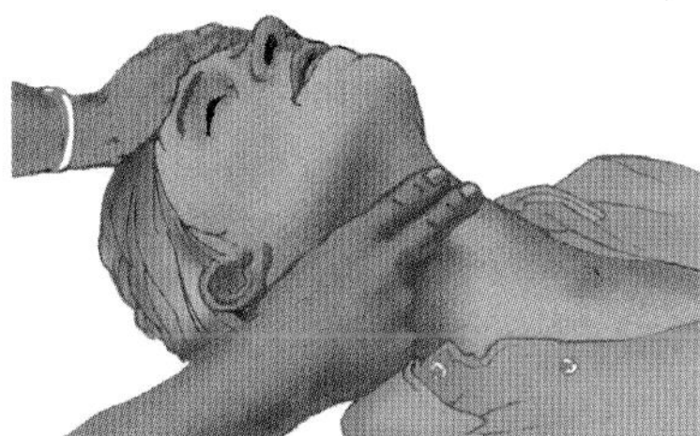

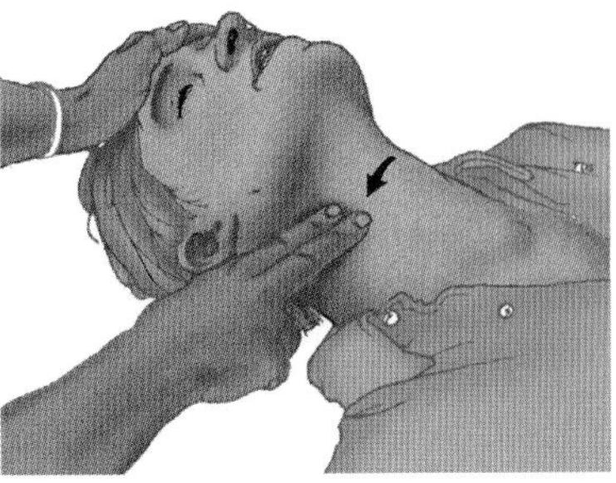

Figure 31-7
Determining pulselessness.

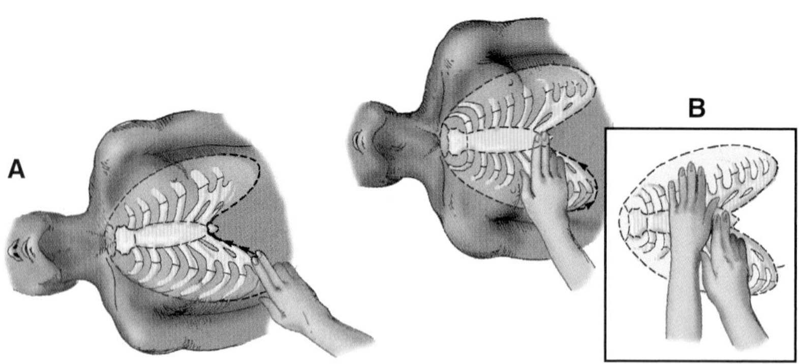

Figure 31-8
Xiphisternal junction. **A,** Locating junction. **B,** Hand position.

is approximately one fourth of normal cardiac output, with arterial systolic blood pressures between 60 and 80 mm Hg. Blood flow during chest compression probably results from both the pump action of the heart and changes in the intrathoracic pressure.

Adults. The procedure for providing chest compressions to adults is as follows (Figures 31-8 and 31-9):

1. Place the victim in a supine position on a firm surface, such as the ground or the floor, because chest compressions are more effective when the victim is on a firm surface. When victims are in bed or on a stretcher, place a board or tray under them. A cardiac arrest board is ideal, but a removable bed piece or food tray may have to be used.
2. Expose the patient's chest to identify landmarks for correct hand position. If the victim is fully clothed, quickly remove or cut off any clothing or underwear.
3. Choose a position close to the patient's upper chest so that the weight of your upper body can be used for compression. If the patient is on a bed or stretcher, stand next to it with the patient close to that side. If the bed is high, or you are short, you may need to lower the bed, stand on a stool or chair, or kneel on the bed next to the victim. If the patient is on the ground, kneel at his or her side.
4. Identify the lower half of the sternum. Locate the lower margin of the patient's rib cage that is closest to you. Palpate upward along the ribs to the midline, locating the notch where the ribs meet the sternum in the center of the lowest part of the chest (see Figure 31-8). Place two fingers on the junction, and the heel of the other hand next to the two fingers. Then place your other hand on top of the hand on the sternum, and lock your elbows.
5. Perform compression with the weight of your body exerting force on your outstretched arms, elbows held straight. Your shoulders should be positioned above the patient so that the thrust of each compression goes straight down onto the sternum, using your upper body weight and the hip joints as a fulcrum (see Figure 31-9). Do not let your hands leave the victim's chest.
6. Compress the sternum 1.5 to 2 inches (3.8 to 5.0 cm). Apply compressions regularly and rhythmically at a rate of 100 per minute, without bouncing or rolling the patient. The compression phase of the cycle should be equal in duration to the upstroke phase.
7. If CPR must be interrupted for transportation or advanced life support measures, chest compression should resume as quickly as possible. Compressions should not cease for more than 5 seconds (30 seconds if the victim is being intubated).

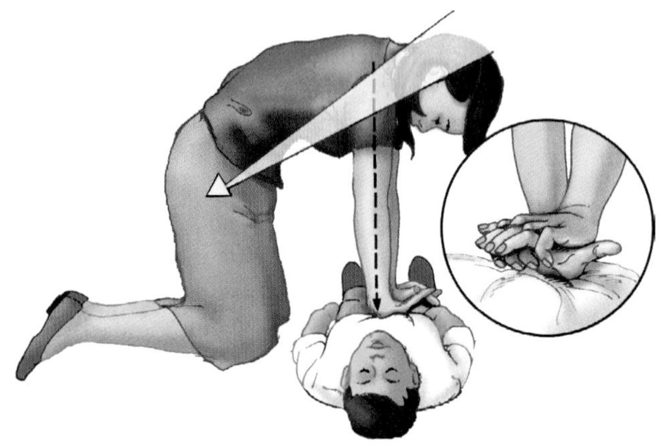

Figure 31-9
Practitioner's position for external cardiac compression. Note interlocked fingers to prevent pressure on rib cage.

Children. Children older than 8 years of age should receive chest compressions as outlined for adults, especially if they are large. The procedure for younger children (1 to 8 years old) is as follows:

1. Place the victim in the supine position on a firm surface. Small children may require additional support under the upper body. This is particularly true when chest compressions are given with mouth-to-mouth ventilation, because extension of

the neck raises the shoulders. The head should be no higher than the body.

2. As with the adult, identify the lower half of the sternum. Because the liver and spleen of younger children lie higher in the abdominal cavity, take special care to ensure proper positioning. Palpate upward along the rib cage toward the midline until you reach the notch where the sternum and ribs meet. Place the heel of the hand you will use for compression two finger widths above this point. However, use the other hand to maintain head position and maintain an airway.
3. Compress the chest approximately 1 to 1.5 inches at a rate of 100 per minute. In general, the heel of one hand is sufficient to achieve compression. As with adults, compression and relaxation times should be equal in length and delivered smoothly.

Infants. The procedure for infants (up to 1 year of age) is as follows (Figure 31-10):

1. Use the lower half of the sternum for compression in the infant. Proper placement is determined by imagining a line across the chest connecting the nipples. Place your index finger along this line on the sternum. Then place your middle and ring fingers next to the index finger. Raise your index finger and perform compressions with the middle and ring fingers. Use the other hand to maintain the infant's head position and airway.
2. Compress the sternum approximately ½ to 1 inch at a rate of at least 120 per minute. Compression and upstroke phases should be equal in length and delivered smoothly. Your fingers should remain on the chest at all times.

Neonates. For neonates, life-threatening emergencies commonly result from hypoxia and hypothermia. Rapid correction of these problems may forestall the need for CPR. However, chest compressions are indicated if the neonate's heart rate falls below 60 beats/min or remains between 60 and 80 beats/min for more than 30 seconds, despite adequate ventilation with 100% oxygen.

Neonatal chest compression can be performed using a "wraparound" technique (Figure 31-11). To use this method, the rescuer encircles the neonate's chest with both hands and positions his or her thumbs on the victim's sternum, using the other fingers of both hands to support the neonate's back. The rescuer should position his or her thumbs just below the victim's intermammary line, making sure not to compress the xiphoid process. He or she should compress ½ to ¾ inch, at a rate of 120 per minute. Compression should be performed smoothly, with downstroke and upstroke times approximately equal. After every third compression, the neonate should receive a breath of 100% oxygen.

Chest Compressions Under Special Circumstances

The following unique circumstances require modification of the normal procedures for applying cardiac compressions: near drowning, electrical shock, and patients with pacemakers or prosthetic heart valves.

Near Drowning. When cardiac arrest occurs as a result of drowning, the victim must be moved as quickly as possible to a firm surface. Cardiac compressions cannot be given while a victim is in the water.

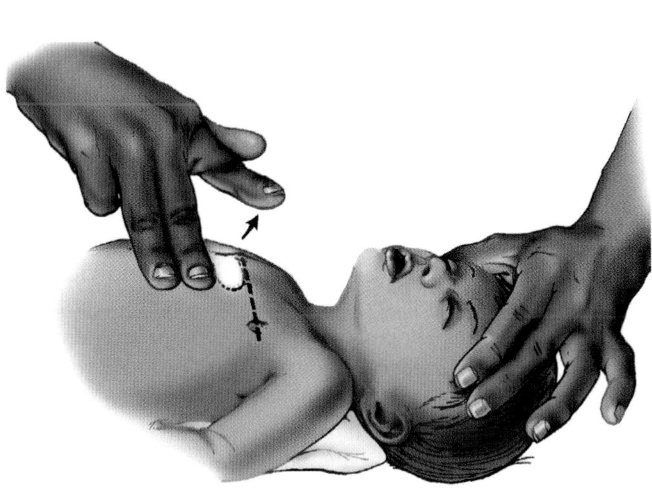

Figure 31-10
Position for chest compression in infants.

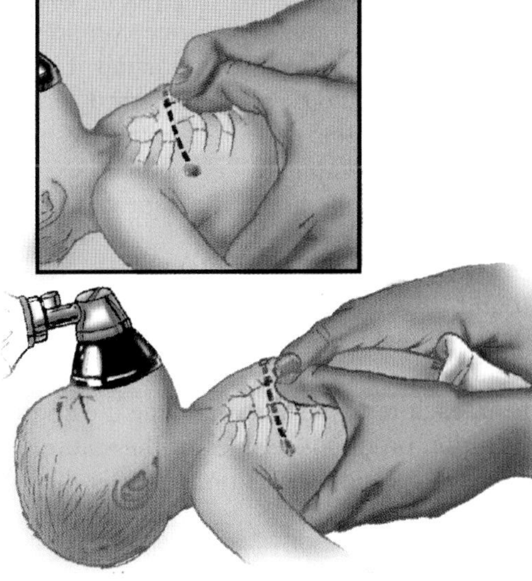

Figure 31-11
Neonatal chest compression using the wraparound technique.

Electrical Shock. Electrical shock can cause either cardiac or respiratory arrest. Cardiac arrest is caused by ventricular fibrillation. Respiratory arrest occurs secondary to paralysis of the ventilatory muscles. Initially, the victim must be removed from contact with the source of electricity and evaluated. *The rescuer must pay special attention to his or her own safety!* A victim who is still connected to an electrical source must not be touched. The power must be turned off. If cardiac arrest has occurred, CPR should be administered immediately.

Pacemakers. Individuals with pacemakers may suffer cardiac arrest as a result of battery failure or other mechanical difficulties. The CPR procedure for a person with a pacemaker is similar to that previously described.

Artificial Heart Valves. Chest compressions can damage the heart of a patient who has recently undergone surgery for artificial heart valve implantation (especially mitral or tricuspid valves). However, the patient will die if nothing is done. For this reason, external cardiac compressions should be done until a qualified surgeon can perform an emergency thoracotomy and internal cardiac compression.

One- Versus Two-Rescuer Adult CPR

Outside the hospital, one-rescuer CPR is common. In such cases, the rescuer must assess the victim, call for help, and begin CPR without assistance from others. This requires the rescuer to remain calm and remember the steps of one-rescuer CPR. The technique for opening the airway, giving mouth-to-mouth breaths, and performing chest compressions is the same, regardless of the number of rescuers.

When performing CPR alone, the rescuer must remember to give two breaths to 15 compressions for adult victims and five breaths to one compression for children and infants. After approximately 1 minute of CPR, the patient should be reassessed for determination of any response. If the patient does not respond and remains pulseless and apneic, CPR should be continued, and the reassessment should be repeated every few minutes until help arrives.

When two rescuers are available, the assessment, rescue, and evaluation can be shared. One rescuer ventilates and evaluates the effectiveness of CPR. The other administers cardiac compressions. To facilitate movement, each rescuer should assume the appropriate rescue position on opposite sides of the victim. For the adult, the compression/ventilation ratio is the same as for the single rescuer (15:2), and the timing for compressions is "one and two and three and four and five" (a rate of 100 times per minute).

When two people provide support, the individual providing compressions briefly pauses after the fifteenth compression so that the other person can administer the ventilation. The cycle is then repeated. After the first minute, the pulse is reassessed. If there is no pulse, CPR is continued. Reassessment is performed every few minutes thereafter. If a pulse returns, the airway must be maintained and ventilations supported as needed.

To provide rest for the individual delivering cardiac compressions, the rescuers may change positions. The individual doing cardiac compressions calls for the change, saying in sequence with compression, "We/will/change/next/time," or words to this effect. The individual providing ventilation gives a breath at the end of the next compression cycle and moves quickly into position for cardiac compression. The individual previously responsible for compressions moves to the head and checks for a carotid pulse. If no pulse is found, he or she should give one breath. The cycle then continues with the two rescuers in their new positions.

Rescue attempts should continue until (1) advanced life support is available, (2) the rescuers note spontaneous pulse and breathing, or (3) a physician pronounces the victim dead. A cardiopulmonary emergency presents a crisis for the victim and his or her family, and appropriate support and intervention should be provided for both. Victims who survive CPR should be transported quickly to tertiary care facilities, ideally only after advanced life support is instituted.

Automated External Defibrillation

Early Defibrillation

Since 1990, the AHA has recommended adding a fourth step to the treatment of cardiac arrest. This step involves early defibrillation, after the airway has been established and CPR has been initiated. The rationale for this is as follows: (1) The most common initial rhythm in witnessed sudden cardiac arrest is ventricular fibrillation, (2) the most effective treatment for ventricular fibrillation is electrical defibrillation, (3) the probability of successful defibrillation diminishes rapidly over time, and (4) ventricular fibrillation tends to convert to asystole within a few minutes.[6] Studies have shown that the survival rate increases significantly when defibrillation is available for use by the initial rescuers.[6,10]

The AHA recommendation is that **automatic external defibrillators (AEDs)** be made available to individuals expected to respond to emergencies, such as police, security personnel, ski patrol personnel, flight attendants, and first-aid volunteers (Figure 31-12). Early defibrillation has already proven to be effective in saving lives of people who otherwise may have not been successfully resuscitated.[10-12] After appropriate training and implementation of the ABCs, this step is inserted as the letter *D,* for Defibrillation. This step should be initiated within 5 minutes of when CPR is begun.

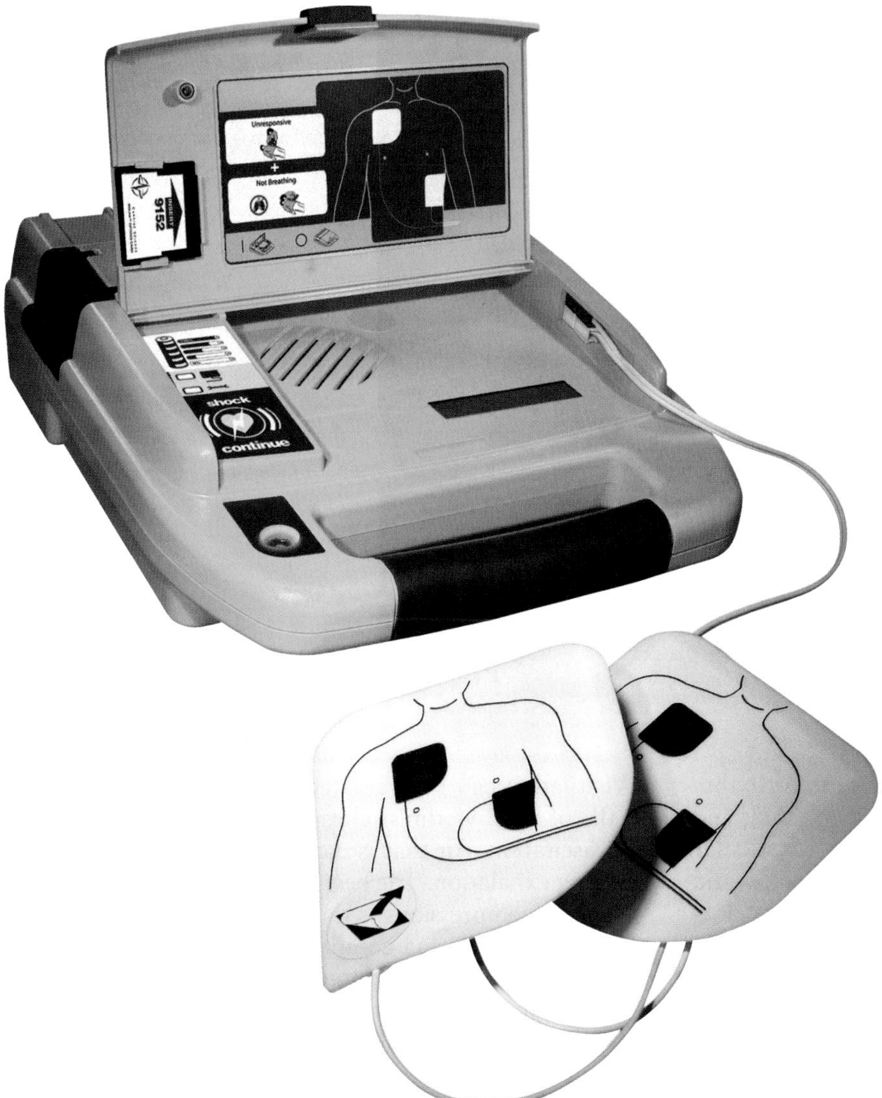

Figure 31-12
Powerheart AED with pads attached. *(Courtesy Cardiac Science Inc., Irvine, California, www.cardiacscience.com.)*

Personnel employed at high-acuity hospitals would not be equipped with AEDs, because access to ACLS is readily available, usually within minutes of the code being called. However, low-acuity hospitals, skilled nursing facilities, and other medical facilities that do not have a code team on the premises would benefit from AEDs. RTs working at such facilities should inquire whether one is on the premises, and if so, where it is located and how it functions. If one is not present, a recommendation should be made to the facility's administration to have one purchased. The AHA recommends that an AED be available wherever CPR is likely to be performed.

Until recently, the AED had received approval by the U.S. Food and Drug Administration (FDA) only for use in adults and children older than 8 years of age. In May 2001, the Heartstream FR2 AED (Agilent Technologies, Inc., Palo Alto, California) was approved for use on infants and children up to age 8 and/or on those weighing up to 55 lb.[13] This device delivers 50 J of energy when pediatric pads are used and 150 J when adult pads are connected. Other AEDs may also receive FDA approval for use in infants and children in the future.

The AHA is also promoting public access defibrillation (PAD) programs. These programs endeavor to place AEDs throughout the community and to train lay rescuers in CPR and in the use of the AED. In the spirit of community service, RTs are encouraged to become involved in these programs and to lend their support and expertise in helping improve survival from sudden, out-of-hospital cardiac arrest.

Automatic External Defibrillators

The AED functions more in a semiautomated fashion; it only recommends that a shock be delivered, rather than initiating one automatically. Fully automatic defibrillators are available but are used only in special circumstances. Adhesive electrodes from the AED are attached to the patient. Once all of the equipment is hooked up, the

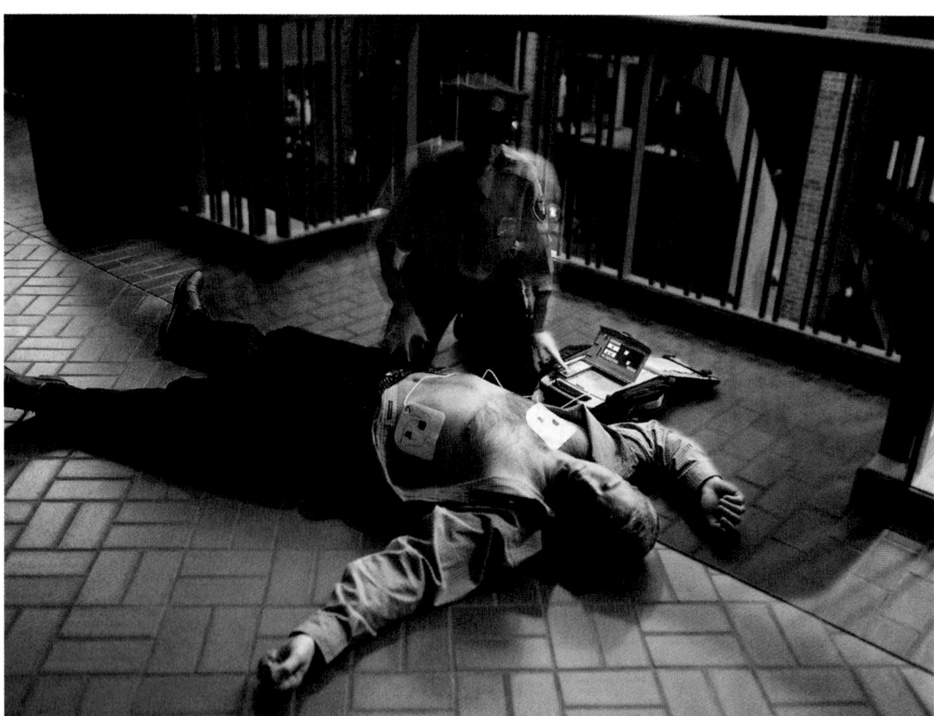

Figure 31-13
Positioning of rescuer and placement of pads when using the AED. *(Courtesy Cardiac Science Inc., Irvine, California, www.cardiacscience.com.)*

"Analyze" button should be pressed to begin. A rhythm recognition program analyzes the patient's rhythm, and if it detects ventricular tachycardia or ventricular fibrillation, it advises the rescuer through voice and visual prompts that a shock be delivered. If a shock is indicated, the rescuer should "Clear" the patient and press the "Shock" button. Once the shock has been delivered, he or she should press the "Analyze" button to determine if another shock is necessary. The victim may be shocked three times in succession, with analysis of rhythm in between, before CPR is resumed. If the AED has the option to increase the strength of each shock, the rescuer should begin with the lowest level for the first shock and then progress to the highest level by the third shock. If it does not have this option, he or she should press the indicated "Shock" button whenever directed by the AED to do so. After the third shock, if there are still no signs of circulation, CPR should be resumed for approximately 1 minute. Then, the rescuer should check for circulation once more, and if no signs are found, he or she should analyze the rhythm again and follow the directions of the AED. If the message reads "No shock indicated," CPR should be performed for 1 to 2 minutes and then the rhythm analysis should be repeated. This should be continued until assistance arrives. Figure 31-13 indicates how the AED is used by the rescuer.

Evaluating the Effectiveness of CPR

It is important for CPR providers to judge continuously both the effectiveness of CPR and the victim's response. Ventilation can be evaluated by observing the rise and fall of the victim's chest during mouth-to-mouth resuscitation. Air that is escaping can be heard and felt during exhalation. The best indicator of the effectiveness of chest compressions is the presence of a peripheral or central pulse during compression. The pulse should be palpable with each compression. The victim's skin color also provides important information. The return of normal color, particularly in the nailbeds and mucous membranes, indicates effective oxygenation.

Hazards and Complications

The most common complications that occur with CPR are as follows: (1) worsening of existing neck or spine injuries, (2) gastric distension and vomiting, and (3) trauma to internal structures during chest compressions.

Neck and Spine Injuries

Healthcare providers can aggravate neck or spine injuries by inappropriately moving the victim's head. This can be avoided by carefully assessing the victim for head, neck, or spine injuries. If this type of injury is apparent, the head should be carefully supported and side-to-side motion must be avoided. In such situations, using the jaw thrust maneuver rather than the head-tilt/chin-lift method to open the airway is recommended. If the jaw thrust is unsuccessful in establishing an airway, the rescuer should try a slight head-tilt.

Resuscitation in Acute Care Hospitals

AARC Clinical Practice Guideline (Excerpts)*

➤ INDICATIONS

Indications for cardiac arrest, respiratory arrest, or conditions that may lead to cardiopulmonary arrest, as indicated by rapid deterioration in vital signs, level of consciousness, and blood gas values, are as follows:

- Airway obstruction
- Acute, unstable MI
- Severe arrhythmias
- Hypovolemic shock
- Severe infections
- Spinal cord or head injury
- Drug overdose
- Pulmonary embolus
- Anaphylaxis
- Pulmonary edema
- Smoke inhalation
- High-risk delivery

➤ CONTRAINDICATIONS

Resuscitation is contraindicated in the following circumstances:

- The patient's desire not to be resuscitated has been clearly expressed and documented in his or her medical record.
- Resuscitation has been determined to be futile because of the patient's underlying condition or disease.

➤ PRECAUTIONS, HAZARDS, AND COMPLICATIONS

The following are airway management hazards and complications:

- Failure to establish airway
- Failure to intubate the trachea
- Failure to recognize intubation of the esophagus
- Dental accidents
- Trauma to the airway or esophagus
- Hypertension and tachycardia
- Aspiration
- Cervical spine trauma
- Unrecognized bronchial intubation
- Arrhythmias
- Eye injury
- Inappropriate tube size
- Facial trauma
- Problems with the endotracheal (ET) tube cuff
- Bronchospasm
- Hypotension and bradycardia
- Laryngospasm

The following are hazards and complications of manual ventilation:

- Hypoventilation or hyperventilation
- Failure to establish adequate functional residual capacity (FRC) (newborns)
- Hypotension caused by reduced venous return
- Prolonged lapse in ventilation for intubation
- Gastric insufflation or rupture

The following are hazards and complications of circulatory maneuvers:

- Ineffective chest compression
- Fractured ribs or sternum
- Laceration of the spleen or liver
- Failure to restore circulation despite functional rhythm

Continued

RESUSCITATION IN ACUTE CARE HOSPITALS—Cont'd

AARC Clinical Practice Guideline (Excerpts)*

The following are hazards and complications of electrical therapy:
- Failure of the defibrillator
- Shock to team members
- Inappropriate countershock
- Fire hazard
- Induction of arrhythmias
- Pacemaker interference

The following are hazards and complications of drug administration:
- Inappropriate drug or dose
- Idiosyncratic or allergic response to a drug
- ET tube drug-delivery failure

➤ ASSESSMENT OF NEED

Assessment of patient condition includes the following:
- Prearrest—identification of patients (including a fetus) in danger of imminent arrest and for whom consequent early intervention may prevent arrest and improve outcome. These patients have conditions that may lead to cardiopulmonary arrest, as indicated by rapid deterioration of vital signs, level of consciousness, blood gas values, or fetal monitoring data.
- Arrest—absence of spontaneous breathing or circulation.
- Postarrest—once a patient has sustained an arrest, the likelihood of additional life-threatening problems is high, and continued vigilance and aggressive action using this guideline are indicated. Control of the airway and cardiac monitoring must be continued, and optimal oxygenation and ventilation must be ensured.

➤ ASSESSMENT OF PROCESS AND OUTCOME

- Timely, high-quality resuscitation improves patient outcome in terms of survival and level of function. Despite optimal resuscitation performance, outcomes are affected by patient-specific factors. Patient condition after cardiac arrest should be evaluated from this perspective.
- Documentation and evaluation of the resuscitation process (e.g., system activation, team member performance, functioning of equipment, adherence to guidelines and algorithms) should occur continuously, and improvements should be made.

➤ MONITORING

Clinical assessment—continuous observation of the patient and repeated clinical assessment by a trained observer provide optimal monitoring of the resuscitation process. Special consideration should be given to the following:
- Level of consciousness
- Adequacy of airway
- Adequacy of ventilation
- Peripheral/apical pulse and character
- Evidence of chest and head trauma
- Pulmonary compliance and airway resistance
- Seizure activity

Assessment of physiological parameters—repeat assessment of physiological data by trained professionals supplements clinical assessment in monitoring patients throughout the resuscitation process. Monitoring devices should be available, accessible, functional, and evaluated periodically for function. These data include the following:
- Arterial blood gas studies, which may have a limited role in the decision-making process during CPR
- Hemodynamic data
- Cardiac rhythm
- Ventilatory frequency, tidal volume, and airway pressure
- Exhaled CO_2
- Neurological status

RESUSCITATION IN ACUTE CARE HOSPITALS—Cont'd

AARC Clinical Practice Guideline (Excerpts)*

Resuscitation process—if properly performed, resuscitation should improve patient outcome. Continuous monitoring of the process will identify the following areas needing improvement:

- Response time
- Equipment function
- Equipment availability
- Team member performance
- Team performance
- Complication rate
- Patient survival and functional status

*For the complete guideline, see Respir Care 38:179, 1993.

Gastric Distension

During prolonged mouth-to-mouth ventilation, air enters the esophagus and stomach. Therefore some gastric distension is not unusual, particularly in children, and appears in approximately 17% of cases.[14] Severe gastric distension puts pressure on the diaphragm, restricting lung expansion. Gastric distension also can increase vagal tone and cause reflex bradycardia and hypotension.

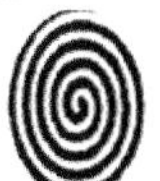

RULE OF THUMB

The best way to avoid gastric distension during artificial ventilation is to provide inspiratory breaths with low to moderate flows.

However, most important is the fact that severe gastric distension prompts regurgitation. Because the unconscious patient lacks normal upper airway reflexes, regurgitated stomach contents can be aspirated easily into the lungs. Massive aspiration of stomach contents into the lungs almost always causes death by making ventilation virtually impossible, or it leads to severe lung injury that causes death days or weeks later.

Vomiting

Vomiting is another complication associated with abdominal thrusts, and one that is impossible to avoid in some victims. Vomiting itself is a minor problem. The hazard is the aspiration of vomitus into the lung. Aspiration can be prevented only by using the accessory airway equipment and the procedures discussed on p. 722.

Internal Trauma

External cardiac compression is hazardous, and every attempt should be made to minimize trauma by using the correct technique. Complications associated with chest compression include the following: gastric perforation, laceration of the liver, contusion of the lung, fractured ribs and/or sternum, pneumothorax, hemothorax, cardiac tamponade, and soft tissue emphysema.[14,15] These complications most often are linked to improper hand position. Placement of the hands too far to either the left or right can cause fractured ribs or lacerated lung. Incorrect placement on the left can injure the heart. Placing the hands too high on the sternum can fracture the sternum; placing the hands too low can cause a fractured xiphoid process or a lacerated liver. Correct identification of landmarks and proper hand placement minimizes the likelihood of these complications.

Internal Organ Damage

The major hazard associated with abdominal thrusts, which are performed when an individual has choked and lost consciousness, is possible damage to internal organs, such as laceration or rupture of abdominal or thoracic viscera.[16] The risk of this complication can be minimized by the rescuer placing his or her arms and fist below the victim's xiphoid process and lower margin of the ribs.

Foreign Object Removal

Manual removal of foreign material from the upper airway also can be hazardous because of the possibility of forcing the object deeper into the airway. This hazard can be minimized by attempting to remove only those objects that are within reach.

Contraindications to CPR

The pulseless, apneic patient will die within 4 to 6 minutes without intervention. Fear of further harm should never influence the decision to begin CPR. CPR is contraindicated only when the patient is obviously biologically dead (as noted by such findings as rigor mortis). In the hospital, CPR is contraindicated when a valid "Do Not Resuscitate" (DNR) order is in effect or when a properly executed living will (advanced directive) specifically requests that CPR not be initiated.

Health Concerns and CPR

Recent concerns have arisen among both laypersons and healthcare professionals regarding possible transmission of infectious diseases, such as acquired immunodeficiency syndrome (AIDS), during CPR.[17,18] In one survey, 45% of the physicians and 80% of the nurses who responded indicated that they would refuse to provide mouth-to-mouth ventilation for a stranger.[19] The actual risk of disease transmission during mouth-to-mouth ventilation is very small. No reports on transmission of human immunodeficiency virus, hepatitis B virus, hepatitis C virus, or cytomegalovirus were found.[20] However, the reluctance to initiate CPR poses a clear threat to the effectiveness of early intervention in life-threatening emergencies, which affects the public as a whole.

Personnel with a duty to provide CPR should follow the guidelines established by the Centers for Disease Control and Prevention (CDC) and the Occupational Safety and Health Administration. These recommendations include the use of latex gloves, masks, and goggles.[6] Mechanical barrier aids to ventilation (e.g., masks, filters, valves) also have been suggested, to allay fear as much as to protect the rescuer. However, these devices require training to be used properly, are not universally available, and may not be as effective as mouth-to-mouth ventilation.

Although, technically, blood or body fluids can be exchanged through mouth-to-mouth ventilation, CDC surveillance of job-related contraction of AIDS has never discovered such an incident.[20]

Other infectious diseases, such as herpes simplex and tuberculosis, may present a higher risk to the rescuer, but few cases have been reported. Although the risk of transmission is believed to be low, healthcare providers who perform mouth-to-mouth ventilation on someone suspected of having tuberculosis should get a follow-up evaluation using standard approaches. In addition, any practitioner who might hesitate to provide mouth-to-mouth ventilation to a victim in need should always carry (and know how to use) an appropriate barrier device for this purpose.

Equipment contaminated with blood or other body fluids during a resuscitation effort should always be discarded in appropriate receptacles or thoroughly cleaned and disinfected according to hospital protocols.

Dealing With an Obstructed Airway

Early recognition of foreign body airway obstruction is critical. Foreign bodies may cause either partial or complete obstruction. Partial obstruction may allow nearly adequate air exchange, in which case the patient remains conscious and coughing. As long as air exchange is present, the patient should be reassured and allowed to clear his or her own airway by coughing.

If partial obstruction persists, or air exchange worsens, the EMS should be activated. Poor air exchange exists when the patient has a weak or ineffective cough, increased inspiratory difficulty, or cyanosis.

With a completely obstructed airway, the patient commonly clutches at his or her throat. This is known as the *universal distress signal* for foreign body obstruction. The person with a complete obstruction cannot talk, cough, or breathe, and is in dire need of emergency intervention using the Heimlich maneuver.

If attempts to open a victim's airway are unsuccessful, or if a foreign body is present in the victim's mouth or pharynx, several procedures can be used to obtain a clear passageway. For adults and children, the procedure of choice for clearing a foreign body is the abdominal thrust, or **Heimlich maneuver.**[6] For infants with an obstructed airway, the rescuer should attempt back blows first and, if unsuccessful, he or she should try chest thrusts. Back blows should not be used on the adult choking victim. However, chest thrusts may be used in place of abdominal thrusts on women in the advanced stages of pregnancy and on markedly obese individuals. Both procedures normally are followed by a manual check and removal of any obstructing foreign material.

Abdominal Thrusts (Heimlich Maneuver)

Forceful thrusts applied to the epigastrium can dislodge an obstruction caused by a food bolus, vomitus, or other foreign body. Quick thrusts to the abdomen rapidly displace the diaphragm upward, thus increasing intrathoracic pressure and creating expulsive expiratory airflow. As with a normal cough, this expulsive airflow may be sufficient to expel the foreign body from the airway. The procedure for performing abdominal thrusts on adults and children is as follows (Figure 31-14):

1. If the victim is sitting or standing, stand behind him or her and wrap your arms around the victim's waist. Make a fist with one hand and place the thumb side midline on the abdomen slightly above the navel and well below the tip of the xiphoid process (see Figure 31-14). Grasp the fist with the

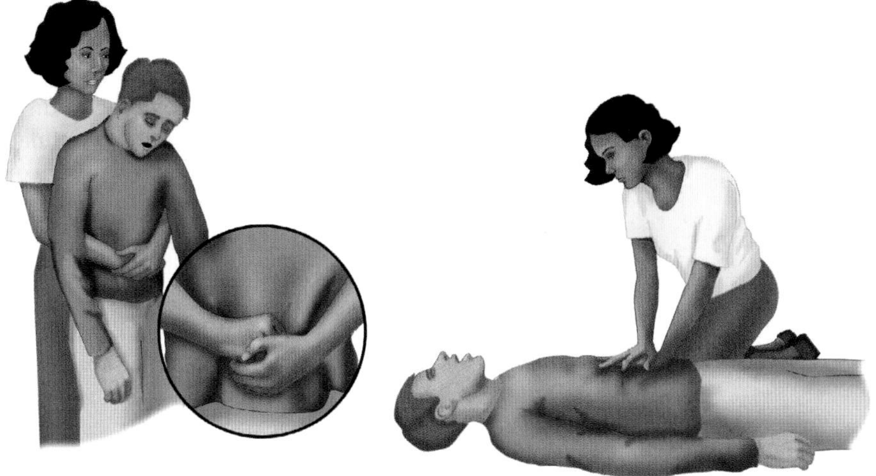

Figure 31-14
Abdominal thrusts. *Left*, Adult victim standing. *Right*, Adult victim lying.

other hand and deliver a quick upward and inward thrust. Each thrust should be a separate and distinct movement. Repeat the process until the obstruction is removed or the victim loses consciousness.

2. If the victim has collapsed or is unconscious, the abdominal thrust can be delivered with the victim in the supine position. Place the victim in the supine position (i.e., face-up), so that the foreign body can be easily expelled. If the victim vomits, quickly turn the victim's head to the side and wipe out the mouth. Kneel astride the victim's hips and place the heel of one hand on the abdomen between the umbilicus and the xiphoid process, and the other hand on top. Then press both hands forward to give a quick upward thrust, repeating five times, or as needed.
3. An alternative approach is to kneel near the victim's hips with your shoulders over the victim, and, using the same hand position, press on the epigastrium (see Figure 31-14). This position is preferred if you also must perform mouth-to-mouth ventilation or external cardiac compression, because you can change position easily. If two rescuers are available, one can give the abdominal thrusts while the other manages the airway and retrieves the foreign body.
4. A conscious victim who is alone can attempt to dislodge the foreign body with self-administered abdominal thrusts, performed by pressing his or her fist into the abdomen or pushing the abdomen against a firm surface such as a counter top, sink, chair back, railing, or tabletop.

After each cycle of abdominal thrusts, the rescuer should check the oral cavity by sweeping it with two or three fingers. After removing any foreign material, he or she should attempt to ventilate the patient again. If ventilation can be provided, breathing and circulation should be assessed and appropriate intervention taken. If the patient cannot be ventilated, another cycle of thrusts should be instituted, followed by an airway check and an attempt to ventilate. This procedure should be repeated until the airway is open and the patient can be ventilated.

Back Blows and Chest Thrusts

Because the Heimlich maneuver can easily cause abdominal injury when applied to infants, a combination of back blows and chest thrusts should be used to clear foreign bodies from the upper airway. Back blows alone may create sufficient force to dislodge trapped objects, but if this is ineffective, the back blows should be followed with five chest thrusts. The rescuer should continue inspecting the airway until the airway is restored. This procedure is as follows (Figure 31-15):

1. Back blows can be administered to infants more efficiently if you hold the child straddled over one arm with the head lower than the body.
2. Use the flat portion of your hand to gently, but quickly, deliver five back blows between the shoulder blades.
3. If the back blows do not clear the infant's airway, turn the infant over and institute a series of five chest thrusts. Like the abdominal thrust, the chest thrust creates a rapid rise in intrathoracic pressure, thereby aiding expulsion of the foreign body. Chest thrusts for infants are performed in the same manner and at the same location as those used for cardiac compressions, but at a slower rate.
4. As for adults, try to clear the airway between attempts to expel the foreign body. To do this, first visually inspect the oral cavity and remove any foreign matter you can see. Deep blind finger sweeps of an infant or child's mouth is not recommended.

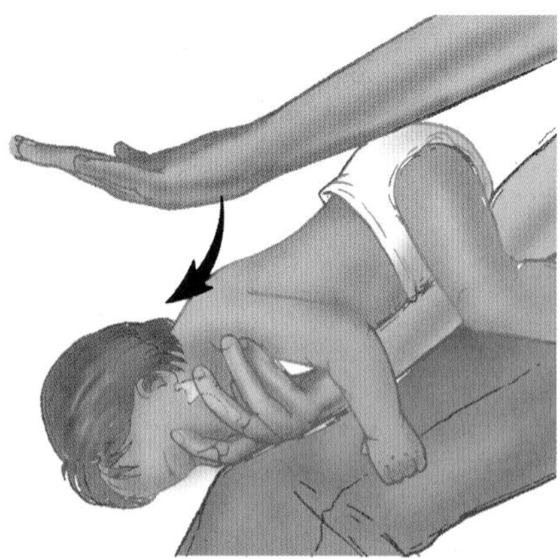

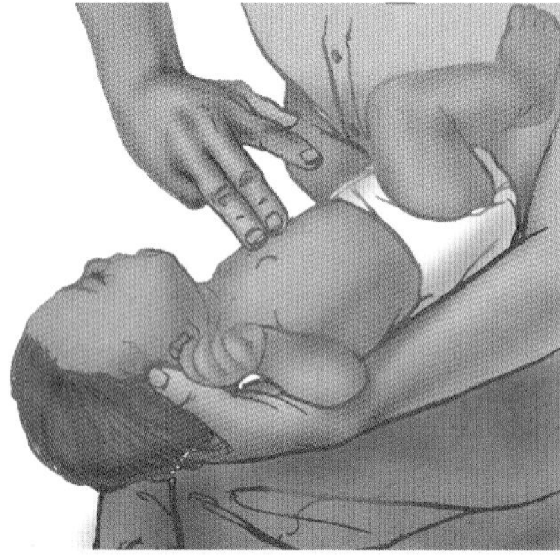

Figure 31-15
Use of back blows and chest thrusts to clear foreign bodies from infant airway.

Evaluating the Effectiveness of Foreign Body Removal

After each airway restoration maneuver, the rescuer must determine whether the foreign body has been expelled and the obstructed airway cleared. If the foreign body has not been dislodged, the appropriate sequence (abdominal thrusts for adults and children, back blows and chest thrusts for infants) should be repeated until successful.

Successful removal of an obstructing body is indicated by the following: (1) confirmed expulsion of the foreign body, (2) clear breathing and the ability to speak, (3) return of consciousness, and (4) return of normal color.

If successive attempts to clear the airway by these means fail, more aggressive techniques are indicated, if available. These include direct laryngoscopy and foreign body removal with Magill forceps, transtracheal catheterization, cricothyrotomy, and tracheotomy. Obviously, these methods require specially trained personnel and equipment, and they are aptly categorized as advanced life support techniques. Transtracheal catheterization and cricothyrotomy are discussed later in this chapter, and laryngoscopy, bronchoscopy, and tracheotomy were described in Chapter 30.

► ADVANCED CARDIAC LIFE SUPPORT

ACLS extends BLS capabilities by providing additional measures beyond immediate ventilatory and circulatory assistance. These measures include using accessory equipment to support ventilation and oxygenation, monitoring the electrocardiogram (ECG), establishing an intravenous (IV) route for drug administration, and applying selected pharmacological agents and electrical therapies (Figure 31-16). However, evidence suggests that in the prehospital setting, defibrillation is the most valuable measure.[8]

During ACLS in the hospital, the RT assumes primary responsibility for supporting oxygenation, establishing and maintaining the airway, and providing ventilation. Practitioners must demonstrate high levels of proficiency in these advanced life support skills.

Support for Oxygenation

Although expired air ventilation provides an acceptable level of oxygenation, low cardiac output, pulmonary shunting, and abnormalities during CPR lead to hypoxia. Hypoxia, in turn, results in anaerobic metabolism and metabolic acidosis. Metabolic acidosis impedes the action of certain drugs and can diminish the effectiveness of electrical therapies. For these reasons, the highest possible concentration of oxygen should be administered as soon as possible. Concerns about oxygen toxicity are not valid during this period of resuscitation.

During ACLS, supplemental oxygen is normally given through accessory devices designed to support ventilation. Thus the ability of these devices to provide a high F_{IO_2} is a key factor in judging their performance.

Airway Control

Accessory equipment designed to provide airway control during ACLS includes a variety of masks and artificial airways.

Masks

A mask that fits the patient well is a useful tool for the application of artificial ventilation by appropriately trained rescuers. It may be used to ventilate the victim with a bag-valve device or simply with the rescuer using his or her own lungs to ventilate the patient. In the latter situation, the mask is connected to an oxygen source, and the procedure is referred to as *mouth-to-mask ventilation.* In general, mouth-to-mask ventilation is easier to perform than ventilation using the bag-valve mask (BVM); however, a higher F_{IO_2} can be delivered with the BVM.

An ideal mask should be made of transparent material, be capable of sealing tightly against the face, provide an

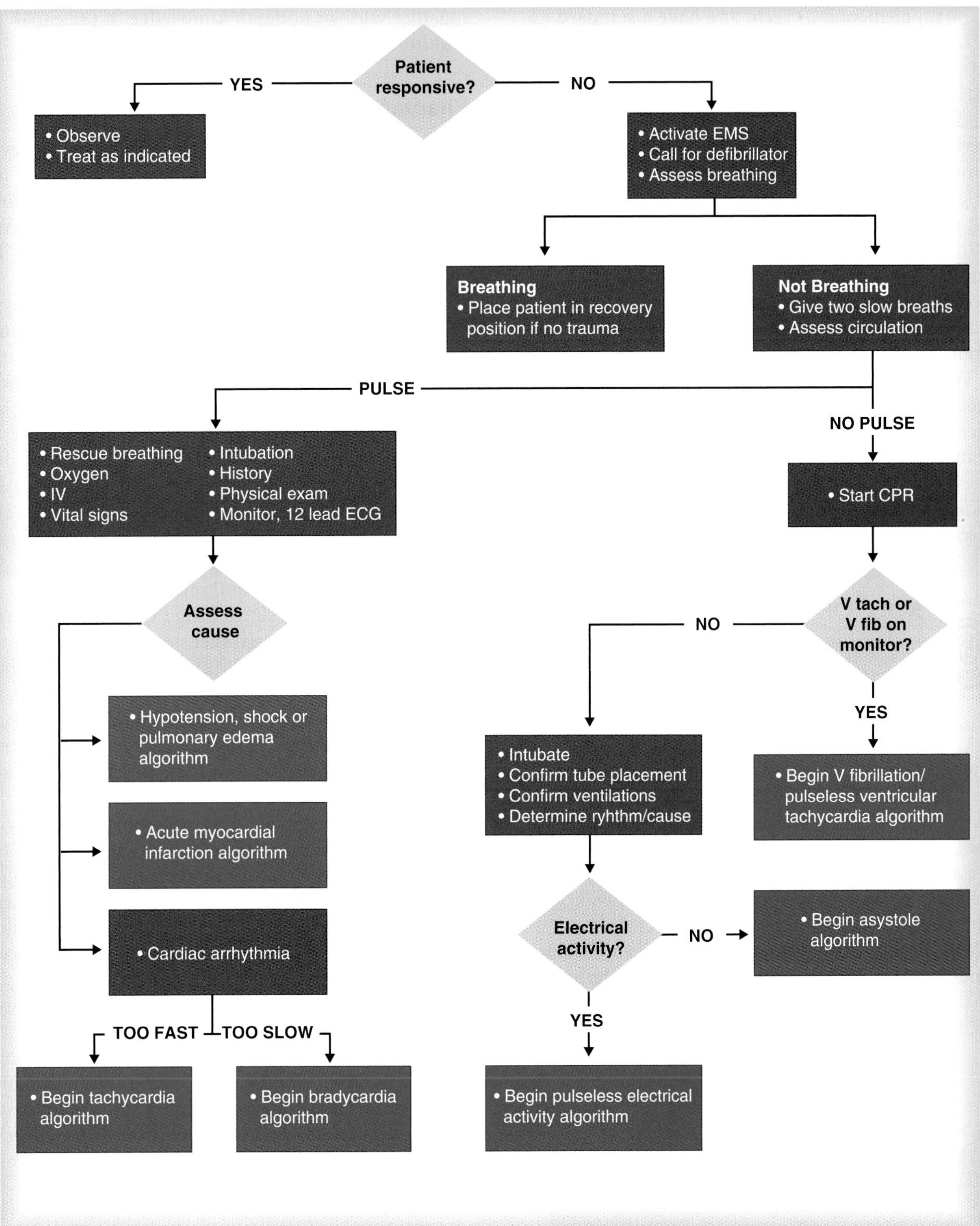

Figure 31-16
American Heart Association universal algorithm for adult emergency cardiac care. *V fib*, Ventricular fibrillation; *V tach*, ventricular tachycardia. *(Courtesy American Heart Association.)*

inlet for supplemental oxygen, and have a standard 15- and 22-mm connection.[6] In addition, it should be available in various sizes to accommodate adults, children, and infants. One-way valves, if provided, should be simple, dependable, and jam free.

The use of masks to support ventilation presumes that the airway can be maintained by conventional BLS techniques. Application of the mouth-to-mask technique is best performed with the practitioner positioned at the head of the victim, using the head-tilt maneuver to maintain the airway (Figure 31-17). Obviously, this approach is possible only when a second person is available to provide chest compressions.

Mouth-to-mask ventilation with supplemental oxygen is a viable alternative to BVM methods of airway maintenance and ventilation. Because masks can serve as barriers, fear of disease transmission can be minimized and rapid response ensured. Thus, in the absence of highly trained personnel, mouth-to-mask ventilation should be considered the procedure of choice until an artificial airway can be properly placed.[6]

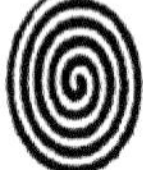

RULE OF THUMB

Mouth-to-mask ventilation often is more effective than using a BVM device, because a better seal is easier to obtain.

After appropriate use of BLS methods to establish the airway, an artificial airway may be used to achieve one or more of the following goals: (1) restoring airway patency, (2) maintaining adequate ventilation, (3) isolating and protecting the airway from aspiration, (4) providing access for clearance of secretions, and (5) providing an alternate route for administration of selected drugs.[6]

Which airway should be used in a given situation depends on careful assessment of the status of the victim, together with an in-depth knowledge of the capabilities and limitations of the equipment at hand.

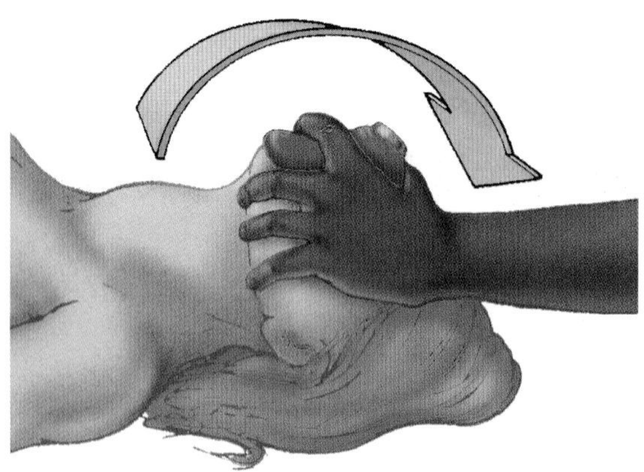

Figure 31-17
Proper placement of hands to hold resuscitator mask to patient's face and perform head-tilt maneuver.

Pharyngeal Airways

Pharyngeal airways can help restore airway patency and maintain adequate ventilation, particularly when using a BVM device. A properly placed pharyngeal airway also may help provide access for suctioning. Pharyngeal airways should be used only after BLS methods have successfully opened and cleared the airway.

Pharyngeal airways restore airway patency by separating the tongue from the posterior pharyngeal wall. Two types of pharyngeal airways are used in clinical practice: (1) the oropharyngeal airway and (2) the nasopharyngeal airway.

Oropharyngeal airways come in many different sizes to fit adults, children, and infants. Figure 31-18 shows the two most common oropharyngeal airway designs: (1) the Guedel airway (see Figure 31-18, *A*) and (2) the Berman airway (see Figure 31-18, *B*). Both types have an external flange, a curved body that conforms to the shape of the oral cavity, and one or more channels. The Guedel airway has a single center channel, whereas the Berman type uses two parallel side channels.

To choose the correct size airway, the clinician should place the devices on the side of the patient's face with the flange even with the patient's mouth. The correct size airway measures from the corner of the patient's mouth to the angle of the jaw following the natural curve of the airway.

Because insertion of an oropharyngeal airway can provoke a gag reflex, vomiting, or laryngeal spasm, these devices generally are contraindicated for conscious or semiconscious patients.[6] They also are contraindicated when there is trauma to the oral cavity or mandibular or maxillary areas of the skull. Moreover, these airways should never be placed when either a space-occupying lesion or a foreign body obstructs the oral cavity or pharynx.

Two techniques may be used to insert an oropharyngeal airway. In the first method, the tongue is displaced away from the roof of the mouth with a tongue depressor. The curved portion of the airway is then slipped over the tongue, following the curve of the oral cavity.

In the second approach, the jaw-lift technique is used to help displace the tongue. The oropharyngeal airway is then rotated 180 degrees before insertion. In this manner, the airway itself helps separate the tongue from the posterior wall of the pharynx. As the tip of the airway reaches the hard palate, it is rotated 180 degrees, aligning it in the pharynx.

In either approach, incorrect placement can displace the tongue, pushing it farther back into the pharynx, worsening the obstruction. Therefore oropharyngeal

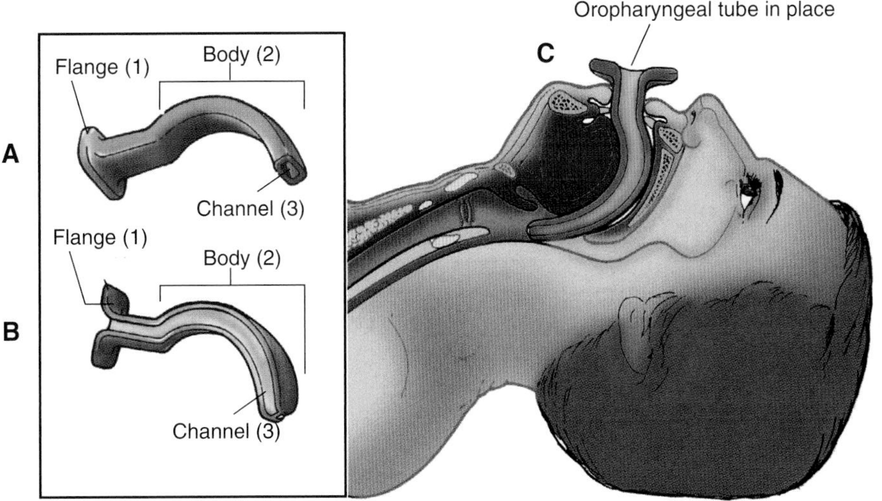

Figure 31-18
Oropharyngeal airways. **A,** Guedel airway. **B,** Berman airway. **C,** Airway in place.

airways must be inserted carefully and by trained personnel only.

As shown in Figure 31-18, C, when properly inserted, the tip of an oropharyngeal airway lies at the base of the tongue above the epiglottis, with its flange portion extending outside the teeth. Only in this position can the device properly maintain airway patency.

Nasopharyngeal Airways

Nasopharyngeal airways are inserted through the nose instead of the mouth. A properly inserted nasopharyngeal airway provides a passageway from the external nares to the base of the tongue. As with the oropharyngeal airway, the nasopharyngeal airway helps restore airway patency by separating the tongue from the posterior pharyngeal wall.

In general, the nasopharyngeal airway is indicated when placement of an oropharyngeal airway is not possible. The nasopharyngeal airway also is used when the jaws of a victim cannot be separated, as may occur with seizures. A nasopharyngeal airway should not be used when there is trauma to the nasal region or when space-occupying lesions or foreign objects block the nasal passages. Moreover, because of the smallness of the nasal passageway in children and infants, the use of nasal airways is generally limited to adults.

Most nasal airways are made from either rubber or plastic polymers and sized by external diameter according to the French scale, with 26 to 32 Fr being the usual range for adults. Anatomically, the length of the airway is more critical than is the diameter. The appropriate length can be estimated by measuring the distance from the patient's earlobe to the tip of the nose.

To insert a nasopharyngeal airway, the clinician tilts the victim's head slightly backward. The airway is lubricated with a water-soluble agent to ease insertion and is positioned perpendicular to the frontal plane of the victim's face. It is slowly advanced through the inferior meatus of either the right or the left nasal cavity, with the bevel edge facing the septum. If an obstruction is felt during insertion, gentle twisting may facilitate placement. If the resistance continues, the most likely cause is a deviated nasal septum. In this case, the clinician should simply attempt to insert the airway through the other naris or try a smaller-diameter tube.

Once the airway is inserted, the clinician should quickly try to visualize and confirm its correct position, using a tongue depressor if necessary. When properly positioned, a nasopharyngeal airway is usually stabilized by its own flange.

Endotracheal Intubation

Endotracheal intubation is the preferred method for securing the airway during CPR. Once positioned properly, an endotracheal tube can maintain a patent airway, prevent aspiration of stomach contents, permit suctioning of the trachea and mainstem bronchi, facilitate ventilation and oxygenation, and provide a route for drug administration.

Attempts to intubate the trachea must never interfere with providing adequate ventilation and oxygenation by other means. Thus only highly trained personnel should perform endotracheal intubation, and each attempt should not exceed 30 seconds, because gas exchange is absent during the procedure. Adequate ventilation and oxygenation must be provided between attempts.[6]

Figure 31-19 shows a cuffed orotracheal tube properly positioned in the trachea. It is being used with a manual bag-valve device to provide ventilation and oxygenation. Adequate ventilation and oxygenation can be provided with 12 to 15 breaths/min.

RTs should be trained in endotracheal intubation techniques, as applied in both emergency life support and prolonged mechanical ventilation situations.

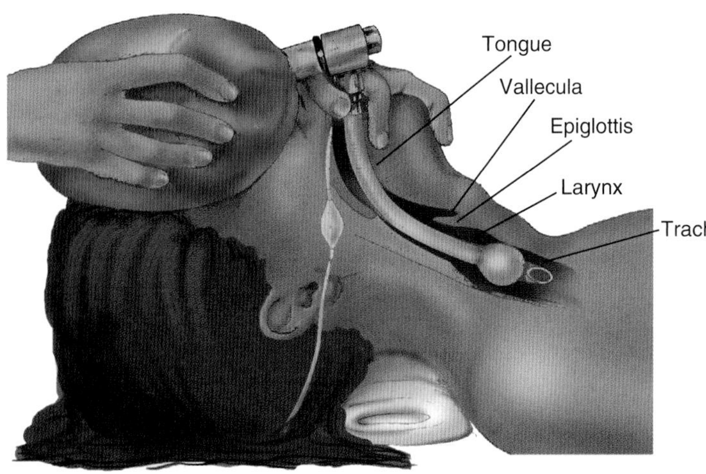

Figure 31-19
Orotracheal tube in place, being used with a bag-valve resuscitator.

Details about the necessary equipment, procedures, and short- and long-term complications of endotracheal intubation are provided in Chapter 30.

Ventilation

Accessory equipment used to support ventilation in advanced life support includes manual and oxygen-powered resuscitators. Manual resuscitators, also called *bag-valve devices,* or *BVMs,* are available for adults, children, and infants. Conversely, oxygen-powered resuscitators are strictly limited to adult application and are not discussed in this chapter.

Bag-Valve Masks

BVMs combine a self-inflating bag with a nonrebreathing valve mechanism. These devices may be used in conjunction with a face mask, endotracheal tube, or esophageal obturator airway. All are capable of providing ventilation with air or with supplemental oxygen. BVMs can provide up to 100% oxygen when properly applied. Although initially designed as adjuncts for emergency life support, BVMs are used extensively in other respiratory care settings, particularly in the areas of airway management and continuous mechanical ventilation.

Design

Figure 31-20 provides a schematic of a typical manual resuscitator, showing gas movement and valve action during both the inhalation-compression and exhalation-relaxation phases. The key components shown in this schematic are the nonrebreathing valve *(left),* the bag itself, the oxygen inlet and bag inlet valve *(to the right of the bag),* and the oxygen reservoir tube *(far right).*

During exhalation (see Figure 31-20, *top*), gas flows out from the patient's lungs through the nonrebreathing valve into the atmosphere. At the same time (while the bag expands), the intake valve opens and 100% oxygen flows into the bag from both the reservoir and oxygen inlet.

During the inhalation phase (see Figure 31-20, *bottom*), the bag is compressed manually, causing bag pressure to rise. This increase in bag pressure simultaneously closes the inlet valve and opens the nonrebreathing valve, forcing gas into the patient. While the bag inlet valve is closed, oxygen coming in through the oxygen inlet goes into the reservoir tube, where it is stored for the next breath.

Use

To use a BVM, the clinician positions himself or herself at the head of the patient's bed. Ideally, an oral airway should be inserted and the head-tilt method used to keep the airway open (assuming there are no neck injuries). While using one hand to keep the patient's head extended and the mask tightly sealed to the patient's face, the clinician uses the other hand to compress the bag (Figure 31-21). For adults, bag compression should deliver a volume of 10 to 15 mL/kg at a moderate flow (lasting approximately 2 seconds).

In addition to providing adequate ventilation, BVMs should provide a high FIO_2. Theoretically, all the BVMs on the market can deliver 100% oxygen; however, the actual FIO_2 provided at the bedside depends on several factors, including oxygen input flow, reservoir volume, delivered stroke volume and rate, and bag refill time. As a guideline to achieve the highest possible FIO_2 with a BVM, clinicians should always do the following: (1) use an oxygen reservoir, (2) provide the highest acceptable oxygen input flow, (3) deliver an appropriate tidal volume for a 2-second period (when using a mask), and (4) ensure the longest possible bag refill time.

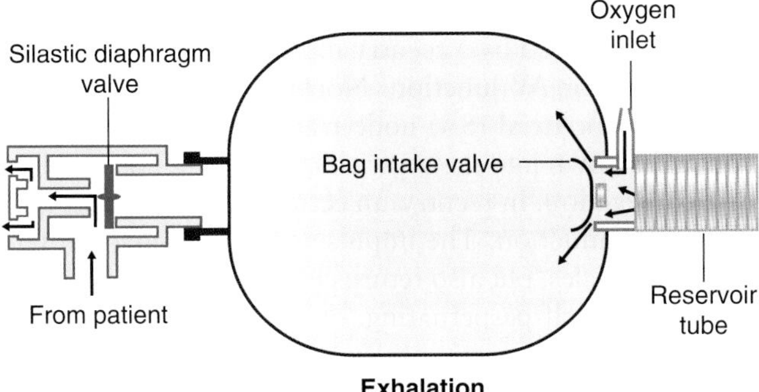

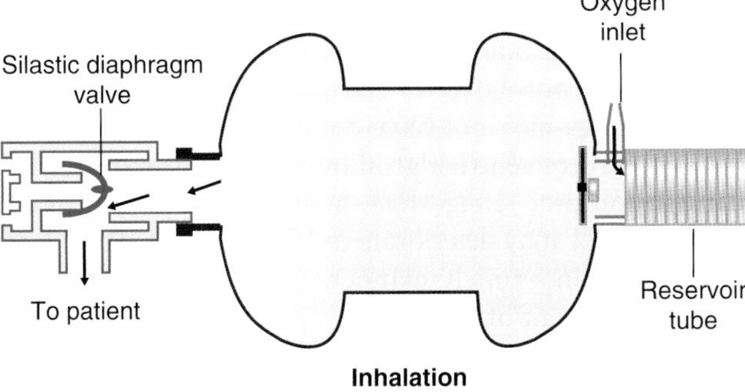

Figure 31-20
Ventilation using a bag-valve mask and head-tilt/chin-lift method.

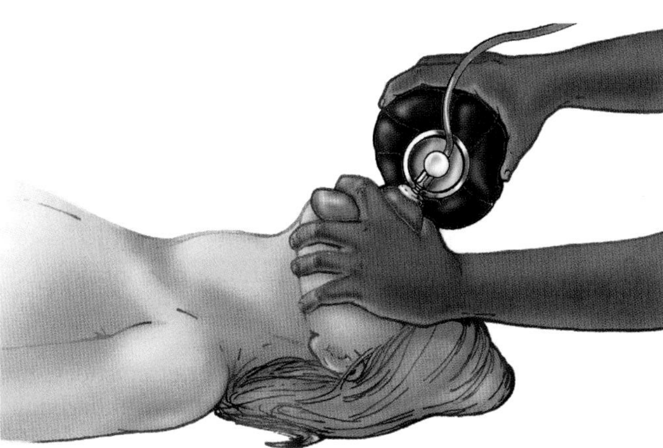

Figure 31-21
Ventilation using a bag-valve mask and the head-tilt/chin-lift method to open the airway.

Hazards and Troubleshooting

BVMs are relatively simple and safe advanced life support devices. However, several major hazards associated with their use bear emphasis. The first and most common problem is *unrecognized equipment failure*. Knowledge of how BVMs operate should help clinicians understand the operational testing of and troubleshooting for these devices.

MINI CLINI

Ventilation During CPR

PROBLEM

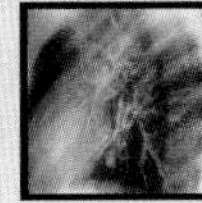

A student is observing a code blue in progress in the intensive care unit. The patient is pulseless, and cardiac compressions are being administered. He notices that the RT is ventilating the patient's lungs with an endotracheal tube at a considerably higher minute ventilation than one would normally establish on a mechanical ventilator for a patient of this size. Is this increased minute ventilation needed?

SOLUTION

During cardiopulmonary arrest, the absence of blood flow and oxygenation leads to severe tissue hypoxia, anaerobic metabolism, and lactic-acid formation. Both bicarbonate and nonbicarbonate ions in the blood buffer the lactic acid, and in the case of the bicarbonate buffer, carbon dioxide is produced as a byproduct, as shown in the following equation:

$$H^+ + HCO_3^- \rightarrow H_2CO_3^- \rightarrow H_2O + CO_2$$

Thus in the cardiopulmonary arrest, carbon dioxide is produced not only by tissue metabolism but also by lactic-acid buffering. Therefore artificial ventilation administered during a code blue should produce larger than "normal" minute ventilation to accommodate the additional carbon dioxide production and to compensate for metabolic lactic acidosis. If sodium bicarbonate were given intravenously, more carbon dioxide would be produced as lactic acid is buffered. This situation also would call for greater alveolar ventilation.

Gastric distension is another common hazard encountered when using a bag-valve device with a face mask. Gastric distension can be minimized by providing low to moderate inspiratory flows. For an adult, this means using a full 2 seconds to deliver the tidal volume.

Barotrauma has long been recognized as a potential hazard of BVM use. However, with the full-bag volume of adult-size BVMs (generally no more than 2000 mL), the potential for barotrauma is small. Obviously, using an adult-size BVM on a child or infant is contraindicated. Some pediatric BVMs have bag volumes of more than 500 mL, which is clearly enough to cause barotrauma if applied to small children or infants.

Restoring Cardiac Function

Perfusion support techniques, such as chest compressions, can restore circulation only temporarily. ACLS must go beyond simple perfusion support to identify, remove, or relieve the underlying cause of cardiac failure. This is done by combining electrocardiographic monitoring with pharmacological and electrical therapies.

Electrocardiographic Monitoring

Because most cases of cardiac arrest are caused by arrhythmias, electrocardiographic monitoring should be started as soon as the necessary equipment and personnel arrive. Monitoring may be done with either standard electrocardiographic equipment or the quick-look paddles now available on most defibrillators.

Given their important role in ACLS, RTs must be skilled in recognizing arrhythmias. Although the experienced RT may be able to quickly interpret gross arrhythmias appearing on electrocardiographic monitors at the bedside, these skills develop only after much practice with actual rhythm strips. Chapter 15 presents a review of ECG interpretation and should be consulted for more information. The reader should concentrate on the following arrhythmias:

- Sinus arrhythmia
- Sinus tachycardia
- Sinus bradycardia
- Sinus arrest
- Premature atrial contractions
- Atrial flutter
- Atrial fibrillation
- Atrioventricular (AV) blocks: first degree, second degree types I and II, and third degree
- Premature ventricular contractions (PVCs)
- Pulseless electrical activity
- Systole

This section briefly covers those arrhythmias closely associated with CPR conditions such as supraventricular tachycardia (SVT), ventricular tachycardia (VT), and ventricular fibrillation (VFib).

Supraventricular Tachycardia (Figure 31-22). The term *supraventricular tachycardia (SVT)* is commonly used to describe any tachycardia not of ventricular origin. This grouping can include sinus tachycardia, atrial tachycardia, junctional tachycardia, atrial flutter, and atrial fibrillation (with rates of more than 100 beats/min). These individual supraventricular arrhythmias should be identified by ECG and treated accordingly.

A more specific form of SVT involves rapid impulse formation caused by a reentry mechanism that develops in the atria or AV junction. Normally, a single impulse from the sinoatrial (SA) node transverses the atria and continues down into the ventricles, causing depolarization and contraction. In reentry, an ectopic focus disrupts this normal conduction. The impulse not only moves down to the ventricles, but also returns to the atria. This pattern repeats in a self-perpetuating, or circular, manner.

Typically, this form of SVT results in heart rates between 160 and 220 beats/min. The rhythm is regular, which distinguishes it from rapid atrial fibrillation. However, because of its rapid rate, P waves may not be seen. If identifiable, the P waves appear abnormal. In addition to the rate and regular rhythm, SVT is characterized by a normal QRS complex. At very high rates, the ventricles may not have enough time to completely fill. Incomplete ventricular filling can result in decreased cardiac output, congestive heart failure, and tissue hypoxia. SVT may deteriorate to VT if it is not recognized and treated in a timely manner.

The treatment of SVT varies according to the clinical situation. If the patient with SVT is ill or unstable, the treatment of choice is immediate synchronized electrical cardioversion (see p. 372). If the patient is stable, other interventions are tried before cardioversion is considered. The most common nonelectrical treatment for SVT is vagal stimulation by carotid artery massage or the Valsalva maneuver. If these attempts are ineffective and the patient remains stable, drugs such as adenosine or verapamil may halt SVT. Other second-line drugs include amiodarone, digoxin, and β-blockers.

Ventricular Tachycardia (Figure 31-23). VT occurs when one or more irritable foci within the ventricle discharge at rapid rates, creating the appearance of a prolonged chain of PVCs. Rates typically range from 140 to 220 beats/min and usually are regular.

Although VT may come and go in brief episodes, or paroxysms, it is always a sign of a serious underlying pathologic condition and should be treated immediately. In general, short, self-limiting runs of VT are managed with lidocaine. If lidocaine does not work, procainamide and amiodarone may be used.[21]

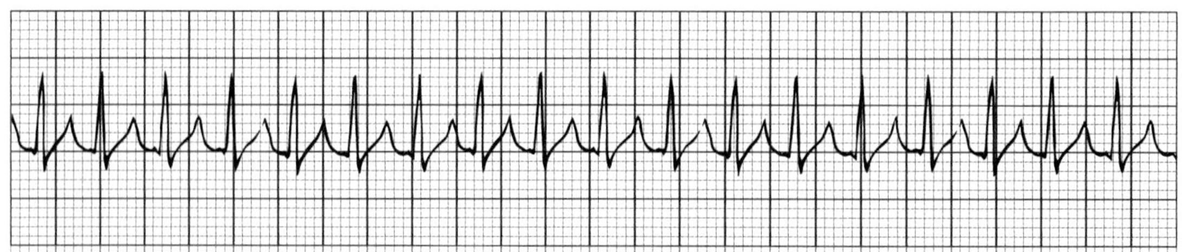

Figure 31-22
Supraventricular tachycardia. Lead II.

For patients with sustained VT who exhibit hypotension, ischemic chest pain, shortness of breath, decreased consciousness, or signs of pulmonary edema, immediate synchronized cardioversion is indicated. Patients with sustained VT in full cardiac arrest are treated similarly to patients with VFib.

Ventricular Fibrillation (Figure 31-24). VFib represents a rapid, sustained, and uncontrolled depolarization of the ventricles. During VFib, the ECG is characterized by irregular, widened, and poorly defined QRS complexes, known as *coarse VFib* (see Figure 31-24, *top*). These complexes then widen further and lose amplitude, resembling a coarse asystole, which now is defined as *fine VFib* (see Figure 31-24, *bottom*). Rather than exhibiting coordinated contractions, the ventricles quiver in a totally disorganized manner. Thus cardiac output during VFib is essentially zero. The rapid fall in cardiac output produces an acute cerebral hypoxia, often manifested by convulsions. Therefore VFib is uniformly fatal if not corrected immediately.

Many conditions can cause VFib. The most common causes include electrical shock, anesthesia, mechanical irritation of the heart, severe hypoxia, MI, and large doses of digitalis or epinephrine.

Regardless of the cause, VFib constitutes a true emergency. Patient survival depends on immediate provision of ACLS, especially electrical defibrillation. Early defibrillation is the major determinant of survival in cardiac arrest caused by VFib.[6]

Pharmacological Intervention

Although the full range of drug use in ACLS is beyond the scope of this chapter, RTs must have a general knowledge of both the various drug categories and the specific agents used in emergency situations.[21] Table 31-2 summarizes the major drug categories and primary agents currently used in ACLS.

Routes of Administration. Unless a central vein is already cannulated, the ideal route for drug administration in

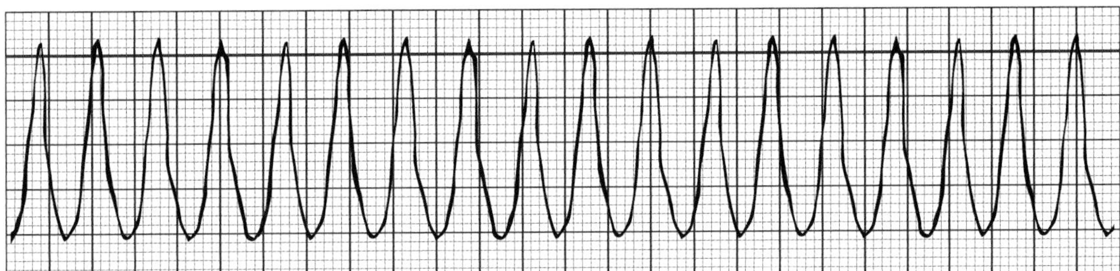

Figure 31-23
Ventricular tachycardia. Lead II.

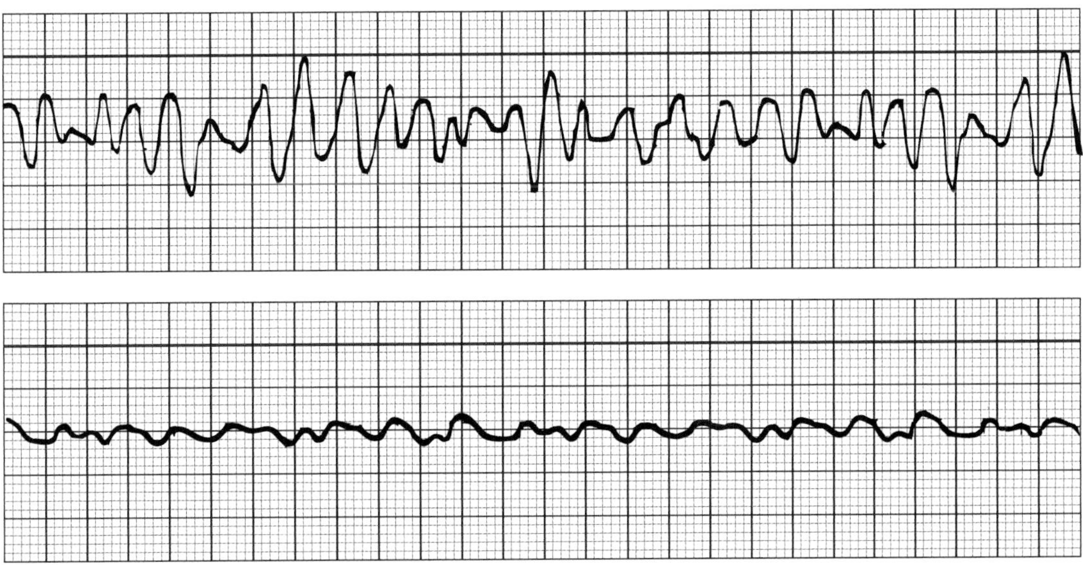

Figure 31-24
Ventricular fibrillation. *Top,* Coarse ventricular fibrillation. *Bottom,* Fine ventricular fibrillation. Lead II.

Table 31-2 ▶▶ Drug Agents Used in Advanced Life Support

Drug	Indications	Contraindications	Preparation	Route	Dosage	Pharmacological Effects
Adenosine	SVT	Use with caution if patient has asthma	3 mg/mL	IV bolus	6-mg rapid IV for 1-2 sec followed by 20-mL saline bolus; repeat with 12 mg in 1-2 min if needed	Conductor decrease AV node
Amiodarone HCl	Atrial and ventricular tachyarrhythmias	Prolonged QT interval; hepatic failure; procainamide procainamide administration	50 mg/mL	IV	150 mg IV over 10 min; may repeat every 10 min to maximum of 2.2 g in 24 hr	Increased PR and QT intervals Depressed sinus node function Inhibited α- and β-adrenergic responses
Atropine sulfate	Idioventricular rhythms; nodal bradycardia; pulseless electrical activity (PEA); escape rhythms; sinus arrest; asystole	Sinus, atrial, and ventricular tachycardia	0.1 mg/mL (10-mL unit)	IV bolus Endotracheal*	0.5- to 1-mg IV repeated every 3-5 min to maximum of 0.04 mg/kg	Increased heart rate Increased force of contractions (mainly affects atrial activity)
Calcium chloride	Hypocalcemia; hyperkalemia; calcium channel-blocker toxicity	Concurrent digitalis use (relative)	100 mg/mL (10% solution)	IV (not to be mixed with other drugs)	2-4 mg/kg for prophylaxis; 8-16 mg/kg for hyperkalemia	Increased force of contractions Increased ventricular excitability May suppress sinus node
Diuretics Lasix (furosemide)	CHF; pulmonary edema	Hypovolemia	100 mg/ 10 mL	IV	0.5-1.0 mg/kg bolus over 1-2 min; slowly increase to 2.0 mg/kg over 1-2 min if no response	Diuresis/venodilation
Dobutamine HCl	Depressed myocardial contractility	Hypertension; PVCs; atrial fibrillation; hypertrophic aortic stenosis	250-mg powder (reconstitute)	IV drip	2.0-20 μg/kg/min Increased heart rate	Increased force of contractions Enhanced AV conduction
Dopamine HCl	Hypotension	Ventricular tachycardia; frequent PVCs; symptomatic bradycardia	40 mg/mL (5-mL unit)	IV drip	1.0-20 mg/kg/min	Increased renal and splenic flow at low doses (1-5 mg/kg/min) β-Adrenergic effects at moderate doses (5-10 mg/kg/min) α-Adrenergic effects at high doses (>10 μg/kg/min)
Epinephrine HCl	Cardiac arrest; ventricular fibrillation; asystole; PEA; sinus arrest; idioventricular rhythm; pulseless ventricular tachycardia	Ventricular tachycardia; frequent PVCs	0.1 mg/mL (1:10000) 1.0 mg/mL (1:1000)	IV bolus Intracardiac Endotracheal† IV drip	1 mg every 3-5 min in cardiac arrest, up to 0.2 mg/kg; 30 mg in 250 mL NS or D_5W at 100 mL/hr	Increased heart rate Increased force of contractions Vasoconstriction Increased coronary perfusion pressures Increased myocardial irritability Increased myocardial O_2 consumption

Table 31-2 ▶▶▶ Drug Agents Used in Advanced Life Support—cont'd

Drug	Indications	Contraindications	Preparation	Route	Dosage	Pharmacological Effects
Isoproterenol HCl	Idioventricular rhythms; bradycardia; heart block	Ventricular tachycardia; frequent PVCs; cardiac arrest	0.2 mg/mL (1:5000)	IV drip with dextrose	2-10 μg/min	Increased heart rate Increased force of contractions Vasodilation Possible decreased coronary perfusion
Lidocaine HCl	Ventricular tachycardia; hyperexcitable myocardium; multifocal PVCs; ventricular fibrillation	Heart block; asystole; PEA	Variable	IV bolus IV drip Intracardiac Endotracheal[†]	1- to 1.5-mg/kg bolus every 5-10 min, up to 3 mg/kg	Raised electrical stimulation threshold Depressed ventricular electrical activity
Norepinephrine	Cardiogenic or vasogenic shock	Hypovolemia	4 mg in 250 mL D_5W or D_5NS	IV drip	0.5-1.0 μg/min titrated to effect, up to 30 μg/min	α-Adrenergic stimulation
Procainamide HCl	Ventricular tachycardia hyperexcitable myocardium; multifocal PVCs; ventricular fibrillation	Heart block; asystole; PEA	100 mg/mL (10-mL unit)	IV bolus IV drip	20 mg/min to maximum of 17 mg/kg 1-4 mg/min	Raised electrical stimulation threshold Depressed ventricular electrical activity May cause hypotension
Propranolol HCl	Angina pectoris; MI; supraventricular arrhythmias; ventricular tachycardia	Hypotension; CHF; reactive airway disease	1 mg/mL	IV drip IV bolus	1-4 mg/min 0.1 mg/kg divided into three equal doses at 2- to 3-min intervals (≤1 mg/min)	Decreased heart rate Decreased stroke volume Decreased myocardial O_2 consumption Increased LVEDP
Sodium nitroprusside	Hypertension	Hypotension; CHF	50-mg powder (reconstitute)	IV drip only	0.1-5.0 μg/kg/min	Direct peripheral vasodilation
Streptokinase	Acute coronary occlusion	Active internal history of CVA/trauma	1.5 million IU powder (reconstitute)	IV	1.5 million IU over 1 hr	Lysis of thrombi clot in coronary artery
Tissue plasminogen activator (tPa)	Acute coronary occlusion	Active internal history of CVA/trauma	50- to 100-mg vials (reconstitute)	IV	15-mg bolus over 5 min	Lysis of thrombi clot in coronary artery
Verapamil HCl	Angina pectoris; MI; supraventricular arrhythmias; mild hypertension	Hypotension; CHF; second- or third-degree heart block, atrial fibrillation, with Wolf-Parkinson-White syndrome	2.5 mg/mL (5-mL unit)	IV bolus	2.5-5 mg over 2 min and 5- to 10-mg bolus every 15-30 min as needed, ≤20 mg total dose	Decreased heart rate Prolonged AV conduction Decreased myocardial contractility Coronary artery vasodilation Peripheral vasodilation

*Dosage is 2.0-3.0 mg diluted in 10 mg normal saline.

[†]Endotracheal dosage is double IV dosage.

AV, Atrioventricular; *CHF*, congestive heart failure; *CVA*, cerebrovascular accident; *D_5NS*, 5% dextrose in normal saline; *D_5W*, 5% dextrose in water; *LVEDP*, left ventricular end-diastolic pressure; *MI*, myocardial infarction; *NS*, normal saline; *PVC*, premature ventricular contraction; *SVT*, supraventricular tachycardia.

emergency situations is a peripheral IV line.[6] IV drugs should be given by rapid bolus injection, followed by a 20-mL bolus of IV fluid and elevation of the extremity.

Selected drugs, such as epinephrine, lidocaine, and atropine, also may be given through an endotracheal tube. Higher doses in larger volumes are necessary if this route is used. For intratracheal instillation, 2 to 2.5 times the usual IV dose, diluted in 10 mL of normal saline or distilled water, should be given.

The intraosseous route also is an option, especially in small children or infants. Direct intracardiac injection is indicated only for epinephrine, and then only if no other route is available.[6] Chapters 29 and 33 provide information about pharmacological agents often used in ACLS.

Electrical Therapy

The following three general types of electrical therapy are used in emergency cardiac care: (1) unsynchronized countershock, or defibrillation; (2) synchronized countershock, or cardioversion; and (3) electrical pacing.

Countershock: Defibrillation and Cardioversion. When an electrical shock of appropriate strength is applied to the myocardium, all myocardial fibers simultaneously depolarize. In theory, once all cells depolarize, those that spontaneously fire at the fastest rate should be able to regain control and pace the heart. Normally, the sinus node spontaneously depolarizes most rapidly. After electrical shock, the sinus node should discharge first, and thus capture all parts of the myocardium as the depolarization wave travels through the still, silent heart.

Defibrillation is an unsynchronized shock used to simultaneously depolarize the myocardial fibers. It is the definitive treatment for both VFib and pulseless VT. If one of these arrhythmias is present and the proper equipment and trained personnel are available, the patient should be defibrillated immediately (see AARC Clinical Practice Guidelines, p. 733).

Currently, the AHA recommends an initial energy level of 200 J for defibrillation of adults and 2 J/kg for children and infants.[6] If 200 J does not restore orderly ventricular depolarization, the second shock should be between 200 and 300 J.[6] Third and subsequent shocks should be 360 J for adults and approximately 4 J/kg for children and infants.

Electrode paddle size and placement are important in ensuring that the full energy of the countershock is applied. For adults, paddles should be approximately 10 cm in diameter; 8 cm is an adequate size for children older than 1 year of age.

Normally, one paddle is placed below the clavicle and just to the right of the upper portion of the sternum, with the other positioned on the midaxillary line to the left of the left nipple. Alternatively, one paddle may be placed on the left precordium, with the other positioned posteriorly under the patient, behind the heart. Paddles should be prepared with conducting gel and applied with firm pressure (approximately 25 lb).

Cardioversion is similar to defibrillation, with two major exceptions. First, the countershock is synchronized with the heart's electrical activity (the R wave). Synchronization is necessary because electrical stimulation during the refractory phase (part of the T wave) can cause VFib or VT. Second, the energy used during cardioversion usually is less than that applied during defibrillation.

Cardioversion is considered when a patient with an organized arrhythmia producing a high ventricular rate exhibits signs or symptoms of cardiac decompensation. These so-called tachyarrhythmias include SVT, atrial flutter, atrial fibrillation, and VT.

If the arrhythmia is not causing serious signs or symptoms, drug therapy is used first. However, if the patient shows hypotension, exhibits signs of decreased consciousness or pulmonary congestion, or complains of chest pain, cardioversion is indicated.

Electrical Pacing. Another application of electrical therapy uses intermittently timed, low-energy discharges to replace or supplement the heart's natural pacemaker. There are

MINI CLINI

Route of Drug Administration

PROBLEM

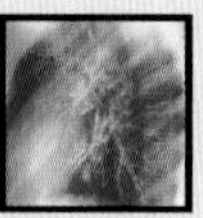

An RT is working in a small, rural hospital and is called to the emergency department where a patient is in cardiac arrest. She is able to intubate and ventilate the patient, using a manual bag-valve device at 100% inspired oxygen concentration.

Nurses are performing cardiac compressions and attempting unsuccessfully to start a peripheral IV line. The ECG monitor reveals a fine VFib pattern. Electrical defibrillation is unsuccessful on the first two attempts. Immediate administration of epinephrine is indicated, but attempts to secure an IV route continue to be unsuccessful. What action is appropriate at this time?

SOLUTION

Because of its strong inotropic and α-adrenergic effects, epinephrine should be the first drug given in cardiac arrest, and it should be administered as soon as possible. Epinephrine can convert fine fibrillation to coarse, vigorous fibrillation (an improvement) and improve the chance for successful electrical defibrillation. In this case, because an IV route is not available, epinephrine should be directly instilled into the endotracheal tube at 2 to 2.5 times the IV dose diluted in 10 mL of normal saline or distilled water. This is an effective route of administration. In addition, lidocaine can be administered through the endotracheal tube.

DEFIBRILLATION DURING RESUSCITATION

AARC Clinical Practice Guideline (Excerpts)*

➤ INDICATIONS

- Cardiac arrest caused by or resulting in ventricular fibrillation
- Pulseless ventricular tachycardia

➤ CONTRAINDICATIONS

Defibrillation is contraindicated in the following circumstances:

- The patient's desire not to be resuscitated has been clearly expressed and documented in his or her medical record or other legal document.
- Continued resuscitation is determined to be futile by the treating physician.
- There is an immediate danger to the rescuers from the environment, the patient's location, or the patient's condition.

➤ PRECAUTIONS, HAZARDS, AND COMPLICATIONS

- AEDs may be hazardous to patients weighing 90 lb or less.
- Superficial arcing of the current along the chest wall can occur as a consequence of the conductive paste or gel between the paddles.
- Malfunction of permanent pacemakers can result from placing defibrillator pads or paddles near the pacemaker.
- Defibrillation in the absence of an ECG rhythm (blind defibrillation) is rarely necessary today because of the almost universal ability of AEDs equipped with monitoring capabilities and diagnostic algorithms. In rare circumstances when electrocardiographic monitoring cannot be implemented in a timely fashion, the experienced practitioner may elect to apply blind defibrillation to a pulseless, comatose patient.
- The aluminized backing on some transdermal systems can cause electrical arcing during defibrillation, with explosive noises, smoke, visible arcing, patient burns, and impaired transmission of current. Therefore patches should be removed before defibrillation.
- A shock can be delivered accidentally to other rescuers.
- Pulse checking between sequential shocks of AEDs delays rapid identification of persistent ventricular fibrillation, interferes with assessment capabilities of the devices, and increases the possibility of operator error.
- The initial three shocks should be delivered in sequence, without interruption for CPR, medication administration, or pulse checks.
- Delays in delivering shocks for ventricular fibrillation and pulseless ventricular tachycardia after defibrillator arrival should be avoided.
- If transthoracic impedance is high, a low-energy shock (<100 J) may fail to generate enough current to achieve successful defibrillation.
- Alcohol should never be used as a conducting material for paddles, because serious burns can result.
- Attention must be paid to factors influencing total and transthoracic impedance.
- AEDs may be hazardous in an oxygen-enriched environment.

➤ ASSESSMENT OF NEED

- Before the arrival of a defibrillator, the patient should be assessed for responsiveness, apnea, and pulselessness, and help should be summoned if needed.
- After the arrival of a defibrillator, the patient should be evaluated immediately for ventricular fibrillation or ventricular tachycardia. This should be done by the operator (conventional) or the defibrillator (automated or semiautomated). Inappropriate defibrillation can cause harm.

➤ ASSESSMENT OF PROCESS AND OUTCOME

- Equipment management issues: use of standard checklists can improve defibrillator dependability
- Defibrillation process issues: system access, response time, first-responder actions, adherence to established algorithms, patient selection and outcome, first-responder authorization to defibrillate

*For the complete guideline, see Respir Care 40:744, 1995.

two primary types of electrical pacing. First, the electrical discharge can be delivered from an external power pack through wires inserted into the patient's chest wall (transcutaneous, or transthoracic, pacing). Alternatively, wire electrodes may be floated through the large veins and implanted directly inside the heart (transvenous pacing). Because it can be started quickly, transcutaneous pacing is the method used most often in emergency cardiac care.

Pacemaker therapy is used to treat sinus bradycardias that produce serious signs and symptoms and that do not respond to atropine. Electrical pacing also is used to manage second-degree type II and third-degree heart block. Electrical pacing also can be used to treat some tachyarrhythmias. In these cases, the pacemaker is set to discharge faster than the underlying rate. After a few seconds, the pacemaker is stopped to allow the heart's intrinsic rate to return. This is called *overdrive pacing*. Although overdrive pacing has shown promise in treating certain types of SVT and VT, pharmacological intervention (when the patient is stable) and cardioversion (when the patient is unstable) remain the treatments of choice.

Because defibrillation can cause damage to permanent pacemakers, care should be taken not to place the electrode paddles near these devices. After a patient with a permanent pacemaker undergoes either cardioversion or defibrillation, the device should be checked for proper functioning.[6]

MINI CLINI

Treating Cardiac Arrhythmias

PROBLEM

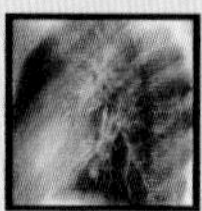

The RT is taking care of a patient who is post-MI and is being supported by mechanical ventilation in the coronary intensive care unit. She has noticed the occurrence of 15 to 20 bizarre ventricular complexes on the ECG during the last minute, as shown in the ECG tracing below. How should the abnormal complex be classified, and what therapy is indicated?

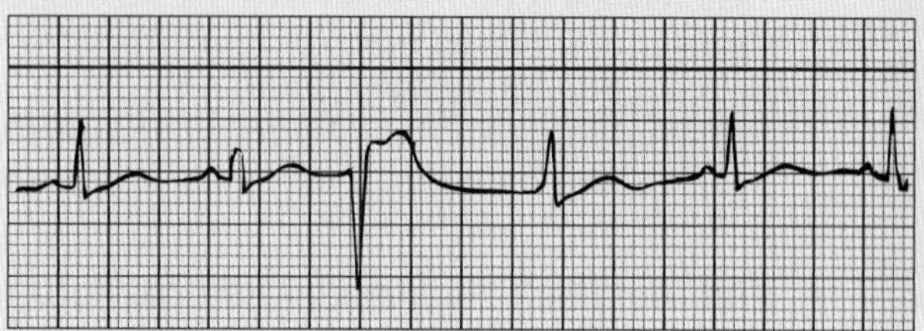

SOLUTION

The ECG tracing reveals a PVC. This means that an irritable focus in the ventricle has fired prematurely. That is, this focus reached its membrane threshold potential earlier than the cells in the SA node, and thus initiated ventricular depolarization. This irritability could be the result of local myocardial hypoxia or electrolyte imbalances. Because the PVCs are occurring at a rate of more than six per minute, aggressive treatment is indicated. Underlying electrolyte imbalances must be corrected, adequate oxygenation must be maintained, and antiarrhythmic drugs should be infused. Lidocaine is the drug of choice for treating PVCs.

Monitoring During Advanced Cardiac Life Support

Although extensive monitoring is used in most critical care settings, monitoring during emergency life support is usually limited to ECG, pulse, blood pressure, and intermittent arterial blood gas (ABG) sampling. Recently, several approaches designed to enhance knowledge of patient status during CPR have been proposed. These include methods to better monitor ventilation, oxygenation, and airway status.

Electrocardiography is the most common and one of the most useful types of monitoring used during ACLS. The ECG provides the basis for selecting various drug and electrical therapies during CPR and helps indicate patient response to these interventions. However, it should be remembered that an acceptable ECG rhythm does not necessarily mean that cardiac output is adequate. Other indexes of perfusion, such as pulse, blood pressure, and skin temperature, are needed to confirm adequate cardiac output.

Postresuscitative Patient Care

The patient in post–cardiac arrest may exhibit an optimal response, in which case he or she will regain consciousness, be responsive, and breathe spontaneously. More often, however, the patient will require support of one or more organ systems.

If the patient is conscious and breathing spontaneously following resuscitation, supplemental oxygen, maintenance of an IV infusion, and continuous cardiac and hemodynamic monitoring may be all that is necessary. A 12-lead ECG, chest x-ray examination, ABG analysis, and clinical chemistry profile should be obtained as soon as possible. Ideally, the patient should be closely supervised, preferably in an intensive care or coronary care unit.

Conversely, patients who remain unconscious, apneic, or hemodynamically unstable must be placed in a special care unit. Only in this setting can underlying organ system insufficiency or failure be properly identified and managed. The organs most likely to exhibit failure after resuscitation are the lung, heart and vasculature, and kidneys. Central nervous system failure is an ominous sign and generally indicates a failed resuscitation attempt.

Respiratory Management

If the patient remains apneic or exhibits irregular breathing after resuscitation, mechanical ventilation should be instituted through a properly positioned endotracheal tube, with an initial oxygen concentration of 100%. ABGs, preferably obtained through an arterial line, should be analyzed as needed until the oxygenation and acid-base status of the patient stabilize. ABG analysis also will help differentiate between pulmonary and nonpulmonary (or cardiac) causes of hypoxemia and tissue hypoxia.[6] For details of the selection and use of mechanical ventilators, as well as appropriate patient monitoring procedures, see Chapters 39 and 43.

Cardiovascular Management

The 12-lead ECG, chest x-ray film, clinical chemistry profile, and cardiac enzyme results should be reviewed, along with current and past drug histories. Where feasible, a flow-directed, balloon-tipped pulmonary artery catheter should be inserted and connected to a thermal dilution cardiac output computer.[6] This will provide needed data on the adequacy of vascular volumes, left ventricular performance, and overall tissue perfusion. Based on these data, sound judgments can be made regarding the need for fluid therapy and the selection and use of appropriate drugs.

KEY POINTS

- The most common cause of sudden death in adults is coronary artery disease; accidents are the most common cause of death in young people.
- The fundamental steps of basic CPR are (1) confirm unresponsiveness, (2) call for help, (3) open the airway, (4) give two quick breaths, (5) check for a pulse, (6) perform 15 cardiac compressions, and (7) initiate automated external defibrillation.
- Evaluating the effectiveness of CPR is important and requires the rescuers to watch for the victim's chest to rise and fall with ventilation and to feel for a peripheral pulse during chest compression.
- Complications of CPR include worsening of potential neck injuries, gastric distension and vomiting, and internal trauma during chest compressions. Correct technique will minimize the risk of such complications.

KEY POINTS—cont'd

- The RT is most often called on to establish an airway and ventilation with an elevated FIO_2 during ACLS of hospitalized patients. Most often, this requires knowledge and skill with BVM devices and oropharyngeal airways.
- Common pharmacological agents used during ACLS include atropine for bradycardia, lidocaine for ventricular arrhythmias, and epinephrine for cardiac arrest and hypotension.
- The RT is often involved in the postresuscitative care of the victim who responds favorably to CPR. In the postresuscitative phase, the RT may need to maintain ventilation and oxygenation and assist the physician and nurses in monitoring the patient's condition.

References

1. Kacmarek RM: The role of the respiratory therapist in emergency care, Respir Care 37:523, 1992.
2. Diem SJ, Lantos JD, Tulsky JA: Cardiopulmonary resuscitation on television: miracles and misinformation, N Engl J Med 334:1578, 1996.
3. Engdahl J et al: Factors affecting short- and long-term prognosis among 1069 patients with out-of-hospital cardiac arrest and pulseless electrical activity, Resuscitation 51:17, 2001.
4. Khalafi K et al: Avoiding the futility of resuscitation, Resuscitation 50:161, 2001.
5. American Heart Association: Heart and stroke facts: 2000 statistical update, Dallas, 1999, American Heart Association.
6. American Heart Association: Basic life support and advanced cardiac life support, Dallas, 2001, American Heart Association.
7. Division of Injury Control, Center for Environmental Health and Injury Control, Centers for Disease Control and Prevention: Childhood injuries in the United States, Am J Dis Child 144:627, 1990.
8. Rainer TH, Marshall R, Cusack S: Paramedics, technicians, and survival from out of hospital cardiac arrest, J Accid Emerg Med 14:278, 1997.
9. Jackson RE, Swor RA: Who gets bystander cardiopulmonary resuscitation in a witnessed arrest? Acad Emerg Med 4:540, 1997.
10. Ross P et al: The use of AED's by police officers in the City of London, Resuscitation 50:141, 2001.
11. White RD et al: High discharge survival rate after out-of-hospital ventricular fibrillation with rapid defibrillation by police and paramedics, Ann Emerg Med 28:480, 1996.
12. White RD et al: Seven years' experience with early defibrillation by police and paramedics in an emergency medical services system, Resuscitation 39:145, 1998.

13. U.S. Food and Drug Administration: FDA talk paper: FDA clears first external defibrillator for use on young children, May 4, 2001. Available at: www.fda.gov/bbs/topics/ANSWERS/2001/ANS01082.html.
14. Oschatz E et al: Cardiopulmonary resuscitation performed by bystanders does not increase adverse effects as assessed by chest radiography, Anesth Analg 93:128, 2001.
15. Sullivan F, Avstreih D: Pneumothorax during CPR training: case report and review of the CPR literature, Prehospital Disaster Med 15:64, 2000.
16. van der Ham AC, Lange JF: Traumatic rupture of the stomach after Heimlich maneuver, J Emerg Med 8:713, 1990.
17. Cardiopulmonary resuscitation, AIDS, and public panic, Lancet 340:456, 1992 (editorial).
18. Michael AD, Forrester JS: Mouth-to-mouth ventilation: the dying art, Am J Emerg Med 10:156, 1992.
19. Brenner BE, Kauffman J: Reluctance of internists and medical nurses to perform mouth-to-mouth resuscitation, Arch Intern Med 153:1763, 1993.
20. Mejicano GC, Maki DG: Infections acquired during cardiopulmonary resuscitation: estimating the risk and defining strategies for prevention, Ann Intern Med 129:813, 1998.
21. American Heart Association: 2000 handbook of emergency cardiovascular care for healthcare providers, Dallas, 2000, American Heart Association.

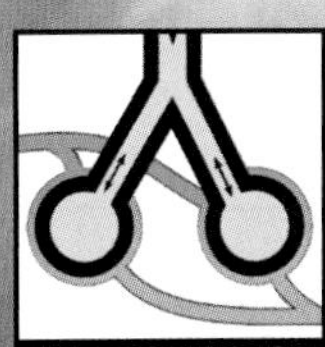

CHAPTER 32

Humidity and Bland Aerosol Therapy

Jim Fink

In This Chapter You Will Learn:

- How airway heat and moisture exchange normally occur
- What effect dry gases have on the respiratory tract
- When to humidify and warm inspired gas
- How various types of humidifiers work
- How to enhance humidifier performance
- How to select and safely use humidifier heating and feed systems
- What indications, contraindications, and hazards pertain to humidification during mechanical ventilation
- How to monitor patients receiving humidity therapy
- How to identify and resolve common problems with humidification systems
- When to apply bland aerosol therapy
- How large-volume aerosol generators work
- What delivery systems are used for bland aerosol therapy
- How to identify and resolve common problems with aerosol delivery systems
- How to perform sputum induction
- How to select or recommend the appropriate therapy to condition a patient's inspired gas

Chapter Outline

Key Terms

American Society for Testing and Materials (ASTM)
baffling
body humidity
heat and moisture exchangers (HMEs)
humidifier
hydrophobic
hygrometer
hygroscopic
hypothermia
inspissated
International Organization for Standardization (ISO)

Continued

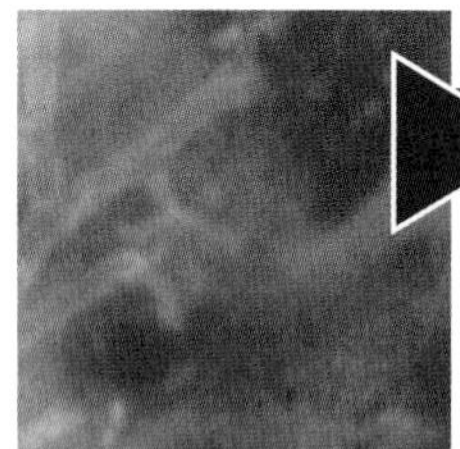

Key Terms—cont'd

isothermic saturation boundary (ISB)
nebulization
piezoelectric crystal
servo-controlled heating system
ultrasonic nebulizer (USN)

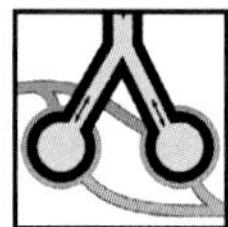

Vapors and mists have been used for thousands of years to treat respiratory disease. Modern respiratory care still uses these treatments at the bedside, in the form of water vapor (humidity) and bland water aerosols. This chapter reviews the principles, methods, equipment, and procedures for using them appropriately.

▶ HUMIDITY THERAPY

Humidity therapy involves adding water vapor and (sometimes) heat to the inspired gas. To understand the need for humidity therapy, clinicians must first understand the normal control of heat and moisture exchange.

Physiological Control of Heat and Moisture Exchange

Heat and moisture exchange is a primary function of the upper respiratory tract, mainly the nose.[1] The nose heats and humidifies gas on inspiration and cools and reclaims water from gas that is exhaled. The nasal mucosal lining is kept moist by secretions from mucous glands, goblet cells, transudation of fluid through cell walls, and condensation of exhaled humidity. The nasal mucosa is very vascular, actively regulating temperature changes in the nose, serving as an active element in promoting effective heat transfer. Similarly, the mucosa lining the sinuses, trachea, and bronchi also aid in heating and humidifying inspired gases.

During inspiration through the nose, the tortuous path of gas through the turbinates increases contact between the inspired air and the mucosa. As the inspired air enters the nose, it warms (convection) and picks up water vapor from the moist mucosal lining (evaporation), cooling the mucosal surface.

During exhalation, the expired gas transfers heat back to the cooler tracheal and nasal mucosa by convection. As the saturated gas cools, it holds less water vapor. Condensation occurs on the mucosal surfaces during exhalation, and water is reabsorbed by the mucus (rehydration). In cold environments, the formation of condensate may exceed the ability of the mucus to reabsorb water (resulting in a "runny nose").

The mouth is a less efficient heat and moisture exchanger than is the nose, because of the relatively low ratio of gas volume to moist and warm surface area and the less vascular squamous epithelium lining the oropharynx and hypopharynx. When a person inhales through the mouth, pharyngeal temperatures are approximately 3°C less than when he or she breathes through the nose, with 20% less relative humidity. During exhalation, the relative humidity of expired gas varies little between mouth and nose breathing, but the mouth is much less efficient in reclaiming heat and water.[2]

As inspired gas moves into the lungs, it achieves BTPS conditions (body temperature, 37°C; barometric pressure; saturated with water vapor [100% relative humidity at 37°C]). This point, normally approximately 5 cm below the carina, is called the **isothermic saturation boundary (ISB)**.[3] Above the ISB, temperature and humidity decrease during inspiration and increase during exhalation. Below the ISB, temperature and relative humidity remain constant (BTPS).

A number of factors can shift the ISB deeper into the lungs. The ISB shifts distally when a person breathes through the mouth rather than the nose; when he or she breathes cold, dry air; when the upper airway is bypassed (breathing through an artificial tracheal airway); or when the minute ventilation is higher than normal. When this shift of ISB occurs, additional surfaces of the airway are recruited to meet the heat and humidity requirements of the lung. If these shifts compromise the body's normal heat and moisture exchange mechanisms, humidity therapy may be indicated.

Indications for Humidification and Warming of Inspired Gases

The primary goal of humidification is to maintain normal physiological conditions in the lower airways. Proper levels of heat and humidity help ensure normal function of the mucociliary transport system. Humidity therapy is also used to treat abnormal conditions. Box 32-1 summarizes the primary and secondary indications for humidity therapy.

Administration of dry medical gases at flows greater than 4 L/min to the upper airway causes immediate heat and water loss and, if prolonged, causes structural damage. As the airway is exposed to relatively cold, dry air, ciliary

Box 32-1 • Indications for Humidification Therapy

PRIMARY
- Humidifying dry medical gases
- Overcoming the humidity deficit created when the upper airway is bypassed

SECONDARY
- Managing hypothermia
- Treating bronchospasm caused by cold air

motility is reduced, airways become more irritable, mucous production increases, and pulmonary secretions become thick and **inspissated.**

The hazard of breathing dry gas is even greater when the normal heat and water exchange capabilities of the upper airway are lost or bypassed, as occurs with endotracheal intubation.[4] Breathing dry gas through an endotracheal tube can cause damage to tracheal epithelium within minutes. However, as long as the inspired humidity is at least 60% of BTPS conditions, no injury occurs in normal lungs.[5,6] Prolonged breathing of improperly conditioned gases through a tracheal airway can result in **hypothermia,** inspissation of airway secretions, mucociliary dysfunction, destruction of airway epithelium, and atelectasis.[7] Figure 32-1 illustrates the level of dysfunction in the airway caused by changes in absolute humidity below BTPS and over hours of exposure. Note that a reduction of 20 mg/L below BTPS (44 mg/L) is less than 60% relative humidity at BTPS.

The amount of heat and humidity that a patient needs depends on the site of delivery (e.g., nose/mouth, hypopharynx, trachea). Table 32-1 summarizes the recommended levels based on current standards.[8]

Warmed, humidified gases are used to prevent or treat a variety of abnormal conditions. For treatment of the

Table 32-1 ▶▶ Recommended Heat and Humidity Levels

Delivery Site	Temperature Range (°C)	Relative Humidity (%)	Absolute Humidity (mg/L)
Nose/mouth	20-22	50	10
Hypopharynx	29-32	95	28-34
Trachea	32-35	100	36-40

From Chatburn RL, Primiano FP: Respir Care 32:249, 1987.

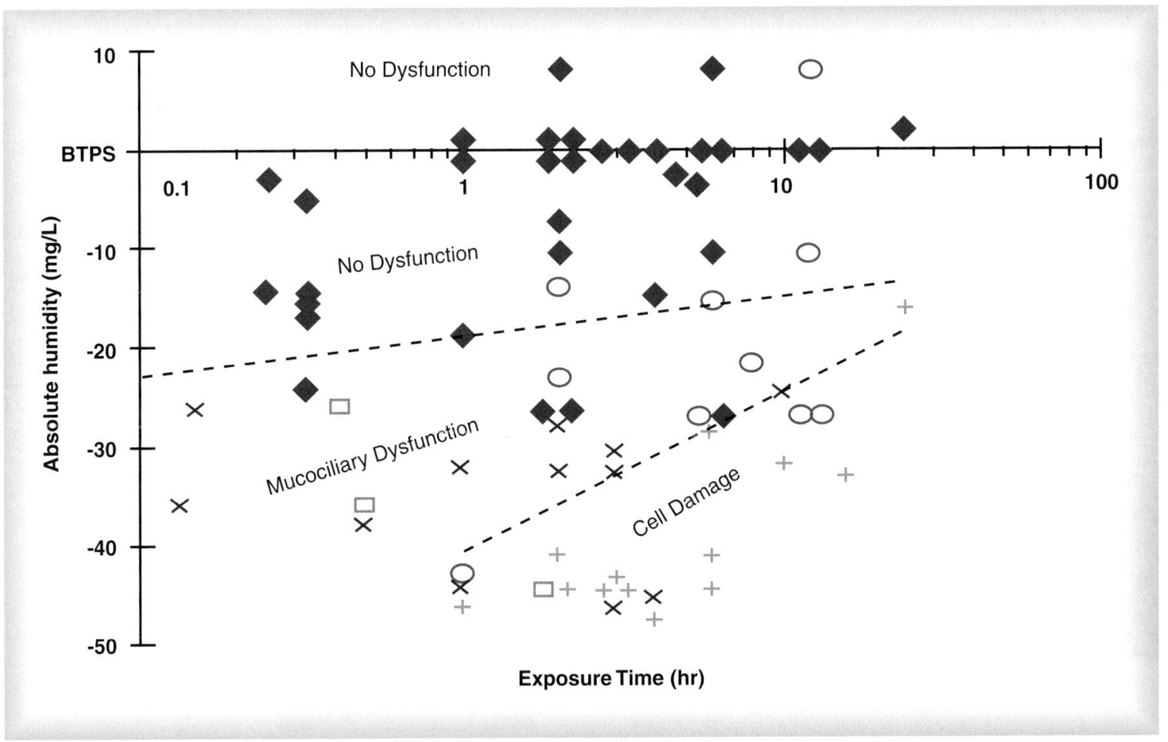

Figure 32-1

A diagram of published data describing the effects of humidity versus exposure time on airway dysfunction. Each point represents a single measurement coded as no dysfunction *(diamond)*, mucus thick or thin *(circle)*, mucociliary transport stopped *(square)*, cilia stopped *(×)*, or cell damage *(+)*. Data are grouped in categories of no dysfunction, mucociliary dysfunction, or cell damage. *(Redrawn from Williams R, Rankin N, Smith T et al: Crit Care Med 24:11, 1996.)*

hypothermic patient, heating and humidifying the inspired gas is one of several techniques used to raise core temperatures back to normal.[9,10] Heated humidification is also used to prevent intraoperative hypothermia.[11] Of possibly greater clinical significance, warming and humidifying the inspired gas can help alleviate bronchospasm in patients who develop airway narrowing after exercise or when they breath cold air. Although the cause of this condition is not known for certain, the primary stimulus is probably a combination of airway cooling and drying, which leads to hypertonicity of airway lining fluid and the release of chemical mediators.[12] Patients may reduce the incidence of cold air–induced bronchospasm by simply wearing a scarf over the nose and mouth when outside in cold weather, because the scarf serves as a passive heat moisture exchanger.

The delivery of cool humidified gas is used to treat upper airway inflammation resulting from croup, epiglottitis, and postextubation edema. This technique is used most often in conjunction with bland aerosol delivery (see p. 751).

Equipment

A **humidifier** is a device that adds molecular water to gas. This occurs by evaporation from a water surface (see Chapter 5), whether the surface of water is in a reservoir or is a sphere of water in suspension (**nebulization**).

Physical Principles Governing Humidifier Function

The following three variables affect the quality of a humidifier's performance: (1) temperature, (2) surface area, and (3) time of contact. These factors are exploited to various degrees in the design of humidification devices.

Temperature. Temperature is an important factor affecting humidifier performance. The greater the temperature of a gas, the more water vapor it can hold (increased capacity). As gas expansion and evaporation cool the water in unheated humidifiers to as low as 10° C below ambient temperature, the humidifiers become less efficient.

Figure 32-2 demonstrates this concept. Because of evaporative cooling, the unheated humidifier on the left is operating at 10° C. Although the humidifier fully saturates the gas, the low operating temperature limits total water vapor capacity to approximately 9.4 mg/L water vapor, equivalent to approximately 21% of **body humidity.** Simply heating the humidifier to 40° C (see Figure 32-2, *right*) increases its output to 51 mg/L, which is more than adequate to meet BTPS conditions.

Surface Area. The greater the area of contact between water and gas, the more opportunity for evaporation to occur. Passover humidifiers pass gas over a large surface area of water. More space-efficient ways to increase the

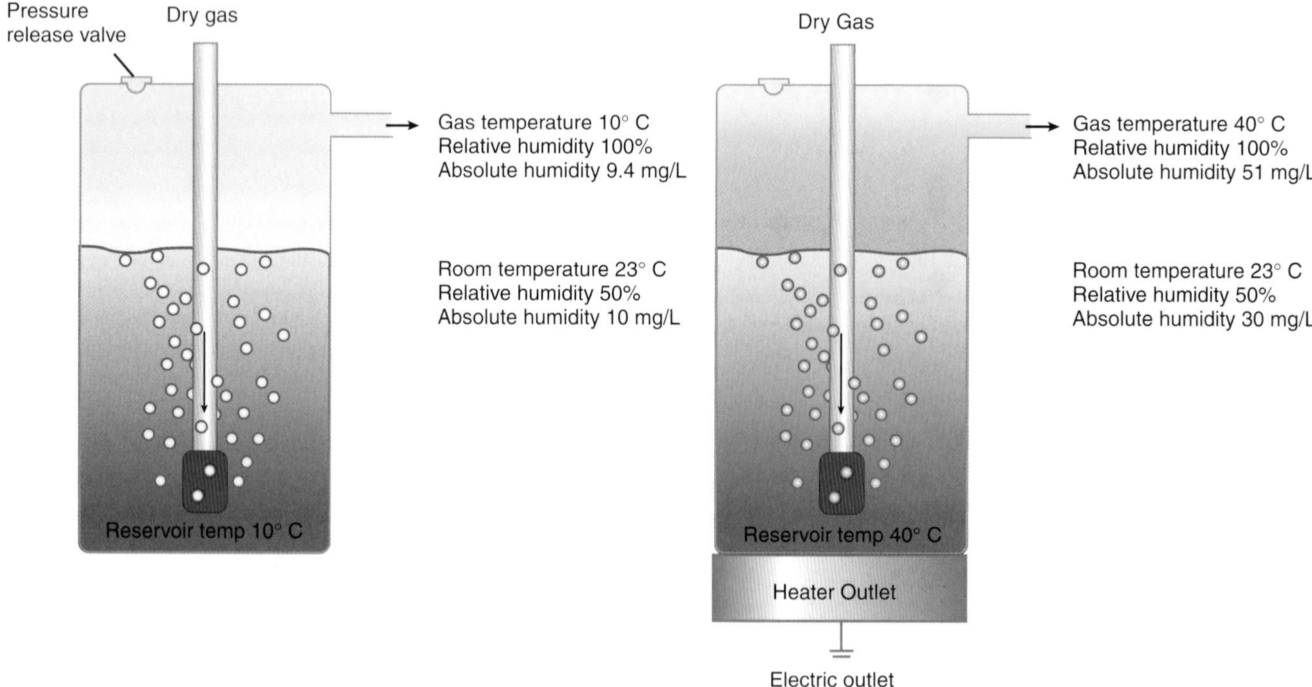

Figure 32-2
The effects of reservoir temperature on humidity output with unheated *(left)* and heated *(right)* bubble-type humidifiers. *(From Fink J, Cohen N: Humidity and aerosols. In Eubank D, Bone R, editors: Principles and applications of cardiorespiratory care equipment, St Louis, 1994, Mosby.)*

water/gas surface-area ratio include bubble diffusion, aerosol, and "wick" technologies.

The bubble-diffusion technique directs a stream of gas underwater, where it is broken up into small bubbles. As the gas bubbles rise to the surface, evaporation increases the water vapor content within the bubble. For a given gas volume, the smaller the bubbles, the greater the water/air surface-area ratio.

An alternative to dispersing gas bubbles in water is spraying water particles into the gas. This is accomplished by generating an aerosol (suspension of water droplets) in the gas stream. The higher the aerosol density (number of particles per volume of gas) the greater the gas/water surface area available for evaporation.

Wick technologies use porous water-absorbent materials to increase surface area. A wick draws water (like a sponge) into its fine honeycombed structure by means of capillary action (see Chapter 5). The surfaces of the wick increase the area of contact between the water and gas, which aids evaporation.

Contact Time. The longer a gas remains in contact with water, the greater the opportunity for evaporation to occur. For bubble humidifiers, contact time depends on the depth of the water column; the deeper the column, the greater the time of contact as the bubbles rise to the surface. In passover and wick-type humidifiers, the flow rate of gas through the humidifier is inversely related to contact time, with high flow rates reducing the time available for evaporation to occur. Aerosols suspended in a gas stream have extended contact time (and opportunity for evaporation) as the aerosol and gas travels to the patient.

Types of Humidifiers

There are three primary types of humidifiers: (1) bubble humidifiers, (2) passover humidifiers, and (3) **heat and moisture exchangers (HMEs)**. These devices are either *active,* actively adding heat and/or water to the device/patient interface, or *passive,* recycling exhaled heat and humidity from the patient. Specifications covering the design and performance requirements for medical humidifiers are established by the **American Society for Testing and Materials (ASTM).**[13]

Bubble. A bubble humidifier breaks (diffuses) an underwater gas stream into small bubbles (see Figure 32-2). Unheated bubble humidifiers are commonly used with oronasal oxygen delivery systems (see Chapter 35). The goal is to raise the water vapor content of the gas to ambient levels.

As indicated in Table 32-2, unheated bubble humidifiers can provide absolute humidity levels between approximately 15 and 20 mg/L.[14-16] At room temperature, 10 mg/L absolute humidity corresponds to approximately

Table 32-2 ▶▶ Absolute Humidity (mg/L) Provided by Four Types of Unheated Bubble Humidifiers

L/min	Aerway	Aquapak	McGaw	Travenol
2	17.2	17.6	20.4	20.4
4	16.0	17.7	18.4	19.5
6	15.6	16.9	16.9	16.2
8	14.6	14.9	14.9	15.7

From Darin J, Broadwell J, MacDonell R: Respir Care 27:41, 1982.

80% relative humidity, but only approximately 25% body humidity (see Chapter 5). As gas flow increases, these devices become less efficient as the reservoir cools and contact time is reduced, limiting their effectiveness at flow rates higher than 10 L/min. Heating the reservoirs of these units can increase humidity content but is not recommended, because the resulting condensate tends to obstruct the small-bore delivery tubing to which they connect.

To warn of flow-path obstruction and to prevent bursting of the humidifier bottle, bubble humidifiers incorporate a simple pressure-relief valve, or *pop-off*. Typically, the pop-off is either a gravity or spring-loaded valve that releases pressures above 2 psi. Humidifier pop-offs should provide both an audible and visible alarm and should automatically resume normal position when pressures return to normal.[13] The pop-off also can be used to test an oxygen delivery system for leaks. If the system is obstructed at or near the patient interface and the pop-off sounds, the system is leak free; failure of the pop-off to sound may indicates a leak (or a faulty pop-off valve).

At high flow rates, bubble humidifiers can produce aerosols. Although not visible to the naked eye, these water-droplet suspensions can transmit pathogenic bacteria from the humidifier reservoir to the patient.[17] Because any device that generates an aerosol poses a high risk of spreading infection, strict infection control procedures must be followed when using these systems (see Chapter 3).

Passover. A passover humidifier directs gas over a water surface. There are two common types of passover humidifiers: (1) the wick type and (2) the membrane type.

Figure 32-3 shows a cross section of a wick-type humidifier designed for placement in a ventilator circuit. The wick (a cylinder of absorbent material) is placed upright in a water reservoir and surrounded by a heating element. Capillary action continually draws water up from the reservoir and keeps the wick saturated. As dry gas enters the chamber it flows around the wick, quickly picking up moisture and leaving the chamber fully saturated with water vapor. No bubbling occurs.

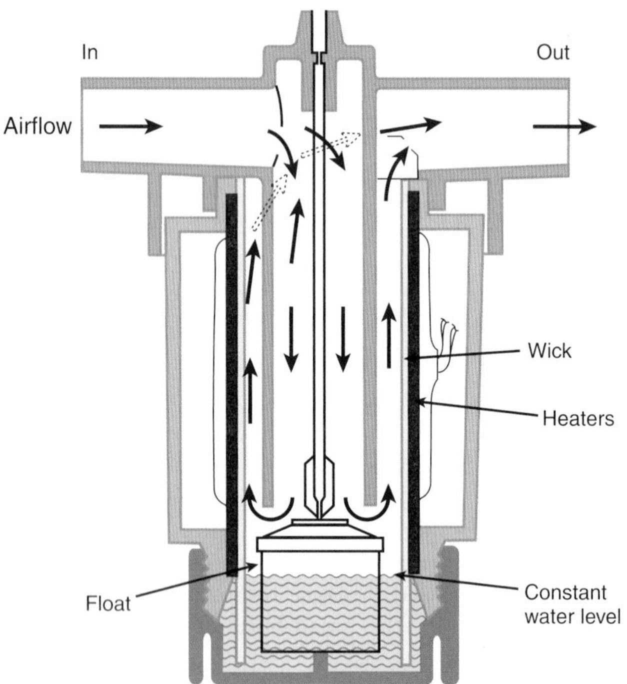

Figure 32-3

Cross section of a wick humidifier designed for placement in a ventilator circuit. *(Modified from McPherson SP: Respiratory therapy equipment, ed 4, St Louis, 1985, Mosby; courtesy Bird Corporation, Palm Springs, Calif.)*

A membrane-type humidifier separates the water from the gas stream by means of a **hydrophobic** membrane (Figure 32-4). Water vapor molecules can easily pass through this membrane, but liquid water cannot. As with the wick-type humidifier, bubbling does not occur. Moreover, if a membrane-type humidifier were to be inspected while it was in use, no liquid water would be seen in the humidifier chamber.

Compared with bubble humidifiers, passover humidifiers using the wick or membrane design offer several advantages.[17,18] First, unlike bubble devices, they can maintain saturation at high flow rates. Second, they add little or no flow resistance to spontaneous breathing circuits. Third, they do not generate any aerosols, and thus pose a minimal risk for spreading infection.

Heat and Moisture Exchangers. An HME is most often a passive humidifier that has been described as an "artificial nose." Like the nose, an HME captures exhaled heat and moisture and uses it to heat and humidify the next inspiration. Unlike the nose, however, most HMEs do not actively add heat or water to the system. The typical HME is a passive humidifier, capturing both heat and moisture from expired gas and returning them to the patient during the next inspiration. Figure 32-5 shows several examples of commercially available HMEs.

Traditionally, HME use has been limited to providing humidification to patients receiving invasive ventilatory support via endotracheal or tracheostomy tubes. More recently, HMEs have been used with success in meeting the short-term humidification needs of spontaneously breathing patients with tracheostomy tubes.[19] Kapadia et al.[20] reviewed airway accidents in their intensive care units for a 4-year period and noted an increasing trend in the incidence of blocked tracheal tubes, which was associated with an increased duration of HME filter use. It is fair to say that there is insufficient evidence to support long-term use of HMEs for spontaneously breathing patients.

There are three types of HMEs: (1) simple condenser humidifiers, (2) **hygroscopic** condenser humidifiers, and (3) hydrophobic condenser humidifiers.

Simple condenser humidifiers contain a condenser element with high thermal conductivity, usually consisting of metallic gauze, corrugated metal, or parallel metal tubes. On inspiration, inspired air cools the condenser element. On exhalation, expired water vapor condenses directly on its surface and rewarms it. On the next inspiration, cool, dry air is warmed and humidified as its passes over the condenser element. Unfortunately, simple condenser humidifiers are able to recapture only approximately 50% of a patient's exhaled moisture (50% efficiency).

Hygroscopic condenser humidifiers provide higher efficiency by (1) using a condensing element of low thermal conductivity (e.g., paper, wool, foam) and (2) impregnating this material with a hygroscopic salt (calcium or lithium chloride). By using an element with low thermal conductivity, hygroscopic condenser humidifiers can retain more heat than simple condenser

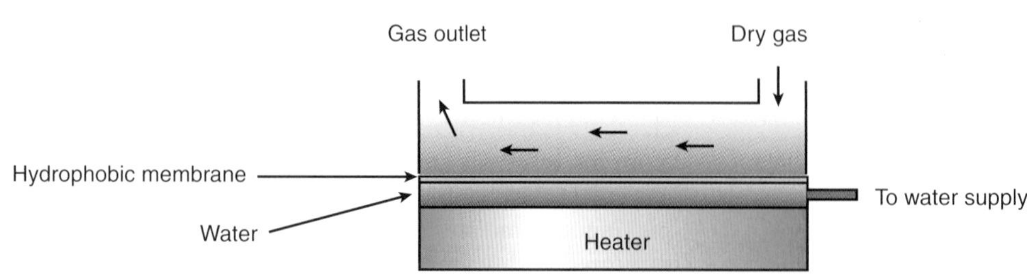

Figure 32-4

Schematic of a membrane-type humidifier. *(From Fink J, Cohen N: Humidity and aerosols. In Eubank D, Bone R, editors: Principles and applications of cardiorespiratory care equipment, St Louis, 1994, Mosby.)*

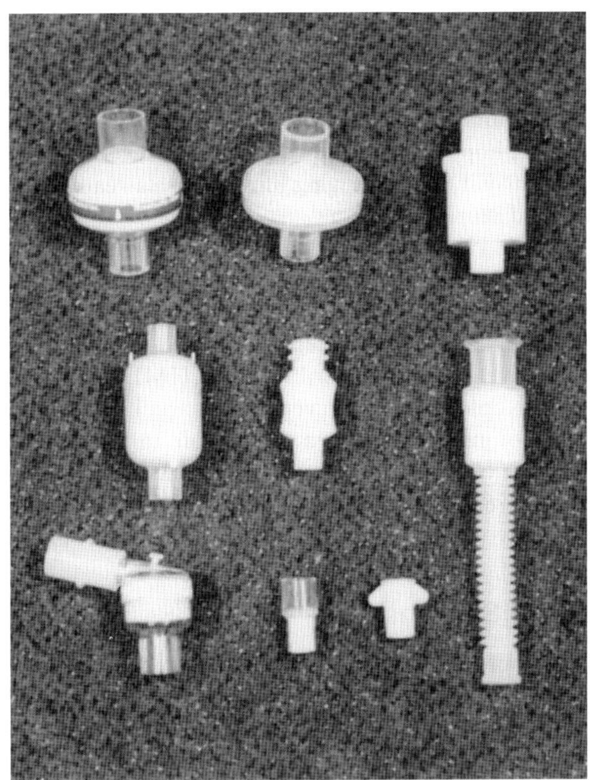

Figure 32-5

Examples of heat and moisture exchangers. *(From Fink J, Cohen N: Humidity and aerosols. In Eubank D, Bone R, editors: Principles and applications of cardiorespiratory care equipment, St Louis, 1994, Mosby.)*

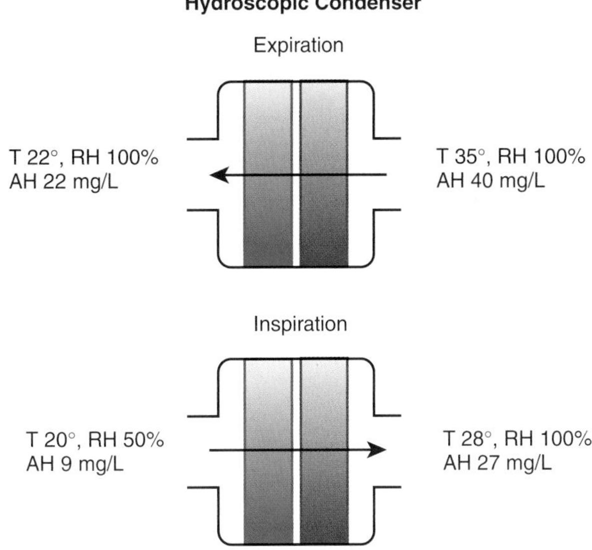

Figure 32-6

Process of humidification with a hygroscopic condenser humidifier. *AH*, Absolute humidity; *RH*, relative humidity; *T*, temperature.

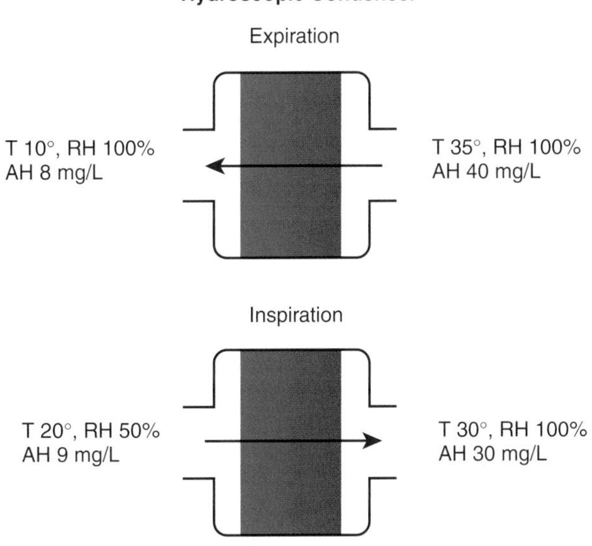

Figure 32-7

Process of humidification with a hydrophobic condenser humidifier. *AH*, Absolute humidity; *RH*, relative humidity; *T*, temperature.

systems can. In addition, the hygroscopic salt helps capture extra moisture from the exhaled gas. During exhalation, some water vapor condenses on the cool condenser element, whereas other water molecules bind directly to the hygroscopic salt. During inspiration, the lower water vapor pressure in the inspired gas liberates water molecules directly from the hygroscopic salt, without cooling. Figure 32-6 depicts the overall process of humidification with a hygroscopic condenser humidifier, showing the changes in temperature and the relative and absolute humidity occurring during the cycle of breathing. As shown, these devices typically achieve approximately 70% efficiency (40 mg/L exhaled, 27 mg/L returned).

Hydrophobic condenser humidifiers use a water-repellent element with a large surface area and low thermal conductivity (Figure 32-7). During exhalation, the condenser temperature rises to approximately 25° C because of conduction and latent heat of condensation. On inspiration, cool gas and evaporation cools the condenser down to 10° C. This large temperature change results in the conservation of more water to be used in humidifying the next breath. The efficiency of these devices is comparable with hygroscopic condenser humidifiers (approximately 70%). However, some hydrophobic humidifiers also provide bacterial filtration[21] (Figure 32-8).

Design and performance standards for HMEs are set by the **International Organization for Standardization (ISO)**.[22] The ideal HME should operate at 70% efficiency or better (providing at least 30 mg/L water vapor); use standard connections; have a low compliance; and add minimal weight, dead space, and flow resistance to a breathing circuit.[23] Table 32-3 compares performance of several commercially available HMEs according to their moisture output, flow resistance, and dead space.[24]

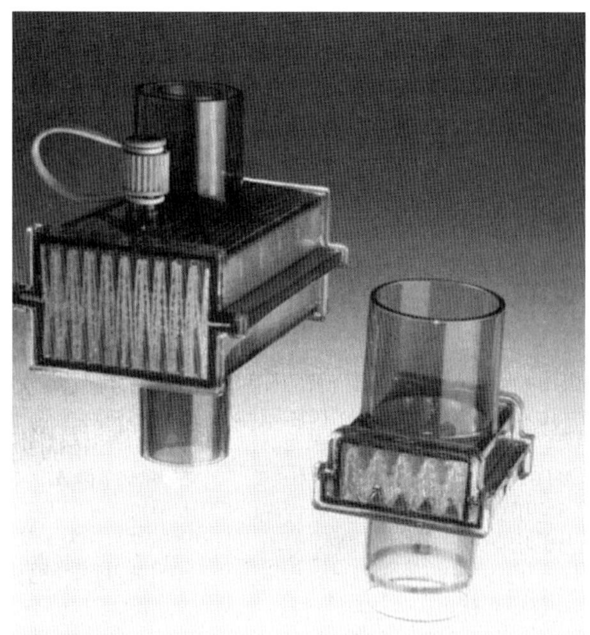

Figure 32-8
Examples of heat and moisture exchanging bacterial filters. *(Courtesy Pall Corp., East Hills, NY.)*

As shown in Table 32-3, the moisture output of HMEs tends to fall at high volumes and rates of breathing. In addition, high inspiratory flows and high F_{IO_2} levels can decrease HME efficiency.[23] Flow resistance through the HME also is important. When an HME is dry, resistance across most devices is minimal. However, because of water absorption, HME flow resistance increases after several hours' use.[24,25] For some patients, the increased resistance imposed by the HME may not be well tolerated, particularly if the underlying lung disease already causes increased work of breathing.

Because HMEs eliminate the problem of breathing-circuit condensation, many consider these devices (especially hydrophobic filter HMEs) to be helpful in preventing nosocomial infections. Indeed, as compared with active humidification systems, HMEs do reduce bacterial colonization of ventilator circuits. However, circuit colonization plays a minor role in the development of nosocomial infections, provided usual maintenance precautions are applied.[26] No evidence to date shows any impact of HME use on patient outcomes.

Heating Systems

Heat improves the water output of bubble and passover humidifiers. Heated humidifiers are used mainly for patients with bypassed upper airways and/or for those receiving mechanical ventilatory support. Although heating a humidifier provides benefits, it also presents additional risks.

An electrical heating element provides the needed energy. Five types of heating elements are common: (1) a "hot plate" element at the base of the humidifier; (2)

Table 32-3 ▶▶ Comparison of 21 Heat and Moisture Exchangers

	Moisture Output (mg H_2O/L) ($V_T \times f$)			Resistance (cm H_2O/L/sec)		
Device	**500 × 20**	**1000 × 10**	**1000 × 20**	**Dry**	**Wet**	**Dead Space**
Aqua H	31.2	28.3	27.1	0.90	1.20	84
Aqua FH*	31.8	29.1	27.1	1.62	1.78	87
ARC	32.0	31.4	30.4	0.70	1.10	89
ARCF*	32.4	32.0	30.6	2.0	2.20	86
Edith	30.6	30.0	28.9	1.48	1.54	82
Engstrom 500	26.7	25.1	24.9	1.60	1.80	19
Engstrom 1000	27.4	26.1	25.8	2.00	2.10	29
Engstrom 1500	29.1	28.4	26.5	3.50	3.67	40
FloCare "L"	30.4	27.1	25.6	1.60	1.78	32
Gibeck HVF*	32.1	30.8	29.7	2.20	2.36	58
Hygrobac*	32.5	31.0	29.4	1.90	2.08	92
Hygrobac S*	29.6	28.0	26.8	2.40	2.57	48
Hygroster*	33.2	31.9	30.6	2.50	2.70	94
Intersurgical*	25.4	22.6	21.8	2.20	2.30	65
Intertech 2841	28.5	27.0	25.5	1.75	1.84	36
Intertech HEP*	24.8	23.6	21.1	1.60	1.79	78
Pall*	24.9	21.2	19.6	2.20	2.38	90
Portex 600	25.2	24.6	22.4	2.70	2.86	10
Portex 1200	27.2	26.4	25.1	1.30	1.50	33
Vital Signs	30.8	28.5	28.1	2.30	2.44	48
Vital Signs*	29.7	28.0	26.9	2.50	2.67	58

Modified from Branson RD, Davis K: Respir Care 41:736, 1996.
*Provides bacterial filtration in addition to humidification.

a "wraparound" type that surrounds the humidifier chamber; (3) a yolk, or collar, element that sits between the water reservoir and the gas outlet; (4) an immersion-type heater, with the element actually placed in the water reservoir; and (5) a heated wire in the inspiratory limb warming a saturated wick or hollow fiber.

Humidifier heating systems also have a controller that regulates the element's electric power. In the simplest systems, *the controller monitors the heating element,* varying the delivered current to match either a preset or an adjustable temperature. In these systems, the patient's airway temperature has no effect on the controller. Conversely, a **servo-controlled heating system** monitors temperature at or near the patient's airway using a thermistor probe. The controller then adjusts heater power to achieve the desired airway temperature. Both types of controller units usually incorporate alarms and alarm-activated heater shutdown.[27] Box 32-2 outlines key features of modern heated humidification systems.[28]

RULE OF THUMB

Place heated humidifier thermistor probes in the inspiratory limb of a ventilator circuit far enough from the patient "wye" to ensure that warm exhaled gas does not fool the controller system. Similarly, never place a thermistor probe in an isolette or radiant warmer, where the probe is warmed externally, and the humidifier is fooled into shutting down, reducing the humidity available to the patient.

Recently, active HMEs have been introduced that add humidity or heat to the inspired gases with chemical or electrical means.[29] The Humid-Heat (Louis Gibeck AB, Upplands Väsby, Sweden) consists of a supply unit with a microprocessor and a water pump and a humidification device, which is placed between the Y-piece and the endotracheal tube. The humidification device is based on a hygroscopic HME, which absorbs the expired heat and moisture and releases it into the inspired gas. External heat and water are then added to the patient side of the HME, so the inspired gas should reach 100% humidity at 37° C (44 mg H_2O/L air). The external water is delivered to the humidification device via a pump onto a wick and then evaporated into the inspired air by an electrical heater. The microprocessor controls the water pump and the heater by an algorithm using the minute ventilation (which is fed into the microprocessor) and the airway temperature measured by a sensor mounted in the flex-tube on the patient side of the humidification device. The active HME is equivalent to mainstream active humidifiers in both in vitro and in vivo use.

Box 32-2 • Key Features for Heated Humidification Systems

- Gas temperature delivered to the patient should not be >40° C. When temperatures of 40° C are reached, audible and visual alarms should indicate an over-temperature condition and interrupt power to the heater.
- Audible and visual alarms should indicate when remote temperature sensors are disconnected, absent, or defective, and power to the heater should be interrupted to prevent overheating.
- Temperature overshoot should be minimized. Overshoot can occur when servo-controlled units warm up without flow through the circuit, when the temperature probe is not inserted in the circuit (or becomes dislodged), or when flow changes during normal operation. Non–servo-controlled units can overshoot when temperature controls are set too high or when gas flow is abruptly reduced.
- Indicators for delivered gas temperature should be accurate to ±3°C of the indicated value.
- Humidifier temperature output should not vary >2° C from the set value (proximal to the patient).
- Warm-up time should not exceed 15 minutes.
- The water level should be readily visible in either the humidifier or the remote reservoir.
- Humidifiers should be able to withstand ventilation pressures of >100 cm H_2O.
- Internal compliance should be low and relatively stable so changes in the water level do not significantly alter the delivered tidal volume.
- The exposed surface of a humidifier should not be too hot to touch during operation. Readily accessible surfaces should not be >37.5° C. A warning label is needed for hotter surfaces.
- Operator, or feed, systems must not be able to overfill the humidifier to the point that water can block gas flow through the humidifier or ventilator circuit. Humidifiers should not be damaged by spilled fluids.
- Electromagnetic interference from other devices should not affect humidifier performance. The unit should not be damaged by 95-135 V rms.
- Fuses or circuit breakers should be clearly labeled and easily reset or replaced. The unit should have adequate overcurrent protection to prevent ventilator shutdown or loss of power to other equipment on the same branch circuit because of internal equipment failures.
- It should be impossible to assemble the unit in a way that would be hazardous to the patient. The direction of gas flow should be indicated on interchangeable components, for which proper direction is essential.
- The humidifier should be assembled and filled in a manner that minimizes the introduction of infectious materials or foreign objects.
- Service and operation manuals should be provided with the humidifier and should cover all aspects of its use and service.

Modified from ECRI: Health Devices 16:223, 1987.

Humidification during Mechanical Ventilation

AARC Clinical Practice Guideline (Excerpts)*

➤ INDICATIONS

Humidification of inspired gas during mechanical ventilation is mandatory when an endotracheal or a tracheostomy tube is present.

➤ CONTRAINDICATIONS

There are no contraindications to providing physiological conditioning of inspired gas during mechanical ventilation. However, a heat and moisture exchanger (HME) is contraindicated in the following circumstances:

- For patients with thick, copious, or bloody secretions
- For patients with an expired tidal volume <70% of the delivered tidal volume (e.g., those with large bronchopleural fistulas or incompetent or absent endotracheal tube cuffs)
- For patients whose body temperature is <32° C
- For patients with high spontaneous minute volumes (>10 L/min)
- An HME must be removed from the patient circuit during in-line aerosol drug treatments.

➤ HAZARDS AND COMPLICATIONS

Hazards and complications associated with the use of heated humidifier (HH) and HME devices during mechanical ventilation include the following:

- High flow rates during disconnect may aerosolize contaminated condensate (HH)
- Underhydration and mucus impaction (HME or HH)
- Increased work of breathing (HME or HH)
- Hypoventilation caused by increased dead space (HME)
- Elevated airway pressures caused by condensation (HH)
- Ineffective low-pressure alarm during disconnection (HME)
- Patient-ventilator dyssynchrony and improper ventilator function caused by condensation in the circuit (HH)
- Hypoventilation or gas tripping caused by mucus plugging (HME or HH)
- Hypothermia (HME or HH); hypothermia (HH)
- Potential for burns to caregivers from hot metal (HH)
- Potential electrical shock (HH)
- Airway burns or tubing meltdown if heated-wire circuits are covered or incompatible with humidifier (HH)
- Possible increased resistive work of breathing caused by mucus plugging (HME or HH)
- Inadvertent overfilling resulting in unintended tracheal lavage (HH)
- Inadvertent tracheal lavage from pooled condensate in circuit (HH)

➤ ASSESSMENT OF NEED

Either an HME or an HH can be used to condition inspired gases:

- HMEs are better suited for short-term use (≤96 hr) and during transport.
- HHs should be used for patients requiring long-term mechanical ventilation (>96 hr) or for patients for whom HME use is contraindicated.

➤ ASSESSMENT OF OUTCOME

Humidification is assumed to be appropriate if, on regular, careful inspection, the patient exhibits none of the listed hazards or complications.

➤ MONITORING

The humidifier should be inspected during the patient-ventilator system check, and condensate should be removed from the circuit as needed. HMEs should be inspected and replaced if secretions have contaminated the insert or filter. The following should be recorded during equipment inspection:

- During routine use on an intubated patient, an HH should be set to deliver inspired gas at 33° C ±2° C and should provide a minimum of 30 mg/L of water vapor.
- Inspired gas temperature should be monitored at or near the patient's airway opening (HH).
- Specific temperatures may vary with the patient's condition; airway temperature should never exceed 37° C.
  - For heated-wire circuits used with infants, the probe must be placed outside the incubator or away from the radiant warmer.

HUMIDIFICATION DURING MECHANICAL VENTILATION—CONT'D

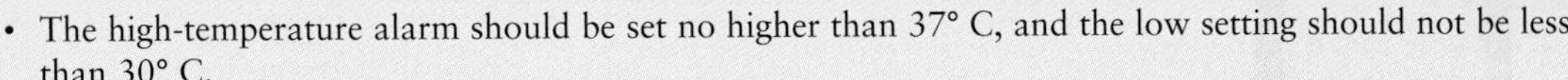

AARC Clinical Practice Guideline (Excerpts)*

- The high-temperature alarm should be set no higher than 37° C, and the low setting should not be less than 30° C.
- Water level and function of automatic feed system (if applicable).
- Quantity and consistency of secretions. Characteristics should be noted and recorded. When using an HME, if secretions become copious or appear increasingly tenacious, an HH should replace the HME.

*For the complete guideline, see Respir Care 37:887, 1992.

Reservoir and Feed Systems

Heated humidifiers operating continuously in breathing circuits can evaporate more than 1 L of water per day. To avoid constant refilling, these devices either incorporate a large water reservoir or use a gravity feed system. An ideal reservoir or feed system should be safe, dependable, and easy to set up and use and should allow for continuity of therapy, even when the reservoir is being replenished.

Simple large reservoir systems are manually refilled (with sterile or distilled water). Unfortunately, this requires a momentary interruption of humidifier operation and mechanical ventilation, if used. Moreover, because the system must be "opened" for refilling, cross contamination can occur. Water levels in manually filled systems are constantly changing, so that changes in the humidifier fill volume alter the gas compression factor and thus the delivered volume during mechanical ventilation. A small inlet that can be attached to a gravity-fed intravenous bag and line allows refilling without interruption of ventilation. Such systems still require constant checking and manual replenishment by opening the line valve or clamp. If not checked regularly, the reservoir in these systems can go dry, placing the patient at considerable risk.

Automatic feed systems avoid the need for constant checking and manual refilling of humidifiers. The simplest type of automatic feed system is the level-compensated reservoir (Figure 32-9). In these systems (Hudson RCI, Temecula, Calif.; Marquest Medical Products, Englewood Colo.), an external reservoir is aligned horizontally with the humidifier, maintaining relatively consistent water levels between the reservoir and the humidifier chamber.

Flotation valve controls are also used to maintain humidifier reservoir fluid volume. In flotation-type systems, a float rises and falls with the water level. As the water level falls below a preset value, the float opens the feed valve; as the water rises back to the set fill level, the float closes the feed valve (see Figure 32-3). An optical sensor can also be used to sense water level, driving a solenoid valve to allow refilling of the humidifier reservoir.

Membrane-type humidifiers do not require a flow control system (see Figure 32-4). Because the liquid water chamber underlying the membrane cannot overfill, these devices require only an *open* gravity feed system to ensure proper function. The Hummax II (Metran Medical Instruments Mfg. Co., Ltd., Saitama, Japan) consists of a heated wire and polyethylene microporous hollow fiber placed in an inspiratory circuit so that water vapor is delivered throughout the circuit (see Figure 32-5).

To guide practitioners in applying humidity therapy during ventilatory support, the American Association for Respiratory Care (AARC) has published *Clinical Practice Guideline: Humidification during Mechanical Ventilation* (p. 746).[7]

MINI CLINI

Selecting the Appropriate Therapy to Condition a Patient's Inspired Gas

PROBLEM

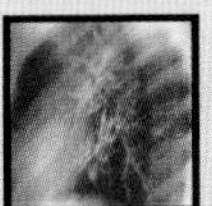

A survivor of near-drowning has just been intubated and placed on mechanical ventilatory support. Her body temperature is 31° C, and her minute ventilation is unknown. What would be the appropriate humidification system to recommend for this patient?

SOLUTION

Normally, patients supported by mechanical ventilation can be started with an HME, unless its use is contraindicated. According to the AARC Clinical Practice Guideline on p. 746, using an HME with this patient is contraindicated because (1) she is hypothermic and (2) she has a high minute ventilation. Based on this assessment and the algorithm in Figure 32-17, the best choice is a heated humidifier, preferably with servo-controlled airway temperature.

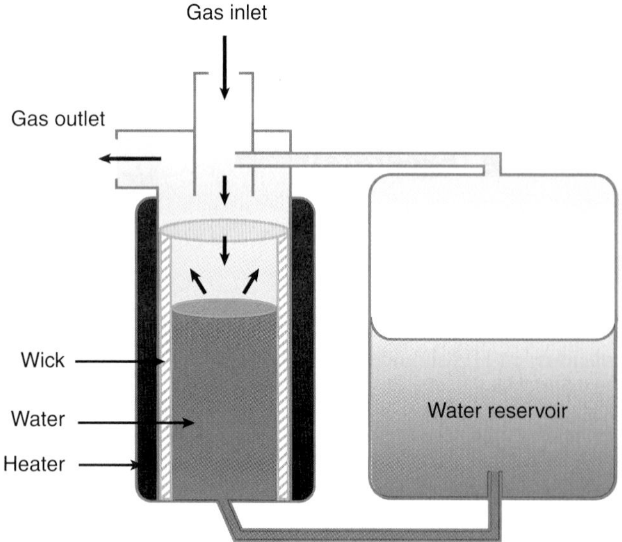

Figure 32-9
Schematic of the Concha-Column wick-type humidifier with level-compensated reservoir feed system (Hudson RCI, Temecula, Calif.) *(From Fink J, Cohen N: Humidity and aerosols. In Eubank D, Bone R, editors: Principles and applications of cardiorespiratory care equipment, St Louis, 1994, Mosby.)*

Setting Humidification Levels

Although the American National Standards Institute (ANSI) recommends minimum levels of humidity for intubated patients (more than 30 mg/L), there is less guidance regarding appropriate settings for optimal humidification. One suggestion is to target the temperature and level of humidity for the normal conditions for the point at which the gas is entering the airway. For example, the humidity of air entering the carina is typically 35 to 40 mg/L. When humidifiers run too cold (less than 32° C), humidity can be reduced to the point of increased airway plugging. Not all active heated humidifiers perform the same under all conditions. Nishida et al.[27] compared the performance of four active humidifiers (MR290 with MR730, MR310 with MR730,* ConchaTherm IV,† and Hummax II‡), which were set to maintain the temperature of the airway opening at 32° and 37° C under a variety of ventilator parameters. The greater the minute ventilation, the lower the humidity delivered with all devices except the Hummax II. When the airway temperature control of the devices was set at 32° C, neither the ConchaTherm IV, the MR 310, nor the MR 730 delivered 30 mg/L of vapor, which is the value recommended by the ANSI. This emphasizes the need to set humidifiers to maintain airway temperatures in the range between 35°and 37°C.

Controversy exists regarding the appropriate temperature and humidity of inspired gas delivered to mechanically ventilated patients with artificial airways. The current AARC *Clinical Practice Guideline* recommends 33°C, within 2°C, with a minimum of 30 mg/L of water vapor. In a comprehensive review, Williams et al.[30] suggest that inspired humidity be maintained at an optimal level, because at humidities higher or lower than this level, mucosal dysfunction will occur. This optimal level is 37°C with 100% relative humidity and 44 mg/L. Theoretically, optimal humidity offers improved mucociliary clearance. The benefits of this strategy are theory based, but have yet to be demonstrated conclusively in the clinical setting. Further controlled studies are needed to better support the need for optimal humidity.

*MR290, MR310, and MR730 from Fisher & Paykel Healthcare Inc., Laguna Hills, Calif.
†ConchaTherm IV from Hudson RCI, Temecula, Calif.
‡Hummax II from Metran Medical Inst. Mfg. Co., Ltd., Saitama, Japan.

Problem Solving and Troubleshooting

Common problems with humidification systems include dealing with condensation, avoiding cross contamination, and ensuring proper conditioning of the inspired gas.

Condensation

In all standard heated humidifier systems, saturated gas cools as it leaves the point of humidification and passes through the delivery tubing en route to the patient. As the gas cools, its water vapor capacity decreases, resulting in condensation or "rain out." Factors influencing the amount of condensation include (1) the temperature difference across the system (humidifier to airway); (2) the ambient temperature; (3) the gas flow; (4) the set airway temperature; and (5) the length, diameter, and thermal mass of the breathing circuit.

Figure 32-10 provides an example of the condensation process. In this case, because of cooling along the circuit, the humidifier temperature has to be set to a higher level (50° C) than that desired at the airway. At 50° C, the humidifier fully saturates the gas to an absolute humidity level of 84 mg/L of water. As cooling occurs along the tubing, the capacity of the gas to hold water vapor decreases. By the time the gas reaches the patient, its temperature has dropped to 37° C, and it is holding only 44 mg/L of water vapor. Although BTPS conditions have been achieved, 40 mg/L, *half* the total output of the humidifier (84 mg/L – 44 mg/L = 40 mg/L), has condensed in the inspiratory limb of the circuit.

The condensation process poses risks to both patients and caregivers and can waste a lot of water. First, condensation can disrupt or occlude gas flow through the circuit, potentially altering FIO_2 and/or ventilator function. Moreover, condensate can work its way toward the patient and be aspirated. For these reasons, circuits must be positioned to drain condensate away from the

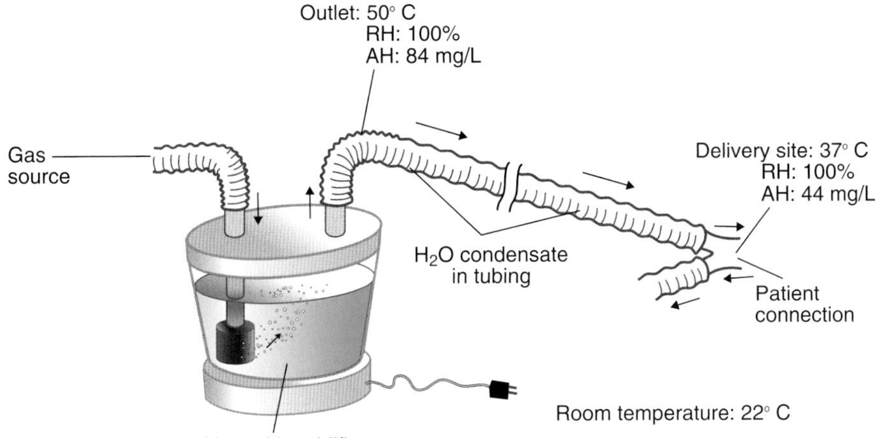

Figure 32-10
Gases leaving a standard heated humidifier are cooled en route to the patient. Although the gas remains saturated (100% relative humidity *[RH]*), cooling reduces its water vapor capacity and condensation forms. Note that almost half of the original water (500 mL/day) is lost to condensation. The temperature at the patient connection (37° C) shown here is for illustrative purposes only. Heated humidifiers should be set to deliver inspired gas at 33° C ± 2° C. *AH,* Absolute humidity.

patient and must be checked often, and excess condensate must be drained from heated humidifier breathing circuits on a regular basis.

Typically, patients contaminate ventilator circuits within hours, and condensate is colonized with bacteria and thus poses an infection risk.[31] To avoid problems in this area, healthcare personnel should treat all breathing-circuit condensate as infectious waste. See Chapter 3 for more detail on control procedures used with breathing circuits, including the AARC Clinical Practice Guideline on changing ventilator circuits.

RULE OF THUMB

Always treat breathing-circuit condensate as infectious waste. Use standard precautions, including wearing gloves and goggles. Always drain the tubing away from the patient's airway into an infectious waste container and dispose of the waste according to the policies and procedures of the institution.

Several techniques are used to minimize problems with breathing-circuit condensate. One common method is to place water traps at low points in the circuit (both the inspiratory and expiratory limbs of ventilator circuits). This aids drainage of condensate and reduces the likelihood of gas flow obstruction. When used in ventilator circuits, water traps should have little effect on circuit compliance, allow emptying without disrupting ventilation, and not be prone to leakage.

One way to avoid condensation problems is to keep it from forming. Because the fall in temperature in gas traveling from the humidifier to the airway causes condensation, maintaining temperature in the circuit can prevent formation of condensate.

Several methods can reduce circuit cooling, by keeping the circuit at a constant temperature, such as insulation or increasing the thermal mass of the circuit. The most common approach uses wire heating elements inserted into the ventilator circuit.

Most heated-wire circuits use dual controllers with two temperature sensors, one monitoring the temperature of gas leaving the humidifier and the other placed at or near the patient's airway (Figure 32-11). The controller regulates the temperature difference between humidifier output and patient airway. When heated-wire circuits are used, the humidifier heats gas to a lower temperature (32° to 40° C) than it does with conventional circuits (45° to 50° C). The reduction in condensate in the tubing results in less water use, reduced need for drainage, and less infection risk for both patient and healthcare workers.

Use of heated-wire circuits in neonates is complicated by the use of incubators and radiant warmers. Incubators provide a warm environment surrounding the child, and radiant warmers use radiant energy to warm objects that intercept radiant light. In both cases, a temperature probe placed in the heated environment will effect humidifier performance, resulting in reduced humidity received by the patient. Figure 32-12 demonstrates the impact of temperature probe placement, in or out of the incubator, on absolute humidity delivered to the neonate. Consequently, temperature probes should always be placed outside of the radiant field or incubator (Figure 32-13).

Cross Contamination

Aerosol and condensate from ventilator circuits are known sources of bacterial colonization.[31] However, advances in both circuit and humidifier technology have reduced the risk of nosocomial infection when these systems are used. Wick- or membrane-type passover humidifiers prevent formation of bacteria-carrying aerosols. Heated-wire circuits reduce production and pooling of condensate within the circuit. In addition, the high reservoir temperatures in humidifiers are bacteriocidal.[32] In fact, in ventilator circuits using wick-type humidifiers with heated-wire systems, circuit contamination usually occurs from the patient to the circuit, rather than vice versa.

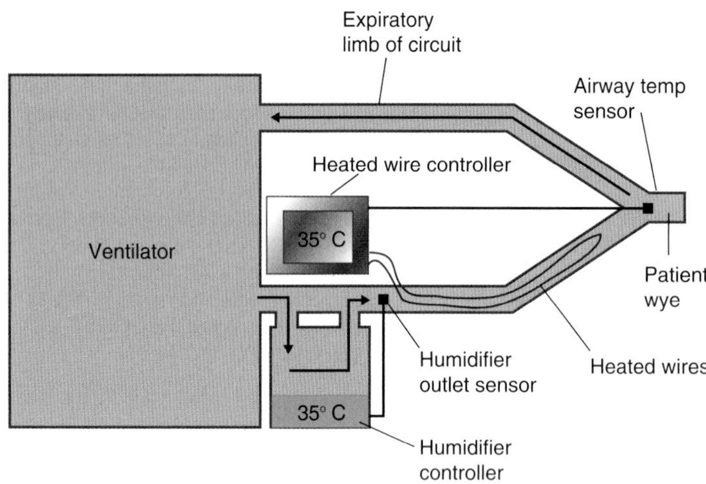

Figure 32-11

Heated-wire humidifier system. Dual sensor system keeps temperature constant throughout inspiratory limb of ventilator circuit, minimizing condensation. Cooling of exhaled gas in the expiratory limb can cause condensation unless it also is heated.

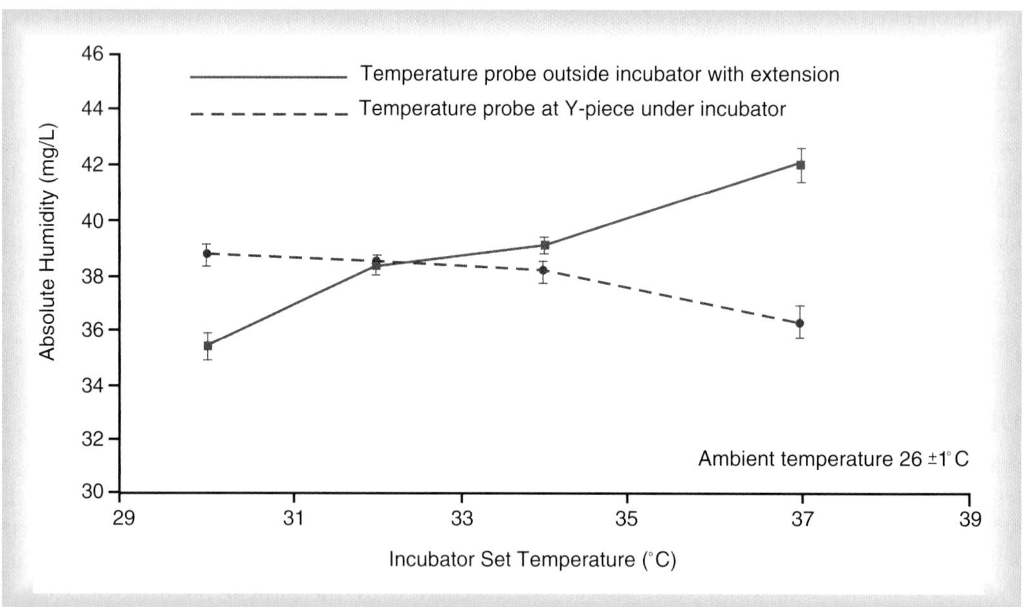

Figure 32-12

Humidity achieved at the Y-piece of a neonatal humidification system when used inside an incubator (*dotted line*), and outside/under an incubator (*solid line*).

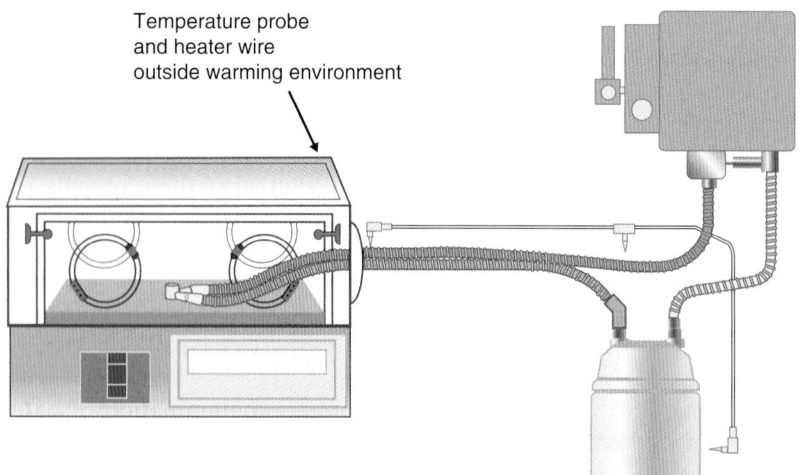

Figure 32-13

Neonatal breathing-circuit configuration used with an incubator, with temperature probe placed outside of the warming environment and an unheated portion of inspiratory circuit delivering the gases to the Y-piece.

For decades, the traditional way to minimize the risk of circuit-related nosocomial infection in critically ill patients receiving ventilatory support was to change the ventilator tubing and its attached components every 24 hours. It is now known that frequent ventilator-circuit changes actually *increase* the risk of nosocomial pneumonia.[33] Current research indicates that there is minimal risk of ventilator-associated pneumonia with weekly circuit changes and that there may be no need to change circuits at all.[34-37] In addition, substantial cost-savings can accrue with decreased frequency of circuit changes.

Proper Conditioning of the Inspired Gas

All respiratory therapists are trained to regularly measure patients' inspired FIO_2 levels and, in ventilatory care, to monitor selected pressures, volumes, and flows. However, few clinicians take the steps needed to ensure proper conditioning of the inspired gas received by their patients.

The most accurate and reliable way to ensure that patients are receiving gas at the expected temperature and humidity level is to measure these parameters. Portable battery-operated digital **hygrometer**-thermometer systems are available for less than $300 and are invaluable in ensuring proper conditioning of the inspired gas. These devices should be as common at the bedside as oxygen analyzers.

Many heated-wire humidification systems have a humidity control. This control does not reflect either absolute or relative humidity, but only the temperature differential between the humidifier and airway sensor. It is possible that, if the heated wires are set warmer than the humidifier, less humidity is delivered to the patient. To ensure that the inspired gas is being properly conditioned, clinicians should always adjust the temperature differential to the point that *a few drops of condensation* form near the patient wye. Lacking direct measurement of humidity, observation of this minimal condensate is the most reliable indicator that the gas is fully saturated at the specified temperature. If condensate cannot be seen, there is no way of knowing the level of relative humidity—it could be anywhere between 99% and 0%! HME performance can be evaluated in a similar manner.[38]

RULE OF THUMB

You can estimate if an HME is performing well at the bedside by visually confirming condensation in the flex tube. Lack of condensate may be a clue that humidification is less than adequate and that alternative systems may be appropriate for use with that particular patient.

▶ BLAND AEROSOL THERAPY

Whereas humidity is simply water in the gas phase, a bland aerosol consists of liquid *particles* suspended in a gas (see Chapter 33 for details on aerosol physics). Bland aerosol therapy involves the delivery of sterile water or hypotonic, isotonic, or hypertonic saline aerosols. Bland aerosol administration may be accompanied by oxygen therapy.

To guide practitioners in applying this therapy, the AARC has published *Clinical Practice Guideline: Bland Aerosol Administration* (p. 752).[39]

Equipment for Bland Aerosol Therapy

The equipment needed for bland aerosol therapy includes an aerosol generator and a delivery system. Devices used to generate bland aerosols include large-volume jet nebulizers and ultrasonic nebulizers (USNs). Delivery systems include a variety of direct airway appliances and enclosures (mist tents).

Aerosol Generators

Large-Volume Jet Nebulizers. The large-volume jet nebulizer is the most common device used to generate bland aerosols. As depicted in Figure 32-14, these devices are pneumatically powered, attaching directly to a flow meter and compressed gas source. Liquid particle aerosols are generated by passing gas at a high velocity through a small "jet" orifice. The resulting low pressure at the jet draws fluid from the reservoir up to the top of a siphon tube, where it is sheared off and shattered into liquid particles. The large, unstable particles fall out of suspension or impact on the internal surfaces of the device, including the fluid surface (**baffling**). The remaining small particles leave the nebulizer through the outlet port, carried in the gas stream. A variable air-entrainment port allows air mixing to increase flow rates and to alter FIO_2 levels (see Chapter 35).

As with humidifiers, if heat is required, a hot-plate, wrap-around, yolk collar, or immersion element can be added. However, unlike heated humidifiers, these devices rarely have sophisticated servo-controlled systems to control delivery temperature. Indeed, many systems do not even shut down when the reservoir empties, resulting in the deliver of hot, dry gas to the patient. Failure of the element can also cause a loss of heating capacity, without warning to the clinician.

Depending on the design, input flow, and air-entrainment setting, the total water output of unheated large-volume jet nebulizers varies between 26 and 35 mg H_2O/L. When heated, output increases to between 33 and 55 mg H_2O/L, mainly because of increased vapor capacity.[40,41]

Bland Aerosol Administration

AARC Clinical Practice Guideline (Excerpts)*

➤ INDICATIONS

- The presence of upper airway edema—cool, bland aerosol
- Laryngotracheobronchitis (LTB)
- Subglottic edema
- Postextubation edema
- Postoperative management of the upper airway
- The presence of a bypassed upper airway
- The need for sputum specimens

➤ CONTRAINDICATIONS

- Bronchoconstriction
- History of airway hyperresponsiveness

➤ HAZARDS AND COMPLICATIONS

- Wheezing or bronchospasm
- Bronchoconstriction when artificial airway is used
- Infection
- Overhydration
- Patient discomfort
- Caregiver exposure to airborne contagions produced during coughing or sputum induction

➤ ASSESSMENT OF NEED

The presence of one or more of the following may be an indication for administration of a water or isotonic or hypotonic saline aerosol:

- Stridor
- Brassy, crouplike cough
- Hoarseness following extubation
- Diagnosis of LTB or croup
- History of upper airway irritation and increased work of breathing (e.g., smoke inhalation)
- Patient discomfort associated with airway instrumentation or insult

Need for sputum induction (e.g., *Pneumocystis carinii* pneumonia or tuberculosis) is an indication for administration of hypertonic saline aerosol.

➤ ASSESSMENT OF OUTCOME

With administration of water or hypotonic or isotonic saline, the desired outcome is one or more of the following:

- Decreased work of breathing
- Improved vital signs
- Decreased stridor
- Decreased dyspnea
- Improved arterial blood gas values
- Improved oxygen saturation, as indicated by pulse oximetry
- With administration of hypertonic saline, the desired outcome is a sputum sample that is adequate for analysis.

➤ MONITORING

The extent of patient monitoring should be determined based on the stability and severity of the patient's condition:

- Patient subjective response—pain, discomfort, dyspnea, restlessness
- Heart rate and rhythm; blood pressure
- Respiratory rate, pattern, mechanics; accessory muscle use
- Sputum production—quantity, color, consistency, odor
- Skin color
- Breath sounds
- Pulse oximetry (if hypoxemia is suspected)

---

*For the complete guideline, see Respir Care 38:1196, 1993.

Larger versions of these devices (with 2- to 3-L reservoirs) are used to deliver bland aerosols into mist tents. These enclosure systems can generate flow rates faster than 20 L/min, with water outputs as high as 5 mL/min (300 mL/hr). Because heat build-up in enclosures is a problem, these systems are always run unheated.

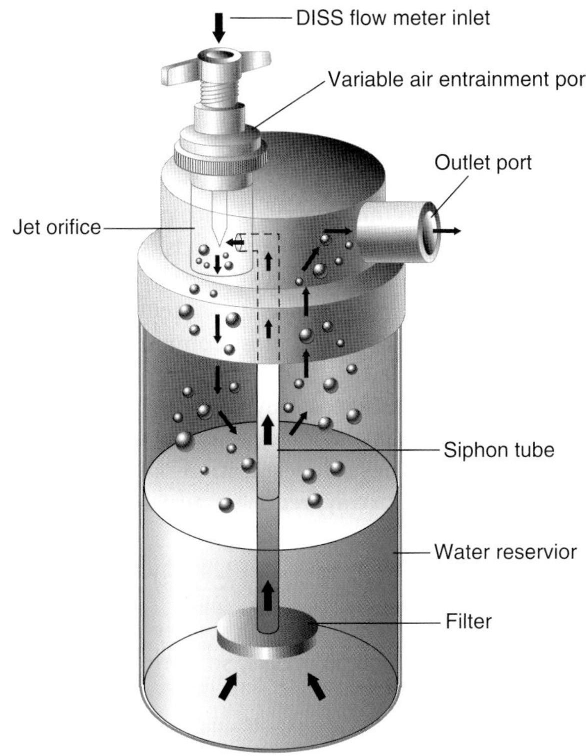

Figure 32-14
All-purpose large-volume jet nebulizer.

Ultrasonic Nebulizers. An **ultrasonic nebulizer (USN)** is an electrically powered device that uses a **piezoelectric crystal** to generate aerosol. This crystal transducer converts radio waves into high-frequency mechanical vibrations (sound). These vibrations are transmitted to a liquid surface, where the intense mechanical energy creates a "geyser" of aerosol droplets. Figure 32-15 provides a functional schematic of a typical large-volume USN. Output from the radiofrequency generator is transmitted over a shielded cable to the piezoelectric crystal. Vibrational energy is transmitted either indirectly through a water-filled couplant reservoir or directly to a solution chamber. Gas entering the chamber inlet picks up the aerosol particles and exits through the chamber outlet.

The properties of the ultrasonic signal determine the characteristics of the aerosol generated by these nebulizers. *Signal frequency,* normally preset by the manufacturer, determines aerosol particle size. Particle size is inversely proportional to signal frequency. For example, a USN operating at a frequency of 2.25 MHz may produce an aerosol with a mass median aerodynamic diameter (MMAD) of approximately 2.5 μm, whereas another nebulizer operating at 1.25 MHz produces an aerosol with a MMAD of between 4 and 6 μm. *Signal amplitude* alters the transducer's vibrational energy and thus directly affects the amount of aerosol produced. Unlike frequency, signal amplitude can be adjusted by the clinician.

Particle size and aerosol density delivered to the patient are also affected by the source and flow of gas through

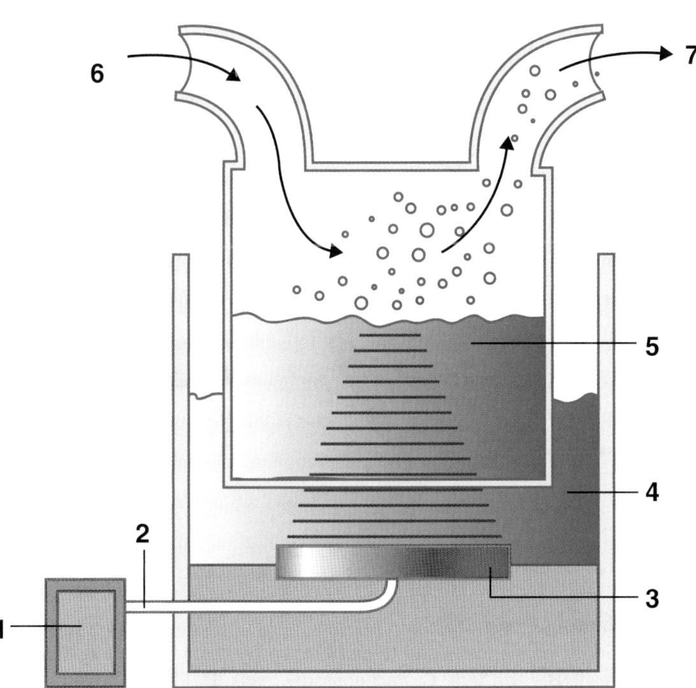

Figure 32-15
Functional schematic of a typical large-volume ultrasonic nebulizer (USN). *(1)* Radiofrequency generator, *(2)* shielded cable, *(3)* piezoelectric crystal transducer, *(4)* water-filled couplant reservoir, *(5)* solution chamber, *(6)* chamber inlet, and *(7)* chamber outlet. *(Modified from Barnes TA: Core textbook for respiratory care practice, ed 2, St Louis, 1994, Mosby.)*

the solution chamber. Large bedside USNs have built-in blowers that deliver room air to the solution chamber. On these systems, airflow may be adjusted by changing the fan speed or using a simple damper valve. Alternatively, compressed gases can be delivered to the chamber inlet through a flow meter. For precise control over delivered oxygen concentrations, clinicians can attach a flow meter with an oxygen blender or air-entrainment system to the chamber inlet.

The flow and amplitude settings interact to determine aerosol density (mg/L) and total water output (mL/min). Amplitude effects water output. At a given amplitude setting, the greater the flow through the chamber, the less the density of the aerosol. Conversely, low flows result in higher-density aerosols. In fact, a USN can produce aerosols with densities as high as 500 mg/L, more than 10 times the amount of water necessary to achieve BTPS conditions! Total aerosol output (mL/min) is greatest when both flow and amplitude are set at the maximum. Using these settings, some units can achieve total water outputs as high as 7 mL/min.

Particle size, aerosol density, and output are also affected by the relative humidity of the carrier gas (see Chapter 33). In addition, unlike jet nebulizers, the temperature of the solution placed in a USN increases during use. Although this affects water vapor capacity, its impact on aerosol output is minimal.

RULE OF THUMB

To produce a high-density aerosol using an ultrasonic nebulizer (useful for sputum induction), set the amplitude high and the flow rate low. To maximize aerosol delivery per minute (when trying to help mobilize secretions), set both the flow rate and the amplitude at the maximum.

Although USNs have some unique capabilities, in most cases of bland aerosol administration, their relative advantages over jet nebulizers are outweighed by their high cost and erratic reliability. Exceptions include the use of a USN for sputum induction. Commercially available USNs (usually marketed as "cool" mist devices) have found a place in the home, being used as room humidifiers. As with any nebulizer, the reservoirs of these devices can easily become contaminated, resulting in airborne transmission of pathogens. Care should be taken to ensure that these units are cleaned according to the manufacturer's recommendations and that water is discarded from the reservoir periodically between cleanings. In the absence of a manufacturer's recommendation, these units should undergo appropriate disinfection at least every 6 days.[42] In general, passover and wick-type humidifiers present less risk than does the USN as a room humidifier.

Airway Appliances

Airway appliances used to deliver bland aerosol therapy include the aerosol mask, face tent, T-tube, and tracheostomy mask (Figure 32-16). The aerosol mask and face tent are used for patients with intact upper airways. The T-tube is used for patients who are orally or nasally intubated or who have a tracheostomy. The tracheostomy mask is used solely for patients who have a tracheostomy. In all cases, large-bore tubing is required to minimize flow resistance and prevent occlusion by condensate.

For short-term therapy to patients with intact upper airways, the aerosol mask is the device of choice. However, some patients cannot tolerate masks and may do better with a face tent. No data support preferential use of an open aerosol mask versus a face tent.

Although the T-tube is the most common application for tracheostomy patients, unless moderate to high F_{IO_2} levels are needed, a tracheostomy mask is a better choice. Unlike T-tubes, tracheostomy masks exert no traction on the airway and they allow secretions and condensate to escape from the airway, reducing airway resistance.

Enclosures (Mist Tents and Hoods)

Infants and small children may not readily tolerate direct airway appliances such as masks, so enclosures such as

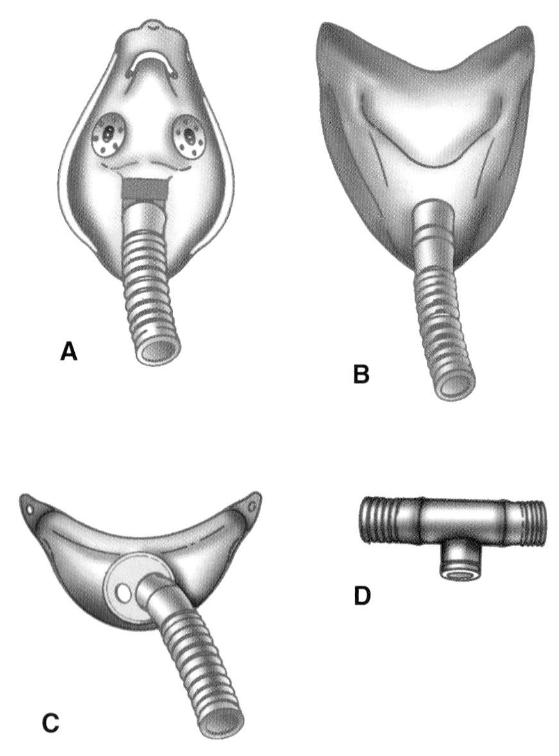

Figure 32-16
Airway appliances used to deliver bland aerosol therapy. **A,** Aerosol mask. **B,** Face tent. **C,** Tracheostomy mask. **D,** T-tube.

mist tents and aerosol hoods are used to deliver bland aerosol therapy to these patients. Because mist tents were used for more than 40 years mainly to treat croup, clinicians still refer to these devices as *croup tents.* The cool aerosol provided through these enclosures promotes vasoconstriction, decreases edema, and reduces airway obstruction.

Any body enclosure poses two problems: CO_2 build-up and heat retention. CO_2 build-up can be reduced by providing sufficiently high gas flow rates. These high flows of fresh gas circulate continually through the enclosure and "wash out" carbon dioxide, while helping maintain desired oxygen concentrations. Heat retention is handled differently by each manufacturer. Some, such as the Maxicool, use high fresh-gas flows to prevent heat build-up. Others incorporate a separate cooling device. The old Air-Shields Croupette used a simple ice compartment to cool the aerosol. New units, such as the Ohmeda Ohio Pediatric Aerosol Tent and the Mistogen CAM-2M Tent, use electrically powered refrigeration units to cool the circulating air.

The cooling from these refrigeration units produces a great deal of condensation, which must be drained into a collection bottle outside of the tent. A newer model, the Mistogen CAM-3M, overcomes some of these problems with its thermoelectric cooling system, in which an electric current passing through a semiconductor augments heat absorption and release. As warm air is taken from the tent, heat is transferred and released in the room while cool air is returned to the tent.

Sputum Induction

As a diagnostic procedure, sputum induction deserves separate attention from other modes of bland aerosol therapy. Over the years, sputum induction has been proven a useful, cost-effective, safe method for diagnosing tuberculosis, *Pneumocystis carinii* pneumonia, and lung cancer.[43-45]

Sputum induction involves short-term application of high-density hypertonic saline (3% to 10%) aerosols to the airway to assist in mobilizing pulmonary secretions for evacuation and recovery. Although high-density aerosols are most easily generated using ultrasonic nebulization, a high-output heated jet nebulizer will suffice. The exact mechanism by which high-density hypertonic aerosols aid mucociliary clearance is unknown. However, an increased volume of surface fluid, combined with stimulation of the irritant (cough) reflex, is the likely factor.

Box 32-3 outlines an example procedure for sputum induction using a 3% saline solution.[46] To ensure a good sputum sample, every effort must be made to separate saliva from true respiratory tract secretions.[47] In some cases, protocols include having patients brush their teeth and tongue surface thoroughly and rinse their mouths before sputum induction. Although the distinction between saliva and sputum can be made in the diagnostic laboratory, care during the collection procedure will eliminate the need for repeat inductions.

Box 32-3 • **Sputum-Induction Procedure**

1. Gather the necessary equipment: ultrasonic nebulizer, aerosol mask, large-bore tubing, specimen container, 3% sterile saline, and stethoscope.
2. Check the chart for order or protocol, diagnosis, history, and other pertinent information.
3. Wash your hands and follow applicable standard, airborne, and tuberculosis precautions.
4. Introduce yourself and identify your department; verify the patient's identity; and explain the procedure and verify that the patient understands it.
5. Have the patient assume an upright, seated position if possible.
6. Have the patient rinse his or her mouth with water, blow his or her nose, and clear any excess saliva.
7. Perform pretreatment assessment, including vital signs, muscle tone, ability to cough, and auscultation.
8. Assemble the nebulizer; fill the couplant chamber with tap water; plug the unit into a grounded electrical outlet; and attach the delivery tubing and mask.
9. Aseptically fill the medication chamber of the nebulizer with 3% sterile saline.
10. Turn the unit on and adjust the output control to achieve adequate flow and high density.
11. Place the mask comfortably on the patient's face and instruct the patient to take slow, deep breaths, with occasional inspiratory hold as tolerated.
12. Periodically reassess the patient's condition (including breath sounds) throughout the application.
13. Modify the technique and reinstruct the patient as needed, based on his or her response.
14. Terminate the treatment after 15-30 min, if significant adverse reactions occur, or when sputum specimen has been obtained.
15. Encourage the patient to cough and expectorate sputum into specimen cup; observe for volume, color, consistency, odor, and presence or absence of blood.
16. Label the specimen container with patient identification and required information and deliver to the appropriate personnel.
17. Chart the therapy according to departmental and institutional protocol.
18. Notify the appropriate personnel of any adverse reactions or other concerns.

Modified from Butler TJ, Close JR, Close RJ: Laboratory exercises for competency in respiratory care, Philadelphia, 1998, FA Davis.

Problem Solving and Troubleshooting

The most common problems with bland aerosol delivery systems are cross contamination and infection, environmental safety, inadequate mist production, overhydration, bronchospasm, and noise.

With regard to cross contamination and infection, rigorous adherence to the infection control guidelines detailed in Chapter 3, especially those covering solutions and equipment processing, should help minimize the risks involved in using these systems. In addition, the water should be changed regularly and the couplant compartments of USNs should be disinfected regularly.

Environmental safety issues arise mainly when aerosol therapy is prescribed for immunosuppressed patients or for those with tuberculosis. To minimize problems in this area, all clinicians should strictly follow Centers for Disease Control and Prevention standards and airborne precautions, including those specified for control of exposure to tuberculosis (see Chapter 3). Additional methods to deal with environmental control of drug aerosols are covered in Chapter 33.

Inadequate mist production is a common problem with all nebulizer systems. With pneumatically powered jet nebulizers, poor mist production can be caused by inadequate input flow, siphon tube obstruction, or jet orifice misalignment. With the exception of inadequate input flow, these problems require unit repair or replacement. If a USN is not functioning properly, the electrical power supply (cord, plug, and fuse or circuit breakers) should be checked first. Then, the clinician should check to confirm that (1) carrier gas is actually flowing through the device and (2) the amplitude, or output, control is set above minimum. If there is still no visible mist output, the clinician should inspect the couplant chamber to confirm proper fill level and the absence of any visible dirt or debris. Finally, the clinician must ensure that the couplant chamber solution meets the manufacturer's specifications (most units will not function properly with distilled water).

Overhydration is a problem with continuous use of heated jet nebulizers and USNs. Indeed, with USNs capable of such extraordinarily high water outputs, *they should never be used for continuous therapy.* The risk of overhydration is highest for infants, small children, and those with preexisting fluid or electrolyte imbalances. Even if used only to meet BTPS conditions, bland aerosol therapy effectively eliminates insensible water loss through the lungs and should thus be equated to a daily water gain (approximately 200 mL/day for the average adult).

In addition to overhydration of the patient, inspissated pulmonary secretions also can swell after high-density aerosol therapy, worsening airway obstruction. Careful patient selection and monitoring can prevent most potential problems with overhydration.

Even bland water aerosols can cause bronchospasm in some patients. Indeed, ultrasonic nebulization of distilled water is used in some pulmonary function laboratories to provoke bronchospasm and to assess bronchial hyperactivity.[45] To avoid this problem at the bedside, the clinician should always carefully review the patient's history and diagnosis before administering any bland aerosol, especially a hypotonic water solution. As indicated in the AARC practice guideline, patients receiving continuous bland aerosol therapy should be initially monitored carefully (including breath sounds and subjective response) and reevaluated every 8 hours or with any change in clinical condition.[39] If bronchospasm occurs during therapy, treatment must be stopped immediately, oxygen must be provided, and appropriate bronchodilator therapy should be initiated as soon as possible. If the physician still requests bland aerosol therapy for such a patient, pretreatment with a bronchodilator may be needed. In addition, isotonic solutions (0.9% saline) may be better tolerated by these patients than water.

A problem unique to large-volume, air-entrainment jet nebulizers is the noise they generate, especially at high flows. The American Academy of Pediatrics recommends that sound levels remain below 58 dB to avoid hearing loss for infants being cared for in incubators and oxygen hoods. Because a number of commercial nebulizers exceed this noise level when in operation, careful selection of equipment is necessary. However, the best way to avoid this problem and further minimize infection risks is to use heated passover humidification instead of nebulization.

▶ SELECTING THE APPROPRIATE THERAPY

Figure 32-17 provides a basic algorithm for selecting or recommending the appropriate therapy to condition a patient's inspired gas. Key considerations include (1) gas flow, (2) presence or absence of an artificial tracheal airway, (3) character of the pulmonary secretions, (4) need for and expected duration of mechanical ventilation, and (5) contraindications to using an HME.

Regarding delivery of oxygen to the upper airway, the American College of Chest Physicians advises *against* using a bubble humidifier at flow rates of 4 L/min or less.[48] For the occasional patient who complains of nasal dryness or irritation when receiving low-flow oxygen, a humidifier should be added to the delivery system. Conversely, the relative inefficiency of unheated bubble humidifiers means that the clinician may need to consider heated humidification for patients receiving long-term oxygen at high flow rates (>10 L/min without air entrainment).

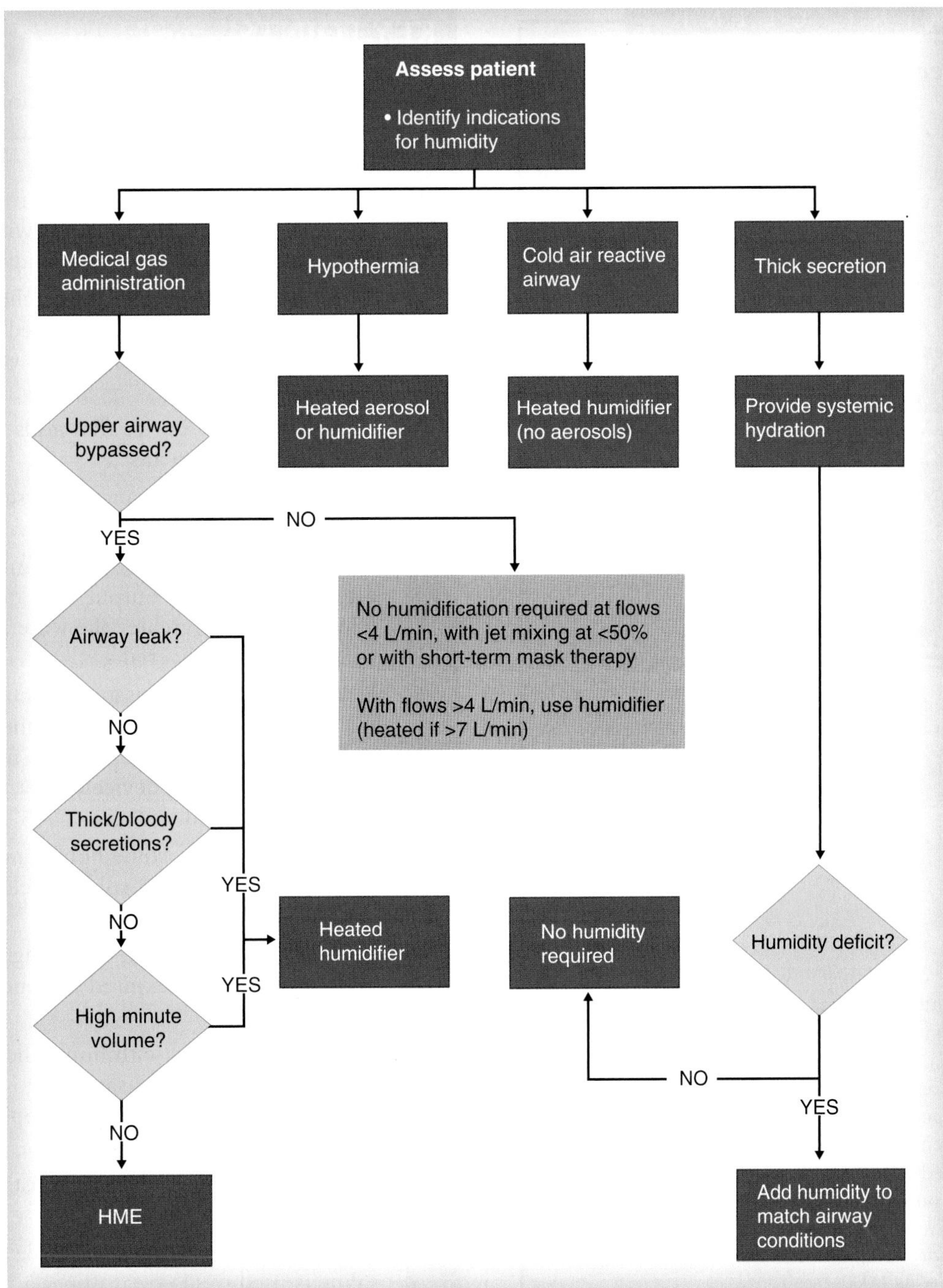

Figure 32-17

Selection algorithm for humidity and bland aerosol therapy.

HMEs provide an inexpensive alternative to heated humidifiers when used for short-term ventilation of patients who do not have complex humidification needs. However, passive HMEs may not provide sufficient heat or humidification for long-term management of certain patients. When an HME is to be used, it should be selected based on individual patient need and ventilatory pattern, as well as the unit's efficiency and size. Moreover, all patients using HMEs should be reevaluated regularly to confirm the appropriateness of continued use.[49]

MINI CLINI

Cost-Effectiveness of Humidification Systems

PROBLEM

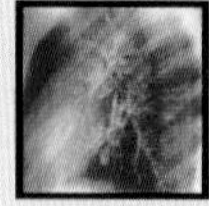

There is a lot of controversy over which is more cost effective—heated water humidifiers or HMEs. How can the cost of passover humidifiers, with standard circuit and heated-wire circuits, be compared with the cost of HMEs?

SOLUTION

First, the daily setup and operating costs must be identified to determine relative break-even costs for the various systems being analyzed. The following table compares the costs associated with three humidification strategies in terms of circuit setup costs, water usage, and labor for a typical patient requiring 12 days of mechanical ventilation at a large, comprehensive acute care hospital.

Components of Circuit Setup Costs	Heated Water Usage of Standard Circuit	Heated Water Usage of Heated-Wire Circuit	Heat and Moisture Exchanger (HME)
Circuit	$3.00	$11.00	$3.00
Humidifier/H_2O	$12.00	$12.00	—
Water traps (2)	$3.00	—	—
HME filter	—	—	$5.00
Setup cost total (with labor)	$18.00	$23.00	$8.00
Daily cost	$11.00	$1.50	$5.00
Total cost (5 days)	$62.00	$29.00	$28.00
Total cost (12 days)	$139.00	$39.50	$63.00

The standard circuit has lower setup costs than the heated-wire circuit, but it has twice the daily water usage and an additional labor cost of $9.50 per day for adding and removing water. The HME has the lowest setup cost, but after ventilator day 5, total costs of daily filter replacement exceed the cost associated with operation of the heated-wire circuit.

The prices used in the comparison include the cost to rent or lease the humidifiers. Even at these prices, it is clear that humidifiers with heated wires are most cost-effective, even with extended change intervals, than conventional, nonheated circuits or HMEs.

KEY POINTS

- Heat and moisture exchange is accomplished primarily by the nose. Bypassing the upper airway without replacing the heat and humidity it provides can cause damage to the respiratory tract.

KEY POINTS—cont'd

- The primary goal of humidification is to maintain normal physiological conditions in the lower airways.
- Gases delivered to the nose and mouth should be conditioned to 20° to 22° C with 10 mg/L water vapor (50% relative humidity).
- When being delivered to the trachea, gases should be warmed and humidified to 32° to 35° C with 36 to 40 mg/L water vapor (100% relative humidity).
- A humidifier is a device that adds invisible molecular water to gas.
- A nebulizer generates and disperses liquid particles in a gas stream.
- Temperature is the most important factor affecting humidifier output. The higher the temperature, the greater the water vapor content of the delivered gas.
- Bubble humidifiers, passover humidifiers, and HMEs are the major types of humidifiers. Bubble and passover humidifiers may incorporate heating devices, as well as reservoir and feed systems.
- At high flow rates, some bubble humidifiers can produce microaerosols particles, which can carry infectious bacteria.
- An HME acts passively, capturing both heat and moisture from expired gas and returning it to the patient.
- Common problems with humidification systems include condensation, cross contamination, and ensuring proper conditioning of the inspired gas.
- Breathing-circuit condensate must always be treated as infectious waste.
- Bland aerosol therapy with sterile water or saline is used to (1) treat upper airway edema, (2) overcome heat and humidity deficits in patients with tracheal airways, and (3) help obtain sputum specimens.
- Large-volume jet nebulizers and USNs are used to generate bland aerosols. Delivery systems include a variety of direct airway appliances and mist tents.
- Common problems with bland aerosol therapy are cross contamination and infection, environmental safety, inadequate mist production, overhydration, bronchospasm, and noise.

References

1. Kapadia FN, Shelley MP: Normal mechanisms of humidification, Probl Respir Care 4:395, 1991.
2. Primiano FP Jr, Montague FW Jr, Saidel GM: Measurement system for water vapor and temperature dynamics, J Appl Physiol 56:1679, 1984.
3. Shelley MP, Lloyd GM, Park GR: A review of the mechanisms and the methods of humidification of inspired gas, Intensive Care Med 14:1, 1988.
4. Ingelstedt S: Studies on the conditioning of air in the respiratory tract, Acta Otolaryngol 131(Suppl):1, 1956.
5. Chalon J, Loew D, Malbranche J: Effects of dry air and subsequent humidification on tracheobronchial ciliated epithelium, Anesthesiology 37:338, 1972.
6. Marfatia S, Donahoe PK, Henderson WH: Effect of dry and humidified gases on the respiratory epithelium in rabbits, J Pediatr Surg 10:583, 1975.
7. American Association for Respiratory Care: Clinical practice guideline: humidification during mechanical ventilation, Respir Care 37:887, 1992.
8. Chatburn RL, Primiano FP: A rational basis for humidity therapy, Respir Care 32:249, 1987.
9. Anderson S, Herbring BG, Widman B: Accidental profound hypothermia, Br J Anaesth 42:653, 1970.
10. Weinberg AD: Hypothermia, Ann Emerg Med 22:370, 1993.
11. Chen TY et al: The effect of heated humidifier in the prevention of intra-operative hypothermia, Acta Anaesthesiol Sin 32:27, 1994.
12. Giesbrecht GG, Younes M: Exercise- and cold-induced asthma, Can J Appl Physiol 20:300, 1995.
13. American Society for Testing and Materials (ASTM): Standard specification for humidifiers for medical use (F1690), Conshohocken, Pa, 1996, ASTM.
14. Gray HSJ: Humidifiers, Probl Respir Care 4:423, 1991.
15. Klein EF et al: Performance characteristics of conventional prototype humidifiers and nebulizers, Chest 64:690, 1973.
16. Darin J, Broadwell J, MacDonell R: An evaluation of water-vapor output from four brands of unheated, prefilled bubble humidifiers, Respir Care 27:41, 1982.
17. Rhame FS et al: Bubbling humidifiers produce microaerosols which can carry bacteria, Infect Control 7:403, 1986.
18. McPherson SP: Respiratory therapy equipment, ed 4, St Louis, 1985, Mosby.
19. Vitacca M et al: Hygroscopic condenser humidifiers in chronically tracheostomized patients who breathe spontaneously, Eur Respir J 7:2026, 1994.
20. Kapadia FN et al: Changing patterns of airway accidents in intubated ICU patients, Intensive Care Med 27:296, 2001.
21. Hedley RM, Allt-Graham J: A comparison of the filtration properties of heat and moisture exchangers, Anaesthesia 47:414, 1992.
22. International Organization for Standardization: Heat and moisture exchangers for use in humidifying respired gases in humans (ISO 9360), Geneva, 1992, International Organization for Standardization.
23. Shelly MP: Inspired gas conditioning, Respir Care 37:1070, 1992.
24. Branson RD, Davis K: Evaluation of 21 passive humidifiers according to the ISO 9360 standard: moisture output, deadspace, and flow resistance, Respir Care 41:736, 1996.
25. Ploysongsang Y et al: Effect of flowrate and duration of use on the pressure drop across six artificial noses, Respir Care 34:902, 1989.
26. Dreyfuss D et al: Mechanical ventilation with heated humidifiers or heat and moisture exchangers: effects on patient colonization and incidence of nosocomial pneumonia, Am J Respir Crit Care Med 151:986, 1995.
27. Nishida T et al: Performance of heated humidifiers with a heated wire according to ventilatory settings, J Aerosol Med 14:43, 2001.
28. Emergency Care Research Institute: Heated humidifiers, Health Devices 16:223, 1987.
29. Larsson A, Gustafsson A, Svanborg L: A new device for 100 per cent humidification of inspired air, Crit Care 4:54, 2000.
30. Williams R et al: Relationship between the humidity and temperature of inspired gas and the function of the airway mucosa, Crit Care Med 24:1920, 1996.
31. Craven DE, Goularte TA, Make BJ: Contaminated condensate in mechanical ventilator circuits: a risk factor for nosocomial pneumonia, Am Rev Respir Dis 129:625, 1984.
32. Gilmour IJ, Boyle MJ, Streifel A: Humidifiers kill bacteria, Anesthesiology 75:A498, 1991.
33. Craven DE et al: Risk factors for pneumonia and fatality in patients receiving continuous mechanical ventilation, Am Rev Respir Dis 33:792, 1986.
34. Hess D et al: Weekly ventilator circuit changes: a strategy to reduce costs without affecting pneumonia rates, Anesthesiology 82:903, 1995.
35. Kollef, MH et al: Mechanical ventilation with or without 7-day circuit changes: a randomized controlled study, Ann Intern Med 123:168, 1995.
36. Fink JB et al: Extending ventilator circuit change interval beyond two days reduces the likelihood of ventilator associated pneumonia (VAP), Chest 113:405, 1998.
37. Dreyfuss D et al: Mechanical ventilation with heated humidifiers or heat and moisture exchangers: effect on patient colonization and incidence of nosocomial pneumonia, Am J Respir Crit Care Med 151:986, 1995.
38. Beydon L et al: Correlation between simple clinical parameters and the in vitro humidification characteristics of filter heat and moisture exchangers, Chest 112:739, 1997.
39. American Association for Respiratory Care: Clinical practice guideline: bland aerosol administration, Respir Care 38:1196, 1993.
40. Mercer TT, Goddard RF, Flores RL: Output characteristics of several commercial nebulizers, Ann Allergy 23:314, 1965.
41. Hill TV, Sorbello JG: Humidity outputs of large-reservoir nebulizers, Respir Care 32:225, 1987.
42. Chatburn RL, Lough MD, Klinger JD: An in-hospital evaluation of the sonic mist ultrasonic room humidifier, Respir Care 29: 893, 1984.
43. Khajotia RR et al: Induced sputum and cytological diagnosis of lung cancer, Lancet 338:976, 1991.

44. Anderson C, Inhaber N, Menzies D: Comparison of sputum induction with fiberoptic bronchoscopy in the diagnosis of tuberculosis, Am J Respir Crit Care Med 152:1570-1574, 1995.
45. Godwin CR, Brown DT, Masur H, et al: Sputum induction: A quick and sensitive technique for diagnosing Pneumocystis carinii pneumonia in immunosuppressed patients, Respir Care 36:33-39, 1991.
46. Butler TJ, Close JR, Close RJ: Laboratory exercises for competency in respiratory care, Philadelphia, 1998, FA Davis.
47. Gershman NH, Wong HH, Liu JT, et al: Comparison of two methods of collecting induced sputum in asthmatic subjects, Eur Respir J 9:2448-2453, 1996.
48. American College of Chest Physicians and NHLBI: National Conference on Oxygen Therapy, Respir Care 29:922, 1984.
49. Branson RD, Chatburn RL: Humidification during mechanical ventilation, Respir Care 38:461–468, 1993 (editorial).

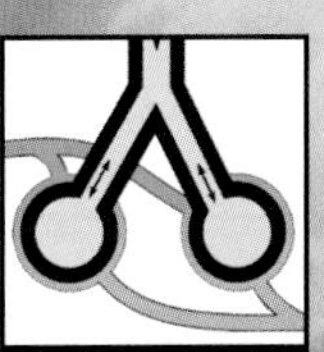

CHAPTER 33

Aerosol Drug Therapy

Jim Fink

In This Chapter You Will Learn:

- What characterizes an aerosol
- How particle size, motion, and airway characteristics affect aerosol deposition
- How aerosols are generated
- What hazards are associated with aerosol drug therapy
- How to select the best aerosol drug delivery system for a given patient
- How to initiate and modify aerosol drug therapy
- What patients need to know to properly self-administer drug aerosol therapy
- How to assess patient response to bronchodilator therapy at the point of care
- How to apply aerosol therapy in special circumstances
- How to protect patients and caregivers from exposure to aerosolized drugs

Chapter Outline

Characteristics of Therapeutic Aerosols
Output
Particle size
Deposition
Aging
Hazards of Aerosol Therapy
Infection
Airway reactivity
Pulmonary and systemic effects
Drug reconcentration
Aerosol Drug Delivery Systems
Metered-dose inhalers
Dry powder inhalers
Pneumatic (jet) nebulizers
Ultrasonic nebulizers
Hand-bulb atomizers
New-generation nebulizers
Advantages and disadvantages
Selecting an Aerosol Drug Delivery System
Assessment-Based Bronchodilatory Therapy Protocols
Sample protocol
Assessing patient response
Patient education
Special Considerations
Continuous nebulization for refractory Bronchospasm
Aerosol administration to intubated patients
Controlling Environmental Contamination
Negative-pressure rooms
Booths and stations
Personal protective equipment

Key Terms

aerosol density
aerosol output
aging
atomizer
baffle
brownian diffusion
breath-enhanced nebulizer
chloroflurocarbons
deposition
emitted dose
fine-particle fraction
geometric standard deviation

Continued

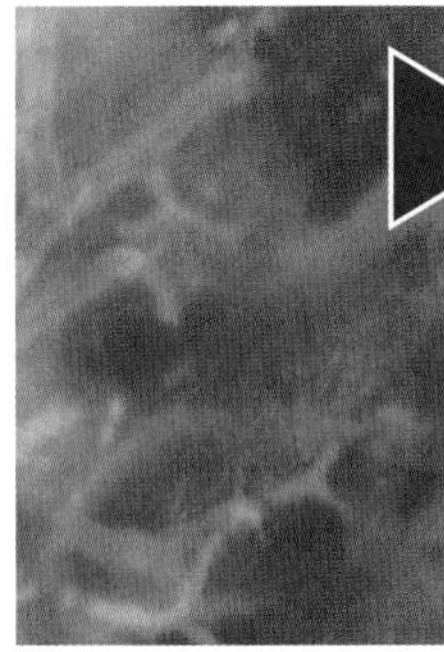

Key Terms—cont'd

heterodisperse
hygroscopic
inertial impaction
inhaled mass
mass median aerodynamic diameter
monodisperse
nebulizer
propellant
residual volume
respirable mass
scintigraphy
sedimentation
therapeutic index
volume median diameter

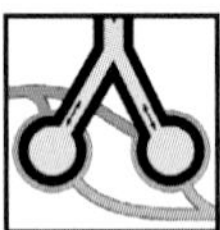

An aerosol is a suspension of solid or liquid particles in gas. Aerosols occur in nature as pollens, spores, dust, smoke, smog, fog, and mist.[1] In the clinical setting, medical aerosols are generated with atomizers, nebulizers, or inhalers—devices that physically disperse matter into small particles and suspend them into a gas. These aerosols can be used to deliver bland water solutions to the respiratory tract (see Chapter 32) or to administer drugs to the lungs, throat, or nose. This chapter focuses on the principles of aerosol drug therapy.

The aim of medical aerosol therapy is to deliver a therapeutic dose of the selected agent to the desired site of action. The indication for any specific aerosol is based on the need for the drug and the targeted site of delivery.[1,2] For patients with pulmonary disorders, administration of drugs by aerosol offers many benefits. Aerosol drugs are delivered directly to the site of action; the result is therapeutic action with minimal systemic side effects (a high **therapeutic index**) and greater efficacy and safety.

▶ CHARACTERISTICS OF THERAPEUTIC AEROSOLS

Effective use of medical aerosols requires an understanding of the characteristics of the aerosol effect of drug delivery to the desired site of action. Key concepts include **aerosol output**, particle size, and **deposition**.

Output

Aerosol output is defined as the weight or mass of aerosol particles produced by a **nebulizer** (usually per minute). For drug delivery systems, *emitted dose* often is used to describe the mass of aerosol leaving the nebulizer. **Aerosol density** is the weight or mass of aerosol per unit volume of gas (mg/L or g/L) leaving the nebulizer.

Aerosol output can be measured by collecting the aerosol that leaves the nebulizer on filters and measuring either the weight (gravimetric analysis) or quantity of drug (assay). Gravimetric measurements of aerosols are less reliable than drug assay techniques, because weight changes due to water evaporation cannot be differentiated from changes in drug mass. A drug assay provides the most reliable measure of aerosol output.

The mass of aerosol leaving a nebulizer tells little about the amount of drug reaching the targeted site of action. A substantial proportion of particles that leave a nebulizer may never reach the lungs. The ability of aerosols to travel through the air, enter the airways, and become deposited in the lungs is based on a number of variables ranging from particle size to breathing pattern.

Particle Size

Aerosol particle size depends on the substance being nebulized, the nebulizer chosen, the method used to generate the aerosol, and the environmental conditions surrounding the particle.[3] It is not possible to visually determine whether a nebulizer is producing an optimal particle size. The unaided human eye cannot see particles less than 50 to 100 μm in diameter (equivalent to a small grain of sand). The only reliable way to determine the characteristics of an aerosol suspension is laboratory measurement. The two most common laboratory methods used to measure aerosol particle size are cascade impaction and laser diffraction. Cascade impactors collect aerosols of different size ranges on a series of stages or plates. The mass of aerosol is quantified by drug assay. In laser diffraction a computer is used to estimate the range and frequency of droplet volumes crossing the laser beam. Because medical aerosols contain particles of many different sizes (are **heterodisperse**), average size is expressed with a measure of central tendency, such as **mass median aerodynamic diameter** (MMAD) for cascade impaction or **volume median diameter** (VMD) for laser diffraction. These measurements of the same aerosol may result in different sizes, so it is important to know which measurement is used. The MMAD and VMD both describe the particle diameter in micrometers (μm). In an aerosol distribution with a specific MMAD, 50% of the particles are smaller and have less mass and 50% are larger and have greater mass.

The **geometric standard deviation** (GSD) describes the variability of particle sizes in an aerosol distribution set at one standard deviation (SD) above or below the median (15.8% and 84.13%). The GSD is divided into or multiplied by the MMAD or VMD to reflect distribution of particle sizes. For an aerosol with an MMAD of 1.8 μm and GSD of 2.0, the range of particle sizes at ±1 SD is 0.9 μm (1.8 ÷ 2) to 3.6 μm (1.8 × 2).

Most aerosols found in nature and used in respiratory care are composed of particles of different sizes, described as heterodisperse. The greater the GSD, the wider is the range of particle sizes and the more heterodisperse is the aerosol. Aerosols consisting of particles of similar size (GSD ≤1.2) are referred to as **monodisperse** aerosols. Nebulizers that produce monodisperse aerosols are used mainly in laboratory research and in nonmedical industries.

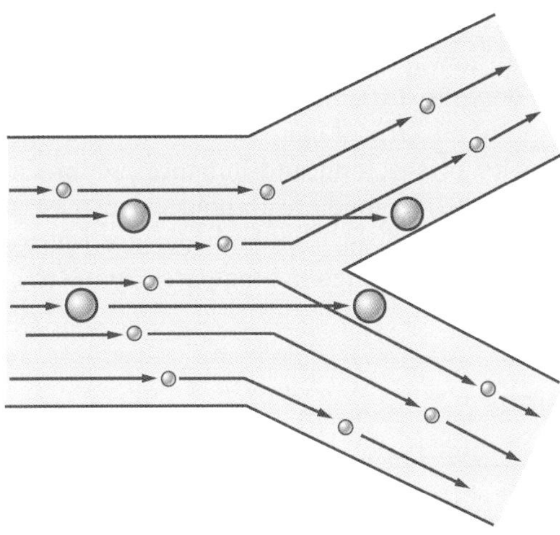

Figure 33-1
Inertial impaction of large particles the masses of which tend to maintain their motion in straight lines. As airway direction changes, the particles are deposited on nearby walls. Smaller particles are carried around corners by the airstream and fall out less readily.

Deposition

Aerosol particles are deposited when they leave suspension in gas. Only a portion of the aerosol generated from a nebulizer (**emitted dose**) may be inhaled (inhaled dose). A smaller fraction of fine particles may be deposited in the lung (respirable dose). **Inhaled mass** is the amount of drug inhaled. The proportion of the drug mass of proper size to reach the lower respiratory tract is the **respirable mass**. Not all aerosol delivered to the lung is retained, or deposited. A significant percentage of inhaled drug may be exhaled. Whether aerosol particles that are inhaled enter and are deposited in the respiratory tract depends on the size, shape, and motion of the particles and on the physical characteristics of the airways and breathing pattern. Key mechanisms of aerosol deposition include **inertial impaction**, gravimetric **sedimentation**, and **brownian diffusion**.[1,3]

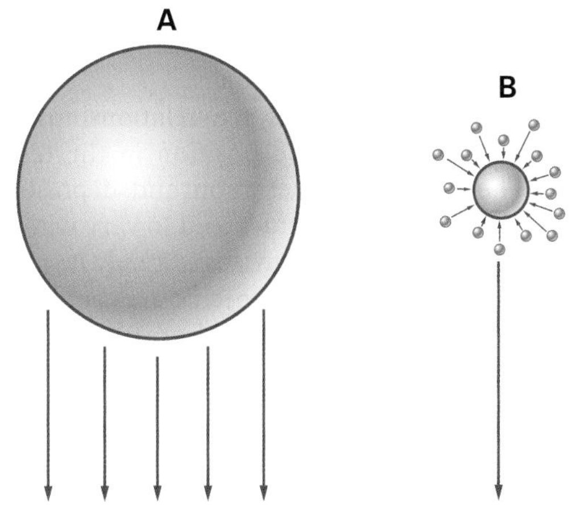

Figure 33-2 · Effect of Mass on Particle Size
Large particles **(A)** are more susceptible to the force of gravity than are smaller particles **(B)**, which are more affected by the bombardment of molecules deposited by diffusion.

Inertial Impaction

Inertial impaction occurs when suspended particles in motion collide with and are deposited on a surface. This is the primary deposition mechanism for particles larger than 5 μm. The greater the mass and velocity of a moving object, the greater is its inertia and the greater is the tendency of that object to continue moving along its set path (Figure 33-1). When a particle of sufficient mass is moving in a gas stream and that stream changes direction, the particle tends to remain on its initial path and collide with the airway surface.

Because inertia involves both mass and velocity, the higher the flow of a gas stream, the greater is the tendency for particles to impact and be deposited in the airways. Turbulent flow patterns, obstructed or tortuous pathways, and inspiratory flow rates greater than 30 L/min are associated with increased inertial impaction. For example, turbulent flow and convoluted passageways in the nose cause most particles larger than 10 μm to impact and become deposited. This process produces an effective filter that protects the lower airway from particulates such as dust and pollen. However, particles in the 5- to 10-μm range tend to become deposited in the oropharynx and hypopharynx, especially with the turbulence created by the transition of air as it passes into the larynx.

Sedimentation

Sedimentation occurs when aerosol particles settle out of suspension and are deposited owing to gravity. The greater the mass of the particle, the faster it settles (Figure 33-2). During normal breathing, sedimentation is the primary mechanism for deposition of particles in the 1- to 5-μm range. Sedimentation occurs mostly in the central airways and increases with time, affecting particles down to 1 μm in diameter. Breath-holding after inhalation of an aerosol increases the residence time for the particles in the lung and enhances sedimentation. For example, a 10-second breath-hold can increase aerosol deposition as much as 10% and increase fourfold the ratio of aerosol deposited in lung parenchyma to central airway.[4]

Diffusion

Brownian diffusion is the primary mechanism for deposition of small particles (<3 μm), mainly in the respiratory region where bulk gas flow ceases and most aerosol particles reach the alveoli by diffusion. These aerosol particles have very low mass and are easily bounced around by collisions with carrier gas molecules. These random molecular collisions cause some particles to contact and become deposited on surrounding surfaces. Particles between 1 and 0.5 μm are so stable that most remain in suspension and are cleared with the exhaled gas, whereas particles smaller than 0.5 μm have a greater retention rate in the lungs.

Figure 33-3 summarizes the relationships between particle size and aerosol deposition in the respiratory tract.[5] The depth of penetration and deposition of a particle in the respiratory tract tend to vary with size and tidal volume. With this knowledge, it may be possible to target aerosol deposition to specific areas of the lung by using the proper particle size and breathing pattern.

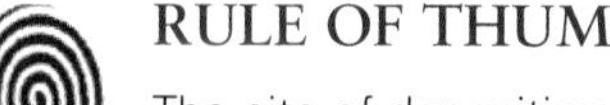

RULE OF THUMB

The site of deposition in the respiratory tract varies with the size of the particle. Use of nebulizers that produce particles in a specific size range improves the targeting of aerosols for deposition to a desired site in the respiratory tract as follows:

Desired Location	Recommended MMAD
Upper airway: nose, larynx, trachea	5 to >50 μm
Lower airways	2-5 μm
Parenchyma: alveolar region	1-3 μm
Parenchyma	<0.1 μm

Aging

Aerosols are dynamic suspensions. Particles constantly grow, shrink, coalesce, and fall out of suspension. The process by which an aerosol suspension changes over time is called *aging*. How an aerosol ages depends on the composition of the aerosol, the initial size of its particles, the time in suspension, and the ambient conditions to which it is exposed.

Aerosol particles can change size as a result of either evaporation or **hygroscopic** water absorption. The relative rate of particle size change is inversely proportional to the size of a particle, so the small particles grow or shrink faster than larger particles. Small water-based particles shrink when exposed to relatively dry gas. Aerosols of water-soluble materials, especially salts,

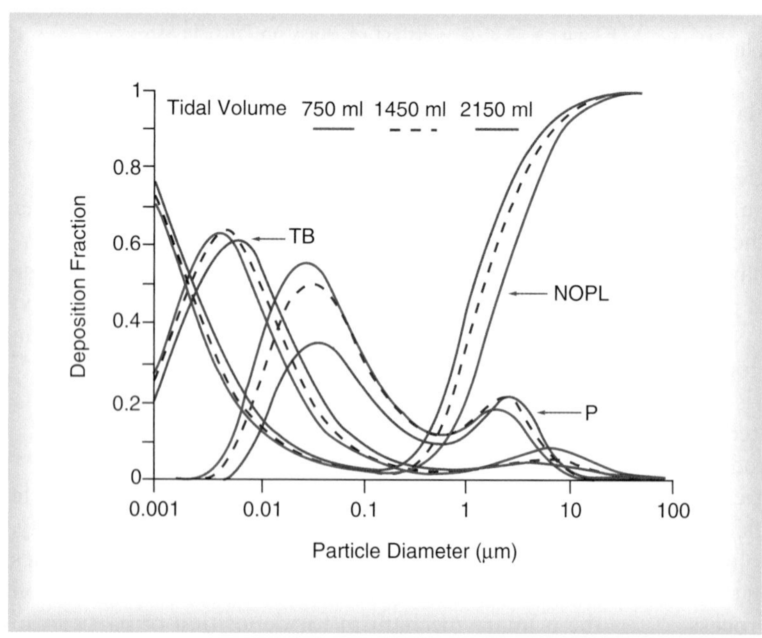

Figure 33-3
Range of particle sizes (MMAD) over which impaction, sedimentation, and brownian diffusion occur in the upper and lower respiratory tract. *NOPL*, Nonpulmonary deposition; *P*, pulmonary; *TB*, terminal bronchials. *(Courtesy Respiratory Care Journal.)*

tend to be hygroscopic, absorbing water and growing when introduced into a high-humidity environment.

Particle size is not the only determinant of deposition. Inspiratory flow rate, flow pattern, respiratory rate, inhaled volume, ratio of inspiratory time to expiratory time (I:E ratio), and breath-holding all influence where a particle of any specific size is deposited. The presence of airway obstruction is one of the greatest factors influencing aerosol deposition. Kim and colleagues have demonstrated that total pulmonary deposition is greater in smokers and patients with obstructive airway disease than in healthy persons (Figure 33-4). Similarly, when inspiratory flow rates are constant, the deposition fraction of monodisperse aerosols increases with increased tidal volume, length of respiratory (inspiratory) period, and particle size (Figure 33-5).

These dynamic variables make it difficult to predict exactly what occurs to aerosol particles once they enter a gas stream and are inhaled. For this reason, prediction of actual aerosol deposition for an individual patient is difficult. At the bedside, quantification of aerosol delivery is based on the patient's clinical response to the drug with either desired therapeutic effects or unwanted adverse effects. For example, inhaled β-agonists are monitored on the basis of changes in pulmonary function (peak flow, forced expiratory volumes or flow), side effects (tremor or tachycardia), or physical changes (reduced wheezing, shortness of breath, or retractions).

Several methods are used to quantify aerosol deposition in vivo. One graphic approach involves scintigraphy in which a drug is tagged with a radioactive substance

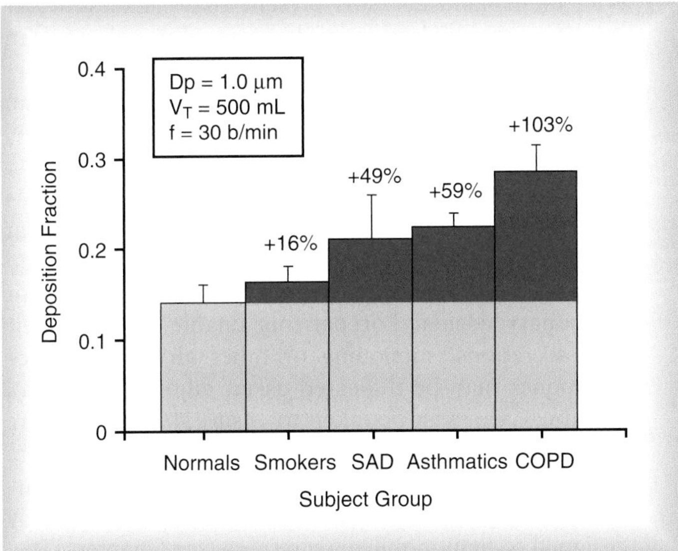

Figure 33-4

Total lung deposition of a fine aerosol of particles 1-μm in diameter in healthy adults and in subjects with obstructive airway disease. Numbers over the bar indicate the percentage increase above normal value. SAD, Smoker with symptoms of small airways disease; COPD, patients with chronic obstructive pulmonary disease. Dp, particle diameter; V_T, tidal volume; f, respiratory rate. *(Modified from Kim CS: Respir Care 45:695, 2000.)*

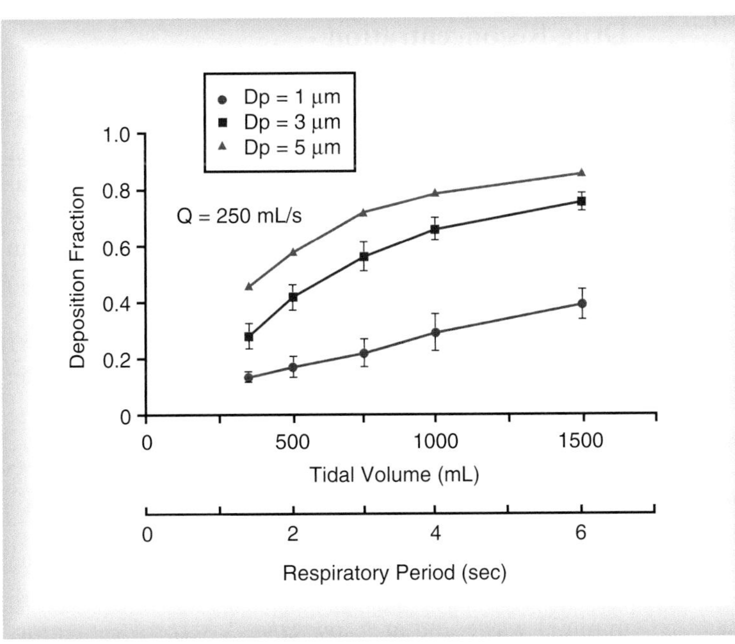

Figure 33-5

Total lung deposition versus tidal volume and respiratory time at a fixed flow: Respiratory flow (Q) = 250 mL/s. Dp, Particle diameter. *(Modified from Kim CS: Respir Care 45:695, 2000.)*

(such as technetium), aerosolized, and inhaled. A scanner (like those used in nuclear medicine) measures the distribution and intensity of radiation across the device and the patient's head and thorax. The result is a radiation map of aerosol deposition in the upper airway, the lungs (central and peripheral airways), and the stomach. This information is used to calculate the percentage of drug retained by the device and delivered to various areas in the patient.

A less direct approach relates the systemic pharmacokinetic profile of a drug delivered by aerosol to an assay of the drug in a patient's blood or urine over time. This method does not estimate actual lung delivery but does provide insight into systemic drug levels achieved after aerosol administration. Care must be taken to differentiate drug absorbed through the lungs from that absorbed through the gastrointestinal tract.

▶ HAZARDS OF AEROSOL THERAPY

The primary hazard of aerosol drug therapy is an adverse reaction to the medication being administered (see Chapter 29). Other hazards include infection, airway reactivity, systemic effects of bland aerosols, and drug reconcentration.

Infection

Aerosol generators can contribute to nosocomial infections by spreading bacteria by the airborne route.[6,7] The most common sources of bacteria are contaminated solutions (i.e., multiple-dose drug vials), caregivers' hands, and the patient's own secretions. Offending organisms are primarily gram-negative bacilli, particularly *Pseudomonas aeruginosa* and *Legionella pneumophila* (the cause of the highly virulent legionnaires' disease).[8,9]

Various procedures can help reduce contamination and infection associated with respiratory care equipment. Guidelines from the Centers for Disease Control and Prevention are that nebulizers be sterilized between patients, frequently replaced with disinfected or sterile units, and rinsed with sterile water (not tap water) every 24 hours (see Chapter 3).

Airway Reactivity

Cold and high-density aerosols can cause reactive bronchospasm and increased airway resistance, especially in patients with preexisting respiratory disease.[10] Medications such as acetylcysteine, antibiotics, steroids, cromolyn sodium, ribavirin, and distilled water have been associated with increased airway resistance and wheezing during aerosol therapy. Administration of bronchodilators before or with administration of these agents may reduce the risk or duration of increased airway resistance.

The risk of inducing bronchospasm always should be considered when aerosols are administered. Monitoring for reactive bronchospasm should include peak flow measurements or percentage forced expiratory volume in 1 second (%FEV_1) before and after therapy; auscultation for adventitious breath sounds and observation of the patient's breathing pattern and overall appearance; and most essentially, communicating with the patient during therapy to determine the perceived work of breathing.[11]

Pulmonary and Systemic Effects

Pulmonary and systemic effects are associated with the site of delivery and the drug being administered. However, even bland aerosols present risk.[12] Excess water can cause overhydration, and excess saline solution can cause hypernatremia. Animal data indicate that long-term, continuous administration of bland aerosols can cause localized inflammation and tissue damage, atelectasis, and pulmonary edema.

Preliminary assessment should balance the need versus the risk of aerosol therapy, especially among patients at high risk, such as infants, those prone to fluid and electrolyte imbalances, and patients with atelectasis or pulmonary edema. For patients unable to clear their own secretions, suctioning or other airway clearance techniques may be indicated as an adjunct to aerosol therapy. Care must be taken to ensure that patients are capable of clearing secretions once the secretions are mobilized by aerosol therapy. Appropriate airway clearance techniques should accompany any aerosol therapy designed to help mobilize secretions (see Chapter 37).

Drug Reconcentration

During the evaporation, heating, baffling, and recycling of drug solutions undergoing jet or ultrasonic nebulization, solute concentration may increase.[13] This process can expose the patient to increasingly higher concentrations of the drug over the course of therapy. The result is that a relatively large amount of drug remains in the nebulizer at the end of therapy. This increase in concentration usually is time dependent, the greatest effect occurring when medications are nebulized over extended periods, as in continuous aerosol drug delivery.

▶ AEROSOL DRUG DELIVERY SYSTEMS

Effective aerosol therapy requires a device that quickly delivers sufficient drug to the desired site of action with minimal waste and at a low cost.[14] Aerosol generators in clinical use include metered-dose inhalers (MDIs), dry powder inhalers (DPIs), jet nebulizers (small- and large-volume), ultrasonic nebulizers (USNs), hand-bulb atomizers (including nasal spray pumps), and a number of emerging technologies.

Clinicians are deluged with competing and often conflicting claims about the different delivery systems and are not provided with the information they need to select the correct system for a given situation. Because device selection can make the difference between successful and unsuccessful therapy,[15] clinicians must have in-depth knowledge of the operating principles and performance characteristics of these various systems and how best to select and apply them.

Metered-Dose Inhalers

The pressurized MDI (pMDI) is the most commonly prescribed method of aerosol delivery in the United States. Pressurized MDIs are portable, compact, and relatively easy to use. A uniform dose of drug is dispensed within a fraction of a second after actuation, and the doses provided are reproducible throughout the canister life.[16] Pressurized MDIs contain drug as micronized powder, either dissolved or suspended in one or more chlorofluorocarbon (CFC) or hydrofluoroalkane (HFA) liquid propellants along with surfactants (oily, viscous, nonvolatile substances used to keep the drug suspended in the propellants and to lubricate the valve mechanism). The volume of the formulation and the amount of drug released per actuation of the pMDI are a function of the size of the metering chamber. Pressurized MDI metering chamber volumes can vary from 30 to 100 μL. Increasing the volume of the metering chamber decreases the rate of evaporation of the increased amount of propellant released. The result is increased loss of drug on the actuator mouthpiece.

Pressurized MDIs are used to administer bronchodilators, anticholinergics, and steroids. More formulations of these drugs are available for use by MDI than for use with other nebulizers. Properly used, pMDIs are at least as effective as other nebulizers for drug delivery.[17] For this reason, pMDIs often are the preferred method for delivering bronchodilators to spontaneously breathing patients as well as those who are intubated and undergoing mechanical ventilation.[11,18]

Equipment Design

An MDI is a pressurized canister that contains the prescribed drug (a micronized powder or aqueous solution) in a volatile propellant combined with a surfactant and dispersing agent (Figure 33-6). When the canister is inverted (nozzle down) and placed in its actuator, or "boot," the volatile suspension fills a metering chamber that controls the amount of drug delivered. Pressing down on the canister aligns a hole in the metering valve with the metering chamber. The high propellant vapor pressure quickly forces the metered dose out through this hole and through the actuator nozzle.

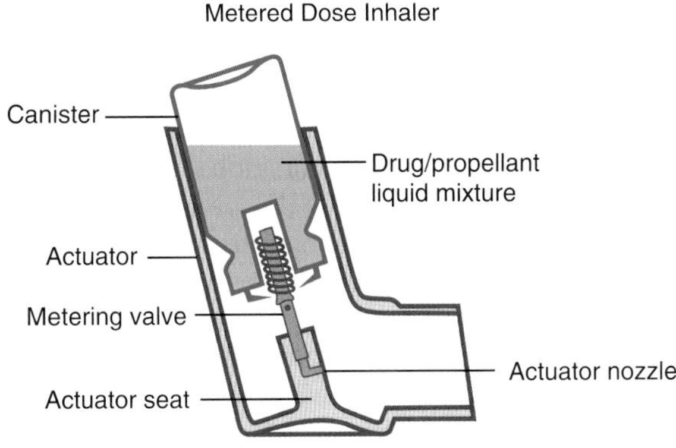

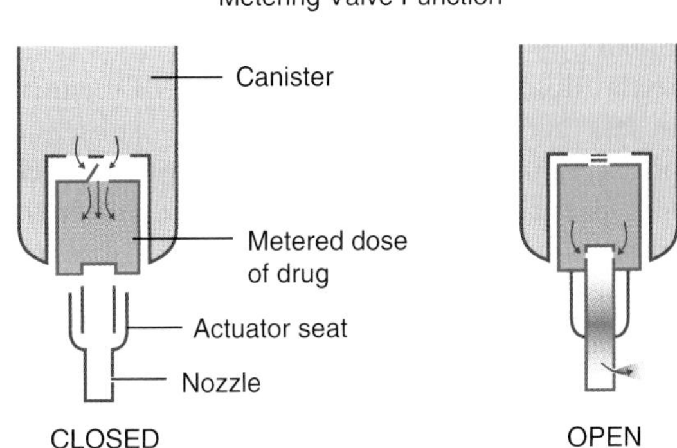

Figure 33-6
Components of a metered-dose inhaler (MDI), including function of the metering valve. *(From Rau JL Jr: Respiratory care pharmacology, ed 6, St Louis, 2002, Mosby.)*

Aerosol production takes approximately 20 milliseconds. As the liquid suspension is forced out of the MDI, it forms a plume, within which the propellants vaporize, or "flash." Initially the velocity of this plume is high (approximately 15 m/s). However, within 0.1 second the plume velocity decreases to less than half its maximum as the plume moves away from the actuator nozzle.[19] At the same time, propellant evaporation causes the initially large particles (35 μm) generated at the actuator orifice to rapidly decrease in size.[20]

The output volume of MDIs varies from 30 to 100 μL. Approximately 60% to 80% by weight of this spray consists of the propellant, only approximately 1% being active drug (50 μg to 5 mg, depending on the drug formulation).[21] For a CFC pMDI used in a standard actuator, loss of drug in the valve stem housing and on the actuator mouthpiece amounts to 10% to 15% of the nominal dose from the metering valve.

Until recently, CFCs such as Freon were the sole propellants used in pMDIs. Because Freon has been associated with adverse responses in some patients[22] and because future use of CFCs is prohibited because of the effect of these compounds on global warming, CFCs are being replaced by other MDI propellants, such as HFA-134a. The new environment-friendly HFA may be clinically safer than CFCs.[23] Redesign of key components of the pMDI has resulted in improved performance.

In addition to the propellant, pMDIs use dispersal agents to improve drug delivery by keeping the drug in suspension. The most common dispersal agents are surfactants, such as soya lecithin, sorbitan trioleate, and oleic acid. These agents help keep the drug suspended in the propellant and lubricate the valve mechanism but may also cause adverse responses (coughing or wheezing) in some patients.[5]

The initial dose actuated from a new pMDI canister contains less active substance than does subsequent actuations.[16] This "loss of dose" from a pMDI occurs when drug particles rise to the top of the canister over time, or "cream." A reduction in emitted dose with the first actuation commonly occurs with a CFC pMDI after storage, particularly with the valve pointed in the downward position. Loss of prime is related to valve design and occurs when propellant leaks out of the metering chamber during periods of nonuse (as short as 4 hours). The result is reduced pressure and drug released with the next actuation.[16] Improved designs of metering valves developed for use with HFA propellants reduce these losses. It is recommended that a single dose be wasted before the next dose is inhaled when a CFC pMDI has not been used for 4 to 6 hours. An HFA pMDI requires no wasting of dose for periods exceeding 1 week or more.[16]

A serious limitation of pMDIs is the lack of a "counter" to indicate the number of doses remaining in the canister. "Tail-off" is variability in the amount of drug dispensed toward the end of the life of the canister. The result of tail-off is swings from normal to almost no dose emitted from one breath to the next with no reliable indicator to the user. New HFA pMDI designs address this issue.

Temperature has been shown to affect CFC pMDIs with decreases in output with decreases in temperature to less than 10° C. Patients with cold air–induced bronchospasm who keep their pMDIs in outer coat pockets when out in cold winter weather may receive only a small percentage of drug compared with that administered with the same pMDI at 25° C. This problem has been less serious with the newer HFA pMDIs.

MINI CLINI

Using Universal MDI Boots

PROBLEM

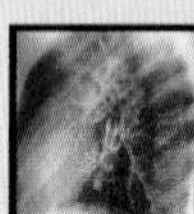

The association of CFCs with degradation of the earth's atmosphere and the ozone layer has resulted in an international treaty banning use of these compounds. As HFAs become the propellants of choice, a problem arises. If the CFC and HFA drug formulations are bioequivalent, can these compounds be used with the same (universal) MDI actuator, or boot?

SOLUTION

In the case of HFA-based albuterol (Proventil HFA), for example, the operating pressure and stem orifice differ from those used for the CFC formulation. The result is different plume geometries. When HFA albuterol is used in a universal adapter designed for CFC albuterol, the MMAD and GSD are greatly increased. The result is that significantly less drug is available to the patient. When possible, select accessory devices are used in the manufacturers' boot with the MDI. If these devices are not available, evaluate the universal adapter device that is available to determine how much additional dose may be required to provide an equivalent dose through a third-party adapter.

Aerosol Delivery Characteristics

Although MDIs produce particles in the respirable range (MMAD 3-6 μm),[20] the initial velocity and dispersion of the aerosol plume cause approximately 80% of the dose leaving the actuator to impact and become deposited in the oropharynx. Significant oropharyngeal deposition may be a factor in systemic absorption of some drugs. Pulmonary deposition ranges between 10% and 20%.[24-26] The exact amount of drug delivered to an individual patient is not predictable because of high variability between patients[24] and because MDI drug administration is technique dependent.

Technique

The successful administration of aerosol drugs by MDI is highly technique dependent. As many as two thirds of both patients and health professionals who teach MDI use do not perform the procedure properly.[27,28] Box 33-1 outlines the recommended steps for self-administering a bronchodilator by simple pMDI.[29,30] Thorough preliminary patient instruction can last 10 to 30 minutes and should include demonstration, practice, and confirmation of patient performance (demonstration MDIs are available for this purpose). Repeated instruction improves performance but must occur several times.[31]

Common hand-breath coordination problems include actuating the MDI before or after the breath. Some patients, especially infants, young children, the elderly, and patients in acute distress may not be able to coordinate actuation of the pMDI with inspiration. Some patients exhibit a "cold Freon effect," which occurs when

Box 33-1 • Optimal Technique for Use of a Metered-Dose Inhaler*

1. Warm the MDI canister to hand or body temperature, and shake it vigorously.
2. Assemble the apparatus, and uncap the mouthpiece, making sure there are no loose objects in the device.
3. Open your mouth wide, keeping your tongue down.
4. Hold the MDI with the canister oriented downward and the outlet aimed at your mouth.†
5. Position the MDI approximately 4 cm (two fingerbreadths) away from your mouth.
6. Breathe out normally.
7. As you slowly begin to breathe in (less than 0.5 L/s), activate (fire) the MDI.
8. Continue inspiration to total lung capacity.
9. Hold your breath for up to 10 seconds.
10. Wait 1 minute between puffs.
11. Disassemble the apparatus, and recap the mouthpiece.

*Bronchodilator only.
†The outlet also may be placed between your lips.

the cold aerosol plume reaches the back of the mouth and the patient stops inhaling. All of these problems reduce aerosol delivery to the lung but can be corrected entirely or in part by use of the proper MDI accessory device. Positioning the outlet of the MDI approximately 4 cm in front of the mouth improves lung deposition by decreasing oropharyngeal impaction.[26] Holding the canister outside the wide open mouth (at two fingerbreadths) provides a space for the particles to decelerate while evaporating. This method enhances the capability of entraining the aerosol into the inspiratory airstream and reduces the amount of propellant inhaled. Use of the open-mouth technique with a low inspiratory flow rate can result in a doubling of the dose delivered to the lower respiratory tract of an adult from approximately 7% to 14%. This technique, however, is even more difficult for patients to perform than is the closed-mouth technique. Although it may reduce oropharyngeal deposition, the technique has not been shown to improve the response to pMDI bronchodilators.[32] Concerns have been raised about use of the open-mouth technique with ipratropium bromide. Use of anticholinergic agents has been associated with increased ocular pressure, which could be dangerous for patients with glaucoma.[33] For avoidance of ocular exposure, the drug manufacturer recommends patients use the closed-mouth technique with ipratropium.

The high percentage of oropharyngeal drug deposition with use of steroid MDIs can increase the incidence of opportunistic oral yeast infection (thrush). Rinsing the mouth after steroid use can help avoid this problem, but most MDI steroid aerosol impaction occurs deep in the hypopharynx, which is not easily rinsed. For this reason, steroid MDIs should not be used alone but always should be used in combination with a spacer or holding chamber.

MDI Accessory Devices

A variety of MDI accessory devices have been developed to overcome the two primary limitations of these systems: hand-breath coordination problems and high oropharyngeal deposition. Accessory devices include flow-triggered MDIs, spacers, and holding chambers.

Flow-Triggered MDIs. The Autohaler is a flow-triggered pMDI developed and marketed by the 3M Corporation (Figure 33-7). The device is designed to eliminate the need for hand-breath coordination by automatically triggering in response to the patient's inspiratory effort.[34] To use the Autohaler, the patient cocks a lever on the top of the unit, which sets in motion a downward spring

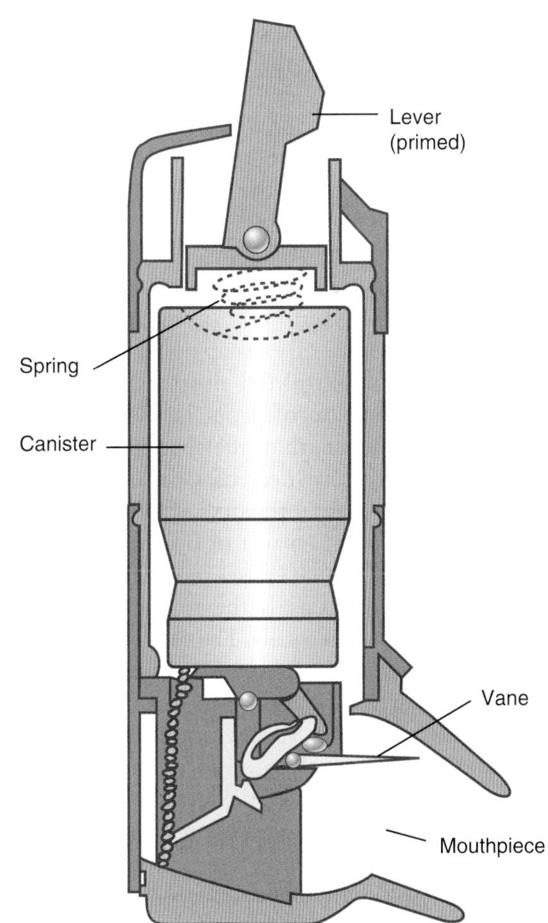

Figure 33-7
Autohaler (3M) flow-triggered MDI. *(From Rau JL Jr: Respiratory care pharmacology, ed 6, St Louis, 2002, Mosby.)*

force. Using the closed-mouth technique, the patient draws through the mouthpiece. When the patient's flow rate exceeds 30 L/min, a vane releases the spring, which forces the canister down and triggers the MDI.

In the United States, the Autohaler is available only with pirbuterol, a bronchodilator similar to albuterol. Current data indicate that the device reduces pharyngeal impaction and enhances lung deposition.[35] A possible limitation of the device is that it can only be breath actuated. Patients experiencing an acute exacerbation of bronchospasm may not be able to generate sufficient flows to trigger the Autohaler. This theoretical concern has not been widely observed in clinical studies of patients with severe exacerbation of asthma receiving treatment in emergency departments. Nevertheless, caution may be appropriate in ordering breath-triggered pMDIs for small children and patients prone to severe levels of airway obstruction.

Spacers and Holding Chambers. A number of accessory devices for use with pMDIs have been developed in response to a variety of administration difficulties encountered by patients (adult and pediatric) with the basic pMDI. It is increasingly common practice to provide asthmatic patients an accessory device to use with the MDI and to teach them to use the MDI with and without the accessory device. The patients are instructed to use the device with the MDI whenever they feel short of breath. Many of these patients find that they get much better relief from the MDI with an accessory device than with the MDI alone.

Spacers and holding chambers are MDI accessory devices designed to reduce both oropharyngeal deposition and the need for hand-breath coordination. Despite differences in design, all spacers reduce the initial forward velocity of the pMDI droplets, which occurs with partial evaporation of propellant in the time the aerosol traverses the length of the spacer. The reduction in initial forward velocity decreases the number of nonrespirable particles exiting the device. With retention of the larger droplets in the spacer or holding chamber, the "cold Freon" effect, which causes many children to stop inhaling, is eliminated, as is the foul taste associated with some of the drug aerosols. The same drug used with different devices demonstrates differences in MMAD, GSD, and fine particle fraction. The quantity of aerosolized drug available at the spacer exit depends on spacer volume and design as well as on formulation factors.

Basic concepts for spacer devices include (1) small volume adapters, (2) open tube designs, (3) bag reservoirs, and (4) valved holding chambers (Figure 33-8). More than a dozen different devices with volumes ranging from 15 to 750 mL have been developed over the last 30 years.

A *spacer* is a simple valveless extension device that puts distance between the MDI and the patient's mouth.

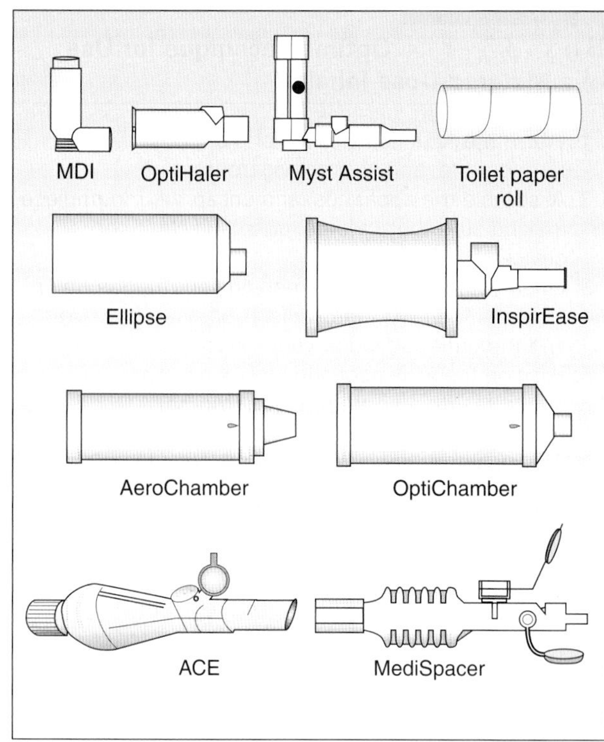

Figure 33-8

Metered-dose inhaler (MDI) and accessory devices consisting of spacer and holding chambers. All of the accessory devices reduce oropharyngeal deposition. Small-volume spacers (OptiHaler and Myst Assist) offer no additional advantage, but large-volume spacers (toilet paper roll and Ellipse) improve inhaled aerosol with delay between actuation and inspiration. Only the bag (InspirEase) and valved holding chambers (AeroChamber, OptiChamber, ACE, and MediSpacer) protect the patient from blowing the dose away when the MDI is actuated during expiration. *(Modified from Wilkes W, Fink J, Dhand R: J Aerosol Med 14:351, 2001.)*

This allows the aerosol plume to expand and the propellants to evaporate before the medication reaches the oropharynx. Larger particles leaving the pMDI tend to impact on the spacer walls. In combination, this phenomenon reduces oropharyngeal impaction and increases pulmonary deposition.[36] Proper use of a simple open-tube spacer still requires some hand-breath coordination because a momentary delay between triggering and inhaling the discharged spray results in a substantial loss of drug and reduced lung delivery. Moreover, exhalation into a simple spacer after MDI actuation clears the aerosol from the device and wastes most of the dose to the atmosphere. This reduction in dose also occurs with small-volume reverse-flow designs if there is no provision for "holding" the aerosol in the device.

Like spacers, *holding chambers* allow the aerosol plume to develop and thus reduce oropharyngeal deposition. A holding chamber also incorporates a valve that prevents the chamber aerosol from being cleared on exhalation. This allows patients with small tidal volumes to empty the aerosol from the chamber over two or three successive breaths. In general, holding chambers provide less oropharyngeal deposition, higher respirable drug dosages, and better protection from poor hand-breath coordination than do simple spacers.[37]

The mass median aerodynamic diameter of the pMDI aerosol exiting a spacer decreases approximately 25% while the fraction containing particles less than 5 μm in diameter increases. With valved holding chambers, this fraction can be augmented by further evaporation of propellant in the finite time between actuation and inhalation. The increase in this fraction appears to depend on the pMDI formulation; the more concentrated the drug, the higher is the fine particle fraction of aerosol exiting the device relative to the original pMDI aerosol.

Holding chambers produce a finer, slower-moving, more "respirable" aerosol with less impaction of drug in the oropharyngeal area than do simple spacers or a pMDI alone. Deposition after inhalation of a radiolabeled pMDI solution aerosol from the AeroChamber compared with that from the same pMDI inhaled with the open-mouth technique showed a 10- to 17-fold decrease in the amount of radioactivity deposited in the oropharyngeal-laryngeal area while a similar lung dose was maintained. This finding was true for both healthy subjects and those with chronic obstructive pulmonary disease (COPD).[38] The advantage of reduced oropharyngeal deposition is fewer side effects from steroid aerosols, as demonstrated in a number of published clinical trials.[39] If multiple actuations of one or more drugs are placed into a spacer, both the total dose and the respirable dose of drug available for inhalation are reduced. The extent of these losses may vary for different drugs and spacer designs.[16]

Box 33-2 • Optimal Technique for Use of a Metered-Dose Inhaler with a Holding Chamber

1. Warm the MDI to hand or body temperature.
2. Assemble the apparatus, making sure there are no objects or coins in the device that could be aspirated or obstruct outflow.
3. Hold the canister vertically and shake it vigorously.
4. Place the holding chamber in your mouth (or place the mask over your nose and mouth), and breathe through your mouth.
5. Breathe normally and actuate at the beginning of inspiration. Continue to breathe through the device for three breaths.*
6. Allow 30 to 60 seconds between actuations.

* For the cooperative patient, larger breaths with breath-holding may be encouraged. This maneuver has not been shown to increase clinical response to inhaled bronchodilators.

Box 33-2 outlines the optimal technique for use of an MDI with a holding chamber.

Holding chambers with masks are available for use in the care of infants, children, and adults (Figure 33-9). These units allow effective administration of aerosol from an MDI to patients who are unable to use a mouthpiece device (because of their size, age, coordination, or mentation).[40] Holding chambers are helpful in administration of MDI steroids because deposition of the drug in the mouth is largely eliminated and systemic side effects can be minimized.[39]

Even with a holding chamber, respirable particles containing drug settle out and become deposited within the device, causing a whitish buildup on the inner chamber walls. This residual drug poses no risk to the patient but may be rinsed out periodically. Drug output from plastic spacers has been shown to decrease owing to the presence of an electrostatic charge.[16] Use of a metal spacer or washing the plastic spacer periodically with deionizing detergent can overcome the loss of fine particle mass due to electrostatic charge. After a chamber or spacer is washed with water, the electrostatic charge is reestablished, making the device less effective for the next few puffs, until the static charge in the chamber (which attracts small particles) is once again reduced. Washing the chamber with conventional dish-washing soap reduces this static charge, the effect lasting up to 30 days.

The addition of a one-way valve to convert an open tube into a reservoir for the aerosol, the incorporation of the actuator in the MDI, the shape of the device, flow of air through the device, edge effects, masks, and manufacturing materials all affect aerosol characteristics and yield. The inhalation valve, which is used to contain the aerosol, also acts as a baffle to reduce oropharyngeal deposition. This valve must be able to withstand the initial pressure from the MDI when the device is triggered and have sufficiently low resistance to open readily when the user inhales, particularly when the user is a child or an infant. Exhalation valves in a face mask attached to a spacer device must provide low resistance. Issues of spacer volume, tidal volume, frequency of breathing and dead space between the spacer and mouth are of particular concern when these devices are used by children. Differences of twofold to threefold in the amount of drug available at the mouth have been measured among spacers currently used to treat infants. Clinicians should determine the delivery efficiencies of spacer devices before using the devices in the care of a particular population.

Accessory devices are used with either the manufacturer-designed boot that comes with the MDI or with a "universal adapter" that triggers the MDI canister. Different formulations of MDI drugs operate at different pressures and have a different-sized orifice in the boot that is specifically designed by the manufacturer

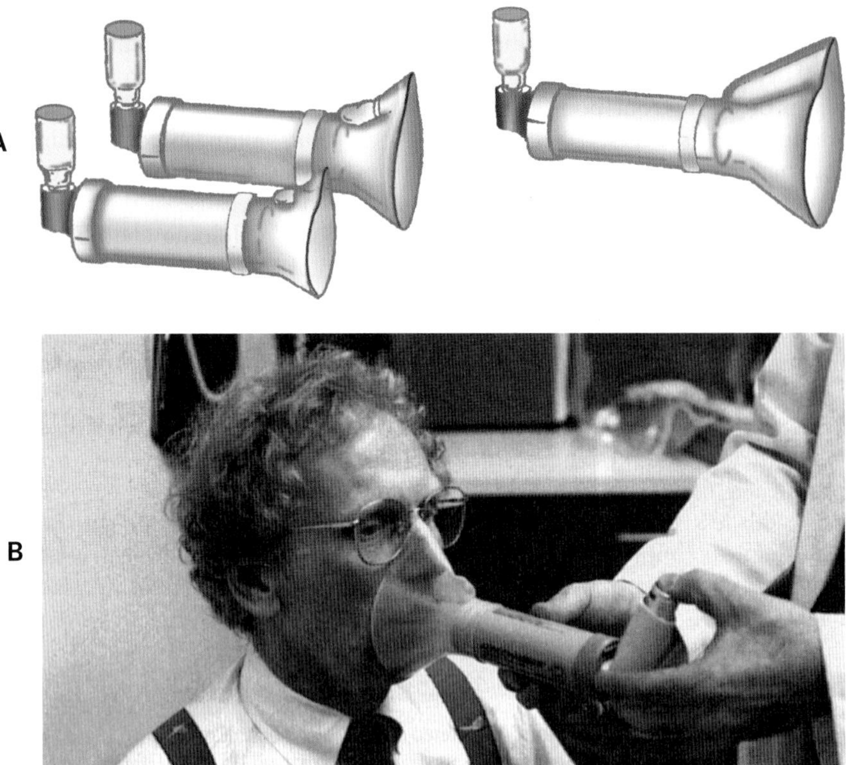

Figure 33-9

A, Sizes of masks used with MDI and holding chamber. **B,** Adult patient receiving medication through a holding chamber with mask. *(From Fink J, Cohen J: Humidity and aerosols. In Eubank D, Bone R: Principles and applications of cardiorespiratory care equipment, St Louis, 1994, Mosby.)*

for use exclusively with that MDI. The output characteristics of an MDI change when an adapter with a different-sized orifice is used. With solution HFA pMDIs, the diameter of the actuator orifice is smaller and the spray predictably finer. When the HFA pMDI is used in an actuator designed for use with CFC pMDIs, output is reduced. When these HFA formulations are used with any particular spacer, it is important to know how comparable the available dose and particle size distribution are to the dose and particle size from an existing CFC pMDI.

Dry Powder Inhalers

A DPI is a breath-actuated metered-dosing system. With a DPI, the patient creates the aerosol by drawing air though a dose of finely milled drug powder. Dry powder inhalers are relatively inexpensive, do not need propellants, and do not require the hand-breath coordination needed for MDIs. However, dispersion of the powder into respirable particles depends on the creation of turbulent flow in the inhaler. Turbulent flow is a function of the ability of the patient to inhale the powder with a sufficiently high inspiratory flow rate (Figure 33-10). In terms of both lung deposition and drug response, DPIs are as effective as MDIs.[41]

Equipment Design and Function

Most passive dry powder dispensing systems require the use of a carrier substance (lactose or glucose) mixed into the drug to enable the drug powder to more readily flow out of the device. Reactions to lactose or glucose appear to be fewer than reactions to the surfactants and propellants used in pressurized MDIs, even though the amount of these substances is substantially greater than that of the drug and can represent 98% or more of the weight per inhaled dose in some blends.

There are a number of DPIs on the market. Early devices such as the Spinhaler or Rotahaler (Figure 33-11) dispense individual doses of drug from punctured gelatin capsules. Multidose systems have been introduced. The Turbuhaler[7] (Astra Draco, Lund, Sweden) is an example of a multidose reservoir powder system preloaded with a quantity of pure drug sufficient for dispensing 200 doses of terbutaline sulphate or budesonide (see Figure 33-11). The Diskhaler (Glaxo Wellcome, Research Triangle Park, N.C.) has drug in four or eight individual blister packets of drug on a disk inserted into the inhaler. The Diskus[7] (Glaxo Wellcome) incorporates a tape system that contains several sealed single doses (Figure 33-12).

The particle size of the dry powder particles of drug ranges from 1 to 2 μm, but the size of the lactose or

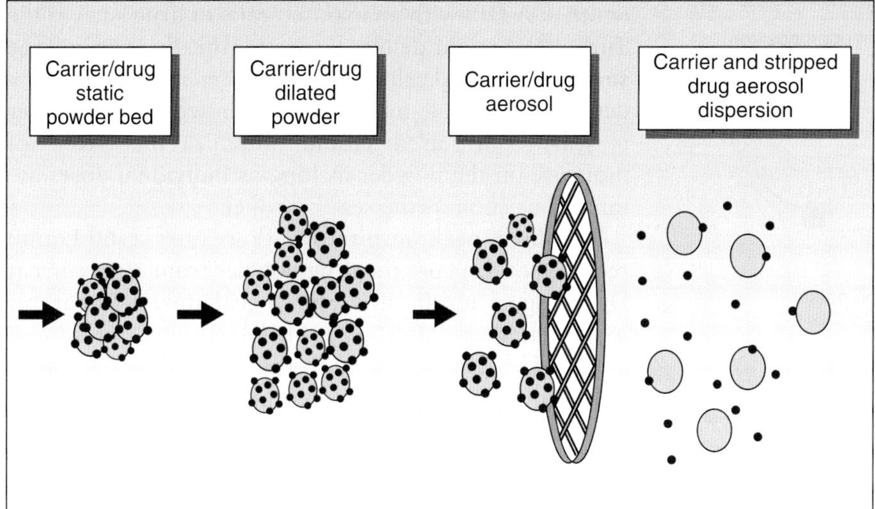

Figure 33-10
Aerosolization of dry powder. *(From Dhand R, Fink J: Respir Care 44:940, 1999.)*

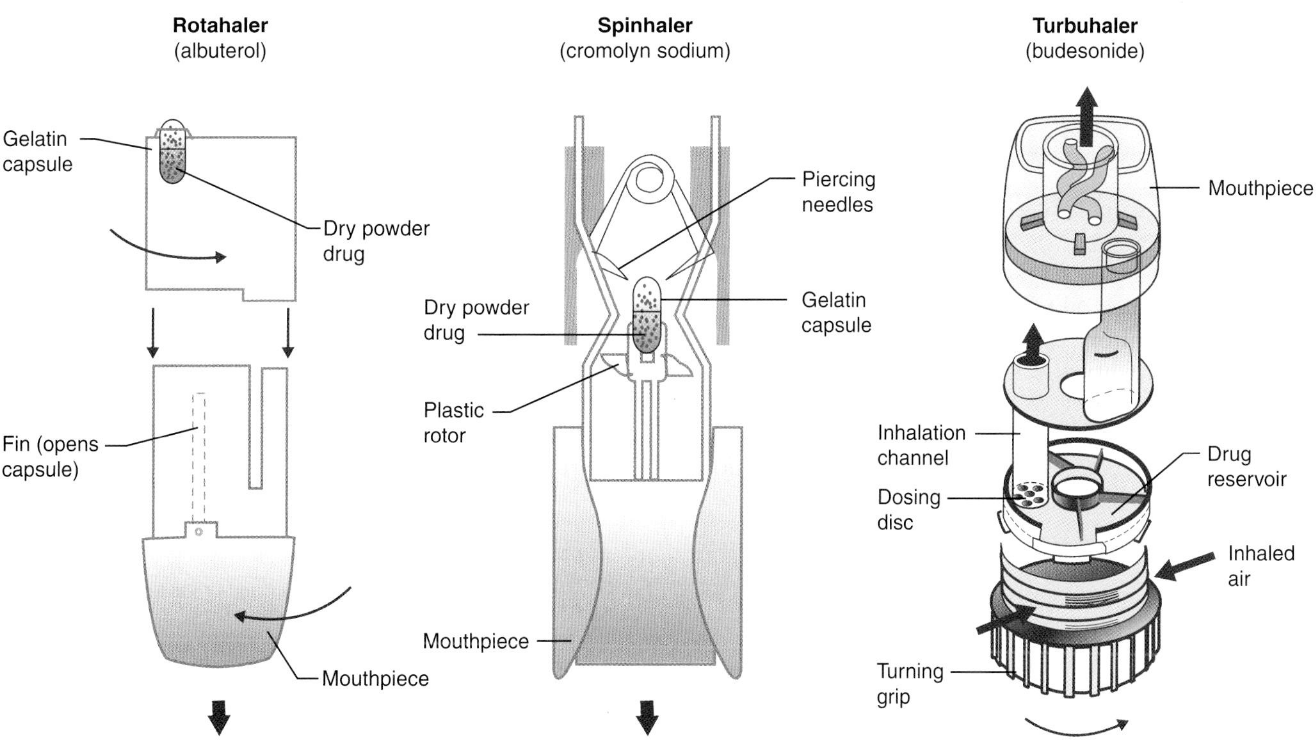

Figure 33-11
Three examples of delivery devices for inhalation of dry powder aerosols: Rotahaler, Spinhaler, and Turbuhaler. *(From Rau JL Jr: Respiratory care pharmacology, ed 5, St Louis, 1998, Mosby.)*

glucose particles can range from approximately 20 to 65 µm, so most of the carrier is deposited in the oropharynx. Performance of DPIs can be affected by the materials used in production and manufacturing. Optimal performance for each DPI design occurs at a specific inspiratory flow rate. The fine particle fraction of respirable drug from existing DPIs ranges from 10% to 60% of the nominal dose. The amount varies with inspiratory flow and device design. The higher the resistance or the greater the flow requirement of a DPI device, the more difficult it is for a compromised or young patient to generate inspiratory flow sufficient to obtain the maximum dose of drug from the device.[42] In contrast, the higher the resistance of the device, the

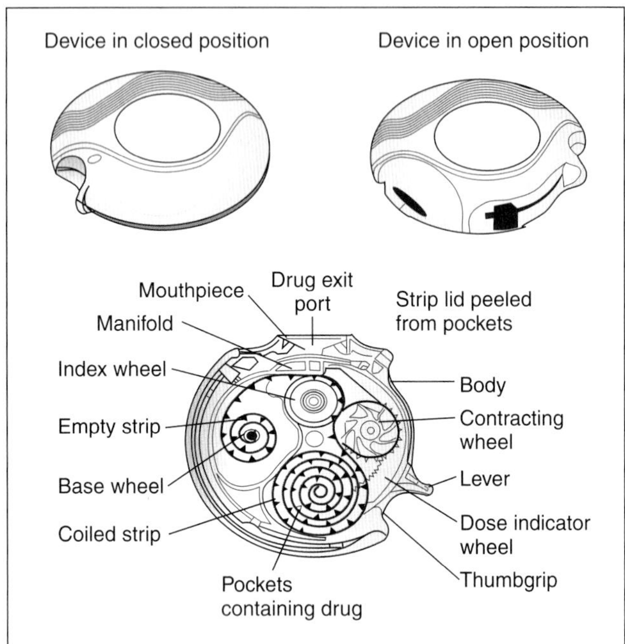

Figure 33-12

The Diskus dry powder inhaler (Glaxo Wellcome, Research Triangle Park, N.C.). The doses are contained in 60 sealed pockets along an aluminum-foil strip that is advanced by the lever. As the drug pocket reaches the mouthpiece, the cover is peeled away, making the drug available for inhalation. A dose counter indicates the number of doses remaining in the device. *(Modified from Dhand R, Fink J: Respir Care 44:940, 1999.)*

greater is the potential for increasing delivery of drug to the lower respiratory tract.

Ambient humidity affects drug delivered from DPIs.[40] The emitted dose decreases in a humid environment, likely because of powder clumping and growth. The longer the exposure to humidity, the lower is the dose emitted. A DPI with an exposed cake of drug such as the Turbuhaler might deliver less respirable drug during the summer in Florida than during winter in Sweden. New designs of multiple-unit-dose DPIs in which the powder is sealed until used should minimize the effects of moisture on the powder as long as individual doses are inhaled as soon as the seal is broken.

The high peak inspiratory flow rates (>60 L/min) required to dispense the drug powder from most current DPI designs result in a pharyngeal dose comparable with that received from a pMDI without an add-on device. The dose delivered to the respiratory tract from the Turbuhaler at 60 L/min has been measured in adults with lung disease and shown to be similar to that from a pMDI: 17% to the lungs and approximately 75% to the oropharynx. If inhalation is not performed at the optimal inspiratory flow rate for a particular device, delivery to the lung decreases as the dose of drug dispensed decreases and the particle size of the powder aerosol increases[40-45] (Figure 33-13).

Despite the foregoing issues, DPIs in general are convenient and easy to use. Newer designs are being developed that provide aerosols with higher fine-particle fractions and more reproducible dosing independent of inspiratory flow rate.

Passive, or patient-driven, DPIs rely on the patient's inspiratory effort to dispense the dose. The result is differences in lung delivery and clinical response. Active, or powered, DPI devices are independent of patient effort. In active DPI designs, such as the Inhale Powder Delivery System (Inhale Therapeutics, San Carlos, Calif.), a storage chamber contains the powder released from the device. These devices are powered by a hand pump that builds up pneumatic pressure, which is blasted through the pierced blister pack immediately before inhalation.

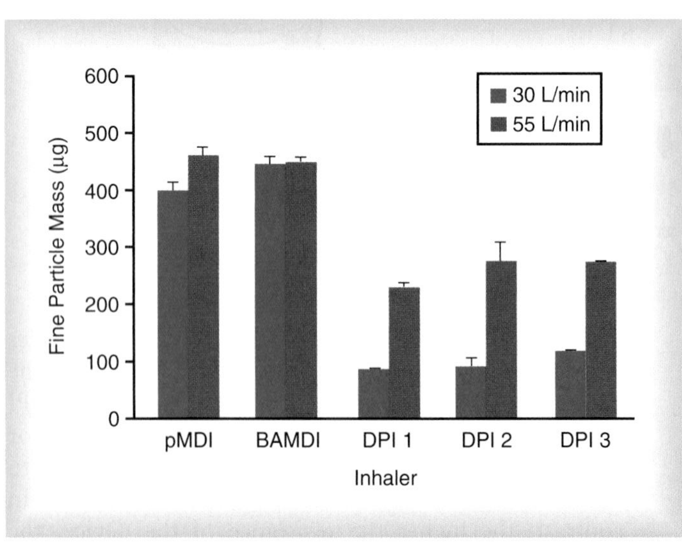

Figure 33-13

Fine particle mass delivered from a 1000-mg dose (±SD) as a function of flow. PMDI, Pressurized metered-dose inhaler; BAMDI, breath-actuated pMDI (Autohaler); DPI, dry powder inhaler; DPI1, Rotahaler; DPI2, Turbuhaler; DPI3, Diskhaler. *(Modified from Smith KJ, Chang H-K, Brown KF: J Aerosol Med 11:231, 1998.)*

Box 33-3 • Optimal Technique for Use of a Dry Powder Inhaler

1. Assemble the apparatus.
2. Load dose.
3. Exhale slowly to functional residual capacity.
4. Seal lips around the mouthpiece.
5. Inhale deeply and forcefully (>40 L/min). A breath-hold is not necessary.
6. Repeat the process until the dosage is completed.
7. Monitor adverse reactions.
8. Assess beneficial effects.

Modified from Pederson S: *Arch Dis Child* 61:11, 1986 and Hansen OR, Pederson S: Eur Respir J 2:637, 1989.

Technique

As with an MDI, to derive the maximum benefit from a DPI, proper technique is essential. Box 33-3 outlines the basic steps for ensuring optimum drug delivery.[43,44]

The most critical factor in using a DPI is the need for *high* inspiratory flow. Patients must generate an inspiratory flow rate of at least 40 to 60 L/min to produce a respirable powder aerosol.[42] Because infants, small children (younger than 5 years) (Figure 33-14), and those not able to follow instructions cannot develop flow this high, these patient groups cannot use DPIs.[44] Patients with severe airway obstruction also may not be able to achieve the required flow[45]; therefore DPIs should not be used in the management of acute bronchospasm.

Although hand-breath coordination is not as important with DPIs as it is with MDIs, exhalation into the device can result in loss of drug delivery to the lung. Some devices also require assembly, which can be cumbersome or difficult for some patients, especially in an emergency. It is important that patients receive demonstrations with their inhalers and have the opportunity to assemble and use the DPI (return demonstration) before self-administration.

Pneumatic (Jet) Nebulizers

Small-Volume Nebulizers

Gas-powered jet nebulizers have been in clinical use for more than 100 years. Most modern jet nebulizers are powered by high-pressure air or oxygen provided by a portable compressor, compressed gas cylinder, or 50-psi wall outlet. Because nebulizers commonly used at home and in the hospital for drug administration have small (≤10 mL) medication reservoirs, they are called *small-volume nebulizers* (SVNs).

Factors Affecting SVN Performance. Nebulizer design, gas pressure and density, and medication characteristics affect SVN performance (Box 33-4).[46,47]

Nebulizer Design. As shown in Figure 33-15, a typical SVN is powered by a high-pressure stream of gas directed through a restricted orifice (the *jet*). The gas stream leaving the jet passes by the opening of a capillary tube immersed in solution. Because it produces low lateral pressure at the outlet, the high jet velocity draws the liquid up the capillary tube and into the gas stream, where it is sheared into filaments of liquid that break up into droplets. This primary spray produces a heterodisperse aerosol with droplets in the 0.1- to 500-μm range.[46]

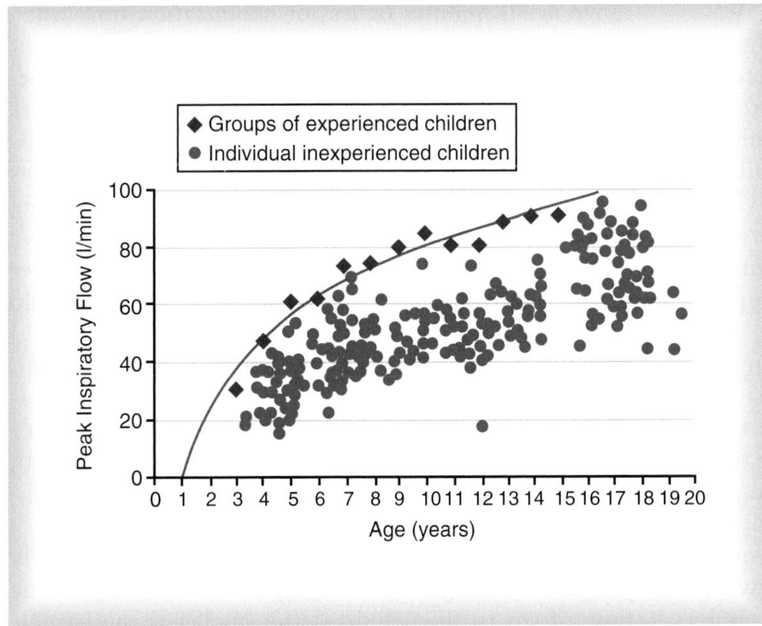

Figure 33-14
Peak inspiratory flows in individual inexperienced children (Pedersen et al, 1990) and groups of experienced children (Agertoft et al, 1995). *(Modified from Pederson S: J Aerosol Med 10:41, 1997.)*

Box 33-4 • Factors Affecting Performance of Small-Volume Nebulizers

NEBULIZER DESIGN
- Baffles
- Fill volume
- Residual volume
- Nebulizer position
- Continuous versus intermittent nebulization
- Reservoirs and extensions
- Vents and gas entrainment
- Tolerances in manufacturing within lots

GAS SOURCE: WALL, CYLINDER, COMPRESSOR
- Pressure
- Flow through nebulizer
- Gas density
- Humidity
- Temperature

CHARACTERISTICS OF DRUG FORMULATION
- Viscosity
- Surface tension
- Homogeneity

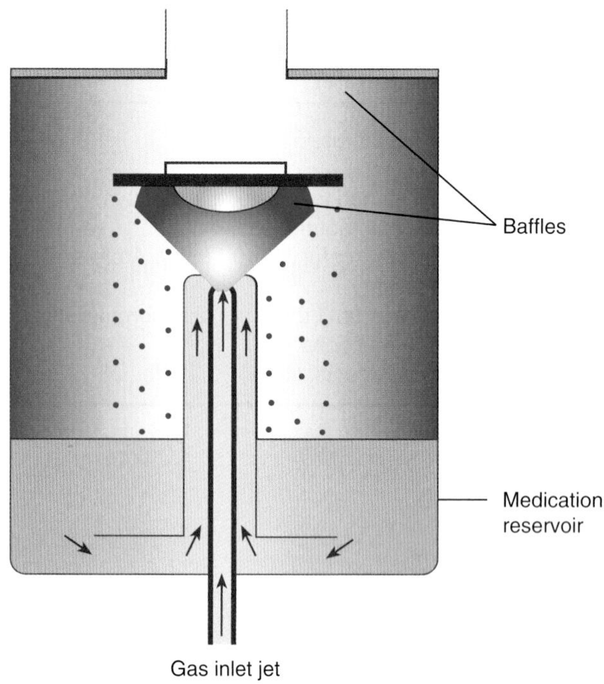

Figure 33-15
Components of a jet nebulizer. *(From Fink J, Cohen J: Humidity and aerosols. In Eubank D, Bone R: Principles and applications of cardiorespiratory care equipment, St Louis, 1994, Mosby.)*

This primary spray is directed against one or more baffles. A **baffle** is simply a surface on which large particles impact and fall out of suspension, a process that decreases the MMAD and GSD of the aerosol. A sphere or plate placed in line with the jet flow can serve as a baffle, as can the internal walls of the nebulizer, the surface of the solution being nebulized, or the internal walls of the delivery system. In many designs, droplets that impact baffles in the SVN return to the medication reservoir to be nebulized again.

Baffles are key elements in SVN design. In jet nebulizers, well-designed baffling systems decrease both the MMAD and the GSD of the generated aerosol. Baffling also can occur unintentionally. **Atomizers** operate with the same basic principles, without baffling, and produce aerosols with larger MMAD and GSD. Unintentional baffles are created by the angles within delivery tubing, by interfaces with other devices outside the aerosol generator, and by the surfaces of the upper airway itself.

Residual or dead volume is the medication that remains in the SVN after the device runs dry.[48,49] The residual volume varies from as little as 0.5 mL to more than 2.2 mL, which can be more than two thirds of the total dose. Of course, the greater the residual volume, the more drug is wasted and the less efficient is the delivery system. Residual volume also depends on the position of the SVN. Some SVNs stop producing aerosol when tilted as little as 30 degrees from vertical. The proportion of drug nebulized by an SVN increases as fill volume increases.[48] In general, SVNs filled to 4 mL deliver more drug than those filled to only 2 mL at a constant input flow of 6 to 8 L/min. This increase in fill volume increases nebulization time. However, varying diluent volumes and flows do not necessarily correlate with differences in clinical responses.

An effective pneumatic nebulizer should deliver more than 50% of its total dose as aerosol in the respirable range in 10 minutes or less of nebulization time when properly used. Nebulizer performance varies with diluent volume, operating flow, pressure, gas density, and nebulizer model. The amount of drug nebulized increases as the volume of diluent is increased. The residual volume of medicine that remains in commercial SVNs varies from 0.2 to 2.2 mL depending on the device. Increasing the fill volume allows a greater proportion of active medication to be nebulized. For example, in a nebulizer with a residual volume of 1.5 mL, a fill of 3 mL would leave only 50% of the nebulizer charge (nominal dose) available for nebulization. In contrast, a fill of 5 mL would make 3.5 mL, or more than 70%, of the medication available for nebulization. To date, no significant difference in clinical response has been shown with varying diluent volumes and flow rates.[49]

Flow. Droplet size and nebulization time are inversely proportional to gas flow through the jet. The higher the flow of gas to the nebulizer, the smaller is the particle size generated and the shorter is the time required to nebulize the full dose. Within the limits of the design of the nebulizer, the higher the gas pressure and flow to the nebulizer, the smaller is the particle generated. Nebulizers that produce smaller particle sizes by use of baffles, such as one-way valves, may reduce total drug output per minute compared with the same nebulizer without baffling and require more time or nominal dose to deliver a standard dose of medication to the lungs.

Gas Source (Hospital versus Home). Gas pressure and flow affect SVN particle size, distribution, and output. Within operating limits, the higher the pressure or flow, the smaller is the particle size, the greater is the output, and the shorter is the treatment time.[47-49] A nebulizer that produces an MMAD of 2.5 μm when driven by a gas source of 50 psi at 6 to 10 L/min may produce an MMAD of more than 5 μm when operated on a home compressor (or ventilator) developing 10 psi. Too low a flow can result in negligible nebulizer output. Consequently, nebulizers used for home care should be matched to the compressor according to data supplied by the manufacturer so that the combination of specific equipment efficiently nebulizes the desired medications prescribed for the patient. In Europe, equipment manufacturers are required to demonstrate that their nebulizer and compressor combinations can nebulize the appropriate fill volume of drug within 10 minutes and deliver more than 50% of the drug in the nebulizer as respirable particles. They must also identify all medications with which the nebulizer and compressor might reliably meet these two criteria. Until such time that similar standards are required in the United States, clinicians should ascertain whether the system prescribed meets these criteria.

Other concerns in the use of disposable nebulizers with compressors at home involve possible degradation of performance of the plastic device over multiple uses. One study showed that repeated use did not alter MMAD or output as long as the nebulizer was cleaned properly. Failure to clean the nebulizer properly resulted in degradation of performance due to clogging the Venturi orifice, reducing the output flow, and buildup of electrostatic charge in the device.

Density. Gas density affects both aerosol generation and delivery to the lungs. The lower the density of a carrier gas, the less turbulent is the flow (i.e. the lower is the Reynolds number), and lack of turbulent flow theoretically decreases aerosol impaction. This phenomenon is most evident with low-density helium-oxygen mixtures. The lower the density of a carrier gas, the less aerosol impaction occurs and the better is the deposition in the lungs.[50] However, when heliox drives a jet nebulizer, aerosol output is substantially less than with air or oxygen, requiring a 300% increase in flow to produce a comparable weight of aerosol per minute. Thus although it increases the amount of aerosol getting into the lungs, helium impairs the actual production of the suspension at the nebulizer.

Humidity and Temperature. Humidity and temperature affect particle size and the concentration of drug remaining in the nebulizer. Evaporation of water and adiabatic expansion of gas can reduce the temperature of the aerosol to as much as 10° C below ambient temperature.[51] This cooling increases the solution viscosity and reduces the nebulizer output while decreasing particle MMAD.[52] Aerosol particles entrained into a warm and fully saturated gas stream increase in size. These particles also can coalesce (stick together), further increasing the MMAD, and, in the case of a DPI, can severely compromise the output of respirable particles. How much these particles enlarge depends primarily on the tonicity of the solution. Aerosols generated from isotonic solutions probably maintain their size as they enter the respiratory tract. Hypertonic solutions tend to enlarge, whereas evaporation can cause hypotonic droplets to evaporate and shrink.

Continuous nebulization with conventional nebulizers wastes medication because the aerosol is produced throughout the respiratory cycle and is largely lost to the atmosphere, as shown in Figure 33-16. Patients with an I:E ratio of 40:60 lose 60% of the aerosol generated to the atmosphere. If only 50% of the total dose is emitted from the nebulizer and 50% of that aerosol is in the respiratory range and only 40% of that is inhaled by the patient, it is clear why less than 12% deposition is commonly measured in adults undergoing nebulizer

MINI CLINI

Home Nebulizer Therapy

PROBLEM

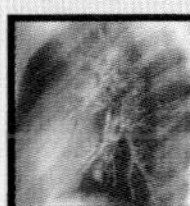

Many patients are sent home with a prescription for home nebulizer therapy prescribed with the intention of giving the patient the same quality of aerosol therapy they received in the hospital. All too often, however, the patient is given the same type of nebulizer used in the hospital because it is inexpensive. These nebulizers provide an aerosol that is too large for optimal deposition in the lungs. What should be done instead?

SOLUTION

Home nebulizers designed for use with compressors should be matched to ensure an MMAD of 1 to 5 μm with the medication being administered. Nebulizer manufacturers such as Pari and Medic-Aid offer matched nebulizer-compressor systems for home use. Although these devices cost a little more, they at least have a chance of meeting therapeutic objectives.

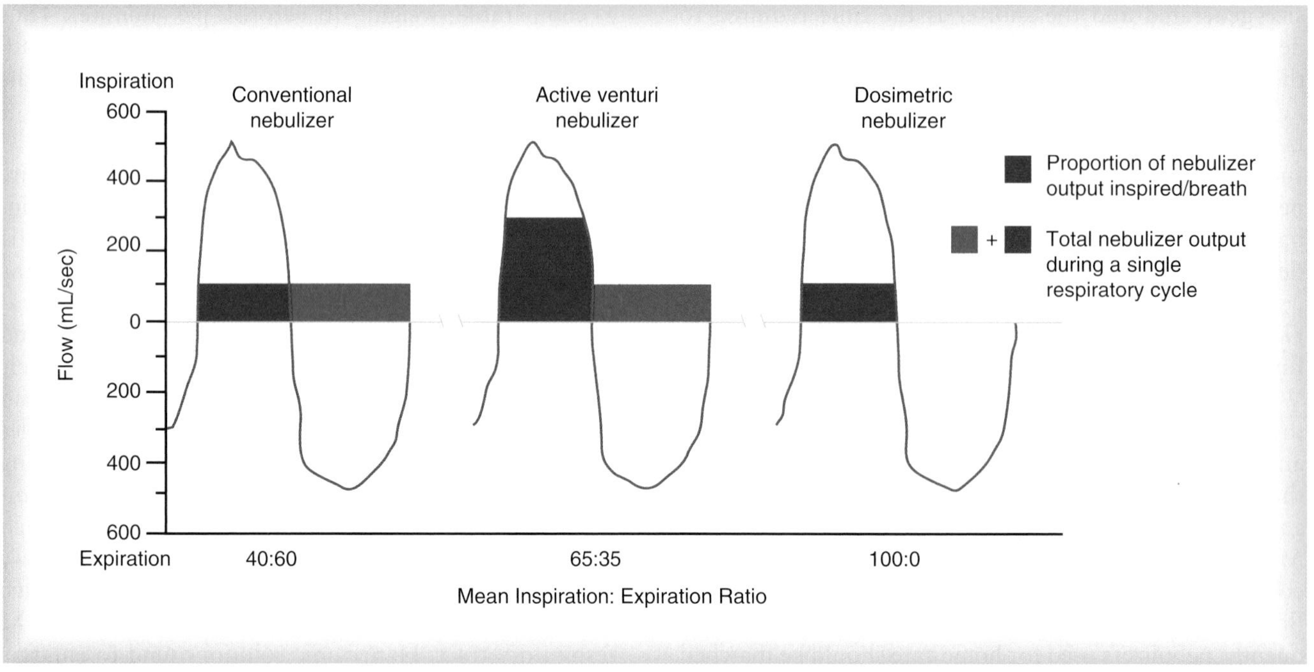

Figure 33-16

Proportions of nebulizer output inhaled with continuous standard jet nebulizer, vented nebulizer, and dosimetric (breath-coordinated) nebulizer. *(Modified from Nikander K: J Aerosol Med 7(suppl 1):S19, 1994.)*

therapy. Given the increased impaction and reduced sedimentation, it is not unexpected that deposition in neonates and infants is less than 2%.

Most SVNs are run continuously until they go dry. With continuous delivery to a patient with an I:E ratio of 1:3, only 25% of the aerosol is inhaled, the remainder being wasted to the atmosphere. Some SVNs have a mechanism for intermittent nebulization. This function usually is accomplished with a patient-controlled finger port that directs gas to the nebulizer only during inspiration. Although this system wastes less aerosol, it can quadruple treatment time. Moreover, this approach requires good hand-breath coordination, something not all patients possess.

Rather than having the patient control when nebulization occurs, a one-way valve system can be used to minimize aerosol waste.[53] In this design (Pari LC Jet Plus), an inspiratory vent allows the patient to draw in air with the aerosolized drug. On exhalation, however, the inlet vent closes, and aerosol exits by a one-way valve near the mouthpiece; this process reduces aerosol waste.

Aerosolized medication can be conserved with reservoirs.[54] Most disposable nebulizers are packaged with a 6-inch (15 cm) piece of aerosol tubing to be used as a reservoir. A reservoir on the expiratory limb of the nebulizer conserves drug aerosol. Bag reservoirs (Piper or Circulaire) hold the aerosol generated during exhalation and allow the small particles to remain in suspension for inhalation with the next breath while larger particles rain out. A device such as the Mizer (Figure 33-17) is designed to hold the aerosol generated during exhalation in a baffled chamber. The small particles remain in suspension for inhalation with the next breath while larger particles rain out.

It can be difficult to determine when a nebulizer treatment is complete. Malone and colleagues[51] found that with three different fill volumes, albuterol delivery from the nebulizer ceased after the onset of inconsistent nebulization (sputtering) (Figure 33-18). Aerosol output declined one half within 20 seconds of the onset of sputtering. The concentration of albuterol in the nebulizer cup increased significantly once the aerosol output declined, and further weight loss in the nebulizer was caused primarily by evaporation. The authors concluded that aerosolization past the point of initial jet nebulizer sputter is ineffective.

Special Medication Delivery Issues for Infants and Children. Children and infants have a smaller airway diameter than do adults. The breathing rate is faster, nose breathing filters out large particles and deposits more medication in the upper airway, and mouthpiece administration often cannot be used. Patient cooperation and ability vary with age and developmental ability.

For patients who can tolerate a mask, a medication nebulizer can be fitted to an appropriately sized aerosol mask. There is no difference in clinical response between mouthpiece and close-fitting mask treatment, so patient compliance and preference should guide selection of the device. There is evidence that the aerosol available is

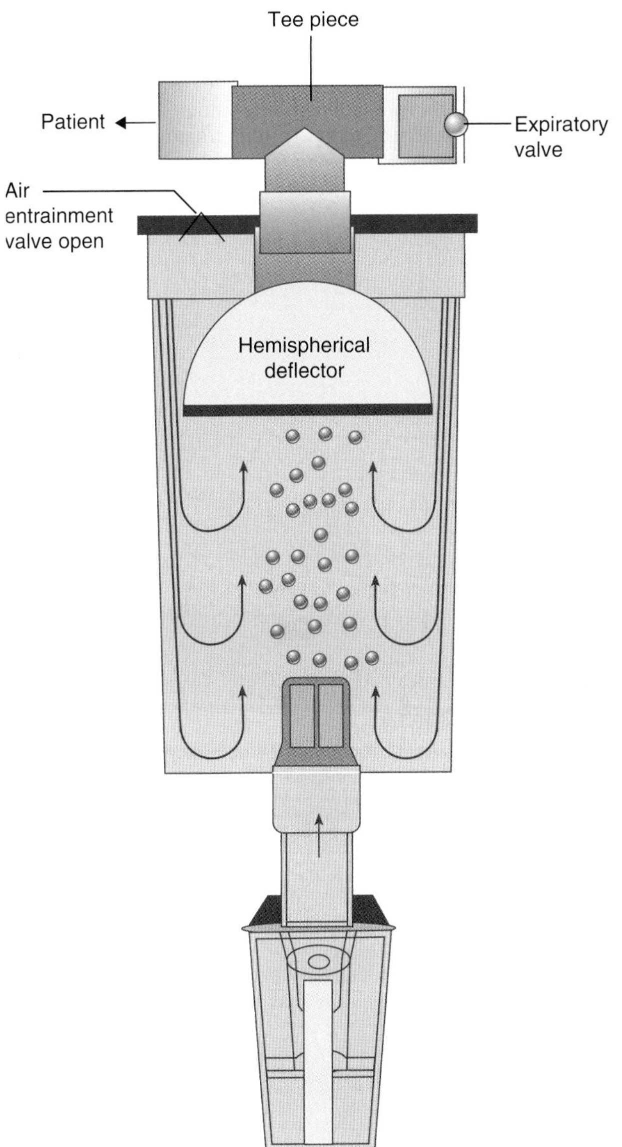

Figure 33-17
Mizer aerosol conservation device attached to a conventional nebulizer. During inspiration, negative pressure inside the holding chamber causes an air entrainment valve to open and air to be drawn in. The entrained air collects aerosol and exits through the Tee piece, delivering aerosol to the patient during inspiration. Expired air is diverted away from the chamber by a valve, and the chamber refills with aerosol.

substantially less when a loosely fitting mask is used than when a mouthpiece is used in the care of patients 5 to 15 years of age.[55] If the patient cannot tolerate mask treatment (e.g., will not wear a close-fitting mask), a commonly used strategy is use of a "blow-by" technique. The practitioner directs the aerosol from the nebulizer toward the patient's nose and mouth. There are no published data supporting the use of the blow-by technique. Results of aerosol deposition studies suggest that almost no drug enters the airway with this method. It may be more efficient to deliver medication with a close-fitting mask when the patient is sound asleep.

Spontaneous breathing results in greater deposition of aerosol from an SVN than occurs with positive-pressure breaths (e.g., intermittent positive-pressure ventilation). This mode of ventilation reduces aerosol deposition more than 30% compared with the effect of spontaneously inhaled aerosols.[56]

Normal tidal breathing is the most effective method for administering aerosols to an infant. Mouth breathing enhances medication delivery to the airways of adults, but there are few data indicating that this holds true for infants, who are preferential nose breathers. Aerosols should never be administered to a crying child. Crying is a long exhalation preceded by a very short and rapid inhalation. Crying greatly reduces lower airway deposition of aerosol medication (Figure 33-19).

Characteristics of Drug Formulation. The viscosity and density of a drug formulation affect both output and particle size. Some drugs, such as antibiotics, are so viscous they cannot be effectively nebulized in some standard SVNs. This also is an issue with suspensions in which some aerosolized particles contain no active drug, whereas other particles, generally larger, carry the active medication. Table 33-1 summarizes some of these key factors for a number of commercially available SVNs.[57] A large number of SVNs are on the market, and they vary widely in design and performance. Unfortunately, SVNs of the same design and lot number can exhibit variable performance, even to the point that some nebulizers of the same model number do not work at all.[58] Managers and clinicians must always carefully evaluate SVNs before purchasing or using them. Manufacturers should provide data on the performance of their nebulizers under common use conditions.

Technique. Box 33-5 outlines the optimal technique for using an SVN for aerosol drug delivery. Use of an SVN is less technique and device dependent than use of an MDI or DPI delivery system. Slow inspiratory flow does improve SVN aerosol deposition. However, deep breathing and breath-holding during SVN therapy do little to enhance deposition over normal tidal breathing.[59] Because the nose is an efficient filter of particles larger than 5 mm, many clinicians prefer not to use a mask for SVN therapy. *As long as the patient is mouth-breathing*, there is little difference in clinical response between therapy given by mouthpiece and that given by mask. The selection of delivery method (mask or mouthpiece) should be based on patient ability, preference, and comfort.

The Centers for Disease Control and Prevention recommendations for nebulizers are that the device be cleaned and disinfected or rinsed with sterile water and air dried between uses. Oie and Kamiya,[60] studying

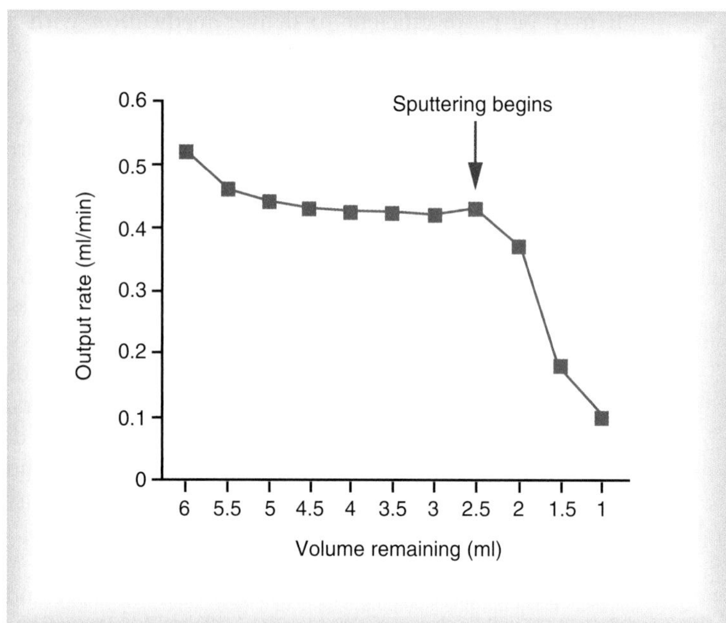

Figure 33-18

The output rate for jet nebulizers is substantially reduced as the nebulizer begins to sputter. The decrease in output rate correlates with reduced drug output. This finding supports a recommendation to end treatment when sputtering begins. *(Modified from Malone RA, Hollie MC, Glynn-Barnhart A, et al: Chest 104:1114, 1993.)*

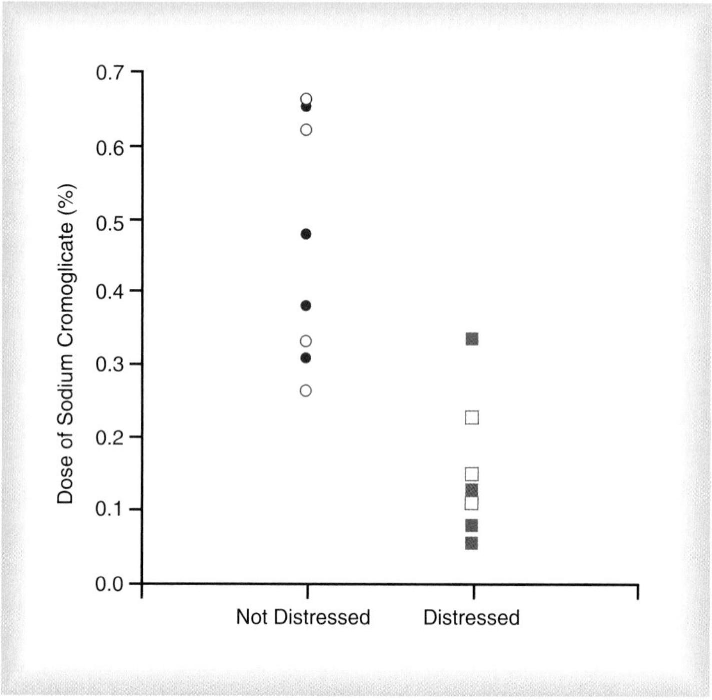

Figure 33-19

Crying substantially reduces the deposition of aerosol inhaled by infants. *(From Iles R, Lister P, Edmunds AT: Arch Dis Child 81:163, 1999.)*

microbial contamination of antibiotic aerosol solutions, found that after 7 days, five of six solutions were contaminated. The contamination appears to have been caused by storage of multiple-dose solutions at room temperature instead of in a refrigerator and reuse of syringes for measuring the solution. Refrigerating solution and disposing syringes every 24 hours eliminated bacterial contamination.

Large-Volume Jet Nebulizers

Large-volume nebulizers are used to deliver aerosolized drugs to the lung. A large-volume nebulizer is particularly useful when traditional dosing strategies are ineffective in the management of severe bronchospasm. For example, when a patient with airway obstruction does not respond to a standard dosage of broncho-

Table 33-1 ▶▶ Selected Nebulizer Performance with Air Compressors

Nebulizer	Residual Volume (mL)	Maximum Fill Volume (mL)	Percentage Nebulized in 5 min	Percentage Nebulized in 10 min	Particles <5 μm (%)	MMAD (μm)
Acorn	1.8	15	30	38	79	3.69
Cirrus	0.9	10	40	46	80	3.50
DeVilbiss 646	2.1	3	26	44	70	2.20
Hudson UD I	2.3	17	—	—	82	4.80
Hudson UD II	1.4	10	25	33	79	3.29
MicroCirrus	1.2	10	—	—	90	1.20
MicroNeb	0.9	13	28	59	78	3.63
MiniNeb	2.3	38	41	51	79	3.54
Pari Boy	2.0	9	50	64	64	4.16
Pari LC Plus	1.0	8	50	50	60	3.80
Respirgard II	1.3	9	—	—	—	1.88
Sidestream	0.7	12	—	—	83	3.18
System 22 Mizer	2.0	15	—	—	73	4.65
Ventstream	1.0	10	—	—	86	3.17

Modified from Kendrick AH, Smith EC, Wilson RSE: Thorax 52(suppl 2):S92, 1997.

Box 33-5 • Optimal Technique for Using a Small-Volume Nebulizer

1. Assess the patient for need (clinical signs and symptoms, breath sounds, peak flow, %FEV_1)
2. Select mask or mouthpiece delivery (noseclips may be needed with mouthpiece).
3. Use conserving system (thumbport or reservoir) if indicated.
4. Place drug in the nebulizer to fill volume ≥4 mL.
5. Set gas flow to nebulizer at 6 to 8 L/min.
6. Coach patient to breathe slowly through the mouth at normal tidal volume.
7. Tap the nebulizer periodically to minimize residual volume.
8. Continue treatment until no aerosol is produced.
9. Rinse the nebulizer with sterile water and run dry.
10. Monitor patient for adverse response.
11. Assess outcome (change in peak flow, %FEV_1).

dilator, it is common practice to repeat the treatment as often as every 15 minutes. To avoid giving separate SVN treatments, some clinicians have adapted an intravenous (IV) infusion pump to drip premixed bronchodilator solution into a standard SVN (Figure 33-20). Although an expensive approach, this technique can provide dosing equivalent to every 15 minutes.[61]

An alternative approach is to provide *continuous* nebulization with a specialized large-volume nebulizer. The high-output extended aerosol respiratory therapy (HEART) and HOPE (B and B) nebulizers are examples of devices designed for this purpose. These nebulizers have a 240-mL reservoir that produces an aerosol with an MMAD between 2.2 and 3.5 μm. Actual output and particle size vary with the pressure and flow at which the nebulizer operates. A potential problem with continuous bronchodilator therapy (CBT) is drug reconcentration. For this reason, patients receiving CBT need close monitoring for signs of drug toxicity.

Another special-purpose large-volume nebulizer is the small-particle aerosol generator (SPAG) (Figure 33-21). The SPAG is manufactured by ICN Pharmaceuticals specifically for administration of ribavirin (Virazole) to infants with respiratory syncytial virus infection. The device is unique in clinical respiratory care practice in that it incorporates a drying chamber with its own flow control to produce a stable aerosol. The SPAG reduces medical gas source from the normal 50 pounds per square inch gauge (psig) line pressure to as low as 26 psig with an adjustable regulator. The regulator is connected to two flowmeters that separately control flow to the nebulizer and drying chamber. The nebulizer is located within the medication reservoir, the fluid surface and wall of which serve as primary baffles. As it leaves the medication reservoir, the aerosol enters a long, cylindrical drying chamber. Here the separate flow of dry gas reduces particle size by evaporation, creating a monodisperse aerosol with an MMAD between 1.2 and 1.4 mm. Nebulizer flow should be maintained at approximately 7 L/min with total flow from both flowmeters no lower than 15 L/min. The latest model operates consistently even with back pressure and can be used with masks, hoods, tents, or ventilator circuits.

Two specific problems arise when the SPAG is used to deliver ribavirin. The first is caregiver exposure to the drug aerosol. Approaches to limit caregiver exposure

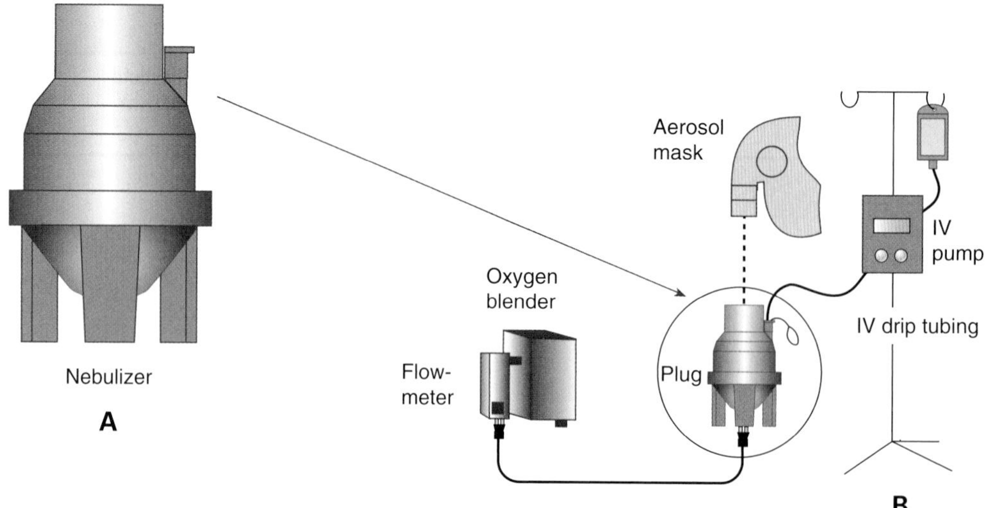

Figure 33-20
Intravenous drip system for continuous nebulization. **A,** Small-volume nebulizer. **B,** Intravenous setup with blender, flowmeter, and drip pump.

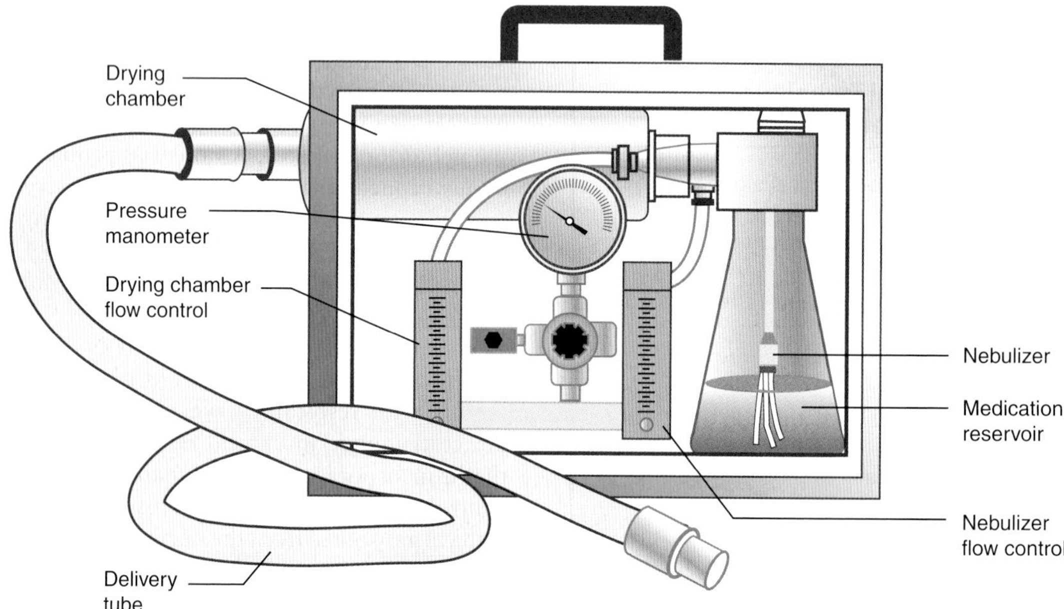

Figure 33-21
Small-particle aerosol generator.

are discussed later (see Controlling Environmental Contamination). The other problem occurs only when the SPAG is used to deliver ribavirin through a mechanical ventilation circuit. Drug precipitation can jam breathing valves or occlude the ventilator circuit. This problem can be overcome by (1) placing a one-way valve between the SPAG and the circuit and (2) filtering out the excess aerosol particles before they reach the exhalation valve.[62, 63]

Ultrasonic Nebulizers

In a USN a piezoelectric crystal is used to produce an aerosol. The crystal transducer converts an electrical signal into high-frequency (1.2 to 2.4 MHz) acoustic vibrations. These vibrations are focused in the liquid above the transducer, where they disrupt the surface and create oscillation waves (Figure 33-22). If the frequency of the signal is high enough and its amplitude strong

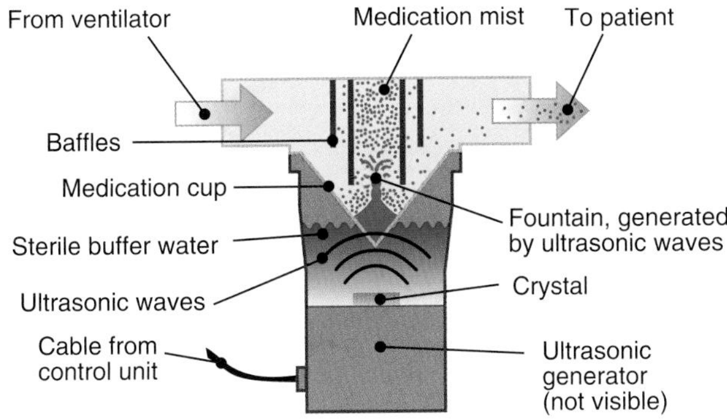

Figure 33-22
Small-volume ultrasonic nebulizer designed for use with mechanical ventilation. A vibrating piezoceramic crystal generates ultrasonic waves that pass through couplant (sterile buffer water) and the medication cup to generate a fountain (or standing wave) of medication that produces aerosol particles. *(Courtesy of Siemens.)*

enough, the oscillation waves form a geyser of droplets that break free as fine aerosol particles.

Ultrasonic nebulizers are capable of higher aerosol outputs (0.2-0.5 mL/min) and higher aerosol densities than are conventional jet nebulizers. Output is determined by the user-selected amplitude setting; the greater the signal amplitude, the greater is the nebulizer output. Particle size is inversely proportional to the frequency of vibrations. Frequency usually is device-specific and is not user-adjustable. For example a DeVilbiss Portasonic nebulizer operating at a frequency of 2.25 MHz produces particles with an MMAD of 2.5 μm, whereas the DeVilbiss Pulmosonic nebulizer operating at 1.25 MHz produces particles in the 4- to 6-μm range. Particle size and aerosol density also depend on the source and flow of gas conducting the aerosol to the patient.

Large-Volume USNs

Large-volume USNs (used mainly for bland aerosol therapy or sputum induction) incorporate air blowers to carry the mist to the patient (see Chapter 32). Low flow is associated with smaller particles and higher mist density. High flow yields larger particles and less density. Unlike jet nebulizers, the temperature of the solution placed in a USN increases during use. As the temperature increases, the drug concentration increases, as does the likelihood of undesired side effects.

Small-Volume USNs

A number of small-volume USNs have been marketed for aerosol drug delivery (see Figure 33-22).[61] Unlike the large units, some of these systems do not use a couplant compartment; the medication is placed directly into the manifold on top of the transducer. The transducer is connected by cable to a power source, often battery-powered to increase portability. These devices have no blower; the patient's inspiratory flow draws the aerosol from the nebulizer into the lung.

Small-volume USNs have been promoted for administration of a wide variety of formulations, ranging from bronchodilators to antiinflammatory agents and antibiotics.[64] Use of a small-volume USN may increase available respirable mass, because most designs have less dead space than do SVNs. This feature reduces the need for a large quantity of diluent to ensure delivery of the drugs. The contained portable power source adds a great deal of convenience in mobility. Both theoretical advantages of the ultrasonic devices are outweighed by the high cost.

Small-volume USNs have been used to administer undiluted bronchodilators to patients with severe bronchospasm.[65] Because the nebulizers have minimal dead space, the treatment time is shortened. Use of undiluted bronchodilator is not new and is typically included in the manufacturer's product dosing information in the *Physician's Desk Reference.*

Some ventilator manufacturers (e.g., Siemens, Nellcor Puritan Bennett) are promoting the use of USNs for administration of aerosols during mechanical ventilation. Unlike SVNs, USNs do not add extra gas flow to the ventilator circuit during use. This feature reduces the need to change and reset ventilator and alarm settings during aerosol administration.[66]

Hand-Bulb Atomizers

The hand-bulb atomizer, or nasal spray pump, is used to administer sympathomimetic, antimuscarinic, antiinflammatory, and anesthetic aerosols to the upper airway (nasal passages, pharynx, larynx). These agents are used to manage upper airway inflammation and rhinitis, to provide local anesthesia, and to achieve systemic effects. Guidelines for the delivery of drugs to the upper airway have been developed by the American Association for Respiratory Care (AARC).[67]

Because it generates relatively low pressure and does not have baffles, the spray pump produces an aerosol suspension with a high MMAD and GSD, which are ideal for upper airway deposition. (Nasopharyngeal deposition is greatest for particles in the range of 5 to 20 μm.) Deposition with the hand-bulb atomizer applied to the nose occurs mostly in the anterior nasal passages with clearance to the nasopharynx. The 100-μL puffs appear to deposit more medication than do 50-μL puffs, and deposition to a greater surface area occurs with a 35-degree spray angle than with a 60-degree angle.

New-Generation Nebulizers

Recent nebulizer designs have increased drug output available to patients. Designs range from breath-enhanced nebulizers that entrain air through the nebulizer during inspiration to breath-actuated nebulizers that reduce or eliminate aerosol generation during the patient's expiratory phase (see Figure 33-16). Use of low-velocity (soft mist) aerosol, improved particle characteristics, and systems that minimize residual volume of medication left in the nebulizer substantially improve aerosol device efficiency. Along with improved performance, some "smart" nebulizers have capability for monitoring patient compliance and aid in managing the patient's treatment schedule.

With pulmonary deposition increased from the old standard of approximately 10% to more than 60% of the nominal dose, these recent device improvements may be accompanied by greater systemic side effects, unless the delivered dose is reduced. The key is to be able to target an effective delivered dose to the lungs.

New Nebulizer Designs for Liquids

The most commonly used jet nebulizer is the constant output design. Supplemental air is entrained across the top of the device and dilutes the aerosol produced within the nebulizer as it exits toward the patient. Aerosol is generated continuously, 30% to 60% of the nominal dose being trapped in the nebulizer, and more than 60% of the emitted dose is wasted to the atmosphere. For reduction of the waste of drug aerosolized during the expiratory phase of the breathing cycle, some nebulizer designs incorporate a thumb control in the compressed air line that allows the patient to divert gas flow to the nebulizer during inspiration only. This feature allows the patient to synchronize inhalation with actuation. Patients with good hand-breath coordination receive a similar amount of aerosol per breath as with a continuous design, but the time required to aerosolize the reservoir contents, or nominal dose, is lengthened up to fourfold. The result is delivery of a substantially greater dose of drug to the lung. Unfortunately, many patients have difficulty coordinating the thumb control with their inspiratory efforts during the course of therapy.

AERx. The AERx device (Aradigm Corp, Hayward, Calif.) is a drug solution in a unit-dose, sterile, preservative-free blister pack containing 25 to 50 μL of fluid. The drug is extruded under pressure through a nozzle containing a number of small, precision-drilled holes that produce a fine, respirable spray on inhalation. The aerosolization nozzle is part of the disposable blister and is not reused. The dose from a single blister is metered in approximately 1.5 seconds. The emitted dose is more than 70% of the dose contained in the blister with an inspiratory flow rate range of 30 to 85 L/min. The AERx device is being tested for use with a number of drugs in liquid form to be used for both topical and systemic therapy. The AERx device has built-in electronic monitoring capabilities for measuring inspiratory flow rate (IFR) during dosing and for triggering the dispensing of the dose at the appropriate IFR for optimal delivery. The dose administered is logged to provide a record of treatments and an indication of patient compliance with therapy. The AERx device is in clinical trials in the United States.

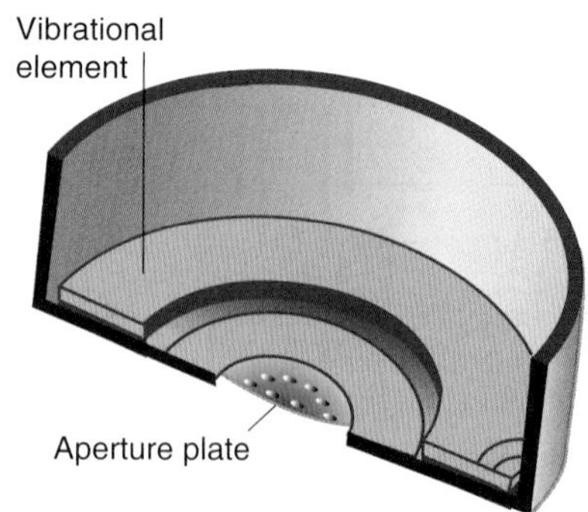

Figure 33-23
Aerosol generator components.

Aeroneb. The Aeroneb nebulizer system (AeroGen, Mountain View, Calif.) (Fig 33-23) is an electric (AC and battery-operated) liquid nebulizer that entails use of vibrating orifice technology for production of a fine aerosol. This nebulizer consists of a dome-shaped plate that contains 1000 tapered apertures. The plate vibrates at ultrasonic frequency and pumps the liquid through the apertures, where it is broken into fine droplets. The exit velocity of the aerosol is low, less than 4 m/s, and the particle size can be 1.5 μm or more (MMAD), varying with aperture size. This technology is used in currently available products for home (Aeroneb) and hospital (Aeroneb Pro). Aerogen is incorporating its proprietary aerosol generator in a breath-actuated inhaler system (Aerodose) currently in clinical trials with drugs such as inhaled insulin.

Respimat. In the Respimat soft-mist inhaler (Boehringer, Ingelheim, Germany), mechanical energy is used to create an aerosol from liquid solutions to produce a low-velocity spray (10 mm/s) that delivers a unit dose of drug in a single actuation. To operate it, patients place the Respimat device in the mouth and press a button to release the drug spray. The Respimat device, as does a pMDI, requires hand-breath coordination on the part of the patient and has not yet been approved for use in the United States.

Breath-Actuated Nebulizers

Breath-actuated nebulizers generate aerosol only during inspiration. This feature eliminates waste of aerosol during exhalation and increases the delivered dose threefold or more over continuous and breath-enhanced nebulizers.

Table 33-2 ▶▶ Advantages and Disadvantages of Aerosol Drug Delivery Systems

Advantages	Disadvantages
MDI	
Convenient Inexpensive Portable No drug preparation required Difficult to contaminate	Patient coordination required Patient activation required High percentage of pharyngeal deposition Risk of abuse Difficult to deliver high doses Not all medications are available Most units still use ozone-depleting CFCs
MDI with Accessory Device	
Less patient coordination required Less pharyngeal deposition No drug preparation required	More complex for some patients More expensive than an MDI alone Less portable than an MDI alone Not all medications available
DPI	
Less patient coordination required Breath activated Breath-hold not required Can provide accurate dose counts No CFCs	Requires high inspiratory flow Most units are single dose Risk of pharyngeal deposition Not all medications are available Difficult to deliver high doses
SVN	
Less patient coordination required High doses possible (even continuous) No CFC release	Expensive Wasteful Drug preparation required Contamination possible if device not cleaned carefully Not all medications available Pressurized gas source required Long treatment times
USN	
Small dead volume Quiet Aerosol accumulates during exhalation	Expensive Prone to electrical or mechanical breakdown Not all medications available Drug preparation required

Modified from Hess D: Respir Care Clin N Am 1:235, 1995.

Dosimeters, used in pulmonary function laboratories, sense inspiration and pulse airflow to the jet orifice and transform a conventional nebulizer into a breath-actuated system.

AeroEclipse (Trudell Medical International, London, Ont., Canada) is a breath-actuated jet nebulizer. A unique, spring-loaded, one-way valve design draws the jet to the capillary tube during inspiration and causes nebulization to cease when the patient's inspiratory flow decreases below the threshold, or the patient exhales into the device. Expiratory pressure on the valve at the initiation of exhalation moves the nebulizer baffle away from its position directly above the jet orifice, reduces the pressure, and stops aerosolization. Drug waste and contamination of the environment during the expiratory phase of the breathing cycle are largely eliminated. The AeroEclipse device is currently marketed in the United States and Europe.

The HaloLite (Medic-Aid, Sussex, U.K.) is a breath-actuated jet nebulizer that monitors pressure changes and inspiratory time for the patient's first three consecutive breaths. Drug is then aerosolized over 50% of the inspiratory maneuver during the fourth and all subsequent breaths. When the patient's preestablished dose has been aerosolized, the system provides an audible signal indicating the treatment should be stopped and the remaining medication discarded. Built-in electronics monitor patient treatment schedules and delivered doses. The goal is improvement of compliance with therapy. The HaloLite, currently sold in the United Kingdom and the rest of Europe, has 510k clearance from the U.S. Food and Drug Administration but has not been marketed in the United States.

Advantages and Disadvantages

Knowledge of the advantages and disadvantages of various aerosol drug delivery systems is critical for proper selection and application. Table 33-2 compares the MDI, DPI, SVN, and USN delivery systems.[68]

▶ SELECTING AN AEROSOL DRUG DELIVERY SYSTEM

To guide practitioners in selecting the best aerosol delivery system for a given clinical situation, the AARC has published clinical practice guidelines for aerosol delivery to the upper airway,[67] lung parenchyma,[69] and neonatal and pediatric patients.[70] For excerpts from the AARC guideline *Selection of Aerosol Delivery Device,*[11] see p. 789.

In selecting the appropriate aerosol delivery device for a given patient, the following must be considered: (1) the available drug formulation, (2) the desired site of deposition, (3) the patient's characteristics (age, acuity of problem, alertness and ability to follow instructions), and (4) the patient's preference.[11,45] For maintenance administration of bronchodilators and antiinflammatory agents to adults, an MDI with a holding chamber is the most convenient, versatile, and cost-effective approach. Dry powder inhalers are gaining popularity as an equivalent to MDIs for maintenance therapy with available drugs for patients capable of generating adequate flow. In acute situations, when high or multiple doses are needed, or when adult patients are not able to follow instructions, an SVN or large-volume continuous nebulizer is an alternative. An adult patient's preference must be considered, because a device that is not favored will not be used.[45] For infants and small children, see the following Rule of Thumb.[70,71] Figure 33-24 is a selection algorithm based on the foregoing discussion.

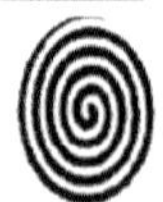

RULE OF THUMB

Guidelines for the Use of Aerosol Devices in the Care of Infants and Children

Device Group	Age
SVN	Neonate
MDI	>5 y
Chamber with mouthpiece	>4 y
Chamber with mask	Neonate/infant/toddler
Endotracheal tube	Neonate
Breath-actuated	>5 y
DPI	≥6 y

Regardless of the device used, the clinician must be aware of the limitations of aerosol drug therapy. First, one must remember that at best only 10% to 20% or less of the output of the device actually is deposited in the lungs (Figure 33-25). As indicated in Box 33-6, additional reductions in lung deposition can occur in many clinical situations that sometimes necessitate the use of higher dosages. Clinical efficacy varies according to both patient technique and device design. For these reasons, the best approach to aerosol drug therapy is to use an assessment-based protocol that emphasizes individually tailored therapy modified according to patient response.

Box 33-6 • Factors Associated With Reduced Aerosol Drug Deposition in the Lung

- Mechanical ventilation
- Artificial airways
- Reduced airway caliber (e.g., infants and children)
- Severe airway obstruction
- Poor patient compliance or technique
- Limitation of specific delivery device

▶ ASSESSMENT-BASED BRONCHODILATOR THERAPY PROTOCOLS

Although the choice of delivery system affects how well an aerosolized drug works, it is ultimately the patient's response that determines the therapeutic outcome. Because patients vary markedly in response to the dose and route of administration of a drug, it makes sense to tailor aerosol drug therapy to each patient. This approach is best made with an assessment-based protocol.

Sample Protocol

Figure 33-26 is an example of an algorithm underlying a bronchodilator therapy protocol for acutely ill adults or children admitted to an emergency department.[72] The protocol relies heavily on bedside assessment of the severity of airway obstruction based on the patient's response to varying drug dosages.

According to the algorithm, a patient with acute airway obstruction (wheezing, cough, dyspnea, and peak expiratory flow rate [PEFR] less than 60% of predicted value) would receive up to three SVN treatments with a standard dose of albuterol, repeated at 20-minute intervals, or 4 puffs of MDI albuterol with a holding chamber (up to 12 puffs). Each treatment is followed by a dose-response assessment to determine the "best" dose. Once determined, this best dose, with the MDI or SVN, would be repeated 1 hour later, then every 4 hours as needed supplemented with patient education. If use of the SVN or MDI with holding chamber were to fail to relieve the symptoms, CBT with 15 mg/h albuterol would be started.

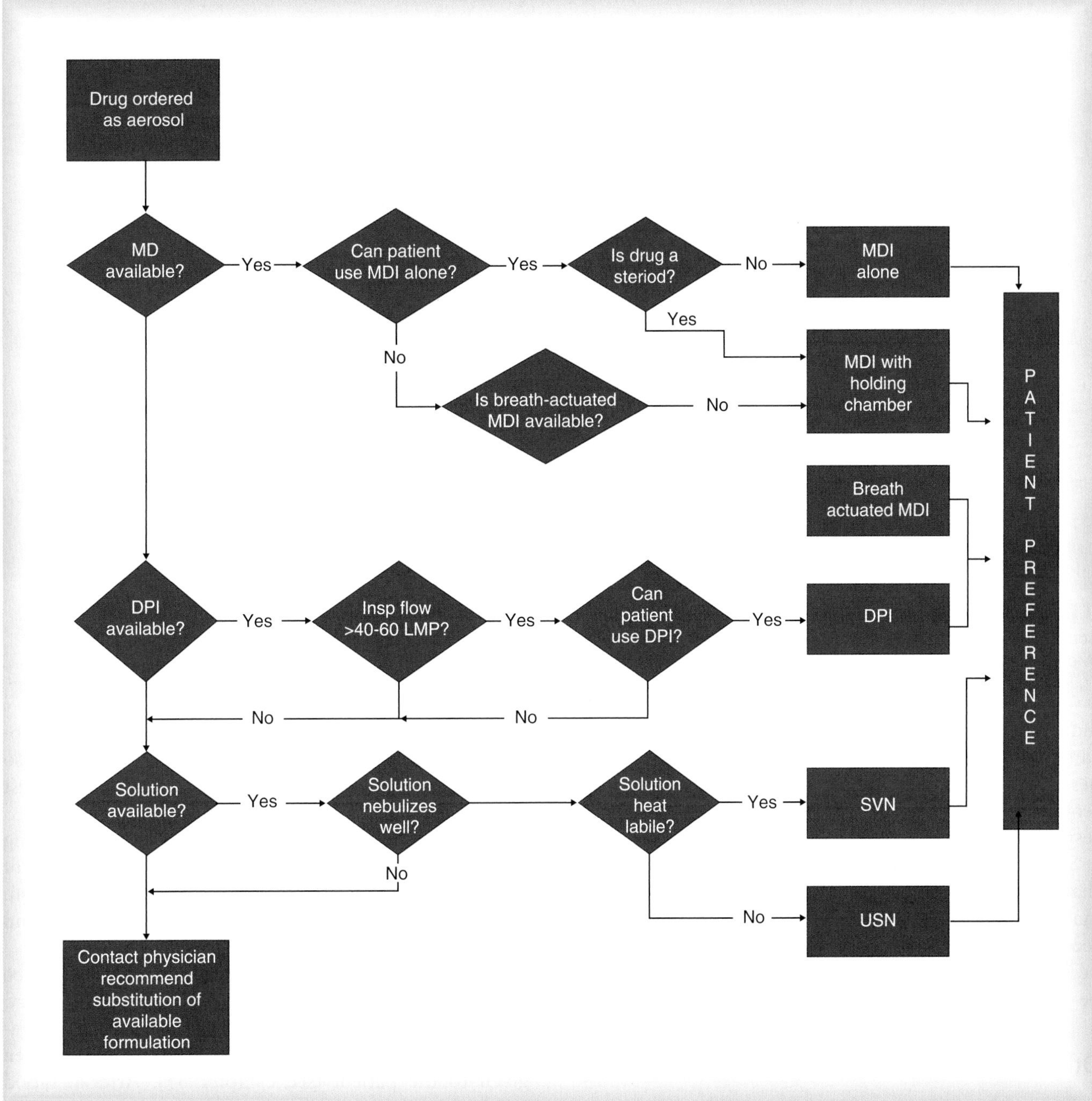

Figure 33-24
Selecting an aerosol drug delivery system. Once the need is established for aerosol drug delivery, determine which formulations are available for the prescribed medication. If an MDI is available, it is the first choice for cost and convenience. The patient's ability to coordinate actuation with inspiration and the need to reduce oropharyngeal deposition (e.g., steroids) determine need for a holding chamber or a breath-actuated unit. Nebulizers are the first choice when the formulation is available only as a solution. When the ordered medication is not available for inhalation use, the RT should recommend a substitution to the ordering physician.

Assessing Patient Response

Careful, ongoing patient assessment is the key to an effective bronchodilator therapy protocol. To guide practitioners in implementing effective bedside assessment, the AARC has published *Clinical Practice Guideline: Assessing Response to Bronchodilator Therapy at Point of Care.*[73] Excerpts appear on p. 790.

Use and Limitations of Peak Flow Monitoring

Because the peak flow measurement is effort and volume dependent, evaluation of patient performance is somewhat subjective, and there are no good acceptability criteria. In addition, agreement between conventional spirometry values, such as forced vital capacity (FVC) and FEV_1, and bedside PEFR values may be poor for

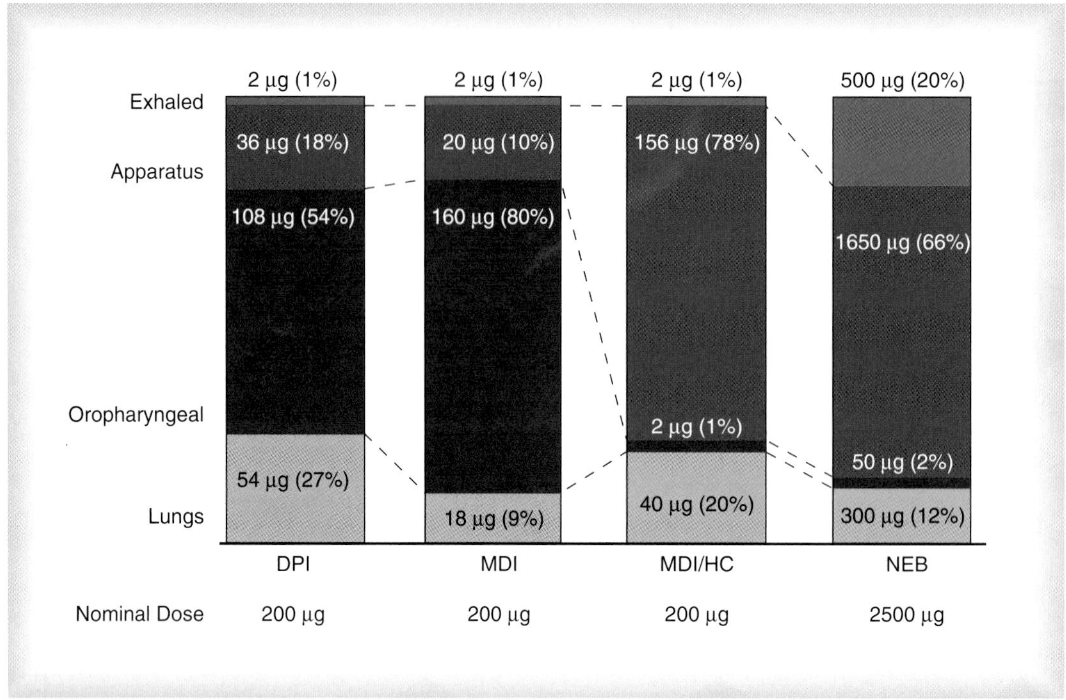

Figure 33-25
Comparison of quality and percentage of nominal dose of albuterol deposited in the lung, oropharynx, and apparatus and exhaled with a DPI. *(Modified from Fink JB: Respir Care 45:623, 2000.)*

individual patients. Although peak flow measurement can be used at the bedside to assess treatment effectiveness and to monitor trends, conventional spirometry remains the standard for determining bronchodilator response.[71,73]

Some peak flowmeters are more accurate and reliable than others. Even different units of the same model may give varied results. For this reason, the AARC recommends that in monitoring of trends, the same unit be used for a given patient and that the patient's range be reestablished if a different flowmeter is used.[73]

Other Components of Patient Assessment

Sole dependence on tests of expiratory airflow for assessing patient response to therapy is unwise, especially because not all patients can perform these maneuvers. Other components of patient assessment useful in evaluating bronchodilator therapy include patient interviewing and observation, measurement of vital signs, auscultation, blood gas analysis, and oximetry.

When possible, the patient should be interviewed to determine the pertinent respiratory history and current level of dyspnea. A validated dyspnea rating scale may be useful for this purpose.[73] Initial determination of patient age and level of consciousness is helpful in selecting both delivery device and starting drug dosage. Observing the patient for signs of increased work of breathing (e.g., tachypnea, accessory muscle use) provides a baseline for assessing status as therapy progresses. Restlessness, diaphoresis, and tachycardia also may indicate severity of airway obstruction but must not be confused with bronchodilator overdose.

In terms of breath sounds, a decrease in wheezing accompanied by an overall decrease in the intensity of breath sounds indicates *worsening* airway obstruction. Improvement is indicated when wheezing decreases and the overall intensity of sounds *increases*.

All patients with acute airway obstruction should be monitored for oxygenation status with pulse oximetry. This value can be used in conjunction with observational assessment to titrate the level of inspired oxygen given to the patient (see Chapter 35). Arterial blood gases are not essential for determining patient response to bronchodilator therapy but may be needed for patients in severe distress to assess for hypercapnic respiratory failure.

Dose-Response Assessment. Poor patient response to bronchodilator therapy often occurs because an inadequate amount of drug dosages reaches the airway. To determine the "best" dosage for patients with moderate obstruction, the respiratory therapist (RT) should conduct a *dose-response titration*.

A simple albuterol dose-response titration involves giving an initial 4 puffs (90 µg/puff) at 1-minute intervals through an MDI with a holding chamber. If after 5 minutes airway obstruction is not relieved, the RT

SELECTION OF AEROSOL DELIVERY DEVICE

AARC Clinical Practice Guideline (Excerpts)*

INDICATIONS

The need to deliver an aerosolized beta-adrenergic, anticholinergic, antiinflammatory, or mucokinetic agent to the lower airway.

CONTRAINDICATIONS

There are no specific contraindications for the administration of aerosols by inhalation. However, there may be contraindications related to the substances being delivered. Consult the package insert for product-specific contraindications.

PRECAUTIONS AND/OR POSSIBLE COMPLICATIONS

- Device malfunction or improper technique may result in underdosing.
- Device malfunction or improper technique (inappropriate patient use) can result in overdosing.
- Complications from a specific pharmacologic agent may occur.
- Cardiotoxic effects of Freon have been reported as an idiosyncratic response to excessive MDI use.
- The detrimental effect of Freon on the ozone layer may affect the environment.
- Repeated exposure to aerosols has been reported to produce asthmatic symptoms in some caregivers.

ASSESSMENT OF NEED

- Based on proven therapeutic efficacy, variety of available medications, and cost-effectiveness, the MDI with an accessory device should be the first choice for aerosol administration to the airway.
- Lack of availability of the prescribed drug in MDI, dry powder, or solution form
- Inability of the patient to use the device properly after coaching and instruction should lead to consideration of other devices.
- Patient preference for a given device that meets therapeutic objectives should be honored.
- When large doses are required, an MDI, SVN, or LVN may be used. Clear superiority of any one method has not been established. Convenience and patient tolerance should be considered.
- When spontaneous ventilation is inadequate, delivery by an intermittent positive pressure breathing (IPPB) device should be considered.

ASSESSMENT OF OUTCOME

- Proper technique is being used.
- Patient response to or compliance with procedure
- Objectively measured improvement (for example, increased %FEV_1 or peak flow)

MONITORING

- Performance of the device
- Technique of device application
- Assessment of patient response, including changes in vital signs

For the complete guideline see Respir Care 39:803, 1994.

gives 1 puff per minute until symptoms are relieved, heart rate increases to more than 20 beats/min, tremors increase, or 12 puffs are delivered. The best dose is that which provides maximum relief of symptoms and the highest PEFR without side effects.

Frequency of Patient Assessment. How frequently patients should undergo assessment for bronchodilator therapy depends primarily on the acuity of the condition. A patient in unstable condition in acute distress should undergo closer and more frequent scrutiny than a patient in stable condition. Box 33-7 provides guidance regarding the frequency of assessment according to acuity.

Patient Education

The desired outcome of all bronchodilator protocols is restoration of normal airflow and cessation of therapy. For patients who need ongoing maintenance therapy after the acute phase of illness, the goal should be effective self-administration. An effective program of aerosol

Assessing Response to Bronchodilator Therapy at Point of Care

AARC Clinical Practice Guideline (Excerpts)*

➤ INDICATIONS

Assessment of airflow and other clinical indicators should be performed when there is a need to:

- Confirm the appropriateness of therapy
- Individualize the patient's medication dose per treatment or frequency of administration
- Determine patient status during acute and long-term pharmacologic therapy
- Change therapeutic dose, frequency, or type of medication

➤ CONTRAINDICATIONS

For patients with acute, severe distress, some assessment maneuvers may be contraindicated or should be postponed until therapy (e.g., bronchodilator treatment) and supportive measures (e.g., oxygen therapy) have been instituted.

➤ HAZARDS AND/OR POSSIBLE COMPLICATIONS

Hazards and complications include those related to the following:

- Deep inhalation and forced exhalation
- Bronchoconstriction
- Airway collapse
- Paroxysmal coughing, with or without syncope
- Specific assessment procedures, such as arterial puncture, esophageal balloons, and forced exhalations

➤ ASSESSMENT OF NEED

- Response to therapy should be evaluated for all patients receiving bronchodilator therapy.
- Patients in severe distress may need immediate treatment, which precludes establishing a quantitative baseline.
- Assessment of patient response must be made with regard for the patient's history, clinical presentation, and results of the physical examination.

➤ ASSESSMENT OF OUTCOME

The following is a guide for determining how assessment affects patient care:

- Action based on the results of assessment, such as an increase or decrease in dosage, change of medication, add medication, continue regimen, or discontinue therapy
- To guide patient management, baseline condition and changes from baseline must be determined.
- Before therapy: establish baseline values, determine the need for therapy, identify contraindications.
- During therapy: identify adverse responses to medication and any clinical change in baseline.
- Following therapy: identify adverse and therapeutic responses (time course for peak varies with different medications).
- For trend analysis: identify change in patient baseline, determine need to modify the dose, change or discontinue therapy, and identify the direction of change in bronchial responsiveness.
- Documentation
  - Patient response to medication
  - Medication type, dose, and time received
  - Measured responses: vital signs, breath sounds, PEFR, FEV_1, $\%FEV_1$, and dyspnea score
  - Observations of time the medication was administered, expected time of onset, and peak response
  - Patient's progress
  - Patient's ability to self-assess, to recognize the need for more aggressive therapy, and to know when and how to communicate with the health professional
  - A record of symptoms and concurrent PEFR measurements should be kept for or by the patient at home.

➤ MONITORING

Monitoring helps establish baseline function and reveals the presence or absence of a desirable response to bronchodilator or other airway medication. It also identifies changes in airway reactivity in response to allergens, exercise, infection, or other causes. Desirable responses are as follows:

- From observation of the patient: general appearance improves, use of accessory muscles decreases, and sputum expectoration increases.

ASSESSING RESPONSE TO BRONCHODILATOR THERAPY AT POINT OF CARE—CONT'D

AARC Clinical Practice Guideline (Excerpts)*

- From auscultation: decreased wheezing and *increased* intensity of breath sounds.
- Vital signs are nearly normal.
- Patient reports improvement.
- From pulmonary function and arterial blood gas analysis:
  - FEV_1, FVC, and $FEF_{25\%-75\%}$ improve (12% increase, calculated from the prebronchodilator response values, *and* a 200-mL increase in either FVC or FEV_1)
  - PEFR increases
  - $Sa{O_2}$ (or $Sp{O_2}$) and arterial blood gas values improve.
- Exercise performance improves, as reflected by a closer to more normal PEFR during or immediately following exercise or an increase in distance achieved during the 6-minute walking test
- Ventilator variables improve: lower peak inspiratory pressure (PIP) during volume ventilation, lower plateau pressure, increased static lung compliance, decreased inspiratory and expiratory resistance, increased expiratory flow, improved flow-volume loop, and decreased auto-PEEP

For the complete guideline, see Respir Care 40:1300, 1995.

Box 33-7 • Frequency of Assessment of Bronchodilator Therapy

For the patient with an acute disorder who is in unstable condition:

- Whenever possible, perform a full assessment and obtain a pretreatment baseline.
- Perform an arterial blood gas analysis if the patient is not responding to bronchodilators and is in severe distress.
- Assess and document all appropriate variables before and after each treatment (breath sounds, vital signs, side effects during therapy, and PEFR or FEV_1).
- The frequency with which physical examination and PEFR or FEV_1 are repeated should be based on the acuteness of the disorder and the severity of the patient's condition.
- $Sp{O_2}$ should be monitored continuously, if possible.
- Assessment should continue as dosages are changed to optimize patient response (e.g., if an asthmatic patient achieves 70% to 90% of predicted or "personal best" or becomes symptom free)

For the stable patient:

- In the hospital, the PEFR should be measured initially before and after each bronchodilator administration. Thereafter, twice daily determinations may be adequate.
- In the home, PEFR should ideally be measured 3 or 4 times a day: on rising, at noon, between 4 PM and 7 PM, and at bedtime.
- For a stable COPD patient at home, measuring PEFR twice a day may be adequate.
- Patients with asthma should adjust the frequency of PEFR measurement according to the severity of symptoms.
- The prebronchodilator and postbronchodilator PEFR levels, medication dosage, date and time, and dyspnea score should be documented.
- The patient should be reevaluated periodically for response to therapy.

Modified from American Association for Respiratory Care: *Respir Care* 40:1300, 1995.

drug self-administration depends on thorough patient education.

The patient's ability to understand the therapy and its goals significantly affects the therapeutic efficacy of any treatment. Whenever possible, patients should be taught to understand the basic administration techniques, to keep track of dosing requirements, to recognize undesirable side effects, and to understand the options and actions required to reduce or eliminate these effects. In addition, patients should be able to demonstrate each technique in aerosol administration that they are expected to perform in self-care. Practitioner demonstration followed by repeated patient demonstration is a must.

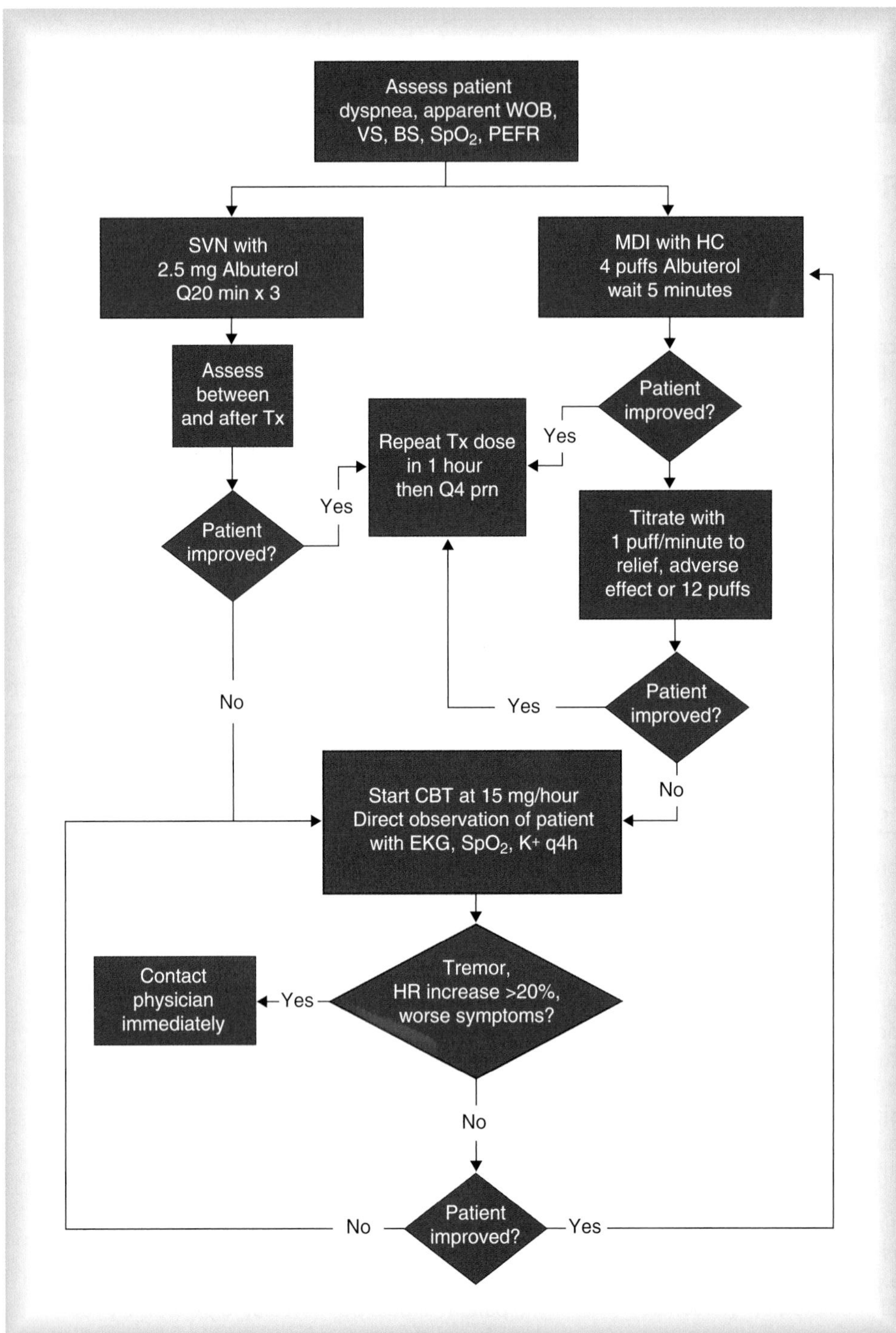

Figure 33-26
Algorithm underlying a bronchodilator therapy protocol for acutely ill adults or children admitted to an emergency department. PEFR, Peak expiratory flow rate; VS, vital signs.

▶ SPECIAL CONSIDERATIONS

Continuous Nebulization for Refractory Bronchospasm

Patients in the emergency department with severe exacerbation of asthma or acute bronchospasm often have been taking standard doses of their bronchodilator before admission without response. Giving nebulizer treatments with standard bronchodilator doses and repeating the treatments until the symptoms are relieved can require hours of staff time. Administering higher doses of albuterol in short time frames can be accomplished by nebulizing undiluted albuterol (8-20 breaths) or by protocol titration with an MDI and holding chamber (up to 12 puffs). If these strategies fail to provide relief, continuous nebulization has proved safe and effective for both adult and pediatric patients.[61,74-81]

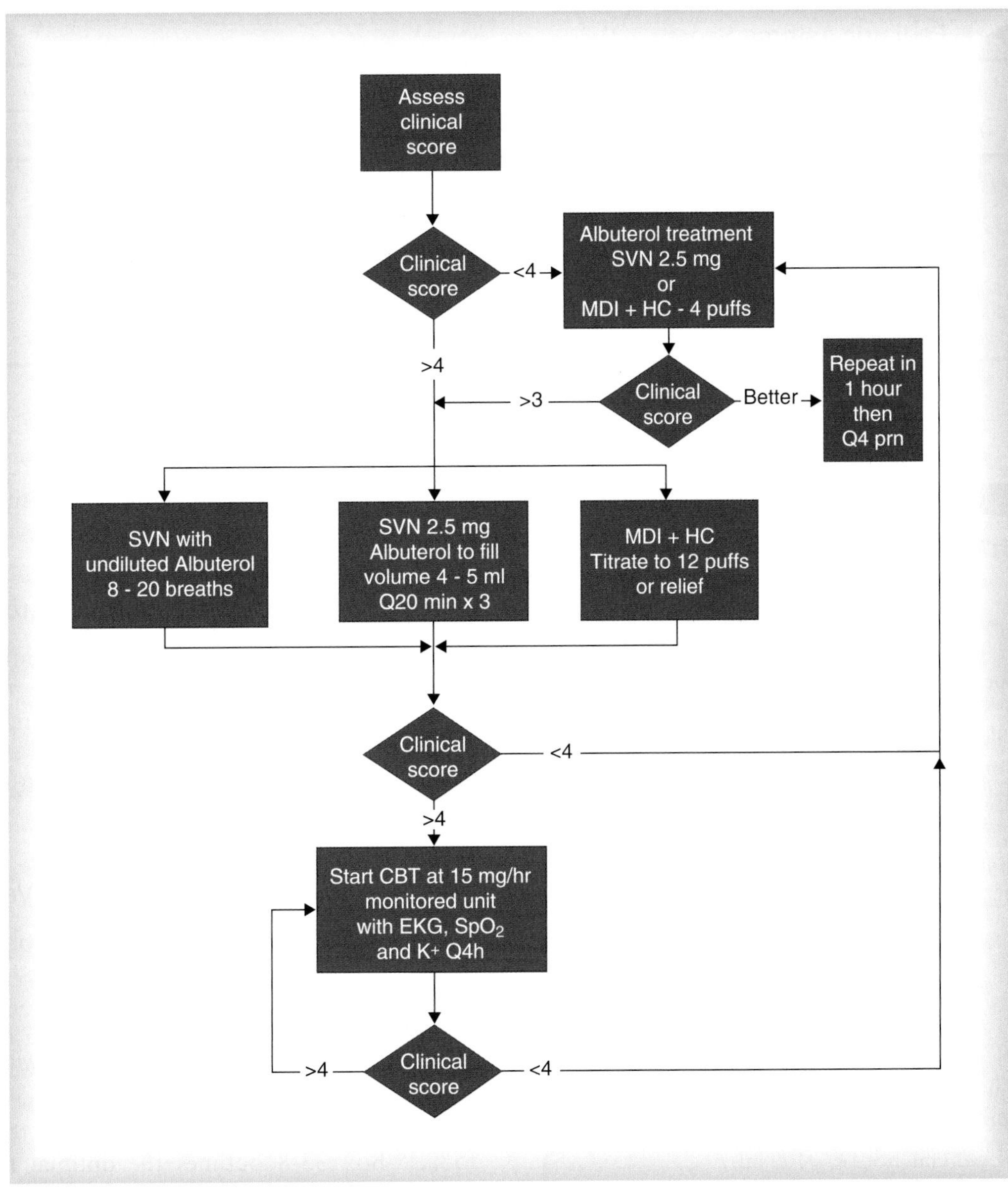

Figure 33-27
Algorithm for CBT for patients younger than 5 years with pediatric asthma in extremis.

Figure 33-27 is a treatment algorithm for high-dose therapy and CBT for pediatric status asthmaticus patients who are unable to perform peak flow maneuvers.[72] Candidates for this protocol are children who, despite frequent β-agonist treatments, remain in extremis with bronchospasm, dyspnea, cough, chest tightness, and diminished breath sounds.

According to this protocol, children older than 6 years with tachypnea, hypoxemia, increased work of breathing, and restlessness who do not respond to standard therapy are given CBT with a large-volume nebulizer or SVN at a dose rate of 15 mg/h (see Mini Clini on p. 794 for dosage computations). A standardized asthma score is used to evaluate children younger than 6 years for the severity of the condition (Table 33-3).[74] Patients with an asthma score of 4 or higher are given CBT.

Once CBT is started, the patient is carefully assessed every 30 minutes for the first 2 hours and thereafter every hour. A positive response is indicated by an increase in PEFR of at least 10% after the first hour of therapy. The goal is at least 50% of the predicted value. For small children, improved oxygenation (oxygen saturation by pulse oximeter [Spo_2] >92% on room air) with evidence of decreased work of breathing indicates a favorable response. Once the patient "opens up," intermittent SVN administration is resumed or an MDI dose-response assessment is conducted.

The patient has responded poorly to CBT if any of

Table 33-3 ▶▶ Pediatric Asthma Score

Indicator	Score 0	1	2
PaO_2	>70 mm Hg (air)	<70 mm Hg (air)	<70 mm Hg (40% O_2)
SpO_2	>94% (air)	<94% (air)	<94% (40% O_2)
Cyanosis	No	Yes	Yes
Breath sounds	Equal	Unequal	Absent
Wheezing	None	Moderate	Marked
Accessory muscles	None	Moderate	Marked
Level of consciousness	Alert	Agitated or depressed	Comatose

Modified from Volpe J: Respir Care Clin N Am 2:117, 1996.

MINI CLINI

CBT Dosage Computations

PROBLEM

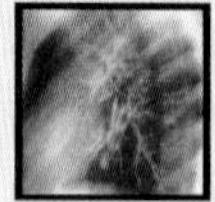

Dosages for CBT are ordered in milligrams per hour, and delivery depends on both drug concentration and nebulizer output. Compute the volume of 1:200 (0.5%) albuterol and the volume of diluent (normal saline solution) needed to provide 4 hours of CBT with 15 mg/h of albuterol in a nebulizer with an output of 25 mL/h.

SOLUTION

Step 1: Compute the volume of albuterol given per hour (mg/h × mL/mg)

15.0 mg/h × 0.2 mL/mg = 3.0 mL/h albuterol

Step 2: Compute the volume of albuterol for the treatment period (hours × mL/h)

4 h × 3.0 mL/h + 12 mL/4 h albuterol

Step 3: Compute the volume of solution nebulized (mL/h nebulizer output × hours)

25 mL/h × 4 h = 100 mL

Step 4: Compute the volume of diluent required

100 mL - 12 mL = 88 mL normal saline solution

To prepare this dosage, mix 12 mL of 0.5% albuterol with 88 mL normal saline solution, for a total nebulizer solution volume of 100 mL. In this example, residual volume of the nebulizer decreases total treatment time and dose.

the indicators listed in Table 33-3 worsens. The patient must be observed for adverse drug responses, including worsening tachycardia, palpitations, and vomiting. In these situations, the attending physician must be contacted immediately.

As an alternative to large-volume drug nebulizers, some protocols are based on high-dose MDI therapy (12-24 puffs per hour).[75] To provide an extra margin of safety, some clinicians recommend that patients receiving CBT undergo continuous electrocardiographic monitoring and measurement of serum potassium level every 4 hours.

Aerosol Administration to Intubated Patients

Many patients undergoing mechanical ventilation receive aerosolized medications, with variable effects. Table 33-4 summarizes the many factors affecting aerosol drug delivery to these patients. The following are techniques to optimize SVN and MDI delivery to patients receiving ventilatory support.

Use of a SVN During Mechanical Ventilation

The aerosol administered by SVN to intubated patients receiving mechanical ventilation tends to be deposited mainly in the tubing of the ventilator circuit. On average, actual pulmonary deposition in these patients ranges between 1.5% and 3.0%.[79,80] When nebulizer output, humidity level, tidal volume, flow, and I:E ratio are optimized, deposition can increase to as much as 15%.[81] Box 33-8 outlines the optimal technique for drug delivery by SVN to intubated patients undergoing mechanical ventilation.

Use of an MDI in the Care of Intubated Patients Underoing Mechanical Ventilation

Results of in vitro studies show effective aerosol delivery by MDIs during mechanical ventilation can range from as little as 2% to as much as 98%. Direct MDI actuation by simple elbow adapters typically results in the least pulmonary deposition, most aerosol impacting in either the ventilator circuit or the tracheal airway. Higher aerosol delivery percentages occur only when a spacer is placed in-line in the ventilator circuit. These spacers allow an aerosol "plume" to develop before the bulk of the particles impact on the surface of the circuit or endotracheal tube. The result is a more stable aerosol mass than can penetrate beyond the artificial airway and be deposited mainly in the lung. This

Table 33-4 ▶ ▶ Factors Affecting Aerosol Drug Delivery During Mechanical Ventilation

Category	Factor
Ventilator-related	Mode of ventilation
	Tidal volume
	Respiratory rate
	Duty cycle
	Inspiratory waveform
	Breath-triggering mechanism
Circuit-related	Size of endotracheal tube
	Type of humidifier
	Relative humidity
	Density and viscosity of inhaled gas
Device-related	
MDI	Type of spacer or adapter used
	Position of spacer in circuit
	Timing of MDI actuation
SVN	Type of nebulizer used
	Fill volume
	Gas flow
	Cycling: inspiration versus continuous
	Duration of nebulization
	Position in circuit
Patient-related	Severity of airway obstruction
	Mechanism of airway obstruction
	Presence of dynamic hyperinflation
	Spontaneous ventilation
	Disease process
Drug-related	Dose
	Aerosol particle size
	Targeted site for delivery
	Duration of action

situation leads to a better clinical response at lower dosages.[82,83] Box 33-9 outlines the optimal technique for drug delivery by MDI to intubated patients undergoing mechanical ventilation.

Regarding dosages, the amount of drug required to achieve the same therapeutic endpoint is substantially larger for medications delivered by MDI to intubated patients than to those who are not intubated.[84] In one study, only 60% of adult patients had *any* significant response to albuterol when given up to 40 puffs.[85] In another study, 4 puffs were shown to produce maximum bronchodilation in stable COPD patients receiving ventilatory support.[86] Differences in response may be due to the level of airway obstruction and the techniques used for assessing response.

Techniques for assessing the response to a bronchodilator in intubated patients undergoing mechanical ventilation differ from those used in the care of spontaneously breathing patients because (1) expiration is passive during mechanical ventilation, (2) forced expiratory values (PEFR, FVC, FEV_1) cannot normally be obtained, (3) a change in the differences between peak and plateau pressures is the most reliable indicator of a change in airway resistance during continuous mecha-

Box 33-8 • Optimal Technique for Drug Delivery by SVN to Intubated Patients Undergoing Mechanical Ventilation

1. Review order, identify patient, and assess need for bronchodilator.
2. Establish dose to compensate for decreased delivery (possibly 2-5 times the normal dose).
3. Place drug in SVN to fill volume of 4-6 mL.
4. Place SVN in the inspiratory line 18 in (46 cm) from the patient wye connector.
5. Turn off flow-by or continuous flow while nebulizing.
6. Remove heat-moisturizer exchanger (HME) from circuit (do not disconnect humidifier).
7. Set gas flow to SVN at 6-8 L/min.
   a. Use a ventilator if it meets the SVN flow needs and cycles on inspiration; otherwise,
   b. Use continuous flow from external source.
8. Adjust ventilator volume or pressure limit to compensate for added flow.
9. Tap SVN periodically until all medication is nebulized.
10. Remove SVN from circuit, rinse with sterile water and run dry, store in safe place.
11. Reconnect humidifier or HME, return ventilator settings and alarms to previous values.
12. Monitor patient for adverse response.
13. Assess outcome and document findings.

Box 33-9 • Optimal Technique for Drug Delivery by MDI to Intubated Patients Undergoing Mechanical Ventilation

1. Review order, identify patient, and assess need for bronchodilator.
2. Establish initial ventilator dose (albuterol 4 puffs).
3. Shake MDI and warm to hand temperature.
4. Place MDI in space chamber adapter in ventilator circuit.
5. Remove heat-moisturizer exchanger (HME). Do not disconnect humidifier.
6. Coordinate firing with beginning of inspiration.
7. Wait at least 15 seconds between actuations; administer total dose.
8. If patient can take a spontaneous breath >500 mL, coordinate firing with breath initiation and encourage 4- to 10-second breath-hold.
9. Monitor for adverse response.
10. Assess response and titrate dosage to achieve desired effect.
11. Reconnect HME.
12. Document clinical outcome.

nical ventilation,[82,83,85,86] (4) automatic positive end-expiratory pressure (auto-PEEP) levels may decrease in response to bronchodilators (see Chapter 41),[87] and (5) breath-to-breath variations make measurements more reliable when the patient is not actively breathing with the ventilator.

▶ CONTROLLING ENVIRONMENTAL CONTAMINATION

Nebulized drugs that escape from the nebulizer into the atmosphere or are exhaled by the patient can be inhaled by anyone in the vicinity of the treatment. Although the risk imposed by this environmental exposure has increased, it remains a subject of controversy. Nonetheless, a variety of techniques are available for protecting patients and caregivers from environmental exposure during aerosol drug therapy. The greatest occupational risk for respiratory care practitioners is believed to be associated with administration of ribavirin and pentamidine. Conjunctivitis, headaches, bronchospasm, shortness of breath, and rashes have been reported among those administering these drugs.[88,89] Patients given aerosolized ribavirin or pentamidine, must be treated in a private room, booth, or tent or at a special station designed to minimize environmental contamination.

Negative-Pressure Rooms

When ribavirin or pentamidine is given, the treatment is provided in a private room. The room should be equipped for negative pressure ventilation with adequate air exchanges (at least 6 per hour) to clear the room of residual aerosols before the next treatment. High-efficiency particulate air (HEPA) filters should be used to filter room or tent exhaust, or the aerosol should be scavenged to the outside.

Booths and Stations

Booths or stations should be used for sputum induction and aerosolized medication treatments given in any area where more than one patient is treated. The area should be designed to provide adequate airflow to draw aerosol and droplet nuclei from the patient into an appropriate filtration system or an exhaust system directly to the outside. Booths and stations should be adequately cleaned between patients.

A variety of booths and specially designed stations are available for delivery of pentamidine or ribavirin. The Emerson containment booth (Figure 33-28) is an example of a system that completely isolates the patient during aerosol administration. All gas is drawn through a prefilter and a HEPA filter. In areas where proper air exchanges do not exist, devices such as the Enviracaire (Figure 33-29) have been used to provide local exhaust ventilation through a HEPA filter medium. Few data exist to support the efficacy of these devices, although they are enjoying increasing popularity in home use.

The AeroStar Aerosol Protection Cart (Respiratory Safety Systems, San Diego, Calif.) is a portable patient isolation station for administration of hazardous aerosolized medication (Figure 33-30). It has been used during sputum induction and for pentamidine treatment. The patient compartment is collapsible with a swing-out counter and three polycarbonate walls. Captured aerosols

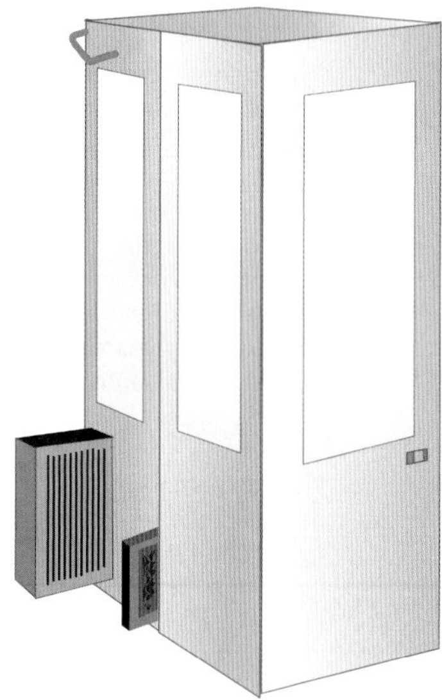

Figure 33-28
Emerson treatment booth provides containment of aerosol during therapy.

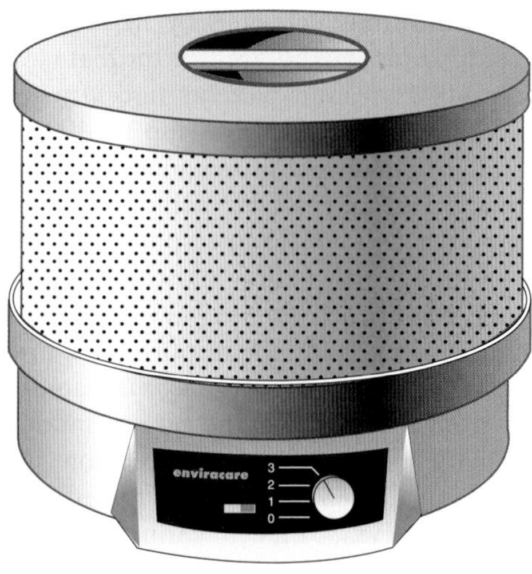

Figure 33-29
Enviracaire room HEPA filter provides local exhaust ventilation.

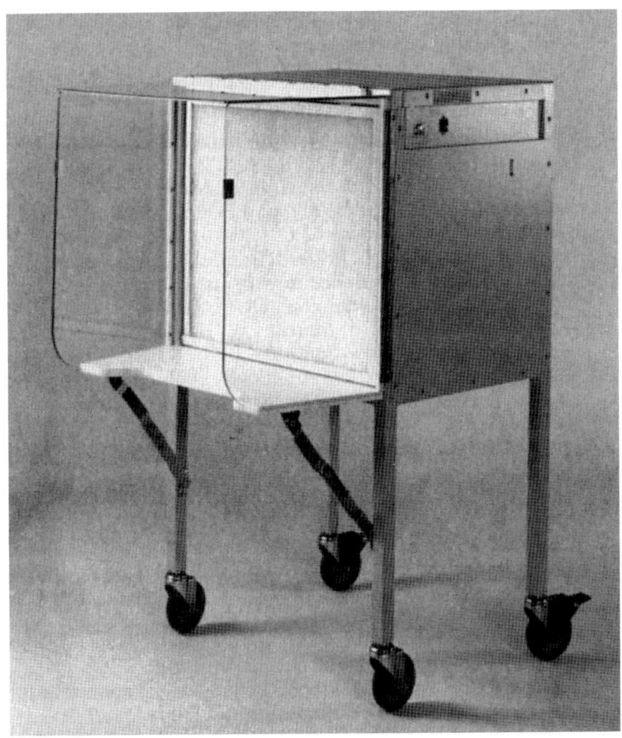

Figure 33-30
BioSafety Systems AeroStar draws gas from the patient through a HEPA filter.

are removed with a HEPA filter. A prefilter is used to retain larger dust particles and to prevent early loading of the more expensive HEPA filter.

Filters and nebulizers used in treatments with pentamidine and ribavirin should be treated as hazardous wastes and disposed of accordingly. Goggles, gloves, and gowns should be used as splatter shields and to reduce exposure to medication residues and body substances. The staff should be screened for adverse effects of exposure to the aerosol medication. The risks and safety procedures should be reviewed regularly.

In addition to the risks associated with administration of aerosol medication, risk of tuberculosis transmission has become a great concern because of an increase in case numbers and the development of multidrug resistant strains of the organism. Tuberculosis is transmitted in the form of droplet nuclei (0.3-0.6 µm) that carry tuberculosis bacilli. Patients with known or suspected tuberculosis need private rooms with negative-pressure ventilation that exhausts to the outside. If environmental isolation is not possible or the healthcare worker must enter the patient's room, personal protective equipment should be used.

Personal Protective Equipment

Personal protective equipment is recommended for caring for any patient with a disease that can be spread by the airborne route.[90-93] The greatest risk is communication of tuberculosis or chickenpox. Although environmental controls should be instituted in the care of these patients, standard and airborne precautions should also be implemented. A variety of masks and respirators have been recommended for use when caring for a patient with tuberculosis or other respiration-transmitted diseases. Traditional surgical masks, particulate respirators, disposable and reusable HEPA filters, and powered air-purifying respirators (PAPR) have been used. No data are available for determining the most effective and most clinically useful device to protect healthcare workers and others, although the U.S. Occupational Safety and Heath Administration requires specific levels of protection (HEPA and PAPRs).

KEY POINTS

- An aerosol is a suspension of solid or liquid particles in gas. In the clinical setting, *therapeutic* aerosols are made with atomizers or nebulizers.
- The general aim of aerosol drug therapy is delivery of a therapeutic dose of the selected agent to the desired site of action.
- Where aerosol particles are deposited in the respiratory tract depends on their size, shape, and motion and on the physical characteristics of the airways. Key mechanisms causing aerosol deposition include inertial impaction, sedimentation, and brownian diffusion.
- For targeting aerosols for delivery to the upper airway (nose, larynx, trachea), particles in the 5- to 20-µm MMAD range are used; for the lower airways, 2- to 5-µm particles; for the lung parenchyma (alveolar region), 1- to 3-µm particles.
- The primary hazard of aerosol drug therapy is an adverse reaction to the medication being administered. Other hazards include infection, airway reactivity, systemic effects of bland aerosols, and drug reconcentration.
- Drug aerosol delivery systems include metered-dose inhalers (MDIs), dry powder inhalers (DPIs), small (SVN)- and large-volume jet nebulizers, ultrasonic nebulizers, and hand-bulb atomizers (nasal spray pumps).

Continued

KEY POINTS—cont'd

- Metered-dose inhalers are the preferred method for maintenance delivery of bronchodilators and steroids to spontaneously breathing patients. Their effectiveness of this therapy is highly technique dependent.
- Accessory devices, spacers, and holding chambers are used with MDIs to reduce oropharyngeal deposition of a drug and to overcome problems with poor hand-breath coordination.
- Effective use of DPIs does not require hand-breath coordination, but it does require high inspiratory flows. Most patients in stable condition prefer DPI delivery systems.
- Compared with MDI and DPI delivery systems, use of a SVN is less technique and device dependent and therefore is the most useful in acute care.
- Large-volume drug nebulizers can be used to provide continuous aerosol delivery when traditional dosing strategies are ineffective in controlling severe bronchospasm.
- Small-volume USNs can be used to administer bronchodilators, antiinflammatory agents, and antibiotics.
- Because patients vary greatly in their response to a particular drug dose and route of administration, aerosol drug therapy should be tailored to each patient with an assessment-based protocol.
- Careful, ongoing patient assessment is the key to an effective bronchodilator therapy protocol. Components of the assessment include patient interviewing and observation, tests of expiratory airflow, measurement of vital signs, auscultation, blood gas analysis, and oximetry.
- Protocols for CBT have proved safe and effective in the management of refractory bronchospasm in both adults and children.
- Many factors decrease the efficiency of aerosol drug delivery during mechanical ventilation. Increased doses, special procedures, and accessory equipment are needed to optimize deposition and achieve the desired clinical outcome.
- A variety of techniques are available for protecting patients and caregivers from environmental exposure during aerosol drug therapy.

References

1. Dolovich MA et al: Consensus statement: aerosols and delivery devices, Respir Care 45:589, 2000.
2. O'Donohue WJ Jr: Guidelines for the use of nebulizers in the home and in domiciliary sites, Chest 109:814, 1996.
3. O'Callaghan C, Barry PW: The science of nebulized drug delivery, Thorax 52(suppl 2):S31, 1997.
4. Heyder J, Gebbart J, Rudolf G, et al: Physical factors determining particle deposition in the human respiratory tract, J Aerosol Sci 11:505, 1980.
5. Newhouse MT, Dolovich M: Aerosol therapy in children. In Chernick V, Mellins RB, editors: Basic mechanisms of pediatric respiratory disease: cellular and integrative, Toronto, 1991, BC Decker.
6. Pierce AK, Sanford JP, Thomas GD, et al: Long-term evaluation of inhalation therapy equipment and the occurrence of necrotizing pneumonia, N Engl J Med 282:528, 1970.
7. Christopher KL, Saravolatz LD, Bush TL, et al: The potential role of respiratory therapy equipment in cross infection: a case study using a canine model for pneumonia, Am Rev Respir Dis 128:271, 1983.
8. Kaan JA, Simoons-Smit AM, MacLaren DM: Another source of aerosol causing nosocomial Legionnaires' disease, J Infect 11:145, 1985.
9. Hamill RJ, Houston ED, Georghiou PR: An outbreak of Burkholderia cepacia respiratory tract colonization and infection associated with nebulized albuterol therapy, Ann Intern Med 122:762, 1995.
10. Wojnarowski C et al: Comparison of bronchial challenge with ultrasonic nebulized distilled water and hypertonic saline in children with mild-to-moderate asthma, Eur Respir J 9:1896, 1996.
11. American Association for Respiratory Care: Clinical practice guideline: selection of aerosol delivery device, Respir Care 37:891, 1992.
12. Stehlin CS, Schare BL: Systemic and pulmonary changes in rabbits exposed to long-term nebulization of various therapeutic agents, Heart Lung 9:311, 1980.
13. Glick RV: Drug reconcentration in aerosol generators, Inhal Ther 15:179, 1970.
14. The Nebuliser Project Group of the British Thoracic Society Standards of Care Committee: Current best practice for nebuliser treatment, Thorax 52(suppl 2):S4, 1997.
15. Newnham DM, Lipworth BJ: Nebulizer performance, pharmacokinetics, airways and systemic effects of salbutamol given by a novel nebulizer system (Ventstream), Thorax 49:762, 1994.
16. Fink JB: Metered-dose inhalers, dry powder inhalers and transitions, Respir Care 45:623, 2000.
17. Lin YZ, Hsieh KH: Metered dose inhaler and nebulizer in acute asthma, Arch Dis Child 72:214, 1995.
18. American Association for Respiratory Care: Aerosol consensus conference statement—1991, Respir Care 36:916, 1991.
19. Dhand R, Malik SK, Balakrishan M, et al: High speed photographic analysis of aerosols produced by metered dose inhalers, J Pharm Pharmacol 40:429, 1988.
20. Kim CS, Trujillo D, Sackner MA: Size aspects of metered-dose inhaler aerosols, Am Rev Respir Dis 132:137, 1985.

21. Moren F: Aerosol dosage forms and formulations. In Moren F, Newhouse MT, Dolovich MB, editors: Aerosols in medicine: principles, diagnosis and therapy, Amsterdam, 1985, Elsevier.
22. Des Jardins T: Freon-propelled bronchodilator use as a potential hazard to asthmatic patients, Respir Care 21:50, 1980.
23. Leach C: Safety assessment of the HFA propellant and the new inhaler, Eur Respir Rev 7:41, 1997.
24. Newman SP: Aerosol generators and delivery systems, Respir Care 36:939, 1991.
25. Newman SP, Pavia D, Moren F, et al: Deposition of pressurized aerosols in the human respiratory tract, Thorax 36:52, 1981.
26. Dolovich M, Ruffin RE, Roberts R, et al: Optimal delivery aerosols from metered dose inhalers, Chest 80(suppl):911, 1981.
27. Larsen JS, Hahn M, Ekholm B, et al: Evaluation of conventional press-and-breathe metered-dose inhaler technique in 501 patients, J Asthma 31:193, 1994.
28. Guidry GG, Brown WD, Stogner SW, et al: Incorrect use of metered dose inhalers by medical personnel, Chest 1010:31, 1992.
29. Newman SP, Pavia D, Clarke SW: Simple instructions for using pressurized aerosol bronchodilators, J Royal Soc Med 73:776, 1980.
30. Rau JL Jr: Respiratory care pharmacology, ed 4, St Louis, 1994, Mosby.
31. De Blaquiere P, Christensen DB, Carter WB, et al: Use and misuse of metered-dose inhalers by patients with chronic lung disease: a controlled randomized trial of two instruction methods, Am Rev Respir Dis 140:910, 1989.
32. Chhabra SK: A comparison of "closed" and "open" mouth techniques of inhalation of a salbutamol metered-dose inhaler, J Asthma 31:123, 1994.
33. Hall SK: Acute angle-closure glaucoma as a complication of combined beta-agonist and ipratropium bromide therapy in the emergency department, Ann Emerg Med 23:884, 1994.
34. Hampson NB, Mueller MP: Reduction in patient timing errors using a breath-activated metered dose inhaler, Chest 106:462, 1994.
35. Terzano C, Mannino F: Probability of particle and salbutamol deposition in the respiratory tract: comparison between MDI and Autohaler, Monaldi Arch Chest Dis 51:236, 1996.
36. Kim CS, Eldridge MA, Sackner MA: Oropharyngeal deposition and delivery aspects of metered-dose inhaler aerosols, Am Rev Respir Dis 135:157, 1987.
37. Wilkes W, Fink J, Dhand R: Selecting an accessory device with a metered-dose inhaler: variable influence of accessory devices on fine particle dose, throat deposition, and drug delivery with asynchronous actuation from a metered-dose inhaler, J Aerosol Med 14:351, 2001.
38. Dolovich M, Ruffin R, Corr D, et al. Clinical evaluation of a simple demand inhalation MDI aerosol delivery device, Chest 84:36, 1983.
39. Salzman GA, Pyszczynski DR: Oropharyngeal candidiasis in patients treated with beclomethasone dipropionate delivered by metered-dose inhaler alone and with Aerochamber, J Allergy Clin Immunol 81:424, 1988.
40. Conner WT, Dolovich MB, Frame RA, et al: Reliable salbutamol administration in 6- to 36-month old children by means of a metered dose inhaler and Aerochamber with mask, Pediatr Pulmonol 6:263, 1989.
41. Dhand R, Fink JB: Dry powder inhalers, Respir Care 44:940, 1999.
42. Pederson S, Hansen OR, Fuglsang G: Influence of inspiratory flowrate upon the effect of a Turbuhaler, Arch Dis Child 65:308, 1990.
43. Pederson S: How to use a Rotohaler, Arch Dis Child 61:11, 1986.
44. Hansen OR, Pederson S: Optimal inhalation technique with terbutaline Turbuhaler, Eur Respir J 2:637, 1989.
45. Pedersen S: Inhalers and nebulizers: which to choose and why, Respir Med 90:69, 1996.
46. Nerbrink O, Dahlback M, Hansson HC: Why do medical nebulizers differ in their output and particle characteristics? J Aerosol Med 7:259, 1994.
47. Dennis JH, Hendrick DJ: Design characteristics for drug nebulizers, J Med Eng Technol 16:63, 1992.
48. Kendrick AH, Smith EC, Denyer J: Nebulizers: fill volume, residual volume and matching of nebulizer to compressor, Respir Med 89:157, 1995.
49. Hess D, Fisher D, Williams P, et al: Medication nebulizer performance: effects of diluent volume, nebulizer flow, and nebulizer brand, Chest 110:498, 1996.
50. Goode ML et al: Improvement in aerosol delivery with helium-oxygen mixtures during mechanical ventilation, Am J Respir Crit Care Med 163:109, 2001.
51. Malone RA et al: Optimal duration of nebulized albuterol therapy, Chest 104:1114, 1993.
52. Phipps PR, Gonda I: Droplets produced by medical nebulisers: effects on particle size and solute concentration, Chest 97:1327, 1990.
53. Nikander K: Drug delivery systems, J Aerosol Med 7(suppl):S19, 1994.
54. Thomas SH, Lanford JA, George RD, et al: Improving the efficiency of drug administration with jet nebulisers, Lancet 1:126, 1988.
55. Rubin BK, Fink JB: Aerosol therapy for children, Respir Care Clin N Am 7:175, 2001.
56. Dolovich MB et al: Pulmonary aerosol deposition in chronic bronchitis: intermittent positive pressure breathing versus quiet breathing, Am Rev Respir Dis 115:397, 1977.
57. Kendrick AH, Smith EC, Wilson RSE: Selecting and using nebuliser equipment, Thorax 52(suppl 2):S92, 1997.
58. Alvine GF, Rodgers P, Fitzsimmons KM, et al: Disposable jet nebulizers: how reliable are they? Chest 101:316, 1992.
59. Zainuddin BM, Tolfree SEJ, Short M, et al: Influence of breathing pattern on lung deposition and bronchodilator response to nebulized salbutamol in patients with stable asthma, Thorax 43:987, 1988.
60. Oie S, Kamiya A: Bacterial contamination of aerosol solutions containing antibiotics, Microbios 82:109, 1995.
61. Colacone A, Wolkove N, Stern E, et al: Continuous nebulization of albuterol (salbutamol) in acute asthma, Chest 97:693, 1990.
62. Demers RR, Parker J, Frankel LR, et al: Administration of ribavirin to neonatal and pediatric patients during mechanical ventilation, Respir Care 31:1188, 1986.

63. Kacmarek RM, Kratohvil J: Evaluation of a double-enclosure double-vacuum unit scavenging system for ribavirin administration, Respir Care 37:37, 1992.
64. Phillips GD, Millard FJL: The therapeutic use of ultrasonic nebulizers in acute asthma, Respir Med 88:387, 1994.
65. Ballard RD, Bogin RM, Pak J: Assessment of bronchodilator response to a beta-adrenergic delivered from an ultrasonic nebulizer, Chest 100:410, 1991.
66. Thomas SH, O'Doherty MJ, Page CJ, et al: Delivery of ultrasonic nebulized aerosols to a lung model during mechanical ventilation, Am Rev Respir Dis 148:872, 1993.
67. American Association for Respiratory Care: Clinical practice guideline: delivery of aerosols to the upper airway, Respir Care 39:803, 1994.
68. Hess D: Aerosol therapy, Respir Care Clin N Am 1:235, 1995.
69. American Association for Respiratory Care: Clinical practice guideline: selection of a device for delivery of aerosol to the lung parenchyma, Respir Care 41:647, 1996.
70. American Association for Respiratory Care: Clinical practice guideline: selection of an aerosol delivery device for neonatal and pediatric patients, Respir Care 40:1325, 1995.
71. National Asthma Education and Prevention Program: Expert panel report II: guidelines for the diagnosis and management of asthma, Bethesda, 1997, National Institutes of Health.
72. Volpe J: Therapist-driven protocols for pediatric patients, Respir Care Clin N Am 2:117, 1996.
73. American Association for Respiratory Care: Clinical practice guideline: assessing response to bronchodilator therapy at point of care, Respir Care 40:1300, 1995.
74. Papo MC, Frank J, Thompson AE: A prospective, randomized study of continuous versus intermittent nebulized albuterol for severe status asthmaticus in children, Crit Care Med 21:1478, 1993.
75. Levitt MA, Gambrioli EF, Fink JB: Comparative trial of continuous nebulization versus metered-dose inhaler in the treatment of acute bronchospasm, Ann Emerg Med 26:273, 1995.
76. Khine H, Fuchs SM, Saville AL: Continuous vs intermittent nebulized albuterol for emergency management of asthma, Acad Emerg Med 3:1019, 1996.
77. Lin RY, Sauter D, Newman T, et al: Continuous versus intermittent albuterol nebulization in the treatment of acute asthma, Ann Emerg Med 22:1847, 1993.
78. Olshaker J, Jerrard D, Barish R, et al: The efficacy and safety of a continuous albuterol protocol for the treatment of acute adult asthma attacks, Am J Emerg Med 11:131, 1993.
79. Dahlback M, Wollmer P, Drefeldt B, et al: Controlled aerosol delivery during mechanical ventilation, J Aerosol Med 4:339, 1989.
80. MacIntyre NR, Silver RM, Miller CW, et al: Aerosol delivery in intubated, mechanically ventilated patients, Crit Care Med 13:81, 1985.
81. O'Riordan TG, Greco MJ, Perry RJ, et al: Nebulizer function during mechanical ventilation, Am Rev Respir Dis 145:1117, 1992.
82. Dhand, R, Jubran A, Tobin MJ: Response to bronchodilator administration by metered dose inhaler in mechanically ventilated patients with COPD, Am Rev Respir Dis 145:A895, 1993 (abstract).
83. Manthous CA, Hall JB, Schmidt Ga, et al: Metered-dose inhaler versus nebulized albuterol in mechanically ventilated patient, Am Rev Respir Dis 148:1567, 1993.
84. Fuller HD, Dolovich MB, Posmituck G, et al: Presurized aerosol versus jet aerosol delivery to mechanically ventilated patients: comparison of dose to the lungs, Am Rev Respir Dis 141:440, 1990.
85. Fink JB, Cohen N, Covington J, et al: Titration for optimal dose response to bronchodilators using MDI and spacer in 120 ventilated adults, Respir Care 36:1321, 1991.
86. Dhand R, Duarte AC, Jubran A, et al: Dose-response to bronchodilator delivered by metered-dose inhaler in ventilator-supported patients, Am J Respir Crit Care Med 154:388, 1996.
87. Leatherman JW: Mechanical ventilation in obstructive lung disease, Clin Chest Med 17:577, 1996.
88. Harrison R: Reproductive risk assessment with occupational exposure to ribavirin aerosol, Pediatr Infect Dis J 9(suppl):S1025, 1990.
89. Oie S, Kamiya A: Exposure to ribavirin aerosol, Appl Occup Environ Hyg 6:271, 1991.
90. Garner JS: Guideline for isolation precautions in hospitals, Infect Control Hosp Epidemiol 17:53, 1996.
91. Centers for Disease Control and Prevention: Guidelines for preventing the transmission of Mycobacterium tuberculosis in health-care facilities, 1994, MMWR Recomm Rep 43(RR-13):1, 1994.
92. Department of Health and Human Services, Department of Labor: Respiratory protective devices: final rule and notice, 60 Federal Register 30336 (1995).
93. ECRI: Tuberculosis, II: respirators and recommendations, Technol Respir Ther 13:14, 1992.

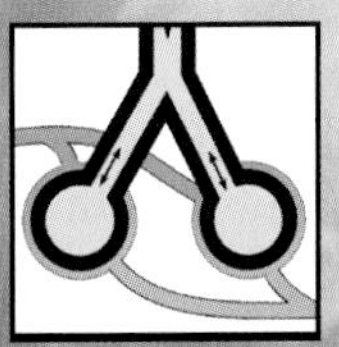

CHAPTER 34

Storage and Delivery of Medical Gases

David L. Vines and Craig L. Scanlan

In This Chapter You Will Learn:

- Which gases and gas mixtures are used clinically and how they are produced
- What differences exist between gaseous and liquid storage methods
- How to determine the contents of liquid and compressed gas cylinders
- How to compute the duration of flow for compressed and liquid gas therapy
- How to properly store, transport, and use compressed gas cylinders
- How to differentiate gas supply systems
- What to do if a bulk oxygen delivery system fails
- What safety systems apply to various equipment connections
- Which device to select to regulate gas pressure and control flow
- How to assemble, check for proper function, and identify malfunctions in gas delivery equipment
- How to correct common malfunctions of gas delivery equipment

Chapter Outline

Key Terms

American standard safety system (ASSS)
Bourdon gauge
cryogenic
diameter-index safety system (DISS)
downstream
flammable
filling density
flowmeter
fractional distillation
heliox
manifold
nonflammable
oxidizing
pin-index safety system (PISS)
psig
reducing valve
regulator
Thorpe tube
upstream
zone valves

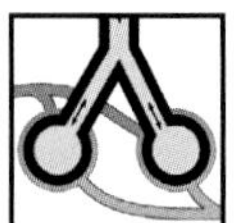

It is from the humble beginning of the hospital "oxygen service" that the present skilled technology of respiratory care evolved. Although respiratory therapists (RTs) have assumed many more challenging duties, ensuring the safe and uninterrupted supply of medical gases is still a key responsibility.

Although there are many commercially produced gases, only a few are used medically (Table 34-1). Medical gases are classified as laboratory gases, therapeutic gases, and anesthetic gases. Laboratory gases are used for equipment calibration and diagnostic testing. Therapeutic gases are used to relieve symptoms and improve patients' oxygenation. Anesthetic gases are combined with oxygen to provide anesthesia during surgery. It is important for RTs to be familiar with all aspects of gases used in the clinical setting, especially the chemical symbols, physical characteristics, ability to support life, and fire risk. In regard to fire risk, medical compressed gases are classified as either **nonflammable** (do not burn), nonflammable but supportive of combustion (also termed **oxidizing**), or **flammable** (burns readily, potentially explosive).[1]

Of the gases listed in Table 34-1, the focus herein is primarily on the therapeutic gases.

▶ CHARACTERISTICS OF MEDICAL GASES

Oxygen (O_2)

Characteristics

Oxygen is a colorless, odorless, transparent, and tasteless gas.[1] It exists naturally as free molecular oxygen and as a component of a host of chemical compounds. Oxygen constitutes almost 50% by weight of the earth's crust and occurs in all living matter in combination with hydrogen as water. At standard temperature, pressure, and dry (STPD), oxygen has a density of 1.429 g/L, being slightly heavier than air (1.29 g/L). Oxygen is not very soluble in water. At room temperature and 1 atm pressure, only 3.3 mL of oxygen dissolves in 100 mL of water. This small amount is sufficient for all aquatic life.

Oxygen is nonflammable, but it greatly accelerates combustion. Burning speed increases with either (1) an increase in oxygen percentage at a fixed total pressure or (2) an increase in total pressure of a constant gas concentration. Thus both oxygen concentration and partial pressure influence the rate of burning.[2]

Production

Oxygen is produced by one of several methods. Chemical methods for producing small quantities of oxygen include electrolysis of water and decomposition of sodium chlorate ($NaClO_3$). Most large quantities of medical oxygen are produced by **fractional distillation** of atmospheric air.[1] Small quantities of concentrated oxygen are produced by physical separation of oxygen from air.

Fractional Distillation. Fractional distillation is the most common and least expensive method for producing oxygen. The process involves several related steps. First, atmospheric air is filtered to remove pollutants, water, and carbon dioxide. The purified air is then liquefied by compression and cooled by rapid expansion (Joule-Thompson effect).

The resulting mixture of liquid oxygen and nitrogen is heated slowly in a distillation tower. Nitrogen, with its boiling point of 195.8° C (320.5° F), escapes first, followed by the trace gases of argon, krypton, and

Table 34-1 ▶▶ Physical Characteristics of Medical Gases

Gas	Chemical Symbol	Color	Taste	Odor	Can Support Life	Flammability
Laboratory Gases						
Nitrogen	N	Colorless	Tasteless	Odorless	No	Nonflammable
Helium	He	Colorless	Tasteless	Odorless	No	Nonflammable
Carbon dioxide	CO_2	Colorless	Slightly acidic	Odorless	No	Nonflammable
Therapeutic Gases						
Air	AIR	Colorless	Tasteless	Odorless	Yes	Supports combustion
Oxygen	O_2	Colorless	Tasteless	Odorless	Yes	Supports combustion
Helium/oxygen (heliox)	He/O_2	Colorless	Tasteless	Odorless	Yes	Supports combustion
Carbon dioxide/oxygen	CO_2/O_2	Colorless	Slightly acidic	Odorless	No	Supports combustion
Nitric oxide	NO	Colorless	Tasteless	Metallic	No	Supports combustion
Anesthetic Gas						
Nitrous oxide	N_2O	Colorless	Tasteless	Slightly sweet	No	Supports combustion

xenon. The remaining liquid oxygen is transferred to specially insulated **cryogenic** (low-temperature) storage cylinders. An alternative procedure is to convert oxygen directly to gas for storage in high-pressure metal cylinders. These methods produce oxygen that is approximately 99.5% pure. The remaining 0.5% is mostly nitrogen and trace argon. United States Food and Drug Administration (FDA) standards require an oxygen purity of at least 99.0%.[3]

Physical Separation. Two methods are used to separate oxygen from air.[4] The first method entails use of molecular "sieves" composed of inorganic sodium aluminum silicate pellets. These pellets absorb nitrogen, "trace" gases, and water vapor from the air, providing a concentrated mixture of more than 90% oxygen for patient use. The second method entails use of a vacuum to pull ambient air through a semipermeable plastic membrane. The membrane allows oxygen and water vapor to pass through at a faster rate than does nitrogen from ambient air. This system can produce an oxygen mixture of approximately 40%. These devices, called *oxygen concentrators*, are used primarily for supplying low-flow oxygen in the home care setting. For this reason, details about the principles of operation and appropriate use are discussed in Chapter 49.

Air

Atmospheric air is a colorless, odorless, naturally occurring gas mixture that consists of 20.95% oxygen, 78.1% nitrogen, and approximately 1% "trace" gases, mainly argon.[1] At STPD, the density of air is 1.29 g/L, which is used as the standard for measuring specific gravity of other gases. Oxygen and nitrogen can be mixed to produce a gas with an oxygen concentration equivalent to that of air.[1] Medical-grade air usually is produced by filtering and compressing atmospheric air.[1,5]

Figure 34-1 shows a typical large medical air compressor system. In these systems an electrical motor is used to power a piston in a compression cylinder. On its downstroke, the piston draws air through a filter system with an inlet valve. On its upstroke, the piston compresses the air in the cylinder (closing the inlet valve) and delivers it through an outlet valve to a reservoir tank. Air from the reservoir tank is reduced to the desired working pressure by a pressure-reducing valve before being delivered to the piping system.

For medical gas use, air must be dry and free of oil or particulate contamination.[5] The most common method used for drying air is cooling to produce condensation. For avoidance of oil or particulate contamination, medical air compressors have air inlet filters and polytetrafluoroethylene (Teflon) piston rings as opposed to oil lubrication. Large medical air compressors must provide high flow (at least 100 L/min) at the standard working pressure of 50 pounds per square inch gauge (**psig**) for all equipment in use.

Smaller compressors (Figure 34-2) are available for bedside or home use. These compressors have a diaphragm or turbine that compresses the air and generally do not have a reservoir. This design limits the pressure and flow capabilities of these devices. For this reason, small

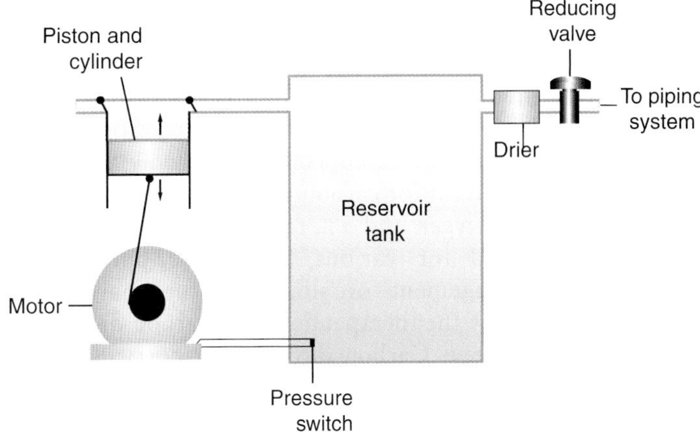

Figure 34-1 · Large Medical Air Compressor

The compressor sends gas to the reservoir at higher than line pressure. When the preset pressure level is reached, the pressure switch shuts off the compressor. Gas leaves the reservoir and passes through the dryer to remove moisture, and the reducing valve reduces gas to the desired line pressure. When reservoir pressure has decreased to near line pressure, the pressure switch turns the compressor back on. *(Modified from McPherson SP, Spearman CB: Respiratory therapy equipment, ed 5, St Louis, 1995, Mosby.)*

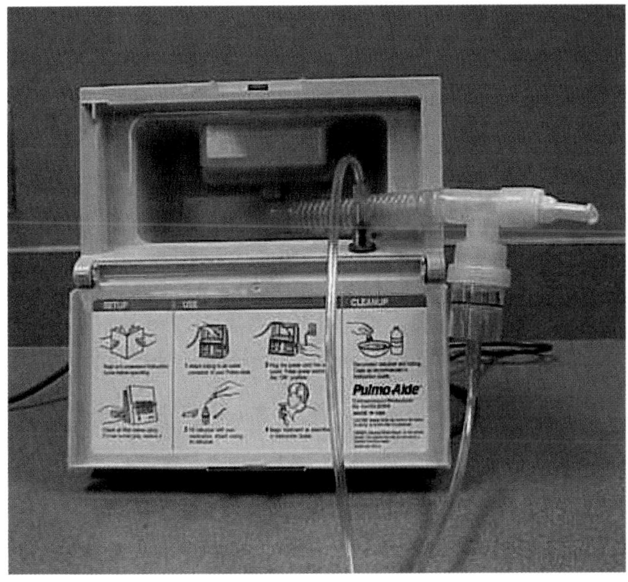

Figure 34-2

Small portable compressor used with a handheld nebulizer to aerosolize medication.

compressors must never be used to power equipment that needs unrestricted flow at 50 psig, such as pneumatically powered ventilators (see Chapter 39). However, small diaphragm or turbine compressors are ideal for powering devices such as small-volume medication nebulizers (see Chapter 33).

Carbon Dioxide (CO_2)

At STPD, carbon dioxide is a colorless and odorless gas with a specific gravity of 1.52 (approximately 1.5 times heavier than air).[1] Carbon dioxide does not support combustion or maintain animal life. For medical use, carbon dioxide usually is produced by heating limestone in contact with water. The gas is recovered from this process and liquefied by compression and cooling.[1] The FDA purity standard for carbon dioxide is 99.0%.[3]

Mixtures of oxygen and 5% to 10% carbon dioxide once were used for various therapeutic purposes, including management of singultus (hiccups) and atelectasis. Today the therapeutic use of carbon dioxide mixtures is limited. Carbon dioxide mixtures still are used in membrane oxygenators (heart-lung machines) and for calibration of blood gas analyzers (see Chapter 16). In addition, CO_2/O_2 mixtures have been used to regulate pulmonary vascular pressures in some congenital heart disorders. However, most medical carbon dioxide is used for diagnostic purposes in the clinical laboratory.

Helium (He)

Helium is second only to hydrogen as the lightest of all gases; it has a density at STPD of 0.1785 g/L. Helium is odorless, tasteless, and nonflammable.[1] It is a good conductor of heat, sound, and electricity but is poorly soluble in water. Although present in small quantities in the atmosphere, helium is commercially produced from natural gas by liquefaction to purity standards of at least 99%.[3]

Being both chemically and physiologically inert, helium cannot support life. Thus breathing 100% helium would cause suffocation and death. For therapeutic use, helium must always be mixed with at least 20% oxygen. Some clinical centers use **heliox** to manage severe cases of large airway obstruction. In these cases, the low density of helium decreases the work of breathing.

> **RULE OF THUMB**
>
> Helium must always be combined with at least 20% oxygen. The higher the concentration of oxygen used in a heliox mixture, the less likely it is that heliox will be beneficial. Rarely are heliox mixtures of less than 60% helium used clinically.

Nitrous Oxide (N_2O)

Nitrous oxide is a colorless gas with a slightly sweet odor and taste that is used clinically as an anesthetic agent.[1] Like oxygen, nitrous oxide can support combustion. However, nitrous oxide cannot support life and causes death if inhaled in pure form. For this reason, inhaled nitrous oxide must always be mixed with at least 20% oxygen. Nitrous oxide is produced by thermal decomposition of ammonium nitrate.[1]

The use of nitrous oxide as an anesthetic agent is based on its central nervous system depressant effect. However, only dangerously high levels of N_2O provide true anesthesia. This is why N_2O/O_2 mixtures almost are always used in combination with other anesthetic agents.

Long-term human exposure to nitrous oxide has been associated with a form of neuropathy. In addition, epidemiological studies have linked chronic nitrous oxide exposure with an increased risk of fetal disorders and spontaneous abortion.[1] On the basis of this knowledge, the National Institute for Occupational Safety and Health (a division of the Occupational Safety and Health Administration) has set an upper exposure limit for hospital operating rooms of 25 ppm nitrous oxide.[1]

Nitric Oxide (NO)

Nitric oxide is a colorless, nonflammable, toxic gas that supports combustion. Nitric oxide is produced by oxidation of ammonia at high temperatures in the presence of a catalyst.[1] In combination with air, nitric oxide forms brown fumes of nitrogen dioxide (NO_2). Together nitric oxide and nitrogen dioxide are strong respiratory irritants that can cause chemical pneumonitis and a fatal form of pulmonary edema. Exposure to high concentrations of nitric oxide alone can cause methemoglobinemia (see Chapter 10). High levels of methemoglobin can cause tissue hypoxia.

Nitric oxide is FDA approved for use in the treatment of term and near-term infants for hypoxic respiratory failure. The American Academy of Pediatrics (AAP) has published a policy statement recommending the use of nitric oxide in the care of term and near-term infants when mechanical ventilation is failing because of hypoxic respiratory failure. The AAP suggests that nitric oxide be used before extracorporeal membrane oxygenation.[6] Additional randomized, controlled studies of the treatment of premature neonates with hypoxic respiratory failure are needed before recommendations can be made for nitric oxide treatment of this patient population.[7] In children and adults with acute hypoxemic respiratory failure, inhalation of nitric oxide has led to transient improvement in arterial oxygenation, but the mortality has not changed in these patient populations.[8]

▶ STORAGE OF MEDICAL GASES

Medical gases are stored either in portable high-pressure cylinders or in large bulk reservoirs. Bulk reservoirs require a separate distribution system to deliver the gas to the patient.

Gas Cylinders

The containers used to store and ship compressed or liquid medical gases are high-pressure cylinders. The design, manufacture, transport, and use of these cylinders are carefully controlled by both industrial standards and federal regulations. Gas cylinders are made of seamless steel and are classified by the federal Department of Transportation (DOT) according to their fabrication method. Department of Transportation type 3A cylinders are made from carbon steel, and DOT type 3AA containers are manufactured with a steel alloy tempered for higher strength.[1]

Markings and Identification

Medical gas cylinders are marked with metal stamping on the shoulders that supplies specific information (Figure 34-3).[1,9] Although the exact location and order of these markings vary, the practitioner should be able to identify several key items of information.

The letters DOT or ICC (Interstate Commerce Commission) are followed by the cylinder classification (3A or 3AA) and the normal filling pressure in pounds per square inch (psi). Below this information usually is the letter size of the cylinder (E, G, and so on) followed by the cylinder serial number. A third line provides a mark of ownership, often followed by the manufacturer's stamp or a mark identifying the inspecting authority. On the opposite side of the cylinder usually is an abbreviation indicating the method of cylinder manufacture. Also in this area is information about the original safety test and dates of all subsequent tests.

Safety tests are conducted every 5 or 10 years, as specified in DOT regulations.[1,9] During these tests, cylinders are pressurized to five thirds of their service pressure. While the cylinder is under pressure, technicians measure cylinder leakage, expansion, and wall stress. The notation "EE" followed by a number indicates the elastic expansion of the cylinder in cubic centimeters under the test conditions. An asterisk (*) next to the test date indicates DOT approval for 10-year testing. A plus sign (+) means the cylinder is approved for filling to 10% above its service pressure. For example, an approved cylinder with a service pressure of 2015 psi can be filled to approximately 2200 psi. After hydrostatic testing, cylinders are subjected to internal inspection and cleaning.

In addition to these permanent marks, all cylinders are color coded and labeled for identification of their

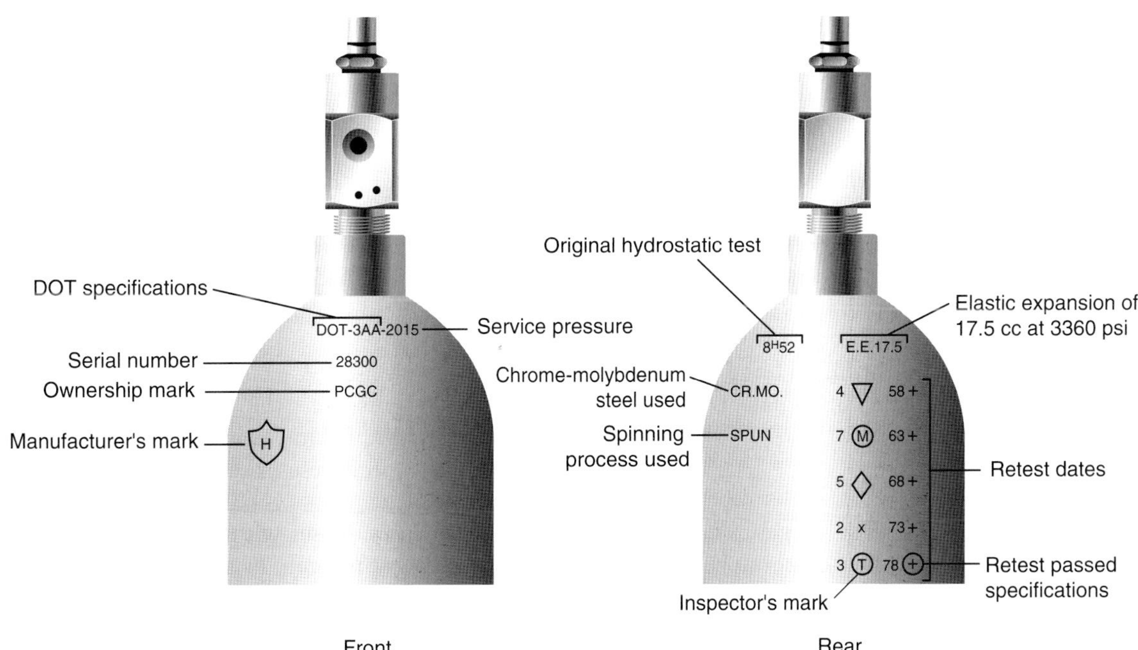

Figure 34-3
Typical markings of cylinders containing medical gases. Front and back views are for illustration purposes only; exact location and order of markings vary.

Table 34-2 ▶ ▶ Color Codes for Medical Gas Cylinders

Gas	United States	Canada
Oxygen	Green	White*
Carbon dioxide	Gray	Gray
Nitrous oxide	Blue	Blue
Cyclopropane	Orange	Orange
Helium	Brown	Brown
Ethylene	Red	Red
Carbon dioxide–oxygen	Gray/green	Gray/white
Helium-oxygen	Brown/green	Brown/white
Nitrogen	Black	Black
Air	Yellow*	Black/white
Nitrogen-oxygen	Black/green	Pink

*Vacuum systems historically are identified as white in the United States and yellow in Canada. For this reason, the Compressed Gas Association (CGA) recommends that white not be used for any cylinders in the United States or that yellow be used in Canada.

contents.[1,10] Table 34-2 lists the color codes for medical gases as adopted by the Bureau of Standards of the U.S. Department of Commerce.[11] For comparison, the color codes adopted by the Canadian Standards Association also are included. Color codes are not standardized internationally. For this reason, cylinder color should be used only as a guide. As with any drug agent, the cylinder contents always must be identified through carefully inspection of the label. To be absolutely sure about the oxygen concentration provided by a cylinder, the user must analyze the gas before administering it (see Chapter 16).[12]

Cylinder Sizes and Contents

Letter designations are used for different sizes of cylinders (Figure 34-4). Table 34-3 is a list of the most common cylinder sizes and contents for therapy gases.

Sizes E through AA are referred to as "small cylinders" and are used most often for transporting patient and anesthetic gases. These small cylinders are easily identified because of their unique valves and connecting mechanisms. Small cylinders have a post valve and yoke connector. Large cylinders (F through H and K) have a threaded valve outlet (Figure 34-5) (see later).

Cylinder Safety Relief Valves

In a closed cylinder, any increase in gas temperature increases gas pressure. Should the temperature increase too much (as in a fire), the high gas pressure could rupture and explode the cylinder. To prevent this type of accident, all cylinders have high-pressure relief valves. These relief valves are of three basic designs: frangible disk, fusible plug, and spring loaded. The frangible metal disk ruptures at a specific pressure. The fusible

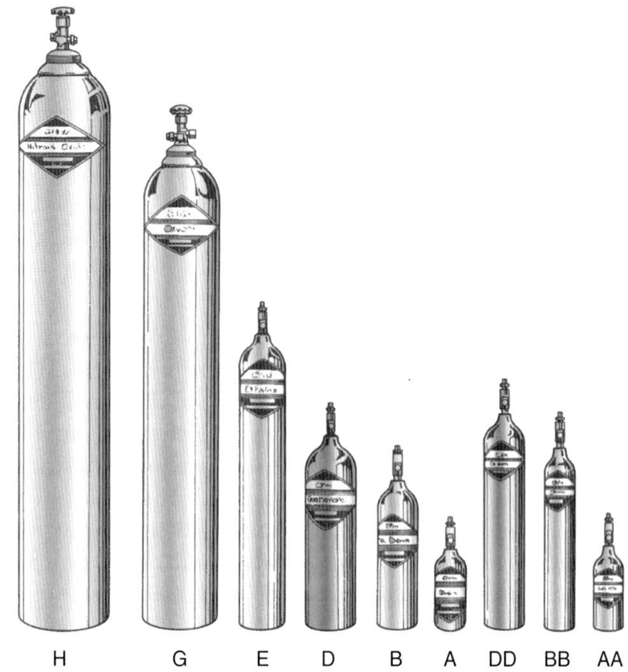

Figure 34-4
Cylinder sizes are identified by letter designations.

plug melts at a specific temperature. The spring-loaded valve opens and vents gas at a set high pressure. In each case, the activated valve vents gas from the cylinder and prevents pressure from becoming too high.

Most small cylinders have a fusible plug relief valve. Most large cylinders have a spring-loaded relief valve. These safety relief valves are always located in the cylinder valve stems.

Filling (Charging) Cylinders

How a cylinder is filled depends on whether its contents will be gaseous or liquid. Among gases stored in liquid form, some can remain at room temperature, but others must be maintained in a cryogenic (low-temperature) state. Cryogenic storage is discussed later.

Compressed Gases. A gas cylinder normally is filled to its service pressure (the pressure stamped on the shoulder) at 70° F. However, approved cylinders can be filled to 10% in excess of service pressure.

Liquefied Gases. Gases with critical temperatures above room temperature can be stored as liquids at room temperature (see Chapter 5). These gases include carbon dioxide and nitrous oxide. Rather than being filled to filling pressure, cylinders of these gases are filled according to a specified **filling density.** The filling density is the ratio between the weight of liquid gas put into the cylinder and the weight of water the cylinder could

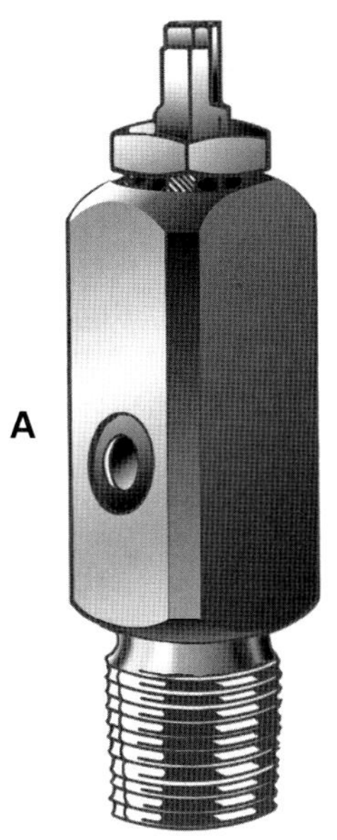

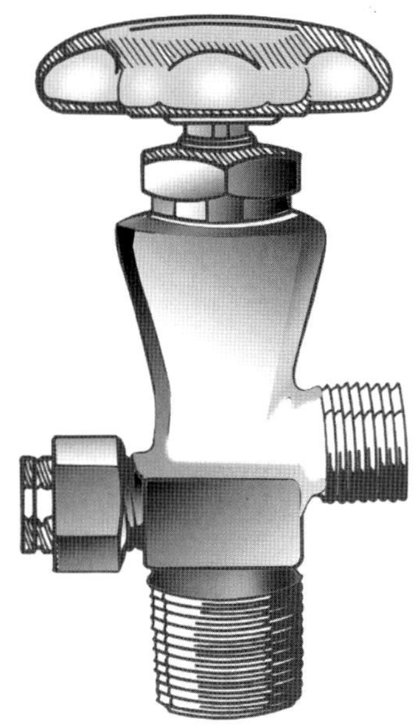

Figure 34-5
A, Post valve for yoke connector used with small cylinders (E-AA). **B,** Large, threaded valve outlet used with large cylinders (H/K, G, M).

Table 34-3 ▶▶ Common Cylinder Sizes and Gases Used in Respiratory Therapy

		Gas (cylinder pressure at 21.11° C [70° F] psig])					
Cylinder Size	**Weight and Volume**	**Carbon Dioxide (840)**	**Helium (1650-2000)**	**Nitrous Oxide (745)**	**Oxygen (1800-2400)**	**Helium-Oxygen Mixtures (1650-2000)**	**Carbon Dioxide Mixtures (1500-2200)**
D	Content weight (lb)	4.0	0.1	4.0	1.0	—	—
	Gas volume at 21.11° C (70° F) and 14.7 psia						
	Cubic feet	33.0	10.6	34.5	12.6	11.0	12.6
	Liters	934.0	300.0	975.0	356.0	310.0	356.0
E	Content weight (lb)	6.6	0.2	6.6	2.0	—	—
	Gas volume at 21.11° C (70° F) and 14.7 psia						
	Cubic feet	56.0	17.0	57.0	22.0	18.0	22.0
	Liters	1585.0	480.0	1610.0	622.0	510.0	622.0
G	Content weight (lb)	50.0	1.5	56.0	16.0	—	—
	Gas volume at 21.11° C (70° F) and 14.7 psia						
	Cubic feet	425.0	146.0	485.0	186.0	150.0	186.0
	Liters	12,000.0	4130.0	13,750.0	5260.0	4250.0	5260.0
H/K	Content weight (lb)	—	—	64.0	20.0	—	—
	Gas volume at 21.11° C (70° F) and 14.7 psia						
	Cubic feet	—	—	557.0	244.0	—	—
	Liters	—	—	15,800.0	6900.0	—	—

From the Standard for Nonflammable Medical Gas Systems (NFPA 56 F), 1973, copyright National Fire Protection Association, Boston, MA.
psig, Pounds per square inch gauge; *psia,* pounds per square inch absolute.

contain if full. For example, the filling density for carbon dioxide is 68%. This system allows the manufacturer to fill a cylinder with liquid carbon dioxide up to 68% of the weight of water that a full cylinder could hold. The filling density of nitrous oxide is 55%.

Cylinder pressures for gases stored in the liquid phase are much lower than for those stored in the gas phase. Because the liquid does not fill the entire volume of a cylinder, the space above the liquid surface contains gas in equilibrium with the liquid. The pressure in a liquid-filled cylinder thus equals the pressure of the vapor at any given temperature.

Pressure in a cylinder depends on the state of its contents. In a gas-filled cylinder, the pressure represents the force required to compress the gas into its smaller volume. In contrast, the pressure in a liquid-filled cylinder is the vapor pressure needed to keep the gas liquefied at the current temperature.

Measuring Cylinder Contents

Because of the previously described differences in the physical state of matter of compressed and liquid gases, different methods are needed to measure the contents of the cylinder.

Compressed Gas Cylinders. For gas-filled cylinders, the volume of gas in the cylinder is directly proportional to its pressure at a constant temperature. If a cylinder is full at 2200 psig, it will be half full when the pressure decreases to 1100 psig. To know how much gas is contained in a compressed gas cylinder, one needs only measure its pressure.

Liquid Gas Cylinders. In a liquid gas cylinder or container, the measured pressure is the vapor pressure above the liquid. This pressure bears no relation to the amount of liquid remaining in the cylinder. As long as some liquid remains (and the temperature remains constant), the vapor pressure and thus the gauge pressure remain constant. When all the liquid is gone and the cylinder contains only gas, the pressure decreases in proportion to a reduction in volume. Monitoring the gauge pressure of liquid gas cylinders is useful only after all the liquid vaporizes. Weighing a liquid-filled cylinder is the only accurate method for determining the contents.

Figure 34-6 compares the behavior of compressed gas and liquid gas cylinders during use. The vapor pressure of liquid gas cylinders varies with the temperature of the contents. For example, the pressure in a nitrous oxide cylinder at 70° F is 745 psig; at 60° F, the pressure decreases to 660 psig. As the temperature increases toward the critical point, more liquid vaporizes, and the cylinder pressure increases. Should a cylinder of nitrous oxide warm to 97.5° F (its critical temperature), all the contents would convert to gas. Only at this temperature and above does the cylinder gauge pressure accurately reflect cylinder contents.

Estimating the Duration of Cylinder Gas Flow

When a cylinder of therapeutic gas is used, it often is necessary to predict how long the contents will last at a given flow. The duration of flow of a cylinder can be estimated if the following are known: (1) the gas flow, (2) the cylinder size, and (3) the cylinder pressure at the start of therapy. For a given flow, the more gas a cylinder holds, the longer it will last. Conversely, the higher the flow, the shorter is the emptying time. The

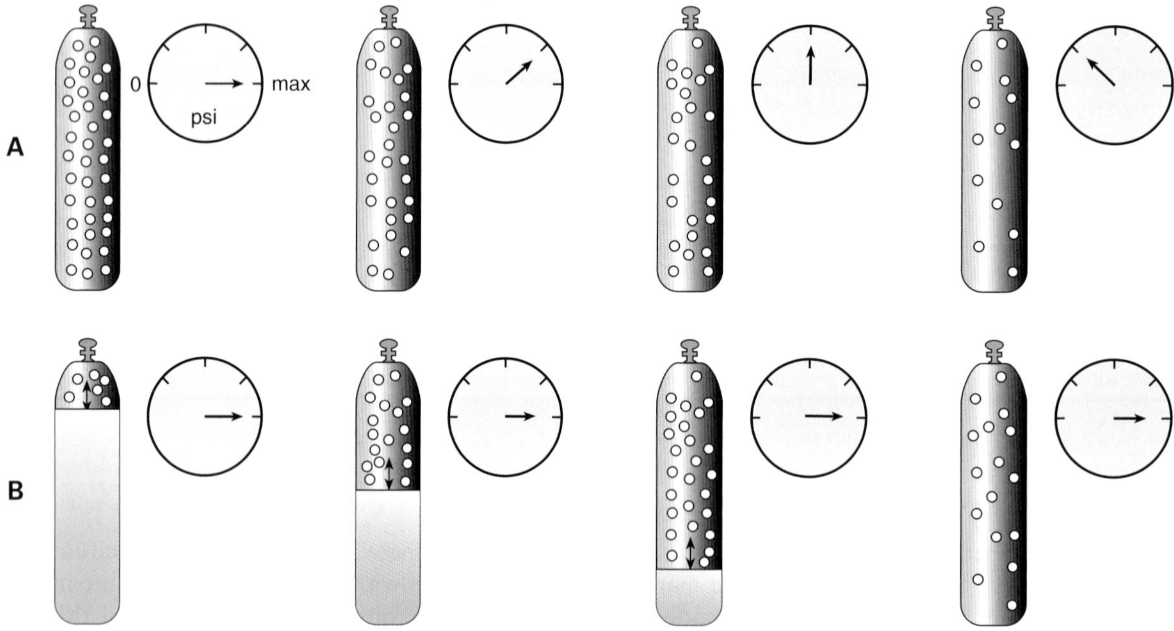

Figure 34-6

The content of a gas-filled cylinder **(A)** is directly proportional to the gas pressure. For example, a pressure decrease of 50% indicates a loss of 50% of the contained gas. In a liquid-gas cylinder **(B)** gauge pressure is a measure of only the vapor pressure of gas in equilibrium with the liquid phase. This value remains constant at a given temperature as long as liquid is present. Only when all the liquid has vaporized, as the cylinder nears depletion, does the gauge pressure decrease proportionately to the terminal volume of remaining gas.

Table 34-4 ▶ ▶ Gas Volume Conversion Factors

Liters	Cubic Feet	Gallons
28.316	1	7.481
1	0.03531	0.2642
3.785	0.1337	1

duration of flow of a cylinder is directly proportional to the contents and inversely proportional to flow, as expressed in the following formula:

$$\text{Duration of flow} = \frac{\text{Contents}}{\text{Flow}}$$

Unfortunately, the units commonly used in the United States for measurement of these quantities are not the same. Cylinder contents are generally specified in cubic feet or gallons, whereas gas flow normally is measured in liters. Table 34-4 provides the factors needed to convert these units.

Rather than memorizing various cylinder contents and constantly converting metric and English units, the user can quickly calculate duration of flow by using cylinder factors. Cylinder factors are derived for each common gas and cylinder size with the following formula:

$$\text{Cylinder factor (L/psig)} = \frac{\text{Cubic feet (full cylinder)} \times 28.3}{\text{Pressure (full cylinder) in psig}}$$

In the numerator of the equation, the English-metric conversion constant (28.3) is used to convert cubic feet to liters. Dividing the resulting volume by the pressure in a full cylinder yields the cylinder factor. The derived factor represents the volume of gas leaving a given cylinder for every 1 psig decrease in pressure. Table 34-5 provides cylinder factors for the therapeutic medical gases and common cylinder sizes.

Once the factors for a given gas and cylinder are known, calculating the duration of flow is a simple matter of applying the following equation:

$$\text{Duration of flow (min)} = \frac{\text{Pressure (psig)} \times \text{Cylinder factor}}{\text{Flow (L/min)}}$$

Table 34-5 ▶ ▶ Factors for Calculation of Cylinder Duration of Flow (minutes)

	Cylinder Size			
Gas	D	E	G	H and K
O_2, O_2/N_2, air	0.16	0.28	2.41	3.14
O_2/CO_2	0.20	0.35	2.94	3.84
He/O_2	0.14	0.23	1.93	2.50

A wide margin of safety must be allowed in estimation of cylinder duration of flow. This principle is especially important if the therapist cannot be present during use and must return with a full cylinder. For example, some clinicians always return 30 to 40 minutes before the calculated time; others compute duration of flow to a level of 300 to 500 psig rather than 0 psig (empty). Assuming the calculations are correct and there is no change in flow, both these methods ensure an uninterrupted supply. The following Rule of Thumb is a shortcut for estimating cylinder duration of flow.

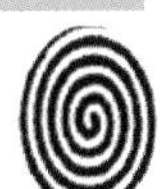

RULE OF THUMB

A full E oxygen cylinder running at 10 L/min lasts approximately 60 minutes (1 h). A full H/K cylinder lasts at least 10 times longer (more than 10 h). Use these two simple rules to estimate flow duration. For example, a half-full E oxygen cylinder running at 10 L/min lasts approximately 30 minutes, whereas a full H cylinder running at 5 L/min last more than 20 hours.

Estimating the Duration of a Liquid Oxygen Cylinder Gas Flow

The only accurate method for determining the volume of gas in a liquid-filled cylinder is by weight. Because 1 L of liquid oxygen weighs 2.5 lb and produces 860 L of oxygen in its gaseous state, the amount of gas in a liquid oxygen cylinder can be calculated with the following formula:

$$\text{Amount of gas in cylinder} = \frac{\text{Liquid } O_2 \text{ weight (lb)} \times 860}{2.5 \text{ lb/L}}$$

MINI CLINI

Computing Cylinder Duration of Flow

PROBLEM

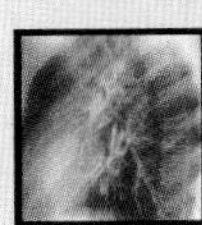

You need to determine how long a G cylinder of oxygen with a gauge pressure of 800 psi set to deliver 8 L/min will last until empty.

SOLUTION

Step 1: Determine the cylinder factor for an oxygen G cylinder (Table 34-5), in this case 2.41.

Step 2: Apply the duration of flow equation:

$$\text{Duration of flow (min)} = \frac{\text{Pressure (psig)} \times \text{Cylinder factor}}{\text{Flow (L/min)}}$$

$$\text{Duration of flow (min)} = \frac{800 \times 2.41}{8} = 241 \text{ minutes (approximately 4 h)}$$

After the amount of oxygen remaining in the cylinder is determined, the duration of the gas in minutes can be calculated with the following formula:

$$\text{Duration of gas (min)} = \frac{\text{Amount of gas in cylinder (L)}}{\text{Flow (L/min)}}$$

As with gaseous oxygen cylinders, a wide margin of safety is needed for estimation of cylinder duration. This margin of safety varies with the size of the portable oxygen unit or large storage container.

Gas Cylinder Safety

The following guidelines for cylinder safety are from the current recommendations of the National Fire Protection Agency (NFPA)[2] and the Compressed Gas Association (CGA).[1] For ease of use, these safety guidelines are divided into cylinder storage, transport, and use.

Cylinder Storage. The following guidelines apply to cylinder storage:

- Store gas cylinders in racks or chain cylinders to the wall to prevent them from falling or becoming damaged.
- Other than the wooden racks used to store the cylinders, store no other combustible material in the vicinity of cylinders or gas supply systems.
- Store gas cylinders away from sources of heat. Keep the cylinder temperature below 125° F (51.7° C).

> MINI CLINI
>
> ### Computing the Duration of a Liquid Oxygen Container
>
> **PROBLEM**
>
> 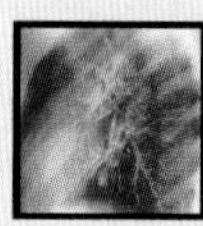
>
> You need to estimate how long Mrs. Jones's portable liquid oxygen container will last if it contains 3 lb of liquid oxygen that supplies an oxygen delivery device running at 2 L/min.
>
> **SOLUTION**
>
> Step 1: Determine the amount of oxygen in the cylinder.
>
> $$\text{Amount of gas in cylinder} = \frac{\text{Liquid } O_2 \text{ weight (lb)} \times 860}{2.5 \text{ lb/L}} = \frac{3 \times 860}{2.5} = 1032 \text{ L}$$
>
> Step 2: Calculate the duration of the gas in the container.
>
> $$\text{Duration of the gas} = \frac{\text{Amount of gas in the cylinder (L)}}{\text{Flow (L/min)}} = \frac{1032 \text{ L}}{2} = 516 \text{ minutes} = 8 \text{ hours and } 36 \text{ minutes}$$

- Store flammable gases separately from gases that support combustion, such as air, oxygen, and nitrous oxide.
- If a cylinder is not in use, keep the protective cylinder cap in place.
- Do not store air compressors and gas cylinders together. A fire involving one or the other can damage both gas delivery systems.
- Contain and store cylinder supply systems in an enclosure constructed of a material with at least a 1-hour fire resistive rating that is well ventilated and well drained.
- Segregate full and empty cylinders; store them separately if possible.
- Place on each door or gate of the enclosure a sign that cautions the presence of an oxidizing gas and alerts against smoking. This sign must be readable from a distance of at least 5 feet (1.5 m).
- Store liquid oxygen containers in a cool, well-ventilated area because of the venting of small amounts of oxygen from these low-pressure containers. The venting of oxygen prevents these containers from over-pressurizing, because liquid oxygen is continuously converting to gaseous oxygen.

Cylinder Transport. The following guidelines apply to cylinder transport:

- Use cylinder carts with a securing mechanism for transportation of cylinders.
- Keep the protective cylinder caps in place in transportation of cylinders.
- Protect gas cylinders from striking other cylinders or objects to avoid damaging the safety devices, valve stems, or the cylinder itself.
- Avoid dropping, dragging, or rolling cylinders in transport.
- Do not transport cylinders for use that are not appropriately labeled.

Cylinder Use. The following guidelines apply to cylinder use.

- Secure gas cylinders at the patient's bedside in a way that prevents them from falling. Secure cylinders to the wall with a chain, bind or chain them to a suitable cart, or support the cylinder with a stand.
- Do not use flammable materials, especially oil or grease, on regulators, cylinders, fittings, or valves. This restriction includes oily hands, rags, and gloves.
- Never cover a cylinder with any material, including bed linens or hospital gowns.
- Open the cylinder valve slightly to remove dust and dirt before attaching the regulator. When slightly opening the valve, make sure no one is in front of

the valve. "Crack" the cylinder before bringing it to the patient's bedside.

- Never use cylinder valves or regulators that need repair.
- Do not alter or deface cylinder markings or color.
- Never place cylinders near sources of heat.
- Never secure cylinders to movable objects unless the object has an apparatus that can contain the cylinder safely.
- Make sure that the connection between the regulator and the cylinder valve is an American standard safety system (ASSS) for H and G cylinders and a pin-index safety system (PISS) for E cylinders.
- When oxygen is in use, post a no smoking sign unless signs in the entrances are posted prohibiting smoking in the facility.

Bulk Oxygen

Large acute care facilities use huge volumes of oxygen every day. To meet these needs, a centralized bulk storage and delivery system is required. By definition, these bulk oxygen storage systems hold at least 20,000 cubic feet of gas, including the unconnected reserves that are on site.[2] Bulk oxygen may be stored in either gaseous or liquid form, but liquid storage is most common. When needed, the oxygen flows from this central source throughout the facility through a piping system with outlets conveniently located.

A bulk oxygen system has several advantages over portable cylinders. First, although initially expensive to construct, bulk oxygen systems are far less expensive over the long term. Second, bulk oxygen systems are less prone to interruption. Third, bulk systems eliminate the inconvenience and hazard of transporting and storing large numbers of cylinders. Fourth, bulk oxygen systems regulate delivery pressures centrally, thereby eliminating the need for separate pressure-reducing valves at each outlet. Last, bulk systems operate at low pressures, making them much safer than high-pressure cylinders.

Safety standards for bulk oxygen systems are set by the NFPA and are subject to further control by local fire and building codes.[2] Respiratory therapists should be familiar with both bulk units in general and the specific gas supply systems used in their facilities.

Gas Supply Systems

There are three types of centrally located gas supply systems: an alternating supply system or cylinder manifold system, a cylinder supply system with reserve supply, and a bulk gas system with a reserve.[2]

The alternating supply or cylinder manifold system consists of large (normally H or K size) cylinders of compressed oxygen banked together in series (Figure 34-7).[2] This alternating supply system has two sides: a primary bank and a reserve bank. When the pressure in the primary bank decreases to a set level, a control valve automatically switches over to the reserve bank. When this occurs, the primary bank is taken off-line, and the empty cylinders are replaced with full ones. The replenished primary bank becomes the reserve bank. Some large alternating supply systems are permanently fixed and are refilled on site by a supply truck. These cylinder manifold systems have pressure-reducing valves for regulation of delivered pressure and normally have low-pressure alarms. These alarms sound when reserve switch-over occurs, and they warn of impending depletion or malfunction. Cylinder manifolds or alternating supply systems are used to supply oxygen from a central location in small facilities or to supply specialty gases, such as nitrous oxide, to operating rooms (Figure 34-8).

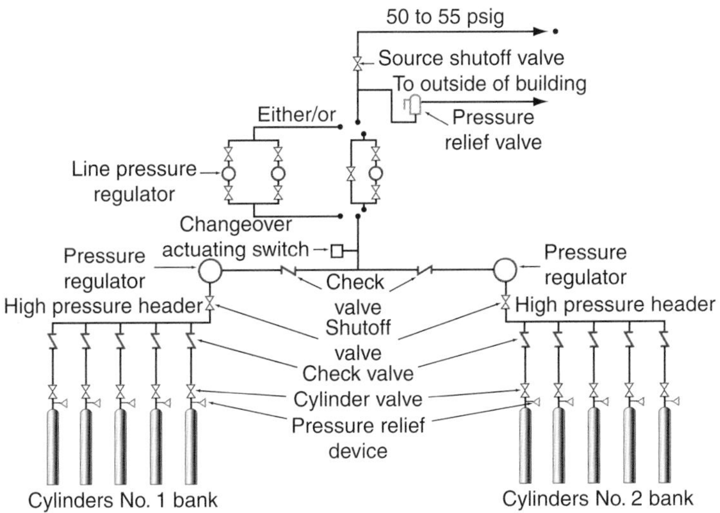

Figure 34-7 · Gas Cylinder Manifold System
Alternating supply system is composed of primary and reserve banks, which alternate to charge the piping system. *(Modified from Standard for nonflammable medical gas systems, NFPA no. 56F. Copyright 1973, National Fire Protection Association, Boston, MA.)*

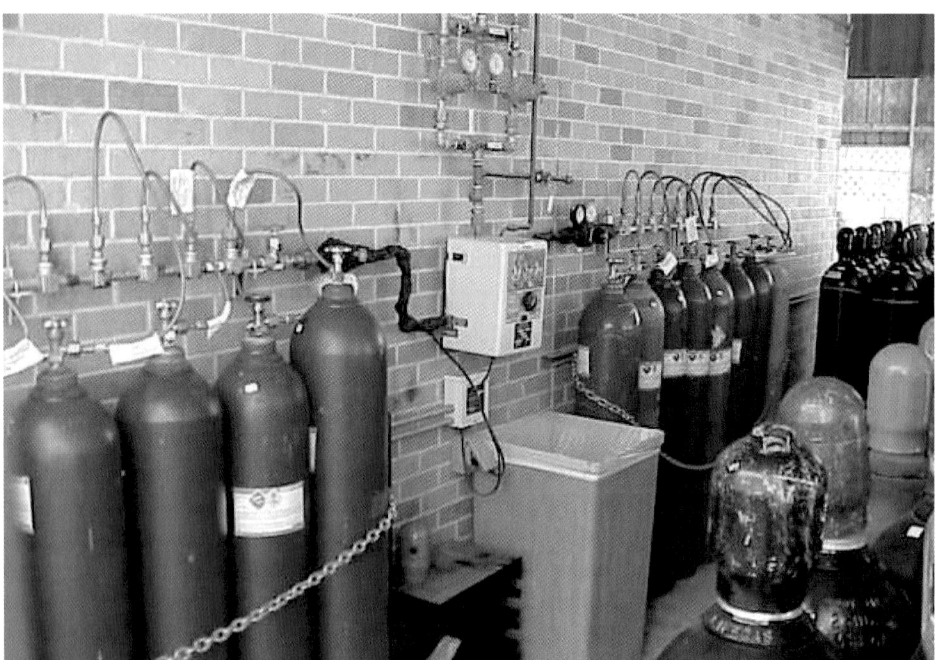

Figure 34-8
Alternating supply system of nitrous oxide.

A cylinder supply system with a reserve consists of a primary supply, a secondary supply, and a reserve supply.[2] When the primary gas supply is depleted by the demand, this supply system automatically switches to the secondary supply. Master signal panels indicate that the changeover has occurred. This supply system operates in a manner similar to that for the alternating system, except this system has a reserve supply if primary and secondary supplies become depleted. Liquid containers may be used as the primary and secondary gas sources, but the reserve supply usually is high-pressure gas cylinders.[2] Gas cylinders are used as the reserve supply because low-pressure liquid containers loose approximately 3% of the supply per day.[2]

For economy, safety, and convenience, most large healthcare facilities use a liquid bulk oxygen system. A small volume of liquid oxygen provides a very large amount of gaseous oxygen and minimizes space requirements. Along with this advantage comes a major problem. Oxygen has a critical temperature well below room temperature (–181.1° F [–118.8° C]). Liquid oxygen must continually be stored below this temperature, or it reverts to its gaseous state.

To stay in liquid form, oxygen is stored in large stand tanks (Figure 34-9) at relatively low pressure (less than 250 psig).[1] These stand tanks are like giant thermos bottles, consisting of inner and outer steel shells separated by an insulated vacuum chamber (Figure 34-10). Because it eliminates heat conduction, the vacuum keeps the liquid oxygen below its critical temperature

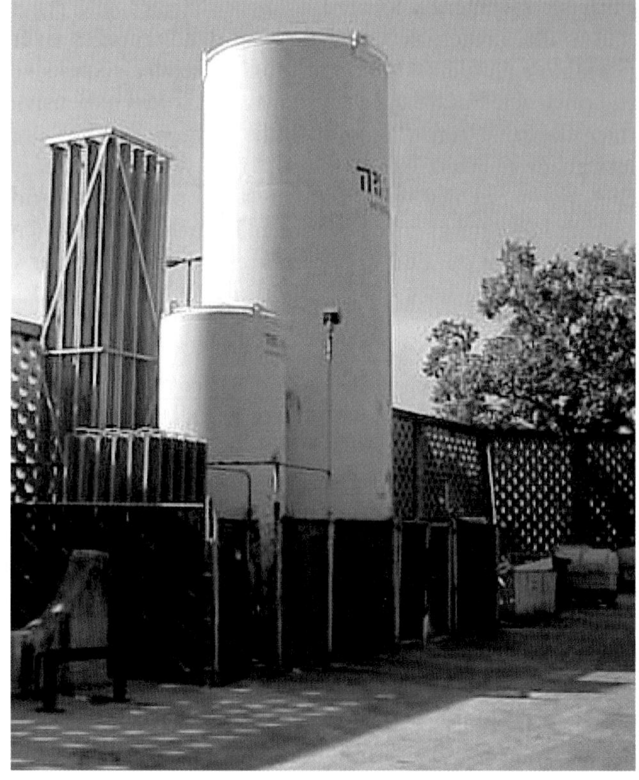

Figure 34-9
Large stand tank and reserve tank of liquid oxygen represents a typical bulk gas system with a reserve.

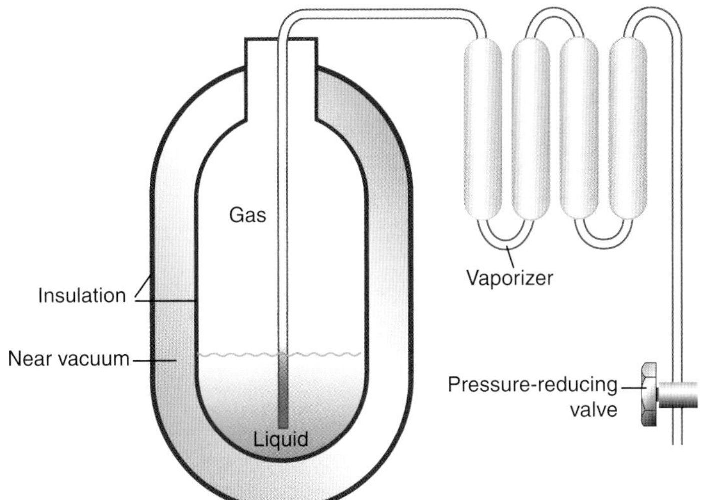

Figure 34-10
Liquid-oxygen stand tank (fixed station). *(From Cairo JM, Pilbeam SP: Mosby's respiratory care equipment, ed 6, St Louis, 1999, Mosby.)*

without refrigeration. When it flows through vaporizer coils exposed to ambient temperature, the liquid oxygen quickly converts back to a gas. With the oxygen in its gaseous form, the pressure is decreased to the standard working pressure of 50 psi by a pressure-reducing valve. A safety vent allows vaporized liquid oxygen to escape if warming causes cylinder pressure to increase above a set limit.

Smaller liquid cylinders are used for home oxygen supply. These cylinders come in several sizes and hold between 2/3 and 1 1/2 cubic feet of liquid oxygen. Small liquid oxygen cylinders are refilled on site by means of transfer of liquid oxygen from a large cylinder. Chapter 49 details the use of these small liquid oxygen cylinders in the home.

Bulk Oxygen Safety Precautions

The NFPA sets standards for the design, construction, placement, and use of bulk oxygen systems.[2] Among the key provisions in these standards is the requirement for a reserve or backup gas supply to equal the average daily gas usage of the hospital. To meet this requirement, most large facilities have a second, smaller liquid stand tank. Smaller facilities may use a cylinder gas manifold as the backup.

Total failure of bulk oxygen supply systems has been reported with resultant major problems.[13-15] Failure of a bulk oxygen supply can be life threatening to any patient receiving oxygen or gas-powered ventilatory support. For this reason, the respiratory care staff must be prepared. Adherence to an established protocol is a quick way to identify and prioritize all affected patients. Once affected patients are identified, staff members move appropriate backup equipment to the bedside (portable cylinders, bag-valve-mask resuscitators, and so on). Trained personnel bypass the failed system and provide needed patient support while engineers determine the cause of the failure and correct it.

▶ DISTRIBUTION AND REGULATION OF MEDICAL GASES

Before it can be administered to a patient, a medical gas must be delivered to the bedside and the pressure reduced to a workable level. This is the primary function of gas distribution and regulation systems. Modern hospital gas distribution systems deliver bulk oxygen and compressed air to patient rooms and special care areas through an elaborate piping network. Included in this network may be a vacuum source and, for surgical areas, nitrous oxide. Patient transport still requires the use of portable cylinders.

Whether delivery occurs by central bulk supply or cylinder, patient safety is always the primary aim. For this reason, RTs must be proficient in the use of both delivery systems.

Central Piping Systems

Structural standards for piping systems are established by the NFPA and are described in more detail elsewhere.[2] Figure 34-11 show a simple central piping gas system. The gas pressure in a central piping system normally is reduced to the standard working pressure of 50 psi at the bulk storage location. A main alarm warns of pressure drops or interruptions in flow from the source. **Zone valves** (Figure 34-12) throughout the system can be closed for system maintenance or in case of fire. Wall or station outlets at the delivery sites allow connection of various types of equipment to the gas distribution system. Because delivery outlets may include not only

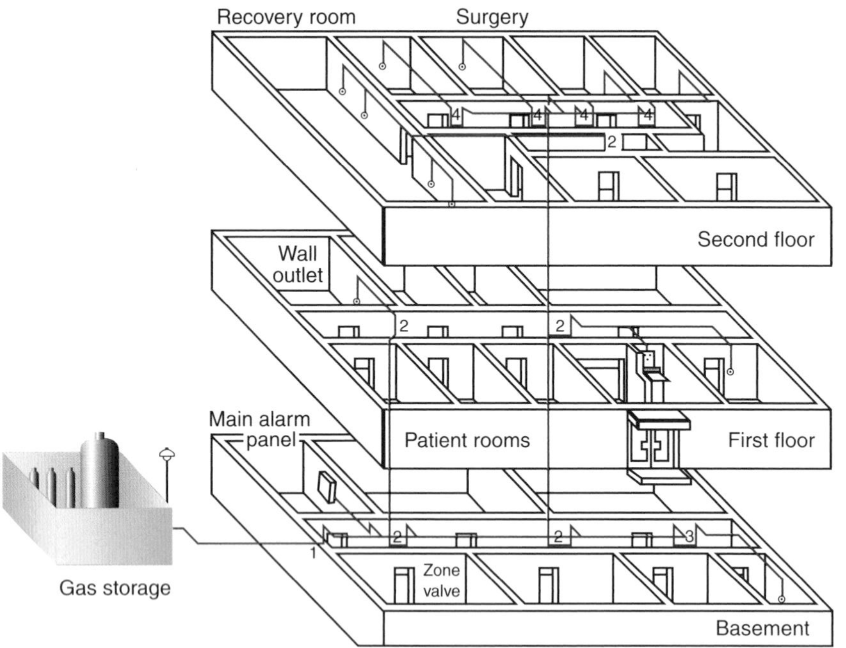

Figure 34-11
A hospital piping system. Numbers indicate zone valves.

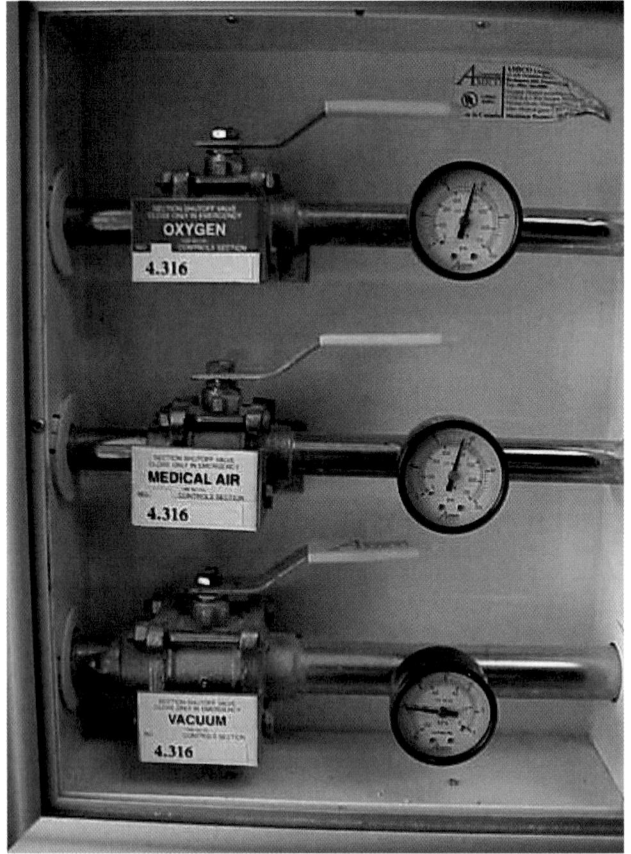

Figure 34-12
Oxygen, air, and vacuum zone valves.

oxygen but also air, vacuum, and possibly nitrous oxide, special safety connectors are used to help prevent accidental misconnections.

Safety Indexed Connector Systems

One of the greatest risks in medical gas therapy is giving the wrong gas to a patient. Carefully reading the cylinder or outlet labels is the best way to avoid these accidents. However, human error does occur. For this reason, the industry has developed indexed safety systems for gas delivery and regulation equipment. These safety systems make misconnection between pieces of equipment nearly impossible. For example, such a system normally prevents connecting a cylinder of nitrous oxide to an oxygen delivery system.

Three basic indexed safety systems are used in the delivery and regulation of medical gases: (1) the American National Standard/Compressed Gas Association Standard for Compressed Gas Cylinder Valve Outlet and Inlet Connections, or American standard safety system (ASSS), (2) the diameter-index safety system (DISS), and (3) the pin-index safety system (PISS).[16,17]

American Standard Safety System (ASSS)

Adopted in the United States and Canada, the ASSS provides standards for threaded high-pressure connections between large compressed gas cylinders (sizes F through H/K) and their attachments.[16] Specifications

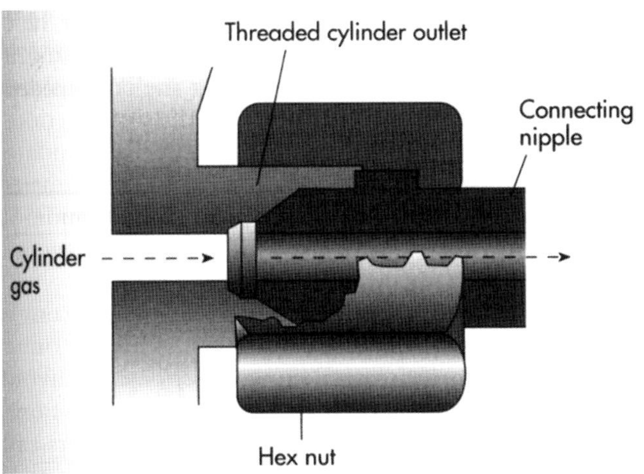

Figure 34-13
A typical ASSS connection used to attach a reducing valve to a large high-pressure cylinder. A hexagonal nut is held on the nipple of the reducing valve by a circular collar. The connection is made by (1) aligning the reducing valve nipple with the conical cylinder valve outlet and (2) tightening the reducing valve hex nut onto the threaded cylinder outlet. Different threading and cylinder outlet sizes make accidental misconnections difficult.

exist for more than 60 gases and gas mixtures. Figure 34-13 shows a typical ASSS connection between a threaded cylinder outlet and a pressure-reducing valve nipple. Because of the size (bore) of the cylinder outlet and its threading, use of the ASSS standards make misconnections difficult.

Because there are only 26 connections for the 62 listed gases and mixtures, each gas may not have a unique connection. This means that some gases have identical connections. Catalogs of cylinder equipment show the connection specifications for each type of cylinder and gas. A typical description for a large cylinder of oxygen is as follows: CGA-540 0.903-14NGO-RH-Ext.

The connection for the threaded outlet of this cylinder is listed by the CGA as connection number 540. The outlet has a thread diameter (bore) of 0.903 inch; there are 14 threads per inch; and the threads are right handed (RH) and external (Ext). It generally is necessary to use only one or two outlet connections, because most of the gases RTs use are grouped within a few connector sizes. However, practitioners should be familiar with the classification scheme in general, because expanding instrumentation and scope of services may bring RTs in contact with other gases and gas systems.

Pin-Index Safety System (PISS)

Pin indexing is part of the ASSS but applies only to the valve outlets of small cylinders, up to and including size E. These cylinders have a yoke type of connection. Figure 34-14 illustrates the general structure of the pin-indexed yoke connection. The upper yoke fits over the

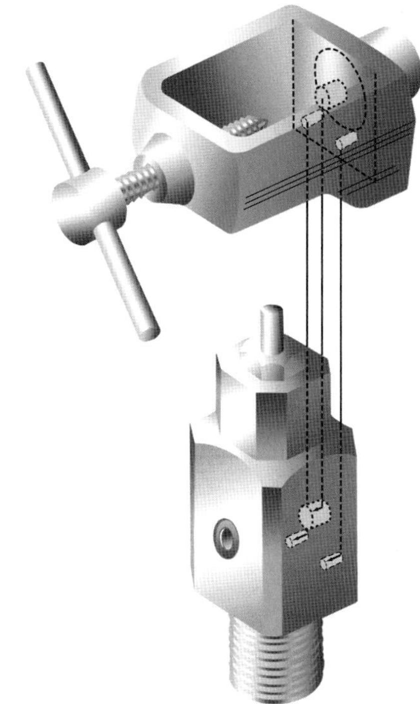

Figure 34-14
Yoke connector showing regulator inlet and pin-indexed safety system (for cylinders size AA to E).

lower valve stem. Two pins, projecting from the inner surface of the yoke connector, mate with two pinholes bored into the valve stem. Proper pin position aligns the small receiving nipple of the yoke with the recessed cylinder valve outlet. Tightening the hand screw on the yoke firmly seats the receiving nipple into the valve outlet. A nylon washer or bushing typically is used to ensure a leak-free connection.

Like the ASSS, the PISS helps prevent accidental misconnections between pieces of equipment. The exact positions of pins and pinholes vary for each gas. Unless the pins and holes align perfectly, the yoke nipple cannot seat in the recessed valve outlet. Six hole and pin positions constitute the total system. Because overlapping holes cannot be used, there are 10 possible pin combinations. Figure 34-15 is a diagram of the location of all six possible holes and their index numbers. Table 34-6 lists the gases included in the PISS system, including their index positions.

Diameter-Index Safety System (DISS)

Whereas the ASSS and the PISS provide standards for high-pressure connections between cylinders and equipment, the DISS was established to prevent accidental interchange of low-pressure (less than 200 psig) medical gas connectors.[17] Respiratory therapists typically find DISS connections (1) at the outlets of pressure-reducing

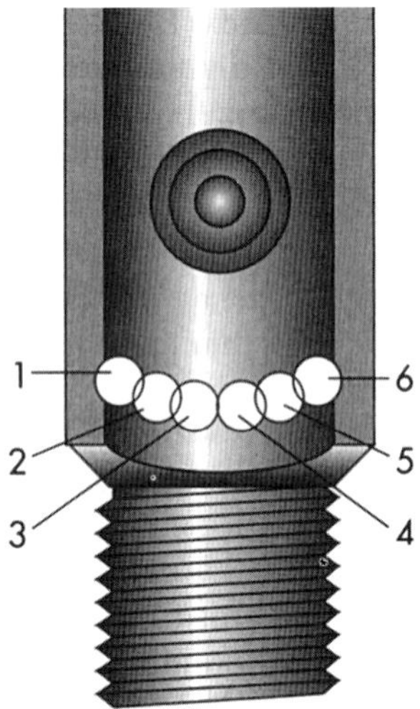

Figure 34-15
Location of the pin-index holes in the cylinder valve face for different gases.

valves attached to cylinders, (2) at the station outlets of central piping systems, and (3) at the inlets of blenders, flowmeters, ventilators, and other pneumatic equipment.

As shown in Figure 34-16, the DISS connection consists of an externally threaded body and a mated nipple with a nut. As the two parts are joined, the shoulders of the nipple and the bores of the body mate, the union held together by a hand-tightened hex nut. Indexing is achieved by varying the dimensions of the borings and shoulders. There are 11 indexed DISS connections and one for oxygen, for a total of 12.[17] The standard threaded oxygen connector (0.5625 inch in diameter and 18 threads per inch) actually preceded adoption of this safety system. Nonetheless it has been assigned a DISS number of 1240.

Table 34-6 ▶ ▶ Pin Index Hole Positions

Gas	Pin Positions
O_2	2-5
O_2/CO_2 (CO_2 not over 7%)	2-6
He/O_2 (He not over 80%)	2-4
C_2H_4	1-3
N_2O	3-5
$(CH_2)_3$	3-6
He/O_2 (He over 80%)	4-6
O_2/CO_2 (CO_2 over 7%)	1-6
Air	1-5

Although oxygen and air are generally used from a central outlet, it may be necessary to administer other gases that have different DISS connections. To avoid stocking a large variety of pressure regulators, flowmeters, and connectors for special gas use, adapters can be used to convert various DISS connections so that they can be used for a different purpose. Using adapters to bypass a safety system carries the increased risk of misconnection. For this reason, RTs should exercise extreme caution when adapting equipment connections. Misconnections can and do occur, with unfortunate patient consequences.[18]

Quick-Connect Systems

Station outlets at the patient's bedside allow quick access to a bulk supply of oxygen and air or a vacuum source. Station outlets have DISS connections or quick-connect systems that are gas or vacuum specific. Various manufacturers have designed specially shaped connectors for each gas (Figure 34-17). Because each connector has a distinct shape, it does not fit into an outlet for another gas, and each manufacturer has its own unique design. For this reason, connectors from different manufacturers are not interchangeable. As long as a facility is standardized for a single quick-connect system, this incompatibility is seldom a problem.

In summary, a variety of safety systems help prevent inadvertent misconnections between medical delivery systems and equipment. Figure 34-18 summarizes the use of and relationships between the ASSS, PISS, and

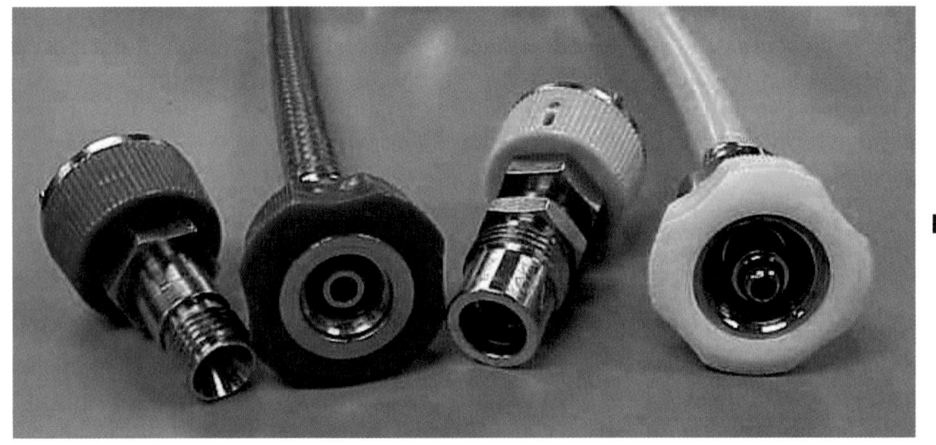

Figure 34-16
Oxygen **(A)** and air **(B)** DISS connections. The two shoulders of the nipple allow the nipple to unite only with a body that has corresponding borings. If the match is incorrect, the nut does engage the body threads. The difference in the shoulders and bore between the oxygen **(A)** and air **(B)** DISS connections is evident.

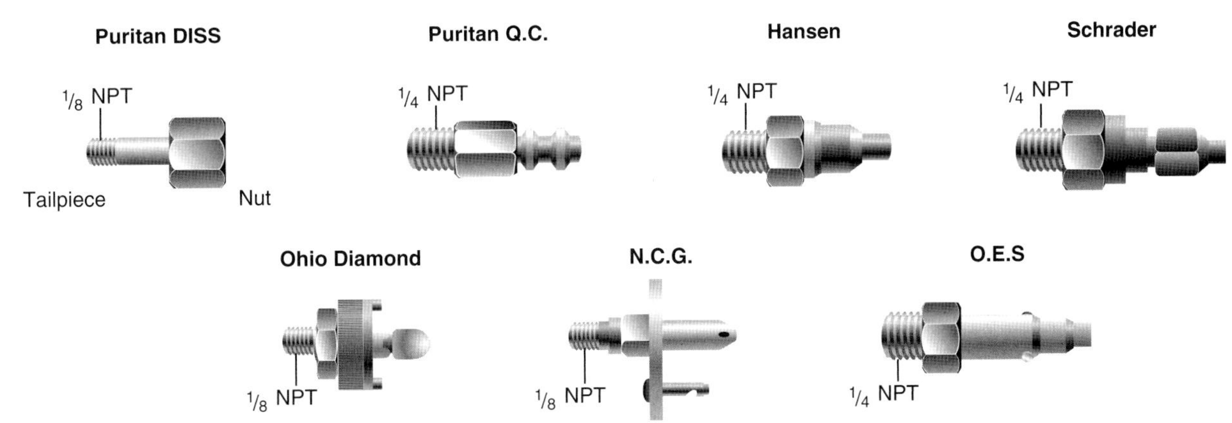

Figure 34-17
Common brands of quick connects. *(Courtesy Nellcor Puritan Bennett, Pleasanton, CA.)*

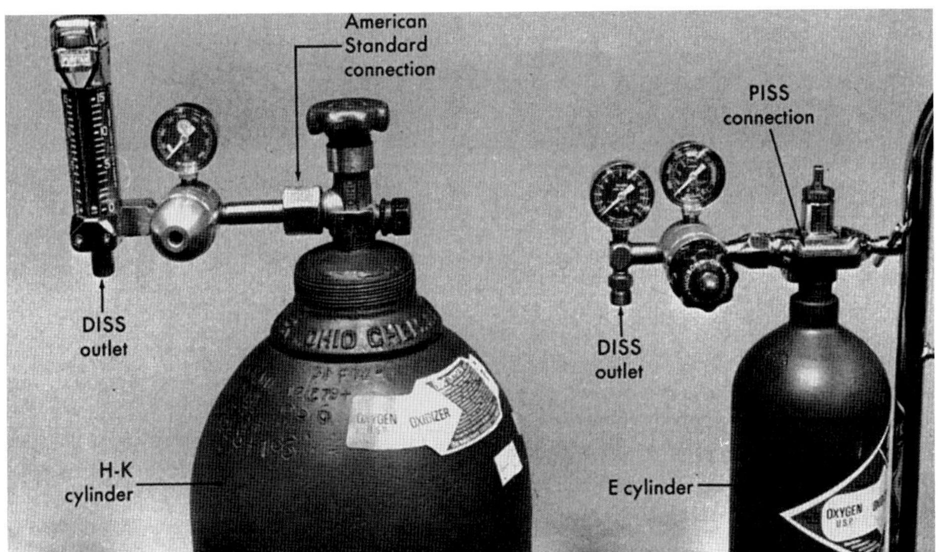

Figure 34-18
Comparison of safety systems used for compressed gases. The DISS connections are for low-pressure outlets (less than 200 psig). The ASSS provides for high-pressure connections with large cylinders. A variation of the ASSS entails a yoke and pin system (PISS) for connecting to small cylinders (AA through E).

DISS systems as applied to cylinder gases. Proficiency in the proper use of these systems is a basic skill of RTs.

Regulating Gas Pressure and Flow

Whatever the source of medical gas, for safe administration to a patient, the pressure and flow must be regulated. If the goal is solely a reduction in gas pressure, a reducing valve is used. For control of gas flow to a patient, a flowmeter is used. If control of both pressure and flow is needed, a regulator is used.

Cylinder gases such as oxygen and air exert a pressure much too high for use with respiratory care equipment. For use at the bedside, these high pressures must be reduced to a lower "working" level. In the United States, this working pressure is 50 psig. For bulk delivery systems with individual station outlets, built-in reducing valves decrease the delivered pressure to 50 psig. This standard pressure can be directly applied to power devices such as ventilators (see Chapter 39). However, if the goal is to control gas delivery to a patient for oxygen therapy or nebulized medication (see Chapters 33 and 35), a flowmeter must also be used.

High-Pressure Reducing Valves

There are two basic types of high-pressure reducing valves: single stage or multiple stage. Reducing valves are available as preset or adjustable.[4] Although all these valves function on the same principle, the design, features, and use are different. The following section differentiates preset reducing valves and adjustable reducing valves and discusses multiple-stage reducing valves.

Preset Reducing Valve. Figure 34-19 shows the basic design of a high-pressure preset reducing valve. High-pressure gas (2200 psig for oxygen) enters through

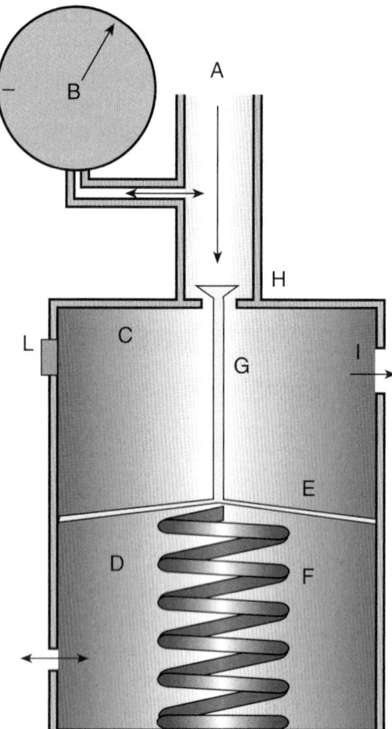

Figure 34-19
Preset high-pressure reducing valve.

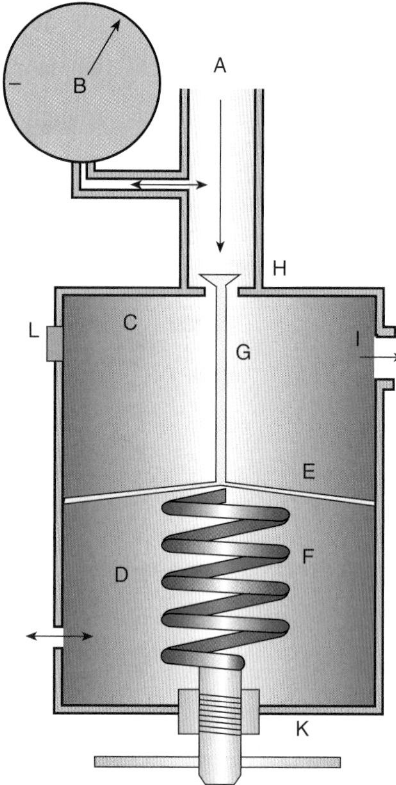

Figure 34-20
Adjustable high-pressure reducing valve.

the valve (A), with the inlet pressure displayed on the pressure gauge (B). The body of the valve is divided into a high-pressure chamber (C) and an ambient-pressure chamber (D) by a flexible diaphragm (E). Attached to the diaphragm in the ambient-pressure chamber is a spring (F), which is fixed to the other side of the chamber. Also attached to the diaphragm, but in the high-pressure chamber, is a valve stem (G) that sits on the high-pressure inlet (H). Gas flows through the valve inlet (H) into the high-pressure chamber and on to the gas outlet (I). The pressure chamber is supplied with a safety vent (L) preset to 200 psig to release pressure in the event of malfunction.

The spring tension is calibrated to give when the pressure on the diaphragm exceeds 50 psig. When this happens, the valve stem is pushed forward and closes the high-pressure inlet, preventing further entry of gas into the reducing valve. However, as long as gas is allowed to escape from the pressure chamber through the outlet (I), the inlet valve remains open and allows gas flow. Thus the regulator maintains a balance between outlet flow and inlet pressure. Automatic adjustment of the diaphragm-spring combination keeps the pressure in the high-pressure chamber at a near-constant 50 psig; thus the name *preset*. Preset reducing valves are normally used in conjunction with high-pressure gas cylinders to lower the pressure to the standard 50 psig used with most respiratory care equipment.

Adjustable Reducing Valve. Although most respiratory care equipment works at the standard 50 psig, some devices need variable pressures. To provide variable outlet pressures from a high-pressure gas source, an adjustable reducing valve is needed. Figure 34-20 shows the basic design of a high-pressure adjustable reducing valve. As with the preset design, the inlet valve (H) remains open until the gas pressure exceeds the spring tension, displacing the diaphragm and blocking further gas entry. However, while the preset reducing valve provides a fixed pressure, the adjustable reducing valve allows a change in outlet pressure. Outlet pressure can be changed with a threaded hand control (K) attached to the end of the diaphragm spring. Changing the tension on the valve spring varies pressure over a wide range, usually between 0 and 100 psig.

The adjustable reducing valve commonly is used in combination with a Bourdon-type flow gauge (see later). The combination of a flowmeter with a reducing valve is called a *regulator*.

Multiple-Stage Reducing Valve. As the name suggests, a multiple-stage reducing valve reduces pressure in two or more steps. Multiple-stage reducing valves can be either preset or adjustable and can be combined with a flow-metering device as a true regulator. Two-stage reducing valves are used occasionally, but rarely are three-stage units needed. A two-stage reducing valve is functionally two single-stage reducing valves working in series. Gas enters the first stage, where the pressure is lowered to an intermediate level (usually 200 to 700 psig). Gas then enters the second stage, where the pressure is decreased to working level (usually 50 psig). Because each pressure chamber has one safety relief vent, the user usually can determine the number of stages in a reducing valve by noting the number of relief vents present. Because they reduce pressure in multiple steps, these valves provide more precise and smooth flow control. However, they are larger and more expensive than single-stage reducing valves. For this reason, a multiple-stage reducing valve should be considered only if minimal fluctuations in pressure or flow are critical factors, as in research activities. For routine hospital work, single-stage reducing valves are satisfactory.

Proper Use of High-Pressure Reducing Valves. When a cylinder attached to a high-pressure reducing valve is open, gas undergoes rapid decompression followed by rapid recompression. Because the recompression is adiabatic (see Chapter 5), the gas temperature quickly increases. These rapid pressure and temperature changes are potentially hazardous. Rapid pressure swings can cause failure of reducing valve components.[19] Failed components can become high-velocity projectiles, endangering practitioner and patient alike. Rapid temperature changes can ignite combustible materials.[20] Ignition of combustible materials in the presence of 100% oxygen can cause an explosion. Box 34-1 provides guidelines for minimizing the risk associated with setting up oxygen cylinders with a high-pressure reducing valve or regulator.[1]

Box 34-1 • Safe Procedure for Setup of an Oxygen Cylinder and Reducing Valve or Regulator

1. Secure the cylinder according to the CGA guidelines. Verify the contents from the label that matches the color code and valve indexing.
2. Remove the protective cap or wrap, and inspect the cylinder valve to be certain that it is free of dirt, debris, and oil.
3. Warn those present that you are about to "crack" the cylinder valve and that it will make some noise. Turn the cylinder valve away from any persons present, stand to the side, and quickly open and close the valve. This removes any dust or small debris from the cylinder valve outlet.
4. Inspect the valve or regulator inlet for debris, dirt, and oil. Check the device label and confirm that it is intended for high-pressure service and for use with the gas to be administered. Oxygen-reducing valves and regulators should have a label stating: OXYGEN: USE NO OIL.
5. Once you confirm that the valve or regulator inlet is free of contaminants, securely tighten (but *do not* force) the device onto the cylinder outlet. When making connections, use appropriate wrenches that are oil and grease free. Never use pipe wrenches. Use only cylinder valve connections that conform to the ASSS and the PISS. Low-pressure connections must comply with the DISS or be noninterchangeable, low-pressure quick connects. Never connect fixed or adjustable orifices or metering devices directly to a cylinder without a pressure-reducing valve.
6. Confirm that the regulator or reducing valve is in the OFF or CLOSED position, and *slowly* open the cylinder valve to pressurize the attached reducing valve or regulator. Once pressurization has occurred, open the cylinder valve completely then turn it back one-fourth to one-half turn (this maneuver prevents a condition known as "valve freeze," in which the valve cannot be turned).

Low-Pressure Gas Flowmeters

As with drugs, giving a medical gas to a patient requires knowledge of the dosage being delivered. Often physicians prescribe oxygen dosage as a flow, in liters per minute. In addition, certain gas-mixing equipment requires accurate knowledge of input flows, sometimes involving two or more gases. Flowmeters are needed to set and control the rate of gas flow to a patient.[4] When the gas source is a high-pressure gas cylinder, a regulator (reducing valve plus flowmeter) is required. However, when the source is a bulk central supply system, the pressure has already been reduced to 50 psig by the time it reaches the outlet stations. This eliminates the need for pressure reduction and requires only a flowmeter.

Three categories of flowmeters are used in respiratory care: the flow restrictor, the Bourdon gauge, and the Thorpe tube. The Thorpe tube has two different designs: pressure compensated or not pressure compensated (uncompensated). Although uncompensated Thorpe tubes are rare, they are still in use in some institutions. For this reason, the principles underlying each of the four types of flow metering devices are compared and contrasted.

Flow Restrictor. The flow restrictor is the simplest and least expensive flow- metering device. As shown in Figure 34-21, a flow restrictor consists solely of a fixed orifice calibrated to deliver a specific flow at a constant pressure (50 psig). The operation of the flow restrictor is based on the principle of flow resistance, as described in Chapter 5. Specifically, the flow of gas through a tube can be quantified with the following equation:

MINI CLINI

Leaky Connections

PROBLEM

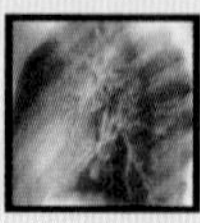

Following standard procedure, you attach a pressure-reducing valve to an oxygen cylinder. When you open the cylinder valve, you hear gas leaking at or near the connection.

SOLUTION

A leak usually indicates that the connection between the pressure-reducing valve and the cylinder outlet is not tight. If the cylinder outlet is a standard ASSS threaded connector, the connection is either cross-threaded or not properly seated and tightened. To solve this problem, close the cylinder valve and remove and reattach the pressure-reducing valve, being careful to properly thread the connection and tighten with a wrench. If the cylinder outlet is a pin-indexed connector, close the cylinder valve and remove the pressure-reducing valve. Check to make sure that the nylon washer is present, in good condition, and properly fitted. Then reattach the pressure-reducing valve, being careful to properly seat the connection, and hand tighten. If the leak continues after these corrective actions, it is likely that the pressure-reducing valve is malfunctioning and should be replaced.

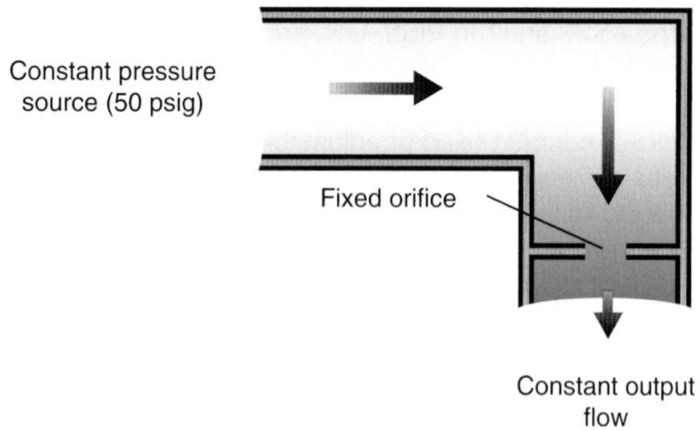

Figure 34-21
Flow restrictor.

$$R = \frac{P_1 - P_2}{V}$$

Rearranging the equation to solve for flow (V) yields the following:

$$V = \frac{P_1 - P_2}{R}$$

where V is the volumetric flow per unit time, P_1 is the pressure at the **upstream** point (point 1), P_2 is the pressure at the **downstream** point (point 2), and R is the total resistance to gas flow.

By design, a flow restrictor requires a source of constant pressure (usually 50 psig). As long as the source pressure remains fixed, $P_1 - P_2$ also should stay constant. With a fixed-size orifice, the flow resistance (R) also remains constant. With both the top and bottom of the equation fixed, the resulting flow is a constant value for any given orifice size. A flow restrictor is thus a fixed-orifice, constant-pressure flow-metering device.[21]

Commercially produced flow restrictors are calibrated at 50 psig. Several models are available, each providing a specific preset flow, usually in the 0.5 to 3 L/min range. Other versions allow the user to select one of several orifice settings, thus providing a range of preset flows. These devices typically are used to provide calibrated low flows of oxygen. They also are common components of some home oxygen delivery systems. Box 34-2 summarizes the advantages and disadvantages of flow restrictors.

Box 34-2 • Advantages and Disadvantages of Flow Restrictors

ADVANTAGES
- Low-cost, simple, reliable (no moving parts)
- Cannot be set to incorrect flow
- Can be used in any position (gravity independent)

DISADVANTAGES
- Different versions required for different flows
- Accuracy varies with changes in source and downstream pressures
- Cannot be used with high-resistance equipment

Bourdon Gauge. A Bourdon gauge (Figure 34-22) is a flow-metering device that is always used in combination with an adjustable pressure-reducing valve. Like the flow restrictor, the Bourdon gauge uses a fixed orifice. Unlike the flow restrictor, the Bourdon gauge operates under variable pressures, as adjusted with the pressure-reducing valve. The Bourdon gauge is thus a fixed-orifice, variable-pressure flow-metering device.[21]

As shown in Figure 34-23, a Bourdon gauge has a calibrated fixed orifice (A), which creates outflow resistance. The gauge itself is attached to the flow stream with a connector (B) located proximal to the orifice. Inside the gauge is a curved, hollow, closed tube (C) that responds to pressure changes by changing shape. The force of gas pressure tends to straighten the tube, causing its distal end to move. This motion is transmitted to a gear assembly and indicator needle (D). A numbered scale is calibrated to read the needle movement in units of flow (liters per minute).

As with the flow restrictor, the fixed orifice of the Bourdon gauge ensures the output flow is proportional to the driving pressure. However, the Bourdon gauge

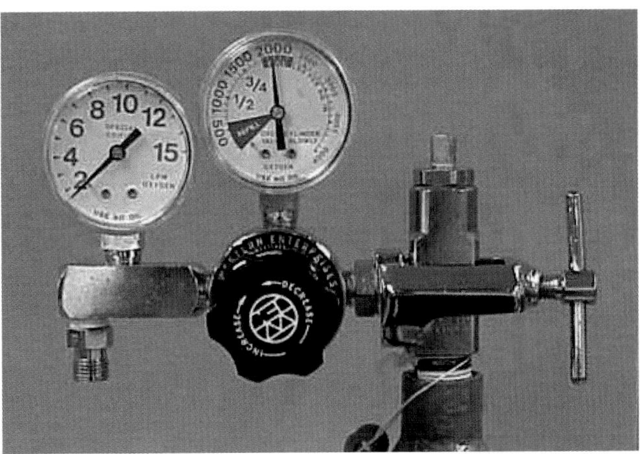

Figure 34-22
A Bourdon gauge regulator.

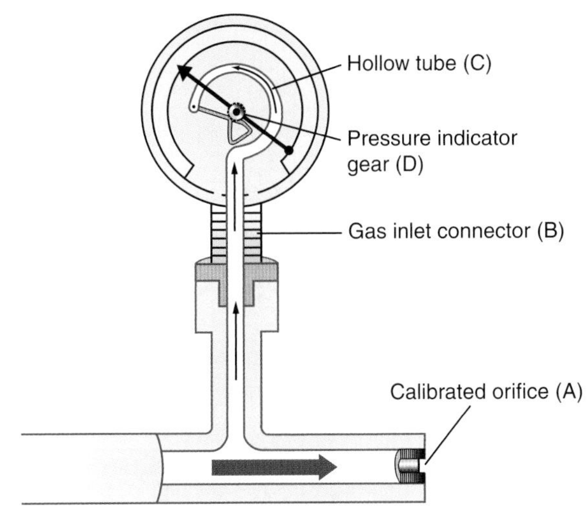

Figure 34-23
Components of a Bourdon pressure gauge.

provides a continuous range of flow, which the user adjusts by altering the pressure on the attached reducing valve. Although the gauge actually measures pressure changes, it displays the corresponding flow.

As with a flow restrictor, gravity does not affect a Bourdon gauge. The Bourdon gauge is the best choice when a flowmeter cannot be maintained in an upright position. This situation is common when a patient is being transported with a portable oxygen source. In these instances, keeping the E cylinder upright is seldom easy, and movement of both the oxygen supply and the patient is common. Combined with its continuous range of flows, this feature makes the Bourdon gauge the metering device of choice for patient transport.

The main disadvantage of the Bourdon gauge is its inaccuracy when pressure distal to the orifice (downstream pressures) changes. Specifically, if downstream pressure increases (as when high-resistance equipment is used), the pressure difference across the orifice and actual output flow decrease. However, the Bourdon gauge flow reading depends on upstream pressure, which stays constant. In this situation the gauge reading is falsely higher than the actual delivered flow.[4] Because it measures upstream pressure, the gauge registers flow even when the outlet is completely blocked (Figure 34-24). A user who needs accurate flow when using a device that creates high resistance should not select a Bourdon gauge. A compensated Thorpe tube should be used instead.

Thorpe Tube. The Thorpe tube flowmeter (Figure 34-25) is always attached to a 50 psig source, either a preset pressure-reducing valve or a bedside station outlet. Compared with the flow restrictor and the Bourdon gauge, the Thorpe tube functions as a variable-orifice, constant-pressure flow-metering device.[21] Figure 34-26 shows how a Thorpe tube works. The key component in this device is a tapered transparent tube that contains a float. The diameter of the tube increases from bottom to top. Gas flow suspends the float against the force of gravity. To read the flow, one simply compares the float position to an adjacent calibrated scale, normally calibrated in liters per minute.

Whereas the Bourdon gauge is used to measure pressure, the Thorpe tube is used to measure true flow. Flow measurement involves the complex interaction of gravity and fluid dynamics. When gas begins to flow into a Thorpe tube, the initial pressure difference lifts the float. As the float rises in the widening tube, the space available for flow around it increases (equivalent to increasing the orifice), and resistance to flow decreases. This decreased resistance allows higher flow for a given pressure difference. The float ultimately stabilizes when the pressure difference across the float (an upward force) equals the opposing downward force of gravity.

As the needle valve of the flowmeter is opened, the increase in flow initially disrupts this balance, causing an increase in the pressure difference across the float. With the upward pressure difference greater than the downward force of gravity, the float rises. However, as the float rises, the available "orifice" increases in diameter. Flow resistance around the float decreases, and the pressure difference once again equilibrates with gravity. The float position thus stabilizes at a higher level, proportionate to the greater flow around it.

Thorpe tubes come in two basic designs: pressure compensated and pressure uncompensated. The term *pressure compensation* refers to a design that prevents changes in downstream resistance, or back pressure, from affecting meter accuracy. For administration of medical gas, all manufacturers now supply only pressure-compensated Thorpe tubes. However, some ventilators and anesthesia machines still use uncompensated Thorpe tubes. For this reason, clinicians using these devices must understand the effect of back pressure

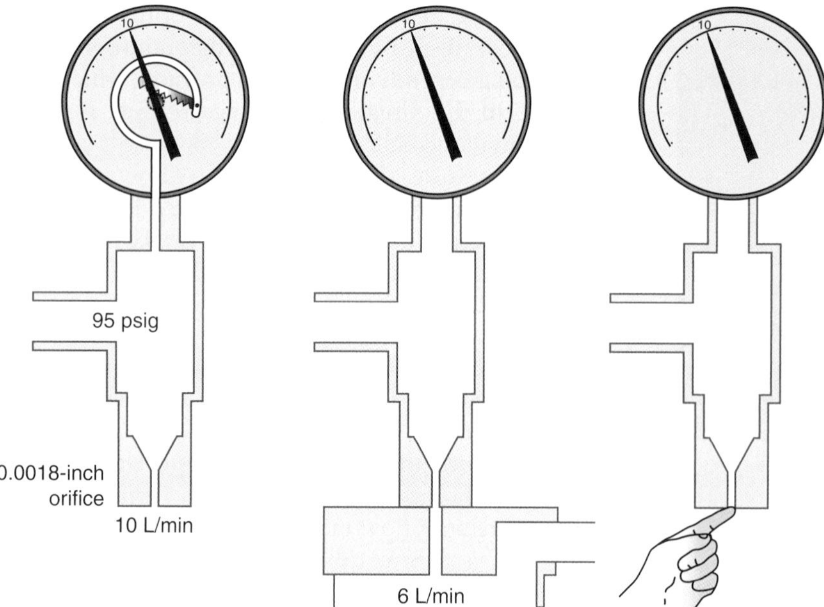

Figure 34-24
Bourdon performance when downstream pressures rise as a result of high-resistance equipment or blockage. Left, Normal state with fixed orifice and no downstream resistance results in an accurate flow reading. Center, High-resistance nebulizer increases downstream pressure, or back pressure. The result is a falsely high reading (10 L/min versus actual flow of 6 L/min). Right, Complete blockage (zero flow) results in flow reading on gauge. *(Courtesy of Nellcor Puritan Bennett, Pleasanton, CA.)*

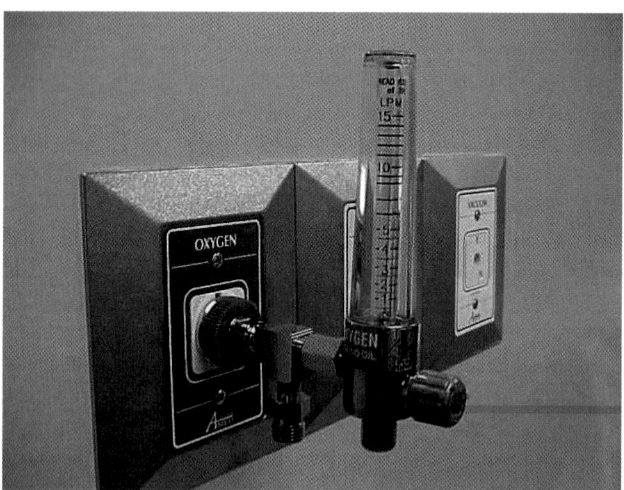

Figure 34-25
Thorpe tube flowmeter.

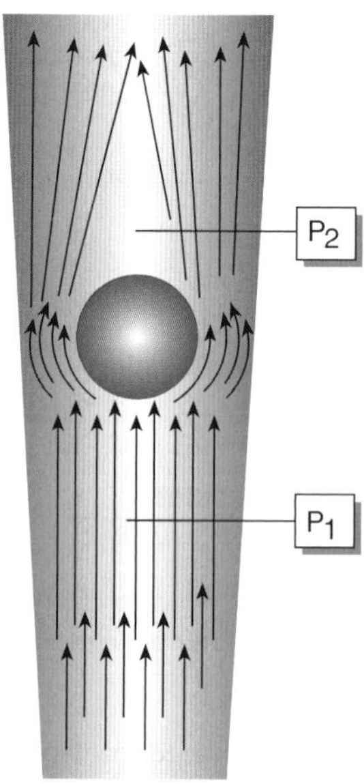

Figure 34-26
The position of the float in a Thorpe tube flowmeter is based on a balance between the force of gravity and the pressure difference ($P_2 - P_1$) across it, as determined by the variable-sized orifice between the float and the tube wall.

on the accuracy of these devices. An increase in downstream resistance occurs when the user connects a flowmeter to certain types of equipment. Almost all therapy gas equipment produces some flow restriction. Devices such as jet nebulizers produce very high downstream resistance. Depending on their design, Thorpe tube flowmeters respond to resistance in one of two ways.

The uncompensated Thorpe tube flowmeter is calibrated in liters per minute, but at atmospheric pressure (without restriction). Gas from a 50 psig source flows into the meter at a rate controlled by a needle valve located before the flow tube (Figure 34-27, *A*). When the user attaches flow-restricting equipment to the meter, downstream resistance increases, raising pressure in the flow tube. As long as this pressure does not exceed 50 psig, gas continues to flow through the tube. However, the added downstream resistance increases the pressure in the flow tube above atmospheric. At higher pressures, a greater amount of gas flows through a given restriction than at atmospheric pressure. Thus with the float at a given height, more gas flows through the tube than is indicated on the scale. Under these conditions, an uncompensated Thorpe tube falsely shows a flow lower than that actually delivered to the patient.[4]

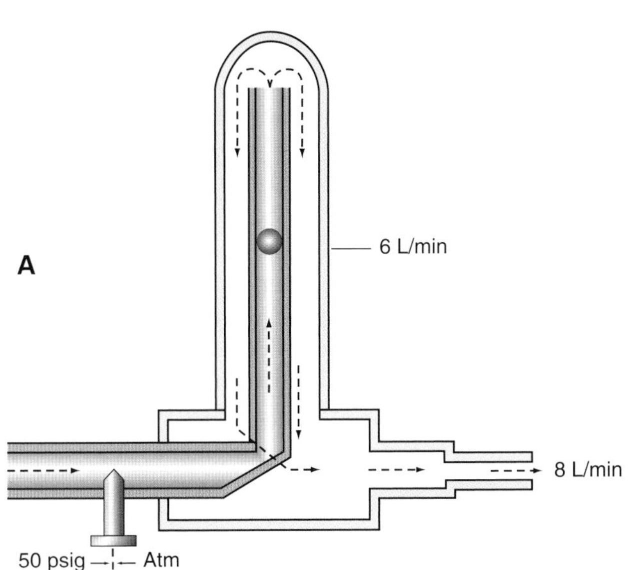

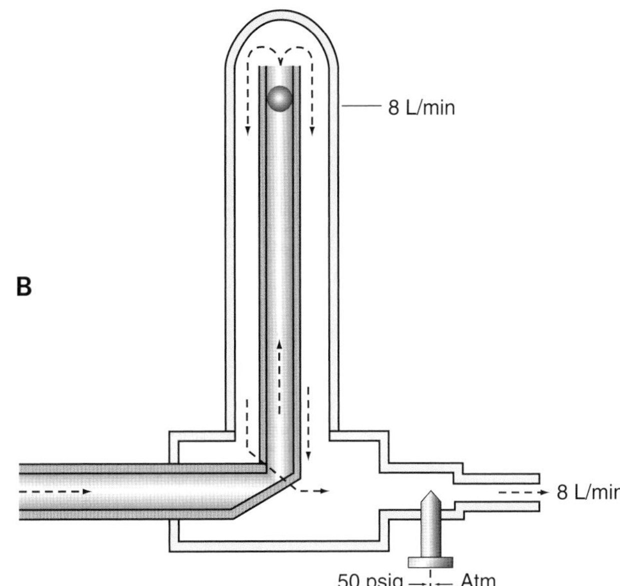

Figure 34-27

Comparison of pressure-uncompensated **(A)**, and pressure-compensated **(B)** Thorpe tube flowmeters. In the former, the flow-control valve is proximal to the meter, and the gauge records less than the actual output. In the latter, location of the valve distal to the meter correlates the gauge reading with the output.

In contrast, the scale of the compensated Thorpe tube flowmeter is calibrated at 50 psig instead of at atmospheric pressure. Its flow control needle valve is placed after (distal to) the flow tube (Figure 34-27, *B*). Thus the entire meter operates at constant 50 psig pressure. Knowing that the compensated Thorpe tube operates at 50 psig helps identify it. When a compensated Thorpe tube is connected to a 50 psig gas source with the needle valve closed, the float "jumps" then returns to zero as the Thorpe tube is pressurized. Because the entire meter operates at constant pressure, an increase in downstream resistance only increases pressure distal to the needle valve. As long as the downstream pressure does not exceed 50 psig (in which case flow ceases), the position of the float accurately reflects actual outlet flow. For this reason, the pressure-compensated Thorpe tube is the preferred instrument in most clinical situations.

The only factor limiting the use of a pressure-compensated Thorpe tube is gravity. Because it is accurate only in an upright position, a Thorpe tube is not the ideal choice for patient transport. In these cases, the gravity-independent Bourdon gauge is a satisfactory alternative.

Figure 34-28 summarizes the effects of downstream resistance, or back pressure, on the Bourdon gauge and the pressure-compensated and uncompensated Thorpe tube flow metering devices.

MINI CLINI

Selection of Devices to Regulate Gas Pressure or Control Flow

PROBLEM

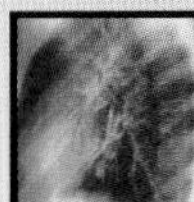

Three staff therapists are given three separate requests to set up oxygen. Mark has an order to transport Ms. Patel to radiology with oxygen. Carmen needs to set up a pneumatically powered ventilator with oxygen in the ambulatory clinic (where there are no oxygen outlets). Monica has to set up oxygen therapy with a jet nebulizer for a patient in the intensive care unit (ICU). What equipment should each therapist select?

SOLUTIONS

(1) Because he has to transport a patient using oxygen, Mark should select an E cylinder with an adjustable regulator that includes a Bourdon gauge (unaffected by gravity). (2) Because pneumatically powered ventilators require 50 psig and no central outlets are available, Carmen needs a preset (50 psig) reducing valve and a large G/H oxygen cylinder. (3) Because all modern ICUs have central wall outlets for oxygen, Monica need only select a flowmeter. A compensated Thorpe tube is required for metering flow through high-resistance equipment such as jet nebulizers.

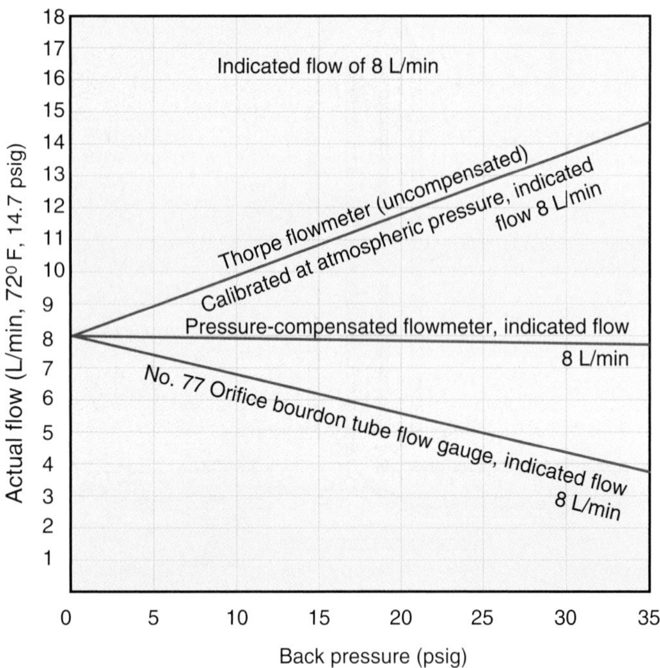

Figure 34-28

Comparative accuracy of flow-metering devices against increasing downstream pressure (back pressure). With the pressure-compensated Thorpe tube, indicated flow equals actual flow, regardless of downstream pressure. With the uncompensated Thorpe tube, indicated flow is progressively lower than actual flow as downstream pressure increases. With the Bourdon gauge, indicated flow is progressively higher than actual flow as downstream pressure increases. *(From McPherson SP, Spearman CB: Respiratory therapy equipment, ed 5, St Louis, 1995, Mosby. Modified from Puritan-Bennett Corp, Los Angeles, CA.)*

KEY POINTS

- All therapy gases must contain at least 20% oxygen; all such gases support combustion.
- Medical gases are stored either in portable high-pressure cylinders or in large centralized bulk reservoirs.
- For positive identification of the contents of a medical gas cylinder, the label must be carefully read.
- The pressure in a gas-filled cylinder indicates its contents; the pressure in a liquid-filled cylinder does not.
- To compute duration of flow (minutes) of a medical gas cylinder, multiply the cylinder pressure (pounds per square inch) by the cylinder factor and divide the result by the set flow (liters per minute).

KEY POINTS—cont'd

- Gas supply systems provide gas at 50 psig to outlets throughout a facility through a network of pipes. Such a system must include both zone valves for repairs or fire and alarms to warn of failure.
- Failure of a bulk gas supply system can threaten the lives of patients receiving oxygen therapy or being supported with pneumatically powered devices. A protocol must exist to deal with this emergency.
- Indexed safety systems help prevent misconnections between equipment. The ASSS provides high-pressure connections with large cylinders; the PISS does the same for small cylinders; and DISS connections are for low-pressure outlets, typically 50 psig.
- A reducing valve is used for reduction of gas pressure. A flowmeter is used for control of gas flow. A regulator is used for control of both pressure and flow.
- A flow restrictor is used to provide fixed low flows of oxygen. A Bourdon gauge is used to meter flow during patient transport. A compensated Thorpe tube is used when accurate flows are needed with high-resistance equipment.

References

1. Compressed Gas Association: Handbook of compressed gas, ed 4, Boston, 1999, Kluwer Academic Publishers.
2. National Fire Protection Association: Health care facilities handbook, ed 6, Quincy, Mass, 1999, National Fire Protection Association.
3. United States Pharmacopeia/National Formulary. Rockville, MD, 2000, United States Pharmacopeial Convention.
4. Cairo JM, Pilbeam SP: Mosby's respiratory care equipment, ed 6, St. Louis, 1999, Mosby.
5. Compressed Gas Association: Compressed air for human respiration (CGA G- 7)/ANSI Z86.1), Arlington, VA, 1989, Compressed Gas Association.
6. American Academy of Pediatrics: Policy statement: use of inhaled nitric oxide, Pediatrics 106:344, 2000.
7. Barrington KJ, Finer NN: Inhaled nitric oxide for respiratory failure in preterm infants (Cochrane review). In: The Cochrane Library, issue 3, Oxford, UK, 2002, Update Software.
8. Sokol J, Jacobs SE, Bohn D: Inhaled nitric oxide for acute hypoxemic respiratory failure in children and adults (Cochrane review). In: The Cochrane Library, issue 3, Oxford, UK, 2002, Update Software.

9. Department of Transportation, 49 Federal Register 100-199 (revised 2001).
10. Compressed Gas Association: Standard color marking of compressed gas containers for medical use (CGA C-9), Arlington, VA, 1989, Compressed Gas Association.
11. Compressed Gas Association: Characteristics and safe handling of medical gases (P-2), Arlington, VA, 1989, Compressed Gas Association.
12. Cylinders with unmixed helium/oxygen, Health Devices 19:146, 1990.
13. Anderson WR: Oxygen pipeline supply failure: a coping strategy, J Clin Monit 7:39, 1991.
14. Feeley TW, Hedley-Whyte J: Bulk oxygen and nitrous oxide delivery systems: design and dangers, Anesthesiology 44:301, 1976.
15. Bancroft ML, duMoulin GG, Headley-Whyte J: Hazards of bulk oxygen systems, Anesthesiology 52:504, 1980.
16. Compressed Gas Association: Compressed gas cylinder valve outlet and inlet connections (ANSI/CGA V-1), Arlington, VA, 1989, Compressed Gas Association.
17. Compressed Gas Association: Diameter index safety systems(CGA V-5), Arlington, VA, 1989, Compressed Gas Association.
18. Mismating of precision brand medical gas fittings, Health Devices 19:333, 1990.
19. Allberry RA: Minireg failure, Anaesth Intensive Care 17:234, 1989 (letter).
20. West GA, Primeau P: Nonmedical hazards of long-term oxygen therapy, Respir Care 28:906, 1983.
21. Ward JJ: Equipment for mixed gas and oxygen therapy. In Barnes TA, editor: Core textbook of respiratory care practice, ed 2, St Louis, 1994, Mosby.

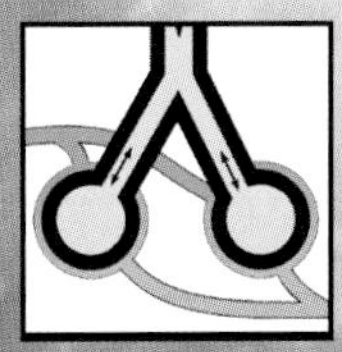

CHAPTER 35

Medical Gas Therapy

Albert J. Heuer and Craig L. Scanlan

In This Chapter You Will Learn:

- When oxygen therapy is needed
- How to assess the need for oxygen therapy
- What precautions and complications are associated with oxygen therapy
- How to select an oxygen delivery system appropriate for the respiratory care plan
- How to administer oxygen to adults, children, and infants
- How to check for proper function and to identify and correct malfunctions of oxygen delivery systems
- How to evaluate and monitor a patient's response to oxygen therapy
- How to modify or recommend modification of oxygen therapy on the basis of patient response
- How to implement protocol-based oxygen therapy
- What indications, complications, and hazards apply to hyperbaric oxygen therapy
- When and how to provide nitric oxide therapy
- When and how to administer helium-oxygen therapy

Chapter Outline

Key Terms

atmospheric pressure absolute (ATA)
bronchopneumonia
bronchopulmonary dysplasia
clubbing
congenital diaphragmatic hernia
croup
cyclic guanosine 3′,5′-monophosphate (cGMP)
exudative
fixed (O_2 delivery)
heliox therapy
high-flow system
hyperbaric oxygen (HBO) therapy

Continued

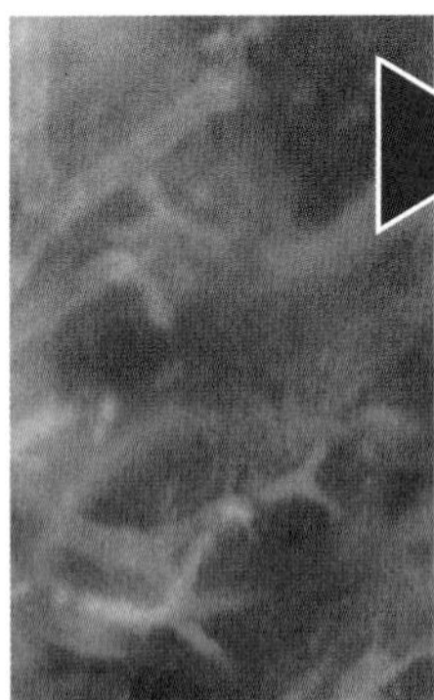

Key Terms—cont'd

hypoxemia
lassitude
low-flow system
myocardial infarction
neovascularization
neutral thermal environment (NTE)
nitric oxide therapy
persistent pulmonary hypertension of the newborn (PPHN)
reservoir system
retinopathy of prematurity (ROP)
variable (O_2 delivery)

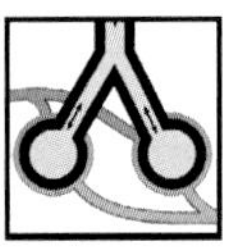

Gas therapy is the most common mode of respiratory care. The origins of the field parallel the introduction of oxygen as a medical treatment. Since that time, understanding of the various medical gases and methods to deliver them have changed. Of particular importance is the growing acknowledgment that medical gases are drugs. As with any drug, respiratory therapists (RTs) recommend and administer a dosage, monitor the response, alter therapy accordingly, and record these steps in relation to the care plan in the patient record. In this context, RTs must have more than technical knowledge of equipment. In consultation with the physician, a skilled clinician should be able to determine the desired goals of therapy, select the mode of administration, monitor the patient's response, and recommend and implement timely and appropriate changes.

▶ OXYGEN THERAPY

Consensus exists among clinicians about the proper use of oxygen therapy.[1-4] As the primary member of the healthcare team responsible for oxygen administration, the RT must be well-versed in the goals and objectives of this therapy and its use in clinical practice.

General Goals and Clinical Objectives

The overall goal of oxygen therapy is to maintain adequate tissue oxygenation while minimizing cardiopulmonary work. Specific clinical objectives for oxygen therapy are to

1. Correct documented or suspected acute **hypoxemia**
2. Decrease the symptoms associated with chronic hypoxemia
3. Decrease the workload hypoxemia imposes on the cardiopulmonary system

Correcting Hypoxemia

Oxygen therapy corrects hypoxemia by raising alveolar and blood levels of oxygen. This is the most tangible objective of oxygen therapy, and the easiest to measure and document.

Decreasing the Symptoms of Hypoxemia

In addition to actually relieving hypoxemia, oxygen therapy can help relieve the symptoms associated with certain lung disorders. Specifically, patients with chronic obstructive pulmonary disease (COPD) and some forms of interstitial lung disease report less dyspnea when receiving supplemental oxygen.[5] Oxygen therapy also may improve mental function among patients with chronic hypoxemia.[6]

Minimizing Cardiopulmonary Workload

The cardiopulmonary system compensates for hypoxemia by increasing ventilation and cardiac output. In cases of acute hypoxemia, supplemental oxygen can decrease demands on both the heart and the lungs. For example, hypoxemic patients breathing air can achieve acceptable arterial oxygenation only by increasing ventilation. Increased ventilatory demand increases the work of breathing. In these cases, oxygen therapy can reduce both the high ventilatory demand and the work of breathing.

Likewise, patients with arterial hypoxemia can maintain acceptable tissue oxygenation only by increasing cardiac output. Because oxygen therapy increases blood oxygen content, the heart does not have to pump as much blood per minute to meet tissue demands. This reduced workload is particularly important when the heart is already stressed by disease or injury, as in myocardial infarction, sepsis, or trauma.

Hypoxemia causes pulmonary vasoconstriction and pulmonary hypertension. Pulmonary vasoconstriction and hypertension increase workload on the right side of the heart. For patients with chronic hypoxemia, this increased workload over the long term can lead to right ventricular failure (cor pulmonale). Oxygen therapy can reverse pulmonary vasoconstriction and decrease right ventricular workload.[7]

Clinical Practice Guideline

To guide practitioners in safe and effective patient care, the American Association for Respiratory Care (AARC) has developed and published clinical practice guidelines for oxygen therapy. Excerpts from the AARC guideline on oxygen therapy in acute care hospitals appear on p. 830.[2] Additional AARC guidelines for oxygen therapy in the home or extended care facility[3] and for selection of oxygen delivery devices for neonatal and pediatric patients[4] are provided in Chapters 45 and 49.

Assessing the Need for Oxygen Therapy

There are three basic ways to determine whether a patient needs oxygen therapy. The first is use of laboratory measures to document hypoxemia. Second, a patient's need for oxygen therapy can be based on the specific clinical problem or condition. Last, hypoxemia has many manifestations, such as tachypnea, cyanosis, and distressed overall appearance. Astute bedside techniques of assessment for these and other symptoms can be used to determine the need for supplemental oxygen.

Laboratory measures for documenting hypoxemia include hemoglobin saturation and partial pressure of oxygen (PO_2), as determined by either invasive or noninvasive means (see Chapter 16). Threshold criteria defining hypoxemia with these measures are described in the AARC clinical practice guideline (see p. 830).[2] As specified in this guideline, the criteria for documenting hypoxemia in newborn infants (younger than 28 days) differ from those used for adults, children, and older infants.[8]

Patients with clinical problems or disorders in which hypoxemia is common need oxygen therapy. Good examples are postoperative patients and those with carbon monoxide poisoning, cyanide poisoning, shock, trauma, or acute myocardial infarction.[1,2]

Careful bedside physical assessment can disclose a patient's need for oxygen therapy. Table 35-1 summarizes the common respiratory, cardiovascular, and neurologic signs used in the detection of hypoxia. The RT combines this information with more quantitative measures to confirm inadequate oxygenation. However, the RT often recommends administration of supplemental oxygen solely on the basis of the clinical signs. Overreliance on quantitative methods such as pulse oximetry can result in dangerous errors.

Table 35-1 ▶▶ Clinical Signs of Hypoxia

Finding	Mild to Moderate	Severe
Respiratory	Tachypnea	Tachypnea
	Dyspnea	Dyspnea
	Paleness	Cyanosis
Cardiovascular	Tachycardia	Tachycardia, eventual bradycardia, arrhythmia
	Mild hypertension, peripheral vasoconstriction	Hypertension and eventual hypotension
Neurologic	Restlessness	Somnolence
	Disorientation	Confusion
		Distressed appearance
	Headaches	Blurred vision
	Lassitude	Tunnel vision
		Loss of coordination
		Impaired judgment
		Slow reaction time
		Manic-depressive activity
		Coma
Other		Clubbing

From Pilbeam SP: Mechanical ventilation, Denver, 1986, Multi-Media Publishing.

MINI CLINI

Conflicting Assessment Information

PROBLEM

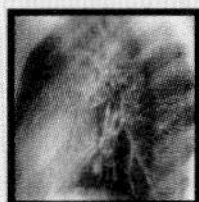

A disoriented postoperative male patient breathing room air exhibits tachypnea, tachycardia, and mild cyanosis of the mucous membranes. Using a pulse oximeter, you measure the patient's oxyhemoglobin saturation as 93%. What should you recommend to the patient's surgeon?

DISCUSSION

This is a classic example of how monitoring data and results of bedside assessment can conflict. Both the patient's condition and the observed clinical signs indicate hypoxemia, but the pulse oximeter indicates adequate oxygenation. In situations such as this, it is always better to err on the side of the patient and recommend oxygen therapy—treat the patient, not the monitor! This concept is particularly important in the use of monitoring technologies known to have limited accuracy, such as pulse oximetry (see Chapter 16).

Precautions and Hazards of Supplemental Oxygen

The AARC clinical practice guideline on p. 830 outlines the major precautions and hazards associated with administration of supplemental oxygen.[2] Four of these hazards are common enough to warrant additional discussion.

Oxygen Therapy in the Acute Care Hospital

AARC Clinical Practice Guideline (Excerpts)*

➤ INDICATIONS

- Documented hypoxemia
  - Adults, children, and infants >28 days old: PaO_2 <60 mm Hg or SaO_2 <90%
  - Neonates, PaO_2 <50 mm Hg, SaO_2 <88%, or capillary PO_2 <40 mm Hg
- Acute care situations in which hypoxemia is suspected
- Severe trauma
- Acute myocardial infarction
- Short-term therapy (e.g., postanesthesia recovery)

➤ CONTRAINDICATIONS

- No specific contraindications to oxygen therapy exist when indications are present.

➤ PRECAUTIONS AND/OR POSSIBLE COMPLICATIONS

- PaO_2 >60 mm Hg may depress ventilation in some patients with chronic hypercapnia.
- FIO_2 >0.5 may cause atelectasis, oxygen toxicity, and/or ciliary or leukocyte depression.
- In premature infants, PaO_2 >80 mm Hg can cause retinopathy of prematurity.
- In infants with ductal heart lesions, high PaO_2 can close or constrict the ductus arteriosus.
- Increased FIO_2 can worsen lung injury in patients with paraquat poisoning or those receiving bleomycin.
- During laser bronchoscopy, minimal FIO_2 should be used to avoid intratracheal ignition.
- Fire hazard is increased in the presence of high FIO_2.
- Bacterial contamination can occur when nebulizers or humidifiers are used.

➤ ASSESSMENT OF NEED

Need is determined by measurement of inadequate PaO_2 and/or SaO_2, by invasive or noninvasive methods, and/or the presence of clinical indicators.

➤ ASSESSMENT OF OUTCOME

Outcome is determined by clinical and physiologic assessment to establish adequacy of patient response to therapy.

➤ MONITORING

- Patient
  - Clinical assessment including cardiac, pulmonary, and neurologic status
  - Assessment of physiologic parameters (PaO_2, SaO_2, SpO_2) in conjunction with the initiation of therapy or:
    Within 12 hours of initiation with FIO_2 >60; 0.40
    Within 8 hours with FIO_2 ≥0.40 (including postanesthesia recovery)
    Within 72 hours in acute myocardial infarction
    Within 2 hours for any patient with principle diagnosis of COPD
    Within 1 hour for the neonate
- Equipment
  - All oxygen delivery systems should be checked at least once per day.
  - More frequent checks are needed in systems:
    Susceptible to variation in FIO_2 (e.g., hood, high-flow blending systems)
    Applied to patients with artificial airways
    Delivering a heated gas mixture
    Applied to patients who are clinically unstable or who require FIO_2 >0.50
  - The standard of practice for newborns appears to be continuous analysis of FIO_2 with a system check at least every 4 hours, but data to support this practice may not be available.

For complete guidelines, see Respir Care 36:1410, 1991.

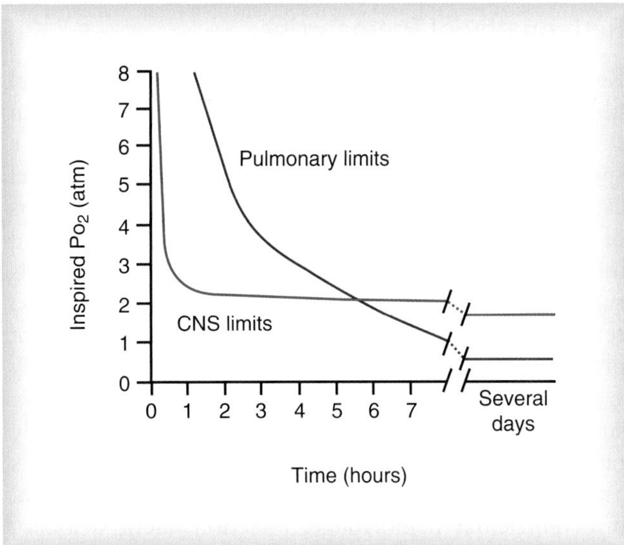

Figure 35-1
Relation between PO_2 and exposure time responsible for oxygen toxicity. *(Modified from Lambertsen CJ: In DiPalma JR, ed: Drill's pharmacology in medicine, New York, 1971, McGraw-Hill.)*

Oxygen Toxicity

Oxygen toxicity primarily affects the lungs and the central nervous system (CNS).[9-11] Two primary factors determine the harmful effects of oxygen: PO_2 and exposure time (Figure 35-1). The higher the PO_2 and the longer the exposure, the greater is the likelihood of damage. Effects on the CNS, including tremors, twitching, and convulsions, tend to occur only when a patient is breathing oxygen at pressures greater than 1 atm (*hyperbaric* pressure). On the other hand, pulmonary effects can occur at clinical PO_2 levels.

Table 35-2 summarizes the physiological response to breathing 100% oxygen at sea level. A patient exposed to a high PO_2 for a prolonged period has signs similar to those of **bronchopneumonia.** Patchy infiltrates appear on chest radiographs and usually are most prominent in the lower lung fields.

Underlying the gross clinical signs is major alveolar injury. Exposure to high PO_2 first damages the capillary endothelium. Interstitial edema follows and thickens the alveolar-capillary membrane. If the process continues, type I alveolar cells are destroyed, and type II cells proliferate. An **exudative** phase follows, resulting from alveolar fluid buildup, which leads to a low ventilation/perfusion ($\dot{V}/\dot{Q}$) ratio, physiological shunting, and hypoxemia. In the end stages, hyaline membranes form in the alveolar region, and pulmonary fibrosis and hypertension develop.

As the lung injury worsens, blood oxygenation deteriorates. If this progressive hypoxemia is managed with additional oxygen, the toxic effects worsen (Figure 35-2). However, if the patient can be kept alive while the fractional inspired oxygen concentration (FIO_2) is decreased, the pulmonary damage sometimes resolves.

The toxicity of oxygen is caused by overproduction of oxygen free radicals. Oxygen free radicals are byproducts of cellular metabolism. If unchecked, these radicals can severely damage or kill cells. Normally, however, special enzymes such as superoxide dismutase inactivate the oxygen free radicals before they can do serious damage. Antioxidants such as vitamin E, vitamin C, and β-carotene also can defend against oxygen free radicals.

These defenses normally are adequate to protect cells exposed to air. In the presence of high PO_2, however, free radicals can overwhelm the antioxidant systems and cause cell damage. Cell damage provokes an immune response and causes tissue infiltration by neutrophils and macrophages. These scavenger cells release inflammatory mediators that worsen the initial injury. At the

Table 35-2 ▶▶ Physiological Responses to Exposure to 100% Inspired Oxygen

Exposure Time (h)	Physiological Response
0-12	Normal pulmonary function Tracheobronchitis Substernal chest pain
12-24	Decreasing vital capacity
25-30	Decreasing lung compliance Increasing $P(A-a)O_2$ Decreasing exercise PO_2
30-72	Decreasing diffusing capacity

Adapted from Jenkinson SG: Respir Care 28:614, 1983.

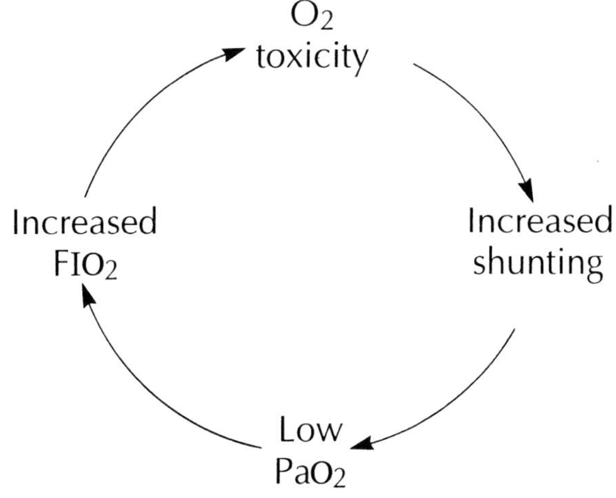

Figure 35-2
The vicious circle that can occur in managing hypoxemia with high FIO_2. High FIO_2 can be toxic to the lung parenchyma and cause further physiological shunting. Increased shunting worsens the hypoxemia, necessitating higher FIO_2. *(Modified from Flenley DC: Respir Care 28:876, 1983.)*

same time, local neutrophils and platelets may release more free radicals, which only continue the process.

Exactly how much oxygen is safe is the subject of heated debate. Results of most studies indicate that adults can breathe up to 50% for extended periods without major lung damage.[12] Rather than applying strict cutoffs, one can weigh both FIO_2 and exposure time in assessing the risks of high PO_2 (see Rule of Thumb).[13] The goal always should be to use the lowest possible FIO_2 compatible with adequate tissue oxygenation.

> **RULE OF THUMB**
>
> **Avoiding Oxygen Toxicity**
>
> Limit patient exposure to 100% oxygen to less than 24 hours whenever possible. High FIO_2 is acceptable if the concentration can be decreased to 70% within 2 days and 50% or less in 5 days.

Because the growing lung may be more sensitive to oxygen, more caution is needed with infants. High PO_2 also is associated with **retinopathy of prematurity** (ROP) and **bronchopulmonary dysplasia** in infants.

Regardless of approach, supplemental oxygen never should be withheld from a hypoxic patient. Although the toxic effects of high FIO_2 can be serious, the alternative is certain death due to tissue hypoxia.

Depression of Ventilation

When breathing moderate to high oxygen concentration, COPD patients with chronic hypercapnia tend to ventilate less.[14] Decreases in ventilation of nearly 20% have been observed among these patients with accompanying 20- to 23-mm Hg elevations in arterial partial pressure of carbon dioxide ($PaCO_2$).[15]

The primary reason some COPD patients hypoventilate when given oxygen is most likely suppression of the hypoxic drive. In these patients, the normal response to high partial pressure of carbon dioxide (PCO_2) is blunted, the primary stimulus to breathe being lack of oxygen, as sensed by the peripheral chemoreceptors. The increase in the blood oxygen level in these patients suppresses peripheral chemoreceptors, depresses ventilatory drive, and elevates the PCO_2.[16,17] High blood oxygen levels may disrupt the normal $\dot{V}/\dot{Q}$ balance and cause an increase in dead space to tidal volume ratio (V_{DS}/V_T) ratio and an increase in $PaCO_2$.[18]

That oxygen therapy can cause some patients to hypoventilate should never stop the RT from giving oxygen to a patient in need. Preventing hypoxia always is the first priority. Avoiding depression of ventilation during oxygen administration is discussed later.

Retinopathy of Prematurity

Retinopathy of prematurity (ROP), also called retrolental fibroplasia, is an abnormal eye condition that occurs in some premature or low-birth-weight infants who receive supplemental oxygen. An excessive blood oxygen level causes retinal vasoconstriction, which leads to necrosis of the blood vessels. In response, new vessels form and increase in number. Hemorrhage of these new vessels causes scarring behind the retina. Scarring leads to retinal detachment and blindness.[19] Retinopathy of prematurity mostly affects neonates up to approximately 1 month of age, by which time the retinal arteries have sufficiently matured. Excessive oxygen is not the only factor associated with ROP. Among the other factors associated with ROP are hypercapnia, hypocapnia, intraventricular hemorrhage, infection, lactic acidosis, anemia, hypocalcemia, and hypothermia.

Because premature infants often need supplemental oxygen, the risk of ROP poses a serious management problem. The American Academy of Pediatrics recommends keeping an infant's arterial PO_2 below 80 mm Hg as the best way of minimizing the risk of ROP.[8]

Absorption Atelectasis

An FIO_2 greater than 0.50 presents a significant risk of absorption atelectasis.[20] Nitrogen normally is the most plentiful gas in both the alveoli and the blood. Breathing high levels of oxygen quickly depletes body nitrogen levels. As blood nitrogen levels decrease, the total pressure of venous gases rapidly decreases. Under these conditions, gases that exist at atmospheric pressure within any body cavity rapidly diffuse into the venous blood. This principle is used for removing trapped air from body cavities. For example, giving patients high levels of oxygen can help clear trapped air from the abdomen or thorax.

Unfortunately, this same phenomenon can cause lung collapse, especially if the alveolar region becomes obstructed (Figure 35-3). Under these conditions, oxygen rapidly diffuses into the blood (Figure 35-3, *A*). With no source for repletion, the total gas pressure in the alveolus progressively decreases until the alveolus collapses. Because collapsed alveoli are perfused but not ventilated, absorption atelectasis increases the physiological shunt and worsens blood oxygenation.[20]

The risk of absorption atelectasis is greatest in patients breathing at low tidal volumes as a result of sedation, surgical pain, or CNS dysfunction. In these cases, poorly ventilated alveoli may become unstable when they lose oxygen faster than it can be replaced. The result is a more gradual shrinking of the alveoli that may lead to complete collapse, even when the patient is not breathing supplemental oxygen (Figure 35-3, *B*). For an

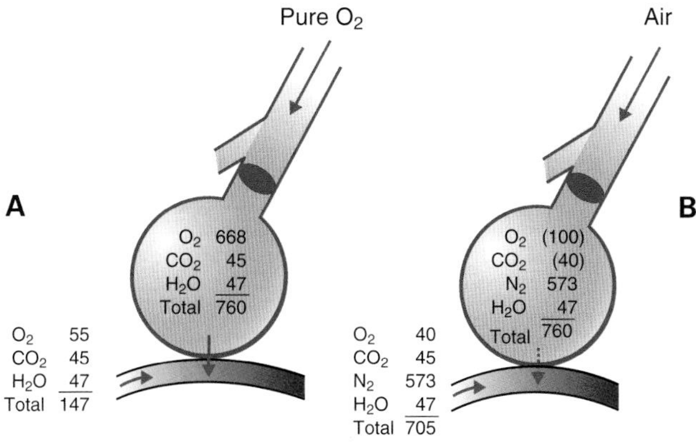

Figure 35-3
The development of atelectasis beyond blocked airways during breathing of oxygen **(A)** and air **(B)**. In both cases, the sum of the gas pressures in the mixed venous blood is less than in the alveoli. **B,** The PO_2 and the PCO_2 are in parentheses because these values change with time. However, the total alveolar pressure remains within a few millimeters of mercury of 760. *(Modified from West JB: Respiratory physiology: the essentials, ed 3, Baltimore, 1985, Williams & Wilkins.)*

alert patient this is not a great risk, because the natural sigh mechanism periodically hyperinflates the lung.

Oxygen Delivery Systems: Design and Performance

Respiratory therapists can select from an array of systems for administering oxygen and other therapeutic gases. Proper device selection requires in-depth knowledge of both the general performance characteristics of these systems and the individual capabilities.[21]

Oxygen delivery devices traditionally are categorized by design. Three basic designs exist: **low flow, reservoir,** and **high flow**. Enclosures, commonly identified as a fourth category, are really head- or body-surrounding reservoirs. The design categories share functional characteristics, capabilities, and limitations.

Although design plays an important role in the selection of these devices, clinical performance ultimately determines how the device is used. The user judges the performance of an oxygen delivery system by answering two key questions. First, how much oxygen can the system deliver (the FIO_2 or FIO_2 range)? Second, does the delivered FIO_2 remain fixed or vary under changing patient demands[22]?

Regarding the FIO_2 range, oxygen systems can be broadly divided into those designed to deliver a low (<35%), moderate (35% to 60%), or high oxygen concentration (>60%). Some designs can deliver oxygen across the full range of concentrations (21% to 100%).

Whether a device delivers a **fixed** or **variable** FIO_2 depends on how much of the patient's inspired gas it supplies. If the system provides *all* the patient's inspired gas, the FIO_2 remains stable, even under changing demands. If the device provides only *some* of the inspired gas, the patient must draw the remainder from the surrounding air. In this case, the more the patient breathes, the more air dilutes the delivered oxygen, and the lower is the FIO_2. If the patient breathes less with this type of device, less air dilutes the oxygen, and the FIO_2 increases. A system that supplies only a portion of

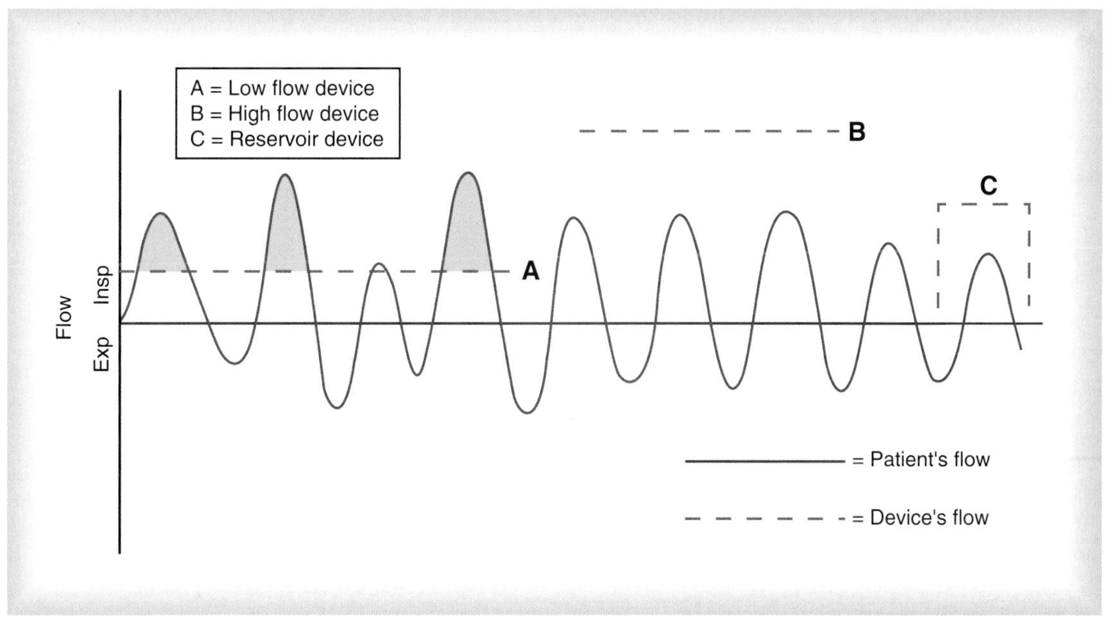

Figure 35-4
Differences between oxygen delivery systems. **A,** Low-flow device; **B,** high-flow device; **C,** reservoir device.

Table 35-3 ▶▶▶ Overview of Oxygen Therapy Systems

Category	Device	Flow	FIO_2 Range	FIO_2 Stability	Advantages	Disadvantages	Best Use
Low flow	Nasal cannula	¼-8 L/min (adults) ≤2 L/min (infants)	22%-45%	Variable	Use on adults, children, infants; easy to use; disposable; low cost; well tolerated	Unstable, easily dislodged; high flow uncomfortable; can cause dryness, bleeding; polyps; deviated septum and mouth breathing may reduce FIO_2	Patient in stable condition who needs low FIO_2; home care patient who needs long-term therapy, low to moderate FIO_2 while eating
	Nasal catheter	¼-8 L/min	22%-45%	Variable	Use on adults, children, infants; good stability; disposable; low cost	Difficult to insert; high flow increases back pressure; needs regular changing; polyps, deviated septum may block insertion; may provoke gagging, air swallowing, aspiration	Procedures in which cannula is difficult to use (bronchoscopy); long-term care of infants
	Transtracheal catheter	¼-4 L/min	22%-35%	Variable	Lower O_2 use and cost; eliminates nasal and skin irritation; improved compliance; increased exercise tolerance; increased mobility; enhanced image	High cost; surgical complications; infection; mucus plugging; lost tract	Home care or ambulatory patients who need increased mobility or do not accept nasal oxygen
Reservoir	Reservoir cannula	¼-4 L/min	22%-35%	Variable	Lower O_2 use and cost; increased mobility; less discomfort because of lower flow	Unattractive, cumbersome; poor compliance; must be regularly replaced; breathing pattern affects performance	Home care or ambulatory patients who need increased mobility
	Simple mask	5-12 L/min	35%-50%	Variable	Use on adults, children, infants; quick, easy to apply; disposable, inexpensive	Uncomfortable; must be removed for eating; prevents radiant heat loss; blocks vomitus in unconscious patients	Emergencies, short-term therapy requiring moderate FIO_2, mouth breathing patients requiring moderate FIO_2
	Partial rebreathing mask	6-10 L/min (prevent bag collapse on inspiration)	35%-60%	Variable	Same as simple mask; moderate to high FIO_2	Same as simple mask; potential suffocation hazard	Emergencies, short-term therapy requiring moderate to high FIO_2
	Nonbreathing mask	6-10 L/min (prevent bag collapse on inspiration)	55%-70%	Variable	Same as simple mask; high FIO_2	Same as simple mask; potential suffocation hazard	Emergencies, short-term therapy requiring high FIO_2
	Nonbreathing circuit (closed)	$3 \times V_E$ (prevent bag collapse on inspiration)	21%-100%	Fixed	Full range of FIO_2	Potential suffocation hazard; requires 50 psi air/O_2; blender failure common	Patients who need precise FIO_2 at any level (21%-100%)

Table 35-3 ▶▶▶ Overview of Oxygen Therapy Systems—cont'd

Category	Device	Flow	F_{IO_2} Range	F_{IO_2} Stability	Advantages	Disadvantages	Best Use
High flow	Air-entrainment mask	Varies; should provide output flow >60 L/min	24%-50%	Fixed	Easy to apply; disposable, inexpensive; stable, precise F_{IO_2}	Limited to adult use; uncomfortable, noisy; must be removed for eating; F_{IO_2} >0.40 not ensured; F_{IO_2} varies with back pressure	Patients in unstable condition who need precise low F_{IO_2}
	Air-entrainment nebulizer	10-15 L/min input; should provide output flow of at least 60 L/min	28%-100%	Fixed	Provides temperature control and extra humidification	F_{IO_2} <0.28 or >0.40 not ensured; F_{IO_2} varies with back pressure; high infection risk	Patients with artificial airways who need low to moderate F_{IO_2}
	Blending system (open)	Should provide output flow of at least 60 L/min	21%-100%	Fixed	Full range of F_{IO_2}	Requires 50 psi air + O_2; blender failure or inaccuracy common	Patients with high $\dot{V}_E$ who need high F_{IO_2}
Enclosure	Oxyhood	≥7 L/min	21%-100%	Fixed	Full range of F_{IO_2}	Difficult to clean, disinfect	Infants who need supplemental oxygen
	Isolette	8-15 L/min	40%-50%	Variable	Provides temperature control	Expensive, cumbersome; unstable F_{IO_2} (leaks); difficult to clean, disinfect; limits patient mobility; fire hazard	Infants who need supplemental oxygen and precise thermal regulation
	Tent	12-15 L/min	40%-50%	Variable	Provides concurrent aerosol therapy	Expensive, cumbersome; unstable F_{IO_2} (leaks); requires cooling; difficult to clean, disinfect; limits patient mobility; fire hazard	Toddlers or small children who need low to moderate F_{IO_2} and aerosol

$\dot{V}_E$, Minute volume.

the inspired gas always provides a variable FIO_2.[23] The FIO_2 supplied with such systems can vary widely from minute to minute and even from breath to breath.

Figure 35-4 demonstrates these concepts as applied to low-flow, reservoir, and high-flow systems. With the low-flow system (Fig. 35-4, *A*) the patient's inspiratory flow often exceeds that delivered by the device; the result is air dilution *(shaded areas)*. The greater the patient's inspiratory flow, the more air is breathed, and the lower is the FIO_2. The high-flow system (Fig. 35-4, *B*) always exceeds the patient's flow and thus provides a fixed FIO_2. A fixed FIO_2 can be achieved with a reservoir system (Fig. 35-4, *C*), which stores a reserve volume (flow × time) that equals or exceeds the patient's tidal volume. For a reservoir system to provide a fixed FIO_2, the reservoir volume must always exceed the patient's tidal volume, and there cannot be any air leaks in the system.

Table 35-3 outlines the general specifications for the common oxygen therapy systems in current use.

Low-Flow Systems

Typical low-flow systems provide supplemental oxygen directly to the airway at a flow of 8 L/min or less. Because the inspiratory flow of a healthy adult exceeds 8 L/min, the oxygen provided by a low-flow device is always diluted with air; the result is a low and variable FIO_2. Low-flow oxygen delivery systems include the nasal cannula, the nasal catheter, and the transtracheal catheter.

Nasal Cannula. The nasal cannula is a disposable plastic device consisting of two tips or prongs approximately 1 cm long connected to several feet of small-bore oxygen supply tubing (Figure 35-5). The user inserts the prongs directly into the vestibule of the nose while attaching the supply tubing either directly to a flowmeter or to a bubble humidifier. In most cases, a humidifier is used only when the input flow exceeds 4 L/min.[2] Even with extra humidity, flow greater than 6 to 8 L/min can cause patient discomfort, including nasal dryness and bleeding.[21] In newborns and infants, flow must be limited to a maximum of 2 L/min.[2] Table 35-3 lists the FIO_2 range, FIO_2 stability, advantages, disadvantages, and best use of the nasal cannula.

Nasal Catheter. A nasal catheter is a soft plastic tube with several small holes at the tip. The therapist inserts the catheter by gently advancing it along the floor of either nasal passage and visualizing it just behind and above the uvula (Figure 35-6). If there is marked resistance to insertion, the other naris is used. Once in position, the catheter is taped to the bridge of the nose. If direct visualization is not possible, the catheter is blindly inserted to a depth equal to the distance from the nose to the tragus (lobe) of either ear. Placed too deep, the catheter can provoke gagging or swallowing of gas, which increases the likelihood of aspiration. Because a it affects production of secretions, a nasal catheter should be removed and replaced with a new one (placed in the opposite naris) at least every 8 hours.

Nasal cannulas have largely replaced catheters for simple oxygen administration. Table 35-3 lists the FIO_2 range, FIO_2 stability, advantages, disadvantages, and best use of the nasal catheter.

Transtracheal Catheter. The transtracheal oxygen catheter was first described by Heimlich in 1982.[24] A physician

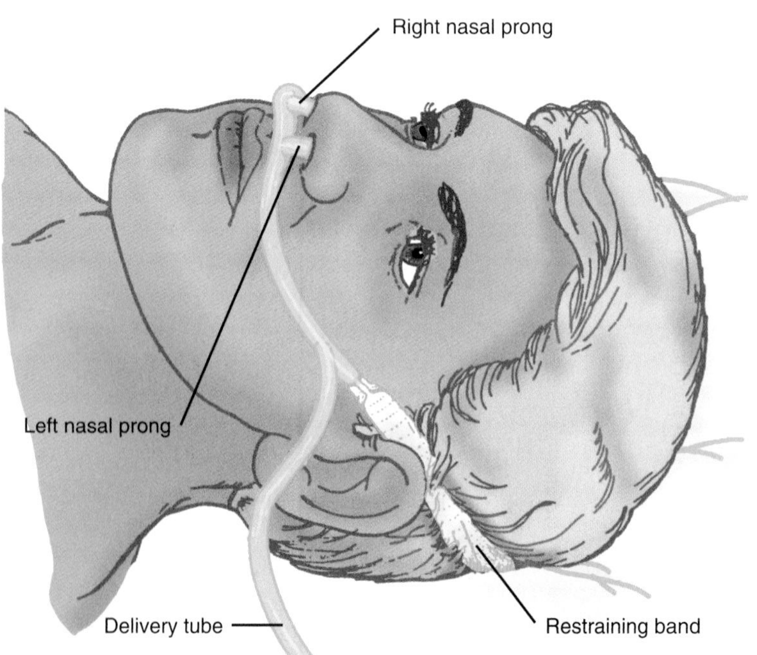

Figure 35-5
Nasal cannula.

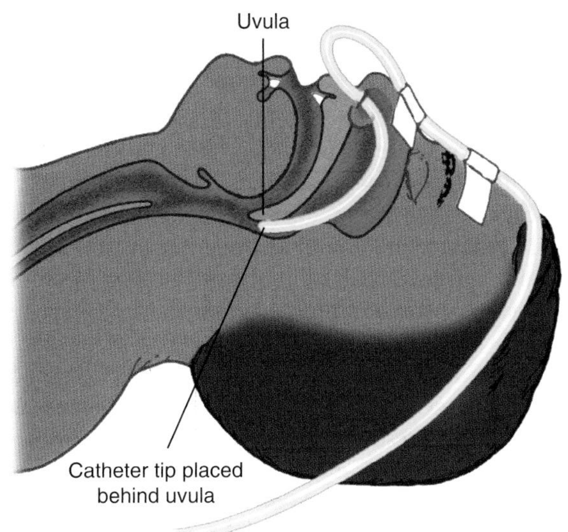

Figure 35-6
Placement of nasal catheter in the nasopharynx.

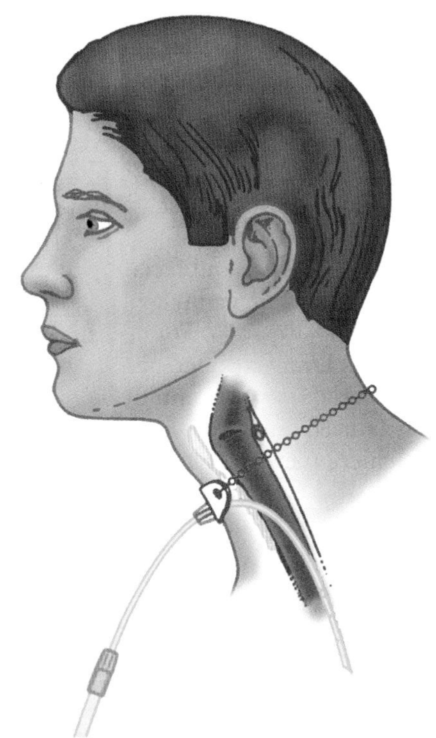

Figure 35-7
Transtracheal oxygen catheter.

surgically inserts this thin polytetrafluoroethylene (Teflon) catheter with a guidewire directly into the trachea between the second and third tracheal rings (Figure 35-7). A custom-sized chain necklace secures the catheter in position. Standard tubing connected directly to a flowmeter provides the oxygen source flow.[25] Because flow is so low, no humidifier is needed.

Because the transtracheal catheter resides directly in the trachea, oxygen builds up both there and in the upper airway during expiration. This process effectively expands the anatomic reservoir and increases the FIO_2 at any given flow. Compared with a nasal cannula, a transtracheal catheter needs 40% to 60% less oxygen flow to achieve a given arterial partial pressure of oxygen (PaO_2).[26] Some patients need a flow of only 0.25 L/min to achieve adequate oxygenation. This can be of great economic benefit to those needing continuous long-term oxygen therapy. In addition, the low flow used with transtracheal delivery increases the duration of flow, or use time, for portable oxygen storage systems. This benefit can dramatically increase patient mobility.

Transtracheal oxygen therapy can pose problems and risks. As a result, these devices have not received widespread acceptance. Careful patient selection, rigorous patient education, and ongoing self-care with professional follow-up evaluation can help minimize these risks. Chapter 49 provides details on these aspects of transtracheal oxygen therapy. Table 35-3 lists the FIO_2 range, FIO_2 stability, advantages, disadvantages, and best use of the transtracheal catheter.

Performance Characteristics of Low-Flow Systems

Research studies on nasal low-flow systems show oxygen concentration ranging from as low as 22% at 1 L/min to as high as 60% at 15 L/min.[21] The range of 22% to 45% cited in Table 35-3 is based on 8 L/min as the upper limit of comfortable flow. These wide FIO_2 ranges occur because the oxygen concentration delivered by a low-flow system varies with the amount of air dilution. The amount of air dilution depends on several patient and equipment variables. Table 35-4 summarizes these key variables and how they affect the FIO_2 provided by low-flow systems.

Simple formulas exist for estimating the FIO_2 provided by low-flow systems (see the Rule of Thumb). Given the

Table 35-4 ▶▶ Variables Affecting the FIO_2 of Low-Flow Oxygen Systems

Increases FIO_2	Decreases FIO_2
Higher O_2 input	Lower O_2 input
Mouth-closed breathing*	Mouth-open breathing*
Low inspiratory flow	High inspiratory flow
Low tidal volume	High tidal volume
Slow rate of breathing	Fast rate of breathing
Small minute ventilation	Large minute ventilation
Long inspiratory time	Short inspiratory time
High I:E ratio	Low I:E ratio

*Cannula only.

large number of variables affecting FIO_2, however, the RT can never know precisely how much oxygen a patient is receiving with these systems. Even if it were possible to measure the exact FIO_2, this value could change from minute to minute and even from breath to breath. Without knowing the patient's exact FIO_2, the RT must rely on assessing the actual response to oxygen therapy.

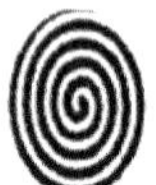

RULE OF THUMB

Estimating the FIO_2 Provided by Low-Flow Systems

For patients with a normal rate and depth of breathing, each liter per minute of nasal oxygen increases the FIO_2 approximately 4%. For example, a patient using a nasal cannula at 4 L/min has an estimated FIO_2 of approximately 37% (21 + 16).

Troubleshooting Low-Flow Systems

Common problems with low-flow oxygen delivery systems include inaccurate flow, system leaks and obstructions, device displacement, and skin irritation.

The problem of inaccurate flow is greatest when low-flow flowmeters (≤3 L/min) are used. Given the trend toward assessment of outcome of oxygen therapy (with either blood gases or pulse oximetry), ensuring the absolute accuracy of oxygen input flow usually is not essential. Nonetheless, like all respiratory care equipment, flowmeters should be subjected to regular preventive maintenance and testing for accuracy. Equipment failing preventive maintenance standards should be removed from service and repaired or replaced.

Table 35-5 provides guidance on troubleshooting the most common clinical problems with nasal cannulas. Details on troubleshooting transtracheal catheters are provided in Chapter 49.

Reservoir Systems

Reservoir systems incorporate a mechanism for gathering and storing oxygen between patient breaths. Patients draw on this reserve supply whenever inspiratory flow exceeds oxygen flow into the device. Because air dilution is reduced, reservoir devices generally provide higher FIO_2 than do low-flow systems. Reservoir devices can decrease oxygen use by providing FIO_2 comparable with that of nonreservoir systems but at lower flow.

Reservoir systems in current use include reservoir cannulas, masks, and nonrebreathing circuits. In principle, enclosure systems, such as tents and hoods, operate as head- or body-surrounding reservoirs.

Reservoir Cannula. Reservoir cannulas are designed to conserve oxygen. There are two types of reservoir cannulas: nasal reservoir and pendant reservoir. Table 35-3 lists the FIO_2 range, FIO_2 stability, advantages, disadvantages, and best use of the reservoir cannula.

The nasal reservoir cannula operates by storing approximately 20 mL of oxygen in a small membrane reservoir during exhalation (Figure 35-8). The patient draws on this stored oxygen during early inspiration. The amount of oxygen available increases with each breath and decreases the flow needed for a given FIO_2. Although the device is comfortable to wear, many patients object to its appearance and may not always comply with prescribed therapy.

The pendant reservoir system helps overcome aesthetic concerns by hiding the reservoir under the patient's clothing on the anterior chest wall (Figure 35-9). Although the device is less visible, the extra weight of the pendant can cause ear and facial discomfort.

At low flow, reservoir cannulas can reduce oxygen use as much as 50% to 75%. For example, a patient at rest who needs 2 L/min through a standard cannula to achieve an arterial oxygen saturation (SaO_2) greater than 90% may need only 0.5 L/min through a reservoir cannula to achieve the same blood oxygenation. During exercise, reservoir cannulas can reduce flow needs approximately 66%; the savings is approximately 50% at high flow.[26]

Although flow savings is fairly predictable, factors such as nasal anatomy and breathing pattern can affect the performance of the device. For these devices to function properly at low flow, patients must exhale through the

Table 35-5 ▶▶ Troubleshooting Common Problems With a Nasal Oxygen Cannula

Problem or Clue	Cause	Solution
No gas flow can be felt coming from the cannula	Flowmeter not on	Adjust flowmeter
	System leak	Check connections
Humidifier pop-off is sounding	Obstruction distal to humidifier	Find and correct the obstruction
	Flow is set too high	Use alternative device
	Obstructed naris	Use alternative device
Patient reports soreness over lip or ears	Irritation or inflammation caused by appliance straps	Loosen straps Place cotton balls at pressure points Use a different device
Mouth breathing	Habitual mouth breathing, blocked nasal passages	Switch to simple mask or ventari mask

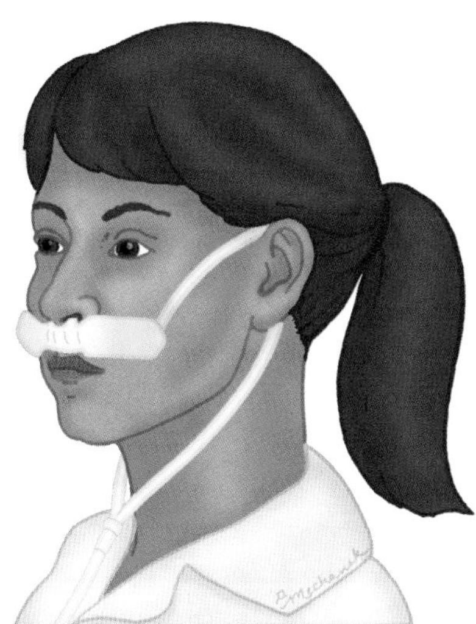

Figure 35-8
Reservoir cannula.

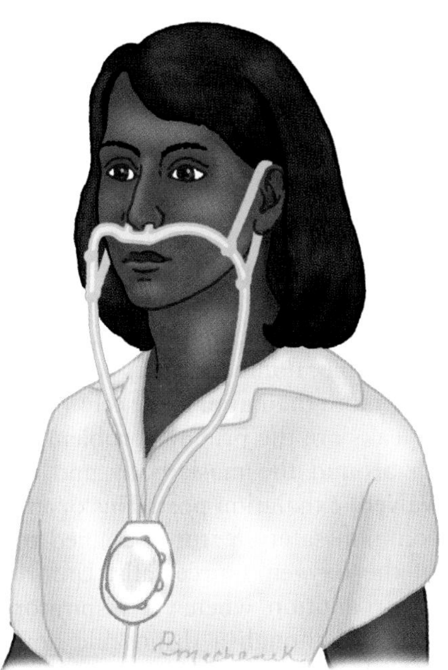

Figure 35-9
Pendant reservoir cannula.

nose (this reopens or resets the reservoir membrane). In addition, exhalation through pursed lips may impair performance, especially during exercise. For these reasons, prescribed flow settings should be individually determined by means of monitoring SaO_2 during both rest and exercise.[26]

The low flow at which the reservoir cannula operates makes humidification unnecessary. Excess moisture can hinder proper action of the reservoir membrane.[26] Even regular use can cause membrane wear. For this reason, patients should replace the reservoir cannula approximately every 3 weeks. Replacement needs partially offset the oxygen cost savings afforded by these devices.

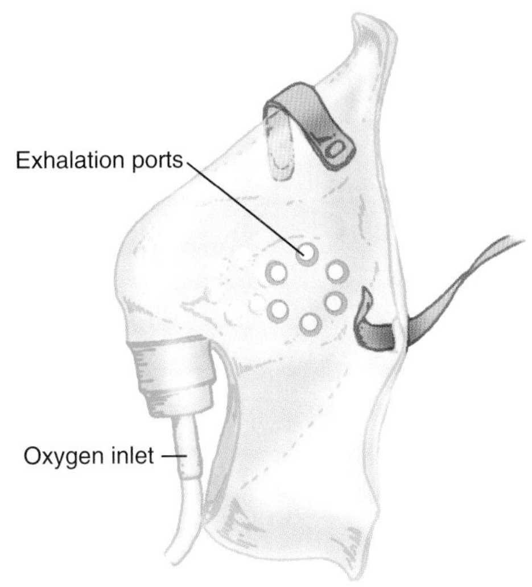

Figure 35-10
Simple oxygen mask.

Reservoir Masks. Masks are the most commonly used reservoir systems. There are three types of reservoir masks: the simple mask, the partial rebreathing mask, and the nonrebreathing mask. Table 35-3 lists the FIO_2 range, FIO_2 stability, advantages, disadvantages, and best use of each of these devices.

The simple mask is a disposable plastic unit designed to cover both the mouth and the nose (Figure 35-10). The body of the mask itself gathers and stores oxygen between patient breaths. The patient exhales directly through open holes or ports in the mask body. Should oxygen input flow cease, the patient can draw in air through these holes and around the mask edge.

The input flow range for an adult simple mask is 5 to 12 L/min. In general, if flow greater than 12 L/min is needed for satisfactory oxygenation, use of a device capable of a higher FIO_2 should be considered. At a flow less than 5 L/min, the mask volume acts as dead space and causes carbon dioxide rebreathing.[27]

Because air dilution easily occurs during inspiration through its ports and around its body, the simple mask provides a variable FIO_2. How much the FIO_2 varies depends on the oxygen input flow, the mask volume, the extent of air leakage, and the patient's breathing pattern.[28]

As shown in Figure 35-11, the partial rebreathing mask and the nonrebreathing mask have a similar design. Each has a 1-L flexible reservoir bag attached to the oxygen inlet. Because the bag increases the reservoir volume, both masks provide higher FIO_2 capabilities than does a simple mask.

The key difference between these designs is the use of valves. A partial rebreather has no valves (Figure 35-11, *A*). During inspiration, source oxygen flows into the

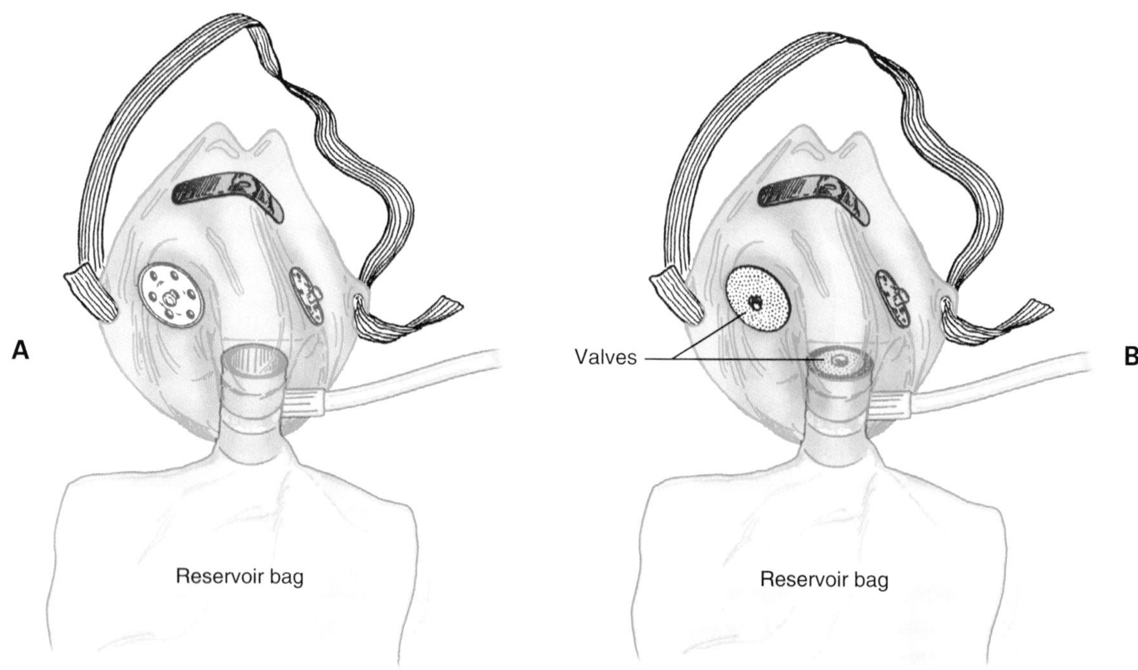

Figure 35-11
A, partial rebreathing mask; **B,** nonrebreathing mask.

mask and passes directly to the patient. During exhalation, source oxygen enters the bag. However, because no valves separate the mask and the bag, some of the patient's exhaled gas also enters the bag (approximately the first third). Because it comes from the anatomic dead space, the early portion of exhaled gas contains mostly oxygen and little carbon dioxide. As the bag fills with both oxygen and dead space gas, the last two thirds of exhalation (high in carbon dioxide) escapes out the exhalation ports of the mask. As long as the oxygen input flow keeps the bag from collapsing during inhalation, carbon dioxide rebreathing is negligible.

Although it can provide higher FIO_2 than a simple mask (see Table 35-3), the standard disposable partial rebreather is subject to considerable air dilution. The result is delivery of a moderate but variable FIO_2 dependent on the same factors as with the simple mask.

A nonrebreathing mask prevents rebreathing with one-way valves (Figure 35-11, *B*). An inspiratory valve sits atop the bag, and expiratory valves cover the exhalation ports on the mask body. During inspiration, slight negative mask pressure closes the expiratory valves, preventing air dilution. At the same time, the inspiratory valve atop the bag opens, providing oxygen to the patient. During exhalation, valve action reverses the direction of flow. Slight positive pressure closes the inspiratory valve, which prevents exhaled gas from entering the bag. Concurrently, the one-way expiratory valves open and divert exhaled gas out to the atmosphere.

Because it is a closed system, a leak-free nonrebreathing mask with competent valves and enough flow to prevent bag collapse during inspiration can deliver 100% source gas. As indicated in Table 35-3, however, modern disposable nonrebreathers normally do not provide much more than approximately 70% oxygen.[21]

Large air leaks are the primary problem. Air leakage occurs both around the mask body and through the open (nonvalved) exhalation port. This open exhalation port is a common safety feature designed to allow air breathing if the oxygen source fails. Unfortunately, it also allows air dilution whenever inspiratory flow or volume is high. Although a disposable nonrebreather can deliver moderate to high oxygen concentration, the FIO_2 still varies with the amount of air leakage and the patient's breathing pattern.

Nonrebreathing Reservoir Circuit. A nonrebreathing circuit operates with the same design principles as a nonrebreathing mask but is more versatile. Unlike nonrebreathing masks, these systems can provide a full range of FIO_2 (21%-100%) and deliver the prescribed concentration to both intubated and nonintubated patients.[21] As shown in Figure 35-12, a typical nonrebreathing circuit incorporates a blending system to premix air and oxygen. The gas mixture is warmed and humidified, ideally with a servo-controlled heated humidifier. Gas then flows through large-bore tubing into an inspiratory volume reservoir, which includes a fail-safe inlet valve. The patient breathes through a

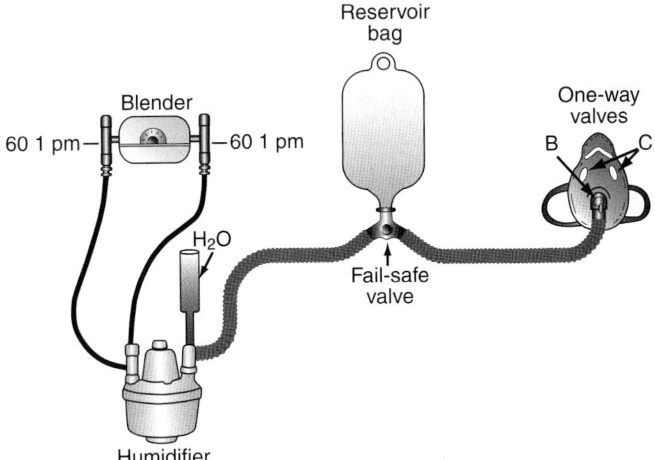

Figure 35-12
Nonrebreathing reservoir circuit with a valved face mask. Reservoir bag in combination with high-flow (0 to 100 L/min) flowmeters ensures delivery of set FIO_2. *(Modified from Foust GN et al: Chest 99:1346, 1991.)*

closed airway appliance, in this case a mask with one-way valves. A valved T tube also can be used in the care of a patient with an endotracheal or tracheostomy tube.

Troubleshooting Reservoir Systems. Common problems with reservoir masks include device displacement, system leaks and obstructions, improper flow adjustment, and skin irritation. Table 35-6 provides guidance on troubleshooting the most common clinical problems with reservoir masks.

High-Flow Systems

High-flow systems supply a given oxygen concentration at a flow equaling or exceeding the patient's peak inspiratory flow. An air-entrainment or a blending system is used. As long as the delivered flow exceeds the patient's flow, both systems can ensure a fixed FIO_2. The following Rule of Thumb can help determine which devices truly qualify as high-flow systems.

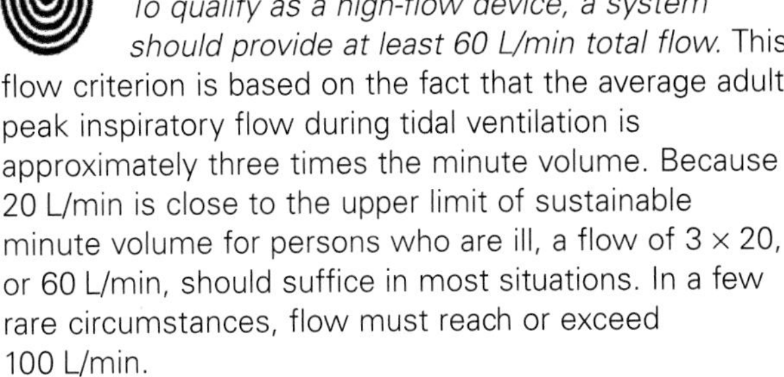

RULE OF THUMB

To qualify as a high-flow device, a system should provide at least 60 L/min total flow. This flow criterion is based on the fact that the average adult peak inspiratory flow during tidal ventilation is approximately three times the minute volume. Because 20 L/min is close to the upper limit of sustainable minute volume for persons who are ill, a flow of 3 × 20, or 60 L/min, should suffice in most situations. In a few rare circumstances, flow must reach or exceed 100 L/min.

Principles of Gas Mixing. All high-flow systems mix air and oxygen to achieve a given FIO_2. These gases are mixed with air-entrainment devices or blending systems. Computations involving mixtures of air and oxygen are based on a modified form of the dilution equation for solutions:

$$V_FC_F = V_1C_1 + V_2C_2$$

In this equation, V_1 and V_2 are the volumes of the two gases being mixed; C_1 and C_2, the oxygen concentration in these two volumes; and V_F and C_F, the final volume and concentration of the resulting mixture.

Box 35-1 shows how to apply variations of this equation to compute (1) the final concentration of a mixture of air and oxygen, (2) the air-to-oxygen ratio needed to obtain a given FIO_2, (3) the total output flow from an air-entrainment device, and (4) the amount of oxygen that must be added to a volume of air to obtain a given FIO_2. The Mini Clinis show clinical examples of these computations.

Table 35-6 ▸▸ Troubleshooting Common Problems With Reservoir Masks

Problem or Clue	Cause	Solution
Patient constantly removes mask	Claustrophobia Confusion	Use alternative device Restrain patient
No gas flow can be detected	Flowmeter not on System leak	Adjust flowmeter Check connections
Humidifier pop-off is sounding	Obstruction distal to humidifier High input flow Jammed inspiratory valve	Find and correct obstruction Omit humidifier if therapy is short term Fix or replace valve
Reservoir bag collapses when the patient inhales	Flow is inadequate	Increase flow
Reservoir bag remains inflated throughout inhalation	Large mask leak Inspiratory valve jammed or reversed	Correct leak Repair or replace mask
Erythema develops over face or ears	Irritation or inflammation due to appliance or straps	Reposition mask or straps Place cotton balls over ear pressure points Provide skin care

Box 35-1 • Equations for Computing Oxygen Percentage, Ratio, and Flow*

1. To compute the oxygen percentage of a mixture of air and oxygen:

$$\%O_2 = \frac{(\text{Air flow} \times 21) + (O_2 \text{ flow} \times 100)}{\text{Total flow}} \quad \textit{Equation 35-1}$$

2. To compute the air-to-oxygen ratio needed to obtain a given oxygen percentage:

$$\frac{\text{Liters air}}{\text{Liters } O_2} = \frac{(100 - \%O_2)}{(\%O_2 - 21)} \quad \textit{Equation 35-2}$$

3. To compute the total output flow from an air-entrainment device (given the oxygen input):
   a. Compute the air-to-oxygen ratio (Equation 35-2).
   b. Add the air-to-oxygen ratio parts.
   c. Multiply the sum of the ratio parts by the oxygen input flow.
4. To compute the flow of oxygen and air needed to obtain a given oxygen percentage at a given total flow:
   a. Compute the oxygen flow:

$$O_2 \text{ flow} = \frac{\text{Total flow} \times (O_2\% - 21)}{79} \quad \textit{Equation 35-3}$$

   b. Compute the air flow:

$$\text{Air flow} = \text{Total flow} - O_2 \text{ flow}$$

*For simplicity, in all equations percentage concentration (0 to 100) is used instead of decimal-based FIO_2. To convert a computed percentage to the corresponding FIO_2, divide by 100.

MINI CLINI

Computing the Total Flow Output of an Air-Entrainment Device

PROBLEM

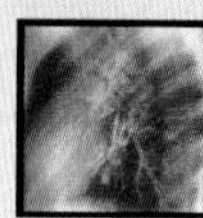

A patient is receiving oxygen through an air-entrainment device set to deliver 50% oxygen. The input oxygen flow is set to 15 L/min. What is the total output flow of this system?

SOLUTION

Step 1: Compute the air-to-oxygen ratio by substituting 50 for the $\%O_2$ in Equation 35-2:

$$\frac{\text{Liters air}}{\text{Liters } O_2} = \frac{(100 - \%O_2)}{(\%O_2 - 21)}$$

$$\frac{\text{Liters air}}{\text{Liters } O_2} = \frac{(100 - 50)}{(50 - 21)}$$

$$\frac{\text{Liters air}}{\text{Liters } O_2} = \frac{50}{29}$$

$$\frac{\text{Liters air}}{\text{Liters } O_2} \approx \frac{1.7}{1}$$

Step 2: Add the air-to-oxygen ratio parts:

$$1.7 + 1 = 2.7$$

Step 3: Multiply the sum of the ratio parts times the oxygen input flow:

$$2.7 \times 15 \text{ L/min} \approx 41 \text{ L/min}$$

An air-entrainment device set to deliver 50% oxygen that has an input flow of 15 L/min provides a total output flow of approximately 41 L/min.

MINI CLINI

Determining the FIO_2 of an Air-Oxygen Mixture

PROBLEM

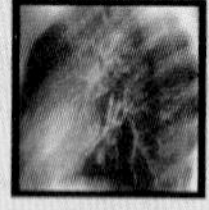

An air-entrainment device mixes at a fixed ratio of three volumes of air to each volume of oxygen (3:1 ratio). What is the resulting FIO_2?

SOLUTION

Substituting air, oxygen, and total (air + oxygen) volumes into Equation 35-1:

$$\%O_2 = \frac{(\text{Air flow} \times 21) + (O_2 \text{ flow} \times 100)}{\text{Total flow}}$$

$$\%O_2 = \frac{(3 \times 21) + (1 \times 100)}{3 + 1}$$

$$\%O_2 = 41$$

An air-entrainment device that mixes three volumes of air with one volume of oxygen provides a gas mixture with an FIO_2 of approximately 0.40.

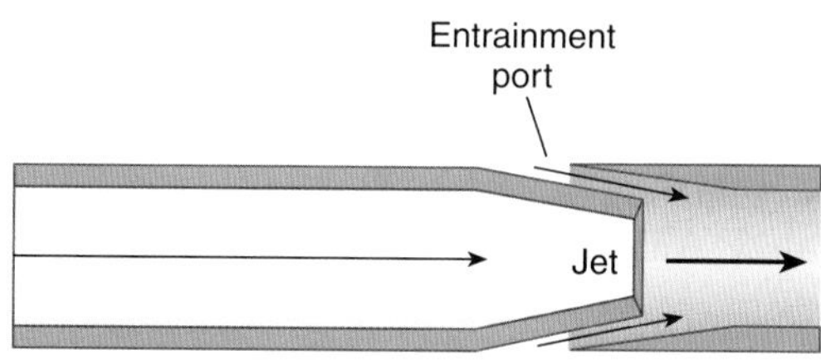

Figure 35-13
Basic components of an air-entrainment system. Pressurized gas passes through a nozzle or jet, beyond which are air-entrainment ports. Shear forces at the jet orifice entrain air into the primary gas stream, diluting the oxygen and increasing the total flow output of the device.

Air-Entrainment Systems. Air-entrainment systems direct a high-pressure oxygen source through a small nozzle or jet surrounded by air-entrainment ports (Figure 35-13). The amount of air entrained at these ports varies directly with the size of the port and the velocity of oxygen at the jet. The larger the intake ports and the higher the gas velocity at the jet, the more air is entrained.

Because they dilute source oxygen with air, entrainment devices always provide less than 100% oxygen.

The more air they entrain, the higher is the total output flow, but the lower is the delivered F_{IO_2}. *High flow is possible only when low oxygen concentration is delivered.* For these reasons, air-entrainment devices function as true high-flow systems only at low F_{IO_2}. If the flow output from an air-entrainment device decreases below a patient's inspiratory flow, air dilution occurs, and the F_{IO_2} becomes variable.

The F_{IO_2} provided by air-entrainment devices depends on two key variables: the air-to-oxygen ratio and the amount of flow resistance downstream from the mixing site. Changing the input flow of an air-entrainment device alters the total output flow but has little effect on delivered F_{IO_2}. In general, F_{IO_2} remains within 1% to 2% of that specified by the manufacturer, regardless of input flow.[29]

The size of the jet and entrainment ports of a device determines the air-to-oxygen ratio and thus the delivered F_{IO_2}. The Mini Clini shows how to compute the F_{IO_2} provided by an air-entrainment system if the air-to-oxygen ratio is known.

A more common clinical problem arises when the total output flow from an air-entrainment system must be determined. As described in the previous Rule of Thumb, the total flow output of a system determines whether it truly performs as a high-flow device. The Mini Clini shows how to determine the total output flow of an air-entrainment system.

Rather than using Equation 35-2 to compute air-to-oxygen ratio, many RTs derive quick estimates by using a simple mathematical aid called the magic box (Figure 35-14). To use the magic box, simply draw a square and place *20* in the top left corner and *100* in the bottom left corner. Place the desired oxygen percentage in the center of the box (in this case 70%). Subtract diagonally from lower left to the upper right (disregard the sign). Subtract diagonally again from upper left to lower right (disregard the sign). The resulting numerator (30) is the value for air, the denominator (50) being the value for oxygen.

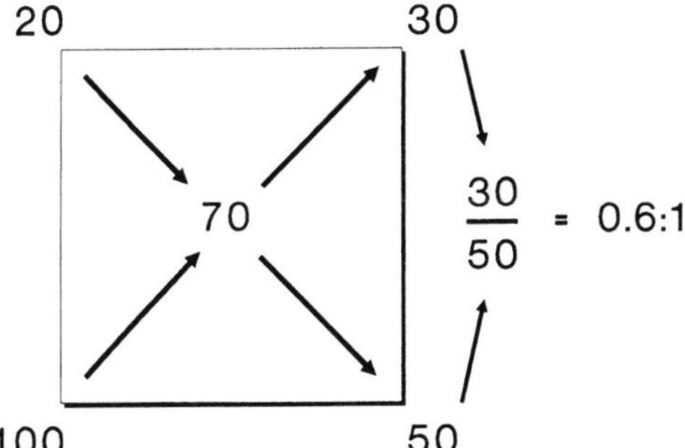

Figure 35-14
The magic box used to estimate air-to-oxygen ratio.

By convention, the air-to-oxygen ratio is expressed with the denominator (liters of oxygen) set to 1. Thus an air-entrainment device with a 7:1 ratio mixes 7 L of air with each liter of oxygen. To reduce any ratio to a ratio of *x*:1, divide both the numerator and the denominator by the denominator. In the magic box example:

$$\frac{30}{50} = \frac{30/50}{50/50} = \frac{0.61}{1}$$

The magic box can be used only for estimation of air-to-oxygen ratio. For absolute accuracy, Equation 35-2 always should be used. Based on Equation 35-2, Table 35-7 lists the approximate air-to-oxygen ratios for several common oxygen percentages.

The other major factor determining the oxygen concentration provided by an air-entrainment device is downstream flow resistance. In the presence of flow resistance distal to the jet, the volume of air entrained always decreases. With less air being entrained, total flow output decreases, and the delivered oxygen concentration increases.

Although the delivered oxygen concentration increases, the actual F_{IO_2} received by the patient may decrease, especially on devices set to deliver 30% to 50% oxygen.[29] This phenomenon is caused mainly by the decrease in total output flow. As the total output flow decreases below that needed to meet the patient's inspiratory needs, room air must be inhaled. A similar event occurs if the air intake ports surrounding the jet are blocked. Under both conditions, these high-flow systems begin to behave as low-flow devices.

The two most common oxygen delivery systems in which air entrainment is used are the air-entrainment mask (AEM) and the air-entrainment nebulizer.

Table 35-7 ▶▶ Approximate Air-to-Oxygen Ratios for Common Oxygen Concentrations*

Approximate Air-to-Oxygen Ratio	Percentage Oxygen	Total Ratio Parts
100	0:1	1
80	0.3:1	1.3
70	0.6:1	1.6
60	1:1	2
50	1.7:1	2.7
45	2:1	3
40	3:1	4
35	5:1	6
30	8:1	9
29	10:1	11
24	25:1	26

*Total output flow (air + oxygen) in L/min can be calculated by multiplying the total ratio parts by the oxygen input flow (L/min).

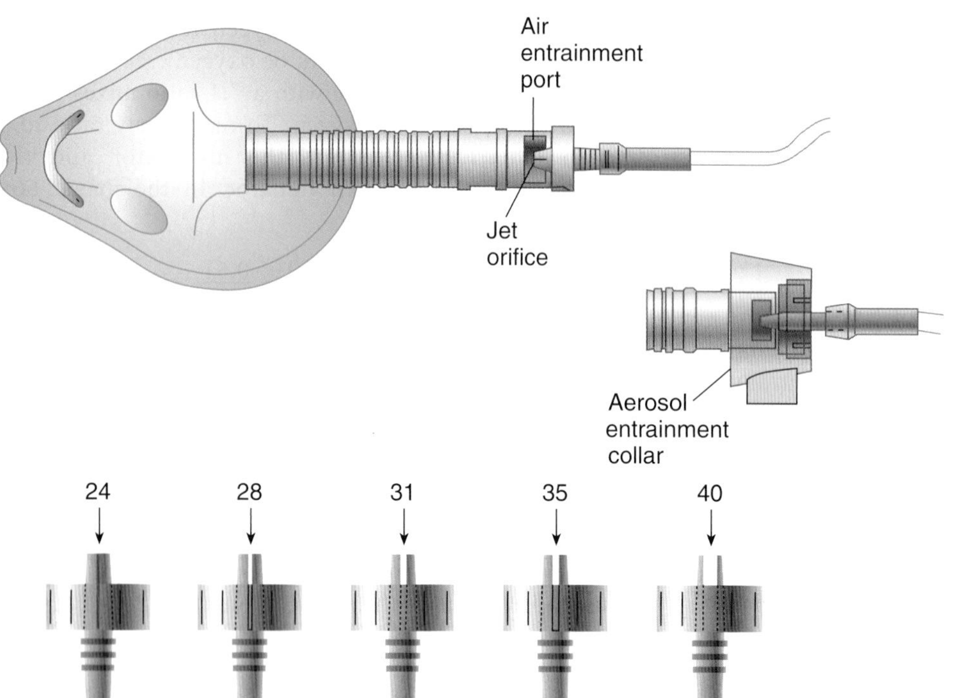

Figure 35-15
Typical air-entrainment mask. The F_{IO_2} is regulated by changing a jet adapter. The aerosol collar allows high humidity or aerosol entrainment from an air source. *(Modified from Kacmarek RM: In-hospital O_2 therapy. In Kacmarek RM, Stoller J, editors: Current respiratory care, Toronto, 1988, BC Decker.)*

Air-Entrainment Mask. The use of an oxygen mask for provision of controlled F_{IO_2} by means of air entrainment was first reported in 1941 by Barach and Eckman.[30] The system provided relatively high F_{IO_2} (greater than 40%) through the use of adjustable air-entrainment ports that controlled the amount of air mixed with oxygen. Some 20 years later, Campbell[31] developed an entrainment mask that provided controlled, low F_{IO_2} and called the device a venti-mask.

As the name *venti-mask* suggests, the operating principle behind these devices has often been attributed to the Venturi principle (see Chapter 5). This assumption is incorrect.[32] Rather than having an actual Venturi tube that entrains air, these devices have a simple restricted orifice or jet through which oxygen flows at high velocity. Air is entrained by shear forces at the boundary of jet flow, not by low lateral pressures. The smaller the orifice, the greater is the velocity of oxygen and the more air is entrained.

Figure 35-15 depicts a typical AEM, designed to deliver a range of low to moderate F_{IO_2} (0.24-0.40). The mask consists of a jet orifice or nozzle around which is an air-entrainment port *(upper drawing)*. The body of the mask has several large ports, which allow escape of both excess flow from the device and exhaled gas from the patient. In this design, the F_{IO_2} is regulated by selection and changing of the jet adapter. The smallest jet provides the highest oxygen velocity and thus the most air entrainment and the lowest F_{IO_2} (0.24).

The largest jet provides the lowest oxygen velocity and thus the least air entrainment and the highest F_{IO_2} (0.40). Other AEM designs may vary both jet and entrainment port size to provide an even broader range of F_{IO_2}. The aerosol entrainment collar fits over the air-entrainment ports (see later).

For controlled F_{IO_2} at flow high enough to prevent air dilution, the total output flow of an AEM must exceed the patient's peak inspiratory flow.[29] With an entrainment ratio exceeding 5:1, an AEM set to deliver less than 35% oxygen has little trouble meeting or exceeding the 60 L/min high-flow criterion (see previous Rule of Thumb). At settings above 35%, however, total AEM flow decreases significantly, and the F_{IO_2} becomes variable.[32-34] For example, when set to deliver 50% oxygen, some AEMs provide an F_{IO_2} as low as 0.39.

Air-Entrainment Nebulizer. Pneumatically powered air-entrainment nebulizers have most of the features of AEMs but have added capabilities, including additional humidification and temperature control. Humidification is achieved through production of aerosol at the nebulizer jet. Temperature control is provided by an optional heating element. In combination, these added features allow delivery of particulate water (in excess of needs for body temperature and pressure, saturated) to the airways.

Because of added humidification and heat control, air-entrainment nebulizers have been the traditional device of choice for delivering oxygen to patients with artificial tracheal airways. The oxygen typically is delivered with a T tube or a tracheostomy mask. An alternative is to use an aerosol mask or a face tent to

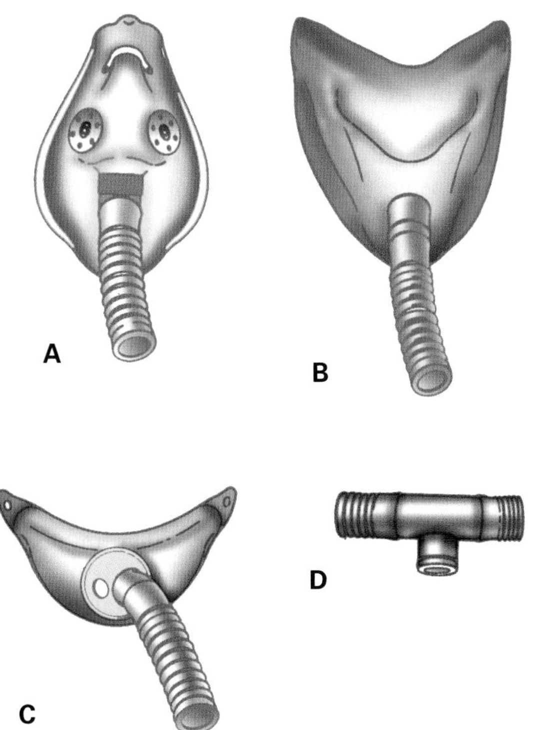

Figure 35-16
Devices for delivery of oxygen mixtures with aerosol. **A,** Aerosol mask; **B,** face tent; **C,** tracheostomy collar; **D,** T tube. *(Modified from Kacmarek RM: In-hospital O_2 therapy. In Kacmarek RM, Stoller J, editors: Current respiratory care, Toronto, 1988, BC Decker.)*

deliver an oxygen mixture with aerosol to patients with intact upper airways (Figure 35-16).[35]

Whereas AEMs can vary both jet and entrainment port size to obtain a given FIO_2, gas-powered nebulizers have a fixed orifice. Thus air-to-oxygen ratios can be altered only by varying entrainment port size. Most nondisposable nebulizers have fixed entrainment settings, such as 100%, 70%, and 40%. Disposable nebulizers usually have a continuous range of settings from 28% to 100%.[21]

As do AEMs, air-entrainment nebulizers perform as fixed-performance devices only when output flow meets or exceeds the patient's inspiratory demand. Unlike AEMs, however, air-entrainment nebulizers do not allow easy increases in nebulizer output flow by means of an increase in oxygen input. With most nebulizer systems, the extremely small size of the jet needed for aerosol production limits the maximum oxygen input flow to 12 to 15 L/min at 50 psig. For example, the total output flow of an air-entrainment nebulizer set to deliver 40% oxygen ranges from 48 to 60 L/min. Although this amount may be adequate for most patients, it is not sufficient for those with very high inspiratory flow or minute volume.

The actual FIO_2 received by patients may be affected by the choice of airway appliance. For example, the FIO_2 delivered by face tent is consistently less than the set nebulizer concentration, especially at higher levels.[36]

Air-entrainment nebulizers should be treated as fixed-performance devices only when set to deliver low oxygen concentration (35% or less).[33] When a nebulizer is used to deliver a higher concentration of oxygen, the RT must determine whether the flow is sufficient to meet patient needs.

There are two ways to assess whether the flow of an air-entrainment nebulizer meets the patient's needs. The first method is simple visual inspection. With this approach (generally used only with a T tube), the RT sets up the device to deliver the highest possible flow at the prescribed FIO_2. After connecting the system to the patient, the RT observes the mist output at the expiratory side of the T tube. As long as mist can be seen escaping *throughout inspiration,* flow is adequate to meet the patient's needs, and the delivered FIO_2 is ensured.

The second way to assess the adequacy of nebulizer flow is to compare it with the patient's peak inspiratory flow. A patient's peak inspiratory flow during tidal breathing is approximately three times minute volume. As long as the nebulizer flow exceeds this value, the delivered FIO_2 is ensured. If the patient's peak flow exceeds that provided by the nebulizer, the device functions as a low-flow system with variable FIO_2 (see the Mini Clini for an example).

MINI CLINI

Computing Minimum Flow Needs

PROBLEM

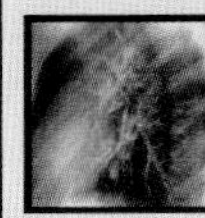

A physician orders 40% oxygen through an air-entrainment nebulizer to a patient with a tidal volume of 0.8 L and a rate of 25 breaths/min. If maximum nebulizer input flow is 12 L/min, will the patient receive 40% oxygen? If not, what total flow is needed to meet this patient's needs?

SOLUTION

1. Estimate the patient's inspiratory flow:

$$\text{Peak inspiratory flow} = \dot{V}_E \times 3 = (0.8 \times 25) \times 3 = 60 \text{ L/min}$$

2. Compute the total flow of the nebulizer:

$$\text{Sum of ratio parts (3:1)} \times \text{Input flow (12 L/min)} = 48 \text{ L/min}$$

3. Compare value 1 with value 2 (patient with nebulizer):

$$60 \text{ L/min (patient)} > 48 \text{ L/min (nebulizer)}$$

Under these conditions, the patient does not receive 40% oxygen. To deliver a stable 40% oxygen concentration, the total flow would have to be at least 60 L/min.

Troubleshooting Air-Entrainment Systems. The major problem with air-entrainment systems is ensuring that the set F_{IO_2} actually is delivered to the patient. Problems usually do not occur when the devices are used to deliver low F_{IO_2} (<0.35). However, the design of these devices makes it difficult to provide even moderate F_{IO_2} at the high flow needed to ensure a set oxygen concentration. The performance of all air-entrainment devices is affected by downstream resistance. The result can be inaccurate F_{IO_2} that makes delivery of a low oxygen concentration difficult with air-entrainment nebulizers.

Providing Moderate to High F_{IO_2} at High Flow. Air-entrainment masks and air-entrainment nebulizers differ in ratio settings and input/output flow capabilities. Most AEMs can be set to deliver no more than 50% oxygen. When set according to the manufacturer's specifications to provide more than 35% oxygen, AEMs simply do not generate enough flow to ensure the set F_{IO_2}. The solution is to boost the total output flow. With AEMs, total output flow can be boosted with a simple increase in input flow. For example, for a 35% AEM (5:1 ratio) with an input flow of 8 L/min, the total output flow is 48 L/min. This flow is not sufficient to ensure 35% oxygen delivery to all patients. Simply increasing the input flow to 12 L/min boosts the output flow of the AEM 50%, to 72 L/min. The new high flow ensures delivery of the set oxygen concentration to essentially all patients.

This solution is not possible with most air-entrainment nebulizers. Because the small jets in these devices limit oxygen flow to 12 to 15 L/min, the input flow cannot be increased above these levels. The five alternatives for boosting the F_{IO_2} capabilities of air-entrainment nebulizers are presented in Box 35-2.

Box 35-2 • Increasing the F_{IO_2} Capabilities of Air-Entrainment Nebulizers

- Add open reservoir to expiratory side of T tube.
- Provide inspiratory reservoir with one-way expiratory valve.
- Connect two or more nebulizers together in parallel.
- Set nebulizer to low concentration; bleed-in oxygen; analyze and adjust.
- Use a commercial dual-flow system.

The simplest approach to achieving higher F_{IO_2} with these devices is to add a 50- to 150-mL aerosol tubing reservoir to the expiratory side of the T tube (Figure 35-17). Given its simplicity, adding an open volume reservoir to the expiratory side of T tubes is standard procedure in most clinical settings. Unfortunately, this approach can be used only in the treatment of intubated patients. Even then, the small reservoir size limits the ability of this system to ensure stable F_{IO_2}, especially greater than 40%, and larger reservoirs can cause rebreathing.

Rather than a simple open reservoir, a closed-reservoir or nonrebreathing system similar to that in Figure 35-12 can be used. These systems combine an inspiratory volume reservoir (usually a compliant 3- to 5-L anesthesia bag) with a one-way expiratory valve. Whenever patient flow exceeds nebulizer flow, the expiratory valve closes, and the patient draws additional gas from the reservoir. Although they can ensure delivery of the set oxygen concentration, these systems pose considerable hazards. Should source flow stop for any reason, the patient can suffocate. For this reason, these systems must be equipped with an emergency inlet valve that allows room air breathing in the event of source gas failure.

The third and most common approach to higher F_{IO_2} with air-entrainment nebulizers is to connect two or more devices together with a wye adapter (Figure 35-18).[21] For example, whereas a single air-entrainment nebulizer set at 60% (1:1 ratio) with a maximum input flow of 15 L/min has a total output flow of only 30 L/min, connecting two of these devices together doubles the total output flow to 60 L/min (the minimum needed for a high-flow device). This approach works well only for delivery of a concentration of 60% or less to patients with a minute volumes less than 10 L/min.[37]

A fourth method for boosting the F_{IO_2} provided by air-entrainment nebulizers is to set the device to a *lower* concentration than that prescribed (to generate high

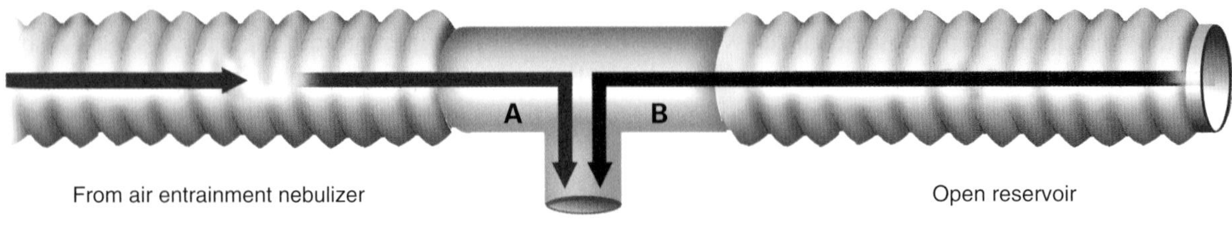

Figure 35-17

Use of an open volume reservoir to enhance delivered oxygen concentration with a T tube. Fifty to 150 mL of aerosol tubing is connected to the expiratory side of the T tube. When the patient inhales, gas at the set F_{IO_2} is drawn first through the inspiratory side of the circuit **(A)**. If the patient's flow exceeds nebulizer flow, gas is drawn from the reservoir side **(B)**. Only after the reservoir volume is fully tapped is room air entrained and does F_{IO_2} decrease.

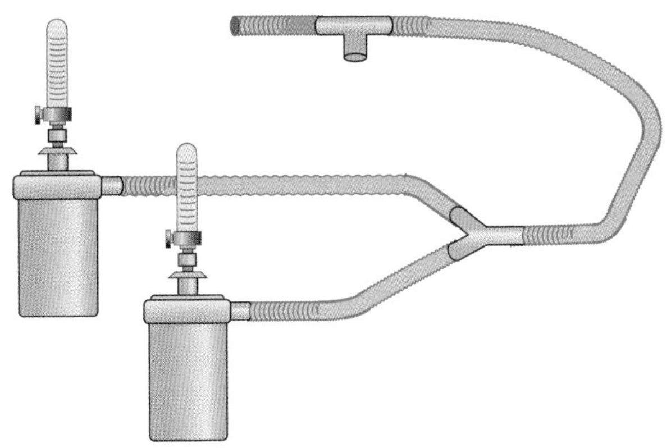

Figure 35-18
Use of two nebulizers in parallel to provide high FIO_2 at high flow.

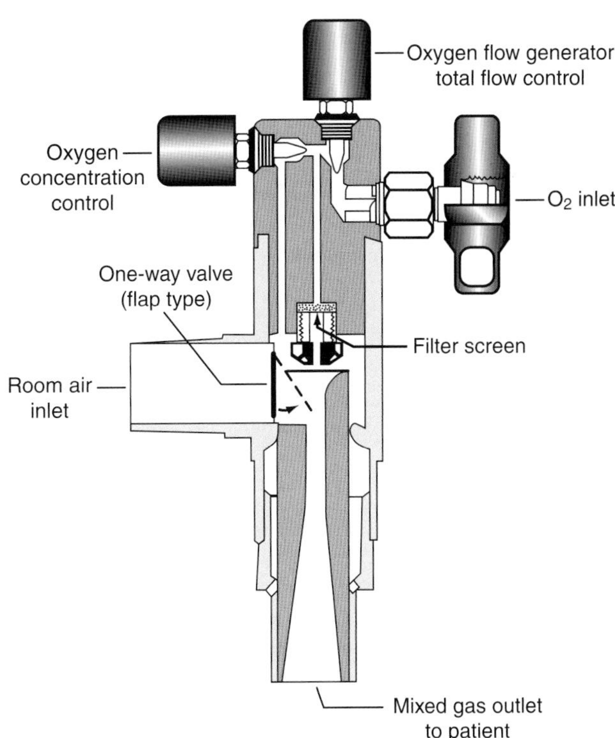

Figure 35-19
Downs adjustable flow generator. Oxygen source gas goes through two needle valves. One powers the jet and determines the amount of air entrained. The other provides supplemental oxygen to boost the FIO_2.

flow) while bleeding supplemental oxygen into the delivery tubing. This increases both FIO_2 and total output flow. To achieve a specific FIO_2 in this type of system, the RT must analyze the delivered concentration and carefully adjust the supplemental oxygen input flow until the concentration is the desired value.[35]

Commercial dual-flow systems entail a similar approach. One flow source powers the jet while another flow source provides supplemental oxygen. The Misty Ox (Medical Moulding Corp.) gas injection nebulizer is a good example. This system can provide an FIO_2 of 0.70 to 0.75 at a flow of 60 L/min or more when oxygen powers the nebulizer at 40 L/min and air is injected. The Misty Ox also can provide an FIO_2 of 0.65 to 0.70 at higher flow (90 to 100 L/min) when air powers the nebulizer and oxygen is injected.

If aerosol is not needed, a simple dual-flow device such as the Downs flow generator (Figure 35-19) can be used. This device is attached to a 50-psig oxygen source and provides oxygen concentration of 30% to 100% at a flow up to 100 L/min.[38]

Problems with Downstream Flow Resistance. Any increase in flow resistance downstream from (distal to) the point of air entrainment alters the performance of all air-entrainment systems. Increased downstream flow resistance increases back pressure. The increase in back pressure decreases both the volume of entrained air and the total flow output of these devices. With less air entrained, the delivered oxygen concentration increases; however, because total flow output also decreases, the effect on FIO_2 varies. High downstream flow resistance usually turns air-entrainment systems from high-flow (fixed) oxygen delivery systems into low-flow (variable) oxygen delivery systems incapable of delivering a precise and constant FIO_2.

This problem explains why it is extremely difficult to deliver *less than* 28% to 30% oxygen with an air-entrainment nebulizer. The 5 to 6 feet (1.5 to 1.8 m) of aerosol tubing normally used with these devices produces enough flow resistance to decrease air entrainment and prevent a lower FIO_2.

A similar situation can occur when the entrainment ports of an air-entrainment device become obstructed (most common with AEMs). Delivered oxygen concentration increases, but total output flow decreases. The net effect usually is a variable FIO_2. The Mini Clini is an example of the effect of increased downstream flow resistance on the performance of an air-entrainment device.

Blending Systems. When air-entrainment devices cannot provide high enough oxygen concentration or flow, use of a gas blending system should be considered. With a blending system, separate pressurized air and oxygen sources are input, and the gases are mixed either manually or with a precision valve (blender). This system allows precise control over both FIO_2 and total flow output. Most blending systems can provide flow well in excess of 60 L/min, qualifying them as true fixed-performance delivery devices. For adults, gas is delivered from the blender either through an open system, such as an aerosol mask or T tube, or with a closed nonrebreathing system.

MINI CLINI

Effect of Downstream Flow Resistance on Performance of an Air-Entrainment Device

PROBLEM

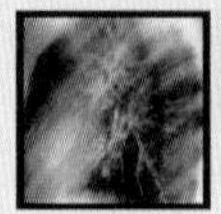

A tracheostomy patient is receiving oxygen therapy through a T tube attached to an air-entrainment nebulizer set at 35% oxygen with an input flow of 10 L/min. Over the last 30 minutes, the patient's Spo_2 has decreased from 93% to 88%. When assessing the patient, you find that the large-bore delivery tubing of the nebulizer is partially obstructed with condensate and that aerosol mist at the T tube is not visible throughout inspiration. What is the likely problem and the best solution?

SOLUTION

The likely problem is a decrease in F_{IO_2} due to the increased downstream resistance caused by the condensate. At 10 L/min input flow, the device was probably delivering approximately 60 L/min of 35% oxygen before the tubing became obstructed. Because aerosol mist is not visible at the T tube throughout inspiration, it is clear that the total output flow is no longer sufficient and that the patient is now diluting the delivered oxygen with room air. Draining the tubing restores the system flow and ensures delivery of the set F_{IO_2}.

MINI CLINI

Manually Mixing Air and Oxygen to Achieve Specified Concentration at a Given Flow

PROBLEM

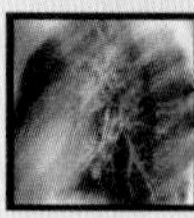

To manually mix air and oxygen to provide a patient with 50% oxygen at a total flow of 60 L/min, what oxygen and air flow would you set?

SOLUTION

1. Use Equation 35-3 to compute the oxygen flow:

$$O_2 \text{ flow} = \frac{\text{Total flow} \times (O_2\% - 21)}{79}$$

$$O_2 \text{ flow} = \frac{60 \times (50 - 21)}{79}$$

$$O_2 \text{ flow} = 22 \text{ L/min}$$

2. Compute the air flow:

$$\text{Air flow} = \text{Total flow} - \text{Oxygen flow}$$

$$\text{Air flow} = 60 - 22$$

$$\text{Air flow} = 38 \text{ L/min}$$

To provide a patient with 50% oxygen at a total flow of 60 L/min, blend 22 L of oxygen with 38 L of air.

Mixing Gases Manually. When gases are mixed manually, separate air and oxygen flowmeters must be adjusted for the desired F_{IO_2} at the needed flow (see Mini Clini). For adults, this approach requires calibrated high-flow flowmeters (at least 60 L/min).

Oxygen Blenders. Rather than manually mixing air and oxygen, the RT can use an oxygen blender. Figure 35-20 shows the major components of a typical oxygen blender. Air and oxygen enter the blender and pass through dual pressure regulators that exactly match the two pressures. Gas then flows to a precision proportioning valve. Because the two gas pressures at this point are equal, varying the size of the air and oxygen inlets provides precise control over the relative concentration.

An alarm system gives an audible warning when either source gas fails or the pressure decreases below a specified value. The alarm system usually has a crossover or bypass feature whereby failure of one gas source causes the blender system to switch to the other. For example, should the air source fail when delivering 60% oxygen, the alarm sounds, and the blender switches over to delivery of 100% oxygen.

Although they allow ideal control over both F_{IO_2} and flow, blenders are prone to inaccuracy and failure.[39,40] To avoid these problems, the RT always should conduct an operational check of any blender before using it on a

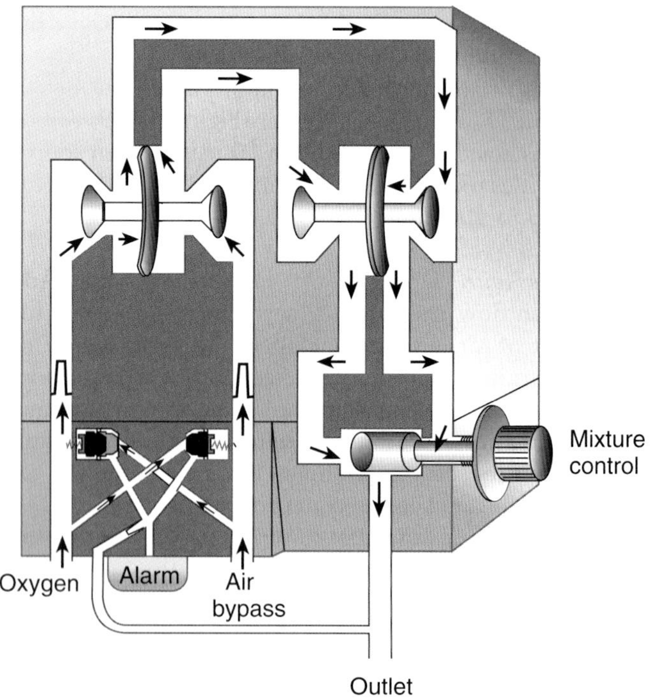

Figure 35-20
Oxygen blending device. *(Modified from McPherson SP: Respiratory therapy equipment, ed 3, St Louis, 1985, Mosby.)*

Box 35-3 • Procedure for Confirming Operation of an Oxygen Blender

1. Confirm that inlet pressures of air and oxygen are within manufacturer's specifications.
2. Test low air and oxygen alarms by disconnecting each source; also confirm safety bypass or crossover system.
3. Analyze oxygen concentration at 100%, 21%, and specified FIO_2.

patient (Box 35-3). The FIO_2 should be checked and confirmed with a calibrated oxygen analyzer at least once per shift.[2] As always, a device that does not perform according to expectations should be replaced immediately. When a blender is used in the care of a neonate, an oxygen analyzer should be kept in-line at all times.

In the use of a nonrebreathing or closed delivery system, (1) all breathing valves should be inspected and tested *before* application to a patient, and (2) a fail-safe inspiratory valve should be included in the delivery system.

Enclosures. The concept of enclosing a patient in a controlled-oxygen atmosphere is among the oldest approaches to oxygen therapy. Entire rooms once were used for this purpose. With today's simpler airway devices, enclosures are generally used only in the care of infants and children. The primary types of oxygen enclosures used for infants and children are tents, incubators, and hoods.

Oxygen Tents. Oxygen tents once were the most common method of oxygen therapy in the treatment of both adults and children. Today, use of oxygen tents in the care of adults is rare, but tents are still used for children. In general, tents are air-conditioned or cooled with ice to provide a comfortable temperature within a plastic sheet canopy (Figure 35-21).

The main problem with tents is that frequent opening and closing of the canopy cause wide swings in oxygen concentration. Moreover, constant leakage makes a high FIO_2 impossible. For example, in large tents oxygen input flow of 12 to 15 L/min can provide only 40% to 50% oxygen levels. Comparable FIO_2 can be achieved in smaller pediatric or **croup** tents with flow between 8 and 10 L/min. Because of these limitations, tents are used primarily for pediatric aerosol therapy in the care of children with croup or cystic fibrosis.

Hoods. An oxygen hood is the best method for administration of controlled oxygen therapy to infants. As shown in Figure 35-22, an Oxyhood covers only the head, leaving the infant's body free for nursing care. Oxygen is delivered to the hood through either a heated air-entrainment nebulizer or a blending system with a heated humidifier. A minimum flow of 7 L/min should be set to prevent accumulation of carbon dioxide.[41] Depending on the size of the hood, flow of 10 to 15 L/min may be needed to maintain stable high oxygen concentration. Higher flow generally is not needed and may produce a harmful noise level and additional stress on neonatal patients.[42]

In the care of premature infants, it is especially important to ensure that the gas mixture is properly warmed and humidified and not directed toward the patient's face or head. Low temperatures or convection

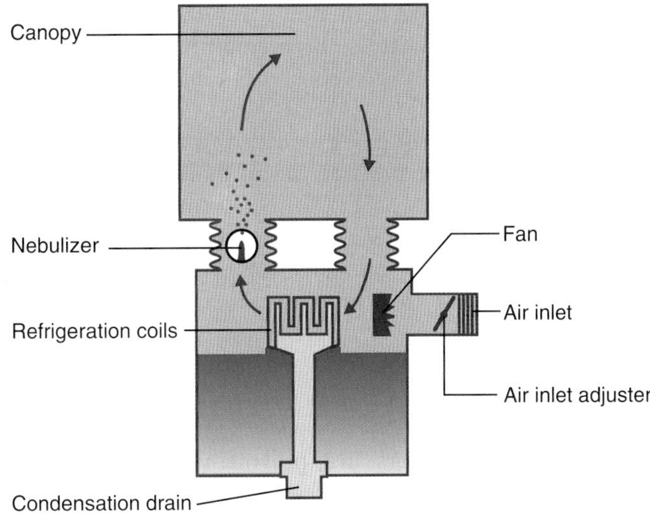

Figure 35-21
Adult oxygen tent incorporating refrigeration coils for cooling. *(From Cairo JM, Pilbeam SP: Mosby's respiratory care equipment, ed 6, St Louis, 1999, Mosby.)*

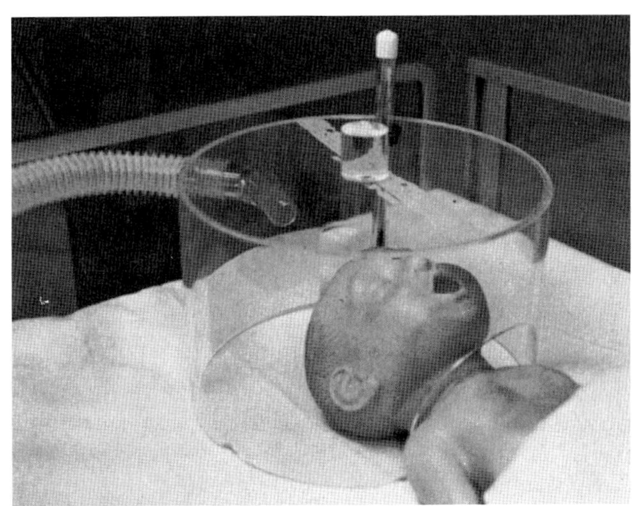

Figure 35-22
Infant oxygen hood.

cooling produced by high flow over the head causes heat loss and cold stress. In premature infants, cold stress can increase oxygen consumption and even cause apnea.[43]

The temperature of gases provided to an infant in an Oxyhood should be precisely set to maintain a **neutral thermal environment** (NTE). The NTE temperature varies according to an infant's age and weight. For example, the NTE temperature for newborns weighing less than 1200 g is 35° C. For older infants weighing 2500 g or more, the NTE is lower, approximately 30° C.[43] More detail on the importance of temperature regulation in infants is provided in Chapter 45.

Incubators. Incubators are polymethyl methacrylate (Plexiglas) enclosures that combine servo-controlled convection heating with supplemental oxygen (Figure 35-23). In older models, humidification was provided with a blow-over water reservoir located under the patient platform. Because of the high infection risk associated with this design, these systems are no longer in common use. When it is needed, supplemental humidity usually is provided with an external heated humidifier or nebulizer.

Supplemental oxygen can be administered with a direct connection between the incubator and a flowmeter that has a heated humidifier. In some units, a filtered air-entrainment device limits the delivered concentration to approximately 0.40. However, leaks and frequent opening of the incubator dilute the oxygen levels well below 40%. On the other hand, blockage of the inlet filter can cause less air entrainment and a higher oxygen concentration.

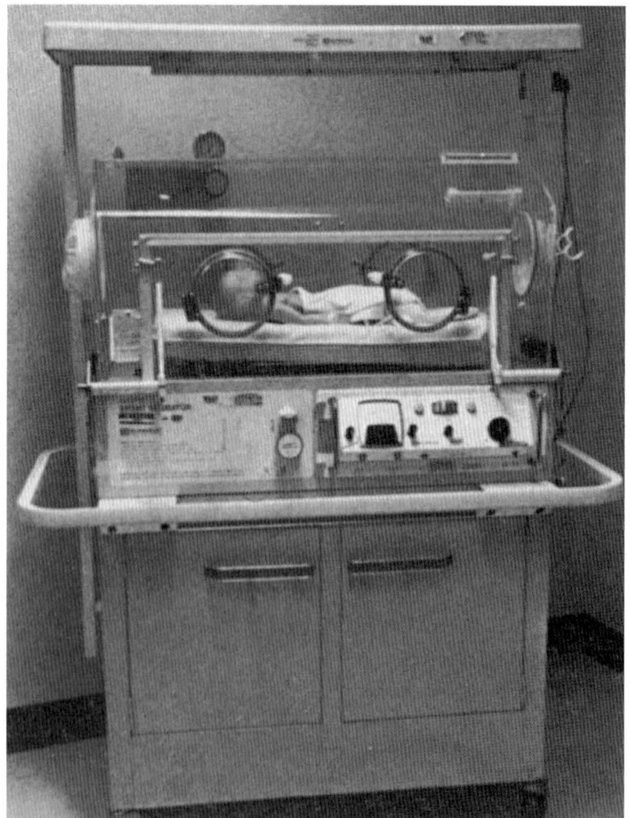

Figure 35-23
Infant incubator.

Given the highly variable oxygen concentration provided by these devices, the best way to control oxygen delivery to infants in an incubator is with an Oxyhood. The Oxyhood is placed over the infant's head inside the incubator. The oxygen concentration and gas temperature within the Oxyhood, not in the incubator, must be assessed. It is ideal to monitor incubator or Oxyhood oxygen concentration continuously (see later).[2,4]

Because hoods allow better FIO_2 control, and because servo-controlled radiant heating warmers are generally more convenient, Plexiglas incubators are not as popular as they used to be. However, these devices are still the best choice for providing infants in stable condition with a neutral thermal environment.

Selecting a Delivery Approach

With the variety of techniques available for giving oxygen, there is no one best delivery method. Although the decision to give oxygen is a medical one, it is not always easy for the physician to know exactly which approach is the best for a given patient. For this reason, the RT should be involved in the initial selection of an appropriate delivery system. The RT also should be responsible for ongoing oversight of the prescribed therapy. This responsibility should include making recommendations—on the basis of sound patient assessment—to change or discontinue the treatment regimen (see later, Protocol-Based Oxygen Therapy).

The three Ps—purpose, patient, and performance—are used in the selection or recommendation of a change in oxygen delivery system. The goal is to match the performance characteristics of the equipment to both the objectives of therapy (purpose) and the patient's special needs.

Purpose

The general purpose or objective of all oxygen therapy is to increase FIO_2 sufficiently to correct arterial hypoxemia. Other objectives, including decreasing hypoxic symptoms and minimizing increased cardiopulmonary work, follow from this primary purpose.

Patient

Key patient considerations in selecting oxygen therapy equipment for use in acute care are summarized in Box

Box 35-4 • Patient Factors in Selecting Oxygen Therapy Equipment

- Severity and cause of hypoxemia
- Patient age group (infant, child, adult)
- Degree of consciousness and alertness
- Presence or absence of a tracheal airway
- Stability of minute ventilation

35-4. Knowledge of these factors helps guide the RT in selecting the appropriate equipment. For example, for a moderately hypoxemic adult patient with an endotracheal tube in place, the selection generally is limited to either an air-entrainment nebulizer or an oxygen blender-humidifier system connected to a T tube (Briggs adapter). An infant with moderate hypoxia and a normal airway usually needs an oxygen enclosure (hood or enclosed incubator).

Equipment Performance

Oxygen systems vary according to actual F_{IO_2} delivered and stability of the F_{IO_2} under changing patient demands. As a rule, the more critically ill the patient, the greater is the need for a stable, high F_{IO_2}. Less acutely ill patients generally need a lower, less exact F_{IO_2}. Table 35-8 lists guidelines for selecting an oxygen delivery system on the basis of the level and stability of the F_{IO_2} needed.

Table 35-8 ▶▶ Selection of an Oxygen Delivery System Based on Desired F_{IO_2} Level and Stability

	Desired F_{IO_2} Stability	
Desired F_{IO_2} Level	**Fixed**	**Variable**
Low (<35%)	AEM	Nasal cannula
	Air-entrainment nebulizer	Nasal catheter
	Blending system	Transtracheal catheter
	Isolette, incubator (infant)	
Moderate (35%-60%)	Air-entrainment nebulizer	Simple mask
	Blending system	Air-entrainment nebulizer
	Oxyhood (infant)	Tent (child)
High (>60%)	Blending system	Partial
rebreather		
	Oxyhood (infant)	Nonrebreather

General Goals and Patient Categories

On the basis of overall consideration of the three Ps, general goals can be set for several patient categories.

In emergencies in which tissue hypoxia is suspected, patients should be given as high an F_{IO_2} as possible, ideally 100%. This level can be achieved with a true high-flow or a closed reservoir system. The goal is the highest possible blood oxygen content. Clinical examples include respiratory or cardiac arrest, severe trauma, shock, carbon monoxide poisoning, and cyanide poisoning. Carbon monoxide and cyanide poisoning may necessitate **hyperbaric oxygen** (HBO) **therapy** (see later).

A critically ill adult patient with moderate to severe hypoxemia needs either a reservoir or a high-flow system capable of at least 60% oxygen. Thereafter, changes in F_{IO_2} (and device) should be based on results of assessment of physiological values. The goal is a Pa_{O_2} greater than 60 mm Hg or a hemoglobin saturation greater than 90%.

In the care of adult patients in more stable condition but who are acutely ill with mild to moderate hypoxemia, a system capable of low to moderate oxygen concentration can be used. In these cases, stability of F_{IO_2} is not critical. Applicable devices include a nasal cannula at moderate flow or a simple mask. Common examples include patients in the immediately postoperative phase or those recovering from acute myocardial infarction.

Adult patients with chronic lung disease and accompanying acute-on-chronic hypoxemia present a special case. In the care of this group, the goal is to ensure adequate arterial oxygenation without depressing ventilation. Adequate oxygenation of these patients generally means an Sa_{O_2} of 85% to 90% with a Pa_{O_2} of 50 to 60 mm Hg.[31,44] These values usually are achieved with either low-flow nasal oxygen or a low-concentration (24% to 28%) AEM. The less stable the patient's condition, the greater is the need for a high-flow AEM.[21]

Because of size, discomfort, and appearance, AEMs are less well tolerated for long-term therapy than are nasal cannulas. Moreover, unlike a cannula, an AEM must be removed for eating and drinking. Because even a short break in oxygen therapy can cause a rapid decrease in Pa_{O_2} in some patients, these patients should be taught to switch to a nasal cannula whenever they must remove the mask.[21]

Protocol-Based Oxygen Therapy

Oxygen therapy is ideally suited for a protocol. Noninvasive bedside assessment of oxygenation has progressed to the point at which it no longer makes sense for a physician to be constantly involved in writing orders to change delivery systems or F_{IO_2}. An order for "oxygen therapy via protocol" ensures the patient (1) undergoes initial assessment, (2) is evaluated for protocol criteria, (3) receives a treatment plan that is modified according

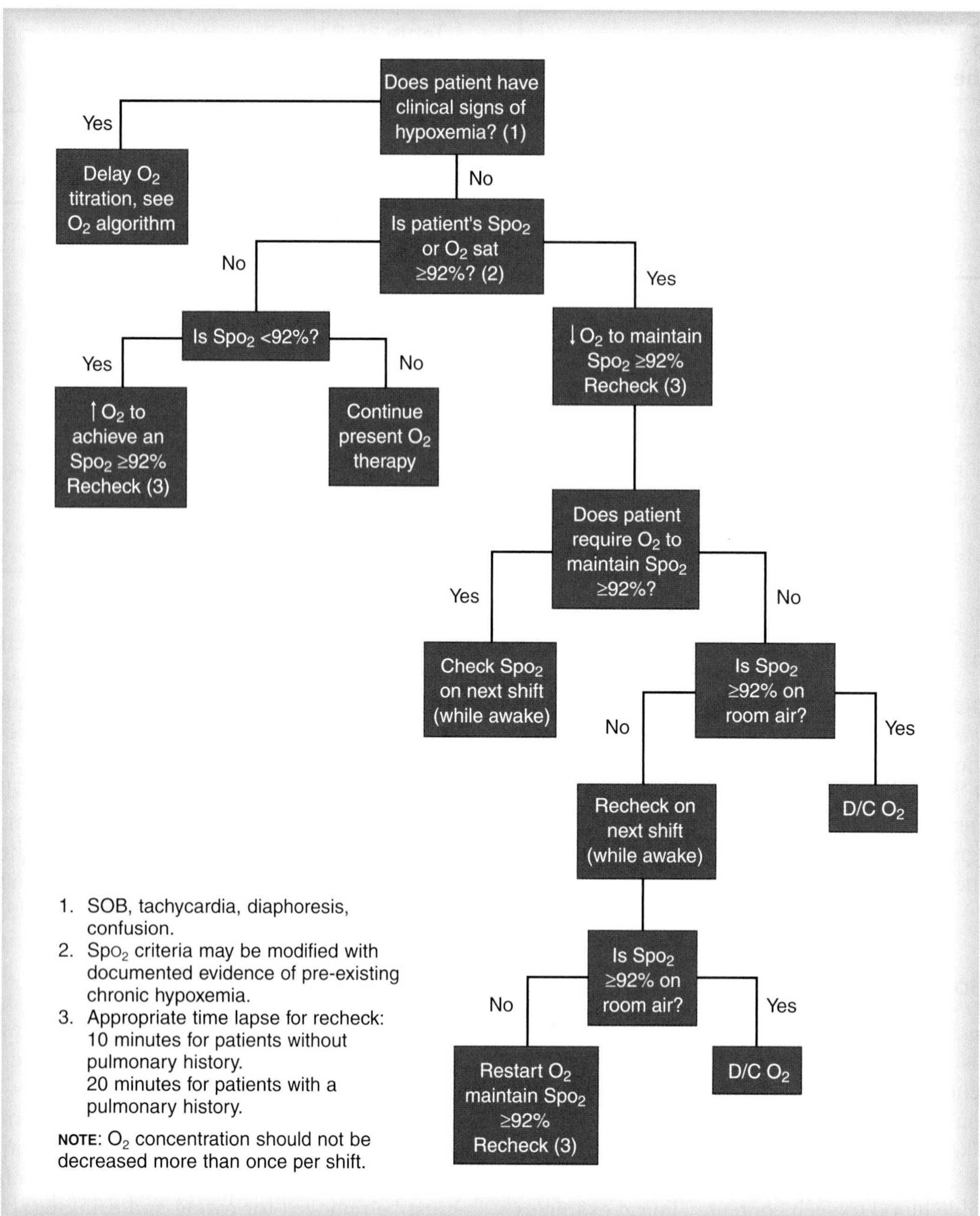

Figure 35-24
Protocol for titration of oxygen therapy.

to need, and (4) stops receiving therapy as soon as it is no longer needed.[45]

Figure 35-24 shows the decision algorithm underlying an oxygen therapy titration protocol developed at the Cleveland Clinic Foundation. In the algorithm, a pulse oximetry saturation (Spo_2) of 92% is the threshold value that indicates the need for therapy. As indicated in the algorithm, the titration process is bypassed if the patient already has signs of hypoxemia. Instead, the patient immediately receives supplemental oxygen. Otherwise, the level of supplemental oxygen is adjusted, and the patient is reassessed on each shift for determination of continuing need. Once the Spo_2 is 92% or higher on room air, therapy is discontinued.

▶ HYPERBARIC OXYGEN THERAPY

Hyperbaric oxygen therapy is the therapeutic use of oxygen at pressures greater than 1 atm.[46-48] Pressures during HBO therapy usually are expressed in multiples of **atmospheric pressure absolute** (ATA). One ATA

Box 35-5 • Physiological Effects of Hyperbaric Oxygen Therapy

- Bubble reduction (Boyle's law)
- Hyperoxygenation of blood and tissue (Henry's law)
- Vasoconstriction
- Enhanced host immune function
- Neovascularization

equals 760 mm Hg (101.32 kPa). Most HBO therapy is conducted at pressures between 2 and 3 ATA, although other pressures may be used and often are based on U.S. Navy diving treatment tables.[47, 49]

Physiological Effects

The known physiological effects of HBO therapy are summarized in Box 35-5.[46] These effects are mainly due to either high pressure or high oxygen tension in body fluids and tissues.

In conditions such as air embolism and decompression sickness, high pressure exerts a physical effect on air or nitrogen bubbles trapped in the blood or tissues. According to Boyle's law, high pressure decreases the size of these bubbles and minimizes potential harm. Because pressure is crucial in these cases, HBO treatments may be conducted at 6 ATA or more.[47]

The second beneficial effect of HBO is hyperoxia. When a patient is breathing room air, only a small amount of oxygen dissolves in the plasma (approximately 0.3 mL/dL). At 3 ATA, plasma contains nearly 7 mL/dL dissolved oxygen, a level exceeding average resting tissue uptake.

Oxygen supply to the tissues affects the immune system, wound healing, and vascular tone. A tissue Po_2 of at least 30 mm Hg is necessary for normal cellular function. Damaged and infected tissues often have a lower Po_2. Increasing oxygen supply to these tissues can help restore both white blood cell function and antimicrobial activity.

Hyperoxia affects the cardiovascular system. Hyperbaric oxygen therapy causes generalized vasoconstriction and a small decrease in cardiac output. Although these changes may decrease blood flow to a region, this effect is more than offset by the increase in oxygen content. In conditions such as burns, cerebral edema, and crush injuries, vasoconstriction may be helpful because it reduces edema and tissue swelling while maintaining tissue oxygenation.

Hyperoxia also helps form new capillary beds, a process called **neovascularization.** Although the exact mechanism is unknown, neovascularization is an essential component of tissue repair, especially in radiation-induced injuries.[47]

Results of studies have suggested that HBO may be useful in the management of stroke, noxious gas exposure, crush injuries, and exercise-induced tissue injuries.[50-52]

Although there are several established and promising indications for HBO, this therapy can be expensive in relation to other treatments. Extensive medical justification often is necessary before reimbursement approval from governmental and private health insurance providers.

Methods of Administration

Hyperbaric oxygen is administered in either a multiplace or a monoplace chamber. A multiplace chamber is a large tank capable of holding a dozen or more people (Figure 35-25, *A*). Because patients are directly cared for by medical staff inside the tank, multiplace chambers have air locks that allow entry and egress without altering the pressure. The multiplace chamber is filled with air. Only the patient breathes 100% oxygen (through a mask or another device). Because they can achieve pressures of 6 ATA or more, multiplace chambers are ideal for the management of decompression sickness and air embolism.[47]

The typical monoplace chamber consists of a transparent Plexiglas cylinder large enough only for a single patient (Figure 35-25, *B*). During therapy, the cylinder oxygen concentration is kept at 100%. Thus the patient need not wear a mask. Because of the high oxygen concentration, most electronic equipment cannot be used in a monoplace chamber. In addition, many ventilators do not function properly under these conditions. However, monitoring systems and ventilators can be adapted to allow treatment of a critically ill patient with hyperbaric pressure.[46]

Indications

Hyperbaric oxygen has long been accepted as the primary treatment of divers with decompression sickness. Other indications for HBO therapy are listed in Box 35-6.[46,47] The two most common acute conditions for which RTs administer HBO are air embolism and carbon monoxide poisoning.

Air Embolism

Air embolism is a complication that can occur with certain cardiovascular procedures, lung biopsy, hemodialysis, and central line placement. Air bubbles that reach the cerebral or cardiac circulation can cause severe neurologic symptoms or sudden death. Hyperbaric oxygen decreases the volume of air bubbles and helps oxygenate local tissues. Typical therapy for air embolism involves immediate pressurization in air to 6 ATA for 15 to 30 minutes. This step is followed by decompression to 2.8 ATA with prolonged oxygen treatment.[47]

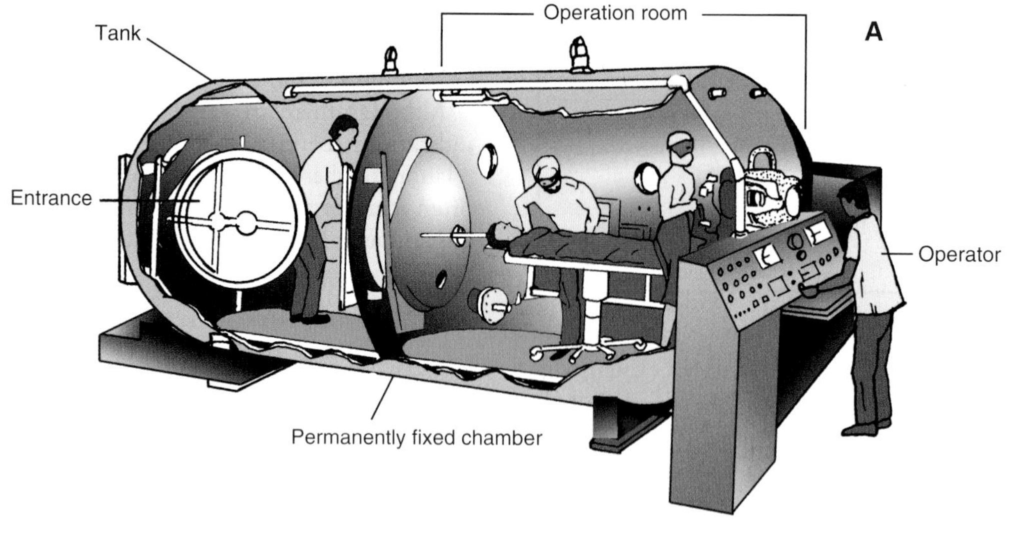

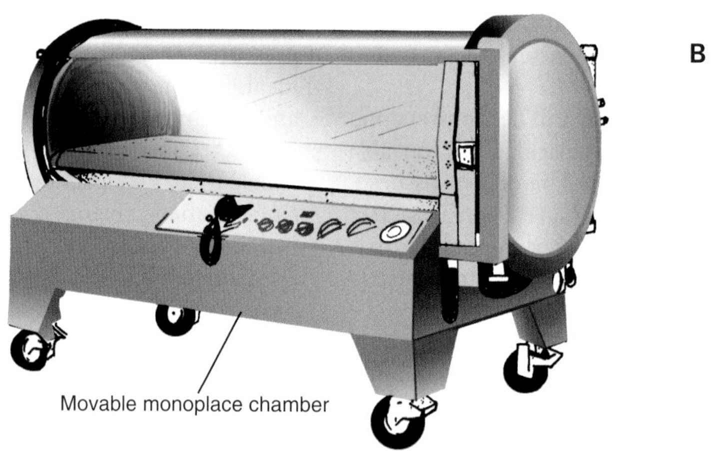

Figure 35-25
A, Fixed hyperbaric chamber. **B,** Monoplace chamber.

Carbon Monoxide Poisoning

Carbon monoxide poisoning accounts for half of all poisoning deaths in the United States. The condition of a patient with carbon monoxide poisoning improves quickly with HBO treatment because this treatment is the fastest way to remove carbon monoxide from the blood.[53] If a patient breathes air, it takes more than 5 hours to remove only one half of the carboxyhemoglobin in the blood. Breathing 100% oxygen reduces this "half-life" to 80 minutes. The half-life of carboxyhemoglobin under HBO at 3 ATA is only 23 minutes. Box 35-7 lists current criteria for selecting patients with acute carbon monoxide poisoning for treatment with HBO.[47]

Complications and Hazards

Although the benefits of HBO are significant, this type of therapy is not without risks. The risks can be serious and therefore must be compared with the potential benefits before therapy is initiated. The common complications of HBO are listed in Box 35-8.[47] These complications are caused by either high pressure or oxygen toxicity. The most frequent problems involve barotrauma to closed body cavities, such as the middle ear or sinuses. Pneumothorax and air embolism also are possible during HBO treatment but are rare in patients with normal lungs.

Oxygen at high pressure can be neurotoxic. Early signs of impending CNS toxicity include twitching,

Box 35-6 • Indications for Hyperbaric Oxygen Therapy

ACUTE CONDITIONS
- Decompression sickness
- Air or gas embolism
- Carbon monoxide and cyanide poisoning
- Acute traumatic ischemia (compartment syndrome, crush injury)
- Clostridial gangrene
- Necrotizing soft-tissue infection
- Ischemic skin graft or flap
- Exceptional blood loss

CHRONIC CONDITIONS
- Nonhealing wounds
- Refractory osteomyelitis
- Radiation necrosis

Box 35-7 • Criteria for HBO Therapy for Acute Carbon Monoxide Poisoning

- History of unconsciousness
- Presence of neuropsychiatric abnormality
- Presence of cardiac instability or cardiac ischemia
- Carboxyhemoglobin level 25% (lower levels for children and pregnant women)

Box 35-8 • Major Complications of Hyperbaric Oxygen Therapy

BAROTRAUMA
- Ear or sinus trauma
- Tympanic membrane rupture
- Pneumothorax
- Air embolism

OXYGEN TOXICITY
- Central nervous system toxic reaction
- Pulmonary toxic reaction

OTHER
- Fire
- Sudden decompression
- Reversible visual changes
- Claustrophobia

sweating, pallor, and restlessness. These signs usually are followed by seizures and convulsions. However, CNS toxicity rarely occurs with the pressures and treatment times commonly used for clinical HBO therapy.

In terms of pulmonary oxygen toxicity, HBO treatments do not normally expose patients to high PO_2 long enough to cause damage. However, HBO may have an additive effect on critically ill patients who receive high FIO_2 between HBO treatments.[47]

Avoiding fire and avoiding sudden decompression are primary safety concerns. Only 100% cotton fabric should be used to avoid static electrical discharge. No alcohol or petroleum-based products should be used, and the patient must not wear sprays, makeup, or deodorant.

Troubleshooting

Although fire hazards restrict the use of certain electronic equipment, some monitors and ventilators with solid-state circuitry can be used within the chamber. This equipment allows intensive care of critically ill patients.[46]

In regard to ventilator use, reductions in delivered tidal volume should be expected and corrected.[46] If not accounted for, this problem can lead to respiratory hypercapnia and acidosis. Hypercapnia can result in respiratory acidosis and can worsen CNS toxicity due to cerebral vasodilation.

Pressure- and flow-regulating equipment used in a hyperbaric chamber must be specifically designed for operation at chamber pressure or appropriately modified to the additional barometric pressure exerted.

▶ OTHER MEDICAL GAS THERAPIES

Oxygen is not the only medical gas administered by RTs. Nitric oxide shows great promise as a potent pulmonary vasodilator, and helium is undergoing renewed emphasis as an adjunct tool in certain forms of airway obstruction.

Nitric Oxide Therapy

Mode of Action

Nitric oxide (NO) gas is a highly diffusible, lipid-soluble free radical that oxidizes quickly to nitrogen dioxide (NO_2) in the presence of oxygen. Endogenous nitric oxide is normally produced from L-arginine in a reaction catalyzed by the enzyme nitric oxide synthase. Nitric oxide activates guanylate cyclase, which catalyzes the production of **cyclic guanosine 3′,5′-monophosphate** (cGMP). Increased cGMP levels cause smooth-muscle relaxation.[53]

Because it relaxes capillary smooth muscle, inhalation of nitric oxide improves blood flow to ventilated alveoli. The result is a reduction in intrapulmonary shunting, improvement in arterial oxygenation, and a decrease in pulmonary vascular resistance and pulmonary arterial pressure.

The effects of nitric oxide are limited to the pulmonary circulation. After diffusing into the capillaries, free nitric oxide immediately binds to hemoglobin, forming nitrosylhemoglobin. Nitrosylhemoglobin is rapidly oxidized to methemoglobin, which eventually undergoes conversion to reduced hemoglobin.

Indications

After several years of clinical testing, inhaled nitric oxide was approved in 1999 by the U.S. Food and Drug Administration (FDA) for widespread use in the care of neonates. Nitric oxide, in conjunction with ventilatory support and other appropriate agents, is indicated for the treatment of term and near-term (>34 weeks) neonates with hypoxic (type I) respiratory failure with associated pulmonary hypertension. Although it was somewhat effective in the management of pulmonary hypertension associated with acute respiratory distress syndrome (ARDS) in adults, nitric oxide was found not to significantly improve mortality and overall outcome. Consequently, nitric oxide has not been approved for widespread use in the treatment of adults. The established and potential clinical uses of nitric oxide are under investigation and are listed in Box 35-9.[54,55]

Dosing

The amount of nitric oxide needed to improve oxygenation or decrease pulmonary vascular pressure in neonates is relatively low. The recommended initial dose of nitric oxide is 20 ppm. Treatment should be continued up to 14 days or until underlying oxygenation desaturation has resolved. Dosages often can be reduced to 5 ppm at the end of 4 hours of initial treatment, as tolerated. At these levels, nitric oxide has minimal toxicity.[54] In clinical trials, higher doses were not shown more effective and placed the patient at higher risk of complications.[55]

Box 35-9 • Potential Uses for Inhaled Nitric Oxide

- ARDS
- Persistent pulmonary hypertension of the newborn
- Primary pulmonary hypertension
- Pulmonary hypertension following cardiac surgery
- Cardiac transplantation
- Acute pulmonary embolism
- COPD and chronic pulmonary fibrosis
- Bronchodilation
- Congenital diaphragmatic hernia
- Congenital heart disease

Toxicity and Adverse Effects

The toxicity of nitric oxide is caused by its own direct action and its chemical byproducts. In high concentration (5000 to 20,000 ppm) nitric oxide causes acute pulmonary edema that can be fatal. Inhalation of a lower concentration has been associated with direct cellular damage and impaired surfactant production.[56]

Most of the toxic effects of nitric oxide are caused its chemical byproducts, especially nitrogen dioxide. Nitrogen dioxide is produced spontaneously whenever nitric oxide is exposed to oxygen. Nitrogen dioxide is more toxic than is nitric oxide. Levels greater than 10 ppm can cause cell damage, hemorrhage, pulmonary edema, and death. The U.S. Occupational Safety and Health Administration has set the safety limit for nitrogen dioxide exposure at 5 ppm. The clinical goal is to keep nitrogen dioxide exposure less than 2 ppm during administration of nitric oxide.

Other harmful chemical byproducts produced in reaction with nitric oxide include methemoglobin and peroxynitrite (produced when nitric oxide reacts with superoxide). Although it can occur with nitric oxide administration, methemoglobinemia probably is not a large problem at the doses commonly used. Peroxynitrite is a potent oxidant that can cause severe cell damage; however, there is no hard evidence supporting its toxic effects during nitric oxide administration.

Potential adverse effects associated with nitric oxide therapy are listed in Box 35-10.[56] A poor or paradoxical response to nitric oxide has been observed in some patients. As many as 40% of ARDS patients do not have initial improvement in oxygenation with nitric oxide therapy, and some patients have experienced more severe hypoxemia (probably due to a worsening $\dot{V}/\dot{Q}$ imbalance when no shunt was present). Nitric oxide inhibits platelet agglutination, and the result is an antithrombotic effect. However, no significant increase in bleeding time has been reported in nitric oxide trials with human subjects. Because it can quickly reduce right ventricular afterload, nitric oxide may increase left ventricular filling pressure in some patients. In the presence of congestive heart failure, this effect could cause or worsen pulmonary edema. Withdrawal of nitric oxide has resulted in development of hypoxemia and pulmonary hypertension worse than they were before

Box 35-10 • Adverse Effects Associated With Nitric Oxide Therapy

- Poor or paradoxical response
- Platelet inhibition
- Increased left ventricular filling pressure
- Rebound hypoxemia, pulmonary hypertension

therapy was started. This phenomenon is known as a *rebound effect*. Although it may improve gas exchange and reduce respiratory failure in ARDS patients, nitric oxide has been shown not to have a favorable effect on mortality among adult patients. Because of the findings of an FDA review of the risk and benefits, inhaled nitric oxide has not been approved for widespread use in the treatment of adults with ARDS.[57]

Although nitric oxide has been used safely with other drugs and treatments such as dopamine, steroids, surfactant, and high-frequency ventilation, extensive studies have not been completed regarding the interaction of nitric oxide with other medications. Likewise, the carcinogenic, mutagenic, and other adverse effects of nitric oxide are still under investigation.[55]

Methods of Administration

Nitric oxide must be delivered through a system with the capability for operator-determined concentration of nitric oxide in the breathing gas, a constant concentration throughout the breathing cycle, and a concentration that does not cause generation of excessive inhaled nitrogen dioxide. Features of an ideal nitric oxide delivery system are listed in Box 35-11. Commercial systems such as the Datex Ohmeda INOvent (Figure 35-26) have been developed to provide these features.[55,57] The current design incorporates a nitric oxide injector and flow controller and flow sensor in the inspiratory limb of the ventilator circuit. Nitric oxide is injected in proportion to the total inspiratory gas flow for administration of a selectable nitric oxide concentration. The set nitric oxide level is stable over a wide range of flow and flow patterns, including spontaneous breathing modes. Nitric oxide, nitrogen dioxide, and oxygen are measured in the inspiratory limb of the circuit, just before the patient wye. A calibration mode verifies proper analyzer function. High and low alarms are provided for all three gases, and there is an automatic cutoff to prevent nitric oxide overdosage.[58]

These systems entail use of cylinder mixtures of nitric oxide (typically 100 to 800 ppm of nitric oxide in nitrogen). This high concentration of nitric oxide is then diluted with nitrogen, air, or oxygen before delivery to the patient. Because adding nitric oxide to the circuit decreases the FIO_2, oxygen concentration must be monitored distal to the titration site.

Box 35-11 • Features of Ideal Nitric Oxide Delivery System

- Dependability and safety
- Delivery of a precise and stable dose of nitric oxide
- Limited production of nitrogen dioxide
- Accurate monitoring of nitric oxide and nitrogen dioxide levels
- Capability for scavenging of nitric oxide
- Maintenance of adequate patient ventilation

Monitoring

Regardless of the delivery method, inhaled nitric oxide and nitrogen dioxide levels must be carefully monitored. The concentration of nitric oxide and nitrogen dioxide can be measured with chemiluminescence or electrochemical analysis. In chemiluminescence measurement, nitric oxide in sample gas reacts with ozone (O_3) to produce activated nitrogen dioxide. As it returns to its basal energy level, the activated nitrogen dioxide emits a photon. This electromagnetic radiation is detected

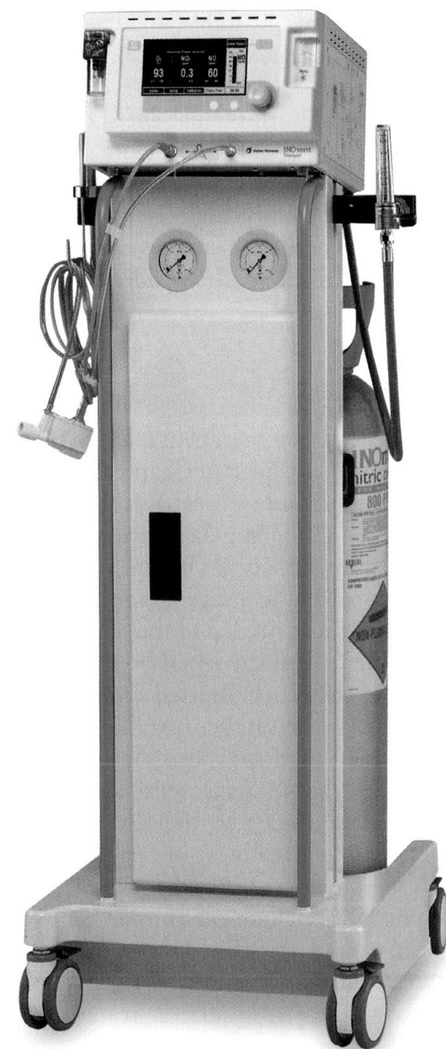

Figure 35-26
INOvent delivery system for administration of nitric oxide to mechanically ventilated patients. *(Courtesy of Datex-Ohmeda, Madison, WI.)*

photoelectrically; its magnitude is proportional to the amount of nitric oxide in the sample. Electrochemical analysis of nitric oxide is similar to electrochemical analysis of oxygen.

The FDA standards for nitric oxide and nitrogen dioxide monitoring devices require accuracy of ±20% (or 0.5 ppm for nitric oxide, whichever is greater). Ten percent to 90% of the full signal response time should occur in less than 30 seconds, and there must be audible and visual alarms in which the upper limit can be set from 2 ppm to the maximum of the range.[58]

Withdrawing Therapy

Care must be taken when nitric oxide therapy is withdrawn to prevent the rebound effect. First, the nitric oxide level should be reduced to the lowest effective dose (ideally ≤5 ppm). Second, the patient's condition should be hemodynamically stable, and the patient should be able to maintain adequate oxygenation while breathing a moderate F_{IO_2} (≤0.4) on low levels of positive end-expiratory pressure Third, the patient should be hyperoxygenated (F_{IO_2}, 0.60 to 0.70) just before discontinuation of nitric oxide inhalation. Last, preparation should be made to provide hemodynamic support should the patient need it. Use of these measures usually avoids any untoward effect of nitric oxide withdrawal.[54]

Helium Therapy

Indications

The value of helium as a therapeutic gas is based solely on its low density. As detailed in Chapter 5, when flow is turbulent, driving pressure varies with the square of the flow. Because flow in the large airways is mainly turbulent, breathing a low-density gas mixture can decrease the driving pressure needed to move gas in and out of this area. With less pressure needed to move gas through the large airways, the patient's work of breathing decreases. However, this effect is limited to large airway obstruction (flow in the small airways is not turbulent).

Helium has been used for more than 65 years as an adjunct tool in the management of large airway obstruction.[59] Helium-oxygen therapy has since been shown effective in the treatment of certain patients with COPD. This treatment decreases the respiratory rate and level of dyspnea.[60,61] Helium-oxygen, or heliox, therapy also has been found effective in the management of acute upper airway obstruction of varying origin,[62,63] postextubation stridor in pediatric trauma patients,[64] and refractory viral croup.[65]

Guidelines for Use

Because it is inert and unable to support life, helium always must be mixed with at least 20% oxygen. The most common combination is 80% helium and 20% oxygen. For practical purposes, this mixture is comparable with air, but helium is used in place of nitrogen. Although air has a density of 1.293 g/L, the density of an 80% helium mixture is 0.429 g/L. For a comparable flow through obstructed large airways, this low-density mixture can dramatically decrease the work of breathing.

Although it is possible to mix helium and oxygen at the bedside, it is much safer and more convenient to use commercially prepared cylinders of premixed gases. In addition to the 80/20 combination, a mixture of 70% helium and 30% oxygen is commonly available (density, 0.554 g/L). This mixture provides additional oxygen, which is helpful in management of the hypoxemia that can occur with large airway obstruction.

Because helium is highly diffusible, mixtures of this gas generally should be administered with a closed system (such as a nonrebreathing mask) or with a small-volume reservoir device, such as a simple mask.[66] Because of leakage, low-flow nasal devices are ineffective for delivering helium mixtures. Large-volume enclosures, such as hoods, also are unsatisfactory because helium tends to concentrate at the top of these devices. Helium mixtures can be given through a cuffed tracheal airway with a positive-pressure ventilator.

When a helium-oxygen mixture is given by mask, the RT should realize that a typical hospital oxygen flowmeter is not accurate. Flowmeters calibrated for helium exist, but they are not required. Correction factors can be used instead. For example, the correction for an 80/20 helium-oxygen mixture is 1.8. This means that for every 10 L/min indicated flow, 10 × 1.8, or 18 L/min, of the 80/20 mixture actually leaves the flowmeter. For delivery of a specific flow from an 80/20 helium-oxygen source, the RT sets the flowmeter to the desired flow divided by 1.8. If a flow of 9 L/min of an 80/20 helium-oxygen mixture is needed, the RT sets the flowmeter to 9/1.8, or 5 L/min. Factors for any other mixture can be calculated if needed. The factor for a 70/30 helium-oxygen mixture is 1.6.

Troubleshooting

The low density of helium mixtures makes them poor vehicles for aerosol transport. High-density bland water aerosols are difficult to deliver with helium mixtures, as are aerosolized drugs.

The low density of helium mixtures also makes coughing less effective. An expulsive cough depends in part on the development of turbulent flow in the large airways. Because helium promotes laminar flow, clearance of secretions by coughing is impaired. If the patient can develop an effective cough, this problem can be rectified by means of washing out the helium before coughing.

The most common side effect of helium is a benign one. When a patient is breathing a helium mixture, the spoken word is badly distorted at a pitch so high as to make it almost unintelligible. This effect is caused by the passage of a low-density gas through the vocal cords on exhalation. The effect is important only to conscious, nonintubated patients, who should be warned of the effect and reassured that it disappears immediately after therapy is stopped.

A more serious problem is hypoxemia associated with breathing helium mixtures.[67] Although this problem may have been caused by using too low an oxygen concentration (20%), there is another possibility. Some commercial cylinders of helium-oxygen have been found to contain these gases in an unmixed, or separated, state. The only way to avoid this potential hazard is to analyze the oxygen concentration coming from the cylinder before administering the gas mixture to a patient.

KEY POINTS

- Oxygen therapy is used to (1) correct acute hypoxemia, (2) decrease the symptoms of chronic hypoxemia, and (3) decrease cardiopulmonary workload.
- The need for supplemental oxygen can be assessed with laboratory measures, clinical history or status, and bedside patient evaluation.
- In the care of adults, children, and infants older than 28 days, oxygen therapy is indicated if the PaO_2 is less than 60 mm Hg or the SaO_2 is less than 90%.
- Exposure to 100% oxygen for more than 24 hours should be avoided whenever possible; high FIO_2 is acceptable if the concentration can be decreased to 0.70 within 2 days and to 0.50 or less in 5 days.
- That oxygen therapy can cause hypoventilation never should preclude administration of oxygen to a patient in need. Prevention of hypoxia always is the first priority.
- If an oxygen delivery system provides *all* a patient's inspired gas, the FIO_2 remains stable. If the device provides only *some* of the inspired gas, air dilutes the oxygen, and the FIO_2 varies with breathing.
- The oxygen provided with low-flow devices such as a nasal cannula always is diluted with air; the result is a low and variable FIO_2.
- Reservoir devices can provide higher FIO_2 than low-flow systems or can be used to conserve oxygen.

KEY POINTS—cont'd

- To avoid rebreathing, the RT must administer at least 5 L/min flow with a reservoir mask; for masks with bags, the flow must be sufficient to prevent bag collapse.
- A nonrebreathing reservoir circuit can provide a full range of FIO_2 (21% to 100%) at any needed flow to both intubated and nonintubated patients.
- High-flow systems supply a given oxygen concentration at a flow of at least 60 L/min.
- Because they dilute source oxygen with air, entrainment devices always provide less than 100% oxygen. The more air entrained, the higher is the total flow, but the lower is the delivered FIO_2.
- Air-entrainment nebulizers should be treated as fixed-performance devices only when set to deliver low oxygen concentration (35% or less).
- The most common way to achieve high FIO_2 with air-entrainment nebulizers is to connect two or more devices together in parallel.
- Back pressure decreases both the volume of entrained air and the total flow output of air-entrainment devices.
- A blending system allows precise control over both FIO_2 and total flow output; most blending systems qualify as true fixed-performance delivery devices.
- An operational check of an oxygen blender always should be conducted before the device is used to treat a patient.
- Oxygen therapy enclosures are used mainly in the care of children and infants. Problems include limited and highly variable FIO_2 and temperature control.
- The three Ps—purpose, patient, and performance of the device—should be considered in the when selection or recommendation of an oxygen delivery system.
- In HBO therapy, oxygen is administered at a pressure greater than 1 atm for management of conditions such as air embolism and carbon monoxide poisoning.
- Inhaled nitric oxide improves blood flow to ventilated alveoli, reduces intrapulmonary shunting, improves arterial oxygenation, and decreases pulmonary vascular resistance and pulmonary arterial pressure.

Continued

KEY POINTS—cont'd

- An ideal nitric oxide delivery system provides precise and stable delivery of the nitric oxide dose, limits nitrogen dioxide production, and allows accurate monitoring, with alarms, of nitric oxide and nitrogen dioxide levels.
- When nitric oxide therapy is being withdrawn, care must be taken to prevent a rebound effect.

References

1. Fulmer JF, Snider GL: American College of Chest Physicians National Heart, Lung and Blood Institute National Conference on Oxygen Therapy, Chest 86:224, 1984.
2. American Association for Respiratory Care: Clinical practice guideline: oxygen therapy in the acute care hospital, Respir Care 36:1410, 1991.
3. American Association for Respiratory Care: Clinical practice guideline: oxygen therapy in the home or extended care facility, Respir Care 37:918, 1992.
4. American Association for Respiratory Care: Clinical practice guideline: selection of an oxygen delivery device for neonatal and pediatric patients, Respir Care 41:637, 1996.
5. Swinburn CR et al: Symptomatic benefit of supplemental oxygen in hypoxemic patients with chronic lung disease, Am Rev Respir Dis 143:913, 1991.
6. Block AJ: Neuropsychologic aspects of oxygen therapy, Respir Care 28:885, 1983.
7. MacNee W et al: The effects of controlled oxygen therapy on ventricular function in patients with stable and decompensated cor pulmonale, Am Rev Respir Dis 137:1289, 1988.
8. American Academy of Pediatrics/American College of Obstetricians and Gynecologists: Guidelines for perinatal care, ed 4, Elk Grove Village, IL, American Academy of Pediatrics, 1997.
9. Lodato RF: Oxygen toxicity, Crit Care Clin 6:749, 1990.
10. Jackson RM: Molecular, pharmacologic, and clinical aspects of oxygen-induced lung injury, Clin Chest Med 11:73, 1990.
11. Durbin CG, Wallace KK: Oxygen toxicity in the critically ill patient, Respir Care 38:739, 1993.
12. Register SD, Downs JB, Stock MC: Is 50% oxygen harmful? Crit Care Med 15:598, 1987.
13. Steinberg KP, Pierson DJ: Clinical approaches to the patient with acute oxygenation failure. In Pierson DJ, Kacmarek RM, editors: Foundations of respiratory care, New York, 1992, Churchill Livingstone.
14. Beachey W: Respiratory care anatomy and physiology: foundations for clinical practice, St Louis, 1997, Mosby.
15. Aubier M et al: Effects of the administration of oxygen on ventilation and blood gases in patients with chronic obstructive pulmonary disease during acute respiratory failure, Am Rev Respir Dis 122:747, 1980.
16. Cullen JH, Kaemmerlen JT: Effect of oxygen administration at low rates of flow in hypercapnic patients, Am Rev Respir Dis 95:116, 1967.
17. Dunn WF, Nelson SB, Hubmayr RD: Oxygen-induced hypercapnia in obstructive pulmonary disease, Am Rev Respir Dis 144:526, 1991.
18. Sassoon CS, Hassell KT, Mahutte CK: Hyperoxic-induced hypercapnia in stable chronic obstructive pulmonary disease, Am Rev Respir Dis 135:907, 1987.
19. Flynn JT: Retinopathy of prematurity, Pediatr Clin North Am 34:1487, 1987.
20. Shapiro BA et al: Changes in intrapulmonary shunting with administration of 100 percent oxygen, Chest 77:138, 1980.
21. Branson RD: The nuts and bolts of increasing arterial oxygenation: devices and techniques, Respir Care 38:672, 1993.
22. Shapiro BA et al: Clinical applications of respiratory care, ed 4, St Louis, 1991, Mosby.
23. Leigh JM: Variation in performance of oxygen therapy devices, Ann R Coll Surg Engl 52:234, 1973.
24. Heimlich HJ: Respiratory rehabilitation with transtracheal oxygen system, Ann Otol Rhinol Laryngol 91:643, 1982.
25. Spofford B et al: Transtracheal oxygen therapy: a guide for the respiratory therapist, Respir Care 32:345, 1987.
26. Hoffman LA: Novel strategies for delivering oxygen: reservoir cannula, demand flow, and transtracheal oxygen administration, Respir Care 39:363, 1994.
27. Jensen AG, Johnson A, Sandstedt S: Rebreathing during oxygen treatment with face mask: the effect of oxygen flow rates on ventilation, Acta Anaesthesiol Scand 35:289, 1991.
28. Goldstein RS, Young J, Rebuck AS: Effect of breathing pattern on oxygen concentration received from standard face masks, Lancet 2:1188, 1982.
29. McPherson SP: Oxygen percentage accuracy of air-entertainment masks, Respir Care 19:658, 1974.
30. Barach AL, Eckman M: A physiologically controlled oxygen mask apparatus, Anesthesiology 2:421, 1941.
31. Campbell EJM: A method of controlled oxygen administration which reduces the risk of carbon dioxide retention, Lancet 1:12, 1960.
32. Cohen JL et al: Air-entrainment masks: a performance evaluation, Respir Care 22:277, 1977.
33. Redding JS, McAfee DD, Parham AM: Oxygen concentrations received from commonly used delivery systems, South Med J 71:169, 1978.
34. Woolner DF, Larkin J: An analysis of the performance of a variable Venturi-type oxygen mask, Anaesth Intensive Care 8:44, 1980.
35. McPherson SP: Respiratory therapy equipment, ed 5, St Louis, 1995, Mosby.
36. Monast RL, Kaye W: Problems in delivering desired oxygen concentrations from jet nebulizers to patients via face tents, Respir Care 29:994, 1984.
37. Foust GN et al: Shortcomings of using two jet nebulizers in tandem with an aerosol face mask for optimal oxygen therapy, Chest 99:1346, 1991.
38. Fried JL et al: A new Venturi device for administering continuous positive airway pressure (CPAP), Respir Care 26:133, 1981.

39. Karmann U, Roth F: Prevention of accidents associated with air-oxygen mixers, Anaesthesia 37:680, 1982.
40. Inaccurate O_2 concentrations from oxygen-air proportioners, Health Devices 18:366, 1989.
41. Gale R, Redner-Carmi R, Gale J: Accumulation of carbon dioxide in oxygen hoods, infant cots, and incubators, Pediatrics 60:453, 1977.
42. Dawes GW, Williams TJ: The oxygen hood as a noise factor in infant care, Respir Care 24:12, 1979 (abstract).
43. Klaus MH, Fanaroff AA, editors: Care of the high risk neonate, ed 3, Philadelphia, 1986, WB Saunders.
44. O'Donohue WJ, Baker JP: Controlled low-flow oxygen for respiratory failure, Chest 63:818, 1973.
45. Smoker JM et al: A protocol to assess oxygen therapy, Respir Care 31:35, 1986.
46. Weaver LK: Hyperbaric treatment of respiratory emergencies, Respir Care 37:720, 1992.
47. Grim PS et al: Hyperbaric oxygen therapy, JAMA 263:2216, 1990.
48. Tibbles PM, Edelsberg JS: Hyperbaric-oxygen therapy, N Engl J Med 334:1642, 1996.
49. Branger AB, Lambertsen CJ, Eckmann DM: Cerebral gas embolism absorption during hyperbaric therapy, J Appl Physiol 90:593, 2001.
50. Gunn B, Wong R: Noxious gas exposure in the outback: two cases of hydrogen sulfide toxicity, Emerg Med (Freemantle) 13:240, 2001.
51. Auer RN: Non-pharmacologic neuroprotection in the treatment of brain ischemia, Ann N Y Acad Sci 939:271, 2001.
52. Harrison BC et al: Treatment of exercise-induced muscle injury via hyperbaric oxygen therapy, Med Sci Sports Exerc 33:36, 2001.
53. Hurford WE: The biologic basis for inhaled nitric oxide, Respir Care Clin North Am 3:357, 1997.
54. Hess D et al: Use of inhaled nitric oxide in patients with acute respiratory distress syndrome, Respir Care 41:424, 1996.
55. Center for Drug Evaluation and Research: NO labeling, Washington, DC, 1999, U.S. Food and Drug Administration.
56. INOmax (nitric oxide) for inhalation package insert. Clinton, NJ, revised June 2001, INO Therapeutics.
57. Hess D, Ritz R, Branson RD: Delivery systems for inhaled nitric oxide, Respir Care Clin North Am 3:371, 1997.
58. Body SC, Hartigan PM: Manufacture and measurement of nitrogen oxides, Respir Care Clin North Am 3:411, 1997.
59. Manthous CA et al: Heliox in the treatment of airflow obstruction: a critical review of the literature, Respir Care 42:1034, 1997.
60. Ishikawa S, Segal MS: Re-appraisal of helium-oxygen therapy on patients with chronic lung disease, Ann Allergy 31:536, 1973.
61. Jolliet P et al: Beneficial effects of helium:oxygen versus air:oxygen noninvasive pressure support in patients with decompensated chronic obstructive pulmonary disease, Crit Care Med 27:2422, 1999.
62. Boorstein JM et al: Using helium-oxygen mixtures in the emergency management of acute upper airway obstruction, Ann Emerg Med 18:688, 1989.
63. Skrinskas GJ, Hyland RH, Hutcheon MA: Using helium-oxygen mixtures in the management of acute upper airway obstruction, Can Med Assoc J 128:555, 1983.
64. Kemper KJ et al: Helium-oxygen mixture in the treatment of postextubation stridor in pediatric trauma patients, Crit Care Med 19:356, 1991.
65. Nelson DS, McClellan L: Helium-oxygen mixtures as adjunctive support for refractory viral croup, Ohio State Med J 78:729, 1982.
66. Stillwell PC et al: Effectiveness of open-circuit and Oxyhood delivery of helium-oxygen, Chest 95:1222, 1989.
67. Cylinders with unmixed helium/oxygen, Health Devices 19:146, 1990.

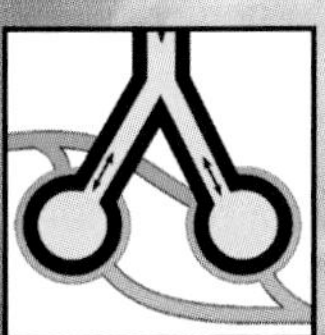

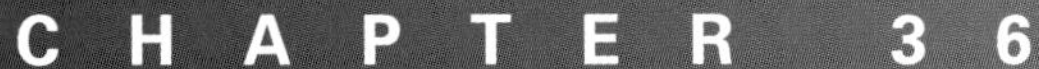

CHAPTER 36

Lung Expansion Therapy

Robert L. Wilkins

In This Chapter You Will Learn:

- What causes the various types of atelectasis
- Who needs lung expansion therapy
- What clinical findings are seen in atelectasis
- How lung expansion therapy works
- What indications, hazards, and complications are associated with the various modes of lung expansion therapy
- What the primary responsibilities of the registered respiratory therapist (RRT) are in planning, implementing, and evaluating lung expansion therapy

Chapter Outline

Key Terms

atelectasis
lobar atelectasis
passive atelectasis
resorption atelectasis

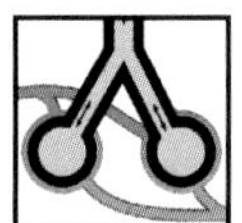

Pulmonary complications are the most common serious problems seen in patients who have undergone thoracic or abdominal surgery.[1] Such complications include atelectasis, pneumonia, and acute respiratory failure. These respiratory problems can be minimized or avoided if proper respiratory therapy is implemented during the perioperative period. The most common form of respiratory therapy utilized in high-risk patients is lung expansion therapy.

Lung expansion therapy includes a variety of respiratory care modalities designed to prevent or correct atelectasis. Historically, intermittent positive pressure breathing (IPPB) was used extensively for this purpose. More recently, incentive spirometry (IS), continuous positive airway pressure (CPAP), and positive expiratory pressure (PEP) have been introduced as alternative lung expansion strategies.

Ongoing research on these methods demonstrates that they can be effective in preventing or correcting atelectasis in select patients.[2] The precise method to apply, however, in any given situation is not always clear because no advantage of any one method has been established. The most efficient use of resources is a primary concern with any plan to apply lung expansion therapy.

In this context, the registered respiratory therapist (RRT) plays a vital role. In consultation with the prescribing physician, the RRT should assist in identifying those patients most likely to benefit from lung expansion therapy, recommend and initiate the appropriate and most efficient therapeutic approach, monitor the patient's response, and alter the treatment regimen as needed.

▶ CAUSES AND TYPES OF ATELECTASIS

Although atelectasis can occur from a large variety of problems, this chapter will focus on the two primary types associated with postoperative or bedridden patients: (1) resorption atelectasis and (2) passive atelectasis. Resorption atelectasis occurs when mucus plugs are present in the airways and block ventilation of the affected region.[3] Gas distal to the obstruction is absorbed by the passing blood in the pulmonary capillaries, which causes the nonventilated alveoli to partially collapse.

Passive atelectasis is primarily caused by persistent use of small tidal volumes by the patient. This is common when general anesthesia is given, with the use of sedatives and bed rest, and when deep breathing is painful as when broken ribs are present or surgery has been performed on the upper abdominal region. Weakening or impairment of the diaphragm also can contribute to passive atelectasis also. Passive atelectasis results when the patient does not periodically take a deep breath and fully expand the lungs. It is a common cause of atelectasis in the hospitalized patient. It may occur in combination with resorption atelectasis in the patient with excessive airway secretions who breathes with small tidal volumes for a prolonged period of time.

A severe form of atelectasis, *lobar atelectasis*, occurs in about 5% of patients who have undergone lung resection.[4] This type of atelectasis significantly lengthens the patient's stay in the intensive care unit (ICU) and hospital. The cause of lobar atelectasis often centers around a large mucus plug but is often the result of multiple factors.

▶ INDICATIONS FOR LUNG EXPANSION THERAPY

Atelectasis can occur in any patient who cannot or does not take deep breaths periodically. Patients who have difficulty taking deep breaths without assistance include those with neuromuscular disorders, those who are heavily sedated, and those who have undergone upper abdominal or thoracic surgery.[5] Patients undergoing lower abdominal surgery are at less risk for atelectasis than those undergoing upper abdominal or thoracic surgery, but still are at significant risk.[6] Patients with spinal cord injury are prone to respiratory complications, the most common of which is atelectasis.[7] Bedridden patients, such as those recovering from major trauma, are prone to develop atelectasis due to their lack of mobility. Clinicians are wise to initiate a prophylactic plan in these high-risk patients to prevent atelectasis.

Postoperative patients are at the highest risk for atelectasis.[5] Patients undergoing upper abdominal surgery with abnormal preoperative spirometry are at greatest risk for postoperative pulmonary complications.[8] Factors contributing to postoperative atelectasis include general anesthesia, shallow breathing, and a transient decrease in surfactant production. In combination, these factors cause a progressive decrease in functional residual capacity (FRC) during general anesthesia and during the first 48 hours following major surgery. The decrease in FRC is associated with alveolar collapse, most often in the basal or dependent portions of the lung.[3] Because perfusion remains unchanged, a ventilation/perfusion ($\dot{V}/\dot{Q}$) mismatch results, causing arterial hypoxemia. Pain further restricts ventilation.[9] Compounding the effects of the pain itself is the tendency of postoperative patients to voluntarily contract or "splint" muscles in the incision area. Splinting further decreases tidal volume and hinders deep breathing. The result is a decrease in ventilatory reserve, as measured by the vital capacity (VC).

MINI CLINI

Risk Factors for Atelectasis

PROBLEM

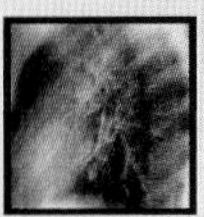

You are called to evaluate a 47-year-old obese man admitted to the hospital for upper abdominal surgery. He has a 60 pack-year smoking history and is scheduled for surgery tomorrow morning. Your examination reveals bilateral inspiratory and expiratory coarse crackles and expiratory wheezes. He is alert and oriented with normal vital signs. His past medical history is positive for diabetes and kidney stones. What factors are present in this patient that predispose him for postoperative atelectasis and what treatment plan do you recommend?

DISCUSSION

Several important risk factors are present in this patient. The three most important are his positive smoking history, obesity, and the site of surgery (upper abdomen). The findings of adventitious lung sounds and positive smoking history are very suggestive of a current pulmonary problem that will probably require bronchial hygiene and humidity therapy and bronchodilators prior to surgery. Delaying the surgery may be necessary if significant secretion retention is present. Postoperatively, this high-risk patient will need careful monitoring and IS to minimize the risk of atelectasis.

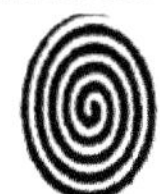

RULE OF THUMB

The closer the incision is to the diaphragm the greater the risk for postoperative atelectasis.

Most postoperative patients also have problems coughing effectively because of their reduced ability to take deep breaths. An ineffective cough impairs normal clearance mechanisms and increases the likelihood of retained secretions and resorption atelectasis in the patient with excessive mucus production. For this reason, patients with a history of lung disease that causes increased mucus production (e.g., chronic bronchitis) are most prone to develop complications in the postoperative period.[10] Similarly, patients with a significant history of cigarette smoking should alert the RRT to the high risk for respiratory complications after surgery. Such patients must be identified in the preoperative period and treated with bronchial hygiene. Elective surgery may need to be postponed in some cases. Lung expansion therapy and chest physical therapy in the postoperative period may help improve clearance of secretions by improving the effectiveness of coughing and secretion removal. One study has demonstrated that chest physical therapy alone is sufficient in minimizing postoperative complications in patients who have had thoracic surgery.[11] In this study, the addition of IS did not further reduce the incidence of postoperative complications. More studies need to be done to further clarify which patients will benefit most from lung expansion therapy.

Patients with a history of inadequate nutritional intake as demonstrated by an albumin level less than 3.2 mg per dL have an increased risk for pulmonary complications in the postoperative period.[12] This is most likely due to inadequate strength of the inspiratory muscles to maintain a normal FRC and VC.

▶ CLINICAL SIGNS OF ATELECTASIS

RRTs must be able to recognize the clinical signs of atelectasis in their patients so appropriate therapy can be implemented in a timely fashion. The patient's medical history often provides the first clue in identifying atelectasis. Recent upper abdominal or thoracic surgery in any patient should suggest possible atelectasis. The history of chronic lung disease and/or cigarette smoking provides additional evidence that the patient is prone to respiratory complications following major surgery or prolonged bed rest.

The physical signs of atelectasis may be absent or very subtle if the patient has minimal atelectasis. When the atelectasis involves a more significant portion of the lungs, the patient's respiratory rate will increase proportionally. Fine, late-inspiratory crackles may be heard over the affected lung region. These crackles are produced by the sudden opening of distal airways with deep breathing. Bronchial-type breath sounds may be present as the lung becomes more consolidated with atelectasis. Diminished breath sounds are common when excessive secretions block the airways and prevent transmission of breath sounds. Tachycardia may be present if the atelectasis leads to significant hypoxemia. Patients with preexisting lung disease will often present with significant abnormalities in respiratory and heart rates, even when the atelectasis is not severe. Atelectasis alone does not cause the patient to develop a fever unless pneumonia is also present.[13]

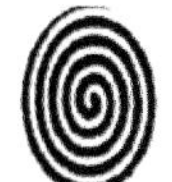

RULE OF THUMB

There is a direct relationship between the spontaneous respiratory rate and the degree of atelectasis present.

The chest film is often used to confirm the presence of atelectasis. The atelectatic region of the lung will demonstrate increased opacity. Evidence of volume loss is present in those patients with significant atelectasis. Direct signs of volume loss on the chest film include displacement of the interlobar fissures, crowding of the pulmonary vessels, and air bronchograms.[3] Indirect signs include elevation of the diaphragm; shift of the trachea, heart, or mediastinum; pulmonary opacification; narrowing of the space between the ribs; and compensatory hyperexpansion of the surrounding lung.

▶ LUNG EXPANSION THERAPY

All modes of lung expansion therapy increase lung volume by increasing the transpulmonary pressure (P_L) gradient. As detailed in Chapter 9, P_L gradient represents the difference between the alveolar pressure (P_{alv}) and the pleural pressure (P_{pl}):

$$P_L = P_{alv} - P_{pl}$$

With all else being constant, the greater the P_L gradient, the more the alveoli expand.

As depicted in Figure 36-1, the P_L gradient can be increased by either: (1) decreasing the surrounding P_{pl} (Figure 36-1, *A*) or (2) increasing the P_{alv} (Figure 36-1, *B*). A spontaneous deep inspiration increases the P_L gradient by decreasing the P_{pl}. On the other hand, the application of positive pressure to the lungs increases the P_L gradient by raising the pressure inside the alveoli.

All lung expansion therapies use one of these two approaches. IS enhances lung expansion via a spontaneous and sustained decrease in P_{pl}. Positive airway pressure techniques increase P_{alv} in an effort to expand the lung. Positive pressure lung expansion therapies may apply pressure during inspiration only (as in intermittent positive pressure breathing [IPPB]), during expiration only (as in positive expiratory pressure [PEP] and expiratory positive airway pressure [EPAP]), or during both inspiration and expiration (CPAP).

Although all these approaches are used in lung expansion therapy, it should be clear that those methods that decrease P_{pl} (e.g., IS) have more of a physiological effect than those that raise P_{alv} and often are most effective. They do, however, require an alert, cooperative patient who is capable of taking a deep breath.

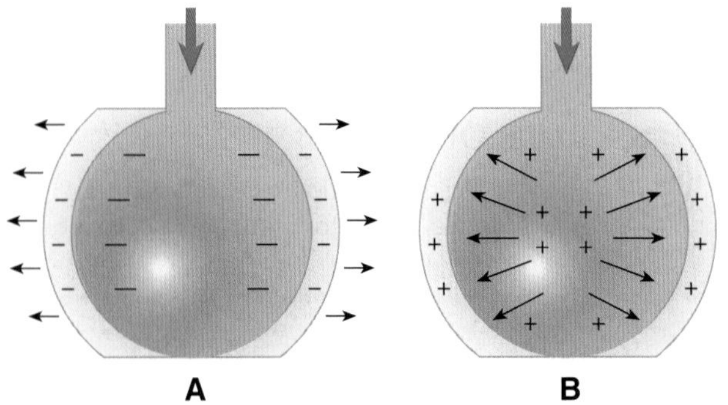

Figure 36-1
Transpulmonary pressure gradients with **(A)** spontaneous inspiration and **(B)** positive pressure inspiration.

The goal of any lung expansion therapy should be to implement a plan that provides an effective strategy in the most efficient manner. Staff time and equipment are the two major issues related to efficiency. For the patient with minimal risk of postoperative atelectasis, deep breathing exercises, frequent repositioning, and early ambulation are usually effective and can be done with minimal coaching and time from clinicians and without equipment. For the patient at high risk for atelectasis (e.g., the upper abdominal surgery patient), IS is usually employed.[14] The additional staff time and equipment is justified in this high risk group. Positive pressure therapy requires significantly more staff time and equipment and is reserved for the high risk patients who cannot perform IS techniques. The remainder of this chapter describes the use of IS and positive pressure therapy for the prevention or correction of atelectasis.

▶ INCENTIVE SPIROMETRY (IS)

IS has been the mainstay of lung expansion therapy for well over a decade. IS is designed to mimic natural sighing by encouraging patients to take slow, deep breaths. IS is performed using devices that provide visual cues to the patients when the desired flow or volume has been achieved.

The desired volume and number of repetitions to be performed is initially set by the RRT or other qualified caregiver. The inspired volume goal is set on the basis of predicted values or observation of initial performance.

Physiological Basis of IS

The basic maneuver of IS is a sustained, maximal inspiration (SMI). An SMI is a slow, deep inhalation from the FRC up to (ideally) the total lung capacity, followed by a 5 to 10 second breath hold. An SMI is thus functionally equivalent to performing an inspiratory capacity (IC) maneuver, followed by a breath hold.

Figure 36-2 compares the alveolar and P_{pl} changes occurring during a normal spontaneous breath and an SMI during IS.

During the inspiratory phase of spontaneous breathing, the drop in P_{pl} caused by expansion of the thorax is transmitted to the alveoli. With P_{alv} now negative, a pressure gradient is created between the airway opening and the alveoli. This transrespiratory pressure gradient causes gas to flow from the airway into the alveoli. Within certain limits, the greater the transrespiratory pressure gradient, the more lung expansion will occur.

INCENTIVE SPIROMETRY

AARC Clinical Practice Guideline (Excerpts)*

➤ INDICATIONS

- Presence of conditions predisposing to the development of pulmonary atelectasis (upper abdominal surgery, thoracic surgery, surgery in patients with COPD)
- Presence of pulmonary atelectasis
- Presence of restrictive lung defect associated with quadriplegia and/or dysfunctional diaphragm

➤ CONTRAINDICATIONS

- Patient cannot be instructed or supervisted to ensure approproate use of the device
- Patient cooperation is absent or patient is unable to understand or demonstrate proper use of the device
- IS is contraindicated in patients unable to deep breathe effectively (e.g., with VC less than about 10 mL/kg or IC less than about one third of predicted)
- The presence of an open tracheal stoma is not a contraindication but requires adaptation of the spirometer

➤ HAZARDS AND COMPLICATIONS

- Ineffective unless closely supervised or performed as ordered
- Hyperventilation
- Exacerbation of brochospasm
- Hypoxia due to break in mask O_2 therapy
- Inappropriate as sole treatment for major lung collapse or consolidation
- Barotrauma (emphysematous lungs)
- Fatigue
- Discomfort secondary to inadequate pain control

➤ ASSESSMENT OF NEED

- Surgical procedure involving upper abdomen or thorax
- Conditions predisposing to atelectasis, including immobility, poor pain control, and abdominal binders
- Presence of neuromuscular disease involving respiratory musculature

➤ ASSESSMENT OF OUTCOME

- Absence of or improvement in signs of atelectasis
- Decreased respiratory rate
- Resolution of fever
- Normal pulse rate
- Absence of crackles or presence of or improvement in previously absent or diminished breath sounds
- Normal chest radiograph
- Improved PaO_2 and decreased PAO_2
- Increased VC and peak expiratory flows
- Return of FRC or VC to preoperative values, in absence of lung resection
- Improved inspiratory muscle performance (e.g., attainment of preoperative flow and volume levels, increased forced vital capacity [FVC])

➤ MONITORING

- Direct supervision of every patient performance is not needed once the patient has mastered technique; however, preoperative instruction, volume goals, and feedback are essential to optimal performance
- Observation of patient performance and use
  - Frequency of sessions
  - Number of breaths/session
  - Inspiratory volume or flow goals achieved and 3- to 5-second breath-hold maintained
  - Effort/motivation
- Periodic observation of patient compliance with technique, with additional instruction as necessary
- Device within reach of patient and patient encouraged to perform independently
- New and increasing inspiratory volumes established each day
- Vital signs

*For complete guidelines, see Respir Care 36:1402, 1991.

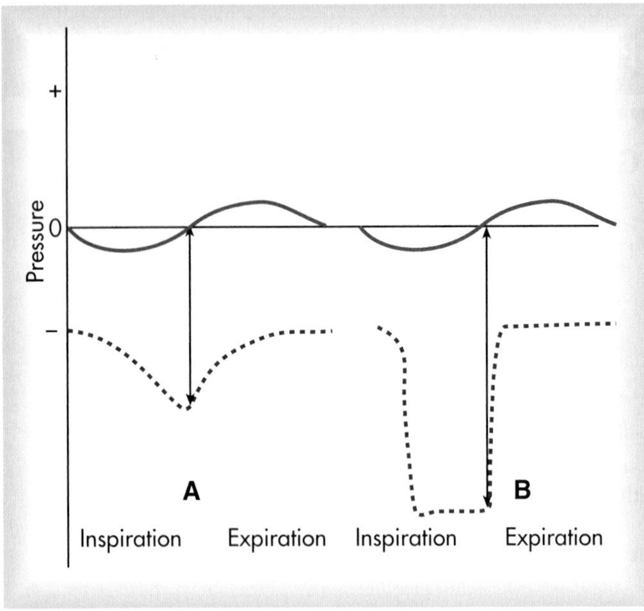

Figure 36-2
Alveolar *(solid lines)* and pleural *(dotted lines)* pressure changes during **(A)** spontaneous breathing and **(B)** sustained maximum inspiration (SMI). Note the difference in P_L gradients *(arrowed lines)*.

Indications for IS

Indications for IS are listed in Box 36-1.[15] The primary indication for IS is to treat existing atelectasis. IS may also be used as a preventive measure when conditions exist that make the development of atelectasis likely. IS devices can be used to monitor lung function in the postoperative period because there is good correlation between IS performance and VC measurement by spirometry.[16] IS with inspiratory muscle training can significantly improve lung function in patients with chronic obstructive lung disease (COPD) undergoing lung resection.[17]

Box 36-1 • Indications for Incentive Spirometry

- Presence of pulmonary atelectasis
- Presence of conditions predisposing to atelectasis:
  - Upper abdominal surgery
  - Thoracic surgery
  - Surgery in patients with COPD
- Presence of a restrictive lung defect associated with quadriplegia and/or dysfunctional diaphragm

Contraindications for IS

IS is a simple and relatively safe modality. For this reason, contraindications are few (Box 36-2).

Box 36-2 • Clinical Situations Contraindicating Incentive Spirometry

- Unconscious patients or those unable to cooperate
- Patients who cannot properly use IS device after instruction
- Patients unable to generate adequate inspiration, for example:
  - VC <10 mL/kg or
  - IC <? predicted normal

Hazards and Complications of IS

Given its normal physiological basis, IS presents few major hazards and complications. Those that can occur are listed in Box 36-3.[15]

Acute respiratory alkalosis is the most common problem and occurs when the patient performs IS too rapidly. Dizziness and numbness around the mouth are the most frequently reported symptoms associated with respiratory alkalosis. This problem is easily corrected with careful instruction and monitoring of the patient.

Discomfort with deep inspiratory efforts secondary to pain is usually the result of inadequate pain control in the postoperative patient. This problem can be rectified by ensuring appropriate analgesia. In addition, pain medication should be coordinated with IS activity.

Box 36-3 • Hazards and Complications of Incentive Spirometry

- Hyperventilation and respiratory alkalosis
- Discomfort secondary to inadequate pain control
- Pulmonary barotrauma
- Exacerbation of bronchospasm
- Fatigue

Equipment

The equipment needed for IS is typically simple, portable, and inexpensive. Although recent advances in technology have produced more complex devices, there is no evidence that they produce any better outcomes than their lower cost, disposable counterparts.

IS devices can generally be categorized as volume- or flow-oriented. True volume-oriented devices actually measure and visually indicate the volume achieved during an SMI. The most popular true volume-oriented IS devices use a bellows that rises according to the inhaled volume. Once the patient reaches a target inspiratory volume, a controlled leak in the device allows the patient to sustain the inspiratory effort for a short period of time (usually 5 to 10 seconds). Because the bellows type of ISs are bulky and large, smaller devices that indirectly indicate volume based on flow through a fixed orifice have been developed. Such devices sacrifice accurate measurement of the inhaled volume to achieve portability and smaller size (Figure 36-3).

Flow-oriented devices measure and visually indicate the degree of inspiratory flow (Figure 36-4). This flow can be equated with volume by assessing the duration of inspiration or time (flow × time = volume). Both flow-oriented and volume-oriented devices attempt to encourage the same goal for the patient: a sustained maximal inspiratory effort to prevent or correct atelectasis. No evidence to date indicates that one type is more beneficial than the other.

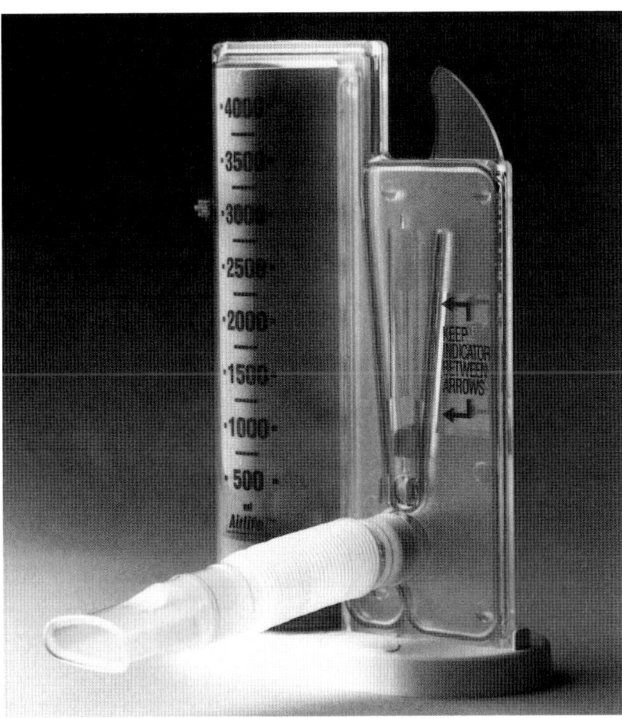

Figure 36-3
Volumetric incentive spirometer. *(Courtesy of Allegiance Health Care, McGaw Park, Illinois.)*

Administering IS

The successful application of IS involves three phases: planning, implementation, and follow-up. Since many of the components of this process are similar to those previously described, we will highlight only the key points and differences in approach.

Preliminary Planning

During preliminary planning, the need for IS should be determined by careful patient assessment. Once the need is established, planning for IS should focus on selecting explicit therapeutic outcomes. Box 36-4 lists

Box 36-4 • Potential Outcomes of Incentive Spirometry

- Absence of or improvement in signs of atelectasis:
- Decreased respiratory rate
- Normal pulse rate
- Resolution of abnormal breath sounds
- Normal or improved chest radiograph
- Improved Pa_{O_2} and decreased Pa_{CO_2}
- Increased SpO_2
- Increased VC and peak expiratory flows
- Restoration of preoperative FRC or VC
- Improved inspiratory muscle performance and cough
- Attainment of preoperative flow and volume levels
- Increased FVC

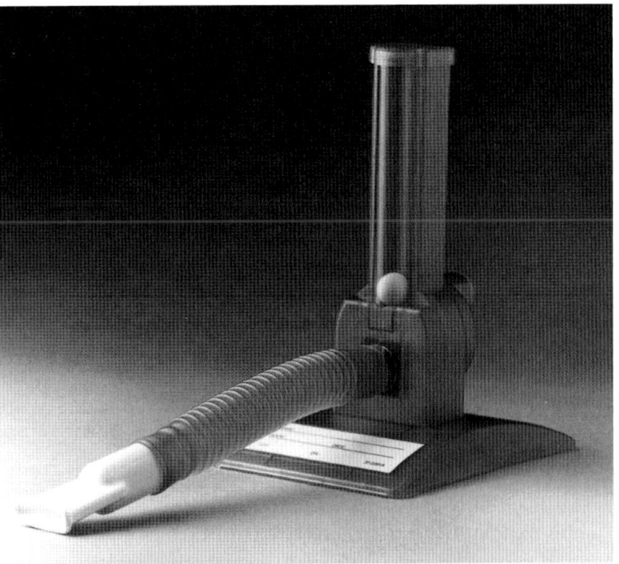

Figure 36-4
Flow-oriented incentive spirometer. *(Courtesy of Allegiance Health Care, McGaw Park, Illinois.)*

potential outcomes that can be considered for patients receiving IS.[15]

Obviously, the outcomes applicable to a given patient depend on the diagnostic information that supports the need for IS. In this regard, the baseline patient assessment is critical. Patients scheduled for upper abdominal or thoracic surgery should be screened prior to undergoing the surgical procedure. Assessment conducted at this point will help identify patients at high risk for postoperative complications and allow determination of their baseline lung volumes and capacities. Moreover, this approach provides an opportunity to orient high-risk patients to the procedure before undergoing surgery, thereby increasing the likelihood of success when IS is provided after surgery.

Implementation

Successful IS requires effective patient teaching. The RRT should set an initial goal (e.g., a certain volume) that is attainable but requires some moderate effort. Setting too low an initial goal for the patient results in little incentive and an ineffective maneuver, at least initially. The patient should be instructed to inspire slowly and deeply to maximize the distribution of ventilation.

The RRT should observe the patient perform the initial inspiratory maneuvers and make sure the patient uses correct technique. Correct technique calls for diaphragmatic breathing at slow-to-moderate inspiratory flows. Demonstration is probably the most effective way to assist patient understanding and cooperation. By using yourself as an example, both the operation of the device and the proper breathing technique can be easily explained, and much trial and error can be avoided.

Instruct the patient to sustain his or her maximal inspiratory volume for 5 to 10 seconds. Many patients have difficulty with this aspect of the maneuver. Adding a one-way valve (which prevents exhalation) to the IS device can increase both inspired volume and breath-hold time, even in uncoached patients.[18] The safety of this modification, however, has not been assessed.

A normal exhalation should follow the breath-hold, and the patient should be given the opportunity to rest as long as needed prior to the next SMI maneuver. Some patients in the early postoperative stage may need to rest for as much as 30 seconds to a minute between maneuvers. This rest period helps avoid a common tendency by some patients to repeat the maneuver at rapid rates, thereby causing respiratory alkalosis. The goal is not rapid, partial lung inflation but intermittent, maximal inspiration.

The exact number of sustained maximal inspirations needed to reverse or prevent atelectasis is not known and probably varies according to the patient's clinical status. However, because healthy individuals average about 6 sighs per hour, an IS regimen should probably aim to ensure a minimum of 5 to 10 SMI maneuvers each hour.[15,19]

Follow-Up

As always, assessing the patient's performance is vital to ensuring achievement of goals. To do so, the RRT should make return visits to monitor treatment sessions until the correct technique and appropriate effort are achieved. Suggested monitoring activities for IS are outlined in Box 36-5.[15]

Once the patient has demonstrated mastery of technique, IS may be performed with minimal supervision.[20] Even when self-administered, records of progress pertaining to the patient's clinical status, must be maintained throughout the course of treatment. The result of this assessment can guide the physician and RRT in revising the respiratory care plan or terminating treatment once the goals are achieved.

▶ INTERMITTENT POSITIVE PRESSURE BREATHING (IPPB)

IPPB was introduced as a clinical modality by Motley in 1947.[21] Since that time, IPPB has had a volatile history. During its early years, IPPB enjoyed widespread use and popularity. Physicians prescribed IPPB for a broad range of clinical conditions. Although clinical evidence supporting its use was lacking, IPPB became the predominant mode of respiratory care by 1970.

Subsequently, IPPB came under attack as both an unvalidated and overused treatment modality. In 1980, the Respiratory Care Committee of the American Thoracic Society (ATS) prepared guidelines for the use of IPPB, supporting its rational application in certain clearly defined clinical situations. Later in that decade, the

Box 36-5 • Monitoring Patients Receiving Incentive Spirometry

Observation of patient performance and use:
- Frequency of sessions
- Number of breaths/session
- Volume/flow goals achieved
- Breath-hold maintained
- Effort/motivation
- Periodic observation of patient compliance, with additional instruction as needed
- Device within reach of patient and patient encouraged to perform independently
- New and increasing inspiratory volumes established each day
- Vital signs/breath sounds

American Association for Respiratory Care (AARC) disseminated a statement asserting the effectiveness of IPPB in several, very specific clinical situations.[22] Most recently, the AARC has established a clinical practice guideline for IPPB therapy.[23]

Clearly, IPPB should neither be totally condemned nor universally applied. Like so many other respiratory care modalities, the proper use of IPPB requires that:

1. Patients be carefully chosen.
2. The indications for therapy be specifically defined.
3. The goals of therapy be clearly understood.
4. The treatment be properly administered and monitored by a trained RRT.

Definition and Physiological Principle

IPPB refers to the application of inspiratory positive pressure to a spontaneously breathing patient as an intermittent or short-term therapeutic modality.[23] IPPB "treatments" usually last 15 to 20 minutes and may be given for a variety of reasons. This chapter will emphasize the intermittent use of IPPB as a modality for the treatment of atelectasis.

Figure 36-5 compares the alveolar and P_{pl} changes occurring during a normal spontaneous breath and during IPPB. As can be seen in Figure 36-5, *B*, IPPB reverses the normal spontaneous pressure gradients. Positive pressure at the airway opening creates the needed pressure gradient to cause gas flow into the lungs. P_{alv} rises during the inspiratory phase of IPPB as flows the gas from the airways into the alveoli.

Positive pressure is transmitted from the alveoli to the pleural space during the inspiratory phase of an IPPB treatment, causing P_{pl} to rise somewhat during inspiration. Depending on the mechanical properties of the lung, P_{pl} may actually exceed atmospheric pressure during a portion of inspiration.

As with spontaneous breathing, the recoil force of the lung and chest wall, stored as potential energy during the positive pressure breath, causes a passive exhalation. As gas flows from the alveoli out to the airway opening, P_{alv} drops to atmospheric level while P_{pl} is restored to its normal subatmospheric range (Figure 36-5, *A*).

Indications for IPPB

IPPB may be useful for patients with clinically diagnosed atelectasis not responsive to other therapies, such as IS and chest physiotherapy. In addition, IPPB may be useful for patients who are at high risk for atelectasis and not able to cooperate with more simple techniques such as IS. In either case, IPPB should not be used as a single treatment modality for the patient with resorption atelectasis due to excessive airway secretions. Applying positive pressure to the lung in such cases is likely to cause overinflation of the lung regions not affected by secretions and minimal or no expansion of the affected lung segments. Bronchial hygiene with humidity therapy must be used in conjunction with IPPB for the most optimal results in such cases.

In concept, a correctly administered IPPB treatment should provide the patient with augmented tidal volumes, achieved with minimal effort. In fact, an aggressive respiratory therapy regimen that includes IPPB has been shown to be as effective as therapeutic bronchoscopy in treating patients with lobar atelectasis.[24] The optimal breathing pattern to reinflate collapsed lung units with IPPB consists of slow, deep breaths that are sustained or held at end-inspiration. This type of inspiratory maneuver increases the distribution of inspired gas to areas of the lung with low compliance, specifically, the atelectatic areas.

Although the application of IPPB to treat atelectasis is well substantiated, its use prophylactically to prevent the occurrence of this postoperative complication is not supported.[25]

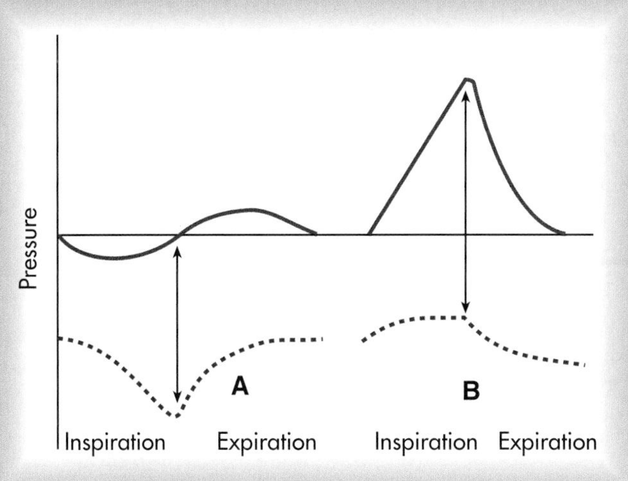

Figure 36-5

Alveolar *(solid lines)* and pleural *(dotted lines)* pressure changes during **(A)** spontaneous breathing and **(B)** IPPB. Note the difference in P_L gradients *(arrowed lines)*.

Intermittent Positive Pressure Breathing

AARC Clinical Practice Guideline (Excerpts)*

➤ INDICATIONS

- The need to improve lung expansion
  - The presence of clinically important pulmonary atelectasis when other forms of therapy (e.g., IS) have been unsuccessful or the patient cannot cooperate
  - Inability to clear secretions adequately because of pathology that severely limits the ability to ventilate or cough effectively and failure to respond to other modes of treatment
- The need for short-term noninvasive ventilatory support for hyercapnic patients (as an alternative to intubation and continuous ventilatory support)
- The need to deliver aerosol medication
  - Although some authors oppose the use of IPPB in the treatment of severe bronchospasm (e.g., acute asthma), we recommend a careful, closely supervised trial of IPPB when treatment using other techniques (metered dose inhaler [MDI] or nebulizer) has been unsuccessful.
  - IPPB may be used to deliver aerosol medications to patients with ventilatory muscle weakness or fatigue or chronic conditions in which intermittent noninvasive ventilatory support is indicated.

➤ CONTRAINDICATIONS

Although no absolute contraindications to the use of IPPB therapy (except tension pneumothorax) have been reported, the patient with any of the following should be carefully evaluated before a decision is made to initiate IPPB therapy:

- ICP >15 mm Hg
- Hemodynamic instability
- Recent facial, oral, or skull surgery
- Tracheoesophageal fistula
- Recent esophageal surgery
- Active hemoptysis
- Nausea
- Air swallowing
- Active, untreated tuberculosis
- Radiographic evidence of bleb
- Singulus (hiccups)

➤ HAZARDS AND COMPLICATIONS

- Increased airway resistance
- Barotrauma, pneumothorax
- Nosocomial infection
- Hyperventilation/hypocapnia
- Hemoptysis
- Hyperoxia when oxygen is the gas source
- Gastric distention
- Secretion impaction (inadequate humidity)
- Psychological dependence
- Impedance of venous return
- Exacerbation of hypoxemia
- Hypoventilation
- Increased $\dot{V}/\dot{Q}$ mismatch
- Air trapping, autoPEEP, overdistended alveoli

➤ ASSESSMENT OF NEED

- Presence of atelectasis
- Reduced timed volumes or VC (e.g., FEV_1 <65% predicted, FVC <70% predicted, maximum voluntary ventilation (MVV) <50% predicted, or VC <10 mL/kg) precluding an effective cough
- Neuromuscular or skeletal disorders associated with decrease in lung volumes and capacities

INTERMITTENT POSITIVE PRESSURE BREATHING—CONT'D

AARC Clinical Practice Guideline (Excerpts)*

- Fatigue or muscle weakness with impending respiratory failure
- Presence of acute, severe bronchospasm or exacerbated COPD that fails to respond to other therapy (consider MDI with spacer/holding chamber first)
- With demonstrated effectiveness, the patient's preference for a positive pressure device should be honored

➤ ASSESSMENT OF OUTCOME

- Tidal volume during IPPB greater than during spontaneous breathing (by at least 25%)
- FEV_1 or peak flow increase
- Cough more effective with treatment
- Secretion clearance enhanced as a consequence of deep breathing and coughing
- Chest radiograph improved
- Breath sounds improved
- Favorable patient subjective response

➤ MONITORING

Items from the following list should be chosen as appropriate for the specific patient:

- Machine performance (trigger sensitivity, peak pressure, flow settings, FIO_2, inspiratory time, expiratory time, plateau pressure, PEEP)
- Respiratory rate and volume
- Peak flow or FEV_1/FVC
- Pulse rate and rhythm from ECG if available
- Patient subjective response to therapy (pain, discomfort, dyspnea)
- Sputum production (quantity, color, consistency, and odor)
- Mental function
- Skin colors
- Breath sounds
- Blood pressure
- Arterial hemoglobin saturation by pulse oximetry (if hypoxemia is suspected)
- ICP in patients for whom ICP is of critical importance
- Chest radiograph

*For complete guidelines, see Respir Care 38:1189, 1993.

MINI CLINI

Importance of Air Bronchograms on the Chest Film

PROBLEM

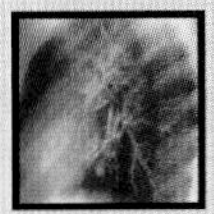

You are called to evaluate a 59-year-old woman admitted to the hospital several days ago for cardiac surgery. The patient underwent surgery two days ago and has developed complications. She is alert but disoriented and has decreased breath sound bilaterally in the bases. The chest radiograph demonstrates elevation of the right hemidiaphragm and air bronchograms in both lower lung fields. The attending physician wants to start IPPB and asks your opinion about the treatment plan.

DISCUSSION

It is clear this patient needs lung expansion therapy, but IPPB alone could be harmful given the evidence of retained secretions. Air bronchograms are seen when air-filled airways are surrounded by portions of the distal lung regions impacted with mucus. The application of positive pressure to the lungs in this situation may be harmful because the pressure will shunt toward the nonobstructed airways and may lead to overinflation of selected regions. This patient needs bronchial hygiene and humidity therapy in addition to lung expansion therapy.

Box 36-6 • Clinical Situations Contraindicating IPPB Therapy

- Tension pneumothorax
- ICP >15 mm Hg
- Hemodynamic instability
- Active hemoptysis
- Tracheoesophageal fistula
- Recent esophageal surgery
- Active, untreated tuberculosis
- Radiographic evidence of blebs
- Recent facial, oral, or skull surgery
- Singultus (hiccups)
- Air swallowing
- Nausea

Contraindications for IPPB

There are several clinical situations in which IPPB should not be used (Box 36-6).[22] With the exception of untreated tension pneumothorax, most of these contraindications are relative. As with all procedures, a sound knowledge of the patient's condition tempered with common sense should guide the RRT in the decision-making process. Thus, a patient with any of the listed conditions should be carefully evaluated before a decision is made to begin IPPB therapy.

Hazards and Complications of IPPB

As with any clinical intervention, certain hazards and complications are associated with IPPB. These potential problems should be addressed in the initial stages of planning for IPPB. In addition, hazards and complications must be considered throughout the course of therapy as part of the process of assessing the patient for unwanted side effects. The most common complication associated with IPPB is the inducement of respiratory alkalosis. This occurs when the patient breathes too rapidly during the treatment. Deep and fast breathing leads to a sharp drop in P_{CO_2} and an equally marked increase in arterial pH. This usually causes the patient to feel light-headed and numb around the mouth. Arrhythmias are also possible if the alkalosis is severe or if the patient's heart is unstable. This problem is easily avoided through proper coaching of the patient prior to and during treatment.

Another potential complication of IPPB is gastric distension. This occurs when gas from the IPPB device passes directly into the esophagus. It is not common in the alert patient but represents a significant risk for the neurologically obtunded patient. Normally, the esophagus does not open until a pressure of about 20 cm H_2O has been reached. Therefore gastric distension represents the greatest risk in patients receiving IPPB at high pressures. The major hazards and complications of IPPB are listed in Box 36-7.[23]

Box 36-7 • Hazards and Complications of IPPB

- Increased airway resistance
- Pulmonary barotrauma
- Nosocomial infection
- Respiratory alkalosis
- Hyperoxia (with O_2 as source gas)
- Impaired venous return
- Gastric distention
- Air trapping, autoPEEP, overdistention
- Psychological dependence

Administering IPPB

Effective IPPB requires careful preliminary planning, individualized patient assessment and implementation, and thoughtful follow-up. In all three phases of the process, the RRT should work closely with the prescribing physician to determine patient need, select the appropriate therapeutic approach, and assess patient progress toward predefined clinical outcomes. Only by ensuring that these elements are combined as part of the overall respiratory care plan can the RRT expect to achieve the desired results.

Preliminary Planning

During preliminary planning, the need for IPPB should be determined, and desired therapeutic outcomes should be set. The outcomes chosen for a given patient should be based on diagnostic information that supports the need for IPPB therapy. In addition, therapeutic outcomes should be as explicit and measurable as possible. Outcomes must also be consistent with the therapeutic indications previously described. Outcomes that are inconsistent with these indications are generally inappropriate. Box 36-8 lists potential accepted and desired outcomes of IPPB therapy.

Obviously, not all these outcomes apply to every patient. As an example, for a patient exhibiting clinical signs and symptoms of postoperative atelectasis, we might set the following outcomes:

1. A spontaneous IC 70% of predicted
2. Improvement in the chest radiograph
3. Remission of auscultatory signs of atelectasis (fine, late-inspiratory crackles)
4. Reduction of the spontaneous respiratory rate to <25/minute

MINI CLINI

Evaluating the Effectiveness of Lung Expansion Therapy

PROBLEM

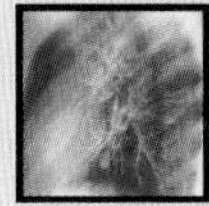

You are the supervisor for the day shift in the surgical ICU. The nursing supervisor asks for your opinion on the best ways to evaluate the effectiveness of lung expansion therapy. She is developing a new documentation form for the nurses to use at the beside and wants your opinion on the parameters to list. What is your response?

DISCUSSION

You should suggest that numerous parameters are useful. One of the best is observation of the patient's spontaneous respiratory rate at rest. There is a strong correlation between respiratory rate and degree of atelectasis. The more atelectasis present, the higher the spontaneous respiratory rate will be. If lung expansion therapy is preventing or correcting atelectasis, the respiratory rate will be at or near normal. Auscultation can also be useful and should document the presence of abnormal breath sounds and adventitious lung sounds. A reduction in late-inspiratory crackles and improvement in breath sounds suggest the treatment is effective. Findings on the most recent chest film can be very useful to document the presence or lack of atelectasis. The signs of volume loss will disappear with effective lung expansion therapy. In addition, the patient may complain of less dyspnea when the lung is expanded to its healthy position.

Box 36-8 • Potential Outcomes of IPPB Therapy

- Improved inspiratory or VC
- Increased FEV_1 or peak flow
- Enhanced cough and secretion clearance
- Improved chest radiograph
- Improved breath sounds
- Improved oxygenation
- Favorable patient subjective response

Evaluating Alternatives

A key component in early planning must be consideration of alternative therapies. Specifically, before starting IPPB, the RRT and prescribing physician must determine whether simpler and less costly methods might be as effective in achieving the desired outcomes. If this is the case, further consideration of IPPB should be postponed until the patient's response to the simpler therapy is assessed.

Box 36-9 • Infection Control Precautions for IPPB Therapy

- Use proper hand-washing technique
- Follow Centers for Disease Control and Prevention (CDC) universal precautions
- Follow CDC guidelines for preventing spread of tuberculosis
- Observe all infection control guidelines posted for patient
- Use only sterile diluents and medications
- Disinfect all reusable equipment between patients
- Change nebulizers or perform high-level disinfection at conclusion of dose administration, every 24 hours with continuous use, or more often when visibly soiled
- Rinse nebulizer with sterile water only

Baseline Assessment

Prior to beginning therapy, the RRT should conduct a baseline patient assessment. This information will help individualize the treatment and allows objective evaluation of the patient's subsequent response to therapy. Together with the patient's medical history, this baseline assessment also alerts the RRT to possible problems or hazards associated with administering IPPB to a specific patient.

The baseline assessment should include both a general evaluation of the patient's clinical status and a specific assessment related to the chosen therapeutic goals. The general assessment, common to all patients for whom IPPB is ordered, should include: (1) measurement of vital signs, (2) observational assessment of the patient's appearance and sensorium, and (3) breathing pattern and chest auscultation. The more focused assessment should be individualized according to the identified clinical goals.

Implementation

Implementation of the IPPB involves infection control, equipment preparation, patient orientation, and careful adjustment of the treatment parameters according to the patient's response.

Infection Control. Standard considerations to avoid transmission of infection between RRT and patient during IPPB therapy are outlined in Box 36-9.

Equipment Preparation. Although all IPPB equipment should undergo a regular schedule of preventive maintenance and calibration, it is the RRT's responsibility to ensure that all components are in proper working order prior to any patient use. Most respiratory care departments have standard protocols for this purpose.

Because pressure-cycled IPPB devices will not end inspiration if leaks in the system occur, it is important to check the patency of the patient's breathing circuit prior to each use. This can be done by aseptically occluding the patient connector and manually triggering a breath at a low-flow setting. If the system pressure rises and the machine cycles off, the circuit is free of any major leak.

Patient Orientation. Successful IPPB therapy depends mainly on the effectiveness of initial patient orientation. Before the first treatment, the RRT must carefully explain to the patient the purpose of the therapy. This explanation should be tailored to the patient's level of understanding and address, at a minimum, the following points: (1) why the physician ordered the treatment, (2) what the treatment does, (3) how it will feel, and (4) what are the expected results.

The IPPB device must not be brought to the bedside until the RRT feels the patient adequately understands the procedure and the importance of cooperation. Once the RRT decides to bring the equipment to the bedside, a simple functional description may allay any fear or anxiety associated with the use of such an unfamiliar device.

A simulated demonstration of the procedure can be particularly useful in this regard. This can be done effectively with a test lung or, if deemed necessary, by self-application using a separate breathing circuit kept for this purpose. For some patients, an effective demonstration can make the difference between success and failure in implementing the treatment regimen.

Patient Positioning. For best results, the patient should be in a semi-Fowler's position. Slouching should be discouraged because it will impair diaphragm movement and decrease inspired volumes. The supine position is acceptable in certain patients in which an upright position is contraindicated.

Initial Application. To eliminate airway leaks in the alert patient, an initial trial of nose clips may be needed until the technique is understood and the treatment can be performed without them. The mouthpiece must be inserted well past the lips, and a tight seal must be encouraged to prevent gas leakage from the site. The use of a mask is fraught with hazards and is suggested only for alert and cooperative patients otherwise unable to accomplish the treatment without leakage from the system.

The machine should be set so that a breath can be initiated with minimal patient effort. A sensitivity or trigger level of 1 to 2 cm H_2O is adequate for most patients. Initially, system pressure is set to between 10 to 15 cm H_2O. Resulting volumes should be measured, and the pressure should be adjusted accordingly after the treatment has begun. If the device has a flow control, the RRT should begin the treatment with a low-to-moderate flow and adjust it according to the patient's breathing pattern. Generally, the goal is to establish a breathing pattern consisting of about 6 breaths/minute, with an expiratory time of at least three to four times longer than inspiration (I:E ratio of 1:3 to 1:4 or lower). Obviously, these settings may need to be adjusted according to individual needs and patient response. Moreover, careful monitoring of the breathing pattern and coaching to maintain it must be conducted throughout the treatment.

Adjusting Parameters. Once the treatment begins and the patient's basic ventilatory pattern is established, the pressure and flow should be individually adjusted and monitored according to the goals of the therapy. IPPB therapy should be volume-oriented when used to treat atelectasis. In these situations, arbitrary pressure settings are not acceptable and tidal volumes must be monitored. A tidal volume goal must be set for each individual patient and the therapy must be delivered on the basis of these goals.

There are various ways of determining these volume goals. Most clinical centers strive to achieve an IPPB tidal volume of 10 to 15 mL/kg of body weight or at least 30% of the patient's predicted IC. If the initial volumes fall short of this goal and the patient can tolerate it, the pressure is gradually raised until the goal is achieved. Pressures as high as 30 to 35 cm H_2O may be needed to achieve this end when lung compliance is reduced.

To achieve the largest inspiratory volumes during IPPB, the RRT should encourage the patient to breathe actively during the positive pressure breath. However, no definitive studies exist that demonstrate the need to have the patient actively participate in inspiration. Regardless of the approach, IPPB is only useful in the treatment of atelectasis if the volumes delivered exceed those volumes achieved by the patient's spontaneous efforts.

Discontinuation and Follow-Up

Depending on the goals of therapy and condition of the patient, IPPB treatments typically last from 15 to 20 minutes. Follow-up activities include posttreatment assessment of the patient, recordkeeping, and equipment maintenance.

Posttreatment Assessment

At the end of a treatment session, the RRT should repeat the patient assessment. As with the baseline assessment, this follow-up evaluation has two components. The general follow-up evaluation of the patient's clinical status should focus on determining any pertinent changes in vital signs, sensorium, and breath sounds, with emphasis on identifying possible untoward effects. The more specific follow-up assessment provides information relevant to evaluating progress toward achieving the chosen goals of therapy.

Treatment frequency should be determined by assessing patient response to therapy. For acute care patients, orders should be reevaluated based on patient response to therapy at least every 72 hours or with any change of patient status.[17]

Recordkeeping

A succinct but complete account of the treatment session, including the results of preassessment and postassessment, must be entered in the patient's medical record according to the approved institutional protocol. Any untoward patient responses must also immediately be reported to responsible personnel, to include at least the prescribing physician and attending nurse.

Monitoring and Troubleshooting

As indicated in Box 36-10, monitoring of IPPB therapy involves both machine performance and patient response.[23] Information derived from monitoring helps the RRT make adjustments to therapy and can aid in the identification of common problems.

Machine Performance

In terms of machine performance, large negative pressure swings early in inspiration indicate an incorrect sensitivity or trigger setting. In this case, the RRT should increase the sensitivity or alter the trigger level until only 1 to 2 cm H_2O are needed to trigger the device into inspiration.

Should system pressure drop after inspiration begins or fails to rise until the very end of the machine breath, the problem is too low a flow. In this situation, the RRT should increase the flow (as tolerated) until system pressure rises steadily and holds near the preset value.

The opposite situation can also occur. Too high a flow will cause the device to cycle off prematurely. A lower flow setting will usually resolve this common problem. Alternatively, an IPPB device may cycle off prematurely when airflow is obstructed. Kinked tubing, an occluded mouthpiece, or active resistance to inhalation by the patient are the most common causes of this problem. Checking the circuit and properly instructing the patient are the best ways to prevent or correct these problems.

Leaks pose a different problem. In the presence of leaks, a pressure-cycled IPPB device will not reach its preset cycling pressure and thus will not cycle off. This problem is evident when inspiration continues well beyond the expected time.

To troubleshoot leaks, the RRT should differentiate between the machine and patient interface. Machine leaks most commonly occur at connection points, such as the nebulizer or exhalation valve. In addition, a torn or improperly seated exhalation valve diaphragm will cause a large system leak. Leaks at the patient interface usually occur at the mouth (loose seal around mouthpiece) or through the nose. If the problem is mouth leaks, additional instruction may help. If not, a flanged mouthpiece may be needed. Leaks through the nose are easily corrected with nose clips.

Box 36-10 • Monitoring IPPB Therapy

MACHINE PERFORMANCE
- Sensitivity
- Peak pressure
- Flow setting
- FIO_2
- I:E ratio

PATIENT RESPONSE*
- Breathing rate and expired volume
- Peak flow or FEV_1/FVC %
- Pulse rate and rhythm (from electrocardiogram [ECG] if available)
- Sputum quantity, color, consistency, and odor
- Mental function
- Skin color
- Breath sounds
- Blood pressure
- SpO_2 (if hypoxemia is suspected)
- ICP (in patients for whom ICP is important)
- Chest radiograph (when appropriate)
- Subjective response to therapy

*Above items should be chosen as appropriate for the specific patient.

Patient Response

In monitoring the patient's response, the RRT must take into account the intended purpose of the therapy and the patient's clinical conditions. These factors will dictate exactly what must be monitored for a given patient. Should any significant problem arise indicating an adverse response, we recommend that RRTs always follow the "triple-S" rule: Stop, stay, and stabilize. Stop the treatment (it may be causing the adverse response); stay with the patient (call for help if needed); and stay with the patient until the patient's condition has stabilized.

▶ POSITIVE AIRWAY PRESSURE (PAP) THERAPY

Like IPPB, PAP adjuncts use positive pressure to increase the P_L gradient and enhance lung expansion. Unlike IPPB, PAP therapy requires no complex machinery. Indeed, some methods do not even need a source of pressurized gas.

Definitions and Physiological Principle

There are three current approaches to PAP therapy: PEP, EPAP, and CPAP.[26] Recent evidence suggests that all three techniques are equally effective in treating atelectasis in most postsurgical patients.[27,28] Noninvasive ventilation on bilevel positive airway pressure has also proven to be effective in treating atelectasis.[29] Because PEP and EPAP are used most often as part of bronchial hygiene, they are described in Chapter 37. This chapter will describe the intermittent use of CPAP for the treatment of atelectasis. Continuous use of CPAP is discussed in Chapter 40.

While PEP and EPAP create expiratory positive pressure only, CPAP maintains a positive airway pressure throughout both inspiration and expiration.[28] Figure 36-6 compares the alveolar and P_{pl} changes occurring during a normal spontaneous breath (Figure 36-6, *A*) and CPAP (Figure 36-6, *B*). As can be seen, CPAP elevates and maintains high alveolar and airway pressures throughout the full breathing cycle. This increases P_L gradient throughout both inspiration and expiration.

Typically, the patient on CPAP breathes through a pressurized circuit against a threshold resistor, with pressures maintained between 5 and 20 cm H_2O.[26] To maintain system pressure throughout the breathing cycle, CPAP requires a source of pressurized gas.

Exactly how CPAP helps resolve atelectasis is unknown. However, the following factors probably contribute to its beneficial effects: (1) the recruitment of collapsed alveoli via an increase in FRC, (2) a decreased work of breathing due to increased compliance or abolition of autopositive end-expiratory pressure (PEEP), (3) an improved distribution of ventilation through collateral channels (e.g., Kohn's pores), and (4) an increase in the efficiency of secretion removal.

Indications for CPAP

Even though evidence exists to support the use of CPAP therapy in the treatment of postoperative atelectasis, the duration of beneficial effects appears limited. Indeed, the corresponding increase in FRC may be lost within 10 minutes after the end of the treatment. For this reason, it has been suggested that CPAP should be used on a continuous, not intermittent basis.

CPAP by mask also has been used to treat cardiogenic pulmonary edema. In such patients, CPAP reduces venous return and cardiac filling pressures and also improves lung compliance and decreases the work of breathing.

Contraindications for CPAP

Intermittent use of CPAP for the correction of atelectasis is contraindicated when certain clinical situations exist. For example, the patient who is hemodynamically unstable is not likely to tolerate CPAP for even a short period of time. The patient who is suspected of having hypoventilation is not a good candidate for CPAP because it does not ensure ventilation. Other problems that may indicate that CPAP is not an appropriate therapy include nausea, facial trauma, untreated pneumothorax, and elevated intracranial pressure (ICP).

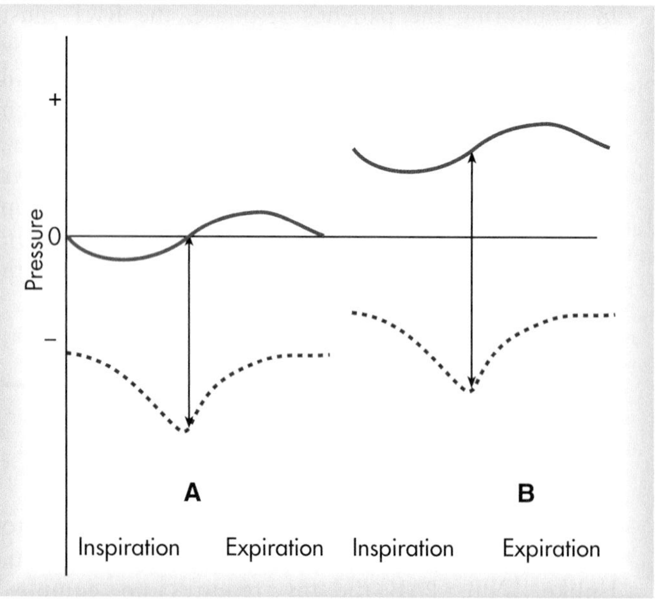

Figure 36-6
Alveolar *(solid lines)* and pleural *(dotted lines)* pressures during **(A)** spontaneous breathing and **(B)** CPAP. Note difference in P_L gradients *(arrows)*.

Hazards and Complications of CPAP

Most hazards and complications associated with CPAP are caused by either the increased pressure or the apparatus. The increased work of breathing caused by the apparatus can lead to hypoventilation and hypercapnia.[28] In addition, because CPAP does not augment spontaneous ventilation, patients with an accompanying ventilatory insufficiency may hypoventilate during application. Barotrauma is a potential hazard of CPAP and is more likely to occur in the patient with emphysema and blebs. Gastric distention may occur especially if CPAP pressures above 15 cm H_2O are needed. This may lead to vomiting and aspiration in the patient with an inadequate gag reflex.

Equipment

Equipment used to deliver CPAP varies substantially in design and complexity. For purposes of illustration, the key elements of a simple continuous flow CPAP circuit are shown in Figure 36-7. A breathing gas mixture from an oxygen blender *(A)* flows continuously through a humidifier *(B)* into the inspiratory limb of a breathing circuit *(C)*. A reservoir bag *(D)* provides reserve volume if the patient's inspiratory flow exceeds that of the system. The patient breathes in and out through a simple valveless T-piece connector *(E)*. A pressure alarm system with manometer *(F)* monitors the CPAP pressure at the patient's airway. The alarm system can warn of either low (usually due to a disconnection) or high system pressure. The expiratory limb of the circuit *(G)* is connected to a threshold resistor, in this case a water column *(H)*.

As can be seen, the CPAP circuit is essentially the same as the EPAP circuit, with the exception of the closed reservoir and monitoring system. Because it is a closed system, the CPAP circuit should also have an emergency inlet valve (not shown). This emergency inlet valve ensures that atmospheric air is available to the patient should the primary gas source fail.

Administering Intermittent CPAP

As with all respiratory care, effective CPAP therapy requires careful planning, individualized patient assessment and implementation, and thoughtful follow-up.

Planning

During planning, the need for PAP therapy should be determined, and desired therapeutic outcomes should be set. Specifically, an improvement in breath sounds, improvement in vital signs (e.g., lower respiratory rate), resolution of abnormal radiograph findings, and restoration of normal oxygenation would all indicate that the therapy has achieved its goal.

Procedures

Whether used on an intermittent or continuous basis, CPAP is a complex and potentially hazardous approach to patient management. As with all therapies, the appropriate CPAP level for a given patient must be determined on an individual basis. Initial application and monitoring require a broader range of knowledge and skill than that required for simpler modes of lung expansion therapy.

Monitoring and Troubleshooting

CPAP poses a real danger of hypoventilation. Experience with long-term CPAP clearly demonstrates that

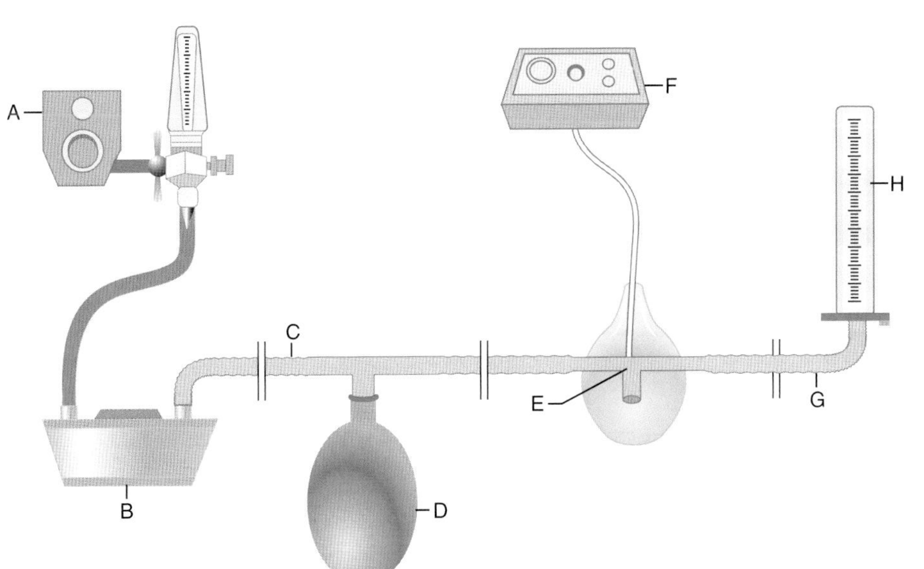

Figure 36-7
Continuous-flow CPAP system. See text for description. *(Modified from Branson Rd, Hurst JM, Dellayen CB: Mask CPAP: state of the art, Respir Care 30:846, 1985.)*

patients must be able to maintain adequate excretion of carbon dioxide on their own if the therapy is to be successful.

For these reasons, patients receiving CPAP must be closely and continuously monitored for untoward effects. In addition, it is vital that the CPAP device be equipped with a means to monitor the pressure delivered to the airways and alarms to indicate the loss of pressure due to system disconnect or mechanical failure. These are essential components of any CPAP device.

The most common problem with PAP therapies is system leaks. When using a mask, a tight seal must be maintained to keep pressure levels above atmospheric levels. Any significant leaks in the system will result in the loss of PAP. Because a tight seal requires a tight-fitting mask, pain and irritation may occur in some patients, especially if the therapy is prolonged.

The development of the new nasal CPAP units has addressed some of the comfort issues as well as correction of leakage associated with CPAP. Its use intermittently for this purpose, however, has not been well documented.

A more serious problem associated with CPAP is the possibility of gastric insufflation and aspiration of stomach contents. As with IPPB by mask, this potential hazard can be eliminated by use of a nasogastric tube.

The RRT must also ensure that the flow is adequate to meet the patient's needs with the use of CPAP systems. Generally, the flow is initially set to 2 to 3 times the patient's minute ventilation. Thereafter, flow

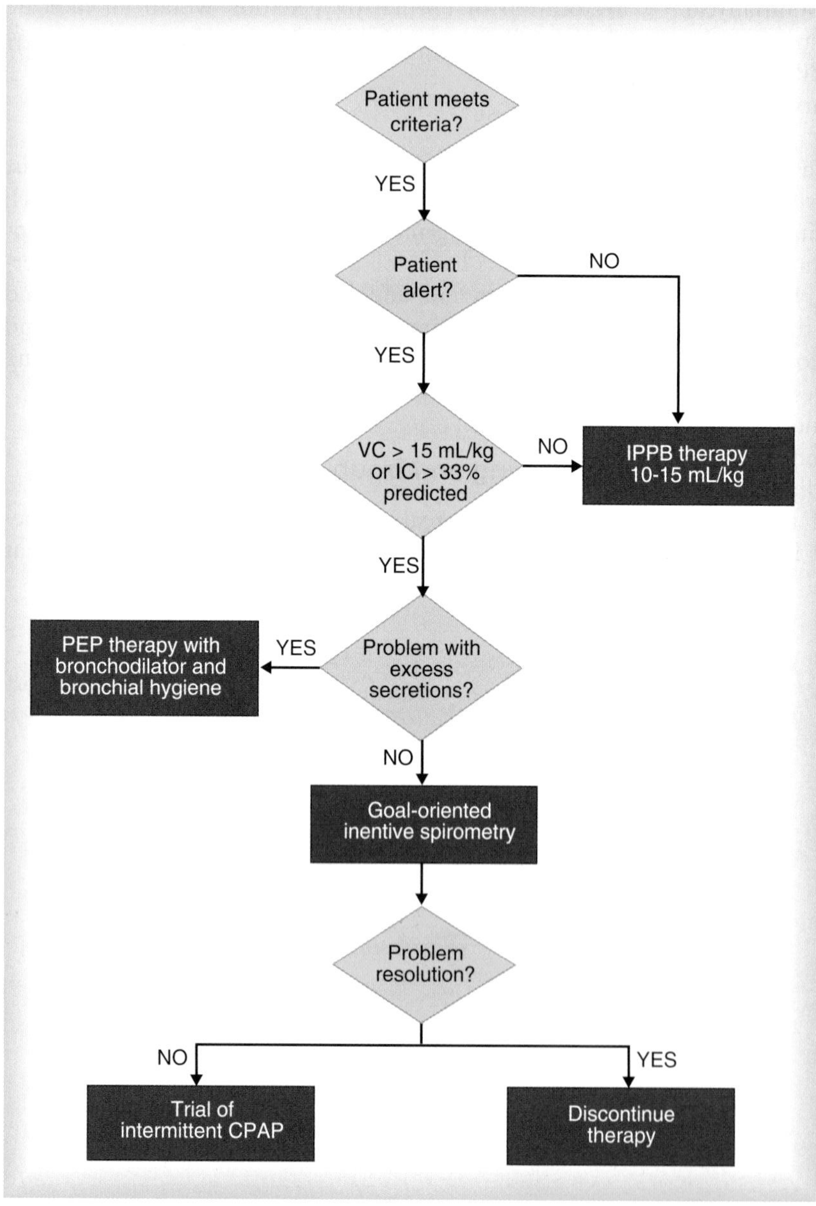

Figure 36-8
Example protocol for selecting an approach for lung expansion therapy (see text for details.)

adjustments are made by carefully observing the airway pressure. Flow is adequate when the system pressure drops no more than 1 to 2 cm H_2O during inspiration.

▶ SELECTING AN APPROACH

The best approach for achieving a given clinical goal is always the safest, simplest, and most effective method for a given patient. Selecting an approach for lung expansion therapy thus requires in-depth knowledge of both the methods available and the specific condition and needs of the patient being considered for therapy.

Figure 36-8 presents a sample protocol for selecting an approach to lung expansion therapy. As indicated in the algorithm, the patient must first meet the criteria for therapy by having one or more of the indications previously specified. For patients meeting the inclusion criteria, the RRT first determines the degree of alertness. Because an obtunded patient cannot be expected to cooperate with IS or PEP/EPAP therapy, IPPB at 10 to 15 mL/kg is initiated with appropriate monitoring.

If, on the other hand, the patient is alert, a bedside assessment is conducted. This assessment should include measurement of either the inspiratory or VC and evaluation of the volume and consistency of the patient's secretions.

For the patient having no difficulty with secretions, if the VC exceeds 15 mL/kg of lean body weight, or the IC is greater than 33% of predicted, IS is given. If either the VC or IC is less than these threshold levels, IPPB is initiated, with the pressure gradually manipulated from the initial setting to deliver at least 15 mL/kg.

If excessive sputum production is a compounding factor, a trial of PEP therapy is substituted for IS. Based on patient response, bronchodilator therapy and bronchial hygiene measures may be added to this regimen.

If monitoring fails to reveal improvement and atelectasis persists, a trial of CPAP should be considered. Because evidence of the effectiveness of CPAP is still contradictory, its current use should be limited to treating atelectasis after alternative approaches have been tried without success.

KEY POINTS

- Atelectasis is caused by persistent ventilation with small tidal volumes or by resorption of gas distal to obstructed airways.
- Patients who have undergone upper abdominal or thoracic surgery are at the greatest risk for atelectasis. A history of lung disease or significant cigarette smoking increases the risk.

KEY POINTS—cont'd

- Patients with atelectasis usually demonstrate rapid, shallow breathing; fine, late-inspiratory crackles; and abnormalities on the chest radiograph. Fever is not associated with atelectasis.
- Lung expansion therapy corrects atelectasis by increasing the P_L gradient. This can be accomplished by deep spontaneous breaths or by the application of positive pressure.
- The most common problem associated with lung expansion therapy is the onset of respiratory alkalosis, which occurs when the patient breathes too fast.
- RRTs have the responsibility of implementing, monitoring, and documenting results of lung expansion therapy.

References

1. Ferguson MK: Preoperative assessment of pulmonary risk, Chest 115:58S, 1999.
2. Thomas JA, McIntosh JM: Are IS, IPPB, and deep breathing exercises effective in the prevention of postoperative pulmonary complications after abdominal surgery? A systematic overview and meta-analysis, Phys Ther 74:8, 1994.
3. Woodring JH, Reed JC: Types and mechanisms of pulmonary atelectasis, J Thoracic Imaging 11:92, 1996.
4. Uzieblo M et al: Incidence and significance of lobar atelectasis in thoracic surgery. Am Surg 66:476, 2000.
5. Rezaiguia S, Jayr G: Prevention of respiratory complications after abdominal surgery, Ann Fr Anesthesia Reanim 15:623, 1996.
6. Lindberg P et al: Atelectasis and lung function in the postoperative period, Acta Anesth 36:546, 1992.
7. Jackson AB, Groomes TE: Incidence of respiratory complications following spinal cord injury, Arch Phys Med Rehabil 75:270, 1992.
8. Kocabas A et al: Value of preoperative spirometry to predict postoperative pulmonary complications, Respir Med 90:25, 1996.
9. Sabanathan S, Eng J, Mearns AJ: Alterations in respiratory mechanics following thoracotomy, J R Coll Surg Edinb 35:144, 1990.
10. Doyle RL: Assessing and modifying the risk of postoperative pulmonary complications, Chest 115: 77S, 1999.
11. Gosselink R: IS does not enhance recovery after thoracic surgery, Crit Care Med 28: 679, 2000.
12. King MS: Preoperative evaluation, Am Fam Physician 62:387, 2000.
13. Engoren M: Lack of association between atelectasis and fever, Chest 107:81, 1995.

14. Hall JC et al: Prevention of respiratory complications after abdominal surgery: a randomized clinical trial, BMJ 312:148, 1996.
15. American Association for Respiratory Care: Clinical practice guideline: IS, Respir Care 36:1402, 1991.
16. Bastin R, Moraine JJ: IS performance. A reliable indicator of pulmonary function in the early postoperative period after lobectomy? Chest 111:559, 1997.
17. Weiner P: The effect of IS and inspiratory muscle training on pulmonary function after lung resection, J Thorac Cardiovasc Surg 113:552, 1997.
18. Baker WL, Lamb VJ, Marini JJ: Breath-stacking increases the depth and duration of chest expansion by IS, Am Rev Respir Dis 141:343, 1990.
19. McConnell EA: Teaching your patient to use an incentive spirometer, Nursing 23:18, 1993.
20. Rau JL, Thomas L, Haynes RL: The effect of method of administering IS on postoperative pulmonary complications in coronary artery bypass patients, Respir Care 33:771, 1988.
21. Motley HL et al: Observations on the clinical use of intermittent positive pressure, J Aviat Med 18:417, 1947.
22. American Association for Respiratory Care: The pros and cons of IPPB: AARC provides an assessment on its effectiveness, AARC Times 10:48, 1986.
23. American Association for Respiratory Care: Clinical practice guideline. Intermittent positive pressure breathing, Respir Care 38:1189, 1993.
24. Darin J: Effectiveness of hyperinflation therapies for the prevention and treatment of postoperative atelectasis, Curr Rev Respir Ther 12:91, 1984.
25. Handelsman H: Intermittent positive pressure breathing (IPPB) therapy, Health Technol Assess Rep 1:19, 1991.
26. American Association for Respiratory Care: Clinical practice guideline: Use of positive airway pressure adjuncts to bronchial hygiene therapy, Respir Care 38:516, 1993.
27. Ingwersen UM et al: Three different mask physiotherapy regimens for prevention of postoperative pulmonary complications after heart and pulmonary surgery, Intensive Care Med 19:294, 1993.
28. Richter LK et al: Mask physiotherapy in patients after heart surgery: a controlled study, Intensive Care Med 21:469, 1995.
29. Matte P et al: Effects of conventional physiotherapy, continuous positive airway pressure and noninvasive ventilatory support with bilevel positive airway pressure after coronary artery bypass grafting, Acta Anaesthesiol Scand 44:75, 2000.

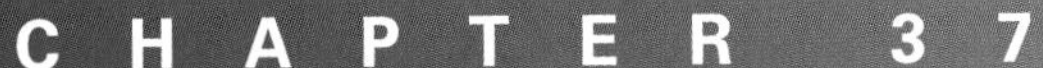

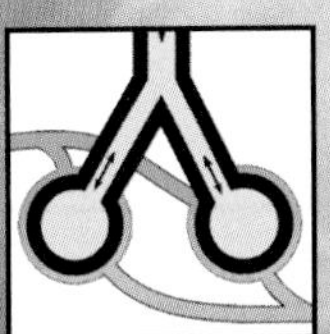

CHAPTER 37

Bronchial Hygiene Therapy

Mary Jane Myslinski and Craig L. Scanlan

In This Chapter You Will Learn:

- How normal airway clearance mechanisms work and what can impair their function
- What diseases are associated with abnormal clearance of secretions
- What goals and indications apply to bronchial hygiene therapy
- How to assess the need for bronchial hygiene therapy
- How to select and perform various bronchial hygiene therapies, including:
  - Postural drainage therapy
  - Directed coughing and related expulsion techniques
  - Positive expiratory pressure (PEP) therapy
  - High-frequency compression/oscillation methods
  - Mobilization and exercise
- How to monitor and evaluate a patient's response to bronchial hygiene therapy
- How to modify bronchial hygiene therapies on the basis of patient response

Chapter Outline

Key Terms

active cycle of breathing
acute respiratory distress syndrome (ARDS)
autogeneic drainage (AD)
bronchiectasis
ciliary dyskinetic syndromes
forced expiration technique (FET)
high-frequency chest wall compression (HFCWC)
"huff" cough
hertz (Hz)
inspissation

Continued

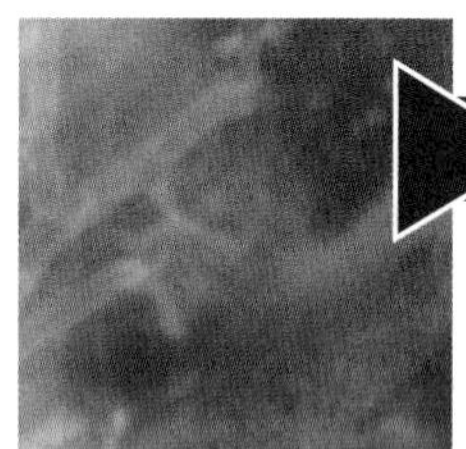

Key Terms—cont'd

intermittent percussive ventilation (IPV)
mucus-plugging
oscillation
positive expiratory pressure (PEP)
spinal shock
splinting
venostasis

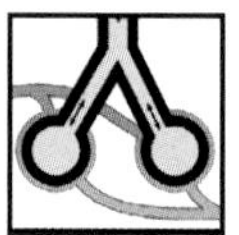

Bronchial hygiene therapy involves the use of noninvasive airway clearance techniques designed to help mobilize and remove secretions and improve gas exchange.[1-6] In the past, bronchial hygiene methods often were grouped under a broad category of techniques called *chest physical therapy* (CPT). CPT involves not only airway clearance techniques but also various exercise protocols and breathing retraining methods.[1] Here our focus is solely on noninvasive airway clearance.

Traditionally, bronchial hygiene therapy involved postural drainage, percussion, and vibration (PDPV), combined with cough training.[5] Over the years, several additional noninvasive clearance methods have been developed to augment or replace this traditional approach. These newer techniques include both modified breathing/coughing routines and mechanical devices designed to augment secretion clearance.[6]

As is common in medical practice, bronchial hygiene methods often have been introduced without firm scientific knowledge of their effectiveness. For example, years ago it was common practice to order PDPV on essentially all postoperative patients, in hopes that its use would prevent the respiratory complications of surgery.[7] We now know that this broad application of bronchial hygiene therapy is both ineffective and costly.[8,9]

On the other hand, bronchial hygiene, when combined with exercise, can actually improve lung function in cystic fibrosis (CF) patients.[10] Thus bronchial hygiene therapy can be a valuable component of comprehensive respiratory care, but only if used when indicated.[11] In a Cochrane Review, it was demonstrated that insufficient evidence exists to support or refute the use of CPT with acute and stable chronic obstructive pulmonary disease (COPD), chronic bronchitis, or bronchiectasis.[12] Successful outcomes require knowledge of normal and abnormal physiology, careful patient evaluation and selection, a clear definition of therapeutic goals, rigorous application of the appropriate methods, and ongoing assessment and follow-up.[13-15]

► PHYSIOLOGY OF AIRWAY CLEARANCE

To properly apply bronchial hygiene methods, one must first understand how normal airway clearance mechanisms work and what can impair their function.

Normal Clearance

Normal airway clearance requires a patent airway, a functional mucociliary escalator, and an effective cough.[6] Airways normally are kept open by structural support mechanisms (see Chapter 7) and kept clear by proper function of their ciliated mucosa. The mucociliary clearance mechanism operates from the larynx down to the respiratory bronchioles.[16] The mucus itself originates from the goblet cells and submucosal glands, although Clara cells and tissue fluid transudation also contribute to airway secretions. Ciliated epithelial cells normally move this mucus via a coordinated wave of ciliary motion toward the trachea and larynx, where excess secretions can be swallowed or expectorated.

Although essentially a reserve clearance mechanism, the cough is one of our most important protective reflexes.[16-18] By ridding the larger airways of excessive mucus and foreign matter, the cough complements normal mucociliary clearance and helps ensure airway patency.

As shown in Figure 37-1, there are four distinct phases to a normal cough: irritation, inspiration, compression, and expulsion. In the initial irritation phase, an abnormal stimulus provokes sensory fibers in the airways to send impulses to the brain's medullary cough center. This stimulus normally is either inflammatory, mechanical, chemical, or thermal. Infection is a good example of cough stimulation due to an inflammatory process. Foreign bodies can provoke a cough through mechanical stimulation. Chemical stimulation can occur when irritating gases are inhaled (e.g., cigarette smoke). Finally, cold air may cause thermal stimulation of sensory nerves and produce a cough.

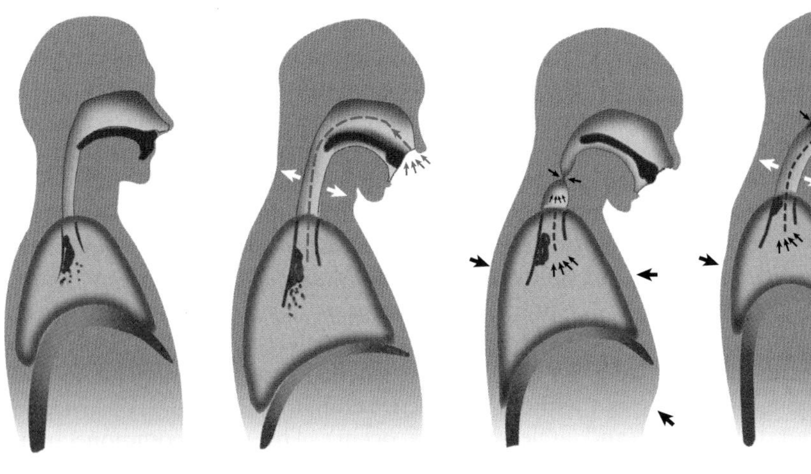

Figure 37-1
The cough reflex. *(Modified from Cherniack RM, Cherniack L: Respiration in health and disease, ed 3, Philadelphia, 1983, WB Saunders.)*

Once these afferent impulses are received, the cough center generates a reflex stimulation of the respiratory muscles to initiate a deep inspiration (the second phase). In normal adults, this inspiration averages 1 to 2 L.

During the third or compression phase, reflex nerve impulses cause glottic closure and a forceful contraction of the expiratory muscles. Lasting about 0.2 seconds, this compression phase results in a rapid rise in pleural and alveolar pressures, often in excess of 100 mm Hg.

At this point the glottis opens, initiating the expulsion phase. With the glottis open, a large pressure gradient is established between the alveoli and the airway opening. Together with the continued contraction of the expiratory muscles, this pressure gradient causes a violent, expulsive flow of air from the lungs, with velocities often as high as 500 miles per hour. High-velocity gas flow, combined with dynamic airway compression, creates huge shear forces that displace mucus from the airway walls into the airstream. This causes mucus and foreign material to be expelled from the lower airways to the upper airway, where they can be expectorated or swallowed.

Abnormal Clearance

Any abnormality that alters airway patency, mucociliary function, or the effectiveness of the cough reflex can impair airway clearance and cause retention of secretions.[6] In addition, some therapeutic interventions, especially those used in critical care, can result in abnormal clearance.

Retention of secretions can result in full or partial airway obstruction. Full obstruction, or mucus plugging, can result in atelectasis and impaired oxygenation due to shunting. By restricting airflow, partial obstruction can increase the work of breathing and lead to air trapping, overdistention, and ventilation/perfusion ($\dot{V}/\dot{Q}$) imbalances.

In the presence of pathogenic organisms, retention of secretions can lead to infection. Infectious processes, in turn, provoke an inflammatory response and the release of chemical mediators. These chemical mediators, including leukotrienes, proteases, and elastases, can damage the airway epithelium and increase mucus production, resulting in a vicious cycle of worsening airway clearance.[6]

Compounding these problems may be failure of the cough reflex. In patients with retained secretions, interference with any one of the cough's four phases can result in ineffective airway clearance. Table 37-1 provides examples of factors that can impair the normal cough reflex, according to the phase affected.

As indicated in Box 37-1, additional factors can impair airway clearance in critically ill patients with artificial airways, the most important of which is the airway itself.[16] The tube presence in the trachea increases mucus secretion, while the tube cuff mechani-

Table 37-1 ▶▶ Mechanisms Impairing the Cough Reflex

Phase	Examples of Impairments
Irritation	Anesthesia CNS depression Narcotic-analgesics
Inspiration	Pain Neuromuscular dysfunction Pulmonary restriction Abdominal restriction
Compression	Laryngeal nerve damage Artificial airway Abdominal muscle weakness Abdominal surgery
Expulsion	Airway compression Airway obstruction Abdominal muscle weakness Inadequate lung recoil (e.g., emphysema)

cally blocks the mucociliary escalator. In addition, movement of the tube tip and cuff can cause erosion of the tracheal mucosa and further impair mucociliary clearance. Last, artificial tracheal airways impair the compression phase of the cough reflex by preventing closure of the glottis (see Table 37-1).

Although suctioning is used to aid secretion clearance, it too can cause damage to the airway mucosa and thus impair mucociliary transport. Inadequate humidification can cause inspissation of secretions, mucus plugging, and airway obstruction. High FIO_2s can impair mucociliary clearance, either directly or by causing an acute tracheobronchitis. Several common drugs, including some general anesthetics and narcotic-analgesics, can depress mucociliary transport. Last, several diseases commonly seen in critical care are associated with poor secretion clearance[16] (see below).

Diseases Associated With Abnormal Clearance

Several diseases are associated with abnormal clearance, including those affecting airway patency, the composition and production of mucus, ciliary structure and function, and the normal cough reflex.[6]

Internal obstruction or external compression of the airway lumen can impair airway clearance. Examples include foreign bodies, tumors, and congenital or acquired thoracic anomalies such as kyphoscoliosis.[6] Internal obstruction also can occur with mucus hypersecretion, inflammatory changes, or bronchospasm, further narrowing the lumen. Examples include asthma, chronic bronchitis, and acute infections.[6]

Diseases that alter normal mucociliary clearance can also cause secretion retention. CF is the most common disorder in this category. In CF, the solute concentration of the mucus is altered because of abnormal sodium and chloride transport.[19] This increases mucus viscosity and impairs its movement up the respiratory tract. Although less common, there are several conditions in which the respiratory tract cilia do not function properly.[20] These ciliary dyskinetic syndromes also can contribute to ineffective airway clearance.

Chronic airway inflammation and infection can lead to bronchiectasis, a common finding in both CF and ciliary dyskinetic syndromes.[6] In bronchiectasis, the airway is permanently damaged, dilated, and prone to constant obstruction by retained secretions.[21] Other conditions that can lead to bronchiectasis include chronic obstructive lung diseases, foreign-body aspiration, and obliterative bronchiolitis.[22]

As previously discussed, any condition that affects the four components of an effective cough will also alter airway clearance. Mucociliary function may be normal, but without an effective cough, mucus plugs, obstruction, and atelectasis can occur.[6] The most common conditions affecting the cough reflex are musculoskeletal and neurological disorders, including muscular dystrophy, amyotrophic lateral sclerosis, spinal muscular atrophy, myasthenia gravis, poliomyelitis, and cerebral palsy.[6]

Box 37-1 • Causes of Impaired Mucociliary Clearance in Intubated Patients

- Endotracheal or tracheostomy tube
- Tracheobronchial suction
- Inadequate humidification
- High FIO_2s
- Drugs
  - General anesthetics
  - Opiates
  - Narcotics
- Underlying pulmonary disease

▶ GENERAL GOALS AND INDICATIONS

The primary goal of bronchial hygiene therapy is to help mobilize and remove retained secretions, with the ultimate aim to improve gas exchange and reduce the

MINI CLINI

Assessing a Patient's Cough Clearance

PROBLEM

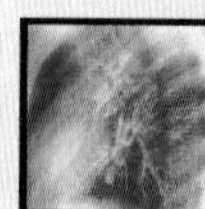

You are called by a nurse to determine why her patient is having difficulty clearing secretions. The patient is an alert, obese, 45-year-old man who underwent general anesthesia and surgery for bowel obstruction 3 hours ago. Physical signs indicate retention of secretions, but there is no history of lung disease. The patient is breathing through an endotracheal tube and receiving 40% oxygen with aerosol via T-tube. Through visual clues, the patient has been indicating severe pain in the epigastric area. The patient was started on IV morphine 1 hour ago.

DISCUSSION

Even without lung disease, it is no wonder that this patient is having difficulty clearing secretions via cough. Recent anesthesia and the narcotic-analgesic potentially are impairing the irritation phase of the cough, while the obesity, abdominal restriction/weakness, and pain are impairing the inspiration, compression, and expulsion phases. Last, the presence of the endotracheal tube further impairs coughing and clearance.

The patient should immediately be started on an aggressive bronchial hygiene regimen. Judicious use of pain medication, coinciding with therapy, should continue. Cough training (with instruction in splinting) should be part of the plan. Last, the sooner the endotracheal tube can be removed, the better (until then, prn suctioning is required).

work of breathing.[1-6] Box 37-2 lists the general indications for bronchial hygiene therapy.[11,23] We describe more specific indications as we discuss each clearance technique.

Bronchial Hygiene Therapy for Acute Conditions

Among the acute conditions for which bronchial hygiene therapy may be indicated are: (1) acutely ill patients with copious secretions, (2) patients in acute respiratory failure with clinical signs of retained secretions (audible abnormal breath sounds, deteriorating arterial blood gases [ABGs], chest radiographic changes), (3) patients with acute lobar atelectasis, and (4) patients with $\dot{V}/\dot{Q}$ abnormalities due to lung infiltrates or consolidation.[13-15]

Acute conditions for which bronchial hygiene therapy is probably not helpful include (1) acute exacerbations of COPD, (2) pneumonia without clinically significant sputum production, and (3) uncomplicated asthma.[11]

Bronchial Hygiene Therapy for Chronic Conditions

Bronchial hygiene therapy has proved effective in aiding secretion clearance and improving pulmonary function in chronic conditions associated with copious sputum production, including CF, bronchiectasis, and in certain patients with chronic bronchitis.[13-15] In general, sputum production must exceed 25 to 30 mL/day for bronchial hygiene therapy to significantly improve secretion removal.[11]

Box 37-2 • Indications for Bronchial Hygiene Therapy

TREATING ACUTE CONDITIONS
- Copious secretions
- Acute respiratory failure with retained secretions
- Acute lobar atelectasis
- $\dot{V}/\dot{Q}$ abnormalities caused by unilateral lung disease

TREATING CHRONIC CONDITIONS WITH COPIOUS SECRETIONS
- Cystic fibrosis
- Bronchiectasis
- Ciliary dyskinetic syndromes
- Chronic bronchitis

PREVENTING RETENTION OF SECRETIONS
- Acute disease
  - Immobile patients
  - Postoperative patients?
  - Exacerbations of COPD?
- Chronic disease
  - Cystic fibrosis
  - Neuromuscular disorders?

? indicates questionable efficacy.

RULE OF THUMB

When obtaining information from patients regarding sputum production, use common measures they can understand. For example, copious production (25 to 30 mL/day) is about a fluid ounce or a "shot glass full."

Bronchial Hygiene Therapy to Prevent Retention of Secretions

Bronchial hygiene therapy has been used as a preventive or prophylactic mode of respiratory care in a variety of patient disorders.[1,2] Current evidence presents a mixed picture regarding the benefits of this approach.

The best-documented preventive uses of bronchial hygiene therapy include (1) body positioning and patient mobilization to prevent retained secretions in the acutely ill[16] and (2) PDPV combined with exercise to maintain lung function in CF.[10] Most other prophylactic applications of bronchial hygiene therapy have not proved useful.[11, 23]

▶ DETERMINING THE NEED FOR BRONCHIAL HYGIENE THERAPY

Effective bronchial hygiene therapy requires proper initial and ongoing patient assessment. Obviously, all the key elements involved in determining the need for respiratory care apply, as detailed in Section 3 of this book. Formulation of the respiratory care plan thus depends on the results of records review and interview, physical assessment, laboratory testing (including pulmonary function tests), and radiologic evaluation.

Box 37-3 lists the key factors you must consider in assessing a patient's need for bronchial hygiene therapy.[2,13-15] In regard to the bedside assessment, an ineffective cough, absent or increased sputum production, labored breathing pattern, decreased breath sounds, crackles or rhonchi, tachypnea, tachycardia, or fever indicates a potential problem with retained secretions.

In combination, comprehensive review and evaluation of these various factors will determine the likelihood of successful outcomes. Such assessment, when incorporated into the respiratory care planning process, clearly distinguishes the "bang, breathe, and cough" approach from an effective and individually tailored treatment plan.[2]

Box 37-3 • Initial Assessment of Need for Bronchial Hygiene Therapy

MEDICAL RECORD
- History of pulmonary problems causing increased secretions
- Admission for upper abdominal or thoracic surgery; consider:
  - Age (elderly)
  - History of COPD
  - Obesity
  - Nature of procedure
  - Type of anesthesia
  - Duration of procedure
- Presence of artificial tracheal airway
- Chest radiograph indicating atelectasis or infiltrates
- Results of pulmonary function testing
- ABG values or oxygen saturation

PATIENT
- Posture, muscle tone
- Effectiveness of cough
- Sputum production
- Breathing pattern
- General physical fitness
- Breath sounds
- Vital signs, heart rate, and rhythm

▶ BRONCHIAL HYGIENE METHODS

There are five general approaches to bronchial hygiene therapy, which can be used alone or in combination. These approaches include (1) postural drainage therapy (including turning, percussion, and vibration), (2) coughing and related expulsion techniques, (3) PAP adjuncts (PEP, continuous PAP [CPAP], expiratory PAP [EPAP]), (4) high-frequency compression/oscillation methods, and (5) mobilization and exercise. Appropriate use of these techniques requires an understanding of their underlying principles, relative efficacy, and methods of application.

Postural Drainage Therapy

Postural drainage therapy involves the use of gravity and mechanical energy to help mobilize secretions, improve $\dot{V}/\dot{Q}$ balance, and normalize the functional residual capacity (FRC).[13] Postural drainage therapy includes turning, postural drainage, and percussion and vibration. Cough methods are used with postural drainage therapy, but are discussed separately.

To guide practitioners in applying these techniques, the American Association for Respiratory Care (AARC) has developed and published a clinical practice guideline on postural drainage therapy. Excerpts from the AARC guideline, including indications, contraindications, hazards and complications, assessment of need, assessment of outcome, and monitoring, appear on pp. 892–893.[13]

Turning

Turning is the rotation of the body around the longitudinal axis.[13] Turning is also referred to as *kinetic therapy* or *continuous lateral rotational therapy*.[24,25] Patients may turn themselves, be turned by a caregiver, or use a special rotational bed. An extreme version of turning is placing the patient in the prone position (known as proning the patient) and is discussed below.

The primary purpose of turning is to promote lung expansion, improve oxygenation, and prevent retention of secretions. Other benefits include a reduction in venostasis and prevention of skin ulcers.[26]

There are only two absolute contraindications to turning: unstable spinal cord injuries and traction of arm abductors.[24] Relative contraindications include severe diarrhea, marked agitation, a rise in intracranial pressure (ICP), large drops in blood pressure (>10%), worsening dyspnea, hypoxia, and cardiac arrhythmias.[24]

Special rotational beds, such as the RotoRest Delta Bed (Kinetic Concepts, Inc., San Antonio, Texas), rotate continuously on their long axis through a 124-degree arc every 3 to 4 minutes (Figure 37-2).[24,25] Trendelenburg and reverse Trendelenburg positions can be used, and

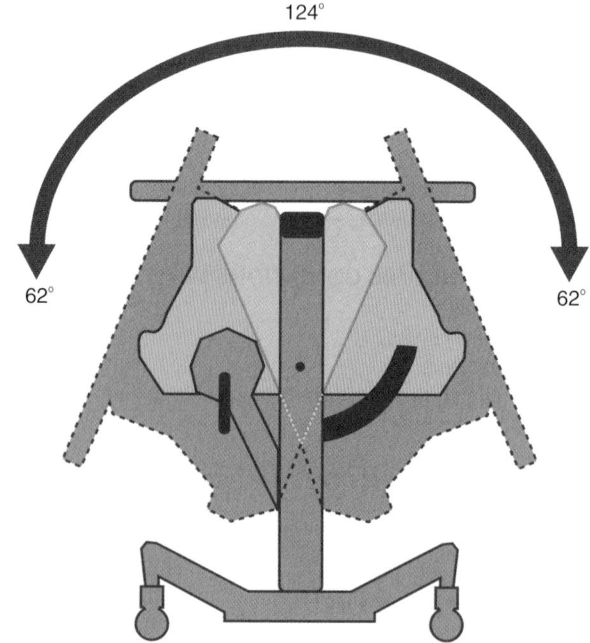

Figure 37-2
Rotation arc of RotoRest® Delta Bed. *(Courtesy of Kinetic Concepts, Inc., San Antonio, Tex.)*

any position locked along the rotation arc. Alternatively, repositioning can be accomplished by using automated inflation and deflation of air-filled mattress compartments.[25]

In addition to the hazards and complications listed in the AARC Clinical Practice Guideline, turning poses significant "plumbing" problems. "Plumbing" problems include ventilator disconnection, accidental extubation, accidental aspiration of ventilator circuit condensate, and disconnection of vascular lines or urinary catheters.[24] Only careful planning and due care during turning procedures can ensure avoidance of these problems.

Proning the patient is a strategy most often applied to the treatment of patients with acute lung injury (ALI) (see Chapter 24). It has been shown to improve oxygenation in patients with ALI without negative effects on hemodynamics.[27-31] This may allow ventilation with a lower FIO_2 and lower pressures. Although proning the patient increases oxygenation in most patients with ALI, it does not appear to improve survival.[32]

Two factors may account for the improvement in oxygenation when proning patients with ALI. First, the transpulmonary pressure generated in the prone position probably exceeds the airway opening pressure in dorsal lung regions (where atelectasis, shunt, and $\dot{V}/\dot{Q}$ heterogeneity are most severe).[33] Second, the prone position probably shifts blood flow away from shunt regions, thus increasing areas with normal $\dot{V}/\dot{Q}$ balance. This redistribution of blood flow is most likely caused by gravity-induced recruitment of previously atelectatic but healthy areas.[34] The prone position also may decrease the likelihood of further lung injury associated with positive-pressure ventilation of patients with ARDS.[35,36]

Postural Drainage

Postural drainage involves the use of gravity to help move respiratory tract secretions from distal lung lobes or segments into the central airways, where they can be removed by cough or suctioning.[13] This is done by simply placing the segmental bronchus to be drained in a vertical position relative to gravity.[1] Positions generally are held for 3 to 15 minutes (longer in special situations) and modified as the patient's condition and tolerance warrant.[13]

Postural drainage is most effective in conditions characterized by excessive sputum production (> 25 to 30 mL/day).[11] For maximum effect, head-down positions should exceed 25 degrees below horizontal.[11,37,38] Postural drainage is not likely to succeed unless and until adequate systemic and airway hydration is ensured.[39] In critical care patients, including those on mechanical ventilation, postural drainage should be performed from every 4 to 6 hours as indicated. In spontaneously breathing patients, frequency should be determined by assessing patient response to therapy.[13]

Technique. On the basis of a preliminary assessment of the patient and review of the physician's order, you should identify the appropriate lobe(s) and segments for drainage. Also on the basis of the preliminary assessment, you should determines if the position(s) chosen need to be modified. You may need to modify head-down positions in patients with unstable cardiovascular status, hypertension, cerebrovascular disorders, or orthopnea.[13]

To avoid gastroesophageal reflux and the possibility of aspiration,[40] you should schedule treatment times before or at least 1½ to 2 hours after meals or tube

MINI CLINI

Patient Positioning

PROBLEM

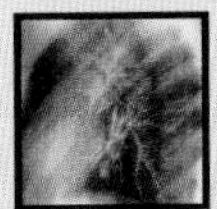

A patient with ARDS is receiving mechanical ventilatory support with 70% oxygen and 15 cm PEEP. Despite this aggressive treatment, the patient's PaO_2 remains dangerously low (45 mm Hg). What might you recommend to the physician to improve this patient's oxygenation?

DISCUSSION

Given that the patient is already near the upper limits of conventional therapy for ARDS, it would be worth seeing if a change to the prone position might provide some improvement in oxygenation. A change to the prone position also may increase the likelihood of further lung injury associated with positive-pressure ventilation. Other alternatives include nitric oxide therapy (Chapter 35) and different modes of ventilatory support (Chapter 41).

MINI CLINI

Postnasal Drainage, Percussion, and Vibration

PROBLEM

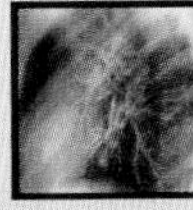

A physician's progress note indicates a potential bacterial pneumonia localized to a patient's right middle lobe. He orders "PDPV qid until radiograph clears." What position(s) would you select for postural drainage, and where would you provide percussion?

DISCUSSION

As shown in Figure 37-3 (p. 890), the correct position for draining the right middle lobe would be head-down (foot of bed raised about 12 inches), with the patient rotated about 45 degrees left from supine (modified left side-lying position). Percussion should be performed on the right anterior chest wall, between the fourth and sixth ribs (see Chapter 14) for external anatomic landmarks).

feedings.[2] If the patient assessment indicates that pain may hinder treatment implementation, you also should consider coordinating the treatment regimen with prescribed pain medication.

Before positioning, you should explain the procedure (including adjunctive techniques) to the patient. As necessary, loosen clothing around the waist and neck. Also, inspect any monitoring leads, intravenous (IV) tubing, and oxygen therapy equipment connected to the patient; if necessary, make adjustments to ensure continued function during the procedure. Since postural drainage positioning predisposes patients to arterial desaturation, pulse oximetry should be considered a routine component of monitoring during postural drainage.[41] Before starting the procedure, measure the patient's vital signs and auscultate the chest. These simple assessments will serve as baseline measurements for monitoring the patient's response during the procedure and can assist in determining its outcomes.

Figure 37-3 depicts the primary positions used to drain the various lung lobes and segments. In head-down positions in general, you must lower the head of the bed by at least 16 to 18 inches to achieve the desired 25-degree angle. In the ambulatory care setting, you can use a "tilt table" in lieu of a hospital bed. A tilt table allows precise positioning at head-down angles up to 45 degrees. When angles this large are used, shoulder supports must be provided to prevent the patient from sliding off the table.

Once you position the patient, you should confirm his or her comfort and ensure proper support of all joints and bony areas with pillows or towels. You should maintain the indicated position for a minimum of 3 to 15 minutes if tolerated, and longer if good sputum production results.[13] Between positions, pauses for relaxation and breathing control are useful and can help prevent hypoxemia.[42] Because postural drainage therapy can increase oxygen consumption, some clinicians recommend giving critically ill patients 100% oxygen during the procedure.[43]

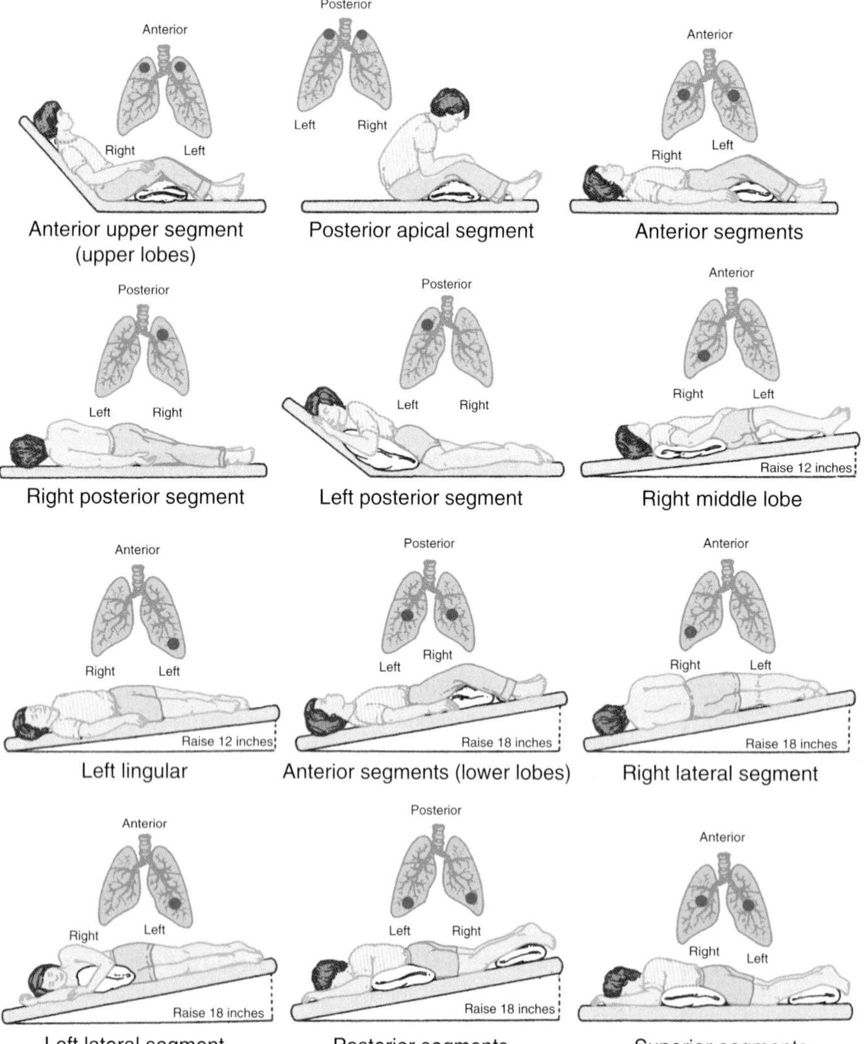

Figure 37-3

Patient positions for postural drainage. *(Modified from Potter PA, Perry AG: Fundamentals of nursing: concepts, process and practice, ed 4, St. Louis, 1997, Mosby.)*

Table 37-2 ▶▶ Complications of Postural Drainage Therapy and Recommended Interventions

Complication	Action to Be Taken/Possible Intervention
Hypoxemia	Administer higher FIO_2 during procedure if potential for or observed hypoxemia exists. If patient becomes hypoxemic during treatment, administer 100% oxygen, stop therapy immediately, return patient to original position, and consult physician.
Increased intracranial pressure	Stop therapy, return patient to original resting position, and consult physician.
Acute hypotension during procedure	Stop therapy, return patient to original resting position, and consult physician.
Pulmonary hemorrhage	Stop therapy, return patient to original resting position, and call physician immediately. Administer oxygen and maintain an airway until physician responds.
Pain or injury to muscles, ribs, or spine	Stop therapy that appears directly associated with pain or problem, exercise care in moving patient, and consult physician.
Vomiting and aspiration	Stop therapy, clear airway and suction as needed, administer oxygen, maintain airway, return patient to previous resting position, and contact physician. immediately.
Bronchospasm	Stop therapy, return patient to previous resting position, and administer or increase oxygen delivery while contacting physician. Administer physician-ordered bronchodilators.
Arrhythmias	Stop therapy, return patient to previous resting position, and administer or increase oxygen delivery while contacting physician.

During the procedure, you should continually observe the patient for any untoward effects or complications (refer to AARC Clinical Practice Guideline excerpts). You should expect moderate changes in vital signs during treatment; however, as indicated in Table 37-2, significant problems may require your immediate intervention.[13]

You should also ensure appropriate coughing technique, both during and after positioning. When using the head-down position, the patient should avoid strenuous coughing, since this will markedly raise intracranial pressure. Rather, you should have the patient use the forced expiration technique (described later). In general, total treatment time should not exceed 30 to 40 minutes. Both the patient and clinician should understand that postural drainage does not always result in the immediate production of secretions. More often, secretions are simply mobilized toward the trachea for easier removal by coughing. If the procedure causes vigorous coughing, you should have the patient sit up until the cough subsides.

After the procedure, you should restore the patient to the pretreatment position, and ensure his or her stability and comfort. Immediate posttreatment assessment should include repeat vital signs, confirmation of satisfactory arterial saturation, chest auscultation, and patient questioning regarding his or her subjective response to the procedure.

> **RULE OF THUMB**
>
> In general, whenever you observe an untoward patient response during postural drainage therapy, follow the "triple S rule": Stop the therapy (return patient to original resting position) and Stay with the patient until Stabilized.

Outcome Assessment. Specific outcome criteria indicating a positive response to postural drainage are listed in the AARC Clinical Practice Guideline excerpts on p. 893. In general, achievement of one or more of these outcomes indicates that the therapy is meeting its objectives and should be continued. Not all criteria are required to justify continuing postural drainage.[13]

Because secretion clearance is affected by patient hydration, you may need to wait for at least 24 hours after optimal systemic hydration has been achieved to see any evidence of increased sputum production.[13] In the interim, you can enhance tracheobronchial clearance in some patients by providing bland aerosol therapy with an unheated jet nebulizer.[44]

In assessing outcomes, you also should be aware that breath sounds may actually seem to "worsen" following therapy.[13] Typically, you may initially note diminished breath sounds and crackles before therapy that change over to coarse rhonchi after treatment. This is due to the loosening of secretions and their movement into the larger airways, an intended purpose of the therapy. These coarse rhonchi should clear after coughing or suctioning.

In terms of the patient's subjective response to therapy, you should encourage the patient to report any pain, discomfort, shortness of breath, dizziness, or nausea during or after therapy.[13] Any of these adverse effects may be grounds for either modifying or stopping treatment. On the other hand, patient reports of easier clearance or increased volume of secretions after therapy support continuing therapy.[13]

On the basis of assessment results, the postural drainage order should be reevaluated at least every 48 hours for critical care patients and at least every 3 days for other hospitalized patients.[13] Home care patients should be reevaluated at least every 3 months, or whenever their status changes.

Postural Drainage Therapy

AARC Clinical Practice Guideline (Excerpts)*

➤ INDICATIONS

- Turning
- Inability or reluctance of patient to change body position
- Poor oxygenation associated with position (e.g., unilateral lung disease)
- Potential for or presence of atelectasis
- Presence of artificial airway
- Postural drainage
- Evidence or suggestion of difficulty with secretion clearance
- Difficulty clearing secretions, with expectorated sputum production greater than 25 to 30 mL/day (adult)
- Evidence or suggestion of retained secretions in the presence of an artificial airway
- Presence of atelectasis caused by or suspected of being caused by mucus plugging
- Diagnosis of diseases such as CF, bronchiectasis, or cavitating lung disease
- Presence of foreign body in airway
- External manipulation of the thorax: sputum volume or consistency suggesting a need for additional manipulation (e.g., percussion and/or vibration) to assist movement of secretions by gravity in a patient receiving postural drainage

➤ CONTRAINDICATIONS

The decision to use postural drainage therapy requires assessment of potential benefits versus potential risks. Therapy should be provided for no longer than necessary to obtain the desired therapeutic results. *Listed contraindications are relative unless marked as absolute (A).*

Positioning: all positions are contraindicated for:

- Head and neck injury until stabilized (A)
- Active hemorrhage with hemodynamic instability (A)
- ICP >20 mm Hg
- Recent spinal surgery or acute spinal injury
- Active hemoptysis
- Empyema
- Bronchopleural fistula
- Pulmonary edema associated with congestive heart failure (CHF)
- Aged, confused, or anxious patients who do not tolerate position changes
- Pulmonary embolism
- Rib fracture, with or without flail chest
- Surgical wound or healing tissue
- Large pleural effusions

Trendelenburg position is contraindicated for:

- Recent gross hemoptysis related to recent lung carcinoma treated surgically or with radiation therapy
- ICP >20 mm Hg
- Uncontrolled hypertension
- Distended abdomen
- Patients in whom increased ICP is to be avoided (e.g., neurosurgery, aneurysms, eye surgery)
- Uncontrolled airway at risk for aspiration (tube feeding or recent meal)
- Esophageal surgery

External manipulation of the thorax (in addition to contraindications previously listed):

- Subcutaneous emphysema
- Recent epidural spinal infusion or spinal anesthesia
- Recently placed transvenous pacemaker or subcutaneous pacemaker
- Lung contusion
- Osteomyelitis of the ribs
- Coagulopathy
- Recent skin grafts, or flaps, on the thorax
- Burns, open wounds, and skin infections of the thorax
- Suspected pulmonary tuberculosis

POSTURAL DRAINAGE THERAPY—CONT'D

AARC Clinical Practice Guideline (Excerpts)*

- Bronchospasm
- Osteoporosis
- Complaint of chest-wall pain

➤ HAZARDS AND COMPLICATIONS

- Hypoxemia
- Increased ICP
- Acute hypotension during procedure
- Pulmonary hemorrhage
- Pain or injury to muscles, ribs, or spine
- Vomiting and aspiration
- Bronchospasm
- Dysrhythmias

➤ ASSESSMENT OF NEED

The following should be assessed *together* to establish a need for postural drainage therapy:

- Excessive sputum production
- Effectiveness of cough
- History of problems treated successfully with postural drainage (e.g., bronchiectasis, CF)
- Decreased breath sounds or crackles or rhonchi suggesting secretions in the airway
- Change in vital signs
- Abnormal chest radiograph consistent with atelectasis, mucus plugging, or infiltrates
- Deterioration in arterial blood gas values or oxygen saturation

➤ ASSESSMENT OF OUTCOME

These represent individual criteria that indicate a positive response to therapy (and support continuation of therapy). Not all criteria are required to justify continuation of therapy (e.g., a ventilated patient may not have sputum production >30 mL/day, but have improvement in breath sounds, chest radiograph, or increased compliance or decreased resistance).

- Change in sputum production
- Change in breath sounds of lung fields being drained
- Patient subjective response to therapy
- Change in vital signs
- Change in chest radiograph
- Change in ABG values or oxygen saturation
- Change in ventilator variables

➤ MONITORING

The following should be chosen as appropriate for monitoring a patient's response to postural drainage therapy before, during, and after therapy:

- Subjective response (pain, discomfort, dyspnea, response to therapy)
- Pulse rate, arrhythmia, and ECG if available
- Breathing pattern and rate, symmetrical chest expansion, synchronous thoracoabdominal movement, flail chest
- Sputum production (quantity, color, consistency, odor) and cough effectiveness
- Mental function
- Skin color
- Breath sounds
- Blood pressure
- Oxygen saturation by pulse oximetry (if hypoxemia is suspected)
- ICP

---

*For complete guidelines see: Respir Care 36:1418, 1991.

Documentation and Follow-Up. Your chart entry should include the position(s) used, time in position, patient tolerance, subjective and objective indicators of treatment effectiveness (including the amount, color, and consistency of sputum produced), and any untoward effects observed. Since the effects of the procedure may not be immediately evident, you should make a return visit within 1 to 2 hours after treatment, or follow up with the patient's nurse.

Percussion and Vibration

Percussion and vibration involve application of mechanical energy to the chest wall by using either the hands or various electrical or pneumatic devices. Both methods are designed to augment secretion clearance.[45] In theory, percussion should help jar retained secretions loose from the tracheobronchial tree, making them easier to remove by coughing or suctioning. Vibration, on the other hand, should aid movement of secretions toward the central airways during exhalation.

The effectiveness of percussion and vibration as an adjunct to postural drainage remains controversial.[11] This is partly due to the fact that there is no consensus as to what represents the "right" force or frequency for either technique.[2,46] In addition, because percussion and vibration are often only a part of the treatment regimen in most clinical studies, it is hard to draw conclusions about the effect of these methods alone. Moreover, both the types of patients studied and the outcome measures used often differ across studies. In studies that focus on patients who produce copious secretions, percussion generally is found effective in increasing sputum production.[47] On the other hand, when the outcome measure is not the volume of secretions by actual tracheobronchial clearance of radioaerosol, results are less positive.[48,49]

For these reasons, and in light of current knowledge, the routine use of these methods cannot be justified.[11] However, since percussion and vibration may increase the volume of sputum production in some patients, the addition of these techniques to postural drainage therapy may be appropriate in selected cases, especially if postural drainage alone fails to mobilize secretions.[13,50]

Manual Percussion and Vibration. You apply percussion over the lobe or segment being drained (see Figure 37-3). You perform manual percussion with the hands in a cupped position, with fingers and thumb closed. This traps a cushion of air between the hand and chest wall. The striking force may be against the bare skin, although a thin layer of cloth, such as a hospital gown or bedsheet, does not significantly impair transmission of the energy wave.

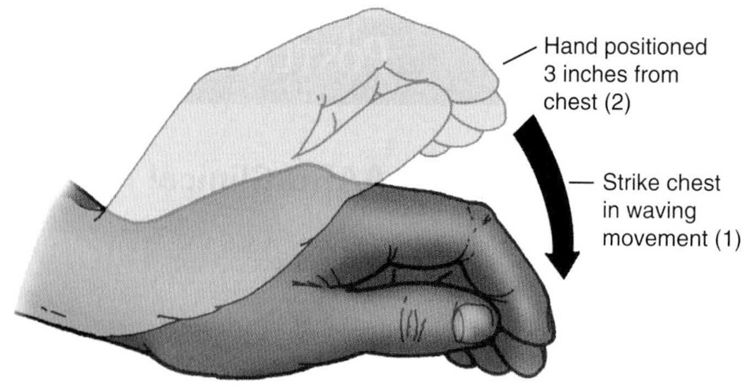

Figure 37-4
Movement of cupped hand at wrist to percuss chest.

Holding your arms with the elbows partially flexed and wrists loose, you rhythmically strike the chest wall in a waving motion, using both hands alternately in sequence (Figure 37-4). Slower, more relaxing rates are better tolerated by patient and clinician alike.[1] It is not a difficult technique to master, but practice is needed to determine the appropriate force and to maintain a rhythmic pattern.

Ideally, you should percuss back and forth in a circular pattern over the localized area for a period of 3 to 5 minutes. You must take care to avoid tender areas or sites of trauma or surgery, and never percuss directly over bony prominences, such as the clavicles or vertebrae.

Vibration sometimes is used together with percussion, but limited to application during exhalation. To vibrate the chest wall, you lay one hand on the patient's chest over the involved area and place the other hand on top of the first (Figure 37-5). Alternatively, you may place your hands on either side of the chest. After the patient takes a deep breath, you exert slight-to-moderate pressure on the chest wall, and initiate a rapid vibratory motion of the hands throughout expiration.

Mechanical Percussion and Vibration. Various electrical and pneumatic devices have been developed to generate and apply the energy waves used during percussion and vibration. Typically, these devices have both a frequency and a percussion force control (Figure 37-6). Most units provide frequencies up to 20 to 30 cycles per second, or 20 to 30 Hz. Noise, excess force, and mechanical failure are all potential problems. Electrical devices also pose a potential shock hazard.

Although no substitute for a skilled clinician, these devices do not tire and can deliver consistent rates, rhythms, and impact forces.[51] However, there is currently no firm evidence that such devices are any more effective than manual techniques.[13] For this reason, the selection of manual or mechanical methods should be left to the patient.[52]

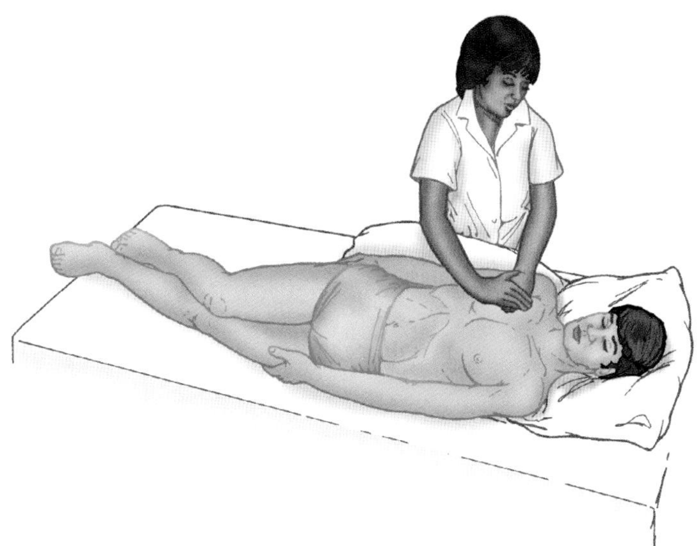

Figure 37-5
Chest vibration.

Coughing and Related Expulsion Techniques

Most bronchial hygiene therapies only help move secretions into the central airways. Actual clearance of these secretions requires either coughing or suctioning. In this respect, an effective cough (or alternative expulsion measure) is an essential component of all bronchial hygiene therapy. These expulsion methods are also useful in obtaining sputum specimens for diagnostic analysis.

> **RULE OF THUMB**
>
> Without an effective cough, most bronchial hygiene techniques cannot succeed in fully clearing secretions. Clinicians must ensure an effective cough regimen in their patients. The reader is referred to the Consensus Panel Report of the American College of Chest Physicians for a more in-depth look at the cough mechanism.[53]

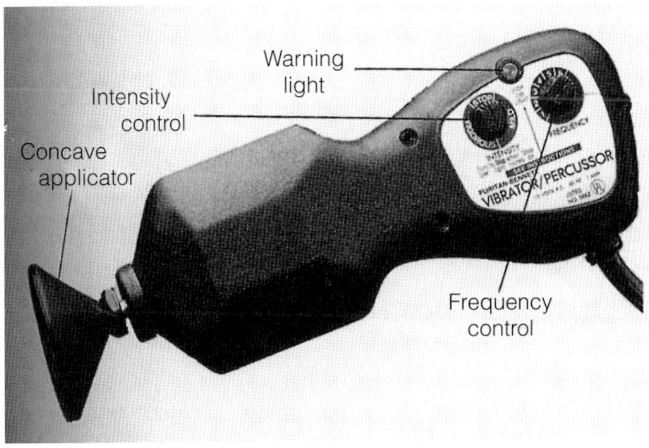

Figure 37-6
Example of an electrically powered mechanical percussor/vibrator. *(Courtesy Nellcor Puritan-Bennett Corp. Manufacturer's Note: This product is no longer being manufactured.)*

Directed Cough

Directed cough is a deliberate maneuver that is taught, supervised, and monitored. Directed cough aims to mimic the features of an effective spontaneous cough, to help provide voluntary control over the reflex, and to compensate for physical limitations that can impair this reflex.[14]

Although it may stimulate mucociliary activity, cough has little direct effect on secretion clearance in individuals who do not produce sputum.[54, 55] On the other hand, in patients with copious secretions directed coughing is at least as good at clearance as more complicated methods.[11,37] It should be noted, however, that coughing is most effective in clearing secretions from the central, but not peripheral, airways.[56,57] This difference is consistent with our understanding of the normal cough mechanism, previously discussed.

To help practitioners apply this important technique, the AARC has developed and published a clinical practice guideline on directed cough. Excerpts from the AARC guideline, including indications, contraindications, hazards and complications, assessment of need, assessment of outcome, and monitoring, appear on pp. 896–897.[14]

Standard Technique. Once the clinical need for directed coughing has been established, the RRT should assess the patient for any factors that could limit the success of directed cough. For example, an effective directed cough regimen is generally not possible with obtunded, paralyzed, or uncooperative patients.[14] In addition, some patients with advanced COPD or severe restrictive disorders (including neurologic, muscular, or skeletal abnormalities) may not be able to generate an effective spontaneous cough.[14] Likewise, pain or fear of pain caused by coughing may limit the success of directed cough. Last, systemic dehydration; thick, tenacious

DIRECTED COUGH

AARC Clinical Practice Guideline (Excerpts)*

➤ INDICATIONS

- The need to aid in the removal of retained secretions from central airways
- The presence of atelectasis
- As prophylaxis against postoperative pulmonary complications
- As a routine part of bronchial hygiene in patients with CF, bronchiectasis, chronic bronchitis, necrotizing pulmonary infection, or spinal cord injury
- As an integral part of other bronchial hygiene therapies, such as postural drainage therapy, PEP therapy, and incentive spirometry
- To obtain sputum specimens for diagnostic analysis

➤ CONTRAINDICATIONS

Directed cough is rarely contraindicated. The contraindications listed must be weighed against potential benefit in deciding to eliminate cough from the care of the patient. Listed contraindications are relative:

- Inability to control possible transmission of infection from patients suspected or known to have pathogens transmittable by droplet nuclei (e.g., *M. tuberculosis*)
- Presence of an elevated ICP or known intracranial aneurysm
- Presence of reduced coronary artery perfusion, such as in acute myocardial infarction
- Acute unstable head, neck, or spine injury
- Manually assisted directed cough *with pressure to the epigastrium* may be contraindicated in the presence of increased potential for regurgitation/aspiration, acute abdominal pathology, abdominal aortic aneurysm, hiatal hernia, pregnancy, a bleeding diathesis, or untreated pneumothorax
- Manually assisted directed cough *with pressure to the thoracic cage* may be contraindicated in presence of osteoporosis or flail chest

➤ HAZARDS AND COMPLICATIONS

- Reduced coronary artery perfusion
- Reduced cerebral perfusion
- Incontinence
- Fatigue
- Rib/costochondral fracture
- Headache
- Visual disturbances, including retinal hemorrhage
- Bronchospasm
- Muscular damage or discomfort
- Incisional pain, evisceration
- Anorexia, vomiting, retching
- Gastroesophageal reflux
- Spontaneous pneumothorax, pneumomediastinum, subcutaneous emphysema
- Cough paroxysms
- Chest pain
- Central line displacement
- Paresthesia

➤ ASSESSMENT OF NEED

- Spontaneous cough that fails to clear secretions from the airway
- Ineffective spontaneous cough as judged by clinical observation, evidence of atelectasis, and/or results of pulmonary function testing
- Postoperative upper abdominal or thoracic surgery patient
- Long-term care of patients with tendency to retain airway secretions
- Presence of endotracheal or tracheostomy tube

➤ ASSESSMENT OF OUTCOME

- The presence of sputum specimen following a cough
- Clinical observation of improvement
- Patient's subjective response to therapy
- Stabilization of pulmonary hygiene in patients with COPD and a history of secretion retention

DIRECTED COUGH—CONT'D

AARC Clinical Practice Guideline (Excerpts)*

➤ MONITORING

Items from the following list should be chosen as appropriate for monitoring a patient's response to cough technique:

- Patient response: pain, discomfort, dyspnea
- Sputum expectorated following cough (note, color, consistency, odor, volume of sputum produced)
- Breath sounds
- Presence of any adverse neurologic signs or symptoms following cough
- Presence of any cardiac dysrhythmias or alterations in hemodynamics following coughing
- Measures of pulmonary mechanics, when indicated, may include vital capacity, peak inspiratory pressure, peak expiratory pressure, PEF, and airway resistance

*For complete guidelines see Respir Care 38:495, 1993.

secretions; artificial airways; or the use of central nervous system (CNS) depressants or antitussives can thwart efforts to implement an effective directed cough regimen.

Should one or more of these limitations exist, it is the responsibility of the RRT to recommend alternative means to help expel secretions. Alternative secretion clearance strategies are discussed subsequently.

Good patient teaching is critical in developing an effective directed cough regimen. The three most important aspects involved in patient teaching are (1) instruction in proper positioning, (2) instruction in breathing control, and (3) exercises to strengthen the expiratory muscles.[17] These activities are modified according to the patient's underlying clinical problem.

You should teach patients to assume a position that aids exhalation and allows easy thoracic compression.[1,17] Because of abdominal muscle tension, it is difficult to generate an effective cough in the supine position. Rather, the patient should assume a sitting position, with shoulder rotated inward, the head and spine slightly flexed, and the forearms relaxed or supported. To provide abdominal and thoracic support, provide support for the feet. If the patient is unable to sit up, raise the head of the bed and make sure that the knees are slightly flexed with the feet braced on the mattress.

Breathing control measures help ensure that the inspiration, compression, and expulsion phases of the cough are maximally effective and coordinated. For effective inspiration, you should teach the patient to inspire slowly and deeply through the nose, using the diaphragmatic method (discussed subsequently). In patients with copious amounts of sputum, such breaths alone may stimulate coughing by loosening secretions in the larger airways.

After you confirm that the patient can take a good, deep inspiration, have the patient bear down against the glottis, in much the same manner as would occur during straining at stool. For patients with pain, or those subject to bronchiolar collapse, it is probably best that they be shown how to "stage" their expiratory effort into two or three short bursts. For these patients, this method is generally less fatiguing and more effective in producing sputum than a single violent expulsion.[1, 17] Effective breathing control is best taught via demonstration. Using demonstration, you should go through the various phases of the cough sequence, emphasize the correct technique, and point out common errors, such as simple throat clearing.

At times, proper positioning and breathing control alone may not ensure an effective cough. More often than not, this limitation is due to weak expiratory muscles. Expiratory muscle weakness is common in patients with neuromuscular disease, patients with COPD, and patients having undergone long-term ventilatory support, during which muscles may atrophy from lack of use. In these cases, either suctioning or mechanical insufflation-exsufflation (MIE) may be required.

Modifications in Technique. As previously discussed, several factors can limit the success of directed cough. To overcome these limitations, you may need to modify the normal directed cough routine, according to the needs of the individual patient. Good clinical examples of the need to modify directed cough are seen in surgical patients, patients with COPD, and patients with neuromuscular disorders.

In surgical patients, preoperative training in breathing control can help prepare the patient for the postoperative regimen. This can minimize the anxiety over pain that commonly impairs an effective cough in these patients. In addition, the postoperative regimen can be enhanced by coordinating the coughing sessions with prescribed pain medication and assisting the patient in splinting the operative site. This may initially be accomplished by the clinician, using the hands to support the area of incision. Later, you can teach the patient to use a pillow to splint the site. The forced expiration technique (FET) (to be discussed subsequently) may also be of value in these patients.

In some patients with COPD, the high pleural pressures during a forced cough may compress the smaller airways and limit the cough's effectiveness. In this case, the patient should be placed in the sitting position previously described.[17] You then instruct the patient to slowly take in a moderate breath through the nose. A moderate, as opposed to full, inspiration reduces the volume of air to be removed by the patient and results in less of a rise in pleural pressure.

To help enhance expulsion, have the patient exhale with moderate force through pursed lips, while bending forward.[17] This forward flexion of the thorax enhances expiratory flow by upward displacement of the abdominal contents. After 3 to 4 repetitions of this maneuver, you encourage the patient to bend forward and initiate short staccato-like bursts of air. This technique relieves the strain of a prolonged hard cough, and the staccato rhythm at a relatively low velocity minimizes airway collapse. This technique has a modification called "huffing" whereby the patient is instructed to make the sound of "huff, huff, huff" rapidly with the mouth open, the sound audibly coming from the throat.[58] Alternatively, either the forced expiration technique or autogenic drainage may be used in these patients. We discuss both these clearance mechanisms subsequently.

Patients with neuromuscular conditions present a special challenge in cough management. These patients typically are unable to generate the forceful expulsion needed to move secretions toward the trachea.[59] If this problem results in retained secretions, there are only three options. The first approach is invasive: placement of an artificial airway and removal of secretions by tracheobronchial suctioning (refer to Chapter 30). Alternative noninvasive strategies include manually assisted cough and MIE. Here we discuss manually assisted cough.

Manually assisted cough or "chest compression" is the external application of pressure to the thoracic cage or epigastric region, coordinated with forced exhalation.[14] In this technique, the patient takes as deep an inspiration as possible, assisted as needed by the application of positive pressure via self-inflating bag or intermittent positive pressure breathing (IPPB) device. At the end of the patient's inspiration, you begin exerting pressure on the lateral costal margin or epigastrium, increasing the force of compression throughout expiration. This mimics the normal cough mechanism by generating an increase in the velocity of the expired air and may be helpful in moving secretions toward the trachea, where they can be removed by nasotracheal suctioning.[60] Manually assisted cough with pressure to the lateral costal margins is contraindicated in patients with osteoporosis or flail chest.[14] Manually assisted cough using epigastric pressure is contraindicated in unconscious patients with unprotected airways; in pregnant women; and in patients with acute abdominal pathology, abdominal aortic aneurysm, or hiatal hernia.[14]

Forced Expiratory Technique

FET is a modification of the normal directed cough. The FET, or huff cough, consists of one or two forced expirations of middle to low lung volume *without closure of the glottis*, followed by a period of diaphragmatic breathing and relaxation.[61] The goal of this method is to help clear secretions with less change in pleural pressure and less likelihood of bronchiolar collapse.[11] To help keep the glottis open during an FET, the patient should be taught to phonate or "huff" during expiration. The period of diaphragmatic breathing and relaxation following the forced expiration is essential in restoring lung volume and minimizing fatigue.

Comparative clinical studies on the effectiveness of this method have demonstrated favorable results. In general, the FET results in better sputum production and radioaerosol clearance than directed coughing, especially when combined with postural drainage.[61-64] The technique is particularly useful in patients prone to airway collapse during normal coughing, such as those with emphysema, CF, or bronchiectasis.[5] However, the FET requires that patients generate high expiratory airflow, which may not be attainable in intubated patients with respiratory failure.[16]

Active Cycle of Breathing

To emphasize that the FET always should include breathing exercises, the originators of the FET modified the procedure and renamed it the *active cycle of breathing* (ACB.)[5] ACB consists of repeated cycles of breathing control, thoracic expansion, and the FET (Box 37-4). Breathing control involves gentle diaphragmatic breathing at normal tidal volumes with relaxation of the upper chest and shoulders. This phase is intended to help

Box 37-4 • Active Cycle of Breathing (ACB) Sequence

1. Relaxation and breathing control
2. Three to four thoracic expansion exercises
3. Relaxation and breathing control
4. Repeat three to four thoracic expansion exercises
5. Repeat relaxation and breathing control
6. Perform one or two FETs (huffs)
7. Repeat relaxation and breathing control

prevent bronchospasm. The thoracic expansion exercises involve deep inhalation with relaxed exhalation, which may be accompanied by percussion, vibration, or compression. The thoracic expansion phase is designed to help loosen secretions, improve the distribution of ventilation, and provide the volume needed for FET. The subsequent FET moves secretions into the central airways.

Although ACB can be performed in the sitting position, it is considered most beneficial when combined with postural drainage therapy. As an added benefit, ACB appears to minimize or prevent the oxygen desaturation so common during postural drainage therapy, at least in patients with CF.[65]

When ACB is compared with similar methods of secretion clearance, preliminary studies indicate that ACB can provide comparable results in terms of both sputum production and distribution of ventilation.[66] Of course, ACB is not useful with young children (younger than 2 years) or the extremely ill. We believe more study of this technique is warranted.

Autogenic Drainage

Autogenic drainage (AD) is another modification of directed coughing, designed as an airway clearance mechanism that can be performed independently by trained patients.[67,68] During AD, the patient uses diaphragmatic breathing to mobilize secretions by varying lung volumes and expiratory airflow in three distinct phases (Figure 37-7).[69] For maximum benefit, the patient should be in the sitting position. Patients are taught to control their expiratory flows to prevent airway collapse while trying to achieve a mucus "rattle" rather than a wheeze. Coughing should be suppressed until all three breathing phases are completed.

In patients with CF, AD provides sputum clearance comparable to PDPV but is less likely to produce oxygen desaturation and may be better tolerated by patients.[70,71] Unfortunately, the technique is difficult to teach patients (especially children) and is probably of little value with the critically ill.[72] A simplified approach has been developed to make the procedure easier to teach and learn,[73] but this modification has not undergone testing by clinical trials.

Mechanical Insufflation-Exsufflation

In the early 1950s, "artificial cough machines" or mechanical exsufflators were used to help patients with polio clear secretions. Their use continued until the mid-

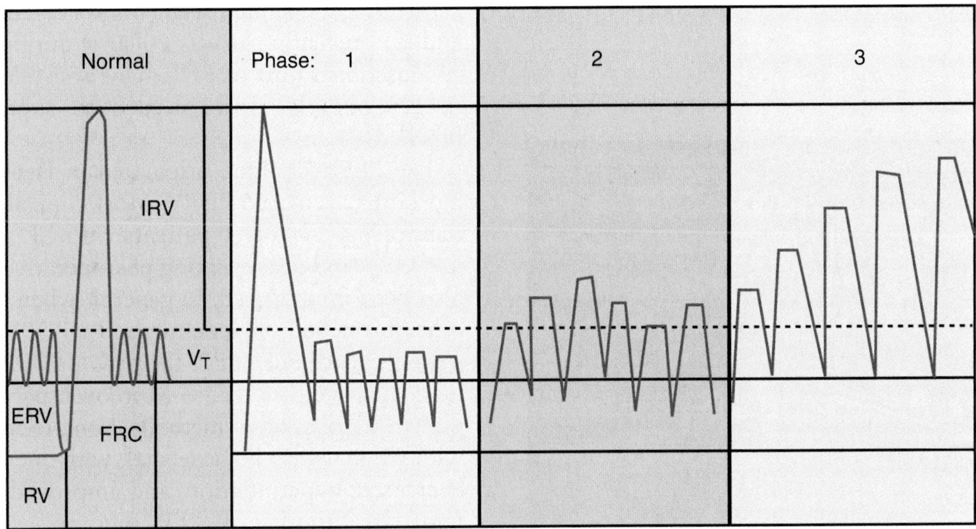

Figure 37-7

Spirogram of lung volumes during three phases of autogenic drainage. Phase 1 involves a full inspiratory capacity maneuver, followed by breathing at low lung volumes. This phase is designed to "unstick" peripheral mucus. Phase 2 involves breathing at low to middle lung volumes in order to collect mucus in the middle airways. Phase 3 is the evacuation phase, in which mucus is readied for expulsion from the large airways. *(Modified from Hardy KA, Anderson BD: Respir Care Clin North Am 2:323, 1996.)*

1960s, when artificial tracheal airways and suctioning became the method of choice for secretion clearance in patients unable to cough.[16]

Recently, an MIE device has been reintroduced and used on patients with neuromuscular disorders (Figure 37-8).[74] The device delivers a positive-pressure breath of 30 to 50 cm H_2O over a 1- to 3-second period via an oral-nasal mask or tracheal airway. The airway pressure is then abruptly reversed to -30 to -50 cm H_2O and maintained for 2 to 3 seconds. Peak expiratory "cough" flows obtained with this device are in the normal range (mean of 7.5 L/second), far better than can be achieved with manually assisted coughing.[74] Moreover, expiratory flows remain high in the immediate postexsufflation period, indicating that MIE does not promote airway collapse.

When MIE is applied via a tracheal airway, the tube cuff should be inflated; when MIE is used via an oral-nasal mask, an abdominal thrust should be timed to the exsufflation cycle.[75,76] A typical treatment session consists of about five cycles of MIE followed by a period of normal spontaneous or assisted breathing (to avoid hyperventilation). This process is repeated five or more times until secretions are cleared and the vital capacity (VC) and Spo_2 return to baseline.[76] Treatments may be required as often as every 10 minutes during acute respiratory tract infections. Prior treatment with bland aerosol can aid clearance when secretions are inspissated. Because airway clearance occurs without the discomfort and trauma of tracheal aspiration, patients tend to prefer MIE to suctioning.[76]

MIE via an oral-nasal interface is effective, provided that there is no fixed airway obstruction or glottic collapse during exsufflation. For patients with severe restrictive disease who have not been receiving deep breaths,

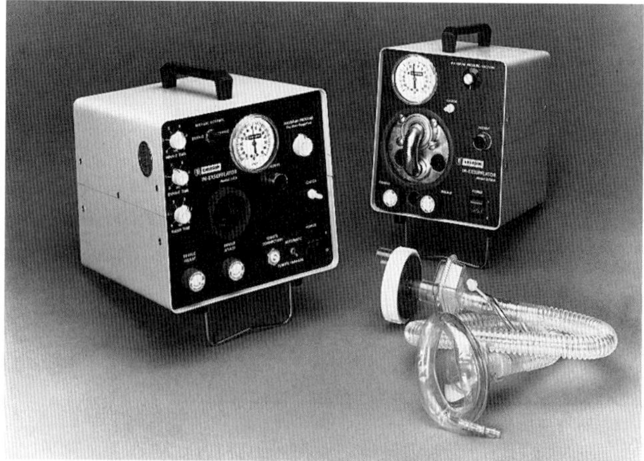

Figure 37-8
In-Exsufflator mechanical insufflation-exsufflation devices. *(Courtesy J.H. Emerson Co., Cambridge, Mass.)*

insufflation pressures should be increased gradually to avoid chest wall muscle pulls. Patients in spinal shock are susceptible to exsufflation-associated bradycardias. Abdominal distention is infrequent and eliminated by decreasing insufflation, not exsufflation, pressures. Otherwise, no untoward effects of MIE have been reported in chronic neuromuscular patients.[76] On the other hand, the effectiveness of MIE for critically ill patients has not yet been determined.[16]

PAP Adjuncts

Positive airway pressure (PAP) adjuncts are used to help mobilize secretions and treat atelectasis. As adjuncts for airway clearance, these methods are never used alone but always combined with directed cough or other airway clearance techniques.[15] One of three different approaches can be used: (1) continuous PAP (CPAP), (2) expiratory PAP (EPAP), and (3) positive expiratory pressure (PEP).

To guide practitioners in applying these techniques, the AARC has developed and published a clinical practice guideline on the use of PAP adjuncts to bronchial hygiene therapy. Excerpts from the AARC guideline, including indications, contraindications, hazards and complications, assessment of need, assessment of outcome, and monitoring, appear on p. 901.[15] The use of these methods to treat atelectasis was reviewed in Chapter 36. Here we will focus on their application as adjuncts in secretion clearance, with an emphasis on PEP therapy.

PEP therapy involves active expiration against a variable flow resistance. In theory, PEP helps move secretions into the larger airways by (1) filling underaerated or nonaerated segments via collateral ventilation and (2) preventing airway collapse during expiration.[6,77] A subsequent huff or FET maneuver allows the patient to generate the flows needed to expel mucus from blocked airways.

The PEP technique originated in Denmark, where it has largely replaced PDPV. Most clinical studies of PEP therapy have involved patients with CF, although its use in COPD and in preventing postoperative atelectasis has also been investigated. In general, when compared with other bronchial hygiene methods (PDPV, AD, ACB) in patients with CF, PEP therapy provides comparable mucociliary clearance.[6,77] Moreover, patients invariably prefer PEP over other methods. Long-term use in patients with CF may also be beneficial, with one report showing decreased hyperinflation and improved lung function with 10 months of PEP therapy.[78] However, PEP therapy does not appear to be as useful in enhancing lung clearance in chronic bronchitis.[79,80] In regard to the prevention of postoperative atelectasis, studies provide conflicting results.[81-83] In addition, PEP therapy cannot be used in young children (younger than 3 years).[6]

Use of PAP Adjuncts to Bronchial Hygiene Therapy

AARC Clinical Practice Guideline (Excerpts)*

➤ INDICATIONS

- To reduce air trapping in asthma and COPD
- To aid in mobilization of retained secretions (in CF and chronic bronchitis)
- To prevent or reverse atelectasis
- To optimize delivery of bronchodilators in patients receiving bronchial hygiene therapy

➤ CONTRAINDICATIONS

Although no absolute contraindications to the use of PEP, CPAP, or EPAP mask therapy have been reported, the following should be carefully evaluated before initiating therapy:

- Patients unable to tolerate increased work of breathing (acute asthma, COPD)
- ICP >20 mm Hg
- Hemodynamic instability
- Acute sinusitis
- Active hemoptysis
- Untreated pneumothorax
- Known or suspected tympanic membrane rupture or other middle ear pathology
- Recent facial, oral, or skull surgery or trauma
- Epistaxis
- Esophageal surgery
- Nausea

➤ HAZARDS AND COMPLICATIONS

- Pulmonary barotraumas
- Increased ICP
- Cardiovascular compromise (myocardial ischemia, decreased venous return)
- Skin breakdown and discomfort from mask
- Air swallowing, vomiting, and aspiration
- Claustrophobia
- Increased work of breathing that may lead to hypoventilation and hypercapnia

➤ ASSESSMENT OF NEED

The following should be assessed together to establish a need for PAP therapy:

- Sputum retention not responsive to spontaneous or directed coughing
- History of pulmonary problems treated successfully with postural drainage therapy
- Decreased breath sounds or adventitious sounds suggesting secretions in the airway
- Change in vital signs (increase in breathing frequency, tachycardia)
- Abnormal chest radiograph consistent with atelectasis, mucus plugging, or infiltrates
- Deterioration in ABG values or oxygen saturation

➤ ASSESSMENT OF OUTCOME

- Change in sputum production
- Change in breath sounds
- Patient subjective response to therapy
- Change in vital signs
- Change in chest radiograph
- Change in ABG values or oxygen saturation

➤ MONITORING

The following items should be chosen as appropriate for a specific patient's response:

- Patient subjective response (pain, discomfort, dyspnea, response to therapy)
- Pulse rate and cardiac rhythm (if ECG is available)
- Mental function
- Breath sounds

Continued

USE OF PAP ADJUNCTS TO BRONCHIAL HYGIENE THERAPY—CONT'D

AARC Clinical Practice Guideline (Excerpts)*

- Pulse oximetry/ABG analysis (if indicated)
- Breathing pattern/rate, symmetrical costal expansion, synchronous abdominal movement
- Sputum production (quantity, color, consistency, and odor)
- Skin color
- Blood pressure
- ICP (if indicated)

*For complete guidelines see Respir Care 38:516, 1993.

The clinical procedure for PAP therapy appears in Box 37-5.[84] Equipment can be easily assembled from available parts in most respiratory care departments. Alternatively, United States Food and Drug Administration (FDA)-approved single-use commercial devices are now available for purchase (Figure 37-9). Regardless of equipment used, it is essential to monitor actual airway pressures (as opposed to set or intended pressures).[85]

Common strategies for PEP therapy vary from twice to four times daily, with frequency determined by assessment of patient response to therapy.[15] During acute exacerbations, therapy should be performed at decreasing intervals rather than extending the length of the therapy sessions. Aerosol drug therapy may be added to a PEP session, using either an in-line handheld nebulizer or a metered-dose inhaler (MDI) attached to the one-way valve inlet of the system (see Figure 37-9).[84] The combination of aerosol drug therapy with PEP appears to improve the efficacy of bronchodilator

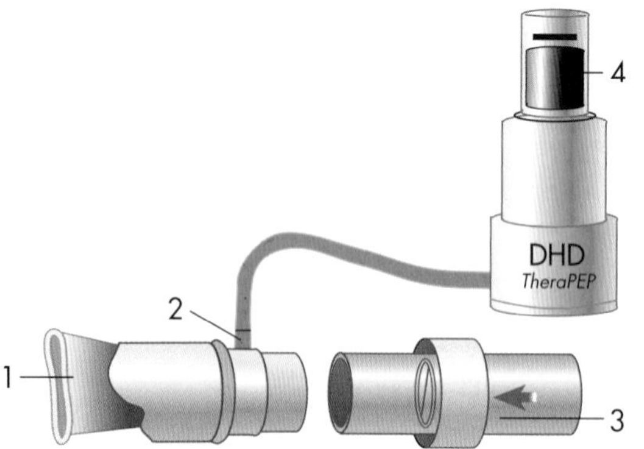

Figure 37-9

Example of commercial single-use PEP device (DHD TheraPEP). *1,* Mouthpiece; *2,* pressure tap; *3,* one-way inlet valve; *4,* pressure generator.

Box 37-5 • Clinical Procedure for PAP Therapy

1. Assess need for PAP therapy and design a treatment program to accomplish treatment objectives.
   a. Bring equipment to bedside and provide initial therapy to patient, adjusting pressure settings to meet patient need.
   b. After initial patient treatment and/or training, communicate treatment plan to physician and nurse, and provide instruction to nursing staff if required.
2. Explain purpose of PAP therapy to patient; teach patient "huff"(directed cough procedure).
3. Instruct the patient to:
   a. Sit comfortably.
   b. If using a mask, apply it tightly but comfortably over the nose and mouth. If mouthpiece is used, place lips firmly around it and breath through mouth.
   c. Take in a breath that is larger than normal, but not to fill lungs completely.
   d. Exhale actively, but not forcefully, creating a PAP of 10 to 20 cm H_2O during exhalation (determined with manometer during initial therapy sessions). Length of inhalation should be approximately one third of the total breathing cycle (I:E ratio of 1:3 to 1:4).
   e. Perform 10 to 20 breaths.
   f. Remove the mask or mouthpiece and perform two or three "huff" coughs, and rest as needed.
   g. Repeat above cycle four to eight times, not to exceed 20 minutes.
4. Evaluate the patient for the ability to self-administer.
5. When appropriate, teach the patient to self-administer. Observations on several occasions of proper technique uncoached should precede allowing the patient to self-administer without supervision.
6. When patients are also receiving bronchodilator aerosol, administer in conjunction with PAP therapy by placing a nebulizer in line with the PAP device.

Box 37-5 • Clinical Procedure for PAP Therapy—cont'd

7. When the PAP device is visibly soiled, rinse it with sterile water and shake/air dry; leave within reach at patient bedside in a clear plastic bag.
8. Send the PAP device (if single-patient use) home with the patient, or discard it on discharge. If it is nondisposable, send in-house for high-level disinfection.
9. Document in the patient's medical record procedures performed (including device, settings used, pressure developed, number of breaths per treatment, and frequency), patient response to therapy, patient teaching provided, and patient ability to self-administer.

administration, probably because of better distribution to the peripheral airways.[84]

High-Frequency Compression/Oscillation

As applied to airway clearance, oscillation refers to the rapid vibratory movement of small volumes of air back and forth in the respiratory tract. At high frequencies (12 to 25 Hz), these oscillations act as a physical "mucolytic," enhancing cough clearance of secretions.[86]

There are two general approaches to oscillation: external (chest wall) application and airway application. External application is often called *high-frequency chest wall compression* (HFCWC). Airway application of oscillation methods include (1) the flutter valve and (2) intrapulmonary percussive ventilation (IPV).

High-Frequency Chest Wall Oscillation

High-frequency chest wall oscillation (HFCWO) is accomplished by using a two-part system: (1) a variable air-pulse generator and (2) a nonstretch inflatable vest that covers the patient's entire torso (The Vest™ airway clearance system), Figure 37-10.[87] Small gas volumes are alternately injected into and withdrawn from the vest by the air-pulse generator at a fast rate, creating an oscillatory motion against the patient's thorax. Typically, patients perform 30-minute therapy sessions at oscillatory frequencies between 5 and 25 Hz. Depending on need and response, between one and six therapy sessions may occur per day.

Oscillation frequency and flow bias (inspiratory versus expiratory) determine the effectiveness of therapy. Animal studies have shown that if the flow bias during treatment is not expiratory, mucus may actually move deeper into the lung.[6] Additionally, the oscillation frequency used affects both patient comfort and efficacy.[88] The current recommendation is to individually identify the frequency that produces the highest flows and largest volumes in a given patient.

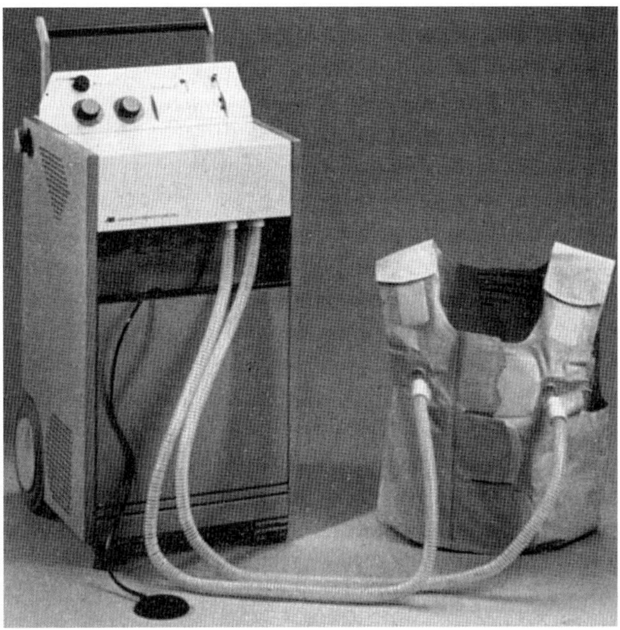

Figure 37-10
The Vest™ airway clearance system, a high-frequency chest wall compression (HFCWC) system. *(Courtesy Advanced Respiratory, Inc.)*

Although preliminary case reports of HFCWC were positive, comparative clinical studies have provided only mixed results. For example, when compared with PDPV in patients with cystic fibrosis hospitalized for acute pulmonary exacerbations, HFCWC did not result in better sputum mobilization, pulmonary function, or weight gain.[89] Given the high expense of HFCWC and the recent availability of other, cheaper methods, more research is needed to determine its efficacy, cost benefits, and optimum treatment strategies.

An alternative device, the Hayek oscillator, is now available in the United States (Breasy Medical Equipment, Stamford, Conn.). Instead of a vest, the Hayak oscillator uses a chest shield (turtle shell) strapped to the anterior chest wall. The shell is connected by a large hose to a negative/positive pressure generator that can provide oscillations at frequencies up to 15 Hz. Currently, there are no published studies demonstrating the effectiveness of this device for airway clearance.

Flutter Valve

Originally developed in Switzerland, the flutter valve combines the techniques of EPAP with high-frequency oscillations (HFO) at the airway opening.[6] The valve consists of a pipe-shaped device with a heavy steel ball sitting in an angled "bowl" (Figure 37-11). The pipe bowl is covered by a perforated cap. When the patient exhales actively into the pipe, the ball creates a positive expiratory pressure of between 10 and 25 cm H_2O. At the same time, the pipe angle causes the ball to flutter

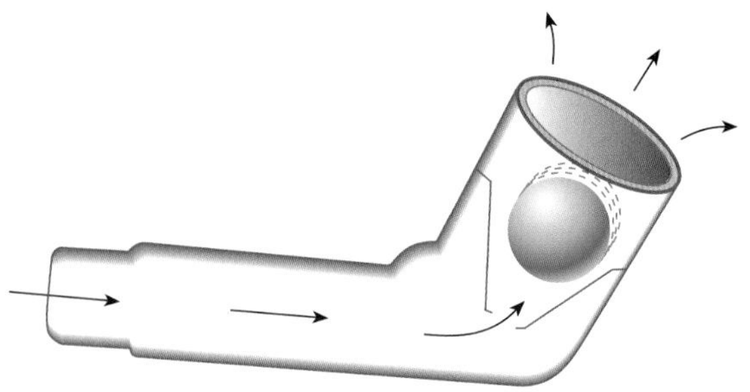

Figure 37-11
Cross section of a flutter valve. Exhalation through the device provides both positive expiratory pressure (PEP) and high-frequency oscillations.

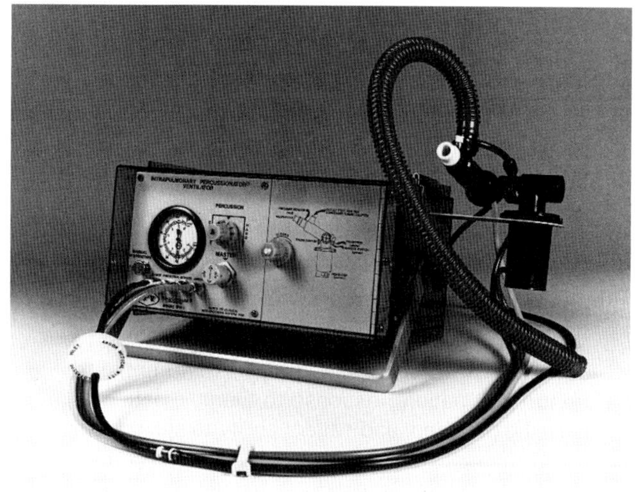

Figure 37-12
Intrapulmonary Percussive Ventilator (IPV). *(Courtesy Percussionaire, Sand Point, Idaho.)*

back and forth at about 15 Hz. When the valve is properly used, the oscillations it creates are transmitted down into the airways. Patients can control the pressure by changing their expiratory flows. Changing the angle of the device alters the oscillations.[6]

Clinical trials of the flutter valve provide mixed results. In patients with CF, the flutter valve has proved less,[90] equally,[91] and more effective[92] in sputum volume when compared with existing methods of airway clearance (PDPV or ACB). The flutter device, however, can decrease mucus viscoelasticity within the airways thus modifying mucus and allowing it to be cleared more easily by cough.[93] Interestingly, use of the flutter valve in patients with hyperproductive allergic asthma improved pulmonary function values (forced expiratory volume in one second [FEV_1], peak expiratory flow [PEF]) after 1 month of treatment.[94] Given that the flutter valve is readily accepted by patients, inexpensive, and fully portable, and does not require caregiver assistance (once instruction is provided), additional short- and long-term clinical trials seem justified.[92]

Intrapulmonary Percussive Ventilation

Intrapulmonary percussive ventilation is an airway clearance technique that uses a pneumatic device to deliver a series of pressurized gas minibursts at rates of 100 to 225 cycles per minute (1.6 to 3.75 Hz) to the respiratory tract, usually via a mouthpiece (Figure 37-12). The device was FDA approved in 1993 and is marketed as the Intrapulmonary Percussive Ventilator, or IPV (Percussionaire, Sand Point, Idaho).

The duration of each percussive cycle is manually controlled by the patient or clinician using a thumb button.[84] During the percussive cycle, constant PAP is maintained at the airway. The device also incorporates a pneumatic nebulizer for delivery of bland or medicated aerosol. The manufacturer recommends a total treatment time of about 20 minutes.

Although current research is limited, two comparative studies show that IPV is as effective as standard aerosol and PDPV in improving short-term pulmonary function test results and enhancing sputum expectoration in patients with CF.[95,96] The therapy is well tolerated by stable patients and has no reported side effects. Further research is needed to confirm the potential benefits of intrapulmonary percussive ventilation.

Mobilization and Exercise

Immobility is a major factor contributing to retention of secretions. Early mobilization and frequent position changes are now standard preventive interventions for atelectasis and postoperative pneumonia.[97] Adding exercise to mobilization and coughing further enhances mucus clearance.[37,98]

Exercise also improves overall aeration and ventilation-perfusion matching. Besides increasing sputum production, it can also improve pulmonary function.[99-102] In addition, exercise can improve a patient's general fitness, self-esteem, and quality of life.[5] For ambulatory patients, exercise not only is socially acceptable, but actually is encouraged as part of a healthy lifestyle. Involvement in exercise activity thus makes patients feel more a part of the mainstream.

On the other hand, exercise can be fatiguing and result in oxygen desaturation among patients with significant pulmonary impairment.[103] For these reasons, it is probably wise to conduct an exercise evaluation on any ambulatory patient with severe lung disease being considered for exercise therapy (see Chapter 48). In addition, young children and patients with neuromuscular limitations are not good candidates for airway clearance via exercise activity.[5]

▶ SELECTING BRONCHIAL HYGIENE TECHNIQUES

Selection Factors

Box 37-6 specifies the key factors clinicians should consider when selecting a bronchial hygiene strategy.[5]

Motivation is key to routine performance of any procedure, especially for chronically ill patients in ambulatory or home care settings. No bronchial hygiene strategy will succeed if it is abandoned by the patient. Likewise, no routine strategy is likely to be followed without tangible results. In this regard, increased sputum production, though frequently shown *not* to be related to improved pulmonary function, is one of the few tangible outcomes clinicians can use to motivate the patient and gain his or her ongoing cooperation.[5]

Age and patient preference often dictate available methods. If a number of methods are deemed equivalent, it makes sense to allow the patient to choose. Patient and caregiver goals for treatment should be discussed jointly, with the intent of choosing the method that best fits the patient's goals and lifestyle.[5] The clinician's skill in teaching a particular technique will also determine success, as will the patient's ease of learning.

Since patients will reject methods that are tiring or fatiguing, this should be considered in selection. In addition, the patient's disease may either suggest the best approach or impose certain limitations that preclude using a particular method. For example, we have seen that patients with certain neuromuscular diseases may not be able to engage in therapeutic exercise. Last, cost is becoming a critical factor in selecting all treatment strategies. Clearly, all else being equal, we should always select the least expensive strategy.[5] More and more, this is coming to mean therapies that are either self-administered or provided by unskilled caregivers outside the acute care setting. In this context, effective patient or caregiver education is going to play an increasingly important role (see Chapter 46).

Box 37-6 • Key Factors in Selecting a Bronchial Hygiene Strategy

- Patient's motivation
- Patient's goals
- Physician/caregiver goals
- Effectiveness of technique
- Patient's age
- Patient's ability to concentrate
- Ease of learning and teaching
- Skill of therapists/teachers
- Fatigue or work required
- Need for assistants or equipment
- Limitations of technique based on disease type and severity
- Costs (direct and indirect)
- Desirability of combining methods

Clearance Strategies for Specific Conditions

Table 37-3 specifies airway clearance techniques for the most common conditions associated with retained secretions. In some cases, a combination of methods may be needed to achieve desired results.

MINI CLINI

Recommending Bronchial Hygiene Strategies

PROBLEM

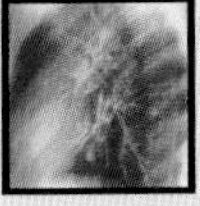

You are asked to evaluate and recommend an appropriate ambulatory bronchial hygiene therapy regimen for a 7-year-old active female patient with CF who is being cared for in her home by elderly grandparents.

DISCUSSION

In general, appropriate secretion clearance strategies for this patient include exercise, PEP, PDPV, ACB, and HFO (Table 37-3). Since PDPV will be difficult to implement in this patient's home setting (elderly caregivers), emphasis should be placed on either PEP with ACB or HFO (flutter valve) with ACB. An exercise plan should also be incorporated into the overall strategy. Of course, dietary and medication considerations are also important.

Table 37-3 ▶▶ Recommended Airway Clearance Techniques in Specific Conditions

Problem Area	Appropriate Techniques
Cystic Fibrosis, ciliary dyskinesia, bronchiectasis	
Infants	PDPV
3-12 years	Exercise, PEP, PDPV, ACB, HFO
>12 years	Exercise, ACB, AD, PEP, PDPV, HFO
Atelectasis	PEP, PDPV, ACB
Asthma (with mucus plugging)	Exercise, PEP, PDPV, HFO (flutter valve)
Neurologic abnormalities (spasticity, bulbar palsy, aspiration-prone)	PDPV, suction, MIE
Musculoskeletal weakness (muscular dystrophy, myasthenia gravis, poliomyelitis)	PEP, MIE

▶ PROTOCOL-BASED BRONCHIAL HYGIENE

A number of therapist-driven protocols have been published for bronchial hygiene therapy. All involve rigorous assessment of the patient, both to establish preliminary need and to determine continuation of or modification in therapy. Figure 37-13 provides an example of the algorithm used in one such protocol. Note that changes in therapy occur throughout and are based on the patient's response and the evaluation of the clinician.

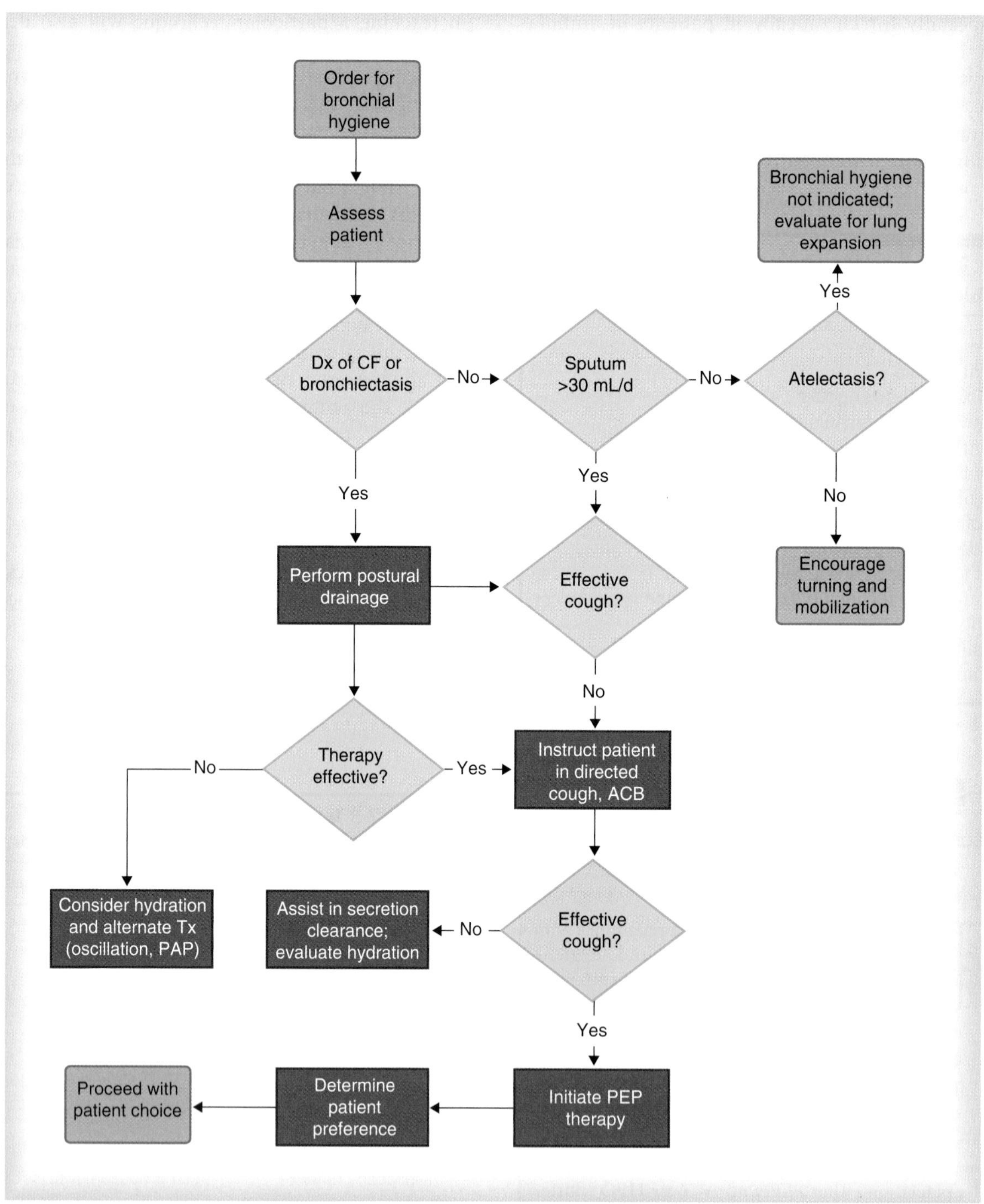

Figure 37-13

Example of algorithm underlying a bronchial hygiene therapy protocol. *(Modified from Sobush DC, Hilling L, Southorn PA: Bronchial hygiene therapy. In Burton GG, Hodgkin JE, Ward JJ: Respiratory care: a guide to clinical practice, ed 4, Philadelphia, 1997, JB Lippincott.)*

KEY POINTS

- Normal airway clearance requires a patent airway, a functional mucociliary escalator, and an effective cough.
- The primary goal of bronchial hygiene therapy is to help mobilize and remove retained secretions, improve gas exchange, and reduce the work of breathing.
- Retained secretions can increase the work of breathing, cause air trapping, worsen $\dot{V}/\dot{Q}$ balance, promote atelectasis and shunting, and increase the incidence of infection.
- Disorders associated with abnormal secretion clearance include foreign bodies, tumors, congenital or acquired thoracic anomalies, asthma, chronic bronchitis, CF, bronchiectasis, and acute infections.
- Musculoskeletal and neurological disorders can impair coughing and lead to mucus plugging, airway obstruction, and atelectasis.
- Both mechanical and treatment factors impair mucociliary clearance in intubated patients.
- Clinical signs indicating retained secretions include ineffective cough, absent or increased sputum production, a labored breathing pattern, decreased breath sounds, crackles or rhonchi, tachypnea, tachycardia, or fever.
- Turning promotes lung expansion, improves oxygenation, and prevents retention of secretions.
- In patients with unilateral lung disease, placing the good lung down can improve oxygenation; exceptions include internal bleeding, abscess, and unilateral pulmonary interstitial emphysema.
- Postural drainage involves placing the segmental bronchus to be drained in a vertical position relative to gravity and holding the position for 3 to 15 minutes.
- Whether percussion and vibration are effective remains controversial.
- In patients with copious secretions, directed coughing is as least as good at clearance as more complicated methods.
- Cough methods must be modified in surgical patients, patients with COPD, and patients with neuromuscular disorders.

KEY POINTS—cont'd

- The FET, or "huff cough," consists of one or two forced expirations of middle to low lung volume *without closure of the glottis*, followed by a period of diaphragmatic breathing and relaxation.
- The ACB consists of repeated cycles of breathing control, thoracic expansion, and the FET.
- During AD, the patient uses diaphragmatic breathing to mobilize secretions by varying lung volumes and expiratory airflow in three distinct phases.
- MIE involves delivery of a positive-pressure breath followed by the quick application of negative pressure; PEFs exceed those developed by manually assisted coughing.
- PEP therapy is a self-administered clearance technique involving active expiration against a variable-flow resistance, followed by an FET; patients invariably prefer PEP over other methods.
- At high frequencies (12 to 25 Hz), airway oscillations enhance cough clearance of secretions.
- Airway oscillations can be created externally (HFCWC) or at the airway opening (flutter valve, intrapulmonary percussive ventilation).
- Adding exercise to mobilization and coughing enhances mucus clearance, improves overall aeration and ventilation-perfusion matching, and improves pulmonary function.
- Numerous factors must be considered in trying to select the best bronchial hygiene strategy for a given patient.

References

1. Frownfelter DL, Dean E: Principles and practice of cardiopulmonary physical therapy, ed 3, St. Louis, 1996, Mosby.
2. Frownfelter D: Chest physical therapy and airway care. In Barnes TA: Core textbook of respiratory care practice, ed 2, St. Louis, 1994, Mosby.
3. Dean E, Ross J: Discordance between cardiopulmonary physiology and physical therapy. Toward a rational basis for practice, Chest 101:1694, 1992.
4. Eid N et al: Chest physiotherapy in review, Respir Care 36:270, 1991.
5. Hardy KA: A review of airway clearance: new techniques, indications, and recommendations, Respir Care 39: 440, 1994.

6. Hardy KA, Anderson BD: Noninvasive clearance of airway secretions, Respir Care Clin North Am 2:323, 1996.
7. MacKenzie CF et al: Chest physiotherapy in the intensive care unit, Baltimore, 1981, Williams & Wilkins.
8. Stiller K et al: Efficacy of breathing and coughing exercises in the prevention of pulmonary complications after coronary artery surgery, Chest 105:741, 1994.
9. Alexander E, Weingarten S, Mohsenifar Z: Clinical strategies to reduce utilization of chest physiotherapy without compromising patient care, Chest 110:430, 1996.
10. Thomas J, Cook DJ, Brooks D: Chest physical therapy management of patients with cystic fibrosis: a meta-analysis, Am J Respir Crit Care Med 151:846, 1995.
11. Kirilloff LH et al: Does chest physical therapy work? Chest 88:436, 1985.
12. Jones AP: Bronchopulmonary hygiene physical therapy for chronic obstructive pulmonary disease and bronchiectasis, Cochrane Review 3:1,2000.
13. American Association for Respiratory Care: Clinical practice guideline: postural drainage therapy, Respir Care 36:1418, 1991.
14. American Association for Respiratory Care: Clinical practice guideline: directed cough, Respir Care 38:495, 1993.
15. American Association for Respiratory Care: Clinical practice guideline: use of PAP adjuncts to bronchial hygiene therapy, Respir Care 38:516, 1993.
16. Judson AM, Sahn SA: Mobilization of secretions in ICU patients, Respir Care 39:213, 1994.
17. Langerson J: The cough: its effectiveness depends on you, Respir Care 24:142, 1979.
18. Irwin RS et al: Cough: a comprehensive review, Arch Intern Med 137:1189, 1977.
19. Hardy KA: Advances in our understanding and care of patients with cystic fibrosis, Respir Care 38:282, 1993.
20. Le Mauviel L: Primary ciliary dyskinesia, West J Med 155:280, 1991.
21. Luce JM: Bronchiectasis. In Murray JF, Nadel JA, editors: Textbook of respiratory medicine, ed 2, Philadelphia, 1994, WB Saunders.
22. Hardy KA, Schidlow DV, Zaeri N: Obliterative bronchiolitis in children, Chest 93:460, 1988.
23. Sutton P et al: Chest physiotherapy: a review, Eur J Respir Dis 63:188, 1982.
24. Hess D, Agarwal NN, Myers CL: Positioning, lung function, and kinetic bed therapy, Respir Care 37:181, 1992.
25. Basham KA, Vollman KM, Miller AC: An overview of continuous lateral rotation therapy, Respir Care Clin North Am 3:109, 1997.
26. Sahn SA: Continuous lateral rotational therapy and nosocomial pneumonia, Chest 99:1263, 1991.
27. Johannigman JA et al: Prone positioning for acute respiratory distress syndrome in the surgical intensive care unit: who, and how long? Surgery 128:708, 2000.
28. Jolliet P, Bulpa P, Chevrolet JC: Effects of the prone position on gas exchange and hemodynamics in severe acute respiratory distress syndrome. Crit Care Med 26:1977, 1998.
29. Voggenreiter G et al: Crit Care Med 27:2375, 1999.
30. Breiburg AN et al: Efficacy and safety of prone positioning for patients with acute respiratory distress syndrome, J Adv Nurs 32:922, 2000.
31. Chatte G et al: Prone position in mechanically ventilated patients with severe acute respiratory failure, Am J Respir Crit Care Med 155:473, 1997.
32. Gattinoni L et al: Effect of prone positioning on the survival of patients with acute respiratory failure, N Engl J Med 345:610, 2001.
33. Lamm WJ, Graham MM, Albert RK: Mechanism by which the prone position improves oxygenation in acute lung injury, Am J Respir Crit Care Med 150:184, 1994.
34. Pappert D et al: Influence of positioning on ventilation-perfusion relationships in severe adult respiratory distress syndrome, Chest 106:1511, 1994.
35. Broccard AF et al: Influence of prone position on the extent and distribution of lung injury in a high tidal volume oleic acid model of acute respiratory distress syndrome, Crit Care Med 25:16, 1997.
36. Du HL et al: Beneficial effects of the prone position on the incidence of barotrauma in oleic acid-induced lung injury under continuous positive pressure ventilation, Acta Anaesthesiol Scand 41:701, 1997.
37. Oldenburg FA et al: Effects of postural drainage, exercise, and cough on mucus clearance in chronic bronchitis, Am Rev Respir Dis 120:739, 1979.
38. Wong JW et al: Effects of gravity on tracheal transport rates in normal subjects and in patients with cystic fibrosis, Pediatrics 60:146, 1977.
39. Chopra SK et al: Effects of hydration and physical therapy on tracheal transport velocity, Am Rev Respir Dis 115:1009, 1974.
40. Taylor CJ, Threlfall D: Postural drainage techniques and gastro-oesophageal reflux in cystic fibrosis, Lancet 31;349 (965):1567, 1997.
41. Ross J, Dean E, Abboud RT: The effect of postural drainage positioning on ventilation homogeneity in healthy subjects, Phys Ther 72:794, 1992.
42. Pryor JA, Webber BA, Hodson ME: Effect of chest physiotherapy on oxygen saturation in patients with cystic fibrosis, Thorax 45:77, 1990.
43. Kigin C: Chest physical therapy. In Pierson DJ, Kacmarek RM, editors. Foundations of respiratory care, New York, 1992, Churchill Livingstone.
44.Conway JH et al: Humidification as an adjunct to chest physiotherapy in aiding tracheobronchial clearance in patients with bronchiectasis, Respir Med 86:109, 1992.
45. Radford R et al: A rational basis for percussion: augmented mucociliary clearance, Respir Care 27:556, 1982.
46. Sutton PP et al: Assessment of percussion, vibratory-shaking and breathing exercises in chest physiotherapy, Eur J Respir Dis 66:147, 1985.
47. Gallon A: Evaluation of chest percussion in the treatment of patients with copious sputum production, Respir Med 85: 45, 1991.
48. Murphy MB, Concannon D, FitzGerald M: Chest percussion: help or hindrance to postural drainage, Ir Med J 76:189, 1983.

49. Wollmer P et al: Inefficiency of chest percussion in the physical therapy of chronic bronchitis, Eur J Respir Dis 66:233, 1985.
50. van der Schans CP, Piers DA, Postma DS: Effect of manual percussion on tracheobronchial clearance in patients with chronic airflow obstruction and excessive tracheobronchial secretion, Thorax 41:448, 1986.
51. Eubanks DH, Bone RC: Comprehensive respiratory care: a learning system, St Louis, 1985, Mosby.
52. Bauer ML, McDougal J, Schoumacher RA: Comparison of manual and mechanical chest percussion in hospitalized patients with cystic fibrosis, J Pediatr 124:250, 1994.
53. Irwin RS et al: Managing cough as a defense mechanism and as a symptom: a consensus panel of the American College of Chest Physicians, Chest 114:133S, 1998.
54. Camnet P: Studies on the removal of inhaled particles from the lungs by voluntary coughing, Chest 80:824, 1981.
55. Bennett WD, Foster WM, Chapman WF: Cough-enhanced mucus clearance in the normal lung, J Appl Physiol 69:1670, 1990.
56. Bateman JR et al: Is cough as effective as chest physical therapy in the removal of excessive bronchial secretions? Thorax 36:683, 1981.
57. Hasani A et al: The effect of unproductive coughing/FET on regional mucus movement in the human lungs, Respir Med 85:23, 1991.
58. Hietpas BG, Roth RD, Jensen WM: Huff coughing and airway patency, Respir Care 24:710, 1979.
59. Szeinberg A et al: Cough capacity in patient with muscular dystrophy, Chest 94:1232, 1988.
60. Braun SR, Giovannoni R, O'Connor M: Improving the cough in patients with spinal cord injury, Am J Phys Med 63:110, 1984.
61. Partridge C, Pryor J, Webber B: Characteristics of the forced expiratory technique, Physiotherapy 75:193, 1989.
62. Pryor S et al: Evaluation of the forced expiration technique as an adjunct to postural drainage in treatment of cystic fibrosis, Br Med Bull 2:417, 1979.
63. Sutton P et al: Assessment of the forced expiration technique, postural drainage, and directed coughing in chest physiotherapy, Eur J Respir Dis 64:62, 1983.
64. Olseni L et al: Chest physiotherapy in chronic obstructive pulmonary disease: forced expiratory technique combined with either postural drainage or positive expiratory pressure breathing, Respir Med 88:435, 1994.
65. Pryor JA, Webber BA, Hodson ME: Effect of chest physiotherapy on oxygen saturation in patients with cystic fibrosis, Thorax 45:77, 1990.
66. Miller S et al: Chest physiotherapy in cystic fibrosis: a comparative study of autogenic drainage and the active cycle of breathing techniques with postural drainage, Thorax 50:165, 1995.
67. Chevalier J: Autogenic drainage. In Lawson D, editor: Cystic fibrosis: horizons, Chichester, 1984, John Wiley.
68. Schoni MH: Autogenic drainage: a modern approach to physiotherapy in cystic fibrosis, J R Soc Med 82:32, 1989.
69. Dab I, Alexander F: The mechanism of autogenic drainage studied with flow volume curves, Monogr Paediatr 10:50, 1979.
70. Pfleger A et al: Self-administered chest physiotherapy in cystic fibrosis: a comparative study of high-pressure PEP and autogenic drainage, Lung 170:323, 1992.
71. Giles DR et al: Short-term effects of postural drainage with clapping vs. autogenic drainage on oxygen saturation and sputum recovery in patients with cystic fibrosis, Chest 108:952, 1995.
72. Anderson JB, Falk M: Chest physiotherapy in the pediatric age group, Respir Care 36:546, 1991.
73. Lindemann H, Boldt A, Kieselmann R: Autogenic drainage: efficacy of a simplified method, Acta Univ Carol 36:210, 1990.
74. Bach JR: Mechanical insufflation-exsufflation. Comparison of peak expiratory flows with manually assisted and unassisted coughing techniques, Chest 104:1553, 1993.
75. Bach JR: Update and perspective on noninvasive respiratory muscle aids. II: The expiratory muscle aids, Chest 105:1538, 1994.
76. Dean S, Bach JR: The use of noninvasive respiratory muscle aids in the management of patients with progressive neuromuscular diseases, Respir Care Clin North Am 2:223, 1996.
77. Malmeister MJ, Fink JB, Hoffman GL: Positive expiratory pressure mask therapy: theoretical and practical considerations and a review of the literature, Respir Care 36:1218, 1991.
78. Oberwaldner B, Evans JC, Zach MS: Forced expirations against a variable resistance: a new chest physiotherapy method in cystic fibrosis, Pediatr Pulmonol 2:358, 1986.
79. van Hengstum M et al: Effect of positive expiratory pressure mask physiotherapy (PEP) versus forced expiration technique (FET/PD) on regional lung clearance in chronic bronchitis, Eur Respir J 4:651, 1991.
80. Olseni L et al: Chest physiotherapy in chronic obstructive pulmonary disease: forced expiratory technique combined with either postural drainage or positive expiratory pressure breathing, Respir Med 88:435, 1994.
81. Frolund L, Madsen F: Self-administered prophylactic postoperative positive expiratory pressure in thoracic surgery, Acta Anaesthesiol Scand 30:381, 1986.
82. Ricksten SE et al: Effects of periodic PAP by mask on postoperative pulmonary function, Chest 89:774, 1986.
83. Ingwersen UM et al: Three different mask physiotherapy regimens for prevention of postoperative pulmonary complications after heart and pulmonary surgery, Intensive Care Med 19:294, 1993.
84. Fink JB: Volume expansion therapy. In Burton GG, Hodgkin JE, Ward JJ: Respiratory care: a guide to clinical practice, ed 4, Philadelphia, 1997, JB Lippincott.
85. Christensen EF et al: Flow-dependent properties of positive expiratory pressure devices, Monaldi Arch Chest Dis 50:150, 1995.
86. Tomkiewicz RP, Biviji A, King M: Effects of oscillating air flow on the rheological properties and clearability of mucus gel simulants, Biorheology 31:511, 1994.

87. Whitman J et al: Preliminary evaluation of high-frequency chest compression for secretion clearance in mechanically ventilated patients, Respir Care 38:1081, 1993.
88. Rubin EM et al: Effect of chest wall oscillation on mucus clearance: comparison of two vibrators, Pediatr Pulmonol 6:122, 1989.
89. Ahrens R et al: Comparative efficacy of high frequency chest compression and conventional chest physiotherapy in hospitalized patients with cystic fibrosis (abstract), Pediatr Pulmonol Suppl 9:267, 1993.
90. Pryor JA et al: The Flutter VRP-1 as an adjunct to chest physiotherapy in cystic fibrosis, Respir Med 88:677, 1994.
91. Ambrosino N et al: Clinical evaluation of oscillating positive expiratory pressure for enhancing expectoration in diseases other than cystic fibrosis, Monaldi Arch Chest Dis 50:269, 1995.
92. Konstan MW, Stern RC, Doershuk CF: Efficacy of the Flutter device for airway mucus clearance in patients with cystic fibrosis, J Pediatr 124:689, 1994.
93. App EM et al: Sputum rheology changes in cystic fibrosis lung disease following two different types of physiotherapy: flutter vs. autogenic drainage, Chest 114:171, 1998.
94. Girard JP, Terki N: The Flutter VRP-1: a new personal pocket therapeutic device used as an adjunct to drug therapy in the management of bronchial asthma, J Investig Allergol Clin Immunol 4:23, 1994.
95. Natale JE, Pfeifle J, Homnick DN: Comparison of intrapulmonary percussive ventilation and chest physiotherapy. A pilot study in patients with cystic fibrosis, Chest 105:1789, 1994.
96. Homnick DN, White F, de Castro C: Comparison of effects of an intrapulmonary percussive ventilator to standard aerosol and chest physiotherapy in treatment of cystic fibrosis, Pediatr Pulmonol 20:50, 1995.
97. Lewis FR: Management of atelectasis and pneumonia, Surg Clin North Am 60:1391, 1980.
98. Wolff RK et al: Effects of exercise and eucapnic hyperventilation on bronchial clearance in man, J Appl Physiol 43:46, 1977.
99. Zach MS, Purrer B, Oberwaldner B: Effect of swimming on forced expiration and sputum clearance in cystic fibrosis, Lancet 2:1201, 1981.
100. Zach M, Oberwaldner B, Hausler F: Cystic fibrosis: physical exercise versus chest physiotherapy, Arch Dis Child 57:587, 1982.
101. Baldwin DR et al: Effect of addition of exercise to chest physiotherapy on sputum expectoration and lung function in adults with cystic fibrosis, Respir Med 88:49, 1994.
102. Olseni L, Midgren B, Wollmer P: Mucus clearance at rest and during exercise in patients with bronchial hypersecretion, Scand J Rehabil Med 24:61, 1992.
103. Henke KG, Orenstein DM: Oxygen saturation during exercise in cystic fibrosis, Am Rev Respir Dis 129:708, 1984.

SECTION VI

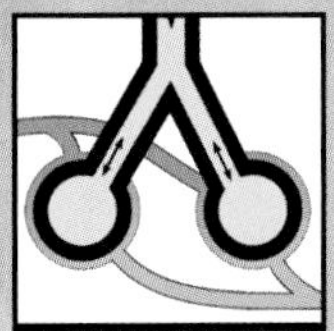

Acute and Critical Care

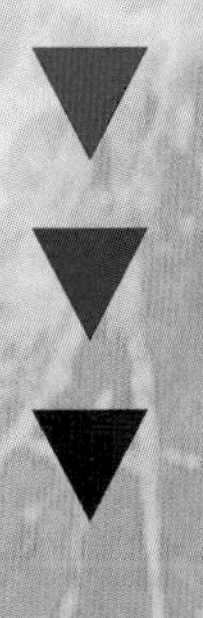

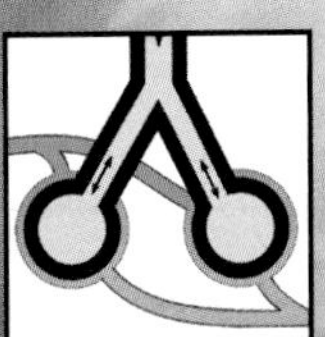

CHAPTER 38

Respiratory Failure and the Need for Ventilatory Support

Howard A. Christie and Lawrence S. Goldstein

In This Chapter You Will Learn:

- How acute respiratory failure is defined
- How hypoxemic respiratory failure (Type I) differs from hypercapnic respiratory failure (Type II)
- What causes acute respiratory failure
- How chronic respiratory failure and acute-on-chronic failure are identified
- How the complications of respiratory failure are identified
- What indicates the need for ventilatory support
- Which general principles should be followed when managing hypoxemic and hypercapnic respiratory failure
- What indications show the need for noninvasive ventilation

Chapter Outline

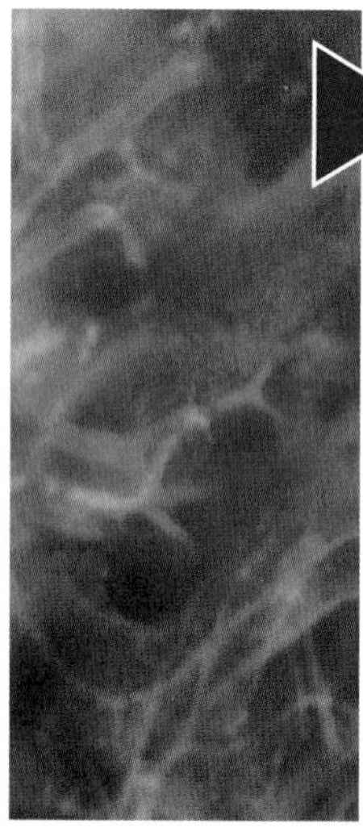

Key Terms

assist control (AC)
auto-PEEP
barotrauma
continuous positive airway pressure (CPAP)
contractile duration
dynamic hyperinflation
high frequency ventilation
hypercapnic respiratory failure (Type II)
hypoxemic respiratory failure (Type I)
maximum expiratory pressure (MEP)
maximum inspiratory pressure (MIP)
maximum voluntary ventilation (MVV)
muscle fatigue
noninvasive positive pressure ventilation (NIPPV)
positive end-expiratory pressure (PEEP)
pressure control ventilation (PCV)
pressure support ventilation (PSV)
respiratory alternans
synchronized intermittent mandatory ventilation (SIMV)
tension-time index
work of breathing

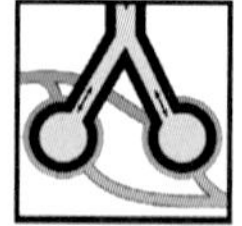

Respiratory failure is a clinical problem that all respiratory care practitioners must be skilled at identifying, assessing, and treating. A 1994 study of over 1400 patients concluded that 44% of patients diagnosed with acute respiratory failure requiring intensive care admission died in the hospital. This figure had not changed significantly in 20 years despite the advances in intensive care monitoring and therapy.[1] A 1999 review shows only marginal improvement, with a 36% hospital mortality.[2] The need for oxygen delivery, mechanical ventilation, and other modalities makes the respiratory therapist indispensable in the treatment of this life-threatening condition.

Put simply, respiratory failure is the "inability to maintain either the normal delivery of oxygen to the tissues or the normal removal of carbon dioxide from the tissues."[3] The advent of arterial blood gas (ABG) sampling has provided objective criteria to evaluate respiratory failure. Generally, failure is marked by a PaO_2 (arterial partial pressure of oxygen) less than 60 mm Hg and/or a $PaCO_2$ (alveolar partial pressure of carbon dioxide) greater than 50 mm Hg in otherwise healthy individuals breathing room air at sea level. These criteria were established as early as 1965 by Campbell.[4] Respiratory failure can be an acute or a chronic process. Additionally and classically, it has also been separated into two other categories to reflect the type of physiologic impairment. Hypoxemic (Type I) respiratory failure occurs when the primary problem is inadequate oxygen delivery. Hypercapnic (Type II) respiratory failure describes "bellows failure" of the lungs resulting in elevated carbon dioxide levels. Hypercapnic respiratory failure is also known as *ventilatory failure*. Patients with baseline acid-base derangement (e.g., chronic obstructive pulmonary disease [COPD], restrictive lung disease) may be chronically hypercapnic and, therefore, in chronic ventilatory failure based on the guidelines. These individuals develop acute failure when their chronic state deteriorates significantly. This is sometimes referred to as acute ventilatory failure superimposed on chronic ventilatory failure.

While ABGs are helpful in distinguishing hypoxemic (Type I) and hypercapnic (Type II) respiratory failure, many patients in acute respiratory failure develop both hypoxemia and hypercapnia. As noted above, patients with chronically elevated arterial $PaCO_2$ levels (chronic ventilatory failure) may develop a sudden, further increase in $PaCO_2$ associated with an acute exacerbation of their chronic condition (acute ventilatory failure superimposed on chronic ventilatory failure).

▶ ACUTE HYPOXEMIC RESPIRATORY FAILURE (TYPE I)

The primary causes of hypoxemia are the following:

- Ventilation/perfusion mismatch
- Shunt
- Alveolar hypoventilation
- Diffusion impairment
- Perfusion/diffusion impairment
- Decreased inspired oxygen

These are discussed in more detail in Chapters 9 and 10 but are briefly discussed here.

Ventilation/Perfusion Mismatch

Even in healthy lungs, there are regions where ventilation and perfusion are not evenly matched, so it seems logical that this is the most common cause of hypoxemia. Respiratory therapists are familiar with this concept, through the work of John West, which described a high ventilation/perfusion ($\dot{V}/\dot{Q}$) ratio at the apex of the lungs and a low ratio at the bases.[5] This can be oversimplified and stated as more air than blood at the apices and more blood than air at the bases.

Pathologic $\dot{V}/\dot{Q}$ mismatch occurs when disease disrupts this balance and hypoxemia results. Most commonly, this is seen as areas of low $\dot{V}/\dot{Q}$ ratio develop in which ventilation is compromised despite adequate blood flow. Obstructive lung diseases are frequent causes. The bronchospasm, mucus plugging, inflammation, and premature airway closure that signal asthmatic or emphysematous exacerbations worsen ventilation and create $\dot{V}/\dot{Q}$ mismatch. Infection, heart failure, and inhalation injury may lead to partially collapsed or fluid filled alveoli, also resulting in decreased ventilation and reduced blood oxygen levels.

Clinical Presentation of $\dot{V}/\dot{Q}$ Mismatch

As patients present with hypoxemia, the initial goal is always to treat the low PaO_2 or SpO_2 (arterial oxygen saturation by pulse oximeter). $\dot{V}/\dot{Q}$ mismatch will respond to supplemental oxygen. Hypoxemia commonly presents with dyspnea, tachycardia, and tachypnea, but these are very nonspecific findings. Patient observation is extremely valuable, however. The use of accessory muscles of respiration (scalene, pectoralis major, and sternomastoid) is an important sign that normal diaphragmatic inspiration is inadequate. In an elderly, cachectic, or barrel-chested individual who is leaning forward on his or her arms, COPD is the likely diagnosis. Nasal flaring may be present. Lower extremity edema is more indicative of cardiac failure as the cause of the hypoxemia. Cyanosis may be peripheral and primarily due to decreased blood flow. Central cyanosis, seen most easily as a bluish tint around the lips, occurs when greater than 5g/dL of unsaturated hemoglobin are present. This is more common in patients with polycythemia, but may be subject to wide observer variability. More severe hypoxemia can lead to significant central nervous system (CNS) dysfunction, ranging from irritability to confusion to coma.

Auscultation is very useful when added to patient observation. Bilateral wheezing, especially in the young patient in respiratory distress, often identifies the bronchospasm of asthma. Upper airway disease or fluid-filled airways may also result in wheezing. Breath sounds that are diminished bilaterally are common in emphysema. Unilateral abnormalities are significant. Wheezing in one lung may identify an endobronchial lesion, while the absence of breath sounds on one side of the chest may reveal collapse, infection, edema, or effusion as potential causes of $\dot{V}/\dot{Q}$ mismatch. Unilateral crackles generally indicate an alveolar filling process (mass, infection, fluid).

Radiographically, $\dot{V}/\dot{Q}$ mismatch can present as a "black" radiograph, with large or hyperinflated lungs as in the case of obstructive disease. A "white" chest radiograph is evident when alveoli are partially occluded. Indeed, the "blackness" or "whiteness" of the lung fields on the plain chest radiograph has important diagnostic value in assessing the patient with acute respiratory failure.

Shunt

Shunt is an extreme version of $\dot{V}/\dot{Q}$ mismatch in which there is no ventilation to match perfusion ($\dot{V}/\dot{Q} = 0$). About 2% to 3% of the blood supply is shunted via the bronchial and thebesian veins that feed the lungs and heart. This is normal anatomical shunt. Pathological anatomical shunt occurs as a result of right-to-left blood flow through cardiac openings (e.g., atrial or ventricular septal defects) or in pulmonary arteriovenous malformations. Physiological shunt leads to hypoxemia when alveoli collapse or are filled with fluid or exudate. Common etiologies may be atelectasis, pulmonary edema, or pneumonia. Unlike $\dot{V}/\dot{Q}$ mismatch, shunt does not respond to supplemental oxygen because the gas exchange unit (the alveolus) is not open.

Clinical Presentation of Shunt

In many ways, the clinical presentation of shunt is very similar to the presentation of $\dot{V}/\dot{Q}$ mismatch. Patient observations are similar, although chest excursion may be asymmetrical in shunt on occasion. Bilateral or unilateral crackles are common due to the alveolar filling process. Unilateral absence of breath sounds may indicate significant collapse, mass, or effusion, which require treatment before oxygenation can improve. Shunt usually presents with a "white" chest radiograph. The most advanced example of this is the diffuse, bilateral haziness in adult respiratory distress syndrome (ARDS).

Alveolar Hypoventilation

This cause of hypoxemia will be discussed under the section Acute Hypercapnic Respiratory Failure (Type II).

Diffusion Impairment

Clinically relevant diffusion refers to movement of gas across the alveolar-capillary membrane due to a pressure gradient. While this is rarely a cause of significant hypoxemia at rest, its effects become more pronounced with exercise.[6,7] In exercise, blood flow increases, which limits the time for gas exchange. This is normally not a problem, but when diffusion impairment is present, hypoxemia results. The most common presentation is in patients with interstitial lung disease (e.g., pulmonary fibrosis, asbestosis, sarcoidosis) in which the thickening and scarring of the interstitium undermine normal gas exchange. Emphysema, with its inherent alveolar destruction, also has subnormal transfer of O_2 and CO_2 between the alveolus and the capillary. The reduced ventilation in both diseases implies that $\dot{V}/\dot{Q}$ mismatch also plays a role in the resulting hypoxemia.

Pulmonary vascular abnormalities can also lead to diffusion impairment. Anemia, pulmonary hypertension, and pulmonary embolus all may reduce capillary blood flow resulting in diminished gas transfer.

Clinical Presentation of Diffusion Impairment

Diffusion impairment rarely presents as an acute hypoxemia in its classic form. Signs and symptoms are related to the specific disease. Interstitial lung disease may be the diagnosis of a dyspneic patient with a dry cough and fine, basilar crackles on auscultation. Patients may have clubbing of the nailbeds. Rheumatological manifestations may be present if the underlying cause is a connective tissue disorder. Joint abnormalities, Raynaud's disease, and telangiectasia (a vascular lesion formed by dilatation of a group of small blood vessels) may be observed. The pallor of anemia can be a clue to poor gas exchange, though chronic hypoxemia may lead to polycythemia and possibly cyanosis. Pulmonary hypertension may present with signs of right heart failure such as edema, jugular vein distension, and a louder pulmonary component of the second heart sound.

Diffusion impairment can also present with multiple, varied radiographic forms. The hyperinflated, dark radiograph of emphysema has been mentioned. Interstitial disease may present with a normal film or demonstrate reduced lung volumes with interstitial markings. Enlarged right ventricle and pulmonary arteries may be evident in pulmonary hypertension.

Perfusion/Diffusion Impairment

Perfusion/diffusion impairment is a rare cause of hypoxemia found in individuals with liver disease complicated by the hepatopulmonary syndrome.[8] In this condition, right-to-left intracardiac shunt combines with dilated pulmonary capillaries resulting in impaired gas exchange. Cirrhosis is the most common liver disease and portal hypertension is usually present. Though shunt is a component of the syndrome, significant supplemental oxygen can overcome the gas transfer reduction due to the dilated vessels, so this is commonly called a *perfusion/diffusion defect.*

Clinical Presentation of Perfusion/Diffusion Impairment

Obvious signs of liver disease (e.g., ascites, jaundice, and spider nevi) may or may not be present. Digital clubbing can be found in the hepatopulmonary syndrome. Platypnea, which is the sensation of dyspnea when moving to the upright position from the supine position, may be a patient complaint. An actual decrease in the measured oxygen level, orthodeoxia, may parallel this subjective sensation.

Decreased Inspired Oxygen

Also clinically uncommon, hypoxemia may develop when the inspired oxygen falls below body requirements. The most common situation is at high altitude where barometric pressure decreases, which results in a decrease in the partial pressure of inspired oxygen. While airlines account for this by pressurizing their cabins, travelers with chronic hypoxemia may still need supplemental oxygen.[9,10] Similarly, mountain climbers at times require oxygen masks. The hopefully rare cases of patient-oxygen disconnects and delivery of an incorrect gas source are also included in this category.

Interestingly, inspired oxygen less than 21% can actually be used therapeutically. A mixture of helium and oxygen (Heliox) may reduce the work of breathing in patients with severe asthma. The low density of the helium gas is the key factor. Infants with certain cyanotic congenital heart defects (e.g., hypoplastic left ventricle) may benefit from an FIO_2 below room air level. In the preoperative state, this will help to prevent pulmonary dilatation and the excessive pulmonary blood flow, which could flood the lungs.

Clinical Presentation of Decreased Inspired Oxygen

The signs and symptoms of hypoxemia may be present, with the cause clearly related to the patient environment such as the altitude.

Differentiating the Causes of Acute Hypoxemic Respiratory Failure

In focusing on the three main causes of hypoxemic respiratory failure (hypoventilation, ventilation/perfusion mismatch, and shunt), it is important to recognize the physiological basis of each. Hypoventilation differs from the other causes in presenting with a normal alveolar-to-arterial PO_2 (partial pressure of oxygen) difference $[P(A\text{-}a)O_2]$ indicating normal lung parenchyma. A clinical determination of this difference is made by subtracting the PaO_2 from the PAO_2 (partial pressure of alveolar oxygen) derived from the alveolar air equation:

$$PAO_2 = FIO_2\ (PB - PH_2O\ ) - PaCO_2\ /\ R$$

where PB is barometric pressure, PH_2O is water vapor tension, and R is the respiratory exchange ratio (0:8).

The $P(A\text{-}a)O_2$ ranges from 10 mm Hg in young patients to approximately 25 mm Hg in the elderly while breathing room air (see following Rule of Thumb.) In patients with hypoxemia due to hypoventilation, treatment can be focused on improving ventilation because the hypoxemia is purely a result of alveolar displacement of oxygen by elevated carbon dioxide.

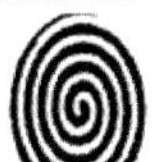

RULE OF THUMB

The mean alveolar-to-arterial difference [$P(A\text{-}a)O_2$] in PO_2 increases slightly with age and can be estimated by the following equation:

$$\text{Mean age-specific } P(A\text{-}a)O_2 = \text{age}/4 + 4$$

For example, a 76-year-old person living at sea level:

$$P(A\text{-}a)O_2 = 76/4 + 4 = 19 + 4 = 23 \text{ mm Hg}$$

A $\dot{V}/\dot{Q}$ mismatch and shunt both result in *elevated* $P(A\text{-}a)O_2$ levels, indicating that the resultant hypoxemia is due to an abnormality of lung tissue, requiring treatment to address that abnormality. When the respiratory therapist encounters an increased $P(A\text{-}a)O_2$, a $\dot{V}/\dot{Q}$ mismatch and shunt can then be differentiated by means of oxygen administration. A significant response to applying even small amounts of oxygen identifies $\dot{V}/\dot{Q}$ mismatch as the cause of hypoxemia because ventilation has not been totally obliterated. On the other hand, true shunt will show little or no improvement in oxygenation even with 100% FIO_2 (fractional inspired oxygen concentration). As a result, treatment of intrapulmonary shunt must be directed toward opening collapsed alveoli or clearing fluid or exudative material before oxygen can be beneficial at below toxic levels. Testing to rule out anatomical shunt should be done in the right clinical setting (e.g., clear or black parenchyma on the chest radiograph).

▶ ACUTE HYPERCAPNIC RESPIRATORY FAILURE (TYPE II)

Hypercapnic respiratory failure ("pump failure," "ventilatory failure") is characterized by an elevated $PaCO_2$, creating an uncompensated respiratory acidosis (whether

MINI CLINI

Differentiating Causes of Hypoxemia

PROBLEM

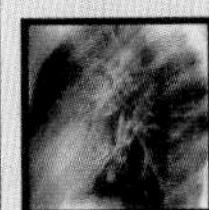

Two patients present with the following ABGs at sea level:

Patient A:		Patient B:	
pH	7.45	pH	7.21
$PaCO_2$	33 mm Hg	$PaCO_2$	72 mm Hg
PaO_2	40 mm Hg	PaO_2	53 mm HG
HCO_3^-	22 mEq/L	HCO_3^-	28 mEq/L
SaO_2	70%	SaO_2	81%
FIO_2	0.21	FIO_2	0.21

1. Define the respiratory condition indicated by each ABG.
2. What is the $P(A\text{-}a)O_2$ for each blood gas?
3. In which case would administration of 100% FIO_2 help determine therapy?

DISCUSSION

1. Patient A exhibits uncompensated respiratory alkalosis with hypoxemia.
   Patient B exhibits partially compensated respiratory acidosis with hypoxemia.
2. **Patient A:** $PAO_2 = 0.21\ (760\text{-}47)\text{-}33/.8 = 108$ mm Hg
   $PaO_2 = 40$ mm Hg
   $P(A\text{-}a)O_2 = 108\text{-}40 = 68$ mm Hg on room air
   Patient B: $PAO_2 = 0.21\ (760\text{-}47)\text{-}72/0.8 = 60$ mm Hg
   $PaO_2 = 53$ mm Hg
   $P(A\text{-}a)O_2 = 60\text{-}53 = 7$ mm Hg on room air
   The normals for $P(A\text{-}a)O_2$ range from 10 mm Hg in young people to approximately 25 mm Hg in the elderly while breathing room air.
3. Patient A is a case of hypoxemic respiratory failure (Type I) as characterized by the below normal PaO_2 (40 mm Hg). The $PaCO_2$ is also below normal (33 mm Hg) indicating hyperventilation is taking place in an effort to improve the oxygenation.
   Patient B is a case of hypercapnic respiratory failure (Type II) as characterized by the above normal $PaCO_2$ (72 mm Hg) indicating hypoventilation (ventilatory failure) is occurring. This is also known as acute ventilatory failure superimposed on chronic ventilatory failure. This patient is also hypoxemic (53 mm Hg). There is a slight elevation of the HCO_3^- (28 mEq/L) indicating an element of chronic respiratory failure may be present, which has now become acute.
4. Patient A has hypoxemic respiratory failure with a $P(A\text{-}a)O_2$ of 68 mm Hg, which is well above normal, indicating an oxygenation defect. The administration of 100% oxygen in this case would help to determine the cause of the defect. Significant response to the 100% FIO_2 would point to $\dot{V}/\dot{Q}$ mismatch as the cause, while shunt would be implicated if the PaO_2 did not respond to the increase in delivered O_2. In the latter, some form of PEEP would be necessary to improve gas exchange by improving FRC.
   Patient B has hypercapnic respiratory failure (ventilatory failure) with hypoxemia, but with a $P(A\text{-}a)O_2$ of 7 mm Hg, which is within the normal range. This indicates a pure ventilatory defect as the cause of the hypoxemia, and administration of 100 % FIO_2 would not help to determine therapy. Depending upon the full patient scenario, this patient may require intubation and mechanical ventilation to restore normal acid-base status.

acute or acute-on-chronic). In fact, $PaCO_2$ and alveolar ventilation ($\dot{V}_A$) are inversely related, meaning that alveolar and arterial $PaCO_2$ levels are doubled when alveolar ventilation is halved. This is illustrated by the relationship:

$$PaCO_2 = (0.863\ \dot{V}CO_2)/\dot{V}_A$$

where $\dot{V}_A$ is alveolar ventilation (L/min) and $\dot{V}CO_2$ is carbon dioxide production (mL/min).

Similarly, this demonstrates that $PaCO_2$ may rise as dead space (VD/VT) rises or as CO_2 production ($\dot{V}CO_2$) increases. Hypoxemia may often accompany pump failure due simply to the displacement of alveolar PO_2 (PAO_2) by the increased $PACO_2$. This situation is identified on a room air ABG by a normal $P(A\text{-}a)O_2$ as discussed above. This situation identifies the fifth cause of hypoxemic respiratory failure as mentioned above: alveolar hypoventilation. The presence of an increased $P(A\text{-}a)O_2$ indicates that concomitant hypoxemia is present, most likely as a result of $\dot{V}/\dot{Q}$ mismatch or shunt.

The three major disorders responsible for hypercapnic respiratory failure (ventilatory failure) will be discussed next.[2,6,10]

Decreased Ventilatory Drive

Inspiratory muscles are innervated by the phrenic and intercostal nerves via spinal cord transmission from the CNS. Both central (medullary) and peripheral (aortic and carotid bodies) chemoreceptors responding to CO_2 tension and O_2 tension stimulate the drive to breathe.[11] This ventilatory drive can be diminished by various factors such as drugs (overdose/sedation), brainstem lesions, hypothyroidism, morbid obesity (e.g., obesity-hypoventilation), and sleep apnea. Significantly, many causes of central depression are easily reversible with treatment, so the clinician should be attentive to reversible causes.

Clinical Presentation of Decreased Ventilatory Drive

The hallmark of this clinical scenario is, of course, bradypnea and perhaps ultimately apnea. A respiratory rate less than 12 breaths per minute is abnormal in adults. Drug overdose or a brain disorder can present with an altered level of consciousness ranging from merely lethargic to obtunded and even comatose, with decreased respirations. Evidence of drug use by history or toxicity screen confirms the diagnosis in the former. Evidence of head trauma or brain computed tomography (CT) abnormalities are important in the latter diagnosis. While hypothyroidism classically presents with fatigue, weight gain, hyporeflexia, and constipation, it can progress to significant hypoventilation and myxedema coma. The overweight, hypersomnolent male who may have a large tongue and crowded oropharynx can suffer with sleep apnea. Patients with obesity-hypoventilation may actually have a rapid, shallow breathing pattern due to the increased work of breathing, which results from decreased compliance and microatelectasis. While they may also have nighttime sleep apnea, their daytime $PaCO_2$ is also elevated.[12]

Respiratory Muscle Fatigue or Failure

The lung is basically a pump that inhales and exhales under the guidance of the CNS. In some patients, the CNS signal does not reach its goal, resulting in neuromuscular dysfunction. Lesions of the anterior horn cells may gradually lead to progressive ventilatory failure in amyotrophic lateral sclerosis (ALS). Peripheral nerve disorders may include Guillain-Barré syndrome and diaphragmatic dysfunction accompanying critical illness polyneuropathy. Abnormalities of neuromuscular transmission characterize myasthenia gravis. Finally, pure muscle disease itself (muscular dystrophy, acid maltase deficiency) can cause hypercapnia, as can respiratory muscle weakness related to connective tissue disorders (e.g., polymyositis).[13] These diseases range from irreversible and usually terminal (e.g., ALS) to reversible and usually self-limiting (e.g., Guillain-Barré syndrome) disease.[14]

Clinical Presentation of Respiratory Muscle Fatigue or Failure

While hypercapnia may be a common endpoint, these diseases have varied clinical presentations. Patient observation is a key skill. Drooling, dysarthria, and weak cough are common signs in ALS. As muscle wasting and weakness become more severe, diaphragmatic insufficiency develops and supine paradoxical breathing is common.[15] Guillain-Barré syndrome can commonly present with lower extremity weakness progressing to the respiratory muscles in one third of patients.[14] Weak cough and gag may be seen, which can threaten airway patency and lead to microatelectasis, hypoxemia, and uncompensated respiratory acidosis. While myasthenia gravis commonly presents with ocular muscle weakness, it also can exhibit bulbar weakness on its path to respiratory muscle fatigue. Myasthenia gravis does not always result in respiratory failure.[16] While these diseases are quite different in clinical course, there is much overlap in their presentations, and they commonly result in respiratory muscle fatigue and elevated $PaCO_2$.

Increased Work of Breathing

Despite normal respiratory drive, nerve transmission, and neuromuscular response, hypercapnic respiratory failure can still occur if the imposed workload cannot be overcome.[3,17,18] Most commonly, this situation occurs when increased deadspace accompanies COPD or elevated airway resistance accompanies asthma. Both of these obstructive airway diseases may raise respiratory work requirements excessively due to the presence of intrinsic positive end-expiratory pressure (PEEP). Increased workload can also result from thoracic abnormalities such as pneumothorax, rib fractures, pleural effusions, and other conditions creating a restrictive burden on the lungs. Finally, requirements for increased minute ventilation can arise when increased CO_2 production accompanies hypermetabolic states, such as in extensive burns.

Clinical Presentation of Increased Work of Breathing

The respiratory therapist must be alert to the possibility of respiratory failure when a heavy load is imposed on the respiratory system. Patients with asthma or COPD should present with hyperventilation in an exacerbation, but if breathing becomes more rapid but shallow it may indicate impending failure. This increased dead-space tidal volume leads to hypercapnia, as the significant airway obstruction does not resolve with treatment. Diminished breath sounds in a young patient with asthma can likewise be an ominous sign. Irritability, confusion, and ultimately coma are possible signs in worsening hypercapnia, as they are in hypoxemic respiratory failure. Subtler findings include muscle tremor due to catecholamine release and papilledema resulting from the cerebral vasodilatation in states of elevated arterial carbon dioxide.[19]

In summary, hypercapnic (Type II) respiratory failure, also known as *ventilatory failure,* develops when ventilation is impaired due to a decreased ventilatory drive, respiratory muscle fatigue, or increased work of breathing (Table 38-1).

▶ CHRONIC RESPIRATORY FAILURE: TYPE I AND TYPE II

For some pulmonary patients with respiratory failure, the condition has developed over weeks to months and has become a chronic state. This has allowed the body to develop compensatory mechanisms to adapt to the disease. Most commonly, chronic hypercapnic respiratory failure accompanying COPD or obesity hypoventilation syndrome would elicit a renal response by which the kidneys retain bicarbonate to elevate the blood pH. This compensatory metabolic alkalosis, however, would not be expected to restore the pH to normal. Chronic hypercapnic respiratory failure is also known as *chronic ventilatory failure.*

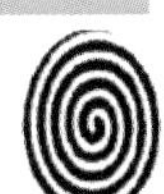

RULE OF THUMB

Chronic and acute hypercapnic respiratory failure can be differentiated by the severity of change in pH.[18]

Acute Hypercapnic Failure (Acute Ventilatory Failure):

pH drops 0.08 for every 10 mmHg rise in $PaCO_2$

Chronic Hypercapnic Failure (Chronic Ventilatory Failure):

pH drops 0.03 for every 10 mmHg rise in $PaCO_2$

Table 38-1 ▶▶ Causes of Respiratory Failure

	Type II (Hypercapnic)		
Type I (Hypoxemic)	**Decreased Ventilatory Drive**	**Increased Work of Breathing**	**Respiratory Muscle Fatigue**
ARDS	Drug overdose	COPD	Guillain-Barré Syndrome
Pulmonary embolism	Central sleep apnea	Asthma	ALS
Pulmonary edema	Brainstem lesions	Obesity	Myasthenia gravis
Septic shock	Hypothyroidism	Pneumothorax	Muscular dystrophy
Pulmonary infection	Metabolic alkalosis CVA	Severe burns	Acid-maltase deficiency
Viral	Primary alveolar hypoventilation	Kyphoscoliosis	Phrenic nerve injury
Bacterial	(Ondine's curse)	Upper airway obstruction	Botulism
Fungal	Infection (encephalitis)	Pleural effusion	Polymyositis
Inhalation		Airway Edema	SLE
Smoke		Infection	Spinal cord injury
Chemical		Ankylosing spondylitis	Muscular weakness
Water			Hypokalemia
Pleural effusion			Hypophosphatemia
Interstitial lung disease			Hypomagnesemia
Obstructive lung disease			Hypocalcemia
Aspiration			
Primary pulmonary hypertension			

Similarly, polycythemia may result from prolonged hypoxemic respiratory failure (e.g., sleep apnea) when oxygen delivery to the tissues is compromised and erythropoietin levels rise to elicit erythrocytosis. Hemoglobin also releases oxygen more easily as the oxygen dissociation curve shifts to the right in the face of acidosis. Finally, oxygen delivery to the brain is enhanced when hypercapnia results in increased cerebral blood flow.[19]

Acute-on-Chronic Respiratory Failure

Chronic respiratory failure can be complicated by acute setbacks that create acute-on-chronic respiratory failure. Patients with chronic hypercapnic respiratory failure (chronic ventilatory failure) are at significant risk for this, as indicated by the fact that COPD is now the fourth leading cause of death in the United States. Most common precipitating factors include bacterial or viral infections, congestive heart failure, pulmonary embolus, chest wall dysfunction, and medical noncompliance.[20,21] It is in these patients that the presence of respiratory failure cannot be judged by the normal blood gas criteria but by a significant change from the baseline $PaCO_2$ to a level having the potential for morbidity and mortality. Treatment goals include normalizing pH (avoiding mechanical ventilation if possible), elevating SaO_2 (arterial oxygen saturation) to 90% (if hypoxemia is also present), improving airflow, treating infection, monitoring and maintaining fluid status, and preventing or treating complications as necessary.[18,20,21] Optimally treated patients with acute-on-chronic respiratory failure have shown improving hospital mortality rates despite the overall stagnant rates for respiratory failure in general.[22,23] Higher death rates are associated with factors such as significant baseline disease, a severe precipitating illness, severity of acidosis, and presence of complications.[23] The use of advance directives regarding a patient's desire for mechanical ventilation will certainly influence short-term mortality. Episodes of acute respiratory failure in these patients seem to have significant long-term influence with mortality rates reaching 49% within 2 years of an acute exacerbation.[22]

Patients with chronic hypoxemic respiratory failure (Type I) are at similar risk for acute deterioration of their hypoxemia. Infection and heart failure can result in worsening of the tenuous oxygenation status of patients with interstitial pulmonary fibrosis or primary pulmonary hypertension.

MINI CLINI

Acute or Chronic Hypercapnic Respiratory Failure

PROBLEM

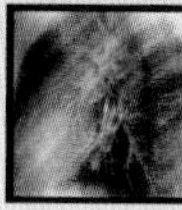

A 55-year-old male presents to the emergency department complaining of increased shortness of breath and yellow-green sputum production for one week. He is alert and oriented. He has a 60 pack-year smoking history.

Vital signs are: BP 165/90 P120/min R 25/min T 100.5° F oral.

ABG values on room air are:		
	pH	7.28
	$PaCO_2$	70 mm Hg
	PaO_2	35 mm Hg
	HCO_3^-	36 mm Hg
	SaO_2	66%

1. Define the respiratory condition indicated by the ABGs.
2. What is the $P(A\text{-}a)O_2$?
3. What type of respiratory failure is present?
4. What kind of therapy is indicated?

DISCUSSION

1. The ABG values indicate a partially compensated respiratory acidosis with hypoxemia:
2. $PAO_2 = 0.21\ (760\text{-}47) - 70/.8 = 62$ mm Hg
   $PaO_2 = 35$ mm Hg
   $P(A\text{-}a)O_2 = 62\text{-}35 = 27$ mm Hg on room air
3. This is hypercapnic respiratory failure (Type II), also known as ventilatory failure. However, according to Rule of Thumb 38-2, in acute failure the pH drops 0.08 for every 10 mm Hg rise in $PaCO_2$. In this patient, the $PaCO_2$ has risen 30 mm Hg (70-40) and the pH has dropped 0.12. The pH would be expected to drop 0.24 (3×0.08) if this were *acute* ventilatory failure. Therefore this is a case of acute-on-chronic failure. The HCO_3^- of 36 mEq/L (normal 22-26 mEq/L) also indicates some renal compensation is in place, which takes days to achieve. The $P(A\text{-}a)O_2$ is 27 mm Hg, which is above normal indicating that the hypoxemia cannot be explained fully by the hypoventilation.
4. Since the patient is alert, conservative therapy to improve lung function is indicated. Oxygen administration to achieve an SaO_2 of at least 90% is required. If the PaO_2 does not respond to oxygen administration, shunt is present and positive airway pressure may be necessary. Antibiotics are indicated for the probable infection (fever, discolored sputum) and bronchopulmonary hygiene (bronchodilators, steroids, chest PT) to improve ventilation.

Complications of Acute Respiratory Failure

Though acute respiratory failure is life-threatening by itself, frequently, complications arise which can add significantly to morbidity and mortality. In fact, especially in patients with ARDS, more deaths are due to complications (e.g., sepsis, multiorgan failure) than due to the primary disease.[24] The modern intensive care unit with sophisticated mechanical ventilation can prolong but may not necessarily preserve life. Pulmonary complications such as emboli, barotrauma, and infection may be secondary to treatment strategies such as catheters, mechanical ventilation, and endotracheal tubes. A wide array of nonpulmonary complications exists, ranging from cardiac disorders (arrhythmias, hypotension) to gastrointestinal ailments (hemorrhage, dysmotility) to renal disturbances (acute renal failure, positive fluid balance). Bacteremia, malnutrition, and even psychosis secondary to prolonged intensive care stays can also seriously complicate an episode of acute respiratory failure.[24]

▶ INDICATIONS FOR VENTILATORY SUPPORT

For each type of oxygenation and ventilatory failure, the goal of mechanical ventilation is to support the patient either until the underlying problem resolves or to maintain support of the patient with chronic ventilatory problems. These goals may be achieved by improving alveolar ventilation and arterial oxygenation, increasing lung volume, or reducing work of breathing.[25] This section will discuss the indications for mechanical ventilation for both hypoxemic (Type I) and hypercapnic (Type II) respiratory failure. Hypoxemic respiratory failure will be divided into processes that require short-term and long-term ventilatory support. Hypercapnic respiratory failure will be broken down into unstable ventilatory drive, muscle fatigue, excessive work of breathing, and alveolar hypoventilation. The relationship between work of breathing and the need for mechanical ventilation will be discussed. Numerical indicators of the need for ventilatory support will be reviewed. Management that is specific for each type of respiratory failure will be described, including the indications for less commonly used modes of ventilation. Finally, the specific management of the patient with obstructive lung disease and the patient with head injury will be discussed.

Parameters Indicating the Need for Ventilatory Support

Although various measurements have been proposed to help decide if a patient needs mechanical ventilation, the clinical status of the patient is clearly the most important criterion. Table 38-2 and the discussion that follows review common physiological indicators for initiating support by the underlying cause of respiratory failure. Specific indications for ventilator initiation are described in Chapter 41.

Hypoxemic Respiratory Failure

Severe, refractory hypoxemia represents a common indication for intubation and ventilator support. Table 38-2 lists different measures of hypoxemia that have been used to assess the need for ventilatory support. Most commonly, PaO_2 is compared with inspiratory oxygen fraction (FIO_2) as with PaO_2/ FIO_2 ratio or the alveolar-arterial oxygen difference [$P(A\text{-}a)O_2$]. Indicators of profoundly impaired oxygenation suggesting the need for intubation, high inspired oxygen administration, and PEEP include a $P(A\text{-}a)O_2$ value of 350 mm Hg on FIO_2 of 1.0 or a PaO_2/FIO_2 value <200. These values are useful for all causes of hypoxemic respiratory failure but cannot help distinguish if the process is a readily

Table 38-2 ▶▶ Physiological Indicators for Ventilatory Support, Classified by the Mechanism Underlying Respiratory Failure

Mechanism	Normal Values	Support Indicated
Inadequate alveolar ventilation		
$PaCO_2$ (torr)	35-45	> 55
pH	7.35-7.45	< 7.20
Inadequate lung expansion		
Tidal volume (V_T) mL/kg	5-8	< 5
Vital capacity (VC) mL/kg	65-75	< 10
Respiratory rate	12-20	> 35
Inadequate muscle strength		
Maximum inspiratory pressure (cm H_2O)	−80-100	≥ −20
Vital capacity (VC, mL/kg)	65-75	< 10
Maximum voluntary ventilation MVV (L/min)	120-180	< 2 x VE
Increased work of breathing		
Minute ventilation ($V_E\dot{V}$)	5-6	> 10
VD/VT (%)	0.25-0.40	> 0.6
Hypoxemia		
$P(A\text{-}a)O_2$ on 100% oxygen (torr)	25-65	> 350
PaO_2 /FIO_2	350-450	< 200

reversible one, such as pulmonary edema or atelectasis, or a process, such as acute lung injury, that will resolve more slowly. Frequently, patients have a combination of hypoxemic and hypercapnic respiratory failure at the same time.

Hypercapnic Respiratory Failure (Ventilatory Failure)

As previously discussed, hypercapnic (Type II) respiratory failure or ventilatory failure can be caused by increased ventilatory dead space, increased CO_2 production or decreased alveolar ventilation. All of these processes cause an increase in $PaCO_2$.[26] Assessment of the pH allows a determination of whether the problem is acute or chronic. Chronic hypoventilation is compensated for by the kidneys' retention of bicarbonate, though this response requires several days. The following example shows the importance of pH in interpreting the significance of an elevated $PaCO_2$.

	Patient A	Patient B
$PaCO_2$	60 mm Hg	60 mm Hg
Serum HCO_3^-	25 mEq/L	36 mEq/L
pH	7.25	7.38

Although both patients have the same level of hypercapnia, only Patient A exhibits acute ventilatory failure with an elevated $PaCO_2$ but normal serum bicarbonate (25 mEq/L). On the other hand, Patient B has a compensated respiratory acidosis from chronic hypercapnic respiratory failure, as indicated by the normal pH and elevated serum bicarbonate (36 mEq/L). This condition is also known as *chronic ventilatory failure.* The distinction between acute and chronic ventilatory failure is very important in respiratory care and emphasizes the need to use both $PaCO_2$ and pH as indicators for ventilatory support. The trend in pH and $PaCO_2$ values is also useful in assessing the effects of therapies in correcting acute ventilatory failure.

Significance of an Elevated $PaCO_2$

Because an elevated $PaCO_2$ increases ventilatory drive in healthy subjects, the very existence of hypoventilation suggests other problems with the respiratory apparatus. Specifically, the presence of acute respiratory acidosis indicates one of three major problems: (1) the respiratory center is not responding normally to the elevated $PaCO_2$, (2) the respiratory center is responding normally, but the signal is not getting through to the respiratory muscles, or (3) despite normal neurological response mechanisms, the lungs and chest bellows are simply incapable of providing adequate ventilation due to parenchymal lung disease or muscular weakness.[27]

► MECHANISMS OF HYPERCAPNIC RESPIRATORY FAILURE

Decreased Ventilatory Drive

Patients at risk of having a decreased ventilatory drive can usually be identified by their clinical situation (e.g., CNS insult, an overdose of sedative medications). As previously discussed, other less common potential causes include metabolic alkalosis, malnutrition, sleep deprivation, and hypothyroidism.[28] Patients with metabolic encephalopathy or elevated intracranial pressure may develop a reduced drive to breathe.

Respiratory Muscle Fatigue and Weakness

For effective ventilation to occur, the respiratory muscles must be capable of bearing the load put on them. Muscle fatigue is defined as a condition in which there is loss of the capacity to develop force and/or velocity of a muscle resulting from muscle activity under load, which is reversible by rest.[29] Fatigue can be caused both by specific demands placed on the muscle and reduced supply of necessary nutrients. The demand on a muscle is increased by increased work of breathing, increased strength of muscle contraction, and decreased muscle efficiency. Hypoxemia, decreased inspiratory muscle blood flow, poor nutrition, and a muscle's inability to extract energy from supplied substrates can lead to fatigue as well.[30]

There are three types of respiratory muscle fatigue: (1) central, which is an exertion-induced, reversible decrease in central respiratory drive; (2) transmission, which is an exertion-induced, reversible impairment in the transmission of neural impulses; and (3) contractile, which is a reversible impairment in the contractile response to a neural impulse in an overloaded muscle.[27] Respiratory muscle weakness, defined as the decreased capacity of a rested muscle to generate force and decreased endurance, can predispose to ventilatory muscle fatigue.[30] This most commonly occurs in patients with neuromuscular disease. Conditions that lead to muscle fatigue by increasing demand include COPD, kyphoscoliosis, and obesity.

Bedside Assessment of Respiratory Muscle Fatigue and Failure

The most commonly used tests to assess respiratory muscle strength at the bedside are maximum inspiratory pressure (MIP) and maximum expiratory pressure (MEP),[31] forced vital capacity, and maximum voluntary ventilation (MVV) (see Table 38-2). An MIP of ≤-30 cm H_2O usually indicates adequate respiratory muscle strength to initiate weaning from mechanical ventilation, but the overall trend needs to be considered. This is especially true in patients with myasthenic crisis or Guillain-Barré syndrome, where values of MIP that are becoming less negative may be the only clue to impending respiratory failure. The MVV maneuver can be performed at the bedside with a handheld spirometer, but its use in the critical care setting is limited because substantial patient cooperation is required. The sniff nasal inspiratory pressure may also be used to assess inspiratory muscle strength but experience with it is limited.[32] The tension-time index, defined as the product of contractile force (ratio of diaphragmatic pressure to maximum diaphragmatic pressure) and the contractile duration (ratio of inspiratory time to total breathing cycle time) is also useful in assessing muscle fatigue but is not routinely measured. Fatigue is likely to occur if the tension-time index exceeds 0.15.[30] Comparing the spontaneous minute ventilation with MVV is also helpful in predicting muscle fatigue. Fatigue is likely to occur if the minute ventilation exceeds 60 percent of MVV.[30]

Clinically, the patient with respiratory muscle fatigue shows an initially increased respiratory rate followed by bradypnea (slowed respiratory rate) and apnea as fatigue ensues. Respiratory alternans, which is a phasic alteration between rib cage and abdominal breathing, may also occur. Opinions vary on the sensitivity and specificity of abdominal motion paradox in patients with respiratory muscle weakness, but at least some investigators suggest that respiratory muscle paradox is an early sign (see Chapter 14). When ventilatory failure is full blown, ABGs will show hypercapnia with acidosis. As mentioned earlier, the presence of hypercapnia with acidosis can also indicate that the respiratory center is not responding properly.[26]

Increased Work of Breathing

Work of breathing is the amount of force needed to move a given volume into the lung with a relaxed chest wall. Excessive work of breathing is the most common cause of respiratory muscle fatigue. Work of breathing is due to physiological work and imposed work. Physiological work involves overcoming the elastic forces during inspiration and overcoming the resistance of the airways and lung tissue. Airway and pulmonary parenchymal abnormalities both can increase the physiological work of breathing. In intubated patients, sources of imposed work of breathing include the endotracheal tube, ventilator circuit, and auto-PEEP due to dynamic hyperinflation with airflow obstruction, as is commonly seen in the patient with COPD.[33]

Tachypnea is the cardinal sign of increased work of breathing. Tachypnea occurs when the respiratory center increases breathing frequency in an attempt to lessen respiratory excursion and therefore lessen the amount of work performed by the respiratory muscles.[33] Overall workload is reflected in the minute volume needed to maintain normocapnia.

Increased work of breathing can also be an impediment to weaning. Recently, measurement of work of breathing with an esophageal balloon catheter and a flow transducer has been used to determine work of breathing and break it down into physiological and imposed components.[34] Kirton et al showed that 96% of patients with a physiological work of breathing under 0.8 joules per liter were successfully weaned and extubated from ventilatory support.[35]

▶ CHOOSING A VENTILATORY SUPPORT STRATEGY FOR DIFFERENT CAUSES OF RESPIRATORY FAILURE

The remainder of this chapter briefly discusses current ventilatory strategies for both hypoxemic and hypercapnic respiratory failure (Table 38-3). The clinical application of specific modes of mechanical ventilation is described in Chapters 39 and 41. Once it has been determined that the patient needs ventilatory support, the initial decision is whether to intubate or to ventilate noninvasively. In the acute setting, this decision is sometimes

Table 38-3 ▶ ▶ Modes of Support for Individual Types of Respiratory Failure

Type of Failure	Recommended Therapy
Rapidly reversible hypoxemic respiratory failure (e.g., congestive heart failure)	Recommended Therapy CPAP
Slowly reversible hypoxemic respiratory failure (e.g., acute lung injury)	High inspired FIO_2 PEEP Inverse ratio ventilation Bi-level mask ventilation If elevated airway pressures, pressure controlled ventilation
Acute alveolar hypoventilation	Assist-control SIMV with high back-up rate Pressure support ventilation with high pressure
Chronic alveolar hypoventilation	Bi-level mask ventilation or assist-control via tracheostomy
Altered mental status	Assist-control SIMV with adequate back-up rate
Acute respiratory muscle fatigue	Bi-level or pressure support mask ventilation if invasive ventilation is required, Assist-control or SIMV with adequate back-up rate
Chronic	Nighttime bi-level mask ventilation or assist-control or SIMV via tracheostomy

based on how rapidly the underlying process can be reversed. Chronic hypercapnic respiratory failure also frequently requires decisions on how and when to ventilate a patient.

Ventilatory Support in Hypoxemic Respiratory Failure

The ventilatory management of the hypoxemic patient is usually determined by the cause of hypoxemia. The patient who has a readily reversible cause of hypoxemia, such as cardiogenic pulmonary edema, can often be managed noninvasively with supplemental oxygen and continuous positive airway pressure (CPAP) or bi-level positive airway pressure. [36]

CPAP is useful in the treatment of hypoxemia due to readily reversible causes. CPAP works by recruiting alveoli and maintaining their patency throughout the respiratory cycle. This causes a reduction in ventilation-perfusion mismatch and shunt.[37] CPAP is thought to decrease work of breathing and mildly improve cardiac function in patients with congestive heart failure.[38] Intermittent or continuous CPAP is frequently combined with bronchodilators and percussive therapy to treat lobar atelectasis.[39] Patients with accompanying hypercapnic respiratory failure can be treated with bi-level or mask ventilation.[40] However, patients with hypoxemia who are unable to protect their airway or handle secretions should be intubated and mechanically ventilated.

Patients with profound hypoxemia from a process that is expected to resolve slowly, such as acute lung injury, usually require intubation and mechanical ventilation, though recent literature has shown that noninvasive ventilation may be useful even in illnesses with a longer time to recovery.[41,42] These patients require a ventilatory strategy that will open alveoli and maintain their patency. High-inspired FIO_2 and PEEP have been the main forms of treatment for these patients. Profound hypoxemic respiratory failure is often due to severe pneumonia and ARDS. Patients with these conditions have very noncompliant lungs. Volume-cycled ventilation in patients with ARDS frequently leads to high peak airway and plateau pressures. It has clearly been established that ventilating these patients with small

MINI CLINI

Indications for CPAP versus CMV With PEEP

PROBLEM

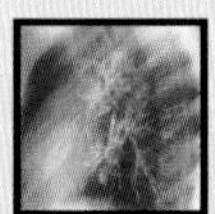

A patient in the intensive care unit is severely tachypneic and hypoxemic. The respiratory rate is 30/minute. On approximately 50% oxygen by mask at sea level, the patient's PaO_2 is 50 mm Hg, $PaCO_2$ is 30 mm Hg, pH is 7.51, and HCO_3^- is 23 mEq/L. The patient is in distress but alert and able to cooperate and follow instructions.

1. What is this person's $P(A\text{-}a)O_2$?
2. What type of respiratory failure is this?
3. What is the appropriate initial therapy?

DISCUSSION

First, the patient does not have hypercapnic respiratory failure as is confirmed by the $PaCO_2$ of 30 mm Hg. The patient does have a serious oxygenation defect, confirmed by the $P(A\text{-}a)O_2$.

$$PAO_2 = 0.50\ (713)\ 30/0.8 = 318 \text{ mm Hg}$$
$$P(A\text{-}a)O_2 = 318 - 50 = 268 \text{ mm Hg}$$

The high $P(A\text{-}a)O_2$ indicates the presence of severe intrapulmonary shunt. Shunts this severe can only occur when significant airway closure and atelectasis are present. The mode of therapy should be aimed at reinflating collapsed alveoli and keeping them open throughout the breathing cycle. In this patient, alveolar ventilation is obviously not impaired ($PaCO_2$ = 30 mm Hg). Therefore, CPAP alone may be effective in reducing shunt. (CPAP does not ventilate the patient; all breaths are patient-initiated and spontaneous.) CPAP may be applied noninvasively by mask, as would be indicated in this alert, cooperative patient. If hypercapnia and acidemia develop, then mechanical ventilation with PEEP would be indicated.

MINI CLINI

Acute Hypercapnic Respiratory Failure

PROBLEM

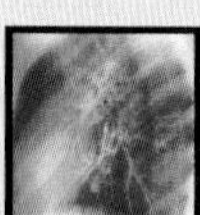

A patient with COPD presents to the emergency department in moderate respiratory distress. He is alert and cooperative. Respiratory rate is 26 breaths/minute. Lung examination shows poor air entry with expiratory wheezing. A room air ABG shows pH of 7.24, $PaCO_2$ of 60 mm Hg, and PaO_2 of 60 mm Hg.

1. What type of respiratory failure is this?
2. How should the patient be managed?

DISCUSSION

The ABG shows an acute respiratory acidosis with a normal PAO_2 - PaO_2 gradient.

$$PAO_2 = 0.21(700) - 60/0.8 = 72$$
$$P(A\text{-}a)O_2 = 72 - 60 = 12 \text{ torr}$$

This patient has hypercapnic respiratory failure related to obstructive lung disease, also known as ventilatory failure. In addition to bronchodilators and corticosteroids, the respiratory therapist should aim to improve ventilation to reverse the respiratory acidosis. In this patient who is alert and cooperative, noninvasive positive pressure ventilation via face mask may be tried. Initial mask ventilation can start in the PSV mode with a level of support of 10 cm H_2O and no PEEP. Efforts should be made to maintain a tidal volume of approximately 7 mL/kg. If this patient deteriorates in spite of therapy, he would need to be intubated and mechanically ventilated.

tidal volumes (6 mL/kg) reduces complications associated with mechanical ventilation and improves survival.[43] Pressure control ventilation (PCV) is a useful mode of ventilation in patients with noncompliant lungs because it limits airway pressures, which reduces the risk of overdistension, called *volutrauma*. Other newer modes and strategies that have been applied to patients with profound hypoxemic respiratory failure include inverse ratio ventilation (IRV), liquid ventilation, prone positioning, and high frequency ventilation. Both PCV and IRV are usually reserved for profound hypoxemia, which is not responding to conventional modes of ventilation.[44]

Ventilatory Support in Hypercapnic Respiratory Failure (Ventilatory Failure)

The goal for patients with hypercapnic respiratory failure is to support ventilation, though the type and duration of therapy in hypercapnic failure depends on the underlying disease. Invasive and noninvasive forms of ventilation are useful in both acute and chronic forms of hypercapnic respiratory failure. This section will discuss the management of hypercapnic respiratory failure due to alveolar hypoventilation and muscle fatigue. The special circumstance of obstructive lung disease is discussed later in this chapter.

Ventilatory Support for Acute Ventilatory Failure

Volume-cycled assist-control ventilation is most commonly used in patients with acute ventilatory failure in order to guarantee minimum minute ventilation. Synchronous intermittent mandatory ventilation (SIMV) with a high backup rate and pressure support ventilation (PSV) with adequate preset pressure can also be used. In treating patients with chronic ventilatory failure, the goal is to normalize the pH but not necessarily the $PaCO_2$. Correction of the $PaCO_2$ in a patient with chronic hypoventilation will lead to respiratory alkalosis, which can produce unwanted side effects such as seizures and arrhythmias.

Ventilatory Support for Respiratory Muscle Fatigue and Weakness

Respiratory muscle fatigue can develop because of imposed forces as well as intrinsic causes, such as muscle weakness. As in hypoxemic respiratory failure, the underlying and exacerbating cause of muscle fatigue determines the therapy. Patients with acute hypercapnic respiratory failure from respiratory muscle fatigue can often be managed with bi-level or PSV via a face mask. Increasing levels of pressure support progressively unload the respiratory muscles and can be useful in cases when respiratory muscle fatigue is due to a reversible cause. Acute exacerbations of COPD represent one such example. Patients who require intubation for respiratory muscle fatigue generally need 24 to 48 hours of full ventilatory support before attempting to wean from the ventilator. Patients with ventilatory failure from neuromuscular disease are often more comfortable with higher tidal volumes, which help lung expansion.

Long-term support of respiratory muscles is commonly required in the management of neuromuscular diseases, such as ALS, and restrictive lung diseases, such as kyphoscoliosis. Such ventilatory support can be noninvasive or invasive via tracheostomy and can lead to improvement in daytime functioning and improvement of daytime ABGs.

▶ SPECIAL CONSIDERATIONS DURING VENTILATORY SUPPORT

Increased Intracranial Pressure

Hyperventilation may be used to reduce intracranial pressure (ICP). The goal is to lower the $PaCO_2$ to between 25 to 30 mm Hg, which causes alkalosis and combines with hypocapnia to reduce cerebral blood flow. Although reducing blood flow can reduce brain swelling and ICP, cerebral ischemia can also result. Another concern in ventilating patients with elevated ICPs is using PEEP to manage hypoxemia. There is a concern that increased intrathoracic pressure due to PEEP will cause decreased cerebral venous return leading to increased ICP and that PEEP can decrease cerebral perfusion by limiting cardiac output. The use of PEEP in patients with elevated ICP may require invasive monitoring of ICP because the combination of decreased cerebral perfusion and elevated ICP can narrow cerebral perfusion pressure.[45]

Obstructive Lung Disease

Patients with obstructive lung disease have markedly increased airway resistance that leads to a decrease in the rate of expiratory flow with resulting hyperinflation. These patients frequently have problems with elevated airway pressure or dynamic hyperinflation (auto-PEEP), which can cause the complication of volutrauma, defined as damage to the lungs caused by overdistension.[46] In addition to causing volutrauma, auto-PEEP can lower cardiac output by increasing intrathoracic pressure and decreasing venous return to the heart. For this reason, lower tidal volumes and ventilator rates are recommended in patients with COPD.

The management goal for patients with COPD with respiratory failure is to successfully oxygenate and ventilate the patient while avoiding volutrauma. There is growing evidence that in the appropriately selected patient, noninvasive positive pressure ventilation (NIPPV) can be used to avoid intubation in patients with COPD[47] and status asthmaticus.[48] Although there are no definitive guidelines as to which patients are best suited for NIPPV, patients should have a normal mental status, the ability to clear tracheal secretions, and they should be hemodynamically stable.

In patients who require intubation and mechanical ventilation due to obstructive lung disease, it is important to minimize dynamic hyperinflation. MacIntyre et al[49] showed that the progressive application of extrinsic PEEP caused a progressive decline in auto-PEEP. Such auto-PEEP can pose an inspiratory threshold that can frustrate weaning by requiring that the patient perform inspiratory work that does not move air. In such patients, lower tidal volumes (8 to 10 mL/kg) and high inspiratory flow rate (60 to 100 L/min) are recommended to avoid volutrauma.[50] Both of these maneuvers minimize inspiratory times, which allows the patient with obstructive lung disease to have a longer time to exhale.

KEY POINTS

- Acute respiratory failure is identified by a PaO_2 <60 mm Hg and/or a $PaCO_2$ >50 mm Hg in otherwise healthy individuals at sea level.
- Hypoxemic respiratory failure is most commonly due to ventilation/perfusion mismatch, shunt, or hypoventilation.
- Hypercapnic respiratory failure, also known as ventilatory failure, results from either decreased ventilatory drive, respiratory muscle fatigue, or increased work of breathing.
- Chronic respiratory failure may present with hypercapnia and evidence of a compensatory metabolic alkalosis (chronic ventilatory failure) or with polycythemia reflecting chronic hypoxemia.
- The clinical status of the patient is the most important factor determining the need for ventilatory support.
- Excessive work of breathing is the most common cause of respiratory muscle fatigue.
- Only patients with a rapidly reversible condition should undergo noninvasive ventilation in the acute setting.
- Increased FIO_2 and PEEP are the main therapies for severe hypoxemia.

KEY POINTS—cont'd

- The goal of therapy in hypercapnic respiratory failure (acute ventilatory failure) is to guarantee a set minute ventilation.
- Fatigued respiratory muscles should be rested for 24 to 48 hours.

References

1. Vasileyev S, Schaap RN, and Mortenson JD: Hospital survival rates of patients with acute respiratory failure in modern respiratory intensive care units. Chest 107: 1083, 1995.
2. Behrendt CE: Acute respiratory failure in the United States: incidence and 31-day survival, Chest 118:1100, 1999.
3. Greene KE, Peters JI: Pathophysiology of acute respiratory failure, Clin Chest Med 15:1,1994.
4. Campbell EJM: Respiratory failure, Br Med Bull 1:1451, 1965.
5. West JB: Respiratory physiology: the essentials, Baltimore, 1990, Williams and Wilkins.
6. Pierson DJ: Normal and abnormal oxygenation: physiology and clinical syndromes, Respir Care Clin N Am 38:587, 1993.
7. George RB et al: Chest medicine, essentials of pulmonary and critical care medicine, ed 3, Baltimore, 1995, Williams and Wilkins.
8. Lange PA, Stoller JK: The hepatopulmonary syndrome, Ann Intern Med 122: 521, 1995.
9. Stoller JK: Travel for the technology-dependent individual, Respir Care Clin N Am 39:347, 1994.
10. Gong H: Air travel and oxygen therapy in cardio-pulmonary patients, Chest 101:1104, 1992.
11. Johnson DC, Kazemi H: Central control of ventilation in neuromuscular disease, Clin Chest Med 15:607, 1994.
12. Epstein SK, Singh N: Respiratory acidosis, Respir Care Clin N Am 46:366, 2001.
13. Mier A: Respiratory muscle weakness, Respir Med 84:351, 1990.
14. Teitelbaum JS, Borel CO: Respiratory function in Guillain-Barré syndrome, Clin Chest Med 15:705, 1994.
15. Kaplan LM, Hollander D: Respiratory dysfunction in amyotrophic lateral sclerosis, Clin Chest Med 15:675, 1994.
16. Zulueta JJ, Fanburg BL. Respiratory dysfunction in myasthenia gravis, Clin Chest Med 15:683, 1994.
17. Schmidt GA et al: Ventilatory failure. In Murray JF and Nadel JA, editors: Respiratory Medicine, ed 2, Philadelphia, 1994, WB Saunders.
18. Curtis JRC, Hudson LD: Emergent assessment and management of acute respiratory failure in COPD, Clin Chest Med 15:481, 1994.
19. Jozefowicz RF: Neurologic manifestations of pulmonary disease, Neurol Clin 7:605, 1989.

20. Derenne JP, Fleury B, Pariente R: Acute respiratory failure of chronic obstructive pulmonary disease, Am Rev Respir Dis 138:1006, 1988.
21. Schmidt GA, Hall JB: Acute on chronic respiratory failure, JAMA 261:3444, 1989.
22. Connors AF et al: Outcomes following acute exacerbation of severe chronic obstructive lung disease: the SUPPORT investigators (Study to Understand Prognoses and Preferences for Outcomes and Risks of Treatments), Am J Respir Crit Care Med 154:959, 1996.
23. Hudson LD: Survival data in patients with acute and chronic lung disease requiring mechanical ventilation, Am Rev Respir Dis 140:S19, 1989.
24. Pingleton SK: Complications of acute respiratory failure, Am Rev Respir Dis 137:1463, 1988.
25. Slutsky A: Consensus conference on mechanical ventilation, Intensive Care Med 20:64, 1994.
26. Roussos C: Respiratory muscle fatigue and ventilatory failure, Chest 97:895, 1990.
27. Mador MJ: Respiratory muscle fatigue and breathing pattern, Chest 100:1430, 1991.
28. Dick CR, Sassoon SH: Patient-ventilator interaction, Clin Chest Med 17:423, 1996.
29. Anonymous: NHLBI workshop summary: respiratory muscle fatigue, report of the respiratory muscle fatigue workshop, Am Rev Respir Dis 142:474, 1992.
30. Stoller JK: Physiologic rationale for resting the ventilatory muscles, Resp Care Clin N Am 36:290, 1991.
31. Gibson GJ: Measurement of respiratory muscle strength, Respir Med 89:529, 1995.
32. Heritier F et al: Sniff nasal inspiratory pressure, Am J Respir Crit Care Med 150:1678, 1994.
33. Banner MJ: Respiratory muscle loading and the work of breathing, J Card Vasc Anes 9:192, 1995.
34. Petros AJ, Lemond CT, Bennett D: The Bicore pulmonary monitor, Anaesthesia 48:985, 1993.
35. Kirton OC et al: Elevated work of breathing masquerading as ventilator weaning intolerance, Chest 108:1021, 1995.
36. Bach JR et al: Non-invasive positive pressure ventilation consensus statement, Respir Care Clin N Am 42:364, 1997.
37. Abou-Shala N, Meduri GU: Noninvasive mechanical ventilation in patients with acute respiratory failure, Crit Care Med 24:705, 1996.
38. Lenique F et al: Ventilatory and hemodynamic effects of continuous positive airway pressure in left heart failure, Am J Resp Crit Care Med 155:500, 1997.
39. Meduri GU: Non-invasive positive pressure ventilation in patients with acute respiratory failure, Clin Chest Med 17:513, 1996.
40. Meduri GU et al: Non-invasive positive pressure ventilation via face mask. First line intervention in patients with acute hypercapnic and hypoxemia respiratory failure, Chest 109:179, 1996.
41. Hilbert G et al: Noninvasive ventilation in immunosuppressed patients with pulmonary infiltrates, fever and acute respiratory failure, N Engl J Med 344:481, 2001.
42. Confalonieri M et al: Acute respiratory failure in patients with severe community-acquired pneumonia, Am J Respir Crit Care Med 160:1585, 1999.
43. The Acute Respiratory Distress Syndrome Network: Ventilation with lower tidal volumes as compared with traditional tidal volumes for acute lung injury and the acute respiratory distress syndrome, N Engl J Med 342:1301, 2000.
44. MacIntyre N: New modes of mechanical ventilation, Clin Chest Med 17:411, 1996.
45. Borel C: Intensive management of severe head injury, Chest 98:180, 1990.
46. Leatherman J: Mechanical ventilation in obstructive lung disease, Clin Chest Med 17:577, 1996.
47. Brochard L et al: Noninvasive ventilation for acute obstructive pulmonary disease, N Engl J Med 333:817, 1995.
48. Meduri GU: Noninvasive positive pressure ventilation in status asthmaticus, Chest 110: 767, 1996.
49. MacIntyre NR, Cheng KCG, McConnell R: Applied PEEP during pressure support reduces the inspiratory threshold of intrinsic PEEP, Chest 111:188, 1997.
50. Corbridge TC, Hall JB: The assessment and management of status asthmaticus, Am J Resp Crit Care Med 151:1296, 1995.

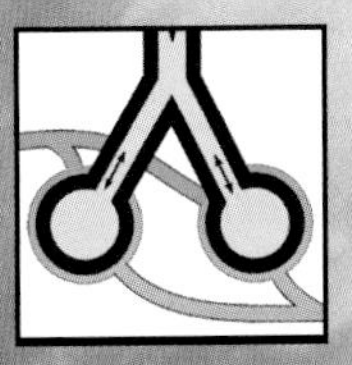

CHAPTER 39

Mechanical Ventilators

Robert L. Chatburn and Teresa A. Volsko

In This Chapter You Will Learn:

- The basic design features of ventilators
- How to classify ventilators and how they work
- What constitutes a mode of ventilation
- How to classify and understand modes of ventilation
- When to use the basic modes of ventilatory support
- How selected modes of ventilatory support are applied

Chapter Outline

Key Terms

breath sequence
breathing pattern
closed loop control
compliance
conditional variable
continuous mandatory ventilation (CMV)
continuous positive airway pressure (CPAP)
continuous spontaneous ventilation (CSV)
control variable
cycle variable
dual controlled ventilation
elastance
elastic load
intermittent mandatory ventilation (IMV)
limit variable
mandatory breath
open loop control
phase variable
positive end expiratory pressure (PEEP)
pressure-controlled ventilation
resistance
resistive load
spontaneous breath
time constant
trigger variable
volume-controlled ventilation

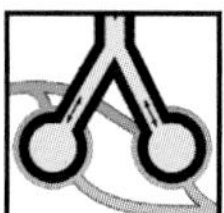

To safely and effectively initiate and manage a mechanical ventilator, the respiratory therapist must thoroughly understand (1) ventilator design, classification, and operation; (2) appropriate clinical application of ventilatory modes (i.e., the proper matching of ventilator capability with physiological need); and (3) the physiological effects of mechanical ventilation, including gas exchange and pulmonary mechanics. This chapter focuses on the first and second of these. It will explain classification terminology and outline a framework for understanding current and future ventilatory support devices.[1-3] The application of ventilators will be dealt with by outlining the specific indications and clinical use of the various modes of full and partial ventilatory support.

▶ HOW VENTILATORS WORK

To understand how ventilators work, one must have some knowledge of basic mechanics. We begin by recognizing that a ventilator is simply a machine. A machine is a system designed to alter, transmit, and direct applied energy in a predetermined manner to perform useful work.[4] Ventilators are provided with energy in the form of either electricity or compressed gas. That energy is transmitted or transformed (by the ventilator's drive mechanism) in a predetermined manner (by the control circuit) to augment or replace the patient's muscles in performing the work of breathing (the desired output). Thus, to understand mechanical ventilators we must first understand their four basic functions:

- Input power
- Power transmission and conversion
- Control system
- Output (pressure, volume, and flow waveforms)

This simple outline format can be expanded to add as much detail about a given ventilator as desired, as shown in Box 39-1.

Box 39-1 • Ventilator Classification System Outline

I. Input power
  A. Electric
  B. Pneumatic
  C. Manual
II. Power conversion and transmission
  A. Drive mechanism
  B. Output control valves
III. Control system
  A. Control variables
    1. Pressure
    2. Volume
    3. Flow
    4. Time
  B. Phase variables
    1. Trigger
    2. Limit
    3. Cycle
    4. Baseline
  C. Conditional variables
  D. Modes of ventilation
    1. Breathing pattern
    2. Control type
    3. Specific control strategy
IV. Output
  A. Control variable waveforms
    1. Pressure
    2. Volume
    3. Flow
  B. Displays
V. Alarms
  A. Input power
  B. Control circuit
  C. Output

Input Power

The power source for a ventilator is either electrical energy (Energy = Volts × Amperes × Time) or compressed gas (Energy = Pressure × Volume).[5]

Electric

An electrically powered ventilator uses voltage from an electrical line outlet. In the United States, this line voltage is normally 110 to 115 volts AC (60 Hz). In addition to powering the ventilator, this AC voltage may be reduced and converted to direct current (DC). This DC source can then be used to power delicate electronic control circuits. Some ventilators, notably infant and transport ventilators, have rechargeable batteries to be used as a back-up source of power if AC current is not available. In the homecare setting, battery backup for electrically powered ventilators is an essential life-saving feature in the event of a power outage.

Pneumatic

A pneumatically powered ventilator uses compressed gas as its power source. Most modern intensive care unit (ICU) ventilators are pneumatically powered. Ventilators powered by compressed gas usually have internal pressure reducing valves so that the normal operating pressure is lower than the source pressure. This allows uninterrupted operation from hospital piped gas sources, which are usually regulated to 50 psi (pounds per square inch) but are subject to periodic fluctuations.

Most pneumatically powered ICU ventilators still require electrical power to support their control functions (see the following section on control mechanisms). However, a few pneumatically powered ventilators can function without electrical power. These devices are ideal in situations where electrical power is unavailable (e.g., during certain types of patient transport) or as a backup to electrically powered ventilators in case of power failures. They are also particularly useful where electrical power is undesirable, as near magnetic resonance imaging (MRI) equipment.

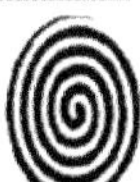

RULE OF THUMB

For patient transport you must use either a pneumatically powered ventilator or one that can run solely on batteries. Always take along a manually powered bag-valve-mask and for long transports be sure to have back-up power available (extra cylinders or batteries).

Power Transmission and Conversion

The power transmission and conversion system consists of the drive and output control mechanisms. The drive mechanism generates the actual force needed to deliver gas under pressure. The output control consists of one or more valves that regulate gas flow to the patient.

Drive Mechanism

The ventilator's drive mechanism converts the input power to useful work. The characteristic flow and pressure patterns the ventilator produces is determined, in part, by the type of drive mechanism it contains. Drive mechanisms can be either: (1) a direct application of compressed gas via a pressure reducing valve or (2) an indirect application via an electric motor or compressor. This chapter will forgo further elaboration on drive mechanisms. Descriptions of these devices can be found in textbooks devoted to respiratory care equipment.[6]

Output Control Valve

The output control valve regulates the flow of gas to the patient. It may be a simple on/off exhalation valve, as in the Newport E100i. Alternatively, the output control valve can shape the output waveform, as in the Siemens Servo 300. Commonly used output control valves include the pneumatic diaphragm, electromagnetic poppet/plunger valve, and the proportional valve. Descriptions of these devices can be found in respiratory care equipment textbooks.[6]

Control System

Knowledge of the mechanics of breathing provides a good foundation for understanding how ventilators work. Specifically, we are interested in the pressure needed to drive gas into the airway and inflate the lungs. The formula that relates these variables is known as *the equation of motion for the respiratory system*[7] (Figure 39-1):

$$\text{Muscle Pressure} + \text{Ventilator Pressure} = (\text{Elastance} \times \text{Volume}) + (\text{Resistance} \times \text{Flow}) \qquad \textit{Equation 39-1, A}$$

$$\text{Muscle Pressure} + \text{Ventilator Pressure} = \text{Elastic Load} + \text{Resistive Load} \qquad \textit{Equation 39-1, B}$$

Muscle pressure is equivalent to the pressure difference generated by the muscles during inspiration. Ventilator pressure is equivalent to the airway pressure generated by the ventilator during inspiration. The combined muscle and ventilator pressures cause gas to flow into the lungs. Elastance (elastance = pressure/volume) and resistance (resistance = pressure/flow) together constitute the impedance or load against which the muscles and ventilator do work. The equation of motion is sometimes expressed in terms of compliance (compliance = volume/pressure) instead of elastance.

Pressure, volume, and flow are all changeable variables measured relative to their baseline or end-expiratory values. When pressure, volume, and flow are plotted as functions of time, characteristic waveforms for volume-controlled ventilation and pressure-controlled ventilation are produced (Figure 39-2). The conventional order of presentation is pressure, volume, and flow, respectively, from top to bottom. Convention also dictates that positive flow values (above the horizontal axis) correspond to inspiration, and negative flow values (below the horizontal axis) correspond to expiration. The vertical axes are in units of the measured variables (usually cm H_2O for pressure, L or mL for volume, and L/minute or L/second for flow). The horizontal axis of these graphs is time. Many ventilators have monitors that display pressure, volume, and flow waveforms providing the clinician with information to evaluate ventilator-patient interaction.

In Figure 39-2 you will note that the expiratory lung pressure curves are the same shape for both volume and pressure control. This shape is called an *exponential decay waveform* (often mistakenly called a "decelerating" waveform[3]), and it is characteristic of passive emptying of the lungs (exhalation). If the equation of motion is solved for lung pressure we get the expression:

$$\textit{lung pressure during passive exhalation} = \frac{\textit{tidal volume}}{\textit{compliance}} e^{-t/RC} \qquad \textit{Equation 39-2}$$

where e is the base of the natural logarithms (approximately 2.72), t is time (in this case the time allowed for

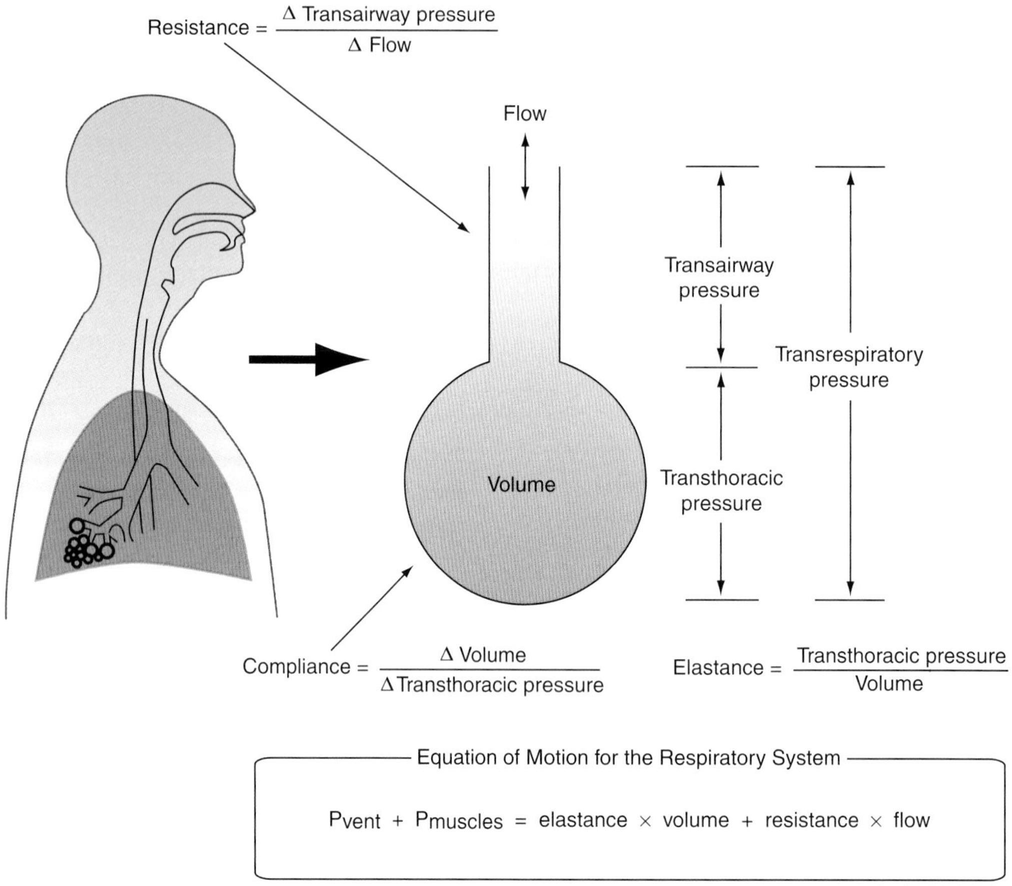

Figure 39-1

The respiratory system can be modeled as a single-flow conducting tube connected to a single elastic compartment. This physical model can be described by a mathematical model called the equation of motion for the respiratory system. In this model, pressure, volume, and flow are variables (i.e., functions of time) whereas resistance and elastance (or compliance) are constants.

exhalation), R is respiratory system resistance and C is respiratory system compliance. The product of R and C has units of time and is called the *time constant.* It is referred to as a "constant" because for any value of R and C, the time constant always equals the time necessary for the lungs to empty by 63%. In other words, when the expiratory time is equal to the time constant, the patient will have passively exhaled 63% of his or her tidal volume. We can demonstrate this using Equation 39-2 by setting t equal to RC:

$$\textit{lung pressure} = \frac{\textit{tidal volume}}{\textit{compliance}}\, e^{-RC/RC}$$

$$= \frac{\textit{tidal volume}}{\textit{compliance}}\, 2.72^{-1} = \frac{\textit{tidal volume}}{\textit{compliance}}\, 0.37$$

Equation 39-3

This expression shows that after an expiratory time equal to one time constant, only 37% of the lung pressure is left. Because volume is equal to pressure times compliance, we can multiply both sides of Equation 39-3 by compliance and see that only 37% of the tidal volume remains in the lungs. This implies that 63% of the tidal volume has been exhaled. After two time constants (i.e., $t = 2RC$), exhalation will be 86% completed and after three time constants, exhalation is 95% complete. After five time constants, exhalation is considered to be 100% complete for all practical purposes (Figure 39-3).

A similar expression can be derived for passive inhalation:

$$\textit{lung pressure during passive inhalation} = \frac{\textit{tidal volume}}{\textit{compliance}}\,(1 - e^{-t/RC})$$

Equation 39-4

When this equation is graphed, it looks like the curved line showing lung pressure and volume during inhalation for pressure-controlled ventilation in Figure 39-2. These same equations govern the passive flow curves for volume- and pressure-controlled ventilation. It is important to understand the concept of time constants in order to make appropriate ventilator setting adjustments. For example, in any mode of ventilation, the expiratory time should be at least three time constants long to avoid clinically important gas trapping. Similarly, in pressure controlled modes, inspiratory time should be

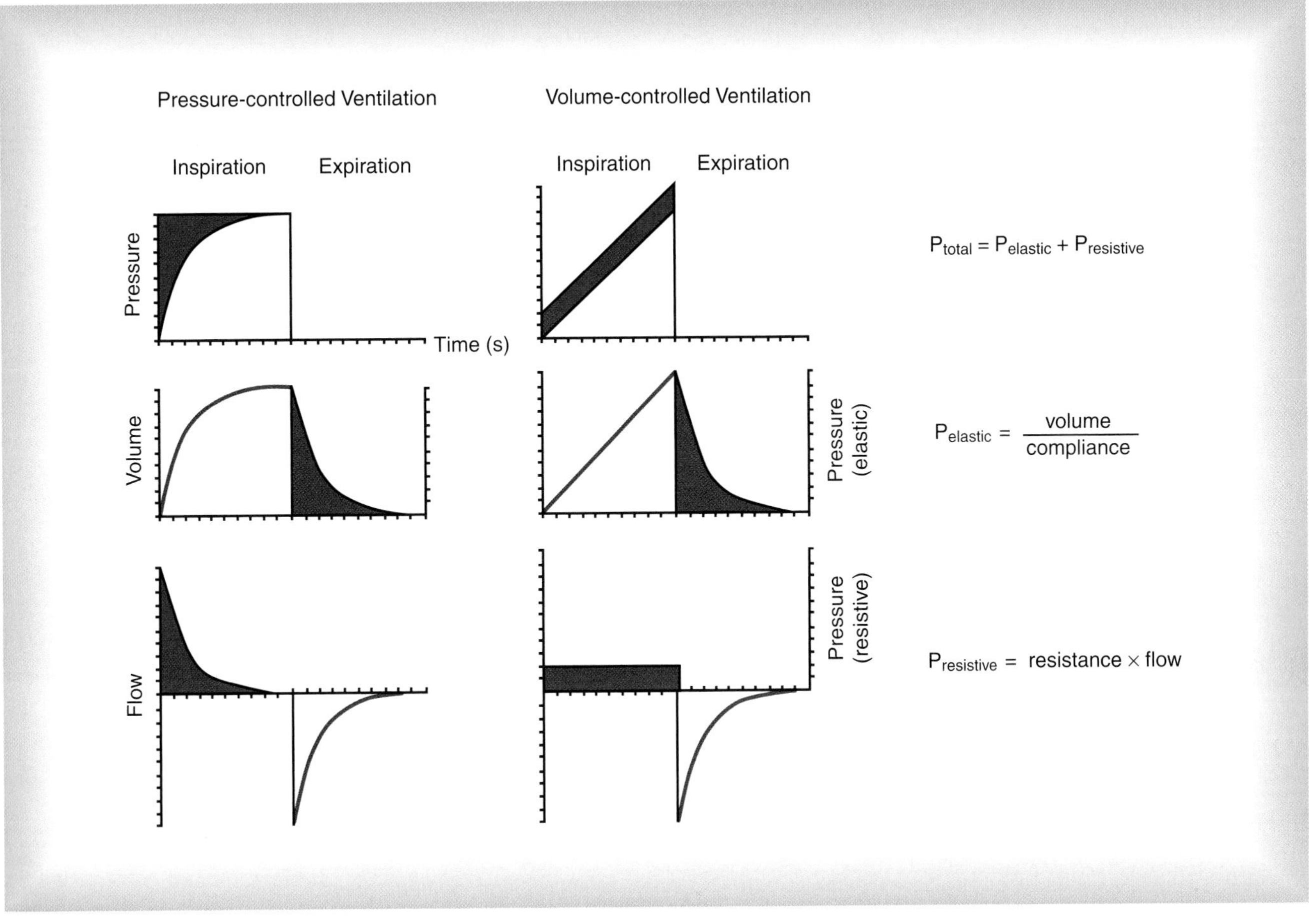

Figure 39-2

Characteristic waveforms for volume-controlled ventilation and pressure-controlled ventilation. Note that the volume waveform has the same shape as the transthoracic or lung pressure waveform (i.e., pressure due to elastic recoil). The flow waveform has the same shape as the transairway pressure waveform (i.e., pressure due to airway resistance). The shaded areas represent pressures due to resistance; the open areas represent pressure due to elastic recoil. The dotted lines represent mean airway pressure. Note that the mean pressure at the airway is the same as that in the lung and that mean pressure for volume-controlled ventilation is less than that for pressure-controlled ventilation.

at least five time constants long to get the maximum tidal volume from the set pressure gradient (i.e., peak inspiratory pressure [PIP] – end expiratory pressure).

Control Circuit

To manipulate pressure, volume, and flow, a ventilator must have a control circuit. A control circuit is a system of components that measures and directs the output of the ventilator to replace or assist the patient's breathing efforts. A ventilator control circuit may include mechanical, pneumatic, electric, electronic, or fluidic components. Most modern ventilators combine two or more of these subsystems to provide user control.

Mechanical control circuits use devices such as levers, pulleys, and cams. These types of circuits were used in the early manually operated ventilators illustrated in history books.[8] Pneumatic control is provided using gas-powered pressure regulators, needle valves, jet entrainment devices, and balloon-valves. Some transport ventilators use pneumatic control systems. The Ohmeda Logic-07 is an example.

Electric control circuits use only simple switches, rheostats (or potentiometers), and magnets to control ventilator operation. Electronic control circuits use devices such as resistors, capacitors, diodes, and transistors as well as combinations of these components in the form of integrated circuits. The most sophisticated electronic systems use preprogrammed microprocessors to control ventilator function.

Fluidic logic-controlled ventilators, such as the Bio-Med MVP-10 and Sechrist IV-100B, also use pressurized gas to regulate the parameters of ventilation. However, instead of simple pressurized valves and timers, these ventilators use fluidic logic circuits that function much like electrical circuit boards.[9] Fluidic control mechanisms have no moving parts. In addition, fluidic circuits are immune to failure from surrounding electromagnetic interference, as can occur around MRI equipment.

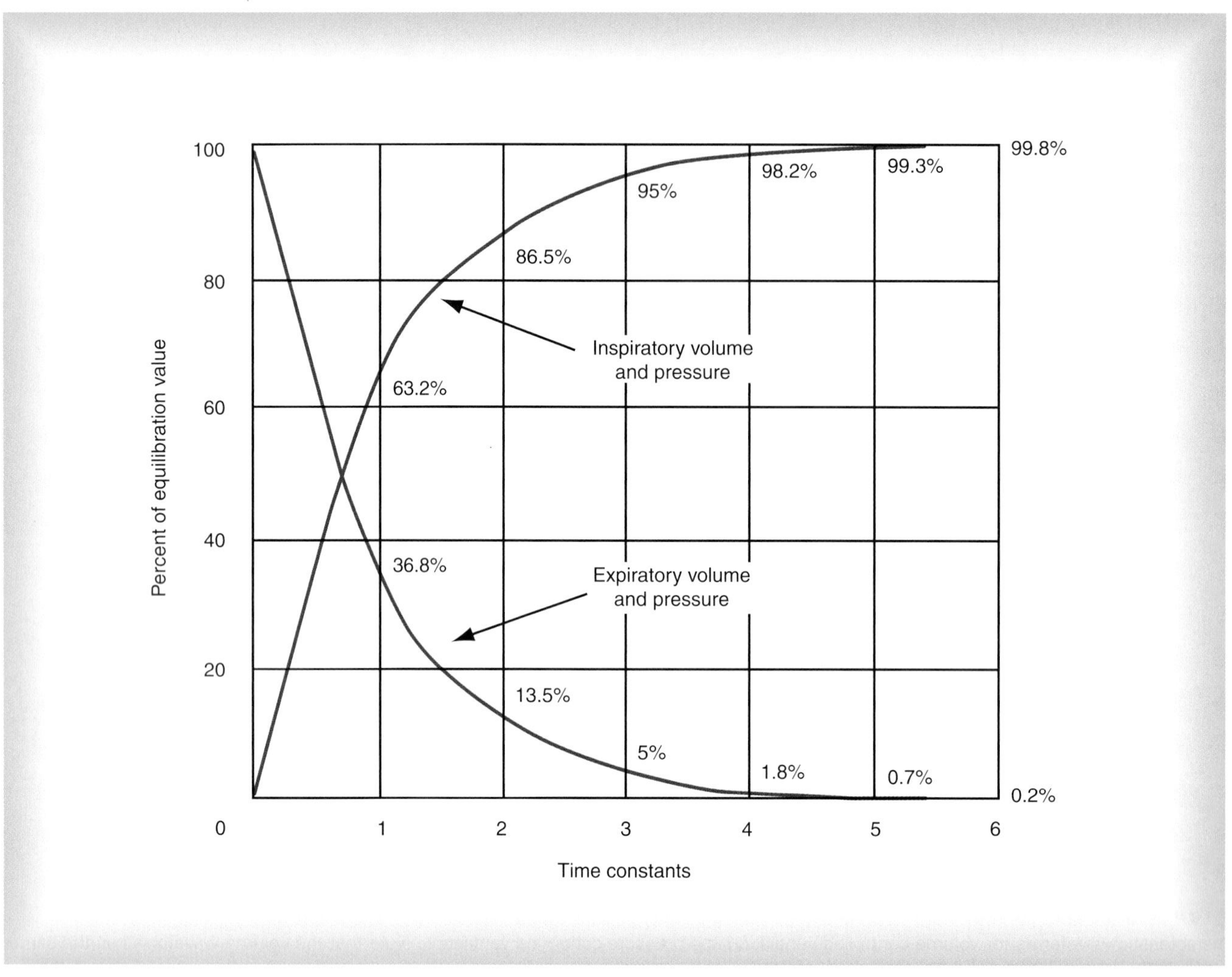

Figure 39-3
The time constant is a measure of how long the respiratory system takes to passively inflate or deflate in response to a sudden change in transrespiratory system pressure. The time constant is calculated as the product of resistance × compliance and is expressed in units of time, usually seconds.

Control Variables

A control variable is the primary variable that the ventilator manipulates to cause inspiration. There are only three variables in the equation of motion that a ventilator can control: pressure, volume, and flow. Because only one of these variables can be directly controlled at a time, a ventilator must function as either a pressure, volume, or flow controller. Time is implicit in the equation of motion and in some cases will serve as a control variable. Figure 39-4 illustrates the criteria for determining what variable the ventilator controls at any given time.

Pressure. If the ventilator controls pressure, the pressure waveform will remain constant but volume and flow will vary with changes in respiratory system mechanics. The ventilator can control either the airway pressure (causing it to rise above body surface pressure for inspiration) or the pressure on the body surface (causing it to fall below airway opening pressure for inspiration). This is the basis for classifying ventilators as being either positive or negative pressure types. For example, the Newport Wave would be classified as a positive pressure controller that generates a rectangular pressure waveform, while the Emerson Iron Lung is a negative pressure controller that produces a quasisinusoidal pressure waveform.

Volume. If the ventilator controls volume, the volume and flow waveforms will remain constant, but pressure will vary with changes in respiratory mechanics. To qualify as a true volume controller, a ventilator must measure volume and use this signal to control the volume waveform. Volume can be controlled directly by

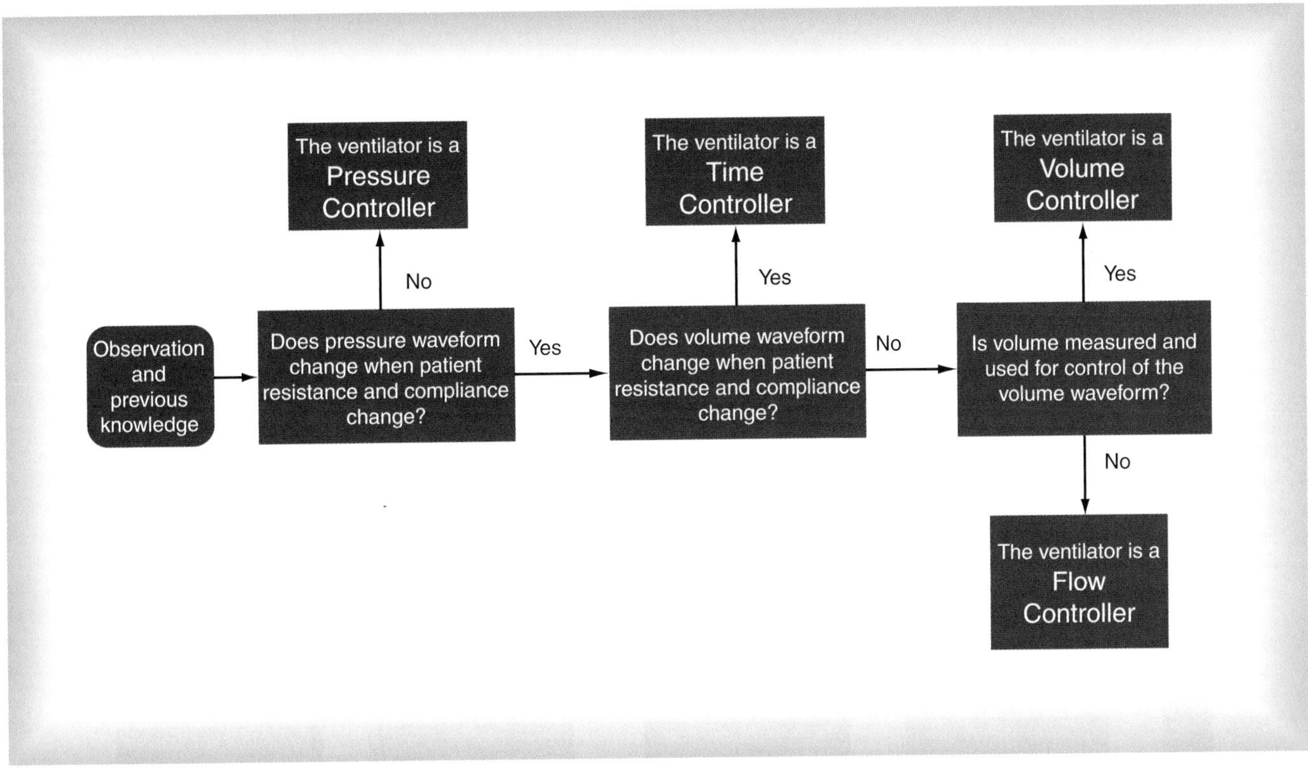

Figure 39-4
Criteria for determining the control variable during a ventilator-assisted inspiration.

the displacement of a device such as a piston or bellows. Volume can be controlled indirectly by controlling flow. This follows from the fact that volume and flow are inverse functions of time (i.e., volume is the integral of flow and flow is the derivative of volume).

Flow. If the ventilator controls flow, the flow and volume waveforms will remain constant, but pressure will vary with changes in respiratory mechanics. Flow can be controlled directly using something as simple as a flowmeter or as complex as a proportional solenoid valve.[6] Flow can be controlled indirectly by controlling volume.

Infant ventilators, such as the Bear Cub, are the simplest examples of flow controllers. In this ventilator, we control flow directly via a flowmeter and electromagnetic plunger valve. As long as the airway pressure does not reach the set pressure limit, the resulting volume waveform remains constant.[10] Most current generation adult ICU ventilators (e.g., Servo 300, Puritan-Bennett 840, the Bear-1000, Hamilton Galileo) can function as flow controllers. However, these systems are much more complex than ventilators like the Bear Cub; flow is measured and adjusted thousands of times per second via sophisticated computerized output control valves.

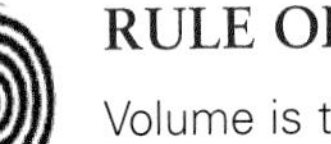

RULE OF THUMB

Volume is the integral of flow. In simple terms: Flow × Time = Volume. Any ventilator that controls flow and time controls volume. Think of using your water faucet to fill the sink: the greater the flow and the longer the time, the greater the volume.

Phase Variables

A complete ventilatory cycle or breath consists of four phases: the initiation of inspiration, inspiration itself, the end of inspiration, and expiration. To understand a breath cycle, you must therefore know how the ventilator starts, sustains, and stops inspiration and you must know what occurs between breaths.

The phase variable is a variable that is measured and used by the ventilator to initiate some phase of the breath cycle. The variable causing a breath to begin is the *trigger variable*. The variable limiting the magnitude of any parameter during inspiration is the *limit variable*. The variable causing a breath to end is the *cycle variable*. To describe what happens during expiration, we must know what *baseline variable* is in effect. Figure 39-5 shows the criteria for determining phase variables.

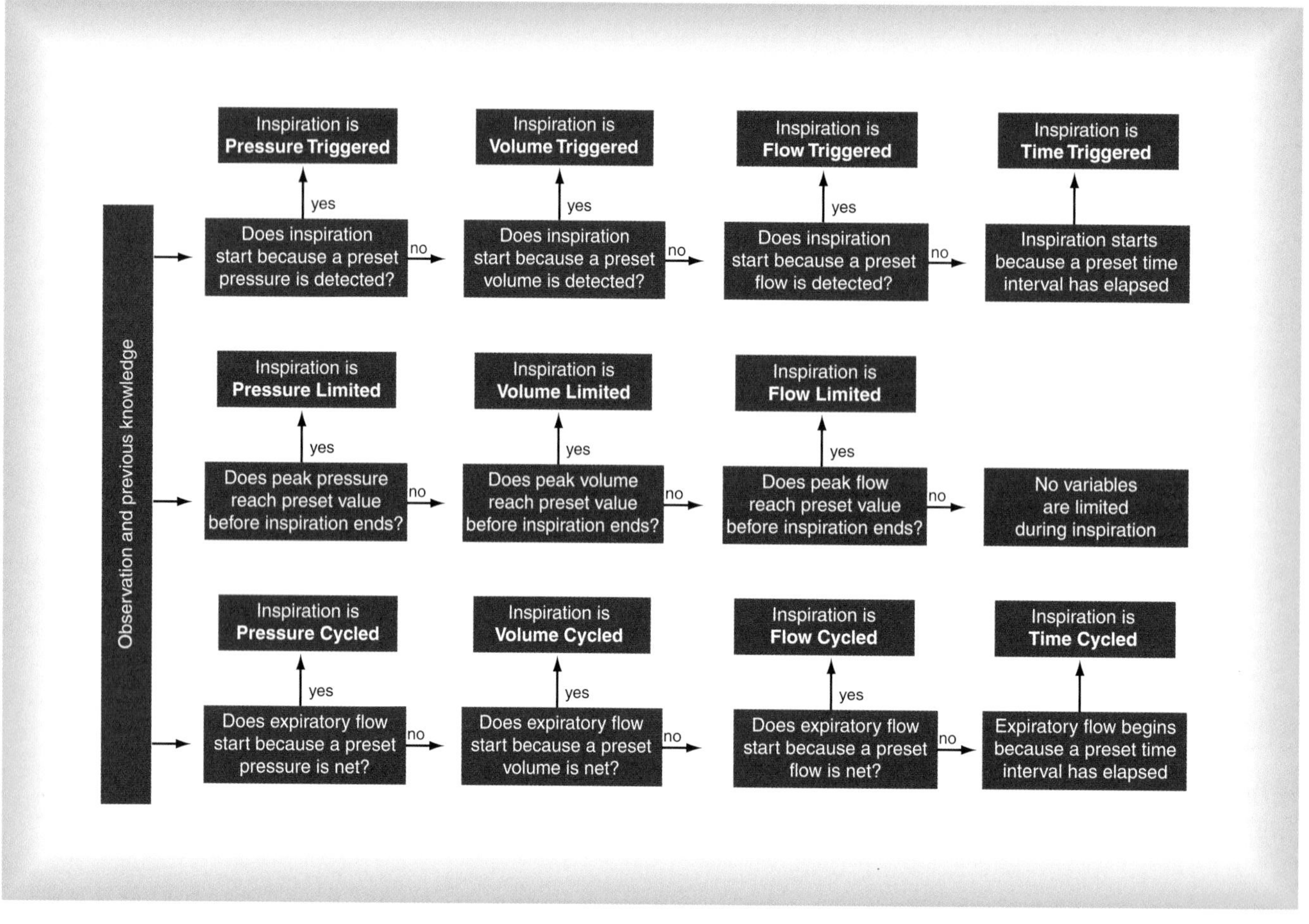

Figure 39-5
Criteria for determining the phase variables during a breath on a mechanical ventilator.

Trigger Variable

On most modern ventilators, either the machine or patient can initiate a breath. If the machine initiates the breath, the trigger variable is time. If the patient initiates the breath, pressure, flow, or volume may serve as the trigger variable. Manual or operator-initiated triggering is also available on most ventilators.

Time Triggering. When triggering by time, a ventilator initiates a breath according to a predetermined time interval, without regard to patient effort. In the past, time triggering was the only method available to initiate a ventilator cycle. Currently time triggering is most commonly seen when using the IMV mode (intermittent mandatory ventilation).

Specific systems for setting a breathing rate vary from ventilator to ventilator. The most common approach is via a *rate control*, which divides each minute into equal time segments, allotting one time segment for each full breath. When a rate control is used, inspiratory and expiratory times will vary according to other control settings, such as flow and volume. An alternative approach is to provide separate timers for inspiration and expiration. Changing either or both of these timers will alter the breathing rate.

Patient Triggering. With patient triggering, the patient's inspiratory effort signals the ventilator to begin inspiration. To do so, the ventilator must "sense" the patient's effort. This is usually done by measuring pressure, flow, or volume.

Pressure triggering occurs when a patient's inspiratory effort causes a drop in pressure within the breathing circuit. When this pressure drop reaches the pressure sensing mechanism, the ventilator triggers on and begins gas delivery. On most ventilators, you can adjust the pressure drop needed to trigger a breath. The trigger level is often called the *sensitivity.* Typically, you set the trigger level 0.5 to 1.5 cm H_2O below the baseline expiratory pressure. Setting the trigger level to a higher number, say 3.0 cm H_2O, makes the ventilator less sensitive and requires the patient to work harder to initiate inspiration. Conversely, setting the trigger level lower makes the ventilator more sensitive. How *fast* the

MINI CLINI

Calculate the Expiratory Time Setting From the Frequency and Inspiratory Time

PROBLEM

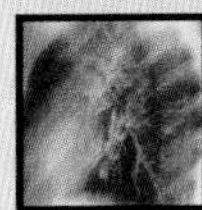

You are assigned to the neonatal intensive care unit (NICU) and have successfully intubated a newborn term infant diagnosed with respiratory distress syndrome. You are manually ventilating the infant with a flow-inflating bag at a frequency of 25 breaths per minute. An inline manometer indicates the PIP is approximately 24 cm H_2O and the PEEP 4 cm H_2O. The infant's vital signs (heart rate, respiratory rate, and blood pressure) are within normal limits and SpO_2 is 95%. The pressure and frequency you are using manually will serve as the initial ventilator settings on a Sechrist infant ventilator. With this particular ventilator, however, setting the inspiratory and expiratory times determines the frequency. The attending physician has requested an inspiratory time (T_I) of 0.7 seconds.

Calculate the expiratory time (T_E) necessary to give the desired frequency.

DISCUSSION

Step 1: Compute the total cycle time (TCT) using the frequency (f):

$$TCT = \frac{1}{f} = T_I + T_E$$

$$f = \frac{25\ breaths}{minute} \times \frac{1\ minute}{60\ seconds} = \frac{25\ breaths}{60\ seconds}$$

$$TCT = \frac{1}{25\ breaths/60\ seconds} = \frac{60\ seconds}{25\ breaths}$$

$$= \frac{2.4\ seconds}{breath}$$

Step 2: Compute the expiratory time:

$$T_E = TCT - T_I = 2.4 - 0.7 = 1.7\ seconds$$

ventilator mechanism responds to patient effort is called the *response time*. It is important for the ventilator to have a short response time to maintain optimal synchrony with the patient's inspiratory efforts. Either a large pressure drop (i.e., low sensitivity setting) or a delay in flow delivery can increase a patient's work of breathing.

Using flow as the trigger variable is a bit more complex. A ventilator that uses flow triggering typically provides a continuous low flow of gas through its circuit. The ventilator measures the flow coming out of the main flow control valve and also the flow through the exhalation valve. Between breaths, these two flows are equal (assuming no leaks in the patient circuit). When the patient makes an inspiratory effort, the flow through the exhalation valve falls below the flow from the output valve. The difference between these two flows is the flow trigger variable.

To adjust the sensitivity of a flow-triggered system, you usually set both a base continuous flow and a trigger flow level. Typically, the trigger flow level is set to 1 to 3 L/minute (below baseline). For example, if you set the base continuous flow at 10 L/minute and the trigger at 2 L/minute, the ventilator will trigger when the output flow falls to 8 L/minute or less. An alternative approach used by some ventilators is to simply measure the flow at the wye connector and trigger on that signal.

When compared with pressure, using flow as the trigger variable decreases a patient's work of breathing.[11,12] However, ventilators that use a flow-triggering mechanism tend to be highly susceptible to circuit leaks or movement caused by turbulence or gas flow through condensed water. Either of these conditions can cause spurious breaths, which can disrupt patient-ventilatory synchrony and increase the work of breathing. Using volume as the trigger can help overcome this problem, but currently only the Drager Babylog uses true volume triggering.

Variables other than pressure, flow, or volume can be used to trigger inspiration. For example, the Infrasonics Star Sync module allows triggering of the Infant Star ventilator by chest wall movement. The Sechrist infant ventilator can be triggered with a chest wall impedance signal.

Limit Variable

A limit variable is one that can reach and maintain a preset level *before* inspiration ends but does not terminate inspiration. Either pressure, flow, or volume can serve as a limit variable.

Clinicians often confuse limit variables with cycle variables. A cycle variable always ends inspiration. A limit variable does not terminate inspiration–it only sets an upper bound for pressure, volume, or flow. The confusion over limit and cycle variables is due, in part, to the nomenclature used by many ventilator manufacturers. They often use the term *limit* to describe what happens when a pressure or time alarm threshold is met (i.e., inspiration is terminated and an alarm is activated). To be consistent with accepted nomenclature, it is best to refer to these threshold alarms as back-up cycling mechanisms rather than limits. Figure 39-6 illustrates the importance of distinguishing between limit and cycle variables.

Cycle Variable

The inspiratory phase always ends when some variable reaches a preset value. The variable that is measured and used to end inspiration is called the *cycle variable.* The cycle variable can be pressure, volume, flow, or time. Manual cycling is also available on some modern ventilators.

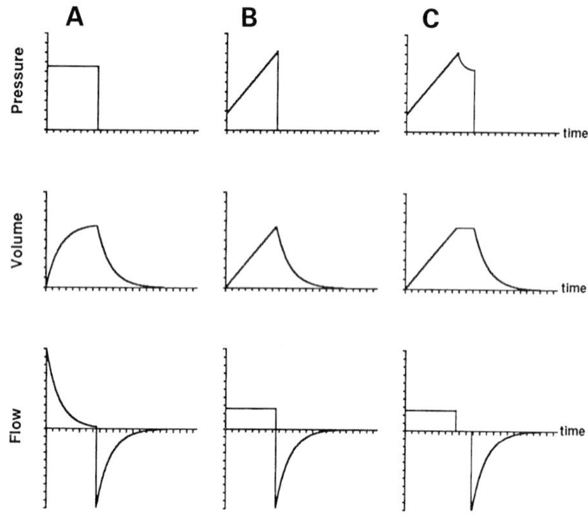

Figure 39-6

This figure illustrates the importance of distinguishing between the terms *limit* and *cycle*. **A,** Inspiration is pressure limited and time cycled. **B,** Inspiration is flow limited and volume cycled. **C,** Inspiration is both flow limited and volume limited (because flow and volume reach preset values before inspiratory time ends) and time cycled (after the preset inspiratory hold time).

Pressure Cycling. When a ventilator is set to pressure-cycle, it delivers flow until a preset pressure is reached. When the set pressure is achieved, inspiratory flow stops and expiratory flow begins. The most common application of pressure-cycling is for alarm settings. Intermittent positive pressure breathing (IPPB) therapy is usually performed with pressure cycled machines.

Volume Cycling. When a ventilator is set to volume-cycle, it delivers flow until a preselected volume has been expelled from the device. As soon as the set volume is met, inspiratory flow stops and expiratory flow begins. Note that the volume that passes through the ventilator's output control valve is never exactly equal to the volume delivered to the patient because of the volume compressed in the patient circuit. Some ventilators use a sensor at the wye connector (e.g., the Hamilton Galileo) for accurate tidal volume measurement. Others measure volume at some point inside the ventilator, and the operator must know whether or not the ventilator compensates for compressed gas in its tidal volume readout.

Flow Cycling. When a ventilator is set to flow cycle, it delivers flow until a preset level is met and then flow stops and expiration begins. The most frequent application of flow cycling is in the pressure control mode.* In this mode, the control variable is pressure and the ventilator provides the flow necessary to meet the inspiratory pressure limit. In doing so, flow starts out at a relatively high value and decays exponentially (see Figure 39-2). Once flow has decreased to a relatively low value (e.g., 25% of peak flow, preset by the manufacturer) inspiration is cycled off. Manufacturers often set the cycle threshold slightly above zero flow to avoid inspiratory times from getting so long that patient synchrony is degraded.

Time Cycling. Time cycling means that expiratory flow starts because a preset time interval has elapsed. There are several time intervals of interest during inspiration. One is the inspiratory flow time. Like the name implies, this is the time during which inspiratory flow is delivered to the patient. Another interval is the inspiratory hold time, during which inspiratory flow has ceased, but expiratory flow is not yet allowed. The sum of these two intervals is the inspiratory time. Therefore time cycling occurs when the inspiratory time has elapsed. Note that an inspiratory hold time may not be used. If it is used, it may be set directly, or it may occur indirectly if the set inspiratory time is longer than the inspiratory flow time (determined by the set tidal volume and flow; time = volume/flow).

Baseline Variable

The baseline variable is the parameter controlled during expiration. Although pressure, volume, or flow could serve as the baseline variable, pressure control is the most practical and is implemented by all modern ventilators.

Baseline or expiratory pressure is always measured and set relative to atmospheric pressure. Thus, when we want baseline pressure to equal atmospheric pressure, we set it at zero. When we want baseline pressure to exceed atmospheric pressure, we set a positive value, called positive end-expiratory pressure (PEEP). Although seldom used, we could also set the baseline below atmospheric pressure, a technique called negative end-expiratory pressure (NEEP).

Zero end-expiratory pressure (ZEEP) is the default baseline value during positive pressure ventilation, meaning that it is normally in effect unless purposely changed. Regardless of the mechanism by which gas is delivered to the lungs, it must leave before the next inspiration. Exhalation normally occurs by virtue of the stored pressure in the expanded lungs and thorax. With ZEEP in effect, when exhalation begins, the ventilator's expiratory valve simply opens to the atmosphere, exposing the patient's airway to a relative pressure of zero. At this point, alveolar pressure exceeds airway pressure, gas moves from alveoli out to the atmosphere, and the lungs and thorax passively recoil down to their resting volume, or functional residual capacity (FRC).

---

*The term pressure control is used to refer to a breathing pattern in which the control variable is pressure and in which the airway pressure waveform is preset. Pressure-limited, flow-cycled breaths are a form of pressure control commonly referred to as *pressure-support ventilation (PSV)*.

MINI CLINI

Calculate Inspiratory Hold Time Given Set Inspiratory Time, Tidal Volume, and Flow as in Siemens Servo

PROBLEM

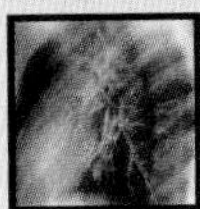

You are performing a ventilator check on an ICU patient with a blunt chest trauma. The ventilator is set to volume controlled SIMV on a Dräger Evita 4. The physician wants the minimum mean airway pressure for the given level of ventilation to preserve the patient's already low cardiac output. She asks you to make sure the night shift therapist removed the inspiratory hold the patient had been on.

Determine from the ventilator settings alone whether there is an inspiratory hold and if so, make the appropriate changes to eliminate it. Ventilator settings are:

Tidal volume: 500 mL = 0.5 L
Inspiratory flow: 60 L/minute = 1 L/second
Inspiratory time: 0.8 seconds
Frequency: 10 breaths per minute

DISCUSSION

Step 1: Calculate the inspiratory flow time (T_F):

$$T_F = \frac{\textit{tidal volume}}{\textit{inspiratory flow}} = \frac{500\ mL}{60\ L/minute} \times \frac{1\ L}{1000\ mL} \times \frac{60\ seconds}{1\ minute} = \frac{0.5\ L}{1\ L/second}\ 0.5\ seconds$$

Step 2: Compare the set inspiratory time (0.8 seconds) with the flow time resulting from the tidal volume and flow settings (0.5 seconds). Inspiratory time lasts longer than inspiratory flow. Because inspiration is time cycled, this means that there is an inspiratory hold of duration equal to 0.8 – 0.5 = 0.3 seconds

Step 3: You could eliminate the inspiratory hold either by decreasing the inspiratory flow or decreasing the inspiratory time. Your goal is to minimize the mean inspiratory pressure. You choose to decrease inspiratory time for two reasons: (1) it decreases the I:E ratio and may allow more time for spontaneous breaths to occur, thus lowering mean intrathoracic pressure; (2) decreasing inspiratory flow may make tidal volume delivery slower than the patient demands, thus decreasing ventilator-patient synchrony.

PEEP is the application of pressure above atmospheric pressure at the airway throughout expiration. By doing this, PEEP elevates a patient's FRC and can help improve oxygenation by preventing collapse of alveolar units that are made unstable by lack of surfactant or disease.

NEEP is the application of *subatmospheric* pressure to the airway during expiration. NEEP was originally developed to overcome the harmful cardiovascular effects of positive pressure ventilation. The assumption was that NEEP could offset the impedance to venous return created by the positive pressure during inspiration. More recently, NEEP (e.g., exhalation assist on the Venturi ventilator) has been promoted as a way to help patients overcome expiratory airway resistance. In this approach, negative pressure is applied only to help return airway pressure to baseline. Given that NEEP can cause airway collapse and decrease the FRC if misapplied, great care must be taken in applying this technique.

Conditional Variables

Ventilators can also use pressure, volume, flow, or time (and their derivatives such as minute ventilation) as conditional variables. A conditional variable is used by a ventilator's control circuit to make decisions. A simple conditional formula takes the form of an "if-then" statement. That is, *if* the value of a conditional variable reaches some preset level, *then* some action occurs to change the ventilatory pattern.

An example of conditional logic is the Puritan-Bennett 7200 sigh function. When activated, the sigh function delivers multiple breaths with supernormal tidal volumes every few minutes. In this case, the conditional variable is time. *If* a preset time interval has elapsed (the sigh interval), *then* the ventilator switches to the sigh pattern. Another good example of conditional logic is the switchover between patient-triggered breaths and machine-triggered breaths that occur during intermittent mandatory ventilation.

Modes of Ventilation[3]

The objective of mechanical ventilation is to ensure that the patient receives the minute volume of appropriate gases required to satisfy respiratory needs while not damaging the lungs, impairing circulation, or increasing the patient's discomfort. A *mode of ventilation* is the manner in which a ventilator achieves this objective. A mode can be identified by specifying a combination of:

- Breathing pattern, which includes the primary breath control variable and the breath sequence
- Control type (e.g., set point, servo, or adaptive control)
- Specific control strategy, including phase variables and operational logic

Box 39-2 gives an outline for describing modes of ventilation.

The key to understanding modes of ventilation is to link simple, defined terms in a way that allows us to build descriptions of varying complexity. This is much more practical than trying to memorize arbitrary names for every new feature a manufacturer wishes to promote. It is analogous to using an alphabet of several dozen letters to build words rather than memorizing tens

Box 39-2 • Mode Classification Scheme

The following elements can be used to characterize modes of ventilator operation. If both mandatory and spontaneous breaths are possible in a given mode, the specification of that mode should begin with, and may just be limited to, a description of the mandatory breaths. However, a complete specification would include descriptions of both mandatory and spontaneous breaths.

I. Breathing pattern
  A. Primary breath control variable
    1. Volume
    2. Pressure
    3. Dual
      a. Within breaths
      b. Between breaths
  B. Breath sequence
    1. Continuous mandatory ventilation (CMV)
    2. Intermittent mandatory ventilation (IMV)
    3. Continuous spontaneous ventilation (CSV)
II. Control type
  A. Setpoint control
  B. Servo control
  C. Adaptive setpoint control
III. Specific control strategy
  A. Phase variables
    1. Trigger
    2. Limit
    3. Cycle
  B. Operational logic
    1. Conditional variables
    2. Output variables
    3. Performance function (e.g., function that is maximized or minimized for adaptive strategies)

of thousands of separate ideographs that each represents a word. One need only compare the English language to the Chinese language to appreciate the analogy.

Box 39-2 shows that three basic components of a mode (breathing pattern, control type, and specific control strategy) make up a complete classification for any mode of ventilation.

Breathing Pattern. As a first step, Box 39-2 shows that a mode can be classified simply on the basis of the breathing pattern it produces. The first component of the breathing pattern is the primary breath control variable. We said earlier that a ventilator can control either pressure, volume, or flow. When we talk about modes of ventilation, we do not need to be so specific. Because control of volume implies control of flow and vice versa, we can simply refer to two basic modes of ventilation: volume control and pressure control. Volume control implies that tidal volume and inspiratory flow are preset and airway pressure is then dependent upon those settings and respiratory system elastance and resistance (according to the equation of motion). On the other hand, pressure control implies that the airway pressure waveform is preset (e.g., PIP and end expiratory pressure) and tidal volume and inspiratory flow are then dependent on these settings and the elastance and resistance of the respiratory system.

There are clinical advantages and disadvantages to each type of control, which will be discussed in the clinical application section later in this chapter. For now, we can simply say that volume control results in a more stable minute ventilation (and hence more stable blood gases) than pressure control if lung mechanics are unstable. On the other hand, pressure control allows better synchronization with the patient because inspiratory flow is not constrained to a preset value. While it is possible to control only one variable at a time, a ventilator can automatically switch between pressure control and volume control in an attempt to guarantee minute ventilation while maximizing patient synchrony. This is called *dual control.*

Currently, there are two approaches to dual control. One approach is to control pressure within a breath but to control tidal volume over several breaths through automatic adjustment of the pressure limit. An example of this is the pressure-regulated, volume-control mode on the Siemens Servo 300 ventilator. Another approach to dual control is to switch between pressure control and volume control within a breath. An example of this is volume-assured, pressure-support mode on the Bird 8400ST ventilator (Figure 39-7).

Specifying only the breath control variable for a mode, we can only distinguish among pressure control, volume control, and dual control modes. Often this is all we need to communicate. For example, at the bedside we might simply have to indicate that the patient's lung mechanics have become unstable and therefore the mode has been changed from volume control to dual control.

The second component of the breathing pattern specification is the breath sequence. A *breath* is defined as a positive change in airway flow (inspiration) paired with a negative change in airway flow (expiration), both relative to baseline flow and associated with ventilation of the lungs. This definition excludes flow changes caused by hiccups or cardiogenic oscillations. But it allows the superimposition of, say, a spontaneous breath on a mandatory breath or vice versa (these breath types are defined below). Traditionally, the flow baseline is taken as Flow = 0 (i.e., end expiration). However, since "breaths" can be superimposed on existing flow in various circumstances (e.g., high frequency ventilation), the inspiratory and expiratory movements of gas must be judged relative to the level of flow existing when these movements occur. Typically, inspiration imme-

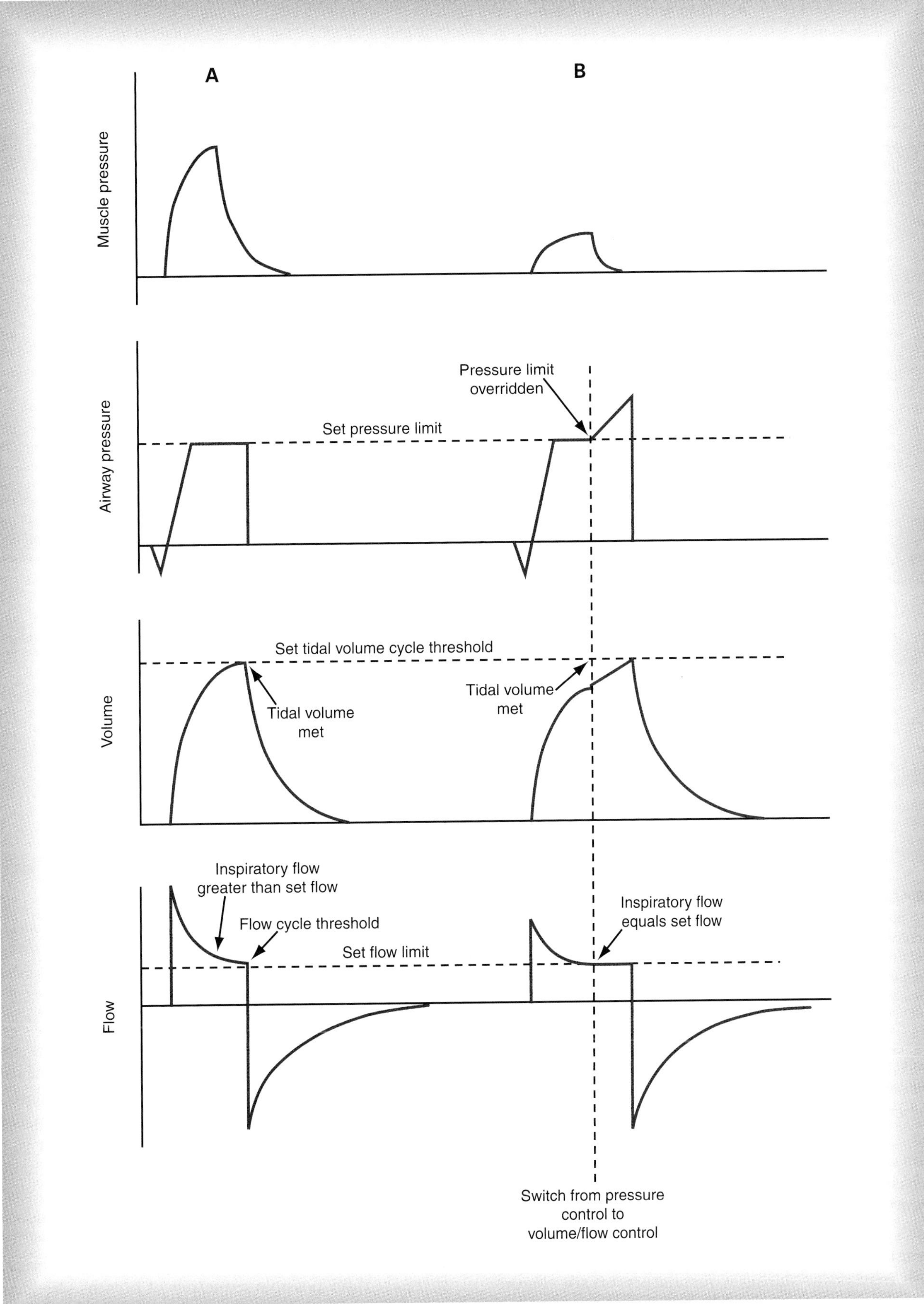

Figure 39-7

Characteristic waveforms for dual control within breaths. **A,** Pressure-controlled breath with large patient effort (muscle pressure). The set tidal volume has been reached before flow has decayed to the set flow limit, so the breath continues in pressure control until the flow cycle threshold is reached. This value may be an arbitrary percentage of the of the peak flow for the pressure controlled portion of the breath (e.g., Pressure Augment on the Bear 1000), or it may be the set flow (e.g., VAPS on the Bird 8400ST). The breath is essentially a pressure support breath. **B,** Switch from pressure control to flow control because flow decayed to the set flow before the set tidal volume was met. This result was caused by a smaller patient effort. Inspiration continues at the set flow and pressure rises as expected for volume control.

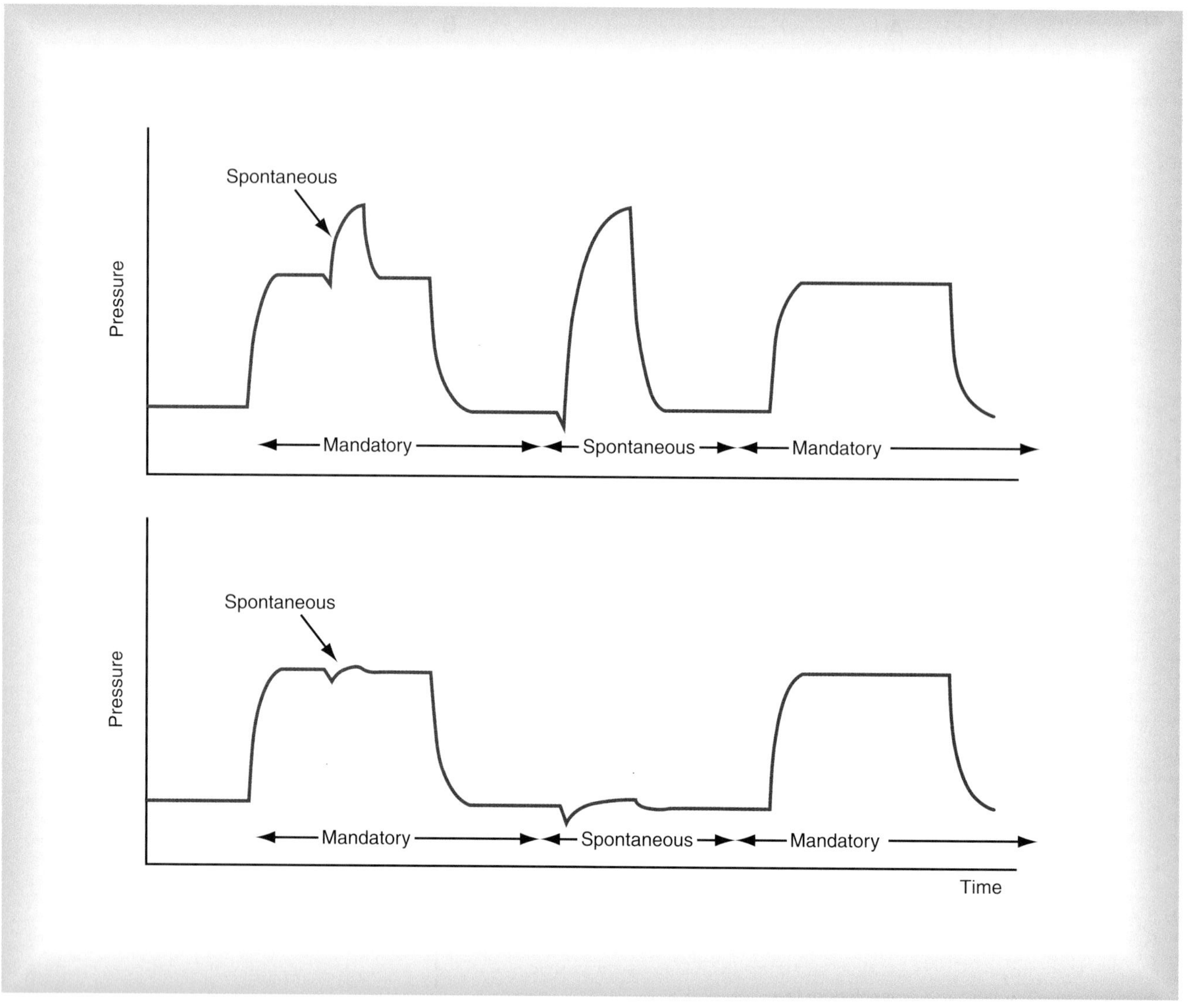

Figure 39-8

These pressure-time curves illustrate how a spontaneous breath (e.g., pressure-triggered, flow-cycled) can occur either between or during mandatory breaths (e.g., time-triggered, time-cycled). Spontaneous breaths may be assisted (pressure support in this figure but could be something else, such as proportional assist or tube compensation) as shown in the top curve, or unassisted, as shown in the bottom curve. As one example of this, the Puritan Bennett 840 ventilator allows all spontaneous breaths to be assisted during the bilevel mode.

diately precedes expiration. However, it is possible for the reverse to occur, such as during manual resuscitation by chest compression or during assisted ventilation using a tilt bed.

The classification of modes requires the definition of two basic types of breaths: spontaneous and mandatory. A *spontaneous breath* is a breath for which the patient decides the start time and the tidal volume. That is, the patient both triggers and cycles the breath. A spontaneous breath may occur during a mandatory breath (Figure 39-8). A spontaneous breath may be assisted or unassisted. An assisted breath is a breath during which all or part of inspiratory or expiratory flow is generated by a change in transrespiratory pressure (i.e., airway pressure minus body surface pressure, P_{aw} - P_{bs}) due to an external agent (e.g., manual or mechanical ventilator).

A *mandatory breath* is a breath for which the machine sets the start time and/or the tidal volume. That is, the machine triggers and/or cycles the breath. All mandatory breaths are, by definition, assisted. Box 39-3 shows an algorithm defining spontaneous and mandatory breaths.

Having defined spontaneous and mandatory breaths, there are three possible sequences of breaths, designated as follows:

- Continuous mandatory ventilation (CMV): All breaths are mandatory.

Box 39-3 • Algorithm Defining Spontaneous and Mandatory Breaths

Note that the patient may cycle inspiration off, either actively (e.g., an active expiratory effort) or passively as the lungs accumulate volume and pressure and flow decays to zero (e.g., flow-cycling in the pressure support mode).

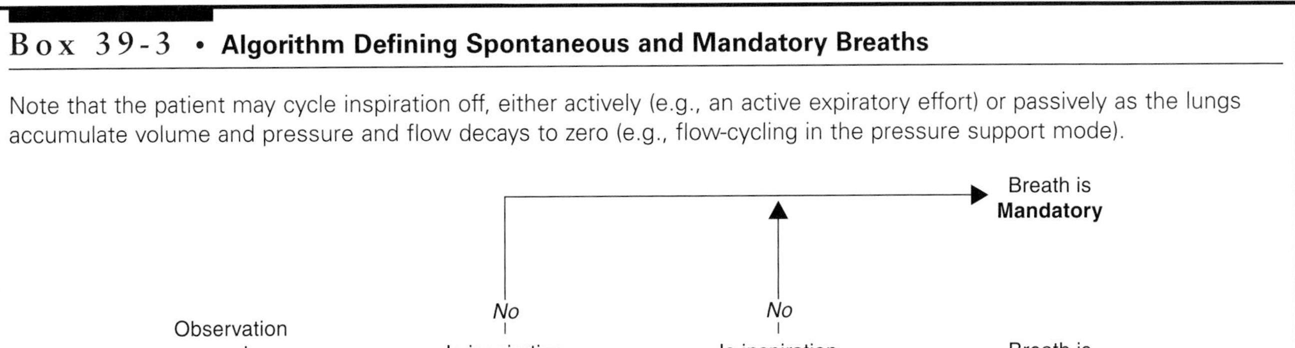

Table 39-1 ▶▶ Possible Breathing Patterns

Breath Control Variable	Breath Sequence	Abbreviation
Volume control	Continuous mandatory ventilation	VC-CMV
	Intermittent mandatory ventilation	VC-IMV
Pressure control	Continuous mandatory ventilation	PC-CMV
	Intermittent mandatory ventilation	PC-IMV
	Continuous spontaneous ventilation	PC-CSV
Dual control	Continuous mandatory ventilation	DC-CMV
	Intermittent mandatory ventilation	DC-IMV
	Continuous spontaneous ventilation	DC-CSV

- Continuous spontaneous ventilation (CSV): All breaths are spontaneous.
- Intermittent mandatory ventilation (IMV): Breaths can be either mandatory or spontaneous.

Breaths can occur separately (e.g., IMV) or breaths can be superimposed on each other (e.g., spontaneous breaths superimposed on mandatory breaths, as in bilevel or airway pressure release ventilation [APRV]; or mandatory breaths superimposed on spontaneous breaths, as in high frequency ventilation administered during breathing). When the mandatory breath is patient triggered, it is commonly referred to as synchronized IMV (SIMV). However, because the trigger variable can be specified in the description of phase variables, we will use IMV instead of SIMV to designate general breath sequences.

When we add the breath sequence to the control variable in classifying a mode, we get a greater ability to discriminate between similar modes. We can distinguish between, say, pressure controlled-IMV (PC-IMV) and pressure controlled-CSV (PC-CSV). If we confine ourselves to classifying modes based solely on the breathing pattern, we see that there are only eight possibilities in three groups (Table 39-1). The utility of this system is immediately obvious. We can explain a new mode, say, APRV, as simply a form of PC-IMV. Assuming we already understand the concept of PC-IMV, it takes little effort to understand the additional nuances of APRV (e.g., different labels for control settings, alarms, etc.). At this level of description, we can avoid the cumbersome verbal ad hoc definition for APRV such as "a mode that allows spontaneously breathing patients to breathe at a positive-pressure level, but drops briefly to a reduced pressure level for CO_2 elimination during each breathing cycle," or the cryptic description of some authors who explain APRV as two levels of CPAP (continuous positive airway pressure).

We can also use PC-IMV and PC-CSV to clarify what *bilevel positive airway pressure ventilation (BiPAP)* means. For example, on the Respironics BiPAP S/T-D ventilator, the "Timed" BiPAP mode is PC-IMV whereas the "Spontaneous" BiPAP mode is PC-CSV. "BiPAP Ventilation" and "Bilevel Ventilation" are particularly ambiguous terms because any form of assisted ventilation can be thought of as using two levels of pressure (see the definition of assisted breath above). To make matters even more confusing, the Mallinckrodt Puritan Bennett 840 ventilator has a "BiLevel" mode that allows for additional pressure support during a pressure-limited, time cycled, mandatory breath. Therefore with PEEP, the mandatory pressure limit and the pressure support limit, the mode actually provides "trilevel" ventilation.

The specification of breathing pattern is also useful for grouping together modes that function the same way but are given different names. For example, both Pressure Augment (Bear 1000) and Volume Assured Pressure Support (Bird 8400ST) are dual controlled IMV (i.e., dual control within breaths). Another example would be Pressure Regulated Volume Control (Siemens 300) and Pressure-Controlled Assist Control + Adaptive Pressure Ventilation (Hamilton Galileo), which are both dual control CMV (i.e., dual control between breaths). It is also possible to group ventilators in terms of the number of breathing patterns they offer; some offer only one or two, others offer all eight. This might be useful as an initial screening tool when planning ventilator purchases.

Here is another example: Dräger calls AutoFlow a "mode extension." But it is simply dual control (between breaths) similar to that type of dual control on other ventilators. What makes AutoFlow an extension on the Evita 4 is that it can be used with different breath sequences to get different breathing patterns (e.g., dual controlled-CMV and dual controlled-IMV). This ability to "build" a mode is consistent with the "increasing detail" approach to mode descriptions shown in Box 39-2, even if the nomenclature is not. On the other hand, the front panel layout of the Dräger Evita 4 would lead one to think that P_{max} is just a pressure-limit control. But activating this feature actually changes the breathing pattern from volume control CMV or IMV to dual control (within breaths) CMV or IMV (Table 39-2). On another ventilator, dual control may be a preset mode by itself (e.g., Volume Support on the Siemens 300).

Control Type. We have discussed "control variables" and the differences between pressure, volume, and dual control but we have not really explained what is meant by "control" in the first place. There are two general ways to control a variable: open loop control and closed loop control.

Open loop control is essentially no control. For example, early high frequency ventilators simply generated pulses of gas flow without measurement or control of pressure, volume, or flow. Flow into the patient was a function of the relative impedances of the respiratory system and the exhalation manifold. Thus, delivered pressures and volumes were affected by any disturbances in the system (e.g., changing lung mechanics, the patient's ventilatory efforts, and leaks).

Closed loop control is an improvement in that the delivered pressure, volume, and flow can be measured and used as feedback information to control the driving mechanism (like speed control in an automobile). Thus, inspiratory volumes, flows, and pressures can be made to match or follow specified input values despite disturbances such as changes in patient load and minor leaks in the system.

Box 39-2 shows that a more detailed mode description would include the type of control scheme used to manipulate the control variables to produce the permissible breaths. For single variable, closed loop control, setpoint, and servo types have been employed. Setpoint control means that the output of the ventilator is forced to match a constant, unvarying, operator preset input value (e.g., the production of a constant inspiratory pressure from breath to breath). Servo control means the output is forced to follow a dynamic, varying, operator-specified input. For example, the tube compensation feature on the Puritan Bennett 840 ventilator measures instantaneous flow and forces instantaneous pressure to be equal to flow multiplied by a constant (representing endotracheal tube resistance).

Dual variable, closed loop control (dual control) has used setpoint and adaptive setpoint control. Adaptive control means that the output of the ventilator is forced to match an operator specified input (such as tidal volume or minute ventilation) as the characteristics of the respiratory system change. The ventilator typically measures pressure, volume, and flow and then uses the equation of motion to monitor lung elastance and resistance on a breath-by-breath basis.[13] This dynamic tracking of respiratory system mechanics makes adaptive control possible by allowing the ventilator to adjust the primary control variables itself to achieve some higher level goal such as a consistent tidal volume or minimum work of breathing. Examples of adaptive (dual) control can be seen in modes like Pressure Regulated Volume Control (on the Siemens 300 ventilator), Adaptive Support Ventilation (Hamilton Galileo ventilator), and Auto Flow (Dräger Evita 4 ventilator).

Control Strategy. So far we have shown how modes of ventilation can be described at various levels of detail, depending on how and with whom we need to communicate. At the highest level of detail, we can fully characterize a mode by adding the specific strategy it employs. This begins with the naming of the phase variables, followed by detailing the operational logic, and, if necessary, giving the parameter values used in the conditional statements. The specification of the breathing pattern that the mode can produce (i.e., breath control variable(s) and breath sequence), the type of control (setpoint, servo, or adaptive control), and the specific strategy (phase variable an operational logic) it uses, for both mandatory and spontaneous breaths, make up a complete classification for any mode of ventilation.

Box 39-4 provides a simple example of how a mode can be described using this system.

A complete description helps us to distinguish between different modes that look the same on graphics monitors and suggests what the operator must do to set the controls. For example, Pressure Support (any ventilator) is PC-CSV for which the operator sets the

Table 39-2 Detailed Description of Modes Available on 5 Intensive Care Ventilators Used in the United States

				Specific Control Strategy					
				Phase Variables					
	Mode Name	**Breathing Pattern**	**Control Type**	**Trigger**	**Limit***	**Cycle***	**A-Cycle**†	**Operational Logic**
Dräger Medical –Evita 4	Continuous mandatory ventilation	VC-CMV	Setpoint	T	F, V	T	P	N/A
	Continuous mandatory ventilation + assist	VC-CMV	Setpoint	T, F	F, V	T	P	N/A
	Continuous mandatory ventilation + autoflow	DC-CMV	Adaptive	T, F	P	T	P, V	If set tidal volume not achieved then adjust pressure limit.
	Continuous mandatory ventilation + pressure-limited ventilation	DC-CMV	Set point	T, F	F, V, P	T	N/A	If pressure hits set value (P_{max}) then switch from flow limit to pressure limit.
	Synchronized intermittent mandatory ventilation + pressure support	VC-IMV	Setpoint	F, T	F, V, P	T	P, T	Switch between mandatory and spontaneous breaths.
	Synchronized intermittent mandatory ventilation + autoflow	DC-IMV	Adaptive	T, F	P	T, F	P, V	If set tidal volume not achieved then adjust pressure limit.
	Synchronized intermittent mandatory ventilation + pressure-limited ventilation	DC-IMV	Setpoint	T, F	F, V, P	T	N/A	If pressure hits set value (P_{max}) then switch from flow limit to pressure limit.
	Pressure-controlled ventilation + (bi-level) positive airway pressure/pressure support	PC-IMV	Setpoint	T, F	P	T, F	N/A	Switch between mandatory and spontaneous breaths.
	Pressure controlled-ventilation + assist	PC-CMV	Setpoint	T, F	P	T	N/A	N/A
	Mandatory minute-volume ventilation + pressure support	VC-IMV	Setpoint	T, F	P, V, F	T, F	P, T	If set minute ventilation not achieved by spontaneous breaths then trigger mandatory breaths.
	Mandatory minute-volume ventilation + autoflow	DC-IMV	Adaptive	T, F	P, V, F	T	P, V	If set minute ventilation not achieved by spontaneous breaths then trigger mandatory breaths. If set tidal volume not achieved then adjust pressure limit.
	Mandatory minute-volume ventilation + pressure limited-ventilation	DC-IMV	Setpoint	T, F	F, V, P	T	P	If set minute ventilation not achieved by spontaneous breaths then trigger mandatory breaths. If pressure hits set value (P_{max}) then switch from flow limit to pressure limit.
	Airway pressure release ventilation	PC-IMV	Setpoint	T, F	P	T, F	N/A	N/A
	Pressure support	PC-CSV	Setpoint	F	P	F	T	N/A
	Continuous positive airway pressure	PC-CSV	Setpoint	F	P	F	N/A	N/A
	Automatic tube compensation	PC-CSV	Servo	F	P	F	N/A	The instantaenous value of pressure is proportional to the instantaneous flow.
Puritan Bennet – 840	Volume control assist control	VC-CMV	Setpoint	T, P, F	F	T	P	N/A
	Pressure control assist control	PC-CMV	Setpoint	T, P, F	P	T	P	N/A
	Synchronized intermittent mandatory ventilation	VC-IMV	Setpoint	T, P, F	F	T	P, T	Switch between mandatory and spontaneous breaths.
	Pressure control synchronized intermittent mandatory ventilation	PC-IMV	Setpoint	T, P, F	P	T, F	P, T	Switch between mandatory and spontaneous breaths.
	Bi-level	PC-IMV	Setpoint	T, P, F	P	T, F	P	Switch between mandatory and spontaneous breaths.
	Spontaneous	PC-CSV	Setpoint	P, F	P	F	T, P	N/A
	Tube compensation	PC-CSV	Servo	F	P	F	N/A	The instantaneous value of pressure is proportional to the instantaneous flow.
Hamilton Medical –Galileo	Assist control (synchronized controlled mandatory ventilation)	VC-CMV	Setpoint	T, P, F	F, V	T	P	N/A
	Pressure-controlled assist control (pressure-controlled, controlled mandatory ventilation)	PC-CMV	Setpoint	T, P, F	P	T	P	N/A
	Pressure-controlled assist control (pressure-controlled, controlled mandatory ventilation) + adaptive pressure ventilation	DC-CMV	Adaptive	T, P, F	P	T	P	If set tidal volume not achieved then adjust pressure limit.

Continued

Table 39-2 ▶▶ Detailed Description of Modes Available on 5 Intensive Care Ventilators Used in the United States—*cont'd*

Ventilator	Mode Name	Breathing Pattern	Control Type	Specific Control Strategy: Phase Variables: Trigger	Limit*	Cycle*	A-Cycle[†]	Operational Logic
Hamilton Medical–Galileo	Synchronized intermittent mandatory ventilation	VC-IMV	Setpoint	T, P, F	F, V	T	P	Switch between mandatory and spontaneous breaths.
	Synchronized intermittent mandatory ventilation + pressure support	VC-IMV	Setpoint	T, P, F	F, V, P	T, F	P, T	Switch between mandatory and spontaneous breaths.
	Pressure-controlled synchronized intermittent mandatory ventilation	PC-IMV	Setpoint	T, P, F	P	T	P	Switch between mandatory and spontaneous breaths.
	Pressure-controlled synchronized intermittent mandatory ventilation + pressure support	PC-IMV	Setpoint	T, P, F	P	T, F	P, T	Switch between mandatory and spontaneous breaths.
	Pressure-controlled synchronized intermittent mandatory ventilation + adaptive pressure ventilation	DC-IMV	Adaptive	T, P, F	P	T	P	If set tidal volume not achieved then adjust pressure limit.
	Adaptive support ventilation	DC-IMV	Adaptive	T, P, F	P	T, F	P	Each breath is pressure-limited but pressure limit and frequency adjusted according to lung mechanics to maintain minute ventilation and lung protective strategy.
	Spontaneous	PC-CSV	Setpoint	P, F	P	F	N/A	N/A
Siemens Medical–300	Pressure control	PC-CMV	Setpoint	T, P, F	P	T	N/A	N/A
	Volume control	VC-CMV	Setpoint	T, P, F	F, V	T	P	N/A
	Pressure regulated volume control	DC-CMV	Adaptive	T, P, F	P	T	N/A	If set tidal volume not achieved then adjust pressure limit.
	Volume support	DC-CSV	Adaptive	P, F	P	F	V, T	If set tidal volume not achieved then adjust pressure limit.
	Synchronized intermittent mandatory ventilation (volume control) + pressure support	VC-IMV	Setpoint	T, P, F	F, V, P	T, F	P, T	Switch between mandatory and spontaneous breaths.
	Synchronized intermittent mandatory ventilation (pressure control) + pressure support	PC-IMV	Setpoint	T, P, F	F, V, P	T, F	P, T	Switch between mandatory and spontaneous breaths.
	Pressure support/continuous positive airway pressure	PC-CSV	Setpoint	P, F	P	F, P	P, T	N/A
Thermo Respiratory Group – Bear 1000	Assist control mechanical ventilation	VC-CMV	Setpoint	T, P	F, V	V, T	P	N/A
	Assist control mechanical ventilation + pressure augment	DC-IMV	Setpoint	T, P	P, F	F, T	N/A	If tidal volume not met when flow decays to set value, switch from pressure limit to flow limit.
	Pressure control	PC-CMV	Setpoint	T, P	P	T	N/A	N/A
	Synchronized intermittent mandatory ventilation + pressure support	VC-IMV	Setpoint	T, P	F, V, P	V, T, F	P, T	Switch between mandatory and spontaneous breaths.
	Synchronized intermittent mandatory ventilation + pressure augment	DC-IMV	Setpoint	T, P, F	P	T, F	N/A	If tidal volume not met when flow decays to set value, switch from pressure limit to flow limit.
	Minimum minute volume	VC-IMV	Setpoint	T, P	F, V, P	V, T, F	P, T	If set minute ventilation not achieved by spontaneous breaths then trigger mandatory breaths.
	Pressure support/continuous positive airway pressure	PC-CSV	Setpoint	P, F	P	F	P, T	N/A

All 8 possible breathing patterns shown in Table 3 are represented here.

*Multiple limit and cycle variables account for mandatory breaths, mandatory breaths with inspiratory hold, and spontaneous breaths. A more detailed description could separate each case.

[†]Additional variables for alarm conditions.

VC = volume control. PC = pressure control. DC = dual control.

CMV = continuous mandatory ventilation. IMV = intermittent mandatory ventilation. CSV = continuous spontaneous ventilation.

T = time. P = pressure. V = volume. F = flow. N/A = not applicable. P_{max} = preset maximum pressure.

Box 39-4 • An Example Classification of a Ventilator Mode

Ventilator Name: Bear 1000
Mode Name: SIMV/CPAP (PSV)
Breathing Pattern: Volume-controlled IMV
Control Type: Hierarchical setpoint
Control Strategy:

Phase Variables for Mandatory Breaths

Trigger: pressure (sensitivity adjustable from 0.2 to 5.0 cm H_2O); time (rate adjustable from 0 to 120 cycles/minute)
Limit: flow (10 to 150 liters/minute); volume (whenever the inspiratory pause time is set >0)
Cycle: volume (tidal volume adjustable from 100 to 2000 mL); time (whenever the inspiratory pause time is set >0); pressure (when inspiratory pressure violates alarm setting)
Baseline: PEEP/CPAP level (adjustable from 0 to 50 cm H_2O)

Phase Variables for Spontaneous Breaths

Trigger: pressure (sensitivity adjustable from 0.2 to 5.0 cm H_2O)
Limit: pressure (0 to 65 cm H_2O above baseline)
Cycle: flow (when inspiratory flow decays to 30% of peak flow); time (when inspiration exceeds preset threshold)
Baseline: PEEP/CPAP level.adjustable from 0 to 50 cm H_2O

Operational Logic

If the patient triggers a breath after the start of a ventilatory period (the time equal to the reciprocal of the set ventilatory rate) then a mandatory breath is delivered. If subsequent breathing efforts are detected during the same period, then spontaneous breaths are delivered. If a breathing effort is not detected during a given ventilatory period, then a mandatory breath is time triggered at the beginning of the next period, and time triggered mandatory breaths will continue at the set rate until a breathing effort is detected and the sequence repeats.

sensitivity (trigger variable) and pressure limit (limit variable). In contrast, Volume Support (Siemens 300) is DC-CSV, which looks similar to Pressure Support on a graphics monitor, but the operator must set a tidal volume (cycle variable) in addition to sensitivity and pressure limit.

Specifying the phase variables and operational logic also helps to distinguish between modes with similar sounding names. For example, on the Bear 1000, Assist Control is VC-CMV but Assist Control + Pressure Augment is DC-IMV, about as different as two modes can get. Most clinicians think of "Assist Control" in traditional terms where every breath is mandatory and volume controlled (although the term says nothing about the control variable or the breathing sequence and only suggests that breaths may be either patient or machine triggered). How can adding Pressure Augment change not only the control type but also the breath sequence designation?

First of all it is necessary to have a clear understanding of the definitions of mandatory versus spontaneous breaths and phase variables (see definitions above). Next we need a description of the phase variables for these two modes:

1. Assist Control (without an inspiratory hold) is patient or time triggered, flow limited, and volume cycled. Because every breath is machine cycled, they are mandatory and thus the breath sequence is CMV.
2. Assist Control + Pressure Augment is patient or time triggered, pressure or flow limited, and flow or volume cycled. If a breath happens to be patient triggered and flow cycled, it is spontaneous. If it is patient or time triggered and volume cycled, it is mandatory. Because both types of breaths are possible, the pattern is IMV.

In a similar manner, specifying the phase variables and operational logic helps to distinguish among the four types of DC-IMV on the Dräger Evita 4 (see Table 39-2).

Table 39-2 gives a detailed description of all the modes found on some of the commonly used ventilators in the United States. It is a sort of Rosetta stone that allows us to interpret the different languages used by various manufacturers. This table has been simplified in that the phase variables for both mandatory and spontaneous breaths have been combined. Ideally, the mandatory and spontaneous phase variables should be separated for a complete and unambiguous description of a mode (see Box 39-4). The Puritan Bennett 840 illustrates one example of why it is important to separate mandatory from spontaneous breath descriptions. This ventilator offers both BiLevel mode and Pressure Control Synchronized Intermittent Mandatory Ventilation mode. Both are forms of PC-IMV and both use the same trigger, limit, and cycle variables and conditional logic (as shown in Table 39-2). If that were all the detail we had, it would seem that the modes were identical. The subtle difference becomes evident when we examine the phase variables for the spontaneous breaths in the two modes. During both BiLevel and Pressure Control Synchronized Intermittent Mandatory Ventilation, spontaneous breaths that occur between mandatory breaths are pressure or flow triggered, pressure limited, and flow cycled. Both modes also permit spontaneous breaths to occur during a mandatory breath cycle. However, during Pressure Control Synchronized Intermittent Mandatory Ventilation, these spontaneous breaths are only pressure triggered, have a factory-set pressure limit, and are flow cycled. In contrast, during BiLevel, spontaneous breaths that are initiated during a mandatory breath cycle are flow or pressure triggered, have an adjustable pressure limit (i.e., Pressure Support can be added), and are flow cycled.

Table 39-2 highlights two important facts about current ventilators. First, they offer far more complex modes than in the past, so understanding how they work is no trivial task. Manufacturers are throwing together combinations of features that are not only difficult to comprehend but also strain rational justification, often with no clinical data to support their efficacy. Second, there is absolutely no agreement among ventilator manufacturers when it comes to nomenclature. The names they create for modes are baffling. Table 39-2 shows 36 different names. And that is only for five ventilators.

Another utility of Table 39-2 is that it unmasks the identical modes. Notice all the different names for a basic mode like VC-CMV. Recognizing redundancies can have simple, practical applications. For example, a table appeared in a recent magazine entitled "Ventilators at a Glance." The table has ventilator models as column headings and specific features as row headings. Ventilators are thus quickly compared by the number of x's in each column, representing the number of features each model has. The table lists "Pressure Ventilation SIMV," along with "Airway Pressure Release Ventilation," yet the two are functionally the same mode. Also "Pressure Ventilation with Volume Guarantee" is listed as separate from "Adaptive Pressure Ventilation," yet they both are dual control. Also, it makes no sense to list a proprietary name for a specific ventilator (like Adaptive Support Ventilation) as a feature to be compared across all ventilators. Nomenclature problems like these limit the usefulness of such a table whose key function is to compare different ventilators by tallying features (i.e., wrong tally, wrong comparison).

▶ OUTPUT WAVEFORMS

To understand heart physiology we study electrocardiograms (ECGs) and blood pressure waveforms. In the same way, to understand ventilator-patient interaction, we must examine output waveforms. Of course, the output waveforms of interest during ventilatory support are pressure, volume, and flow. For each control variable, there are a limited number of waveforms produced by current ventilators. Basic waveforms are shown in Figure 39-9.

Because the waveforms in Figure 39-9 are models, they do not show the minor deviations or "noise" often seen during actual ventilator use. Such noise can be caused by many factors, including vibration and turbulence. These waveforms also do not show the effect of expiratory circuit resistance because this varies depending on the ventilator and type of circuit. Nor do the waveforms show the various indicators of problems with ventilator-patient synchrony (e.g., improper sensitivity setting and gas trapping), which are beyond the scope of this chapter. Lastly, one must remember that waveform appearances change when the time scale is altered. A faster sweep (shorter time scale) will tend to widen a given waveform, while a slower sweep speed (longer time scale) will compress the waveform.

Most ventilator waveforms are either rectangular, exponential, ramp, or sinusoidal in shape. Although a variety of subtypes are possible, we will describe only the most common. Waveforms are listed according to the shape of the control variable waveform. Any new waveforms produced by future ventilators can easily be accommodated by this system.

Pressure

Rectangular

Mathematically, a rectangular waveform is referred to as a step or instantaneous change in transrespiratory pressure from one value to another (Figure 39-9, *A*). In response, volume rises exponentially from zero to a steady state value equal to compliance times the change in airway pressure (i.e., PIP–PEEP). Inspiratory flow falls exponentially from a peak value (at the start of inspiration) equal to (PIP–PEEP) divided by resistance.

Exponential

Exponential pressure waveforms are common outputs of neonatal ventilators and also can be produced by adjusting the pressure rise control on some newer adult ventilators. The resulting pressure and volume waveforms can take on a variety of shapes ranging from an exponential rise (same shape as the volume waveform in Figure 39-9, *A*) to a linear rise (same shape as the volume waveform in Figure 39-9, *B*). In general, the flow waveform is similar to that seen in Figure 39-9, *A*, except that peak inspiratory flow is reached gradually rather than instantaneously (resulting in a rounded rather than peaked waveform), and peak flow is lower than with a rectangular pressure waveform.

Sinusoidal

As previously described, a sinusoidal pressure waveform can be created by attaching a piston to a rotating crank. In addition, a linear drive motor driven by a microprocessor can produce a sine wave pressure

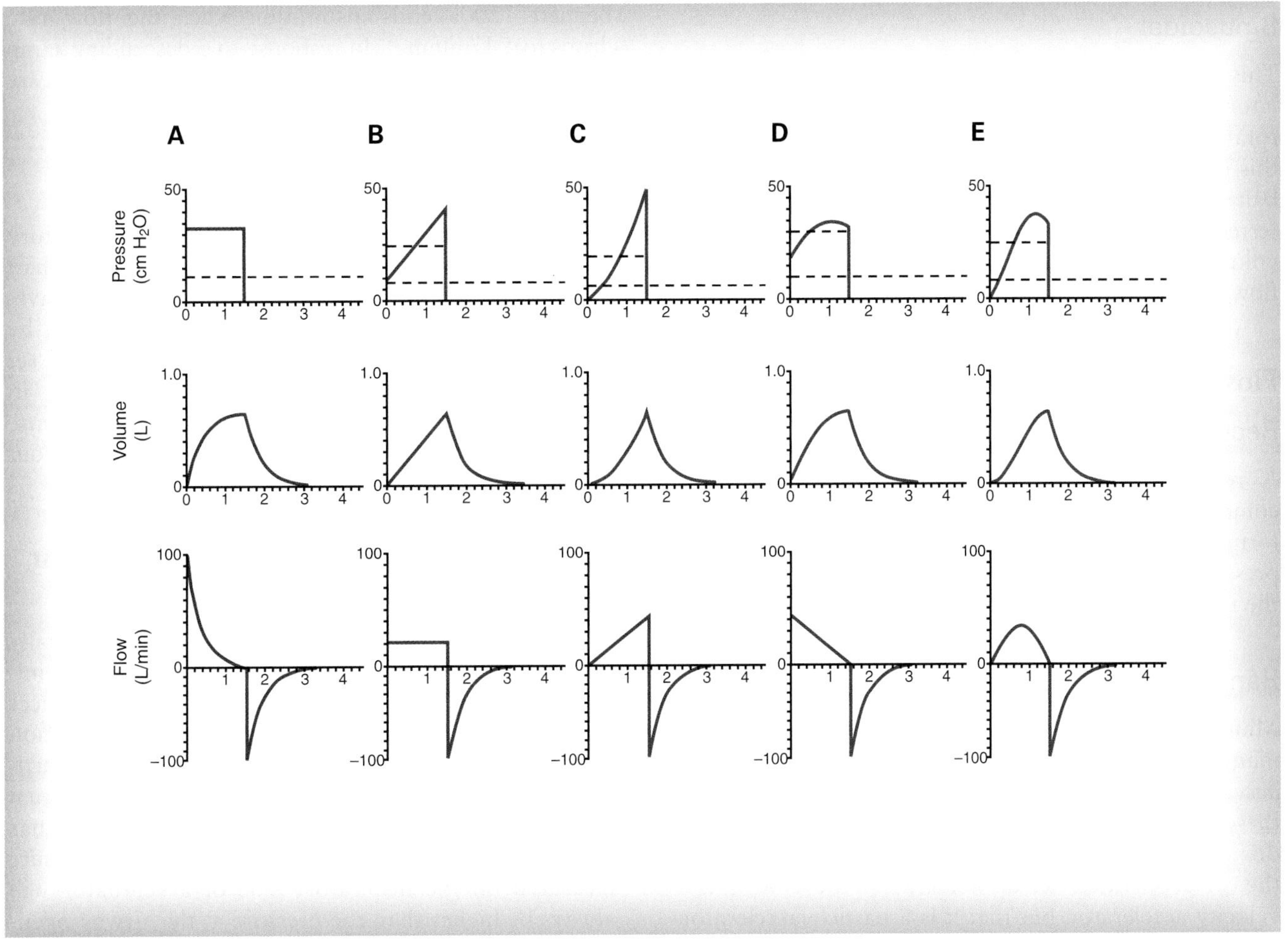

Figure 39-9
Model pressure, volume, and flow waveforms generated with a computer using the equation of motion. **A,** Pressure-controlled inspiration with a rectangular pressure waveform (identical to flow-controlled inspiration with an exponential decay flow waveform). **B,** Flow-controlled inspiration with a rectangular flow waveform (identical to volume-controlled inspiration with an ascending ramp volume waveform). **C,** Flow-controlled inspiration with an ascending ramp flow waveform. **D,** Flow-controlled inspiration with a descending ramp flow waveform. **E,** Flow-controlled inspiration with a sinusoidal flow waveform. The short dotted lines represent mean inspiratory pressure while the long dotted lines represent mean airway pressure (assuming zero PEEP). Note that for the rectangular pressure waveform in **A,** the mean inspiratory pressure is the same as the PIP. For all waveforms, V_T = 644 mL, compliance = 20 mL/cm H_2O, and resistance = 20 cm H_2O/L/s.

pattern. In response, the volume and flow waveforms are also sinusoidal, but they attain their peak values at different times (Figure 39-9, *E*).

Oscillating

Oscillating pressure waveforms can take on a variety of shapes, from sinusoidal to ramp (SensorMedics 3100 Oscillator), to roughly triangular (Infrasonics Star Oscillator). The distinguishing feature of a ventilator classified as an oscillator is that it can generate negative transrespiratory pressure. That is, if the mean airway pressure is set equal to atmospheric pressure, then the airway pressure waveform oscillates above and below zero.

If the pressure waveform is sinusoidal, volume and flow will also be sinusoidal but out of phase with each other (i.e., their peak values occur at different times).

Volume

Ramp

Volume controllers that produce an ascending ramp waveform (that is, the Bennett MA-1) produce a linear rise in volume from zero at the start of inspiration to the peak value, or set tidal volume, at end-inspiration (Figure 39-9, *B*). In response, the flow waveform is rectangular. The pressure waveform rises instantaneously from zero to a value equal to resistance times flow at the start of inspiration. From here it rises linearly to its peak value (PIP) equal to (Tidal Volume × Elastance) + (Flow × Resistance).

Sinusoidal

This volume waveform is most often produced by ventilators whose drive mechanism is a piston attached to a rotating crank (e.g., Emerson). The output waveform of this type of ventilator can be approximated by the first half of a cosine curve, whose shape in this case is referred to as a *sigmoidal curve* (Figure 39-9, *E*). Because volume is sinusoidal during inspiration, pressure and flow are also sinusoidal.

Flow

Rectangular

A rectangular flow waveform is perhaps the most common output (Figure 39-9, *B*). When the flow waveform is rectangular, volume is a ramp waveform and pressure is a step followed by a ramp as described for the ramp volume waveform.

Ramp

Many respiratory care practitioners (and ventilator manufacturers) refer to ramp waveforms as either *accelerating* or *decelerating* flow patterns. But the use of these terms is usually inappropriate. If a car slows, we do not say that its velocity decelerates, we say that the car decelerates. We do not say that a cyclotron is a velocity accelerator, but that it is a particle accelerator. The rate of change of position of an object is the velocity of the object; analogously, the rate of change of volume is flow. The rate of change of velocity of an object is the acceleration of the object; likewise, the rate of change of flow is the acceleration of volume, *not* the acceleration of flow. So if we want to say that flow changes, we should simply talk about an increasing flow or a decreasing flow (or an accelerating volume or a decelerating volume), *not* an accelerating flow or a decelerating flow.

Ascending Ramp. A true ascending ramp waveform starts at zero and increases linearly to the peak value (Figure 39-9, *C*). Ventilator flow waveforms are usually truncated. Inspiration starts with an initial instantaneous flow (e.g., the Bear-5 starts inspiration at 50% of the set peak flow). Flow then increases linearly to the set peak flow rate. In response to an ascending ramp flow waveform, the pressure and volume waveforms are exponential with a concave upward shape.

Descending Ramp. A true descending ramp waveform starts at the peak value and decreases linearly to zero (Figure 39-9, *D*). Ventilator flow waveforms are usually truncated; inspiratory flow rate decreases linearly from the set peak flow until it reaches some arbitrary threshold where flow drops immediately to zero (e.g., the Puritan Bennett 7200a ends inspiration when the flow rate drops to 5 L/minute). In response to a descending ramp flow waveform, the pressure and volume waveforms are exponential with a concave downward shape.

Sinusoidal

Some ventilators offer a mode in which the inspiratory flow waveform approximates the shape of the first half of a sine wave (Figure 39-9, *E*). As with the ramp waveform, ventilators often truncate the sine waveform by starting and ending flow at some percentage of the set peak flow rather than start and end at zero flow. In response to a sinusoidal flow waveform, the pressure and volume waveforms will also be sinusoidal but out of phase with each other.

Effects of Calibration Errors and the Patient Circuit

The pressure, volume, and flow the patient actually receives are never precisely the same as what the clinician sets on the ventilator. Sometimes these differences are caused by instrument inaccuracies or calibration error. In addition, the patient delivery circuit contributes to discrepancies between the desired and actual patient values. This is because the patient circuit has its own compliance and resistance. Thus, the pressure measured on the inspiratory side of a ventilator will always be higher than the pressure at the airway opening due to patient circuit resistance. In addition, the volume and flow coming out of the ventilator will exceed that delivered to the patient because of the compliance of the patient circuit.

▶ CLINICAL APPLICATION OF MODES

Volume Control Versus Pressure Control

Figure 39-10 illustrates the important variables for *volume control* modes. It shows that the primary variable we wish to control is the patient's minute ventilation. A particular ventilator may allow the operator to set minute ventilation directly. More frequently, minute ventilation is adjusted by means of a set tidal volume and frequency. Tidal volume is a function of the set inspiratory flow and the set inspiratory time. Inspiratory time is affected by the set frequency and, if applicable, the set I:E ratio. The mathematical relations among all these variables are shown in Table 39-3.

With *pressure control* modes, the goal is also to maintain adequate minute ventilation. However (as the equation of motion shows), when pressure is controlled, tidal volume and thus minute ventilation are determined not only by the ventilator's pressure settings but also by

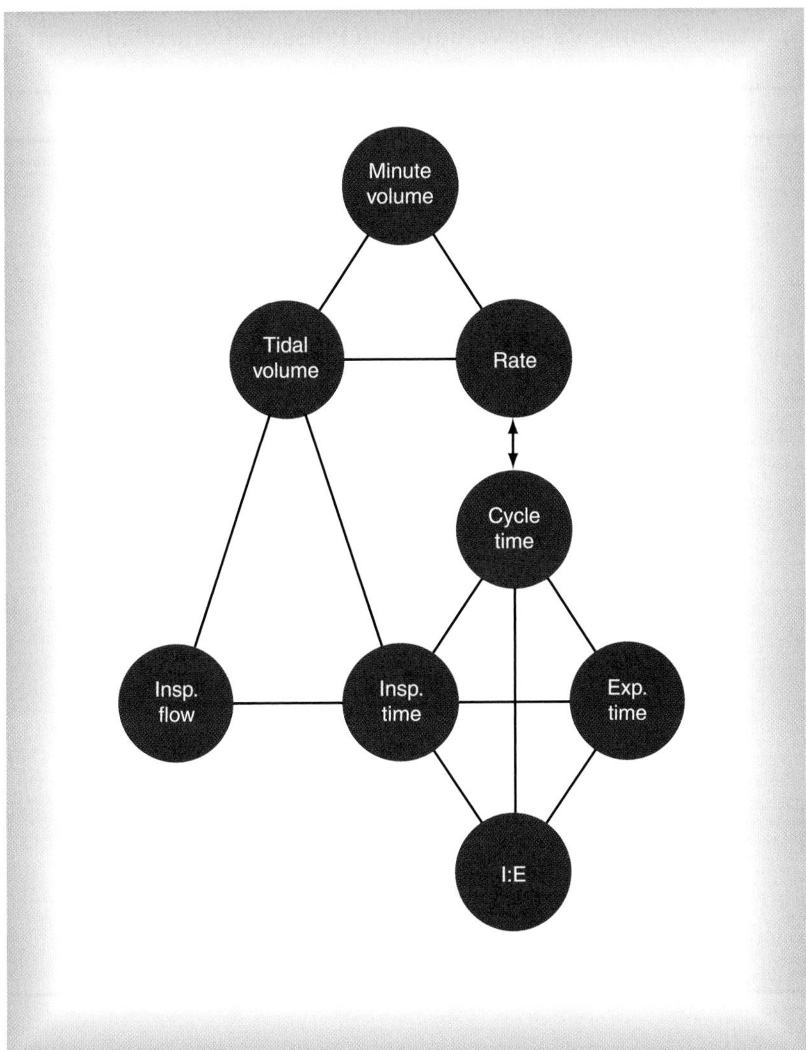

Figure 39-10
Influence diagram for volume-controlled ventilation. Variables are connected by straight lines such that if any two are known, the third can be calculated (see Table 39-3).

the elastance and resistance of the patient's respiratory system. This makes minute ventilation (and hence gas exchange) less stable in pressure control modes than volume control modes. Figure 39-11 shows the important variables for *pressure control* modes. Tidal volume is not set on the ventilator. It is the result of the pressure settings and the patient's lung mechanics as well as the inspiratory time. On some ventilators, the speed with which the PIP is achieved (i.e., the pressure rise time) is adjustable. That adjustment affects the shape of the pressure waveform and thus the mean airway pressure. Mean airway pressure is important because, within reasonable limits, as the mean airway pressure rises, arterial oxygen tension rises. As shown in Figure 39-2, mean airway pressure is higher for pressure controlled modes than volume controlled modes (at the same tidal volume) due to the differences in the shapes of the airway pressure waveforms.

Continuous Mandatory Ventilation (CMV)

CMV (sometimes referred to as *Assist/Control*) is a mode of ventilation in which total ventilatory support is provided by the mechanical ventilator. All breaths are mandatory and delivered by the ventilator at a preset volume or pressure, breath rate, and inspiratory time.

If the patient has spontaneous respiratory efforts, the ventilator will deliver a patient triggered breath. If patient efforts are absent, the ventilator delivers time triggered breaths. It is important for the clinician to set an appropriate trigger level and flow rate for the patient in this mode of ventilation. There is a potential for the ventilator to autotrigger when the trigger level is set too sensitive. As a result, hyperventilation, air trapping, and patient anxiety often ensue. However, if the trigger level is not sensitive enough, the ventilator will not respond to the patient's inspiratory efforts, which results in an increased work of breathing.

Table 39-3 ▶▶ Equations Relating the Important Parameters for Volume and Pressure-Controlled Ventilation

Mode	Parameter	Symbol	Equation
Volume controlled	Tidal volume (L)	V_T	$V_T = \dot{V}_E \div f$ $V_T = \overline{V}_I \times T_I$
	Mean inspiratory flow (L/minute)	$\overline{V}_I$	$\overline{V}_I = 60 \times V_T \div T_I$ $\overline{V}_I = \frac{\dot{V}_E \times TCT}{T_I}$
Pressure controlled	Tidal volume (L) VT	VT	$V_T = \Delta P \times C \times (1 - e^{-t/\tau})$
	Instantaneous inspiratory flow (L/minute)	$\dot{V}_I$	$\dot{V}_I = \left(\frac{\Delta P}{R}\right) e^{-t/\tau}$
	Pressure gradient (cm H_2O)	ΔP	$\Delta P = PIP - PEEP$
Both modes	Exhaled minute ventilation (L/minute)	$\dot{V}_E$	$\dot{V}_E = V_T \times f$
	Total cycle time or ventilatory period (seconds)	TCT	$TCT = T_I + T_E = 60 \div f$
	I:E ratio	I:E	$I : E = T_I : T_E = \frac{T_I}{T_E}$
	Time constant (seconds)	τ	$\tau = R \times C$
	Resistance (cm H_2O/L/second)	R	$R = \frac{\Delta P}{\Delta \dot{V}}$
	Compliance (L/cm H_2O)	C	$C = \frac{\Delta V}{\Delta P}$
	Elastance	E	$E = \frac{1}{C}$
	Mean airway pressure (cm H_2O)	$\overline{P}_{aw}$	$P_{aw} = \left(\frac{1}{TCT}\right) \int_{t=0}^{t=TCT} P_{aw} dt$
Primary variables	Pressure (cm H_2O)	P	
	Volume (L)	V	
	Flow (cm H_2O/L/s)	$\dot{V}$	
	Time (seconds)	τ	
	Inspiratory time (seconds)	T_I	
	Expiratory time (seconds)	T_E	
	Frequency (breaths per minute)	f	
	Base of natural logarithm (≈ 2.72)	e	

There may be an occasion where all attempts to optimize patient comfort, reduce work of breathing, and achieve the goals of this mode of ventilation are futile. In the case where this mode is poorly tolerated and spontaneous triggering is counterproductive to the goals set for a particular patient, sedation or paralysis may be required. These agents may be used to minimize patient effort and normalize the work of breathing.

Volume Control

Indications. Volume controlled CMV is indicated when a precise minute ventilation or blood gas parameter, such as $Pa{CO_2}$, is therapeutically essential to the care of patients with normal lung mechanics.[14] Theoretically, volume control (with a constant inspiratory flow) results in a more even distribution of ventilation (compared to pressure control) among lung units with different time constants where the units have equal resistances but unequal compliances (e.g., acute respiratory distress syndrome [ARDS]).[15,16]

During volume controlled CMV, changes in the patient's lung mechanics result in changes in airway pressure. A reduction in lung compliance and/or an increase in resistance will cause higher peak airway pressures (see Equation 39-1).[17] Care should also be taken when setting the inspiratory flow. Avoid setting a flow that fails to match patient needs or exceeds their demand. An insufficient flow rate would result in an imposed increase in the patient's work of breathing and a concomitant increase in oxygen consumption. The inspiratory phase may be prematurely shortened if the set inspiratory flow exceeds patient demands. Meticulous patient monitoring and use of volume control CMV allow the clinician to achieve precise and predictable physiological results.

Example. Perhaps the most common application of this mode of ventilation is its use to facilitate therapeutic hyperventilation in the patient with traumatic brain injury. Patients are often sedated to reduce oxygen consumption, minimize the patient's response to noxious stimuli, and ventilator asynchrony. VC-CMV can achieve fairly precise regulation of $Pa{CO_2}$ and support efforts to alleviate intracranial hypertension and reduce the likelihood of secondary complications from cerebral ischemia.[18]

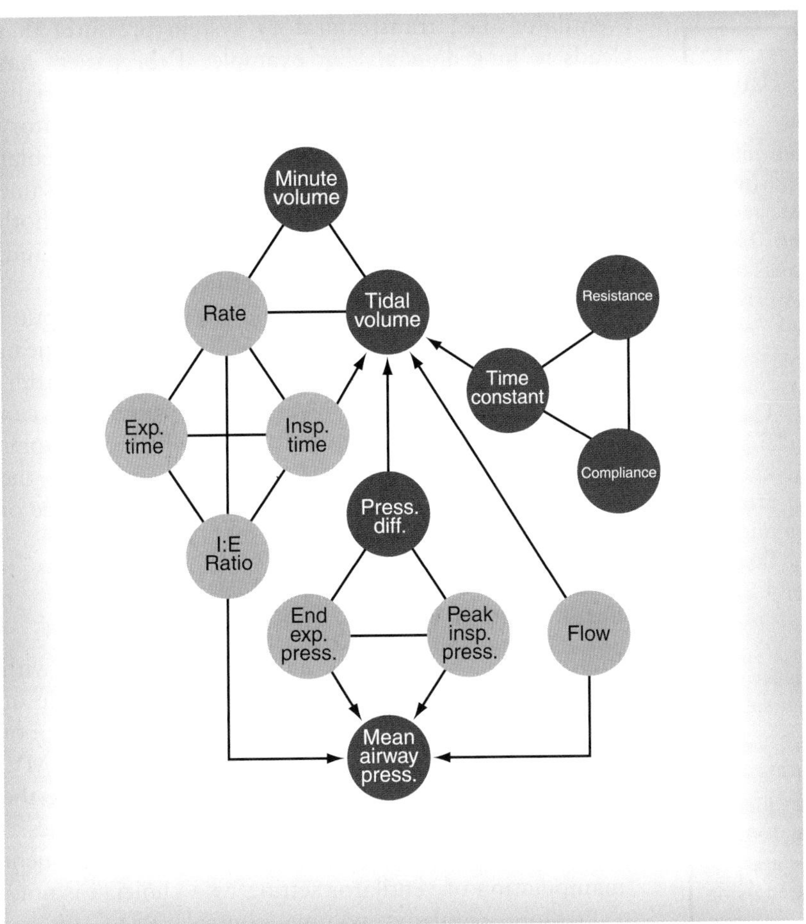

Figure 39-11

Influence diagram for pressure-controlled ventilation. Variables are connected by straight lines such that if any two are known, the third can be calculated (see Table 39-3). Arrows represent relations that are more complex. Shaded circles represent variables that are directly controlled by ventilator settings. Open circles show indirectly controlled variables.

Pressure Control

Indications. Pressure controlled CMV is indicated when adequate oxygenation has been difficult to achieve in other modes of ventilation.[19,20] Theoretically, pressure control (with a constant inspiratory pressure) results in a more even distribution of ventilation (compared to volume control) among lung units with different time constants when units have equal compliances but unequal resistances (e.g., status asthmaticus).[15] The instability of tidal volume caused by airway leaks can be minimized by using pressure-controlled ventilation rather than volume controlled ventilation. Increased tidal volume stability may lead to better gas exchange and lower risk of pulmonary volutrauma.[21]

Use of a rectangular pressure waveform opens alveoli earlier in the inspiratory phase during PC-CMV and results in a higher mean airway pressure than VC-CMV with a rectangular flow waveform, allowing more time for oxygenation to occur.[22] As with VC-CMV, physiological outcomes, such as gas exchange, are more predictable than modes that provide partial ventilatory support. In PC-CMV however, inspiratory flow is not a parameter set by the clinician. It is variable and dependent on patient effort and lung mechanics, thus improving patient comfort and patient-ventilator synchrony. However, as lung mechanics and/or patient effort change, volume delivery (tidal volume and minute ventilation) changes, leading to poor control of blood gases.

Because tidal volume is not directly controlled, the pressure gradient (PIP – PEEP) is the primary parameter used to alter the breath size and hence carbon dioxide tensions. Typically the PIP is adjusted to provide the patient with a tidal volume within the desired range. PIPs may be adjusted to achieve a tidal volume of 5 to 7 mL/kg.[23] As with VC-CMV, the mandatory breath rate set by the clinician is dependent upon the presence of ventilatory muscle activity and the severity of lung disease. When higher mandatory breath rates are needed (30 to 60 breaths per minute), it is essential for the clinician to provide a sufficient expiratory time and prevent air-trapping.

As long as lung mechanics and patient effort remain constant, the volume and peak flow delivered to the patient will remain unchanged.[24] Should a decrease in patient effort, decrease in compliance, or increase in resistance occur, less volume will be delivered for the preset pressure for each breath. Conversely, improvements in patient effort and mechanics can dramatically

MINI CLINI

Determining Appropriate Ventilator Rate

PROBLEM

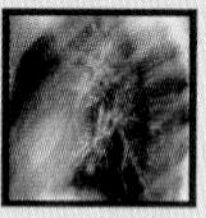

A 6-year-old child with traumatic brain injury was intubated in the emergency department with a 6.0 endotracheal tube and transferred to you in the pediatric intensive care unit. He is paralyzed and sedated. His current ventilator settings are:

Mode: VC-CMV
Tidal volume: 250 mL
Frequency: 15 breaths per minute
FIO_2: 1.0

His pulse oximeter displays 97% and his end-tidal CO_2 monitor is reading 38. His weight is estimated at 25 kg. His end-tidal CO_2 is stable and within ±1 mm Hg of arterial blood gas value for $PaCO_2$. The clinical goal is to minimize intracranial pressure. Because intracranial blood flow is inversely proportional to $PaCO_2$, we would like to increase ventilation to maintain a $PaCO_2$ of about 27 mm Hg.

Make appropriate ventilator changes to achieve the target $PaCO_2$.

DISCUSSION

The current tidal volume is already large at 10 mL/kg. The increase in ventilation must come by increasing frequency. Because the patient is paralyzed, the ventilation level is controlled by the set frequency and thus the $PaCO_2$ is predictable. The new frequency required is calculated using the following equation*:

$$required\ frequency = \frac{current\ P_aCO_2 \times current\ frequency}{desired\ P_sCO_2}$$

$$required\ frequency = \frac{38\ torr \times 15\ breaths/minute}{27\ torr} = 21\ breaths/minute$$

*Wojciechowski WV. Respiratory Care Sciences, Albany: Delmar Publishers, 1996:27-29.

increase the volume delivery to the patient in this mode. Close tidal volume monitoring is required to avoid ventilator-induced hypoventilation or volutrauma.

Example. Perhaps the most common use of PC-CMV, has been in patients with ARDS whose oxygenation status has failed to improve with the application of VC-CMV. Pressure-controlled ventilation is often touted as being superior to volume controlled ventilation because it results in lower peak airway pressure. But this concept is often misunderstood. Peak airway pressure during volume control is higher because of the resistive pressure drop across the endotracheal tube and upper airways (i.e., Flow × Resistance in the equation of motion). However, it is transalveolar pressure (Alveolar Pressure – Pleural Pressure), not airway pressure displayed by the ventilator (i.e., transrespiratory system pressure) that leads to lung damage. For example, if the patient has severely decreased chest wall compliance or a partially blocked endotracheal tube, the peak transrespiratory system pressures may be very high, but the transalveolar pressures might be normal. If tidal volumes are the same for pressure control and volume control, then both would produce the same peak alveolar pressure and, presumably, the same risk for overdistension.

The patient's cardiac index and oxygen consumption should be closely monitored as well. The higher mean airway pressures may impair cardiac output. Additionally, PC-CMV with inverse ratio ventilation can lead to the development of auto-PEEP which can impair venous return, compromise oxygen delivery to the tissues, and result in air-trapping and the occurrence of volutrauma.[25]

Dual Control

Indications. DC-CMV is indicated in patients with moderate to severe lung disease, in which unstable or changing pulmonary mechanics make precise control of minute ventilation difficult to achieve.[26] In DC-CMV, the ventilator adjusts the pressure limit (and hence the tidal volume) in response to changes in lung mechanics.[27] Although patient monitoring is still necessary, frequent manipulation of ventilator setting by a clinician is not.

Pressure regulated volume control (PRVC) is an example of a DC-CMV mode. See Table 39-2 for a complete listing. When a clinician places a patient in PRVC, a tidal volume, breath rate, and maximum (i.e., alarm) pressure limit are operator set. Once connected to the ventilator, the patient-ventilator interaction that occurs in the first few breaths is critical. Initially, the ventilator calculates a total system compliance. On the succeeding three or four breaths, the ventilator monitors the peak airway pressures and expiratory tidal volume. The ventilator then determines the pressure limit necessary to deliver the clinician set "target" tidal volume, for the given total system compliance. (We say "target" because the ventilator aims to deliver it, over the course of several breaths, but may not hit the mark if the maximum pressure limit is set too low.) The patient-ventilator interaction is monitored on a breath-by-breath basis. Should the patient's lung compliance improve (or patient effort increase), the ventilator delivers subsequent mandatory breaths at a lower pressure limit to maintain the target tidal volume. This reduces the risk of alveolar overdistension and volutrauma. Conversely, the ventilator responds to worsening pulmonary compliance (or decreasing patient effort) by increasing the pressure limit until the tidal volume is achieved. In PRVC, the ventilator makes pressure limit changes in small increments, 3 to 4 cm H_2O per breath, and will not exceed the maximum pressure limit set by the operator.

MINI CLINI

Using Pressure Control Ventilation

PROBLEM

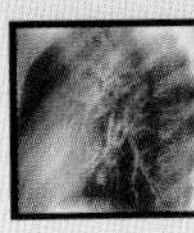

You are caring for a 10-year-old patient with ARDS. The patient has no respiratory effort. Current ventilator settings are:

Mode: VC-CMV
Tidal volume: 350 mL

Frequency: 25 breaths per minute
PEEP: 14 cm H_2O
F_{IO_2}: 1.0
PIPs monitored on the ventilator: 60-70 cm H_2O
Mean airway pressure: 28-30 cm H_2O
Plateau pressure: 40 cm H_2O

An arterial blood gas is obtained, which reveals:

pH: 7.28
P_{CO_2}: 41 torr
P_{O_2}: 50 torr

The physician would like to employ pressure control ventilation.

Select appropriate initial settings in PC-CMV mode to maintain the current minute ventilation.

DISCUSSION

Initial ventilator setting would be as follows:

Ventilator frequency, PEEP, and F_{IO_2}: the same.
Frequency: 25 breaths per minute
PEEP: 14 cm H_2O
F_{IO_2}: 1.0

To keep the minute ventilation constant, we need to set the PIP high enough to deliver the same tidal volume as in volume control (350 mL).

Step 1: Calculate the patient's respiratory system compliance:

$$\text{static compliance} = \frac{\text{tidal volume}}{\text{plateau pressure} - \text{PEEP}}$$

$$= \frac{350\ mL}{40\ cm\ H_2O - 14\ cm\ H_2O}$$

$$= 13.5\ mL \cdot cm\ H_2O^{-1}$$

Step 2: Calculate the pressure limit in PC-CMV mode to achieve the target tidal volume. Because the pressure limit is measured relative to PEEP on this ventilator, the equation is:

$$pressure\ limit = \frac{desired\ tidal\ volume}{compliance}$$

$$= \frac{350\ mL}{13.5\ mL/cm\ H_2O}$$

$$= 25.9\ cm\ H_2O \approx 26\ cm\ H_2O$$

Notice that a shortcut is to realize that the required pressure limit is the plateau pressure on VC-CMV. The PIP (relative to atmospheric pressure) will thus be 40 cm H_2O.

MINI CLINI

PIP Response to Surfactant Therapy

PROBLEM

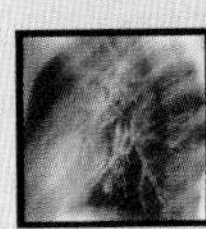

A 27-week-old, 1700-gram infant with severe RDS is intubated and placed on the Siemans Servo 300 ventilator in the pressure regulated volume control mode.

The nurse noted that 10 minutes after surfactant administration, the PIP is 10 cm H_20 higher than what she documented before surfactant administration. She has been sitting by the bedside charting and knows that no ventilator setting changes have been made. She believes the ventilator is malfunctioning.

DISCUSSION

You confirmed that the desired tidal volume is still being delivered. You explain to the nurse that pressure regulated volume control is a form of dual control ventilation. In this case the operator sets the desired V_T and the ventilator adjusts the pressure limit, based on the patient's compliance. Usually after surfactant administration, compliance drops transiently so the pressure limit is automatically increased to maintain a constant V_T.

Later, after compliance improves, the pressure limit will be automatically adjusted down.

These automatic ventilator responses to changes in a patient's lung mechanics minimizes the risk of ventilator-induced hypoventilation or volutrauma. The outcome of this is a stable or consistent minute ventilation and enhanced patient comfort.

Example. DC-CMV has been used in infants with respiratory distress syndrome (RDS) after instillation of artificial surfactant. Rapidly changing pulmonary mechanics from surfactant administration are associated with complications such as pulmonary air leaks, intraventricular hemorrhage, and bronchopulmonary dysplasia. DC-CMV responds to changes in a patient's lung mechanics and results in a lower incidence of these common complications.[26,27]

Intermittent Mandatory Ventilation (IMV)

As a partial support mode, IMV allows or requires the patient to sustain some of the work of breathing. The level of mechanical support needed is dependent upon the specific physiological process causing the need for mechanical ventilation, presence and/or degree of ventilatory muscle weakness, and presence and severity of lung disease. In this mode mandatory breaths are delivered at a set rate. Between the mandatory breaths, the patient can breathe spontaneously at his or her own tidal volume and rate. Breaths can occur separately (e.g., IMV) or breaths can be superimposed on each other (e.g., spontaneous breaths superimposed on mandatory breaths, as in BiLevel or APRV); or mandatory breaths superimposed on spontaneous breaths, as in high frequency ventilation administered during spontaneous breathing. Spontaneous breaths may be assisted (e.g., Pressure Support) or unassisted (e.g., CPAP/PEEP).

When the mandatory breath is patient triggered, it is commonly referred to as synchronized IMV (SIMV). With SIMV, the ventilator will deliver the mandatory breath in synchrony with the patient's inspiratory effort. If no spontaneous efforts occur, the ventilator will deliver a time-triggered breath.

Because spontaneous breaths decrease pleural pressure, ventilatory support with IMV usually results in a lower mean intrathoracic pressure than CMV, which can result in a higher cardiac output.[28]

When used to wean a patient from mechanical ventilation, the intent of IMV is to provide respiratory muscle rest during the mandatory breaths and exercise during spontaneous breaths. However, studies have demonstrated that IMV weaning prolongs the duration of mechanical ventilation when compared to pressure support ventilation and spontaneous breathing trials.[29,30] Since there are a variety of factors that determine the need for ventilatory support, there is not one weaning method that will benefit all mechanically ventilated patients.

Volume Control

Indications. VC-IMV is indicated for patients with relatively normal lung function recovering from sedation or rapidly reversing respiratory failure.[31]

As the patient is capable of providing more work, the level of ventilatory support can be decreased accordingly. Weaning from VC-IMV usually involves the gradual reduction of the mandatory breath rate, while maintaining a constant tidal volume. Frequency is decreased rather than tidal volume because the patient's spontaneous breaths tend to be shallow at first, and relatively large mandatory breaths tend to prevent atelectasis and preserve oxygenation. Another reason is that as the patient's spontaneous efforts begin to support a normal tidal volume it would cause an increased work of breathing if the ventilator delivered small breaths. As the breath rate is reduced, the patient assumes more of the load. When the mandatory breath rate has been reduced enough (typically less than or equal to four breaths per minute) the patient is assessed for either a spontaneous breathing trial or extubation.

Example. VC-IMV is usually selected for patients with neuromuscular disorders, such as Guillain-Barré syndrome. Typically, normal lung function and an intact ventilatory drive characterize this patient population. As the disease progresses, ascending muscle weakness eventually affects the patient's ventilatory muscles. Mechanical ventilation is considered when it is difficult for the patient to sustain tidal volumes and minute ventilation. The degree of support is dependent upon the patient's inherent muscle strength. Large tidal volumes (12 to 15 mL/kg) and high peak flows (> 60 L/minute) may be needed to alleviate dyspnea and maximize patient comfort.[32] As respiratory muscle function improves, mandatory breath support can be reduced.

Pressure Control

Indications. PC-IMV is indicated when preservation of the patient's spontaneous efforts is important, but adequate oxygenation has been difficult to achieve with

MINI CLINI

Weaning With Pressure Support

PROBLEM

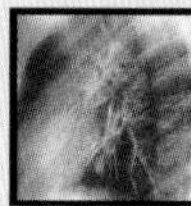

You are asked to wean a 37-year-old patient with Guillain-Barré syndrome from the ventilator. He is currently on a partial support mode of ventilation (VC-IMV).

Current ventilator settings are as follows:

Tidal volume: 1.2 L
Frequency: 8 breaths per minute
Inspiratory flow rate: 70 L/minute
FIO_2: 45
Pressure support : 25 cm H_2O

He has spontaneous respiratory efforts, with a total breath rate of 14 breaths per minute. His minute ventilation is 16.8 L/minute.

What set ventilator parameter would you change to wean this patient?

DISCUSSION

Step 1: Assessment of the patient's current ventilatory status.

The patient's minute ventilation is 16.8 L/minute.

9.8 L/minute is provided by the IMV rate (1.2 L/breath × 8 breaths per minute).

Spontaneous V_T

Minute ventilation = (Set V_T × IMV frequency) + (Spontaneous V_T × Spontaneous breath rate)

$$16.8 \text{ L/minute} = (1.2 \times 8) + (\text{Spontaneous } V_T \times \text{Spontaneous breath rate})$$
$$16.8 \text{ L/minute} = 9.6 \text{ L/minute} + (\text{Spontaneous } V_T \times 6)$$
$$16.8 \text{ L/minute} - 9.6 \text{ L/minute} = \text{Spontaneous } V_T \times 6$$
$$7.2 \text{ L/minute} = \text{Spontaneous } V_T \times 6$$
$$\frac{7.2 \text{ L/minute}}{6 \text{ breaths per minute}} = \text{Spontaneous } V_T$$
$$1.2 \text{ L/ breath} = \text{Spontaneous } V_T$$

The level of pressure support is providing tidal volumes identical to that provided on mandatory breaths. Reducing the frequency would not facilitate weaning, since it would not affect minute ventilation. Instead, the level of pressure support should be reduced, to allow the patient to assume more of the load.

volume control modes.[33] PC-IMV has been traditionally associated with mechanical ventilation of infants not only because of their oxygenation problems, but also because traditionally it had been difficult to control tidal volumes at such small values.[34]

Liberation from this mode involves the gradual reduction of the PIP, as well as the mandatory breath rate. As lung compliance improves, adjustments in PIP and set mandatory breath rate are critical to prevent volutrauma and hyperventilation.

Example. Perhaps the most familiar scenario is the application of PC-IMV in premature infants with RDS. Initially, because of a noncompliant lung, compliant chest wall, and poor respiratory effort, the infant may require a relatively high PIP and mandatory breath rate to achieve acceptable tidal volumes and acid base balance. Mandatory breath rates are set to provide adequate minute ventilation.

With PC-IMV, the infant can breathe spontaneously between or during the mandatory breaths, at his or her own rate and tidal volume. Liberation from this mode of partial support ventilation involves the gradual reduction of the PIP, as well as the mandatory breath rate. As the infant's lung compliance improves and spontaneous ventilatory efforts become more effective, lower PIPs and mandatory breath rates are needed to deliver adequate minute ventilation.

Dual Control

Indications. As a partial support mode of ventilation, DC-IMV is useful in stabilizing tidal volume on spontaneous and mandatory breaths in patients with changing pulmonary mechanics or inconsistent respiratory efforts.[35] The key point with this mode of ventilation, as with any partial ventilatory support mode, is to allow spontaneous breaths to occur.

In DC-IMV the clinician sets the mandatory breath rate, maximum inspiratory pressure limit, and target tidal volume (and for some dual control modes, inspiratory flow). In the case of volume assured pressure support (VAPS) or pressure augment (PA), Branson and colleagues[36] suggest setting the level of pressure support equal to the plateau pressure obtained during a mandatory or controlled breath at the desired tidal volume for the patient.

Caution should be taken with setting the peak flow for dual control within breaths. As with any volume control mode, the clinician should adjust the flow to match the patient's inspiratory demands. Care should be taken to ensure appropriate inspiratory times and I:E ratios are achieved. Failure to do so, on mandatory breaths, will result in flows that fail to meet or exceed a patient's demands. An increased work of breathing and concomitant increase in oxygen consumption will result.[37] Furthermore, inappropriate flow settings will defeat the benefits of dual control (i.e., if flow is too high, the breath is essentially volume controlled and if too low, inspiratory time may be prolonged).

It is important for the clinician to take the time to carefully select and set the ventilator parameters. The outcome of these efforts is improved patient-ventilator synchrony, consistent tidal volumes, and a decreased work of breathing.

Example. A clinical application of this mode of ventilation would be in acute respiratory failure in the patient with severe airway obstruction. In VC-IMV the constant inspiratory flow (operator set) may fail to match a patient's inspiratory demands and lead to patient-ventilator asynchrony. Asynchrony may lead to

MINI CLINI

Using the Star Sync Feature

PROBLEM

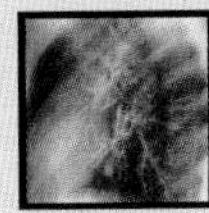

You are assigned to the NICU and have successfully intubated an infant diagnosed with respiratory distress syndrome (RDS). You need to choose a ventilator to provide PC-IMV. There are two ventilators remaining in the equipment room, both are Infant Star ventilators. However, one ventilator has the Star Sync option, which you choose. The physician would like you to explain how the Star Sync feature works and why you chose it.

DISCUSSION

The Star Sync option provides a means for the patient to trigger the ventilator and thereby to synchronize mandatory breaths. This is accomplished by taping a skin sensor, consisting of a thin, plastic-covered foam rubber disk, to the upper portion of the infant's diaphragm. The sensor is connected by small bore tubing to a pressure transducer. The sensor is compressed each time a diaphragmatic movement occurs. Each time the sensor is compressed a signal is transmitted to the Star Sync unit, and inspiration is triggered.

You selected a ventilator that could synchronize IMV breaths because studies in premature infants with RDS have demonstrated that mechanical breaths synchronized with an infant's spontaneous breathing efforts results in larger, more stable tidal volumes,* and increased and more consistent tidal volumes during synchronized intermittent mandatory ventilation in newborn infants.† Other studies have demonstrated an improvement in oxygenation and risk of the complications of mechanical ventilation, such as a lower incidence of severe intraventricular hemorrhage and bronchopulmonary dysplasia when compared to infants ventilated with conventional IMV.‡

*Bernstein G, Heldt GP, Mannino FL. *Acta Paediatr.* 1997 Nov; 86(11):1275-6.

†Bernstein G, Heldt GP, Mannino FL. *Am J Respir Crit Care Med.* 150(5):1444-8, 1994.

‡Chen JY, Ling UP, Chen JH: Comparison of synchronized and conventional intermittent mandatory ventilation in neonates, *Acta Paediatr Jpn* 39(5):578,1997.

MINI CLINI

Use of Time Constants

PROBLEM

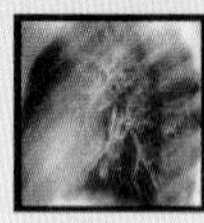

A 47-year-old patient is being ventilated for acute respiratory failure. On VC-CMV, the patient is agitated, tachypneic, and generating enough auto-PEEP to cause the high pressure alarm to sound intermittently. Bedside measurements show respiratory system resistance of 46 cm $H_2O \cdot s \cdot L^{-1}$ and compliance of 23 mL/cm H_2O. The patient is switched to a Hamilton Galileo ventilator in the Adaptive Support mode. This is a form of DC-IMV where mandatory breaths are time triggered, pressure limited, and time cycled. Spontaneous breaths are patient triggered, pressure limited, and flow cycled. Ventilator-patient synchrony improves, but the attending physician thinks the expiratory time (2.5 seconds) still seems to be short enough to cause gas trapping in this patient. You consult the operator's manual and discover that the ventilator will not allow the expiratory time to fall below two time constants. The physician asks you to explain the significance of this and check that the ventilator is operating properly.

Explain what a time constant is and how it relates to gas trapping. Calculate the minimum expiratory time the ventilator will allow for this patient and assess whether gas trapping may be occurring.

DISCUSSION

A time constant is the amount of time required for the patient to passively exhale 63% of his tidal volume. After two time constants, the patient has exhaled about 86% of the tidal volume and after three time constants, 95% of his tidal volume.

Mathematically, the time constant is calculated as resistance times compliance. For this patient:

$$\textit{time constant} = \textit{resistance} \times \textit{compliance} =$$

$$\frac{46\ cm\ H_2O \cdot second}{L} \times \frac{0.023\ L}{cm\ H_2O} = 1.058\ seconds$$

The ventilator will not allow the expiratory time to be less than two time constants, which for this patient is 2 × 1.058 = 2.1 seconds. The patient's current expiratory time is 2.5 seconds. Thus the ventilator is operating properly, but the patient may be gas trapping between 5% and 14 % of the exhaled tidal volume. You judge this to be clinically insignificant. The actual value is calculated as:

$$\%\ \text{gas}\ exhal = 100 \times (1 - e^{-t/RC})$$

where e is the base of the natural logarithms (about 2.72), t is the actual expiratory time, and RC is the time constant. For this example:

$$\%\ \text{gas}\ exhal = 100 \times (1 - 2.72^{-2.5/1.058}) = 100 \times (1 - 0.094) \approx 91\%$$

So for this patient, we expect that no more than about 9% of his tidal volume is left in the lung at the time of the next inspiration.

increased work of breathing, tachypnea, and respiratory muscle fatigue.[38,39] DC-IMV matches inspiratory flow to the patient's needs and maintains adequate tidal volumes. This facilitates synchronous patient-ventilator interaction and minimizes the risk of hypoventilation and patient anxiety.

Continuous Spontaneous Ventilation (CSV)

Pressure Control

Spontaneous breath modes include those in which all breaths are initiated and ended by the patient. The level of support this mode of ventilation provides determines the amount of work of breathing the patient will ultimately assume. CPAP, PSV, automatic tube compensation, and proportional assist ventilation are continuous spontaneous breath modes. We will focus on the two most commonly used forms of CSV: CPAP and PSV.

Indications. PC-CSV ventilation is indicated to reduce the work of breathing and improve or stabilize oxygenation by reducing alveolar derecruitment in intubated patients who do not require full ventilatory support.[40,41]

CPAP provides no inspiratory muscle unloading. Rather, it reduces abnormalities in gas exchange that can be associated with the presence of an artificial airway in patients requiring no assisted mechanical ventilatory support. Low levels of CPAP, 3 to 5 cm H_2O, maintain physiological PEEP and prevent alveolar collapse at end expiration.[41]

However, if CPAP levels are set inappropriately high, alveolar overdistension, rather than alveolar recruitment, and air-trapping result.[42] In addition to deleterious pulmonary effects, circulatory impairment may result from a decrease in left ventricular stroke volume. The reduction in cardiac output and arterial blood pressure will also hinder adequate oxygen delivery.[43]

Pressure support ventilation is a form of PC-CSV that assists the patient's inspiratory efforts. At very low levels of support this mode unloads the work of breathing the ventilator circuitry imposes on the respiratory muscles.[44] If the level of support is maximized, the ventilator may assume all of the work of breathing.[45] The result of high levels of support is a reduction in the respiratory rate, reduction in respiratory muscle activity and fatigue, reduction in oxygen consumption, and improvement or stabilization of spontaneous tidal volumes.[46,47] However, the positive attributes of this mode of ventilation can be negated if ventilator parameters are not properly set. The ventilator must be able to detect spontaneous patient effort. Therefore it is critical for the clinician to adjust the trigger sensitivity correctly. Of equal importance is the clinician set rise time (i.e., the time required for the ventilator to reach the inspiratory pressure limit). Ventilator graphics are often helpful

MINI CLINI

Overcoming Endotracheal Tube Resistance During Weaning

PROBLEM

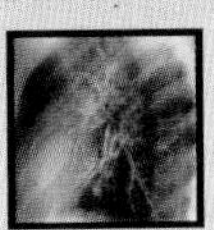

You are weaning an adult patient in the ICU on VC-IMV with pressure support. The plan for the patient is to initiate a spontaneous breathing trial. To do this, you place him in a PC-CSV mode with just enough support to overcome the resistance in the endotracheal tube. The current settings are:

VC-IMV mode
Frequency: 4 breaths per minute
V_T: 750 mL
Inspiratory flow: 60 L/minute = 1 L/second
Pressure support: 26 cm H_2O
PEEP: 4 cm H_2O
FIO_2: 0.40
PIP: 38 cm H_2O
Plateau Pressure: 25 cm H_2O

Select the level of pressure support needed to overcome the resistant in the endotracheal tube.

DISCUSSION

From the equation of motion we know that:

Ventilator pressure = Elastic load + Resistive load = (Tidal volume/Compliance) + (Flow × resistance)

We would like the patient to do the work to overcome the elastic load but want to use the ventilator to support the work of breathing through the increased airway resistance caused by the endotracheal tube. In essence, we will use the ventilator to make the patient feel like the tube has been removed, then observe whether he has the strength and endurance to breathe. This is what the Automatic Tube Compensation mode on the Draeger or Puritan Bennett ventilators attempts to do.

To approximate this with pressure support, we need to know the elastic load, which is equivalent to the patient's average inspiratory flow during spontaneous breaths times the airway resistance (including the endotracheal tube). One way to estimate mean inspiratory flow for spontaneous (unassisted) breaths is to switch the ventilator to CPAP for a few breaths and measure the actual spontaneous tidal volume (assuming the ventilator has this capability). Dividing the spontaneous tidal volume by the approximate inspiratory time gives average inspiratory flow. Alternatively, you could just use peak inspiratory flow, which would be easier but would slightly overestimate the pressure support needed. Another way is to just estimate a spontaneous tidal volume and inspiratory time based on body weight, expected spontaneous breathing frequency, and I:E ratio. In this case we will estimate the patient's mean inspiratory flow as 25 L/minute or 0.42 L/second.

Step 1: Calculate airway resistance.
From the equation of motion we get the equation for airway resistance using the mandatory breath settings:

$$\textit{airway resistance} = \frac{\textit{peak inspiratory pressure} - \textit{plateau pressure}}{\textit{inspiratory flow}}$$

$$\textit{airway resistance} = \frac{38\ cm\ H_2O - 25\ cm\ H_2O}{1\ L/s}$$

$$= 13\ cm\ H_2O \cdot s \cdot L^{-1}$$

Step 2: Calculate the ventilator pressure (i.e., pressure support) required to generate the average spontaneous flow through the resistance:

pressure support = mean spontaneous inspiratory flow × airway resistance

$$\textit{pressure support} = \frac{0.42\ L}{s} = \frac{13\ cm\ H_2O \cdot s}{L}$$

$$\approx 6\ cm\ H_2O$$

So, you set the pressure support level to 6 cm H_2O (above PEEP) and the patient should have enough ventilatory assistance to avoid the work of breathing through the endotracheal tube. If the spontaneous breathing trial is successful, you can confidently extubate the patient expecting him to be liberated from the ventilator.

when adjusting this parameter and optimizing patient-ventilator synchrony.

Regardless of the level of support provided, the patient has primary control over the breath rate, and inspiratory time and flow rate delivered during this mode of assisted ventilation.

Example. An example of the use of PC-CSV is noninvasive CPAP in the preterm, surfactant-deficient infant with RDS to prevent the need for intubation. CPAP holds open collapsible small airways and surfactant-deficient alveoli. As a result, alveolar gas exchange is enhanced.

Dual Control

Indications. DC-CSV is indicated to stabilize minute ventilation in spontaneously breathing patients with an intact ventilatory drive and normal pulmonary mechanics.[48] As a spontaneous breathing mode of ventilation, all breaths are patient triggered, flow cycled, and pressure limited. The patient controls the inspiratory time, flow, and frequency. The clinician sets a target tidal volume. The ventilator monitors exhaled volume and frequency and regulates, on a breath-by-breath basis, the level of pressure support needed to meet the set volume. The volume support ventilation mode on the Siemans Servo 300 is an example of DC-CSV. Should a patient become apneic in the volume support mode, the ventilator switches to DC-CMV.

MINI CLINI

Application of Volume Support Ventilation

PROBLEM

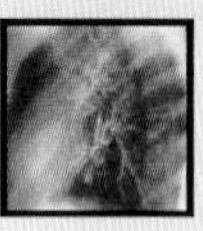

You are managing a mechanically ventilated postoperative pediatric patient. Currently he is on the Siemens Servo 300 in the VC-IMV mode. He is alert with stable vital signs. His current ventilator settings are as follows:

IMV: 6
Total frequency: 18 breaths per minute
V_T: 400 mL
FIO_2: 0.40
Spontaneous V_T: 100-300 mL

The physician orders a spontaneous breathing trial.

Although the patient is alert and has an intact ventilatory drive, you recognize the patient has inconsistent tidal volumes because of the lingering effects of anesthesia. Therefore PC-CSV may not be appropriate for this patient. You want to ensure that the patient maintains a minimally acceptable tidal volume. What mode could you use and why?

DISCUSSION

The Siemens Servo 300 provides a DC-CSV mode called Volume Support Ventilation. You select the following settings:

Target V_T: 80% of current volume = 320 mL
FIO_2: 0.40

Now each breath is flow-triggered, pressure-limited, and flow-cycled. The ventilator automatically adjusts the pressure limit so that the patient maintains a tidal volume equal to or larger than the set target of 320 mL. As the patient recovers from the effects of anesthesia, his inspiratory efforts become stronger and more consistent. In response, the ventilator gradually decreases the pressure limit.

In a case series of 20 pediatric patients weaned in the DC-CSV mode, Keenan and Martin[49] suggest initially setting the target tidal volume to achieve as 75% to 90% of the minute ventilation the current mode of ventilation provides to the patient. Care should be taken to avoid hypoventilation or hyperventilation by setting the target minute ventilation too low or too high, respectively.

Example. The application of volume support ventilation may be best appreciated in postoperative patients. Because of anesthesia, these patients may require intubation for airway protection and short-term mechanical ventilation to support inconsistent spontaneous minute ventilation.

KEY POINTS

- To understand mechanical ventilators you must first understand their four basic functions: power input, power conversion, control mechanism, and output.
- The equation of motion for the respiratory system relates the key variables (pressure, volume, flow, and time) and parameters (elastance or compliance and resistance) that describe the mechanical interaction of the patient with the ventilator.
- The time constant describes the time necessary for the lungs to passively inflate or deflate during mechanical ventilation. It is an important concept in selecting appropriate inspiratory and expiratory times.
- Given that only one variable can be controlled at a time, all ventilators must function as either pressure, volume, or flow controllers.
- There have been three major types of control schemes used in ventilators, open loop control, closed loop control of a single control variable, and closed loop control of two control variables, also known as *dual control.*
- To understand ventilator operation, we must also examine output waveforms. The output waveforms of interest during ventilatory support are pressure, volume, and flow. For each control variable there are a limited number of waveforms produced by current ventilators.
- A spontaneous breath is one in which the patient controls the start time and the tidal volume. In terms of the ventilator's phase variables, the patient both triggers and cycles the breath.
- A mandatory breath is a breath for which the ventilator sets the start time and/or the tidal volume. In terms of the ventilator's phase variables, the ventilator triggers and/or cycles the breath.
- There are three possible sequences of breaths that can occur during patient-ventilator interaction: (1) continuous mandatory ventilation (CMV) in which all breaths are mandatory, (2) continuous spontaneous ventilation (CSV) in which all breaths are spontaneous, and (3) intermittent mandatory ventilation (IMV) in which breaths can be either mandatory or spontaneous.

KEY POINTS—cont'd

- A mode of ventilation can be completely described by specifying: (1) the breathing pattern, including the control variable (pressure, volume, or dual control), and breath sequence (CMV, IMV, or CSV); (2) the control type (set point, servo, or adaptive); and (3) the specific control strategy including phase variables and operational logic.
- If any input, control, or output functions fail, a life-threatening situation may result. Thus, ventilators are equipped with various types of alarms, which may be classified in the same manner as the other major ventilator characteristics.

References

1. Consensus statement on the essentials of mechanical ventilators 1992, Respir Care Clin N Am 37:1000, 1992.
2. Chatburn RL: Classification of mechanical ventilators, Respir Care Clin N Am 37:1009, 1992.
3. Chatburn RL, Primiano FP Jr: A new system for understanding modes of mechanical ventilation, Respir Care Clin N Am 46:604, 2001.
4. Morris W: The American heritage dictionary of the English language, Boston, 1975, American Heritage and Houghton Mifflin.
5. Barnes TA: Core textbook of respiratory care practice, ed 2, St. Louis, 1994, Mosby.
6. Branson RD, Hess DR, Chatburn RL: Respiratory care equipment, ed 2, Philadelphia, 1999, Lippincott Williams & Wilkins.
7. Chatburn RL: Classification of mechanical ventilators. In Tobin MJ: Principles and practice of mechanical ventilation, New York, 1994, McGraw-Hill Inc.
8. Morch ET: History of mechanical ventilation. In Kirby RR, Smith RA, Desautels DA, editors: Mechanical ventilation, New York, 1985, Churchill Livingstone.
9. Russell DF, Ross DG, Manson HJ: Fluidic cycling devices for inspiratory and expiratory timing in automatic ventilators, J Biomech Eng 5:227, 1983.
10. Hess D, Lind L: Nomograms for the application of the Bourns Model BP200 as a volume-constant ventilator, Respir Care Clin N Am 25:248, 1980.
11. Sassoon CS et al: Inspiratory work of breathing on flow-by and demand-flow continuous positive airway pressure, Crit Care Med 17:1108, 1989.
12. Branson RD: Flow-triggering systems, Respir Care Clin N Am 39:138, 1994.
13. Branson RD, MacIntyre NR: Dual-control modes of mechanical ventilation, Respir Care Clin N Am 41:294, 1996.
14. Rattenborg CC, Via-Reque E: Clinical use of mechanical ventilation, Chicago, 1981, Mosby.
15. Chatburn RL, El-Khatib MF, Smith PG: Respiratory system behavior during mechanical inflation with constant inspiratory pressure and flow, Respir Care Clin N Am 39:979,1994.
16. Gillette MA, Hess DR: Ventilator-induced lung injury and the evolution of lung protective strategies in acute respiratory distress syndrome, Respir Care Clin N Am 46:130, 2001.
17. Rau JL: Inspiratory flow patterns: the "shape" of ventilation, Respir Care Clin N Am 38:132, 1993.
18. Demling R, Riessen R: Pulmonary dysfunction after cerebral injury, Crit Care Med 18:768, 1990.
19. Natalini G et al: Pressure-controlled verses volume controlled ventilation with mask airway, J Clin Anesth 13:436, 2001.
20. Stoller JK, Kacmarek RM: Ventilatory strategies in the management of adult respiratory distress syndrome, Clin Chest Med 11:755,1990.
21. Chatburn RL, Volsko TA, El-Khatib M: The effect of airway leak on tidal volume during pressure- or flow-controlled ventilation of the neonate: a model study, Respir Care Clin N Am 41:728, 1996.
22. Greaves TH et al: Inverse ratio ventilation in a 6-year old with severe post-traumatic adult respiratory distress syndrome, Crit Care Med 17:588, 1989.
23. Mammel MC, Bing DR: Mechanical ventilation of the newborn: an overview, Clin Chest Med 17:603, 1996.
24. Marini JJ: Paying the piper: the linkage of alveolar ventilation to alveolar pressure, Intensive Care Med 16:73, 1990 (editorial).
25. McCarthy MC et al: Pressure control inverse ratio ventilation in the treatment of adult respiratory distress syndrome in patients with blunt chest trauma, Am Surg 6:1027, 1999.
26. Piotrowski A, Sobala W, Kawczynski P: Patient-initiated, pressure-regulated, volume-controlled ventilation compared with intermittent mandatory ventilation in neonates: a prospective, randomized study, Intensive Care Med 23:975, 1997.
27. Raneri VM: Optimizing patient ventilator interactions: closed loop technology, Intensive Care Med 23:936, 1997.
28. Weisman JM et al: Intermittent mandatory ventilation, Am Rev Respir Dis 127:641, 1983.
29. Brochard L et al: Comparison of three methods of gradually withdrawal from ventilatory support during weaning from mechanical ventilation, Am J Respir Crit Care Med 150: 896, 1994.
30. Hummler H et al: Influence of different modes of synchronized mechanical ventilation on ventilation, gas exchange, patient effort, and blood pressure fluctuations in premature neonates, Pediatr Pulmonol 22:305, 1996.
31. Calzia E et al: Stress response during weaning after cardiac surgery, Br J Anaesth 87:490, 2001.
32. Hahn AF: The challenge of respiratory dysfunction in Guillain-Barré syndrome, Arch Neurol 58:893, 2001.
33. Roze JC et al: Oxygen cost of breathing and weaning process in newborn infants, Eur Respir J 10:2583, 1997.
34. Sinha SK, Donn SM: Volume-controlled ventilation: variations on a theme, Clin Perinatol 28:547, 2001.

35. Amato MBP et al: Volume assured pressure support ventilation: a new approach for reducing muscle workload during acute respiratory failure, Chest 102:1225, 1992.
36. Branson RD, Campbell RS: Modes of ventilator operation. In MacIntyre NR, Branson RD, editors: Mechanical ventilation, Philadelphia, 2001, Saunders.
37. Haas CF: Patient determined inspiratory flow during assisted mechanical ventilation, Respir Care Clin N Am 40:716, 1995.
38. Davis K, Jr et al: Comparison of volume control and pressure control ventilation: is flow waveform the difference? J Trauma 41:808, 1996.
39. Eros B, Powner D, and Grenvik A: Common ventilatory modes: terminology, Int Anesthesiol Clin 18:11, 1980.
40. MacIntyre NR: Respiratory function during pressure support ventilation, Chest 89:677, 1986.
41. Tunsmann G et al: Alveolar recruitment strategy improves arterial oxygenation during general anesthesia, Br J Anaesth 82:8, 1999.
42. Klerk AM, Klerk RK. Nasal continuous positive airway pressure and outcomes or preterm infants, Neonatal Intensive Care 14:58, 2001.
43. Dinger J et al: Effect of positive end expiratory pressure on functional residual capacity and compliance in surfactant-treated preterm infants, Neonatal Intensive Care 14:26, 2001.
44. Brochard L, Pluskwa F, and Lemaire F: Improved efficacy of spontaneous breathing with inspiratory pressure support, Am Rev Respir Dis 136:411, 1987.
45. MacIntyre NR: Pressure support ventilation: effects on ventilatory reflexes and ventilatory muscle workload, Respir Care Clin N Am 32:447, 1987.
46. Brochard L et al: Pressure support decreases work of breathing and oxygen consumption during weaning from mechanical ventilation, Am Rev Respir Dis 135:A51, 1987 (abstract).
47. Grande CM, Kahn RC. The effect of pressure support ventilation on ventilatory variables and work of breathing, Anesthesiology 65:A84, 1986 (abstract).
48. Branson RD, Davis K: Dual control modes, combining volume and pressure breaths, Respir Care Clin N Am 7(3):397, 2001.
49. Keen HT, Martin LD: Volume support ventilation in infants and children: analysis of a case series, Respir Care Clin N Am 42:281, 1997.

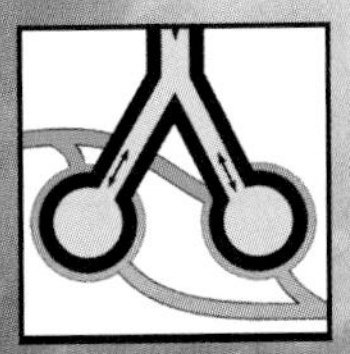

CHAPTER 40

Physiology of Ventilatory Support

Timothy B. Op't Holt

In This Chapter You Will Learn:

- What are the effects of mechanical ventilation on oxygenation, ventilation, and lung mechanics
- What are the effects of positive pressure ventilation on other body systems
- What are complications and hazards of providing mechanical ventilatory support
- How to minimize the adverse effects of mechanical ventilation

Chapter Outline

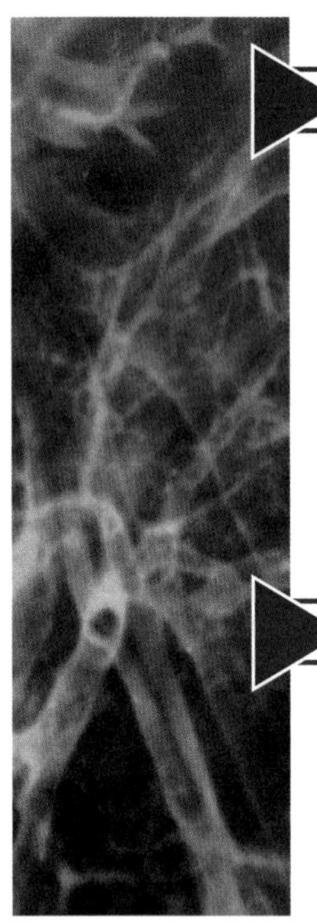

Chapter Outline—cont'd

Key Terms

aerophagia
autoregulation
barotrauma
intrinsic PEEP
mean airway pressure
patient-ventilator asynchrony
time constant
transairway pressure
transpulmonary pressure
transrespiratory pressure
transthoracic pressure
volutrauma
work of breathing

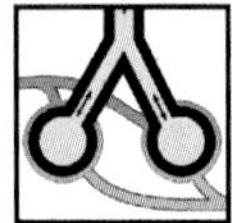

Mechanical ventilation can be beneficial or detrimental to the patient depending on how it is initially applied and modified as the patient's condition changes. Respiratory therapists must be able to anticipate potential physiological effects of mechanical ventilation and respond appropriately when complications arise. The purpose of this chapter is to familiarize the reader with (1) the physiological effects of mechanical ventilation on lung and cardiovascular function and other body systems and (2) the complications and hazards of mechanical ventilation. A solid understanding of the normal physiology of breathing is essential for all respiratory therapists, especially when working with patients receiving mechanical ventilation. Respiratory therapists must understand intrathoracic pressure changes associated with spontaneous, negative pressure, and positive pressure breathing. Intrathoracic pressure changes result in ventilation and may induce a variety of physiologic changes in other systems.

▶ PRESSURE AND PRESSURE GRADIENTS

For gas to flow through an airway, a pressure gradient must exist. The airways begin at the mouth and end at the alveoli, so mouth pressure (pressure at the airway opening [P_{awo}]) and alveolar pressure (P_{alv}) are important in describing gas flow, as are intrapleural pressure (P_{pl}) and body surface pressure or atmospheric pressure (P_{bs}). The P_{pl} is the pressure in the pleural space, between the visceral and parietal pleurae and is usually negative in relation to P_{alv}. Four pressure gradients exist and help describe airflow in the lungs. They are transpulmonary pressure (P_L or P_{tp}), transthoracic pressure (P_w or P_{tt}), transairway pressure (P_{ta}), and transrespiratory pressure (P_{tr}). These pressures and their gradients are described in Figure 40-1.

Transpulmonary pressure is the difference between alveolar pressure and pleural pressure ($P_L = P_{alv} - P_{pl}$). Transpulmonary pressure maintains alveolar inflation. Transpulmonary pressure in the three types of ventilation discussed later (spontaneous, negative pressure, and positive pressure) is the result of an increase in P_{awo} or a decrease in P_{pl}. Transthoracic pressure is the difference between alveolar pressure and body surface pressure ($P_{alv} - P_{bs}$). Transthoracic pressure is the pressure necessary to expand the lungs and chest wall concurrently. Transairway pressure (P_{ta}) is the difference between airway pressure and alveolar pressure ($P_{aw} - P_{alv}$). Transairway pressure causes airflow in the conducting airways and is the pressure resulting from airway resistance. Transrespiratory pressure is the difference between airway opening pressure and body surface pressure ($P_{awo} - P_{bs}$). Once these pressures and pressure gradients are understood, the differences between spontaneous, positive, and negative pressure ventilation become evident.

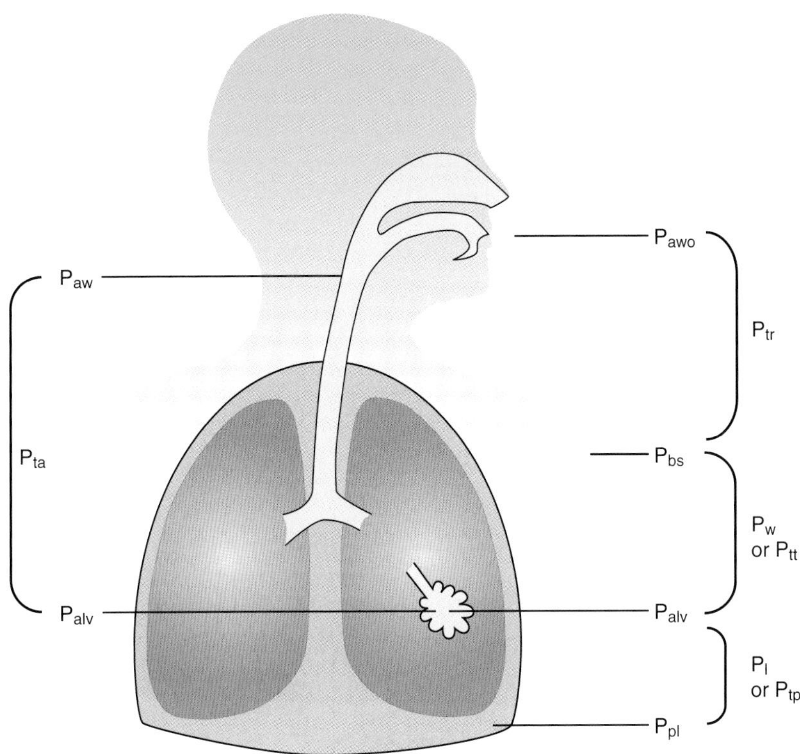

Figure 40-1

Pressures and pressure gradients in the lung. Airflow is a function of the transairway pressure (P_{ta}), which is the pressure gradient between the airway (P_{aw}) and the alveoli (P_{alv}). Transpulmonary pressure (P_{tp}) maintains alveolar inflation, and transthoracic pressure (P_{tt}) is the pressure needed to expand the lungs and chest wall.

P_{awo} - Mouth or airway opening pressure
P_{alv} - Alveolar pressure
P_{pl} - Intrapleural pressure
P_{bs} - Body surface pressure
P_{aw} - Airway pressure (=P_{awo})

P_L or P_{tp} = Transpulmonary pressure ($P_L = P_{alv} - P_{pl}$)
P_w or P_{tt} = Transthoracic pressure ($P_{BS} - P_{alv}$)
P_{ta} = Transairway pressure ($P_{aw} - P_{alv}$)
P_{tr} = Transrespiratory pressure ($P_{awo} - P_{bs}$)

Table 40-1 ▶▶ Changes in Airway Pressure Gradients During Spontaneous, Negative, and Positive Pressure Ventilation

Pressure (cm H_2O) Ventilation Type	Transpulmonary Pressure	Transthoracic Pressure	Transairway Pressure	Transrespiratory Pressure
Spontaneous				
Inspiration	Small (–) increase	Increase (–)	Increase (–)	Constant at 0
Expiration	Small (+) increase	Increase (+)	Increase (+)	Constant at 0
Negative (NPV)				
Inspiration	Small (–) increase	Increase (–)	Increase (–)	Increase (–)
Expiration	Small (+) increase	Increase (+)	Increase (+)	Increase (+)
Positive (PPV)				
Inspiration	Small (+) increase	Increase (+)	Increase (+)	Increase (+)
Expiration	Small (–) increase	Decrease	Decrease	Decrease

Airway, Alveolar, and Intrathoracic Pressure, Volume, and Flow During Spontaneous Ventilation

Breathing usually is an autonomic phenomenon. Not until our breathing is stressed do we think about the effort to breathe or the energy expended. At end-exhalation, intrapleural pressure is slightly negative. Alveolar, mouth, and body surface pressures are zero. The diaphragm contracts in response to stimulation of the phrenic nerve by the respiratory center in the medulla of the brain. When the diaphragm contracts, it descends into the abdominal cavity, which further decreases intrapleural pressure. When intrapleural pressure becomes more negative, alveolar pressure becomes negative as well. The effects of spontaneous breathing on the pressure gradients are shown in Table 40-1. Under normal circumstances, a decrease in intrapleural pressure results in decreased

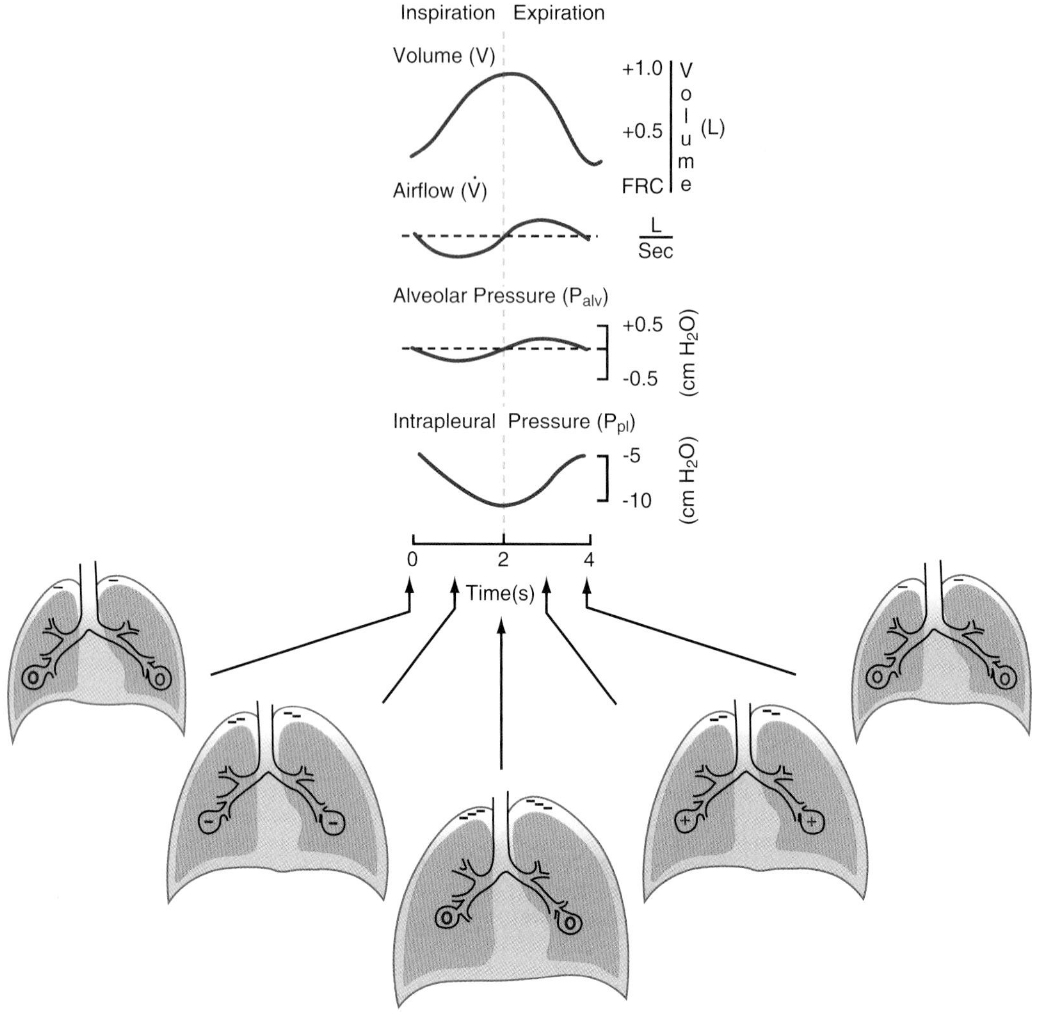

Figure 40-2
Changes in pressure, volume, and flow during a single spontaneous breath. FRC, Functional residual capacity. *(Modified from Martin L: Pulmonary physiology in clinical practice: the essentials for patient care and evaluation, St Louis, 1987, Mosby.)*

alveolar pressure, increased transairway pressure, and inspiration of the tidal volume (Figure 40-2).

At end-inspiration, alveolar pressure returns to zero when the muscles of inspiration stop contracting. Lung recoil causes a sudden increase in alveolar pressure in relation to pressure at the mouth, reversing the transrespiratory pressure gradient, and air flows out of the lungs. Normally, there is a short end-expiratory pause before the next inspiration.

Tidal volume and flow during spontaneous ventilation may be described by the equation of motion.[1] The equation of motion describes the relation between muscle pressure (analogous to pleural pressure in spontaneous breathing), compliance, resistance, flow, and volume as follows:

$$P_{musc} = \frac{\text{Volume}}{\text{Compliance}} \times (\text{Resistance} \times \text{Flow})$$

where P_{musc} is muscle pressure, volume is tidal volume, compliance is lung-thorax compliance, resistance is airway resistance, and flow is airway flow. When the equation is rearranged, volume inhaled during spontaneous ventilation is proportional to muscle pressure and lung-thorax compliance and inversely related to the product of airway resistance and flow:

$$\text{Volume} = \frac{P_{musc}}{(\text{Resistance} \times \text{Flow})} \times \text{Compliance}$$

Airway, Alveolar, and Intrathoracic Pressure, Volume, and Flow During Negative Pressure Mechanical Ventilation

Mechanical negative pressure ventilation (NPV) is similar to spontaneous breathing. Negative pressure ventilation decreases pleural pressure (P_{pl}) during inspiration by exposing the chest to subatmospheric pressure. Negative pressure at the body surface (P_{bs}) is transmitted first to the pleural space and then to the alveoli (P_{alv}).

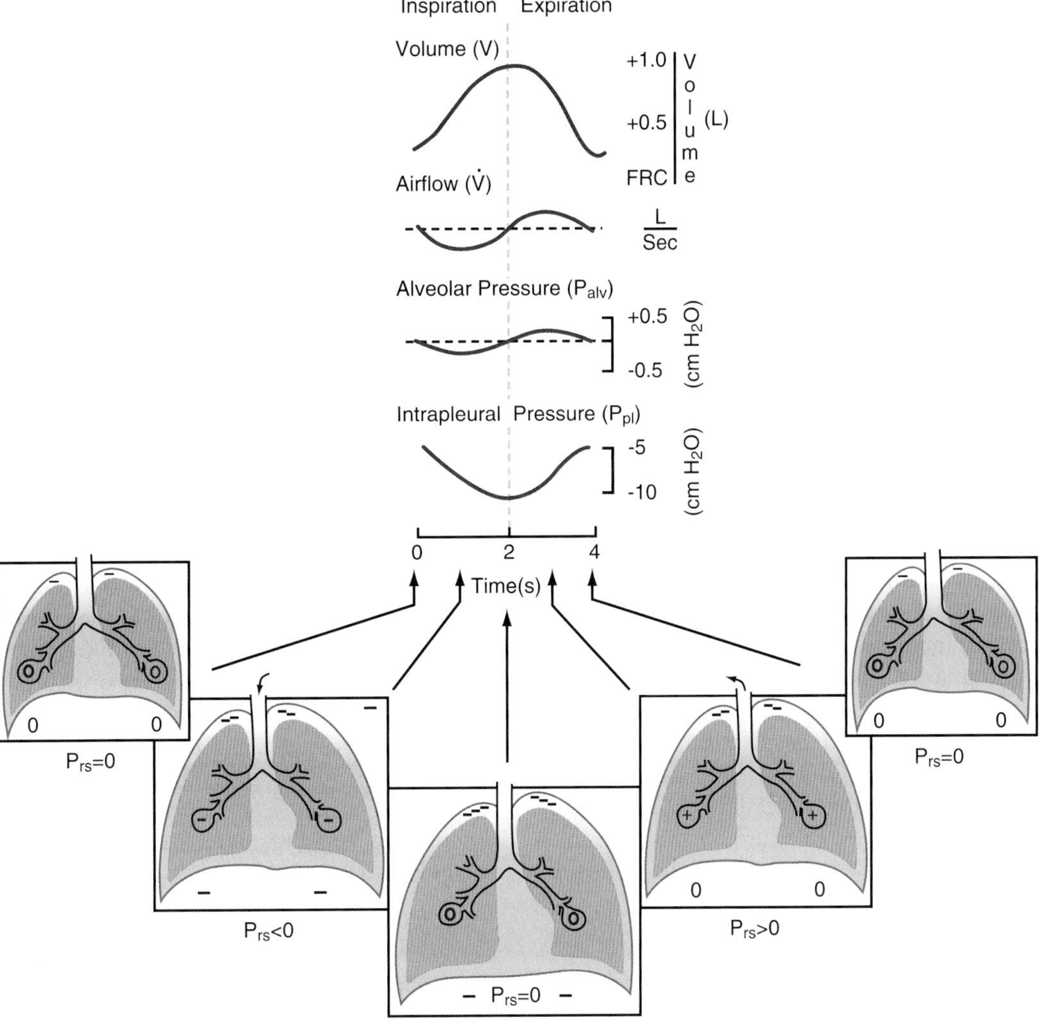

Figure 40-3

Changes in pressure, volume, and flow during a single mechanical negative pressure breath. The box surrounding the lungs represents the enclosure formed by the negative pressure ventilator. P_{rs}, Pressure of the respiratory system. *(Modified from Martin L: Pulmonary physiology in clinical practice: the essentials for patient care and evaluation, St Louis, 1987, Mosby.)*

Because the airway opening remains exposed to atmospheric pressure during NPV, a transrespiratory pressure gradient is created. Thus gas flows from the relatively high pressure at the airway opening (zero) to the relatively low pressure in the alveoli (negative). As with spontaneous breathing, alveolar expansion during NPV is determined by the magnitude of the transrespiratory pressure gradient. During expiration in both spontaneous breathing and NPV, the lungs and chest wall passively recoil to their resting end-expiratory levels. As this recoil occurs, pleural pressure becomes less negative, and alveolar pressure increases above atmospheric pressure (Figure 40-3). This increase in alveolar pressure reverses the transrespiratory pressure gradient. As P_{alv} becomes greater than P_{awo}, gas flows from the alveoli to the airway opening. The effects of negative pressure ventilation on the pressure gradients are shown in Table 40-1.

Volume and flow during NPV also are described by the equation of motion, except the pressure developed by the ventilator fully or partially replaces the patient's respiratory muscle pressure as follows:

$$P_{musc} + P_{vent} = \frac{\text{Volume}}{\text{Compliance}} \times (\text{Resistance} \times \text{Flow})$$

In this version, P_{vent} is the pressure the ventilator develops to overcome the patient's lung-thorax elastance and airway resistance to deliver the tidal volume. In this case P_{vent} is negative but is the driving force behind decreasing the intrapleural pressure and increasing the transairway pressure.

Physiological complications associated with NPV are uncommon because NPV simulates normal spontaneous breathing. The most common problems with NPV are related to interference with caring for the patient caused by the device surrounding the chest (the iron lung or chest cuirass). Systems that enclose the entire thorax and lower body, such as the iron lung and Porta-Lung, may impede venous return and result in a phenomenon known as "tank shock."

Airway, Alveolar, and Intrathoracic Pressure, Volume, and Flow During Positive Pressure Mechanical Ventilation

Positive pressure ventilation (PPV) reverses the pressure gradients that occur during spontaneous breathing and NPV. Gas flows into the lungs because pressure at the airway opening (P_{awo}) is positive, whereas alveolar pressure (P_{alv}) initially is zero. However, alveolar pressure rapidly increases during the inspiratory phase of PPV. The increased alveolar pressure expands the airways and alveoli. Because alveolar pressure is greater than pleural pressure (P_{pl}) during PPV, positive pressure is transmitted from the alveoli to the pleural space, causing pleural pressure to increase during inspiration. Depending on the compliance and resistance of the lungs, pleural pressure may actually exceed atmospheric pressure during a portion of inspiration. The main changes in pleural pressure during PPV can lead to significant physiological changes (see later). Changes in the pressure gradients during PPV are shown in Table 40-1. All the pressure gradients change in the opposite direction between NPV and PPV.

As with spontaneous breathing, the recoil force of the lungs and chest wall, stored as potential energy during the positive pressure breath, causes passive exhalation. As gas flows from the alveoli to the airway opening, alveolar pressure decreases to atmospheric level while pleural pressure is restored to its normal subatmospheric range (Figure 40-4).

Volume and flow during PPV also are described by the equation of motion. In PPV, however, P_{vent} is positive. The magnitude of P_{vent} to supply the patient's ventilatory needs depends on the P_{musc} of the patient. If the patient makes no effort, P_{vent} is responsible for all volume and flow. As muscle strength increases, P_{vent} can be decreased. The result is liberation from the ventilator and resumption of spontaneous breathing.

▶ EFFECTS OF MECHANICAL VENTILATION ON OXYGENATION

Increased Inspired Oxygen

Mechanical ventilators may deliver a fractional inspired oxygen concentration (FIO_2) of 0.21 to 1.0. As a result, the alveolar (PAO_2) and arterial (PaO_2) partial pressure of oxygen may be restored to normal with appropriate management. The effectiveness of increased FIO_2 in the management of hypoxemia depends on the cause of the hypoxemia. Hypoxemia caused by a decrease in ventilation/perfusion ($\dot{V}/\dot{Q}$) ratio is more responsive to increased FIO_2 than is hypoxemia caused by hypoventilation, diffusion defect, or shunt. Hypoxemia caused by hypoventilation responds well to restoration of alveolar ventilation. Hypoxemia caused by diffusion defect and shunt often responds to an increase in alveolar positive end-expiratory pressure (PEEP) and an increase in FIO_2. That PaO_2 responds to increased FIO_2 helps the therapist determine that a low $\dot{V}/\dot{Q}$ ratio is the cause of hypoxemia. If the patient is receiving mechanical ventilation and has adequate alveolar ventilation, failure of the PaO_2 to respond to increased FIO_2 likely means that the hypoxemia is due to diffusion defect or shunt.

In summary, mechanical ventilation increases alveolar ventilation, which increases PaO_2 if the underlying problem is hypoventilation. An increase in PaO_2 after an increase in FIO_2 likely means that the cause of the hypoxemia is a low $\dot{V}/\dot{Q}$ ratio. In the event that the PaO_2 is not restored by an increase in FIO_2, the hypoxemia is probably due to diffusion defect or shunt.

Alveolar Oxygen and the Alveolar Air Equation

Increasing the FIO_2 increases PAO_2, according to the alveolar air equation:

$$PAO_2 = [FIO_2\,(P_B\text{-}47)] - PaCO_2 \times [FIO_2 + \frac{1 - FIO_2}{R}]$$

where PAO_2 is the partial pressure of oxygen in the alveoli.

FIO_2 is the fraction of inspired oxygen.

P_B is the barometric pressure in millimeters of mercury.

47 is the partial pressure of water vapor in the alveoli in millimeters of mercury.

$PaCO_2$ is the partial pressure of carbon dioxide in arterial blood in millimeters of mercury.

R is the respiratory exchange ratio ($\dot{V}CO_2/\dot{V}O_2$), normally, 0.8.

When FIO_2 is increased, PAO_2 increases as well, if there is no change in $PaCO_2$ or respiratory exchange ratio. The $PaCO_2$ may change with a change in alveolar ventilation or metabolic rate. Oxygen consumption and carbon dioxide production increase with an increase in metabolic rate, such as with fever or overfeeding. If metabolic rate and alveolar ventilation are constant, an increase in FIO_2 results in a proportional increase in PAO_2.

Arterial Oxygenation and Oxygen Content

Mechanical ventilation at an FIO_2 of 0.21 may restore arterial oxygenation if the only cause of hypoxemia was hypoventilation. This may be the case with central

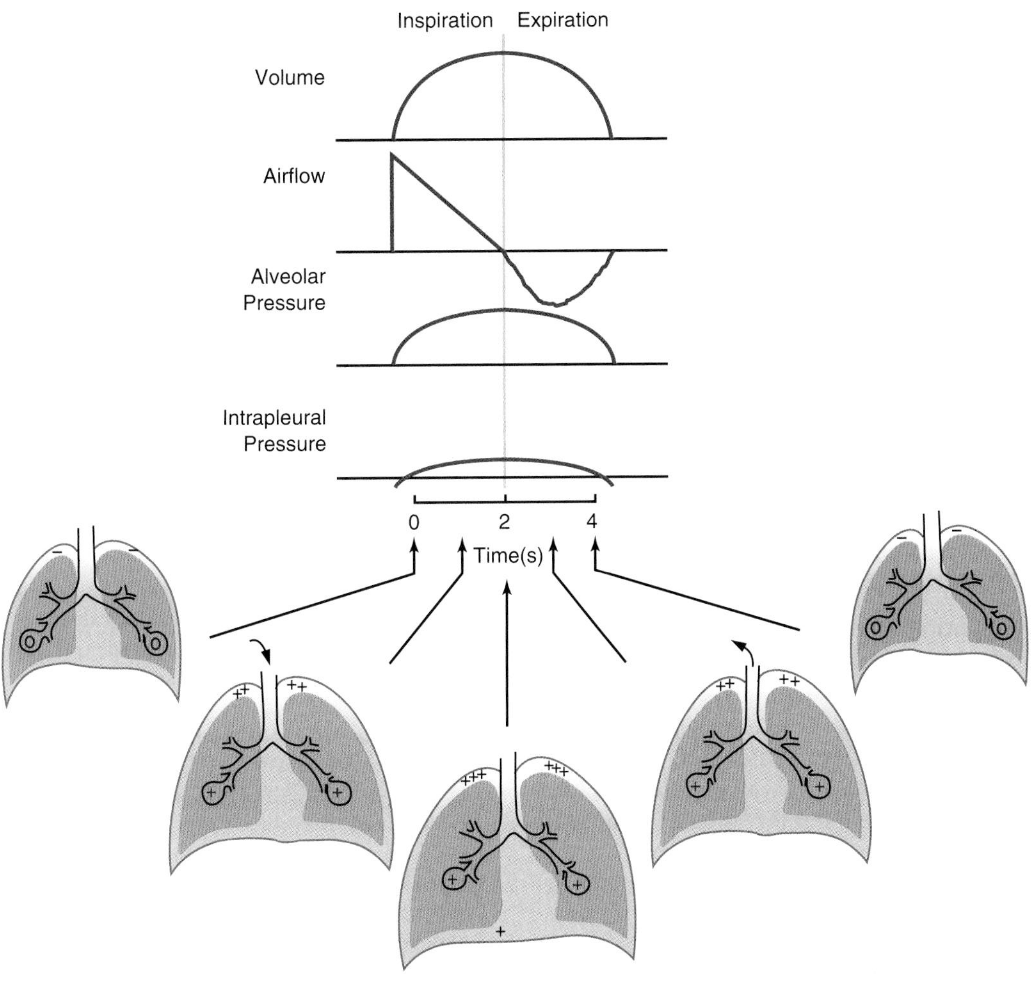

Figure 40-4
Changes in pressure, volume, and flow during a single decelerating flow, positive pressure breath. Arrows into and out of the trachea represent airflow. *(Modified from Martin L: Pulmonary physiology in clinical practice: the essentials for patient care and evaluation, St Louis, 1987, Mosby.)*

nervous system depression, apnea, and neuromuscular disease. With other causes of hypoxemia, an increase in F_{IO_2} is needed to increase arterial oxygenation and content.

Arterial oxygenation is determined with Fick's law of diffusion:[2]

$$\text{Diffusion} = \frac{A \times D \times (P_1 - P_2)}{T}$$

where A is the surface area available for diffusion (alveolar surface area).

D is the diffusion coefficient of the gas.

$P_1 - P_2$ is the partial pressure difference across the membrane ($P_{AO_2} - P_cO_2$).

T is the membrane thickness.

Under normal circumstances, oxygen readily diffuses across the alveolar-capillary (A-C) membrane owing to the large alveolar surface area, alveolar to pulmonary arterial oxygen pressure gradient (approximately 60 mm Hg), and the very thin A-C membrane (approximately 1 mm). In hypoventilation and low $\dot{V}/\dot{Q}$ abnormalities, P_{AO_2} is decreased. The result is decreased diffusion and a decrease in Pa_{O_2}. When P_{AO_2} is restored, Pa_{O_2} normalizes. In diffusion defects, the thickness of the membrane increases, and diffusion decreases. In shunt, because the alveoli are flooded or collapsed, surface area and P_{AO_2} are decreased. With acute lung injury (ALI), the permeability of the capillary endothelium to fluid is increased. The results are fluid filling of the interstitial and alveolar space and an increase in the thickness of the A-C membrane. These factors contribute to the marked hypoxemia that accompanies shunt. The use of PEEP and control of membrane permeability accompany the management of shunt. These factors also explain why an increase in P_{AO_2} alone often does not increase diffusion and arterial oxygenation in these disorders.

Oxygen content is directly related to arterial oxygenation and hemoglobin concentration, defined by the equation for arterial oxygen content (Ca_{O_2}):

$$Ca_{O_2}\ (vol\%) = (1.34 \times Hb \times Sa_{O_2}) \times (Pa_{O_2} \times 0.003\ mL\ O_2/mm\ Hg)$$

where 1.34 is a constant for the amount of oxygen carried by each fully saturated gram of hemoglobin (1.34 mL oxygen per gram of hemoglobin).

Hb is the hemoglobin concentration in grams per deciliter.

Sa_{O_2} is the oxygen saturation of hemoglobin.

0.003 is the amount of oxygen carried in the plasma in milliliters per millimeter of mercury Pa_{O_2}.

Under circumstances of normal diffusion, F_{IO_2}, and hemoglobin concentration, the arterial content is normal at approximately 19.8 mL O_2/100 mL blood. As defined by this equation, Ca_{O_2} decreases if hemoglobin concentration, arterial saturation, or Pa_{O_2} decreases.

Decreased Shunt

Mechanical ventilation alone does not decrease shunt. Otherwise it would be much easier to restore Pa_{O_2} in patients with acute respiratory distress syndrome (ARDS). Administration of PEEP with mechanical ventilation or to a spontaneously breathing patient in the form of continuous positive airway pressure (CPAP) helps to open or recruit and stabilize small, collapsed, or fluid-filled alveoli. The results are an increase in alveolar surface area for diffusion and improvement in $\dot{V}/\dot{Q}$ matching and arterial oxygenation.

Positive end-expiratory pressure or CPAP must be used judiciously (see Chapter 41). High pressure can overdistend alveoli and redistribute pulmonary blood flow to capillaries surrounding poorly ventilated alveoli; the result is increased shunt.

Increased Tissue Oxygen Delivery

When a mechanical ventilator is used to improve arterial oxygenation by increasing the F_{IO_2} or PEEP, Ca_{O_2} increases. However, the increase in Ca_{O_2} represents only part of tissue oxygen delivery, because oxygen delivery is defined by Ca_{O_2} and cardiac output, as follows:

$$D_{O_2}\ (\text{tissue oxygen delivery in mL/min}) = Ca_{O_2}\ (\text{mL } O_2/100\ \text{mL blood}) \times \text{Cardiac output (L/min)} \times 10$$

where 10 is a constant for converting deciliters to milliliters.

Normal D_{O_2} is approximately 1000 mL/min, because the normal Ca_{O_2} is approximately 20 vol% and the normal cardiac output is approximately 5 L/min. When Pa_{O_2}, Ca_{O_2}, and cardiac output are adequate, so is tissue oxygen delivery. When it is needed for improving the Pa_{O_2}, PEEP must be used with caution. Positive end-expiratory pressure increases intrathoracic pressure. When intrathoracic pressure is increased, the pleural pressure around the heart also increases, and the increase can impede venous return and decrease cardiac output. As discussed in Chapter 41, therapists generally use enough PEEP to increase the Pa_{O_2} to 60 mm Hg while not depressing cardiac output. This "optimal PEEP" provides adequate arterial oxygenation and tissue oxygen delivery. Another goal of PEEP is to decrease the F_{IO_2} to a value less than that thought to promote oxygen toxicity. This approach to PEEP seeks to achieve an adequate Pa_{O_2} with a safe F_{IO_2}. In general a Pa_{O_2} of

MINI CLINI

Oxygen Delivery (D_{O_2})

PROBLEM

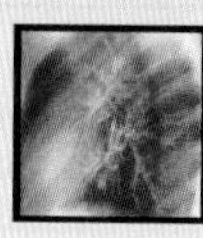

Oxygen delivery depends on Pa_{O_2}, hemoglobin concentration, and cardiac output. The formula for D_{O_2} follows:

$$D_{O_2} = Ca_{O_2} \times \text{Cardiac output (L/min)} \times 10$$

where Ca_{O_2} is the arterial oxygen content, and 10 is the conversion factor between deciliters and milliliters. Normal D_{O_2} is 990 mL/min. This is true when the hemoglobin concentration is 15 g/dL, cardiac output is 5.0 L/min, and Pa_{O_2} is 100 mm Hg:

$$D_{O_2} = [15\ g\ Hb \times 1.34\ mL\ O_2/g\ Hb \times 0.97\ (Sa_{O_2}) + 0.003 \times 100\ mm\ Hg] \times (5.0\ L/min) \times 10 = 19.8\ (Ca_{O_2}) \times 5\ (L/min) \times 10 = 990\ mL/min$$

Oxygen delivery also can be indexed to body surface area (BSA) and therefore referred to as the *oxygenation index* (D_{O_2}/BSA). When the practitioner calculates the D_{O_2} and determines it to be low, the component of the formula that is low denotes the problem and the therapeutic target. If the Ca_{O_2} is low because of a low hemoglobin concentration, increasing the hemoglobin concentration with blood transfusion is indicated. If Ca_{O_2} is low because of low Pa_{O_2} or Sa_{O_2}, increasing the Pa_{O_2} and Sa_{O_2} with oxygen or PEEP as indicated. If cardiac output is low, the cause (decreased preload, increased afterload, decreased contractility, or bradycardia) is determined, and appropriate therapy is initiated. In the event of a decrease in Ca_{O_2}, cardiac output may compensate to restore D_{O_2}.

For example, given a Pa_{O_2} of 65 mm Hg, hemoglobin concentration of 10 g/dL, Sa_{O_2} of 91%, and cardiac output of 4.8 L/min, what increase in cardiac output is necessary to maintain a D_{O_2} of 900 mL/min?

$$D_{O_2} \text{ at the given values is } [(1.34 \times 10 \times 0.97) + (0.003 \times 65)] \times 4.8 \times 10 = 633\ mL/min$$

An increase in cardiac output to 6.8 L/min results in a D_{O_2} that is close to normal: $[(1.34 \times 10 \times 0.97) + (0.003 \times 65)] \times 6.8 \times 10 = 897$ mL/min. An increase in cardiac output to 6.8 L/min increases myocardial work. Because the cause of the decreased D_{O_2} in this patient is hypoxemia and anemia, the goal of therapy should be increasing the hemoglobin concentration and restoring the Pa_{O_2}. This strategy allows cardiac output and work to return to normal while an adequate D_{O_2} is maintained.

60 mm Hg or greater with an F_{IO_2} of 0.40 to 0.50 or less is considered an appropriate goal.

▶ EFFECTS OF MECHANICAL VENTILATION ON VENTILATION

Increased Minute Ventilation

One indication for mechanical ventilation is hypercapnic respiratory failure, also known as *ventilatory failure*. For patients with acute ventilatory failure, the initiation of mechanical ventilation must improve alveolar ventilation to compensate for the patient's inability to maintain a normal Pa_{CO_2}. The Pa_{CO_2} is the result of the alveolar ventilation, which is related to minute ventilation. Minute ventilation is the product of tidal volume (V_T) and ventilatory rate (f): $\dot{V}_E = V_T \times f$. Use of a mechanical ventilator usually implies a change in tidal volume, ventilatory rate, or both from preintubation values. A normal spontaneous tidal volume is approximately 5 to 7 mL/kg. The currently accepted tidal volume for mechanical ventilation is 5 to 8 mL/kg for patients with ARDS, 8 to 12 mL/kg for patients with COPD, 10 to 12 mL/kg for patients with normal lungs, and 12 to 15 mL/kg for patients with neuromuscular disease.[3] These volumes are based on ideal body weight. In most cases, tidal volume increases with the initiation of mechanical ventilation. The increase in tidal volume depends on the tidal volume delivered for volume-controlled ventilation or the set pressure for pressure-controlled ventilation. The mechanical ventilatory rate depends on the patient's status. For postoperative ventilation, a rate of 10 to 12 breaths/min is adequate. Conditions that may necessitate a higher initial rate include acutely increased intracranial pressure (ICP) (with caution; see later) and metabolic acidosis. Conditions that may necessitate a lower rate include COPD and acute asthma exacerbation to allow an increased expiratory time to avoid air trapping. Once an adequate tidal volume is established, the set rate is adjusted to achieve the desired Pa_{CO_2}.

In summary, mechanical ventilation increases minute ventilation by increasing tidal volume, ventilatory rate, or both.

Increased Alveolar Ventilation

Alveolar ventilation ($\dot{V}_A$) is inversely related to Pa_{CO_2} as defined by the relation:

$$\dot{V}_A = \frac{\dot{V}CO_2 \times 0.863}{PaCO_2}$$

where $\dot{V}_{CO_2}$ is carbon dioxide production.

As alveolar ventilation decreases, Pa_{CO_2} increases. As carbon dioxide production increases, alveolar ventilation must increase to maintain the same Pa_{CO_2}. Mechanical ventilation may be needed in either case. It is more useful to look at this equation solved for Pa_{CO_2}, because changes in Pa_{CO_2} usually correlate with the need for mechanical ventilation:

$$PaCO_2 = \frac{\dot{V}CO_2 \times 0.863}{\dot{V}_A}$$

If $\dot{V}_A$ decreases or $\dot{V}_{CO_2}$ increases, Pa_{CO_2} increases, and hypercapnic respiratory failure follows. If the patient is unable to compensate for these changes, ventilatory failure results, and mechanical ventilation may be indicated. Because mechanical ventilation increases ventilation, Pa_{CO_2} decreases to the desired level depending on the mandatory $\dot{V}_E$ set by the therapist and the patient's contribution to the $\dot{V}_E$.

Decreased Ventilation/Perfusion Ratio

Early studies with COPD patients showed increases in the difference between alveolar and arterial partial pressure of oxygen [$P(A\text{-}a)O_2$] during positive pressure breathing. The findings suggested that inspired gas was not being normally distributed throughout the lung. The early notion that PPV might alter the distribution of gases in the lungs has been confirmed with healthy subjects. The reasons for this alteration in gas distribution are apparent when spontaneous ventilation is compared with positive pressure breathing.

Spontaneous ventilation results in gas distribution mainly to the dependent and peripheral zones of the lungs. Positive pressure ventilation tends to reverse this normal pattern of gas distribution, and most of the delivered volume is directed to nondependent lung zones (Figure 40-5). This phenomenon is caused in part by the inactivity of the diaphragm and chest wall. Although these structures actively facilitate gas movement during spontaneous breathing, their inactivity during PPV impedes ventilation to dependent lung zones. An increase in ventilation to the nondependent zones of the lung, where there is less perfusion, increases the $\dot{V}/\dot{Q}$ ratio, effectively increasing physiologic dead space. Therefore the increase in $P(A\text{-}a)O_2$ often observed with PPV is caused by areas of low $\dot{V}/\dot{Q}$ ratio, primarily in the bases and dependent lung zones.

Positive pressure ventilation decreases the $\dot{V}/\dot{Q}$ ratio in the bases and dependent lung zones mainly by its effect on the pulmonary circulation. Positive pressure ventilation can compress the pulmonary capillaries. This compression increases pulmonary vascular resistance and decreases perfusion. Minimal blood flow perfuses the areas with the greatest pressure and contributes to a further increase in dead space. Conversely, blood intended for these areas is diverted to regions with lower vascular resistance, which are those receiving the least pressure and ventilation. Thus pulmonary blood flow

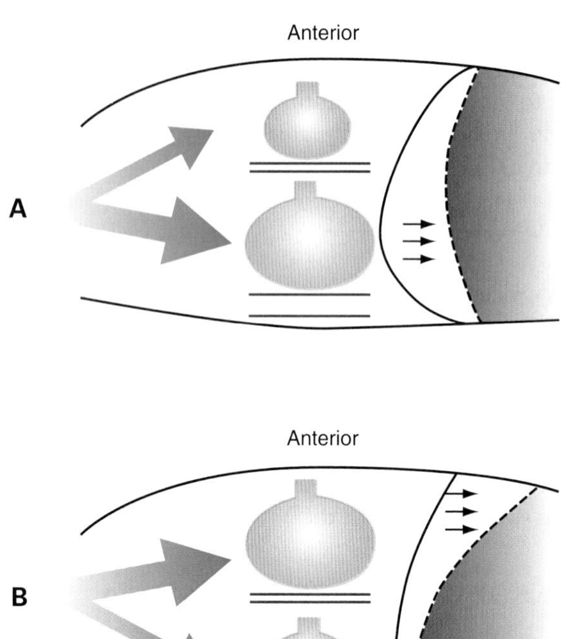

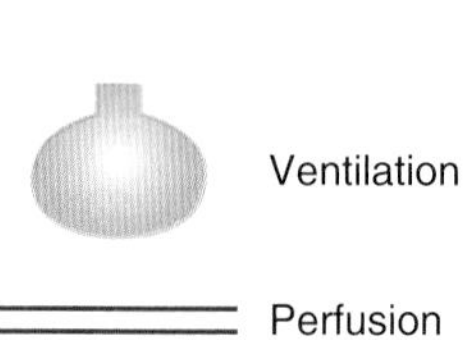

Figure 40-5

Effect of spontaneous ventilation and PPV on gas distribution in a supine subject. During spontaneous ventilation **(A),** diaphragmatic action distributes most ventilation to the dependent zones of the lungs, where perfusion is greatest. The result is a nearly normal $\dot{V}/\dot{Q}$ ratio. Partly because of diaphragmatic inactivity, PPV reverses this normal pattern of gas distribution, and most delivered volume is directed to the upper lung zones. **B,** An increase in ventilation to the upper lung zones, where there is less perfusion, increases the $\dot{V}/\dot{Q}$ ratio, effectively increasing physiological dead space. At the same time, higher alveolar pressure in the better-ventilated upper lung zones diverts blood flow away from these areas to those receiving the least ventilation. The result is areas of low $\dot{V}/\dot{Q}$ ratio and impaired oxygenation. *(Modified from Kirby RR: Clinical application of ventilatory support, New York, 1990, Churchill Livingstone.)*

during PPV tends to perfuse the least well-ventilated lung regions. This decreases the $\dot{V}/\dot{Q}$ ratio in those areas and increases the $P(A\text{-}a)O_2$.

Alveolar and Arterial Carbon Dioxide

Normal alveolar carbon dioxide tension (P_ACO_2) is 40 mm Hg; mixed venous blood has a $P\bar{v}CO_2$ of 45 mm Hg. Under normal circumstances, carbon dioxide moves out of the blood at the pulmonary capillary interface; the result is a $PaCO_2$ of 40 mm Hg. In the event of a decrease in alveolar ventilation or an increase in carbon dioxide production, $PaCO_2$ increases. Mechanical ventilation can increase minute volume and alveolar ventilation and reduce $PACO_2$ and $PaCO_2$.

With an increase in dead space to tidal volume ratio (V_{DS}/V_T), $PaCO_2$ increases if there is no change in minute volume. This may happen when alveolar blood flow is decreased by acute pulmonary embolism, an excessive level of PEEP, or advanced dead space–producing disease, such as emphysema.

When excessive PEEP is used, blood flow is diverted from ventilated alveoli to hypoventilated alveoli; the result is an increased $\dot{V}/\dot{Q}$ ratio. In emphysema, formation of bullae is coincident with the destruction of pulmonary capillaries; the result is large areas of poorly perfused, ventilated alveoli. Pulmonary emboli may completely occlude pulmonary vessels; the result is lack of perfusion to alveoli distal to the blockage.

Changes in Acid-Base Balance

Respiratory acidemia, defined by a $PaCO_2$ greater than 45 to 50 mm Hg and a pH less than 7.35, occurs when minute ventilation and alveolar ventilation per minute ($\dot{V}_A$) are inadequate. This may be the result of setting the tidal volume and mandatory ventilator rate too low in the absence of spontaneous breathing. Respiratory acidemia also can occur when the tidal volume is set too low, even though an accompanying mandatory rate is high enough to maintain the desired minute ventilation. This situation can occur with volume loss due to tubing compliance when a small tidal volume is used. An increase in V_{DS}/V_T ratio can cause a reduction in alveolar ventilation per minute, even though minute ventilation may be normal or increased. These problems emphasize the importance of proper selection of ventilator values. When respiratory acidemia exists, the patient may become restless and anxious; the result is patient-ventilator asynchrony. A communicative patient may indicate he or she is dyspneic. If the symptoms are observed, especially when $PaCO_2$ is increased, the minute ventilation must be increased appropriately.

Another physiologic effect of respiratory acidemia is a right shift of the oxyhemoglobin dissociation curve. This shift decreases the ability of hemoglobin to bind with oxygen at the alveoli and facilitates oxygen dissociation to the tissues.

In prolonged hypoventilation and acidosis, hyperkalemia occurs as a compensatory response to maintain ionic balance in the cells. Hyperkalemia may result in cardiac arrhythmia (elevated and peaked T waves, S-T segment depression, widened QRS complexes, and a long P-R interval).

Unless permissive hypercapnia is desired (as in the management of ARDS), ventilation to achieve the patient's normal $PaCO_2$ and pH should be implemented with appropriate tidal volume and mandatory rate settings.

Respiratory alkalemia occurs if the minute ventilation is too high. It is recognized when $PaCO_2$ is less than 35 mm Hg and pH is greater than 7.45. The patient may cause this condition if dyspneic, anxious, or in pain; the usual manifestations are an increased ventilatory rate or patient-ventilator asynchrony. The ventilator can cause respiratory alkalemia due to an inappropriately high tidal volume, mandatory rate, or trigger sensitivity setting. Regardless, the result is excessive minute ventilation and alveolar ventilation per minute. This condition requires that the therapist adjust the ventilator appropriately and address the patient's pain or anxiety. Respiratory alkalemia causes a left shift of the hemoglobin dissociation curve, which increases the binding of oxygen to hemoglobin at the alveoli. Unfortunately, this shift inhibits oxygen dissociation at the tissues, which can cause tissue hypoxia. Prolonged hyperventilation may result in hypokalemia as potassium is excreted in the renal tubules as a compensatory response to maintain cellular ionic balance. The cardiac effects of hypokalemia include prolonged Q-T interval, S-T segment depression, negative T-wave deflection, inverted P waves, atrioventricular block, premature ventricular contractions, paroxysmal tachycardia, and atrial flutter.

Metabolic acidemia in a patient receiving mechanical ventilation is recognized by a normal $PaCO_2$, with a decreased pH (<7.35), decreased bicarbonate level (<22 mEq/L), and decreased base deficit (< −2 mEq/L). The problem with metabolic acidemia is that the patient must try to compensate by increasing minute ventilation to blow off carbon dioxide in an effort to increase the pH. The resulting increase in the work of breathing leads to ventilatory muscle fatigue and continued respiratory failure. The best therapy for metabolic acidosis is to manage the underlying cause while supporting the patient's ventilation as needed. Many patients cannot be liberated from mechanical ventilation until the underlying acidosis is controlled. Bicarbonate has been advocated as therapy for metabolic acidosis. If it is administered, bicarbonate quickly combines with hydrogen ions and dissociates to form carbon dioxide and water, a reaction that may increase the work of breathing. In general, bicarbonate administration is not recommended until the acidosis is severe (pH <7.2). When necessary, bicarbonate is administered according to the following formula:

$$\text{NaHCO}_3^- \text{ required} = \frac{(^1/_4 \times \text{Body weight in kg} \times \text{Base deficit})}{2}$$

A temporary measure to partially compensate for metabolic acidosis is to increase minute ventilation during therapy to control the acidosis with the goal of a pH greater than 7.2.

Metabolic alkalemia is defined as a normal $PaCO_2$ with an elevated pH (>7.45) and an increased bicarbonate level (>26 mEq/L) and base excess (> +2 mEq/L). The problem with metabolic alkalemia is that in an effort to compensate for the increased pH, the patient tries to decrease minute ventilation. In an effort to retain carbon dioxide, the patient receiving mechanical ventilation does not breathe spontaneously or may not spontaneously trigger ventilator breaths. If weaning is attempted when the patient has metabolic alkalemia, the patient may continue to hypoventilate, and weaning may fail. As with metabolic acidemia, the underlying cause should be determined and managed. Common causes of metabolic alkalosis include hypochloremia or hypokalemia due to gastrointestinal loss, diuretics, or steroid administration. The respiratory therapist should recognize these abnormalities and report them to the physician, but therapy relies on medical management.

▶ EFFECTS OF POSITIVE PRESSURE MECHANICAL VENTILATION ON LUNG MECHANICS

Time Constants

The time necessary for adequate inflation of each alveolus is determined by the product of compliance and resistance. This product is the time constant of the alveolar unit. The compliance of a "normal" alveolus is 0.1 L/cm H_2O, and its resistance is 1 cm H_2O/L per second. Therefore the time constant for normal alveoli is 0.1 second (0.1 L/cm $H_2O \times 1$ cm H_2O/L per second). For patients with normal lungs, 95% of the alveoli are inflated within three time constants, that is, within 0.3 seconds. If four time constants are used (0.4 s), 98% of alveoli are inflated, and if five time constants are used (0.5 s), 99.3% of alveoli are inflated. The same numbers apply for exhalation.

Two major factors affect alveolar time constants: changes in compliance and changes in resistance. If compliance or resistance decreases, the time constant for a given alveolus decreases, and the alveolus fills and empties faster. If compliance or resistance increases, the time constant increases, and it takes more time to fill and empty the alveolus.

There are clinical implications for patients with disorders consistent with abnormal time constants. A longer inspiratory time may be needed for patients with ARDS, because the alveoli have a decrease in compliance. Attempting to ventilate these patients with a normal inspiratory time may result in inadequate volume to affected alveoli, because these alveoli are stiff, and volume is likely to travel to more compliant alveoli. Hypothetically, if a patient has a compliance of 0.02 L/cm H_2O and normal resistance, the time constant is 0.02 seconds. However, because the alveolus is stiff, even five time constants (0.1 s) would be inadequate for complete inflation. To prolong the inspiratory phase, the therapist can increase the inspiratory time directly, use an end-inspiratory pause (inflation hold), or decrease the inspiratory flow. All these methods increase the ratio of inspiratory time to expiratory time (I:E ratio). As the I:E ratio increases beyond 1:1, a condition called inverse I:E ratio exists (see Chapter 39). The use of inverse I:E ratios often is reserved for patients with severe ARDS. An inflation hold provides additional time for gas redistribution among lung units with different time constants. This step should improve gas distribution and oxygenation. Stiff alveoli deflate quickly, so time is easily "borrowed" from expiration to allow for an increase in inspiratory time within a given total cycle time.

Because of the marked increase in airway resistance, a longer expiratory time may be needed in the care of patients with COPD. Patients with COPD have a loss of elastic function, which allows airways to collapse during expiration. In addition, secretions clogging the airways inhibit expiratory flow. For example, a patient with an increased resistance of 10 cm H_2O/L per second and normal or increased compliance has a time constant of 1.0 second or greater. An alveolar unit with an increased time constant requires more time for expiration than do normal alveoli. In the care of patients with COPD, it is best to prolong the available expiratory time to allow adequate alveolar emptying. Methods of increasing expiratory time include increasing the inspiratory flow, directly increasing the expiratory time, decreasing the mandatory ventilator rate, or decreasing the tidal volume. When airway resistance is increased and compliance is low, alveoli fill quickly, so time may be borrowed from inspiration to allow for a longer expiratory time within the given total cycle time. Ventilator management in the care of patients with COPD, asthma, and ARDS is described in Chapters 20, 24, and 41.

Increased Pressure

Peak inspiratory pressure (PIP) is the highest pressure produced during the inspiratory phase. It is the sum of the pressures necessary to overcome airway resistance and inflate the alveoli ($P_{ta} + P_{alv}$). Peak inspiratory pressure is also known as peak pressure or peak airway pressure.

Plateau pressure (P_{plat}) is the pressure observed on the manometer during a period of inflation hold or end-inspiratory pause. To obtain a plateau pressure, the therapist initiates an inspiratory pause time of 0.5 to 1.0 second. During inspiration, the peak pressure is reached and immediately followed by the inspiratory pause. During the pause, pressure decreases to a pressure plateau (P_{plat}). Once a valid plateau pressure value is obtained, the inspiratory pause time is returned to zero. Plateau pressure represents the pressure necessary to inflate the alveoli (P_{alv}). In volume-controlled ventilation, plateau pressure is always lower than peak pressure, because the peak pressure is the sum of the alveolar pressure and the pressure needed to overcome airway resistance. The difference between plateau pressure and peak pressure is the pressure necessary to overcome airway resistance. If the tidal volume is divided by the difference between the plateau pressure and the PEEP, the quotient is the static compliance:

$$C_{static} = V_T/(P_{plat} - PEEP)$$

Airway resistance (Raw) during volume ventilation is estimated by the difference between PIP and P_{plat} divided by the inspiratory flow rate ($\dot{V}_I$) in liters per second:

$$Raw = (PIP - P_{plat})/\dot{V}_I$$

During mechanical ventilation, the plateau pressure should be maintained at less than 30 to 35 cm H_2O. At levels greater than 30 to 35 cm H_2O, alveolar damage from excessive shear forces can occur. This trauma can result in air leakage from alveoli, the release of inflammatory mediators, and multisystem organ failure. When the plateau pressure approaches 30 to 35 cm H_2O during volume-controlled ventilation, pressure-controlled ventilation may be considered. If this value is approached during pressure-controlled ventilation, the pressure limit should be reduced, and tidal volume decreases. This is the "lung protective strategy" referred to in the literature about mechanical ventilation of patients with ARDS.[4]

Mean Airway Pressure

As shown in Figure 40-6, mean airway pressure is the area under the pressure-time curve during inspiration and expiration. Because expiratory (baseline) pressure is lower than inspiratory pressure, the mean pressure is between peak and baseline pressure. Mean airway pressure is computed as the integral of the pressure signal over the total cycle time. The many variables affecting mean pleural and mean airway pressure are summarized in Box 40-1. In terms of ventilatory support, the greater the ratio of spontaneous to mandatory breaths, the lower is the mean airway pressure. Thus for a given minute volume, partial ventilatory support modes such as synchronized intermittent mandatory ventilation (SIMV) result in lower mean airway and pleural pressures than do full support modes such as continuous mandatory ventilation (CMV). For a mandatory breath, the higher the peak pressure, the greater is the area under the pressure curve and the higher is the mean pressure. In Figure 40-7, pressure waveform E has the highest applied pressure over a constant time and the greatest mean pressure. Likewise, long inspiratory times increase the area under the pressure curve (Figure 40-8). With an increase in inspiratory time, mean airway pressure increases. Expiratory time has an opposite

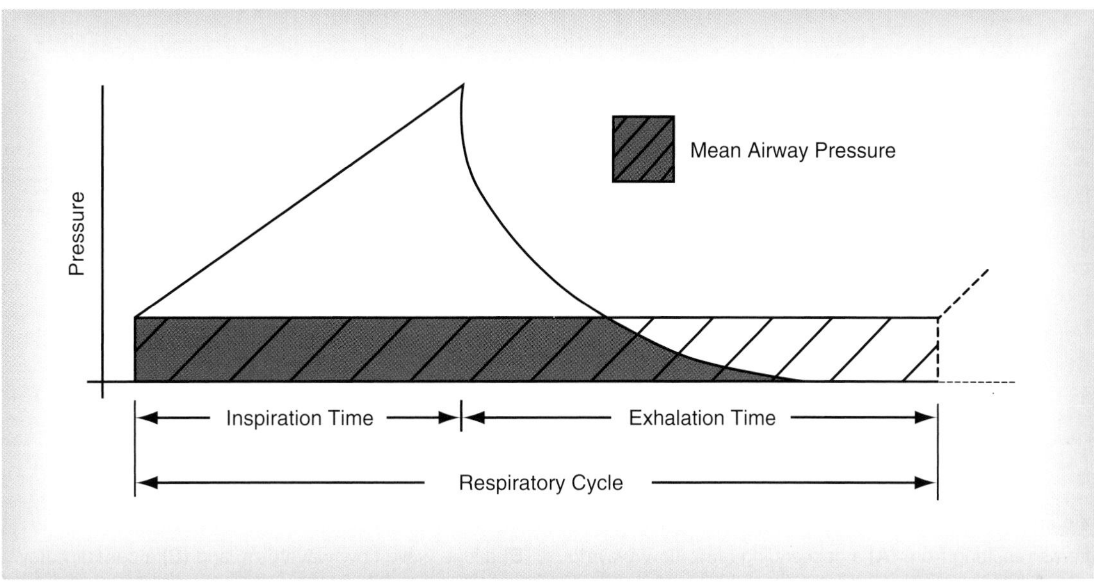

Figure 40-6
Mean airway pressure is defined as the area under the pressure curve for the duration of the respiratory cycle *(purple area)*. Most microprocessor ventilators calculate and display this value.

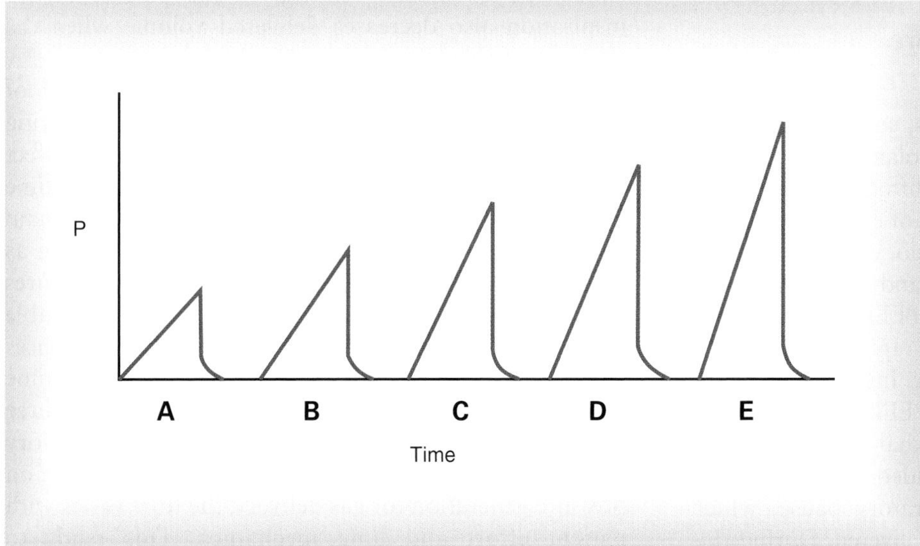

Figure 40-7
Effect of changes in peak pressure on mean airway pressure (P_{aw}). If the inspiratory time remains constant, mean airway pressure increases as peak airway pressure increases. Waveform **E** has the greatest mean pressure.

Box 40-1 • Factors That Increase Mean Pleural Pressure

- Mandatory breath modes
- Increasing positive pressure
- Increasing duration of inspiration
- Decreasing duration of expiration
- Nature of the inspiratory waveform
- Increasing level of PEEP
- Decreasing compliance, increasing resistance

effect on mean airway pressure. In general, harmful cardiovascular effects of PPV are most likely to occur when the I:E ratio is greater than 1:2 (e.g., 2:1).

The pressure waveform of a mandatory breath affects mean pressure. In Figure 40-8, for a given inspiratory time, the constant pressure pattern (curve A) results in the greatest area and thus the highest mean airway pressure. A constant pressure pattern is normally produced by a pressure controller that provides decreasing (descending ramp) flow. However, this same pattern can be produced by a nonconstant flow controller.

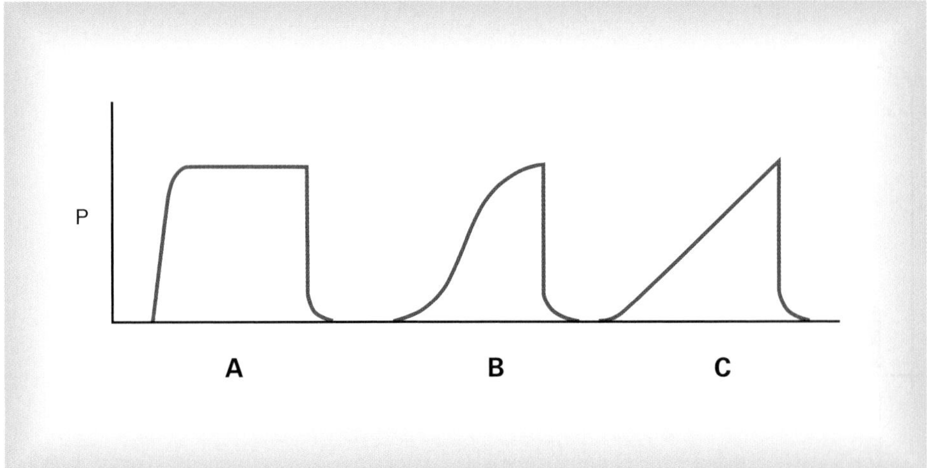

Figure 40-8
Pressure patterns resulting from **(A)** a descending ramp flow waveform, **(B)** a sine wave flow waveform, and **(C)** a constant flow waveform. Since waveform **A** has the highest pressure for the longest inspiratory time, it also has the greatest mean airway pressure.

The effect of PEEP on mean airway pressure is simple: every 1 cm H_2O of applied PEEP increases the mean airway pressure 1 cm H_2O.

Effect of Mean Airway Pressure on Oxygenation

As mean airway pressure increases, so does functional residual capacity (FRC). At the alveolar level, this means that the surface area available for diffusion is increased. As a result, PaO_2 increases. The use of extrinsic PEEP or the implementation of inverse ratio ventilation (IRV) increases mean airway pressure and PaO_2. Extrinsic PEEP is controlled directly by the PEEP control on the ventilator control panel, and the therapist always knows how much extrinsic PEEP is present. Inverse ratio ventilation may add intrinsic or auto-PEEP by starting the next breath before the previous exhalation has ended. The amount of intrinsic PEEP added by IRV can be measured by adding an end-expiratory pause, which stops the next breath from being delivered. During this end-expiratory pause, alveolar and mouth pressures equilibrate, and the total PEEP registers on the ventilator manometer. The amount of auto-PEEP present is the difference between the total PEEP and the extrinsic PEEP:

$$\text{Intrinsic PEEP (auto-PEEP)} = \text{Total PEEP} - \text{Extrinsic PEEP}$$

Increased Lung Volume

Tidal Volume

The volume delivered during pressure-controlled modes varies with changes in set pressure, patient effort, and lung mechanics. For all pressure-targeted modes, the volume delivered at a given pressure decreases as compliance declines. An increase in resistance on active exhalation or muscle tensing by the patient during inspiration also decreases delivered volume when the cycling variable is pressure.

If pressure serves as the limit variable instead of the cycle variable, changes in airway resistance during pressure-limited ventilation may or may not affect delivered volume. In this case, the key factor is the time available for pressure equilibration. Volume can remain constant even if airway resistance increases, as long as there is sufficient time for alveolar and airway pressures to equilibrate. However, if insufficient time is available for pressure equilibration, delivered volume decreases as airway resistance increases. The length of time needed for pressure equilibration is usually at least three times greater than the time constant for the respiratory system. Because all pressure-controlled modes rely on pressure generation for gas delivery, the flow varies with patient effort and lung mechanics. This tends to enhance patient-ventilator synchrony, as argued by proponents of these modes.[5]

Increased Functional Residual Capacity

The FRC is not known to change significantly with the application of PPV alone, because passive exhalation allows the FRC to return to baseline with each breath. If an increase in FRC is to be achieved, the baseline pressure must be increased. This increase is commonly achieved with PEEP or CPAP. The magnitude of increase in FRC is proportional to lung-thorax compliance near the existing FRC. With acute restriction, as PEEP is increased, lung compliance improves. Initially,

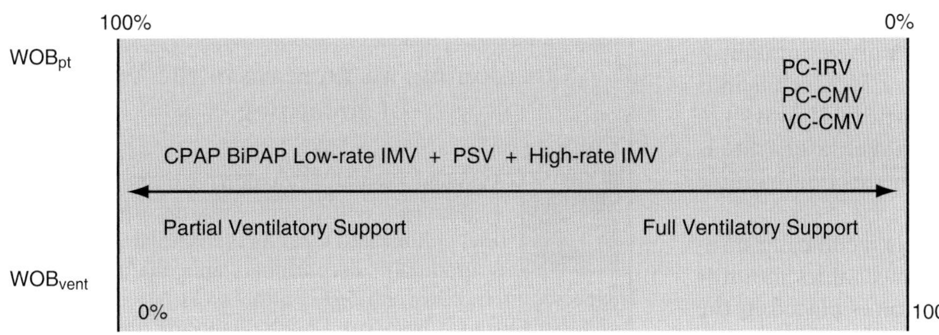

Figure 40-9
Continuum of ventilatory support illustrating the relative work of breathing between patient and ventilator, depending on mode of ventilation. *PSV*, Pressure-supported ventilation; *BiPAP*, bilevel positive airway pressure; *PC*, pressure-controlled.

the FRC gain as PEEP is added is small. However, as FRC and compliance increase, additional increments of PEEP tend to result in larger increases in FRC up to the point at which overdistension occurs. At that point, as PEEP is increased, increases in FRC decline. There is no practical way of measuring FRC at the bedside, so other methods of determining an increase in FRC are used, such as improving PaO_2 at a constant FIO_2, increasing PaO_2/FIO_2 ratio, decreasing shunt fraction, or decreasing FIO_2 and maintaining PaO_2. Positive end-expiratory pressure sometimes is titrated by observation of the effect of increases in PEEP on lung compliance or adjustment of the PEEP level such that it is above the lower inflection point on a static pressure-volume curve. The management of PEEP is described in more detail in Chapter 41.

Increased Dead Space

The dead space fraction is increased with the institution of mechanical ventilation owing to inspiratory mechanical bronchodilation and the preferential ventilation of more apical, nondependent alveoli with the continued perfusion of basilar or dependent alveoli (Figure 40-5). This increase is concurrent with a decrease in $\dot{V}/\dot{Q}$ ratio.

Decreased Work of Breathing

Positive pressure ventilation can significantly reduce the work of breathing in patients with actual or impending respiratory muscle fatigue. Therapists frequently see the gratifying physical relaxation enjoyed by patients as the ventilator assumes a major portion of their work of breathing. To lessen the work of breathing, ventilation must be sufficient to meet the patient's needs. Otherwise, a spontaneously breathing patient tends to resist the ventilator, and an asynchronous breathing pattern develops. Inappropriately applied PPV can result in alveolar hypoventilation and, as a result of patient struggling, a considerable increase in the work of breathing.

Mode, trigger variable, and inspiratory flow have an effect on the work of breathing. Work of breathing consists of two components: (1) ventilator work (WOB_{vent}) occurring as the ventilator forces gas into the lungs, and (2) patient work (WOB_{pt}) as the inspiratory muscles draw gas into the lungs. The magnitude of WOB_{pt} depends on patient variables such as compliance, resistance, and ventilatory drive and on ventilator variables, such as trigger sensitivity, peak flow, and tidal volume.[6]

Several reports have demonstrated that flow triggering decreases the WOB_{pt} and the pressure-time product necessary to start a breath, compared with pressure triggering at -2 cm H_2O, to the extent that flow triggering is recommended.[7]

Mechanical ventilation modes may be thought of as being on a continuum from assuming very little to assuming all the work of breathing (Figure 40-9). As the mode is changed from CPAP to pressure-supported ventilation (PSV) to SIMV to time-triggered CMV, the ventilator assumes more of the work. When all breaths are time triggered, as when the patient is pharmacologically paralyzed, all work performed is WOB_{vent}. Although it may be advantageous for the ventilator to assume all of the work of breathing for a while, extended periods of controlled ventilation may cause diaphragmatic atrophy, which unnecessarily prolongs the need for mechanical ventilation. At initiation of assisted pressure- or volume-controlled modes, WOB_{pt} resumes. With volume ventilation, this work is primarily associated with triggering the ventilator and inspiring the tidal volume at the set inspiratory flow rate. If the sensitivity and inspiratory flow rate are set appropriately, WOB_{pt} is negligible. If flow is set too low, patient-ventilator asynchrony often occurs, and an increased WOB_{pt} results.

Once the ventilator mode is changed to SIMV, most clinicians add PSV to spontaneous breaths to overcome the imposed work of breathing due to ventilator demand flow systems, ventilator circuits, and the artificial airway. There is vast literature on the unloading and reloading of the patient's muscles of ventilation when PSV is used.[8] As the PSV level is increased, the muscles are unloaded, tidal volume increases for a given amount of patient effort, and WOB_{pt} decreases. Most clinicians increase PSV until the breathing pattern is closer to normal, that is, until the spontaneous ventilatory rate is 15 to 25 breaths/min and the spontaneous tidal volume is normal.

Measuring the work of breathing is technically difficult, necessitating the use of a lung mechanics monitor specifically for that purpose. A balloon is placed in the distal third of the esophagus, and a pneumotachometer is attached to the airway. The work of breathing is calculated with the monitor as the integral of the esophageal pressure and tidal volume. Normal work of breathing is 0.6 to 0.8 J/L. One approach to PSV is titration of the PSV level on the basis of measured work of breathing. If work is greater than 0.8J/L, PSV is increased until work decreases to within normal limits (unloading the muscles of ventilation). If work is less than 0.6 J/L, PSV is decreased until work increases to within normal limits (loading the muscles of ventilation). Use of PSV in this manner maintains muscle work at a normal level, and muscle fatigue or atrophy may be prevented. Although it may be useful to titrate PSV to level WOB_{pt}[9] on the basis of bedside measurement of work of breathing, not every hospital has the capability of measuring WOB_{pt}. Respiratory rate and frequency and patients' answers to questions about their breathing comfort help the therapist determine whether WOB_{pt} is excessive. Once the patient's tidal volume is adequate, PSV may be gradually discontinued with spontaneous respiratory rate as a guide. If the patient's spontaneous respiratory rate increases, PSV has been decreased excessively, and a slower approach should be adopted.

An alternative to measuring the work of breathing at the bedside is calculation of the rapid shallow breathing index (RSBI), which is the quotient of spontaneous respiratory rate (f) and tidal volume (V_T), which is measured in liters. The formula for RSBI is

$$RSBI = f/V_t$$

The RSBI is commonly used for prediction of successful liberation from mechanical ventilation. If the RSBI is greater than 105, there is decreased likelihood that the patient may be successfully weaned from the ventilator.[10] If the spontaneous respiratory rate is high or tidal volume low, the work of breathing may be increased. For example, if the patient is breathing 15 breaths/min with a tidal volume of 0.55 L, the RSBI is 27. If the patient meets other criteria for liberation from the ventilator, extubation should be successful. If the patient has a respiratory rate of 35 breaths/min with a tidal volume of 0.28 L, the RSBI is 125, indicating a high work of breathing and the probability of weaning failure.

MINI CLINI

Overcoming an Increase in the Work of Breathing

PROBLEM

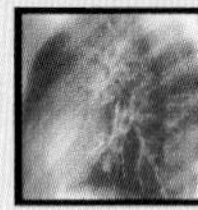

A patient's work of breathing is minimal during mechanical ventilation with an appropriate tidal volume and rate. As the ventilator support is gradually discontinued and the patient is expected to take over more of the work of breathing, airway resistance associated with breathing through an endotracheal tube may become clinically important. The therapist must be able to readily recognize this problem and know how to correct it.

PROBLEM

A patient has received mechanical ventilation in a volume-controlled CMV mode for the past week. The patient's condition is now clinically stable, and weaning has begun with SIMV. As the SIMV rate is decreased to less than 5 breaths/min, the patient begins using the accessory muscles to breathe, the spontaneous respiratory rate increases to 30 breaths/min, and the patient reports shortness of breath. Blood gas values are acceptable, and no abnormal lung sounds are present. What is the problem, and what should the therapist do?

SOLUTION

The patient is probably experiencing excessive work of breathing due to airway resistance associated with the endotracheal tube. Other possibilities that should be considered include deterioration in the patient's cardiopulmonary disease, but the normal blood gas values and lung sounds suggest the problem is outside the lungs. The addition of pressure support at 5 to 10 cm H_2O is useful in such situations to overcome the excessive resistance that often occurs when the patient breathes through an endotracheal tube. Automatic tube compensation also may be used. Once the patient is extubated, the excessive work imposed by the endotracheal tube no longer is present.

▶ MINIMIZING ADVERSE PULMONARY EFFECTS OF POSITIVE PRESSURE MECHANICAL VENTILATION

Decreasing Pressure

The main objective of mechanical ventilation is a minute ventilation adequate to provide the patient with adequate alveolar ventilation. Supplemental oxygen and PEEP are provided for adequate arterial oxygenation.

Peak pressure is the result of the pressure required to overcome system resistance and elastance. Although there is no absolute maximum pressure, most practitioners try to avoid peak pressures greater than 40 cm H_2O. As the peak pressure approaches 40 cm H_2O, it is important to consider the causes. Factors that increase airway resistance include airway edema, bronchospasm, and secretions. The therapist can manage or avoid these problems by assuring adequate humidity, bronchial hygiene (suctioning, airway care), and administration of bronchodilators and antiinflammatory drugs. Factors that increase the pressure needed to inflate the lung and overcome decreased compliance include alveolar and interstitial edema, fibrosis, and chest wall restriction. These conditions may be difficult to control, and the therapist must rely on the medical staff to prescribe drugs that decrease the pulmonary vascular load, such as pulmonary vasodilators and diuretics, and drugs that increase cardiac contractility in the case of cardiogenic pulmonary edema. There is little the therapist can do if the patient has pulmonary fibrosis. Chest wall restriction may be caused by restrictive bandaging, which can be removed if no longer needed.

Plateau pressure reflects alveolar pressure. Alveolar pressures of 30 to 35 cm H_2O or greater are associated with alveolar damage. If alveolar pressure approaches 30 to 35 cm H_2O during volume-controlled ventilation, the tidal volume should be decreased so the alveolar pressure is 30 to 35 cm H_2O or less, or the mode should be changed to pressure controlled with a pressure of 30 to 35 cm H_2O or less.[11]

Mean airway pressure is increased by an increase in inspiratory time, tidal volume, respiratory rate, PEEP, or PIP. A decrease in any of these settings may be effective in reducing mean airway pressure. Increases in mean airway pressure are associated with improvements in PaO_2; however, increased mean airway pressure reduces venous return and may reduce cardiac output in compromised patients.

Positive End-Expiratory Pressure/Continuous Positive Airway Pressure

Positive end-expiratory pressure is the use of positive pressure to change the baseline pressure during either CMV or IMV (see Chapter 41). Positive end-expiratory pressure is used primarily to improve oxygenation in patients with refractory hypoxemia. As a rule, refractory hypoxemia exists when a patient's PaO_2 cannot be maintained above 50 to 60 mm Hg with an FIO_2 of 0.40 to 0.50 or more. Positive end-expiratory pressure improves oxygenation in these patients by opening collapsed alveoli (recruitment), restoring the FRC, and decreasing physiological shunting. As a result, the improved alveolar volume provided by PEEP allows use of a lower FIO_2. Other values such as lung compliance, shunt fraction, and PaO_2/FIO_2 ratio also may improve when PEEP is appropriately applied. Positive end-expiratory pressure may be indicated in the care of patients with COPD who have dynamic hyperinflation (auto-PEEP) during mechanical ventilatory support after other efforts to decrease auto-PEEP fail.[12] Appropriate PEEP levels to overcome auto-PEEP are described in Chapter 41.

There are beneficial as well as harmful effects associated with the use of PEEP (Table 40-2). The most important factor in PEEP management is to not use too much. Detrimental effects of inappropriately high levels of PEEP include barotrauma, decreased cardiac output, increased pulmonary vascular resistance, and increased dead space. When one or more of these problems occurs, the PEEP usually is decreased to the previous level or to a value between the current level and the previous level. If cardiac output decreases and the increase in PEEP is absolutely necessary to maintain oxygenation, intravenous fluid, inotropic cardiac drugs, or both sometimes are administered for restoration of cardiac output.

Positive end-expiratory pressure is contraindicated in the presence of an unmanaged bronchopleural fistula or pneumothorax. Application of PEEP to both lungs is contraindicated in severe unilateral lung disease, because PEEP tends to overinflate the lung with higher compliance. The result is lung overdistension and compression of adjacent pulmonary capillaries. Independent lung ventilation can be used to apply separate inspiratory and baseline pressures to the right and the left lung when unilateral lung disease is present.[13] Positive end-expiratory pressure also is contraindicated in the care of patients with an increase in ICP when the application of PEEP further increases ICP.

Table 40-2 ▶ ▶ Physiological Effects of Positive End-Expiratory Pressure

Beneficial Effects of Appropriate PEEP	Detrimental Effects of Inappropriate PEEP
Restored FRC, alveolar recruitment	Increased incidence of pulmonary barotrauma
Decreased shunt fraction	Potential decrease in venous return and cardiac output
Increased lung compliance	Increased work of breathing (with overdistension)
Decreased work of breathing	Increased pulmonary vascular resistance
Increased PaO_2 for a given FIO_2	Increased ICP
	Decreased renal and portal blood flow
	Increased dead space
	Increased mean airway pressure

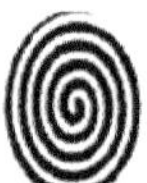

RULE OF THUMB

Refractory hypoxemia exists when a patient's PaO_2 cannot be maintained above 50 to 60 mm Hg with an FIO_2 of 0.40 to 0.50 or greater. This situation is an indication for PPV with PEEP or CPAP, because PPV with either of these modalities improves oxygenation by decreasing physiological shunting.

Effects of Ventilatory Pattern

Modern positive pressure ventilators have an assortment of inspiratory flow patterns, including square, increasing (accelerating), decreasing (decelerating), sine, and others. In mechanical and computer models, a decelerating flow pattern improves gas distribution to lung units with long-time constants. Similar findings in humans have been reported. Compared with a square flow waveform, decreasing flow has been shown to reduce peak pressure, inspiratory work, V_{DS}/V_T ratio, and $P(A - a)O_2$ without affecting hemodynamic values.[14] Compared with volume-controlled ventilation with a square flow waveform, pressure-controlled ventilation with decreasing flow may result in a higher PaO_2, lower $PaCO_2$, and lower peak inspiratory and plateau pressures. However, mean airway pressure is higher with the decreasing flow waveform, even if inspiratory time remains constant. The popularity of the decreasing flow waveform may be due to its ability to deliver most of the tidal volume at a time when the lungs are most compliant. As a breath ends, flow is least, and the volume being pushed into the lungs is least. The result is a lower peak airway pressure for any given tidal volume.

In most spontaneously breathing persons, lower inspiratory flows improve gas distribution. However, during PPV, low inspiratory flow may lead to air trapping if expiratory time is too short. High ventilator inspiratory flow allows more time for exhalation and reduces the incidence of air trapping. Avoidance of air-trapping improves gas exchange and reduces the work of breathing in patients with severe airflow obstruction.[15]

An inflation hold also affects gas exchange. By momentarily maintaining lung volume under conditions of no flow, an inflation hold allows additional time for gas redistribution between lung units with different time constants. This step should improve gas distribution and oxygenation. As applied clinically, however, an inflation hold has a greater effect on the efficiency of ventilation than on oxygenation. In both animal and human studies, increasing the length of an inflation hold decreases the V_{DS}/V_T ratio, $PaCO_2$, and inert gas washout time. Adding an inflation hold effectively increases total inspiratory time, thereby shortening the time available for exhalation. This step predisposes patients with airway obstruction to intrinsic PEEP. In practice, inflation hold is rarely used other than to obtain P_{plat} values. Because the technique does not seem natural to the patient, asynchrony can occur. Inflation hold also increases mean airway pressure, and the high airway pressure decreases cardiac output in compromised patients.

Trigger Site and Work of Breathing

Studies have examined the effects of sensing the patient's inspiratory effort at the tip of the endotracheal tube rather than in the ventilator circuit, as is done with most ventilators. Tidal volume and peak inspiratory flow were significantly higher with the sensor at the tip of the endotracheal tube, and the pressure time product and RSBI were significantly lower.[16] The investigators recommended moving the site of trigger sensing to the tip of the endotracheal tube, although this would require modifications by the manufacturers of both the endotracheal tube and the ventilator.[17]

▶ PHYSIOLOGICAL EFFECTS OF VENTILATORY MODES

Volume-Controlled Modes

Volume-controlled modes include volume-controlled continuous mandatory ventilation (VC-CMV) and volume-controlled intermittent mandatory ventilation (VC-IMV). Volume-controlled CMV includes what has been called for years *assist/control ventilation* and time-triggered volume-controlled ventilation. In assist/control, the patient may flow or pressure trigger (assist) mandatory breaths in addition to time-triggered breaths. Volume-controlled IMV may include pressure-controlled spontaneous breaths as pressure-supported breaths (PSV) (see Chapter 39).

Volume-controlled CMV provides all of the patient's minute ventilation as mandatory breaths. Each tidal volume is nearly the same. In time-triggered CMV, the patient may be sedated and is sometimes paralyzed. Time-triggered CMV affords greatest control over the patient's ventilatory pattern, PaO_2, $PaCO_2$, and acid-base balance because the patient is not permitted to initiate or limit breaths. Because every breath is volume controlled, mean airway pressure tends to be greater compared with the mean airway pressure with SIMV and PSV, and pulmonary arterial pressure and cardiac output may be lower.[17] High airway pressure can cause cardiovascular complications and barotrauma or volutrauma. Another complication of time-triggered CMV is that paralyzed or sedated patients do not use their muscles of ventilation. Over a few days, muscle atrophy develops and prolongs weaning.

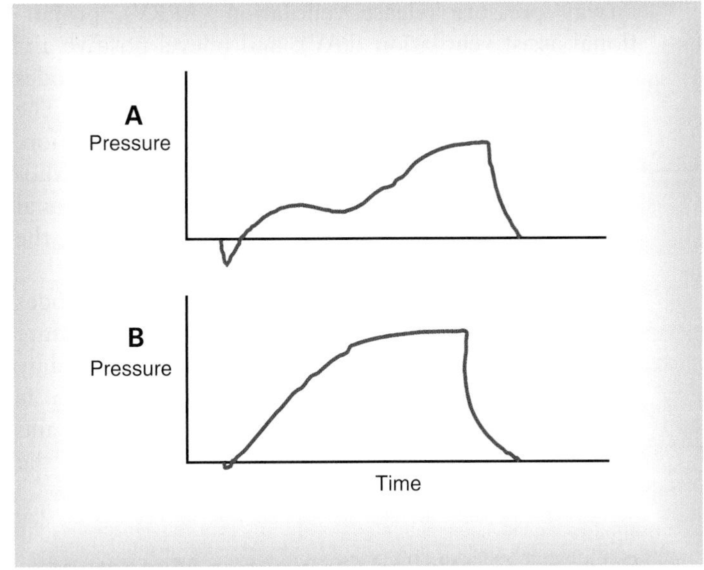

Figure 40-10
Pressure waveforms. **A,** Sensitivity set such that inspiratory effort must be excessive. Flow set such that it does not meet patient demand. Both result in increased work of breathing and patient-ventilator asynchrony. **B,** Appropriate settings for sensitivity and flow result in a normal pressure-time curve for a mandatory breath.

In pressure-triggered CMV, sensitivity and inspiratory flow must be set to correspond to patient inspiratory effort. If sensitivity is set too low, such that considerable effort is necessary to trigger the ventilator, patient-ventilator asynchrony occurs. A pressure sensitivity of −0.5 to −1.5 cm H_2O is regarded as optimal. Inspiratory flow must be set to meet the patient's inspiratory demand. An insufficient inspiratory flow can cause patient-ventilator asynchrony and increased work of breathing. By using waveform graphics, the practitioner can determine sufficient sensitivity and flow. At the beginning of inspiration, a small negative deflection on the manometer suggests an appropriate sensitivity setting. Likewise, the inspiratory pressure waveform should have a smooth appearance without any sharp spikes or dips (Figure 40-10).

Most patients are capable of providing at least part of their ventilation. In these cases, IMV is recommended. Advantages of IMV include patients' use of their own muscles of ventilation to help prevent muscle atrophy and lower mean airway pressure, which can assist in avoiding cardiovascular compromise.

With volume-controlled, flow-limited ventilation, the breath-to-breath volume delivered by the ventilator remains relatively constant, and the airway pressure varies according to the patient's lung mechanics. For example, should compliance decrease or airway resistance increase, the pressure needed to deliver the volume increases. Only if the pressure exceeds a set alarm threshold does inspiration end.

The volume delivered to a patient during volume-controlled, flow-limited ventilation (as with any positive pressure ventilator) is always less than that generated by the machine. Two factors account for this volume loss. First, gases are compressed when delivered under pressure. Thus the generated volume (at atmospheric pressure) occupies less space when delivered under pressure. Second, most ventilator circuits are somewhat compliant. Expansion of the tubing under pressure takes some of the volume that would otherwise go to the patient. In combination, these factors contribute to the compressed volume loss during PPV (see Chapter 39). In general, compressed volume loss is critical only when the delivered volume is small, as in infant, pediatric, and high-frequency applications. As a rule, the smaller the tidal volume required, the smaller is the compression factor needed. To achieve the lowest possible compression factor, the therapist uses (1) a ventilator with minimal internal volume, (2) low-volume, low-compliance tubing, and (3) a low-volume humidifier. Compressed volume loss must be accounted for in certain monitoring functions, such as bedside estimation of compliance and resistance (see Chapter 43). As the tidal volume required to ventilate the patient decreases (as in the care of children), a circuit with a lower compressible volume is recommended.

An additional factor that can cause a patient to receive less volume than the ventilator delivers is a leak. Because the cycle variable during volume-targeted modes is the volume generated by the machine (as opposed to that actually received by the patient), a system leak decreases the volume reaching the patient. For this reason, volume-targeted ventilators are said to compensate poorly for leaks in the system. A low exhaled volume or low inspiratory pressure alarm must be incorporated into the design.

Last, when spontaneous breathing is part of a given mode (as during partial ventilatory support with SIMV), volume-targeted breaths make up only a portion of the patient's total minute ventilation. Because the level of spontaneous breathing varies according to patient effort, total minute ventilation is not constant. Thus the main advantage of the volume-targeted approach (a consistent minute volume) does not apply during partial ventilatory support.

A volume-targeted approach may not provide a constant minute volume under all conditions. In addition, physiological changes that cause pressure to vary also may change gas distribution and the $\dot{V}/\dot{Q}$ ratio within the lung. Thus even if volume targeting were to provide the same overall ventilation against changing lung mechanics, the resulting arterial blood gases could vary. All these factors make it important to monitor physiological and arterial blood gas values as well as exhaled volume and to make ventilator adjustments accordingly.

Adaptive Support Ventilation

Adaptive support ventilation (ASV) is a dual-controlled mode of ventilation in which an automated increase or decrease in ventilatory support is based on patient effort and time constants. The system is based on the minimum work of breathing advanced by Otis in the 1950s. Otis proposed that there is an "ideal" ventilatory pattern that results in the lowest work of breathing based on compliance and resistance and that the pattern optimizes the tidal volume and respiratory rate. This mode, available only on the Hamilton Galileo ventilator, is perhaps the most "automatic" mode because most of the ventilation is left to microprocessor algorithms. In ASV, the therapist inputs the patient's ideal body weight, high pressure limit, PEEP, F_{IO_2}, inspiratory increase time, and flow cycle time. The ventilator continuously measures system compliance, airway resistance, and auto-PEEP and determines the desired mandatory rate. Ideal body weight is used by the ventilator to calculate the minute volume, which is divided by the rate for determination of tidal volume.[18] The ventilator attempts to deliver 100 mL/kg per minute of minute ventilation for adults or 200 mL/kg per minute for children. Adaptive support ventilation is time or patient triggered, pressure limited, and time or flow cycled at the calculated tidal volume. It has been shown clinically that ASV provides an adequate minute volume. The algorithm provides slightly higher rates and lower tidal volume than chosen by clinicians but with no difference in arterial blood gas values. Adaptive support ventilation also adapts to changes in patient position. Adaptive support ventilation is not intended to be an automatic weaning mode.[19]

Pressure-Controlled Modes

Included in this category are pressure-controlled CMV (PC-CMV), pressure-controlled IMV (PC-IMV), volume-assured pressure-supported ventilation (VAPS), PSV, CPAP, airway pressure release ventilation (APRV), proportional assist ventilation (PAV), and bilevel positive airway pressure (BiPAP). Most pressure-controlled modes include the use of the decreasing flow waveform. The extent to which any of these modes affects ventilation, and the extent to which any of them affects the cardiovascular system or leads to barotrauma, is proportional to the pressure gradient during inspiration or to the level of baseline pressure.

The physiological benefits of pressure-limited modes are based on the limitation of peak alveolar pressure and on the good patient-ventilator synchrony offered by the decelerating flow pattern. Other benefits, such as improved gas mixing, distribution of ventilation, and improved oxygenation remain unproved owing to the number of extraneous variables in available studies.

Pressure-Controlled Continuous Mandatory Ventilation

Pressure-controlled CMV may be used to reduce airway and alveolar pressures in patients with ALI and ARDS. When airway pressure is limited, shear forces that may damage alveoli whenever plateau pressure during VC-CMV exceeds 30 to 35 cm H_2O can be avoided.[4]

Pressure-controlled CMV may be used in conjunction with permissive hypercapnia as part of a lung protective strategy in the management of ALI/ARDS. Permissive hypercapnia is an increase in Pa_{CO_2} through a planned reduction in PPV. The resultant reduction in transpulmonary pressure should reduce the incidence of barotrauma and other complications associated with PPV (see later). A gradual increase in Pa_{CO_2} is accomplished by reduction of the mechanical tidal volume and usually does not reduce oxygenation. Permissive hypercapnia is generally well tolerated and does not adversely affect pulmonary vascular resistance, systemic vascular resistance, cardiac index, or systemic oxygen delivery or consumption.[20] Severe hypercapnia can have adverse effects. These may include increased ICP, depressed myocardial function, increased pulmonary arterial pressure, and decreased renal blood flow.[21] Permissive hypercapnia is contraindicated in the care of patients with cerebral disorders and should be used with caution in the care of patients with left ventricular failure, myocardial ischemia, pulmonary hypertension, or right heart failure.

Pressure-Controlled Inverse Ratio Ventilation

Pressure-controlled CMV may be used for PC-IRV. Pressure-controlled IRV is defined as pressure-controlled ventilation with an I:E ratio greater than 1:1. With PC-IRV, mean airway pressure increases with the I:E ratio. Pressure-controlled IRV has been suggested for severe hypoxemia when high F_{IO_2} and high PEEP have failed

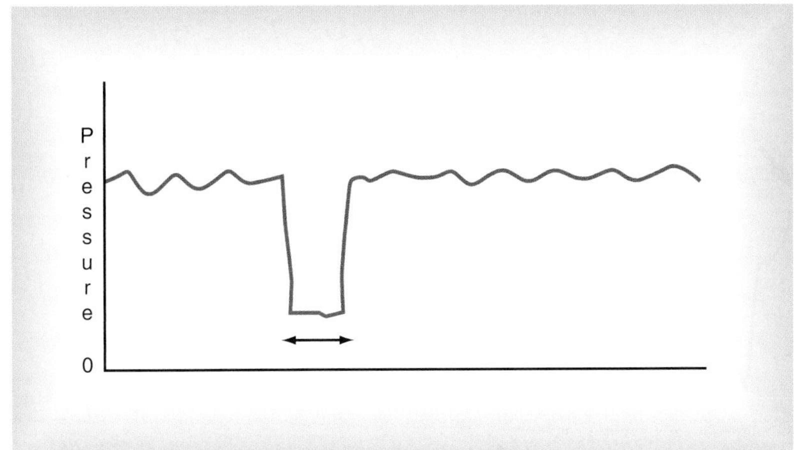

Figure 40-11
Airway pressure release ventilation is a simple modification of CPAP. During APRV, the CPAP pressure is intermittently released or decreased for a short period, usually less than 1.5 seconds *(bidirectional arrow)*. This intermittent pressure release helps eliminate carbon dioxide.

to improve oxygenation. Because alveoli affected by ARDS have short time constants, more time is allotted to inspiration and less time is allotted to expiration. The result is intrinsic PEEP and an increase in mean airway pressure, which is the mechanism for alveolar recruitment and improved arterial oxygenation in this mode.[22] Although some studies have shown improvement in oxygenation with PC-IRV versus CMV with PEEP, others have shown concurrent decreases in cardiac output.[23,24] Although PC-IRV may improve oxygenation at the lung level, a decrease in cardiac output may result in an overall decrease in tissue oxygenation.

Airway Pressure Release Ventilation

A related mode is APRV, in which the patient breathes spontaneously throughout periods of raised and lowered airway pressure (Figure 40-11). Airway pressure release ventilation intermittently decreases or "releases" the airway pressure from an upper CPAP (inspiratory positive airway pressure) to a lower level (expiratory positive airway pressure). The pressure release usually lasts 1.5 seconds or less, enough time for gas to passively leave the lungs and for carbon dioxide to be eliminated. The I:E ratio during APRV usually is greater than 1:1, which is similar to that for PC-IRV but offers the advantage of allowing spontaneous breathing. Airway pressure release ventilation may provide sufficient ventilation and oxygenation without significant differences in hemodynamic values. Because patients undergoing APRV are breathing spontaneously, the need for sedation is much less than during PC-IRV, possibly because of improved oxygenation during APRV compared with PC-IRV. In addition, peak airway pressure during APRV may be less than with PC-IRV for comparable oxygenation and ventilation.[25] One study of patients with ALI compared VC-IRV with APRV. During APRV, peak airway pressure and venous admixture were lower than during VC-IRV, a finding that indicated progressive alveolar recruitment.[26]

Specific indications for APRV remain unclear. This modality was originally proposed as therapy for severe hypoxemia; however, it has not been shown to markedly improve oxygenation in humans with ALI. Airway pressure release ventilation may be more effective in improving oxygenation than improving alveolar ventilation. Airway pressure release ventilation has the physiological benefits of CPAP and has the advantage of enhanced ventilation. Airway pressure release ventilation has not been extensively studied, perhaps because few ventilators offer this mode.[27] As with bilevel CPAP, controlled studies of APRV are still needed.

Pressure-Supported Ventilation

Pressure-supported ventilation consists of patient-triggered, pressure-limited, flow-cycled breaths that provide supplemental pressure at the beginning of inspiration. Pressure-supported ventilation is designed to overcome airway resistance caused by an endotracheal tube, secretions, bronchospasm, or other imposed mechanical resistance. Regardless of the pressure-support level provided, the patient has primary control over the frequency of breathing, the inspiratory time, and flow. Thus the tidal volume resulting from a PSV breath depends on the pressure level set, the patient effort, and the mechanical forces opposing ventilation. Since the early description in 1982, PSV has been used either to overcome the imposed resistance associated with the artificial airway or to ensure an acceptable spontaneous tidal volume.

Clinical studies have shown that compared with spontaneous breathing (including that occurring during IMV), PSV can result in a decreased respiratory rate, increased tidal volume, reduced respiratory muscle activity, and decreased oxygen consumption. Moreover, heart rate, blood pressure, hemoglobin saturation, and end-tidal carbon dioxide levels achieved with PSV are comparable with those realized with SIMV. Last, PSV may be preferred by patients over more traditional modes of ventilatory support.

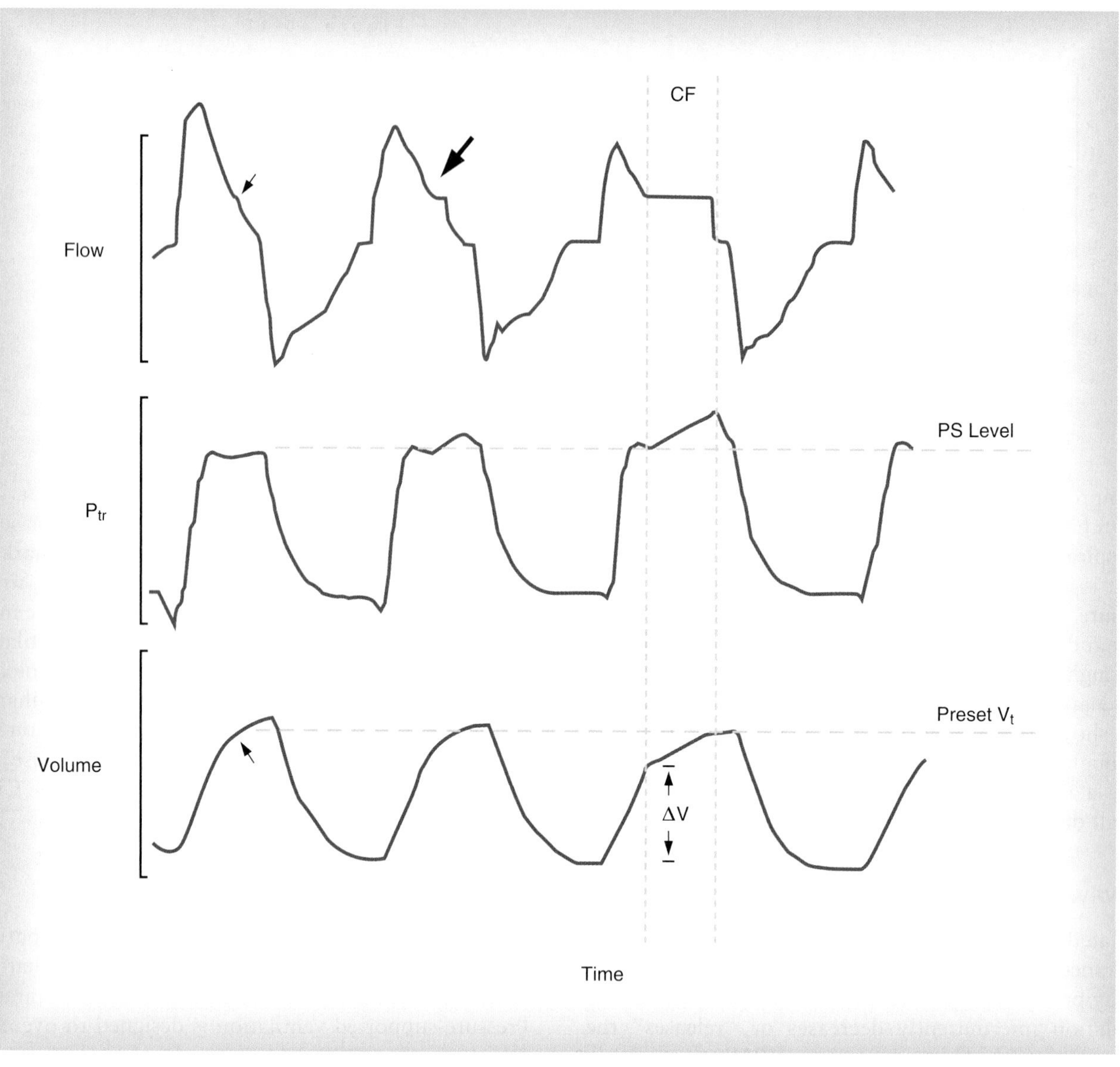

Figure 40-12

Pressure, volume, and flow waveforms in VAPS. Large arrow on the flow waveform indicates the progressive increase in continuous flow *(CF)* as the patient's inspiratory effort decreases (on the pressure waveform). Tidal volume remains constant despite decreased inspiratory effort. *(Modified from Amato MB et al: Chest 102:1225, 1992.)*

Volume-Assured Pressure-Support Ventilation

Pressure-supported ventilation with a volume guarantee is the goal of VAPS. This dual-control mode has two sources of gas flow. The first source provides flow with a rectangular pattern set by the clinician (10-120 L/min), and a constant volume is provided. The second source of flow (up to 200 L/min) is set to reach a preset pressure limit. When the patient initiates a breath, both flow sources are activated. The second flow source rapidly delivers gas into the circuit until a preset pressure limit (set by the pressure-support control) is reached. This flow decreases for maintenance of constant pressure. If delivered tidal volume is greater than the preset minimum tidal volume, the breath is a pressure-supported breath. Although a minimum tidal volume is guaranteed, VAPS allows tidal volume to exceed the set tidal volume according to patient demand (Figure 40-12). Physiological effects of VAPS include improved patient-ventilator synchrony and reduced pressure-time product, which is an indicator of decreased work of breathing. Improved patient-ventilator synchrony occurs when ventilator flow output is matched to patient demand

and when airway pressure is reduced through delivery of high flow during early inspiration and lower flows at end expiration.[28]

Continuous Positive Airway Pressure

Continuous positive airway pressure increases alveolar pressure and causes alveolar recruitment. However, unlike NPV and PPV, airway pressure with CPAP is theoretically constant (±2 cm H_2O) throughout the respiratory cycle. Because airway pressure does not change, CPAP does not provide ventilation. For gas to move into the lungs during CPAP, the patient must create a spontaneous transrespiratory pressure gradient. Thus although NPV and PPV produce the pressure gradients needed for gas flow into the lungs, CPAP only maintains alveoli at greater inflation volume. An important physiological feature of CPAP is that as alveoli are recruited, the FIO_2 needed to maintain adequate PaO_2 may decrease. Therefore oxygenation becomes more efficient at any given FIO_2, as measured by PaO_2/FIO_2 ratio and shunt fraction. The potential side effects associated with PPV also exist for CPAP but usually to a lesser degree.

Bilevel Continuous Positive Airway Pressure

Bilevel CPAP is a spontaneous breathing mode in which PSV is combined with CPAP. Bilevel CPAP is referred to as BiPAP by Respironics, Inc. Unlike CPAP, bilevel CPAP allows separate regulation of inspiratory and expiratory pressures.[29] The system is adjusted to switch between a high inspiratory positive airway pressure (IPAP) and a lower expiratory positive airway pressure (EPAP). The volume displacement caused by the difference between IPAP and EPAP contributes to the total ventilation. The duration of IPAP and EPAP can be independently adjusted to yield a phase ratio much like an I:E ratio. Although it was originally developed to enhance the capabilities of home CPAP systems used for management of obstructive sleep apnea, bilevel CPAP has since been successfully used in the home and the hospital for nocturnal ventilatory support of patients with chronic restrictive and obstructive disorders.[30] This mode has been found useful in the prevention of intubation in acute exacerbation of COPD.[31] In ARDS, bilevel CPAP has been shown to significantly reduce peak-inspiratory and end-expiratory pressures at a lower FIO_2 while maintaining oxygenation and carbon dioxide removal.[32]

Automatic Tube Compensation

Automatic tube compensation (ATC) is not a mode of ventilation. It is an adjunct that automatically adjusts the pressure-support level to compensate for endotracheal tube diameter and flow demand on the basis of calculation of tracheal pressure. The goal is to decrease work of breathing during inspiration. At an arbitrary pressure-support setting (5-10 cm H_2O), the patient's work of breathing due to the endotracheal tube or flow demand may be over or under compensated. In ATC, the therapist inputs into the ventilator (Drager Evita 4) the type of artificial airway (endotracheal tube or tracheostomy tube) and the percentage compensation desired (10%-100%). The ATC program calculates a tracheal pressure on which the "automatic" setting of the PSV is based. Automatic tube compensation also may decrease the PEEP during expiration to compensate for expiratory resistance imposed by the endotracheal tube. Clinical data indicate that ATC is superior to an arbitrary setting of PSV to overcome endotracheal tube resistance, may help eliminate auto-PEEP,[33] and may improve patient comfort owing to prevention of hyperinflation caused by PSV.[34]

Proportional Assist Ventilation

Proportional assist ventilation is a mode of ventilation designed to vary inspiratory pressure in proportion to patient effort. This mode should improve patient-ventilator synchrony while maintaining a constant work of breathing. This change in support may be useful as the characteristics of the lungs change with the progression of respiratory failure. Proportional assist ventilation is based on the equation of motion described earlier. The equation of motion states that airway pressure is related to lung elastance and resistance, tidal volume, and flow as follows:

$$\text{Paw} = \text{Elastance}\ (V_t) + \text{Resistance}\ (\text{flow})$$

With PAV, the therapist sets volume and flow "gains" at approximately 80%. The ventilator measures elastance and resistance and provides airway pressure, flow, tidal volume, and inspiratory time that vary with elastance and resistance. Each breath in PAV is patient triggered, pressure limited, and flow cycled. This mode has not been approved by the Food and Drug Administration, so it is not available in the United States. Two problems are apparent with PAV. First, there is no minute volume guarantee. Second, there is difficulty with the accuracy of measuring elastance and resistance. Because they vary with secretions, elastance and resistance vary breath to breath in ventilated patients. Overestimation of elastance and resistance can result in runaway ventilation, which also can be caused by leaks in the system. The clinical data on PAV indicate that the muscles of ventilation are unloaded, as they are in PSV. The flow gain unloads the resistive load (which helps overcome airway resistance), and the volume gain unloads elastance loads (alveolar stiffness).[35]

Patient Positioning to Optimize Oxygenation and Ventilation

Patients receiving mechanical ventilation are turned frequently, usually at least every 2 hours, unless turning is contraindicated. New kinetic beds continually rotate patients and are designed to help prevent atelectasis, hypoxemia, secretion retention, and pressure sores. When patients are kept immobile, pooling of secretions in dependent lung zones can promote nosocomial pneumonia, and shrinking of dependent alveoli leads to decreases in ventilation and hypoxemia. However, the use of rotating kinetic beds remains an unresolved issue in the prevention of nosocomial pneumonia.[36]

Patients with unilateral lung disease or ARDS benefit from being placed in positions that promote improved ventilation and perfusion. In unilateral lung disease, only one lung is affected by atelectasis or consolidation. If the affected lung is placed in the dependent position, blood flow follows. The resultant $\dot{V}/\dot{Q}$ ratio in the affected lung may contribute to venous admixture and hypoxemia. However, if the patient is rotated so that the good lung is in the dependent position, these relations are reversed. With the good lung down, blood flows to well-ventilated alveoli, and $\dot{V}/\dot{Q}$ matching and arterial blood gas values improve. An added benefit of this maneuver is that the affected lung is placed in a postural drainage position, which promotes gravity drainage of retained secretions so the fluid can be removed.

A similar phenomenon has recently been described in ARDS. In a supine patient with ARDS, dependent alveoli in the bases and posterior segments become atelectatic. Shunt increases, and the patient needs a high FIO_2 and PEEP for adequate oxygenation. If the patient is rotated into the prone position, the dependent, fluid-filled alveoli are placed in the nondependent position, and functioning alveoli are placed in the dependent position, where they are adequately perfused. Previously closed alveoli in the dependent lung zones are recruited. The result is improved oxygenation and the ability to decrease the FIO_2.[3] In a review of 20 clinical studies of 297 patients, Curley[37] found that oxygenation improved within 2 hours in 69% of cases, and improvements were cumulative and persistent. However, factors predictive of patients' responses were inconsistent, and patients' initial responses were not predictive of subsequent responses. An improvement in PaO_2 of 10 mm Hg within 30 minutes may differentiate responders from nonresponders. Patient positioning is not without complications. Several persons are needed to "flip" the patient while ensuring monitoring lines and catheters are not disrupted. Wound dehiscence, facial or upper chest wall necrosis despite extensive padding, cardiac arrest immediately after achievement of the prone position, dependent edema of the face, and corneal abrasion have been reported.[38]

> **RULE OF THUMB**
>
> Patients who have unilateral or dependent consolidation or atelectasis may benefit from positioning with the affected lung or segments in the nondependent position to promote improvement in $\dot{V}/\dot{Q}$ relations. Prone positioning may be hazardous, so take great care while rolling the patient.

► CARDIOVASCULAR EFFECTS OF POSITIVE PRESSURE MECHANICAL VENTILATION

Thoracic Pump and Venous Return During Spontaneous and Mechanical Ventilation

With the close functional relation between the lungs and heart, it is not surprising that impaired performance of one affects the other. For this reason, the therapist must fully understand what happens to cardiovascular function when a patient receives PPV support.

Early studies of the effect of PPV on the cardiovascular system showed an early, small, and transient increase in cardiac output that was followed almost immediately by a marked reduction in left ventricular outflow. In general, the reduced cardiac output in these cases was directly related to the amount of pressure applied. More specifically, the decrease in left ventricular output corresponded to the increase in pleural pressure that occurred with PPV. Figure 40-13 compares the effects of a spontaneous inspiration with the effect observed during PPV. Negative pleural pressure during inspiration normally enhances venous return, increases right atrial filling, and improves pulmonary blood flow (Figure 40-13, *A*). In combination these factors increase left atrial and left ventricular filling and left ventricular stroke volume.

When the lung is ventilated with positive pressure, pleural pressure can become positive (Figure 40-13, *B*). Positive pleural pressure compresses the intrathoracic veins and increases central venous (CVP) and right atrial filling pressures. As these pressures increase, venous return to the heart is impeded, and right ventricular preload and stroke volume decrease, as does pulmonary blood flow. Blood already in the pulmonary circulation initially is displaced into the left side of the heart and causes a transient increase in filling pressure and output. This initial effect lasts for but a few heart strokes. If positive pressure is continued, flow both to and from the left side of the heart decreases.

The high impedance encountered by blood returning to the right heart causes venous pooling, mainly in the capacitance vessels of abdominal viscera. This process effectively removes a large volume of blood from the

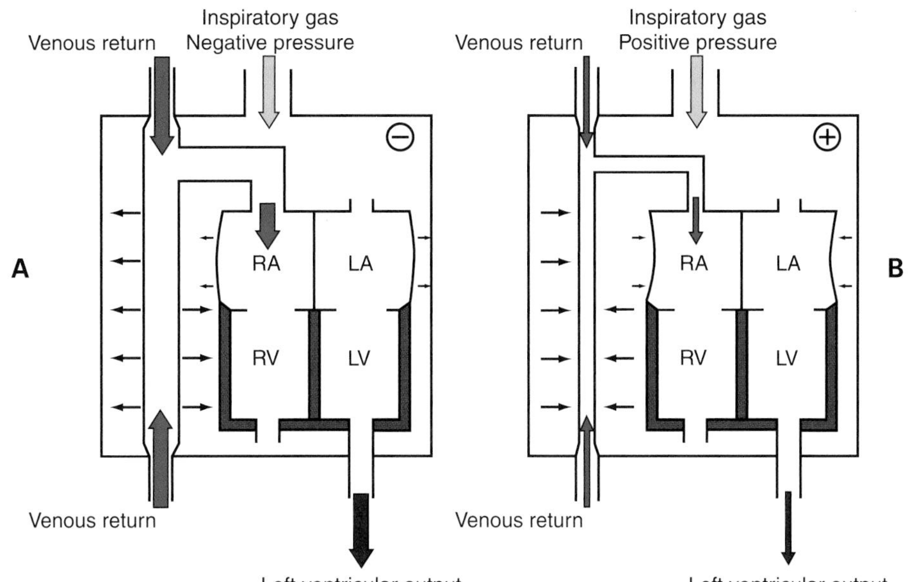

Figure 40-13
Relation between pleural pressure and cardiac output in spontaneous **(A)** and positive pressure **(B)** breathing. *RA*, Right atrium; *LA*, left atrium; *RV*, right ventricle; *LV*, left ventricle.

circulation, which can further impair left ventricular output. These interactions are magnified when pleural pressure is further increased or circulating blood volume is low.[39] The venous impedance caused by PPV is not limited to blood flow coming from the abdomen. An increase in CVP can restrict return flow from the brain. Impedance to venous return from the brain can increase ICP and reduce cerebral perfusion pressure. In combination with a decrease in left ventricular output, an increase in ICP during PPV can significantly impair cerebral perfusion and possibly result in cerebral ischemia and cerebral hypoxia.

In healthy persons, the effects of PPV on cerebral blood flow (CBF) are minimized by autoregulatory mechanisms that maintain cranial perfusion pressures within a narrow range. Patients with preexisting cerebrovascular problems, however, and those who already have an elevation in ICP may be at risk of decreased cerebral perfusion with PPV. Examples include neurosurgical patients and those with head injuries, intracranial tumors, or cerebral edema from any cause. In the care of these patients, ICP monitoring may be necessary.

Compensation in Healthy Persons

A decrease in cardiac output or blood pressure is rare among persons with a normal cardiopulmonary system who are receiving mechanical ventilation. Compensatory mechanisms used to counter the decrease in stroke volume include an increased heart rate, an increase in systemic vascular and peripheral venous resistance, and shunting of blood away from the kidneys and lower extremities, which results in a consistent blood pressure. Because these compensatory mechanisms function by reflexes, the reflexes must be intact. Factors that block or blunt these vascular reflexes include sympathetic blockade, spinal anesthesia, spinal cord transection, and polyneuritis.

Pulmonary Vascular Pressure, Blood Flow, and Pulmonary Vascular Resistance

In patients with a normal cardiopulmonary system who are receiving mechanical ventilation, there is no significant increase in pulmonary vascular pressure or pulmonary vascular resistance and no decrease in pulmonary blood flow. When, however, alveoli are distended by increased tidal volume or high PEEP, pulmonary blood flow is impeded because the alveoli press against the pulmonary capillaries. The pressure increases right ventricular afterload and volume and decreases right ventricular output. The ventricular septum may be shifted to the left, but this effect is more consistent with a high PEEP. Such a condition decreases left ventricular filling and output. The magnitude of these changes is proportional to lung compliance. As lung compliance decreases, the stiffer lungs can retain the increased pressure imposed by PEEP. In other words, the increased pressure in the lung is not transmitted to the vasculature to impede right ventricular output. An increase in intrapleural pressure due to an increase in lung pressure impedes venous return and further decreases cardiac output.

Right and Left Ventricular Function

Under conditions of a normal cardiovascular system with normal ventilation values, there are no significant changes in right or left ventricular function. Otherwise, mechanical ventilation would be difficult to manage, and the mortality and morbidity among patients receiving ventilation would be much higher. It appears that right or left ventricular dysfunction occurs if the patient is hypovolemic, receiving an excessive tidal volume, or receiving more than optimum PEEP. The common factor is excessive alveolar pressure, enough to overcome or impede pulmonary blood flow or venous return.

Effect With Left Ventricular Dysfunction

Positive pressure ventilation can improve cardiac output in some patients. In patients with left ventricular failure, application of PPV can increase both the left ventricular ejection fraction and cardiac output. These improvements occur because PPV decreases left ventricular afterload in these patients. Afterload is an important factor in determining cardiac output, as is the resistance of the systemic vasculature. When afterload increases, cardiac output decreases (heart failure). When afterload is decreased by PPV or pharmacologic therapy, cardiac output may increase. This phenomenon explains why the cardiovascular status of some patients deteriorates when PPV is discontinued or treatment is changed from full to partial ventilatory support.

Endocardial Blood Flow

Blood flow in the coronary arteries depends on the gradient between the systemic diastolic pressure and the left ventricular end diastolic pressure (represented by the pulmonary capillary wedge pressure). Any factor that decreases systemic diastolic pressure or increases wedge pressure decreases endocardial perfusion pressure. The factors of PPV that may decrease the systemic diastolic pressure are high mean airway pressure, due to a high PEEP, high tidal volume, or long inspiratory time. Factors that may increase the wedge pressure include excessive PEEP and left ventricular failure.

Cardiac Output, Cardiac Index, and Systemic Blood Pressure

When the cardiovascular system is normal with normal ventilation values, there are no significant changes in cardiac output, cardiac index, or systemic blood pressure. Cardiac output can be affected by a decrease in stroke volume with PPV, but this decrease is compensated by an increase in heart rate. Because the cardiac index is the quotient of cardiac output and body surface area (Cardiac index = Cardiac output in liters per minute/Body surface area in square meters), a change in cardiac output would be reflected in the cardiac index. Systemic arterial pressure remains stable because of reflex compensation, which increases systemic vascular resistance. Only when mean airway pressure is high and intrapleural pressure increases precipitously does cardiac output, and therefore cardiac index and arterial pressure, decrease. Hypotension due to PPV alone is rare, because therapists and the medical staff do all that is necessary to prevent it: adequate fluid administration, proper management of mean airway pressure and PEEP, and use of vasoconstricting drugs. Most cases of hypotension during mechanical ventilation are caused by sepsis and the accompanying vascular collapse.

▶ MINIMIZING THE CARDIOVASCULAR EFFECTS OF POSITIVE PRESSURE MECHANICAL VENTILATION

The effect of PPV on the circulatory system depends primarily on two major factors: mean pleural pressure and cardiovascular status.

Mean Pleural Pressure

Mean pleural pressure is the average pressure in the pleural "space." At the bedside, pleural pressure usually is measured indirectly as the esophageal pressure through an esophageal balloon connected to a pressure transducer. Because the esophagus is close to the pleurae, separated by only a flexible esophageal wall, esophageal and pleural pressures are nearly the same.

An alternative to measuring mean pleural pressure is measuring mean airway pressure. Mean airway pressure is linearly related to mean pleural pressure and can be used clinically for monitoring of pressure changes.[40]

The effect of PEEP on mean pleural pressure is complex and depends on the patient's lungs and thoracic mechanics. Some of the pressure generated by a ventilator eventually reaches the alveoli, where it is transmitted across the alveolar walls to the pleural space. How much of this alveolar pressure is transmitted to the pleural space depends on lung and thoracic mechanics.

In general, for a given alveolar pressure, the more compliant the lung, the greater is the increase in pleural pressure. Thus a patient with a disease causing a loss of elastic tissue, such as emphysema, is more subject to the cardiovascular effects of positive pressure than is a person with normal lungs. In contrast, a lung with low compliance transmits less pressure to the pleural space. This explains, in part, why high levels of PEEP often are used with minimal cardiovascular effects on patients with low lung compliance (e.g., ARDS).

On the other hand, when the compliance of the chest wall is reduced, expansion of the thorax is limited, and more alveolar pressure is transmitted to the pleural space. Thus patients who have normal lungs but have thoracic restriction, as caused by kyphoscoliosis and spondylitis, are more subject to the cardiovascular effects of positive pressure than are persons with normal chest wall compliance. A similar effect can occur in patients with normal thoracic compliance who actively oppose a mandatory breath by contracting the expiratory muscles (as might occur in patient-ventilator asynchrony). Contraction of the expiratory muscles effectively decreases thoracic compliance and causes more alveolar pressure to be transmitted to the pleural space.

If resistance to airflow is high, less of the pressure generated at the airway reaches the alveoli. Thus the high airway pressure common in patients with obstructive disorders is not necessarily reflected in high pleural pressure.

The effects of moderate increases in pleural pressure on cardiac output in healthy persons are minimal. In healthy persons, as left ventricular stroke volume decreases, compensatory responses increase both the cardiac rate and the tone of the venous capacitance vessels. These normal responses ensure adequate blood flow and perfusion pressure. However, if the patient already is hypovolemic or has lost peripheral venomotor tone, cardiovascular compensation may be impossible. In these cases, even a small increase in pleural pressure may result in a marked decrease in cardiac output.

Decreasing the Mean Airway Pressure

Mean airway pressure is affected by respiratory rate, tidal volume, inspiratory time, inspiratory pause, expiratory time, I:E ratio, peak pressure, baseline pressure (PEEP/CPAP), and inspiratory flow waveform. If a decrease in mean airway pressure is necessary, altering any factor that contributes to mean airway pressure has an effect. The arterial blood gas values are a determining factor. If the PaO_2 is high, one of the most effective changes is a decrease in PEEP, because it has a 1:1 relation with mean airway pressure. If a decrease in PEEP is indicated, the therapist must assure that desaturation does not occur once the decrease has been accomplished. If the patient is being hyperventilated, a decrease in mandatory rate or tidal volume also decreases mean airway pressure. The best way to determine the magnitude of the change is to use the mean airway pressure monitor on the ventilator. The peak pressure usually decreases with a decrease in tidal volume. In pressure control modes, the peak pressure may be decreased directly. The plateau pressure is the result of distension of the alveoli. In volume-controlled ventilation, a decrease in tidal volume decreases plateau pressure. In pressure-controlled ventilation, the pressure limit may be reduced to limit plateau pressure. Efforts that increase lung compliance, such as PEEP or administration of diuretics to decrease interstitial edema, also may be effective.

Inspiratory time, expiratory time, and I:E ratio affect mean airway pressure. As inspiratory time lengthens or expiratory time decreases, mean airway pressure increases. This is the mechanism of action of IRV.

Changing the mode of ventilation to one that provides fewer mandatory breaths also decreases mean airway pressure. For example, if a patient is capable of assuming some ventilation, SIMV with pressure support should be used instead of volume-controlled, time- and patient-triggered ventilation (assist control). Addition of pressure support to the SIMV mode or an increase in PSV level increases mean airway pressure.

Fluid Management and Cardiac Output

The relation between cardiac output and preload (end-diastolic volume) is described by the Frank-Starling phenomenon, which states, "in the normal heart, the diastolic volume (preload) is the principle force that governs the strength of ventricular contraction."[41] In other words, as preload (stretch) increases, so do force and presumably stroke volume (Figure 40-14). Stroke volume continues to increase with preload until the heart is distended by excess preload, after which stroke volume decreases. Another cause of a decrease in stroke volume is the decrease in ventricular contractility that occurs when afterload increases as the result of hypertension. With hypertension come dilation and distension of the ventricles, which make the heart structurally abnormal. In an abnormal heart, it takes much less preload to put the heart into failure. Failure in this case is defined as decreased stroke volume despite increased preload (Figure 40-15).

When a patient receives PPV, there is risk of a decrease in venous return (preload) because of the increase in intrapleural pressure. Stroke volume may decrease, but

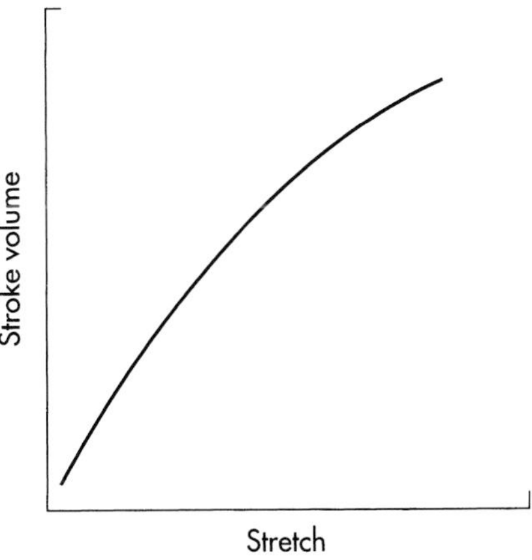

Figure 40-14 · Frank-Starling Law
Stroke volume is a function of ventricular end-diastolic stretch. An increase in the stretch of the ventricles immediately before contraction (end diastole) results in an increase in stroke volume. Ventricular end-diastolic stretch is synonymous with the concept of preload.

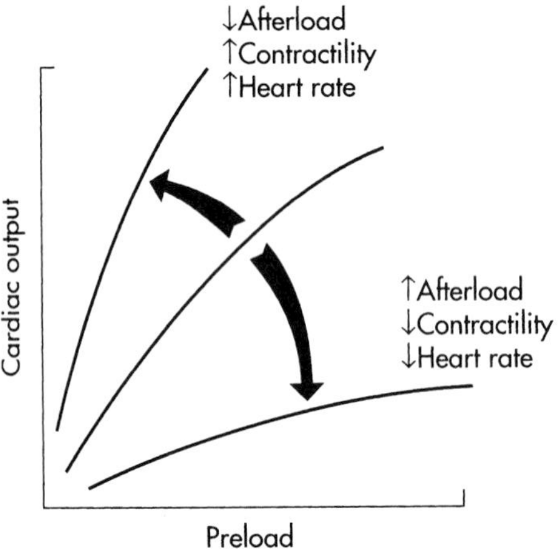

Figure 40-15

Effects of preload, afterload, contractility, and heart rate on cardiac output function curve. *(Modified from Green JF: Fundamental cardiovascular and pulmonary physiology, ed 2, Philadelphia, 1987, Lea & Febiger.)*

the decrease is compensated for by a reflex increase in heart rate and vasomotor tone. Because of these compensatory mechanisms, most patients with a normal cardiopulmonary status who receive mechanical ventilation do not need additional fluid to maintain cardiac output. However, certain conditions can increase the risk of relative or actual hypovolemia, and the increase can decrease stroke volume, even if normal reflex compensation is present. These conditions include hypovolemic shock (due to trauma and blood loss), sepsis (in which the normal reflex compensation is not present), and high PEEP and high mean airway pressure. In these conditions, fluid or blood administration may be necessary to maintain cardiac output and end-organ perfusion. In some patients who receive PPV with PEEP, an increase in PEEP can decrease cardiac output. In this case, the outcome of PEEP in terms of improved tissue oxygenation ($Do_2 = Cao_2 \times$ Cardiac output) should be determined. If Do_2 decreases because of a decrease in cardiac output, but Cao_2 increases, fluid administration may be indicated to restore cardiac output by increasing preload.

Pharmacological Maintenance of Cardiac Output and Blood Pressure

First-line therapy for decreased cardiac output and blood pressure is fluid administration, unless the patient has congestive heart failure. In heart failure, inotropic therapy is indicated for decreased myocardial contractility, and vasodilators and diuretics are used to control hypertension, which decreases afterload. Diuretics are used to control fluid overload and to decrease preload to the distended heart. These factors in combination may return the heart to a more optimal portion of the Frank-Starling curve and improve stroke volume.

In shock, fluid should be administered to achieve a CVP of 8 to 10 mm Hg or wedge pressure of 18 mm Hg. If fluid management is optimal, and the patient remains in shock, dobutamine is administered until the cardiac index is restored (>3.0 L/min per square meter). If blood pressure is low, dopamine is administered, starting at 5 μg/kg per minute. The goal is to restore Do_2 to normal (1000 mL/min).[41]

► EFFECTS OF POSITIVE PRESSURE MECHANICAL VENTILATION ON OTHER BODY SYSTEMS

Increased Intracranial Pressure

Perfusion of the brain is quantified with the cerebral perfusion pressure (CPP). The CPP is the difference between mean arterial pressure (MAP) and ICP. Cerebral perfusion pressure may decrease in any case in which MAP decreases or ICP increases. Should CPP decrease, cerebral blood flow (CBF) decreases. The result is cerebral ischemia and a decrease in cerebral oxygen metabolism. The cerebral circulation has the ability to maintain CBF even when CPP changes, a process called *cerebral autoregulation.* Cerebral autoregulation is a function of cerebral vascular resistance (CVR). If CPP decreases, CVR decreases to maintain CPP. Cerebral autoregulation functions as long as the CPP is in the 60 to 150 mm Hg range and is limited by the ability of the cerebral arterioles to constrict and dilate. Under normal conditions, cerebral oxygen delivery and CPP exceed the metabolic needs of the brain for oxygen and glucose.

Normal MAP is 93 mm Hg if arterial pressure is 120/80 mm Hg. Normal ICP is 0 to 5 mm Hg, so normal CPP is 88 to 93 mm Hg. Cerebral perfusion pressure decreases when MAP decreases or ICP increases. Conditions leading to a decrease in MAP are shock, high PEEP, and a high mean airway pressure. Increases in ICP are caused by traumatic brain injury (TBI), cerebral hemorrhage, cerebrovascular accident (stroke), and masses. Data have shown that a CPP greater than 60 mm Hg maintains CBF and cerebral oxygen metabolism.

Carbon dioxide is a potent cerebral vasodilator. The response of the cerebral arteriolar diameter is called *carbon dioxide reactivity.* As $Paco_2$ decreases from 40 mm Hg, systemic pH increases. Carbon dioxide concurrently diffuses across the blood-brain barrier. The result is an increased CSF pH. Even though $Paco_2$ is monitored when the patient is hyperventilated in TBI, it is the CSF pH that modulates CVR in an effort to decrease the ICP. When mechanical hyperventilation is used, CVR increases, and the result is decreased ICP. This is why hyperventilation has been used in the management of TBI and increased ICP. In the presence of an already decreased CPP, CBF decreases to the point at which cerebral ischemia is likely. Herein lies the problem with immediate hyperventilation of a patient with TBI. In addition, prolonged hyperventilation allows for the time needed for renal excretion of bicarbonate, which allows the CSF pH to return to normal and negates any positive effect of hyperventilation on ICP. The effect of hyperventilation on the reduction of ICP lasts as little as 1 hour. If hyperventilation is withdrawn and arterial pH and $Pa{CO_2}$ return to normal values, the CSF pH decreases. Subsequent CSF acidosis leads to cerebral vasodilation and a rebound increase in CBF and ICP that exceeds the values before hyperventilation. It is for these reasons that hyperventilation must be used cautiously in the treatment of patients with TBI.[42]

Treatment of the Patient With Closed Head Injury

Guidelines for the management of severe TBI were developed by neurosurgeons in the Joint Section on Neurotrauma and Critical Care.[43] The recommendation is as follows: "The use of prophylactic hyperventilation ($Pa{CO_2}$ <35 mm Hg) during the first 24 hours after TBI should be avoided because it can compromise cerebral perfusion during a time when CBF is reduced." Further, "hyperventilation therapy may be necessary for brief periods when there is acute neurologic deterioration or for longer periods if there is intracranial hypertension refractory to sedation, paralysis, CSF drainage, and osmotic diuretics." The Joint Section further noted that "in the absence of increased ICP, chronic, prolonged hyperventilation therapy ($Pa{CO_2}$ ≤25 mm Hg) should be avoided after TBI."

These findings have resulted in several recommendations regarding the care of patients with TBI:

1. *Patients with a transient increase in ICP*. Patients with TBI may have transient, short periods of increased ICP, called *plateau waves*. Plateau waves may be caused by suctioning, repositioning, or other noxious stimuli. During a plateau wave, acute hyperventilation with a manual resuscitator or with an increase ventilator rate can control ICP until the pressure returns to baseline, at which time ventilation is resumed at the previous rate.
2. *Hyperventilation as an immediate temporizing measure*. Hyperventilation should be used temporarily after TBI until other methods can be used to decrease elevated ICP. These methods include ventriculostomy for drainage of CSF, craniotomy for removal of mass lesions, osmotic diuretics, sedation, placing the patient in the semi-Fowler's position, and paralysis. Cerebral perfusion pressure is maintained at more than 70 mm Hg.

Hyperventilation is instituted with a moderate tidal volume (10-12 mL/kg) and an increased rate. A moderate tidal volume is used to avoid an increase in intrathoracic pressure, which can decrease MAP. Intubation should be attempted only after the patient has been sedated, to prevent the associated increase in ICP. Exhaled carbon dioxide ($P_{ET}CO_2$) should be monitored to maintain a constant $Pa{CO_2}$ after arterial blood gas values are determined to find the correlation between $Pa{CO_2}$ and $P_{ET}CO_2$.

Once ICP is less than 20 mm Hg, hyperventilation may be gradually discontinued through decreasing the mandatory rate. The rate of weaning must be individualized by means of monitoring the response to an increase in $Pa{CO_2}$. If there is a subsequent increase in ICP, the new respiratory rate can be maintained until the CBF readjusts and ICP decreases.[43]

Effect on Renal Function

Some patients receiving long-term PPV retain salt and water. Among critically ill patients, water retention usually is evident when rapid weight gain occurs. In addition, such patients may have a reduced hematocrit, which is also consistent with hypervolemia due to water retention. These early observations are now attributed to both the direct and indirect effects of PPV on renal function.

In terms of direct effect, PPV can reduce urinary output as much as 30% to 50%. This reduced urinary output during PPV is associated with a simultaneous reduction in renal blood flow, glomerular filtration rate, and sodium and potassium excretion.

Decreases in MAP to less than 75 mm Hg reduce renal blood flow, glomerular filtration rate, and urinary output. However, MAP this low seldom is caused by PPV alone, and kidney autoregulatory mechanisms generally can keep renal perfusion pressure within normal limits over a wide range of arterial pressures. Moreover, because restoring cardiac output to normal does not entirely restore urinary output compromised by PPV, other mechanisms must be involved. Early evidence suggested that the decreased urinary output that occurred with PPV was due to redistribution of rather than reduction in renal blood flow. Results of more recent analysis tend to refute this explanation, instead showing that impaired renal function during PPV is better associated with a decrease in intravascular volume.

The indirect effect of PPV on renal function may be most important. Positive pressure ventilation has a marked effect on the water- and sodium-retaining hormonal

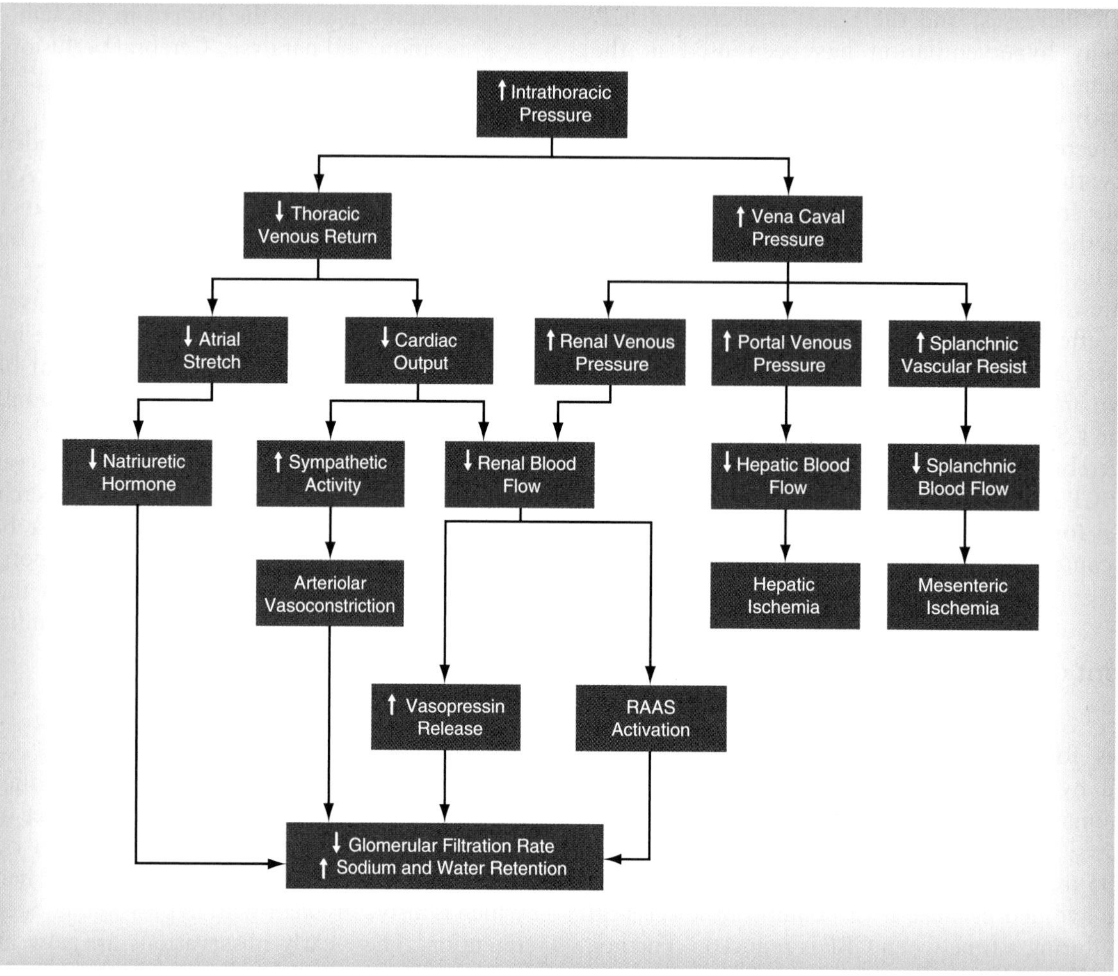

Figure 40-16

Cardiac, renal, hepatic, and splanchnic effects associated with increased intrathoracic pressure due to PPV. *RAAS*, Renin-angiotensin-aldosterone system; ↑, increased; ↓, decreased. *(Modified from Florete OG, Gammage GW: Complications of ventilatory support. In Kirby RR, Banner MI, Downs JB, editors: Clinical applications of ventilatory support, New York, 1990, Churchill Livingstone.)*

systems. Specifically, long-term PPV increases plasma renin activity, plasma aldosterone level, and the level of vasopressin (urinary antidiuretic hormone [ADH]). In addition, PPV decreases atrial natriuretic hormone levels (Figure 40-16).

Decreased right atrial transmural pressure is primarily responsible for the decrease in atrial natriuretic hormone, which leads to sodium retention. Similarly, vasopressin secretion may be enhanced by stimulation of the left atrial stretch receptors, which innervate the posterior pituitary gland. Increased secretion of vasopressin (ADH) and activation of the renin-angiotensin-aldosterone system lead to a decrease in urine output.

Decreased Liver and Splanchnic Perfusion

Related to its effects on the cardiovascular system are the effects of PPV on the liver and intestine. Hepatic dysfunction with PPV can occur in patients with otherwise normal livers and manifests as an increase in serum bilirubin level. These effects appear to be directly related to the reduction in hepatic blood flow that occurs with PPV. Regardless of cause, these effects are aggravated by PEEP but can be reversed when cardiac output is returned to pre-PEEP levels with intravascular volume infusions.

Decreased Gastrointestinal Function

An increase in splanchnic resistance can contribute to gastric mucosal ischemia and helps explain the high incidence of gastrointestinal bleeding and stress ulceration in patients receiving long-term PPV. Stress ulcers (erosions of the gastric mucosa) are common among patients with life-threatening illness. Impaired blood flow inhibits the ability of the gastric mucosa to normally replace itself every 2 or 3 days. Therefore stress ulcers are caused by impaired blood flow, not gastric acidity.

Gastroduodenal motility also is severely impaired in mechanically ventilated patients.[44] These factors may result in translocation of bacteria from the intestine to the blood and nosocomial septicemia. Mechanical ventilation for more than 48 hours and most other conditions necessitating intensive care admission are considered indications for stress ulcer prophylaxis. Optimal prophylaxis for stress ulcers is restoration of mesenteric blood flow. Second-line prophylaxis is the provision of enteral nutrition. Pharmacologic approaches include administration of a cytoprotective agent (sucralfate) and an acid suppression agent (cimetidine or ranitidine).[41]

Gastric distension can be caused by aerophagia due to an artificial airway cuff leak or by the use of mask ventilation (pressure >20 cm H_2O). The therapist prevents this complication by taking great care to assure that the cuff is properly inflated. If patients being ventilated with a mask are swallowing air, an artificial airway may be considered. In the case of aerophagia and gastric distension, a nasogastric tube may be inserted to evacuate the air.

Bleeding from erosion through the surface vessels of the gastric mucosa is one consequence of stress ulceration. The incidence of bleeding from stress ulcers is almost 100%, but the incidence is only approximately 5% for clinically apparent hemorrhage and 1% to 2% for hemorrhage necessitating blood transfusion.

Because patients receiving mechanical ventilation often have an artificial airway or are obtunded, a nutritional deficit may exist. Intravenous solutions of saline solution and dextrose provide only a fraction of the required calories, even in a normal metabolic state. Patients in the intensive care unit (ICU) often are hypermetabolic and need 2 to 3 times the normal calories. In the absence of enteral or parenteral nutrition, the patient is malnourished. Malnutrition results in muscle wasting that leads to difficulty with weaning, slowed wound healing, immunosuppression, and a delayed response to hypoxemia and hypercapnia. Detection of acute malnutrition and monitoring of the adequacy of nutritional therapy are accomplished by monitoring prealbumin level. The caloric requirements can be calculated by use of the Harris-Benedict equation and compensatory factors for activity, temperature, and injury or by calorimetry. Feeding usually begins within 24 hours of admission to the ICU. The preferred route for nutrition is the gastrointestinal tract. Preferably, the patient is fed whole nutrients, that is, carbohydrates, fats, and proteins, which are contained in some canned supplements. If the patient cannot tolerate whole nutrients, micronutrient supplements containing amino acids, sugars, and lipids are administered. Patients who cannot tolerate any gastrointestinal feeding receive total parenteral nutrition (TPN). Total parenteral nutrition consists of amino acids, sugars, lipids, and micronutrients and is administered intravenously. As soon as the patient can tolerate it, enteral feeding should be begun for prophylaxis against stress ulceration and bacterial translocation.

Effect on the Central Nervous System

Patients in the ICU are placed into an artificial environment over which they have little control. From the start, the patient loses autonomy. When mechanical ventilation is introduced, the patient is sedated and possibly paralyzed, and may never return to a normal, awake level of consciousness. Instead, the patient is kept somnolent (easily aroused and aware) or is stuporous (arousable with difficulty and impaired awareness) or comatose (arousable but unaware).[41] The presence of an artificial airway makes communication difficult. Caregivers should make a paper tablet and pen, communication board, or communication cards available to patients who are aware enough to write or use them.

Sedatives, Hypnotics, and Neuromuscular Blocking Agents

Sedation is necessary for the management of the nearly inevitable agitation, fear, and anxiety associated with the ICU environment, pain, invasive and noninvasive procedures, and loss of normal sleep pattern. The Society of Critical Care Medicine (SCCM) has published the following guidelines for sedation and analgesia in the care of critically ill patients:[45]

1. Midazolam (Versed) or propofol for the short term (<24 hours) management of anxiety
2. Lorazepam (Ativan) for the prolonged management of anxiety
3. Morphine for analgesia in hemodynamically stable patients
4. Fentanyl for analgesia in hemodynamically unstable patients
5. Haloperidol for the management of delirium

The level of sedation is monitored with the Modified Ramsay Scale (Box 40-2). Sedation is titrated to achieve a level of 3 on the Ramsay scale. This way the patient is responsive yet not restless or agitated and not paralyzed or comatose.

Box 40-2 • Modified Ramsay Scale

1. Agitated, anxious, restless
2. Calm, cooperative, oriented, tranquil
3. Responds to verbal commands
4. Brisk response to light touch
5. Unable to be assessed (paralyzed)

According to the SCCM, facilitation of mechanical ventilation is the most common reason for prolonged neuromuscular blockade. Neuromuscular blocking agents (NMBAs) are used with pressure control and IRV to avoid ICP spikes and to prevent bodily injury. Because they paralyze but do not sedate, NMBAs always are used in conjunction with appropriate sedative or analgesic agents (see earlier). In the absence of a sedative, a patient under the influence of an NBMA is paralyzed and fully aware of the surroundings. The SCCM recommends pancuronium (Pavulon) for prolonged neuromuscular blockade in the care of most critically ill patients. In patients with cardiac disease, hemodynamic instability, or in whom tachycardia (caused by pancuronium) may be deleterious, vecuronium (Norcuron) is recommended. During neuromuscular blockade, patients should be assessed for the degree of blockade that is being sustained.[45] The patient is observed for ventilatory effort, and train-of-four stimulation is performed. Although it is commonly used in the operating room, train-of-four stimulation is uncommon in the ICU. Neuromuscular blockade should be allowed to dissipate daily so that clinical evaluation, assessment of concomitant sedation and analgesia, and evaluation of the need for continued paralysis can be conducted.

Some patients who have undergone ventilation for a long time become psychologically dependent on mechanical ventilation. Despite meeting the physiologic criteria for weaning, when they are taken off the ventilator, these patients become restless and agitated. Patient reassurance, attendance at the bedside by the nurse or therapist, and administration of anxiolytic drugs may be helpful.

▶ COMPLICATIONS OF MECHANICAL VENTILATION

Negative Pressure Ventilation

Pulmonary

Hypoventilation during NPV can be caused by a decrease in the transairway pressure due to inadequate negative pressure or leaks in the ventilator or patient-ventilator interface. Iron lung negative pressure ventilators rely on a tight seal at the patient's neck and at all access ports in the tank. Chest cuirass ventilators rely on a tight seal between the cuirass and thorax. Poncho-type ventilators must remain free of leaks or tears. When there is a leak at any of these points, transairway pressure decreases, and the result is a decrease in minute ventilation.

Hyperventilation can occur if the pressure is more negative than is necessary. The results are increased transairway pressure, increased tidal volume, and increased minute ventilation.

Cardiovascular

Abdominal blood pooling can occur in patients receiving NPV in an iron lung. The negative pressure exerted on the thorax also is exerted on the more compliant abdominal wall. When the pressure in the iron lung becomes negative, the abdominal wall is pulled outward and with it the viscera and associated blood supply. Venous return to the heart, cardiac output, and systemic blood pressure decrease; the result is a condition called *tank shock*.

Patients undergoing ventilation in an iron lung often experience isolation due to the presence of the tank surrounding the thorax and extremities. The tank also interferes with patient care. One can access the patient's body for care only by placing one's arms through an access port lined with a foam gasket to prevent leaks.

Advances in artificial airways and the change in patient population from those with neuromuscular to those with lung disease have led to a decline in the use of NPV.

Positive Pressure Ventilation

Artificial Airway Complications

Chapter 30 describes complications related to artificial airways. Major complications are summarized here. During intubation, the patient's eyes may be injured because the practitioner is working over the face. The laryngoscope blade may break teeth or lacerate soft tissue if it is advanced haphazardly.

Nasal endotracheal tubes can cause epistaxis. For this reason, the tube used for nasal intubation is 1.0 mm smaller than that used for oral intubation. Other nasal tube complications include sinusitis from sinus blockage, ischemia and necrosis of the nares, increased resistance (due to the decreased tube size), and difficulty with suctioning.

An oral endotracheal tube resting against the lips can cause pressure necrosis if left in one place for more than 48 to 72 hours. The patient may bite on the tube, necessitating placement of a bite block, which can cause a pressure sore. During insertion, the tube can be inserted too far and cause endobronchial intubation or not be inserted far enough and cause ventilation leaks due to the presence of the cuff in the larynx. Esophageal intubation results in no ventilation. Inadequate cuff inflation can result in a ventilation leak, aspiration of pharyngeal contents, and possible nosocomial pneumonia. Excessive cuff pressure results in tracheal edema and ischemia, which eventually result in necrosis of the tracheal wall. Excessive cuff pressure can rupture the cuff and necessitate reintubation. Inadequate humidification and airway care can result in occlusion of the endotracheal tube by mucus. These complications are avoided by skilled intubation in which the endotracheal tube is properly secured and periodically relocated at the mouth and proper cuff care and adequate humidity are provided.

When it appears that prolonged mechanical ventilation or long-term use of an artificial airway is indicated, tracheotomy is performed, and a tracheostomy tube is inserted (see Chapter 30). Immediate complications include hemorrhage, cannulation of the pretracheal space, subcutaneous emphysema, and pneumothorax. Long-term complications include innominate artery erosion, hemorrhage, and tracheal stenosis. In addition, all complications related to the artificial airway cuff should be considered.

Complications Related to Pressure

High ventilation pressure has long been associated with barotrauma. Barotrauma is categorized as pneumothorax, pneumomediastinum, pneumopericardium, and subcutaneous emphysema (Figure 40-17). All these complications are descriptions of extraalveolar air. High ventilatory pressure can cause gas to escape through ruptured alveoli and alveolar bases. The eventual location of the escaping gas defines the type of barotrauma. If gas escapes through ruptured alveoli into the pleural space, pneumothorax occurs. Gas escaping along perivascular sheaths to the mediastinum produces pneumomediastinum. Further dissection from the mediastinum to tissue planes in the neck and chest wall results in subcutaneous emphysema. Should air cross the diaphragm after pneumomediastinum, pneumoperitoneum is established.

Pneumothorax is identified by observation of a decrease in chest movement, hyperresonance on percussion, and decreased or absent breath sounds over the affected side. In nonintubated patients, there may also be a decrease in vocal fremitus over the affected side. A line separating lung tissue from air is observed on the chest radiograph, although the line sometimes is difficult to see in a small (<20%) pneumothorax. Respiratory distress increases with increasing pneumothorax, as does hypoxemia. Normally, in spontaneously breathing patients, intrapulmonary and pleural pressures are equal in pneumothorax. Positive pressure ventilation can cause intrapleural pressures to increase (tension pneumothorax). Tension pneumothorax is life threatening, because it shifts the mediastinum, heart, and great vessels; the results are a decrease in cardiac output and hypotension. A medical emergency, tension pneumothorax is relieved by insertion of a large-bore needle into the pleural space through the anterior second or third interspace above the rib. This maneuver is followed by chest tube insertion. While waiting for needle decompression, the patient may be ventilated with 100% oxygen with a manual resuscitator at a low tidal volume and pressure. Pneumomediastinum and pneumoperitoneum are identified on a chest radiograph by the presence of air in these locations.

Complications Related to Volume Are the Result of Alveolar Overdistension

Alveolar distension occurs when the lungs are stiff and the chest wall is normal, or when one or both lungs are ventilated with a high tidal volume. An excellent method of detection of overdistension is observation of the pressure-volume loop on a ventilator graphics display. If a beak in the waveform occurs toward end inspira-

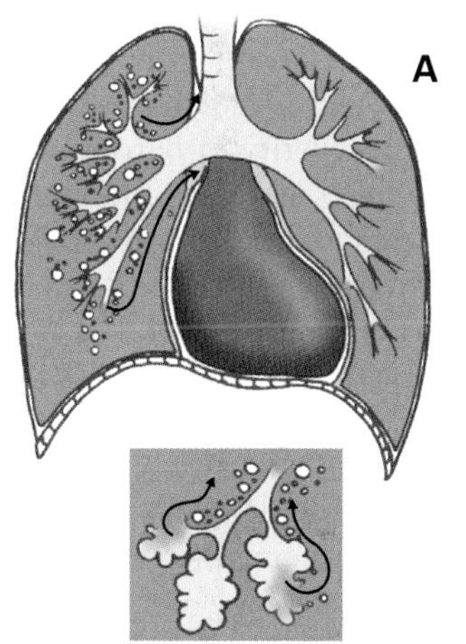

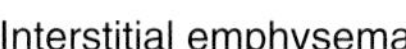

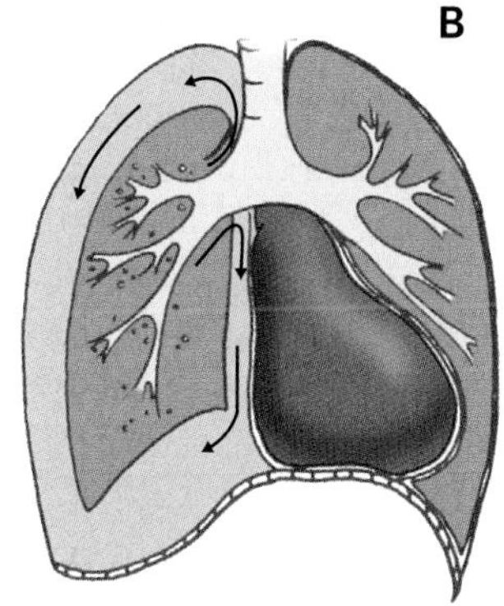

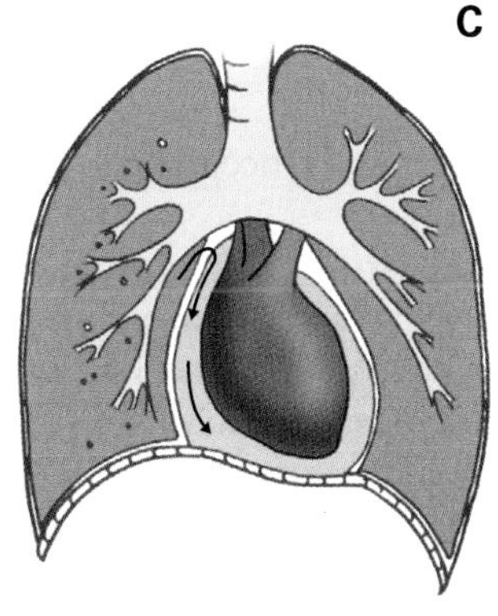

Figure 40-17 · Pulmonary Barotrauma

A, Ruptured alveoli are indicated in framed alveoli at bottom. Air dissects from alveoli along vascular sheaths to the hilum and then to the pleural space. **B,** Pneumothorax. Origin of air in lung tissue and its pathway to inflate pleural space are indicated. The heart shifts to the left because of high pressure in the right side of the chest **C,** Course of air from lung to pericardial space. Distended pericardial space causes cardiac tamponade. *(Modified from Korones SB: High-risk newborn infants, ed 4, St Louis, 1986, Mosby.)*

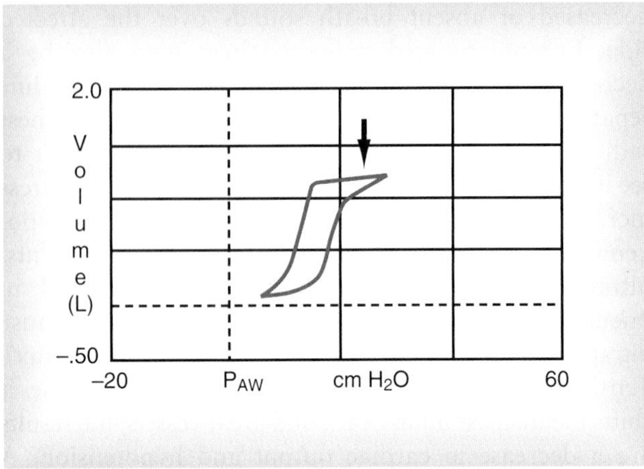

Figure 40-18
Pressure-volume loop for a patient receiving a volume-targeted breath of 1.2 L with peak inspiratory pressure of approximately 30 cm H_2O. The extended upper flat portion of the "beaked" appearance of the curve indicates overdistension.

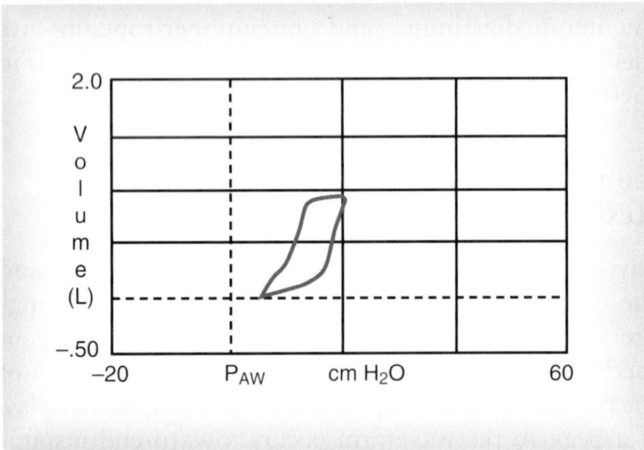

Figure 40-19
The pressure-volume loop "beak" is no longer present, a sign of reduction in unnecessary pressure.

tion, overdistension is occurring (Figures 40-18 and 40-19).

Experimental studies in animals, reviewed by Knudsen and Falkerson,[46] have shown that when the lungs are ventilated with high tidal volume, congestion and pulmonary edema result. This ALI is associated with surfactant alteration, terminal lung unit instability, and tissue injury. Because these abnormalities are related more to a high tidal volume than to a high distending pressure, the term *volutrauma* has been applied. In ALI, such as ARDS, when patients are ventilated with a high tidal volume, regional differences in compliance result in distension of lung units of a higher compliance, which become overdistended and damaged. At the same time, small lung units are subjected to opening and closing with each breath and are subject to shear stress damage (Figure 40-20).

Human studies of low tidal volume in ARDS have resulted in "lung protective strategies." Results of studies by Hickling,[47] Amato,[48] and Stewart[49] and their associates and by the National Institutes of Health have substantiated the use of low tidal volume as a way to limit volutrauma. The resulting recommendation is the use of tidal volume of 6 to 8 mL per kilogram of ideal body weight in patients with ARDS, even in the presence of hypercapnia.[50] Plateau pressure should be limited to 30 cm H_2O or less. Optimal PEEP may be used to assist in maintaining and recruiting alveoli so they do not open and collapse with each breath. The lower inflexion point in a static pressure-volume curve can be used to determine the best PEEP level, but the method is difficult.

Auto–Positive End-Expiratory Pressure

Air trapping occurs with incomplete emptying of lung units. Lung units prone to air trapping are those with long-time constants (i.e., with high resistance or high compliance). Air trapping during PPV is often referred to as *dynamic hyperinflation*, *auto-PEEP*, *occult PEEP*, or *intrinsic PEEP*. The terms *occult* and *intrinsic* are more descriptive because this form of air trapping can not be discerned with simple observation of airway pressure. Thus auto-PEEP often goes unrecognized.

Figure 40-21, *A*, shows the generation of auto-PEEP. As long as airway resistance is normal and expiratory time is sufficiently long, distal airway pressure and lung volume return to normal during PPV breaths. Alone or in combination, two factors account for the development of auto-PEEP. First, by effectively increasing the time constant of the lung, high expiratory resistance prolongs exhalation to the point at which air trapping begins (Figure 40-21, *B*). Any shortening of the expiratory time (Figure 40-21, *C*) aggravates the problem and increases both distal airway pressure and lung volume (auto-PEEP).

By increasing FRC and alveolar pressure, auto-PEEP increases the risk and severity of barotrauma and volutrauma. Auto-PEEP also increases the work of breathing and impedes venous return, the result being a decrease in cardiac output. Auto-PEEP also can increase pulmonary vascular resistance.

Patients at greatest risk of development of auto-PEEP are those with high airway resistance who are being supported by modes that limit expiratory time. High-risk patient groups include those with obstructive disease, any disease producing increased secretions, and any disease that increases lung compliance. High-risk ventilatory support techniques include any method that increases the I:E ratio, especially CMV at a high rate or in the assist-control mode, and approaches that purposefully shorten expiratory time, such as IRV or the use of low inspiratory flow. Techniques for detecting, preventing, and minimizing auto-PEEP are discussed in Chapter 43.

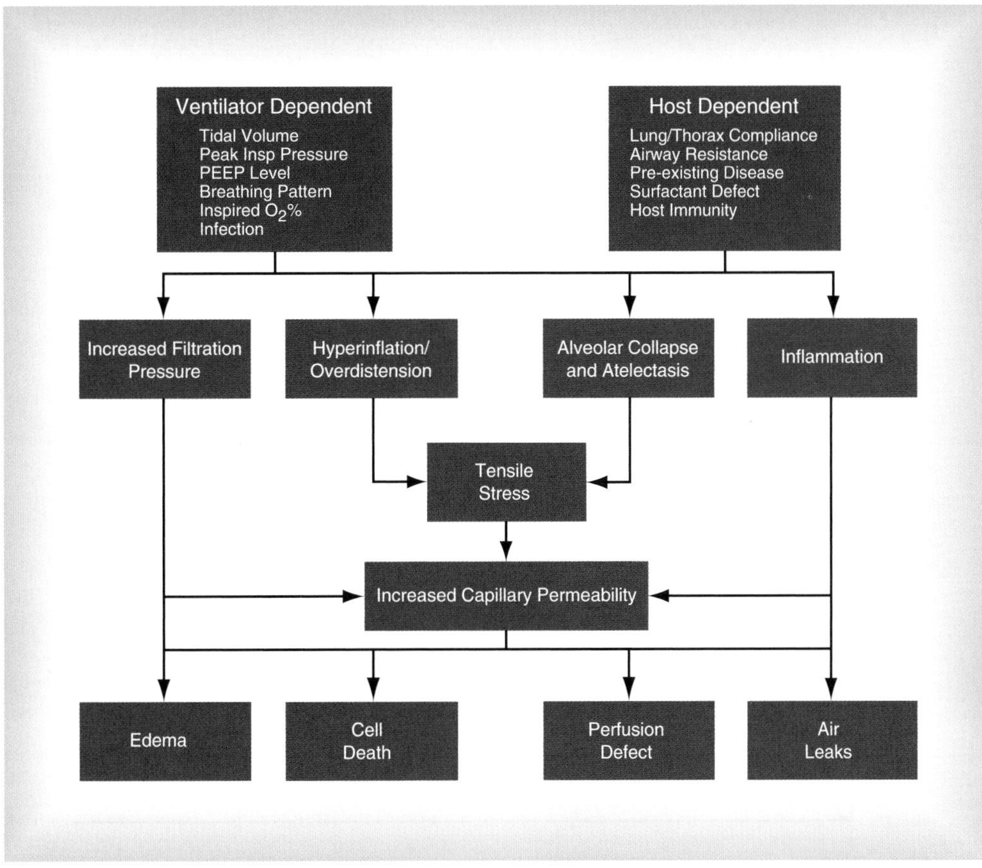

Figure 40-20

Ventilator and patient- and host-dependent factors involved in lung injury during ventilatory support. These factors can cause inflammation, atelectasis, overdistension, or increased capillary filtration pressure. Increased tensile stress on lung tissue and increased capillary permeability result in one or more of the following lung injuries: air leak, perfusion defect, edema, and cell death. *(Modified from Parker JC et al: Crit Care Med 21:141, 1993.)*

Auto-PEEP can increase the work of breathing. This increase in work is due to two factors. First, hyperinflation caused by auto-PEEP stretches the lung, and the stretching impairs the contractile action of the diaphragm. Second, in pressure- or flow-triggered breaths, the high alveolar pressure caused by auto-PEEP must be overcome before any airway pressure change can occur. This situation effectively reduces machine sensitivity and increases response time. Increased effort is required by the patient before the ventilator recognizes the flow or pressure change and triggers to inspiration.

Oxygen Toxicity

Oxygen toxicity causes lung tissue damage and an increase in the permeability of the A-C membrane as a result of an excessive FIO_2. Factors associated with the development of oxygen toxicity include FIO_2, duration of exposure, and the patient's susceptibility. An FIO_2 of 0.5 or more for longer than 24 to 48 hours is associated with the development of oxygen toxicity. In the presence of a high concentration of oxygen, oxygen free radicals are produced. These radicals are the hydroxyl (OH^-), perhydroxyl (HO_2), and superoxide (O_2^-) radicals. Free radicals normally are rapidly detoxified by the enzyme superoxide dismutase, which is produced by alveolar type II cells. The higher the FIO_2, the greater is the presence of free radicals and the less likely are type II cells to produce superoxide dismutase. The presence of the free radicals increases the permeability of the A-C membrane. The combination of direct injury by free radicals and decreased surfactant production leads to exudation of fluid into the alveoli and a subsequent decrease in compliance. Every effort should be made to decrease the FIO_2 whenever it exceeds 0.5. The decrease usually is accomplished with application of end-expiratory pressure, such as PEEP or CPAP.

Ventilator-Associated (Nosocomial) Pneumonia

Pneumonia is the second most common nosocomial infection, primarily affecting infants and young children, adults older than 65 years, persons with severe underlying disease, and those who are immunosuppressed, have depressed sensorium or cardiopulmonary disease, or have had thoracoabdominal surgery. It is no wonder

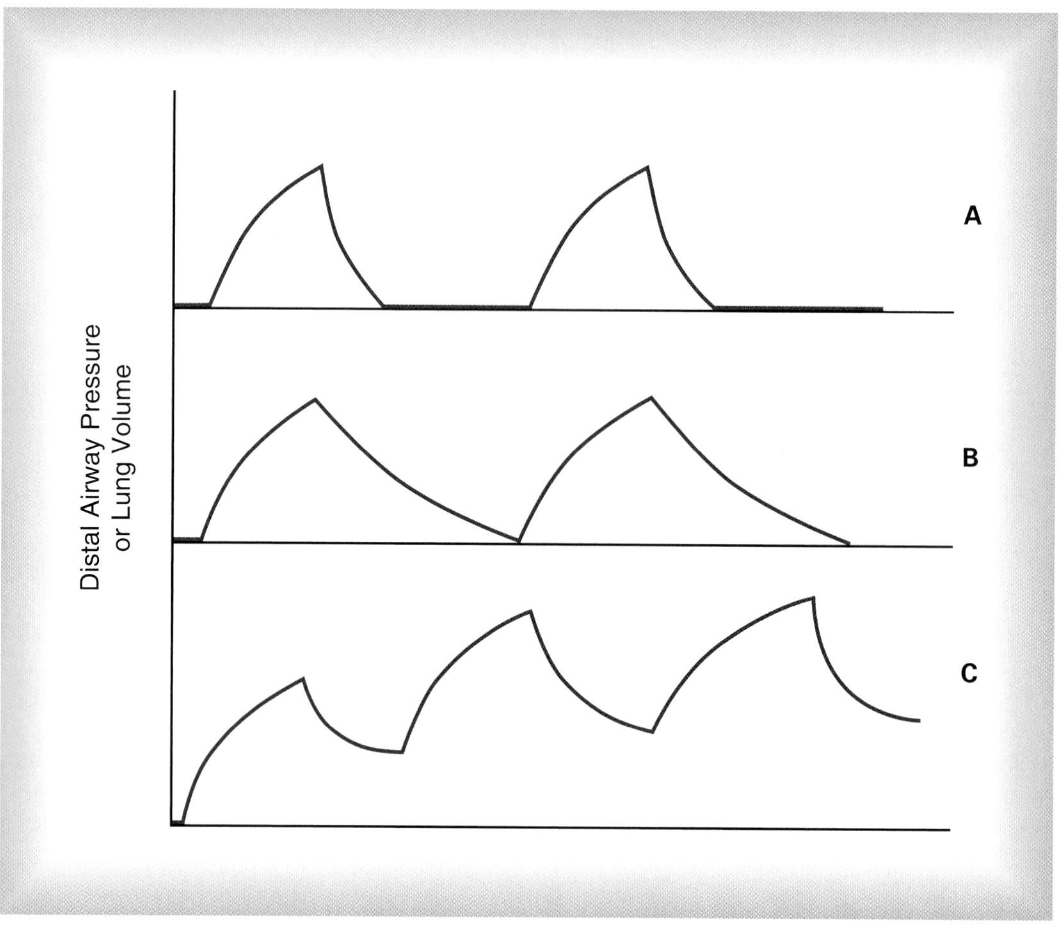

Figure 40-21 · Causes of auto-PEEP.

A, When airway resistance is normal and expiratory time is long enough, distal airway pressure and lung volume return to normal after a positive pressure breath. **B,** High expiratory resistance prolongs exhalation to the point at which air trapping begins and causes auto-PEEP. **C,** Shortening the expiratory time aggravates the problem and worsens auto-PEEP. *(Modified from Benson MS, Pierson DJ: Respir Care 33:557, 1988.)*

that respiratory therapists should be prepared to prevent this threat to our patient population, which is 6 to 21 times more susceptible to the development of nosocomial pneumonia than is the general population. Most of these cases of pneumonia are caused by aspiration of bacteria that have colonized the upper gastrointestinal tract or oropharynx. Intubation and mechanical ventilation greatly increase the risk of nosocomial pneumonia, because the lower airway is left exposed and normal protective mechanisms are bypassed. Most cases of pneumonia are polymicrobial, consisting of gram-negative organisms. However, methicillin-resistant *Staphylococcus aureus* has been common in the past 10 years.

In addition to standard precautions, specific infection control procedures apply to the use of endotracheal tubes and ventilators. These include gentle suctioning (presumably to help prevent coughing and aspiration), placing the patient in a semirecumbent position (30- to 45-degree head elevation), not routinely changing ventilator circuits more often than every 48 hours, draining and discarding inspiratory tube condensate (or prevent its formation by using heated wire circuits), or using a heat and moisture exchanger, if indicated. Suctioning of secretions that pool around the top of the endotracheal tube cuff can delay the onset of pneumonia, but additional studies are needed to determine the cost-benefit ratio of a special endotracheal tube for this purpose. Hand-washing between patients remains essential. The routine use of gloves is recommended but is not an absolute method of preventing nosocomial pneumonia. Other measures that may decrease the likelihood of nosocomial infection include the use of closed suction systems (although the benefit remains unproved), disposable resuscitation bags, and high-level disinfection of adjunct devices, such as respirometers and oxygen analyzers, between patients. When a heat-moisturizer exchanger (HME) is used, it should be changed according to the manufacturer's specifications and whenever it is contaminated or malfunctioning. The ventilator circuit attached to the HME need not be changed while attached to the patient. Small-volume nebulizers should be disinfected and rinsed with sterile water or air dried between treatments. Because condensate in the inspiratory side of the circuit should be avoided, the spacer chambers of metered-dose inhalers should be removed or collapsed between treatments.[36]

Aberrant Work of Breathing

Muscle atrophy can occur if the patient is ventilated longer than necessary, once the underlying indications for mechanical ventilation have been reversed. If the patient is ventilated such that the muscles of ventilation are underused, the diaphragm becomes deconditioned. Once the original reason for mechanical ventilation is reversed in these patients, weaning becomes difficult because the deconditioned diaphragm is unable to resume normal function. This iatrogenic failure is avoided when a mode of ventilation is used that assures the patient is providing some level of ventilation spontaneously without fatigue. The therapist should use measures of ventilatory mechanics (rate, tidal volume, RSBI, and vital capacity) and measures of ventilatory muscle strength (maximum inspiratory pressure) to determine whether the patient's ventilatory muscles are becoming fatigued.

Muscle fatigue occurs when the demand on the muscles of ventilation exceeds the mechanical ability to sustain ventilation (demand > capacity). This condition occurs when compliance decreases or when resistance increases to the point at which ventilation causes the patient to become exhausted. The therapist observes an increase in respiratory rate, a decrease in tidal volume, and increased RSBI (>105), anxiety, air hunger, and accessory muscle use. Arterial blood gas results show hypoxemia, hypocapnia early, and hypercapnia late. Muscle fatigue can occur during mechanical ventilation if the patient is already deconditioned and the ventilator fails to provide an adequate minute ventilation. The therapist must assure an adequate minute ventilation, as evidenced by normal blood gas values for the patient. The patient's clinical appearance should be relaxed without dyspnea or air hunger.

▶ VENTILATOR MALFUNCTION

Malfunction can be categorized as a failure in the patient circuit or a failure in the ventilator. Failures in the patient circuit include those related to the endotracheal tube: cuff rupture, mainstem intubation, laryngeal intubation, esophageal intubation, soft-tissue erosion because the cuff pressure is too high, and disconnection from the circuit. Failures in the tubing circuit include leaks anywhere there is a tubing connection, a leak at the site of a nebulizer or metered-dose inhaler, humidifier malfunctions that include failure to fill the reservoir, overheating or mechanical failure, and exhalation valve failure. These failures are recognized by the ventilator as changes in respiratory rate, airway pressure, or tidal volume outside the limits set on the alarms. Alarms are described in Chapter 39.

Airway and ventilator malfunctions can be avoided with proper care of the endotracheal tube cuff, moving the oral endotracheal tube from side to side every 24 hours and taping it snugly, assuring equal breath sounds, checking to ensure the tubing is patent and free of leaks, and assuring that all connections are firmly made. If patient activity is the cause of ventilator disconnection, sedation or restraint may be necessary. Hospital policy and state laws regulate the use of restraints.

Failures related to the ventilator include electrical failure, microprocessor failure, exhalation valve failure, internal volume leakage, gas supply failure, and any failure that could result in an increase or decrease in minute ventilation or FIO_2. Ventilators have alarms that alert the therapist to these dysfunctions. Problems than can occur with the ventilator, the possible causes, and corrective actions are described in Chapter 43.

Sometimes a ventilator is working as expected, but the patient appears to be in distress. Signs of distress include dyspnea, tachypnea, tachycardia, hypotension, diaphoresis, use of accessory muscles, retractions, and a paradoxical breathing pattern. These ventilatory efforts result in patient-ventilator asynchrony, a problem commonly termed "fighting the ventilator." The acute problems that cause asynchrony and a brief description of the remedies are listed in Table 40-3. The management of artificial airway problems is discussed in Chapter 30.

Patient safety is always the primary concern when a malfunction is detected. For this reason, a manual resuscitator always should be placed near the bedside. If the reason for the patient's distress is clear, such as disconnection at the endotracheal tube, the connection is reestablished, and patient comfort and ventilation are assured. If the reason is not obvious, the patient is ventilated with the resuscitator while the cause of the malfunction is investigated. The steps for managing sudden distress in a patient receiving ventilatory support are listed in Table 40-3.

RULE OF THUMB

Always have a manual resuscitator at the bedside of a patient receiving mechanical ventilation. Assure that the resuscitator is connected to an oxygen source. If the patient is receiving PEEP, be sure the resuscitator is equipped with a PEEP valve that provides the PEEP equivalent of that being administered to the patient with the ventilator. Keep the patient connection of the resuscitator clean and the valve free of secretions.

Table 40-3 ▶▶ Causes of Sudden Respiratory Distress and Their Remedies in a Patient Receiving Ventilatory Support

Cause	Remedy
Patient Related	
Artificial airway problems	Assessment of cuff, airway position (see Chapter 30)
Pneumothorax	Chest tube insertion
Bronchospasm	Bronchodilator therapy
Secretions	Suctioning, mucolytic therapy, other tracheobronchial hygiene
Pulmonary edema	Therapy directed at the cause of the pulmonary edema
Auto-PEEP	Tracheobronchial hygiene, decrease in I:E
Abnormal respiratory drive	Therapy directed at cause, possible sedation or paralysis
Alteration in body posture	Repositioning of the patient
Abdominal distension	Therapy directed at cause, insertion of nasogastric tube
Anxiety	Reassurance, anxiolytics, assessment of minute ventilation
Patient-ventilator asynchrony	Assessment of flow and sensitivity, auto-PEEP, change of mode to accommodate patient's pattern of ventilation
Ventilator Related	
System leak	Assessment of connections in the ventilator circuit
Circuit malfunction	Assessment of circuit with test lung, replace if necessary
Inadequate FIO_2	Assessment of SpO_2, assessment of FIO_2 with analyzer, increase in FIO_2 or replacement of blender or ventilator if malfunction is found
Inadequate ventilatory support	Review of therapeutic strategy for the patient (see Chapter 43)
Improper flow-trigger setting	Adjust trigger and flow to patient demand

KEY POINTS

- Response to an increase in FIO_2 helps determine the cause of hypoxemia. Hypoxemia responsive to an increase in FIO_2 is likely caused by a low $\dot{V}/\dot{Q}$ ratio. Hypoxemia unresponsive to increased FIO_2 is likely caused by a diffusion defect or shunt.
- Alveolar ventilation and carbon dioxide production determine the arterial PCO_2. Mechanical ventilation should increase alveolar ventilation and may decrease carbon dioxide production when the work of breathing is relieved. These factors decrease $PaCO_2$.
- Mechanical ventilation with positive pressure increases dead space and decreases $\dot{V}/\dot{Q}$ ratio.
- Inspiratory or expiratory time can be manipulated to improve oxygenation and alveolar emptying in disorders that effect alveolar time constants
- Physiological benefits of PPV include improved oxygenation and ventilation, alveolar expansion, decreased work of breathing and cardiac work, and improved oxygen delivery.
- Because of vast differences in the characteristics of modes of ventilation, no one statement can summarize the physiologic effects of all modes. The mode should be matched to the patient's lung characteristics to optimize patient-ventilator synchrony and improve acid-base and oxygenation status while protecting against alveolar damage, oxygen toxicity, muscle atrophy, and fatigue.
- No single flow pattern has been demonstrated to be the most physiologically beneficial. Research results indicate better oxygenation, ventilation, and patient-ventilator synchrony with the decreasing flow in relation to the square wave flow pattern. A decreasing flow waveform tends to have a lower peak and a higher mean airway pressure, whereas a square wave tends to have a higher peak and a lower mean airway pressure.
- Flow triggering appears to decrease work of breathing when compared with pressure triggering.
- Positive end-expiratory pressure is used to restore FRC in acute restrictive disease and to splint the airways in obstructive disease. In restrictive disease, optimal PEEP allows the respiratory therapist to decrease the FIO_2 and avoid the complications associated with oxygen toxicity.

KEY POINTS—cont'd

- Work of breathing is decreased by the appropriate application of mode, trigger variable, and flow. Monitoring of the work of breathing allows the therapist to titrate work to an acceptable level.
- Positive pressure ventilation is detrimental to the $\dot{V}/\dot{Q}$ ratio primarily by shifting ventilation to areas that are less perfused. Positive pressure ventilation can cause hyperventilation, tissue damage, and barotrauma if not carefully managed.
- Positive pressure ventilation can decrease venous return and cardiac output, especially when it increases the intrapleural and mean airway pressures.
- Positive pressure ventilation can cause renal, hepatic, and gastrointestinal malfunction primarily owing to decreased perfusion of those capillary tissue beds.
- Elevation of the head, osmotic diuretics, and CSF drainage are effective means of decreasing ICP in traumatic brain injury. Acute hyperventilation should be used only temporarily until other more effective means can be used.

References

1. Chatburn RL: Classification of mechanical ventilators. In Branson RD et al, editors: Respiratory care equipment, 2nd ed, Philadelphia, 1999, Lippincott Williams & Wilkins.
2. Beachy W: Respiratory care anatomy and physiology: foundations for clinical practice, St Louis, 1998, Mosby.
3. Pilbeam SP: Mechanical ventilation: physiological and clinical applications, 3rd ed, St Louis, 1998, Mosby.
4. Slutsky AS: Consensus conference on mechanical ventilation, Intensive Care Med 20:64, 1994.
5. MacIntrye NR: Patient-ventilator interactions. In MacIntyre NR, Branson RD, editors: Mechanical ventilation, Philadelphia, 2001, Saunders.
6. Haas CF et al: Patient-determined inspiratory flow during assisted mechanical ventilation, Respir Care 40:716, 1995.
7. Sassoon CS et al: Influence of pressure and flow triggered synchronous intermittent mandatory ventilation on inspiratory muscle work, Critical Care Med 22:1933, 1994.
8. MacIntryre NR: Respiratory system mechanics. In MacIntyre NR, Branson RD, editors. Mechanical ventilation, Philadelphia, 2001, Saunders.
9. Banner MJ et al: Partially and totally unloading respiratory muscles based on real-time measurements of work of breathing: a clinical approach, Chest 106:1835, 1994.
10. Lee KH et al: Rapid shallow breathing (frequency tidal volume ratio) did not predict extubation outcome, Chest 105:540, 1994.
11. MacIntyre NR: Mechanical ventilation strategies for parenchymal lung injury. In MacIntyre NR, Branson RD, editors: Mechanical ventilation, Philadelphia, 2001, Saunders.
12. Ranieri VM et al: Physiologic effects of positive end-expiratory pressure in patients with chronic obstructive pulmonary disease during acute ventilatory failure and controlled mechanical ventilation, Am Rev Respir Dis 147:5, 1993.
13. Ost D, Corbridge T: Independent lung ventilation, Clin Chest Med 17:591, 1996.
14. Al Saady N, Bennett ED: Decelerating inspiratory flow waveform improves lung mechanics and gas exchange in patients on intermittent positive-pressure ventilation, Intensive Care Med 11:68, 1985.
15. Tuxen DV, Lane S: The effects of ventilatory pattern on hyperinflation, airway pressures, and circulation in mechanical ventilation in patients with severe airflow obstruction, Am Rev Respir Dis 136:872, 1987.
16. Messinger G, Banner MJ: Tracheal pressure triggering a demand flow continuous positive airway pressure system decreases patient work of breathing, Crit Care Med 24:1829, 1996.
17. Sternberg R, Sahebjami H: Hemodynamic and oxygen transport characteristics of common ventilatory modes, Chest 105:1798, 1994.
18. Hamilton Medical: Adaptive support ventilation, www.hamilton-medical.com.
19. Campbell RS, Branson RD, Johannigman JA: Adaptive support ventilation, Respir Care Clin N Am 7:425, 2001.
20. MacIntyre RC et al: Cardiopulmonary effects of permissive hypercapnia in the management of adult respiratory distress syndrome, J Trauma 37:433, 1994.
21. Tobin MJ: Medical progress: advances in mechanical ventilation, N Engl J Med, 344:1986, 2001.
22. Lessard MR et al: Effects of pressure-controlled ventilation with different I:E ratios versus volume-controlled ventilation on respiratory mechanics, gas exchange and hemodynamics in patients with adult respiratory distress syndrome, Anesthesiology 80:983, 1994.
23. Mancebo J et al: Volume controlled ventilation and pressure controlled inverse ratio ventilation: a comparison of their effects in ARDS patients, Monaldi Arch Chest Dis 49:201, 1994.
24. Chan K, Abraham E: Effects of inverse ratio ventilation on cardiorespiratory parameters in severe respiratory failure, Chest 102:1556, 1992.
25. Davis K et al: Airway pressure release ventilation, Arch Surg 128:1348, 1993.
26. Sydow M et al: Long term effects of two different ventilatory modes on oxygenation in acute lung injury, Am J Resp Crit Care Med 149:1550, 1994.
27. Sassoon CSH, Mahutte CK, Light RW: Ventilator modes: old and new, Crit Care Clin 6:605, 1990.
28. Amato MB et al: Volume assure pressure support ventilation: a new approach for reducing muscle workload during acute respiratory failure, Chest 102:1225, 1992.

29. Kacmarek RM: Characteristics of pressure-targeted ventilators used for noninvasive positive pressure ventilation, Respir Care 42:380, 1996.
30. Wunderink RG, Hill NS: Continuous and periodic applications of noninvasive ventilation in respiratory failure, Respir Care 42:394, 1996.
31. Hess D: Noninvasive positive pressure ventilation: Predictors of success and failure for adult and acute care applications, Respir Care 42:424, 1996.
32. Kiehl M et al: Volume controlled vs. biphasic positive airway pressure ventilation in leukopenic patients with severe respiratory failure, Crit Care Med 24:780, 1996.
33. Stocker R, Fabry B, Haberthur C: New modes of ventilatory support in spontaneously breathing intubated patients. In Vincent JL, editor, Yearbook of intensive care and emergency medicine, New York, 1997, Springer-Verlag.
34. Guttman J et al: Respiratory comfort of automatic tube compensation and inspiratory pressure support in conscious humans, Intensive Care Med 23:1119, 1997.
35. Branson RD, Campbell RS: Modes of ventilator operation. In MacIntyre NR, Branson RD, editors: Mechanical ventilation, Philadelphia, 2001, Saunders.
36. Guidelines for prevention of nosocomial pneumonia, MMWR Recomm Rep 46:1, 1997.
37. Curley MA: Prone positioning of patients with acute respiratory distress syndrome: a systematic review, Am J Crit Care 8:397, 1999.
38. Offner PJ et al: Complications of prone ventilation in patients with multisystem trauma with fulminant acute respiratory distress syndrome, J Trauma 48:224,2000.
39. Pinsky MR: The effects of mechanical ventilation on the cardiovascular system, Crit Care Clin 6:663, 1990.
40. Marini JJ, Ravenscraft SA: Mean airway pressure: physiologic determinants and clinical importance, I: physiologic determinants and measurements, Crit Care Med 20:1461, 1992.
41. Marino PL: The ICU book, 2nd ed, Philadelphia, 1998, Lippincott Williams & Wilkins.
42. Yundt KD, Diringer MN: The use of hyperventilation and its impact on cerebral ischemia in the treatment of traumatic brain injury, Crit Care Clin 13:163, 1997.
43. Bullock R et al: The use of hyperventilation in the acute management of severe traumatic brain injury. In Bullock R et al, editors: Guidelines for the management of severe head injury, New York, 1995, Brain Trauma Foundation.
44. Dive A et al: Gastroduodenal motility in mechanically ventilated critically ill patients: a manometric study, Crit Care Med 22:441, 1994.
45. Shapiro BA et al: Practice parameters for intravenous analgesia and sedation for adult patients in the intensive care unit: an executive summary, Crit Care Med 23:1596, 1995.
46. Knudsen NW, Fulkerson WJ: Lung injury from mechanical ventilation. In MacIntyre NR, Branson RD, editors: Mechanical ventilation, Philadelphia, 2001, Saunders.
47. Hickling KG et al: Low mortality rate in adult respiratory distress syndrome using low volume pressure limited ventilation with permissive hypercapnia: a prospective study, Crit Care Med 22:1568, 1994.
48. Amato MBP et al: Beneficial effects of the "open lung approach" with low distending pressures in the acute respiratory distress syndrome, Am J Respir Crit Care Med 152:1835, 1995.
49. Stewart TE et al: Evaluation of a ventilation strategy to prevent barotrauma in patients at high risk for acute respiratory distress syndrome, N Engl J Med 338:355, 1998.
50. Ventilation with lower tidal volumes as compared with traditional tidal volumes for acute lung injury and the acute respiratory distress syndrome. The Acute Respiratory Distress Syndrome Network, N Engl J Med 342:1301, 2000.

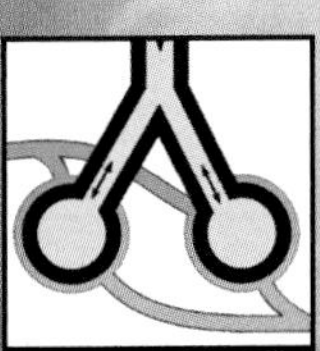

CHAPTER 41

Initiating and Adjusting Ventilatory Support

David C. Shelledy and Jay I. Peters

In This Chapter You Will Learn:

- What are the indications for mechanical ventilation
- How to identify and assess patients who need ventilatory support
- How to choose an appropriate ventilator to begin ventilatory support
- How to select an appropriate mode of ventilation given a patient's specific condition and ventilatory requirements
- What are the appropriate initial ventilator settings, based on a patient assessment, for beginning mechanical ventilation
- How to assess a patient after initiation of ventilation
- How to adjust the ventilator on the basis of the patient's response

Chapter Outline

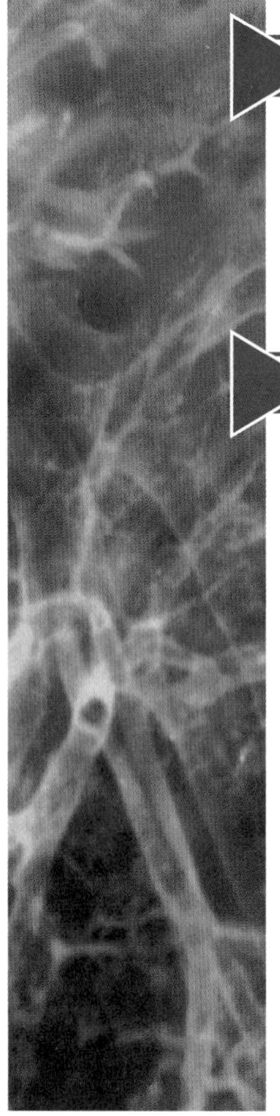

Chapter Outline—cont'd

Key Terms

acute ventilatory failure
adaptive pressure ventilation
adaptive support ventilation
airway pressure release ventilation
apnea
assist-control ventilation
automatic tube compensation
auto-PEEP
bilevel ventilation
continuous mandatory ventilation
continuous positive airway pressure
intermittent mandatory ventilation
mandatory minute volume ventilation
negative pressure ventilation
noninvasive positive pressure ventilation
permissive hypercapnia
positive end-expiratory pressure
pressure augmentation
pressure controlled
pressure-controlled ventilation
pressure-limited ventilation
pressure-regulated volume control
pressure-support ventilation
proportional assist ventilation
proportional pressure support
respiratory failure
synchronous intermittent mandatory ventilation
ventilatory failure
volume-assured pressure support
volume controlled
volume-limited ventilation
volume support

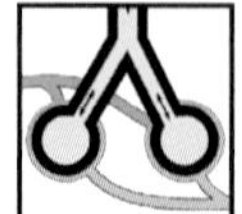

Mechanical ventilation entails the use of sophisticated life support technology aimed at maintaining tissue oxygenation and removal of carbon dioxide. At its most basic level, mechanical ventilation supports or replaces the normal ventilatory pump in moving air into and out of the lungs. To put it simply, the primary function of a mechanical ventilator is to ventilate. It follows that the main indication for mechanical ventilation is inadequate or absent spontaneous breathing.

Mechanical ventilation is not without risk, and the complications and hazards can be life threatening. The decision to initiate mechanical ventilatory support is a serious one that requires sound clinical judgment and a clear understanding of the indications and associated clinical goals.

This chapter reviews the indications for mechanical ventilation and describes the initial setup of the ventilator. After ventilator initiation, adjustments in ventilatory support are made on the basis of the patient's response. Techniques for patient stabilization and methods for optimizing oxygenation, ventilation, and acid-base balance are described, as are methods for minimizing harmful side effects.

INDICATIONS FOR MECHANICAL VENTILATORY SUPPORT

Definitions

The most common reason for initiation of mechanical ventilatory support is respiratory failure.[1] Respiration can be defined as gas exchange across the lung (external respiration) and at the tissue level (internal respiration). Respiration is primarily concerned with delivery of oxygen (O_2) to the tissues and removal of carbon dioxide (CO_2). *Respiratory failure* is a general term defined as an inability of the heart and lungs to provide adequate tissue oxygenation or removal of carbon dioxide.[2] Acute respiratory failure may be defined as a sudden decrease in arterial blood oxygen levels (arterial partial pressure of oxygen [Pao_2] <60 mm Hg; arterial oxygen saturation [Sa_{O_2}] <90%), with or without carbon dioxide retention (arterial partial pressure of carbon dioxide [Pa_{CO_2}] >45 mm Hg).[2,3] Acute respiratory failure may be further classified by the primary disorder present. Hypoxemic respiratory failure, or "lung failure," is present when the primary problem is oxygenation of the arterial blood.[4] Hypercapnic respiratory failure, also known as ventilatory failure or "pump failure," is present when the primary defect is in ventilation.[4]

Ventilation is defined as the bulk movement of gas into and out of the lungs. Ventilation may be assessed by measurement of tidal volume (V_T), respiratory rate (f), total volume per minute, or minute ventilation ($\dot{V}_E$), and calculation of the patient's physiologic dead space and alveolar ventilation ($\dot{V}_A$). The single best index of the effectiveness of ventilation, however, is Pa_{CO_2}. The relation of Pa_{CO_2}, $\dot{V}_A$, and carbon dioxide production ($\dot{V}_{CO_2}$) is as follows:

$$Pa_{CO_2} = \frac{0.863 \times \dot{V}_{CO_2}}{\dot{V}_A}$$

where $\dot{V}_{CO_2}$ is carbon dioxide production in milliliters per minute.

Ventilatory failure may be defined as an elevated Pa_{CO_2} (>45 mm Hg).[5] Acute ventilatory failure is defined as a sudden increase in arterial Pa_{CO_2} with a corresponding decrease in pH. Chronic ventilatory failure, on the other hand, is defined as a chronically elevated Pa_{CO_2} with a normal or near normal pH owing to metabolic compensation.

Table 41-1 ▶▶ Most Common Diagnoses Requiring Mechanical Ventilatory Support

	Rank		Percentage	
Condition	**U.S. and Canada**	**Total**	**U.S. and Canada**	**Total**
Acute respiratory failure	1	1	74	66
COPD exacerbation	2	3	16	13
Coma	3	2	7	15
Neuromuscular disease	4	4	3	5

Modified from Esteban A et al: Am J Respi Crit Care Med 161:1450, 2000.

Table 41-2 ▶▶ Most Common Causes of Acute Respiratory Failure Requiring Mechanical Ventilation in the United States and Canada

Condition	Rank	Percentage
Postoperative respiratory failure	1	17
Sepsis	1	17
Other	2	16
Heart failure	3	13
Pneumonia	3	13
Trauma	3	13
ARDS	4	9
Aspiration	5	3

Modified from Esteban A et al: Am J Respir Crit Care Med 161:1450, 2000.

Disease States or Conditions Necessitating Mechanical Ventilation

The respiratory therapist must be alert to the disease states or conditions that may predispose patients to the development of acute respiratory failure and to the clinical manifestations of ventilatory failure and ventilatory muscle fatigue. Disease states or conditions that predispose patients to the development of respiratory failure are described in Chapter 38. These include acute lung injury (ALI), acute respiratory distress syndrome (ARDS), pneumonia, pulmonary edema, pulmonary embolism, heart failure, shock, sepsis, trauma, smoke or chemical inhalation, aspiration, and near drowning. Decreased ventilatory drive may be caused by excessive sedation, general anesthesia, narcotic or sedative drug overdose, head trauma, and stroke. Respiratory muscle fatigue and increased work of breathing are associated with acute exacerbation of chronic obstructive pulmonary disease (COPD), acute severe asthma, obesity, severe burns, upper airway obstruction, and thoracic deformity. Neuromuscular disease associated with respiratory failure includes Guillain-Barré syndrome, amyotrophic lateral sclerosis, myasthenia gravis, polio, spinal cord injury, botulism, and tetanus. Patients recovering from abdominal or thoracic surgery also may need mechanical ventilatory support.

Table 41-1 describes the most common diagnoses necessitating mechanical ventilation in the United States and Canada and a sample of six other countries. Worldwide the most common condition necessitating mechanical ventilatory support is acute respiratory failure, followed by coma, acute exacerbation of COPD, and neuromuscular disease.[1] The most common causes of acute respiratory failure that necessitate mechanical ventilation include postoperative complications, sepsis, pneumonia, heart failure, trauma, ARDS, and aspiration[1] (Table 41-2).

Clinical Manifestations of Respiratory Failure

The clinical manifestations of respiratory failure include restlessness, tachycardia, headache, hypotension, poor chest expansion, confusion, cyanosis, and depressed respirations. Patients in acute respiratory distress who need mechanical ventilatory support may have signs of increased work of breathing and ventilatory muscle fatigue. Accessory muscle use, intercostal retractions, nasal flaring (especially by children), and asynchronous chest wall to diaphragm movement or inward move-

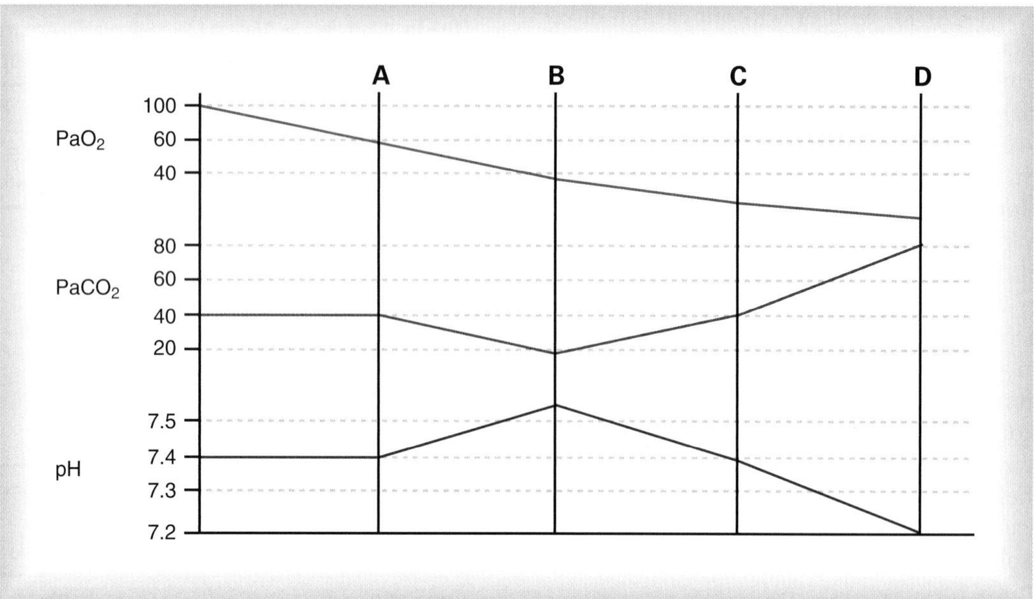

Figure 41-1

The typical progression of acute respiratory failure. Initially there is a decline in arterial oxygen tension and saturation. When the PaO_2 decreases to approximately 60 mm Hg **(A)**, the patient begins to breathe more, $PaCO_2$ decreases, and pH increases. Early in the progression, arterial blood gas results show acute alveolar hyperventilation (uncompensated respiratory alkalosis) secondary to hypoxemia. As the patient's condition worsens, increases in ventilatory workload typically lead to the adoption of a rapid shallow breathing pattern, and although minute ventilation may remain high, effective ventilation decreases, $PaCO_2$ begins to increase, and pH begins to decrease **(B)**. At point **C,** arterial blood gas results may show normal $PaCO_2$ and pH with moderate to severe hypoxemia. If mechanical ventilation is not initiated, the patient's condition may progress to acute ventilatory failure, severe hypoxemia, and corresponding severe respiratory acidosis **(D)**.

ment of the abdominal wall during inspiration (abdominal paradox) are associated with increased work of breathing and ventilatory muscle fatigue. Other signs associated with acute respiratory failure include rapid, shallow breathing, dyspnea, anxiety, sweating, alteration of mental status, and oxygen desaturation as assessed with oximetry. With acute respiratory failure, hypoxemia often develops first and is followed by hyperventilation and respiratory alkalosis. As failure progresses, the patient begins to tire, and $PaCO_2$ increases with a corresponding decrease in pH. Severe hypoxemia and hypercapnia may result in hypotension, ventricular arrhythmia, or profound bradycardia that may progress to cardiopulmonary arrest. The typical progression of acute respiratory failure is described in Figure 41-1. Clinical manifestations of acute hypoxemia and acute ventilatory failure are listed in Table 41-3.

Physiologic Values Associated With the Need for Mechanical Ventilatory Support

Critical values for specific physiologic processes associated with the need for mechanical ventilatory support are described in Chapter 38. In particular, in adults a respiratory rate (f) greater than 30 breaths/min; tidal volume (V_T) less than 300 mL; rapid, shallow breathing index (f/V_T) greater than 105; maximum inspiratory pressure greater than –30 cm H_2O; vital capacity less than 15 to 20 mL/kg or 1.0 L all are associated with impaired ventilation or ventilatory capacity.

Arterial blood gas values consistent with the need for mechanical ventilatory support include an elevated $PaCO_2$ (>45-50 mm Hg) with a corresponding decrease in pH, and severe hypoxemia with supplemental oxygen (PaO_2 <50-60 mm Hg on a fractional inspired oxygen concentration [FIO_2] >0.40-0.50).

Indications for Mechanical Ventilation

The decision to begin mechanical ventilatory support should be made with sound clinical judgment and based on multiple factors, including diagnosis, clinical status, physiologic values (including blood gas results, if available), and the expected progression of the patient's disease or condition. However, the primary indications for mechanical ventilation can be simplified into the Big Four:

1. Apnea
2. Acute ventilatory failure
3. Impending ventilatory failure
4. Severe oxygenation problems

Table 41-3 ▶▶ Clinical Manifestations of Hypoxia and Acute Ventilatory Failure

	Mild to Moderate	Severe
Hypoxia		
Respiratory findings	Tachypnea Dyspnea Paleness	Slowed, irregular breathing Respiratory arrest Dyspnea Cyanosis
Cardiovascular findings	Tachycardia Mild hypertension Peripheral vasoconstriction	Tachycardia, eventual bradycardia, arrhythmias Hypertension and eventual hypotension followed by cardiac arrest
Neurological findings	Restlessness Disorientation Headache Lassitude	Somnolence Confusion Blurred vision Tunnel vision Loss of coordination Impaired judgment Slow reaction time Coma
Acute Ventilatory Failure (Hypercapnia)		
Respiratory findings	Tachypnea Dyspnea	Tachypnea and eventual bradypnea
Cardiovascular findings	Tachycardia Hypertension Vasodilatation	Tachycardia, hypertension and eventual bradycardia and hypotension
Neurological findings	Headache Drowsiness	Hallucinations Convulsions Coma
Other signs	Sweating Redness of the skin	

Apnea

In the absence of spontaneous breathing, mechanical ventilatory support is required if the patient is to survive. Common causes of apnea include cardiac arrest, severe hypoxia, sedative or narcotic drug overdose, paralytic drugs or deep anesthesia, high cervical spinal injury, head trauma, and certain neuromuscular diseases. Regardless of the cause, in the absence of ventilatory support, apnea leads to cardiac arrest and brain death in minutes, although cold water immersion may extend the time during which resuscitation is practical.

Acute Ventilatory Failure

Acute ventilatory failure refers to a sudden increase in arterial Pa_{CO_2} with a corresponding decline in pH. In general, a Pa_{CO_2} greater than 45 to 50 mm Hg resulting in a pH of 7.25 or less represents a critical point at which mechanical ventilation should be seriously considered.

Impending Ventilatory Failure

Acute ventilatory failure can serve as a clear indication for the initiation of mechanical ventilatory support. However, the decision to intubate and begin mechanical ventilation sometimes is made before the appearance of significant respiratory acidosis. In these cases, a clinical judgment is made that the patient's condition will progress to acute ventilatory failure in the near future, and initiation of mechanical ventilatory support before the appearance of significant hypercapnia is prudent.

Some patients have severe air hunger, a respiratory rate greater than 35 breaths/min, diaphoresis, and use accessory muscles for breathing. The clinical appearance of impending respiratory arrest may necessitate intubation and mechanical ventilation before assessment with blood gas values.

Another example of impending ventilatory failure is the patient with Guillain-Barré syndrome. Guillain-Barré syndrome typically manifests as ascending neuromuscular paralysis, often after a flu-like illness in an otherwise healthy adult. As the muscle weakness ascends from the legs toward the thorax, one can see a rapid decline in vital capacity. Patients with Guillain-Barré syndrome consequently are admitted to the hospital, and careful monitoring is conducted for declines in vital capacity and inspiratory muscle strength. When the vital capacity declines to less than 1 L or the maximum inspiratory pressure declines to –20 to –30 cm H_2O, endotracheal intubation may be performed and mechanical ventilatory support begun. Because mechanical ventilation is started before the patient's condition has deteriorated to the point of acute ventilatory failure, the process of establishing the artificial airway and beginning ventilatory support can proceed in an orderly and controlled way. Thus mechanical ventilation may be initiated before the onset of acute ventilatory failure, when, in the judgment of the clinician, acute failure is impending and to delay intubation and initiation of ventilatory support would place the patient at risk.

Severe Oxygenation Problems

Refractory hypoxemia sometimes is defined as an increase in PaO_2 of less than 10 mm Hg after an FIO_2 increase of 0.20 or more. Refractory hypoxemia also may be defined as inadequate arterial oxygenation with an acceptable level of oxygen or, more simply put, a PaO_2 less than 60 mm Hg (SaO_2 <90%) with an FIO_2 greater than 0.40 to 0.50. The PaO_2/FIO_2 ratio often is used to assess the severity of hypoxemia. Acute lung injury is defined as a PaO_2/FIO_2 ratio of 300 or less with bilateral pulmonary infiltrates on a chest radiograph and no evidence of elevated left atrial pressure (normal cardiac function or a pulmonary capillary wedge pressure of 18 mm Hg or less).[6] Acute respiratory distress syndrome (ARDS) is defined as a PaO_2/FIO_2 ratio of 200 or less with bilateral infiltrates and a pulmonary capillary wedge pressure of 18 mm Hg or less.[6] Refractory hypoxemia often requires the use of positive end-expiratory pressure (PEEP), continuous positive airway pressure (CPAP), or another ventilatory support technique, such as prolonged inspiratory time or elevated mean airway pressure, to achieve adequate oxygenation.

Positive end expiratory pressure usually is administered after pressure- or volume-control inspiration. Indications for PEEP are a PaO_2 less than 50 to 60 mm Hg with an FIO_2 greater than 0.40 to 0.50. Disease states or conditions that may require the use of PEEP include ALI/ARDS, chest trauma, postoperative atelectasis, and pulmonary edema.[7] In addition, PEEP has been suggested for maintaining functional residual capacity (FRC) when an endotracheal or tracheotomy tube is used .[7] Small increments of PEEP may be used to overcome auto-PEEP.[7]

Continuous positive airway pressure may be defined as spontaneous breathing with an elevated baseline pressure. The indications for CPAP include refractory hypoxemia (PaO_2 <60 mm Hg, SaO_2 <90%, FIO_2 >0.40-0.50) in the presence of adequate ventilatory status ($PaCO_2$ <45 mm Hg, pH 7.35-7.45). Continuous positive airway pressure has been shown to reduce the work of breathing and improve outcome among patients with severe congestive heart failure (CHF). Continuous positive airway pressure may be applied through a spontaneous breathing apparatus and face mask without the use of a mechanical ventilator.

Patients with severe oxygenation problems often have a marked increase in work of breathing. Although these patients may maintain adequate ventilation while receiving CPAP alone for some period of time, they often eventually tire, and carbon dioxide levels increase. Consequently, in the face of refractory hypoxemia with an elevated work of breathing and respiratory distress, many clinicians choose to begin mechanical ventilatory support. This type of support allows incorporation of the sophisticated alarm and monitoring systems that are a part of modern critical care ventilators. It also allows application of PEEP, pressure support, and if indicated, pressure-control ventilation (PCV). There is evidence that CPAP alone by face mask is ineffective in avoiding intubation or improving outcome among patients with ALI and hypoxemia, even if carbon dioxide levels are not elevated.[8]

In summary, the most common reasons for initiating mechanical ventilatory support are acute respiratory failure, acute exacerbation of COPD, coma, and neuromuscular disease. The clinical manifestations of acute respiratory failure include restlessness, confusion, anxiety, diaphoresis, accessory muscle use, dyspnea, tachypnea, and tachycardia. Physiologic markers associated with the need for mechanical support include an elevated respiratory rate (f >30 breaths/min), a decrease in spontaneous tidal volume (V_T <300 mL), an elevated rapid shallow breathing index (V_T/f >105), a decline in vital capacity (<15-20 mL/kg, or 1.0 L), a decline in inspiratory force (maximum inspiratory pressure >–20 mm Hg), inadequate arterial oxygenation (PaO_2 <60 mm Hg, SaO_2 <90%) while the patient is receiving supplemental oxygen, and the development of respiratory acidosis ($PaCO_2$ >45-50 mm Hg, pH ≤7.25). Regardless of the cause, the four primary indications for initiation of mechanical ventilatory support remain

1. Apnea
2. Acute ventilatory failure
3. Impending ventilatory failure
4. Severe oxygenation problems

Goals of Mechanical Ventilatory Support

The goals of mechanical ventilatory support are to maintain adequate alveolar ventilation and oxygen delivery, restore acid-base balance, and reduce the work of breathing with minimum harmful side effects and complications.[9] Mechanical ventilation also may reduce increased myocardial work secondary to hypoxemia and an increased work of breathing.[9] Other physiologic objectives of mechanical ventilatory support may include increasing or maintaining lung volume with the appropriate use of end-inspiratory or expiratory pressure and with promotion, improvement, or maintenance of lung recruitment.[9] Specific clinical objectives may include reversal of hypoxemia, hypercapnia, and the associated respiratory acidosis and prevention or reversal of ventilatory muscle fatigue.[9,10] Mechanical ventilation may be used to allow sedation or paralysis for certain procedures, to decrease myocardial and ventilatory muscle oxygen consumption to maximize oxygen delivery to the tissues, to decrease intracranial pressure (ICP) in the presence of closed head injury or cerebral edema (by reducing the $Pa{CO_2}$ to 25-30 mm Hg and thus promoting cerebral vasoconstriction), to prevent or reverse atelectasis, and to stabilize the chest wall in the case of a massive flail or chest wall resection.[9,10] Hazards of mechanical ventilation include decreased venous return and cardiac output, increased work of breathing and ventilatory muscle fatigue due to inappropriate ventilator settings, and ventilator-induced lung injury.[11,12] Nosocomial pneumonia poses a significant risk for intubated patients. Box 41-1 lists the goals of ventilatory support. Box 41-2 lists specific objectives of mechanical ventilation.

Alveolar damage may be caused by elevated transpulmonary pressure during positive pressure breathing. Transpulmonary pressure is the difference between alveolar pressure and pleural pressure. Normal lungs are not overdistended as long as transpulmonary pressure is less than 30 to 35 cm H_2O.[12] High transpulmonary pressure is associated with alveolar overdistension and lung injury.[9,12] Plateau pressure (P_{plat}) during mechanical ventilation reflects alveolar pressure, and limiting P_{plat} may reduce ventilator-induced lung injury, although patients with decreases in thoracic compliance may have an alveolar pressure greater than 35 cm H_2O without overdistension.[12]

Box 41-1 • Physiological Goals of Ventilatory Support

- To support or manipulate gas exchange
  - Alveolar ventilation ($Pa{CO_2}$ and pH)
  - Arterial oxygenation ($Pa{O_2}$, $Sa{O_2}$, $Sp{O_2}$, $Ca{O_2}$, and $D{O_2}$)
- To increase lung volume
  - End-inspiratory and end-expiratory lung inflation
  - Functional residual capacity (FRC)
- To reduce or manipulate the work of breathing
- To minimize cardiovascular impairment

From Slutsky AS: Chest 104:1833, 1993.

Box 41-2 • Specific Clinical Objectives of Ventilatory Support

- To reverse hypoxemia
- To reverse acute respiratory acidosis
- To relieve respiratory distress
- To prevent or reverse atelectasis
- To reverse ventilatory muscle fatigue
- To allow sedation and neuromuscular blockade
- To decrease systemic or myocardial oxygen consumption
- To maintain or improve cardiac output
- To reduce ICP
- To stabilize the chest

From Slutsky AS: Chest 104:1833, 1993.

VENTILATORY MANAGEMENT STRATEGIES FOR SPECIFIC DISORDERS

The basic principles of maintaining oxygenation, ventilation, and acid-base homeostasis while minimizing harmful side effects apply across patient types and disorders. Specific ventilatory strategies may differ depending on the patient's disease state or condition. Care of patients with normal pulmonary mechanics, ARDS, COPD, acute severe asthma exacerbation, postoperative state, myocardial infarction, CHF, neuromuscular disease, head trauma, unilateral lung disease, and bronchopleural fistula (BPF) is described briefly.

Normal Pulmonary Mechanics

Patients with normal lung function sometimes need mechanical ventilatory support because of apnea or severe hypoventilation caused by a nonpulmonary problem. Examples of such problems include recovery from major abdominal or thoracic surgery, sedative or narcotic drug overdose (without pulmonary aspiration), high spinal cord injury, cardiac arrest after myocardial infarction, electric shock, or related trauma, neuromuscular disease, head trauma, and certain central nervous system (CNS) disorders. As a rule, patients with normal compliance, airway resistance, and lung function can be easily ventilated with volume ventilation in the assist-control or synchronous intermittent mandatory ventilation (SIMV) mode. Tidal volume usually is started at 10 to 12 mL/kg of ideal body weight (IBW) with a machine rate of 10 to 12 breaths/min. Larger tidal volume (12-15 mL/kg) and a slower rate (6-10 breaths/min) may be used in the SIMV mode if there are concerns about maintaining lung volume or satisfying patients' air hunger. Inspiratory flow in the range of 60 to 80 L/min generally is used and results in a ratio of inspiratory time to expiratory time (I:E ratio) of 1:2 or better. Low to moderate inspired oxygen concentration usually is sufficient for adequate arterial oxygenation for these patients. Care is taken to ensure a plateau pressure of 30 cm H_2O or less, if possible. Small tidal volume

(<7 mL/kg) is avoided in patients with normal lung function, because atelectasis can develop.[13,14]

Acute Respiratory Distress Syndrome

Acute respiratory distress syndrome is characterized by a diffuse, uneven alveolar injury that leads to hypoxemic respiratory failure (see Chapter 24). Most ARDS patients can be effectively ventilated with volume ventilation in the assist-control or SIMV mode. Patients with ARDS typically receive ventilation with lower tidal volume and a higher respiratory rate than used with other types of patients who need mechanical ventilation. Initial tidal volume is set at 8 mL/kg and adjusted downward to 6 mL/kg.[12,15,16] The goal is to limit transpulmonary pressure and the resultant barotrauma caused by overdistending portions of the lung. Maintaining a plateau pressure of 30 cm H_2O or less is preferred, and tidal volume may be decreased to as low as 4 mL/kg. The ventilator rate is increased up to 35 breaths/min to maintain minute volume.[15,16] Positive end-expiratory pressure must be used with a low tidal volume to reduce atelectasis. The $Paco_2$ may be allowed to increase (permissive hypercapnia), but this is not a therapeutic goal. Rather, hypercapnia is a tradeoff and may be accepted as a lung protective strategy when necessary to decrease airway pressure.[17] In general, an increase in rate can offset the decreased tidal volumes used in the management of ARDS. In no case should $Paco_2$ be allowed to increase to the point of a severe acidosis, and a minimal pH of 7.20 or more should be maintained. Positive end-expiratory pressure and CPAP are important adjuncts in the management of ARDS. Positive end-expiratory pressure and CPAP increase FRC, recruit alveoli, and allow Fio_2 to be reduced to a nontoxic level. Positive end-expiratory pressure and CPAP generally begin in the range of 5 to 8 cm H_2O and are then titrated to optimal levels (see later, Oxygenation).

Chronic Obstructive Pulmonary Disease

Patients with COPD tend to have lungs with high compliance and high airway resistance. The lungs of these patients are easy to inflate, but air trapping and auto-PEEP can be problems if expiratory time is too short. Most COPD patients who need mechanical ventilatory support can be easily treated with volume ventilation in the assist-control or SIMV mode.[7,9] Noninvasive positive pressure ventilation (NPPV) by nasal or full face mask is a good alternative during acute exacerbation of COPD. Noninvasive positive pressure ventilation also may be useful in avoiding intubation and conventional mechanical ventilation. A good starting point for most patients is 10 mL/kg and a rate of 10 to 12 breaths/min with an inspiratory flow of at least 60 L/min. A smaller tidal volume (8-10 mL/kg) and slightly lower rate (8-10 breaths/min) with increased inspiratory flow (60-100 L/min) can be used in the care of COPD patients to allow adequate expiratory time and lung emptying.[7,14,18] Assist-control mode should be used with caution in the care of these patients, because the ventilator can be triggered at a rate that results in a shortened expiratory time. Care must be taken to avoid overventilating COPD patients, especially those with chronic carbon dioxide retention, to prevent posthypercapnic alkalosis.

Auto-PEEP may be present when the patient has difficulty triggering a machine breath.[12,14] An expiratory pause should be used to measure auto-PEEP, and the PEEP level can be set below the auto-PEEP level to splint the airways as an aid to complete exhalation.[14] The preferred method of managing auto-PEEP is to increase expiratory time. Inspiratory flow up to 100 L/min may be helpful in decreasing inspiratory time and increasing expiratory time.[14,18] Tidal volume or rate may be decreased to reduce inspiratory time; however, one must ensure that the resultant level of ventilation is adequate for the patient. In general, COPD patients are not difficult to ventilate, and attention to adequate expiratory time and an I:E ratio of 1:2 or less (e.g., 1:3) is effective for most patients.[14]

Acute Severe Asthma Exacerbation

Successful intubation and safe, effective ventilation of a patient with acute, severe asthma who needs mechanical ventilatory support can be a challenge. As with COPD, air trapping and auto-PEEP are a problem; however, patients with severe asthma are especially prone to pneumothorax and cardiovascular compromise secondary to dynamic hyperinflation of the lungs.[19] Consequently, the decision to initiate mechanical ventilation in the care of an asthmatic patient should not be made lightly. Coma or impending or actual respiratory arrest necessitates immediate intubation and mechanical ventilation.[20] Severe exacerbation of asthma (peak expiratory flow or forced expiratory volume in 1 second [FEV_1] <50% of personal best) with severe symptoms at rest, accessory muscle use, and the presence of retractions may help identify the at-risk patient.[20] Wheezing intensity cannot be used to infer the severity of an asthma attack. The absence of wheezing in the face of other indicators of acute severe asthma may indicate that airflow is so reduced that arrest is imminent.[20,21] A history of intubation or mechanical ventilation is an ominous sign.[20] Oxygen therapy and administration of inhaled short-acting β_2-agonists combined with inhaled anticholinergic drugs and systemic corticosteroids are begun. A poor response to therapy (peak expiratory flow or FEV_1 <50%), worsening fatigue, declining mental clarity, drowsiness, and confusion all are indications for admission of the patient to the intensive care unit (ICU).[20,21] Continued poor response despite maximal bronchodilator therapy and failure of $PaCO_2$ to normalize ($PaCO_2$ ≥42 mm Hg) indicate the need for intubation and mechanical ventilation.[20] Intubation should be performed semielectively, not when the patient is in extreme distress.[21] The process of intubation may worsen bronchospasm, and the use of topical lidocaine may be helpful, although sedation and paralysis may be required.[21] The preferred ventilator strategy for acute severe asthma exacerbation includes permissive hypercapnia to minimize high airway pressure and barotrauma.[20,21]

Tidal volume may begin in the range of 8 to 10 mL/kg with an initial ventilator rate of 10 to 12 breaths/min. The SIMV mode is suggested to avoid patient triggering at an increased rate, which may result in a decrease in expiratory time and possible further overinflation. A lower rate and tidal volume (as low as 5-6 mL/kg) may be required.[7,21] Although external PEEP should be avoided, with severe asthma the development of auto-PEEP may be inevitable. With controlled ventilation, a small amount of PEEP to overcome auto-PEEP may be cautiously applied. It is generally best to sedate the patient until apnea is produced.[21] Neuromuscular blocking agents should be avoided, if possible, because there have been reports of prolonged paralysis, especially among patients receiving corticosteroids.[7] Oxygen should be started at 100% and adjusted as indicated on the basis of oximetric findings and arterial blood gas values.[7] If paralytics are required, pancuronium, vecuronium, or rocuronium is preferred, because histamine release is associated with other neuromuscular blocking agents. Bronchodilators and corticosteroids remain the primary elements in treatment of patients with severe asthma. Often two to four times the usual dose of bronchodilators is required for nebulization in patients receiving mechanical ventilation because of the reduction in drug delivery caused by the endotracheal tube. The rate, inspiratory flow, and expiratory time are balanced to avoid auto-PEEP while effective ventilation is maintained and airway pressure is minimized. An initial inspiratory flow of 60 L/min or more with a decelerating flow waveform has been suggested.[7]

Postoperative Ventilatory Support

After coronary artery bypass graft surgery, heart valve replacement, and heart transplantation, patients are routinely transported from the operating room directly to the ICU undergoing mechanical ventilatory support. In many instances, patients who have undergone other thoracic or abdominal surgery also are maintained in the ICU with mechanical ventilatory support immediately after the operation. These patients frequently have normal lungs, and ventilation and FIO_2 can be adjusted accordingly. A tidal volume of 10 to 12 mL/kg is appropriate for most patients; however, a larger volume (12-15 mL/kg) and slower rate (6-10 breaths/min) may be used to maintain lung volume.[7,14] Synchronized intermittent mandatory ventilation with pressure support or assist-control volume ventilation are acceptable mode choices. Positive end-expiratory pressure of 3 to 5 cm H_2O may be applied to help prevent the development of atelectasis.[7] Ventilation usually can be discontinued expeditiously, and extubation may be possible after a few hours in the ICU.

Lung resection and lung transplantation patients may need special attention. A smaller volume and more rapid rate may be necessary. Care should be taken to maintain plateau pressure at 30 cm H_2O or less.[7]

Myocardial Ischemia and Congestive Heart Failure

Most patients with myocardial ischemia, myocardial infarction, or CHF can be ventilated and oxygenated adequately with a conventional approach. With hypotension or cardiovascular instability, however, care must be taken to ensure that elevated mean airway pressure does not further impede venous return and reduce cardiac output. Steps to decrease mean airway pressure include decreasing peak pressure, decreasing tidal volume, decreasing inspiratory time, increasing expiratory time, reducing respiratory rate, and switching from a down-ramp to a square or accelerating flow waveform. In addition, one should minimize the work of breathing to reduce oxygen consumption of the ventilatory muscles, ensure adequate arterial oxygen content (CaO_2), and reduce cardiac work.[9]

In patients with severe CHF, positive pressure ventilation may decrease ventricular preload and improve myocardial efficiency.[9] With cardiogenic pulmonary edema, positive pressure ventilation and the application of PEEP should be used to improve oxygenation.

Neuromuscular Disorders

Patients with neuromuscular disease often have normal lung function, the primary problem being neuromuscular transmission. These patients may prefer high volume (12-15 mL/kg) and flow.[9] Patients with neuromuscular disorders often do well with a reduced FIO_2 (even down to 0.21). However, it is best to start at 40% to 50% oxygen or even 100% when in doubt and to titrate the FIO_2 as needed. Positive end-expiratory pressure may be set at zero or 3 to 5 cm H_2O to prevent atelectasis.

Head Trauma

As noted in Chapter 40, patients with closed head trauma or who have undergone a neurosurgical procedure may have cerebral edema and elevated ICP. In the care of these patients, care should be taken to minimize PEEP and mean airway pressure. In addition, as a temporary measure, hyperventilation may be used with a target $PaCO_2$ of 28 mm Hg (range 25-30 mm Hg[9]) to reduce ICP. This treatment results in cerebral vasoconstriction, reduced cerebral blood volume, and transiently lower ICP for 12 to 24 hours. Hyperventilation to decrease ICP should be adjusted gradually to return partial pressure of carbon dioxide (PCO_2) to the normal level over 24 to 48 hours, if the ICP level allows.[9] If the PCO_2 is allowed to climb too quickly, the ICP may rebound and climb to unacceptably high levels, which could compromise cerebral perfusion.

Unilateral Lung Disease

In the presence of unilateral lung disease, positive pressure ventilation tends to go to the healthy lung. Techniques to overcome this problem include use of a double-lumen endotracheal tube to isolate the bad lung combined with independent lung ventilation and differential application of PEEP, placing the good lung down to promote matching of gas and blood, and use of a prolonged inspiratory time to maximize distribution of inspired gas.[9,14]

Bronchopleural Fistula

A BPF is a persistent air leak into the pleural space. Bronchopleural fistula and an associated chest tube air leak are commonly caused by a tear in the lung tissue caused by trauma, surgery, or an invasive procedure, such as placement of a central line.[9] Bronchopleural fistula also can occur as a complication of diffuse lung disease, such as *Pneumocystis carinii* pneumonia, COPD, or ARDS.[9] Most air leaks are minor.[9] Large air leaks may, however, impair ventilation. Measurement of inspired versus expired tidal volume can help with assessment of the size of an air leak. Patients with BPF need chest tube placement. If the patient cannot be successfully treated with conventional volume ventilation, options include high-frequency ventilation (HFV) and independent lung ventilation.[9] Ventilation to minimize airway pressure, including use of a smaller tidal volume (4-8 mL/kg) and use of minimal or no PEEP, may be helpful.[9] The presence of a BPF may necessitate surgical intervention.[9]

▶ VENTILATOR INITIATION

Once the decision to begin mechanical ventilatory support is made, one must choose the mode of ventilation, select an appropriate device, and establish the initial ventilator settings.

In the selection of initial ventilator settings, the goal is to optimize the patient's oxygenation, ventilation, and acid-base balance while avoiding harmful side effects. This goal is achieved by choosing an appropriate mode of ventilation, FIO_2, tidal volume, rate, PEEP/CPAP, and pressure-support level. Appropriate trigger sensitivity, inspiratory flow (or time), pressure limit, alarms, backup ventilation, and humidification then must be selected. After initial ventilator setup, adjustments must be made on the basis of the patient's response and specific clinical goals.

Most patients who need mechanical ventilatory support receive positive pressure ventilation; however, negative pressure ventilation may be considered under certain circumstances. Once the decision for use of positive pressure ventilation is made, the clinician may consider NPPV as an alternative to traditional positive pressure ventilation administered through an endotracheal tube or tracheostomy tube. Next the clinician must choose the mode of ventilation (e.g., assist control, SIMV, pressure-support ventilation [PSV], PCV) and initial ventilator settings (e.g., rate, tidal volume, PSV, FIO_2, PEEP/CPAP). Last, the clinician must choose appropriate alarm and apnea value settings. Box 41-3 summarizes key decisions that must be made as a part of initial ventilator setup.

Negative Pressure Ventilation

Negative pressure ventilation, in the form of the first "iron lung" used clinically on a widespread basis, was developed by Drinker, McKhann, and Shaw at Harvard in 1928.[14] John H. Emerson developed a commercial version of the iron lung that became available in 1932. Today a number of iron lungs remain in use in the United States, and the Porta-Lung, chest cuirasse, and body suit are sometimes called upon for use in the care of patients with chronic neuromuscular or chest wall disease who need intermittent or continuous negative pressure ventilatory support.[14] The advantages of negative pressure breathing devices include the lack of need for an artificial airway and the relative simplicity and ease of use of the devices. Consequently, negative pressure ventilation may have a useful role in the care of patients with chronic problems such as neuromuscular disease or other chronic restrictive disorders.[14,22] Problems with negative pressure devices include difficulty gaining access to the patient, difficulty moving the device owing to its bulk, difficulty maintaining ventilation because of leaks, and the presence of only control mode in older devices. Negative pressure devices function by producing negative pressure around the thorax during inspiration. The result is negative intrathoracic and intrapleural pressure, not unlike normal spontaneous breathing. However, when the entire body is placed in a negative pressure environment, as is the

Box 41-3 • Initial Ventilator Setup

Initial ventilator setup includes the following key decisions:

- Indications for ventilatory support present
- Negative pressure versus positive pressure ventilation
- Noninvasive versus invasive positive pressure ventilation
- Type and method of establishment of an airway
- Pressure versus volume ventilation
- Partial versus full ventilatory support
- Choice of ventilator
- Mode of ventilation
  - Assist-control ventilation versus SIMV (with or without pressure support)
  - Pressure support
  - Pressure control
  - Mixed or dual-control modes
  - Other newer modes and adjuncts

Next, the clinician must consider key ventilatory values. These include the following:

- Trigger method (pressure or flow trigger) and sensitivity
- Tidal volume (volume ventilation) or pressure limit (pressure support and pressure control)
- Rate
- Inspiratory flow, inspiratory time, expiratory time, and I:E ratio
- Inspiratory flow waveform
- FIO_2
- PEEP/CPAP

Last, the clinician must choose appropriate alarm and backup values to include the following:

- Low pressure, low PEEP alarms
- High pressure limit and alarm
- Volume alarms (low tidal volume, high and low minute ventilation)
- High rate alarm
- Apnea alarm and apnea values
- High/low oxygen alarm
- High/low temperature alarm
- I:E ratio limit and alarm

case with the iron lung and the newer Porta-lung, abdominal venous blood pooling, reduced venous return, and tank shock are possible complications. Although it is unlikely that one would consider negative pressure ventilation an alternative to positive pressure ventilation in the critical care setting, negative pressure devices can be useful in the long-term care of patients with chronic respiratory failure.[14,22]

Noninvasive Positive Pressure Ventilation

Continuous positive airway pressure and biphasic (also called bilevel) positive airway pressure (BiPAP) by nasal mask have long been used in the home for the management of sleep apnea. In recent years, there has been an increase in the use of NPPV in the acute care setting in an attempt to avoid endotracheal intubation and conventional mechanical ventilation.[14,23] In the acute care setting, NPPV should be considered in the management of acute exacerbation of COPD[23] and in the treatment of patients who are prematurely extubated after conventional mechanical ventilation, in an attempt to avoid reintubation. Noninvasive ventilation may decrease the need for intubation, the frequency of complications, length of stay, and mortality among selected patients with acute exacerbation of COPD.[23] Noninvasive positive pressure ventilation has been effective in reducing the need for endotracheal intubation in the care of patients with acute respiratory failure and may be useful in the management of CHF.[14,24,25] Contraindications include inability to tolerate the nasal or oral mask, poor mask fit, secretion problems, severe hypoxemia, severe acidosis, hypotension, and upper airway obstruction. Noninvasive positive pressure ventilation should not be used in the care of patients who are prone to aspiration or who otherwise need intubation to protect the airway. Noninvasive positive pressure ventilation may be ineffective in the care of patients who need higher airway pressure than is available with current devices to maintain adequate ventilation. Advantages and disadvantages of NPPV are listed in Box 41-4. The clinical application of NPPV is discussed in detail in Chapter 42.

Establishment of the Airway

Conventional mechanical ventilatory support requires the establishment of an artificial airway. Approximately 75% of patients receiving positive pressure ventilation are intubated, and of these, 95% have oral tubes and approximately 5% have nasal tubes.[1] Approximately 25% of patients receiving mechanical ventilation have a tracheotomy performed at some point.[1] Airway management is described in detail in Chapter 30.

Pressure-Control Versus Volume-Controlled Ventilation

The next decision to be made regarding initiation of mechanical ventilation is whether to use a primarily pressure-controlled* (pressure-limited) or volume-controlled (volume-limited) mode of ventilation. In the

*The term *pressure-controlled* refers to systems that control pressure to cause inspiration. Pressure-support ventilation (PSV) and pressure-control ventilation (PCV) are pressure controlled. Volume-control ventilators control volume to achieve inspiration. For a more thorough explanation of pressure- and volume-controlled ventilation, see Chapter 39.

Box 41-4 • Advantages and Disadvantages of NPPV

ADVANTAGES
- Avoidance of intubation and associated complications in some instances
- Preservation of natural airway defenses
- Patient comfort
- Maintenance of speech and swallowing
- Less need for sedation
- Intermittent use

DISADVANTAGES
- Patient cooperation needed
- Limited access to airway and suctioning
- Mask discomfort
- Facial ulcers, eye irritation, rhinitis, dry nose
- Air leak
- Transient hypoxemia from accidental mask disconnection
- BiPAP limited to 20 to 30 cm H_2O
- Time consuming procedure

past, pressure-controlled, pressure-cycled ventilation was common with ventilators such as the Bird Mark series or Bennett PR-2, particularly for meeting a short-term need, such as postoperative recovery or emergency department care, and when no other more sophisticated ventilators were available. Today, pressure-controlled ventilation often is used in the form of PSV or PCV. These newer modes of pressure-limited ventilation can be used alone or in combination with SIMV.[26,27] In the use of pressure-controlled ventilation, as the patient's compliance and resistance change, the volume delivered varies. Volume-controlled ventilation ensures that volume constant breaths are delivered within the functional limitations of the ventilator and set pressure limit. With volume-controlled ventilation, as compliance decreases or resistance increases, the pressure increases, and the volume remains constant. With pressure-controlled ventilation, if compliance decreases or resistance increases, pressure remains constant, and delivered volume may decline. The two pressure-controlled modes of ventilation in common use today are PCV and PSV. With PSV, the ventilator is patient triggered to inspiration (assist), pressure limited during the inspiratory phase, and flow cycled to expiration.[26] With PCV, the ventilator may be time or patient triggered (assist or control) to inspiration, pressure limited during the inspiratory phase, and time cycled to expiration.[27] Pressure-support ventilation may be used as a stand-alone mode or in conjunction with SIMV.[26] Pressure-control ventilation may be used as an assist-control mode or in combination with SIMV in the form of SIMV pressure control with pressure support.[27] The primary advantage of volume-controlled ventilation is maintenance of a stable constant tidal volume in the face of changing lung mechanics. Pressure-control ventilation is useful in limiting airway pressure and providing a decreasing (decelerating) flow, which may improve gas distribution, patient comfort, and synchrony.

Full Ventilatory Support Versus Partial Ventilatory Support

Full ventilatory support can be defined as the application of mechanical support such that all of the energy necessary for effective alveolar ventilation is provided. When a ventilator is set up to deliver full ventilatory support, adequate ventilation and $PaCO_2$ are maintained, even if the patient makes no spontaneous breathing efforts. Full ventilatory support may be accomplished with the ventilator set in the SIMV or assist-control mode. The key to providing full ventilatory support is to set an appropriate machine rate and tidal volume, usually in the range of 10 to 12 breaths/min with a tidal volume of 10 to 12 mL/kg of IBW. In the event of apnea, these values should ensure a minimum effective level of alveolar ventilation for most adult patients. Lower initial tidal volume and higher rate may be selected for patients with ALI or ARDS.[15,16]

Partial ventilatory support entails use of ventilator settings that require the patient to provide a portion of the ventilation needed to maintain an acceptable $PaCO_2$. Partial ventilatory support is typically provided in the SIMV mode with machine rates of less than 8 to 10 breaths/min. Under these circumstances, the patient must provide a portion of the required alveolar ventilation through spontaneous breathing efforts. With partial ventilatory support, if spontaneous breathing ceases or becomes inadequate, as may be the case with the development of rapid shallow breathing or apnea, alveolar ventilation may decrease, and $PaCO_2$ may increase above an acceptable level. In addition, work of breathing usually is greater with SIMV than with assist-control ventilation.[28,29] Other modes of ventilation that require effective spontaneous breathing include pressure support, volume support, adaptive pressure ventilation (APV), and proportional pressure support. Adaptive support ventilation (ASV) and mandatory minute volume ventilation (MMV) vary the level of mechanical ventilatory support as patient effort varies from full ventilatory support to partial ventilatory support as the patient's spontaneous minute volume increases. Partial ventilatory support strategies may be appropriate in the care of spontaneously breathing patients with primarily hypoxemic respiratory failure and of patients who are able to comfortably provide a portion of their required minute volume. Partial ventilatory support techniques may be especially useful for weaning patients from mechanical ventilatory support, and PSV and SIMV have been advocated as partial support strategies for weaning. Partial ventilatory support should be avoided in the care of patients with ventilatory muscle fatigue or a high-level of work of breathing.

Choice of a Ventilator

After the decision is made to initiate mechanical ventilatory support, the clinician must select an appropriate ventilator. This decision should be guided by considering the features, modes available, pressure and flow capabilities, alarms and monitoring systems included, reliability, cost, and familiarity of the clinician with the equipment. Pressure and flow capabilities of specific ventilators become a concern in the care of patients with low compliance, high resistance, or markedly increased inspiratory demands. The ventilator chosen should adequately ventilate the patient under changing conditions. Table 41-4 compares the pressure and flow capabilities of common ventilator systems.

▶ INITIAL VENTILATOR SETTINGS

Initial ventilator settings are chosen for maintenance and improvement of oxygenation and ventilation with minimum harmful side effects. Attention to the patient's work of breathing, comfort, and adjustment to mechanical support should be considered. Initial ventilator settings include choice of mode, tidal volume, rate, FIO_2 and PEEP. The respiratory therapist must set the trigger level, inspiratory flow or time, alarms and limits, backup ventilation, and humidification.

Choice of Mode

Most modern critical care ventilators include assist control, SIMV, PEEP/CPAP, PSV, and PCV.[14,26,27]

Table 41-4 ▶▶ Pressure and Flow Capabilities of Common Ventilator Systems

Ventilator	Maximum Pressure (cm H_2O)	Maximum Flow (L/min)
Bird Mark 7	40-50	80 (50 on 100%)
Bird Mark 14	190	High
Bennett PR-2	40-50	80
MA-1	80	100
MA-2	100	125
Bennett 7200	120	120
Bennett 740	90	150 (300 spontaneous)
Bennett 840	90	150
Hamilton Veolar	110	I:E of 1:4
Hamilton Galileo	110	180
Bird 8400 STi	140	120
Bird T Bird	120	140
Drager Evita-4	100	120 (180 for auto flow)

Terminology describing various modes of ventilation on specific ventilators can be confusing. For the purposes of this chapter, assist-control volume ventilation also can be described as volume-control continuous mandatory ventilation (VC-CMV). Synchronized intermittent mandatory ventilation is properly classified as a form of volume-control intermittent mandatory ventilation (VC-IMV), and PSV is a form of pressure-control continuous spontaneous ventilation (PC-CSV). For a more complete discussion of ventilator modes, see Chapter 39.

Newer dual-control modes allow for pressure-limited breaths with a volume guarantee. Systems that adjust the pressure level automatically to maintain tidal volume from breath to breath include volume support (VS), pressure-regulated volume control (PRVC) (Siemens Servo 300), and adaptive pressure ventilation (APV) (Hamilton Galileo). Dual-control systems that switch from a pressure-control breath to a volume breath within the breath as necessary to maintain tidal volume include volume-assured pressure support (VAPS) (Bird 8400 ST) and pressure augmentation (PA) (Bear 1000). Other newer modes maintain minimum minute ventilation by means of automatic adjustment of the number of machine breaths, pressure-support level, or pressure-control level. These modes include mandatory minute volume ventilation (Bear 1000, Evita-4) and adaptive support ventilation (Hamilton Galileo). Proportional assist ventilation (PAV) and proportional pressure support (PPS) (Evita-4) automatically vary the pressure support provided as patient effort changes to maintain a "normal" work of breathing. Proportional assist ventilation and PPS are intended to compensate for abnormally increased ventilatory workloads as patient effort varies.[30] Last, adjunctive techniques to minimize imposed work of breathing (WOB_I) include flow trigger, flow by, and automatic tube compensation (ATC) (Evita-4). Chapter 39 describes modes of ventilation available on common mechanical ventilators.

Negative pressure ventilation should be reserved for special circumstances, such as the long-term care of patients with chronic respiratory failure. Noninvasive ventilation should generally be reserved for spontaneously breathing patients who do not need a high level of ventilatory support (see Chapter 42). Noninvasive positive pressure ventilation may be of value in the care of patients with acute exacerbation of COPD in an attempt to avoid intubation and conventional ventilation. Noninvasive positive pressure ventilation also may be useful for avoiding reintubation in patients prematurely extubated after conventional ventilation. In the care of critically ill patients, the most common method of ventilatory support is conventional, volume-control ventilation in the assist-control or SIMV mode (including SIMV with pressure support).[1]

Box 41-5 • Typical Values for Ventilator Initiation for Adults Receiving Assist-Control Volume Ventilation

- Trigger sensitivity: –0.5 to –1.5 cm H_2O or flow trigger set to minimize trigger work without autocycle
- Tidal volume: 10 to 12 mL/kg IBW
- Rate: Backup rate of 10 to 12 breaths/min
- Inspiratory flow: 40 to 80 L/min to achieve an inspiratory time of approximately 1 second (0.8-1.2 s) and an I:E ratio of 1:2 or better. Inspiratory flow of 80 L/min or more may be required in the care of some patients to meet or exceed the patient's spontaneous inspiratory flow demand.
- PEEP: 0 cm H_2O (3-5 cm H_2O may be used as "physiologic" PEEP)
- Pressure limit: Start at 50 cm H_2O and adjust after patient connection to 10 to 20 cm H_2O above the peak inspiratory pressure (PIP)
- Humidification: Begin with heated humidifier to provide a temperature of 35°C at the airway connection and at least 30 mg/L absolute humidity

Assist Control Ventilation (Patient- or Time-Triggered Continuous Mandatory Ventilation)

With assist-control mode, every breath is supported by the ventilator. Breaths are patient- or time-triggered to inspiration and may be volume or pressure limited.[9,10] Inspiration may be volume, pressure, or time cycled to the expiratory phase.[9] Assist-control ventilation typically is delivered in VC-CMV.[14] Suggested initial settings for assist-control volume ventilation in the care of adults are listed in Box 41-5.

Advantages of assist-control volume ventilation include the assurance that a minimum, safe level of ventilation is achieved. Every breath is a volume breath, yet the patient can set his or her own breathing rate. In the event of sedation or apnea, a minimum, safe level of ventilation is guaranteed by the selection of an appropriate backup rate, usually approximately 2 to 4 breaths/min below the patient's assist rate.[10] Because assist-control ventilation usually provides full ventilatory support, it may result in a lower work of breathing than do partial support modes. A lower work of breathing, however, should *not* be assumed just because the patient is in assist-control mode. Trigger work may be significant if inappropriate sensitivity settings are selected. In addition, once a breath is triggered, inspiratory muscle activity persists.[31,32] If the inspiratory flow rate of the ventilator does not meet or exceed the patient's inspiratory demand, the patient's work may be high, equaling or even exceeding the work of achieving a spontaneous unassisted breath.[31,32] If properly applied, however, assist-control ventilation may provide ventilatory muscle rest that allows the ventilatory muscles to recover in the event of ventilatory muscle fatigue. Disadvantages of assist-control mode include an increase in the work of breathing with inappropriate sensitivity and flow settings.[12,14] Assist control also may be poorly tolerated by awake, nonsedated patients. The patient may fight the ventilator, or asynchronous patient-to-ventilator breathing patterns may develop. Patients with a high ventilatory drive may trigger the ventilator at a rapid rate that results in hyperventilation and respiratory alkalosis. In this event, the first step is to attempt to identify the cause of increased respiratory rate and correct it, if possible. Common causes of an increased respiratory rate include anxiety, pain, hypoxemia, metabolic acidosis, and inappropriate ventilator settings. If methods of correcting the problem fail, one may try the SIMV mode, which should be helpful in preventing respiratory alkalosis. Other options include administration of analgesics, sedatives, tranquilizers, and as a last resort, the use of paralytic drugs. Patients with COPD are at special risk of air trapping in the assist-control mode, especially if they attempt to breathe at an increased rate. Consequently, many clinicians prefer to use SIMV with an increased expiratory time to avoid air trapping and auto-PEEP in these patients. With assist-control ventilation, every breath is a "machine" breath, and consequently the mean airway pressure may be higher than that delivered with SIMV. This may be a cause for concern in the care of patients with hypovolemia, hemodynamic instability, or hypotension.

Controlled Ventilation (Time-Triggered Continuous Mandatory Ventilation)

Controlled ventilation, often in the volume-control mode (VC-CMV), is achieved when the patient is apneic because of a medical condition, anesthesia, or use of sedative drugs or paralytic agents. Advantages of controlled ventilation include eliminating the work of breathing entirely and achieving complete control over the patient's inspiratory and expiratory time, flow, and pressure. In cases in which the work of breathing is high, controlled ventilation may allow for ventilatory muscle rest, reduce the oxygen consumption of the ventilatory muscles, and "free up" oxygen for delivery to the tissues.[10] Controlled ventilation may allow prolonged inspiratory times and the use of I:E ratios of 1:1, 1.5:1, and 2:1 in cases in which other methods have failed to improve oxygenation. Disadvantages of controlled ventilation include the need for sedatives and perhaps paralytic drugs in the care of patients with spontaneous breathing efforts. The administration of paralytic agents has been associated with the development of prolonged neuropathy in some patients.[10] Paralytic agents have no effect on the patient's level of consciousness and should not be given without concurrent and appropriate sedation. In addition, in the care of apneic patients, ventilator malfunction or disconnection can lead to a ventilator catastrophe.[10]

Controlled ventilation should *not* be achieved by setting the ventilator sensitivity control at a level at which the patient cannot trigger the ventilator. This practice sometimes is called "locking out" the patient. Although it is possible to set the ventilator so that even with a maximal effort, no patient trigger occurs, this practice should be avoided. If a patient is locked out and begins making spontaneous efforts, large swings in pressure may result. In addition, spontaneous efforts against a closed system can result in patient anxiety, agitation, and even panic at not being able to breathe. Last, controlled ventilation for an extended time may lead to ventilatory muscle atrophy and loss of ventilatory muscle strength and coordination.[10]

Intermittent Mandatory Ventilation

Intermittant mandatory ventilation (IMV) and SIMV may be used as partial or full ventilatory support techniques.[9,14] Patients breathe spontaneously between mandatory machine breaths.[9,14] The machine breath may be time cycled (IMV) or patient triggered (SIMV) to inspiration. The inspiratory phase usually is delivered with a specific inspiratory flow waveform, which may be adjustable.

With SIMV, the machine breath is typically volume cycled to expiration; however, the breath may be pressure limited and time cycled on some ventilators, such as the Siemens Servo 300 in the SIMV pressure control with pressure-support mode. Synchronized intermittent mandatory ventilation often is combined with pressure support to overcome the WOB_I during spontaneous breathing due to demand flow systems, ventilator circuits, and artificial airways. Synchronized intermittent mandatory ventilation allows the clinician to vary the amount of support provided from minimal to full ventilatory support. Further, SIMV is easy to apply, and weaning protocols with SIMV have been effective in removing patients from mechanical support. Synchronized intermittent mandatory ventilation also may be slightly better than assist-control ventilation in preventing hyperventilation and respiratory alkalosis.[14,33,34] Synchronized intermittent mandatory ventilation may provide lower mean airway pressure than assist-control ventilation and may help maintain ventilatory muscle strength and coordination.[14] Disadvantages of SIMV include the possible development of respiratory muscle fatigue, especially in patients with rapid shallow spontaneous breathing patterns; acute hypoventilation with use of low rates if patients do not continue to do their share of breathing; and an increase in work of breathing due to the demand flow system, ventilator circuit, and artificial airway or due to inappropriate trigger sensitivity or ventilator peak flow settings.[14,31] There is also evidence that SIMV may be slower for weaning patients than are spontaneous breathing trials or pressure support.[12,14] The advantages and disadvantages of assist-control and SIMV modes are found in Table 41-5.

Pressure Support

Pressure support assists the patient's spontaneous inspiration with a clinician-selected level of positive pressure.[26] Pressure support is patient triggered, pressure limited, and flow-cycled.[26] Pressure-support ventilation can reduce work of breathing and may improve patient-ventilator synchrony and comfort while limiting the pressure applied to the airway.[26] Pressure support to

Table 41-5 ▶▶ Advantages and Disadvantages of SIMV

Advantages	Disadvantages
Lower mean airway pressure may result than is achieved with assist-control ventilation.	SIMV with PSV may increase mean airway pressure.
Ventilatory muscle activity, strength, and coordination are maintained.	Ventilatory muscle fatigue may occur.
The level of support to maintain adequate levels of alveolar ventilation is easy to titrate.	Acute hypoventilation may occur, especially with lower machine rates (<8-10 breaths/min).
Weaning protocols are easy to apply.	Weaning may be prolonged.
Spontaneous breathing, which is physiologic, is incorporated.	The addition of pressure support often is required to overcome the WOB_I.
Patients tend not to hyperventilate and may not fight the ventilator, as they may do with assist mode.	Patients may have difficulty adjusting to the ventilator; breath stacking is possible with IMV.
Sedation or paralysis is not required, as it is in control mode.	Patients may experience or continue a rapid shallow breathing pattern or continue to make spontaneous breathing efforts during delivery of a "machine breath."
Full or partial ventilatory support and level of support can be titrated according to the patient's need.	Patient workload increases considerably when SIMV rate decreases to approximately 50% of the full ventilatory support value.

overcome WOB_I should be considered in the care of all spontaneously breathing patients in the SIMV mode.[14,26] Synchronized intermittent mandatory ventilation, as originally developed, allowed spontaneous breathing interspersed with volume-limited, patient- or time-triggered machine breaths. The WOB_I during spontaneous breathing due to slow demand flow systems, ventilator circuitry, and the artificial airway prompted the addition of pressure support. Today it is suggested that all spontaneous breaths during SIMV be supported with an appropriate level of pressure support, usually in the range of 5 to 10 cm H_2O, to overcome the WOB_I.[9,26] The PSV level needed to overcome (WOB_I) may be estimated as follows:

$$PSV = \frac{(PIP - P_{plat}) \times \dot{V}_I \text{ spontaneous}}{\text{Ventilator inspiratory flow}}$$

where PSV is the pressure-support level needed to overcome WOB_I, PIP is the peak inspiratory pressure during a volume-control machine breath, P_{plat} is the plateau pressure following an inspiratory pause (usually approximately 1 second), ventilator inspiratory flow rate (L/s) is the inspiratory flow set on the ventilator with a square wave inspiratory flow waveform, and $\dot{V}_I$ is the patient's spontaneous peak inspiratory flow in liters per second. An example of the calculations for the PSV needed to overcome WOB_I is found in Box 41-6.

Stand-Alone PSV

Pressure-support ventilation may be used as a stand-alone mode, either for maximal unloading of the ventilatory muscles (PSV_{max}), simply to eliminate the WOB_I during spontaneous breathing trials, or during weaning to provide partial ventilatory support.[9,26]

Maximal unloading of the ventilatory muscles refers to application of the level of pressure support needed to minimize the ventilatory muscle work.[26] In general, this is the pressure level required to achieve an inspired tidal volume of 10 to 12 mL/kg.[26] For initial ventilator setup, one begins with a pressure of 12 to 15 cm H_2O. Pressure-support ventilation is then rapidly titrated to achieve a target tidal volume, usually 10 to 12 mL/kg IBW with a spontaneous breathing rate of 20 breaths/min or less.[26] Pressure support is an assist mode of ventilation and PSV_{max} should be reserved for spontaneously breathing patients with stable, intact respiratory drives.[26] As compliance and resistance change, delivered volume varies. A small resulting delivered tidal volume (<7 mL/kg) may lead to progressive alveolar collapse.[13,14] For weaning from PSV, the level of support is reduced, generally in increments of 2 to 4 cm H_2O followed by patient assessment. Pressure-support ventilation may be used as an adjunct for overcoming the WOB_I due to artificial airways and breathing circuits during spontaneous breathing trials.[9,26] The PSV level required to overcome WOB_I varies with the size of the endotracheal or tracheostomy tube and the patient's spontaneous inspiratory flow rate.

Problems with PSV include the fact that patients with unreliable ventilatory drive may not trigger the ventilator frequently enough to maintain adequate ventilation.[14,26] Changes in compliance and resistance cause the patient's tidal volume to vary. Pressure-support ventilation also increases mean airway pressure, and the increased pressure may impede venous return and cardiac output in patients whose condition is hemodynamically unstable.[26]

Box 41-6 • Calculation of the PSV Level Needed to Overcome the WOB_I in the SIMV With PSV Mode

- Machine delivered tidal volume: 800 mL
- Machine inspiratory flow rate: 60 L/min (1 L/s)
- Flow pattern: Square wave
- Peak inspiratory pressure (PIP): 40 cm H_2O
- Plateau pressure: 30 cm H_2O
- Patient's spontaneous inspiratory flow rate: 30 L/min (0.5 L/s)

$$PSV = \frac{(PIP - P_{plat}) \times \dot{V}_I \text{ spontaneous}}{\text{Ventilator inspiratory flow}}$$

$$= \frac{(40 - 30 \text{ cm } H_2O) \times 0.5 \text{ L/s}}{1 \text{ L/s}} = \frac{10 \text{ cm } H_2O \times 0.5 \text{ L/s}}{\text{L/s}} = 5 \text{ cm } H_2O$$

Pressure-Control Ventilation

Pressure-control breaths may be time or patient triggered to inspiration (assist or control). The inspiratory phase is pressure limited, and the ventilator breath is cycled to expiration by time. As in pressure support, as system compliance and resistance vary, so does the delivered volume. Pressure-control ventilation may be used as an assist-control mode or in combination with SIMV. With PCV, airway pressure is limited, and this limitation may help guard against the development of barotrauma, especially in patients with ALI and ARDS.[15,27] Pressure-control ventilation also allows application of an extended inspiratory time, which may be beneficial to patients with severe oxygenation problems.[27]

Pressure-control ventilation usually is reserved for patients who have poor results with a conventional ventilation strategy of volume ventilation. However, PCV may be used immediately upon ventilator initiation when limiting the plateau pressure is a concern and in the care of patients expected to need prolonged inspiration or an increased I:E ratio (1:1, 1.5:1, 2:1). These patients typically have ALI or ARDS. In these patients, tidal volumes of 6 mL/kg IBW and plateau pressures of

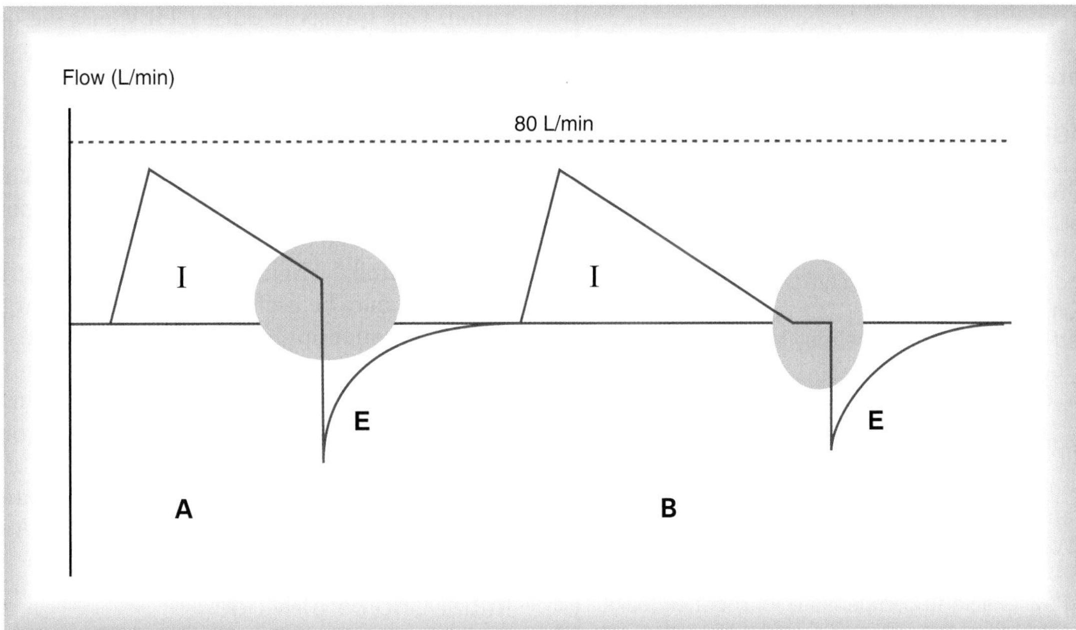

Figure 41-2
Flow versus time waveform during PCV. Curve **A** demonstrates a flow pattern during PCV in which an inadequate inspiratory time (*I*) has been set. During inspiration, flow does not decrease to zero before exhalation occurs, so the preset pressure has not equilibrated to that in the lung. Curve **B** demonstrates an increase in *I* from curve **A**. Inspiratory flow reaches zero and allows the preset pressure to equilibrate in the lungs. Exhaled tidal volume is greater for curve **B** than for curve **A**.

30 cm H_2O or less may reduce barotrauma and improve mortality rate.[12,15] In the care of patients with ALI/ARDS, initial inspiratory pressure should be set to deliver a tidal volume of approximately 8 mL/kg IBW. We suggest beginning with an I:E ratio of 1:1 in these patients with a beginning PEEP level of 5 to 8 cm H_2O. This treatment should result in a period of no flow at end inspiration, as monitored with a ventilator graphics package (Figure 41-2). If the resultant pressure is greater than 30 to 35 cm H_2O, tidal volume may be gradually reduced in intervals of 1 mL/kg every 1 to 2 hours until the pressure is 30 cm H_2O or less and tidal volume is 6 mL/kg.[16] If a pressure of 30 cm H_2O or less cannot be achieved at a volume of 6 mL/kg, tidal volume may be further reduced in a gradual manner to no lower than 4 mL/kg.[16]

Because PCV is administered with lower than conventional tidal volume, careful attention should be paid to maintaining an adequate total minute volume and preventing acute, severe respiratory acidosis. In general, the respiratory rate is initially adjusted to maintain an appropriate baseline minute ventilation ($\dot{V}_E$). For example, a 75-kg IBW adult might have an initial target minute ventilation of approximately 7.5 L/min (100 mL/kg). With a tidal volume of 8 mL/kg, the initial tidal volume might be 600 mL with a rate of approximately 12 to 13 breaths/min. As tidal volume is gradually decreased to 6 mL/kg, rate is increased with a goal of a pH in the range of 7.30 to 7.45. The maximum suggested rate to achieve the desired pH in adult patients is 35 breaths/min, and acidosis may be accepted to maintain the desired pressure limit of 30 cm H_2O or less (permissive hypercapnia).[14,16] Advantages and disadvantages of PCV are described in Box 41-7.

An alternative to PCV in the assist-control mode is the use of SIMV with pressure control and pressure support. An algorithm for initial setup of SIMV with PCV and PSV is found in Figure 41-3. This approach may allow for the benefits of an extended inspiratory time in spontaneously breathing patients without the need for paralysis or the problems of air trapping sometimes associated with PCV in the assist-control mode. For this approach, inspiratory pressure limits are set at the same level for pressure-control and pressure-support breaths, usually with an initial target tidal volume of 8 mL/kg. An initial SIMV rate of 12 breaths/min, a starting I:E ratio of 1:1, and an initial PEEP of 5 to 10 cm H_2O are used, and F_{IO_2} is titrated to maintain an Sa_{O_2} of 90% or more.[27]

High-Frequency Ventilation

High-frequency ventilation entails use of a very rapid rate (60-2400 breaths/min) and small tidal volume, often approaching anatomic dead space.[35] High-frequency positive pressure ventilation (HFPPV), high-frequency jet ventilation (HFJV), and high-frequency oscillation (HFO) all entail different approaches to support venti-

Box 41-7 • Advantages and Disadvantages of PCV

ADVANTAGES

- Variable flow results in a square pressure waveform and improves gas distribution.
- All alveoli are placed under the same sustained inspiratory pressure, which decreases hyperinflation of the more compliant alveoli compared with volume ventilation.
- Sustained inspiration pressure may result in more alveolar recruitment.
- Improved gas distribution allows for a lower tidal volume.
- Lower PIP is achieved in comparison with that achieved with volume ventilation with a square flow waveform.
- The patient may tolerate a longer inspiratory time in SIMV-PCV because flow is variable compared with that in SIMV volume ventilation.
- Variable flow is able to compensate for most air leaks.

DISADVANTAGES

- Higher mean airway pressure can decrease venous return and decrease cardiac output if preload is not adequate.
- Tidal volume varies depending on lung compliance, resistance, and patient effort.
- If tidal volume or minute ventilation alarms are not set properly, alveolar hypoventilation and acidosis may not be detected.

From Vines DL, Peters JI: Clin Pulm Med 8:231, 2001.

lation. Gas transport during HFV may be due to conventional bulk flow, longitudinal (Taylor) dispersion, pendelluft, asymmetric velocity profiles, cardiogenic mixing, or enhanced molecular diffusion.[35] Although HFV has been shown to be safe and effective in maintaining oxygenation and ventilation in a variety of patients,[35,36] whether HFV is superior to conventional ventilation for specific conditions has not been clearly demonstrated. High-frequency jet ventilation, in particular, may be useful in patients with large air leaks due to bronchopulmonary fistula. High-frequency oscillation may be beneficial in infants with respiratory distress syndrome,[35] and results of preliminary studies of HFO for adult ARDS have been promising.[35,36] High-frequency ventilation may allow for a reduction in airway pressure and may have value as part of a lung protective strategy for the management of ARDS.[36]

Initial Choice of Mode

Most patients who need mechanical ventilation in the acute care setting initially are given volume ventilation in the assist-control or SIMV with pressure support mode.[1,14] There is little evidence suggesting either mode is more beneficial in terms of patient outcomes.[14,37] Consequently, the choice of assist-control mode versus SIMV is primarily one of clinician preference and patient tolerance. Synchronized intermittent mandatory ventilation should generally be used with a minimal level of

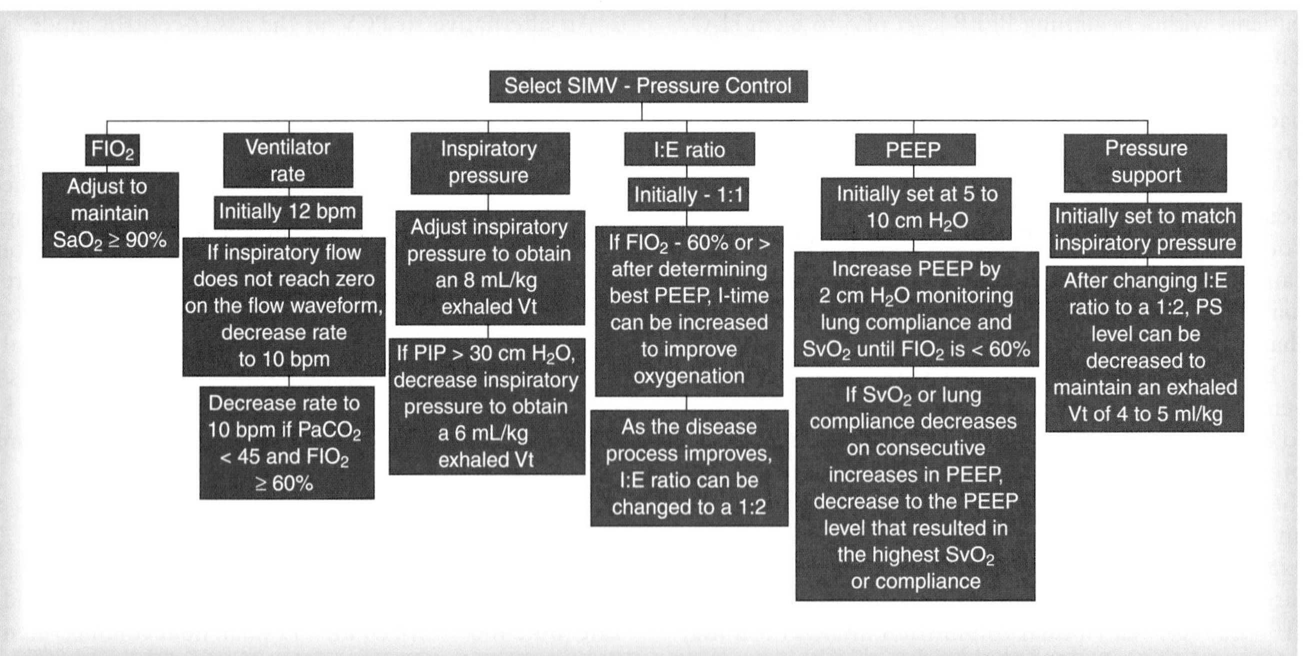

Figure 41-3

Algorithm for initial ventilator setup in the management of ALI/ARDS with SIMV pressure control and pressure support in spontaneously breathing patients. Decreasing rate while maintaining a constant I:E ratio increases inspiratory time, which increases mean airway pressure.

pressure support to overcome the WOB_I performed by spontaneously breathing patients.

Other mode choices for ventilator initiation include PSV, PCV, and the newer dual-control modes, including volume support, adaptive pressure ventilation (APV), and pressure-regulated volume control (PRVC). Techniques that automatically guarantee a minimum minute ventilation include adaptive support ventilation and mandatory minute volume ventilation. Evidence currently available does not suggest that any of these newer modes are superior to assist-control mode or SIMV with PSV for initial ventilator setup in terms of patient outcomes.[9,10,14] Ventilator initiation for most patients usually begins with volume ventilation in assist-control mode or SIMV with pressure support mode to provide full ventilatory support. Partial ventilatory support in the SIMV mode may be considered in the care of spontaneously breathing patients who do not exhibit excessive work of breathing and who are able to contribute to their own ventilation without ventilatory muscle fatigue.

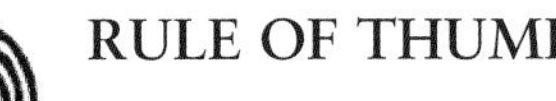

RULE OF THUMB

For most patients, begin mechanical ventilatory support with volume ventilation in the assist-control mode or SIMV with PSV mode. For spontaneously breathing patients in the SIMV mode, pressure support should be initially set at 5 to 10 cm H_2O and adjusted to ensure that the patient's spontaneous work of breathing is not excessive.

Tidal Volume and Rate

Tidal volume and machine rate should be chosen concurrently because these are the two major determinants of minute ventilation. Normal spontaneous tidal volume for adults is approximately 5 to 7 mL/kg with a respiratory rate of 12 to 18 breaths/min for a minute ventilation of approximately 100 mL/kg IBW per minute. In the past, the Radford nomogram was used to estimate tidal volume and rate on the basis of estimated

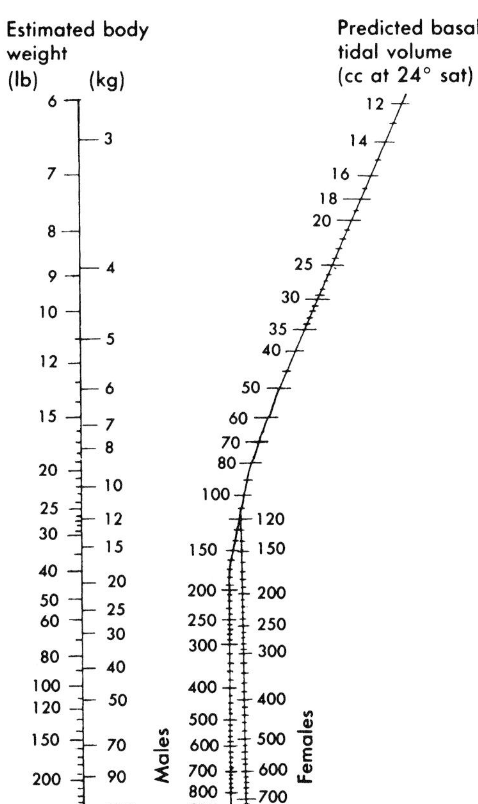

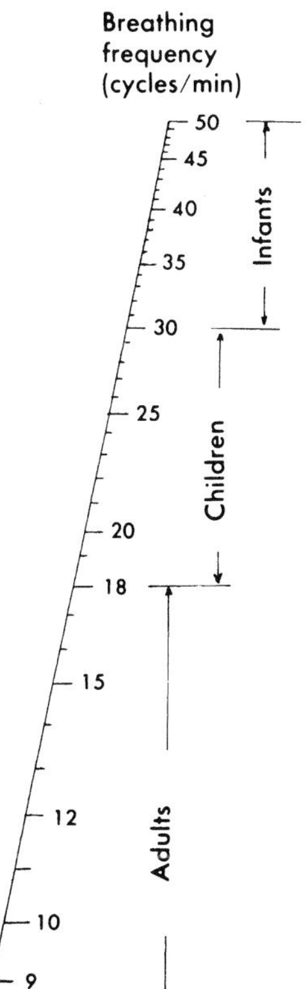

Corrections of predicted basal tidal volumes.
For patients not in coma: add 10%
Fever: add 5% for each °F above 99 (rectal)
add 9% for each °C above 37 (rectal)
Altitude: add 5% for each 2000 feet above sea level
add 8% for each 1000 meters above sea level
Intubation: subtract volume equal to one-half body weight in pounds
subtract 1 cc/kg of body weight
Dead space: add equipment dead space

Figure 41-4 Radford nomogram. *(Modified from Radford EP Jr: J Appl Physiol 7:451, 1955.)*

body weight (Figure 41-4). In modern practice, acceptable tidal volume for mechanical ventilation can range from 5 to 15 mL/kg IBW.[9] In general, for assist-control or SIMV mode, we suggest an initial tidal volume of 10 to 12 mL/kg with a rate of 10 to 12 breaths/min for most patients. After initiation of ventilation, the static or plateau pressure can be assessed, and tidal volume adjusted downward, as needed, for maintenance of a plateau pressure less than 30 to 35 cm H_2O. A larger tidal volume and lower rate (12-15 mL/kg and 6-10 breaths/min) may be considered for maintaining lung volume for patients with neuromuscular disease or postoperative patients with normal lungs. A slightly smaller tidal volume (8-10 mL/kg IBW) has been suggested for patients with obstructive lung disease, including COPD and asthma, to allow for a shorter inspiratory time and longer expiratory time to avoid further air trapping. A smaller initial tidal volume (6-8 mL/kg IBW) is appropriate for patients with ALI or ARDS.[15,16] Table 41-6 lists suggested tidal volumes for men and women according to calculated IBW. With the exception of ALI/ARDS, tidal volume should exceed at least 7 mL/kg for most patients to prevent the development of microatelectasis.[13,14]

Table 41-6 ▶▶ Tidal Volume Based on Ideal Body Weight*

Men

Height (in)	Height (ft)	Weight (lb)	Weight (kg)	6 mL/kg	8 mL/kg	10 mL/kg	12 mL/kg	15 mL/kg
58	4′10″	94	43	260	340	430	520	650
59	4′11″	100	45	270	360	450	540	680
60	5′0″	106	48	290	380	480	580	720
61	5′1″	112	51	310	410	510	610	770
62	5′2″	118	54	320	430	540	650	810
63	5′3″	124	56	340	450	560	670	840
64	5′4″	130	59	350	470	590	710	890
65	5′5″	136	62	370	500	620	740	930
66	5′6″	142	65	390	520	650	780	980
67	5′7″	148	67	400	540	670	800	1010
68	5′8″	154	70	420	560	700	840	1050
69	5′9″	160	73	440	580	730	880	1100
70	5′10″	166	75	450	600	750	900	1130
71	5′11″	172	78	470	620	780	940	1170
72	6′0″	178	81	490	650	810	970	1220
73	6′1″	184	84	500	670	840	1010	1260
74	6′2″	190	86	520	690	860	1030	1290
75	6′3″	196	89	530	700	890	1070	1340
76	6′4″	202	92	550	740	920	1100	1380
77	6′5″	208	95	570	760	950	1140	1430

Women

Height (in)	Height (ft)	Weight (lb)	Weight (kg)	6 mL/kg	8 mL/kg	10 mL/kg	12 mL/kg	15 mL/kg
55	4′7″	80	36	220	290	360	430	540
56	4′8″	85	39	230	310	390	470	590
57	4′9″	90	41	250	330	410	500	620
58	4′10″	95	43	260	340	430	520	650
59	4′11″	100	45	270	360	450	540	680
60	5′0″	105	48	290	380	480	580	720
61	5′1″	110	50	300	400	500	600	750
62	5′2″	115	52	310	416	520	620	780
63	5′3″	120	55	330	440	550	660	830
64	5′4″	125	57	340	460	570	680	860
65	5′5″	130	59	350	470	590	710	890
66	5′6″	135	61	370	490	610	730	920
67	5′7″	140	64	380	510	640	770	960
68	5′8″	145	66	400	530	660	790	990
69	5′9″	150	68	410	540	680	820	1020
70	5′10″	155	70	420	560	700	840	1050
71	5′11″	160	73	440	580	730	876	1095
72	6′0″	165	75	450	600	750	900	1125

* Ideal body weight (lb): Men, 106 + [6(H – 60)]; women, 105 + [5(H – 60)], where H is height in inches.

Tidal volume (V_T) and rate (f) determine minute ventilation ($\dot{V}_E$). As a rule, for adult patients the resultant minute ventilation should be approximately 80 to 100 mL/kg IBW per minute.[14] Thus a 70-kg adult (IBW) would have a minute ventilation of approximately 7000 mL/min. Volume ventilation might be initiated in the assist-control or SIMV mode with a rate of 10 to 12 breaths/min and a tidal volume of 700 mL (10 mL/kg) resulting in a minute ventilation of approximately 7 L/min. Patients with elevated carbon dioxide production ($\dot{V}CO_2$) or physiologic dead space (V_{Dphys}) may need a larger minute ventilation to maintain acceptable $PaCO_2$.

During patient- or time-triggered (assist-control) VC-CMV, every breath is a volume breath, and the total minute ventilation is simply rate multiplied by tidal volume:

$$\dot{V}_E = f \times V_T$$

In IMV and SIMV modes, the total minute ventilation is made up of spontaneous tidal volume (V_{Tsp}), spontaneous rate (f_{sp}), machine tidal volume (V_{Tmach}), and machine rate (f_{mach}). For SIMV mode, total minute ventilation ($\dot{V}_{ETOT}$) is described as follows:

$$\dot{V}_{ETOT} = \dot{V}_E \text{ machine} + \dot{V}_E \text{ spontaneous}$$

and

$$\dot{V}_{ETOT} = (V_{Tmach} \times f_{mach}) + (V_{Tsp(average)} \times f_{sp})$$

For pressure-control continuous mandatory ventilation (PC-CMV), the delivered tidal volume depends on the pressure limit, inspiratory time, and the patient's lung mechanics. In general, the pressure limit is increased or decreased to achieve a target V_T while a plateau pressure of 30 cm H_2O or less is maintained. A good initial pressure setting is to start at 15 cm H_2O (above baseline pressure) and observe the resulting tidal volume. Pressure is then increased or decreased to achieve the desired volume. As with VC-CMV, with PC-CMV minute ventilation is simply rate multiplied by tidal volume ($\dot{V}_E = f \times V_T$). Recommended initial tidal volume and frequency for various patient types are described in Table 41-7.

> **RULE OF THUMB**
>
> When starting ventilatory support for most adult patients, use an initial tidal volume of 10 mL/kg (IBW) and a respiratory rate of 12 breaths/min.

Patients with ALI or ARDS may need lower tidal volume and a higher rate to maintain effective alveolar ventilation while plateau pressure is maintained at 30 cm H_2O or less. Results of a multicenter study suggested a tidal volume of 6 mL/kg for patients with ARDS.[15] In that study, patients receiving a tidal volume of 6 mL/kg had a lower mortality and morbidity than did patients receiving a volume of 12 mL/kg.[15] Thus in the care of ALI/ARDS patients, one may begin with a lower tidal volume (8 mL/kg) and decrease the volume as needed to maintain plateau pressure of 30 cm H_2O or less.[15,38] In ALI/ARDS patients, machine rates of 15 to 30 breaths/min may be needed to maintain an adequate minute ventilation. Box 41-8 summarizes the ARDSNet guidelines for initial ventilator setup.[15,16]

Trigger Sensitivity

Trigger sensitivity for patient-triggered ventilation should be set at the lowest possible level to minimize trigger work while avoiding ventilator autocycling. With pressure

Table 41-7 ▶▶ Suggested Initial Tidal Volume and Frequency for Mechanical Ventilation Based on Disease State or Condition

Patient Type	Tidal Volume (mL/kg)	Frequency (breaths/min)
Adults		
Normal lungs	10-12	10-12
Neuromuscular disease, postoperative period, or with normal pulmonary mechanics in which maintaining lung volume is a concern	12-15	6-10
Acute restrictive disease, ALI, ARDS	6-8*	12-20
Obstructive lung disease (COPD, asthma exacerbation)	8-10	10-12†
Children		
Age 8-16 y	8-10	20-30
Age 0-8 y	6-8	25-35

*For ALI/ARDS, maintain plateau pressure at 30 cm H_2O or less. Volume begins at 8 mL/kg and is gradually reduced to 6 mL/kg. Volume as low as 4 mL/kg may be required in the care of these patients to avoid ventilator-induced lung injury.

†For patients with obstructive disease, ensure a short inspiratory time and long expiratory time to avoid air-trapping and minimize auto-PEEP. Lower tidal volume and rate may be necessary in acute asthma to avoid further lung overinflation. Some clinicians have recommended a lower initial rate (6-8 breaths/min) for COPD patients.[7]

Box 41-8 • NIH NHLBI ARDS Clinical Network Initial Ventilator Setup and Management of Oxygenation, Plateau Pressure, and pH

1. Calculate predicted body weight as follows:
   - Male patients: Weight in kilograms = 50 + 2.3 (Height in inches – 60)
   - Female patients: Weight in kilograms = 45.5 + 2.3 (Height in inches – 60)
2. Select assist-control mode.
3. Set V_T to 8 mL/kg of predicted body weight.
4. Reduce V_T by 1 mL/kg at intervals of 2 hours or less until V_T is 6 mL/kg.
5. Set initial rate to achieve baseline minute ventilation ($\dot{V}_E$). Do not exceed 35 breaths/min.
6. Adjust V_T and rate to achieve a pH of 7.30 to 7.45 while maintaining a P_{plat} of 30 cm H_2O or less.
7. Set inspiratory flow rate above patient demand (may exceed 80 L/min).
8. For oxygenation to achieve Pa_{O_2} of 55 to 80 mm Hg or Sp_{O_2} 88% to 95%, use incremental F_{IO_2} and PEEP in the following combinations:

F_{IO_2}	0.3	0.4	0.4	0.5	0.5	0.6	0.7	0.7	0.7	0.8	0.9	0.9	0.9	1.0	1.0	1.0
PEEP	5	5	8	8	10	10	10	12	14	14	14	16	18	20	22	24

9. Check P_{plat}, Sp_{O_2}, respiratory rate, V_T, and pH (if available) at least every 4 hours and after each change in PEEP or V_T:
   - If P_{plat} is greater than 30 cm H_2O, decrease V_T by 1-mL/kg steps (minimum, 4 mL/kg).
   - If P_{plat} is less than 25 cm H_2O and V_T is less than 6 mL/kg, increase V_T by 1 mL/kg steps until P_{plat} is greater than 25 cm H_2O or V_T is 6 mL/kg.
   - If P_{plat} is less than 20 and breath stacking occurs, V_T may be increased in 1-mL/kg increments (maximum, 8 mL/kg).
10. The pH goal is 7.30 to 7.45.
    For acidosis management (pH <7.30):
    - If pH is 7.15 to 7.30, increase the rate until pH is greater than 7.30 or Pa_{CO_2} is less than 25 (maximum rate, 35). If rate is 35 and Pa_{CO_2} is less than 25, $NaHCO_3$ may be given.
    - If pH is less than 7.15, increase rate to 35. If pH remains less than 7.15 and $NaHCO_3$ is considered or infused, V_T may be increased in 1-mL/kg steps until pH is greater than 7.15 (P_{plat} target may be exceeded).

    For alkalosis management (pH >7.45), decrease ventilator rate, if possible.

Adapted from National Institutes of Health (NIH) National Heart Lung and Blood Institute (NHLBI) ARDS Clinical Network Mechanical Ventilation Protocol Summary.

triggering, the range is generally –0.5 to –1.5 cm H_2O; however, some ventilators autocycle in this range, and the sensitivity must be adjusted to as much as –2 cm H_2O on these machines. The increased use of ventilator graphics packages has led to the recognition that patients' inspiratory efforts often are insufficient to trigger the ventilator.[12] Factors that can prolong ventilator response time include low trigger sensitivity, auto-PEEP, high bias flow in the circuit, abdominal paradox, and mechanical factors (Box 41-9).

Box 41-9 • Factors That Can Prolong Ventilator Response Time

- Low trigger sensitivity
- Abdomen–rib cage paradox
- Auto-PEEP (dynamic hyperinflation)
- High tubing compliance
- High circuit dead space
- Transducer variability
- High bias flow in the circuit
- Unresponsive demand valves

Modified from Tobin MJ: Respir Care 36:395,1991, and Gurevitch MJ, Gelmont D: Crit Care Med 17:354, 1989.

Many ventilators offer the option of a pressure or a flow trigger. In general, flow triggering offers slightly lower trigger work than does pressure triggering,[39-41] although the gain in terms of the patient's total work of breathing may be slight. Newer ventilators with fast pressure-triggering capabilities can be as sensitive as flow-triggering devices.[42] Flow triggering may not be effective in reducing work of breathing because of the presence of a small endotracheal tube or auto-PEEP.[41] Flow-trigger settings vary by ventilator. For example, the flow-trigger and flow-by recommendations for adult patients with the Bennett 7200 are a base flow of 5 to 6 L/min with a flow sensitivity of 3. In general, for flow-triggering the trigger flow should be set 1 to 3 L/min below baseline or bias flow. Initial flow-trigger recommendations for several critical care ventilators are listed in Box 41-10.

Inspiratory Flow, Time, and I:E Ratio for Volume Ventilation

Most modern critical care ventilators allow the clinician to select peak flow, tidal volume, and rate or inspiratory time (or percentage inspiratory time), tidal volume, and rate. For most adults an initial inspiratory time of approximately 1 second (0.8-1.2 seconds) with a resultant I:E ratio of 1:2 or better is a good starting point. This value corresponds to an initial peak flow setting of approximately 60 L/min with a range of 40 to 80 L/min and a down ramp or square flow waveform.[7,9,10] Higher flow (up to 100 L/min) may improve gas exchange in COPD patients, probably because of the resulting increase in expiratory time.[10] Inspiratory flow rate should be adjusted to ensure that the flow provided meets

Box 41-10 • Flow Trigger Recommendations for Specific Mechanical Ventilators

BENNETT 7200
- Base flow: 5 to 6 L/min (range, 5-20 L/min)
- Flow sensitivity:
  - >50 kg: 3 L/min
  - 25 to 50 kg: 2 L/min
  - <25 kg: 1 L/min

BENNETT 840
Flow sensitivity (range, 0.5-20 L/min):
- >24 kg IBW: 3 L/min
- ≤24 kg IBW: 2 L/min

SERVO 300/300A
- Trigger sensitivity: 2 to 32 mL/s set in "green range" on the knob scale
- Preset trigger bias flow:
  - Neonate, 8 mL/s (0.5 L/min)
  - Pediatric, 16 mL/s (1 L/min)
  - Adult, 32 mL/s (2 L/min)

HAMILTON GALILEO
- Automatic base flow: 4 to 30 L/min
- Flow trigger: 2 to 15 L/min set to minimize trigger work without autocycle

DRAGER EVITA-4
- Trigger sensitivity (adults): 0.3 to 15 L/min set to minimize trigger work without autocycle

BEAR 1000
- Base flow: 2 to 20 L/min
- Flow trigger: 1 to 10 L/min set to minimize trigger work without autocycle

Box 41-11 • Calculation of Inspiratory Flow Rate From Percentage Inspiratory Time for the Servo 900C Ventilator

The effect of percentage inspiratory time on inspiratory flow rate can be estimated as follows:

$$\text{Inspiratory flow rate} = \frac{\text{Set minute ventilation}}{\text{Percentage inspiratory time} \times 0.01}$$

For example, a patient being treated with a Siemens Servo 900C ventilator may have the following ventilator settings:
- Set minute ventilation = 16 L/min
- Set CMV rate = 20 breaths/min
- Resulting V_T = 16 L/20 breaths/min = 0.8 L or 800 mL
- Set time inspiratory percentage = 25
- Set pause time percentage = 0
- Set SIMV rate = 10 breaths/min

$$\text{Inspiratory flow rate} = \frac{16\text{ L/min}}{25\% \times 0.01} = \frac{16\text{ L/min}}{0.25} = 64\text{ L/min}$$

or exceeds the patient's spontaneous inspiratory flow.[10] This rate can be achieved by observing the resultant pressure-time curve contour on a graphics monitor. Ideally, the curve should show a smooth increase and convex appearance during inspiration.[10,43] A large negative deflection indicates inadequate trigger sensitivity, and excessive scalloping of the wave form indicates inadequate ventilatory flow settings (Figure 41-5).[10] A less sensitive trigger level and lower ventilator inspiratory flow tend to increase the patient's work of breathing. Common ventilator configurations and related controls that determine inspiratory flow, time, and I:E ratio are described in Figure 41-6.

For ventilators with tidal volume, peak flow, and rate controls (including the Bennett MA-1, MA-2, 7200, 740, 760, and 840 and Bear 1, 2, 3, 5, and 1000), inspiratory time is determined by the tidal volume, peak flow, and flow pattern. To decrease inspiratory time, one may increase the peak flow, decrease the tidal volume, or change from a down ramp or sine wave to a square wave flow pattern. Expiratory time and I:E ratio are determined by inspiratory time and rate. To increase expiratory time (and decrease I:E ratio), one may decrease the inspiratory time as described earlier or increase the expiratory time by decreasing the rate.

For ventilators with tidal volume (or minute ventilation), inspiratory time (or percentage inspiratory time), and rate controls (including the Servo 900C, 300, and 300A, Hamilton Veolar and Galileo, and Drager Evita-4), the inspiratory time and tidal volume determine the inspiratory flow rate. On these ventilators, one can directly increase or decrease the inspiratory time. As inspiratory time (or percentage inspiratory time) decreases, inspiratory flow rate increases. Box 41-11 demonstrates the calculation of inspiratory flow rate based on percentage inspiratory time settings.

To increase expiratory time (and decrease I:E ratio), one may decrease inspiratory time or increase expiratory time by decreasing rate. Changing the inspiratory flow waveform on these ventilators (Hamilton Veolar and Galileo) has no effect on inspiratory time, expiratory time, or I:E ratio; however, flow waveform changes affect peak and mean airway pressure.

Flow Waveform

Flow waveform options on mechanical ventilators vary from a preset square wave (Servo 300) to as many as seven adjustable waveforms on older models of the Hamilton Veolar. Common choices available for waveform include the square, down ramp (decreasing

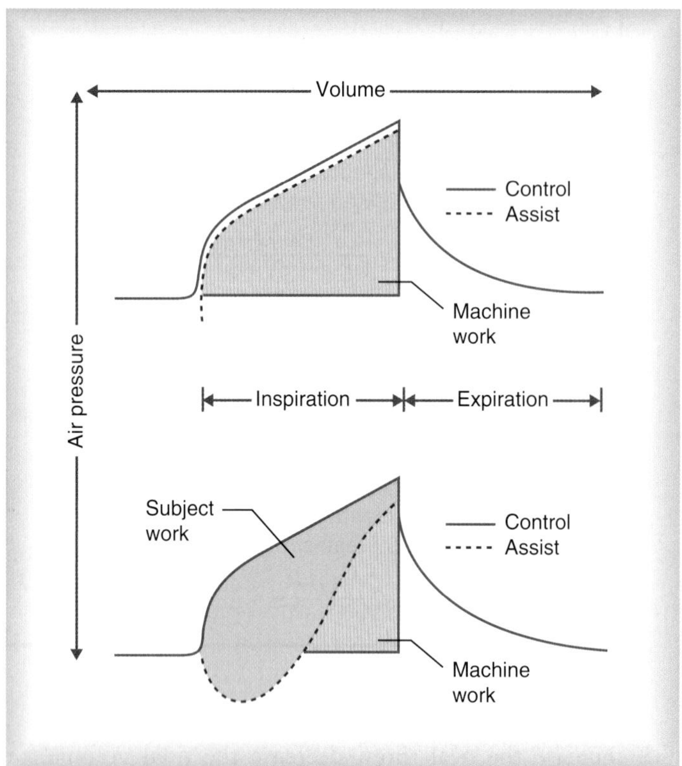

Figure 41-5
Plot of an ideal pressure-time waveform during volume-targeted ventilation (*top*). Plot of actual pressure-time curve (*dotted line*) is superimposed on the ideal curve (*bottom*). The scooped-out actual pressure waveform is evident. The green area reflects the work performed by the patient during assisted volume-targeted ventilation. This type of actual pressure waveform is indicative of inadequate peak inspiratory flow or too lengthy an inspiratory time. The peak flow should be increased, normally to between 60 and 90 L/min to minimize patient effort during volume-limited ventilation. *(Modified from Marini JJ, Rodriguez M, Lamb V: Am Rev Respir Dis 134:902, 1986.)*

or "decelerating" waveform), and sine wave. Pressure-support and pressure-control modes also deliver decreasing flow waveforms. The literature on clinical application of specific waveforms is mixed.[44] However, it seems to be clear that as one moves from an increasing ("accelerating") flow waveform to a square wave to a decreasing flow waveform while holding inspiratory time constant, there tends to be a predictable decrease in peak airway pressure and a corresponding increase in mean airway pressure.[44] Increases in mean airway pressure may improve oxygenation while further impeding venous return to the heart.[44] Thus at least as far as inspiratory flow patterns are concerned, what is good for the lungs may be bad for the heart. We suggest a decreasing, or down ramp, flow waveform when the goal is optimization of the distribution of inspired air and improvement in oxygenation. A square or even accelerating waveform may be useful in reducing mean airway pressure in patients with severe hypotension or cardiovascular instability. Figure 41-7 compares the effect of ventilator flow waveforms on peak and mean airway pressure. Box 41-12 describes guidelines for selecting flow waveform during volume ventilation.

During pressure ventilation (PCV, PSV), a decreasing flow waveform is delivered. The initial peak flow typically is rapidly reached. Flow then decreases throughout inspiration until the breath is terminated. With PSV, inspiration ends when the flow decreases to a preset value, typically 25% of the peak flow, or 5 L/min. With PCV, flow continues to decrease until the inspiratory time has elapsed. With PCV and an adequate inspiratory time, flow reaches zero at end inspiration, and an inspiratory pause (no flow) follows. In the PCV mode, increasing inspiratory time tends to increase tidal volume until zero flow is reached at end inspiration. Further increases in inspiratory time do not increase tidal volume, although distribution of inspired air may improve, and mean airway pressure does increase.

Inspiratory Pause

In addition to inspiratory time or flow, most ventilators have an option for setting an inspiratory pause or hold in the volume-control mode. A brief inspiratory pause (up to 10%) has been recommended in the past for improving the distribution of the inspired air and arterial PaO_2.[45,46] The use of a longer inspiratory pause (up to 30 seconds) has been advocated in the management of ALI/ARDS as a lung recruitment maneuver, and the results have been mixed.[47,48] Use of an inspiratory pause has been suggested for administration of bronchodilators to improve medication delivery. In the treatment of COPD patients, however, a 5-second inspiratory pause did not result in significant improvement in measures related to the effectiveness of the bronchodilator.[49] If a brief inspiratory pause is used, I:E ratio and mean airway pressure increase. An extended inspiratory pause is used for measurement of plateau pressure (P_{plat}) and in estimation of airway resistance

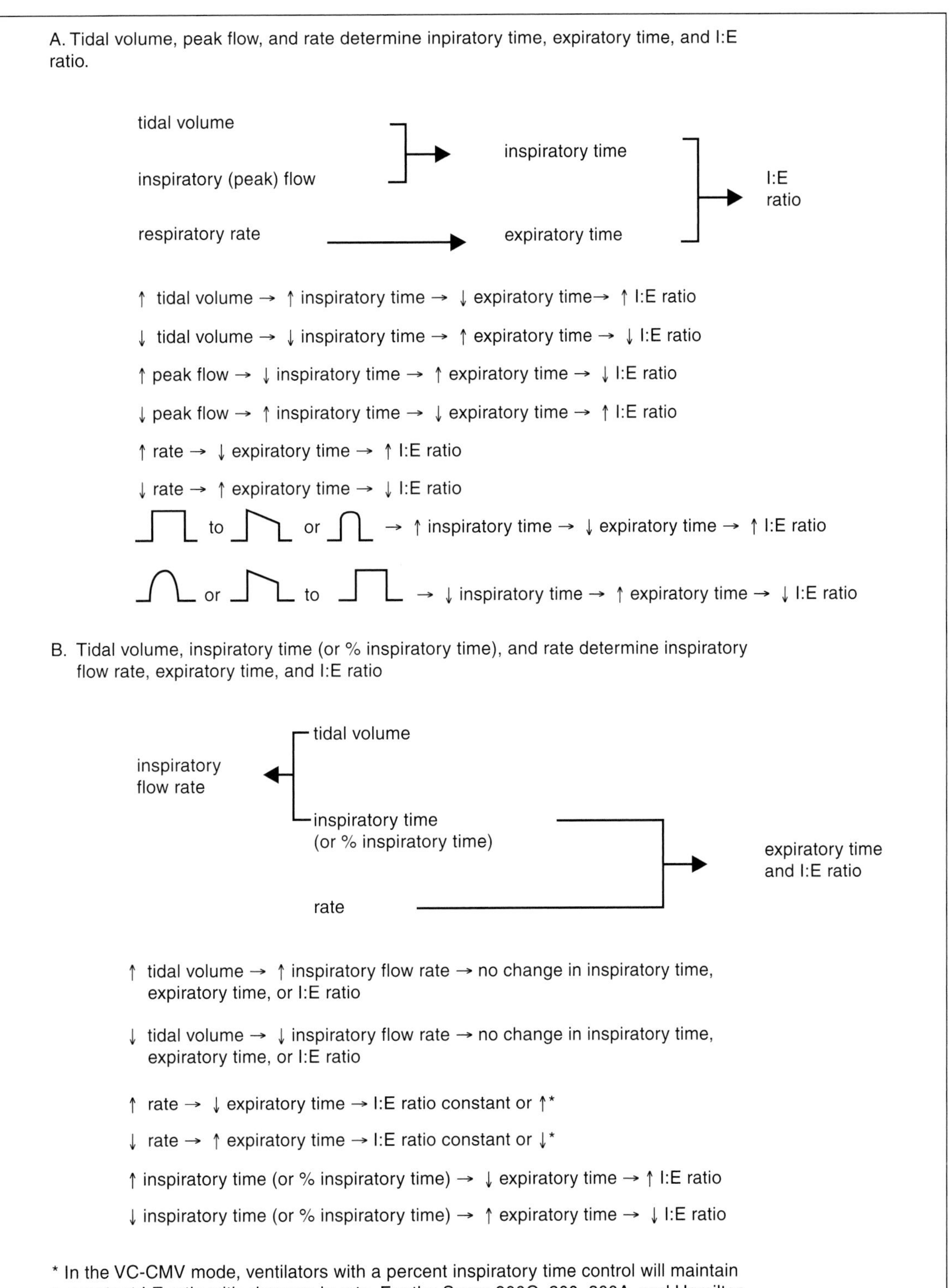

Figure 41-6 · Relation Between Tidal Volume, Inspiratory Flow, Inspiratory Time, Expiratory Time, and I:E Ratio in Various Ventilator Systems

A, Effects of tidal volume, flow, and respiratory rate on inspiratory time, expiratory time, and I:E ratio. Ventilators providing a tidal volume, inspiratory flow, and rate control in the VC-CMV and VC-IMV modes include the Bennett MA-1, MA-2, 7200, 740, and 840 and the Bear 1, 2, 3, 5, and 1000. **B,** Effects of volume, inspiratory time, and rate on inspiratory flow, expiratory time, and I:E ratio. Ventilators that provide controls for inspiratory time (or percentage inspiratory time), tidal volume (or minute ventilation), and rate in the VC-CMV and VC-IMV modes include the Servo 900C, 300, and 300A, the Hamilton Veolar and Galileo, and the Drager Evita-4. In the volume-control mode (controlled ventilation), ventilators with a percentage inspiratory time control (Servo, Hamilton, and Drager) maintain a constant I:E ratio with changes in respiratory rate. In the SIMV mode, changes in SIMV rate alter I:E ratio on these machines.

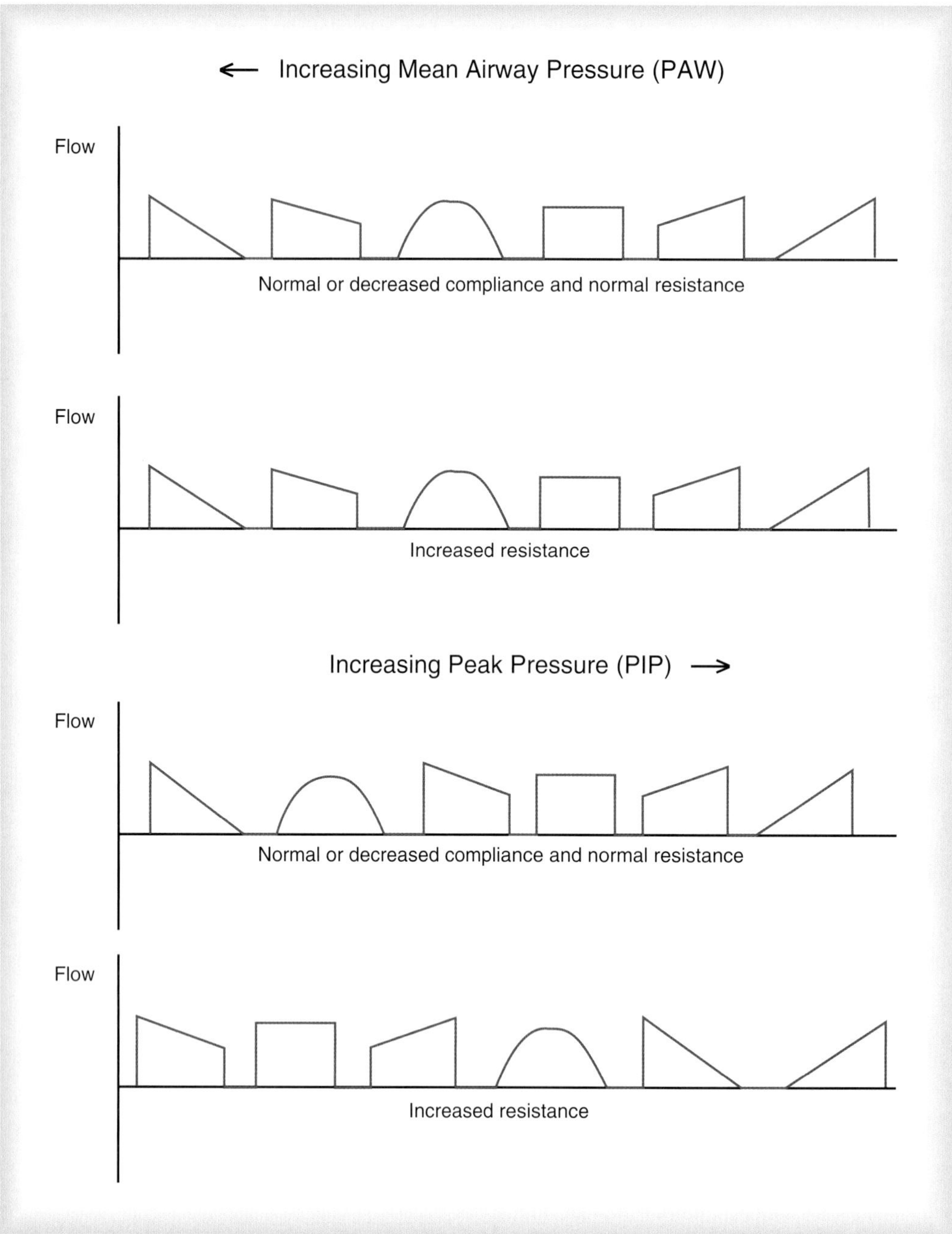

Figure 41-7
The effect of ventilator flow waveform on peak and mean airway pressure with changing lung mechanics. In general, flow waveforms that tend to increase mean airway pressure also decrease peak pressure (PIP) and vice versa. Consequently, if increasing mean airway pressure is the goal, decelerating (down ramp) flow waveforms may be helpful. However, in the care of patients with cardiovascular compromise in which reducing mean airway pressure may be helpful, a square wave or accelerating flow (up ramp) may be of value. Accelerating flow waveforms are no longer available on newer critical care ventilators. *(Modified from Rau JL, Shelledy DC: Respir Care 36:347, 1991.)*

(Raw) where

$$\text{Raw} = \frac{\text{PIP} - P_{plat}}{\text{Inspiratory flow (L/s)}}$$

For this calculation, an inspiratory pause of approximately 1 second is used and is removed as soon as the measurement is satisfactorily completed. An inspiratory pause can be used to ensure a full inspiration before a chest radiograph is obtained, and this step may improve the quality of the resulting radiograph.[50] With the possible exception of ALI/ARDS patients, use of an extended inspiratory pause should be limited because of the resultant increase in mean airway pressure and risk of impeding venous return and cardiac output, especially in patients who are hypovolemic or hypotensive or whose condition is hemodynamically unstable.

Box 41-12 • Guidelines for Selecting Inspiratory Flow Waveform During Volume Ventilation (VC-CMV and VC-IMV)

CONSTANT FLOW WAVEFORM

- Alternative terms: Square wave, rectangular wave, constant flow generator
- Advantages: High flow provided with a reduced inspiratory time and improved I:E ratio. May decrease mean airway pressure, which may be helpful in terms of venous return and cardiac output in compromised patients.
- Disadvantages: Increased PIP may lead to excessive pressure. Lower mean airway pressure may affect oxygenation.

DECREASING FLOW WAVEFORM

- Alternative terms: Down ramp, decelerating flow, descending ramp
- Advantages: Lower PIP and higher mean airway pressure. This flow waveform may improve gas distribution, oxygenation, and patient-ventilator synchrony.
- Disadvantages: Increased mean airway pressure may impede venous return and cardiac output in compromised patients. In ventilators that have a peak flow control, the down ramp increases inspiratory time and I:E ratio and decrease expiratory time.

SINE WAVE

- Alternative terms: Sine wave–like, modified sine wave, one-half sine wave
- Advantages: Flow waveform is similar to that during spontaneous breathing; thus some experts have claimed that the sine wave is more "physiologic," although there is no evidence that this feature is clinically important.
- Disadvantages: Initial flow is slow and could be less than patient spontaneous demand. In ventilators with peak flow controls, the sine wave increases inspiratory time and I:E ratio and reduces expiratory time. The sine wave also tends to result in higher peak and lower mean airway pressures than a does a down ramp when inspiratory time is held constant.

INCREASING FLOW WAVEFORM

- Alternative terms: Accelerating flow pattern, increasing flow, up ramp, and modified sine wave. Increasing flow waveforms that have been available in the past include the modified sine (one-fourth sine wave) and the up ramp. Newer critical care ventilators do not have the selectable increasing flow waveform as an option.
- Advantages: Increasing flow waveforms tend to result in lower mean airway pressure than do other waveforms. This feature may be of value in the care of patients with cardiovascular compromise for minimizing the decrease in venous return associated with mechanical ventilatory support.
- Disadvantages: Initial flow may not meet the patient's inspiratory demand. Decreased mean airway pressure may affect oxygenation. Higher peak pressure may be excessive. Distribution of inspired air may be less effective than with a decreasing flow waveform.

Oxygen Percentage

The F_{IO_2} setting at the beginning of mechanical ventilation varies with the patient's condition. If little is known about the patient or if the patient's condition appears to be grave, 100% oxygen is the preferred starting point. Examples of disease states or conditions that typically warrant an initial F_{IO_2} of 1.0 include acute pulmonary edema, ARDS, near drowning, cardiac arrest, severe trauma, suspected aspiration, severe pneumonia, carbon monoxide poisoning, and any disease state or condition resulting in a large right to left shunt. After initiation of mechanical ventilation with an F_{IO_2} of 1.0, the F_{IO_2} should be reduced to 0.40 to 0.50 or less as soon as is practical to avoid oxygen toxicity and absorption atelectasis.

Patients who have undergone previous blood gas measurement or oximetry who are doing well clinically and patients with disease states or conditions that normally respond to low to moderate concentrations of oxygen may begin ventilation with 40% to 50% oxygen. These typically are patients with normal $\dot{V}/\dot{Q}$ or a $\dot{V}/\dot{Q}$ imbalance without shunt ($\dot{V}/\dot{Q} < 1$ but > 0). Patients who often do well with low to moderate concentrations of oxygen include those with acute exacerbation of COPD, asthma, emphysema, chronic bronchitis, drug overdose without aspiration, or neuromuscular disease and postoperative patients with normal lungs. For example, a patient with an acute exacerbation of COPD who needs mechanical ventilatory support may have had an arterial Pa_{O_2} of 50 mm Hg with a nasal cannula at 4 L/min before intubation and mechanical ventilation. This patient will probably do well with an F_{IO_2} of 0.40 to 0.50 or less once adequate ventilation is restored. The patient can begin to receive 40% to 50% oxygen and be immediately assessed with oximetry for assurance of an adequate oxygen saturation by pulse oximeter (Sp_{O_2}). The F_{IO_2} can then be adjusted according to the patient's response.

In summary, if previous blood gas values or results of oximetry indicate the patient is likely to respond well to low to moderate concentrations of oxygen, or if the patient has a disease state or condition that typically does not require a high concentration of oxygen, the patient may begin therapy with 40% to 50% oxygen. In these cases, the patient should be immediately assessed by means of oximetry and clinical observation for adequate oxygenation, and the FIO_2 should be adjusted accordingly. If there is any doubt about the patient's condition, or if the patient is doing poorly, 100% oxygen should be the starting point. It is best to err on the high side regarding the patient's oxygenation needs and titrate the FIO_2 down on the basis of findings at oximetry, blood gas measurement, and clinical assessment.

Positive End-Expiratory Pressure and Continuous Positive Airway Pressure

Positive end-expiratory pressure and CPAP are effective techniques for improving and maintaining lung volume and improving oxygenation for patients with acute restrictive disease such as ALI, pneumonia, pulmonary edema, and ARDS. Positive end-expiratory pressure and CPAP should probably not be routinely used in the treatment of patients with an already elevated FRC, such as those with COPD or acute asthma, except in small amounts that may be helpful to overcome auto-PEEP and air trapping. In general, the indications for PEEP or CPAP in the critical care setting are an inadequate arterial oxygen level with moderate to high concentrations of oxygen. A PaO_2 less than 50 to 60 mm Hg with an FIO_2 greater than 0.40 to 0.50 is a good general starting place for considering use of PEEP or CPAP.

In terms of ventilator initiation, initial PEEP/CPAP levels usually are between 0 and 8 cm H_2O. Some experts have advocated the use of 3 to 5 cm H_2O of "physiologic" PEEP for all patients who have an artificial airway in place. Intubation may result in small reductions in FRC,[7] which can be balanced with the application of PEEP or CPAP. Whether the application of physiologic PEEP has important benefits in terms of patient outcome is not known.

Positive end-expiratory pressure has been advocated in small increments (2-3 cm H_2O) for overcoming auto-PEEP, particularly in the care of patients with obstructive lung disease.[18] These patients may be unable to exhale completely before the next machine breath begins. The resultant air trapping may cause problems for patient triggering of the machine and contribute to lung overinflation.[18] We suggest that use of PEEP for overcoming auto-PEEP be reserved for patients in whom auto-PEEP can be demonstrated, preferably by the application of a brief expiratory pause and observation of the resultant pressure increase. The amount of PEEP applied should be approximately one-half the measured auto-PEEP (adjusted for the baseline PEEP level). Auto-PEEP ideally should be rechecked to assure intrinsic PEEP decreases rather than increases. Box 41-13 summarizes methods for minimizing the effects of auto-PEEP.

Box 41-13 • Techniques for Minimizing the Effects of Auto-PEEP

- Decrease airflow obstruction
  - Secretion management
  - Aggressive bronchodilation
- Use larger endotracheal tube
- Modify ventilatory pattern
  - Decrease inspiratory time
    - Increase inspiratory flow (on ventilators with inspiratory peak flow control)
    - Use square flow waveform (not down ramp, sine wave)
    - Decrease percentage inspiratory time (on ventilators with $\%T_i$ control)
    - Decrease tidal volume
  - Increase expiratory time
    - Decrease inspiratory time while maintaining rate (see above)
    - Decrease rate
- Use low-compressed volume circuit
- Use low-rate SIMV (not assist-control)
- Consider permissive hypercapnia (decrease V_T, allow $PaCO_2$ to increase)
- Apply PEEP or CPAP to balance auto-PEEP

Modified from Tobin MJ: Respir Care 36:395, 1991.

Last, in the care of patients with ALI or ARDS, it is probably wise to initiate mechanical ventilation with PEEP levels of 5 to 8 cm H_2O.[6] An open lung ventilation strategy in early-stage ARDS may improve outcome.[51] Such a strategy may incorporate pressure-limited ventilation with a tidal volume of 6 mL/kg or less and a PEEP level set at 2 cm H_2O above the lower inflection point on a static pressure-volume curve or adjusted according to the FIO_2.[51] Overall, approximately 30% of patients with ALI do not benefit from PEEP, and those with pulmonary (versus nonpulmonary) causes of ALI/ARDS, such as pneumonia, are less likely to benefit.[12] Nonpulmonary causes of ALI/ARDS that may be more likely to be relieved with PEEP include extrathoracic trauma and intra-abdominal sepsis.[12] Contraindications to PEEP include hypotension, elevated ICP, and uncontrolled pneumothorax.

Pressure Support

Pressure support to overcome WOB_I should be included for most spontaneously breathing patients in the SIMV mode. Pressure-support ventilation to overcome WOB_I can be calculated and usually is in the range of 5 to 10 cm H_2O.

Pressure Rise Time or Slope

Many newer critical care ventilators include an inspiratory pressure rise time or pressure slope. This control

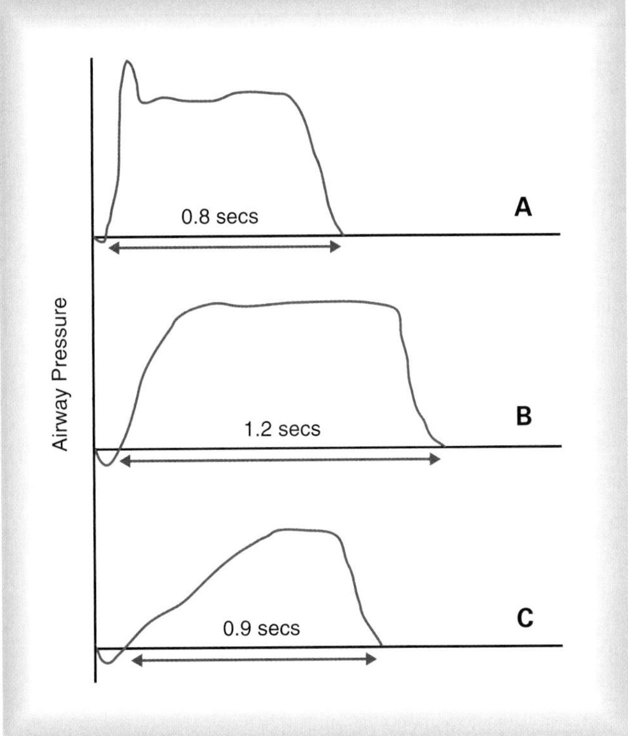

Figure 41-8

Effect of changing inspiratory rise time during pressure-limited breaths for a patient who prefers a moderate flow. **A,** Flow exceeds patient demand, and a pressure spike and short inspiratory time result. **B,** As flow is decreased, inspiratory time lengthens, and the pressure spike disappears. Machine output matches patient demand. **C,** When flow is further reduced, patient demand exceeds machine flow; the result is deformation of the pressure waveform and a decrease in inspiratory time. *(Modified from Branson RD et al:* Respir Care 35:1056, 1990.)

may function only with pressure-limited breaths (PSV, PCV) or may be available in all modes. The purpose of this control is to slow the rate at which the inspiratory pressure limit is reached for PCV and PSV breaths. In general, rise time should be set at a value that assures adequate inspiratory gas flow (meeting or exceeding patient demand) without an excessive "overshoot" of the pressure at the beginning of inspiration. An excessively slow rise time may increase the patient's work of breathing.[43,52] The effect of changing inspiratory rise time is described in Figure 41-8.

Limits and Alarms

Ventilator alarms and limits warn of ventilator malfunction and changes in patient status. Ventilator malfunction alarms include power or gas supply loss and electronic or pneumatic malfunction. These alarms usually are preset by the manufacturer.

Patient status alarms usually are set by the respiratory therapist. These include maximum inspiratory pressure limit, low pressure and low PEEP alarms, high- and low-volume alarms, oxygen and humidification alarms, and apnea alarms. After initiation of ventilation, alarms and limits are readjusted as needed. Alarms usually are set so that they warn the clinician of important changes or problems without becoming a nuisance by falsely signaling problems that are not real.

Pressure Limits

In the volume-limited mode, a backup pressure limit should be set. In general, before the patient is connected to the ventilator, the limit should be set at 50 cm H_2O to avoid overpressuring the system when the patient is connected. After the patient is connected to the ventilator, the peak and plateau pressures should be assessed. If the plateau pressure is greater than 30 cm H_2O, consideration should be given to decreasing the set tidal volume. If the plateau pressure is 30 cm H_2O or less, the high pressure limit can be adjusted to 10 to 20 cm H_2O above the peak inspiratory pressure (PIP). One can decrease peak pressure by decreasing the peak flow rate, increasing the inspiratory time, changing the inspiratory flow waveform from a square to a down ramp, or decreasing the delivered tidal volume. For spontaneously breathing patients, inspiratory flow and time must remain such that the patient's inspiratory demand is met or exceeded to ensure one does not further increase the patient's work of breathing.

Alarms and Apnea Values

Alarms, which may be preset or adjustable, common to many ventilators include pressure (high-low), volume (tidal volume, minute ventilation), apnea, oxygen percentage, and temperature. Suggested initial settings for these alarms and backup ventilator settings are described in Table 41-8.

Humidification

Humidification is required during mechanical ventilation when an artificial airway is present. A heated humidifier or a heat and moisture exchanger (HME) should provide a minimum of 30 mg/L of water with a temperature of 30° C or higher.[53] Use of HMEs should be avoided in the care of patients with secretion problems and those with low body temperature (<32° C), high spontaneous minute ventilation (>10 L/min), or air leaks in which exhaled tidal volume is less than 70% of delivered tidal volume.[53] Heated humidifiers may be used to deliver up to 100% body humidity at 37° C. Current clinical practice guidelines suggest an inspired gas temperature of 33 ± 2° C, although inspiratory gas temperatures of 37° C or lower are acceptable.[53] We prefer an optimal humidity approach and use a heated humidifier to deliver gas in the range of 35° C to 37° C at the airway.

MINI CLINI

Selecting Initial Ventilator Settings

PROBLEM

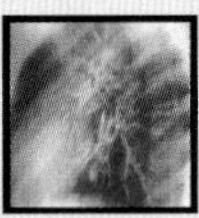

A 52-year-old, 5 ft 10 in (178 cm), 200-lb (91 kg) man is being returned from the operating room after coronary artery bypass surgery. He is being manually (bag-tube) ventilated with supplemental oxygen by the anesthesiologist en route to the ICU. He is apneic at this time. The patient has no history of lung disease and has never smoked cigarettes. Heart rate and blood pressure are stable, and the patient's SpO_2 during manual ventilation is 99%. What initial mode, V_T, rate, and FIO_2 would you select when starting ventilatory support for this patient?

SOLUTION

The patient is apneic at this time but probably will resume spontaneous breathing as the anesthetic wears off and sedation is reduced. Because the patient is expected to resume breathing spontaneously, volume ventilation in either the assist-control (VC-CMV) or SIMV mode (VC-IMV) is appropriate.

An initial tidal volume and rate should be selected to provide full ventilatory support. In general, an initial tidal volume of approximately 10 mL/kg with a rate of 12 breaths/min provides an adequate starting minute ventilation for most adult patients. The formulas for estimating IBW are

$$\text{IBW in kilograms (men)} = [106 + 6(H - 60)]/2.2$$
$$\text{IBW in kilograms (women)} = [105 + 5(H - 60)]/2.2$$

where H is height in inches.

For this patient:

$$\text{IBW} = [106 + 6(70 - 60)]/2.2 = 75.5 \text{ kg}$$

On the basis of an IBW of 75.5 kg, initial V_T can be set at 750 to 900 mL. Initial inspiratory flow should be set at 60 L/min to achieve an inspiratory time of approximately 1 second. Trigger sensitivity (assist-control or SIMV) should be set so that minimal patient effort triggers the ventilator without autocycling.

Initial FIO_2 may be set at 40%, because of the patient history and the presence of normal lung function. If there is doubt, an initial FIO_2 of 1.0 is acceptable, followed by rapid titration of the FIO_2 downward to maintain an SpO_2 of 92% or more.

Initial PEEP may be set at 0 or 2 to 3 cm H_2O (physiologic PEEP). If the SIMV mode is chosen, PSV should be started at 5 cm H_2O and adjusted as needed when the patient resumes spontaneous breathing.

In summary, appropriate initial ventilator settings for this patient are

Mode: SIMV with PSV (VC-IMV) or assist-control (VC-CMV)
V_T: 10 to 12 cc/kg, or 750 to 900 mL
f_{mach}: 10 to 12 breaths/min (Note: A rate of 12 breaths/min with a tidal volume of 750 to 800 mL would be an appropriate starting place for this patient.)
PSV: 5 cm H_2O (SIMV mode only)
FIO_2: 0.40 followed by immediate assessment and SpO_2 observation (1.0 is an acceptable starting point if there is doubt)
Inspiratory flow and time: 60 L/min or approximately 1 second
Flow waveform: square or down ramp (Note: Observe effect of waveform on peak and mean airway pressures and I:E ratio.)
Pressure limit: 50 cm H_2O and adjust to 10 to 20 cm H_2O above the PIP after patient connection
Humidification: Heated humidifier to achieve a temperature of 35°C at the airway

Table 41-8 ▶▶ Alarm and Backup Ventilation Settings for Initial Ventilatory Setup (Adults)

Low Pressure	8 cm H2O or 5-10 cm H2O below PIP
Low PEEP/CPAP	3-5 cm H_2O below PEEP
High pressure limit	50 cm H_2O, which is adjusted to 10-20 cm H_2O above PIP
Low exhaled tidal volume	100 mL or 10%-15% below set V_T
Low exhaled minute ventilation	2-5 L/min or 10%-15% below minimum SIMV or assist-control backup minute ventilation
High minute ventilation	5 L/min or 10%-15% above baseline minute ventilation
Oxygen percentage (FIO_2)	5% above and below set oxygen percentage
Temperature	2° above and below set temperature; high temperature not to exceed 37° C
Apnea delay	20 s
Apnea values	Tidal volume and rate set to achieve full ventilatory support (V_T, 10-12 mL/kg; rate 10-12 breaths/min) with 100% O_2

Periodic Sighs

Constant, monotonous tidal ventilation at a small volume (<7 mL/kg) results in progressive atelectasis.[13,14] Periodic deep breaths or sighs taken every 6 to 10 minutes reverse this trend.[13,14] During the 1960s and 1970s, it was common to ventilate patients with a smaller tidal volume (5-7 mL/kg), and an intermittent sigh function was incorporated into most volume ventilators. Sighs were programmed at $1^1/_2$ to 3 times the set tidal volume at an interval of every 6 to 10 minutes. Sometimes multiple sighs of two or three deep breaths were included at a preset interval of up to 10 times per hour. Because a larger tidal volume (>7 mL/kg) commonly is used for most patients receiving mechanical ventilation, sighs are no longer routinely included. Indications for sigh breaths are listed in Box 41-14.

MINI CLINI

Humidification of the Airways During Mechanical Ventilation

PROBLEM

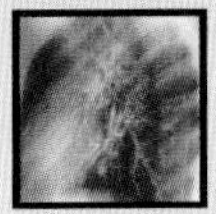

A mechanically ventilated patient is in the medical ICU recovering from acute respiratory failure secondary to aspiration pneumonia. The patient currently needs airway suctioning every 30 to 60 minutes, according to the respiratory therapist and staff nurse caring for the patient. Both caregivers note that the secretions are thick and copious. Current ventilator settings are as follows:

Mode: assist-control volume ventilation (VC-CMV)
V_T: 900 mL
Preset rate: 12 breaths/min
Total rate: 20 breaths/min
F_{IO_2}: 0.50
PIP: 46 cm H_2O
$\dot{V}_E$: 18.1 L/min

The respiratory therapist is asked to place an HME unit with high efficiency bacterial filtration on the ventilator circuit at the wye so that the circuit will not have to be changed as frequently. Is this an appropriate action?

SOLUTION

Humidification can be provided with either a heated humidifier or an HME unit. Although useful in some instances, placement of an HME would be contraindicated in this case for several reasons. Adequate humidification for a patient with an artificial airway is critical in preventing inspissation of airway secretions, injury to and destruction of the airway epithelium, atelectasis, and possible hypothermia.

The patient information in this clinical scenario points to several potential problems with use of an HME, the most obvious one being copious, thick airway secretions. The HME may not provide sufficient water vapor and heat output, and secretions could be retained. The airway secretions could be coughed into the HME, causing increased resistance to flow and possible obstruction. Because the patient has high ventilatory requirements, as evidenced by an elevated exhaled minute ventilation, it is important that the humidification system be able to maintain adequate heat and moisture output when demands dictate.

Other situations in which an HME should not be used are administration of aerosol treatments through the ventilator tubing circuit, high spontaneous minute ventilation (>10 L/min), and body temperature less than 32° C.

To summarize, initial ventilator setup for conventional mechanical ventilation usually includes assist-control ventilation or SIMV with pressure support, according to clinician preference and experience. Synchronized intermittent mandatory ventilation may be preferred for patients with obstructive disease for avoidance of further air trapping, and PCV may be considered for patients with ALI or ARDS. For assist control or SIMV, the initial ventilator rate is typically 10 to 12 breaths/min with a tidal volume of 10 to 12 mL/kg. A larger tidal volume (12-15 mL/kg) and lower rate (6-10 breaths/min) may be considered for the SIMV mode in the care of patients with normal lungs or neuromuscular disease for maintenance of lung volume. A smaller initial tidal volume should be the goal in the management of ALI/ARDS. Therapy begins at 8 mL/kg and is gradually adjusted to 6 mL/kg while the respiratory rate is titrated for maintenance of a pH of 7.30 to 7.45, if possible. For all patients, plateau pressure should be maintained at 30 cm H_2O or less, if possible.

For initial oxygen concentration, in cases in which little is known about the patient or the patient is not doing well, 100% oxygen is a good starting point. In cases in which previous blood gas values or results of oximetry indicate moderate concentrations of oxygen will suffice or in which the patient's condition typically responds to a low to moderate concentration of oxygen, 40% to 50% oxygen is a reasonable beginning point. However, if there is doubt, it is better to err on the high side in terms of initial oxygen concentration and then titrate the F_{IO_2} downward. The goal is to maintain an Sa_{O_2} of 90% or more and Sp_{O_2} of 92% or more on an F_{IO_2} of 0.40 to 0.50 or less for most patients.

Box 41-14 • Appropriate Times for Sigh Breaths

- Before and after suctioning
- During chest physiotherapy
- During and after bronchoscopy
- Before and during extubation
- During use of a small tidal volume (<7 mL/kg)
- During lung reexpansion

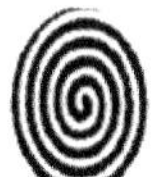

RULE OF THUMB

If a patient's oxygenation status is unknown, or if the patient's condition is unstable or critical, begin ventilatory support with an F_{IO_2} of 1.0 until Pa_{O_2}, Sa_{O_2}, or Sp_{O_2} can be assessed.

Positive end-expiratory pressure and CPAP may be started at zero or 3 to 5 cm H_2O, although patients with ALI/ARDS may begin with a PEEP/CPAP level of 5 to 8 cm H_2O. Trigger sensitivity for SIMV or assist breathing should be adjusted to minimize trigger work and avoid autocycling. Inspiratory flow, time, and I:E ratio should be adjusted to exceed the spontaneously breathing patient's inspiratory demand. Typically, an inspiratory flow rate of 60 L/min with an inspiratory time of approximately 1 second is a good starting point for most adult patients. This setting should result in an

Box 41-15 • General Guidelines for Initial Ventilator Settings for Adult Patients

MODE

- Assist-control (VC-CMV)
- SIMV with pressure support (VC-IMV)

TIDAL VOLUME (V_T)

- 8 to 12 mL/kg IBW
- Avoid overdistension
- Prefer volume on the steep part of the pressure-volume curve
- Maintain P_{plat} at 30 cm H_2O or less
- 10 to 12 mL/kg IBW is a good starting point for most patients
- 12 to 15 mL/kg IBW may be considered to maintain lung volume in patients with normal lungs (e.g., those with neuromuscular disease or recovering from a surgical procedure)
- For COPD and acute asthma exacerbation, a volume of 8 to 10 mL/kg in SIMV mode with adequate expiratory time for reducing air trapping is suggested
- For ALI/ARDS, begin at 8 mL/kg; reduce gradually to 6 mL/kg to maintain P_{plat} at 30 cm H_2O or less

RATE (F)

- 6 to 20 breaths/min
- Minimize auto-PEEP
- Set initial rate and tidal volume to maintain baseline minute ventilation (approximately 100 mL/kg IBW for most adults). Appropriate initial rate and tidal volume combinations, mode, F_{IO_2}, PEEP/CPAP, PSV, sensitivity, and flow settings may include the following:

Mode	V_T	f (breaths/min)	Comments
Assist-control or SIMV	10-12 mL/kg	10-12	Adequate for most patients except those with ALI/ARDS
	8 mL/kg down to 6 mL/kg	12-16	ALI/ARDS. Goal is to keep P_{plat} at 30 cm H_2O or less. Begin at 8 mL/kg and reduce volume in increments of 1 mL/kg every 1-2 h until 6 mL/kg and P_{plat} of 30 cm H_2O or less is reached (may continue to reduce V_T to 4 mL/kg, if necessary, while maintaining an acceptable PH).
SIMV only	12-15 mL/kg	6-10	Normal lungs, neuromuscular disease in which maintaining lung volume is a concern
	8-10 mL/kg	10-12	Obstructive disease in which air trapping is a concern
F_{IO_2} (titrate to obtain Pa_{O_2} ≥60 mm Hg; Sa_{O_2} ≥90%; Sp_{O_2} ≥92%)	1.0		For patients with demonstrated poor response to oxygen therapy, large right to left shunt, or in whom little is known or the situation appears to be grave
	0.40-0.50		Previous blood gas values or patient condition indicate probable good response to low to moderate concentrations of oxygen
PEEP/CPAP	0		Acceptable for most patients
	3-5		For prevention of atelectasis or compensation for auto-PEEP
	5-8		ALI/ARDS
PSV	5-10 cm H_2O		For overcoming WOB_I in spontaneously breathing patients in the SIMV mode. Higher values may be required with increased airway resistance or high spontaneous inspiratory flow.
	12-30 cm H_2O		PSV_{max} to obtain a target tidal volume (10-12 mL/kg) with assist rate less than 20 breaths/min as an assist mode of ventilation
Trigger sensitivity	–0.5 to –1.5 cm H_2O or flow trigger		Minimize trigger work without autocycle
Inspiratory flow and time	60 L/min (40-80 L/min) 1 s (0.80-1.2)		Inspiratory flow must meet or exceed patient's spontaneous inspiratory flow demand. Resultant I:E ratio should be 1:2 or better.

I:E ratio of 1:2 or better, although an I:E ratio starting at 1:1 may be appropriate for ALI/ARDS patients. Inspiratory flow rate is then adjusted to ensure that flow satisfies the patient's inspiratory demand and maintains an acceptable I:E ratio. General guidelines for initial ventilator settings for most adult patients are described in Box 41-15.

▶ ADJUSTING VENTILATORY SUPPORT

After ventilator initiation, the patient should be carefully assessed and the ventilator adjusted so that patient-ventilator synchrony is assured, work of breathing is minimized, and oxygenation, ventilation, and acid-base balance are optimized while harmful cardiovascular effects are minimized. Initial patient evaluation should include physical assessment, assessment of ventilatory values, cardiovascular assessment, oximetry, and measurement of arterial blood gases (Box 41-16).

Physical assessment should include general appearance, level of consciousness, signs of anxiety or dyspnea, color, extremities (temperature, edema, capillary refill), heart rate and blood pressure, respiratory rate and pattern, and inspection of the neck for jugular venous distension and chest examination. Cyanosis is associated with hypoxemia. Use of accessory muscles, tachypnea, retractions, or chest to abdomen asynchrony may indicate increased work of breathing. Unilateral or unequal lung expansion is associated with bronchial intubation, pneumothorax, and other unilateral disorders.

Breath sounds should be assessed for good aeration, and absent, diminished, or abnormal breath sounds should be documented. Palpation should be performed as appropriate for tracheal position, chest wall motion, and presence of subcutaneous air. Percussion of the chest should be performed in an assessment for resonance, dullness, or hyperresonance. Key findings at initial assessment of a patient undergoing ventilation are described in Table 41-9.

Box 41-16 • Initial Assessment of Ventilatory Support

- Inspection, palpation, and auscultation
- Assessment of the position of the artificial airway and cuff inflation
- Assessment of pulse, blood pressure, and electrocardiogram
- Inspection of the patient-ventilator system breathing circuit, humidifier, ventilator settings, and findings
- Analysis of arterial blood gas values
- Inspection of chest radiograph

Ventilatory values that should be assessed after initiation of mechanical ventilation include peak, plateau, and mean airway pressures, exhaled volumes (spontaneous and machine tidal volumes, minute ventilation), respiratory rate (spontaneous and machine rate), baseline pressures (PEEP, CPAP, auto-PEEP), trigger effort, oxygen concentration, inspiratory time, flow, I:E ratio, humidification, and airway temperature. In addition, patient-ventilator interaction should be assessed to ensure that the spontaneously breathing patient is able to easily trigger a breath and that inspiratory flow and time are such that work of breathing is minimized. Factors that may affect patient-ventilator interaction are listed in Box 41-17.

The artificial airway should be assessed for proper placement, patency, and cuff inflation. Size, position, and depth of the endotracheal tube and cuff pressure, including volume used to inflate the cuff, should be recorded. An extra endotracheal tube or tracheostomy tube of the correct size should be placed at the patient's bedside, and the equipment needed to replace the airway must be available and easily accessible. A clean, functioning manual resuscitator with oxygen supply and suction equipment, including an appropriate supply of suction catheters, sterile water or saline solution, and sterile gloves also must be placed near the bedside.

Cardiovascular assessment should include observation of heart rate, blood pressure, and electrocardiogram (ECG) for the presence of arrhythmias. Tachycardia, ST-segment elevation and frequent premature ventricular contractions may indicate myocardial hypoxia. If the patient has a central venous line or pulmonary arterial catheter, hemodynamic variables may be assessed, including central venous pressure, pulmonary arterial pressure, wedge pressure, and cardiac output.

Continuous monitoring with pulse oximetry is recommended for patients receiving mechanical ventilatory support in the intensive care setting, and arterial blood gases should be measured 20 to 30 minutes after initiation of mechanical ventilation, although 10 minutes may be adequate in the care of patients without obstructive disease. A chest radiograph should be obtained to verify proper endotracheal tube placement and to evaluate the chest. After the initial assessment, including blood gases, the method and level of ventilatory support are adjusted to optimize oxygenation, ventilation, work of breathing, acid-base balance, and cardiovascular status. The following discussion describes the ventilatory adjustments for each of these areas.

Patient-Ventilator Interaction

Patient-ventilator interaction refers to patient comfort, work of breathing, and synchrony during ventilator-assisted breaths. In general, ventilatory support should be initially adjusted to minimize the work of breathing

Table 41-9 ▶ ▶ Assessment of Ventilatory Support: Key Findings

Ancillary equipment in room	Crash cart (patient's condition unstable), cardiac monitor, chest tubes (pneumothorax, chest drainage, thoracic surgery), aortic balloon pump (heart failure), cooling blanket (fever), other
General appearance	Resting quietly, calm, relaxed (no distress); restless, anxious, distressed (pain, anxiety, inadequate oxygenation or ventilation)
Level of consciousness	Alert, awake and oriented to person, place, and time (good mental status, neurologic function); confused (neurologic problems, hypoxia, low cardiac output, drugs); sleepy (tired, sedatives, narcotics); lethargic (exhaustion, impaired CNS status, sedation); somnolent (CNS impairment, sedation); coma (CNS malfunction, heavy sedation, severe hypoxia)
Extremities	Cyanosis (hypoxemia), pale, cold, and clammy (poor cardiac output, low blood pressure, shock), edema (fluid overload)
Respiratory rate and pattern	Normal (good cardiopulmonary status); tachypnea (pain, anxiety, hypoxemia, acidosis, CNS problems); bradypnea or apnea (severe hypoxia, CNS problems, heavy sedation, paralysis)
Head, eyes, ears, nose, and throat	Cyanotic lips and gums (hypoxemia); pupils dilated (drugs, severe hypoxia, low cardiac output, cardiac arrest); pupils dilated and fixed (brain death); pupils contracted (drugs, light); response to light (good if responsive)
Neck	Accessory muscle use (increased work of breathing, respiratory distress); jugular vein distension (right side heart failure, positive pressure impeding venous return)
Chest inspection	Right-left chest wall synchrony (normal); right-left chest wall asynchrony (right mainstem intubation, pneumothorax, large unilateral pleural effusion, flail on one side); chest-diaphragm synchrony (normal); chest-diaphragm asynchrony—abdominal paradox (increased work of breathing, diaphragmatic fatigue)
Chest auscultation	Good bilateral breath sounds (normal); decreased breath sounds unilaterally (right mainstem intubation, pneumothorax, unilateral lung disease); bilaterally decreased or absent breath sounds (inadequate or decreased ventilation, large leak, ventilator malfunction or disconnect, misplaced endotracheal tube); air leak around cuff (under inflation, cuff malfunction); wheezing (bronchospasm, tumor, narrowing of the airway); bibasilar crackles in patients with CHF (pulmonary edema); rhonchi, course crackles (secretions in the larger airways); bronchial breath sounds (consolidation or microatelectasis)
Palpation	Subcutaneous air (pneumothorax, pneumomediastinum), tracheal shift (tension pneumothorax, large area of atelectasis), right-left chest motion symmetry (normal), right-left asymmetrical breathing (unilateral disease, pneumothorax, bronchial intubation)
Percussion	Resonant over lung tissue (normal), dull (pleural effusion, lobar infiltrates, consolidation, atelectasis), hyperresonant (pneumothorax, overinflation-COPD, asthma exacerbation)
Vital signs	Normal heart rate and rhythm (normal), tachycardia (hypoxemia, pain, anxiety, distress), hypertension (anxiety, cardiovascular disease, head trauma), bradycardia (severe hypoxia, severe hypercapnia, cardiac disease), hypotension (blood loss, shock, gram negative sepsis, heart failure)

Box 41-17 • Factors Affecting Patient-Ventilator Interaction

- Artificial airway
- Mode of ventilation
- Level of ventilatory support
- Inspiratory flow
- Trigger sensitivity
- Flow-triggered system function
- Demand valve function
- PEEP valve function
- Presence of auto-PEEP
- Humidification systems

Modified from Tobin MJ: Respir Care 36:395, 1991; Kacmarek RM: Optimizing ventilatory muscle function during mechanical ventilation. In Pierson DJ, Kacmarek RM, editors: Foundations of respiratory care, New York, 1992, Churchill-Livingstone.

and to allow the ventilatory muscles to rest.[54] Diaphragmatic fatigue often accompanies ventilatory failure, and a sustained increase in workload can lead to structural injury to the muscle.[12] Once the ventilatory muscles become fatigued, at least 24 hours is required for recovery.[55] Complete rest of the diaphragm, as in controlled ventilation, may lead to diaphragmatic deconditioning, weakness, and atrophy in as little as 48 hours.[54] In the presence of spontaneous breathing, inappropriate ventilator settings may further increase patient work and fatigue.[12] Careful selection of ventilator settings, however, can reduce the workload to a normal range without resulting in deconditioning and atrophy of the respiratory muscles.[12]

Synchronized intermittent mandatory ventilation, assist-control, and pressure-support modes can reduce inspiratory effort without eliminating respiratory muscle activity. The ideal is perfect synchronization of the positive pressure breath with the patient's inspiratory effort.[12,43] The expiratory phase of the ventilator also should match that of the patient.[12] Patient work to trigger the ventilator should be minimal, and the clinician must be alert to patient efforts not recognized by the ventilator. This situation can occur when trigger sensitivity is too great or in the presence of auto-PEEP.

If inspiratory flow from the ventilator does not meet the patient's ventilatory needs, patient work increases.[12,43]

Excessive inspiratory flow, however, can cause immediate and persistent tachypnea.[12,43] In general, the lowest inspiratory flow setting that meets the patient's inspiratory needs should be used.

Mode of ventilation can affect patient-ventilator interaction. Assist-control mode may result in an excessive trigger rate, hyperventilation, and patient-ventilator asynchrony. Synchronized intermittent mandatory ventilation allows continued spontaneous breathing efforts and in the absence of pressure support may worsen ventilatory muscle fatigue. During volume ventilation, the patient may attempt to exhale before the machine has completed the inspiratory phase. Pressure-support ventilation may continue to provide inspiratory gas flow even though the patient has begun to exhale.[12] Patients with COPD who have higher levels of PSV (20 cm H_2O) may recruit the expiratory muscles in an attempt to cycle the ventilator to the expiratory phase, and the work of breathing is increased.[12]

Careful patient observation for trigger effort, accessory muscle use, chest-to-diaphragm synchrony, respiratory rate, and signs of distress should identify patients needing attention. Trigger sensitivity, inspiratory flow and flow waveform, tidal volume, pressure limit and mode should be adjusted as needed to minimize patient work, provide for patient comfort, and ensure patient-ventilatory synchrony.

▶ OXYGENATION

Oxygenation Concentration

Initiation of treatment of most patients in the acute care setting is with 100% oxygen or 40% to 50% oxygen, depending on the patient's condition. The F_{IO_2} is then titrated to achieve a Pa_{O_2} in the range of 60 to 100 mm Hg with an Sa_{O_2} of 90% or more or an Sp_{O_2} of 92% or more.* Pulse oximetry values always should be compared by means of simultaneous measurement of Sa_{O_2} to ensure correlation. Estimates of oxygen needs can be derived as follows:

$$F_{IO_2} \text{ required} = \left(\frac{Pa_{O_2} \text{ desired}}{Pa_{O_2}/PA_{O_2} \text{ ratio}} + Pa_{CO_2} \times 1.25\right) \times \frac{1}{P_B - P_{H_2O}}$$

where F_{IO_2} required is the F_{IO_2} needed to achieve a desired Pa_{O_2}, Pa_{O_2}/PA_{O_2} is the initial Pa_{O_2} divided by the initial alveolar partial pressure of oxygen (PA_{O_2}), Pa_{CO_2} is the initial Pa_{CO_2}, P_B is barometric pressure, and P_{H_2O} is water vapor pressure. A simpler, but less accurate calculation is

$$\underset{\text{Initial}}{Pa_{O_2}/F_{IO_2}} = \underset{\text{Desired}}{Pa_{O_2}/F_{IO_2}}$$

*Recommended Sp_{O_2} is 95% or higher in patients with deeply pigmented skin.

Instead of a formula, a nomogram can be used to predict a patient's required F_{IO_2} (Figure 41-9). In either case, it is suggested that oxygen levels be titrated down from 100% to 50% oxygen in decrements not to exceed 20%; titration is followed by oximetry or measurement of blood gases. When titrating F_{IO_2} downward, the clinician should wait at least 10 minutes between changes in F_{IO_2} to allow oxygen levels to stabilize. Patients with obstructive disease need a longer period for to equilibration after a change in F_{IO_2}.

For reducing oxygen concentration from 50% to 21%, oxygen changes should be in steps of 5% to 10% followed by oximetry or measurement of blood gases. Once the patient has reached the desired F_{IO_2}, and if the Sp_{O_2} is at least 92%, a blood gas sample should be drawn to ensure that actual Pa_{O_2}, Sa_{O_2}, ventilation, and acid-base balance are acceptable. Box 41-18 lists a conservative method of titrating oxygen concentration down from an initial F_{IO_2} of 1.0 on the basis of Pa_{O_2}.

Once the desired Pa_{O_2} and saturation are reached, monitoring should be continued. In general, oxygen levels are titrated up and down as needed with adjustments in F_{IO_2} by units of 0.05 to 0.10 to maintain a Pa_{O_2} of 60 to 100 mm Hg with an Sp_{O_2} of 92% to 97%. Titration is followed by oximetry or measurement of blood gases. An Sa_{O_2} of 88% to 90% may be acceptable for patients who need an F_{IO_2} of 0.80 or more for an extended time.

Positive End-Expiratory Pressure and Continuous Positive Airway Pressure

Various approaches to adjusting PEEP/CPAP have been suggested over the years, including minimum PEEP, optimal or best PEEP, and PEEP titrated by compliance or pressure-volume curves. With acute restrictive disease, as PEEP or CPAP levels are increased, Pa_{O_2}, Sa_{O_2}, and static compliance tend to improve until the point at which lung overinflation occurs. As mean airway pressure increases, venous return decreases. The result may be a decrease in cardiac output. Figure 41-10 shows the physiologic factors that change during application of PEEP/CPAP. Four approaches to adjusting PEEP/CPAP levels are described.

Minimum Positive End-Expiratory Pressure

Minimum PEEP can be defined as the minimal PEEP needed to achieve an adequate Pa_{O_2} (and Sa_{O_2}) with a safe F_{IO_2}. In general,, the PEEP level needed to achieve a Pa_{O_2} of at least 60 mm Hg (Sa_{O_2} ≥90, Sp_{O_2} ≥92) with an F_{IO_2} of 0.40 to 0.50 or less is the minimum PEEP. With this approach, the least PEEP or CPAP level needed to achieve this therapeutic endpoint is applied.[7]

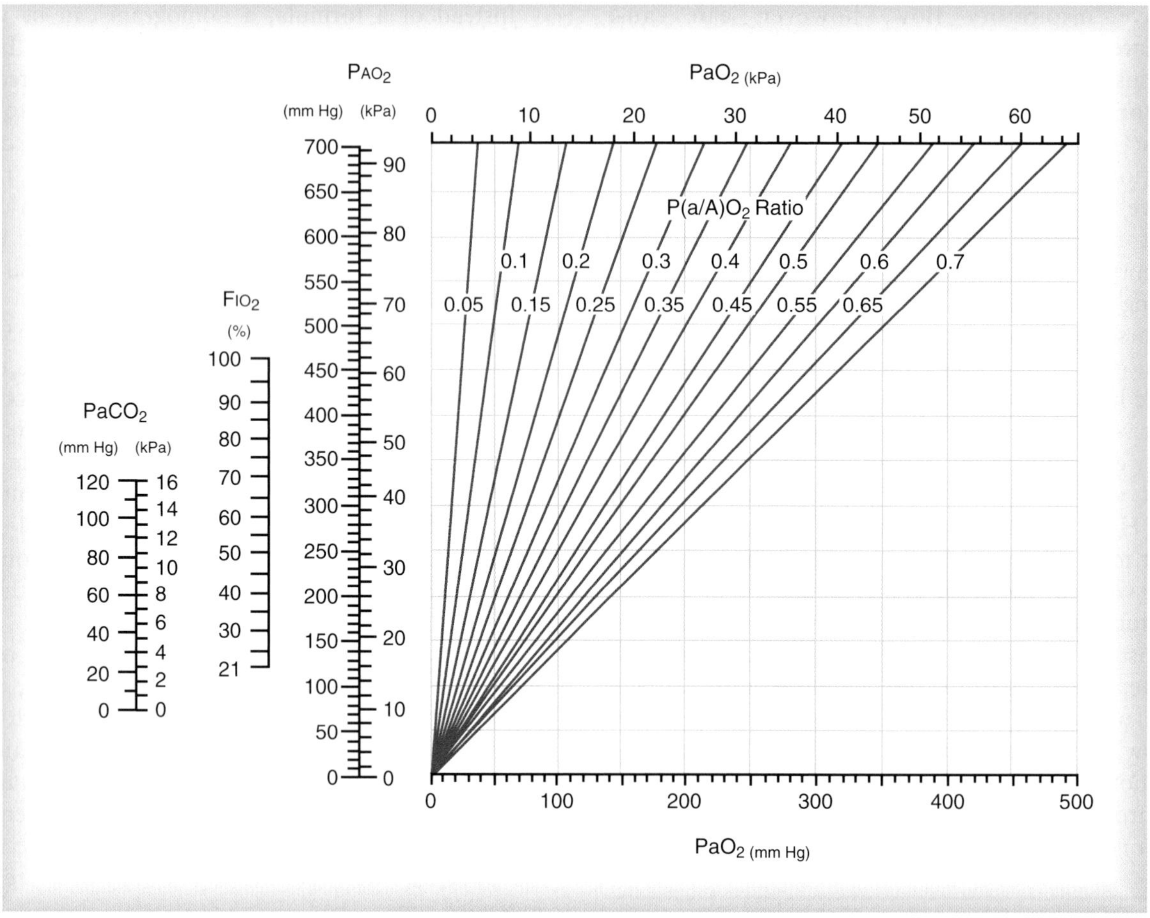

Figure 41-9

Nomogram for computing $Pa{O_2}/PA{O_2}$ ratio and predicting the $FI{O_2}$ needs of patients. To use the nomogram, first align the patient's current $FI{O_2}$ and $Pa{CO_2}$ (*left*) with a straight edge. This line will intersect the vertical lines corresponding to the patient's current $PA{O_2}$ and $Pa{O_2}$. Intersecting the $Pa{O_2}$ vertical line at this point will be a diagonal line corresponding to the patient's $Pa{O_2}/PA{O_2}$ ratio. Next, move along this diagonal line to a point above the desired $Pa{O_2}$. From this point (the patient's $Pa{O_2}/PA{O_2}$ ratio and desired $Pa{O_2}$), draw a horizontal line to the left until you intersect the $PA{O_2}$ vertical line. Last, connect this point (the needed $PA{O_2}$) to the patient's $Pa{CO_2}$. Where this line intersects the $FI{O_2}$ vertically is the needed $FI{O_2}$.

Optimal or Best PEEP

Optimal or best PEEP usually is defined as the PEEP that maximizes oxygen delivery ($D{O_2}$). Oxygen delivery is calculated as cardiac output ($\dot{Q}_T$) times oxygen content ($Ca{O_2}$):

$$D{O_2} = \dot{Q}_T \times Ca{O_2}$$

For the optimal PEEP level, PEEP is increased in increments of 3 to 5 cm H_2O. Blood pressure, mixed venous oxygen levels (partial pressure of oxygen in mixed venous blood [$P\bar{v}{O_2}$], mixed venous oxygen saturation [$S\bar{v}{O_2}$]), arteriovenous oxygen contents difference [$C(a\text{-}v){O_2}$], cardiac output, and cardiac index are then assessed. Positive end-expiratory pressure is increased incrementally until there is a decline in oxygen delivery, at which point the best or optimal PEEP has been exceeded. The PEEP is then adjusted down to the previous level that represents the "best" PEEP. Table 41-10 shows an example of a PEEP study for determining the optimal PEEP based on oxygen delivery ($D{O_2}$). In the table, as PEEP is increased from 0 to 5 to 10 cm H_2O, $P\bar{v}{O_2}$, $S\bar{v}{O_2}$, and $D{O_2}$ increase with no decline in cardiac output ($\dot{Q}_T$) or blood pressure. However, when PEEP is increased to 15 cm H_2O, $Sv{O_2}$, $D{O_2}$, $\dot{Q}_T$ and blood pressure decline, indicating that the optimal PEEP for this patient has been exceeded. The best PEEP for this patient would be 10 cm H_2O.

Compliance-Titrated PEEP

With this technique, PEEP is increased in increments of 3 to 5 cm H_2O, and the patient's static compliance (Cs) is measured where

$$Cs = \frac{\text{Volume delivered (mL)}}{P_{plat} - P_{baseline}\ \text{(PEEP/CPAP)}}$$

MINI CLINI

Adjustment of Oxygen Concentration Down From 100% for a Ventilated Patient According to F_{IO_2} and Blood Gas Values

PROBLEM

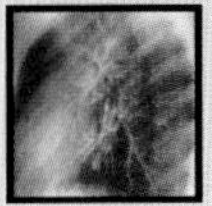

At 9:00 AM, mechanical ventilation is initiated with the following settings for a 70-kg patient:

Mode: SIMV
V_T (machine): 700 mL
Rate (machine): 10 breaths/min
F_{IO_2}: 1.0
PEEP/CPAP: +5 cm H_2O
PSV: +5 cm H_2O

Twenty minutes after ventilator initiation, an arterial blood gas is obtained:

F_{IO_2}: 1.0
Pa_{O_2}: 225 mm Hg
pH: 7.42
Pa_{CO_2}: 40 mm Hg
HCO_3: 24 mEq/L
Base excess (BE): +1 mEq/L

Calculated alveolar PA_{O_2} and Pa_{O_2}/PA_{O_2} ratios are:

$$PA_{O_2} = F_{IO_2}\,(P_B - P_{H_2O}) - Pa_{CO_2} \times 1.25 = 663$$
$$Pa_{O_2}/PA_{O_2} = 225/663 = 0.34$$

What F_{IO_2} is needed to achieve a target Pa_{O_2} of 80 mm Hg?

SOLUTION

The first equation and normal barometric pressure (P_B = 760), lead to the following calculation:

$$F_{IO_2}\text{ required} = \left(\frac{Pa_{O_2}\text{ desired}}{Pa_{O_2}/PA_{O_2}\text{ ratio}} + Pa_{CO_2} \times 1.25\right) \times \frac{1}{P_B - P_{H_2O}}$$
$$= \left(\frac{80}{0.34} + (40 \times 1.25)\right) \times \frac{1}{760 - 47} = 0.40$$

An alternative calculation would be:

$$\text{Initial} \quad \text{Desired}$$
$$Pa_{O_2}/F_{IO_2} = Pa_{O_2}/F_{IO_2}$$
$$225/1.0 = 80/F_{IO_2}\text{ desired}$$
$$F_{IO_2}\text{ desired} = 80 \times (1.0/225) = 80/225 = 0.36$$

What should the clinician do now?

The target oxygen concentration to achieve a Pa_{O_2} in the range of 60 to 100 mm Hg (with 80 mm Hg as the specific target for the purpose of this calculation) would be approximately 40%. However, it is suggested that for adjusting down from 100% after initial ventilator setup, changes in F_{IO_2} be limited to 0.20 in the range of F_{IO_2} 1.0 to 0.50 and 0.10 to 0.05 below an F_{IO_2} of 0.50. Each change in F_{IO_2} should be followed by oximetry and patient assessment.

In this example, we may see the F_{IO_2} decreased in a stepwise manner, as follows:

Time	F_{IO_2}	Sp_{O_2} (%)	Pa_{O_2} (mm Hg)
9:30	1.0	99	225
9:45	0.80	99	177
10:00	0.60	98	129
10:15	0.50	97	104
10:30	0.45	97	92
10:45	0.40	95	80

Box 41-18 • Titrating F_{IO_2} Down From an Initial Starting Point of 1.0 According to Initial Pa_{O_2} and Pulse Oximetric Findings

Initial Pa_{O_2} on F_{IO_2} 1.0 (mm Hg)	F_{IO_2} Step 1	Step 2	Step 3	Step 4	Step 5
>300	0.80	0.60	0.50	0.40	0.35*
200-300	0.80	0.60	0.50	0.40*	—
150-199	0.80	0.60*	—	—	—
100-149	0.80*	—	—	—	—

Decrease F_{IO_2} to the target value in steps and perform pulse oximetry or arterial blood gas measurements. Patients should continue to receive a given F_{IO_2} long enough to ensure equilibration and an acceptable Sp_{O_2} before further reductions are made in F_{IO_2}. This procedure takes 5 to 10 minutes per F_{IO_2} change for most patients, up to 30 minutes for patients with obstructive disease. It usually is safe to continue to decrease F_{IO_2} as long as Sp_{O_2} is greater than 97% (which should correspond to a Pa_{O_2} >90 mm Hg) for most patients. When Sp_{O_2} less than 97% but greater than 95%, increase or decrease F_{IO_2} in steps of 0.05 per change. When the target F_{IO_2} is reached, an arterial blood gas should be obtained to verify an acceptable Pa_{O_2} and Sa_{O_2}.

*Target F_{IO_2} based on initial Pa_{O_2}.

Best PEEP has been exceeded at the point at which an increase in PEEP is followed by a decrease in compliance. Positive end-expiratory pressure is then reduced to the previous level, and this is the optimal PEEP based on compliance. For the example shown in Table 41-10, the best PEEP based on compliance would be 10 cm H_2O. Unfortunately, regional lung overdistension and declines in cardiac output can occur below the compliance-titrated best PEEP, and consequently compliance-titrated PEEP should be used with caution.

Positive End-Expiratory Pressure Titrated With Pressure-Volume Curves

Another approach to determining the best PEEP in patients with ALI/ARDS is the use of static pressure-volume curves. To obtain a static pressure-volume curve, the therapist passively inflates the patient's lungs with varying volumes in increasing increments of 50 to 100 mL. At each endpoint, static pressure is obtained by means of application of an end-inspiratory pause, and the resultant pressure-volume curve is plotted (Figure 41-11). An upper and a lower inflection point typically can be determined. The lower inflection point is thought to be the point at which significant alveolar recruitment

MINI CLINI

Adjusting F_{IO_2}

PROBLEM

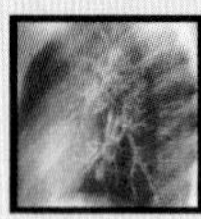

A 70-kg patient in the ICU is receiving mechanical ventilation in the volume-control mode (VC-CMV). The patient's arterial blood gas values and related ventilator settings are

Mode: VC-CMV
F_{IO_2}: 0.40
Pa_{O_2}: 50 mm Hg
V_T: 700 mL
pH: 7.4
f: 12 breaths/min
Pa_{CO_2}: 40 mm Hg
PEEP: +5 cm H_2O
HCO_3: 24 mEq/L
BE: +1 mEq/L

What F_{IO_2} would be required to raise this patient's Pa_{O_2} to 60 mm Hg?

SOLUTION

First, calculate the patient's current P_{AO_2} and Pa_{O_2}/P_{AO_2} ratio:

$$P_{AO_2} = F_{IO_2}(P_B - P_{H_2O}) - Pa_{CO_2}/0.8$$
$$= 0.40\,(760 - 47) - 40/0.8$$
$$= 285 - 50 = 235 \text{ mm Hg}$$
$$Pa_{O_2}/P_{AO_2} = 50/235 = 0.21$$

Next, calculate the F_{IO_2} needed to achieve the desired Pa_{O_2} of 60 mm Hg:

$$F_{IO_2} \text{ required} = \left(\frac{Pa_{O_2} \text{ desired} + Pa_{CO_2} \times 1.25 \times 1}{Pa_{O_2}/P_{AO_2} \text{ ratio } P_B - P_{H_2O}}\right)$$
$$= \left(\frac{60 + (40 \times 1.25) \times 1}{0.21\ 760 - 47}\right)$$
$$= \frac{335.7 \times 1}{713} = 0.47$$

For this patient, if the F_{IO_2} is increased from 0.40 to 0.47, the Pa_{O_2} should increase from 50 to 60 mm Hg. An alternative calculation, based on Pa_{O_2}/F_{IO_2} ratio, would be

$$\text{Actual } Pa_{O_2}/F_{IO_2} = \text{Desired } Pa_{O_2}/F_{IO_2}$$

Solving for F_{IO_2}, this becomes

$$F_{IO_2} \text{ required} = Pa_{O_2} \text{ desired} \times (F_{IO_2} \text{ actual}/Pa_{O_2} \text{ actual})$$
$$= 60 \times (0.40/50) = 0.48$$

To increase this patient's Pa_{O_2} more than 60 mm Hg requires increasing the F_{IO_2} to approximately 0.50. Although an F_{IO_2} of 0.50 or less is acceptable, as an alternative, the respiratory therapist may consider increasing the PEEP to +8 cm H_2O and perform a clinical assessment, including evaluation of the effect of the increase on blood pressure, and measure arterial blood gases.

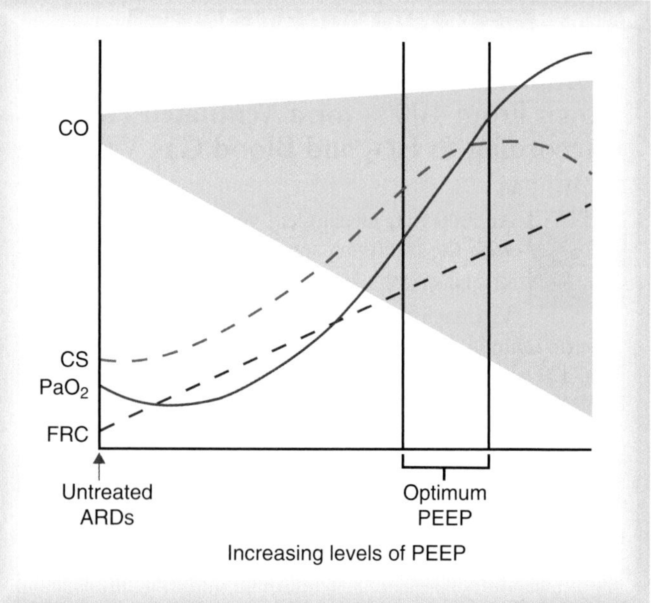

Figure 41-10
Curves represent the physiological factors that change during the application of PEEP and CPAP. As the PEEP level is increased, Pa_{O_2}, FRC, and static compliance (Cs) normally increase. Cardiac output (CO), represented by the shaded area, can increase slightly, stay the same, or decrease. The optimum PEEP level can be expected to occur when Pa_{O_2}, FRC, and Cs are high. Cardiac output should be maintained near normal so that oxygen transport to the tissues remains high. *(Modified from Pilbeam SP: Mechanical ventilation: physiological and clinical applications, ed 3, St. Louis, 1998, Mosby.)*

occurs. The upper inflection point may indicate lung overdistension. The PEEP is then set at approximately 2 cm H_2O above the lower inflection point. Tidal volume may be adjusted to assure that the upper inflection point is not exceeded during inspiration.

Calculating the static pressure-volume curve is technically difficult and time consuming.[12] An alternative to use of the static pressure-volume curve is use of the slow-flow pressure-volume curve. A slow-flow curve (≤15 L/min) may indicate the lower inflection point for the purposes of setting PEEP (Figure 41-12). In either case, however, some patients do not have a lower inflection point. In addition, observer variability in identifying the lower inflection point can be significant.[56]

Regardless of the approach to setting PEEP, it is suggested that the PEEP level be titrated to allow reduction of the F_{IO_2} to 0.40 to 0.50. After reduction of the F_{IO_2} to 0.40, PEEP can be reduced gradually as the patient improves. In general, an F_{IO_2} of 0.40 or less with a PEEP/CPAP of 5 cm H_2O or less should be obtained before discontinuance of mechanical ventilation is considered (see Chapter 44).

Table 41-10 ▶▶ Example of a PEEP Study Including Ventilation, Oxygenation, and Hemodynamic Data*

Value	PEEP = 0	PEEP = 5	PEEP = 10	PEEP = 15	PEEP = 20
Time (min)	0	20	40	60	80
V_T (L)	0.6	0.6	0.6	0.6	0.6
f (breaths/min)	16	16	16	16	16
FIO_2 (%)	80	80	80	80	80
PEEP (cm H_2O)	0	5	10	15	20
I:E ratio	1:2.7	1:2.7	1:2.7	1:2.7	1:2.7
P_{peak} (cm H_2O)	30	32	35	42	50
P_{plat} (cm H_2O)	25	27	29	36	43
Cs (mL/cm H_2O)	24	27	32	29	26
$PaCO_2$ (mm Hg)	43	42	43	42	44
pH	7.38	7.37	7.39	7.35	7.32
PaO_2 (mm Hg)	52	66	87	90	97
SaO_2 (%)	86	92	96	97	98
$P\bar{v}O_2$ (mm Hg)	32	35	37	37	36
$S\bar{v}O_2$ (mm Hg)	61	66	71	69	64
Blood pressure	131/78	133/82	130/79	125/74	110/69
Cardiac output (L/min)	5.9	5.7	5.9	5.4	4.8
DO_2 (mL/min)	989	1022	1105	1021	917

*When first reviewing a PEEP study, observe changes in the following: (1) airway pressure, (2) blood pressure, (3) arterial oxygen (PaO_2, SaO_2) and mixed venous oxygenation ($P\bar{v}O_2$, $S\bar{v}O_2$), and (4) oxygen transport (DO_2). With increases in PEEP, PaO_2 and saturation improve; airway pressure increases; compliance improves and then decreases at higher levels of PEEP; and oxygen transport (DO_2) improves and then declines. The optimum PEEP for this patient is 10 cm H_2O because it provides the best arterial oxygenation (PaO_2, SaO_2) without a decline in DO_2 or cardiac output.

MINI CLINI

Use of PEEP

PROBLEM

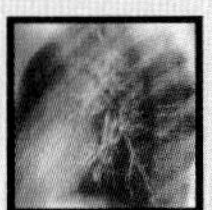

A 30-year-old, 80-kg (IBW) man is in the critical care unit because of blunt trauma to the chest after a motor vehicle accident. The patient's initial mechanical ventilatory support machine settings are as follows:

Mode: = Assist-control volume ventilation (VC-CMV)
V_T: 500 mL
Rate: 20 breaths/min
FIO_2: 0.70
PIP: 35 cm H_2O
P_{plat}: 30 cm H_2O
PEEP: 0

Arterial blood gas analysis yielded the following results:

pH: 7.38 PaO_2: 48 mm Hg
$PaCO_2$: 36 mm Hg SaO_2: 81%

The respiratory therapist considers a recommendation that PEEP be instituted. What are the goals of this type of adjunctive therapy, and what are some of the potential adverse effects of PEEP of which the respiratory therapist should be aware?

SOLUTION

The general goals of PEEP are to recruit and stabilize atelectatic alveolar units to achieve adequate oxygenation and to avoid potentially unsafe levels of FIO_2 and inflation pressure. Improvement is most commonly assessed with arterial blood gas analysis (PaO_2 or SaO_2) and measurement of blood pressure and cardiac output.

The use of PEEP in this situation is appropriate because the PaO_2 and SaO_2 values indicate poor arterial oxygenation despite an elevated FIO_2. When the PaO_2 does not respond to a high FIO_2, the condition is referred to as *refractory hypoxemia*. Precise determination of an optimum PEEP can be difficult unless measures of oxygen transport and utilization are available. The procedure would require placement of a pulmonary arterial catheter, measurement of cardiac output, and acquisition of mixed venous blood. An appropriate initial PEEP for this patient would be +5 cm H_2O, and arterial blood gases, plateau pressure, blood pressure, and if possible, cardiac output should be assessed. As the level of PEEP is increased, the respiratory therapist must be alert for signs of the following potential complications: barotrauma (indicated by high inflation hold pressure and mean airway pressure); decreased cardiac output and oxygen transport (despite an improvement in PaO_2 and SaO_2), which results from decreased venous return; and increased pulmonary vascular resistance caused by intrathoracic pressure.

In the absence of a pulmonary arterial catheter, assessment of arterial blood pressure, heart rate, and sensorium would be helpful.

Measurement of effective compliance and inflation hold pressure (P_{plat}) may be useful when higher levels of PEEP are indicated and alveolar overdistension is possible. In all cases, the lowest PEEP level that provides acceptable oxygenation should be selected.

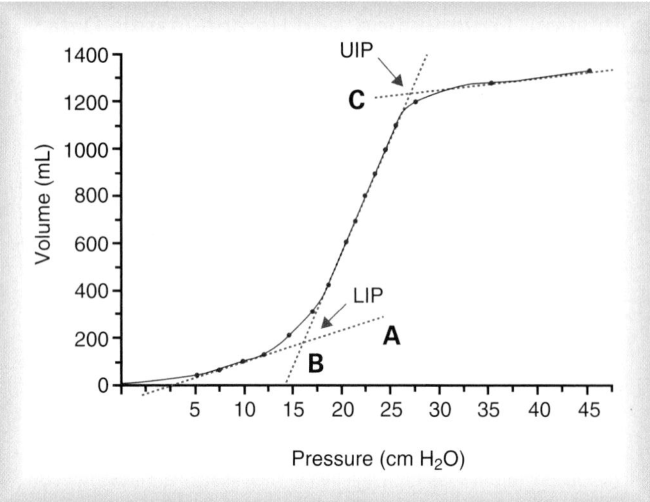

Figure 41-11

Static pressure-volume curve of a patient with ARDS. Volume is increased in increments of approximately 100 mL, inspiratory plateau pressure (P_{plat}) is measured, and a pressure-volume curve is plotted. Straight lines (**A, B,** and **C**) are drawn tangent to the curve, and the lower inflection point (*LIP*) and upper inflection point (*UIP*) are identified. Positive end-expiratory pressure is then adjusted to approximately 2 cm H_2O above the LIP.

Other Techniques for Improving Oxygenation

The primary techniques for optimizing oxygenation in patients receiving mechanical ventilatory support are adjusting FIO_2 and PEEP/CPAP. Other techniques that may be helpful in improving arterial oxygen levels include the use of PCV with a prolonged inspiratory time, use of an inspiratory pause, inverse I:E ratio ventilation, prone positioning, and open lung techniques.[6] In addition, appropriate use of bronchial hygiene, humidification, suctioning, and airway care and administration of bronchodilator therapy can be helpful to most patients.

Pressure-Control Ventilation With Prolonged Inspiratory Time

Pressure-control ventilation with prolonged inspiratory time has been associated with improvement in PaO_2 in patients with ALI/ARDS.[6,27] The mechanism may include the improvement in $\dot{V}/\dot{Q}$ associated with prolonged inspiratory time, the inspiratory plateau achieved with a prolonged inspiratory phase during pressure-limited ventilation, or the effects of auto-PEEP resulting from a short expiratory time.[6,27] Regardless of the mechanism, pressure control can be an effective mode for ventilating ALI/ARDS patients and may improve oxygenation while limiting alveolar pressure to avoid barotrauma.[6] In general, the inspiratory time is increased in the control mode until a period of no flow results at the end of inspiration. We suggest an initial I:E ratio of 1:1. If resultant arterial oxygen levels are inadequate (and PEEP levels are optimized), the I:E ratio may then be increased from 1:1 to 1.5:1. Assessment of the patient that includes measurement of arterial blood gases, blood pressure, and hemodynamic variables should follow each increase in I:E ratio. If there are no adverse effects and further improvement in PaO_2 is needed, the I:E ratio may be increased to 2:1. The maximum benefit of inverse ratio ventilation may take several hours to achieve.[27]

Prolonged inspiratory time and inverse I:E ratio ventilation may result in reductions in venous return and cardiac output. In addition, most spontaneously breathing patients do not tolerate a prolonged inspiratory phase in the assist-control mode and may need sedation or paralysis. Synchronized intermittent mandatory ventilation–pressure control with pressure support may be better tolerated by these patients.[6] Another alternative to sedation and paralysis is the use of airway pressure release ventilation or bilevel ventilation.[14]

Bronchial Hygiene

Turning, sitting up, and getting the patient out of bed into a chair can be helpful in improving oxygenation in many patients. Upright positioning appears to be beneficial for ventilated patients, and supine positioning may increase the risk of pneumonia, especially in patients receiving enteral feeding or with a decreased level of consciousness.[57] Special roto-beds can be used to optimize PaO_2 and SaO_2. Postural drainage and chest percussion, adequate humidification, and bronchodilator therapy all may improve oxygenation and should be considered in the care of ventilator patients when not specifically contraindicated.

Prone Positioning

Prone positioning may be an effective technique for improving oxygenation in patients with ALI/ARDS.[58-60] Prone positioning is a relatively low-risk maneuver and may improve PaO_2 by 30 to 50 mm Hg and decrease shunt fraction from 25% to 12%.[58] Although improvement in PaO_2 may be dramatic and sustained (up to 12 hours), not all patients benefit from prone positioning. The procedure is not without risk. Care must be taken to ensure that endotracheal tubes, intravenous lines, and catheters are not blocked or dislodged. The patient may also have skin breakdown at specific pressure points (face, sternum, hips, knees), and facial or eyelid edema may occur, although the latter is primarily a cosmetic concern that resolves quickly when the patient returns to a supine or sitting position.[59] The most serious complication is corneal abrasion necessitating corneal transplantation.[59,60] Prone positioning is labor intensive, often requiring two nurses, a respiratory therapist, and a physician to "flip" the patient.

The mechanism of action of prone positioning is unclear. In ARDS, dorsal lung injury tends to increase shunt and decrease $\dot{V}/\dot{Q}$, resulting in hypoxemia. Supine positioning tends to increase regional pressure in the dependent, or dorsal, portions of the lungs. Prone positioning may improve $\dot{V}/\dot{Q}$ and reduce shunting by removing the pressure of the heart on the dorsal regions and causing regional dorsal traction, which may promote lung opening. The recommended technique for prone positioning is outlined in Box 41-19.

In summary, prone positioning can be safe and effective in improving Pa_{O_2} in ALI/ARDS patients, although survival has not been shown to improve. Research is being conducted to determine whether the benefits of prone positioning are enhanced by combining the technique with administration of pulmonary vasodilators, including nitric oxide.[61,62]

Open Lung Techniques

Various lung recruitment maneuvers have been suggested for improving $\dot{V}/\dot{Q}$ and reducing shunting in ALI/ARDS patients. These include several variations that incorporate a prolonged end-inspiratory pause, which is applied at intervals to open dependent areas of the lung.[38,63] For example, one experimental technique is to apply 40 cm H_2O pressure for 30 seconds to maximally inflate the lung. The procedure is repeated at regular intervals. Inspiratory recruitment maneuvers are combined with PEEP above the lower inflection point on a pressure-volume curve, and these combined techniques may improve oxygenation and other patient factors.[27,38,63] Because these procedures remain experimental, routine application in clinical practice should await clear guidelines based on research findings. In addition, misapplication of recruitment techniques involving increased airway pressure can cause barotrauma or result in cardiovascular compromise.

Box 41-19 • Prone Positioning

Preparation for flipping includes the following:
- Adequate sedation of the patient
- Clear assignment of responsibilities between the team members
- Moving the patient to one side of the bed
- Checking all lines for length
- Checking the security of the endotracheal tube
- Endotracheal suctioning
- Preoxygenation with 100% oxygen
- Checking all vital signs

The turn includes
- Tipping the patient to the side
- Unhooking ECG leads
- Turning the patient prone
- Turning the patient's head toward the ventilator
- Reattaching ECG leads

Care after the turn includes
- Checking all lines
- Checking ventilator pressure and volume
- Monitoring vital signs
- Repositioning and recalibrating pressure transducers

The patient needs supports (pillows) for each side of chest and forehead so the endotracheal tube and head are not compressed.

▶ VENTILATION

Alveolar ventilation is determined by respiratory rate, tidal volume, and dead space and is described by the following equation:

$$\dot{V}_A = (V_T - V_{Dsphys})f$$

where $\dot{V}_A$ is alveolar ventilation, V_T is tidal volume, V_{Dsphys} is physiologic dead space, and f is respiratory frequency or rate. The relation between arterial Pa_{CO_2}, alveolar ventilation ($\dot{V}_A$), and carbon dioxide production ($\dot{V}_{CO_2}$) is described as follows:

$$Pa_{CO_2} = \frac{0.863 \times \dot{V}_{CO_2}}{\dot{V}_A}$$

Arterial Pa_{CO_2} is considered the single best index of effective ventilation. Increases in $\dot{V}_A$ or decreases in $\dot{V}_{CO_2}$ result in a decrease in Pa_{CO_2}, whereas increases in $\dot{V}_{CO_2}$ or decreases in $\dot{V}_A$ result in an increase in Pa_{CO_2}. If there is no change in $\dot{V}_{CO_2}$, the following relations can be used to estimate the effect of changes in $\dot{V}_A$ on Pa_{CO_2}:

Initial Desired

$$Pa_{CO_{2(1)}} \times \dot{V}_{A(1)} = Pa_{CO_{2(2)}} \times \dot{V}_{A(2)}$$

Box 41-20 gives an example of the effect of a change in $\dot{V}_A$ on Pa_{CO_2}.

The foregoing predictive equation can be used during mechanical ventilation with the following modifications:

Initial Desired

$$Pa_{CO_{2(1)}} \times \dot{V}_{A(1)} = Pa_{CO_{2(2)}} \times \dot{V}_{A(2)}$$

and

$$Pa_{CO_{2(1)}}(V_{T(1)} - V_{Dsphys(1)})f_{(1)} = Pa_{CO_{2(2)}}(V_{T(2)} - V_{Dsphys(2)})f_{(2)}$$

For changes in rate alone, if there is no change in $\dot{V}_{CO_2}$ or physiologic dead space (V_{Dsphys}), this becomes

Initial Desired

$$Pa_{CO_{2(1)}} \times f_{(1)} = Pa_{CO_{2(2)}} \times f_{(2)}$$

Box 41-20 • Example of the Effect of Change in $\dot{V}_A$ on $Paco_2$

If a patient has an initial $Paco_2$ of 50 mm Hg with a corresponding alveolar ventilation ($\dot{V}_A$) of 4 L/min, what level of alveolar ventilation is required to decrease the $Paco_2$ to 40 mm Hg (if there is no change in $\dot{V}co_2$)?

Initial Desired

$$Paco_{2(1)} \times \dot{V}_{A(1)} = Paco_{2(2)} \times \dot{V}_{A(2)}$$

$$50 \times 4 = 40 \times \dot{V}_{A(2)}$$

$$\dot{V}_{A(2)} \text{ desired} = (50 \times 40)/40 = 5 \text{ L/min}$$

If the patient's $\dot{V}_A$ is increased from 4 L/min to 5 L/min, the $Paco_2$ should decrease from 50 to 40 mm Hg.

For changes in tidal volume alone, this becomes

Initial Desired

$$Paco_{2(1)} \times V_{T(1)} = Paco_{2(2)} \times V_{T(2)}$$

A major goal of mechanical ventilatory support is optimization of the patient's ventilation and $Paco_2$. Acceptable arterial pH and alveolar pressure are maintained as assessed by plateau pressure. For many patients, this means adjusting the level of ventilatory support to achieve a $Paco_2$ of 35 to 45 mm Hg with a pH of 7.35 to 7.45. In the care of patients with acute exacerbation of chronic carbon dioxide retention, such as those with long-standing COPD and accompanying chronic ventilatory failure, the clinician may target ventilatory support to achieve the patient's "normal" $Paco_2$ and pH. For COPD patients with chronic hypercapnia, this may mean a target $Paco_2$ of 50 to 60 mm Hg with a pH of 7.35 to 7.38.

Regardless of the patient's condition, optimizing pH is more important than targeting a specific $Paco_2$ value.[10]

Adjusting Tidal Volume and Rate

Tidal volume and rate may be adjusted for a desired level of ventilation as assessed by $Paco_2$. Tidal volume usually is based on specific patient considerations, and respiratory rate is adjusted to achieve a desired $Paco_2$. For example, larger tidal volume may be chosen in the SIMV mode for patients with normal lungs (neuromuscular disease, postoperative state) to maintain lung volume. A smaller tidal volume may be the target in the care of patients with ALI/ARDS to ensure plateau pressure is 30 cm H_2O or less or in patients with acute, severe asthma exacerbation to avoid barotrauma and auto-PEEP. A large tidal volume may improve Pao_2 and help prevent the development of atelectasis. Small tidal volume (<7 mL/kg) has been associated with the development of progressive microatelectasis.[13,14] Because of this association, intermittent lung hyperinflation or sighs have been used in the past when smaller tidal volume was used.

Once an appropriate tidal volume has been selected, rate is increased or decreased to achieve a target $Paco_2$. Options for altering $Paco_2$ for ventilator patients include changing rate, changing tidal volume, and changing mechanical dead space. Three types of patients frequently are encountered for whom $Paco_2$ may be adjusted. These are apneic patients, spontaneously breathing patients receiving ventilation in the SIMV mode, and spontaneously breathing patients receiving ventilation in the assist-control mode. Optimizing ventilation and $Paco_2$ in each of these situations is discussed.

Apnea (Controlled Ventilation)

In the apneic patient, precise control of $Paco_2$ usually can be achieved with volume ventilation (VC-CMV) because the ventilator rate and tidal volume are determined by the clinician.

Rate. In the care of apneic patients, the clinician has complete control over the patient's rate, and changes in ventilator rate can be used to precisely alter $Paco_2$. For rate changes alone (tidal volume held constant):

Initial Desired

$$Paco_{2(1)} \times f_{(1)} = Paco_{2(2)} \times f_{(2)}$$

For example, if a patient's initial rate was 8 breaths/min and the resultant $Paco_2$ was 50 mm Hg, the rate change needed to decrease the patient's $Paco_2$ to 40 mm Hg could be calculated:

Initial Desired

$$Paco_{2(1)} \times f_{(1)} = Paco_{2(2)} \times f_{(2)}$$

$$50 \times 8 = 40 \times f_{(2)}$$

$$f_{(2)} = (50 \times 8)/40 = 10 \text{ breaths/min}$$

For this patient, an increase in machine rate from 8 to 10 breaths/min would decrease $Paco_2$ from 50 to 40 mm Hg. Two warnings must be kept in mind in the use of this predictive equation. First, it is assumed that $\dot{V}co_2$ is constant. If there is an increase or decrease in $\dot{V}co_2$, the resultant $Paco_2$ is different form the predicted value. Common causes of increased $\dot{V}co_2$ in the ICU include pain, agitation, anxiety, fever, overfeeding, increased activity, and fighting the ventilator. Decreases in $\dot{V}co_2$ may be caused by decreased activity, sedation, paralysis, anesthesia, or sleep. Second, the equation is based on the assumption that the patient is apneic. Patients who are triggering the ventilator in the assist-control mode determine their own $Paco_2$ on the basis of the assist rate. Patients in the IMV or SIMV mode who are spontaneously breathing may simply increase or decrease their level of spontaneous breathing and make $Paco_2$ prediction difficult.

Tidal Volume. Changes in tidal volume can be used to alter $PaCO_2$. For example, for a 70-kg (IBW) patient receiving ventilation in the control mode with a tidal volume of 800 mL (12 mL/kg) and a resultant $PaCO_2$ of 30 mm Hg, the tidal volume change to achieve a PaO_2 of 40 mm Hg would be calculated as follows:

Initial Desired

$$PaCO_{2(1)} \times V_{T(1)} = PaCO_{2(2)} \times V_{T(2)}$$

$$30 \times 800 = 40 \times V_{T(2)}$$

$$V_{T(2)} = (30 \times 800)/40 = 600 \text{ mL}$$

For this patient, a decrease in V_T from 800 to 600 mL results in an increase in $PaCO_2$ from 30 to 40 mm Hg. Again, several warnings should be kept in mind for changes in tidal volume. First, the tidal volume should be within the preferred range for a given patient condition. Tidal volume should be large enough to prevent atelectasis and maintain lung volume, but small enough to avoid barotrauma, and maintain plateau pressure at 30 cm H_2O or less. Second, in this equation $\dot{V}CO_2$ and physiologic dead space (V_{DSphys}) are assumed to be constant, and changes in $\dot{V}CO_2$ or V_{DSphys} affect $PaCO_2$. Activity, agitation, fever, and overfeeding may increase $\dot{V}CO_2$, whereas sedation, paralysis, or sleep may decrease $\dot{V}CO_2$. Physiologic dead space changes with changes in airway pressure and increases in ventilator tidal volume may result in increased dead space. Development of pulmonary emboli may abruptly increase physiologic dead space. Last, in the equation, apnea (control mode) is assumed, so the equation cannot be used in the treatment of patients who are triggering the ventilator in the assist-control mode or patients who are breathing spontaneously in the SIMV mode.

Mechanical Dead Space. Mechanical dead space is defined as the volume of gas rebreathed as the result of use of a mechanical device. Large-bore tubing attached between the patient wye and the patient connection serves as mechanical dead space, and 6 inches (15 cm) of large-bore tubing represents a volume of approximately 50 to 70 mL.

Six inches (15 cm) of mechanical dead space often is used for ventilation of tracheostomy patients to keep the weight of the wye connection and tubing off of the tracheostomy tube and to give additional flexibility to the circuit for patient movement. Mechanical dead space usually is not used for endotracheally intubated patients, and the addition of mechanical dead space can serve as a reservoir for secretions and bacteria. In the care of apneic patients, however, the addition of mechanical dead space can be used to increase $PaCO_2$. In general, $PaCO_2$ increases 2 to 3 mm Hg for each 6 inches (15 cm) of dead space added. The exact amount of mechanical dead space to add is calculated as follows:

Box 41-21 • Mechanical Dead Space

A patient is receiving mechanical ventilation in the control mode with the following ventilator settings and related physiologic values:

V_T: 800 mL
f: 12 breaths/min
V_{Dmech}: 0 mL
V_{Dphys}: 400 mL
$V_D/V_T = 0.50$*
$PaCO_2$: 30 mm Hg

How much additional mechanical dead space is needed to increase the $PaCO_2$ to 40 mm Hg?

$$V_{Dmech(2)} = V_T - V_{Dphys} - \left[\frac{PaCO_{2(1)}\ (V_T - V_{Dphys} - V_{Dmach(1)})}{PaCO_{2(2)}}\right]$$

$$V_{Dmech(2)} = 800 - 400 - \left[\frac{30\ (800 - 400 - 0)}{40}\right]$$

$$= 100 \text{ mL}$$

* $V_{DS}/V_T = (PaCO_2 - P\bar{E}CO_2)/PaCO_2$ and $V_{DSphys} = V_{DS}/V_T \times V_T$

Initial Final

$$PaCO_{2(1)}\ (V_{T(1)} - V_{Dphys(1)} - V_{Dmech(1)})f_{(1)} = PaCO_{2(2)}\ (V_{T(2)} - V_{Dphys(2)} - V_{Dmech(2)})f_{(2)}$$

or

$$V_{Dmech(2)} = V_T - V_{Dphys} - \left(\frac{PaCO_{2(1)}\ (V_T - V_D - V_{Dmech(1)})}{PaCO_{2(2)}}\right)$$

An example of the calculation of the amount of mechanical dead space to add in the control mode in the treatment of an apneic patient is found in Box 41-21.

V_{DSphys} is calculated as follows:

$$V_{Dphys} = \left(\frac{PaCO_2 - P\bar{E}CO_2}{PaCO_2}\right) \times V_T$$

where $P\bar{E}CO_2$ is the partial pressure of expired carbon dioxide.

In healthy persons, physiologic and anatomic dead space are approximately the same and can be estimated at approximately 1 mL per pound of IBW. Although healthy persons have a dead space to tidal volume ratio (V_{DS}/V_T) of approximately 0.20 to 0.40, a V_{DS}/V_T ratio of 0.50 or higher is not uncommon among ventilator patients. As with the predictive equations for tidal volume and rate changes, in this equation it is assumed that $\dot{V}CO_2$ and physiologic dead space are constant and that the patient is apneic (control mode).

Control of $PaCO_2$ in the Synchronized Intermittent Mandatory Ventilation Mode

In the SIMV mode, machine breaths are interspersed with spontaneous breathing, and the spontaneous

MINI CLINI

Adjusting $PaCO_2$ During Volume Ventilation

PROBLEM

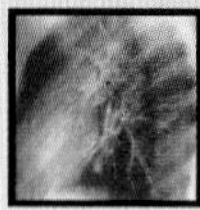

A 22-year-old, 5 ft 10 in (178 cm) man being treated for a drug overdose is being ventilated with the following settings:

Mode: SIMV with PSV (VC-IMV)
FIO_2: 0.40
V_T: 750 mL
SIMV rate: 15 breaths/min
Total rate: 15 breaths/min
PIP: 30 cm H_2O
P_{plat}: 25 cm H_2O
PEEP/CPAP: +3 cm H_2O
PSV: +5 cm H_2O

The patient's lungs are clear to auscultation, and there is no evidence of aspiration.

Arterial blood gas values obtained 15 minutes ago were:

PaO_2: 80 mm Hg	$PaCO_2$: 30 mm Hg
SaO_2: 95%	HCO_3: 24 mEq/L
pH: 7.52	BE: +2 mEq/L

The physician asks the respiratory therapist to normalize this patient's oxygenation and ventilatory status. What should the respiratory therapist do?

SOLUTION

At this time, the patient is making no spontaneous breathing efforts. In the absence of spontaneous breathing in the volume-control mode, $PaCO_2$ can be adjusted by changing machine rate (f), tidal volume (V_T), and mechanical dead space (V_{DSmach}).

For prediction of the needed change in tidal volume to increase the $PaCO_2$ to 40 mm Hg, the following calculation could be performed:

Actual Desired

$$V_{T(1)} \times PaCO_{2(1)} = V_{T(2)} \times PaCO_{2(2)}$$
$$V_{T(2)}\text{ Desired} = (V_{T(1)} \times PaCO_{2(1)})/PaCO_{2(2)}$$
$$V_{T(2)}\text{ Desired} = (750 \times 30)/40 = 563\text{ mL}$$

If V_T is decreased to 550 to 600 mL, $PaCO_2$ and pH should normalize. However, the patient's IBW is 166 lb (75 kg; 166 lb/2.2). The current V_T is 750 mL, or 10 mL/kg. If V_T is decreased to 550 mL, the result is only approximately 7 mL/kg (550 mL/75 kg). Peak inspiratory pressure and plateau pressure are acceptable (P_{plat}, 25 cm H_2O). The patient's lungs are clear, and most likely this patient has normal lung function. Preferred tidal volume for patients with normal lungs is in the range of 10 to 12 mL/kg. A larger volume (up to 15 mL/kg) with a slower rate sometimes is used to maintain lung volume and satisfy air hunger. A reduction in V_T of less than 10 mL/kg is not indicated for this patient.

The alternative for increasing this patient's $PaCO_2$ would be to decrease the rate. The rate change needed to increase this patient's $PaCO_2$ from 30 to 40 mm Hg can be calculated as follows:

Initial Desired

$$f_{(1)} \times PaCO_{2(1)} = f_{(2)} \times PaCO_{2(2)}$$
$$f_{(2)}\text{ desired} = (f_{(1)} \times PaCO_{2(1)})/PaCO_{2(2)}$$
$$f_{(2)}\text{ desired} = (15 \times 30)/40 = 11.25$$

A decrease in SIMV rate from 15 to 11 or 12 breaths/min should result in an increase in $PaCO_2$ and a pH that is closer to normal. It is assumed that the patient does not resume spontaneous breathing when the SIMV rate is decreased.

The third option for increasing $PaCO_2$ for this patient would be to add V_{DSmach}. This option is not recommended for patients undergoing ventilation in the SIMV or assist-control mode. However, one can expect approximately a 2 to 3 mm Hg increase in $PaCO_2$ for each 6 inches (15 cm) of dead space added when the patient is in the control mode. The V_{DSmach} needed can be calculated more accurately should this be desired.

The best decision for this patient would be to decrease the SIMV rate to 12 breaths/min and to monitor for the beginning of spontaneous breathing.

breaths may be pressure supported (PSV). The $PaCO_2$ can be decreased by increasing tidal volume, increasing PSV for spontaneous breaths, or increasing the machine rate. Levels of $PaCO_2$ may be increased by reducing the machine rate, decreasing tidal volume, or decreasing the level of PSV for spontaneous breaths. As with apneic (control) ventilation, we suggest that an appropriate tidal volume be selected on the basis of the patient's condition and with the goal of keeping plateau pressure at 30 cm H_2O or less. Pressure-support ventilation level in the SIMV mode should be adjusted to overcome WOB_I, and the usual range is 5 to 10 cm H_2O, although higher levels may be needed by patients with high resistance or a high spontaneous inspiratory flow rate. Pressure-support ventilation should be adjusted to ensure that during spontaneous breathing, the work of breathing is not excessive. Accessory muscle use or suprasternal, intercostal, or substernal retractions during spontaneous breathing would indicate the need to increase the PSV level. Once an appropriate tidal volume and PSV level are selected, the primary method for adjusting $PaCO_2$ is to increase or decrease the SIMV rate.

After ventilator initiation, two different approaches may be taken. For full ventilatory support, an initial SIMV rate and tidal volume are selected to provide 100% of the patient's ventilatory requirements. For most adults, this means starting with a tidal volume of 10 to 12 mL/kg with an SIMV rate of 10 to 12 breaths/min. In general, a minute ventilation of approximately 100 mL/kg IBW is achieved with these initial settings.

Arterial blood gas values are obtained 20 to 30 minutes after initiation of mechanical ventilation, and the SIMV rate is titrated up or down in increments of 2 breaths/min until the desired $Paco_2$ is achieved. Monitoring is continued, and adjustments are made by increasing or decreasing the SIMV rate to maintain full ventilatory support until the patient's condition improves and ventilator weaning is considered.

Partial ventilatory support in the SIMV mode requires a different initial approach. Ventilation begins with a tidal volume and machine rate sufficient to provide full ventilatory support, and arterial blood gases are measured. If $Paco_2$ is adequate, the patient is immediately challenged with a decrease in the SIMV rate of 2 breaths/min. This procedure is followed by patient assessment and measurement of arterial blood gases. If the resultant blood gas values remain adequate, the patient continues to be challenged with decreases in the SIMV rate until $Paco_2$ increases. At that point, the patient's ventilatory capacity has been exceeded, and the SIMV rate is returned to the previous value. Box 41-22 provides an example of titration of the SIMV rate for partial ventilatory support after ventilator initiation in a spontaneously breathing patient.

Box 41-22 • Partial Ventilatory Support With SIMV

Mechanical ventilation is initiated in the SIMV mode for a 70-kg, spontaneously breathing 38-year-old male patient. Before initiation of ventilation, the patient's spontaneous rate was 30 breaths/min with a spontaneous tidal volume of 200 mL. Initial ventilator settings are

V_T: 700 mL
SIMV rate: 10 breaths/min
Fio_2: 0.40
PSV: +8 cm H_2O
PIP: 36 cm H_2O
P_{plat}: 28 cm H_2O

Arterial blood gases are obtained in 20 minutes, with the following results:

Pao_2: 88 mm Hg
Sao_2: 97%
pH: 7.38
$Paco_2$: 40 mm Hg
HCO_3: 24 mEq/L
BE: +1 mEq/L

The decision is made to provide partial ventilatory support for this patient, and the SIMV rate is titrated as follows:

Time	Tidal Volume (mL)	SIMV Rate (breaths/min)	Total Rate (breaths/min)	$Paco_2$ (mm Hg)
9:00 AM	700	10	20	40
9:30 AM	700	8	15	38
10:00 AM	700	6	18	38
10:30 AM	700	4	24	46
11:00 AM	700	6	18	42

The patient's condition should now be stabilized at a rate of 6 breaths/min with titration of SIMV to the patient's needs with observation and measurement of arterial blood gases. When the rate is decreased to 4 breaths/min, $Paco_2$ begins to increase. The rate is then increased to the previous setting of 6 breaths/min. Titrating the level of SIMV support to the patient's needs is not the same as weaning the patient. After improvement in the patient's condition, weaning may be tried (see Chapter 44) with a daily spontaneous breathing trial or further reductions in the SIMV rate.

Assist-Control Mode Volume Ventilation and $Paco_2$

Ventilator initiation in the assist-control mode begins with selection of an initial tidal volume and backup control rate to ensure a safe minimum level of ventilation. The patient is allowed to trigger the machine as often as desired above this backup rate, and the resultant assist rate is determined by the patient's ventilatory drive. If the respiratory drive is intact, patients tend to trigger the ventilator at an appropriate rate to achieve an adequate $Paco_2$ and pH. By allowing patients to set their own rates, the level of ventilation increases or decreases on the basis of the patient's physiologic needs. Should the patient become apneic owing to sedation or sleep, a minimum backup control rate is provided.

Because the patient determines the level of ventilation, $Paco_2$ levels are regulated by the patient. This is a simple and physiologically sound approach to mechanical ventilation. Problems arise, however, when the patient triggers the ventilator at an inappropriately rapid rate. Pain, anxiety, hypoxemia, secretions in the airway, and metabolic acidosis may contribute to an excessive trigger rate. The result can be an inappropriate I:E ratio and an inadequate expiratory time. These abnormal values may increase mean airway pressure, reduce venous return, and result in auto-PEEP and overinflation, especially in patients with obstructive disease. Patients may fight the ventilator, the result being high inspiratory pressure. In the event that a patient receiving ventilation in the assist-control mode is triggering the ventilator at an inappropriately high rate, the first step the therapist should take is to identify the problem. Patient anxiety may be diminished with simple reassurance and encouragement to relax and "let the machine breathe for you." Hypoxemia should be managed with appropriate oxygen therapy and PEEP or CPAP, if indicated. Secretions should be removed by suctioning, and bronchial hygiene techniques should be applied. The cause of metabolic acidosis should be identified and managed, if possible. If correcting the cause of an inappropriately high trigger rate fails, the SIMV mode can be considered. Synchronized intermittent mandatory ventilation is the preferred mode for patients with COPD or acute, severe asthma exacerbation to avoid overinflation and auto-PEEP. For these patients, expiratory times should be increased as needed to avoid air trapping.

Patients who begin fighting the ventilator after a previous period of calm may have a new and potentially life-threatening complication. If a patient begins fighting the ventilator, a careful assessment should be made to identify the problem. Often, careful attention to the ventilator trigger sensitivity, flow rate, volume, and pressure is helpful, and administration of analgesic and sedative agents may be needed.[10] A last resort is pharmacological paralysis and controlled ventilation.[10] In the presence of metabolic acidosis, a sudden change from assisted ventilation at a rapid rate with the associated hyperventilation to controlled ventilation at a slower rate can result in severe acidosis, which can be life threatening. Other problems with controlled ventilation include patient safety, ventilatory muscle atrophy, and prolonged muscle weakness after discontinuance of paralytic agents.

Pressure-Support Ventilation and $Pa{CO_2}$

With the use of SIMV with PSV, the PSV usually is set at the level needed to overcome WOB_I and is not routinely increased or decreased to effect ventilation. The PSV_{max}, however, is an assist mode of ventilation. With PSV_{max}, PSV levels are titrated for an appropriate tidal volume and at a level that allows the patient trigger rate to decrease to the range of 10 to 20 breaths/min while acceptable $Pa{CO_2}$ and pH are maintained. To increase or decrease tidal volume, the clinician simply increases or decreases the PSV level and observes the resultant tidal volume on the ventilator exhaled volume monitoring screen or window. Because PSV_{max} is an assist mode, the patient is allowed to trigger the ventilator as desired. The result should be adequate $Pa{CO_2}$ and pH. In patients with an unstable ventilatory drive or periods of apnea, PSV_{max} should be avoided .

Pressure-Control Ventilation and $Pa{CO_2}$

Management of ventilation and $Pa{CO_2}$ during PCV can be challenging. Pressure-control ventilation is time or patient triggered to begin inspiration, pressure limited, and time cycled to expiration. Most ventilators offering PCV allow the clinician to set machine rate (f), trigger sensitivity, pressure limit, and percentage inspiratory time ($\%T_i$) or I:E ratio.

In PCV mode, as the difference between inspiratory pressure and baseline pressure (ΔP) increases, tidal volume increases. As ΔP decreases, tidal volume decreases. In general, baseline pressure (PEEP/CPAP) is set to optimize oxygenation and lung volume. The pressure limit is adjusted up or down to deliver a desired tidal volume. To increase or decrease $Pa{CO_2}$ in the PCV mode, the therapist can simply increase or decrease the pressure limit while observing the exhaled tidal volume on the ventilator display monitor until the desired tidal volume is obtained. The most important problem with the use of tidal volume to adjust $Pa{CO_2}$ in the PCV mode is that the pressure should not be increased above 30 cm H_2O, if possible, to avoid ventilator-induced lung injury. In the management of ALI/ARDS, it is recommended that tidal volume be limited to 6 mL/kg. On the other hand, in patients without acute restrictive lung disease, delivered tidal volume should be at least 7 mL/kg to avoid the development of atelectasis. Consequently, the range of acceptable tidal volume in the PCV mode may be limited.

The alternative to tidal volume for altering $Pa{CO_2}$ in the PCV mode is to change the rate. If tidal volume remains constant, an increase in rate decreases $Pa{CO_2}$ and vice versa. However, in the PCV mode, $\%T_i$ and I:E ratio may be fixed. If $\%T_i$ is constant and respiratory rate is increased, actual inspiratory time decreases, and tidal volume also may decrease. Decreases in rate ($\%T_i$ and pressure limit constant) may result in an increase in delivered tidal volume. The following example demonstrates this principle.

A patient receiving ventilation in the PCV mode has an inspiratory pressure of 25 cm H_2O, PEEP of +5 cm H_2O, %Ti of 50%, I:E ratio of 1:1 , and rate of 15 breaths/min. In this example, respiratory cycle time can be calculated as follows:

$$\text{Respiratory cycle} = 60/f = 60/15 = 4 \text{ s}$$

Inspiratory time (T_i) would be

$$T_i = \%T_i \times \text{Respiratory cycle} = 0.50 \times 4 = 2 \text{ s}$$

A pressure of 25 cm H_2O applied for 2 seconds might achieve a tidal volume of 600 mL for this patient.

If the rate were increased to 20 breaths/min, what would happen to respiratory cycle time, inspiratory time, and delivered tidal volume? Respiratory cycle and inspiratory time are calculated for a rate of 20 breaths/min as follows:

$$\text{Respiratory cycle} = 60/f = 60/20 = 3 \text{ s}$$

$$T_i = \%T_i \times \text{Respiratory cycle} = 0.50 \times 3 = 1.5 \text{ s}$$

At a constant inspiratory pressure of 25 cm H_2O, a decrease in inspiratory time from 2 seconds to 1.5 seconds may reduce delivered tidal volume to 500 mL. Thus an increase in respiratory rate may actually reduce delivered tidal volume and increase (rather than decrease) $Pa{CO_2}$.

A

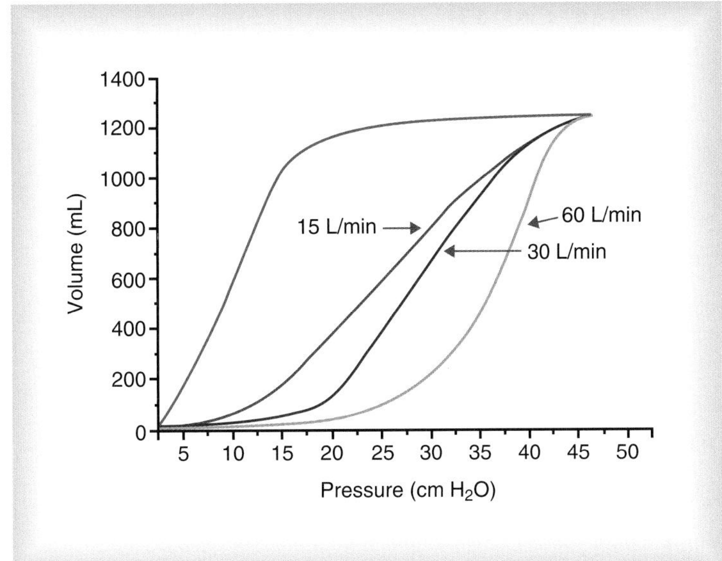

B

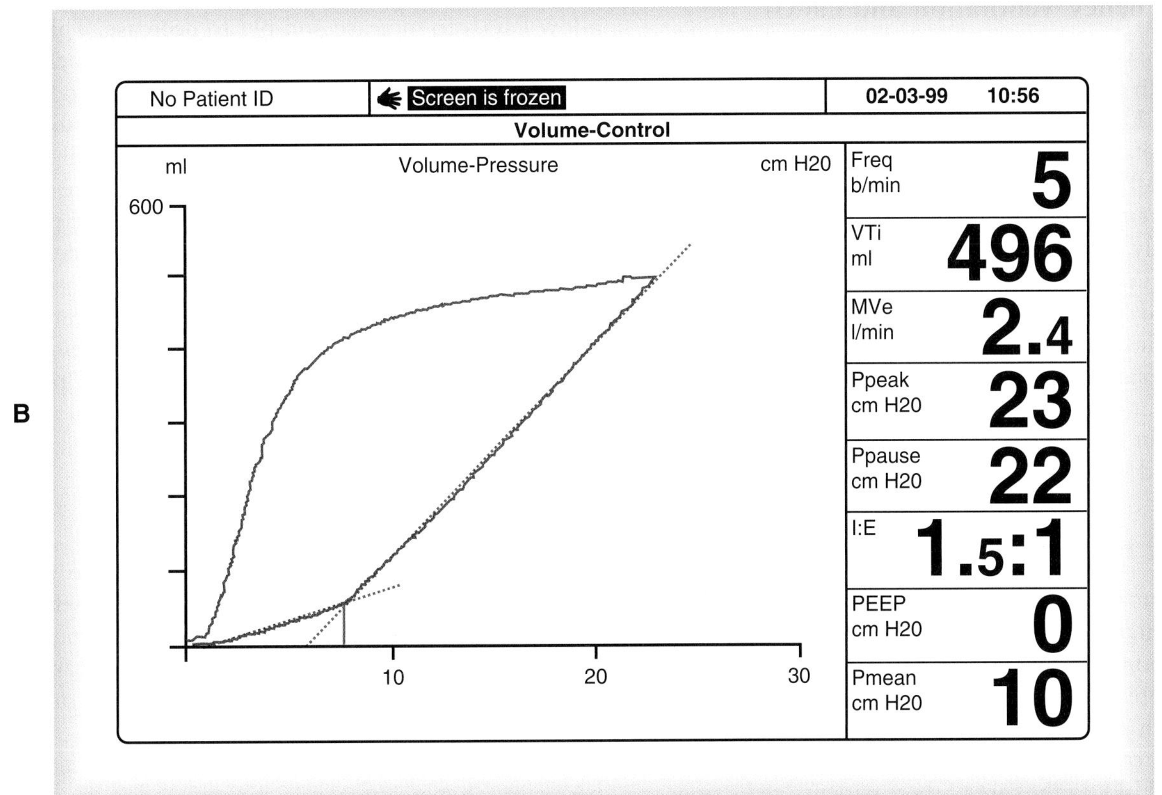

Figure 41-12

A, Pressure-volume curves generated by a ventilator graphics package with the flow set at 60, 30, and 15 L/min. As flow is decreased, the curve shifts to the left and more closely approximates a static pressure-volume curve. Flow of less than 15 L/min is recommended for substituting the lower inflection point (*LIP*) from a slow-flow pressure-volume curve for the static curve value. **B,** Slow-flow (<10 L/min) pressure-volume curve with use of a set rate of 5 breaths/min, I:E ratio of 1.5:1, and V_T of 500 mL. The LIP is approximately 8 cm H_2O. The respiratory cycle time is 12 seconds (Cycle time = 60/f = 60/5 = 12 s). An I:E ratio of 1.5:1 results in an inspiratory time of 4.8 seconds. Inspiratory flow is V_T/T_i = 0.5 L/4.8 s = 0.104 L/s, or approximately 6 L/min. *(Modified from Haas C: AARC Times 24:64, 2000.)*

When using PCV, the respiratory therapist should observe the effect of inspiratory time and pressure limit on the patient's flow and volume curves as displayed by a ventilator graphics monitoring package. In general, as inspiratory time increases at a given pressure, volume also increases until an inspiratory plateau or hold is reached. This point can be identified by observing the inspiratory flow curve. If the curve decreases to zero and holds that value for a time before exhalation begins, an inspiratory plateau is present (Figure 41-12). Further increases in inspiratory time do not result in additional tidal volume. Conversely, if an inspiratory plateau or hold is present, a decrease in inspiratory time does not decrease tidal volume (at the same pressure limit) until the inspiratory plateau is no longer present (Figure 41-13).

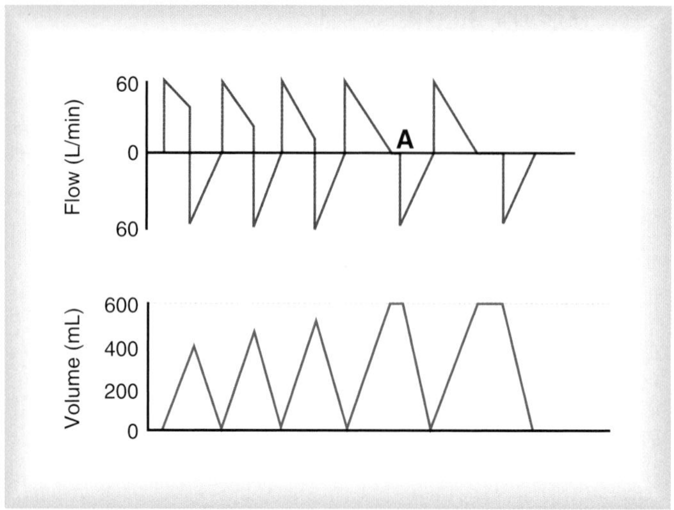

Figure 41-13
The effect of inspiratory time and inspiratory plateau on delivered tidal volume (V_T) in the PCV mode. Initially, as inspiratory time is increased, V_T increases. Once an inspiratory plateau **(A)** is achieved, a further increase in inspiratory time does not result in increased V_T. The same effect occurs as inspiratory time is decreased. Initially, with small decreases in inspiratory time, there would be no change in V_T as long as an end-inspiratory plateau were maintained. Once the inspiratory time is less than that needed for an inspiratory plateau, further decreases in inspiratory time will result in a decrease in V_T at the same pressure.

High-Frequency Ventilation and $Pa{CO_2}$

Management of $Pa{CO_2}$ during HFV presents special challenges. In general, HFV allows for setting a baseline pressure (PEEP/CPAP) and an inspiratory pressure. The difference between the inspiratory pressure and baseline pressure (ΔP) determines tidal volume. As ΔP is increased, ventilation improves, and $Pa{CO_2}$ decreases. Consequently, changes in ΔP can be used to affect $Pa{CO_2}$. Frequency and $\%T_i$ determine inspiratory time. With a fixed $\%T_i$, decreases in frequency result in an increase in inspiratory time and an increase in ventilation (at the same ΔP). Consequently, unlike in conventional mechanical ventilation, in HFV a decrease in rate may result in an *increase* in ventilation and a *decrease* in $Pa{CO_2}$ and vice versa.

Permissive Hypercapnia

Most patients who need mechanical ventilatory support can be adequately maintained with an acceptable $Pa{CO_2}$ and corresponding pH by appropriate adjustments in ventilator rate and tidal volume. However, in the care of patients with ALI/ARDS, a tidal volume of 6 mL/kg or less may be required to maintain plateau pressure of less than 30 cm H_2O. In the care of these patients, reductions in tidal volume may be compensated for by increasing the ventilator rate. For example, a 70-kg patient with ARDS may need a tidal volume of 400 mL (6 mL/kg) to maintain a plateau pressure of 30 cm H_2O or less. This may require a respiratory rate of approximately 18 breaths/min to maintain a target minute ventilation of approximately 100 mL/kg IBW and normal $Pa{CO_2}$ and pH. With a low tidal volume, patients with increased $\dot{V}{CO_2}$ or increased V_{DS}/V_T may need a respiratory rate as high as 25 to 30 breaths/min or the administration of sodium bicarbonate to maintain a normal pH and $Pa{CO_2}$.[16] For these patients, the decision may be made to allow $Pa{CO_2}$ to increase and pH to decrease. This technique is known as permissive hypercapnia.[6] An elevated $Pa{CO_2}$ resulting in a pH in the range of 7.25 to 7.35 is well tolerated by most patients. In the presence of cardiac ischemia, left ventricular compromise, pulmonary hypertension, or right heart failure, permissive hypercapnia should be used with caution.[17] In addition, patients with head trauma, intracranial disease, or metabolic acidosis may be at greater risk, and an intracranial lesion is considered an absolute contraindication to permissive hypercapnia.[17] Permissive hypercapnia may be instituted rapidly; however, most clinicians prefer a gradual approach, allowing $Pa{CO_2}$ to increase incrementally over a period of hours.

Open Lung Approach

The open lung approach, described by Amato et al,[38] combines permissive hypercapnia, PCV, PEEP set above the lower inflection point of the pressure-volume curve, and the use of reduced tidal volume (<6 mL/kg).[38,63] Although open lung techniques may improve outcome in ARDS, additional studies are needed.[64]

In addition to being recommended for ARDS patients, permissive hypercapnia is a recommended ventilatory strategy for patients with acute, severe asthma exacerbations necessitating mechanical ventilation.[20] Signs of impending ventilatory failure in these patients include declining mental clarity, worsening fatigue, and $Pa{CO_2}$ of 42 mm Hg or more.[20,21] For these patients, intubation and mechanical ventilation may be instituted, and the ventilator adjusted to minimize airway pressure and allow a prolonged expiratory time to avoid auto-PEEP and barotrauma. Tidal volume of 10 mL/kg or less and a rate of 8 breaths/min or less along with sufficient sedation to avoid ventilator dyssynchrony have been recommended.[7]

MINI CLINI

Adjusting Ventilation in PCV Mode

PROBLEM

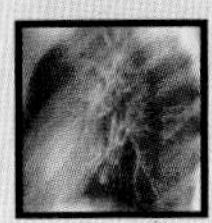

A 70-kg (IBW) ARDS patient is receiving PCV in the control mode with the following ventilator settings:

Pressure: 25 cm H_2O
Rate: 15 breaths/min
$\%T_i$: 50%
I:E ratio: 1.1
FIO_2: 0.60
PEEP: +8 cm H_2O
V_T (exhaled): 425 mL

Arterial blood gas values with these ventilator settings are as follows:

PaO_2: 60 mm Hg
SaO_2: 90%
pH: 7.30
$PaCO_2$: 50 mm Hg
HCO_3: 23 mEq/L
BE: –2 mEq/L

The inspiratory and expiratory flow curves on the ventilator graphics display are as follows:

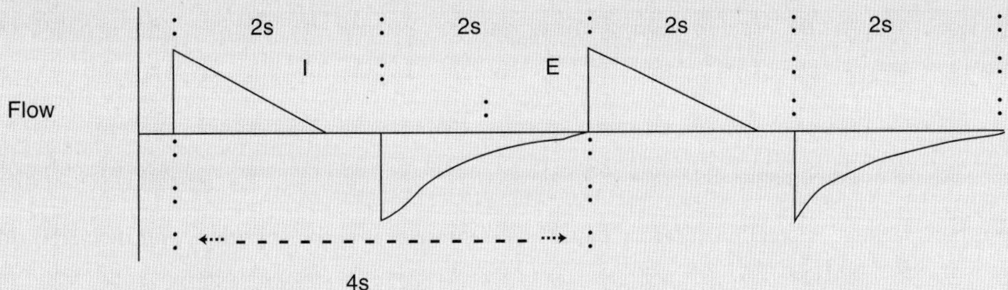

The physician requests that the respiratory rate be increased to 18 breaths/min to decrease the patient's $PaCO_2$ to 40 mm Hg and normalize the pH. What should the respiratory therapist do?

SOLUTION

This patient has a PaO_2/FIO_2 ratio of 100 (60/0.60), which is consistent with the diagnosis of ARDS. Special considerations for the ventilatory management of ARDS include maintaining the plateau pressure at 30 cm H_2O or less. Tidal volume is started at 8 mL/kg and then gradually reduced to 6 mL/kg to achieve this goal and minimize ventilator-induced lung injury. Respiratory rate may be increased to maintain $PaCO_2$ and pH closer to normal, as long as volume and plateau pressure are acceptable. The $PaCO_2$ may be allowed to increase if necessary to maintain plateau pressure at 30 cm H_2O or less and as long as pH is 7.25 or higher. Oxygenation problems are managed initially with PEEP to achieve a PaO_2 of 60 mm Hg or more with an acceptable FIO_2. If PEEP fails to improve PaO_2, alternative techniques may be tried, including inverse ratio ventilation and prone positioning.

For this patient, the tidal volume is acceptable at approximately 6 mL/kg (70 kg × 6 mL/kg = 420 mL), and P_{plat} is 25 cm H_2O. The $PaCO_2$ (50 mm Hg) and pH (7.30) are acceptable, and a PEEP of +8 cm H_2O with an I:E ratio of 1:1 is appropriate for an ARDS patient. To decrease $PaCO_2$, the rate could be increased as follows:

Initial Desired

$$f_{(1)} \times PaCO_{2(1)} = f_{(2)} \times PaCO_2$$

$$15 \times 50 = f_{(2)} \times 40$$

$$f_{(2)} \text{ Desired} = (15 \times 50/40 = 18.75$$

If tidal volume is maintained at 425 mL, a rate of 18 to 19 breaths/min should bring the $PaCO_2$ and pH into normal range. However, with PCV and a fixed $\%T_i$, if rate is changed, respiratory cycle time, inspiratory time, and expiratory time also change. In this case, the current inspiratory time (T_i) can be calculated as follows:

$$\text{Respiratory cycle time} = 60/f = 60/15 = 4 \text{ s}$$

$$T_i = \%T_i \times (60/f) = 0.50 \times 4 \text{ s} = 2 \text{ s}$$

If respiratory rate is increased to 18 breaths/min, T_i becomes the following:

$$T_i = \%T_i \times (60/f) = 0.50 \times (60/18) = 0.50 \times 3.33 = 1.67 \text{ s}$$

Continued

MINI CLINI—cont'd

With PCV, if pressure is held constant, tidal volume may change with changes in inspiratory time. Specifically, a decrease in inspiratory time may decrease tidal volume at the same pressure level. However, tidal volume tends *not* to change as long as an end-inspiratory pause is still present. In this case, the machine rate is increased from 15 to 18 breaths/min with the following results:

PaO_2 = 62 mm Hg
V_T = 425 mL
SaO_2 = 91%
f = 18 breaths/min
pH = 7.38
FIO_2 = 0.60
$PaCO_2$ = 44 mm Hg
PEEP = +8 cm H_2O
HCO_3 = 24 mEq/L
BE = −1 mEq/L

The ventilator graphics display for flow is as follows:

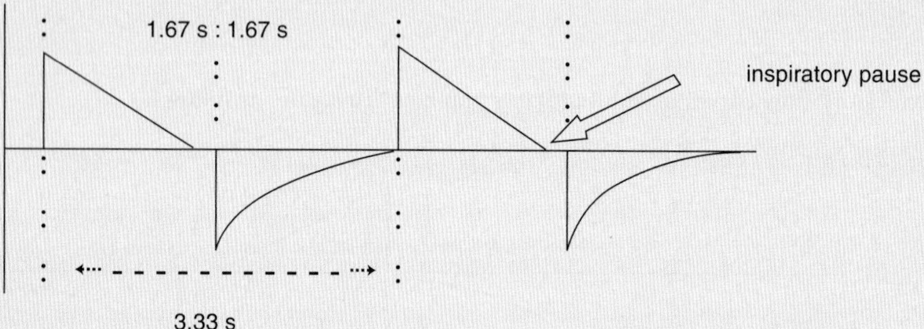

As noted on the graphics package, a small inspiratory pause is still present at end inspiration, and delivered tidal volume does not change.

Alternative Lung Protective Strategies for Acute Lung Injury and Acute Respiratory Distress Syndrome

Alternative techniques for facilitating carbon dioxide removal while lung protective strategies are implemented in the management of ARDS include extracorporeal carbon dioxide removal, extracorporeal membrane oxygenation (ECMO), reduction of carbon dioxide production by control of fever, avoidance of overfeeding, neuromuscular paralysis, intravascular membrane oxygenation (IVOX, IMO), HFV, and tracheal gas insufflation.[6,12,17] Tracheal gas insufflation involves insertion of a tracheal catheter for injection of fresh gas into the central airways to improve alveolar ventilation and reduce the level of mechanical ventilatory support required.[65]

A very rapid rate and small tidal volume are used in HFV. Types of HFV include high-frequency jet ventilation (HFJV), high-frequency percussive ventilation (HFPV), and high-frequency oscillation (HFO).[35] The smaller tidal volume and ability to better maintain adequate $PaCO_2$ levels during HFV make HFV an attractive option for ALI/ARDS patients as part of a lung protective strategy. More research, however, is needed to demonstrate the value of HFV in the care of adult patients with severe respiratory failure.[35] There is evidence that HFO, in particular, may be safe and effective in significantly improving gas exchange and reducing FIO_2 in adult patients with severe ARDS for whom conventional mechanical ventilation is unsuccessful.[36]

Extracorporeal membrane oxygenation is effective in supporting newborns with acute respiratory failure; survival rates of 80% have been achieved.[66] The results of early studies of ECMO in the treatment of adult patients with ARDS were disappointing.[9] The use of new, advanced ECMO technology may be beneficial in the care of adults with ARDS; however, randomized, controlled studies are needed to demonstrate the value of ECMO to adults in respiratory failure.[66]

The first intravascular oxygenation and carbon dioxide removal device (IVOX) was capable of removing up to 30% of carbon dioxide produced in normocapnic patients and allowed reduction in ventilatory requirements.[67] In the future, IVOX-type devices may be beneficial in implementing lung protective ventilatory strategies in the management of severe respiratory failure.[67]

Table 41-11 ▶▶▶ Changing Ventilation and $Paco_2$

Mode Increase	Ventilation (↓$Paco_2$)	Decrease Ventilation (↑$Paco_2$)
Volume-Control Ventilation		
VC-CMV control	↑ V_T; ↑ f; remove V_{Dmach}	↓ V_T; ↓ f; add V_{Dmach}
VC-CMV assist control	↑ V_T; ↑ f (to greater than assist rate); remove V_{Dmach}	↓ V_T; ↓ f (may require sedation, control mode)
SIMV	↑ V_T; ↑ f; add/increase PSV	↓ V_T; ↓ f; reduce PSV
Pressure-Control Ventilation		
PCV*	↑ ΔP; ↑ f (maintaining same T_i)	↓ ΔP; ↓ f (maintaining same T_i)
PSV	↑ ΔP	↓ ΔP
BiPAP	↑ IPAP (↑ ΔP)	↓ IPAP (↓ ΔP)
APRV	↑ ΔP ↑ release frequency	↓ ΔP ↓ release frequency

In assist (patient-triggered) mode, the patient may simply alter the trigger rate after a ventilator change, and it becomes difficult to predict the results of a ventilator change on $Paco_2$ in the assist mode.
*In PCV, %T_i is preset; an increase in respiratory rate results in a decrease in inspiratory time and may reduce tidal volume (V_T). For example, if %T_i is set at 50% in PCV mode, an increase in rate from 15 to 20 breaths/min causes inspiratory time to decrease from 2 seconds (50% of 4 seconds) to 1.5 seconds (50% of 3 seconds). If the pressure limit is not changed, tidal volume will probably decrease.
APRV, airway pressure release ventilation; *IPAP,* inspiratory positive airway pressure.

In summary, adjustments to alter patients' ventilatory status vary depending on the mode of ventilation and the presence of spontaneous breathing. With control mode (apnea), $Paco_2$ can be precisely adjusted with changes in delivered tidal volume, respiratory rate, or mechanical dead space. For patients receiving ventilation in the SIMV mode, including SIMV with pressure support, $Paco_2$ adjustments are made by increasing or decreasing the SIMV rate, usually by 2 breaths/min and performing blood gas analysis. For assist-control modes, including PSV as a stand-alone mode (PSV_{max}), patients are allowed to set their own respiratory rate, as determined by their ventilatory drive. Because the patient's ventilatory drive determines rate, appropriate $Paco_2$ and pH levels should be achieved with minimal intervention by the clinician. In the event that the assist rates are too high, other modes of ventilation may be considered. Table 41-11 summarizes methods of altering $Paco_2$ during volume-control and pressure-control ventilation.

Acid-Base Homeostasis

An acceptable pH is a more desirable endpoint than a specific $Paco_2$. A normal pH (7.35-7.45) should be the clinician's goal; however, hypercapnia and mild respiratory acidosis will probably be well tolerated by most critically ill patients. Exceptions include patients with cardiovascular or neurologic problems, including myocardial ischemia, ventricular failure, head trauma, cerebrovascular accident, or neurosurgery.

Respiratory alkalosis caused by providing a higher level of mechanical support than needed may be desirable in patients with neurologic problems. Targeting a $Paco_2$ in the range of 25 to 30 mm Hg may be helpful in the care of these patients by causing cerebral vasoconstriction and reducing ICP.

Because changes in the level of ventilation result in an almost immediate change in $Paco_2$, the effect of a change in $Paco_2$ on pH can be estimated.[68] Estimating the effect of a change in ventilation on acid-base balance and pH can have important implications. As a rough rule, for an immediate change in $Paco_2$ of 10 mm Hg, pH changes in the opposite direction approximately 0.08.[21] For example, a patient with metabolic acidosis in the assist-control mode may be able to hyperventilate with the assistance of a ventilator; the result is a $Paco_2$ of 20 mm Hg with a pH of 7.30. Should sedation, paralysis, or a change to IMV mode eliminate the patient's ability to continue to hyperventilate, $Paco_2$ increases and pH decreases. In this example, if $Paco_2$ suddenly increases from 20 mm Hg to 40 mm Hg, pH decreases to approximately 7.14. The respiratory therapist must consider the effect of a ventilator change on overall acid-base balance to avoid harmful, even catastrophic results. Table 41-12 compares the effect of acute changes in $Paco_2$ on pH.

Metabolic acid-base disorders are common in the ICU. A common cause of metabolic acidosis is lactic acidosis due to severe hypoxia, often after cardiac arrest or severe hypotension. Renal failure and diabetic or alcoholic ketoacidosis also are common causes of metabolic acidosis in the ICU. In the event of severe metabolic acidosis, patients receiving mechanical ventilation may be hyperventilated to maintain a viable pH until the underlying cause of the acidosis can be addressed. Administration of sodium bicarbonate remains controversial; however, we believe that it should be considered in the event of severe acidosis as long as adequate ventilation and circulation are present. Current ARDSNet

Table 41-12 ▶▶ Effect of Acute Changes in Pa_{CO_2} on pH

Pa_{CO_2}	pH
80	7.16
70	7.22
60	7.28
50	7.34
40	7.40
35	7.45
30	7.50
25	7.55
20	7.60

From Malley JW: Clinical blood gases: applications and noninvasive alternatives, Philadelphia, 1990, WB Saunders.

guidelines for ventilation of patients with ALI/ARDS are to consider administration of sodium bicarbonate if a respiratory rate of 35 breaths/min is ineffective in maintaining a pH of at least 7.30.

Metabolic alkalosis is a common occurrence in the ICU. Common causes include electrolyte disturbances (hypokalemic and hypochloremic alkalosis), vomiting, and nasogastric suctioning. Treatment should be aimed at correcting the underlying cause of the alkalosis. In the case of severe metabolic alkalosis, administration of acetazolamide or ammonium chloride may be considered.

KEY POINTS

- The four main indications for mechanical ventilation are apnea, acute ventilatory failure, impending ventilatory failure, and severe oxygenation problems.
- Severe oxygenation problems are identified by an inadequate arterial oxygen level (Pa_{O_2} <60, Sa_{O_2} <90) with a moderate to high F_{IO_2} (>0.40-0.50).
- Goals of mechanical ventilatory support include maintaining ventilation, oxygenation, and acid-base balance while reducing work of breathing and minimizing harmful side effects and complications.
- Mechanical ventilation may be used to allow sedation or paralysis for certain procedures, decrease myocardial and ventilatory oxygen consumption, decrease ICP after closed head injury, and to stabilize the chest wall in the case of a massive flail or chest wall resection.
- Transpulmonary pressure of more than 30 to 35 cm H_2O is associated with alveolar overdistension and lung injury.

KEY POINTS—cont'd

- Plateau pressure should be maintained at less than 30 cm H_2O, if possible, to prevent ventilator-induced lung injury.
- Negative pressure ventilation may be useful to patients with chronic respiratory failure.
- Noninvasive positive pressure ventilation may be considered for acute exacerbation of COPD, to avoid intubation and conventional mechanical ventilation.
- Ventilator initiation includes choice of mode, tidal volume, rate, F_{IO_2}, and PEEP levels.
- Positive end-expiratory pressure is used primarily to improve oxygenation and lower F_{IO_2} in patients with severe oxygenation problems and refractory hypoxemia.
- Mechanical ventilatory support for most patients includes volume ventilation in either the assist-control or the SIMV mode.
- When SIMV is used, pressure support of 5 to 10 cm H_2O should be included to overcome WOB_I.
- For PSV_{max}, adjust the pressure limit to achieve a tidal volume of 10 to 12 mL/kg with a rate of 10 to 20 breaths/min.
- Pressure-control ventilation with a prolonged inspiratory time may be useful in limiting pressure and improving oxygenation in ALI/ARDS patients.
- The pathophysiological status of the patient determines the optimal ventilatory settings for each patient.
- Initial tidal volume of 10 to 12 mL/kg with a rate of 10 to 12 breaths/min is appropriate for most patients.
- Patients with ALI/ARDS may begin mechanical ventilation with a tidal volume of 8 mL/kg and have volume adjusted to 6 mL/kg to maintain plateau pressure at 30 cm H_2O or less.
- Lung protective strategies in the management of ALI/ARDS include use of lower tidal volume (6 mL/kg), maintaining plateau pressure at 30 cm H_2O or less, permissive hypercapnia, and PEEP set above the lower inflection point on the static pressure-volume curve.
- Trigger sensitivity should be set to achieve minimal trigger work without autocycling.

KEY POINTS—cont'd

- Inspiratory flow should be initially set at approximately 60 L/min to achieve an inspiratory time of approximately 1 second and an I:E ratio of 1:2 or better.
- When in doubt, set the initial FIO_2 at 1.0.
- An initial PEEP level of 3 to 5 cm H_2O may help maintain lung volume and prevent atelectasis.
- Auto-PEEP can be a problem in patients with obstructive lung disease (COPD, asthma).
- Appropriate setting of ventilator alarms is vital for warning clinicians of a device malfunction or changes in the patient's condition.
- FIO_2 and PEEP levels are adjusted to optimize oxygenation without harmful side effects.
- An appropriate goal of PEEP would be to achieve a PaO_2 of 60 to 100 mm Hg with an FIO_2 of 0.40 to 0.50 or less.
- Rate and tidal volume are adjusted to optimize ventilation and $PaCO_2$.
- Mode of ventilation, trigger sensitivity, and inspiratory flow settings should be adjusted to optimize the patient-ventilator interaction.
- Other techniques to improve oxygenation in ventilator patients include bronchial hygiene, optimal humidification, bronchodilators, turning, sitting up in bed, suctioning, and airway care.
- Prone positioning may improve oxygenation in ALI/ARDS patients.
- Alternative lung protective strategies in ALI/ARDS may include ECMO, IVOX, HFV, and tracheal gas insufflation.
- Careful attention to acid-base homeostasis and the effect of $PaCO_2$ on pH is an essential part of ventilator management.

References

1. Esteban A et al: How is mechanical ventilation employed in the intensive care unit? an international utilization review, Am J Respir Crit Care Med 161:1450, 2000.
2. Cherniack RM, Cherniack L: Pathophysiology of respiratory failure. In: Respiration in health and disease, ed 3, Philadelphia, 1983, WB Saunders.
3. West JB: Acute respiratory failure. In: Pulmonary physiology and pathophysiology: an integrated, case-based approach, Philadelphia, 2001, Lippincott, Williams & Wilkins.
4. Weinberger SE: Classification and pathophysiologic aspects of respiratory failure. In: Principles of pulmonary medicine, ed 3, Philadelphia, 1998, WB Saunders.
5. Shapiro BA, Peruzzi WT, Kozelowski-Templin R: Clinical application of blood gases, ed 5, St. Louis, 1994, Mosby.
6. Kollef MH, Schuster DP: Medical progress: the acute respiratory distress syndrome, N Engl J Med 332:27, 1995.
7. Hess DR, Kacmarek RM: Essentials of mechanical ventilation, New York, 1996, McGraw-Hill.
8. Delclaux C et al: Treatment of acute hypoxemic nonhypercapnic respiratory insufficiency with continuous positive airway pressure delivered by a face mask: a randomized controlled trial, JAMA 284:2352, 2000.
9. American College of Chest Physicians: ACCP consensus conference: mechanical ventilation, Chest 104:1833, 1993.
10. Tobin M et al: Current concepts: mechanical ventilation, N Engl J Med 330:1056, 1994.
11. Tobin MJ, et al: Update in critical care medicine, Ann Intern Med 125:909, 1996.
12. Tobin MJ et al: Advances in mechanical ventilation, N Engl J Med 344: 1986, 2001.
13. Bendixen HH et al: Respiratory care, St. Louis, 1965, Mosby.
14. Tobin MJ et al: Principles and practice of mechanical ventilation, New York, 1994, McGraw-Hill.
15. Ventilation with lower tidal volumes as compared with traditional tidal volumes for acute lung injury and the acute respiratory distress syndrome. The Acute Respiratory Distress Syndrome Network, N Engl J Med 342:1301, 2000.
16. NIH/NHLBI ARDS Clinical Network: Mechanical ventilation protocol summary, 2000.
17. Gillette MA, Hess DR: Ventilator-induced lung injury and the evolution of lung-protective strategies in acute respiratory distress syndrome, Respir Care 46:130, 2001.
18. Sethi J et al: Mechanical ventilation in chronic obstructive lung disease, Clin Chest Med 21:799, 2000.
19. Georgopoulos D, Kondili E, Prinianakis G: How to set the ventilator in asthma, Monaldi Arch Chest Dis 55:74, 2000.
20. National Institutes of Health, National Heart, Lung and Blood Institute: Guidelines for the diagnosis and management of asthma: expert panel report 2, NIH publication no. 98-4051, 1997.
21. George RB et al: Chest medicine: essentials of pulmonary and critical care medicine, Philadelphia, 2000, Lippincott Williams & Wilkins.
22. Gammon RB et al: Mechanical ventilation: a review for the internist, Am J Med 9:553, 1995.
23. Brochard L et al: Noninvasive ventilation for acute exacerbations of chronic obstructive pulmonary disease, N Engl J Med 333:817, 1995.
24. Martin TJ et al: A randomized, prospective evaluation of noninvasive ventilation for acute respiratory failure, Am J Respir Crit Care Med 161:807, 2000.
25. Kramer N et al: Randomized, prospective trial of noninvasive positive pressure ventilation in acute respiratory failure, Am J Respir Crit Care Med 151:1799, 1995.
26. Dekel B, Segal E, Perel A: Pressure support ventilation, Arch Intern Med 156:369, 1996.

27. Vines DL, Peters JI: Pressure control ventilation in acute lung injury, Clin Pulm Med 8:231, 2001.
28. Mecklenburgh JS et al: Excessive work of breathing during intermittent mandatory ventilation, Br J Anaesth 58:1048, 1986.
29. Marini JJ, Smith TC, Lamb VJ: External work output and force generation during synchronized intermittent mechanical ventilation: effect of machine assistance on breathing effort, Am Rev Respir Dis 138:1167, 1988.
30. Grasso S, Puntillo F, Mascia L, et al: Compensation for increase in respiratory workload during mechanical ventilation: pressure-support versus proportional-assist ventilation, Am J Respir Crit Care Med 161:819, 2000.
31. Marini JJ, Rodriguez RM, Lamb V: The inspiratory workload of patient-initiated mechanical ventilation, Am Rev Respir Dis 134:902, 1986.
32. Marini JJ, Capps JS, Culver BH: The inspiratory work of breathing during assisted mechanical ventilation, Chest 87:612, 1985.
33. Hudson LD et al: Does intermittent mandatory ventilation correct respiratory alkalosis in patients receiving assisted mechanical ventilation? Am Rev Respir Dis 132:1071, 1985.
34. Culpepper JA, Rinaldo JE, Rodger RM: Effect of mechanical ventilator mode on tendency towards respiratory alkalosis, Am Rev Respir Dis 132:1075, 1985.
35. Krishman J, Brower R: High-frequency ventilation for acute lung injury and ARDS, Chest 118:795, 2000.
36. Fort P et al: High frequency oscillatory ventilation for adult respiratory distress syndrome: a pilot study, Crit Care Med 25:937, 1997.
37. Groeger JS, Levinson MR, Carlon GC: Assist-control versus synchronized intermittent mandatory ventilation during acute respiratory failure, Crit Care Med 17:607, 1989.
38. Amato, MBP et al: Effect of a protective-ventilation strategy on mortality in the acute respiratory distress syndrome, N Engl J Med 338:347, 1998.
39. Hill LL, Pearl RG: Flow triggering, pressure triggering and auto triggering during mechanical ventilation, Crit Care Med 28:579, 2000.
40. Sassoon CSH: Mechanical ventilator design and function: the trigger variable, Respir Care 37:1056, 1992.
41. Branson RD: Flow-triggering systems, Respir Care 39:138, 1994.
42. Holbrook PJ, Guiles SP: Response time of four pressure support ventilators: effect of triggering method and bias flow, Respir Care 42:952, 1997.
43. Jubran A: Inspiratory flow rate: more may not be better, Crit Care Med 27:670, 1999.
44. Rau JL, Shelledy DC: The effect of varying inspiratory flow waveforms on peak and mean airway pressures with a time-cycled volume ventilator: a bench study, Respir Care 36:347, 1991.
45. Pilbeam SP: Mechanical ventilation: physiological and clinical applications, St. Louis, 1998, Mosby.
46. Lindahl S: Influence of an end inspiratory pause on pulmonary ventilation, gas distribution, and lung perfusion during artificial ventilation, Crit Care Med 7:540, 1979.
47. Mercat A et al: Extending inspiratory time in acute respiratory distress syndrome, Crit Care Med 29:40, 2001.
48. Lim CM et al: Mechanistic scheme and effect of "extended sigh" as a recruitment maneuver in patients with acute respiratory distress syndrome: a preliminary study, Crit Care Med 29:1255, 2001.
49. Mouloudi E et al: Bronchodilator delivery by metered-dose inhaler in mechanically ventilated COPD patients: influence of end-inspiratory pause, Eur Respir J 12:165, 1998.
50. Langevin PB et al: Synchronization of radiograph film exposure with the inspiratory pause: effect on the appearance of bedside chest radiographs in mechanically ventilated patients, Am J Resp Crit Care Med 160:2067, 1999.
51. Amato MB et al: Beneficial effects of the open lung approach with low distending pressures in acute respiratory distress syndrome. A prospective randomized study on mechanical ventilation, Am J Respir Crit Care Med 152:1835, 1995.
52. Bonmarchand G, Chevron V, Menard JF, et al: Effects of pressure ramp slope values on the work of breathing during pressure support ventilation in restrictive patients, Crit Care Med 27:715, 1999.
53. AARC clinical practice guideline: Humidification during mechanical ventilation, American Association for Respiratory Care, Respir Care 37:887, 1992.
54. MacIntyre N: Of Goldilocks and ventilatory muscle loading, Crit Care Med 28:588, 2000.
55. Burns SM et al: Weaning from long-term mechanical ventilation, Am J Crit Care 4:4, 1995.
56. O'Keefe GE et al: Imprecision in lower "inflection point" estimation from static pressure-volume curves in patients at risk for acute respiratory distress syndrome, J Trauma 44:1064, 1998.
57. Drakulovic MB, Mm Hges A, Bauer TT, et al: Supine body position was a risk factor for nosocomial pneumonia in mechanically ventilated patients: a randomized trial, Lancet 354:1851, 1999.
58. Voggenreiter G et al: Intermittent prone positioning in the treatment of severe post-traumatic lung injury, Crit Care Med 27:2375, 1999.
59. Curley MA: Prone positioning in patients with acute respiratory distress syndrome: a systematic review, Am J Crit Care 8(6):397, 1999.
60. Hirvela E: Advances in the management of acute respiratory distress syndrome: protective ventilation, Arch Surg 135:126, 2000.
61. Papazian I et al: Respective and combined effects of prone position and inhaled nitric oxide in patients with acute respiratory distress syndrome, Am J Respir Crit Care Med 157:580, 1998.
62. Germann P et al: Additive effects of nitric oxide inhalation on the oxygenation benefit of the prone position in the acute respiratory distress syndrome, Anesthesiology 89:1401, 1998.
63. Medoff BD, Harris SR, Kesselman H, et al: Use of recruitment maneuvers and high positive end expiratory pressure in a patient with acute respiratory distress syndrome, Crit Care Med 28:1210, 2000.
64. Bulger EM et al: Current clinical options for the treatment and management of acute respiratory distress syndrome, J Trauma 48:562, 2000.

65. Hess DR, Gillette MA: Tracheal gas insufflation and related techniques to introduce gas flow into the trachea, Respir Care 46:119, 2001.
66. Lewandowski K: Extracorporeal membrane oxygenation for severe acute respiratory failure, Crit Care 4:156, 2000.
67. Zwischenberger JB, Tao W, Bidani A: Intravascular membrane oxygenation and carbon dioxide removal devices: a review of performance improvements, ASAIO J 45:41,1999.
68. Malley JW: Clinical blood gases: applications and noninvasive alternatives, Philadelphia, 1990, WB Saunders.

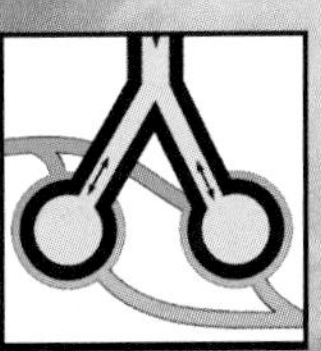

CHAPTER 42

Noninvasive Positive Pressure Ventilation

David L. Vines

In This Chapter You Will Learn:

- How noninvasive positive pressure ventilation (NPPV) is defined
- What are the goals of and indications for NPPV
- How to select patients for NPPV
- What factors are predictive of success during NPPV
- How to differentiate patient interfaces, types of ventilators, and their modes of ventilation
- How to initiate and manage NPPV in the acute care setting
- What complications are associated with NPPV and the possible solutions
- How much staff time is associated with NPPV

Chapter Outline

Key Terms

acute cardiogenic pulmonary edema
asthma
chronic obstructive pulmonary disease (COPD)
community-acquired pneumonia
continuous positive airway pressure (CPAP)
expiratory positive airway pressure (EPAP)
hypoxic respiratory failure
intrinsic PEEP
intermittent abdominal pressure ventilator
inspiratory positive airway pressure (IPAP)

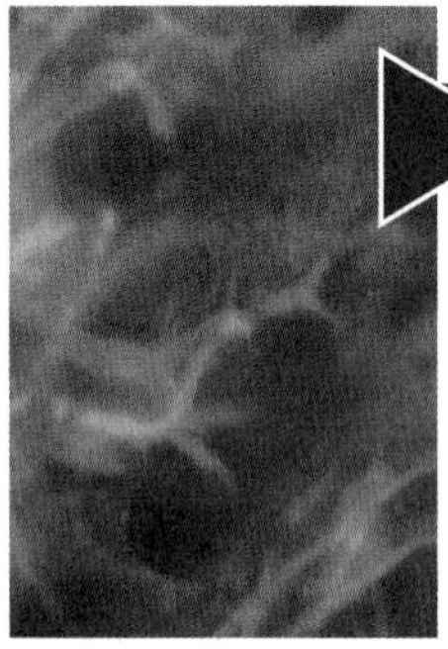

Key Terms—cont'd

negative pressure ventilator
nocturnal hypoventilation
noninvasive positive pressure ventilation (NPPV)
noninvasive ventilation
positive end-expiratory pressure (PEEP)
restrictive thoracic diseases
rocking bed
Trendelenburg position

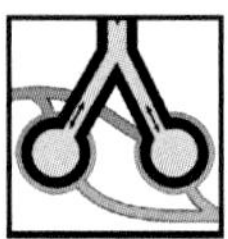

Noninvasive positive pressure ventilation (NPPV, sometimes abbreviated NIPPV) is defined as "the application of positive pressure via the upper respiratory tract for the purpose of augmenting alveolar ventilation."[1] Unlike invasive positive pressure ventilation, which is delivered through an endotracheal or tracheostomy tube, NPPV typically is administered through a nasal or an oral mask. The use of NPPV in the acute care setting has been increasing in recent years because of continued development of new or improved patient interfaces and noninvasive ventilators and because of reports of success in the literature.[2] This chapter reviews the literature and recommendations regarding the use of NPPV in the management of various disease processes. It also provides insight into the different methods of applying **noninvasive ventilation** and focuses on the application of NPPV in the acute care setting.

▶ TYPES OF NONINVASIVE VENTILATION

Noninvasive ventilation can be provided with a negative pressure ventilator, positive pressure ventilator, rocking bed, or intermittent abdominal pressure ventilator (IAPV). The IAPV, or "pneumobelt," was invented in the 1930s.[3] The IAPV has a rubber bladder that is strapped around the abdomen. When inflated, the rubber bladder compresses the abdomen, pushes the diaphragm upward in the thorax, and causes exhalation. The rubber bladder is deflated, and the abdominal contents and diaphragm move down, facilitating inspiration. Because this device requires gravity to be effective, the patient must be sitting up at a 30-degree angle or greater.[4] It has been reported that patients dependent on a ventilator for extended periods can be safely and effectively supported with IAPV for daytime ventilatory support. Some patients who are ventilator-dependent for a long time prefer IAPV to NPPV while in a wheelchair.[5]

A **rocking bed** works by the same principle as an IAPV. Rather than a rubber bladder that inflates and deflates, a bed that rocks from **Trendelenburg position** to reverse Trendelenburg position produces exhalation and inspiration. Rocking beds were used in the 1950s to wean patients from negative pressure ventilators and provide long-term ventilatory support to postpolio patients.[3]

Negative pressure ventilators provide noninvasive ventilation by surrounding the chest wall with negative pressure on inspiration. This negative pressure causes the chest wall to rise, and inspiration occurs. When the negative pressure is released, exhalation occurs passively owing to the elastic recoil of the lung and chest wall. The first electrically powered, negative pressure ventilator, known as the "iron lung," surrounded the entire body except for the head and neck. This device and similar versions were widely used from the late 1920s through the 1960s during the polio epidemic.[3] During this period, a portable negative pressure ventilator, known as the *chest cuirass*, also was used. This device covered only the patient's chest and made a seal with an air-filled rubber edge.[3] The use of negative pressure ventilators decreased greatly in the 1960s because of higher reported survival rates with invasive positive pressure ventilation, the development of intensive care units (ICUs), and the increased availability of inexpensive, easy to operate positive pressure ventilators.[3]

In 1780, the first device to provide NPPV was a bag-mask apparatus used during resuscitation instead of mouth-to-mouth ventilation.[2] Widespread clinical use of NPPV began with the introduction of intermittent positive pressure breathing (IPPB) in 1947.[2,3] Intermittent positive pressure breathing was widely used to deliver aerosolized medicines for 10 to 15 minutes several times a day. The use of IPPB declined significantly in the mid 1980s[3] after a randomized, controlled trial revealed no benefit, compared with results of the use of a small-volume nebulizer, in the treatment of patients with **chronic obstructive pulmonary disease.**[6] Around this time, nasal mask **continuous positive airway pressure** (CPAP) was suggested as a therapy for obstructive sleep apnea.[7] Nasal masks also were used nocturnally in conjunction with positive pressure ventilators to provide rest for the respiratory muscles in the care of some patients with neuromuscular disorders.[8] In

1989, NPPV was used successfully to support 8 of 10 patients with acute respiratory failure.[9] Since that time, numerous studies have investigated the use of NPPV in the management of various clinical conditions and settings with various apparatuses and outcome. There also has been a significant increase in the technology of NPPV ventilators and advances in noninvasive patient interfaces.

▶ GOALS OF AND INDICATIONS FOR NONINVASIVE POSITIVE PRESSURE VENTILATION

This section describes the goals and potential benefits of NPPV in the management of the various types of respiratory failure. With the onset of respiratory failure, the likelihood of intubation and invasive positive pressure ventilation increases dramatically. There are complications associated with the intubation process, with the introduction of microorganisms into the lungs, and with the extubation process. Details on these complications can be found in Chapter 30. Avoiding intubation and invasive positive pressure ventilation is a major goal of NPPV in the acute care setting (emergency department, ICU, or hospital ward). In the chronic care setting, major goals of NPPV are to relieve symptoms associated with hypoventilation and improve quality of life. The goals of NPPV in the acute and chronic care settings are listed in Box 42-1. Noninvasive positive pressure ventilation may be indicated in the management of numerous disease processes in the acute and chronic care settings (Box 42-2).

Box 42-1 • Goals of Noninvasive Positive Pressure Ventilation

ACUTE CARE SETTING
- Avoid intubation
- Relieve symptoms
- Enhance gas exchange
- Improve patient-ventilator synchronization
- Maximize patient comfort
- Decrease length of stay

CHRONIC CARE SETTING
- Relieve or improve symptoms
- Enhance quality of life
- Increase survival
- Improve mobility

Modified from Mehta S, Hill NS: Am J Respir Crit Care Med 163:540, 2001.

Box 42-2 • Acute and Chronic Disease Processes for Which NPPV May Be Indicated

ACUTE CARE SETTING
- COPD exacerbations
- Asthma
- Acute cardiogenic pulmonary edema*
- Community-acquired pneumonia†
- Hypoxemic respiratory failure
- Immunocompromised state
- Do-not-intubate orders
- Postoperative status
- Difficulty weaning

CHRONIC CARE SETTING
- Restrictive thoracic disease
- COPD
- Nocturnal hypoventilation

*Only if hypercapnia develops during CPAP therapy.
†Beneficial only to patients with underlying COPD.

Acute Care Setting

Chronic Obstructive Pulmonary Disease

The management of hypercapnic respiratory failure due to COPD exacerbation with NPPV has been the subject of numerous studies. Several randomized, controlled trials involving patients with COPD exacerbations have shown a reduction in the need for intubation compared with the results of standard medical treatment.[10-13] Other studies have shown a reduction in in-hospital mortality,[11,13-15] reduced length of hospital stay,[11,12] and significantly fewer complications compared with the results of standard therapy.[11] Only one randomized, controlled trial that compared NPPV to standard therapy in the care of patients with acute COPD exacerbation failed to show significant improvement in the measured variables.[16] The average pH of the patients in this study[16] was higher (7.33) than the pH in other studies (7.27[11] and 7.28[12]). This difference in pH may have been reflective of the severity of illness. The differences in reported outcome between these studies suggests that NPPV should be reserved for COPD patients at risk of intubation.[3] Noninvasive positive pressure ventilation appears to be an acceptable alterative to invasive positive pressure ventilation in the care of patients with acute COPD exacerbations if selection and exclusion criteria are met. Selection and exclusion criteria for NPPV are discussed later.

RULE OF THUMB

Patients with acute COPD exacerbations should be evaluated for NPPV as an alternative to intubation and conventional mechanical ventilation.

Asthma

Although no results of randomized, controlled trials are available, Meduri et al[17] reported positive results in the care of 17 patients with status asthmaticus. The initial average arterial partial pressure of carbon dioxide ($PaCO_2$) was 65 mm Hg, and pH was 7.25. The $PaCO_2$ decreased and pH increased significantly within the first 2 hours of NPPV. During this period, the ratio of arterial partial pressure of oxygen to fractional inspired oxygen concentration (PaO_2/FIO_2) increased from an average of 315 to 403. Respiratory rate also was significantly reduced from an average of 29 to 22 breaths/min. These positive physiologic changes were accomplished with an average inspiratory pressure of 18 cm H_2O and never more than 25 cm H_2O. All but two of the patients avoided intubation. Although the results from this pilot study are promising, a randomized, controlled trial is needed to validate these results.

Acute Cardiogenic Pulmonary Edema

In 1991, mask CPAP was shown to improve gas exchange and reduce the need for intubation in the care of patients with severe cardiogenic pulmonary edema.[18] In 1997, nasal CPAP of 10 cm H_2O was compared with nasal NPPV with an inspiratory positive airway pressure (IPAP) of 15 cm H_2O and an expiratory positive airway pressure of 5 cm H_2O.[19] Nasal NPPV improved ventilation and vital signs faster than nasal CPAP in this study, although the study has been criticized because of problems related to the type of patients in the treatment group.[3] A prospective study showed that NPPV effectively improved ventilation and vital signs and relieved dyspnea in patients with cardiogenic pulmonary edema who met clinical criteria for intubation.[20] These results must be validated with further studies before a conclusion can be drawn regarding the safety of NPPV for patients with acute cardiogenic pulmonary edema. A review suggested that CPAP of 10 to 12.5 cm H_2O be considered first in the management of acute pulmonary edema; if the patient is hypercapnic or has persistent dyspnea, inspiratory pressure may be added.[3]

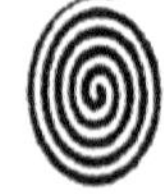

RULE OF THUMB

A CPAP of 10 to 12.5 cm H_2O should be considered before NPPV is used in the care of patients with acute pulmonary edema.

Community-Acquired Pneumonia

A randomized, controlled trial compared NPPV and standard treatment with standard treatment alone in the care of patients with severe community-acquired pneumonia.[21] In a subgroup analysis of the data, it was found that a significant reduction in intubation rate and duration of stay in the ICU occurred only among the patients with underlying COPD. These findings were not evident in patients without COPD. Patients with COPD and community-acquired pneumonia also had a significant reduction in 2-month mortality and nursing care workload.[21] Further studies are needed to confirm these findings. The current recommendation for the use of NPPV in the care of patients with community-acquired pneumonia is to limit its routine use to patients with underlying COPD.[3]

Hypoxemic Respiratory Failure

Hypoxemic respiratory failure usually is defined by a PaO_2/FIO_2 ratio of less than 200, but many disorders are grouped under this heading. One study showed that NPPV reduced intubation rate, length of ICU stay, and mortality rate compared with the results of conventional therapy in the care of patients with respiratory failure when $PaCO_2$ was greater than 45 mm Hg. When, however, all patients with respiratory failure were grouped together, there was no difference in this outcome, and COPD patients were excluded from this study.[22] Another study compared NPPV with endotracheal intubation by means of mechanical ventilation in the care of patients with hypoxemic respiratory failure.[23] Both methods of ventilation improved gas exchange, but NPPV resulted in fewer complications and shorter ICU stays.[23] Other investigators have reported a reduced intubation rate in the same patient population.[24] Not all use of NPPV has been associated with improved outcome. In a small, randomized, controlled trial including patients with various causes of respiratory distress, investigators found a greater mortality rate in the NPPV group. The high mortality may have been related to the marked delays in endotracheal intubation that occurred in this group.[25] A randomized, controlled trial showed that mask CPAP significantly improved PaO_2/FIO_2 ratio within the first hour but failed to reduce the intubation rate, length of ICU stay, or hospital mortality compared with the results of standard therapy in the care of patients with hypoxemic respiratory failure without hypercapnia.[26] These conflicting reports limit clinical recommendations at this time. Additional randomized, controlled trials are needed to identify which types of patients with hypoxemic respiratory failure will benefit from NPPV.

Other Indications

Other indications for NPPV in the acute care setting may include providing ventilatory support for immunocompromised, do-not-intubate, and postoperative patients; assisting in weaning from mechanical ventilation; and avoiding reintubation. A lower risk of nosocomial infection has been reported with the use of NPPV compared with invasive positive pressure ventilation.[27,28] This potential benefit has created interest in the use of NPPV in the treatment of immunocompromised patients. Two prospective, randomized trials showed reductions in intubation rate, rate of serious complications, and ICU mortality for NPPV as opposed to standard medical treatment of immunocompromised patients with acute hypoxemic respiratory failure.[29,30] The current recommendation for immunocompromised patients with moderate to severe respiratory distress is to use NPPV unless contraindications exist.[31]

The use of NPPV in the care of do-not-intubate patients with irreversible disease remains controversial. There is evidence that NPPV offers patients with end-stage disease an effective method of support and provides them with some relief from associated symptoms.[32] The current recommendation is that the use of NPPV is justified in the care of do-not-intubate patients if the patient understands that NPPV is a form of life support and that the *acute* disease process is reversible.[3]

Short-term use of NPPV in postoperative care has shown some promise. The use of NPPV after lung resection increased $Pa{O_2}$ without increasing dead space or worsening air leaks.[33] Prophylactic use of NPPV in the care of obese patients after gastroplasty has been shown to markedly improve the pulse oximetry oxygen saturation ($Sp{O_2}$) and forced vital capacity (FVC), which allowed faster recovery of preoperative pulmonary function.[34] Larger randomized, controlled trials are needed to identify outcome and potential applications in postoperative care.

The use of NPPV to facilitate weaning from mechanical ventilation has been evaluated in the care of patients with acute superimposed on chronic respiratory failure. It was found that NPPV reduced weaning time, length of ICU stay, incidence of nosocomial pneumonia, and 60-day mortality compared with the results of conventional weaning with invasive pressure support ventilation (PSV).[15] Noninvasive positive pressure ventilation has been shown to reduce the amount of daily ventilatory support, but the duration of ventilatory support in this study was greater with NPPV than with conventional weaning with invasive PSV.[35] Three-month mortality and duration of ICU and hospital stays were similar for both groups.[35] A prospective study of difficult-to-wean COPD patients showed that both NPPV and invasive PSV significantly reduced the diaphragmatic work of breathing and improved ventilation compared with the results in a T-piece trial.[36] This study also showed that NPPV was associated with greater respiratory pump efficiency and lower overall dyspnea scores than was invasive PSV in this patient population.[36] Although the results of these studies supported the use of NPPV in facilitating weaning of COPD patients from invasive mechanical ventilation, caution is needed in patient selection. For NPPV to be successful, patients must be cooperative, able to maintain a patent upper airway, and able to clear secretions. Patients who are difficult to reintubate should not be extubated early to receive NPPV.[3]

Reintubation has been associated with increased mortality, longer hospital stay, and a greater need for a long-term care than is the case for patients successfully extubated.[37] If NPPV can prevent reintubation, outcome may improve. When extubation failed in the care of COPD patients, NPPV improved gas exchange and reduced the need for reintubation to 20% compared with 67% among historically matched controls.[38] Further studies are needed to validate these results and identify which patients will benefit from NPPV when extubation fails. Patients who may benefit from NPPV after extubation include those with COPD, those with acute pulmonary edema, and those with postextubation stridor.[3]

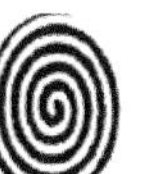

RULE OF THUMB

Before using NPPV in the management of acute respiratory failure, be sure the process causing respiratory failure is reversible within several days, selection criteria are met, and exclusion criteria are absent.

Chronic Care Setting

Restrictive Thoracic Diseases

Restrictive thoracic diseases successfully managed with NPPV include postpolio syndrome, neuromuscular diseases, chest wall deformities, spinal cord injuries, and severe kyphoscoliosis.[39] Three mechanisms have been proposed to explain the benefits gained by patients with restrictive thoracic disease. The first mechanism is the ability of NPPV to rest the respiratory muscles. Second, NPPV lowers the $Pa{CO_2}$, and the decrease is believed to reset the central ventilatory controller and establish a new baseline $Pa{CO_2}$ for the patient. The third mechanism is the improvement in lung compliance, lung volume, and dead space that result from NPPV.[39]

A study of nocturnal NPPV in the care of patients with severe kyphoscoliosis showed benefits in improved night and daytime gas exchange, relief of symptoms of hypoventilation, and improved tidal volume and FVC.[40] Several studies of patients with amyotrophic lateral sclerosis (ALS) have shown that NPPV improves survival.[41-43] The most recent of these studies showed improved quality of life, but NPPV had no effect on the rate of lung function decline in these ALS patients.[43] In contrast, other investigators have reported that ALS patients with tracheostomy and mechanical ventilation had increased survival compared with patients receiving NPPV.[44] Further studies are needed to clarify which method of ventilation is best for ALS patients.

The prophylactic use of NPPV has been discouraged. One study of patients with Duchenne muscular dystrophy, a rapidly progressive neuromuscular disorder, compared prophylactic nocturnal NPPV with conventional treatment. Nocturnal NPPV failed to slow disease progression and was associated with a higher mortality rate.[45] The current recommendation for patients with restrictive thoracic disorders is to first document the onset of symptoms (daytime hypersomnolence, morning headache, fatigue, dyspnea, and cognitive dysfunction) associated with nocturnal hypoventilation before starting NPPV.[39] The need for careful and continuous follow-up care as well as mandatory reassessment by a physician within 60 days to assess patient adherence and benefit must be emphasized.[39]

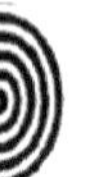

RULE OF THUMB

Patients with restrictive thoracic disorders should have symptoms of nocturnal hypoventilation before NPPV is considered.

Long-term Care of Patients With Chronic Obstructive Pulmonary Disease

There are two proposed hypotheses to explain how patients with severe COPD benefit from the use of NPPV.[39] First, positive inspiratory pressure may improve gas exchange and unload the respiratory muscles, allowing these muscles to recover, gain strength, and reduce fatigue. These benefits should reduce symptoms associated with hypoventilation and improve quality of life. Second, patients with severe COPD have poor sleep quality, shorter sleep time, and nocturnal hypoventilation. When nocturnal NPPV is used, sleep quality and time should improve. Noninvasive positive pressure ventilation also should relieve nocturnal hypoventilation, which may reset the respiratory center to respond to a lower carbon dioxide level. These benefits may improve sleep quality, daytime gas exchange, and quality of life.[39]

Current studies of NPPV in the management of severe COPD have had conflicting results. Two studies showed little or no benefit from 3 months of nocturnal NPPV in the care of patients with severe COPD who were in stable condition.[46,47] In both studies, a higher number of patients withdrew from the NPPV group than from the control group. Another study, however, showed significant improvement in gas exchange, sleep quality, sleep time, and quality of life in patients with stable, hypercapnic COPD after 3 months of nocturnal NPPV.[48] Differences between these studies may provide insight as to which COPD patients are likely to benefit from nocturnal NPPV. Patients with hypercarbia and nocturnal desaturation may be more likely to benefit from nocturnal NPPV.[39]

Noninvasive positive pressure ventilation has been shown to improve gas exchange and the functional ability of patients with severe COPD and restrictive ventilatory disorders, both immediately and after 6 months of use, although patient compliance may be a problem.[49] Another study of severe COPD compared NPPV and long-term oxygen therapy with long-term oxygen therapy alone in the assessment of patient outcome for 1 year.[50] Noninvasive positive pressure ventilation, compared with oxygen therapy alone, improved the Borg dyspnea rating and the results of one psychomotor coordination test.[50] The NPPV group had a significantly lower number of hospital admissions at 3 months, but there was no difference between the groups at 6 months. There were also no differences in the occurrence of acute exacerbations or in survival at 1 year.[50] The use of NPPV in the management of stable, severe COPD remains controversial. The current recommendation from a consensus conference is to use NPPV in the care of patients with severe COPD with symptoms of nocturnal hypoventilation and one of the following: Pa_{CO_2} of 55 mm Hg or greater, a Pa_{CO_2} between 50 to 54 mm Hg with nocturnal desaturation, or more than two hospital admissions related to hypercapnic respiratory failure.[39]

Nocturnal Hypoventilation

Nocturnal hypoventilation has been associated with other disorders besides restrictive lung disease and COPD, such as central sleep apnea, obstructive sleep apnea, and some lung parenchymal diseases.[39] A study of patients with obesity hypoventilation syndrome showed improved gas exchange and relief of symptoms associated with chronic hypoventilation after 4 months of nocturnal NPPV.[50] Nocturnal NPPV is currently recommended for nocturnal hypoventilation when nasal CPAP and other first-line therapies fail to alleviate the hypoventilation.[1,39]

▶ PATIENT SELECTION AND EXCLUSION CRITERIA FOR NONINVASIVE POSITIVE PRESSURE VENTILATION

Acute Care Setting

In the selection of patients for NPPV in the acute care setting, the need for ventilatory assistance must be established. This need generally is established when the patient has signs and symptoms of respiratory distress and abnormal gas exchange.[1,3] Signs and symptoms of respiratory distress include use of accessory muscles, paradoxical breathing, a respiratory rate of 25 breaths/min or more, and the presence of moderate to severe dyspnea. The feeling of dyspnea should be worse than usual for COPD patients. Abnormal gas exchange is confirmed when $Pa{CO_2}$ is greater than 45 mm Hg with a pH less than 7.35 or the $Pa{O_2}/F{IO_2}$ ratio is less than 200.[1,3]

Once the need for ventilatory assistance is established, exclusion criteria must be addressed. Exclusion criteria include apnea, hemodynamic or cardiac instability, lack of cooperation by the patient, facial burns, facial trauma, copious amounts of secretions, high risk of aspiration, and any anatomic abnormalities that interfere with gas delivery.[1,3] The underlying disease causing the acute respiratory failure must be taken into consideration in the selection of patients for NPPV. In the acute care setting, most evidence supports the use of NPPV in the care of patients with COPD exacerbations. There is less evidence supporting the use of NPPV for the other indications for NPPV discussed earlier. If the selection criteria (Box 42-3) are met and exclusion criteria (Box 42-4) are absent, NPPV may be justified if the acute respiratory failure is reversible within several days.[3] Further randomized, controlled trials are needed to identify and validate selection criteria for other disease processes. For now, sound clinical judgment should be used in the selection of patients for NPPV.

Box 42-3 • Selection Criteria for NPPV in the Care of Patients With Acute Respiratory Failure

Two or more of the following should be present:

- Use of accessory muscles
- Paradoxical breathing
- Respiratory rate ≥25 breaths/min
- Dyspnea (moderate to severe or increased in COPD patients)
- $Pa{CO_2}$ >45 mm Hg with pH <7.35
- $Pa{O_2}/F{IO_2}$ ratio <200

Box 42-4 • Exclusion Criteria for NPPV in Patients With Acute Respiratory Failure

- Apnea
- Hemodynamic or cardiac instability
- Uncooperative behavior on the part of the patient
- Facial burns
- Facial trauma
- High risk of aspiration
- Copious secretions
- Anatomic abnormalities that interfere with gas delivery

Predictors of Success During Noninvasive Positive Pressure Ventilation

Several studies have identified potential predictors of success during NPPV (Box 42-5). Successful outcome during NPPV includes improving gas exchange and preventing endotracheal intubation. Successful outcome also includes decreasing length of stay and decreasing mortality. Among patients with hypercapnic respiratory failure, factors associated with success during nasal NPPV include minimal air leak through the mouth (100 ± 70 mL), ventilator-patient synchronization, decreased severity of illness, and rapid improvement in baseline $Pa{CO_2}$, pH, and respiratory rate.[51] Patients with COPD with acute on chronic respiratory failure are less likely to have successful NPPV if severe illness or pneumonia is present.[52] Severe hypercapnia and severe acidosis have been identified as predictors of failure, and early institution of NPPV is encouraged.[52] Significant improvement in $Pa{CO_2}$ and pH after 30 minutes of NPPV is predictive of success in the care of various patients with acute respiratory failure.[53-55] In the use of NPPV to manage acute respiratory failure, there appears to be a "window of opportunity."[3] The window begins with the onset of acute respiratory distress and ends when endotracheal intubation is required.[3] Clinical experience and use of the selection criteria will help identify this window of time, which may increase the success of NPPV in the acute care setting.

Chronic Care Setting

The currently recommended selection guidelines for NPPV in restrictive thoracic disease may be separated into two parts. One is identifying symptoms of chronic hypoventilation and lack of sleep quality. The other

Box 42-5 • Predictors of Success During NPPV in the Acute Care Setting

- Minimal air leak
- Low severity of illness
- Respiratory acidosis ($Pa{CO_2}$ >45 mm Hg but <92 mm Hg)
- pH <7.35 but >7.22
- Improvement in gas exchange within 30 minutes to 2 hours of initiation
- Improvement in respiratory rate and heart rate

Modified from Mehta S, Hill NS: Am J Respir Crit Care Med 163:540, 2001.

is one of the following: $PaCO_2$ 45 mm Hg or greater, nocturnal oxygen saturation less than 88% for 5 minutes, or maximal inspiratory pressure less than 60 cm H_2O or FVC less than 50% of predicted value.[39] Although a decline in pulmonary function has been associated with carbon dioxide retention, more evidence is needed to support the use of a declining maximal inspiratory pressure or FVC as an indication for NPPV.[3] Once NPPV has been initiated, follow-up examinations are suggested for the first month or so to assist the patient with acclimation to the device. It is also recommended that patients be reassessed within 60 days to determine compliance with the NPPV therapy and establish benefit.[39]

Recommendations for use of NPPV in the management of nocturnal hypoventilation due to disorders other than restrictive lung disease and COPD include documentation of a disorder that causes hypoventilation and failure of the disorder to respond to "first-line therapy."[39] First-line therapy includes weight loss, oxygen therapy, respiratory stimulants, and CPAP. Noninvasive positive pressure ventilation is recommended as the initial therapy for moderate to severe cases of nocturnal hypoventilation.[39]

In the care of COPD patients with signs and symptoms of chronic hypoventilation and poor quality of sleep, it is important to establish that the patient has received optimal medical treatment before NPPV is recommended.[39] Once it is assured that management is optimal and symptoms remain, the presence of one of the following selection criteria indicates the need for NPPV: $PaCO_2$ 55 mm Hg or greater or $PaCO_2$ of 50 to 54 mm Hg with recurrent hospitalizations or nocturnal desaturation.[39] Recurrent hospitalization is defined as two or more hospitalizations for hypercapnic respiratory failure in a 12-month period. Nocturnal desaturation is defined by a pulse oximeter reading of less than 89% for 5 minutes with administration of at least 2 L/min of oxygen.[39] These patients should undergo follow-up evaluation within 60 days for assessment of compliance with the NPPV therapy and for benefit. A review pointed out that unless patients have symptoms of hypoventilation and poor quality of sleep (dyspnea, morning headache, fatigue, hypersomnolence) when selected for NPPV, their compliance with the therapy and benefit usually are low.

Exclusion Criteria for the Chronic Care Setting

Exclusion criteria for restrictive thoracic disease, nocturnal hypoventilation, and chronic COPD are similar to the exclusion criteria in the acute care setting. The exclusion criteria include an unsupportive family, lack of financial resources, required ventilator assistance for most of the day, copious amounts of secretions, uncooperative behavior on the part of the patient, high risk of aspiration, and any anatomic abnormality that interferes with gas delivery.[3] These exclusion criteria are considered relative contraindications.

▶ EQUIPMENT USED IN THE APPLICATION OF NONINVASIVE POSITIVE PRESSURE VENTILATION

After it has been identified that a patient may benefit from NPPV, the type of patient interface, ventilator, mode of ventilation, and initial ventilator settings must be chosen. All play a role in determining whether NPPV is successful in a given patient. This section addresses the equipment and modes of ventilation used in the application of NPPV.

Patient Interfaces

Nasal mask, full-face mask, and mouthpiece are the general types of NPPV patient interfaces. These devices provide a delivery mechanism for moving the pressurized gas from the ventilator circuit to the patient's upper airway. Nasal and full-face masks are used most often in the acute care setting. Nasal masks may be better tolerated than full-face masks by patients with claustrophobia. Full-face masks usually are less prone to leaking than are nasal masks because both the nose and mouth are covered. Mouthpieces are used to provide IPPB to patients in the acute care setting but are rarely used for today's application of NPPV (see Chapter 36).

Nasal masks (Figure 42-1) usually are triangular and are made to fit around the nose. The body of these devices is made of clear, hard plastic. On the bottom of the hard plastic is a material that cushions the mask around the nose. The material used to make the cushion may be soft plastic or a plastic cuff filled with air or silicone. Used in conjunction with straps around the head, this cushion forms an airtight seal around the nose (Figure 42-2). Caution must be taken not to overtighten the straps on the mask, because excessive pressure on the bridge of the nose can cause tissue necrosis. A small leak around the mask can be tolerated. Foam bridges that attach to the end of the nasal mask and rest on the forehead can help prevent the cushion from collapsing onto the bridge of the nose. Use of an appropriately sized foam bridge can help obtain a better seal. The nasal mask should be sized so that the cushion starts at the dorsum of the nasal bridge and fits closely around the nasal alae and rests in the mid philtrum (Figure 42-3).

Sizes of nasal masks range from small to large in wide and narrow designs. Trying several different sizes of mask can be expensive. Sizing gauges can be used to

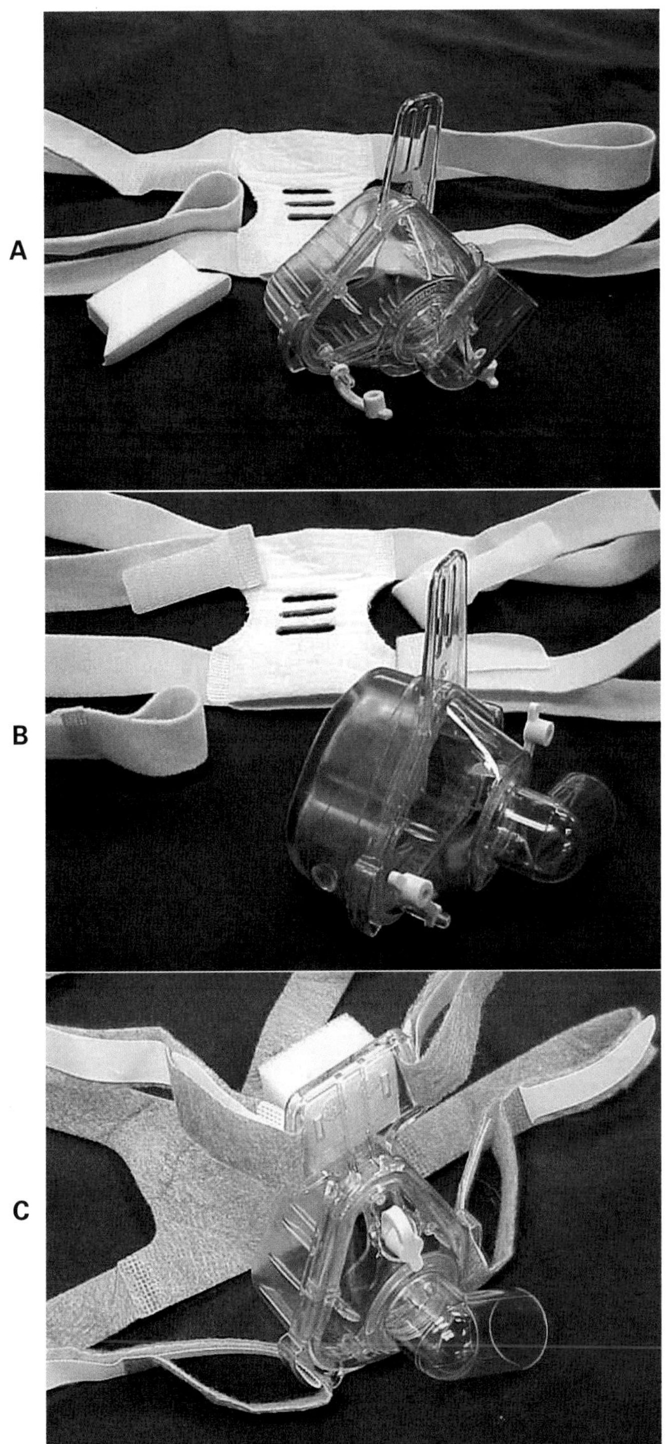

Figure 42-1
A, Disposable nasal mask. **B,** Gel nasal mask. **C,** New disposable Contour Deluxe nasal mask (Respironics, Murrysville, PA.).

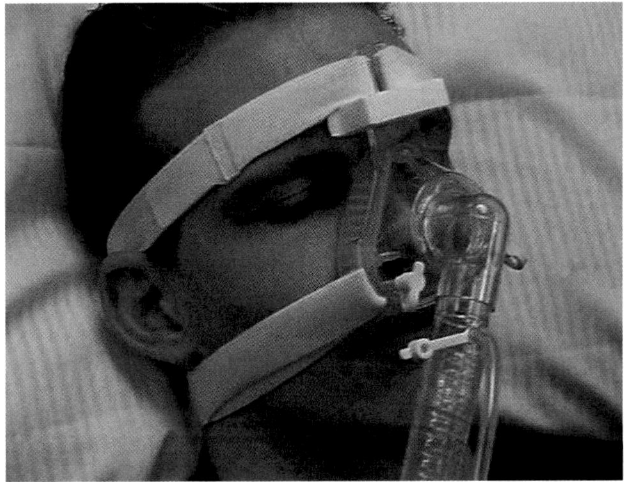

Figure 42-2
Nasal mask applied with a foam bridge.

find an appropriate nasal mask and foam bridge for the patient (Figure 42-3). Use of a sizing gauge should save money and provide a better fit. Use of an appropriately sized nasal mask may result in better patient compliance with therapy. Compared with full-face masks, nasal masks are more prone to air leaks, especially for patients who are mouth breathers. Chin straps may help prevent oral leaking in some patients by providing tension to help keep the mouth closed.

Alterations have been made in nasal masks in an effort to provide patients more comfort and to promote a higher compliance with NPPV. One is the mini nasal mask that is shaped like a wedge and covers the end of the nose. Another is nasal pillows or nasal prongs. Nasal prongs are round, soft cushions that fit directly in the nares. Specially designed headgear holds the prongs in place. These devices are used most often to provide nasal CPAP to patients with chronic disease who do not tolerate a nasal mask or have skin necrosis on the bridge of the nose.

Full-face masks generally are oval and made of clear, hard plastic with a plastic air-filled cushion surrounding the bottom of the mask (Figure 42-4). A full-face mask should start at the dorsum of the nasal bridge, surround the nose and mouth, and rest below the lower lip. If the mask is too large or small, it will be difficult to obtain an adequate seal. A sizing gauge can be used in choosing an appropriately sized full-face mask (Figure 42-5). Caution must be taken to position the straps to avoid contact around the eyes and overtightening the straps. When excessive pressure is used to seal the mask, tissue necrosis may occur on the bridge of the nose. Once the mask is sized, the headgear and straps hold the mask in place (Figure 42-6). When a resuscitation mask is used with a critical care ventilator, crisscrossing the straps as depicted in Figure 42-6 can help avoid contacting the area around the eyes. Compared with nasal masks, full-face masks are associated with an increase in dead

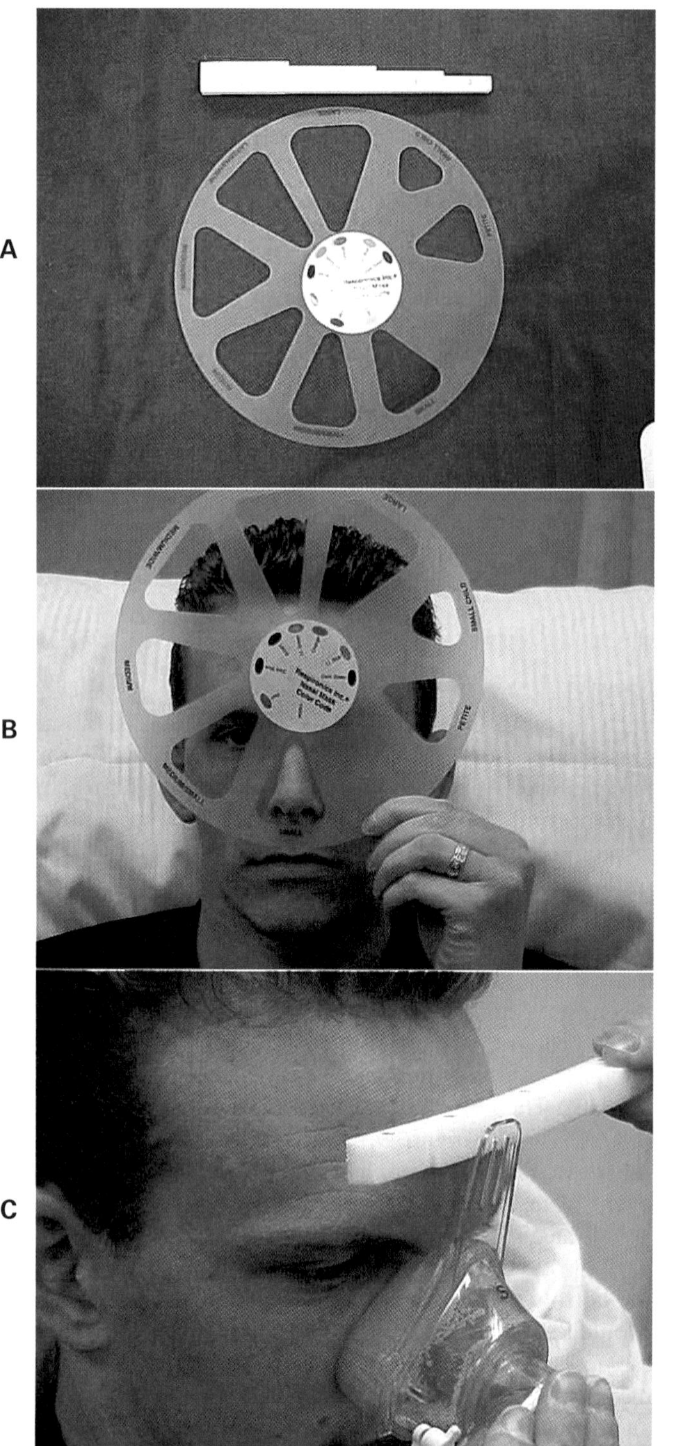

Figure 42-3

A, Nasal mask and foam bridge sizing gauge. **B,** In the use of the sizing gauge, the slot that starts at the dorsum of the nasal bridge, fits closely around the nasal alae, and rests in the mid philtrum should reveal the appropriately sized nasal mask. **C,** To determine the size of foam bridge needed, place the mask on the patient and slide the sizing gauge between the forehead and the lip of the nasal mask until the gauge stops. The number on the sizing gauge corresponds to a number on one of the foam bridges included with the nasal mask. Select the appropriate number and slide it over the lip of the nasal mask.

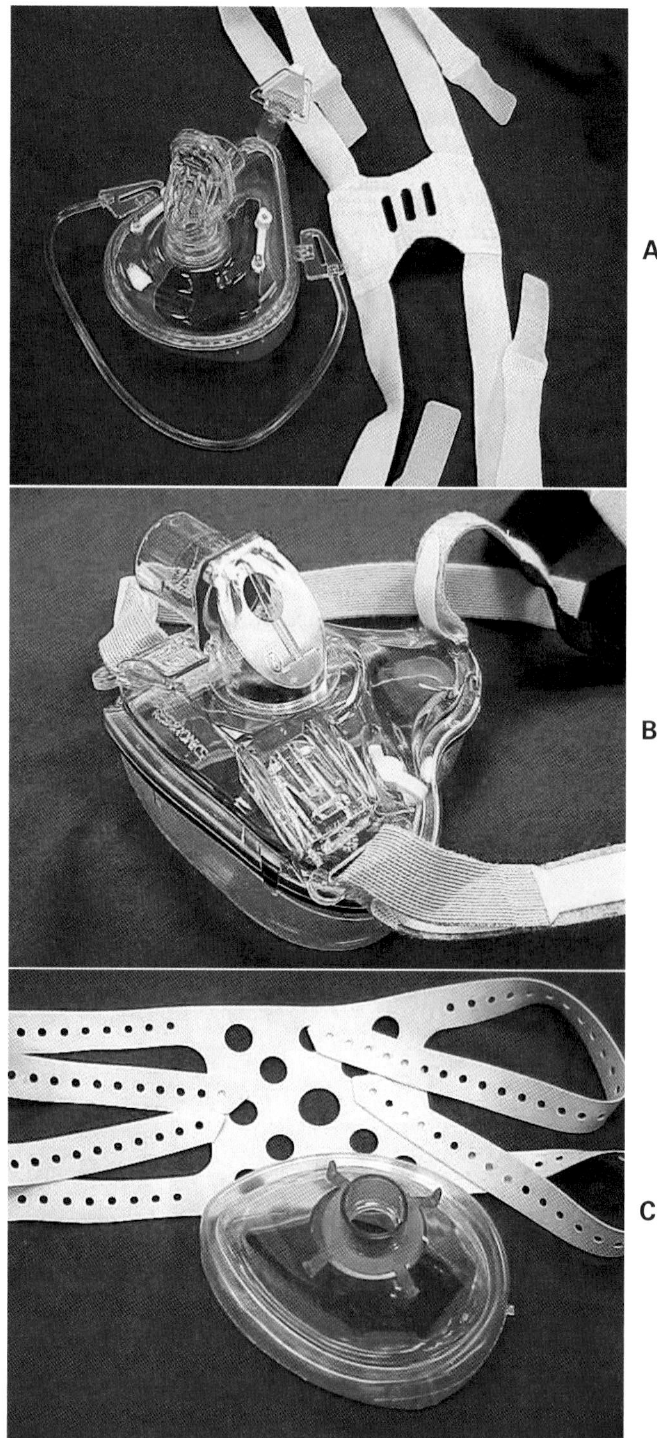

Figure 42-4

A, Spectrum disposable full-face mask (Respironics, Murrysville, PA). **B,** Image 3 disposable full-face mask (Respironics, Murrysville, PA.). **C,** Resuscitator mask. **A** and **B** are used with a noninvasive ventilator. **C** is used with a critical care ventilator.

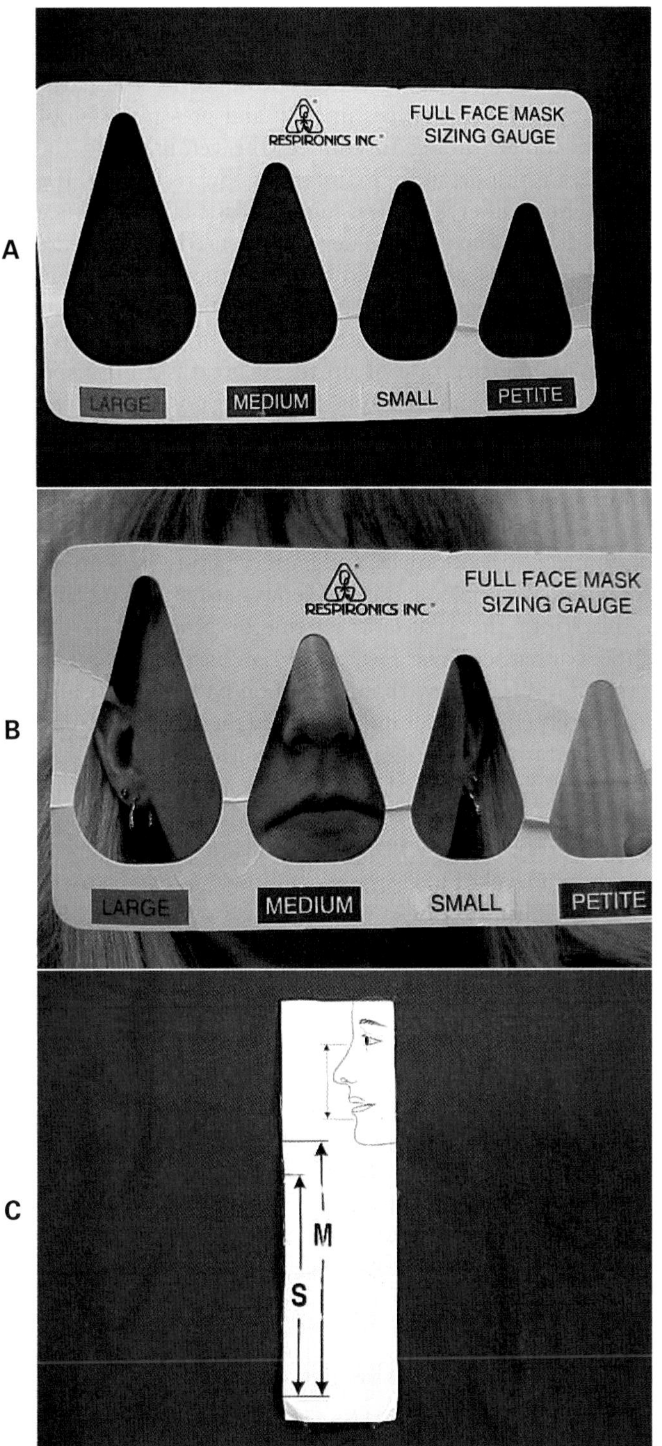

Figure 42-5

A, Sizing gauge for a full-face mask. **B,** The slot on the sizing gauge that starts at the dorsum of the nasal bridge, surrounds the nose and mouth, and rests below the lower lip should reveal the appropriately sized full-face mask. **C,** Sizing gauge on the package of every Image 3 disposable full-face mask (Respironics, Murrysville, PA.).

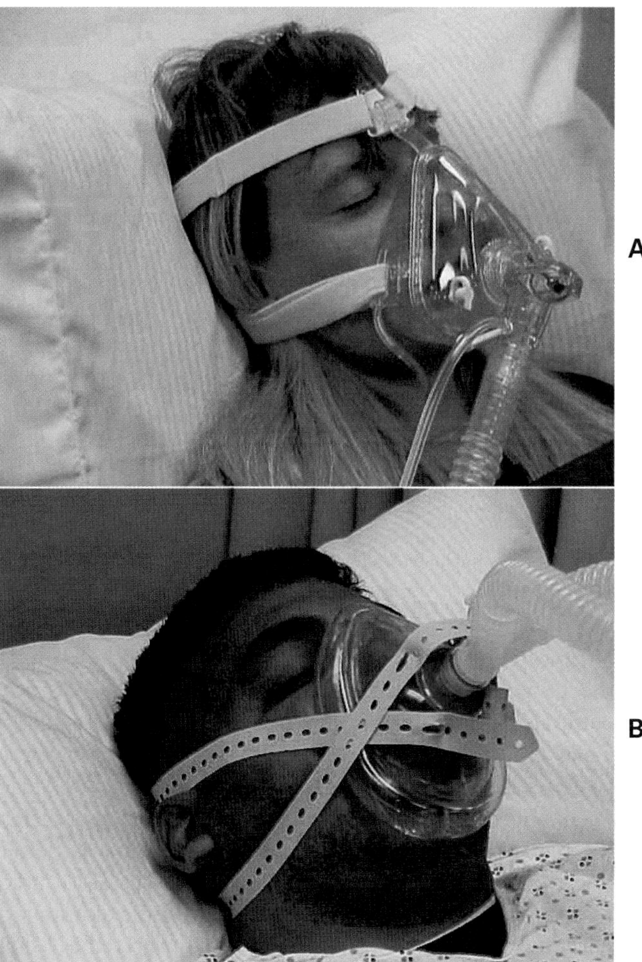

Figure 42-6

A, Application of a full-face mask used with a noninvasive ventilator. **B,** Application of a full-face mask used with a critical care ventilator.

space, risk of aspiration, and claustrophobia. Full-face masks also interfere with expectoration of secretions, with communication, and with eating. Most patients wearing a nasal mask can clear secretions and communicate.

Advances in mask design have incorporated quick-release straps that allow rapid removal of the mask if the patient vomits and entrainment valves that prevent asphyxia if the ventilator fails or the tubing becomes disconnected. The newest version of the full-face mask is a total face mask, which surrounds the entire face (Figure 42-7). A soft, flexible layer around the edge of this mask forms a seal and prevents leaking when the mask is pressurized. The total face mask comes in one size, which allows quick application in the emergency department or critical care unit. Because it does not obstruct the patient's vision, this mask may help patients who feel claustrophobic when wearing other full-face masks or nasal masks.

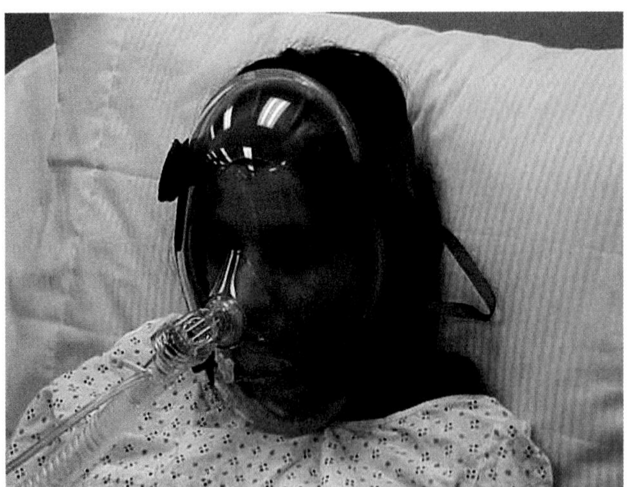

Figure 42-7
Total face mask (Respironics, Murrysville, PA.).

Few data are available in the literature to help guide the choice of a patient interface for NPPV. A study compared 30 minutes of full-face mask, nasal mask, and nasal pillows applied in random order to hypercapnic patients. The investigators reported that the full-face mask and nasal pillows improved ventilation more than the nasal mask did but that the nasal mask was better tolerated.[56] Use of a full-face mask also was associated with a significant increase in tidal volume compared with the nasal mask. This finding supports the belief that full-face masks may be more effective for dyspneic patients in the acute care setting.[3] If an acute care patient cannot tolerate a full-face mask, a nasal mask should be tried.

Ventilators Used for Noninvasive Positive Pressure Ventilation

Three types of ventilators are used for NPPV. They include noninvasive ventilators, critical care ventilators, and portable volume ventilators. This section describes the differences between the three types of ventilators and the modes of ventilation.

Noninvasive Ventilators

Most noninvasive ventilators are electrically powered, blower driven, and microprocessor controlled (Figure 42-8). These devices have a single-circuit design for delivering a constant flow of gas to the patient interface. A small leak is required in the circuit or patient interface for these ventilators to work correctly. The most important advantage of noninvasive ventilators over other types is the ability to trigger and cycle appropriately when small to moderate air leaks are present. Flow and pressure are measured in the device, and this information is used by the microprocessor to control gas delivery to the patient. Resistance between the patient and the ventilator must be kept low, so the ventilator can rapidly sense changes in flow and pressure. Use of smooth-lumen tubing to connect the ventilator to the interface is important in maintaining low resistance. If a heated humidifier is used, it must provide low resistance to gas flow. When NPPV devices are used in the acute care of patients who would otherwise need intubation, a few minimum performance characteristics must be met. Noninvasive positive pressure ventilators should provide a mandatory rate of up to 30 breaths/min, inspiratory pressure up to 30 cm H_2O, end positive airway pressure (EPAP) up to 15 cm H_2O, inspiratory flow of at least 60 L/min at 20 cm H_2O, FIO_2 from 0.21 to 0.50, minimal rebreathing potential, and antiasphyxia capabilities.[1] The ventilator must have alarms for circuit disconnect, loss of power, and battery failure if a battery is present. If supplemental oxygen is needed, the oxygen is bled into the ventilator circuit or attached to the patient interface. The FIO_2 rarely is constant owing to varying levels of flow that depend on patient effort and leaks. Difficulty obtaining an FIO_2 higher than 0.50 can be a limitation in the management of hypoxemic respiratory failure. The manufacture's recommendations should be consulted for an approximate FIO_2 range with a given oxygen flow rate and limitations on the maximum level of bled-in oxygen flow that can be used. Caution must be observed in the use of low baseline pressure levels. Low baseline pressure settings have been associated with significant rebreathing of carbon dioxide.[57,58] These reports suggest use of a nonrebreathing valve to prevent rebreathing of carbon dioxide, but use of this device produces greater expiratory resistance,[58] which may cause increased expiratory work of breathing or a higher baseline pressure. Increasing the baseline pressure may eliminate the problem of rebreathing carbon dioxide. When a baseline pressure of 5 cm H_2O was used in one study, the work of breathing and gas exchange were similar for a noninvasive ventilator and a critical care ventilator with the same settings.[59]

Modes on noninvasive ventilators usually include CPAP, spontaneous (pressure assist), and timed (pressure-limited, time-cycled) modes. Continuous positive airway pressure mode is a baseline pressure that is elevated above atmospheric pressure in a spontaneously breathing patient (Figure 42-9). With CPAP, there is no additional increase in pressure to alleviate the work of breathing when the patient inspires. The patient simply breathes with an elevated baseline. During the spontaneous or timed mode, the baseline pressure at end expiration is referred to as *expiratory positive airway pressure* (EPAP), and the increase in airway pressure that occurs during inspiration is referred to as *inspiratory positive airway pressure* (IPAP) (Figure 42-9). This increase in airway pressure during inspiration is

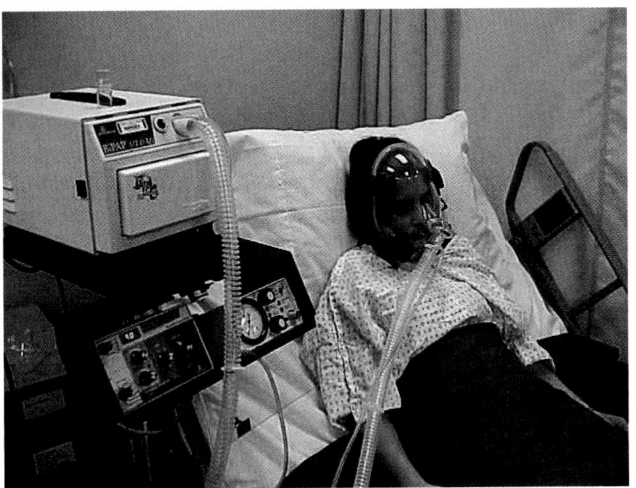

Figure 42-8
Noninvasive ventilator providing NPPV.

patient triggered in the spontaneous mode and time triggered in the timed mode. Inspiratory positive airway pressure usually is pressure limited and flow or time cycled.

Newer noninvasive ventilators for use in acute care include advances in monitoring, control of F_{IO_2}, and mode options. Graphics can be used for adjusting the ventilator settings. A blender is incorporated into the gas delivery system so that an accurate F_{IO_2} can be delivered, ranging from 0.21 to 1.0. Besides the pressure-limited modes of ventilation, the newer noninvasive ventilators have the option of a volume-limited mode. The platforms also allow the addition of new modes as they become approved by the U.S. Food and Drug Administration.

Critical Care Ventilators

Critical care ventilators usually are pneumatically powered and microprocessor controlled (Figure 42-10). These ventilators are available in most hospital critical care areas, and most of the staff is familiar with their general operation. The ventilators have a dual-limbed circuit with a separate exhalation valve, which limits the potential for rebreathing of carbon dioxide. Critical care ventilators have internal blenders that allow precise F_{IO_2} delivery, ranging from 0.21 to 1.0. The ability to

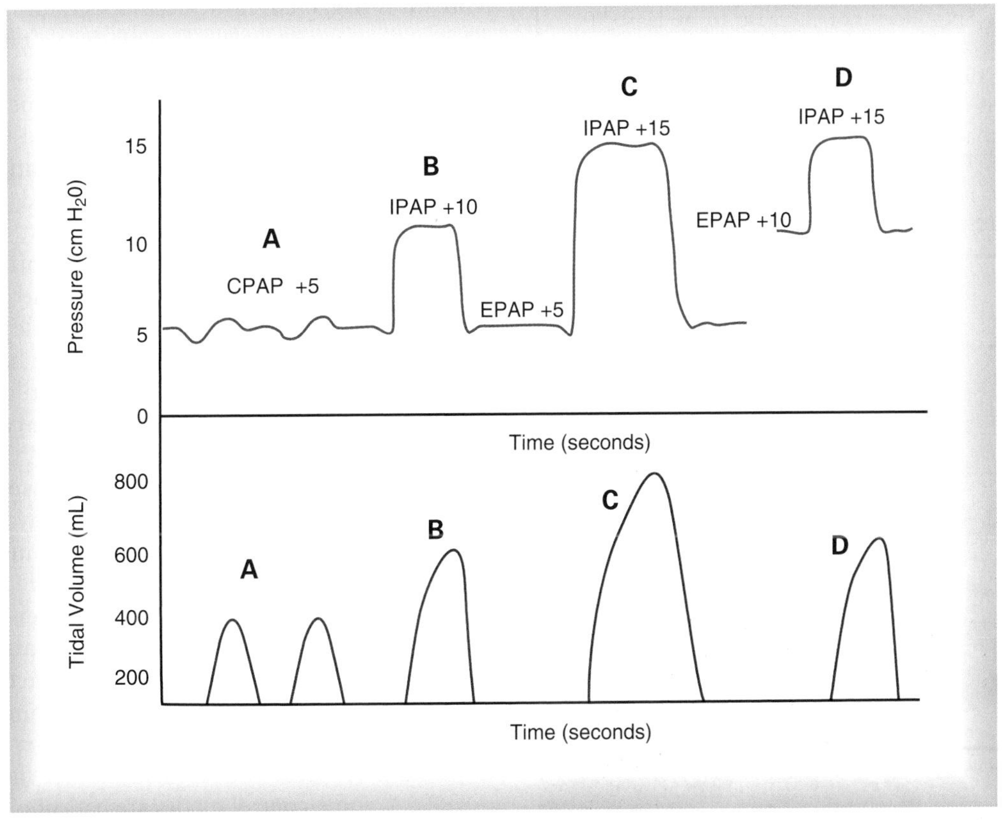

Figure 42-9
A, Continuous positive airway pressure of 5 cm H_2O with a patient breathing spontaneously and the resulting tidal volume. **B,** Patient-triggered breath during NPPV with an IPAP of 10 cm H_2O and EPAP of 5 cm H_2O and the resulting tidal volume. **C,** Inspiratory positive airway pressure has been increased to 15 cm H_2O. The corresponding increase in tidal volume is evident. **D,** Inspiratory positive airway pressure remains 15 cm H_2O, but EPAP has been increased to 10 cm H_2O. The corresponding decrease in tidal volume is evident.

MINI CLINI

Initiation of NPPV

PROBLEM

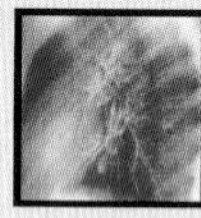

A patient with hypoxic respiratory failure is receiving nasal NPPV with a noninvasive ventilator. The ventilator is set on the spontaneous mode with an IPAP of 12 cm H_2O and EPAP of 5 cm H_2O. An oxygen flow of 6 L/min is going to a port on the nasal mask. The patient is having some difficulty keeping his mouth closed and breathing through his nose. The patient's PaO_2 is 50 mm Hg, and the patient continues to have signs of severe respiratory distress (dyspnea, respiratory rate of 30 breaths/min, heart rate of 130 beats/min, and cyanosis). The patient also reports nasal and oral dryness.

SOLUTION

For patients who cannot keep their mouths closed, nasal NPPV usually is not beneficial. A chin strap can be tried for keeping the patient's mouth closed, but dyspneic patients tend to breathe through their mouths. The best solution is to change to a full-face mask. Because the patient reports nasal and oral dryness, a low-resistance, heated humidifier should be added to the setup. Adding heated humidity should improve the patient's compliance with the therapy. The FIO_2 can be increased to the highest flow recommended by the manufacturer of the noninvasive ventilator. If the patient's SpO_2 does not increase to at least 90%, the noninvasive ventilator could be changed to a critical care ventilator or noninvasive ventilator with an internal blender to allow an FIO_2 of up to 1.0 to be delivered. If the FIO_2 is greater than 0.60, EPAP can be increased to improve oxygenation. If EPAP is increased, IPAP may have to be increased to maintain delivered tidal volume because the difference in pressure decreases when EPAP is increased.

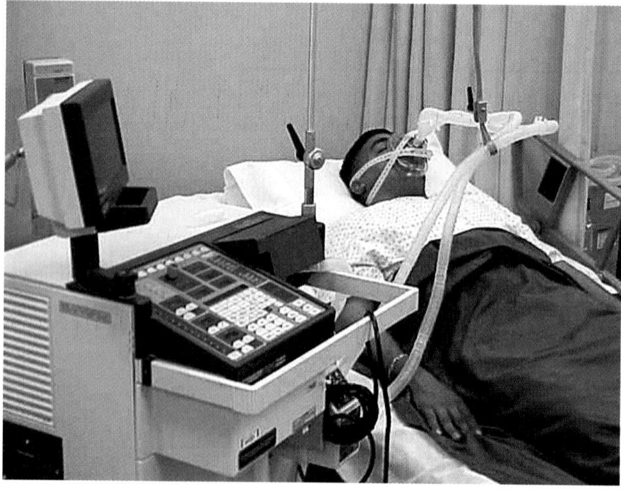

Figure 42-10
Critical care ventilator providing NPPV.

deliver a precise FIO_2 at high concentration can be the difference between success and failure of NPPV in some patients. Most critical care ventilators provide high inspiratory flow capabilities to patients with high demand. They also provide extensive monitoring and alarm capabilities. These alarms can become a nuisance during air leaks. The main problem with critical care ventilators used for NPPV is the inability to function smoothly in the presence of air leaks. Air leaks can cause problems with synchronization and termination of various modes of ventilation. These ventilators may be used in critical care areas with a full-face mask to limit the leaks that occur. The cost of these ventilators and the requirement of external gas sources for air and oxygen limit their usefulness in the home care environment.

Critical care ventilators have both pressure- and volume-limited modes of ventilation, which may be combined with positive end-expiratory pressure (PEEP) to provide an elevated baseline pressure. In general these modes can be patient or time triggered to inspiration and time or flow cycled to expiration. The mode of ventilation most used for NPPV on these ventilators is PSV, which is a pressure-limited, flow-cycled mode. Inspiratory pressure level is set during PSV. When the breath is triggered, flow increases rapidly to achieve this targeted pressure level. The amount of flow delivered depends on the patient's lung mechanics and breathing effort. Once the pressure level is achieved, the flow begins to decrease until a predetermined level of flow is reached, cycling the breath to exhalation. This predetermined flow level usually is a fixed value, such as 5 L/min, or a percentage of peak flow, such as 25%. The flow-cycling of PSV can cause problems during NPPV. When air leaks are present, the flow may not decrease to a low enough level to cycle the breath to expiration. In this case, the patient may have to actively exhale against the flow to cycle the ventilator to exhalation. This process may create unnecessary work for the patient, leading to the failure of NPPV. To correct this problem in the presence of air leaks, inspiration can be time cycled instead of flow cycled by changing the mode. As the set rate is increased, the inspiratory time decreases. Time-cycled (instead of flow-cycled), pressure-limited ventilation in the presence of air leaks may markedly improve respiratory rate and patient comfort.[60] Time-cycled pressure-limited ventilation, therefore, may improve patient compliance with therapy in the presence of air leaks.

Volume-control modes also can be used to deliver NPPV. Volume-control modes are patient or time triggered to inspiration. Instead of a targeted pressure, as with pressure-limited modes, a predetermined tidal volume is set during volume-control ventilation. Pressure varies

MINI CLINI

Improving Patient-Ventilator Synchronization During NPPV

PROBLEM

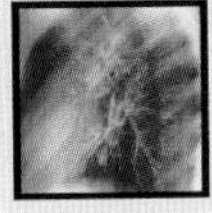

A do-not-intubate oncology patient is receiving NPPV from a critical care ventilator with a full-face mask using a Servo 300 ventilator. The ventilator is set on the PSV mode with an inspiratory pressure of 10 cm H_2O, PEEP of 5 cm H_2O, and a flow trigger of 2 L/min with a baseline flow of 5 L/min. The patient has a nasogastric (NG) tube in place to help protect against aspiration. The NG tube is causing a large leak. The ventilator is autocycling and failing to cycle into expiration when the patient exhales. The patient is fighting the ventilator and is completely asynchronous.

SOLUTION

Patient-ventilator asynchrony results form the large leak around the mask caused by the NG tube. Repositioning the mask and using a flat piece of petroleum gauze between the mask and the NG tube and between the NG tube and the patient's face will help produce a better seal. If an adequate seal cannot be obtained, instead of flow triggering, pressure triggering should be used to prevent autocycling due to the air leak. During PSV, the breath normally cycles into expiration after the flow decreases to a predetermined level or percentage of peak flow. If a large leak is present, the flow during PSV will not decrease to the level needed to cycle the ventilator into exhalation. As a default means of cycling, this ventilator is designed to also cycle at 80% of the set TCT in the PSV mode. Total cycle time is calculated by dividing 60 seconds by the set rate. If the rate setting increases, TCT decreases. Adjusting the rate knob can determine the maximum inspiratory time allowed during a PSV breath. For example, if the rate control is set on 30 breaths/min, 60 seconds divided by 30 would give a TCT of 2 seconds. When 2 seconds is multiplied by 0.80, an inspiratory time of 1.6 seconds is obtained. If the set rate is increased to 60 breaths/min, TCT is 1 second and inspiratory time is limited to 0.8 seconds. Another possible solution is to use a noninvasive ventilator instead of a critical care ventilator. Most noninvasive ventilators can better synchronize with leaks than can critical care ventilators.

with lung mechanics, patient effort, and air leak with volume ventilation. During pressure-control ventilation,* inspiratory pressure is kept constant, and the volume varies with patient's effort and lung mechanics. Air leaks during volume-control ventilation can result in hypoventilation due to loss of minute volume.

*Pressure support ventilation is a form of pressure-control ventilation (see Chapter 39).

Several studies have shown no difference in success or gas exchange between volume-control and pressure-control modes.[56,61,62] In two of these studies, patients preferred the pressure-control mode (PSV) to the volume-control mode of ventilation.[61,62] The current recommendation by an international consensus conference on NPPV in acute respiratory failure (ARF) is as follows: "Choice of mode should be based on local expertise and familiarity, tailored to the etiology and severity of the pathophysiological process responsible for ARF."[63]

In the chronic care setting, volume ventilation has been recommended for patients with neuromuscular weakness.[4] Volume ventilation may allow a patient to stack breaths; this process can increase lung volume to near inspiratory capacity to improve peak cough flow. High peak cough flow may enhance secretion clearance. In patients with limited muscle strength, pressure-control ventilation does not allow breath stacking because inspiratory pressure is held constant, unlike volume ventilation, in which delivered tidal volume is constant. There is no proven advantage of one mode versus another in the chronic care setting.[3]

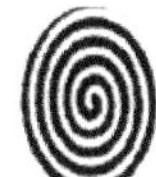

RULE OF THUMB

The choice of ventilator and mode of ventilation is determined primarily by the clinician's and staff's familiarity and experience.

Home Care or Portable Volume Ventilator

Most portable volume ventilators are electrically powered and microprocessor controlled. These devices can operate from alternating current (AC) or direct current (DC) power sources. Direct current power sources can be internal or external batteries that provide power for several hours. The DC power source provides backup if AC power fails and makes these devices portable. The devices have a single-limb ventilator circuit with a true exhalation valve. This exhalation valve should prevent rebreathing of carbon dioxide. These ventilators operate only with pressure triggering, which has been associated with increased inspiratory work to trigger a breath during NPPV.[64] Flow delivery is limited to a sine wave flow pattern. This flow pattern may limit the available flow to a patient with a strong drive to breathe, especially initially. These ventilators are primarily used in the chronic care setting and provide patient- or time-triggered volume ventilation. Home care ventilators are currently recommended for patients who need continuous ventilatory support or high ventilating pressures, such as those with severe chest wall deformities or obesity.[3]

Humidification

During nasal CPAP an increase in nasal resistance and congestion has been reported in patients with mouth leaks.[65,66] The application of heated humidity relieves nasal resistance and congestion.[65,66] The use of cold passover humidification does not significantly relieve nasal resistance.[65] The use of heated humidity during nasal CPAP in the care of patients with sleep apnea and nasal symptoms (sneezing, nasal draining, nasal and oral dryness, and nasal obstruction) has significantly improved patients' compliance with this therapy.[67,68] If nasal symptoms are present during NPPV, using heated humidity should relieve symptoms and improve compliance, as reported in the studies cited. Because the upper airway is not bypassed during NPPV, the current recommendation is no humidity for short-term applications (less than 1 day), unless a large air leak is present.[3]

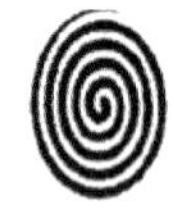

RULE OF THUMB

If the patient reports nasal and oral dryness, a heat humidifier with low resistance should be used.

▶ INSTITUTING AND MANAGING NONINVASIVE POSITIVE PRESSURE VENTILATION

Initiation of Noninvasive Positive Pressure Ventilation

At the initiation of NPPV, the type of ventilator and an appropriately sized interface must be selected and set up. The patient should be seated in a chair or bed at a 30-degree angle or greater. Before the mask is attached to the patient, the initial ventilator settings should be set. Initial pressure or volume should be low in a patient-triggered mode with a backup rate.[3] The recommended initial settings for NPPV in the spontaneous/timed mode are an IPAP of 8 to 12 cm H_2O and EPAP of 3 to 5 cm H_2O with a backup rate.[3] One manufacturer recommends that the initial backup rate be set at 8 breaths/min, which means that a timed breath will be delivered if the patient does not trigger a spontaneous breath every 7.5 seconds. As long as the patient is breathing at a rate higher than the rate set on the machine, all breaths will be patient triggered. In the absence of periodic apnea (daytime or nocturnal), the need for a backup rate in spontaneously breathing patients remains unclear (Box 42-6).

Initial NPPV settings for critical care ventilators may include pressure support of 5 to 8 cm H_2O, PEEP of 0 to 5 cm H_2O, and flow triggering set between 2 and 5 L/min. For volume ventilation with a critical care or home care ventilator in the assist-control mode, an initial tidal volume of 10 mL/kg, flow setting of 60 L/min, and inspiratory time of approximately 1 second are suggested. Patients with COPD exacerbation and hypoxic respiratory failure may need a flow as high as 100 L/min. The initial PEEP is set from 0 to 5 cm H_2O.

After the initial ventilator settings are determined, the patient interface is held in place by the patient or clinician. This procedure allows the patient to become comfortable with the initial settings. As the patient becomes more comfortable breathing with the ventilator, the inspiratory pressure or tidal volume should gradually be increased until dyspnea is relieved, respiratory rate decreases, and exhaled tidal volume is at least 7 mL/kg.[3] If tidal volume is monitored, it can be misleading or inaccurate in the presence of air leaks. If symptoms and vital signs improve, gas exchange should be assessed with blood gas analysis after approximately 1 hour. Supplemental oxygen should be used to maintain an Spo_2 at 90% or higher. Continuous positive airway pressure or PEEP should be adjusted to improve oxygenation or to improve triggering with counter-

Box 42-6 • Initiation of NPPV

1. Choose a location with appropriate monitoring on the basis of the severity of the patient's condition.
2. Place the patient at an angle ≥30 degrees.
3. Select a ventilator and an appropriately sized interface.
4. Connect the ventilator to the patient interface.
5. Turn on the ventilator.
6. Set initial settings depending on the choice of ventilator:
   - Noninvasive ventilator (NPPV): Spontaneous timed mode with IPAP of 8 to 12 cm H_20, EPAP of 3 to 5 cm H_2O, and backup rate of 8 breaths/min
   - Critical care ventilator: PSV with an inspiratory pressure of 5 to 8 cm H_20, PEEP of 0 to 5 cm H_20, and flow triggering set between 2 and 5 L/min
   - Assist-control mode with a tidal volume of 10 mL/kg, flow of 60 L/min, rate of 10 breaths/min, and PEEP of 0 to 5 cm H_20 with flow triggering set between 2 and 5 L/min
7. After setting initial settings, encourage the patient to hold the mask in place while the headgear is applied.
8. Adjust Fio_2 or bleed-in oxygen flow to keep Spo_2 >90%.
9. After the patient becomes comfortable with the initial settings, increase the inspiratory pressure or tidal volume until an exhaled tidal volume of 5 to 7 mL/kg is achieved or signs of respiratory distress improve.
10. Check for air leaks; adjust strap tension as needed.
11. Obtain arterial blood gas values within 1 hour.

balancing of intrinsic PEEP.[3] Estimating the amount of intrinsic PEEP during NPPV can be difficult without the use of an esophageal balloon. If the patient has obstructive disease and is having difficulty synchronizing with the ventilator on an appropriate sensitivity setting, increasing PEEP or CPAP until the patient can trigger the ventilator and improve synchronization may be indicated. In the process of fine-tuning the ventilator settings, the patient must be assessed continually for air leaks, the straps on the mask must be adjusted to maintain comfort, and the patient must be encouraged and reassured.[3]

Noninvasive Ventilator Adjustments

After NPPV is initiated and arterial blood gas analysis has been performed, the ventilator settings may have to be adjusted. Increasing IPAP increases the change in pressure (IPAP − EPAP) and should increase the delivered tidal volume. Increasing tidal volume usually decreases $Paco_2$. Decreasing IPAP decreases the change in pressure, which decreases delivered tidal volume and usually increases $Paco_2$. For patients with chronic hypercapnia, IPAP should be adjusted to maintain an acceptable pH. No attempt should be made to normalize the $Paco_2$ in such patients, but an appropriate pH should be the target.

Increasing EPAP should increase the patient's functional residual capacity (FRC), mean airway pressure, and Pao_2. Increasing EPAP also decreases the change in pressure; the possible result is a decrease in delivered tidal volume and an increase in $Paco_2$. If a patient has intrinsic PEEP due to obstructive disease, increasing EPAP can improve patient-ventilator synchronization. In theory, decreasing EPAP should decrease FRC, mean airway pressure, and Pao_2. In clinical practice, decreasing EPAP may not decrease Pao_2. As the disease process is relieved and alveolar stability improves, Pao_2 should not change significantly when EPAP is decreased. When EPAP is decreased, the change in pressure increases. This increased pressure difference may increase tidal volume and decrease $Paco_2$. If EPAP is decreased to less than 4 cm H_2O, rebreathing of carbon dioxide may occur because baseline flow to maintain the EPAP is not high enough to flush the exhaled carbon dioxide from the circuit.

Increasing Fio_2 usually increases the Pao_2. The Fio_2 is generally increased or decreased to maintain an Spo_2 of 90% or greater. New noninvasive ventilators have internal blenders that allow a precise Fio_2 up to 1.0 to be set. Other noninvasive ventilators require that the oxygen be bled in, and Fio_2 varies depending on the liter flow of oxygen and the ventilator settings. When oxygen is bled into the system, an Fio_2 of more than 0.50 to 0.55 usually is not possible. Bled-in oxygen flow never should exceed the manufacturer's recommendation. High Fio_2 percentages or oxygen flow rates may result in upper airway dryness because of the introduction of a dry medical gas rather than atmospheric air into the system.

Rate control is used to provide a backup rate during the spontaneous/timed mode. When this mode is used, the rate is set at 8 or 10 breaths/min and usually is not changed. In the care of some patients with neuromuscular disease, the timed mode is used, and the patient's ventilation may be greatly dependent on the set rate. In these cases, the set rate has a direct relation to minute ventilation and an inverse relation to $Paco_2$. Increasing rate increases minute ventilation and decreases $Paco_2$ and vice versa. In clinical practice and in the presence of spontaneous breathing, this may not always be the case. Table 42-1 summarizes ventilator adjustments during NPPV.

Monitoring

In acute care or chronic care applications, clinicians must not lose sight of the goals of NPPV.[3] Clinicians must assess the patient for leaks, accessory muscle use, ventilator synchronization, comfort, and improvement

Table 42-1 ▶▶ Noninvasive Positive Pressure Ventilator Adjustments

Setting	Adjustment	Anticipated Result
IPAP	↑	Increased tidal volume: ↑ ventilation and ↓ $Paco_2$
	↓	Decreased tidal volume: ↓ ventilation and ↑ $Paco_2$
EPAP	↑	Increased FRC, ↑ Pao_2, ↓ tidal volume Improved synchronization if intrinsic PEEP is present
	↓	Decreased FRC: ↓ Pao_2, ↑ tidal volume Possible rebreathing of CO_2 if EPAP <4 cm H_2O
Fio_2	↑	Increased Pao_2 Possible oral and nasal drying due to high flow of titrated O_2 or high Fio_2
	↓	Decreased Pao_2
Rate control*	↑	Increased minute volume in timed modes, ↓ $Paco_2$
	↓	Decreased minute volume in timed modes, ↑ $Paco_2$

*Rate control is generally used as a backup during the spontaneous timed mode. In this case the rate usually is set at 8 to 10 breaths/min and is not changed.

MINI CLINI

Problems with Triggering During NPPV

PROBLEM

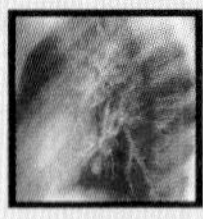

A COPD patient is receiving NPPV with a noninvasive ventilator using a full-face mask. The ventilator settings are as follows: IPAP, 12 cm H_2O; EPAP, 2 cm H_2O; and backup rate, 10 breaths/min in spontaneous/timed mode. You notice that the ventilator is not triggering with every patient effort. The patient's $Pa{CO_2}$ has decreased from 78 to only 75 mm Hg, and respiratory distress has not improved after 30 minutes of NPPV. What should you do to correct these problems with triggering and failure to improve ventilation?

SOLUTION

The failure to trigger and improve ventilation could be related to a poor mask seal, which results in excessive air leaking. You should first assess the patient for an adequate mask seal. If excessive leaking is occurring, refit the mask and adjust strap tension to obtain an adequate seal. If the noninvasive ventilator allows for adjustment of inspiratory sensitivity, the sensitivity setting should be adjusted so that the ventilator triggers with every patient effort. The failure to trigger and improve ventilation in this patient may be due to intrinsic PEEP and rebreathing of carbon dioxide. Increasing the EPAP to 6 or 8 cm H_2O in an effort to match the patient's intrinsic PEEP should improve the patient's ability to trigger the breath and the ability of the ventilator to sense the patient effort. Remember that if the baseline pressure or EPAP is increased, the sensitivity level of the ventilator and the IPAP setting may have to be readjusted. If the ventilator begins to autocycle, decrease sensitivity until autocycling stops. When EPAP is increased from 2 to 8 cm H_2O, the change in pressure (IPAP – EPAP) decreases from 10 to 4 cm H_2O. This decrease in pressure difference usually decreases the delivered tidal volume. If exhaled tidal volume decreases, IPAP should be increased until the exhaled tidal volume is 5 to 7 mL/kg or signs of respiratory distress decrease.

in vital signs and gas exchange. In the acute care setting, respiratory rate, heart rate, and gas exchange should improve within 30 minutes to 2 hours after initiation of NPPV. If the patient's vital signs and blood gas values are worsening after 30 minutes on optimal settings, intubation should be considered.[54] The severity of the patient's illness should determine the need for continuous monitoring of heart rate, blood pressure, and $Sp{O_2}$. A current consensus conference recommendation calls for a higher level of monitoring in the care of patients with acute hypoxemia, worsening condition, involvement of nonrespiratory organ systems, or persistent acidosis.[63] In the chronic care setting, improvement in gas exchange may require weeks to several months depending on daily use and overall compliance with the prescribed therapy.[3] Clinicians providing follow-up treatment in the chronic care setting need to assess usage with the elapsed time indicator on the ventilator. The patient should be assessed for complications, signs and symptoms, and factors that affect compliance and sleep quality.

Location

In the acute care setting, NPPV can be initiated in the emergency department, critical care unit, intermediate care unit, or hospital ward in an effort to prevent further deterioration of the patient's respiratory status.[63] Once NPPV is initiated, these patients should be transferred to an ICU or location that can provide continuous monitoring, skilled staff, and access to endotracheal intubation if needed.[3,63] Currently the only patient population for whom initiation and management of NPPV on a hospital ward are recommended are hypercapnic COPD patients with a pH of 7.30 or greater.[63] This recommendation is based on results of a study that showed NPPV initiated and managed on the general ward compared with standard therapy reduced the need for intubation and decreased in-hospital mortality among hypercapnic COPD patients with a pH of 7.30 or greater.[13] It is important that the staff be adequately trained before they use NPPV on the general hospital ward. Another current consensus conference recommendation calls for one-to-one monitoring of NPPV patients for the first few hours by a trained, experienced respiratory therapist, nurse, or physician.[63]

Weaning From NPPV

Currently there is no proven or broadly accepted standard for weaning from NPPV in the acute care setting. If high levels of inspiratory pressure or baseline pressure are required to maintain acceptable gas exchange and relieve symptoms of respiratory distress, these settings would be lowered to minimal settings as the disease process were to resolve. Patients are periodically given time off the mask to eat and expectorate secretions. As the disease process resolves and the settings are lowered, the amount of time the patient spends on NPPV is decreased. As long as respiratory distress does not develop, NPPV can remain on standby. If NPPV is successful, the patient usually needs 2 or 3 days of support.

▶ COMPLICATIONS OF NONINVASIVE POSITIVE PRESSURE VENTILATION

The reported failure rate of NPPV ranges from 7% to 42%.[3] The causes of failure of NPPV include mask-related complications, flow-related complications, large air leaks, patient-ventilator asynchrony, and failure to improve gas exchange.[3] Table 42-2 is a list of the complications, the rate of occurrence, and possible remedies. Mask-related complications include discomfort, claustrophobia, redness or inflammation around the mask, nasal bridge ulceration, and acneiform rash. An appropriately sized mask, adjustment of strap tension, and encouragement alleviate most of the problems associated with mask discomfort. If the patient continues to report mask discomfort, a new or different type of mask should be tried. Redness around the mask and nasal bridge ulcerations may be prevented by avoiding excessive strap tension and using a forehead spacer on the nasal mask. If redness or skin breakdown continues, application of a wound care dressing or artificial skin should be considered. Skin breakdown also can be prevented by mens of removing the mask every 4 to 6 hours for 15 minutes, as long as respiratory distress does not markedly increase. An air entrainment nebulizer or a nasal cannula can be used to maintain oxygenation during the rest period. Claustrophobia may be relieved by allowing the patient to hold the mask in place while the therapy is initiated, providing adequate inspiratory flow, encouraging the patient, and by using sedation judiciously. Different or newer mask designs also may relieve claustrophobia.

Air pressure and flow-related complications include nasal congestion, upper airway dryness, sinus and ear pain, eye irritation, and gastric insufflation.[3] Nasal congestion can be relieved with antihistamines and decongestants. The upper airway dryness caused by high gas flow may be alleviated with the addition of a heated humidifier. If the high flow causing the dryness is caused by air leaking through the mouth during nasal NPPV, use of a chin strap to help keep the mouth closed or use of a full-face mask should be helpful. Sinus and ear pain may be related to high inspiratory pressure; use of the lowest effective inspiratory pressure may prevent or alleviate this problem. Eye irritation usually is caused by air blowing into the eye as the results of a leak. This problem may be alleviated by use of a forehead spacer, application of an appropriately sized mask, and avoidance of excessive strap tension. Gastric insufflation occurs in as many as 10% of patients using NPPV. Use of the lowest effective pressure may prevent gastric insufflation. Routine use of a nasogastric (NG) tube is not recommended. An NG tube usually causes a large air leak. If an NG tube must be used, petroleum jelly gauze on top of and under the tube may lessen the air leak.

Small air leaks should be expected during noninvasive ventilation. However, large air leaks can lead to failure of NPPV by causing ventilator synchronization problems and reducing delivered tidal volume during volume ventilation. Refitting or changing the mask type, using appropriate mask tension, and using a chin strap and forehead spacer during nasal NPPV should improve the air leaks. To improve the cycling of the ventilator to expiration in the presence of an air leak, time-cycled, pressure-control ventilation can be used instead of flow-cycled, pressure-limited ventilation. Use of time cycling rather than flow cycling requires close attention from

Table 42-2 ▶▶ Frequency of Adverse Side Effects and Complications of NPPV With Possible Remedies

Side Effect	Occurrence (%)	Possible Remedy
Mask related		
Discomfort	30-50	Check fit, adjust strap, change new mask type
Facial skin erythema	20-34	Loosen straps, apply artificial skin
Claustrophobia	5-10	Use a smaller mask, administer sedative
Nasal bridge ulceration	5-10	Loosen straps, apply artificial skin, change mask type
Acneiform rash	5-10	Administer topical steroids or antibiotics
Air pressure– or flow-related		
Nasal congestion	20-50	Administer nasal steroids and decongestant or antihistamines
Sinus or ear pain	10-30	Reduce pressure if the pain is intolerable
Nasal or oral dryness	10-20	Apply nasal saline solution or emollient, add humidifier, decrease leak
Eye irritation	10-20	Check mask fit, readjust straps
Gastric insufflation	5-10	Reassure the patient, administer simethicone, reduce pressure if the pain is intolerable
Air leaks	80-100	Encourage mouth closure, try chin straps, try oronasal mask if using nasal mask, reduce pressure slightly
Major complications		
Aspiration pneumonia	<5	Select patients carefully
Hypotension	<5	Reduce inflation pressure
Pneumothorax	<5	Stop ventilation if possible, reduce airway pressure; insert a thoracostomy tube if indicated

From Mehta S, Hill NS: Am J Respir Crit Care Med 163:540, 2001.

the clinician to determine the patient's optimal inspiratory time. In general, 1 second is a good starting point, but adjustments must be made on the basis of lung mechanics and respiratory rate. Adjusting the trigger sensitivity can improve synchronization of the ventilator with the patient's effort. In the presence of a large air leak, flow triggering may result in autocycling of the ventilator. If autocycling occurs, use of a low level of pressure triggering should improve the patient's synchronization. During volume ventilation, loss in tidal volume due to air leaks usually is corrected with an increase in inspired tidal volume.

Major complications such as aspiration pneumonia, hypotension, and pneumothorax occur less than 5% of the time.[3] Most major complications can be avoided with careful patient selection and use of the lowest inspiratory pressure that improves the patient's gas exchange and relieves the symptoms. Noninvasive positive pressure ventilation should be avoided in the care of patients at risk of aspiration or hemodynamic instability. For do-not-intubate patients at risk of aspiration who choose NPPV, minimizing inspiratory pressure and maintaining the head of the bed at 30 degrees should reduce the risk of aspiration. If these or any other patients experience excessive gastric distention or nausea, an NG tube should be inserted and placed on low suction.

TIME AND COST ASSOCIATED WITH NONINVASIVE POSITIVE PRESSURE VENTILATION

The cost-effectiveness of NPPV is linked to appropriate patient selection, the staff's familiarity with associated procedures, and judicious use of supplies. An analysis showed that NPPV was less expensive and more effective than standard therapy in the care of patients with severe COPD exacerbations,[69] although this study has been criticized because of the lack of well-defined selection criteria in the analysis.[70] Staff time is one of the most valuable and expensive resources in hospitals. One study showed that the time required by nurses and physicians during the first 48 hours of NPPV was similar to the time they required for invasive mechanical ventilation, but the time required by respiratory therapists for NPPV was considerably greater than it was for invasive mechanical ventilation.[71] Another study, however, showed that the time required by respiratory therapists was significantly greater for the first 8 hours but significantly lower during the next 8 hours.[10] This increased time requirement early in the initiation of NPPV is due to mask fitting, application, and adjustment of ventilator settings. After stabilization, the time required to maintain NPPV should decrease significantly. As the experience of the staff increases, the amount of time required for initiation, stabilization, and maintenance should decrease.

KEY POINTS

- Noninvasive positive pressure ventilation is the application of positive pressure to the upper airway with a mask or mouthpiece to improve gas exchange.
- The use of NPPV to manage acute respiratory failure has increased in an effort to avoid the complications associated with intubation and to improve patient outcome.
- Most current evidence supports the use of NPPV in the care of patients with COPD exacerbations. There is less evidence supporting other indications for NPPV.
- Noninvasive positive pressure ventilation may be justified in the management of acute respiratory failure if selection criteria (Box 42-2) are present, exclusion criteria (Box 42-3) are absent, and the disease process is reversible within several days.
- Acute, cardiogenic pulmonary edema should be managed initially with CPAP of 10 to 12.5 cm H_2O. Noninvasive positive pressure ventilation should be considered only if hypercapnia develops or persistent dyspnea exists.
- Noninvasive positive pressure ventilation is most successful in the acute care setting when air leaks are minimal, the patient's severity of illness is low, respiratory acidosis is present but not severe, and gas exchange and vital signs improve within 30 minutes to 2 hours after initiation.
- There currently is no proven advantage of one mode of NPPV ventilation over another. The mode generally is chosen on the basis of the clinician's expertise and familiarity.
- Assessment for risk of complications is important in determining the success of NPPV.
- The time required by staff is lengthy during the initiation of NPPV owing to mask fitting, application, and adjustment of ventilator settings. After stabilization, the time required to maintain NPPV should decrease significantly.

References

1. ARCF Consensus Conference: noninvasive positive pressure ventilation: consensus statement, Respir Care 42:362, 1997.
2. Pierson DJ: Noninvasive positive pressure ventilation: history and terminology, Respir Care 42:370, 1997.
3. Mehta S, Hill NS: Noninvasive ventilation, Am J Respir Crit Care Med 163:540, 2001.
4. Bach JR: The prevention of ventilatory failure due to inadequate pump function, Respir Care 42:403, 1997.
5. Bach JR, Alba AS: Intermittent abdominal pressure ventilator in a regimen of noninvasive ventilatory support, Chest 99:630, 1991.
6. Intermittent positive pressure breathing therapy of chronic obstructive pulmonary disease, Intermittent Positive Pressure Breathing Trial Group, Ann Intern Med 69:612, 1983.
7. Sullivan CE et al: Reversal of obstructive sleep apnoea by continuous positive airway pressure applied through the nares, Lancet 1:862, 1981.
8. Rideau Y et al: Prolongation of life in Duchenne's muscular dystrophy. Acta Neurol Belg 5:118, 1983.
9. Meduri GU et al: Noninvasive face mask ventilation in patients with acute respiratory failure, Chest 95:865, 1989.
10. Kramer N et al: Randomized, prospective trial of noninvasive positive pressure ventilation in acute respiratory failure, Am J Respir Crit Care Med 151:1799, 1995.
11. Brochard L et al: Noninvasive ventilation for acute exacerbations of chronic obstructive pulmonary disease, N Engl J Med 333:817, 1995.
12. Celikel T et al: Comparison of noninvasive positive pressure ventilation with standard medical therapy in hypercapnic acute respiratory failure, Chest 114:1636, 1998.
13. Plant PK, Owen JL, Elliott MW: Non-invasive ventilation for acute exacerbations of chronic obstructive pulmonary disease on general respiratory wards: a multicentre randomized, controlled trial, Lancet 355:1931, 2000.
14. Bott J et al: Randomized, controlled trial of nasal ventilation in acute ventilatory failure due to chronic obstructive airways disease, Lancet 341:1555, 1993.
15. Nava S et al: Noninvasive mechanical ventilation in the weaning of patients with respiratory failure due to chronic obstructive pulmonary disease: a randomized, controlled trial, Ann Intern Med 128:721, 1998.
16. Barbe F et al: Noninvasive ventilatory support does not facilitate recovery from acute respiratory failure in chronic obstructive pulmonary disease, Eur Respir J 9:1240, 1996.
17. Meduri GU et al: Noninvasive positive pressure ventilation in status asthmaticus, Chest 110:767, 1996.
18. Bersten AD et al: Treatment of severe cardiogenic pulmonary edema with continuous positive airway pressure delivered by face mask, N Engl J Med 325:1825, 1991.
19. Mehta S et al: Randomized prospective trial of bilevel versus continuous positive airway pressure in acute pulmonary edema, Crit Care Med 25:620, 1997.
20. Wigder HN et al: Pressure support noninvasive positive pressure ventilation treatment of acute cardiogenic pulmonary edema, Am J Emerg Med 19:179, 2001.
21. Confalonieri M et al: Acute respiratory failure in patients with severe community acquired pneumonia, Am J Respir Crit Care Med 160:1585, 1999.
22. Wysocki M et al: Noninvasive pressure support ventilation in patients with acute respiratory failure: a randomized comparison with conventional therapy, Chest 107:761, 1995.
23. Antonelli M et al: A comparison of noninvasive positive-pressure ventilation and conventional mechanical ventilation in patients with acute respiratory failure, N Engl J Med 339:429, 1998.
24. Martin TJ et al: A randomized prospective evaluation of noninvasive ventilation for acute respiratory failure, Am J Respir Crit Care Med 161:807, 2000.
25. Wood KA et al: The use of noninvasive positive pressure ventilation in the emergency department, Chest 113:1339, 1998.
26. Delclaux C et al: Treatment of acute hypoxemic nonhypercapnic respiratory insufficiency with continuous positive airway pressure delivered by a face mask: a randomized, controlled trial, JAMA 284:2352, 2000.
27. Nourdine N et al: Does noninvasive ventilation reduce the ICU nosocomial infection risk? A prospective clinical survey, Intensive Care Med 25:567, 1999.
28. Girou E et al: Association of noninvasive ventilation with nosocomial infections and survival in critically ill patients, JAMA 285:2361, 2000.
29. Antonelli M et al: Noninvasive ventilation for treatment of acute respiratory failure in patients undergoing solid organ transplantation, JAMA 283:235, 2000.
30. Hilbert G et al: Noninvasive ventilation in immunosuppressed patients with pulmonary infiltrates, fever, and acute respiratory failure, N Engl J Med 344:481, 2001.
31. Hill N: Noninvasive ventilation for immunocompromised patients, N Engl J Med 344: 522, 2001.
32. Meduri GU et al: Noninvasive mechanical ventilation via face mask in patients with acute respiratory failure who refused endotracheal intubation, Crit Care Med 22:1584, 1994.
33. Aguilo R et al: Noninvasive ventilatory support after lung resectional surgery, Chest 112:117, 1997.
34. Joris JL et al: Effect of bi-level positive airway pressure nasal ventilation on the postoperative pulmonary restrictive syndrome in obese patients undergoing gastroplasty, Chest 111:665, 1997.
35. Girault C et al: Noninvasive ventilation as a systematic extubation and weaning technique in acute-on-chronic respiratory failure, Am J Respir Crit Care Med 160:86, 1999.
36. Vitacca M et al: Physiological response to pressure support ventilation delivered before and after extubation in patients not capable of totally spontaneous autonomous breathing, Am J Respir Crit Care Med 164:638, 2001.
37. Epstein SK, Ciubotaru RL, Wong JB: Effect of failed extubation on the outcome of mechanical ventilation, Chest 112:186, 1997.
38. Hilbert G et al: Noninvasive pressure support ventilation in COPD patients with postextubation hypercapnic respiratory insufficiency, Eur Respir J 11:1349, 1998.

39. Clinical indications for noninvasive positive pressure ventilation in chronic respiratory failure due to restrictive lung disease, COPD, and nocturnal hypoventilation: a consensus conference report, Chest 116:521, 1999.
40. Ferris G et al: Kyphoscoliosis ventilatory insufficiency: noninvasive management outcomes, Am J Phys Med Rehab 79:24, 2000.
41. Pinto AC et al: Respiratory assistance with a noninvasive ventilator (BiPAP) in MND/ALS patients: survival rates in a controlled trial, J Neurol Sci 129:19, 1995.
42. Aboussouan LS et al: Effect of noninvasive positive pressure ventilation on survival in amyotrophic lateral sclerosis, Ann Intern Med 127:450, 1997.
43. Aboussouan LS et al: Objective measures of the efficacy of noninvasive positive-pressure ventilation in amyotrophic lateral sclerosis, Muscle Nerve 24:403, 2001.
44. Cazzolli PA, Oppenheimer EA: Home mechanical ventilation for amyotrophic lateral sclerosis: nasal compared to tracheostomy–intermittent positive pressure ventilation, J Neurol Sci 139(suppl):123, 1996.
45. Raphael JC et al: Randomized trial of preventive nasal ventilation in Duchenne muscular dystrophy, French Multicentre Cooperative Group on Home Mechanical Ventilation Assistance in Duchenne de Boulogne Muscular Dystrophy, Lancet 343:1600, 1994.
46. Strumpf DA et al: Nocturnal positive-pressure ventilation via nasal mask in patients with severe chronic obstructive pulmonary disease, Am Rev Respir Dis 144:1234, 1991.
47. Gay PC et al: Nocturnal nasal ventilation for treatment of patients with hypercapnic respiratory failure, Mayo Clinic Proc 66:695, 1991.
48. Meecham-Jones DJ, Paul EA, Jones PW: Nasal pressure support ventilation plus oxygen compared with oxygen therapy alone in hypercapnic COPD, Am J Respir Crit Care Med 152:538, 1995.
49. Criner GJ et al: Efficacy and compliance with noninvasive positive pressure ventilation in patients with chronic respiratory failure, Chest 116:667, 1999.
50. Casanova C et al: Long-term controlled trial of nocturnal nasal positive pressure ventilation in patients with severe COPD, Chest 118:1582, 2000.
51. Masa JF et al: The obesity hypoventilation syndrome can be treated with noninvasive mechanical ventilation, Chest 119:1102, 2001.
52. Soo Hoo GW, Santiago S, Williams AJ: Nasal mechanical ventilation for hypercapnic respiratory failure in chronic obstructive pulmonary disease: determinants of success and failure, Crit Care Med 22:1253, 1994.
53. Ambrosino N et al: Non-invasive mechanical ventilation in acute respiratory failure due to chronic obstructive pulmonary disease: correlates for success, Thorax 50:755, 1995.
54. Poponick JM et al: Use of a ventilatory support system (BiPAP) for acute respiratory failure in the emergency department, Chest 116:166, 1999.
55. Meduri GU et al: Noninvasive positive pressure ventilation via face mask: first line intervention in patients with acute hypercapnic and hypoxemic respiratory failure, Chest 109:179, 1996.
56. Navalesi P et al: Physiologic evaluation of noninvasive mechanical ventilation delivered with three types of mask in patients with chronic hypercapnic respiratory failure, Crit Care Med 28:1785, 2000.
57. Ferguson GT, Gilmartin M: CO_2 rebreathing during BiPAP ventilatory assistance, Am J Respir Crit Care Med 151:1126, 1995.
58. Lofaso F et al: Evaluation of carbon dioxide rebreathing during pressure support ventilation with airway management system (BiPAP) devices, Chest 108:772, 1995.
59. Patel RG, Petrini MF: Respiratory muscle performance, pulmonary mechanics, and gas exchange between the BiPAP S/T-D system and the Servo ventilator 900C with bilevel positive airway pressure ventilation following gradual pressure support weaning, Chest 114:1390, 1998.
60. Calderini E et al: Patient-ventilator asynchrony during noninvasive ventilation: the role of expiratory trigger, Intensive Care Med 25:662, 1999.
61. Vitacca M et al: Non-invasive modalities of positive pressure ventilation improve the outcome of acute exacerbations in COLD patients, Intensive Care Med 19:450, 1993.
62. Girault C et al: Comparative physiologic effects of noninvasive assist-control and pressure support ventilation in acute hypercapnic respiratory failure, Chest 111:1639, 1997.
63. Evans TW: International consensus conference in intensive care medicine: non-invasive positive pressure ventilation, Intensive Care Med 27:166, 2001.
64. Nava S et al: Physiological effects of flow and pressure triggering during non-invasive mechanical ventilation in patients with chronic obstructive pulmonary disease, Thorax 52:249, 1997.
65. Richards GN et al: Mouth leak with nasal continuous positive airway pressure increases nasal airway resistance, Am J Respir Crit Care Med 154:182, 1996.
66. Hayes MJ et al: Continuous nasal positive airway pressure with a mouth leak: effect on nasal mucosal blood flux and nasal geometry, Thorax 50:1179, 1995.
67. Massie CA et al: Effects of humidification on nasal symptoms and compliance in sleep apnea patients using continuous positive airway pressure, Chest 116:403, 1999.
68. Rakotonanahary D et al: Predictive factors for the need for additional humidification during nasal continuous positive airway pressure therapy, Chest 119:460, 2001.
69. Keenan SP et al: Noninvasive positive pressure ventilation in the setting of severe, acute exacerbations of chronic obstructive pulmonary disease: more effective and less expensive, Crit Care Med 28:2094, 2000.
70. Jasmer RM, Matthay MA: Cost-effectiveness of noninvasive ventilation for acute chronic obstructive pulmonary disease: cashing in too quickly, Crit Care Med 28:2170, 2000.
71. Nava S et al: Human and financial costs of noninvasive mechanical ventilation in patients affected by COPD and acute respiratory failure, Chest 111:1631, 1997.

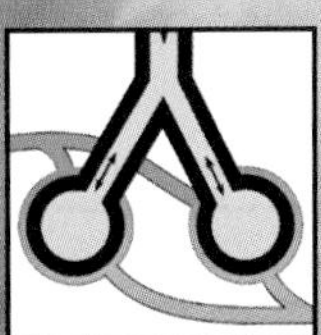

CHAPTER 43

Monitoring and Management of the Patient in the Intensive Care Unit

Alexander B. Adams and Sungchul Lim

In This Chapter You Will Learn:

- The principles of monitoring the respiratory system, cardiovascular system, neurological status, renal function, liver function, and nutritional status in the intensive care setting
- How to judge the risks and benefits of intensive care unit (ICU) monitoring techniques
- Why the caregiver is the most important monitor in the ICU
- How to evaluate measures of patient oxygenation in the ICU
- Why $Paco_2$ is the single best index of ventilation for critically ill patients
- How to evaluate changes in respiratory rate, tidal volume, minute ventilation, $Paco_2$, and end-tidal Pco_2 values for monitoring purposes
- The monitoring techniques used in the ICU to evaluate lung and chest wall mechanics and work of breathing
- The importance of monitoring peak and plateau pressures in patients receiving mechanical ventilatory support
- How to interpret the results of ventilator graphics monitoring
- The cardiovascular monitoring techniques used in the care of critically ill patients and how to interpret the results of hemodynamic monitoring
- The importance of neurological status monitoring in the ICU and the values that should be monitored
- How to evaluate renal function, liver function, and nutritional status in the intensive care setting
- How to use composite and global scores to measure patient status in the ICU, such as the Murray lung injury score and the APACHE II severity of illness scoring system
- How to monitor and troubleshoot the patient-ventilator system in the ICU

Chapter Outline

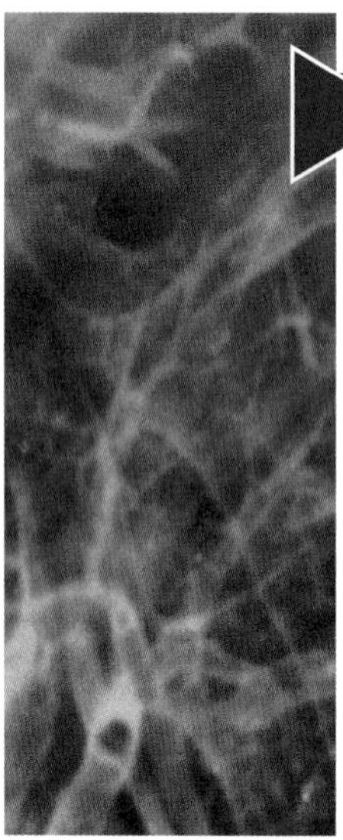

Key Terms

afterload
alveolar-arterial oxygen tension difference [$P_{(A-a)}O_2$]
APACHE scoring
artifacts
capnometry
contractility
dead space/tidal volume ratio (V_D/V_T)
esophageal pressure
factitious events
Fick equations
frequency/tidal volume ratio (f/V_T)
Glasgow coma score
Harris-Benedict equation
intracranial pressure
maximum inspiratory pressure
maximum voluntary ventilation
mean airway pressure
Murray lung injury scoring
oxygen consumption ($\dot{V}O_2$)
PaO_2/FIO_2 ratio
peak and plateau pressures
point-of-care testing
preload
pressure-time product
pressure-volume curve
shunt ($\dot{Q}s/\dot{Q}t$)
Swan-Ganz catheter
systematic errors
venous admixture
ventilatory drive
vital capacity
work of breathing

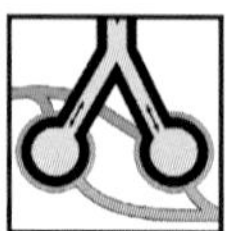

The concept and purpose of monitoring have evolved over the past 50 years. The importance of monitoring was established with the advent of the intensive care unit (ICU) during the polio epidemic in the 1950s.[1] Enhanced monitoring represents the main difference between a hospital bed and the ICU. The general purpose is simple and clear—to measure in "real time" certain physiological values that can change rapidly. Those values can be analyzed and interpreted with the expectation that interventions such as fluid resuscitation, medication administration, or changes in ventilator settings can be made in time to prevent adverse consequences. For the purposes of this chapter, monitoring emphasizes real-time measurements in the ICU and not intermittent diagnostic procedures such as chest radiography, electroencephalographic evaluations, and angiography. The distinction between monitoring and diagnostic testing is not always well defined, and monitoring can be broadly defined in this era of management of chronic disease. For example, pulmonary function values are monitored over years in outpatient clinics. The ICU exists to track the more acute changes in status discussed in this chapter. This chapter describes monitoring of the respiratory system, cardiovascular system, neurological status, renal function, liver function, and nutritional status in the ICU.

▶ PRINCIPLES OF MONITORING

Each monitoring test, procedure, and instrument carries certain risks and provides information that has value. There is an important balance between the risks and the benefit of monitoring techniques and procedures, especially as new monitoring techniques become available. Every test or monitoring method is continually judged for usefulness. Figure 43-1 depicts a continuum for judging the risk and benefit of tests, diagnostic procedures, and monitoring techniques. The better or best tests have little or no risk and high potential value. Poor tests carry higher risk with little potential value. For example, use of a pulse oximeter probe carries little physical risk, and the study provides valuable information about blood oxygenation (a low risk/benefit ratio), yet there is risk in obtaining incorrect numbers with the instrument. On the other hand, hemodynamic monitoring requires placement of a highly invasive **Swan-Ganz catheter** in the pulmonary artery to provide numbers that must be correctly interpreted. This type of monitoring should be undertaken only with the expectation of collection of important (high value) information. Thus the risk/benefit ratio for Swan-Ganz catheterization may be high. There is controversy over the widespread use of pulmonary arterial catheterization for this reason.[2]

The measurements made in monitoring must be critically considered through evaluation of certain characteristics of the data. The measurements define boundaries for acceptable values and indicators of abnormality that may require immediate attention. The fidelity of a measurement—the degree to which the instrument is actually correct in measuring the value—must be known. There often is nearly complete trust in a digital value displayed, yet the monitor might be "displaying" an incorrect value. When something looks wrong, the patient or the monitor could be considered the source of aberrant values. Signals or values are susceptible to variability due to **artifacts**, **factitious**

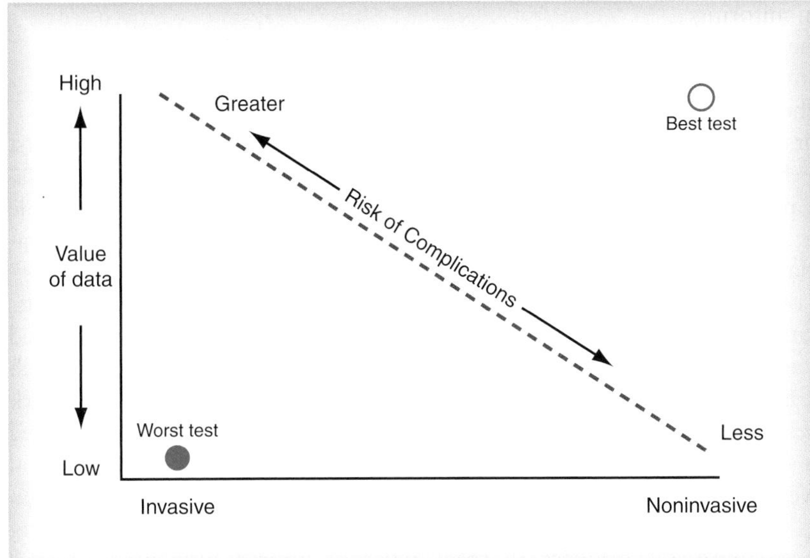

Figure 43-1 · Balancing the Value and Risks of Monitoring

A test or monitoring technique provides valuable data, but acquisition of the information may carry some risks. In general, more invasive techniques have an increasing risk of complications. At the same time, the value of the data should be greater. The best monitoring test would be noninvasive, have little risk, and provide valuable data. In contrast, a poor test would be invasive with high risk and low value.

events, physiological variation, and instrument drift. Artifacts are frequently seen, for example, when the patient or monitoring lines are moved. The artifacts usually are spikes or major shifts in values that are not real; that is, they are nonphysiological values. Factitious events are values that are real and "out-of-range" but often are temporary, such as the elevation in airway pressure during a cough.[3] Factitious events, being real, may require attention, whereas artifacts usually are self-resolving. In addition, the signal itself can exhibit a random variability related to the inherent imprecision of the signal or normal physiological variability in the patient. Blood pressure, for example, changes within a certain range for many reasons. Or the measuring instrument can produce values that are shifted in a systematic way—consistently high or low *or* in error in relation to the magnitude of the signal.[4] These shifts are referred to as either *parallel* or *slope shifts* (Figure 43-2). In general, all values must be interpreted with a background of training and experience so that one may understand when a value is normal and when to be concerned about abnormal values.

Monitored values should be accurate; that is, the measured values should correctly reflect the real values. Values should be precise; that is, measurements should not vary widely when repeated (the standard deviation of repeating the measurements should be low). Systematic errors, such as parallel or slope errors, must be corrected with calibration of the instrument. The "truth" of the data is values that are accurate and precise with minimal errors and are understood in the context of normal physiology or recent pathophysiological changes in the patient.

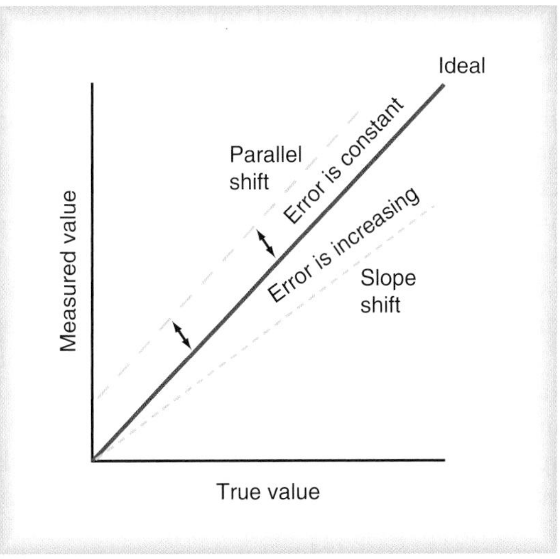

Figure 43-2 · Errors in Data Obtained With a Monitoring Instrument

Under ideal circumstances, the measured values obtained with a monitoring instrument are correct, and the instrument displays the true values. In reality, there are two forms of shifting from the true values—a parallel shift and a slope shift. Parallel shifts have a constant difference from the true value; therefore a one-point calibration brings all values into line. A slope shift occurs when measured values have an increasing (or decreasing) difference from the true values. Slope shifts require two-point calibration.

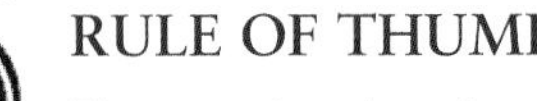

RULE OF THUMB

The caregiver has the ability to interpret a number of monitored values and to intervene. Monitors can run continuously and be used to measure values that caregivers cannot "see." The best monitor is the caregiver who understands the monitoring equipment, alarms, and resulting data.

Instruments and monitors used for ICU monitoring are of several types. The equipment is either at the bedside or brought to the bedside (**point-of-care testing**), or specimens are transported from the patient to instruments in a laboratory. The monitors can be noninvasive, connected to the surface of the body, or invasive, connected to lines or catheters that penetrate the body.

With the responsibility of detecting variations in physiological data comes the responsibility of setting the alarms appropriate to the monitor. The alarms should be set to detect monitored values that require attention. Monitors also are used to detect the artifacts, factitious events, and random variation often seen in the ICU. The ICU is a noisy environment with many alarms sounding that do not require immediate attention. Ventilators respond to coughs, and electrocardiographs (ECGs), oximeters, and vascular pressure monitors sound alarms with physical movements by the patient. Practitioners must develop mental filtering skill to evaluate true and false alarms and to know when to correct the alarm settings, when to wait for multiple alarms, and when to be concerned about an alarm signal (Box 43-1).

The best monitors continue to be the caregivers: the respiratory therapist, nurse, and physician. Changes in the patient's condition are detected and monitored most directly by means of patient assessment in the ICU. Chapter 14 describes the important details and bedside assessment skills required of caregivers in the ICU. This assessment is so valuable because the information is obtained by a potential decision-maker: the caregiver can act, but the monitor is passive. The art of the physical examination is being lost to the use of monitoring instruments. A common observation is a group of caregivers starring intently at monitors while a patient is waving for attention. Nevertheless, monitors have improved and replaced many of the skills of observation. Monitors are needed for two main reasons: (1) continuous assessment (humans need breaks) and (2) measurement of values that caregivers cannot detect such as ECG findings and airway pressure.

Box 43-1 • Monitors and Monitoring Data

- Monitored values can exhibit physiological and instrument variability.
- Monitoring devices can be noninvasive or invasive.
- Alarm systems should be set to properly alert caregivers yet avoid false alarms.
- The best monitors are caregivers who can assess and make decisions, but monitors can run continuously and measure what caregivers cannot see.

▶ PATHOPHYSIOLOGY AND MONITORING

Monitoring produces numbers from measurements. Fixing the numbers rather than managing the dysfunction often becomes the treatment goal. An example is increasing the fractional inspired oxygen concentration (FIO_2) to increase the oxygen saturation "numbers" as read with a pulse oximeter. Whenever possible, the goals of monitoring and treatment should be based on managing the pathophysiological process. For each organ or organ system, there is a conceptual framework for the disease process, and treatment should be based on correcting or adapting to the pathophysiological condition. The lungs, for example, contain 300 million alveoli, but a basic model of lung injury reduces a lung disorder to three types of injured lung units (Figure 43-3): (1) alveoli that are ventilated but not perfused (dead space units), (2) alveoli that are perfused but not ventilated (shunt units) and, (3) alveoli that are receiving either partial ventilation or partial perfusion ($\dot{V}/\dot{Q}$ mismatch). In terms of treatment options, $\dot{V}/\dot{Q}$ mismatching is more receptive to oxygen therapy than are shunt or dead space units. Yet all three forms of lung injury units display reduced oxygen saturation. Within the context of this injury model, treatment should be aimed at the source of the disorder and not be an attempt to "fix" the arterial partial pressure of oxygen (PaO_2) or oxygen saturation by pulse oximeter (SpO_2) value.

▶ RESPIRATORY MONITORING

Gas Exchange

The most important function of the lungs is uptake of oxygen from air into the arterial blood and disposal of carbon dioxide from the mixed venous blood into the environment. Arterial blood gas (ABG) values contain this gas exchange information. A typical report includes PaO_2, oxygen saturation (SaO_2), arterial partial pressure of carbon dioxide ($PaCO_2$), pH, and estimated base excess or deficit. For critically ill patients, ABG specimens can be obtained quickly and sent to the laboratory for analysis. The technology has become available for monitoring ABGs at the bedside (point-of-care testing) and invasively or continuously with indwelling sensors. The typical absolute values, their predicted values, derangements including compensation, and basic interpretation of ABGs are described in Chapter 16. The ABGs do not tell the complete story, however; other values that are actively obtained or calculated are discussed in this section.

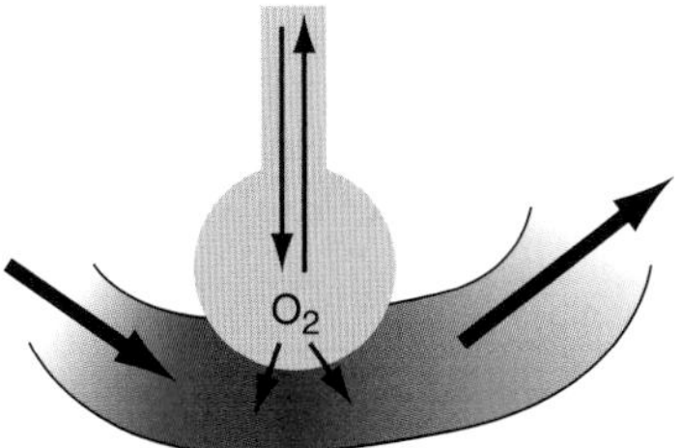

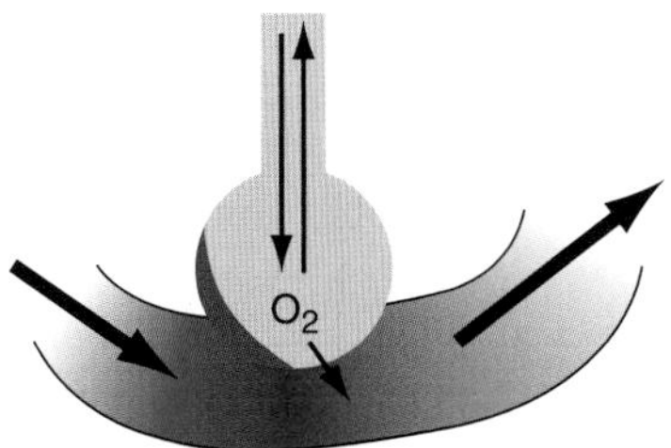

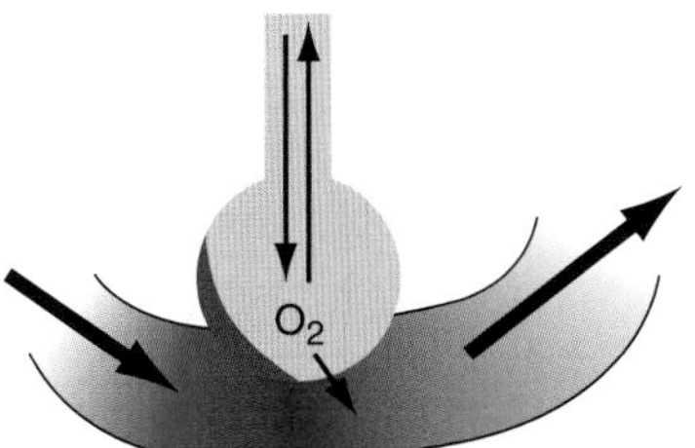

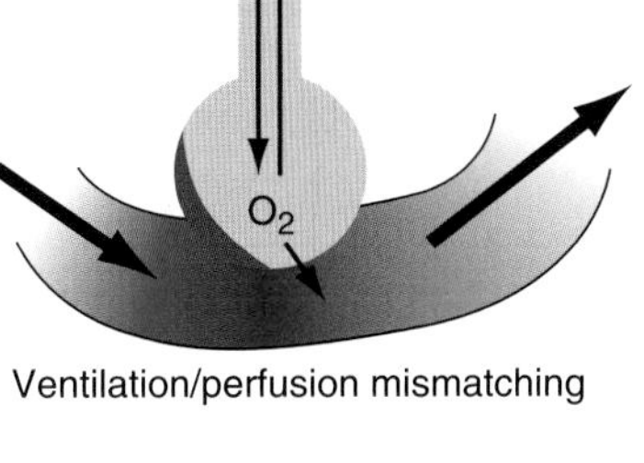

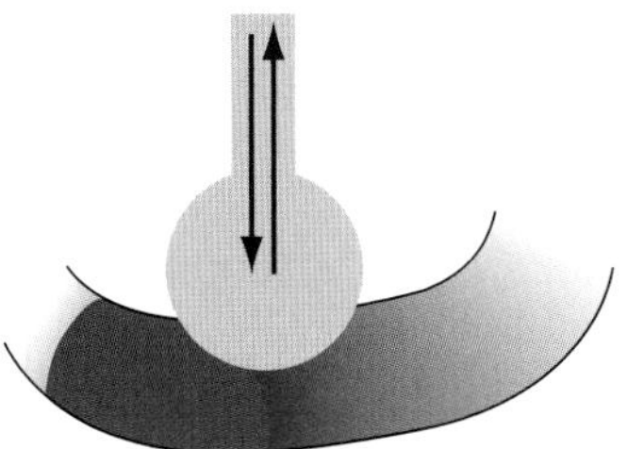

Figure 43-3
A model for the causes of uneven matching of gas and blood in the lung.

Monitoring Oxygenation

Tissue oxygenation depends on inspired oxygen levels (FIO_2, inspired partial pressure of oxygen [PIO_2]), alveolar oxygen tension (PAO_2), arterial oxygenation (PaO_2, SaO_2, oxygen content of arterial blood [CaO_2]), oxygen delivery (DO_2), and tissue perfusion and oxygen uptake.

Arterial Pulse Oximetry. The goal of breathing and circulation is tissue oxygenation. All organs need adequate oxygen delivery with particularly high requirements for the brain and kidneys. An important innovation in monitoring has been the use of oximetry, in which color spectrum measurement is used for continuous assessment of arterial oxygenation (SpO_2). The human eye is not good at detecting or quantifying arterial hypoxemia.[5] Frank cyanosis does not develop until the deoxyhemoglobin level is at least 5 g/dL, which corresponds to an SaO_2 of approximately 67%.[6] Furthermore, the threshold at which cyanosis becomes apparent is affected by skin perfusion, skin pigmentation, and hemoglobin concentration.[7] Blood gas analysis has been the accepted method of detecting hypoxemia in the care of critically ill patients, but ABG analysis is painful, has complications, and does not provide immediate or continuous data.[8] For these reasons, pulse oximetry has become the standard for continuous and noninvasive assessment of SaO_2. Pulse oximetry does not measure $PaCO_2$, and patients breathing an elevated FIO_2 may have increases in $PaCO_2$ before oximetry values are affected. Ventilatory failure may then go unnoticed unless ABGs are measured.

Oximetric measurements are based on spectrophotometric principles, which are based on the law of Beer-Lambert.[9] Lightweight probes direct filtered light of specific wavelengths, usually two, onto the surface of a digit, the nasal bridge, or an earlobe. The relative absorption of these spectrophotometric beams as they pass through the tissue (which differs for oxygen saturated and desaturated blood) is converted into the appropriate saturation value with computer-stored algorithms.

RULE OF THUMB

Pulse oximetric values have been considered a fifth vital sign. There are two very important problems with relying on oximetry to monitor adequate respiratory function: (1) Oximetric values reflect oxygenation, not ventilation, and (2) SpO_2 measurement is susceptible to a number of factors that can produce false values.

Although pulse oximetry has been universally accepted, it does have limitations (Box 43-2). Motion artifact is an important problem, resulting in inaccurate readings and false alarms.[10] Artifacts are commonly caused by motion due to shivering, seizure activity, pressure on the sensor, or transport of the patient. The choice of probe site may also affect accuracy. Finger probes appear more accurate than forehead, nose, or earlobe probes during low perfusion states.[11] Intense daylight and fluorescent, incandescent, xenon, and infrared light sources have caused errors in pulse oximetric readings.[7] Anemia and deeply pigmented skin can affect the accuracy of pulse oximetry; however, the effect of anemia is not clinically significant until the hemoglobin level is less than 5 g/dL.[12] Carboxyhemoglobin and methemoglobin[6] can produce falsely high saturation values and some colors of nail polish, particularly blue, green, and black, interfere with light transmission and absorbency, as do some blood-borne dyes, such as indocyanine green and methylene blue,[13] which tend to produce falsely low oxygen saturation values.

Oxygen Consumption. Oxygen consumption ($\dot{V}O_2$) is the volume of oxygen used by the body (in milliliters per minute). Normal resting oxygen consumption is approximately 250 mL/min, and oxygen consumption increases with activity, stress, and temperature. Although a seemingly valuable measurement, oxygen consumption often is difficult to measure accurately at the bedside in the care of patients receiving mechanical ventilation. Two primary methods are in general use: the Fick method and analysis of inspired and expired gases. Neither method reflects average oxygen consumption when the patient's metabolic rate fluctuates during data collection. The **Fick equations** are as follows:

$$\dot{Q}t = \dot{V}O_2/(CaO_2 - C\bar{v}O_2)$$

$$\dot{V}O_2 = \dot{Q}t \times (CaO_2 - C\bar{v}O_2)$$

in which $\dot{Q}t$ is cardiac output and CaO_2 and $C\bar{v}O_2$ are the arterial and mixed venous oxygen contents, respectively. If the values for $\dot{Q}t$, CaO_2, and $C\bar{v}O_2$ are normal, this becomes

$$\dot{V}O_2 \text{ in mL/min} = \dot{Q}t \times (CaO_2 - C\bar{v}O_2)$$

$$= 5000 \text{ mL/min} \times (20 \text{ mL/100 mL} - 15 \text{ mL/100 mL})$$

$$= 5000 \text{ mL/min} \times 5 \text{ mL/100 mL} = 250 \text{ mL/min}$$

An alternative calculation for oxygen consumption that does not require an arterial or mixed venous blood sample or measurement of cardiac output is

$$\dot{V}O_2 = [FIO_2 \times \dot{V}_I] - [F\bar{E}O_2 \times \dot{V}_E]$$

where FIO_2 and $F\bar{E}O_2$ are the mean inspired and expired fractional concentrations of oxygen and $\dot{V}_I$ and $\dot{V}_E$ are the inspired and expired minute ventilations. If $\dot{V}_I$ equals $\dot{V}_E$ (normally $\dot{V}_I$ is slightly greater than $\dot{V}_E$, but the difference is small), this becomes

$$\dot{V}O_2 = (FIO_2 - F\bar{E}O_2)\dot{V}_E$$

If the values for minute ventilation and inspired and expired gas concentrations are normal, this becomes

$$\dot{V}O_2 = (0.21 - 0.168)6 \text{ L/min} = 0.252 \text{ L/min, or approximately } 250 \text{ mL/min}$$

A normal resting oxygen consumption of 250 mL/min represents approximately 25% of normal oxygen delivery (1000 mL/min); therefore the blood carries a large reservoir of oxygen that can be extracted under conditions of stress.

Oxygen consumption may be useful in determining nutritional requirements and adequacy of oxygen delivery and may occasionally help determine the cause of a high ventilation requirement. If there is a stable tissue demand for oxygen, measurements of oxygen consumption may be used to follow the hemodynamic response to therapeutic interventions. Unfortunately, serial oxygen consumption measurements often are highly variable and are subject to sudden changes in underlying metabolic requirements.

Alveolar-Arterial Oxygen Tension Difference. The difference between alveolar and arterial oxygen tension [$P(A - a)O_2$] is a useful measure of the efficiency of gas exchange. A healthy person breathing room air has a $P(A - a)O_2$ of approximately 5 to 15 mm Hg. This value increases with age to approximately 10 to 20 mm Hg in

Box 43-2 • Values Affecting Pulse Oximetry

- Motion artifact
- Environmental light (e.g., sunlight, fluorescence)
- Anemia
- Deeply pigmented skin
- Carboxyhemoglobin, methemoglobin
- Nail polish
- Blood-borne dyes

MINI CLINI

Trusting the Pulse Oximeter

PROBLEM

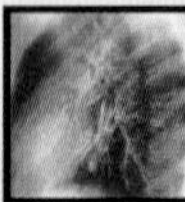

A 32-week-gestation newborn is intubated and receiving continuous positive airway pressure (CPAP) therapy. The patient appears to be in mild to moderate respiratory distress, yet the pulse oximeter displays an SpO_2 of 98%. Hurricane spray (20% benzocaine) had been used to reduce the irritation of the endotracheal tube. Analysis of ABGs reveals a PaO_2 of 325 mm Hg, and the co-oximeter shows a methemoglobin value of 38%.

SOLUTION

The most common problems with the fidelity of pulse oximeter readings are motion artifacts, interference by external light sources, or malposition of the sensor. Each of these problems can be easily and quickly assessed. In this case, the clinical symptoms did not correlate with an acceptable pulse oximetric value. Because adequate oxygen delivery is the ultimate goal, cardiac output and oxygen-carrying ability must be considered as causes of the respiratory distress. The high methemoglobin value necessitates immediate therapy with methylene blue dye. Whereas the pulse oximeter has provided an excellent, safe means of monitoring blood oxygenation, there must be a wary vigilance about trusting the values.

the elderly. The $P(A - a)O_2$ also increases normally with an increasing FIO_2. For example, a healthy person has a $P(A - a)O_2$ of 5 to 15 mm Hg while breathing room air; however, $P(A - a)O_2$ increases to 100 to 150 mm Hg when the person is breathing 100% oxygen.

An abnormally increased $P(A - a)O_2$ is associated with gas exchange problems. For example, if PaO_2 is 80 mm Hg while the patient is breathing 100% oxygen, a significant gas exchange problem is apparent after $P(A - a)O_2$ is determined, according to the following calculation.

If PaO_2 is 80 mm Hg, $PaCO_2$ is 40 mm, FIO_2 is 1.0, and barometric pressure (P_B) is 760 mm Hg, then

$$PAO_2 = PIO_2 - (PaCO_2 \times 1.25) = [(P_B - P_{H_2O})FIO_2] - (PaCO_2 \times 1.25) = [(760\text{-}47)\ 1.0] - (40 \times 1.25) = 663 \text{ mm Hg}$$

$$P(A - a)O_2 = PAO_2 - PaO_2 = 663 - 80 = 583 \text{ mm Hg}$$

where P_{H_2O} is water vapor pressure. This level is markedly elevated considering that normal $P(A - a)O_2$ is 100 to 150 mm Hg while the patient is breathing 100% oxygen. The $P(A - a)O_2$ while the patient is breathing 100% oxygen also can be used to give a rough estimate of percentage shunt where

$$\text{Percentage shunt} \cong \frac{P(A - a)O_2\ (100\%\ O_2)}{20}$$

In this example, percentage shunt would be approximately 29%: $P(A - a)O_2/20 = 583/20 = 29.2\%$).

The $P(A - a)O_2$ takes into account $PaCO_2$ and therefore eliminates hypoventilation and hypercapnia from consideration as the sole cause of hypoxemia.

Arterial-Alveolar Oxygen Tension Ratio. Unlike $P(A - a)O_2$, the arterial-alveolar oxygen tension ratio (PaO_2/PAO_2) has been reported to be relatively stable with changing levels of FIO_2. This index also can be used to predict the FIO_2 needed to achieve a desired PaO_2[14,15] where

$$PAO_2 \text{ required} = \frac{PaO_2 \text{ desired}}{PaO_2/PAO_2 \text{ calculated}}$$

PaO_2/FIO_2 Ratio. The arterial-inspired oxygen concentration ratio (PaO_2/FIO_2) has become important for the determination of acute lung injury (ALI) and acute respiratory distress syndrome (ARDS) in multicenter collaborative studies.[16] A normal PaO_2/FIO_2 ratio is 380 or greater. In the absence of an elevated left atrial pressure, this ratio defines ALI as a PaO_2/FIO_2 ratio less than 300 mm Hg and ARDS as a PaO_2/FIO_2 less than 200 mm Hg. The PaO_2/FIO_2 ratio is easy to calculate and the most reliable index of gas exchange when FIO_2 is greater than 0.5 and PaO_2 is less than 100 mm Hg, values often observed in critically ill patients.

Respiratory Index. Another respiratory index has been defined by $P(A - a)O_2/PaO_2$ ratio. Several studies have shown this index to be an unreliable index of gas exchange efficiency.[17,18] Only one study showed this index to be useful as a predictor of severity and prognosis in ARDS.[19]

Quantification of Shunt. The most accurate and reliable measure of oxygenation efficiency is direct computation of physiological shunt ($\dot{Q}s/\dot{Q}t$). The physiological shunt in the lungs is computed with the following equation:

$$\dot{Q}s/\dot{Q}t = (Cc'O_2 - CaO_2)/(Cc'O_2 - C\bar{v}O_2)$$

where $Cc'O_2$ is the oxygen content of alveolar capillary blood, CaO_2 is the oxygen content of arterial blood, and $C\bar{v}O_2$ is the oxygen content of mixed venous blood, all expressed in milliliters of oxygen per 100 mL of blood. When the patient is breathing 100% oxygen, $\dot{Q}s/\dot{Q}t$ can be estimated with the following alternative calculation:

$$\dot{Q}s/\dot{Q}t = (P(A - a)O_2 \times 0.003)/[(P(A - a)O_2 \times 0.003) + (CaO_2 - C\bar{v}O_2)]$$

For measurement of the physiological shunt, both an arterial and a mixed venous blood sample must be obtained. A true mixed venous blood sample can be obtained only from the distal sample port of an indwelling pulmonary arterial catheter. The total oxygen content of the arterial, mixed venous blood, and pulmonary capillary blood (CaO_2, $C\bar{v}O_2$, $Cc'O_2$) is calculated in the same manner as the oxygen consumption calculations, as follows:

$$\text{Oxygen content} = (1.34 \times Hb \times SO_2) + (0.003 \times PO_2)$$

where Hb is the hemoglobin concentration, SO_2 is the oxygen saturation, and PO_2 is the partial pressure of oxygen. If the patient is breathing 100% oxygen, the capillary saturation is 100%, the $Pc'O_2$ being the calculated PAO_2 value. Samples should be obtained and analyzed in a manner that reduces the time lapse effects of sampling and analysis. Like $P(A - a)O_2$, $\dot{Q}s/\dot{Q}t$ is influenced by variations in $\dot{V}/\dot{Q}$ mismatching and by fluctuations in mixed venous oxygen saturation ($S\bar{v}O_2$) and FIO_2. A "shunt" calculation when FIO_2 is less than 1.0 is a measure of percentage venous admixture. If venous admixture is abnormally high but all alveoli are patent, calculated venous admixture diminishes toward the normal physiological value (<5%) as FIO_2 is increased. Conversely, if increased venous admixture results when blood bypasses patent alveoli through intrapulmonary communications or through an intracardiac defect, there is no change in venous admixture as FIO_2 is increased.

Murray Lung Injury Score. Acute respiratory distress syndrome is the syndrome of severe lung injury that was originally described by Ashbaugh and Petty in 1970.[20] To monitor the severity of this disease, Murray et al

Box 43-3 • Murray Lung Scoring

COMPONENT	VALUE	
1. Chest radiograph		
No alveolar consolidation		0
Alveolar consolidation confined to 1 quadrant		1
Alveolar consolidation confined to 2 quadrants		2
Alveolar consolidation confined to 3 quadrants		3
Alveolar consolidation in all 4 quadrants		4
2. Hypoxemia score		
Pao_2/Fio_2	>300	0
Pao_2/Fio_2	225-299	1
Pao_2/Fio_2	175-224	2
Pao_2/Fio_2	100-174	3
Pao_2/Fio_2	<100	4
3. PEEP score (when ventilated)		
PEEP	>5 cm H_2O	0
PEEP	6-8 cm H_2O	1
PEEP	9-11 cm H_2O	2
PEEP	12-14 cm H_2O	3
PEEP	>15 cm H_2O	4
4. Respiratory system compliance score (when available)		
Compliance	>80 mL/cm H_2O	0
Compliance	60-79 mL/cm H_2O	1
Compliance	40-59 mL/cm H_2O	2
Compliance	20-39 mL/cm H_2O	3
Compliance	<19 mL/cm H_2O	4

The final value is obtained by dividing the aggregate sum by the number of components used.

	Score
No lung injury	0
Mild-to moderate lung injury	0.1-2.5
Severe lung injury (ARDS)	>2.5

developed a lung injury score that often is calculated in studies of ALI and ARDS.[21] The **Murray lung injury score** quantifies the injury level with four factors: chest radiographic findings, Pao_2/Fio_2 ratio, positive end-expiratory pressure (PEEP) setting, and compliance. The lung injury score is an example of a composite score that allows quantification of lung status according to different aspects of the injury—gas exchange, radiographic findings, and mechanics. The Murray lung injury score is reported in many studies of new therapies[21] as an index of the effectiveness of therapy or for interstudy comparisons. The method for calculating the Murray lung injury score is shown in Box 43-3. Other measures of lung injury are listed in Box 43-4.

Monitoring Ventilation

As can oxygenation, the adequacy and efficiency of ventilation can be evaluated (Box 43-5). Routine monitoring of patients receiving mechanical ventilatory support in the ICU includes measurement of the

Box 43-4 • Measures of Decreased Blood Oxygenation or Lung Injury

- ↓ Spo_2
- ↓ Pao_2
- ↑ $P(A - a)o_2 - (PAo_2 - Pao_2)$
- ↓ P/F ratio – (Pao_2/Fio_2)
- ↑ Shunt/venous admixture
- ↑ Murray lung injury score

Box 43-5 • MONITORING THE ADEQUACY OF VENTILATION

- Respiratory volume and rate (V_T, f, $\dot{V}_E$)
- $Paco_2$
- V_{DS}/V_T
- Capnometry (not for routine use but in special situations, such as assuring tracheal intubation and cardiac blood flow in resuscitation efforts)

patient's tidal volume (V_T), respiratory rate (f), and minute ventilation ($\dot{V}_E$) where

$$\dot{V}_E = f \times V_T$$

However, effective ventilation depends on alveolar ventilation ($\dot{V}_A$), as follows:

$$\dot{V}_A = (V_T - V_{DSphys})f$$

where V_{DSphys} is physiological dead space, and

$$\dot{V}_A = \frac{0.863 \times \dot{V}co_2}{Paco_2}$$

where $\dot{V}co_2$ is carbon dioxide production in milliliters per minute, and 0.863 is a conversion factor. With a normal $Paco_2$ and $\dot{V}co_2$ this becomes

$$\dot{V}_A = \frac{0.863 \times 200 \text{ mL/min}}{40 \text{ mm Hg}} = 4.3 \text{ L/min}$$

Because of the relation between alveolar ventilation and $Paco_2$, the single best index of effective ventilation is measurement of the $Paco_2$. Thus $Paco_2$ is the standard for assessment of the adequacy of ventilation in the ICU. Ventilation is adequate if the $Paco_2$ results in a normal arterial pH. For healthy persons, this is a $Paco_2$ between 35 and 45 mm Hg, resulting in an arterial pH of 7.35 to 7.45.

Dead Space. The **dead space/tidal volume ratio** (V_{DS}/V_T) is a measure of the efficiency of gas exchange. This ratio is an estimate of the proportion of ventilation participating in diffusion of carbon dioxide and can be calculated from the Enghoff modification of the Bohr equation as follows:

$$V_D/V_T = (PaCO_2 - P\bar{E}CO_2)/PaCO_2$$

where $P\bar{E}CO_2$ is the carbon dioxide concentration in mixed expired gas. Exhaled gas is collected in a large, airtight collection bag, traditionally called a *Douglas bag*. Exhaled gas should be collected for at least 3 minutes, and a specimen for ABG analysis should be drawn during the collection. The gas and blood samples are analyzed, and the respective PCO_2 values are applied in the foregoing formula. In lieu of measurement of V_{DS}/V_T ratio by means of simultaneous intermittent collection of expired gases and ABG sampling, estimation of physiological dead space can be performed with a capnometer. The mean expired carbon dioxide value is either computed from the $P\bar{E}CO_2$-volume tracing or obtained directly from a collection bag.

In healthy persons who are sitting, the V_{DS}/V_T ratio is 0.20 to 0.40. This value varies little with age, position, exercise, tidal volume, or breath holding.[22] In the setting of critical illness, however, it is not uncommon for the V_{DS}/V_T ratio to increase to values greater than 0.7. Frequently the V_{DS}/V_T ratio is increased in patients with congestive heart failure, pulmonary embolism, ALI, or pulmonary hypertension and in patients undergoing mechanical ventilation. The V_{DS}/V_T ratio has been used to evaluate patients being considered for liberation from mechanical ventilation. A V_{DS}/V_T ratio greater than 0.60 is predictive of lack of success at discontinuance of ventilation.[23]

Monitoring of Inspired and Exhaled Gas. The single best index of effective ventilation is measurement of $PaCO_2$. However, measurement of inspired and expired gas volumes is an important aspect of monitoring of patients receiving mechanical ventilatory support.

For patients receiving ventilation in the assist-control or control mode, minute ventilation ($\dot{V}_E$), respiratory rate (f), and tidal volume (V_T) are assessed where

$$\dot{V}_E = V_T \times f$$

and

$$V_T \text{ average} = \dot{V}_E/f$$

For patients receiving ventilation in the intermittent mandatory ventilation or synchronized intermittent mandatory ventilation (SIMV) mode, total minute ventilation ($\dot{V}_{ETOT}$) is the sum of the patient's spontaneous minute ventilation ($\dot{V}_{Esp}$) and the machine minute ventilation ($\dot{V}_{Emach}$) provided

$$\dot{V}_{ETOT} = \dot{V}_{Esp} + \dot{V}_{Emach}$$

and

$$\dot{V}_{ETOT} = V_{Tmach} \times f_{mach} + V_{Tpatient} \times f_{patient}$$

Increases in minute ventilation tend to increase alveolar ventilation and decrease $PaCO_2$, whereas decreases in minute ventilation tend to have the opposite effect. However, in the presence of rapid shallow breathing with normal or elevated minute ventilation, a decrease in effective ventilation can result in an increase in $PaCO_2$. This effect is caused by ineffective shallow tidal breaths that are at or near dead space volume. Spontaneous respiratory rate often is a sensitive indicator for evaluating the need for mechanical ventilation. Rates greater than 20 breaths/min may indicate distress and a rate greater than 30 breaths/min with a spontaneous tidal volume of less than 300 mL may indicate the need for mechanical ventilatory support in adults.

Inspired versus Expired Tidal Volume. Normal inspired (V_{TI}) and expired tidal volume (V_{TE}) should be nearly the same. However, in the presence of an air leak, inspired tidal volume may be larger than expired tidal volume and measurement of inspired tidal volume versus expired tidal volume may be useful in detecting and quantifying the size of the leak.

Capnography. Capnometry is the measurement of carbon dioxide at the airway opening during the ventilatory cycle.[24] *Capnography* refers to plotting carbon dioxide concentration against time or, more usefully, against exhaled volume. The normal carbon dioxide waveform is displayed in Figure 43-4. The height of the capnogram (the peak value) indicates the end-tidal carbon dioxide value. The $PETCO_2$ normally is 1 to 5 mm Hg less than the $PaCO_2$, ranging between 35 and 43 mm Hg. Because the $PETCO_2$ in healthy persons closely approximates the $PaCO_2$, this measure is a potentially useful noninvasive index of the adequacy of ventilation. Abnormal waveform contours can indicate changes in the distribution of ventilation and perfusion, or airway obstruction. These changes typically are an irregular increase in carbon dioxide level and a lower than normal end-tidal carbon dioxide level. The frequency and rhythm of the capnogram breaths correspond to the frequency and rhythm established by either the patient (spontaneous breathing) or the ventilator. Positive pressure ventilation (especially with PEEP), pulmonary embolism, cardiac arrest, and pulmonary hypoperfusion also may cause an increase in $PaCO_2$ to $PETCO_2$ gradient [$P(a - ET)CO_2$]. Exercise and large tidal volume can reverse the $P(a - ET)CO_2$ gradient, the $PETCO_2$ actually exceeding the $PaCO_2$.

Patients for whom capnometry may be a useful monitoring tool include those with unstable ventilatory drive who are breathing spontaneously or receiving low-level ventilatory support. In these patients, capnometry readings should initially be validated by comparison with the measured $PaCO_2$. Changes in $PETCO_2$ can

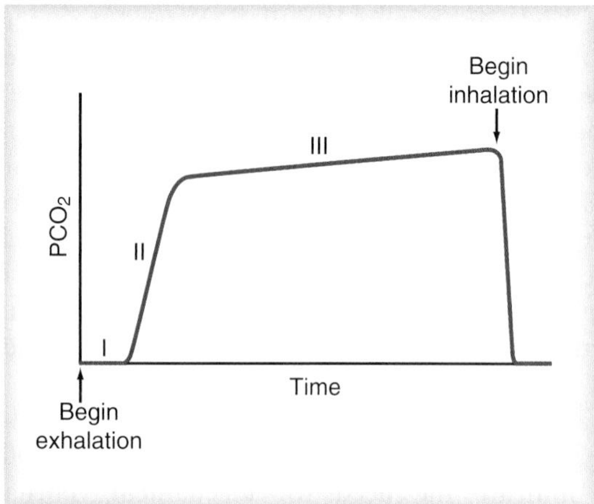

Figure 43-4 · Time-Based Capnograph

Phase I, anatomic dead space. Phase II, transition from anatomic dead space to alveolar plateau. Phase III, the alveolar plateau.

> **Box 43-6 • Causes of Increased and Decreased End Tidal Carbon Dioxide ($PETCO_2$) Values**
>
> **INCREASED $PETCO_2$**
> - Decreased effective ventilation ($\downarrow V_T$, $\downarrow \dot{V}_E$, $\downarrow \dot{V}_A$, $\uparrow PaCO_2$)
> - Increased carbon dioxide production ($\dot{V}CO_2$) (agitation, stress, shivering, fighting the ventilator, pain, anxiety, recovery from sedation or paralysis)
>
> **DECREASED $PETCO_2$**
> - Increased effective ventilation ($\uparrow V_T$, $\uparrow \dot{V}_E$, $\uparrow \dot{V}_A$, $\downarrow PaCO_2$)
> - Marked decrease in effective ventilation ($\downarrow\downarrow V_T$ approaching dead space volume; rapid shallow breathing)
> - Decreased carbon dioxide production ($\dot{V}CO_2$) (sedation, sleep, cooling)
> - Decrease in lung perfusion (pulmonary embolus, decreased cardiac output)
>
> **ABSENT $PETCO_2$**
> - Apnea
> - Cardiac arrest
> - Ventilator disconnect or malfunction
> - Airway obstruction

then be used to alert the clinician to potential changes in patient ventilation. Thereafter periodical reevaluation should be performed as the patient's clinical state changes. Capnometry has been extremely useful in emergency situations such as detection of esophageal intubation and assessment of blood flow during cardiac arrest.

Although the $PETCO_2$ and $PaCO_2$ tend to have a high correlation at single points in time, correlation between changes in $PETCO_2$ and changes in $PaCO_2$ tend to be much weaker.[24] For example, decreases in ventilation tend to be reflected in increased $PETCO_2$ and $PaCO_2$. However, with very small tidal volumes, $PaCO_2$ increases, whereas $PETCO_2$ may be reduced. This phenomenon has led some clinicians to advise against using capnometry as a routine bedside monitoring tool, at least as related to weaning. The appropriate role of capnometry in critical care therefore is not clear. Capnometry is not indicated for every intubated or mechanically ventilated patient. Box 43-6 lists common causes of changes in monitored $PETCO_2$ values.

Monitoring Lung and Chest Wall Mechanics

Ventilation of the lungs involves overcoming the flow-resistive, inertial, and elastic properties of the respiratory system. A reasonable model for the mechanics of the respiratory system is an analogy to an electrical circuit.[25] The circuit for gas flow is the pathway to the lungs with resistive elements interposed in series. The gas is collected or stored in a capacitor (the lungs) and discharged (exhaled) through the circuitry. Several assumptions are made with the acceptance of this model (one value for resistance and compliance and nonturbulent flow), yet this model serves to simplify and explain the dynamics of ventilation for, at least, a mechanical lung model. In vivo measurements of resistance and compliance of the lungs are not constant throughout the respiratory cycle. Resistance varies throughout the cycle, and **compliance** is a function of the pressure-volume (P-V) relation of the respiratory system.

A mechanical test lung displays a straight line during a P-V determination. An actual in vivo P-V relation is curvilinear and displays hysteresis (Figure 43-5). For measurement of the P-V curve from the resting volume of the respiratory system (at functional residual capacity) to the estimated total lung capacity, a calibrated syringe, referred to as a *supersyringe*, ranging from 1.5 to 3.0 L is used. The syringe is filled with humidified oxygen and connected to the endotracheal tube to start measurement. Gas volume is injected in 50- to 100-mL increments with the plunger while airway pressure is recorded. Patients usually are sedated and paralyzed. The measurements are performed after PEEP is set at 0 cm H_2O (zero PEEP).

A P-V curve may, but does not always, reveal two points at which the slope of the curve changes. The lower point at which the slope changes is called the *lower inflection point*. As depicted in Figure 43-5, a lower inflection point may occur over the lower range of volumes, indicating theoretically that total respiratory system compliance has improved owing to alveolar recruitment. A recommended strategy for setting PEEP is to set a level slightly above the lower inflection point with the goal of recruitment and stabilization of dependent alveoli that would otherwise sustain injury

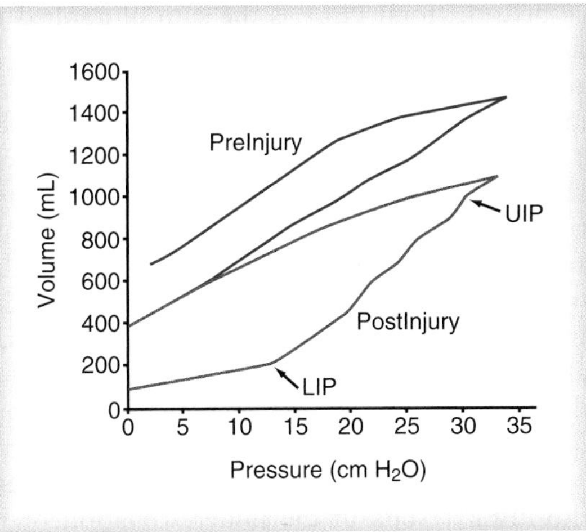

Figure 43-5

Pressure-volume curves generated by a normal lung *(preinjury)* and after oleic acid injury *(postinjury)*. In the preinjury curve, the linear relationship between pressure and volume with minimal hysteresis is evident. The postinjury curve displays marked hysteresis and two changes in compliance on the inspiratory limb: a lower inflection point *(LIP)* and upper inflection point *(UIP)*.

from repetitive opening, closing, and reopening during tidal ventilation. The other change in the slope, called a *deflection point*, may be seen at a higher volume, indicating that compliance has decreased owing to alveolar overdistension. Although the risk of alveolar overdistension is generally reduced if the end-inspiratory hold pressure is kept less than 30 to 35 cm H_2O, deflection points in ARDS patients may occur at pressures as low as 25 cm H_2O. In these cases, the pressure needed to recruit some alveoli may overdistend others.[26-28]

A lung protective strategy of ventilating between the inflection and deflection points is considered beneficial, although there is no consensus in clinical practice on the best technique for measuring P-V curves or on their relevance to tidal ventilation or to the selection of the level of PEEP. Two problems exist: (1) The measurement of P-V curves involves application of zero PEEP in a patient in possibly unstable condition, and (2) there is a potential lack of agreement between the static P-V state and the dynamic state of mechanical ventilation. Therefore the use of static P-V curves cannot be recommended in settings other than research protocols.[29]

Respiratory System Compliance

Respiratory system compliance (C) is an important measure of the stiffness of the lungs. Compliance calculations should be routinely monitored for all ventilated patients. To attain an accurate assessment of compliance, two maneuvers must be performed because the alveolar pressures at end inspiration and end expiration are not available under dynamic conditions. An end-inspiratory hold maneuver allows reading of a plateau pressure (P_{plat}). Because compliance (C) is calculated with $C = \Delta V/\Delta P$, tidal volume (corrected for tubing compliance) is ΔV and ($P_{plat} - PEEP_T$) is ΔP. If auto-PEEP is present, it must be accounted for by adding the auto-PEEP level to the applied PEEP to attain a $PEEP_T$ value.

Normal compliance ranges between 60 and 100 mL/cm H_2O. Diseases of the lung parenchyma, such as pneumonia, pulmonary edema, and any chronic disease causing fibrosis, cause decreased effective compliance. Acute changes, such as atelectasis, pulmonary edema, ARDS, and lung compression, caused by tension pneumothorax cause a rapid decrease in compliance. Compliance can be less than 25 to 30 mL/cm H_2O in ARDS. Common causes of changes in respiratory system compliance are listed in Box 43-7.

Box 43-7 • Common Causes of Changes in Compliance and Resistance in Mechanically Ventilated Patients

DECREASED COMPLIANCE

↓ Lung compliance (atelectasis, pneumonia, pulmonary edema, ALI/ARDS, pneumothorax, fibrosis, bronchial intubation)
↓ Thoracic compliance (obesity, ascites, chest wall deformity)

INCREASED COMPLIANCE

↑ Lung compliance (improvement in any of the above, pulmonary emphysema)
↑ Thoracic compliance (improvement in any of the above; flail chest; position change—sitting patient up)

INCREASED RESISTANCE

Small endotracheal tube, plug in endotracheal tube, biting on endotracheal tube
↑ Bronchospasm, mucosal edema
↑ Secretions
↑ Airway obstruction
High gas flow rate (or ↑ gas flow)

DECREASED RESISTANCE

↑ Improvement in any of the above
↑ Bronchodilator administration
↑ Suctioning and airway care
↑ Use of lower inspiratory gas flow rate

Resistance

Depending on the driving pressure measured, various resistances can be calculated, including airway, pulmonary, chest wall, and total respiratory resistance. Airway resistance (Raw) is determined dynamically from simultaneous measurements of airflow and the pressure difference between the airway opening (P_{ao}) and the alveoli (P_{alv}), R = (P_{ao} − P_{alv})/flow. Because resistance changes throughout inspiration and expiration with, generally, expiratory resistance greater than inspiratory resistance, instantaneous measurement of resistance usually is not performed. Alveolar pressure can be instantaneously measured with an interrupter method that allows such measurements, but this estimate of resistance usually is reserved for research protocols. Inspiratory resistance can be calculated simply during constant flow ventilation for monitoring of airway status over time or after the effects of bronchodilator therapy occur by dividing the pressure change (ΔP) by the flow change (ΔF) [$Raw = \Delta P/\Delta F = (P_{peak} - P_{plat})/\dot{V}(flow)$]. Automated methods of measuring early expiratory resistance have been integrated into some ventilators.

In ventilated patients, a significant component of the total flow resistance may be added with endotracheal tubes, which have highly curvilinear flow-resistive properties. In healthy persons, flow is laminar during tidal ventilation and becomes turbulent only with increasing ventilatory demands. The flow resistance offered by the endotracheal tube increases markedly with increasing flow and varies with the size of the tube. Normal Raw is approximately 1 to 2 cm H_2O/L per second; however, intubated patients receiving mechanical ventilatory support typically have a Raw of 5 to 10 cm H_2O/L per second or more. Tube compensation modes have been added to mechanical ventilators to adjust flow to account for the added resistance of the endotracheal tube. Common causes of changes in airway resistance in mechanically ventilated patients are listed in Box 43-7.

Peak and Plateau Pressures

The maximum value of airway pressure at the airway opening during a ventilatory cycle is routinely monitored in the ICU. Peak airway pressure greater than 50 to 60 cm H_2O is generally discouraged,[30] because high values of P_{peak} carry increased risk of barotrauma and hypotension. An increase in P_{peak} must result from increased resistive pressure or increased elastic pressure from decreased lung or chest wall compliance. Measurement of end-inspiratory plateau pressure (P_{plat}) differentiates the resistive and elastic components. The P_{plat} level should be monitored for all ventilated patients. The P_{plat} levels should not exceed 30 to 35 cm H_2O because higher levels not only would indicate decreased compliance but also could expose the lungs to the risk of ventilator-induced lung injury.

Auto–PEEP (Intrinsic PEEP)

Positive end-expiratory pressure is the pressure applied to the airway by the clinician during exhalation. An alveolar pressure that exists above the applied PEEP at end exhalation is termed *intrinsic PEEP* or *auto-PEEP*. At the bedside, total PEEP is the sum of applied PEEP and auto-PEEP.

A number of factors, both internal and external to the patient, contribute to the development of auto-PEEP. Expiratory muscle activity has been shown to increase auto-PEEP and may interfere with attempts at assessment of auto-PEEP based solely on dynamic hyperinflation.[31] Patients receiving mechanical ventilation for obstructive airways disease have a large degree of inhomogeneity in the emptying of lung units, and auto-PEEP can develop even at relatively low minute ventilation. Auto-PEEP is common in mechanically ventilated patients with high minute ventilation and thus occurs among patients with ARDS. The presence of auto-PEEP results in the underestimation of mean alveolar pressure when mean airway pressure is being monitored to reflect mean alveolar pressure.[32] An increase in mean alveolar pressure due to auto-PEEP may exacerbate the hemodynamic effects of positive pressure ventilation and increase the likelihood of barotrauma in a manner similar to that seen with the application of PEEP. In addition, auto-PEEP alters the effective trigger sensitivity of the ventilator, making it more difficult for the patient to trigger a ventilator-assisted inspiration. Finally, if unrecognized, auto-PEEP leads to erroneous calculation of static lung compliance. Increasing expiratory time is the most important way in which auto-PEEP can be reduced or eliminated. The use of extrinsic PEEP can partially overcome the trigger sensitivity problem seen with auto-PEEP.

Methods for Determining Auto-PEEP. Assessment of auto-PEEP involves first its detection and then its measurement. Auto-PEEP can be suspected if flow is present throughout expiration. In this case, auto-PEEP is present unless there is active contraction of the expiratory muscles. Expiratory muscle activity can be assessed, for example, by inspection and palpation of the thorax and abdomen. The following methods can be used to estimate auto-PEEP level.[33]

Esophageal Balloon. An esophageal balloon is used to measure the esophageal pressure deflection required to trigger the ventilator. This is an important measure of the potential effect of auto-PEEP on inspiratory efforts by the patient.

End-Expiratory Hold by the Ventilator. Either automated or manual, this method closes the expiratory valve at end exhalation. The hold period must extend until the total PEEP is stabilized, or the value will be an underestimate of auto-PEEP.

End-Expiratory Port Occlusion. End-expiratory port occlusion is a manual method that depends on timing the occlusion correctly. It is not recommended.

Pressure at Zero Inspiratory Flow. Pressure at zero inspiratory flow is an automated method in which the ventilator detects the precise pressure during early inspiration when flow "passes" 0 cm H_2O.

Matching Auto–PEEP with PEEP. Positive end-expiratory pressure is applied to a level (in some patients) that results in flow reaching zero at end exhalation. The applied PEEP level is the auto-PEEP estimate.

Mean Airway Pressure

Mean airway pressure represents the average airway pressure over the total ventilatory cycle. Correct measurement of this value requires continuous sampling of airway pressure at the airway opening. However, values computed with pressure devices inside microprocessor-equipped ventilators also are accepted in clinical practice. The mean airway pressure can reflect mean lung volume, which correlates with oxygenation.[34,35] As mean airway pressure increases, arterial oxygen levels may improve, but venous return may be reduced.

Monitoring Breathing Effort and Patterns

Work of Breathing

Work of breathing often is increased in critically ill patients. Measurement of respiratory work once was confined to research laboratories because the necessary equipment can be quite complex. A commercially available monitor has been developed, validated, and used clinically for measuring work of breathing in patients undergoing mechanical ventilation.[36-38] For computation of the spontaneous work of breathing, changes in transpulmonary pressure must be measured. The procedure requires measurement of pleural pressure, normally estimated on the basis of esophageal pressure by means of placement of an esophageal balloon. The measurement is estimated from the esophageal pressure-volume area (Figure 43-6).

For healthy persons, the average total work of breathing ranges between 0.030 and 0.050 kg·m/L (0.3-0.5 J/L). Patients with severe obstructive or restrictive lung disease "work" at levels two to three times this normal value at rest, with marked increases in work at higher minute ventilation. How much work a patient can tolerate before the ventilatory muscles fatigue is not entirely clear. Maintaining adequate spontaneous ventilation probably is not possible when the work load exceeds 0.15 kg·m/L (1.5 J/L). This threshold level surely varies according to the patient's condition.

Monitoring the work of breathing may be of value in certain situations, such as the weaning period. Clinicians are expected to monitor the patient's work of breathing and to take appropriate action if work becomes excessive. Because direct measurement of the work of breathing is difficult, simpler indicators are sought. Monitoring the patient's spontaneous breathing rate and ratio of rate to tidal volume (f/V_T) provides a reliable indicator of the work of breathing.

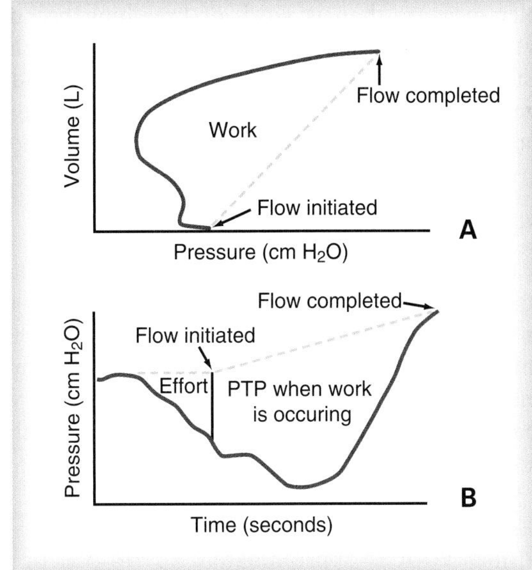

Figure 43-6
Work of breathing and pressure-time product *(PTP)*. Work **(A)** and PTP **(B)**. The work and PTP from the same spontaneous breath of a patient receiving intermittent ventilatory support. *Dashed lines* represent a tracing of passive inflation by a ventilator-supported breath. Areas of work and PTP are not directly comparable because work units (pressure-volume) and PTP units (pressure-time) differ. The area of effort in the total PTP area occurs before (and in addition to) the work measurement.

Esophageal Pressure Monitoring

Esophageal pressure recording is the only realistic method for clinical measurement of intrapleural pressure, or the distending pressure of the lungs and chest wall. Esophageal pressure monitoring allows calculation of work of breathing. The thin esophageal catheter (approximately 2-mm diameter) used for monitoring esophageal pressure is relatively comfortable, is simple to insert, and poses little risk of esophageal perforation. Appropriate placement is achieved by first inflating the 10-cm long balloon with approximately 1 mL of air and passing it into the stomach. The catheter is carefully withdrawn until the final position of the balloon is within the lower third of the esophagus, as assessed by occluding the airway and measuring the simultaneous deflections in pressure at the airway opening and esophageal pressure.

Pressure-Time Product. The pressure-time product (PTP) is the area encompassed by the esophageal pressure-time tracing as shown in Figure 43-6. The PTP is a simpler measure than is work of breathing because it does not require simultaneous measurement of volume. Pressure-time product values parallel effort and the oxygen cost of breathing because PTP also is a measure of the "isometric" component of muscle contraction.[38]

Oxygen Cost of Breathing

The amount of oxygen consumed by the ventilatory muscles ($\dot{V}O_2R$) is an estimate of respiratory effort at its most basic level. The $\dot{V}O_2R$ can be estimated as follows by means of measurement of oxygen consumption during active breathing and oxygen consumption while the patient is apneic and being supported on a ventilator in the control mode:

$$\dot{V}O_2R = \dot{V}O_2 \text{ active breathing} - \dot{V}O_2 \text{ apnea}$$

Normal $\dot{V}O_2R$ is approximately 2% to 5% of total oxygen consumption; however $\dot{V}O_2R$ increases to up to 30% of total oxygen consumption with hyperventilation. In theory, $\dot{V}O_2R$ accounts for all factors that tax the respiratory muscles, that is, the external workload and the efficiency of the conversion between cellular energy and useful work. Unfortunately, $\dot{V}O_2R$ is difficult to measure if the patient's condition is unstable. Thus other measures of respiratory muscle effort are sought.

Assessing Ventilatory Drive

Remarkably little attention has been paid to measurement of respiratory drive during critical illness. During machine-assisted breathing, ventilatory drive plays an important role in determining the energy expenditure of the patient. One study showed that patients not weaned from mechanical ventilation often have elevated drive to breathe and limited ability to respond to increases in ventilatory load (e.g., increased $PaCO_2$).[39]

Two measures are used to index drive: $P_{0.1}$ and V_T/T_i. The $P_{0.1}$ is the pressure recorded 100 ms after initiation of an inspiratory effort against an occluded airway.[30] The V_T/T_i is spontaneous tidal volume divided by inspiratory time, or mean inspiratory flow. The $P_{0.1}$ has been shown to be helpful in prediction of weaning success.[30] The $P_{0.1}$ is influenced by muscle strength and lung volume but does not depend on respiratory mechanics. However, measurement of this index requires a sensitive pressure recording system with a very rapid recording rate.

Rapid Shallow Breathing Index: f/Vt Ratio

When muscular strength is limited, patients tend to meet minute ventilation (V_E) requirements by increasing frequency (f) while decreasing tidal volume (V_T). Although smaller breaths require less effort, the effect of rapid, shallow breathing may be increased dead space ventilation and the need for a higher minute ventilation to eliminate carbon dioxide. A very high and continuously increasing frequency (>30 breaths/min) is a sign of ventilatory muscle decompensation and impending fatigue.

Considerable attention has been focused on the f/V_T ratio, a simply computed bedside index that indicates whether mechanically ventilated patients can breathe without mechanical assistance.[39-41] The rapid shallow breathing index (f/V_T) is easy to measure and is independent of the patient's effort and cooperation. Discontinuation of ventilator support is likely to prove successful if f/VT is less than 100 breaths/min per liter within the first minute of a brief trial of fully spontaneous breathing.

Respiratory Inductive Plethysmography

Respiratory inductive plethysmography is a noninvasive means of monitoring frequency, tidal volume, fractional duration of inspiration (T_i/T_{tot}), and respiratory muscle coordination. With this technique, loose elastic bands encircle the chest and abdomen. Changes in compartmental volume produce proportional changes in the cross-sectional areas of electrical inductance loops. The change in compartmental motion during the respiratory cycle can be summed for estimation of overall lung volume changes. Respiratory inductive plethysmography also can be used as an apnea detector in the care of nonintubated patients and may prove helpful in monitoring of volume changes during pressure-cycled modes of ventilation.[42,43]

Monitoring Strength and Muscle Endurance

The two values most commonly used for bedside assessment of respiratory muscle strength are vital capacity (VC) and maximal inspiratory pressure (MIP). The vital capacity (VC) maneuver can be performed at the bedside with a respirometer connected to the patient's airway. Because the VC maneuver is effort dependent, accurate measurements can be obtained only when the patient is conscious and cooperative. Given the variability in bedside results, two or three measurements should be obtained and the best result reported. Healthy persons are able to generate a VC of approximately 70 mL/kg. A VC less than 10 to 15 mL/kg indicates considerable muscle weakness, which may inhibit the ability to breathe spontaneously.

The MIP is a more specific measure than is VC. The MIP provides information based solely on maximum output of the inspiratory muscles. A maximum stimulus is provided by total occlusion of the airway. Unlike the VC maneuver, the MIP maneuver can be performed on unconscious or uncooperative patients. Measurement of MIP at the bedside usually is done with an aneroid manometer with a maximum value indicator. In an effort to make the measurements more reliable, Marini

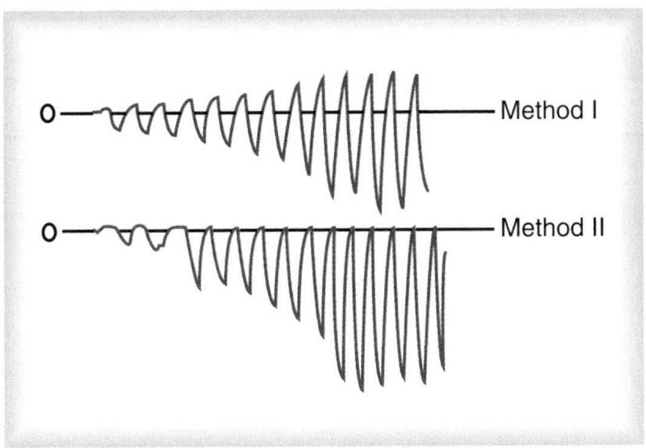

Figure 43-7
Measurement of MIP during 25 seconds of airway occlusion. Method I is occlusion by sealing the airway to allow no movement of air. Method II occludes inspiratory flow but allows expiratory flow through a unidirectional valve.

et al[44] described a modified technique. A one-way valve is attached to the airway to ensure that inspiratory effort is made at a low lung volume. A period of occlusion is maintained for 20 seconds. The MIP gradually increases over the 20 seconds of occlusion, and values with the one-way valve are approximately one-third more negative than values without it (Figure 43-7).

Endurance: Maximum Voluntary Ventilation

Respiratory muscle fatigue (lack of endurance) may be a cause of respiratory failure. A measure used to assess respiratory muscle reserve, endurance, or fatigue is maximum voluntary ventilation (MVV). Whereas VC is measured to assess the patient's coordinated muscle function from a single breath, MVV is measured to determine the ability of a patient to sustain an increased respiratory load over time. As with the VC maneuver, the MVV procedure can be performed with a respirometer attached to the patient's airway. As when the procedure is performed in a pulmonary function test laboratory, the patient is encouraged to breathe as deeply and as fast as possible over a predefined time interval, such as 10 or 15 seconds. The value is then extrapolated to a full minute.

RULE OF THUMB

To wean from mechanical ventilation, the patient must have adequate gas exchange, respiratory muscle strength and endurance, and work of breathing that is not excessive. The original cause of respiratory failure must be partially if not completely resolved. Although a number of values have been studied to indicate the probability of successful weaning, a frequency to tidal volume ratio less than 100 has been the best single index of ability to wean.

Normal MVV values for adults range from 120 to 180 L/min. Values less than twice the spontaneous minute ventilation are associated with difficulty in maintaining spontaneous ventilation without mechanical assistance.[45]

Monitoring the Patient-Ventilator System

Monitoring of a patient receiving mechanical ventilatory support should include physical assessment (inspection, palpation, percussion), assessment of oxygenation and ventilation, and assessment of ventilatory load and capacity. Table 43-1 lists key physiological monitoring data and acceptable values for patients receiving mechanical ventilation. Monitoring of all aspects of the patient-ventilator system is an important responsibility that must be clearly delineated within the ICU. Monitoring a ventilated patient often is the primary responsibility of the respiratory therapist. Important areas of this responsibility include

- The integrity of the airway and circuitry, including secretion clearance
- Maintaining the prescribed settings and assessing their appropriateness
- Assuring acceptable gas exchange values
- Monitoring of respiratory system mechanics
- The comfort and synchrony of breathing of the patient
- Setting of alarms
- Care for any other safety issues, such as the risk of extubation

A system of assuring and documenting all aspects of safe and appropriate care must be in place. This system usually includes a manual or electronic entry monitoring form or spreadsheet for recording of all important settings, alarms, and ABG values at regular intervals. This monitoring process often is called *patient-ventilator checks*. An example of a recording form used for this purpose is shown in Figure 43-8. The respiratory therapist's responsibility is clearly much greater than the task of recording values on a flow chart. The responsibility is care of a critically ill, vulnerable patient with respiratory failure who is being treated with a life-saving machine. The procedure for performing a patient-ventilator system check is outlined in Table 43-2.

Graphics Monitoring. Monitoring of graphic tracings generated during mechanical ventilation has become widely available and accepted in the ICU. A visual display of pressure, flow, and volume tracings is available on all modern ventilators. Graphic displays are possible through the development of improvements in sensing technology, integrated circuitry, and video monitors. Ventilators "sense" inspiratory and expira-

Table 43-1 ▶▶ Physiological Monitoring Data (Respiratory Values)

Function Assessed	Description of Value	Symbol/Formula	Acceptable Value
Oxygenation			
Lung exchange (external)			
Adequacy	Arterial oxygen pressure	PaO_2	60-100 mm Hg
	Arterial oxygen saturation	SaO_2	≥90%
	Oxygen saturation by pulse oximeter	SpO_2	≥90%
	Transcutaneous oxygen partial pressure	$PtcO_2$	60-100 mm Hg
Efficiency	Alveolar to arterial oxygen tension gradient	$P(A - a)O_2$	<350 mm Hg (100% O_2)
	Arterial to alveolar	PaO_2/PAO_2	>0.6
	Respiratory index	$P(A - a)O_2/PaO_2$	<5.0
	P/F ratio	PaO_2/FIO_2	>200
	Percentage shunt	$\dot{Q}s/\dot{Q}t$	<15%-20%
Time exchange (internal)	Mixed venous oxygen content	$C\bar{v}O_2$	>10.0 mL/dL
	Mixed venous oxygen partial pressure	$P\bar{v}O_2$	>30 mm Hg
	Mixed venous oxygen saturation	$S\bar{v}O_2$	>65%
	Arterial-venous oxygen content difference	$C(a - \bar{v}O_2)$	<7.0 mL/dL
Ventilation			
Adequacy	Minute ventilation	$\dot{V}_E$	5-10 L/min
	Arterial carbon dioxide	$PaCO_2$	35-45 mm Hg (normal pH)
	Transcutaneous carbon dioxide partial pressure	$PtcCO_2$	35-45 mm Hg (normal pH)
	End-tidal carbon dioxide partial pressure	$PETCO_2$	35-43 mm Hg (4.6%-5.6%)
Efficiency	Dead space to tidal volume ratio	V_D/V_T	<0.6
	Minute ventilation versus carbon dioxide partial pressure	$\dot{V}_E$ versus $PaCO_2$	$\dot{V}_E$ <10 L/min with $PaCO_2$ <40 mm Hg
Ventilatory Load			
Total impedance	Dynamic "compliance"	$(V_T - V_C)/(PIP - PEEP)$	35-50 mL/cm H_2O
Compliance	Effective compliance	$C_{eff} = \frac{(V_T - V_C)}{(P_{plat} - PEEP)}$	600-100 mL/cm H_2O
Work of breathing	Work = kg × m/L or J/L	Work = P × V	<0.15 kg × m/L <1.5 J/L
Ventilatory Capacity			
Drive	Occlusion pressure	P0.1	<6 cm H_2O
	Mean inspiratory flow	V_T/T_i	Not established
Strength	Vital capacity	VC	>10-15 mL/kg
	Maximal inspiratory pressure	MIP; PI_{max}	<–20 to –30 cm H_2O
Endurance	Maximum voluntary ventilation	MVV	>20 L/min or 2 × $\dot{V}_E$
	Ratio of minute ventilation to MVV	$\dot{V}_E$/MVV	<1:2
	Pressure-time index	$(Pdi/Pmax)*TI/T_{tot}$	<0.15

tory flow and circuit pressure with pneumotachometers and transducers. The volume displays are generated through calculation of an integral of the flow tracings. Thus all three values (flow, pressure, and volume) can be displayed and plotted against time or each other (Figure 43-9).

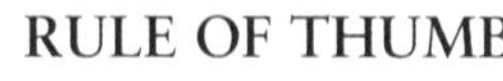

RULE OF THUMB

Modern mechanical ventilators routinely display tracings of flow, pressure, and volume versus time. Ventilator graphics monitoring is a convenient visual method for monitoring patient-ventilator interaction. The graphic patterns allow rapid determination of mode of ventilation, breathing pattern, auto-PEEP, excessive pressure, secretions in the airway, synchrony, and triggering efforts.

Ventilator manufacturers have developed, ingeniously, the graphic displays that allow astute clinicians to base decisions on many more factors than gas exchange values (Box 43-8). Unfortunately, study and verification of features observed in ventilator graphics have not developed at the pace of the technology. Ventilator graphics clearly show many important patient-ventilator interactions, such as presence of auto-PEEP, elevated airway pressure, presence of secretions, and the general pattern and dependability of supported ventilation (Figure 43-10). Nevertheless, although the information may be available through graphic displays, certain aspects of the patient-ventilator interaction have not been clarified systematically, such as the level or adequacy of ventilator-patient synchrony and the level or adequacy of triggering or terminating flow. The potential for expanded use of ventilator graphics awaits further investigation of the clinical importance of the graphic displays.

The University of Texas Health Science Center at San Antonio
Department of Respiratory Care
Adult Mechanical Ventilation Flow Sheet

Patient ______	Cuff pressure (volume) ______
Physician ______	☐ M.O.V. ☐ Minimal leak
Diagnosis ______	Ventilator ______ Vent. day ______
Age ______ Height ______	Circuit change (Date / Time) ______
Weight ______ Ideal body weight ______	Tape change (Date / Time) ______
ET tube / trach tube size ______	Other therapy ______
Tube Position (length) ______	______

Patient ID

Date							
Time							
Mode (A/C; SIMV, PSV, PCV, etc.)							
Set Tidal Volume / Delivered Tidal Volume							
Spontaneous Tidal Volume							
Machine Rate / Total Rate							
Minute Volume							
Peak Pressure / Static Pressure							
Mean Airway Pressure							
PEEP / CPAP [IPAP / EPAP]							
Auto PEEP							
Support / Pressure Control Level (cmH_2O)							
Sensitivity or Flowtrigger (Flowby)							
FIO2 Set / Analyzed							
Inspiratory Flow / Time							
Wave Form (⎍ |\ ⎍)							
I : E Ratio							
Sigh Volume / Sigh Frequency							
Airway Temperature							
Static Compliance / Dynamic Compliance							
Airway Resistance [(PIP - PLAT / Insp. Flow L/Sec)]							
Apnea Parameters Check (Y / N)							
ALARMS	Pressure High / Low						
	Low VT						
	High / Low VE						
	High rate						
BLOOD GASES	pH						
	PaO2						
	PaC02						
	Sa02 / Oximetry (Sp02)						
	Hb						
	HC03-						
	B.E.						
	Ca02						
	Pv02						
	Sv02						
	Ca02 - Cv02						
	Qs / Qt						
	Vd / Vt						
	P (ET) C02						
HEMO DYNAMICS	Pulse						
	Blood Pressure (Systolic / Diastolic)						
	CVP						
	PAP (Systolic / Diastolic)						
	PCWP						
	Cardiac Output / Cardiac Index						
	SVR						
	PVR						
SPONTANEOUS	MIP / MEP						
	Vital Capacity (VC)						
	Spontaneous Volumes (VT / VE)						
	Spontaneous Rate (f)						
	RSBI (f/VT)						
Other							
Initials							

A

Figure 43-8
Ventilator flow sheet.

Continued

The University of Texas Health Science Center at San Antonio
Department of Respiratory Care
Adult Mechanical Ventilation Flow Sheet

Respiratory Care Progress Notes

S: (pt Awareness, response, sedations / paralytics) Responds ☐ Non-responsive ☐ Sedated Paralytics ☐ See comment ☐ ☐

O: (WOB, Color, Chest Expansion, BBS, Sputum Production, latest x-ray, pertinent pt assessment concerns, lab values, fluids)

General Skin Color
- ☐ Pink
- ☐ Ashy
- ☐ Cyanotic
- ☐ Jaundice

Skin Characteristics
- ☐ Warm
- ☐ Dry
- ☐ Diaphoretic
- ☐ Cool
- ☐ Moist

Mucous Membranes
- ☐ Pink
- ☐ Ashy
- ☐ Cyanotic

Work of Breathing
- ☐ Normal
- ☐ Mild
- ☐ Moderate
- ☐ High
- ☐ Absent

Chest Excursion
- ☐ Bilateral
- ☐ Unilateral
- ☐ Diminished
- ☐ Paradoxical/Flail

Chest Configuration
- ☐ Normal
- ☐ Other____________ ____
- ☐ Subcutaneous Emphysema
- ☐ Tactile Fremitus
- ☐ Tracheal Deviation
- ☐ Abdominal Distention

Nailbeds
- ☐ Pink
- ☐ Ashy
- ☐ Cyanotic

Capillary Refill
- ☐ Rapid
- ☐ Sluggish

Auscultation
1) Clear
2) Wheeze
3) Crackles
4) Rhonchi

Anterior

Posterior
A. Good Aeration
B. Diminished
C. Absent

B

A: (Pt history, Admit dx. & date, events leading to intubation/trach/ventilation, significant problems, etc.

P: (Care plan , standing orders, treatments)

WEANING MECHANICS		
TIME		
VC		
I/E FORCES		
VT		
RR		
VE		
f/VT		

Pt. EVENTS/CHANGES	Time	(Reasons for changes, significant pt. events, CT Scan, chest tube placement, BP problems, codes, etc.)

Signature ____________________ Initials ________

____________________ ________

____________________ ________

Figure 43-8, cont'd

Ventilator flow sheet.

Table 43-2 ▶▶ Performing a Patient-Ventilator System Check

Step	Key Points
Gather correct equipment and supplies.	Respirometer, oxygen analyzer, stethoscope, watch with second indicator. Note: Most modern ventilators incorporate volume-measuring devices into the system. Additional auxiliary equipment may include pulse oximeter, cuff pressure manometer, suction and airway equipment, and sterile distilled water.
Review the patient record.	Note the patient's admitting diagnosis or problem list, physician orders, medications, vital signs, history and physical findings, progress notes, results of laboratory studies, chest radiograph, blood gases, and respiratory care notes.
Enter the patient area. Wash hands and put on gloves.	Inattention to proper hand washing and poor aseptic technique are associated with nosocomial infection.
Identify the patient.	Wristbands sometimes may be attached to the patient's leg or to the foot of the bed. If there is no attached name band, check with the patient's nurse.
Explain what you are doing.	Communication with the patient is important. Even patients who appear unaware of their surroundings may be able to hear and understand. Use broad terms, such as "I'm here to assess your breathing."
Observe the overall situation and note general patient condition, including level of consciousness, condition of extremities, presence of pallor, skin color, capillary refill, airway patency, circuit connection and patency, and ECG findings.	Note general appearance, sensorium, color, and level of activity. Note equipment in use, including ventilator, circuit, airway type, humidification, manual resuscitation bag, and related equipment and supplies. Ensure that the patient's condition appears stable and that ventilation is adequate. Note auxiliary equipment in use, including chest drains, intravenous lines, ECG and pressure monitors, catheters, cooling blanket, aortic balloon pumps, pulse oximeters, and end tidal gas monitors.
Drain tubing and service the humidifier, if needed.	This procedure should be done before the actual ventilator check, if possible.
Attend to the patient's airway, if necessary.	Suctioning, cuff deflation, and other airway manipulation should be done before the actual ventilator check, if possible. After suctioning, note volume and character of secretions. Note endotracheal or tracheostomy tube stability and position. Measure tube cuff pressure and volume to inflate. If the ventilator check is performed first and the patient circuit or airway is disrupted, errors may not be caught, and one of the purposes of ventilator monitoring, patient safety, is defeated.
Inspect the chest and note accessory muscle use, retractions, jugular vein engorgement, bilateral symmetrical chest wall movement, symmetrical diaphragm–chest wall movement, respiratory rate and rhythm, and chest wall stability (flail).	Be alert for signs of respiratory distress, increased work of breathing or patient-ventilatory asynchrony. Observe patient effort to ensure adequate trigger sensitivity and inspiratory flow rate.
Auscultate the chest.	Always move the stethoscope from side to side to compare right and left chest. Note adventitious breath sounds (crackles, rhonchi, wheezing, and bronchovesicular breath sounds). Note diminished or absent breath sounds. If breath sounds are absent, attempt to ascertain cause immediately. Water in the tubing, use of chest tubes, or PEEP may result in adventitious sounds.
Percuss the chest for dullness, resonance, or hyperresonance.	Dullness may be caused by pleural effusion, atelectasis, or consolidation. Resonance is the percussion note found over normal lung tissue. Hyperresonance is associated with excess air in the chest (pneumothorax, pulmonary hyperinflation).
Note location of trachea.	Tracheal shift is associated with severe atelectasis and tension pneumothorax, among other things.
Note peak pressure, static or plateau pressure (P_{plat}), baseline pressure (PEEP/CPAP), pressure support level, mean airway pressure, and presence of auto-PEEP.	A sudden increase in peak airway pressure is associated with pneumothorax, secretions in the airway, bronchospasm, fighting the ventilator, biting the endotracheal tube, occlusion of the airway, and bronchial intubation. A sudden decrease in peak airway pressure is associated with reversal of any of the above conditions, a leak in the system, or patient disconnection. Mean airway pressure may be useful in predicting a decrease in cardiac output or barotrauma. The lowest possible mean airway pressure needed to achieve adequate ventilation and oxygenation should be used. Plateau pressure greater than 30-35 cm H_2O is associated with barotrauma. If P_{plat} is ≥30-35 cm H_2O, consider reducing delivered tidal volume.

Continued

Table 43-2 ▶ ▶ Performing a Patient-Ventilator System Check—cont'd

Step	Key Points
Measure exhaled volume and respiratory frequency.	A respirometer should be used. With continuous flow systems, the respirometer must be placed between the patient connection and the patient wye. If volume is measured at the exhalation valve, volume loss due to tubing compliance may be calculated and subtracted from the measured volume.
If an IMV/SIMV system is in use, calculate delivered volume per machine breath, spontaneous volume between machine breaths, machine rate, total rate, patient spontaneous rate, and minute ventilation.	For IMV/SIMV: $V_{isp} = \frac{\dot{V}_{Etot} - \dot{V}_{Emech}}{f_{tot} - f_{mach}}$ For assist control: Average $V_T = \frac{\dot{V}_{Etot}}{f_{tot}}$
If a ventilator graphics package is in use, observe the pressure-time, flow-time, volume-time, and pressure-volume curves.	Mode of ventilation, patient trigger, adequacy of machine inspiratory flow, and patient-ventilator synchrony can be evaluated with a ventilator graphics package. A slow flow pressure-volume curve can be used to assess lower and upper inflection points. Overdistension can be elevated with use of the dynamic pressure-volume curve. The flow-volume curve may be helpful in assessing the effect of a bronchodilator.
Note delivered F_{IO_2}.	The F_{IO_2} should be analyzed.
Record other ventilatory values.	Ventilatory values include inspiratory flow, inspiratory time, ratio of inspiratory time to expiratory time (I:E ratio), inspiratory and expiratory positive airway pressures (IPAP and EPAP), sigh volume and rate, airway temperature, compliance and resistance, and alarm settings. Many departments chart endotracheal tube size, tube length, cuff pressure or volume, use of minimal occluding volume or minimal leak, ventilator day, circuit change, and other therapy.
Record blood gas values and related data, as appropriate.	These data may include pH, Pa_{O_2}, Pa_{CO_2}, Sa_{O_2}, hemoglobin level, HCO_3^- level, IPAP, base excess, and Ca_{O_2}. Blood gas data should be recorded in such a way that the corresponding F_{IO_2}, PEEP, V_T, f, mode, and other ventilator settings on which the sample was obtained are noted.
Record results of other physiological monitoring of the cardiopulmonary system, as appropriate.	These values may include results of pulse oximetry, P_{ETCO_2}, Ptc_{CO_2}, Pt_{CO_2}, $\dot{Q}s/\dot{Q}t$, and V_{DS}/V_T.
Record hemodynamic data, as appropriate.	These values may include heart rate, blood pressure, central venous pressure, pulmonary arterial pressure , PCWP, $\dot{Q}t$, cardiac index, $S\bar{v}_{O_2}$, $P\bar{v}_{O_2}$, $Ca_{O_2} - C\bar{v}_{O_2}$, pulmonary vascular resistance (PVR), and systemic vascular resistance (SVR).
Record weaning values as appropriate.	These values may include spontaneous f, V_T, f/V_T ratio, $\dot{V}_E$, VC, and inspiratory force (MIP).
Return all alarm systems to optimal condition. Complete charting using appropriate departmental forms or computer entry systems.	Alarms include low pressure, high pressure, disconnection, and volume. Apnea values should be reviewed. Apnea values usually are set to deliver an adequate V_T, f_{mach}, and F_{IO_2} (100%) in the event of apnea development.

▶ CARDIAC AND CARDIOVASCULAR MONITORING

The cardiovascular system is routinely monitored in the critical care setting because patient survival depends on reliable, competent cardiac and cardiovascular performance. There is little question about the importance of monitoring ECG, a noninvasive, continuous assessment of the performance of the conduction system of the heart. In the care of acutely ill patients, there may be clear justification for continuous monitoring of arterial blood pressure. More controversial has been assessment of left ventricular function by right heart catheterization

Box 43-8 • Purposes of Graphics Monitoring

- To confirm mode functions
- To detect auto-PEEP
- To determine patient-ventilator synchrony
- To assess and adjust trigger levels
- To measure the work of breathing
- To adjust tidal volume and minimize overdistension
- To assess the effect of administration of bronchodilators
- To detect equipment malfunction
- To determine appropriate PEEP level

Patient-Ventilator System Check

AARC Clinical Practice Guideline (Excerpts)*

➤ INDICATIONS

A patient-ventilator system check must be performed on a scheduled basis, which is institution specific, for any patient requiring mechanical ventilation for life support. A check also should be performed in the following circumstances:

- Before obtaining blood samples for analysis of blood gases and pH
- Before obtaining hemodynamic or bedside pulmonary function data
- After any change in ventilator settings
- As soon as possible after an acute deterioration of the patient's condition. This may or may not be heralded by a violation of ventilator alarm thresholds
- Anytime that ventilator performance is questionable

➤ CONTRAINDICATIONS

There are no absolute contraindications to performance of a patient-ventilator system check. If disruption of PEEP or F_{IO_2} results in hypoxemia, bradycardia, or hypotension, portions of the check requiring disconnection of the patient from the ventilator may be contraindicated.

➤ HAZARDS AND COMPLICATIONS

- Disconnecting the patient from the ventilator during a patient-ventilator system check may result in hypoventilation, hypoxemia, bradycardia, or hypotension.
- Before disconnection, preoxygenation and hyperventilation may minimize these complications.
- When disconnected from the patient, some ventilators generate a high flow through the patient circuit, which may aerosolize contaminated condensate, putting both the patient and clinician at risk for nosocomial infection.

➤ ASSESSMENT OF NEED

Because of the complexity of mechanical ventilators and the large number of factors that can adversely affect patient-ventilator interaction, routine checks of patient-ventilator system performance are mandatory.

➤ ASSESSMENT OF OUTCOME

Routine patient-ventilator system checks should prevent untoward incidents; warn of impending events; and ensure that proper ventilator settings, according to the physician's orders, are maintained.

➤ FREQUENCY

A patient-ventilator system check should be performed at regularly scheduled intervals, as well as in the following circumstances:

- After any change in ventilator settings
- Before obtaining any blood gas samples
- Before obtaining hemodynamic or pulmonary function data
- As soon as possible after an acute deterioration of the patient's condition, particularly when this occurs after a violation of the ventilator alarm threshold.

➤ INFECTION CONTROL ISSUES

- Condensation for the patient circuit should be considered infectious waste and disposed of according to hospital policy.
- The patient circuit should be changed at regularly scheduled intervals according to hospital policy.
- Universal precautions should be observed.

---

*For the complete guideline see Respir Care 37:882, 1992.

A

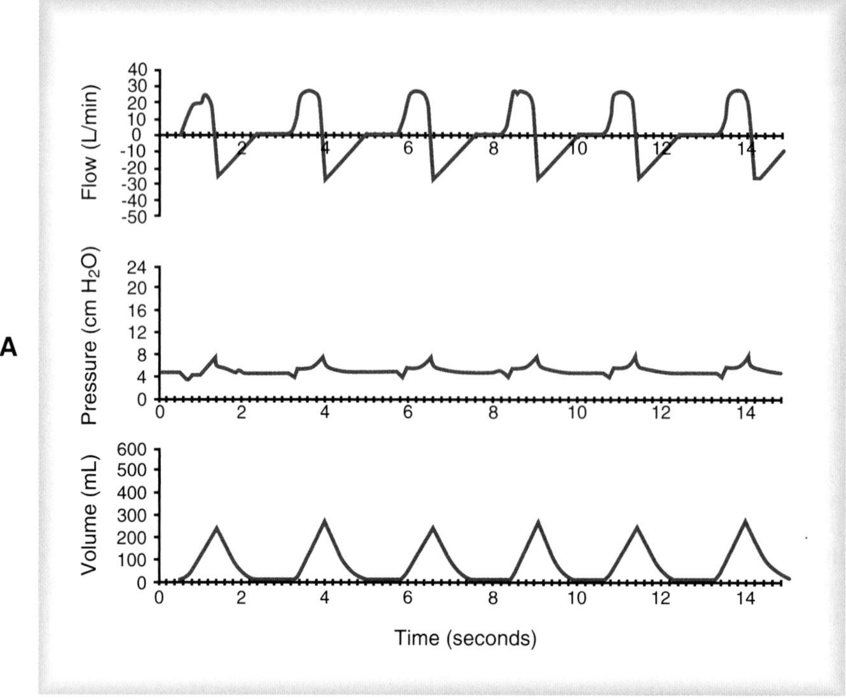

B

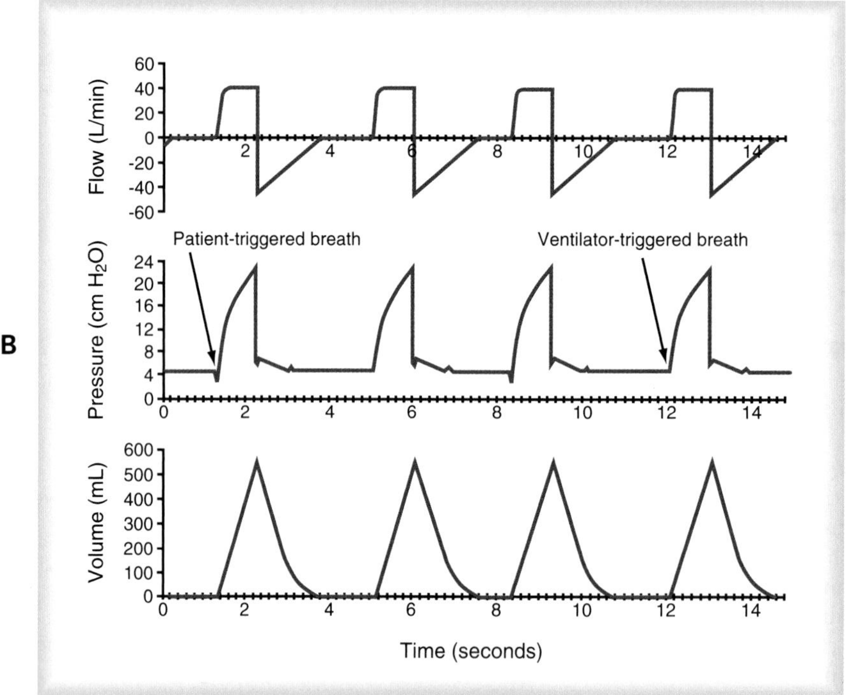

Figure 43-9 · Ventilator Graphics: Flow, Pressure, and Volume Tracings

A, Spontaneous breathing at an elevated baseline pressure (CPAP). The flow, pressure, and volume curves show spontaneous breathing with a CPAP level of approximately 5 cm H_2O. The flow curve is somewhat sinusoidal, the pressure curve fluctuates approximately 1 to 3 cm H_2O around the baseline pressure, and the volume delivered varies. These are typical observations during spontaneous breathing. **B,** Volume ventilation in the assist-control mode. Some breaths are time triggered and others are patient triggered. There is a square wave flow pattern, and volume is constant, breath to breath.

C

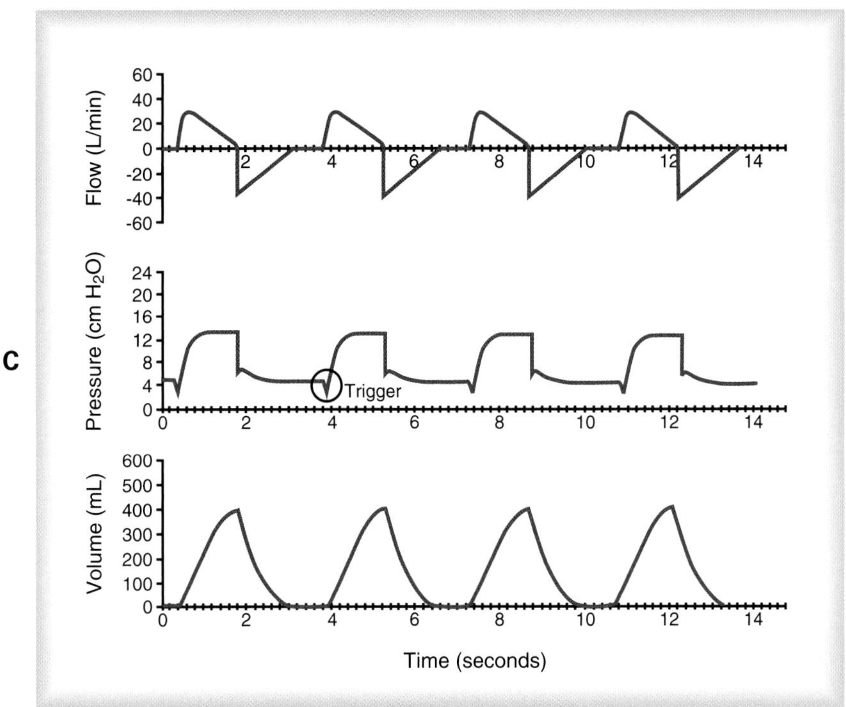

D

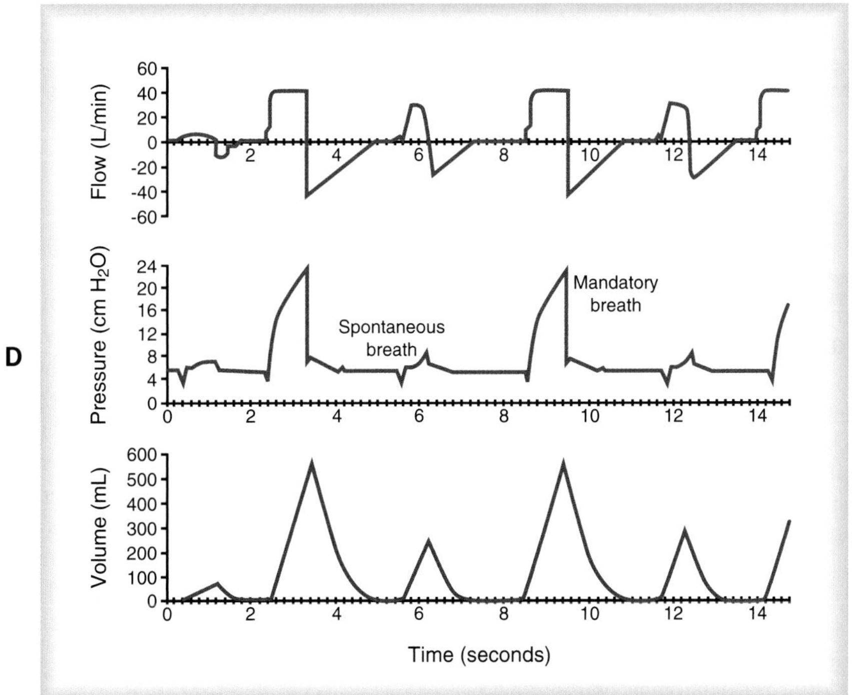

Figure 43-9 · Ventilator Graphics: Flow, Pressure, and Volume Tracings—cont'd

C, Pressure support breaths (PSV). The patient trigger for each breath is evident. Flow is decelerating, and the pressure waveform approaches a square wave. **D,** Synchronized intermittent mandatory ventilation with an elevated baseline (PEEP/CPAP). Spontaneous breathing and machine mandatory breaths are interspersed. Spontaneous volume varies, but the SIMV breaths are constant at 600 mL. The square wave flow pattern for mandatory breaths and the somewhat sinusoidal flow during spontaneous breathing are evident. The baseline pressure (CPAP) is elevated at approximately 5 cm H_2O.

Continued

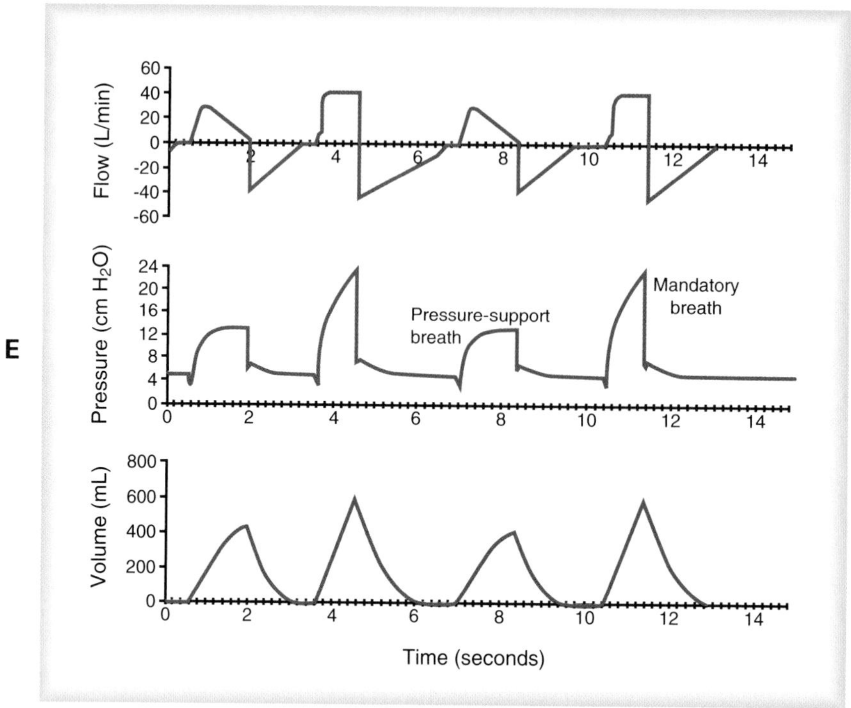

Figure 43-9 · **Ventilator Graphics: Flow, Pressure, and Volume Tracings—cont'd**

E, Synchronized intermittent mandatory ventilation with pressure support. Mandatory breaths have a square flow waveform with a constant volume of 600 mL. The pressure support breaths have a decelerating flow waveform and a pressure pattern approaching a square wave. In this example, there is also an elevated baseline of approximately +5 cm H_2O (PEEP).

MINI CLINI

Ventilator Graphics

PROBLEM

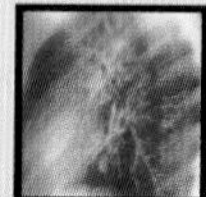

The ventilator-graphic display of a COPD patient receiving mechanical ventilation is showing two distinct features: (1) a pressure-time tracing with spikes and dips that is, generally, irregular and (2) a flow-time tracing that does not reach zero flow at end expiration.

SOLUTION

The irregular tracing implies the presence of airway secretions. Auscultation of the lungs should be performed to assess the need for endotracheal suctioning. Without an active expiratory effort, the existence of flow at end expiration confirms the presence of auto-PEEP. Auto-PEEP can be detected in a large number of COPD patients receiving mechanical ventilation. Yet intervention to reduce or eliminate auto-PEEP may not be necessary. Auto-PEEP should be estimated regularly. More important, the effects of auto-PEEP on the ability to trigger the ventilator or on cardiovascular dynamics (caused by reduced venous return) should be monitored. For reduction or elimination of auto-PEEP, adjusting the ventilator settings or bronchodilator therapy may be required.

with measurement of pulmonary capillary wedge pressure (PCWP) and continuous monitoring of pulmonary arterial pressure. Nevertheless, more complete hemodynamic assessment to evaluate preload, contractility, and afterload (Figure 43-11) may be necessary to guide therapy. Although direct monitoring of cardiac and cardiovascular function is performed at the bedside, assessment of cardiac enzymes or other serological indicators of heart damage usually is conducted in the clinical laboratory. Table 43-3 is a summary of cardiovascular monitoring criteria with normal ranges and abnormal values.

Electrocardiography

The conduction system of the heart is monitored in the ICU with a purpose different from that of the standard 12-lead ECG examination (see Chapter 15). The standard 12-lead ECG can be used to analyze disturbances in the conductive pathway that allow location and extent of injury or the source of dysrhythmia. The ECG in the ICU is used primarily to detect and manage dysrhythmias such as tachycardia, bradycardia, atrioventricular dissociation, ventricular tachycardia, atrial

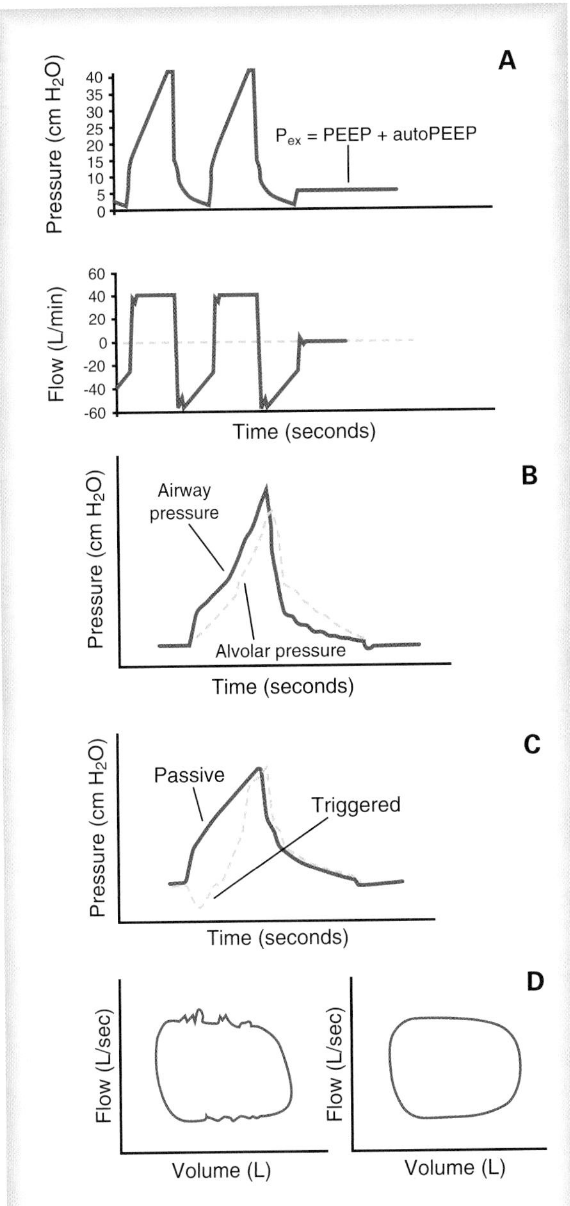

Figure 43-10

Patient-ventilator interactions easily identified from tracings of continuous monitoring of pressure, volume, and flow. **A,** Auto-PEEP. Flow and pressure tracings during ventilator-supported breaths and during end-expiratory occlusion. The airway pressure during the end-expiratory occlusion is an auto-PEEP estimate. **B,** Overdistension. The upper concavity of the airway pressure-time tracing is indicative of overdistension. This example also shows alveolar pressure and its corresponding overdistension. **C,** Patient effort. This is an example of mechanically ventilated passive inflation pressure and the airway pressure-time tracing deformation caused by effort by the patient. **D,** Presence of secretions. Pressure-volume tracing of a ventilator-supported breath displays the presence of secretions. The inspiratory and expiratory limbs are irregular (not smooth) when secretions are present. An irregular airflow-time tracing also can indicate the presence of secretions.

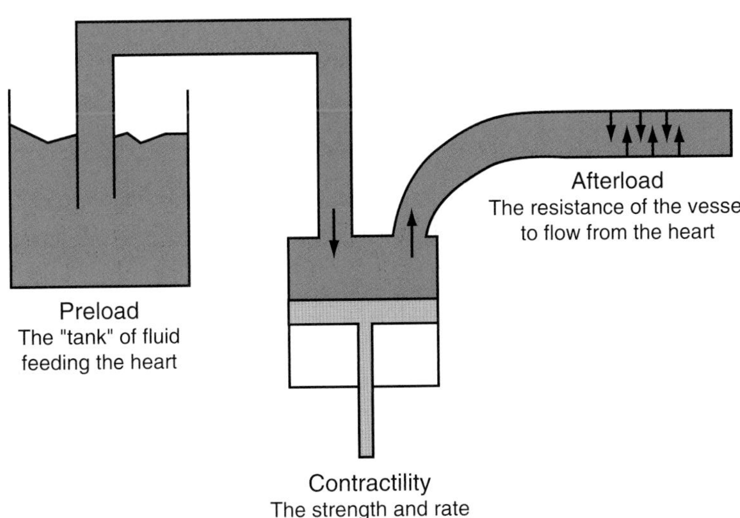

Figure 43-11

Preload contractility and afterload.

Table 43-3 ▶▶ Cardiovascular Monitoring Criteria

Criterion	Normal Value (Range)	Abnormal Value
Heart rate (HR)	80 beats/min (60-100)	>100 beats/min (tachycardia) <60 beats/min (bradycardia)
Arterial blood pressure (ABP)	120/80 mm Hg (90-140/60-90)	>140/90 mm Hg (hypertension) <90/60 mm Hg (hypotension)
Mean arterial blood pressure ($\overline{MAP}$)	90 mm Hg (80-100)	<80 mm Hg (hypotension) >100 mm Hg (hypertension)
ECG	Normal heart rate and rhythm	PR interval >0.2 s; tachycardia, bradycardia, first-, second-, or third-degree heart block, premature ventricular contractions, premature atrial contractions, atrial fibrillation, atrial flutter, elevated ST segment, inverted T wave, ventricular tachycardia, ventricular fibrillation, asystole
Central venous pressure (CVP)	2-6 mm Hg	>6 mm Hg (fluid overload, right ventricular failure, pulmonary hypertension, valvular stenosis, pulmonary embolus, cardiac tamponade, pneumothorax, positive pressure ventilation, PEEP, left ventricular failure) <2 mm Hg (hypovolemia, blood loss, shock, peripheral vasodilation, cardiovascular collapse)
Pulmonary arterial pressure (PAP)	25/10 mm Hg (20-35/5-15)	>35/15 mm Hg (pulmonary hypertension, left ventricular failure, fluid overload) <20/5 mm Hg (pulmonary hypotension, hypovolemia, cardiovascular collapse)
Mean pulmonary arterial pressure ($\overline{PAP}$)	15 mm Hg (10-20)	>20 mm Hg (same as ↑ PAP) <10 mm Hg (same as ↓ PAP)
Pulmonary capillary wedge pressure (PCWP)	5-10 mm Hg (<18)	>18 mm Hg (left ventricular failure, fluid overload) >20 mm Hg (interstitial edema) >25 mm Hg (alveolar filling) >30 mm Hg (frank pulmonary edema) <5 mm Hg (hypovolemia, shock, cardiovascular collapse)
Cardiac output ($\dot{Q}t$ or CO)	5 L/min (4-8)	>8 (elevated) (see Cardiac index) <4 (decreased) (see Cardiac index)
Cardiac index (CI)	2.5-4.0 L/min per m^2	>4 L/min per m^2 (elevated due to stress, septic, shock, fever, hypervolemia, or drugs such as dobutamine, dopamine, epinephrine, isuprel, and digitalis) <2.5 L/min per m^2 (left ventricular failure, myocardial infarction, pulmonary embolus, high levels of positive pressure ventilation, PEEP, pneumothorax, blood loss, hypovolemia)
Systemic vascular resistance (SVR)	900-1400 dynes-sec/cm^5 (11.25-17.5 mm Hg/L per minute)	>1400 dynes-sec/cm^5 (increased due to vasoconstrictors such as dopamine, norepinephrine, and epinephrine, hypovolemia, late septic shock) <900 dynes-sec/cm^5 (decreased due to vasodilators such as nitroglycerin, nitroprusside, and morphine or early septic shock)
Pulmonary vascular resistance (PVR)	110-250 dynes-sec/cm^5 (1.38-3.13 mm Hg/L per minute)	>250 dynes-sec/cm^5 (hypoxemia, ↓ pH, ↑ $Paco_2$, vasopressors, emboli, emphysema, interstitial fibrosis, pneumothorax) <110 dynes-sec/cm^5 (pulmonary vasodilators, nitric oxide, oxygen, calcium blockers)

CI = $\dot{Q}t$/Body surface area.
SVR = [($\overline{MAP}$ − CVP)/CO] × 80 = dynes-sec/cm^5
PVR = [$\overline{PAP}$ − PCWP)/CO] × 80 = dynes-sec/cm^5

flutter, premature ventricular contractions, and ventricular fibrillation. For this purpose there is a need for only three electrodes: right arm (or shoulder or right upper chest), left arm (or shoulder or left upper chest), and left lower chest. The deflections represent, usually, lead II of a standard 12-lead ECG. The direction or amplitude of the waves is of lesser concern than are the rhythms being displayed.

When any dysrhythmia is detected, therapy or intervention can be considered. The source of the dysrhythmia often necessitates management of the underlying cause, such as oxygen therapy for hypoxia or changes or addition to infusion therapy for fluid and electrolyte disturbances. In the ICU, certain interventions may be necessary and must be immediately available. For example, a defibrillator must be available when ventricular fibrillation is detected.

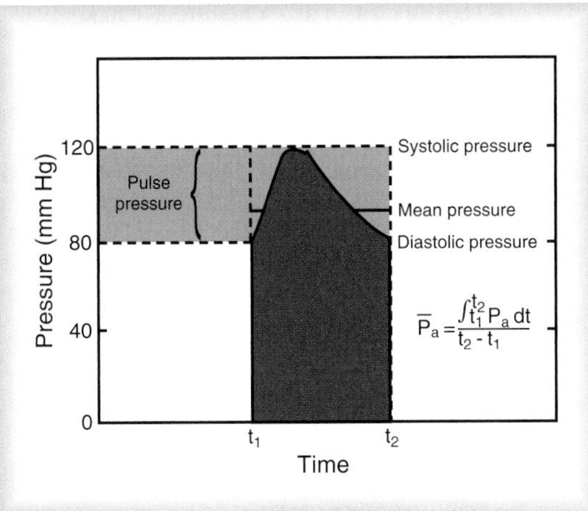

Figure 43-12
Arterial pressure wave form shows anacrotic limb, systolic peak, dicrotic notch, and diastolic pressure.

Arterial Blood Pressure Monitoring

Arterial blood pressure is a crucial measurement for assessing the integrity of cardiovascular tone and the probability that oxygen delivery is dependable. Regulation of cardiovascular tone is under the influence of the autonomic nervous system, but there are other factors that affect blood pressure, such as fluid status or the effects of medications. Major concerns include the adequacy of oxygen delivery during hypotension and the risks of hypertension, such as increased hydrostatic pressure or stroke. Continuous monitoring of the actual blood pressure level is performed by placement of a catheter in, usually, the femoral or radial artery. Because fluid is not compressible, the catheter and connecting tubing are filled with saline solution so that the arterial pressure is transmitted to a transducer that allows display of the arterial pressure tracing (Figure 43-12). The transducer must be properly zeroed and calibrated to reflect the true values of the deflections. The arterial line also provides access for obtaining arterial blood for blood gas analysis.

Central Venous–Right Atrial Pressure Monitoring

Right atrial or central venous pressure often is monitored in the ICU by means of placement of a central venous catheter. Right atrial (RA) pressure normally is the lowest of all the heart chamber pressures, ranging from 2 to 6 mm Hg. Mean RA pressure is the same as central venous pressure (CVP). Central venous pressure is a measure of RA preload. Atrial preload is determined by the balance between the capacity of the cardiovascular system, its circulating volume, and the amount of venous return to the heart (see Chapter 8). Right atrial pressure also is a reflection of right ventricular preload under normal circumstances. As a result, abnormally low RA pressure suggests inadequate filling of the right ventricle and is common in hypovolemia. Causes of abnormal RA pressure/CVP are summarized in Box 43-9.

Box 43-9 • Causes of Increased Right Atrial/Central Venous Pressure

- Right ventricular failure (myocardial infarction, cardiomyopathy)
- Pulmonary valvular stenosis
- Tricuspid stenosis and regurgitation
- Pulmonary hypertension
- Pulmonary embolism
- Volume overload
- Compression around the heart, constrictive pericarditis, cardiac tamponade
- Increased large-vessel tone throughout the body, resulting in venoconstriction
- Arteriolar vasodilation, which increases the blood supply to the venous system
- Increased intrathoracic pressure (positive pressure breath or pneumothorax)
- Placement of the transducer below the patient's right atrial level
- Infusion of solution, especially with pressure infusion pumps, into the CVP line
- Left-sided heart failure

Pulmonary Arterial Pressure Monitoring

Routine monitoring of pulmonary arterial pressure (PAP) began in the 1970s, when the importance of understanding left heart failure became known.[46] Placement of a right heart/pulmonary arterial catheter (Swan-Ganz catheter) is relatively invasive and carries risk of pneumothorax, hemothorax, and, commonly, arrhythmia. Placement of the balloon-tipped 7.5 Fr catheter (Figure 43-13) must be performed aseptically by an experienced clinician. The catheter is guided into the pulmonary artery while the clinician visualizes waveforms with a fluid-filled system identical to the arterial pressure monitoring system (Figure 43-14).

Placement of a Swan-Ganz catheter allows determination of CVP, PAP, and PCWP. Data gathered with a Swan-Ganz catheter can be used to calculate thermodilution cardiac output, pulmonary and arterial vascular resistance, and other associated indices (Table 43-3). Pulmonary arterial pressure monitoring may be helpful in the presence of shock (cardiogenic, hypovolemic, septic), left ventricular failure, myocardial infarction, pulmonary vascular disease, pulmonary edema, and ARDS. Measurement of PCWP is especially helpful in discriminating between cardiogenic and

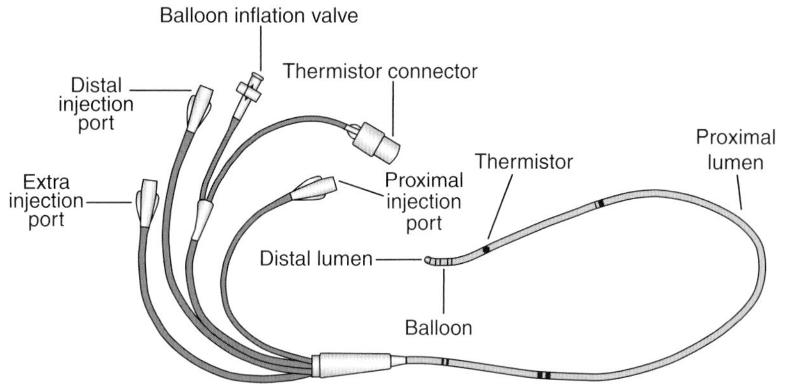

Figure 43-13 · Quadruple-Channel Pulmonary Arterial Catheter

The most distal channel (distal injection port) is for measurement of PAP. Blood can be aspirated from this channel for mixed venous oxygen measurements. A second channel (balloon inflation valve) is used to inflate or deflate the distal balloon. A third channel (proximal injection port), which exits 30 cm from the catheter tip, is used for central venous (right atrial) pressure monitoring and fluid infusion. The fourth channel (extra injection port), which is not present on all catheters, can be used for continuous infusion of hyperalimentation fluid.

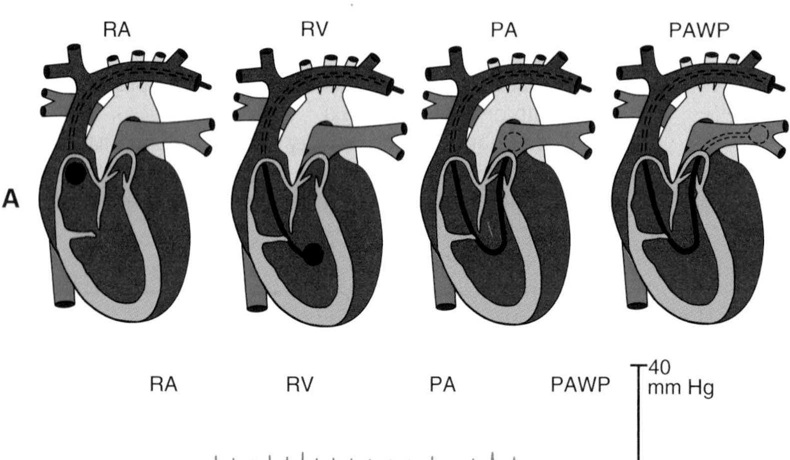

Figure 43-14

A, Position of pulmonary arterial catheter in heart. **B,** As monitored by pressure tracings. *RA*, Pressure tracing from right atrium; *RV*, pressure tracing from right ventricle; *PA*, pressure tracing from pulmonary artery; *PAWP*, pulmonary artery wedge pressure tracing.

noncardiogenic pulmonary edema (e.g., ARDS). In ALI/ARDS, PCWP is generally less than 18 mm Hg, whereas PCWP is elevated in cardiogenic pulmonary edema. It must be noted that the reading and interpretation of Swan-Ganz catheter tracings can be inconsistent. There has been some controversy considering the risk/benefit ratio of the procedure.[2]

An injury model that justifies the use of a pulmonary arterial catheter is the heart as a pump with three factors that affect function: preload, contractility, and afterload (see Figure 43-11).

Preload

Preload is defined as the pressure that stretches the ventricular walls at the onset of ventricular contraction. Preload can be approximated by measurement of PCWP. Pulmonary capillary wedge pressure is an estimate of left atrial pressure, which reflects left ventricular end-diastolic pressure. During left-sided heart failure, preload increases; the increase is reflected in an elevated PCWP. Symptoms of congestive heart failure usually can be controlled with diuretic therapy.

Contractility

Contractility is the forcefulness of the heart muscle contracting under a constant load condition. Digoxin is an agent widely used to cause a modest increase in ejection fraction (contractility) that is associated with improvement in symptoms in patients with congestive heart failure.

Afterload

Afterload usually is defined as the load against which the ventricles must contract. An increase in systemic vascular resistance increases left ventricular afterload. Although increased afterload usually is equated with increased blood pressure, the cause is better understood as the muscle tension required by the left ventricle to generate blood flow. Table 43-4 lists common

MINI CLINI

Hemodynamic Monitoring

PROBLEM

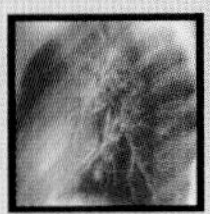

A 55-year-old man with a history of congestive heart failure is admitted to the ICU in acute cardiorespiratory distress. A Swan-Ganz catheter is placed for continuous monitoring of hemodynamic status. Initial cardiac output is 3.2 L/min (↓), cardiac index is 1.6 L/min per m^2 (↓), heart rate is 135 beats/min (↑), stroke volume is 24 mL (↓), SVR is 19.4 mm Hg/L per minute (↔), PVR is 2.3 mm Hg/L per minute (↔), ABP is 90/60 mm Hg (↓), PAP is 38/22 mm Hg (↑), PCWP is 20 mm Hg (↑), and CVP is 8 mm Hg or 11 cm H_2O (↑).

SOLUTION

The patient is being monitored for management of an exacerbation of congestive heart failure. The decreased cardiac output, cardiac index, stroke volume, and ABP accompanied by increases in PCWP and CVP indicate congestive heart failure caused by fluid overload to a weakened heart. Heart rate has increased to compensate for the reduction in stroke volume. The initial conservative treatment is preload reduction by fluid restriction, a diuretic such as furosemide and CPAP therapy. The goals of this treatment are to reduce PCWP and CVP with an expected improvement in cardiac output and index. A question currently under investigation is whether this management plan can be implemented and safely monitored with CVP, ABP data, and clinical signs and symptoms alone.

conditions and associated alterations in hemodynamic variables. Table 43-5 summarizes steps to take in troubleshooting changes in monitored cardiovascular values and vital signs, including possible causes and appropriate corrective action.

▶ NEUROLOGICAL MONITORING

The nervous system is the major organ system the monitoring of which is most frequently overlooked in the ICU. There are several reasons why neurological monitoring in the ICU is so frequently poor. The first and most important is lack of knowledge of proper assessment of the nervous system of a ventilated, restrained, and often sedated ICU patient. Neurological dysfunction is difficult to recognize in a sedated patient. Proper clinical assessment of the nervous system emphasizes the neurological history and examination (Box 43-10).[47,48]

Box 43-10 • Neurological Monitoring

One of the most important, and frequently overlooked, areas of monitoring is the neurological examination, which includes the following:

- History
- Assessment of mental status
- Pupillary response
- Eye movement assessment
- Corneal response
- Gag reflex
- Respiratory rate and pattern
- General motor and sensory evaluations

History

Obtaining historical information from critically ill patients, particularly those with altered states of consciousness, can be difficult. However, attempting to obtain a history by speaking with the patient or family members can provide extremely useful information in the ICU.

Medical conditions with neurological symptoms can be revealed through history and appropriate clinical tests. A history of an evolving focal deficit occurring over days to weeks before loss of consciousness suggests abscess, tumor, or subdural hematoma, whereas a progresion to coma over minutes to hours favors a metabolic cause. Problems such as hypothyroidism, renal failure, cirrhosis, or psychiatric illness suggest greater likelihood of a metabolic cause. Uncontrolled hypertension can induce metabolic (e.g., hypertensive encephalopathy) or structural (e.g., intracerebral hemorrhage) coma.

Neurological Examination

The neurological examination of an ICU patient should address several key issues. In addition to determination of level of consciousness, the primary goal is to determine the presence of focal neurological signs. The clinician can then localize the lesion anatomically and generate a differential diagnosis and treatment plan.

Mental Status

The mental status examination should determine whether the patient has an altered state of consciousness. Terms such as *lethargy*, *confusion*, and *disorientation* lack precise definitions. A brief description of the applied stimulus and arousal pattern is preferred. The mental status examination in the ICU varies if the patient is intubated and cannot vocalize responses or speak. The earliest sign of abnormal mental status often is the patient's inability to follow a conversation or complex commands. Subtle changes in mental status often are the earliest signs of central nervous system dysfunction.

Table 43-4 ▶▶ Common Alterations in Hemodynamic Variables

Condition	Variable							
	Infiltrate on Chest Radiograph	BP	Cardiac Output	CVP	PAP	PCWP	$P\bar{v}O_2$ and $S\bar{v}O_2$	$C(a - \bar{v}O_2)$
Shock								
Hypovolemic	—	↓	↓	↓	Variable	↓	↓	↑
Septic	None, one, or both sides	↓	↑	↓	N or ↓	N or ↓	N or ↑	N or ↑
Cardiogenic	One or both sides	↓	↓	↑↓	↑↑	↑↑	↓	↑
Left ventricular failure								
Mild	One or both sides	N or ↓	↓	N	↑	↑↑	↓	↑
Severe	One or both sides	↓	↓	N or ↑	↑↑	↑↑	↓	↑
Hypervolemic—fluid overload	One or both sides	N or ↑	N or ↑	N or ↑	↑	↑	N or ↑	N or ↓
Pulmonary embolus	None	N	Variable	↑	↑↑	N or ↓	Variable	Variable
ARDS	Both sides	Variable	Variable	Variable	Variable	N or ↓	Variable	Variable
Mechanical ventilation/ PEEP	Variable	N or ↓	N or ↓	N or ↑	N or ↓	↑	N or ↓	N or ↑
Pulmonary hypertension	None	N or ↓	N or ↓	↑↑	↑↑	N	Variable	Variable

BP, Blood pressure; *N*, normal or little or no change.

Table 43-5 ▶▶ Troubleshooting Changes in Vital Signs

Clue	Possible Problem	Advice
Hypotension	Hypovolemia, pump failure	Evaluate fluid balance and possible need for intravenous fluids or inotropic agents.
Hypertension	Anxiety; response to decreased PaO_2, decreased $PaCO_2$ or pain	Reassure, alleviate fear, check patient-ventilator system; if not easily correctable obtain/evaluate ABGs.
Alteration of blood pressure with breathing	Decreased venous return (caused by changes in intrathoracic pressure)	If systolic/diastolic pressures are below adequate perfusion levels, evaluate fluid balance; consider intravenous fluids.
New arrhythmias, tachycardia, bradycardia	Anxiety	Reassure, alleviate fear.
	Decreased PaO_2, decreased $PaCO_2$, increased $PaCO_2$	Check patient-ventilator system; if not quickly correctable, obtain/evaluate ABGs.
	Decreased venous return	Evaluate other hemodynamic values for adequacy of perfusion.
Large swings in CVP or PCWP	Decreased venous return	Evaluate other hemodynamic values for adequacy of perfusion.
Decreased urinary output	Decreased cardiac output Hypovolemia	Evaluate other hemodynamic values for adequacy of perfusion.
Fever	Infection	Control infection; review preventive measures.
	Atelectasis	Check patient-ventilator system for secretions, plugs, slippage of tube into right mainstem bronchus.
	Overheated humidifier	Check humidifier heater temperature.
Weight gain	Fluid retention	Evaluate hemodynamic values for adequacy of perfusion; consider diuresis.
Changes in respiratory rate	Altered settings	Check patient-ventilator settings.
	Change in metabolic needs	Evaluate metabolic rate.
	Anxiety	Reassure, alleviate fear
	Sleep	Normal; metabolic rate is decreased.
Use of accessory muscles or paradoxical breathing	Increased work of breathing	Increase support level; check and change inspiratory flow.
	Patient-ventilator asynchrony	Provide pressure support ventilation. Increase sensitivity.
	Auto-PEEP	Eliminate auto-PEEP.

Pupillary Response

Pupil size, congruency, and response to light and accommodation should be described. Pupillary light reflexes provide information regarding the status of the brain and of the sympathetic and parasympathetic nervous systems. Pupillary function is controlled by the midbrain. If pupil function is normal, the cause of coma is either metabolic or a structural lesion located above the midbrain. Small "pinpoint" pupils usually result from pontine hemorrhage or from ingestion of narcotics or organophosphates. Pupillary responses almost always remain intact in metabolic causes of coma. Dilated and fixed (unresponsive to light) pupils are seen in patients who have been given atropine. Midposition and fixed pupils often indicate severe cerebral damage.

Eye Movements

Abnormalities of extraocular movement have prognostic importance in the ICU. Normal movement of the eyes requires an intact pontomedullary-midbrain connection. The resting position of the gaze, the presence of nystagmus, and the response to head movements and cold tympanic membrane stimulation should be identified. Cervical spine stability must be ensured before oculocephalic maneuvers are performed. If rotation of the head (oculocephalic) and vestibular stimulation (calorics) produces no change in eye position, the pons is nonfunctional. If only the eye ipsilateral to the stimulus abducts, a lesion of the medial longitudinal fasciculus should be suspected.

Corneal Responses

The corneal reflex is used to test the afferent fifth nerve and the efferent seventh nerve. One performs this test by lightly touching the cornea with a cotton swab. The normal response is that the patient should blink both eyes. The presence of this response implies an intact ipsilateral fifth nerve, intact central pons, and intact bilateral seventh nerves. Testing must be performed bilaterally to evaluate both afferent components of the fifth nerve.

Gag Reflex

One tests the gag reflex by using a tongue blade to stimulate one side of the posterior pharynx of an intubated patient . Each side should be tested separately. A normal response demonstrates bilateral movement of the posterior pharyngeal muscles and implies intact ninth and tenth cranial nerves. The ability to cough on suctioning can be tested in an intubated patient and implies an intact tenth nerve. This test should not be attempted on nonintubated patients in the ICU because of the risk of aspiration.

Respiratory Rate and Pattern

The brainstem is the primary site of the central control of respiration. This control occurs at a subconscious level and results in rhythmic contraction and relaxation of the respiratory muscles. The most common abnormal respiratory pattern seen in patients with neurological disorders is Cheyne-Stokes respiration, which consists of phases of hyperpnea that regularly alternate with episodes of apnea. Breathing waxes in a smooth crescendo and once a peak is reached wanes in an equally smooth decrescendo. Cheyne-Stokes respiration usually has an intracranial cause, although hypoxemia and cardiac failure also can be causal. Ataxic breathing is a marker of severe brainstem dysfunction. Despite the nonspecificity of most breathing patterns, the respiratory rate can provide valuable clues to the cause of coma.

Motor Evaluation

A thorough motor evaluation should be performed for all patients. The systematic approach described earlier is key to localization of the site of a pathologic process. The symmetry and pattern of the motor response to noxious stimuli as well as associated neurological symptoms should be documented for all patients.

Sensory Evaluation

The assessment of light touch, pinprick, and temperature sensation can be achieved by respectively applying a cotton swab, clean pin, and a cold or warm object to various parts of the upper and lower extremities. Symmetry of responses between sides and between upper and lower extremities should be documented and is of value in localizing the site of a pathologic process.

Intracranial Pressure Monitoring

There are three primary reasons to measure intracranial pressure (ICP): (1) to monitor patients at risk of life-threatening intracranial hypertension, (2) to monitor for evidence of infection, and (3) to assess the effects of therapy aimed at reducing ICP.

Mean ICP of a supine patient is normally 10 to 15 mm Hg, and the ICP waveform normally undulates gently in time with the cardiac cycle. Fluctuations of the ICP waveform (>10 mm Hg) suggest a position near the critical inflection point of the cranial pressure-volume curve. Elevations in ICP to 15 to 20 mm Hg compress the capillary bed and compromise microcirculation. At ICP levels of 30 to 35 mm Hg, venous drainage is impeded and edema develops in uninjured tissue. Even when autoregulatory mechanisms are intact, cerebral perfusion cannot be maintained if ICP increases to within 40 to 50 mm Hg of the mean arterial pressure.

When ICP approximates mean arterial pressure, perfusion stops and the brain dies.

Currently available ICP monitoring techniques fall into two categories: fluid-filled systems with external transducers, such as intraventricular catheter and subarachnoid bolts, and solid-state systems with miniature pressure transducers that can be inserted in the lateral ventricle, brain parenchyma, or subarachnoid or epidural space.

Glasgow Coma Score

The most widely used scoring system for acute neurological disorders is the Glasgow coma scale (GCS) (Table 43-6). The GSC is used to test best motor response, best verbal response, and the opening of the eyes. The scale goes from 3 to 15 and can be used for rapid triage. Head-injured patients with GCS scores of 13 to 15 often are admitted to a non-ICU observational unit unless neurological examination or a computed tomographic scan reveals a lesion or abnormality that warrants ICU admission. Scores of 9 to 13 on the GCS signify a significant insult with depressed level of consciousness. Head-injured patients with GCS scores of 8 and less need monitoring of ICP.

▶ MONITORING RENAL FUNCTION

The kidney is the main filter of waste products and the principal regulator of the volume and electrolyte composition of body fluid. Because the kidney is the primary excreter of nitrogenous waste, plasma concentrations of blood urea nitrogen (BUN) and creatinine are used to track renal function. As a general guideline, the BUN level increases 10 to 15 mg/dL per day, and the creatinine level increases 1 to 2.5 mg/dL per day after abrupt renal failure. The serum potassium level usually increases 0.5 mEq/L per day and bicarbonate (HCO_3^-) level decreases approximately 1 mEq/L per day. Under the catabolic stress of burns, trauma, rhabdomyolysis (an acute and sometimes fatal disease in which products of skeletal muscle destruction produce acute renal failure), sepsis, or starvation, the rates of change in these values can double. Unlike that of BUN, daily production of creatinine is relatively constant. An increasing creatinine level indicates that the rate of production exceeds its clearance by means of glomerular filtration. Therefore a stable elevation in creatinine level implies a new steady state has been achieved at a decreased glomerular filtration rate (GFR). Until the creatinine level stabilizes, the severity of acute renal dysfunction cannot be assessed reliably. The most common method of estimating GFR (renal function) is measurement of plasma creatinine and creatinine clearance rate. Although calculation of creatinine clearance is more accurate, the procedure entails 24-hour urine collection, and the most important factor is whether GFR is changing or stable; therefore plasma creatinine level is tracked for most patients.

Urine volume usually reflects kidney perfusion. *Polyuria* and *oliguria* refer to a daily urine output of, respectively, more than 3 L and less than 0.4 L in average-sized adults. Anuria is present when urine output is less than 50 mL/d. Polyuria should not be confused with urinary frequency, in which multiple small voidings occur but total output is less than 3 L/d.

▶ MONITORING LIVER FUNCTION

Adequate liver function is essential for survival of critically ill patients. The liver must detoxify wastes from metabolism and digestion and process poisons.

Table 43-6 ▶ ▶ Glasgow Coma Score

Eyes	Open	Spontaneous	4
		To verbal command	3
		To pain	2
		No response	1
Best motor response	To verbal command	Obeys	6
	To painful stimulus	Localized pain	5
		Flexion—withdrawal	4
		Flexion—decorticate	3
		Flexion—decerebrate	2
		No response	1
Best verbal response		Oriented, converses	5
		Disoriented, converses	4
		Inappropriate words	3
		Incomprehensible sounds	2
		No response	1
Total			**3-15**

Elevated results of liver function tests reflect the occurrence of liver parenchymal damage. Hepatic dysfunction may precipitate or worsen ALI.[49] Routine indications for liver function testing in the treatment of critically ill patients include abdominal pain, jaundice, unexplained fever, nausea, malaise, failure to thrive, weight loss, and leukocytosis.[50] Additional indications are facilitation of acuity scoring and definition of the contribution of the liver to multiple-system organ failure.

Batteries of biochemical studies are routine in the evaluation of critically ill patients, but they reflect liver function minimally. Acute liver disease can develop in critically ill patients receiving total parenteral nutrition.[51] The liver disease may manifest as increased liver size and tenderness. Once abnormal results of liver function tests have been obtained, it is essential to determine the cause. Elevations in levels of canalicular enzymes and bilirubin necessitate a search for mechanical obstruction and appropriate radiographic investigations. Elevations of transaminase levels are unusual in cholestatic processes unless there is a superimposed ischemic event, a confounding factor in many critically ill patients. Elevated levels of aspartate aminotransferase and alanine aminotransferase suggest hepatic inflammation. Ischemia, viral hepatitis, and autoimmune hepatitis should be considered in the differential diagnosis.

▶ NUTRITIONAL MONITORING

Assessment and monitoring of nutrition are required in the care of some critically ill patients because nutritional disorders are frequent and important determinants of outcome. Nutritional support is commonly needed by critically ill patients with increased metabolic demands and limited nutritional reserve.

Assessment of Nutritional Status

Early detection of malnutrition in critically ill patients, whether preexisting or a result of acute illness, enables prompt and aggressive intervention with supplemental nutrition. No single measurement or assessment tool can adequately characterize nutritional status, and the diagnosis of malnutrition remains somewhat subjective. However, both functional and biochemical factors should be examined to identify whether a patient is at increased risk of malnutrition and its complications.

Functional Assessment

The functional nutritional assessment consists of the medical history, physical examination, and appraisal of muscle and organ function. Identification of preexisting malnutrition should be attempted by careful attention to the history of present illness, the relevant medical and surgical history, medications, social habits, and a dietary history. Obtaining this information from a critically ill patient is frequently not possible, but a patient's family may be able to provide data on recent dietary habits and weight loss. Historical data should be used to estimate the nutritional consequences of the current hospitalization. Prehospitalization weight should be documented, and any weight changes since hospitalization should be documented and evaluated in the context of diuresis or fluid supplementation. Critically ill patients frequently have volume overload, which makes changes in dry weight difficult to assess.

The findings at physical examination may suggest the presence of nutritional and metabolic deficiencies. Temporal muscle wasting, sunken supraclavicular fossae, and decreased adipose stores are easily recognized signs of starvation. Careful inspection of the hair, skin, eyes, mouth, and extremities can reveal protein calorie malnutrition or vitamin and mineral deficiencies. An assessment of muscle mass and function can provide information about a patient's protein reserves and overall nutritional status. An estimation of muscle mass and fat stores can be obtained from anthropometric measurements such as arm circumference.

The function of the cardiovascular, respiratory, and gastrointestinal systems should be evaluated both for evidence of malnutrition-related dysfunction and because functional deficits may affect the ability of the patient to tolerate nutritional supplementation. For example, the large fluid volumes associated with parenteral nutrition may not be tolerated in the setting of impaired cardiovascular function, and a distended abdomen makes tolerance of enteral supplementation less likely.

Metabolic Assessment

Serum albumin concentration is the most frequently used laboratory measure of nutritional status, a value less than 2.2 g/dL generally reflecting severe malnutrition. Although albumin level is popular as an indicator of nutritional status, the reliability of albumin as a marker of visceral protein status is compromised by its long half-life of 14 to 20 days, making it less responsive to acute changes in nutritional status. Furthermore, serum albumin concentration increases rapidly in response to exogenously administered albumin and is altered irrespective of nutritional status in conditions such as dehydration, sepsis, trauma, and liver disease.[52]

Serum chemistry values are important in determining the specifics of nutritional support but do not directly reflect nutritional status. Sodium, potassium, chloride, total carbon dioxide, blood urea nitrogen, glucose, prothrombin time, partial thromboplastin time, iron, magnesium, calcium, and phosphate should be measured at admission and rechecked periodically.

Estimating Nutritional Requirements

The first step in calculating the nutritional prescription is to estimate the energy or caloric needs of the patient. Determining energy needs requires calculating basal energy expenditure (BEE). The BEE is the amount of energy required to perform metabolic functions at rest and is influenced by both body size and illness. The BEE classically is estimated with the Harris-Benedict equation, as follows:[53]

$$\text{Men: BEE} = 66 + (13.7 \times \text{Weight}) + (5 \times \text{Height}) - (6.8 \times \text{Age})$$

$$\text{Women: BEE} = 65 + (9.6 \times \text{Weight}) + (1.8 \times \text{Height}) - (4.7 \times \text{Age})$$

where weight is expressed in kilograms, height in centimeters, and age in years.

The weight in these equations should be the usual or actual weight of the patient for those without significant weight loss, current weight for those with marked weight loss, and ideal body weight for obese patients. The use of this measurement in the care of the critically ill has traditionally involved multiplication by a stress factor of 0.5 to 2.5.[54] The use of the stress factor may result in overfeeding and may predispose the patient to fatty degeneration of the liver (steatosis), hyperglycemia, electrolyte imbalances, respiratory embarrassment due to increased carbon dioxide production, and macrophage dysfunction. Use of the baseline Harris-Benedict equation without the stress factor in determining the BEE of critically ill patients yields an average estimate of 25 kilocalories per kilogram body weight.

▶ GLOBAL MONITORING INDICES

Organizing the flood of information made available by monitoring instruments is a skill and responsibility of critical care practitioners. In the ICU the immediate concern is the welfare of the patient. Decisions frequently are based on prognosis with respect to the appropriate tests, treatments, and medications prescribed. Guiding those decisions is the weighing of risks and benefits to the patient and the responsible use of resources. Although the physician makes such decisions with all current information, specific data on the probability of survival can be estimated. In the past 30 years, prognostic indices have been derived from large clinical data sets that provide an indication of the seriousness of the patient's condition. These indices (Acute Physiology and Chronic Health Evaluation [APACHE I, II, and III], Acute Physiology Score [APS], Therapeutic Intervention Scoring System [TISS], and Burns Weaning Assessment Program [BWAP]) are determinations of scores from a number of monitored values obtained from snapshots of the patient's condition, usually during the first 24 hours after hospital admission.[55,56] A score may be assigned for that patient at that time, and risk of mortality can be calculated.

Use of severity of illness scoring for individual patients is limited in value, and the accuracy and usefulness of physiology scoring often are questioned. Imposing a scoring system to judge intent to treat places too much emphasis on the validity of the system. Scoring systems, for example, have not been clearly associated with important outcomes such as length of stay or time on mechanical ventilation. At this time, as a bedside tool in the care of an individual patient, scoring systems have limited value. For example, a specific condition may "score" a 17% risk of death, but that patient has possible two outcomes, life (0%) and death (100%). The decision to withdraw or limit care would rarely be based on a "score" because many other factors are involved in such a decision. Inaccuracies in predicting mortality are frequently reported. Discrepancies are probably due to patient mix differences, hospital factors, admission policies, data collection methods, and differences in quality of care. At this time the global indices have limited use in individual patients' care.

Global monitoring does have a definite role in research. Global indices are valuable in the study of the effectiveness of new medications or therapy and the establishment of guidelines for care. When control and experimental (new treatment) groups are compared in a randomized, controlled trial, the severity scores of the groups must be similar, or differences in baseline condition may account for differences in results. As a tracking tool, scoring has important value; for example, the increasing severity of causes of ICU admissions can be followed over time with severity of illness scoring. The consequences of changes in services or policies or interhospital comparisons can be crudely tracked with the use of expected mortality calculations from APACHE scores. Some institutions calculate severity of illness scores for all patients.

Acute Physiology and Chronic Health Evaluation (APACHE)

The **APACHE scoring** system often is used to monitor severity of illness in clinical studies. Studies can then be referenced to a risk of mortality estimate as calculated with APACHE score, and the studies can be compared with similar studies in which the APACHE scoring system is used. The APACHE II scoring system assigns points to physiological variables on the basis of whether the values are high abnormal, low abnormal, or normal. Variables rated include temperature, mean arterial pressure, heart rate, respiratory rate, PaO_2 [or $P(A - a)O_2$], pH, sodium level, potassium level, creatinine level, hematocrit, white blood cell count, and Glasgow coma score. Assigned points are added to derive a total APS. The APACHE II score is derived according to the patient's age, chronic health points, and APS. There is an imprecision to estimating a risk of mortality, yet confidence in the estimates has been reported.[56-58] To emphasize the importance of the neurological examination, the scoring system is weighted toward the importance of the Glasgow coma score. Refinements of APACHE are up to APACHE III,[58] although the APACHE II system continues to be used more often than other systems (Box 43-11).[57-59]

▶ TROUBLESHOOTING

Identification and correction of patient-related and ventilator-related problems during mechanical ventilatory support are primary responsibilities of the respiratory therapist. Under ideal circumstances, potential problems are identified before they occur, or before they can cause harm to the patient. Potential problems with the patient include anxiety, agitation, altered mental status, fighting the ventilator, hypoxemia, hypoventilation, and the development of metabolic acidosis. The patient may experience acute changes in respiratory rate, heart rate, blood pressure, and cardiac output.

Other common patient-related problems include excessive secretions, bronchospasm, and other causes of decreased compliance or increased resistance. Recognition of signs of pneumothorax, pneumomediastinum or subcutaneous emphysema, airway malfunction or leaks, and chest tube leaks should lead to prompt attention to the problem.

Problems associated with the ventilator include leaks or malfunctions in the system, inappropriate ventilator settings (including trigger sensitivity and inspiratory flow rate), development of auto-PEEP, and improper humidification. Box 43-12 lists causes of sudden respiratory distress in patients receiving mechanical ventilatory support. Box 43-13 lists steps for managing sudden distress on the part of ventilator patients. Table 43-7 summarizes troubleshooting of the patient-ventilator system.

Box 43-11 • Global Monitoring Indices

- Indices (scores) have been developed that take into account several monitored values.
- These scoring systems provide an estimate of illness acuity level and an estimate of the risk of mortality.
- For clinical studies, scoring systems are required to assure that the control and experimental groups are similar.
- Scoring systems can be useful as a longitudinal monitor of acuity or a means of evaluating the effect of changes in services.
- At this time, scoring systems have little value in the care of individual patients. The most commonly used acuity of illness scoring system is APACHE II.

Box 43-12 • Causes of Sudden Respiratory Distress in a Patient Receiving Ventilatory Support

PATIENT-RELATED CAUSES

- Artificial airway problems
- Pneumothorax
- Bronchospasm
- Secretions
- Pulmonary edema
- Dynamic hyperinflation
- Abnormal respiratory drive
- Alteration in body posture
- Drug-induced problems
- Abdominal distension
- Anxiety
- Patient-ventilator asynchrony

VENTILATOR-RELATED CAUSES

- System leak
- Circuit malfunction
- Inadequate FIO_2
- Inadequate ventilatory support
- Improper trigger sensitivity
- Improper inspiratory flow setting
- Patient-ventilator asynchrony

From Tobin MJ: Respir Care 36:395, 1991.

Box 43-13 • Steps for Managing Sudden Distress in a Patient Receiving Ventilatory Support

1. Remove the patient from the ventilator.
2. Initiate manual ventilation with 100% oxygen using a self-inflating bag.
3. Perform a rapid physical examination and assess monitoring indices.
4. Check patency of the airway and try to insert a suction catheter.
5. If death appears imminent, consider and manage the most likely causes, such as airway obstruction and pneumothorax.
6. Wait until the patient's condition is stable before attempting more detailed assessment and management.

From Tobin MJ: Respir Care 36:395, 1991.

Table 43-7 ▶▶▶ Troubleshooting the Patient-Ventilator System

Clue to Problem	Possible Cause	Corrective Action
Decreased minute ventilation or tidal volume	Leak around the endotracheal or chest tube	Check all connections for leaks.
	Decreased patient-triggered respiratory rate	Evaluate patient. Check sensitivity. Measure auto-PEEP. Increase set rate. Change mode.
	Decreased lung compliance	Evaluate patient.
	Airway secretions	Clear airway of secretions.
	Altered settings	Check patient-ventilator system.
	Malfunctioning volume monitor	Check with external respirometer.
Increased minute ventilation or tidal volume	Increased patient-triggered respiratory rate	Check respiratory rate. Check sensitivity. Change mode.
	Altered settings	Check patient-ventilator system.
	Hypoxia	Evaluate patient. Consider ABG and Sp_{O_2} values.
	Increased lung compliance	Decrease pressure. Decrease inspiratory time.
	Malfunctioning volume monitor	Check with external respirometer.
Change in respiratory rate	Altered setting	Check patient-ventilator system.
	Increased metabolic demand	Evaluate patient.
	Hypoxia	Evaluate patient. Consider ABG and Sp_{O_2} values.
Sudden increase in peak airway pressure	Coughing	Alleviate uncontrolled coughing.
	Airway secretions or plugs	Clear airway secretions.
	Ventilator tubing kinked or filled with water	Check for kinks and water.
	Changes in patient position	Consider repositioning patient.
	Endotracheal tube in right mainstem bronchus	Verify position.
	Patient-ventilator asynchrony	Correct asynchrony. Check for adequate peak flow. Verify with waveforms.
	Bronchospasm	Identify cause and treat.
	Pneumothorax	Insert chest tubes.
Gradual increase in peak airway pressure	Diffuse, reactive, or obstructive process	Evaluate for problems, such as atelectasis, increasing lung water, bronchospasm.
Sudden decrease in peak airway pressure	Volume loss from leaks in the system	Check patient-ventilator systems for leaks. Verify with waveforms. Check for active inspirations. Evaluate patient.
F_{IO_2} drift	Oxygen analyzer error	Calibrate analyzer. Change oxygen sensor.
	Blender piping failure	Correct failure.
	Oxygen source failure	Correct failure.
	Oxygen reservoir leak	Check ventilator reservoir.
I:E ratio too high or too low	Altered inspiratory flow	Check flow setting and correct.
	Alteration in other settings that control I:E ratio	Check settings and correct.
	Alteration in sensitivity setting	Check setting and correct.
	Airway secretions (pressure ventilator)	Clear airway of secretions.
	Subtle leaks	Measure minute ventilation.
Inspired gas temperature too high	Addition of cool water to humidifier	Wait.
	Altered settings	Correct temperature control setting.
	Adding cool gas by small-volume nebulizer treatment	Turn off heater during treatment.
	Thermostat failure	Replace heater.
Changes in PEEP	Change in tidal volume	Adjust PEEP level.
	Change in compliance	Adjust PEEP level.
	Altered settings	Check settings and correct.
Changes in static pressure	Changes in lung compliance	Evaluate patient and correct if possible.
Changes in ventilator setting	Changes in these settings resulting from deliberate or accidental adjustment of dials or knobs	Determine whether current settings are the intended ones.

Modified from Martz K, Joiner JW, Shepherd RM: Management of the patient-ventilator system: a team approach, ed 2, St Louis, 1994, Mosby.

If medical and mechanical problems have been excluded and the patient continues to fight the ventilator or exhibit high levels of agitation or distress, sedation should be considered. Agents commonly used for sedation in the ICU include benzodiazepines (lorazepam, midazolam), opiates (fentanyl, morphine), haloperidol, and propofol.

Pharmacologic paralysis should be considered only when no other alternatives are effective. The use of neuromuscular blocking agents can mask other patient problems, and ventilator malfunction or disconnection in the care of a paralyzed patient can be catastrophic. In addition, some patients receiving neuromuscular blocking agents in the ICU may experience prolonged neuropathy. Pharmacologic agents used to produce sedation or paralysis in the ICU are listed in Box 43-14.

Box 43-14 • Pharmacologic Agents Used to Produce Sedation or Paralysis

I. Benzodiazepine Tranquilizing Agents
   A. Diazepam (Valium)
   B. Lorazepam (Ativan)
   C. Midazolam (Versed)
II. Sedative Hypnotics and Miscellaneous Agents
   A. Sodium thiopental (Pentothal)
   B. Etomidate (Amidate)
   C. Haloperidol (Haldol)
   D. Propofol (Diprivan)
III. Narcotic Analgesics
   A. Morphine
   B. Fentanyl (Sublimaze)
IV. Neuromuscular Blocking Agents
   A. Nondepolarizing (competitive)
      1. Steroidal agents
         Pancuronium (Pavulon)
         Pipecuronium (Arduan)
         Rocuronium (Zemuron)
         Vecuronium (Norcuron)
      2. Benzylisoquinolinium esters
         Atracurium (Tracrium)
         Cisatracurium (Nimbex)
         Doxacurium (Nuromax)
         Metocurine (Metubine)
         Mivacurium (Mivacron)
         Tubocurarine (Tubarine)
   B. Depolarizing
      1. Succinylcholine (Anectine, Quelicin)
      2. Decamethonium (Syncurine)

KEY POINTS

- The purpose of monitoring is to detect acute changes in patient status. Interpretation of monitored values can lead to prompt initiation of or changes in treatment.
- Caregivers must be experienced at filtering from the noise in the ICU changes that require attention. Caregivers need to recognize when monitors are producing false alarms. They also need to discriminate real pathophysiological changes from normal physiological variations and from variations inherent in the data.
- Because only caregivers can make choices about altering care, caregivers continue to be the most important monitors.
- Monitoring of the respiratory system includes assessment of ventilation, gas exchange, and respiratory system mechanics and function.
- Ventilation is monitored by measurement of tidal volume, respiratory rate, and minute ventilation and by assessment of dead space and alveolar ventilation.
- The single best index of alveolar ventilation is measurement of arterial $PaCO_2$.
- Gas exchange is routinely monitored with ABG analysis and pulse oximetry. Derived values such as V_{DS}/V_T, $P(A - a)O_2$ difference, PaO_2/FIO_2 ratio, shunt, and lung injury score can clarify the nature and severity of gas exchange abnormality.
- Respiratory system mechanics are routinely monitoring by tracking peak and plateau pressures, auto-PEEP, compliance, and resistance.
- Factors such as work of breathing, f/V_T, VC, MIP, and MVV can be extremely helpful in assessing the need to increase ventilatory support or in assessing the potential for weaning.
- The most important responsibility of the respiratory therapist in the ICU is monitoring of the patient-ventilator system.
- Monitoring of the patient-ventilator system includes overall assurance of the integrity and safety of the system. Such monitoring requires complete knowledge and documentation of the ventilator settings, all aspects of ventilator function, the circuitry, airway status, gas exchange, ventilator graphics, lung mechanics, alarms, and the overall care, safety, and comfort of the patient.

Continued

KEY POINTS—cont'd

- Acute changes in cardiac performance, cardiovascular status, or impulse conduction (ECG) can be life threatening, therefore some form of monitoring of the heart, vascular system, and ECG is necessary in the care of nearly all patients in the ICU.
- Hemodynamic monitoring requires the use of invasive pulmonary arterial and other arterial catheters. Values obtained with these monitoring lines must be carefully interpreted by experienced caregivers. Most ICU patients receive ECG monitoring.
- Monitoring of changes in neurological status is extremely important and is more often overlooked than monitoring of other organ systems.
- The Glasgow coma score is one of the most important predictors associated with a greater risk of mortality.
- The neurological examination includes assessment of mental status, pupillary response, eye movements, corneal response, gag reflex, and respiratory rate and pattern and a general motor and sensory evaluation.
- Intracranial pressure monitoring may be needed to detect or manage elevated ICP.
- Global index monitoring is calculation of an illness level score that is an estimate of the risk of mortality from a number of monitoring values. Illness scores are not used in the care plan for an individual patient, but scoring systems are widely used in clinical studies. The APACHE II system is among the most popular of these estimates.
- Troubleshooting the patient-ventilator system is aimed at identifying and correcting problems before they harm the patient.

References

1. Colice GL: A historical perspective on intensive care monitoring. In Tobin MJ, editor. Principles and practice of intensive care monitoring, New York, 1998, McGraw Hill.
2. Swan HJC: Pulmonary artery catheterization: development. In: Tobin MJ, editor. Principles and practice of intensive care monitoring, New York, 1998, McGraw Hill.
3. Pierson DJ: Goals and indications for monitoring. In: Tobin MJ, editor. Principles and practice of intensive care monitoring, New York, 1998, McGraw Hill.
4. Chatburn RL: Principles of measurement. In: Tobin MJ, editor. Principles and practice of intensive care monitoring, New York, 1998, McGraw Hill.
5. Jubran A, Tobin MJ: Monitoring during mechanical ventilation, Clin Chest Med 17:453, 1996.
6. Grace RF: Pulse oximetry: gold standard or false sense of security? Med J Aust 160:638, 1994.
7. Hanning CD, Alexander-Williams JM: Pulse oximetry: a practical review, BMJ 311:367, 1995.
8. Pierson DJ: Pulse oximetry versus arterial blood gas specimens in long-term oxygen therapy, Lung 168:782, 1990.
9. Jubran A, Tobin MJ: Monitoring gas exchange during mechanical ventilation. In: Tobin MJ, editor. Principles and practice of mechanical ventilation, New York, 1994, McGraw-Hill.
10. Mendelson Y: Pulse oximetry: theory and applications for noninvasive monitoring, Clin Chem 38:1601, 1992.
11. Mengelkoch LJ, Martin D, Lawler J: A review of the principles of pulse oximetry and accuracy of pulse oximeter estimates during exercise, Phys Ther 74:40, 1994.
12. Schnapp LM, Cohen NH: Pulse oximetry: uses and abuses, Chest 98:1244, 1990.
13. Ralston AC, Webb RK, Runciman WB: Potential errors in pulse oximetry, Anaesthesia 46:291, 1991.
14. Hess D: Prediction of the change in PaO_2, Crit Care Med 7:568, 1979.
15. Maxwell C, Hess D, Shefet D: Use of the arterial/alveolar oxygen tension ratio to predict the inspired oxygen concentration needed for a desired arterial oxygen tension, Respir Care 29:1135, 1984.
16. Bernard GR et al: The American-European consensus conference on ARDS: definitions, mechanisms, relevant outcomes, and clinical trial coordination, Am J Respir Crit Care Med 1994, 149:818.
17. Zetterstrom H: Assessment of the efficiency of pulmonary oxygenation: the choice of oxygenation index, Acta Anaesthesiol Scand 32:579, 1988.
18. Dean JM, Wetzel RC, Rogers MC: Arterial blood gas derived variables as estimates of intrapulmonary shunt in critically ill children, Crit Care Med 13:1029, 1985.
19. Laghi F et al: Respiratory index/pulmonary shunt relationship: quantification of severity and prognosis in the post-traumatic adult respiratory distress syndrome, Crit Care Med 17:1121, 1989.
20. Petty TL, Ashbaugh DG: The adult respiratory distress syndrome: clinical features, factors influencing prognosis and principles of management, Chest 60:233, 1971.
21. Murray JF et al: An expanded definition of the adult respiratory distress syndrome, Am Rev Respir Dis 138:720, 1988.
22. West JB, Wagner PD: Ventilation-perfusion relationships. In: Crystal RG, West JB, editors. The lung: scientific foundations, New York, 1991, Raven Press.
23. Pontoppidan H, Geffin B, Lowenstein E: Acute respiratory failure in the adult, N Engl J Med 287:743, 1972.
24. Mogue LR, Rantala B: Capnometers, J Clin Monit 4:115, 1988.
25. Bergman NA: Fourier analysis of effects of varying pressure waveforms in electrical lung analogs, Acta Anaesthesiol Scand 28:174, 1984.

26. Benito S, Lemaire F: Pulmonary pressure-volume relationship in acute respiratory distress syndrome in adults: role of positive end expiratory pressure, J Crit Care 5:27, 1990.
27. Beydon L et al: Respiratory mechanics in patients ventilated for critical lung disease, Eur Respir J 9:262, 1996.
28. Roupie E et al: Titration of tidal volume and induced hypercapnia in acute respiratory distress syndrome, Am J Respir Crit Care Med 152:121, 1995.
29. Adams AB, Cakar N, Marini JJ: Static and dynamic pressure-volume curves reflect different aspects of respiratory mechanics in experimental acute respiratory distress syndrome, Respir Care 46:686, 2001.
30. Marini JJ: Controlled ventilation: targets, hazards and options. In: Marini JJ, Roussos C, editors. Ventilatory failure: update in intensive care and emergency medicine, Berlin, 1991, Springer-Verlag.
31. Lessard MR, Lofaso F, Brochard L: Expiratory muscle activity increases intrinsic positive end-expiratory pressure independently of dynamic hyperinflation in mechanically ventilated patients, Am J Respir Crit Care Med 151:562, 1995.
32. Valta P et al: Mean airway pressure as an index of mean alveolar pressure, Am J Respir Crit Care Med 153:1825, 1996.
33. Adams A: Pulmonary function in the mechanically ventilated patient, Respir Care Clin N Am 3:322, 1997.
34. Boros SJ: Variations in inspiratory: expiratory ratio and airway pressure waveform during mechanical ventilation: the significance of mean airway pressure, J Pediatr 94:114, 1979.
35. Brazelton PB et al: Identification of optimal lung volume during high-frequency oscillatory ventilation using respiratory inductive plethysmography, Crit Care Med 29:2349, 2001.
36. Blanch PB, Banner MJ: A new respiratory monitor that enables accurate measurement of work of breathing: a validation study, Respir Care 39:897, 1994.
37. Kallet RH et al: The effects of pressure control versus volume control assisted ventilation on patient work of breathing in acute lung injury and acute respiratory distress syndrome, Respir Care 45:1085, 2000.
38. Marini JJ: Mechanics of the respiratory system. In: Ed: Martin Tobin. Respiratory monitoring, Churchill Livingston, 1991, New York.
39. Purro A et al: Physiologic determinants of ventilator dependence in long-term mechanically ventilated patients, Am J Respir Crit Care Med 161:1115, 2000.
40. Zeggwagh AA et al: Weaning from mechanical ventilation: a model for extubation, Intensive Care Med 25:1077, 1999.
41. Yang K, Tobin M: A prospective study of indexes predicting outcome of trials of weaning from mechanical ventilation, N Engl J Med 324:1445, 1991.
42. Tobin MJ: Noninvasive monitoring of ventilation. In: Tobin MJ. Principles and practice of intensive care monitoring, New York, 1994, McGraw Hill.
43. Marini JJ, Wheeler AP: Critical care medicine: the essentials, ed 2, Baltimore, 1997, Williams & Wilkins.
44. Marini JJ, Smith TC, Lamb V: Estimation of inspiratory muscle strength in mechanically ventilated patients: the measurement of maximal inspiratory pressure, J Crit Care 1:32, 1986.
45. Adams A: Pulmonary function in the mechanically ventilated patient, Respir Care Clin N Am 3:313, 1997.
46. Swan HJC et al: Catheterization of the heart in man with use of a flow-directed balloon-tipped catheter, N Engl J Med 283:477, 1970.
47. Sloan TB: Neurologic monitoring, Crit Care Clin 4:543, 1988.
48. Bleck TP et al: Neurologic complications of critical medical illnesses, Crit Care Med 21:98, 1993.
49. TenHoor T, Mannino DM, Moss M: Risk factors for ARDS in the United States: analysis of the 1993 National Mortality Followback Study, Chest 119:1179, 2001.
50. Kramer DJ: Liver function monitoring in the critically ill patient. In: Tobin MJ, editor. Principles and practice of mechanical ventilation, New York, 1994, McGraw-Hill.
51. Baker AL, Rosenberg IH: Hepatic complications in adults receiving nutrition support, Dig Dis 12:191, 1994.
52. Gianino S, St John RE: Nutritional assessment of the patient in the intensive care unit, Crit Care Nurs Clin North Am 5:1, 1993.
53. MacArthur C: Indirect calorimetry, Respir Care Clin N Am 3:322, 1997.
54. Ackerman MH, Evans NJ, Ecklund MM: Systemic inflammatory response syndrome, sepsis, and nutritional support, Crit Care Nurs Clin North Am 6:321, 1994.
55. Burns SM, Ryan B, Burns JE: The weaning continuum use of APACHE III, BWAP, TISS, and wean index scores to establish stages of weaning, Crit Care Med 28:2259, 2000.
56. Livingston BM et al: Assessment of the performance of five intensive care scoring models within a large Scottish database, Crit Care Med 28:2145, 2000.
57. Knaus WA et al: APACHE II: A severity of disease classification system, Crit Care Med 13:818, 1985.
58. Polderman KH et al: An intra-observer variability in APACHE scoring, Intensive Care Med 27:1550, 2001.
59. Beck DH, Smith GB, Taylor BL: The impact of low-risk intensive care unit admissions on mortality probabilities by SAPS II, APACHE II and APACHE III, Anaesthesia 57:21, 2002.

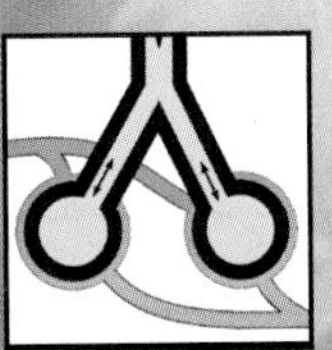

CHAPTER 44

Discontinuing Ventilatory Support

David C. Shelledy

In This Chapter You Will Learn:

- What factors are associated with ventilator dependence
- How to evaluate a patient before attempting ventilator discontinuation or weaning
- What values are recommended for specific weaning indices used to predict a patient's readiness for discontinuation of ventilatory support
- What factors should be optimized before an attempt is made at ventilator discontinuation or weaning
- What techniques are used in ventilator weaning, including traditional T-tube weaning, intermittent mandatory ventilation and synchronized intermittent mandatory ventilation, pressure support ventilation, single, daily spontaneous breathing trials, and other newer methods
- What advantages and disadvantages are associated with various weaning methods and techniques
- How to assess a patient for extubation
- Why some patients cannot be successfully weaned from ventilatory support

Chapter Outline

Continued

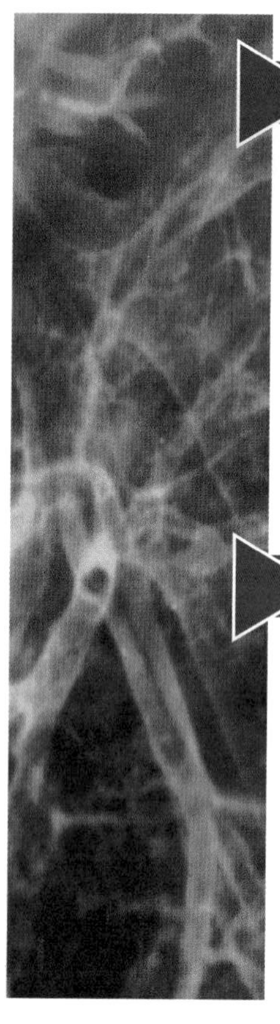

Chapter Outline—cont'd

Key Terms

adaptive support ventilation (ASV)
airway occlusion pressure
automatic tube compensation (ATC)
continuous positive airway pressure (CPAP)
intermittent mandatory ventilation (IMV)
mandatory minute volume ventilation (MMV)
maximum inspiratory pressure (MIP)
maximum voluntary ventilation (MVV)
pressure-support ventilation (PSV)
rapid, shallow breathing index (RSBI)
spontaneous breathing trial (SBT)
synchronized intermittent mandatory ventilation (SIMV)

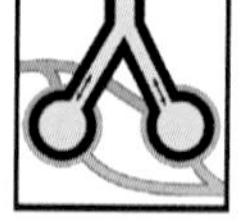

The purpose of mechanical ventilation is to support the patient until the disease state or condition that caused the need for support is alleviated or resolved.[1-3] Ventilatory support can sustain life until relief occurs, but it cannot cure disease. Further, many complications and hazards are associated with mechanical ventilation. Consequently, ventilatory support should be withdrawn as soon as the patient is able to adequately resume spontaneous breathing.[1-4]

Once the problem or condition that caused the need for mechanical ventilation is resolved, most patients can be quickly and easily removed from the ventilator.[1,5] For example, patients who need mechanical ventilation owing to drug overdose or severe asthma, those recovering from postoperative anesthesia, and patients who have received ventilation for 72 hours or less often simply may discontinue ventilation once the precipitating condition has resolved.[1,5] Some patients, however, need mechanical ventilation for longer periods. The term *ventilator dependent* usually is reserved for patients who need ventilatory support for more than 24 hours or who have not responded to attempts at ventilator discontinuation.[3] For these patients, a more formal ventilator discontinuation process should be used.[3]

Ventilator discontinuation should be carefully timed.[4] Premature removal from the ventilator may severely stress the cardiopulmonary system and delay the patient's recovery.[4] Premature discontinuation also exposes the patient to the hazards of reintubation. Delays in discontinuing ventilation, however, expose the patient to increased risk of complications, including nosocomial pneumonia, myocardial infarction, and death.[6]

Weaning refers to the gradual reduction of mechanical ventilatory support that allows the patient to resume spontaneous breathing in an incremental manner.[1,7,8] The need for a gradual, stepwise reduction in the level of ventilatory support is limited to a small number of patients.[1,3,9] The process of removing the ventilator is termed *ventilator discontinuation*.

There are four basic methods for discontinuing ventilatory support: (1) increasing periods of spontaneous breathing (often with a T tube) alternating with mechanical ventilation, (2) intermittent mandatory ventilation (IMV) or synchronized intermittent mandatory ventilation (SIMV), (3) pressure support ventilation (PSV), and (4) a single, daily spontaneous breathing trial (SBT).[4]

Other techniques that may facilitate ventilator discontinuation include the use of mandatory minute volume ventilation (MMV), volume-support ventilation, adaptive support ventilation (ASV), automatic tube compensation (ATC), proportional assist ventilation (PAV), also known as proportional pressure support (PPS), and continuous positive airway pressure (CPAP).[4,7,9]

Techniques for predicting when patients are ready for ventilator discontinuation and weaning have been studied extensively.[6] Many weaning indices have been used, and a number of different weaning methods have been advocated. In spite of this, there are no universally applicable rules for choice of method or predicting success. Although SBTs and PSV have been shown to be more effective than other methods, assessment for ventilator discontinuation and weaning technique should be individualized to the patient. Protocols for ventilator discontinuation administered by respiratory therapists and other healthcare workers can be highly effective, and the use of weaning protocols has been recommended.[3,6,10] Regardless of the method used, success is unlikely unless the precipitating problems causing ventilator dependency have been resolved.[1,3,7] Once these problems are resolved, an organized plan or protocol should be followed, and variations should be based on each patient's response.[3,6,10]

Some patients cannot be successfully removed from mechanical ventilatory support. This group of ventilator-dependent patients poses clinical, economic, and ethical concerns.[11]

▶ DEFINITIONS

Many clinicians use the term *weaning* as a general term to refer to the process of discontinuing ventilatory support, regardless of the time frame or method involved.[7,8,12] *Weaning* also has been used to refer to reductions in fractional inspired oxygen concentration (F_{IO_2}), positive end-expiratory pressure (PEEP), and CPAP.[8] The term *ventilator discontinuation*, on the other hand, has been used to refer to the process of disconnecting a patient from mechanical ventilatory support. For the purposes of this chapter, *weaning* is defined as a gradual reduction in the level of ventilatory support.[1,7-9] *Discontinuing ventilatory support* refers to the overall process of removing the patient from the ventilator, regardless of method used.[3]

Categories for Discontinuing Ventilatory Support

In general, patients being considered for removal from ventilatory support fall into one of three categories: (1) those for whom removal is quick and routine, (2) those who need a more systematic approach to discontinuing ventilatory support, and (3) ventilator-dependent or "unweanable" patients.

▶ REASONS FOR VENTILATOR DEPENDENCE

Patients may need mechanical ventilation because of apnea, acute or impending ventilatory failure, or severe oxygenation problems necessitating high levels of PEEP or CPAP. Common causes of apnea or acute ventilatory failure include drug overdose, trauma, cardiac arrest, severe pneumonia, acute exacerbation of chronic obstructive pulmonary disease (COPD), acute respiratory distress syndrome (ARDS), and neuromuscular disease and spinal cord injury, to name just a few. Impending ventilatory failure and severe oxygenation problems also may necessitate mechanical ventilatory support. Regardless of the reason for initiating mechanical ventilation, patients may remain dependent on the ventilator because of respiratory, cardiovascular, neurologic, or psychological factors.[3]

Ventilatory Workload, or Demand

Patients who need mechanical ventilation often have a ventilatory workload, or demand, that exceeds the patient's ventilatory capacity. This is the most common cause of ventilator dependence.[1,2] *Ventilatory workload* refers to the amount of work the respiratory muscles are asked to perform to provide an appropriate level of ventilation. A patient's total ventilatory workload is primarily determined by (1) the level of ventilation needed, (2) compliance of the lungs and thorax, (3) resistance to gas flow through the airways, and (4) any imposed work of breathing (WOB_I) due to mechanical factors.[1,7]

The level of ventilation required is determined by (1) metabolic rate, (2) central nervous system (CNS) drive, and (3) ventilatory dead space. Common causes of an increased demand for ventilation include increased carbon dioxide production (fever, shivering, agitation, trauma, sepsis) and increased dead space (pulmonary emboli, COPD). Other common causes of increased ventilatory demand include metabolic acidosis, severe hypoxemia, pain, and anxiety.

Compliance is determined by the elastic nature of the lung-thorax system. Resistance is largely related to the nature of the conducting airways. Common causes of decreased lung compliance include atelectasis, pneumonia, pulmonary edema, acute lung injury, and ARDS. Thoracic compliance may be reduced because of obesity, ascites, or abdominal distension. Airway resistance increases with bronchospasm, excessive secretions, and mucosal edema.

Mechanical factors that can increase the WOB_I include artificial airways (endotracheal and tracheotomy tubes), ventilator circuits, demand flow systems, auto-PEEP, and inappropriate ventilator flow and sensitivity

Box 44-1 • Factors That May Increase Ventilatory Workload

INCREASED VENTILATORY DEMAND: INCREASED LEVEL OF VENTILATION REQUIRED
- Increased CNS drive: hypoxia, acidosis, pain, fear, anxiety, and stimulation of J receptors (e.g., pulmonary edema)
- Increased metabolic rate: increased carbon dioxide production, fever, shivering, agitation, trauma, infection, and sepsis
- Increased dead space: COPD, pulmonary embolus

DECREASED COMPLIANCE
- Decreased lung compliance: atelectasis, pneumonia, fibrosis, pulmonary edema, and ARDS
- Decreased thoracic compliance: obesity, ascites, abdominal distension, and pregnancy

INCREASED RESISTANCE
- Increased airway resistance: bronchospasm, mucosal edema, and secretions
- Artificial airways: endotracheal tubes, tracheostomy tubes
- Other mechanical factors: ventilator circuits, demand flow systems, and inappropriate ventilator flow or sensitivity settings

Box 44-2 • Factors That May Reduce Ventilatory Drive

- Decreased $Paco_2$ (respiratory alkalosis)
- Metabolic alkalosis
- Pain (visceral)
- Electrolyte imbalance
- Pharmacologic depressants (narcotics, sedatives)
- Fatigue
- Decreased metabolic rate
- Increased $Paco_2$ associated with chronic carbon dioxide retention
- Neurologic or neuromuscular disease

settings. Factors that may increase ventilatory workload are summarized in Box 44-1.

Ventilatory Capacity

Ventilatory capacity is determined by (1) CNS drive, (2) ventilatory muscle strength, and (3) ventilatory muscle endurance.[13] Most patients being withdrawn from ventilatory support have a normal or increased drive to breathe. Patients with neuromuscular disorders and those receiving sedatives, narcotics, or neuromuscular blocking agents may have a reduced drive to breathe or impaired neuromuscular transmission. Patients with metabolic alkalosis, hypothyroidism, and sleep deprivation also may have reduced ventilatory drive. Box 44-2 summarizes factors that may reduce ventilatory drive.

Muscle strength is influenced by age, sex, muscle bulk, and overall health. Malnutrition, starvation, and electrolyte imbalances (especially calcium, magnesium, potassium, and phosphate) can lead to ventilatory muscle weakness.[13] Controlled ventilation for prolonged periods can cause ventilatory muscle atrophy.[13] Ventilatory muscle endurance is a function of energy supply versus demand. Energy supply is related to nutrition, perfusion, and cell use. Demand is related to the amount of work performed and is a function of minute ventilation, compliance, and resistance. Figure 44-1 summarizes the relations between ventilatory demands and capabilities.

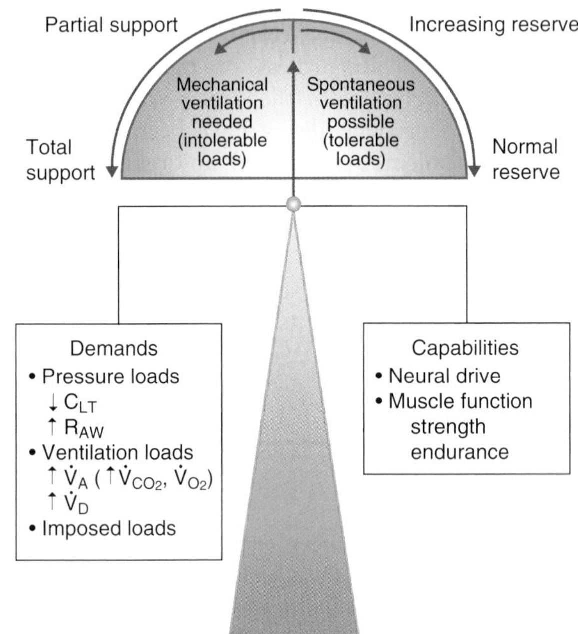

Figure 44-1
Ventilatory failure and the need for ventilatory support depend on the balance between ventilatory muscle demands (loads) and ventilatory muscle capabilities. C_{LT}, Lung-thorax compliance; *Raw*, airway resistance, $\dot{V}_A$, minute alveolar ventilation; $\dot{V}_D$, minute dead space ventilation. *(Modified from MacIntyre NR: Resp Care 40:244, 1995.)*

Discontinuing Ventilatory Support

Success in discontinuing ventilatory support is related to the patient's condition in four main areas: (1) ventilatory workload versus ventilatory capacity, (2) oxygenation status, (3) cardiovascular function, and (4) psychological factors.[1,2,7]

Simply put, when ventilatory workload or demand exceeds ventilatory capacity, successful ventilator discontinuation is unlikely.[1,2] Excessive ventilatory workload may lead to ventilatory muscle fatigue. Once the ventilatory muscles fatigue, they must be rested for at least 24 hours to recover.[3,4,14] Ventilatory workload increases with decreased compliance, increased airway resistance, or an increased level of ventilation. Ventilatory capacity can be reduced by ventilatory muscle fatigue and loss of muscle strength and endurance.

Other factors that may contribute to ventilator dependence include inadequate arterial oxygenation, poor tissue oxygen delivery, myocardial ischemia, arrhythmias, low cardiac output, and cardiovascular instability.[7,12] Neurologic problems that may contribute to ventilator dependence include decreased central drive to breath and impaired peripheral nerve transmission.[3] Psychological issues that may contribute to ventilatory dependence include fear of removal of the life support system, anxiety, stress, depression, and sleep deprivation.[3] Box 44-3 summarizes major factors contributing to ventilator dependence.

Box 44-3 • Factors Contributing to Ventilator Dependence

RESPIRATORY FACTORS

Ventilatory workload exceeds ventilatory capacity
- Decreased compliance: lung tissue or chest wall
- Increased resistance: artificial airways, bronchospasm, mucosal edema, secretions, mechanical demand flow systems
- Increased dead space: pulmonary embolus, COPD
- Ventilatory muscle weakness or fatigue

Oxygenation problems: $\downarrow \dot{V}/\dot{Q}$, $\uparrow \dot{Q}s/\dot{Q}t$, $\downarrow D_{O_2}$, $\uparrow$ oxygen extraction ratio (O_2ER)

NONRESPIRATORY FACTORS
- Cardiovascular factors
  - Myocardial ischemia
  - Heart failure
  - Hemodynamic instability, hypotension, arrhythmias
- Neurologic factors
  - Decreased or increased central drive to breathe
  - Decreased peripheral nerve transmission
- Psychological factors
  - Fear and anxiety
  - Stress
  - Confusion, altered mental status
  - Depression
- Poor nutrition
- Multiple-system organ failure
- Equipment shortcomings

Modified from MacIntyre N: Respir Care 40:244, 1995; American College of Chest Physicians: Chest 104:1833, 1993; Pierson DJ: Respir Care 40:263-270, 1995; Chest 120:375S, 2001; Respir Care 47:69, 2002.

▶ PATIENT EVALUATION

Careful patient assessment is required to determine which patients are ready to be removed from the ventilator quickly, which patient may need a prolonged ventilator discontinuation phase, and which patients are not yet ready for discontinuation of ventilatory support.

An important factor to consider in this assessment is the length of time the patient has been receiving mechanical ventilation. In general, those receiving support for 72 hours or less often can be removed quickly from the ventilator.[1,5,15] Those who need a longer period of support may need a more structured approach. Current guidelines recommend that patients who need mechanical ventilation for more than 24 hours be carefully assessed to determine all of the possible causes of ventilator dependence.[3] These include the respiratory, cardiovascular, neurologic, and psychological causes of ventilator dependence listed in Box 44-3. This recommendation is especially important in the care of patients who have had unsuccessful attempts at discontinuation of ventilation.[3] Factors associated with readiness for discontinuation of ventilatory support are summarized in Box 44-4.

The Most Important Criterion

The single most important criterion to consider when evaluating a patient for ventilator discontinuation or weaning is whether there has been significant alleviation or reversal of the disease state or condition that necessitated use of the ventilator in the first place.[3,7] The clinician should determine whether the patient's condition is improving, whether the initial reason for providing ventilatory support is resolved or relieved, and whether the patient's clinical condition is stable. The following specific questions for patient evaluation have been suggested:[3]

Box 44-4 • Factors Associated With Readiness for Discontinuation of Ventilatory Support

- Reason for instituting mechanical ventilation
- Patient's baseline functional status
- Ventilatory workload versus ventilatory capacity
- Oxygenation status
- Cardiovascular performance
- Current functional status of other organs and systems
- Duration of the critical illness
- Duration of mechanical ventilation
- Psychological factors

Modified from Pierson DJ: Respir Care 40:263, 1995.

1. Is there evidence of alleviation or reversal of the disease state or condition that caused the need for mechanical ventilation?
2. Is the patient's oxygenation status adequate? Specific criteria may include a arterial partial pressure of oxygen (PaO_2) of 60 mm Hg or more with an FIO_2 of 0.40 to 0.50 or less and PEEP of 5 to 8 cm H_2O or less; PaO_2/FIO_2 ratio greater than 150 to 200; and pH of 7.25 or greater.
3. Is the patient's condition hemodynamically stable? Specific criteria may include the absence of acute myocardial ischemia or marked hypotension. Patients should have adequate blood pressure without vasopressor therapy or only low-dose vasopressor therapy (<5 μg/kg min of dopamine or dobutamine).
4. Can the patient initiate an inspiratory effort? The patient must be able to breath spontaneously if ventilator discontinuation is being considered.

If the patient's condition is improving, alleviation or reversal of the precipitating disease state or condition has occurred, the patient is capable of spontaneous breathing, and oxygenation status and hemodynamic values are stable, a formal evaluation for ventilator discontinuation should be performed.[3]

Weaning Indices

Mechanical ventilation is hazardous, and unnecessary delays in ventilator discontinuation increase the complication rate.[3,4] Unfortunately, premature ventilator discontinuation may also cause serious problems, including difficulty in reestablishing the artificial airway and serious compromise of the patient's clinical status.[3,4] Clinical judgment has been found to be a poor guide to determining whether a patient is ready for ventilator discontinuation, and more specific indicators have been sought.[4] Ideally, specific indicators, or weaning indices, would clearly show whether a patient is ready to have the ventilator removed and would help avoid inappropriate ventilator discontinuation.

Traditional weaning indices include PaO_2/FIO_2 ratio, alveolar to arterial oxygen difference ($PAO_2 - PaO_2$), **maximal inspiratory pressure** (MIP) (also known as PI_{max} and negative inspiratory force [NIF]), vital capacity (VC), spontaneous minute ventilation ($\dot{V}_{Esp}$), and **maximum voluntary ventilation** (MVV).[5,15] Newer indices include the rapid, shallow breathing index (f/V_T), airway occlusion pressure ($P_{0.1}$), and measures of WOB.[6-8] Although all these values can be useful, there are enormous discrepancies in the literature regarding the accuracy of these indices in prediction of "weanability"[6,7] With respect to the more traditional weaning indices, vital capacity can be highly variable, whereas MIP, minute ventilation, respiratory rate (f), and f/V_T tend to be more reliable.[16] However, these measures may not correlate well with weaning success among patients receiving long-term ventilatory support, the elderly, or those with major pulmonary abnormalities.[5,14,17]

A comprehensive evidence-based review identified a possible role for 66 specific measurements as predictors of weaning success.[6] Of these, eight values were found consistently predictive of successful ventilator discontinuation.[3,6] Useful predictive measures included spontaneous respiratory rate, spontaneous tidal volume, f/V_T, minute ventilation, MIP, $P_{0.1}$, $P_{0.1}$/MIP, and a combined index—the compliance, rate, oxygenation, and PI_{max} (CROP) score.[3,6] Unfortunately, these measures all have generally low predictive power as assessed with likelihood ratios (LRs).

The LR is a measure of weaning predictor performance. An LR of 1 means the pretest and posttest probabilities are the same, and the test is completely unhelpful.[6] An LR greater than 1 indicates the probability of success increases, and an LR less than 1 indicates the probability of failure increases.[3] Likelihood ratios of 2 to 5 and 0.3 to 0.5 correlate with small but possibly important changes in probability.[3] Likelihood ratios of 5 to 10 or 0.1 to 0.3 correlate with more clinically important changes in probability. Likelihood ratios greater than 10 or less than 0.1 correlate with very large changes in probability.[3] Likelihood ratios for MIP, or NIF, ranged from 0.23 to 2.45.[3] Respiratory rate and tidal volume were slightly better predictors, LRs ranging from 1.00 to 3.89 for respiratory rate and 0.71 to 3.83 for tidal volume.[3] The f/V_T had an LR of 0.84 to 4.67, making it one of the best of the basic indicators.[3,6]

It is doubtful that a single index will be found that can be used for consistent discrimination between success and failure.[7] Moreover, none of these traditional indicators has proved useful in improvement of patient outcome or in selection of a particular weaning method.[7,10] The likely explanation for this failure of research to identify any consistently powerful weaning predictors is that clinicians already fully consider information from predictors in choosing patients for trials of reduction or discontinuation of ventilatory support.[10]

Not withstanding the limitations, measurement of weaning indices, as a part of a comprehensive patient evaluation, can be helpful in assisting the clinician in making sound decisions, and many of these tests perform better than the sum of the data suggests.[10] For example, acceptable values for bedside indices may allow the clinician to discontinue ventilatory support earlier than had otherwise been anticipated.

Critically ill patients have great variation in condition over time, and the patient's ability to resume spontaneous breathing should be reevaluated frequently.[3,6] Specific values for respiratory indices used to predict success in discontinuing ventilatory support are found in Table 44-1. The important specific indices are discussed.

Ventilation

Respiratory rate and pattern, tidal volume, spontaneous minute ventilation, vital capacity, MVV, MIP, $P_{0.1}$, $P_{0.1}$/MIP, f/V_T, and various measures of WOB have been used to assess patients' ability to spontaneously breathe without a ventilator.[6,7]

Table 44-1 ▶▶ Indices Used to Predict Success for Weaning and Ventilator Discontinuation

Measurement	Criterion
Oxygenation	
FIO_2	≤0.40-0.50
PEEP (cm H_2O)	≤5-8
PaO_2 (mm Hg)	≥60
SaO_2 (%)	≥90
$S\bar{v}O_2$ (%)	≥60
PaO_2/PAO_2 ratio	≥0.35
PaO_2/FIO_2 ratio	>150-200
$P(A-a)O_2$ (mm Hg)	<350
$\dot{Q}s/\dot{Q}t$ (% shunt)	<15%-20%
No lactic acidosis, adequate $\dot{Q}t$, blood pressure	
Ventilation	
$PaCO_2$ (mm Hg)	<50
pH	≥7.35
Ventilatory Mechanics	
Respiratory rate (f) (breaths/min)	6-30
Tidal volume (V_T) (mL/kg)	>5
Vital capacity (VC) (mL/kg)	>10-15
Static compliance (mL/cm H_2O)	>25
f/V_T	<105
Respiratory Muscle Strength	
Maximum inspiratory force (MIF) (cm H_2O)	<–20 to –30
Ventilatory Drive (Demand)	
Minute ventilation ($\dot{V}_E$) for	
Normal PCO_2 (L/min)	<10
V_{DS}/V_T	<0.55-0.60
$P_{0.1}$ (cm H_2O)	<6
$P_{0.1}$/MIP	<0.30
Work of Breathing	
Spontaneous work of breathing	<1.6 kg·m/min (<0.14 kg·m/L)
Pressure time index	<0.15-0.18
Ventilatory reserve	
Maximum voluntary ventilation (MVV) (L/min)	>20; more than twice $\dot{V}_E$

Data from Chest 120:375S, 2001; AHRQ publication no. 01-E010, Rockville, MD, 2000, Agency for Healthcare Research and Quality; American College of Chest Physicians: Chest 104:1833, 1993; Burns SM et al: Am J Crit Care 4:4, 1995; Sharar S: Resp Care 40:239, 1995; Bassili HR, Deitel M: JPEN J Parenter Enteral Nutr 5:161, 1981.

Increased thoracic cage movement during spontaneous breathing or asynchronous chest wall to diaphragm movement are related to an increased workload that may lead to ventilatory muscle fatigue and failure.[14] Tachypnea (f ≥30 breaths/min) is a sensitive marker of respiratory distress but can prolong intubation if it is used as an exclusive criterion.[18] Irregular spontaneous breathing or periods of apnea are not good signs of weaning success. Asynchronous and rapid, shallow breathing patterns, although not definitive, suggest respiratory decompensation.[14]

Evaluation of patients for the presence of palpable scalene muscle use during inspiration, an irregular ventilatory pattern, palpable abdominal muscle tensing during expiration, and inability to alter ventilatory pattern on command can be helpful in assessment of the potential for prolonged spontaneous ventilation. Patients with none of these signs have a 90% chance of success.[19] Patients with one or two of these signs usually need continued support. The presence of three or more of these signs can mean the patient's condition is unstable and the patient has a poor prognosis for ventilator removal.

Airway occlusion pressure ($P_{0.1}$) is the inspiratory pressure measured 100 milliseconds after airway occlusion.[15] The $P_{0.1}$ is effort independent and correlates well with central respiratory drive.[14] Ventilator-dependent patients with COPD who have a $P_{0.1}$ greater than 6 cm H_2O tend to be difficult to wean.[15]

MINI CLINI

Calculating and Interpreting the Rapid, Shallow Breathing Index

PROBLEM

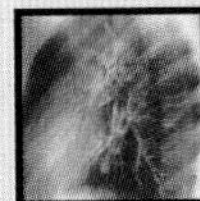

You measure the following spontaneous breathing values for two patients being considered for weaning from mechanical ventilation:

Patient	Rate (f) (breaths/min)	V_T (L)
A	32	0.30
B	28	0.40

For which patient is successful weaning least likely?

SOLUTION

First, compute the rapid, shallow breathing index for each patient as follows:

Patient	Rate (f) (breaths/min)	V_T (L)	f/V_T
A	32	0.30	107
B	28	0.40	70

Patient A clearly exceeds the threshold criterion of 105 breaths/min per liter, whereas patient B falls well below this criterion. All else being equal, patient A is least likely to be successfully weaned.

Rapid, shallow breathing index (f/V_T) is the ratio of spontaneous breathing frequency (breaths/min) to tidal volume (liters), and has been found to be a good predictor of weaning success in the care of many patients who need mechanical ventilation.[4,6,17] The f/V_T has less predictive power in the care of patients who need ventilatory support for more than 8 days and may be less useful in predicting weaning success among the elderly.[8,17] Adjusting the threshold value for f/V_T to 130 or less measured at 3 hours was very effective in predicting weaning success among patients 70 years and older.[20] In spite of these limitations, an f/V_T less than 105 can be an accurate and early predictor of weaning outcome, and an f/V_T of 80 is associated with an almost 95% posttest probability of successful weaning.[4,17] The ratio must be calculated during spontaneous breathing, and the addition of pressure support significantly reduces the predictive value of the ratio.[4]

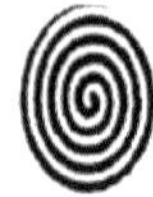

RULE OF THUMB

Adult patients with respiratory rates in excess of 30 breaths/min and tidal volumes less than 300 mL will be difficult to wean.

The $P_{0.1}$/MIP ratio has been found to be a good early predictor of weaning success[3,14] and may be more useful than MIP by itself. The LR values for $P_{0.1}$/MIP range from 2.14 to 25.3, making this one of the better indices in terms of prediction. The f/V_T also has been found to be a better predictor of weaning success than MIP alone.[2,3] However, even with f/V_T, as many as 20% of patients have false-positive results due to unpredictable factors such as congestive heart failure, aspiration, or the development of a new pulmonary lesion.[21] Some patients can be successfully weaned in spite of poor f/V_T values.[22] $P_{0.1} \times f/V_T$ slightly improves specificity over f/V_T alone.[14]

Work of breathing would seem to be an excellent way to gauge spontaneous ventilatory workload. Successful weaning has been found to be less likely among patients with spontaneous work levels greater than 1.6 kg·m/min (16 J/min) or 0.14 kg·m/L (1.4 J/L).[5] However, WOB may not be predictive of weaning success for specific patients.[7] This may be because WOB does not take into account ventilatory muscle capacity or fatigue. Consequently, WOB may be less accurate than other conventional weaning indices.[23]

Percentage oxygen cost of breathing (OCB) is the difference between oxygen consumption during spontaneous breathing and oxygen consumption during apnea (during full ventilatory support), as follows:

$$OCB = \dot{V}O_{2sp} - \dot{V}O_2 \text{ (controlled ventilation)}$$

Once OCB is estimated, the relative proportion of oxygen consumed by the respiratory muscles, compared with the body as a whole, can be calculated as follows:

$$\%\dot{V}O_2 \text{ (resp)} = OCB/\dot{V}O_{2sp}$$

Both OCB and $\%\dot{V}O_2$ have been correlated with the number of days required to wean patients.[14] Patients with an OCB of 15% or less of the total $\dot{V}O_2$ may be more likely to achieve weaning success. In one study, OCB was a better predictor of weaning success than was f/V_T.[24]

Pressure-time product (the area under the inspiratory pressure-time curve) and pressure-time index (PTI) may be the best measures of ventilatory workload in the care of patients receiving mechanical support.[1] The PTI can be calculated as follows:

$$PTI = (\text{mean inspiratory pressure/MIP}) \times T_i/T_{tot}$$

where MIP is maximum inspiratory pressure, T_i is the inspiratory time (seconds), and T_{tot} is the total respiratory cycle. The T_{tot} can be calculated by dividing the respiratory rate (f) into 60 (60/f). A PTI greater than 0.15 to 0.18 has been associated with diaphragmatic fatigue,[25] and a PTI greater than 0.15 cannot be sustained indefinitely.[1] There currently is no well accepted and reliable way to measure ventilatory muscle fatigue for patients receiving mechanical ventilation.[5]

Oxygenation

Poor oxygenation status is associated with weaning failure.[3,7] Arterial blood gas (ABG) analysis, pulse oximetry, and continuous mixed venous oximetry have been used to monitor and assess the oxygenation status of patients before and during weaning.[5,26,27] In general, a PaO_2 of at least 60 mm Hg (50 mm Hg for COPD patients with carbon dioxide retention) with an FIO_2 of 0.40 to 0.50 or less with a PEEP/CPAP level of 5 to 8 cm H_2O or less should be adequate.[3,7] The PaO_2/FIO_2 ratio should be greater than 150 to 200 mm Hg.[3] With these values, normal hemoglobin level, oxygen saturation (SaO_2), and adequate cardiac output and tissue perfusion are assumed. Specific indices used to assess oxygenation status are found in Table 44-1.

Acid-Base Balance

The patient ideally has a normal acid-base balance (pH, 7.35-7.45), and abnormalities should be corrected, if possible, before weaning.[3,5,26] Patients with metabolic acidosis often have an increased ventilatory drive that can make weaning difficult.[12] Patients who have metabolic alkalosis or those who have been mechanically hyperventilated for several days may have reduced ventilatory drive.[12] In these cases, a gradual method of discontinuing ventilatory support should be considered.

Metabolic Factors

Nutrition should be assessed to ensure that it is adequate to maintain respiratory muscle mass and contractile force.[12] Feeding should be adjusted according to individual patient needs; most patients need 1.5 to 2.0 times their resting energy expenditure.[27] In addition, protein intake should be between 1 and 1.5 g/kg per day. Excessive carbohydrate feeding can increase carbon dioxide production and may precipitate acute hypercapnic respiratory failure.[12] Parenteral nutrition solutions containing amino acid formulations (arginine/lysine) can cause metabolic acidosis and thus increase ventilatory demand.[27] Metabolic rate can increase owing to fever or sepsis. Increased WOB, shivering, seizures, or agitation also can increase oxygen demand and should be evaluated.

Renal Function and Electrolytes

Adequate renal function is required to maintain acid-base homeostasis, electrolyte concentrations, and fluid balance.[28] The patient ideally should have an adequate urine output (>1000 mL/d), and there should be no inappropriate weight gain or edema.

Renal insufficiency can lead to metabolic acidosis, which increases respiratory drive. Electrolyte disorders can impair ventilatory muscle function.[3,12] Key electrolytes should be normal (magnesium, 1.8 to 3.0 mEq/L; phosphate, 2.5 to 4.8 mEq/L; potassium, 3.5 to 5.0 mEq/L). Fluid overload can lead to congestive heart failure and pulmonary edema, which may impair pulmonary gas exchange.

Cardiovascular Function

Adequate cardiovascular function is needed to provide sufficient oxygen delivery to the tissues. Cardiac rate and rhythm and blood pressure should be evaluated.[3,12] Tachycardia (heart rate more than 100 to 120 beats/min) and bradycardia (heart rate less than 60 to 70 beats/min) are not positive signs. The presence of arrhythmias, hypotension (blood pressure less than 90/60 mm Hg), and severe hypertension (blood pressure greater than 180/110 mm Hg) should be evaluated carefully before discontinuation of ventilatory support is considered.[3,14]

Cardiac output and index measurements as well as central line and pulmonary arterial pressures (central venous pressure, pulmonary arterial pressure, pulmonary capillary wedge pressure) may be helpful in the evaluation of cardiovascular function. Left ventricular dysfunction, myocardial ischemia, and cardiovascular instability are associated with decreased weaning success.[3,15] Table 44-2 provides criteria for confirming cardiovascular stability.

Psychological Factors and Central Nervous System Assessment

Adequate CNS function is needed to ensure stable ventilatory drive, adequate secretion clearance (cough and deep breathing), and protection of the airway (gag reflex and swallow). Level of consciousness, dyspnea, anxiety, depression, and motivation can affect weaning success.[3,5]

The patient ideally is awake and alert, free of seizures, and able to follow instructions.[3,26,28] Patients should have an intact central drive to breathe and peripheral nerve function. Brainstem strokes, electrolyte disturbances, sedation, and narcotic drugs can impair central neurologic control of ventilation.[3] Obtunded patients should, at a minimum, have an adequate gag reflex and cough. Decreased levels of consciousness are associated with aspiration after extubation. Drugs with depressant effects should be discontinued, if possible, before withdrawal of ventilatory support and extubation.[12] Psychological factors may be among the most important nonrespiratory contributing factors leading to ventilator dependence.[3] Fear, anxiety, and stress should be minimized, and frequent communication among the staff, patient, and patient's family can be

Table 44-2 ▶▶ Criteria for Confirming Cardiovascular Stability

Criterion	Normal Value	Value That May Be Inconsistent With Weaning
Heart rate (beats/min)	60-100	<60, >120
Blood pressure (mm Hg)	90/60-150/90	<90/60, >180/110
$\dot{Q}t$ (L/min)	4.0-8.0	
Cardiac index ($L/min^{-1} \cdot m^2$)	2.5-4.0	<2.1
Cardiac rhythm	No major arrhythmias present	Tachycardia, bradycardia, multiple premature ventricular contractions, heart block
Hemoglobin (g/dL)	12-15	Anemia, <10
Hematocrit	40%-50%	
No angina present		
No lactic acidosis		

Box 44-5 • Nonrespiratory Factors to Evaluate Before Weaning

- Acid-base status
  - Respiratory alkalosis: decreased ventilatory drive
  - Metabolic alkalosis: decreased ventilatory drive
  - Metabolic acidosis: increased ventilatory demand
- Mineral and electrolyte balance
  - Hypophosphatemia: ventilatory muscle weakness
  - Hypomagnesemia: ventilatory muscle weakness
  - Hypokalemia: ventilatory muscle weakness
  - Hypothyroidism: decreased ventilatory drive, impaired muscle function
- Medical stability of other organs and systems
  - Cardiac: excessive preload (e.g., overall volume overload, increased preload on discontinuation of positive pressure ventilation), impaired contractility
  - Renal: renal insufficiency, metabolic acidosis
  - Hepatic: encephalopathy, protein synthesis
  - Gastrointestinal: stress-related hemorrhage, ability to take enteral nutrition
  - Neurologic: level of consciousness, ability to protect airway and clear secretions
  - Effects of drugs: narcotics, benzodiazepines, other sedatives and hypnotics, muscle relaxants, aminoglycosides
- Nutritional status
  - Ventilatory muscle function
  - Ventilatory drive
  - Immune defense system
- Psychological and motivational factors

Modified from Pierson DJ: Respir Care 40:289, 1995.

helpful.[3] Box 44-5 summarizes nonrespiratory factors that should be evaluated before weaning.

Integrated Indices

Many factors are associated with weaning success. Integrated indices may improve prediction by combining several measures of weanability. Examples include the CROP score, the Adverse Factor/Ventilator Score, the weaning index, and the Burns Weaning Assessment Program (BWAP).[7,14]

The CROP score combines measures of ventilatory load, respiratory muscle strength, and gas exchange.[7,17] The CROP score has been shown to be one of the more useful predictors of weaning success, the LR ranging from 1.05 to 19.74.[3]

The Adverse Factor/Ventilator Score combines ratings of 15 adverse factors, including hemodynamic values, infection, nutrition, and neurologic/psychiatric state, with ratings of six ventilator factors, including FIO_2, compliance, minute ventilation, and rate.[14] The weaning index combines measures of ventilatory strength, endurance, and efficiency of gas exchange.[14] A weaning index less than 4 suggests successful weaning from mechanical ventilation.[14,25] The BWAP is a 26-item assessment that includes 12 general and 14 respiratory factors into a single score.[14] Although integrated indices appear promising, no single index has emerged as superior for use in diverse patient populations.[14]

Evaluation of the Airway

The ability to maintain a patent natural airway and the likelihood of aspiration should be evaluated as a part of the process of discontinuing ventilatory support.

It is important for the clinician to separate the decision to discontinue ventilatory support from the decision to extubate.[22] The clinician must also be aware that most weaning indices do not evaluate airway patency or protection (see later, Extubation). The inability to protect or maintain the natural airway is a contraindication to extubation. Some patients who can be successfully removed from a ventilator should not be extubated.[22] Tracheotomy may be considered in the care of patients who need long-term ventilation.

Tracheotomy may improve patient comfort, allow for more effective suctioning, decrease airway resistance, enhance mobility, and allow the patient to eat and speak.[3] Some patients also need high levels of sedation to tolerate the endotracheal tube.[3] Consequently, tracheotomy should be considered in the care of patients likely to benefit and of those who need prolonged mechanical ventilatory support.[3]

Other patients with good airway patency and protection may be unable to maintain spontaneous breathing for prolonged periods without assistance.[22] These patients may be candidates for noninvasive positive pressure ventilation (NPPV) or negative pressure ventilation with a body wrap, chest cuirass, or Port-a-Lung.[14,29]

▶ PREPARING THE PATIENT

Optimizing the Patient's Medical Condition

Before removal of ventilatory support is attempted, the patient's oxygenation status, ventilation, cardiovascular status, and overall medical condition should be optimized. Disease-imposed ventilatory load is minimized with management of infection, bronchospasm, and airway edema.[1] Bronchodilator therapy should be maximized and appropriate use of antiinflammatory agents considered.[1,22] Techniques to facilitate secretion clearance (suctioning, adequate humidification, bronchial hygiene techniques), good nutrition, and optimal positioning should be used.[22] The patient should be rested and not fatigued or sleep deprived, as is common in the intensive care unit (ICU). The patient should be

Box 44-6 • Factors That Should Be Optimized Before Discontinuation of Ventilatory Support Is Attempted

- Oxygenation
  - PaO_2, SaO_2
  - Anemia, if present
  - Atelectasis, pneumonia, acute pulmonary disease
- Ventilation
  - Humidification
  - Secretion clearance (bronchial hygiene, suctioning, chest physiotherapy)
  - Bronchodilator therapy
  - Respiratory alkalosis
  - Imposed work of breathing
  - Respiratory muscle fatigue or atrophy
- Acid-base balance and electrolytes
  - Metabolic acidosis (lactic, ketoacidosis)
  - Metabolic alkalosis (decreased potassium ion, decreased chloride ion, nasogastric tube, vomiting)
  - Low phosphate
  - Low magnesium
- Cardiac, cardiovascular status
  - Blood pressure and cardiac output
  - Arrhythmias, if present
  - Myocardial ischemia
  - Left ventricular function
- Renal factors
  - Kidney function
  - Fluid balance
- Fever, infection, sepsis
- Pain (minimize without oversedation)
- Sleep deprivation
- Exercise tolerance (up in chair, if possible)
- Drugs (narcotics, sedatives, tranquilizers, hypnotics, aminoglycosides, and neuromuscular blocking agents can depress or block ventilatory drive)
- Psychological status
  - Level of consciousness (delirium, coma)
  - Agitation
  - Motivation
  - Fear and anxiety
  - Psychological dependence on the ventilator
  - Depression
  - ICU psychosis
- Hypothyroidism
- Nutritional factors
  - Overfeeding (increased carbon dioxide production)
  - Malnutrition, protein loss
  - Consider high-fat, low-carbohydrate diet to minimize carbon dioxide production
- Gastrointestinal bleeding or obstruction
- Abdominal distension, ascites
- Procedural factors that should be optimized
  - Time of day (avoid evenings, nights, shift change)
  - Adequate staffing
  - Interruptions and disruptions
- Technical factors to consider
  - Appropriate level of PSV to overcome endotracheal tube resistance
  - Flow trigger or flow-by
  - PEEP/CPAP to balance intrinsic PEEP

Modified from Burns SM et al: Am J Crit Care 4:4, 1995; Pierson DJ: Respir Care 40:263, 1995; Goodnough Hanneman SK, Ingersoll GL, Knebel AR, et al: Am J Crit Care 3:421, 1994; Hess DR: Mechanical ventilation of the adult patient: INITIATION, management and weaning. In Burton GG, Hodgkin JE, Ward JJ, editors: Respiratory care: a guide to clinical practice, Philadelphia, 1997, Lippincott Williams & Wilkins; Kacmarek RM, Mack CW, Dimus S: Essentials of respiratory care, ed 3, St Louis, 1990, Mosby.

allowed to sleep at night, and the level of ventilatory support should be increased at that time.[12,30]

The patient's imposed ventilatory workload should be minimized with PSV or a T tube.[22] Flow trigger, flow-by, or ATC also may be helpful in minimizing WOB_I. Intrinsic PEEP during mechanical ventilation may increase trigger work, and small amounts of PEEP or CPAP can help overcome this problem.[1,2] Box 44-6 lists factors that should be optimized before ventilatory support is discontinued.

Patients' Psychological and Communication Needs

As many as 47% of patients who spend more that 5 days in an ICU may experience psychological disturbances.[30] The cause may be the stress of critical illness, interruption of nighttime sleep, or the use of sedatives, tranquilizers, hypnotics, narcotics, and other drugs that affect the CNS.[30] The patient's environment should be optimized, anxiety and depression evaluated, and communication maximized.[3,14,15,30]

Environmental considerations that may improve the patient's sense of well-being and outlook include reducing extraneous noise and providing clocks, calendars, pictures, radio, television, and if possible, a room with windows.[30] Daily mobility should be considered, including getting the patient up in a chair or placing the patient in the hall in a chair.[30] Patients whose condition has been stable long term can sometimes even be helped to walk using an E-cylinder for oxygen, manual resuscitator bag, and two or more healthcare workers for support.

A method for the patient to communicate with staff and visitors should be devised, if possible. Writing tablets, picture boards, and alphabet boards have been used effectively by patients to communicate with staff and visitors.

Anxiety and agitation should be minimized, and communication and encouragement may be helpful.[30] The patient should be told what is planned and be given some control over the situation. Patients should be asked to participate and help in the weaning process. Depression or lack of motivation may increase weaning time.[5,30] If depression is present, assessment and treatment by an appropriate healthcare provider should be considered.[30]

▶ METHODS

There are four basic methods of discontinuing ventilatory support: (1) increasing periods of spontaneous breathing (usually with a T tube) alternating with mechanical ventilatory support, (2) IMV or SIMV, (3) PSV, and a (4) single daily SBT.[4] Box 44-7 summarizes evidence-based criteria and related conclusions regarding methods for ventilator discontinuation.

Rapid Ventilator Discontinuation

Once the precipitating disease state or condition necessitating support has been significantly alleviated or reversed, most patients can be rapidly removed from mechanical ventilation.[12,15] These patients typically have acceptable blood gas levels with mechanical ventilation, adequate myocardial function, and no underlying cardiovascular, pulmonary, neurologic, or neuromuscular disorders.[15]

After a careful evaluation, patients in stable condition who have been treated with a ventilator for less than 72 hours and who have a good spontaneous respiratory rate, minute ventilation, MIP, and f/V_T may undergo a trial of T-tube use for 30 to 120 minutes.[3,7] If the patient does well, ABG analysis may be performed to confirm success. The endotracheal tube then is removed.

Rather than using a T-tube trial, some clinicians prefer to treat the patient with a low level of PSV (5-10 cm H_2O) to overcome the resistance caused by the ventilator circuit, demand flow system, and artificial airway.[2] Others may prefer simply using CPAP (5-7 cm H_2O) or flow-by with the ventilator to provide these modes.[2,3] These methods have the advantage of allowing the clinician to maintain ventilator alarm settings that can provide a margin of safety in the event of apnea or severe hypoventilation. Low levels of CPAP may be useful in maintaining lung volumes and overcoming intrinsic PEEP, if present.[2] Some experts recommend PSV in combination with PEEP/CPAP.[2] Regardless of the method used, a brief trial of successful spontaneous breathing is followed by extubation.

Box 44-7 • Agency for Healthcare Research and Quality Summary of Evidence for Criteria for Weaning for Mechanical Ventilation

- Differences in clinicians' intuitive threshold for reduction or discontinuation of ventilatory support have a far greater impact on failure of spontaneous breathing trials (SBTs) and on reintubation than do modes of weaning. When clinicians set a high threshold, many patients who could tolerate weaning remain on mechanical support longer than is necessary.
- There may be an interaction between threshold and mode of weaning; that is, one mode may be superior when the threshold is high and another when the threshold is low.
- Research to date suggests the best answer to "when to start weaning" is to develop a protocol implemented by nurses and respiratory therapists that begins testing for the opportunity to reduce support very soon after intubation and reduces support at every opportunity.
- For stepwise reductions in mechanical support, pressure support mode or multiple daily T-tube trials may be superior to intermittent mandatory ventilation (IMV).
- For trials of unassisted breathing, low levels of pressure support may be beneficial.
- There may be substantial benefits to early extubation and institution of noninvasive positive pressure ventilation (NPPV) for patients who are alert, cooperative, and ready to breathe without an artificial airway.
- After cardiac surgery, early extubation is unequivocally achieved with a variety of anesthetic interventions and ICU protocols; however, the corresponding reduction in ICU stay is generally small and the effect on complications, though rare, remains unclear.
- The role of computerized weaning protocols has not been established.
- Although steroids can reduce postextubation stridor in children, the impact of steroids on reintubation in children and adults remains uncertain.
- Most theoretically plausible predictors of weaning and extubation success have no predictive power. Those with some predictive power include the rapid, shallow breathing index, which has been most intensively studied, the occlusion pressure/maximum inspiratory pressure ($P_{0.1}$/MIP) ratio, and the compliance, rate, oxygenation, and pressure (CROP) index. However, these are relatively weak predictors of weaning success.
- Tests are rarely useful in increasing the probability of weaning success; on occasion, the results can lead to moderate reductions in the probability of success.
- In general, weaning predictors were probably found to perform poorly because physicians have already considered the results when they select patients for studies.

Modified from Agency for Healthcare Research and Quality, Evidence Report/Technology Assessment Number 23, (AHRQ Publication No. 01-E010), Rockville, MD, 2000.

Patients Who Need Progressive Weaning of Ventilatory Support

Patients who have been receiving mechanical ventilation for longer than 72 hours and those with marginal oxygenation, ventilatory, cardiovascular, or medical status may need a more prolonged period for ventilator discontinuation.[14,15] The most common methods for accomplishing this are T-tube trials interspersed with time on the ventilator, IMV or SIMV, PSV, and a single daily SBT.[4] Each of these methods is described.

Traditional T-Tube Trials

The oldest weaning method is T-tube trials, which allow spontaneous breathing several times per day interspersed with periods of mechanical ventilatory support. For gradual weaning, initial T-tube trials usually last 5 to 30 minutes.[4,7] Full ventilatory support is resumed for a 1- to 4-hour rest period, usually in the assist-control mode. The time off the ventilator is gradually increased until the patient is able to stay off the ventilator for an extended period. T-tube trials can progress rapidly to ventilator removal.

When weaning is very difficult, the process can last weeks or even months. When the ventilator is not being used, the patient is carefully monitored. If distress occurs, mechanical ventilation is resumed. In no case should the patient be overstressed while the T tube is in use, because stress can delay weaning.[2,8] Most patients should resume ventilatory support at night, to rest. An example of a traditional schedule for T-tube weaning is presented in Box 44-8.

In one major multicenter study, one or more daily trials of spontaneous breathing with a T tube were three times faster to extubation than was IMV and two times faster than was PSV.[31] In another study, T-tube trials were more effective than SIMV in weaning quadriplegic patients.[32] Advantages of T-tube weaning include early and frequent testing of the patient's ability to breath spontaneously without support, and this may speed weaning.[2,3] The T tube itself adds little or nothing to the patient's WOB. However, the T tube has no alarms for apnea or acute hypoventilation.[2] The use of traditional T-tube trials several times per day has became unpopular because it requires a great deal of time on the part of ICU staff, and a single, daily SBT may be as effective.[3,4,10] Pressure-support ventilation and CPAP sometimes are used in place of a T tube for spontaneous breathing, and patients who tolerate spontaneous breathing with a low level of PSV should be able to tolerate extubation.

Box 44-8 • Steps for Gradual T-Tube Weaning

1. Prepare the patient psychologically.
2. Perform manual ventilation with a resuscitation bag (optional).
3. Set oxygen/aerosol apparatus at the same FIO_2 or 10% above the FIO_2 setting on the ventilator with the Briggs (T tube) adaptor.
4. Disconnect the ventilator and connect the oxygen/aerosol apparatus with the T-tube adaptor.
5. Monitor the patient's appearance, respiratory rate, pulse, SpO_2, and blood pressure; observe cardiac monitor for arrhythmia.
6. Start with 5 minutes off the ventilator (or less, if the patient does poorly).
7. Work up to 20 or 30 minutes with appropriate rest intervals on the ventilator as necessary. At the end of 20 or 30 minutes, obtain an ABG sample, and reassess the patient's condition while he or she is breathing spontaneously.
8. A schedule for a patient who is having difficulty may be as follows:
   - 5 minutes off and 55 minutes on
   - 10 minutes off and 50 minutes on
   - 15 minutes off and 45 minutes on
   - 20 minutes off and 40 minutes on (obtain samples for ABG analysis after 20 minutes off)
   - 30 minutes off and 30 minutes on
9. Individualize the patient's schedule, depending on his or her condition. Some patients may tolerate the initial time off the ventilator so well that they do not have to resume ventilator use at all. Others may take several days to complete the process. In general, the weaning schedule should be stopped during the night so that the patient can rest and sleep.
10. A variation of this procedure is to turn the ventilator machine rate to zero rather than using a T tube. This procedure allows the therapist to add pressure support (5-7 cmH_2O) or CPAP ($\leq$5 cm H_2O), and it maintains the advantage of use of the sophisticated monitoring alarms available on many ventilators.

Continuous Positive Airway Pressure

Continuous positive airway pressure has been used as an alternative to T-tube weaning in many facilities. Continuous positive airway pressure has the advantage of maintaining lung volume during the weaning phase and thus of improving the patient's oxygenation status. Minimal levels of CPAP may be useful in reducing WOB and compensating for auto-PEEP, particularly in patients with obstructive lung disease.[2] Continuous positive airway pressure is usually provided through the use of the CPAP mode available on most mechanical ventilators. By using the ventilator in the CPAP mode, the clinician can take advantage of the alarm systems available. This may provide an improved margin of safety compared with the use of a T tube alone. However, in one study CPAP was no more effective than T-tube trials in weaning of patients recovering from coronary artery bypass graft surgery.[33]

Intermittent Mandatory Ventilation and Synchronized Intermittent Mandatory Ventilation

Intermittent mandatory ventilation has been advanced since the early 1970s as a method that can speed weaning and ventilator discontinuation.[8] Intermittent mandatory ventilation and SIMV can be used to provide full or partial ventilatory support. Weaning from IMV/SIMV involves gradual reduction of machine rate on the basis of results of ABG analysis and patient assessment.[7] Early claims that IMV allowed faster weaning times[8] were not substantiated in subsequent studies.[34] However, because it is easy to use and is as effective as other methods of ventilation for most patients, IMV/SIMV has become a commonly used mode throughout the United States and the rest of the world.[35]

Some patients receiving ventilation in the SIMV mode may uncouple their breathing effort from the support provided by the machine.[2] When this occurs, the patient continues to make spontaneous breathing efforts during delivery of a "machine breath." Evidence also suggests that once the machine cycling rate is reduced to approximately 50% of the full ventilatory support value, the patient breathes approximately as hard per cycle as when ventilatory support is completely withdrawn.[2] Intermittent mandatory ventilation/SIMV may be preferred over assist control for preventing respiratory alkalosis and reducing mean airway pressure.[14,28] These advantages, however, may not be clinically important.[36] Intermittent mandatory ventilation/SIMV may provide a higher-level WOB than control[37] or assist-control[38] ventilation, although the increase in WOB is not always evident.[36] The demand flow systems used during SIMV may impose a considerable WOB.[37,38] This additional work can be overcome by the use of pressure support (5-10 cm H_2O) and to an extent, the use of flow-by.[10,14]

For initial ventilator setup, the IMV rate and tidal volume usually are set at values designed to achieve full ventilatory support (typically a tidal volume of 10-12 mL/kg ideal body weight and a respiratory rate 10-12 breaths/min for adults). Once the patient's condition has been stabilized, one of two approaches can be used. Some clinicians prefer to continue full ventilatory support until the patient's precipitating disease state or condition has improved considerably.[2] At that point, the rate is reduced in a stepwise manner until complete spontaneous breathing can be achieved.[2] When weaning is delayed until the patient's condition improves, physiological stress is minimized, the ventilatory muscles may recover if they have been fatigued, and ventilator discontinuation may be achieved more quickly, at least in theory.

Other clinicians prefer to immediately reduce the level of mechanical ventilation, providing only partial ventilatory support.[1,2] From the beginning, attempts are made to reduce the IMV rate, and the patient is challenged to provide a portion of the required ventilation.[2] The clinician adjusts the ventilator to make up the difference between what the patient is able to do and the total ventilation needed.[2] The rationale for this partial ventilatory support approach is the idea that only the minimal level of mechanical support needed should be given. The level of partial ventilatory support is titrated up or down the entire time the patient is using the ventilator on the basis of changes in the patient's condition.

The SIMV rate is adjusted in increments of 2 breaths/min. Each adjustment is followed by patient assessment and blood gas analysis, if indicated. This is not weaning per se but is a philosophy of ventilation.[2] Once the precipitating illness has resolved, the rate is then rapidly reduced until complete spontaneous breathing has been achieved.

It once was thought that if patients were required to bear as much of the ventilatory load as they were able, the ventilatory muscle discoordination and atrophy that could occur with prolonged, controlled ventilation would be avoided. Today few patients receive controlled ventilation for extended periods. Consequently, ventilatory muscle discoordination and atrophy due to the use of control mode is probably rare.

Another potential advantage to a partial ventilatory support approach is that when the IMV rate is decreased as soon as possible, mean airway pressure is reduced. This technique may reduce barotrauma and could improve venous return in patients whose cardiac output is compromised by high mean intrathoracic pressure. In addition, it is possible that some patients challenged to breathe more on their own early in the course of mechanical ventilation may be weaned more quickly. Unfortunately, research indicates that IMV may be a slower method of discontinuing ventilatory support than either PSV or T-tube trials.[6,10] It would also seem that partial support may be an unwise strategy in the presence of ventilatory muscle fatigue. An example of titrating the patient's SIMV rate to achieve partial ventilatory support followed by SIMV weaning can be found the Mini Clini on page 1135.

Pressure Support Ventilation

Pressure support ventilation is a mode of ventilatory support that assists the patient's spontaneous inspiratory effort with a clinician-selected level of positive airway pressure. This pressure can range from 1 to 100 cm H_2O and is designed to be held constant throughout the inspiratory cycle.[39] Pressure support breaths can be flow or pressure triggered to inspiration. Pressure support

MINI CLINI

IMV and Partial Ventilatory Support

PROBLEM

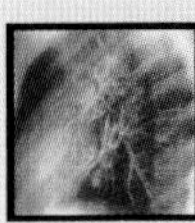

You have a patient with acute ventilatory failure following a motor vehicle accident. The patient is undergoing mechanical ventilation in the SIMV mode. The patient is breathing spontaneously and is able to provide some of the required ventilation. The physician asks that you adjust the ventilator to provide partial ventilatory support.

SOLUTION

Synchronized intermittent mandatory ventilation provides the patient with a preset number of machine breaths. The system allows the patient to take as many or as few breaths spontaneously between the machine breaths as needed or desired. Consequently, the management philosophy is somewhat different from that of assist control.

In general, with SIMV you initiate ventilation at a level needed to provide 100% of the patient's needs, for example:

V_T = 10 to 12 mL/kg*
f = 10 to 12 breaths/min

or

V_T = 12 to 15 mL/kg*
f = 6 to 10 breaths/min

After obtaining a blood gas sample and assuming the presence of spontaneous breathing, you immediately turn down the rate in increments generally of 2 per minute.

For example, the condition of a patient with an ideal body weight of 70 kg (155 lb) and a spontaneous rate of 30 breaths/min would be stabilized with the following titration of IMV rate:

Time of Initial Setting (AM)	Machine Tidal Volume (mL)	Machine Rate (breaths/min)	Total Rate (breaths/min)	Pa_{CO_2} (mm Hg)
9:00	800	10	20	40
9:30	800	8	15	38
10:00	800	6	18	38
10:30	800	4	24	46
11:00	800	6	18	42

With titration of the IMV rate to the patient's needs by means of observation and ABG analysis, the patient's condition should now be stabilized at a rate of 6 breaths/min. This is *not* the same as weaning the patient. Two days later, after significant improvement in the patient's condition and achievement of satisfactory values of various weaning indices, weaning might be tried as follows:

Time of Initial Setting (AM)	Machine Tidal Volume (mL)	Machine Rate (breaths/min)	Total Rate (breaths/min)	Pa_{CO_2} (mm Hg)
9:00	800	6	12	38
9:30	800	4	14	38
10:00	800	2	14	38
11:00	500 (spontaneous)	0	14	38

At this point, the patient is weaned from the ventilator. The endotracheal tube may be removed or a T tube used, *depending on the patient's condition.*

*Current guidelines for treatment suggest that lower tidal volume (5-7 mL/kg) is more appropriate in the treatment of patients with ARDS.[5] A larger tidal volume (12-15 mL/kg) should be reserved for patients with normal lungs or neuromuscular disorders.

ventilation cycles to the expiratory phase when flow decreases to a preset level (usually 5 L/min or 25% of the peak flow) or the set pressure support level is exceeded by 1 to 2 cm H_2O.[39] In at least one large study, pressure support was found superior to T-tube trials and SIMV in achieving weaning from ventilatory support.[40]

For initial ventilator setup in the PSV mode, the beginning pressure level can be adjusted to deliver an appropriate tidal volume, usually 10 to 12 mL/kg of ideal body weight. This is sometimes referred to as *PSVmax*. This level of support can be maintained until it is time to wean the patient. Pressure support ventilation is then gradually reduced to a minimal value to compensate for the artificial airway.[7,8] Once this reduction is accomplished, a T-tube trial may be conducted for 30 to 120 minutes, or extubation can be performed directly from low level pressure support.[2,3]

With PSV, the patient determines the respiratory rate and, to an extent, the inspiratory time and flow. Because of the patient involvement, it is thought that pressure support is a more comfortable mode of ventilation.[1] However, results of some studies indicate that PSV may be no better than IMV in terms of patient comfort, dyspnea, and anxiety.[5]

Pressure support ventilation allows the clinician to manipulate the level of patient work, but the application of this ability to weaning is speculative.[1,2] The OCB has been used to optimize PSV during weaning,[41] although the benefits of this method in terms of speeding weaning are unclear. Pressure support ventilation may be less likely to lead to the uncoupling of the patient's breathing efforts that sometimes occurs with the IMV mode.[2,9]

Low levels of PSV (5-10 cm H_2O) often are used to overcome the WOB_I due to the presence of artificial airways, demand flow systems, and ventilatory circuits. In general, patients who can breath comfortably at this level of PSV can be extubated without problems.[4] However, if upper airway edema is present, WOB following extubation may be about the same as that caused by the endotracheal tube.[4] In these cases, low levels of pressure support may give a false impression about the patient's ability to tolerate extubation.[4]

Pressure support ventilation may produce a greater mean airway pressure than does IMV, and this may be a concern in the care of patients with hemodynamic instability. Pressure support ventilation also does not guarantee a minimum tidal volume. A small tidal volume without intermittent deep breaths could lead to atelectasis.[2,39] Because PSV is an assist mode, in the event of apnea, no machine breaths are delivered. A PSV weaning protocol appears in Box 44-9.

Box 44-9 • Protocol for Pressure Support Weaning

1. Verify that the patient is a candidate for ventilator discontinuation with PSV:
   - Evidence of alleviation or reversal of the disease state or condition necessitating ventilatory support
   - Stable, spontaneous breathing pattern without irregular breathing or periods of apnea
   - Optimization of the patient's medical condition
   - Adequate oxygenation, ventilation, and acid-base balance
2. Begin with a PSV level that achieves a respiratory rate of 20 to 25 beats/min or less. Typically, pressure is adjusted to achieve a tidal volume of 10 to 12 mL/kg. A PSV greater than 30 cm H_2O rarely is needed. The need for a high level of PSV indicates that the patient may not be ready for ventilator discontinuation.
3. Reduce PSV 2 to 4 cm H_2O at least twice daily and reassess the patient for signs of tolerance:
   - Rate >25-30 breaths/min
   - 20% or greater increase in heart rate or heart rate >120 beats/min
   - 20% or greater increase in systolic blood pressure or systolic blood pressure >180 mm Hg or <90 mm Hg
   - Agitation, anxiety, diaphoresis
5. If the patient does not tolerate a reduction in PSV, return to the previous value and reassess.
6. Continue to reduce PSV as tolerated at least twice per day and more frequently if the patient does not have signs of distress.
7. Consider extubation when the patient is able to tolerate a PSV of 5 to 8 cm H_2O for 2 hours with no apparent distress.

Modified from Esteban A, Frutos F, Tobin MJL: N Engl J Med 332:345, 1995; Brochard L, Rauss A, Benito S, et al: Am J Respir Crit Care Med 150:896, 1994.

Intermittent Mandatory Ventilation/Synchronized Intermittent Mandatory Ventilation with Pressure Support Ventilation

With IMV/SIMV the addition of pressure support can overcome the WOB_I during "spontaneous" breaths because of the presence of endotracheal and tracheostomy tubes, demand flow systems, and ventilator circuits. Consequently, it is recommended that during SIMV, pressure support be added to overcome the WOB_I resulting from these mechanical factors. The pressure support level needed to overcome the WOB_I during IMV weaning can be estimated as follows:

$$PSV = [(PIP - P_{plat}) \div \dot{V}_{mach}] \times \dot{V}_{Imax}$$

where PIP is the peak inspiratory pressure during a machine-delivered, volume-cycled breath, P_{plat} is the static airway pressure (plateau pressure) during a mechanical inspiratory volume hold, $\dot{V}_{mach}$ is the flow during the machine breath in liters per second, and $\dot{V}_{Imax}$ is the patient's spontaneous peak inspiratory flow in liters per second. As an alternative, direct measurement of WOB_I can be used to adjust the PSV level.

Although it is clear that the addition of PSV during IMV can reduce or eliminate the WOB_I caused by mechanical factors, it has not been shown how this affects weaning. In one study, SIMV with PSV increased tidal volume and reduced respiratory rate, but did not significantly reduce weaning time or success compared with the results with SIMV alone.[42]

Daily Spontaneous Breathing Trials

A collective task force representing the American College of Chest Physicians, the American Association

MINI CLINI

Setting Pressure Support Levels

PROBLEM

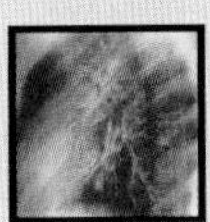

An intubated patient is receiving mechanical ventilation in the SIMV mode with the following settings:

V_T = 800 mL
Rate = 8 breaths/min
Peak inspiratory pressure (PIP) = 50 cm H_2O
Plateau pressure (P_{plat}) = 30 cm H_2O
Ventilatory inspiratory flow ($\dot{V}_{mach}$) = 60 L/min (1 L/s)

The patient is breathing spontaneously with a spontaneous rate of 12 breaths/min and a spontaneous peak inspiratory flow of 30 L/min (0.5 L/s). Find the level of PSV needed to overcome the WOB_I.

SOLUTION

$$PSV = [(PIP - P_{plat}) \div \dot{V}_{mach}] \times \dot{V}_{Imax}$$

$$PSV = \frac{50 \text{ cm } H_2O - 30 \text{ cm } H_2O}{1 \text{ L/s}} \times 0.5 \text{ L/s} = 10 \text{ cm } H_2O$$

$$PSV = 10 \text{ cm } H_2O$$

The calculated PSV level to overcome the WOB_I for this patient is 10 cm H_2O.

Table 44-3 ▶▶ Criteria Used to Determine Whether Patients Receiving High Levels of Ventilatory Support Can Be Considered for Spontaneous Breathing Trials

Criteria	Description
Objective measurements	Adequate oxygenation (e.g., Po_2 ≥60 mm Hg with Fio_2 ≤0.40-0.50; PEEP ≤5-8 cm H_2O; Po_2/Fio_2 ≥150-300) Stable cardiovascular system (e.g., heart rate ≤140; stable blood pressure; no [or minimal] pressors) Afebrile (temperature <38° C) No significant respiratory acidosis Adequate hemoglobin (e.g., ≥8-10 g/dL) Adequate mentation (e.g., arousable, Glasgow coma score ≥13, no continuous sedative infusions) Stable metabolic status (e.g., acceptable electrolyte levels)
Subjective clinical assessments	Resolution of acute phase of disease; physician believes discontinuation possible; adequate cough

Modified from *Chest* 120:375S, 2001; Respir Care 47:69, 2002.

for Respiratory Care, and the American College of Critical Care Medicine published evidence-based guidelines for weaning and discontinuing ventilatory support[3] (Box 44-10). These guidelines were based in part on a comprehensive review of the evidence collected under the direction of the U.S. Agency for Health Care Policy and Research.[6]

The task force made 12 specific recommendations (see Box 44-10). These include the regular use of formal, carefully monitored SBTs to guide clinical decision making regarding the discontinuation of ventilatory support.[3] Specifically, the task force recommended that in the care of patients who need mechanical ventilation for more than 24 hours, a search for all possible causes of ventilatory dependence be conducted and that an attempt be made to reverse or optimize each condition. Spontaneously breathing patients with evidence of reversal of the underlying condition necessitating ventilatory support, adequate oxygenation, and hemodynamic stability should next be assessed with an SBT. Table 44-3 lists criteria to be used in determining whether patients receiving high levels of ventilatory support can be considered for SBTs.

One suggested approach is an initial, brief screening SBT of approximately 3 minutes.[31] During that time, spontaneous tidal volume, respiratory rate, and MIP are assessed. If tidal volume is greater than 5 mL/kg, respiratory rate is less than 30 to 35 breaths/min, MIP is less than –20 cm H_2O (two of three criteria must be met), the patient is entered into a formal SBT of at least 30 minutes but not more than 120 minutes.[3,31] The SBT may be performed with a T tube or in combination with low levels of PSV (5-7 cm H_2O) or CPAP (≤5 cm H_2O).[3] During the SBT, the patient is carefully observed for breathing comfort and signs of anxiety, agitation, dyspnea, or diaphoresis. Respiratory rate, heart rate, blood pressure, and Spo_2 are monitored. The SBT is terminated if any of the following signs of distress are observed:

- Agitation, anxiety, diaphoresis, or change in mental status
- Respiratory rate greater than 30 to 35 breaths/min
- Spo_2 less than 90%
- More than 20% increase or decrease in heart rate or heart rate more than 120 to 140 beats/min
- Systolic blood pressure greater than 180 mm Hg or less than 90 mm Hg

Patients with unsuccessful results of an SBT are returned to full ventilatory support for 24 hours to allow the ventilatory muscles to recover. During this period, the causes of failure are identified and corrected, if possible. The patient is then reevaluated. If the criteria listed in Table 44-3 continue to be met, SBTs are repeated every 24 hours.[3] Patients who tolerate the formal SBT for 30 to 120 minutes remain off the ventilator, and extubation is considered. Box 44-11 is a sample protocol of an SBT for discontinuation of ventilatory support.

Box 44-10 • Evidence-Based Guidelines for Weaning and Discontinuing Ventilatory Support

Recommendation 1: In patients who need mechanical ventilation for >24 h, a search for all the causes that may be contributing to ventilatory dependence should be undertaken. This is particularly true in the patient who has failed attempts at withdrawing the mechanical ventilator. Reversing all possible ventilatory and nonventilatory issues should be an integral part of the ventilatory discontinuation process.

Recommendation 2: Patients receiving mechanical ventilation for respiratory failure should undergo a formal assessment of discontinuation potential if the following criteria are satisfied:

1. Evidence for some reversal of the underlying cause for respiratory failure;
2. Adequate oxygenation (e.g., $Pa{O_2}/F{IO_2}$ ratio >150 to 200; requiring positive end-expiratory pressure [PEEP] ≤5 to 8 cm H_2O; $F{IO_2}$ ≤0.4 to 0.5) and pH ≥7.25;
3. Hemodynamic stability, as defined by the absence of active myocardial ischemia and the absence of clinically significant hypotension (ie, a condition necessitating no vasopressor therapy or therapy with only low-dose vasopressors such as dopamine or dobutamine, <5 μg/kg/min); and
4. The capability to initiate an inspiratory effort.

The decision to use these criteria must be individualized. Some patients not satisfying all of the above criteria (e.g., patients with chronic hypoxemia values below the thresholds cited) may be ready for attempts at the discontinuation of mechanical ventilation.

Recommendation 3: Formal discontinuation assessments for patients receiving mechanical ventilation for respiratory failure should be performed during spontaneous breathing rather than while the patient is still receiving substantial ventilatory support. An initial brief period of spontaneous breathing can be used to assess the capability of continuing onto a formal SBT. The criteria with which to assess patient tolerance during SBTs are the respiratory pattern, the adequacy of gas exchange, hemodynamic stability, and subjective comfort. The tolerance of SBTs lasting 30 to 120 minutes should prompt consideration for permanent ventilatory discontinuation.

Recommendation 4: The removal of the artificial airway from a patient who has successfully been discontinued from ventilatory support should be based on assessments of airway patency and the ability of the patient to protect the airway.

Recommendation 5: Patients receiving mechanical ventilation for respiratory failure who fail an SBT should have the cause for the failed SBT determined. Once reversible causes for failure are corrected, and if the patient still meets the criteria listed in Table 44-3, subsequent SBTs should be performed every 24 h.

Recommendation 6: Patients receiving mechanical ventilation for respiratory failure who fail an SBT should receive a stable, nonfatiguing, comfortable form of ventilatory support.

Recommendation 7: Anesthesia/sedation strategies and ventilatory management aimed at early extubation should be used in postsurgical patients.

Recommendation 8: Weaning/discontinuation protocols that are designed for nonphysician health care professionals (HCPs) should be developed and implemented by ICUs. Protocols aimed at optimizing sedation also should be developed and implemented.

Recommendation 9: Tracheotomy should be considered after an initial period of stabilization on the ventilator when it becomes apparent that the patient needs prolonged ventilatory assistance. Tracheotomy then should be performed when the patient appears likely to gain one or more of the benefits ascribed to the procedure. Patients who may derive particular benefit from early tracheotomy are the following:

- Those who need high levels of sedation to tolerate translaryngeal tubes;
- Those with marginal respiratory mechanics (often manifested as tachypnea) in whom a tracheostomy tube having lower resistance might reduce the risk of muscle overload;
- Those who may derive psychological benefit from the ability to eat orally, communicate by articulated speech, and experience enhanced mobility; and
- Those in whom enhanced mobility may assist physical therapy efforts.

Recommendation 10: Unless there is evidence for clearly irreversible disease (e.g., high spinal cord injury or advanced amyotrophic lateral sclerosis), a patient who needs prolonged mechanical ventilatory support for respiratory failure should not be considered permanently ventilator-dependent until 3 months of weaning attempts have failed.

Recommendation 11: Critical care practitioners should familiarize themselves with facilities in their communities, or units in hospitals they staff, that specialize in managing patients who need prolonged dependence on mechanical ventilation. Such familiarization should include reviewing published peer-reviewed data from those units, if available. When medically stable for transfer, patients who have failed ventilatory discontinuation attempts in the ICU should be transferred to those facilities that have demonstrated success and safety in accomplishing ventilator discontinuation.

Recommendation 12: Weaning strategies in the prolonged mechanical ventilation (PMV) patient should be slow-paced and should include gradually lengthening self-breathing trials.

From Chest 120:375S, 2001; Respir Care 47:69, 2002.

Box 44-11 • Weaning Protocol for a Spontaneous Breathing Trial With a T Tube

1. Verify that the patient is a candidate for ventilator discontinuation.
   a. Is there evidence of reversal or alleviation of the disease state or condition necessitating mechanical ventilatory support?
   b. Is the patient able to breathe spontaneously?
   c. Has the patient's medical condition been optimized (afebrile, adequate hemoglobin, acceptable electrolyte levels)?
   d. Are oxygenation, ventilation, and blood gas values adequate?
      - Pa_{O_2} ≥60 mm Hg with F_{IO_2} ≤0.40 to 0.50 with PEEP/CPAP ≤5 to 8 cm H_2O
      - Pa_{O_2}/F_{IO_2} >150 to 200 mm Hg
      - Pa_{CO_2} <50; pH >7.35
   e. Are other indices of readiness for spontaneous breathing positive?
      - f/V_T <105
      - f <30 and >6 breaths/min
      - V_T >5 mL/kg
      - MIP <–20 cm H_2O
      - VC >10 to 15 mL/kg
      - $\dot{V}_{Esp}$ <10 L/min
   f. Is the patient awake and alert, free of seizures, and able to follow instructions?
   g. Is there evidence of hemodynamic stability?
2. Prepare for T-tube trial.
   a. Adequate personnel present
   b. No other ongoing procedures or other major activities
   c. Eliminate or minimize respiratory depressants (sedatives/narcotics).
   d. Prepare equipment.
      - T tube, aerosol tubing, aerosol generator set at same F_{IO_2} as patient is receiving with the ventilator or 10% higher
      - Suction apparatus
      - Monitoring equipment (oximeter, ECG, respirometer, other)
   e. Suction airway as needed
   f. Sit patient up in bed, if possible.
3. Begin 3-minute screening T-tube trial and monitor patient for tolerance.
   a. Measure tidal volume and respiratory rate with a respirometer.
   b. Measure MIP three times in succession, selecting the best (most negative) value.
4. If at least two of the following three criteria are met, begin a formal SBT of up to 2 hours. If criteria are not met, return the patient to full ventilatory support.
   a. MIP <–20 cm H_2O
   b. V_{Tsp} >5 mL/kg
   c. f_{sp} <35 breaths/min
5. Continue to monitor the patient and return the patient to mechanical ventilatory support for 24 hours if any of the following signs of distress is present:
   a. f >35 breaths/min
   b. Sp_{O_2} <90% to 92%
   c. 20% increase or decrease in heart rate or heart rate >120 to 140 beats/min
   d. Systolic blood pressure >180 mm Hg or <90 mm Hg
   e. Agitation, diaphoresis, or anxiety
6. Continue the trial for at least 30 minutes but not more than 2 hours. If no signs of intolerance develop (see step 5), consider extubation.

Modified from Esteban A et al: N Engl J Med 332:345, 1995; Respir Care 47:69, 2002; Pierson DJ: Respir Care 28:646, 1983.

▶ NEWER TECHNIQUES

Mandatory Minute Volume Ventilation

Mandatory minute volume ventilation was developed by Hewlett, Platt, and Terry and introduced in 1977 in Great Britain.[43] This mode has since proliferated on newer mechanical ventilators. Mandatory minute volume ventilation is available on the Ohmeda CPU-1, Ohmeda Advent, Engstrom Erica, Bear 5, Bear 1000, Hamilton Veolar, and Drager Evita 4 ventilators.

During initial development, MMV was considered a novel approach to the problems associated with weaning patients from mechanical ventilation by means of traditional IMV.[43] Hewlett et al were concerned that traditional IMV did not ensure that patients would receive a constant level of ventilation during the weaning process in the presence of minute-to-minute changes in their ability to breathe spontaneously.[43] It was thought that a system providing a constant level of minute ventilation would allow patients whose ventilation was precarious to be safely maintained during the weaning process.[43] If at any time the patient's spontaneous ventilation decreased, the system would automatically increase the level of mechanical support. Conversely, patients who recovered the ability to breathe spontaneously would automatically move to lower and lower levels of mechanical support without alteration of specific ventilator settings. Mandatory minute volume ventilation was developed for implementation of such a system. Box 44-12 lists the advantages of MMV.

Hewlett warned that great care should be taken in the use of MMV in the care of patients whose spontaneous breathing is shallow and fast.[43] The typical physiological response to a declining ability to maintain adequate spontaneous alveolar ventilation, whether due to a decrease in lung or thoracic compliance or a decrease in ventilatory muscle strength, is an increase in spontan-

Box 44-12 • Advantages of Mandatory Minute Volume Ventilation

- For some patients, MMV should offer greater control over Pa_{CO_2} than does IMV alone.
- Acute hypoventilation or apnea should not result in sudden hypercapnia or resultant acute acidemia.
- The fear of acute hypoventilation after administration of sedatives, narcotics, or tranquilizers for pain, anxiety, or agitation is eliminated.
- Mandatory minute volume ventilation allows a smooth transition from mechanical support to spontaneous ventilation in the care of patients recovering from a drug overdose or anesthesia.

Modified from Shelledy DC, Mikles SP: Respir Manage 18:21, 1988.

eous rate and decrease in tidal volume. As spontaneous tidal volume declines and respiratory frequency increases, physiological dead space begins to assume a larger proportion of the total minute ventilation.

It is theoretically possible for a patient to meet the set MMV level with an effective alveolar ventilation of zero. This value could be achieved with very rapid spontaneous rates and a tidal volume at or near physiological dead space. In addition to the risk of acute hypoventilation, a spontaneous tidal volume less than 7 mL/kg without an intermittent deep breath may promote progressive collapse of alveoli.[43]

It is important to differentiate the methods by which the current generation of ventilators can be used to achieve a constant minute ventilation (MMV) with varying levels of spontaneous ventilation. The CPU-1, Advent, Engstrom Erica, Evita 4, Bear 5, and the Bear 1000 ventilators work in a similar manner.[43] These ventilators "compare" the level of the patients' spontaneous breathing with the desired MMV level and then increase, decrease, or maintain the frequency of mechanical breaths as indicated. The mechanical tidal volume is preset in each case.

The Hamilton Veolar system (Hamilton Medical, Reno, NV) takes a unique approach to maintaining a constant MMV level. Rather than increasing or decreasing the number of mechanical breaths to achieve a desired MMV, the Hamilton Veolar ventilator maintains a preset minute ventilation by automatically adjusting the level of pressure support.[43] As the level of pressure support is increased, the patient receives a larger and larger "spontaneous" breath at the same level of ventilatory work. This method should compensate for any tendency on the part of a patient to take shallow spontaneous tidal breaths. No "machine breaths" with a preset tidal volume are delivered to the patient in the MMV mode when the Hamilton Veolar system is used.

Whether MMV provides a smoother transition from mechanical ventilatory support to spontaneous breathing than other methods of weaning needs further substantiation. However, at least one prospective study[44] has shown that MMV can be safe and effective and has the potential to markedly accelerate weaning in some patient settings. Adaptive support ventilation, which was introduced with the Hamilton Galileo ventilator, also targets a minimum minute ventilation and thus might be considered to be a more sophisticated form of MMV (see later).

Adaptive Support Ventilation

Adaptive support ventilation is a newer mode of ventilation available on the Hamilton Galileo system that maintains a minimum minute ventilation with an optimal breathing pattern (tidal volume and rate).[45,46] Adaptive support ventilation automatically adjusts inspiratory pressure and ventilator rate breath by breath to achieve a target minute ventilation of 100 mL/kg ideal body weight per minute for adults and 200 mL/kg in pediatric patients at the 100% setting.

The ASV software incorporates algorithms designed to choose a target respiratory rate and tidal volume associated with the least WOB and based on the formula of Otis.[45,46] In the event of apnea, ASV provides time-triggered, pressure-control breaths that deliver a calculated tidal volume and a machine rate that maintains minute ventilation. As the patient begins to breathe spontaneously, patient-triggered breaths are pressure supported and volume targeted. Mandatory pressure control breaths continue to be given as needed to ensure an optimal respiratory rate. In theory at least, ASV automatically reduces ventilatory support as the patient's ability to breathe spontaneously improves, and this may facilitate weaning.

A preliminary study of ASV in the care of patients recovering from cardiac surgery showed a reduction in the duration of mechanical ventilation compared with the outcome with an SIMV weaning protocol.[46] The ASV weaning protocol used in the study incorporated two 50% reductions in minute ventilation. Each reduction was followed by an assessment of patient tolerance according to criteria similar to those suggested for SBTs.

Computer-Based Weaning

Current versions of MMV and ASV are examples of computer-controlled mechanical ventilation. Several more complex systems have been developed, including Ventilation Manager, VQ-attending, ESTER, Continuous Respiratory Evaluator (CORE), KUSIVAR, and WEAN-PRO.[14] The desire to develop computer-based weaning protocols is based on two factors. First, weaning is a time-consuming, labor-intensive process. If computer control can expedite or simplify this process, considerable time and money can be saved. Second, because most weaning decisions are based on objective data, computer-based weaning protocols are relatively easy to develop. In one study in which physician-directed weaning was compared with computer-based weaning, the computer-based system resulted in less-frequent assessment of ABGs and shorter wean times.[14] Unfortunately, computer-based systems have not been widely tested to date.[14]

Flow-By, Flow Trigger, Tracheal Pressure Sensing

Flow-by and flow trigger are newer additions to many modern mechanical ventilators. Flow-by typically involves setting an adjustable base flow through the ventilator circuit of 5 to 6 L/min and a flow sensitivity of 1 to 3 L/min, depending on the patient's body weight. Some ventilators have an automatic or preset base flow, and only the flow sensitivity is set.[9] In ventilators with an adjustable base flow, there is some evidence that higher base flow settings may actually increase trigger work in some patients.[9] The purpose of flow-by with flow triggering is to reduce the work associated with spontaneous breathing through a demand flow system in the SIMV, CPAP, or spontaneous mode.[9] Flow triggering also may reduce the work to trigger an SIMV or assist breath.[9,15]

Flow-by can be used in conjunction with pressure support on many newer ventilators. In theory, the combination of flow-by and pressure support allows the clinician to compensate completely for the WOB_I due to demand flow systems, the ventilator circuit, and the artificial airway.[9,15] Results of one study indicated that flow-by may be less expensive than T-tube weaning and just as effective.[47]

An alternative approach to reducing trigger work in ventilator patients has been the use of tracheal pressure sensing.[9] Unfortunately, practical problems with secretions and airway care have limited the value of this technique.[9]

Automatic Tube Compensation

Automatic tube compensation is an option on newer mechanical ventilators that compensates for the flow-dependent pressure decrease across the endotracheal tube during both inspiration and expiration. Automatic tube compensation reduces WOB and may improve patient comfort.[48] Because it compensates for the WOB_I due to the artificial airway, ATC has been referred to as "electronic extubation." Patients able to breathe adequately with the addition of ATC should tolerate extubation. Automatic tube compensation is similar to pressure support in that an inspiratory pressure is used to compensate for WOB_I; however, ATC varies the pressure depending on the size of the endotracheal tube and the patient's inspiratory flow rate. Pressure support ventilation, on the other hand, delivers a preset inspiratory pressure, which may overcompensate or undercompensate for WOB_I at any given point in time. Whether ATC facilitates weaning in terms of patient outcome is not known.

Volume Support and Volume-Assured Pressure Support

Volume support is a newer dual-control mode of ventilation available on the Siemens Servo 300 ventilator (Siemens-Elema, Solna, Sweden).[49] Volume support combines aspects of pressure support and volume ventilation by allowing a level of pressure support that is automatically adjusted to maintain a preset tidal volume.[49] In the volume-support mode, inspiration is initiated by patient trigger. During the inspiratory phase, the pressure level is regulated to a value based on the previous breath's pressure-volume calculation compared with a preset tidal volume and minute ventilation. The pressure-support level is automatically adjusted in a stepwise manner ±3 cm H_2O from one breath to the next to maintain the preset tidal volume.[49]

Inspiratory flow varies depending on the pressure support level, and a decelerating flow waveform is maintained. As in the pressure-support mode, inspiration is terminated when flow has decreased to 5% of the peak flow or after 80% of the set cycle time. Volume support may offer a sort of automatic weaning from pressure support similar to MMV as provided with the Hamilton Veolar ventilator. As the patient's spontaneous tidal volume improves, the level of pressure support is automatically reduced. The potential advantage of using volume support to speed weaning has not been documented in clinical trials.

Volume-assured pressure support (VAPS) is available on the Bird 8400ST system. Volume-assured pressure support is similar to volume support in that a minimum preset tidal volume is maintained by means of automatic adjustment of the ventilator. With VAPS, however, the flow characteristics of the ventilator are adjusted during the breath, thus it is ensured that every breath achieves a minimum desired tidal volume.

Proportional Assist Ventilation and Proportional Pressure Support

Proportional assist ventilation and PPS are newer modes of ventilation designed to normalize a patient's WOB in the face of increased resistance or decreased compliance.[50,51] Proportional assist ventilation and PPS provide partial ventilatory support in proportion to the patient's effort.[51] The greater the patient effort, the higher is the pressure generated by the ventilator. The goal of PAV and PPS is to allow patients to comfortably

Box 44-13 • Advantages and Limitations of NPPV

ADVANTAGES	LIMITATIONS
• Avoids endotracheal intubation and related complications	• Requires patient cooperation
• Preserves airway defense mechanisms	• Limits airway access and suctioning of secretions
• May reduce nosocomial pneumonia	• Causes mask discomfort and feeling of suffocation (face mask)
• Improves patient comfort	• Causes mask-related complications such as facial ulcer from mask pressure, eye irritation, rhinitis, dry nose
• Preserves speech and swallowing	• Causes aerophagia, increased risk of aspiration in the event of vomiting (face mask)
• Reduces the need for sedation	• Air leak, transient hypoxemia from accidental mask removal
• Allows intermittent application	
• May improve weaning outcome	

Modified from Sassoon CSH: Respir Care 40:282, 1995.

breathe as much as desired on the basis of their respiratory control centers. Proportional assist ventilation and PPS may better match patients' spontaneous breathing than does pressure support and may provide a more comfortable mode of ventilation. Whether PAV or PPS is useful in improving outcome in terms of discontinuing ventilatory support is not known.

Noninvasive Positive Pressure Ventilation

Noninvasive positive pressure ventilation by mask can be used to support ventilation without the use of an artificial airway.[29] The most commonly used form of NPPV is BiPAP (Respironics, Murrayville, PA) by nasal mask.[14] BiPAP is a form of bilevel airway pressure that combines aspects of pressure support and CPAP.[14] Noninvasive positive pressure ventilation by mask should be reserved for patients who are able to maintain a natural airway. Patient's at risk of obstruction or aspiration should not be considered for NPPV by mask.[29] Further, patients who are likely to be unsuccessful at weaning are not good candidates for NPPV.[29] Noninvasive positive pressure ventilation, however, can be useful as an alternative to reintubation in the care of patients who have been weaned and extubated and are now doing poorly.[29] Results of two small but sound studies have indicated that NPPV with pressure support (with or without CPAP) may improve mortality, decrease the incidence of nosocomial pneumonia, and reduce ICU stay by almost as much as 9 days.[6] Box 44-13 lists advantages and limitations of NPPV.

Other Techniques for Facilitating Weaning

Biofeedback, the use of standardized weaning protocols, care plans, and development of critical pathways have been shown to have potential for expediting weaning.[3,6,14] An example of a respiratory therapist–directed weaning protocol with SIMV is presented in Box 44-14. Inter-

Box 44-14 • Respiratory Therapist–Directed Weaning Protocol

- The physician's written order identifies the patient as eligible for the respiratory therapist (RT)-directed weaning protocol.
- Timing of weaning initiation is at the discretion of the nurse and RT.
- All patients must undergo continuous oxyhemoglobin saturation monitoring by pulse oximetry; the Spo_2 must be within 5% of that determined with ABG and pH analyses performed at admission and 4 hours later.
- Arterial blood gas samples drawn at the start of weaning must have a Pao_2 greater than 60 mm Hg and a $Paco_2$ less than 50 mm Hg on an Fio_2 less than 0.6 and a PEEP $\leq$ 5 cm H_2O.
- When the patient is awake, obeying simple commands, and in stable condition, the RT may reduce the breathing rate in the SIMV mode but no more than 6 breaths/min at one time and no more than 6 breaths/min in a single hour.
- The breathing rate is reduced, and a T tube is used for a minimum of 20 minutes before extubation if none of the following weaning failure conditions is present: Sao_2 less than 90%, Pao_2 less than 60 mm Hg, $Paco_2$ greater than 50 mm Hg, diaphoresis, spontaneous respiratory rate greater than 20 breaths/min, agitation or decreased level of consciousness, heart rate increase more than 20%, blood pressure change more than 20%, cardiac output reduction more than 30%, or ventricular arrhythmia.
- If the T-tube trial is well tolerated (ABG values are within prespecified limits) and the findings at the physician's examination are unremarkable, the order to extubate the patient is given.

Modified from Wood G, MacLeod B, Moffatt S: Respir Care 40:219, 1995.

disciplinary care teams and specialized weaning centers have been successful in treating difficult-to-wean ventilator patients.[14]

▶ SELECTING AN APPROACH

Current evidence suggests that for progressive weaning from mechanical support, it may be best to avoid IMV and SIMV.[6,10] It is wise, however, not to be dogmatic about the use of other modes.[10] It has been suggested, regardless of the mode of weaning used, that protocols administered by respiratory therapists and other health-care workers be developed.[3,6,10] These protocols should be designed to begin testing for the opportunity to reduce support very soon after intubation and to reduce the level of ventilatory support at every opportunity.[6] With respect to most methods of weaning, the effect of a particular method may be small compared with the effect of the criteria used for selecting patients for the reduction and discontinuation of support.[6] Noninvasive positive pressure ventilation may prove the exception to the rule, and further research is needed to determine whether the positive trends in reducing mortality and improving the complication rates observed with NPPV hold up under further examination.[6]

One large study showed that a once-daily SBT (T-tube trial) led to extubation about three times more quickly than did IMV and about twice as fast as PSV (Figure 44-2).[31] Results of another study favored PSV over T-tube trials or IMV (Figure 44-3).[40] Current recommendations suggest a single, daily trial of spontaneous breathing may be preferred to other methods of weaning. Results of randomized, controlled studies have shown SBTs to be faster than SIMV and at least as effective as PSV.[3,4,10] Further, performing a SBT one time per day is as effective as performing SBTs several times per day, and 30-minute trials were as effective as 120-minute trials in one study.[4]

There may be no one best weaning technique for all situations, and different patients may respond differently to different techniques.[8] Other factors may be more important than the weaning technique used.[6,8] These

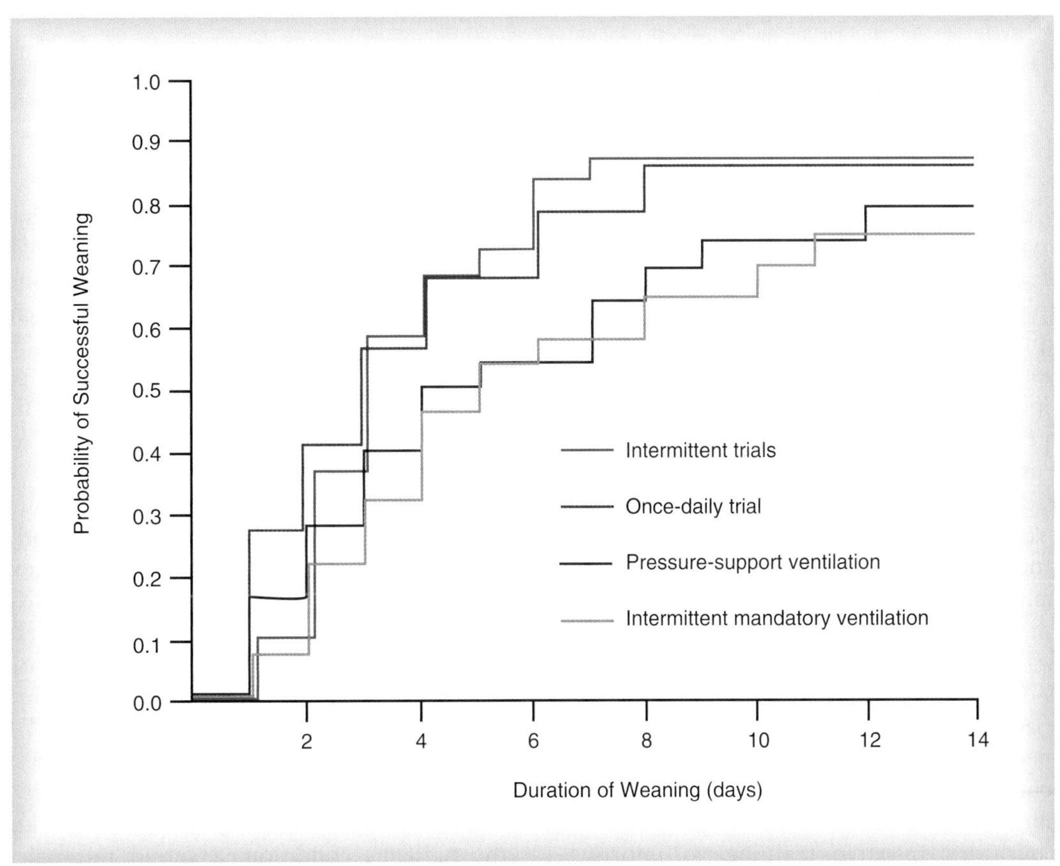

Figure 44-2
Kaplan-Meier curves of the probability of successful weaning with IMV, PSV, intermittent trials of spontaneous breathing, and a once-daily trial of spontaneous breathing. After adjustment for baseline characteristics, the rate of successful weaning with a once-daily trial of spontaneous breathing was 2.83 times higher than that with IMV ($P < .006$) and 2.05 times higher than that of pressure support ($P < .04$). *(Modified from Esteban A, Frutos F, Tobin MJ, et al: N Engl J Med 332:345, 1995.)*

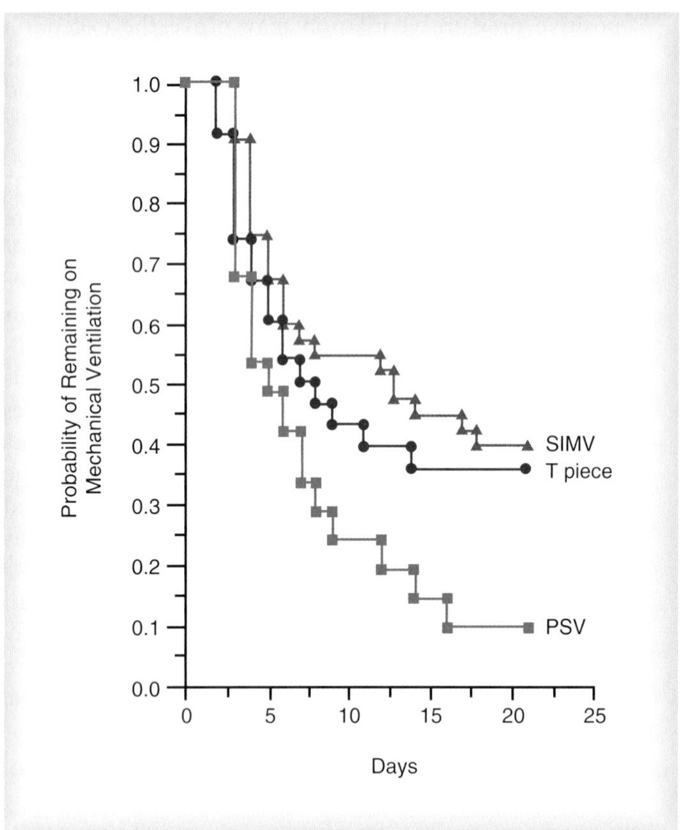

Figure 44-3
Probability of continuing mechanical ventilation in the care of patients with prolonged difficulties in tolerating spontaneous breathing. This probability was significantly lower for PSV than for T tube or SIMV (cumulative probability for 21 d, $P < .03$ with the log-rank test). *(Modified from Brochard L, Rauss A, Bentio S, et al: Am J Respir Crit Care Med 150:896, 1994.)*

include the clinical setting, reason for mechanical ventilation, type of patient, disease state or condition, and type of weaning protocol used.[8] For example, properly applied protocol weaning by a respiratory therapist can be more effective than physician-directed weaning in some circumstances.[52]

With traditional T-tube weaning and SBTs, full ventilatory support (usually assist control) is alternated with no support at all. For SIMV and PSV the level of support is gradually withdrawn, and the patient receives only partial ventilatory support.

One area needing additional research is the role of ventilatory muscle conditioning in patients with acute ventilatory failure. Endurance conditioning of the ventilatory muscles can be achieved by continuous repetition of low levels of ventilatory work.[39] Strength conditioning can be achieved by maximal ventilatory effort for shorter periods.[39] In theory, PSV would allow for improving ventilatory muscle endurance, whereas intermittent T-tube trials would favor developing muscle strength. Inspiratory resistive training to improve ventilatory muscle strength has been tried as an adjunct to weaning in the care of patients undergoing long-term ventilation.[14] The use of drugs (aminophylline) to enhance diaphragmatic strength has been explored.[14] Unfortunately, the role of ventilatory muscle rest and load in the care of difficult-to-wean patients has not been established.[14] Partial ventilatory support may prevent ventilatory muscle atrophy, decrease mean airway pressure, and decrease alveolar overdistension.[1,2] On the other hand, full ventilatory support may be the most appropriate approach in the care of patients with ventilatory muscle fatigue to allow the diaphragm to rest. Once fatigued, the ventilatory muscles may take 24 hours or more to recover.[14]

In summary, a single, daily T-tube trial lasting up to 2 hours has been recommended over more traditional approaches.[3,4] If the trial is successful, extubation is considered. If the trial is unsuccessful, at least 24 hours of full ventilatory support is provided before another trial is attempted.[3] There are advantages and disadvantages to each of the methods used to conduct ventilator patient weaning. Table 44-4 compares T tube, IMV, PSV, and MMV as weaning techniques. The best approach may be the one with which a given clinician is most familiar.[8] It should be based on knowledge of the patient's condition, a sound rationale, and good clinical experience.[2,8] The method chosen should include careful patient assessment, and the patient's condition should be optimized before weaning. A well-thought-out plan or protocol individualized to the patient should be used.

Table 44-4 ▶▶ Comparison of Available Weaning Methods

Method	Advantages	Disadvantages
T tube	Tests patient's true spontaneous ability Allows periods of work and rest Minimal WOB_I May allow strength conditioning of the ventilatory muscles Tests the patient's ability to breathe spontaneously early and often Ambient pressures used May be faster than IMV/SIMV A single, daily SBT may be as effective as multiple trials	More staff time Abrupt transition difficult for some patients No alarms Does not overcome resistance due to endotracheal tubes May overstress the patient, causing diaphragmatic fatigue Requires careful supervision
IMV/SIMV	Less staff time Gradual transition Easy to use Minimum minute ventilation guaranteed Sophisticated alarm systems may be used May be used in combination with PSV or CPAP	Patient-ventilator asynchrony Potentially high WOB May prolong weaning May worsen fatigue
PSV	Less staff time Gradual transition Reduced WOB (versus IMV/SIMV) Prevents fatigue Maintains activity of diaphragm Increased patient comfort Work level can be varied—may allow reconditioning of the diaphragm May be faster than IMV/SIMV Overcomes WOB_I due to • Endotracheal and tracheostomy tubes • Ventilator circuits • Demand flow systems Patient can control cycle length, rate, inspiratory flow Retains machine-patient synchrony or coupling Every breath is supported May help reintegrate coordination of the respiratory muscles Patient can increase supported rate as much as needed (IMV cannot) PSV defers reloading of the respiratory muscles until final stage of weaning	Backup ventilation uncertain Large changes in minute ventilation can occur Increased mean airway pressure (versus IMV or T tube) Tidal volume not guaranteed—low tidal volumes possible
MMV	Less staff time Maintains activity of diaphragm May be more efficient approach to weaning Backup ventilation assured Potential to speed weaning compared with IMV	May not assure efficient pattern of breathing Rapid, shallow breathing possible with MMV on the basis of machine rate

▶ MONITORING THE PATIENT DURING WEANING

Ventilatory Status

Respiratory rate and pattern are easy to monitor and may be the most reliable indicators of patient progress during weaning.[1,5] Weaning may proceed as quickly as the patient's respiratory rate and subjective tolerance allow.[1] In no case, however, should patients be overtired or pushed beyond their physiological limits. To do so may result in diaphragmatic fatigue and further delay the weaning process.[2,4,6] Dyspnea should be monitored during weaning and may be quantified with a visual analog scale or modified Borg scale (Table 44-5).[53] Onset or worsening of discomfort, sweating, signs of increased WOB (accessory muscle use, abdominal paradox), or change in mental status (agitation, anxiety, somnolence, coma) may be signs of intolerance of a weaning trial.[3]

It may be useful to monitor the patient's spontaneous minute ventilation and spontaneous tidal volume. Spontaneous tidal volume in the IMV mode can be estimated as follows:

$$V_{Tsp} = (\dot{V}_{ETOT} - \dot{V}_{Emach}) \div (f_{tot} - f_{mach})$$

where V_{Tsp} is the patient's average spontaneous tidal volume between machine breaths, $\dot{V}_{ETOT}$ is the total

Table 44-5 ▶▶ Modified Borg Scale for Dyspnea

Grade	Degree of Dyspnea
0	None
0.5	Very, very slight (just noticeable)
1	Very slight
2	Slight
3	Moderate
4	Somewhat severe
5	Severe
6	Very severe
7	
8	
9	Very, very severe (almost maximal)
10	Maximal

Modified from Mahler DA: Dyspnea, Mt Kisco, NY, 1990, Futura.

minute ventilation (machine + patient), $\dot{V}_{Emach}$ is the machine minute ventilation, f_{tot} is the total rate (machine + patient), and f_{mach} is the machine set rate. Machine minute ventilation ($\dot{V}_{Emach}$) can be estimated by multiplication of the delivered machine tidal volume V_{Imach} by the preset machine rate (f_{mach}).

The single best index of ventilation remains measurement of $PaCO_2$. Patients who appear to be doing poorly should have an ABG sample drawn before the weaning period is extended. An ABG study also is recommended to verify that a patient is doing well before extubation.

Results of capnography probably should not be used to guide weaning of patients with pulmonary parenchymal disease.[54] End-tidal PCO_2 values can be highly misleading as an estimate of effective ventilation in sick patients.[54] Gastric pH has been used as a predictor of patient status, and gastrointestinal acidosis may be an early sign of weaning failure.[55]

One final note with respect to monitoring ventilatory status during weaning: It has been recommended that the clinician be cautious early with SIMV and late with PSV.[2] It appears that the total work begins to approach that of spontaneous breathing when the SIMV rate is reduced to approximately one half of the full ventilatory support value. For PSV, on the other hand, WOB remains low until the pressure support level is markedly reduced.[2] Consequently, patients undergoing SIMV may have higher workloads early in the weaning process. Patients receiving PSV may have higher workloads late in the weaning process and should be monitored accordingly.[2] In one study, gradual reduction of PSV in increments of 5 cm H_2O did not facilitate recognition of impending ventilatory failure during weaning.[56] With any form of partial ventilatory support, patients should be monitored carefully.

MINI CLINI

Calculation of Spontaneous Tidal Volume in the IMV Mode

PROBLEM

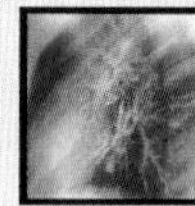

The following data have been collected about a patient being weaned in the IMV mode:

Time	8 AM	9 AM	10 AM	11 AM
Machine rate (f_{mach}) (breaths/min)	4	4	4	4
Total rate (f_{tot}) (breaths/min)	16	28	38	44
Machine tidal volume (V_{Tmach}) (mL)	800	800	800	800
Total minute ventilation ($\dot{V}_{ETOT}$) (L/min)	8	8	8.25	6

Calculate the patient's spontaneous rates and spontaneous tidal volumes for each time recorded.

SOLUTION

The patient's spontaneous rate is the total rate minus the machine rate ($f_{tot} - f_{mach}$). The patient's spontaneous tidal volume is as follows: $V_{Tsp} = (\dot{V}_{ETOT} - \dot{V}_{Emach}) \div (f_{tot} - f_{mach})$. Performing these calculations, we get the following:

Time	8 AM	9 AM	10 AM	11 AM
Patient's spontaneous rate	12	24	34	40
Patient's spontaneous tidal volume (mL)	400	200	150	70

From these data, we can see that although the total minute ventilation remained fairly stable at 6 to 8 L/min, there was a dramatic decrease in the patient's spontaneous tidal volume from 400 to 70 mL. The weaning process should have been reconsidered early in the process, probably at 9 or 10 AM.

Oxygenation

Continuous pulse oximetric (SpO_2) monitoring can provide a sensitive indicator of oxygenation status during weaning.[5] Arterial blood gas analysis for PaO_2, SaO_2, and calculation of the oxygen content of arterial blood (CaO_2) should be performed if doubt exists in assessing a patient's oxygenation status during weaning. Continuous monitoring of mixed venous oxygen saturation ($S\bar{v}O_2$) with a fiberoptic Swan-Ganz catheter has been shown to be helpful during weaning.[5]

Cardiovascular Status

Pulse, blood pressure, and cardiac rhythm should be monitored, and arrhythmias should be assessed to determine whether weaning should be continued.

Table 44-6 ▶▶ Changes During Withdrawal of Ventilatory Support

Expected Change	Deleterious Change
Respiratory	
Increased respiratory rate, up to 14 breaths/min	Respiratory rate ≥30 breaths/min
Stable $\dot{V}_E$	Large increase or decrease in $\dot{V}_E$
Spo_2 ≥90%	Decrease in Spo_2 to ≤85%-90%
5-10 mm Hg swing in Pao_2	Pao_2 <60 mm Hg
5-10 mm Hg swing in $Paco_2$	$Paco_2$ >50 mm Hg
pH >7.30 and <7.50	pH <7.30
Minimal use of accessory muscles	Increased use of accessory muscles
No paradoxical breathing	Paradoxical breathing
	Diaphoresis
	Dyspnea
Cardiovascular	
Heart rate increased 15-20 beats/min	Persistent tachycardia ≥120-140 beats/min
Blood pressure increased 10-15 mm Hg	Hypotension (blood pressure <90/60 mm Hg)
Increased cardiac index	Hypertension (systolic blood pressure >180 mm Hg)
Increased stroke volume	Decreased cardiac index
	Decreased stroke volume
	Angina
	New arrhythmias
	Increased pulmonary capillary wedge pressure
Other	
Mental status good (awake, alert, responsive)	Anxiety, agitation, somnolence, coma

Tachycardia, bradycardia, and abnormalities in blood pressure should be promptly evaluated and the patient returned to full ventilatory support, if indicated. Silent myocardial ischemia may occur frequently in some postoperative patients during weaning.[57] Table 44-6 summarizes changes that may occur during withdrawal of ventilatory support.

▶ EXTUBATION

Effects of Artificial Airways Related to Weaning

The presence of an artificial airway may increase airway resistance nearly threefold, although some evidence calls into question the assumption that breathing through an endotracheal tube offers a greater WOB than does breathing through a natural airway. In a study with 14 successfully extubated patients, at the end of a 2-hour SBT there was no difference in WOB before and after extubation.[58]

There is little difference in the airway resistance of healthy adults at low minute ventilation (8 L/min) whether the endotracheal tube is 7, 8, or 9 mm in internal diameter (ID).[59] Decreases in ID and increases in minute ventilation increase WOB. Adults have a critical increase in workload when the tube is narrower than 7 mm ID.[59] It is thought that the added work due to the presence of an artificial airway may contribute to ventilator dependency among patients with borderline pulmonary function or ventilatory muscle weakness.[59]

Endotracheal tubes themselves can cause reflex bronchoconstriction. Consequently, some experts believe routine use of bronchodilators is justified in the care of intubated patients. Dried secretions in the endotracheal tube can cause dramatic increases in airway resistance, especially in infants and children.[59] Care to provide adequate humidification can help avoid this problem.

Tracheotomy may substantially reduce the WOB of patients who need mechanical ventilatory support.[60] The short length of tracheotomy tubes results in an overall decrease in resistance compared with the resistance of an endotracheal tube, even though the curvature of the tracheotomy tube is greater.[3] It appears that performance of tracheotomy improves airway resistance and reduces the load of the ventilatory muscles. The clinical benefit of this improvement in terms of weaning has not been established.[3]

The dead space of an 8-mm ID tracheostomy tube is 6 to 8 mL, whereas the dead space of an 8-mm endotracheal tube is 12 to 15 mL.[59] The dead space of the natural upper airway is approximately 70 mL. Thus there is a small decrease in dead space in patients who are intubated. The role of an artificial airway in reducing anatomical dead space as it relates to weaning is not known.[59]

The important fact to remember is that the presence of an artificial airway may increase WOB. Pressure support ventilation can be very effective in overcoming this imposed work.[2] Table 44-7 lists the PSV level needed

Table 44-7 ▶▶ Pressure Support Level ($cm\ H_2O$) Necessary to Overcome the Imposed Work of Breathing of the Endotracheal Tube

	Minute Ventilation (L/min)		
Endotracheal Tube Size (mm)	**12**	**16**	**20**
6	11	17	47
7	5	8	20
8	5	5	9

Modified from Sharar SR: Respir Care 40:257, 1995.

to overcome the resistance of various endotracheal tubes at different minute ventilation values. Automatic tube compensation and PAV have been suggested as methods of reducing the WOB of spontaneously breathing patients.

Weaning and extubation should be separate decisions.[22] Weaning indices are not predictive of adequacy of airway patency or the need for protection of the airway in patients with neurologic, anatomical, or secretion problems.[22] The reintubation rate among patients with prolonged postoperative ventilation due to respiratory failure can range from 5% to 20%.[22]

Patients successfully extubated generally have (1) resolution of the disease state or condition, (2) hemodynamic stability, (3) absence of sepsis, (4) adequate oxygenation status with a decreased FIO_2 and decreased PEEP/CPAP, and (5) adequate ventilatory status and $PaCO_2$.[22] The decision to extubate should be based on assessment of adequate ventilatory function as predicted by standard weaning indices *and* assessment of upper airway patency and protection.[22] No one indicator is 100% sensitive and specific in prediction of successful extubation.[22] Practical guidelines for extubation are presented in Box 44-15. Regardless of the weaning technique used, a T-tube trial is recommended before extubation to ensure that the patient has an adequate ventilatory reserve.[2]

Some patients may be successfully extubated even if extubation criteria are not met.[22] If the patient is at risk, trained personnel able to perform reintubation must be immediately available before extubation is attempted.[22] At a minimum, those who perform the extubation must be prepared to provide an airway and ventilatory support in the event of problems immediately after extubation.[22] Extubation should be postponed when myocardial ischemia is present, the patient has upper gastrointestinal hemorrhaging, or a procedure that necessitates reintubation is impending. If difficult reintubation is anticipated, trained personnel should be immediately available, and a bronchoscope and needle cricothyrotomy supplies should be placed at the bedside.[22]

Box 44-15 • Practical Guidelines for Extubation

- No immediate need for mechanical ventilation or intubation
  - The medical course does not suggest impending respiratory failure or other indications for mechanical ventilation.
  - Procedures necessitating intubation and general anesthesia are not immediately planned.
- Achievement of adequate oxygenation and ventilation with spontaneous ventilation
  - The patient's FIO_2 requirement can be achieved with a mask or nasal cannula.
  - The patient no longer needs mechanical ventilatory assistance.
  - Weaning values are positive.
- Minimal risk of upper airway obstruction
  - The patient has minimal edema or mass encroachment of the oropharynx and upper airway; oral and upper airway anatomy is otherwise normal.
  - The result of a "cuff-leak" test is positive.
- Adequate airway protection and minimal risk of aspiration
  - Level of consciousness and neuromuscular function allows gag reflex and adequate cough.
  - Gastric contents are minimized by discontinuation of tube feedings for 4 to 6 hours before extubation.
  - A positive gag reflex is helpful.
- Adequate clearance of pulmonary secretions
  - Level of consciousness and muscular strength allow effective cough.
  - Secretion volume and thickness are not worsening.

Modified from Sharar SS: Respir Care 40:239, 1995.

Many patients report hoarseness and sore throat after extubation. Patients should be advised that these symptoms may occur. Other common problems following extubation include airway obstruction, increased risk of aspiration, and difficulty with secretion clearance.[22] Patients with neurologic or neuromuscular disorders and those with excessive secretions are at increased risk after extubation.[22] Compression of the airway due to traumatic or postoperative hematoma of the neck, infectious masses or abscesses, and malignant tumors or compression after major head or neck surgery can lead to upper airway obstruction after extubation.[22] The cuff leak test is recommended to detect airway obstruction before extubation. The test has 100% sensitivity and 70% specificity among healthy adults.[22] Box 44-16 describes the cuff leak test.

After extubation, glottic edema can result in partial airway obstruction, which can cause mild to severe stridor.[22] Postextubation stridor should be viewed with concern. Severe edema following extubation can lead to complete airway obstruction.[22] Children, patients with

Box 44-16 • Cuff Leak Test

1. Assess the patient to ensure that he or she can breathe spontaneously off the ventilator.
2. Suction the mouth and upper airway.
3. Deflate the cuff.
4. Briefly occlude the endotracheal tube.
5. If the patient is unable to breathe around the occluded endotracheal tube with the cuff deflated, suspect laryngeal edema.

Modified from Sharar S: Respir Care 40:239, 1995.

epiglottitis or angioedema (dermal, subcutaneous, or submucosal edema of the face or larynx), and patients who have sustained smoke inhalation are at greater risk.[22] Postextubation edema occurs in as many as 47% of children suffering from trauma or burns.[22]

Management of postextubation stridor includes the use of a cool aerosol with supplemental oxygen by mask. Nebulized racemic epinephrine (0.5 mL 2.25% epinephrine in 3 mL normal saline solution)[22,26] or dexamethasone (1 mg in 4 mL normal saline solution) by nebulizer has been recommended.[26] Helium-oxygen mixtures (60% helium, 40% oxygen) by nonrebreathing mask may be helpful in decreasing the severity of stridor and reducing the need for reintubation.[22]

Patients are at special risk of postextubation aspiration if they have an impaired cough or gag reflex.[22] Periglottic sensation is reduced for 4 to 8 hours after extubation in patients who have been intubated for more than 8 hours. Glottic function may be impaired in as many as 28% of patients who have been intubated for longer than 6 days.[22] After extubation, patients may have a reduced cough and impaired lower airway protection.[22] Marginal muscle strength (MIP > 33 cm H_2O) has been associated with increased risk of aspiration.[22] Withholding feeding 4 to 6 hours before extubation and clamping feeding tubes may be prudent.[22]

▶ FAILURE

As many as 25% of patients who have been removed from ventilatory support experience respiratory distress severe enough to necessitate reinstitution of mechanical ventilation.[4] In patients unlikely to be successfully weaned, rapid, shallow breathing begins almost immediately after the ventilator is disconnected.[4] As spontaneous breathing continues, respiratory mechanics worsen in these patients for reasons that are not clearly understood.[4] Approximately one half of patients who have poor results after discontinuation of ventilation experience marked hypercapnia due to rapid, shallow breathing.[4] An unsuccessful SBT also causes considerable cardiovascular stress.[4] Myocardial ischemia may occur frequently among ventilator-dependent patients and has been associated with weaning failure.[61] Critical illness polyneuropathy has been cited as a frequent cause of neuromuscular weaning failure among critically ill patients.[14,62] Unsuspected neuromuscular disease may be an important factor in ventilator dependency.[14]

Box 44-17 • Common Causes of Weaning Failure

OXYGENATION PROBLEMS
- Decreased $\dot{V}/\dot{Q}$ (asthma, emphysema, chronic bronchitis, bronchospasm)
- Increased shunt (atelectasis, pneumonia, ARDS, pulmonary edema)
- Low oxygen content of mixed venous blood ($C\bar{v}O_2$) caused by increased O_2ER ($\downarrow \dot{Q}t$, $\uparrow \dot{V}O_2$)

VENTILATION PROBLEMS
- Central hypoventilation (neurologic injury, drugs)
- Impaired neuromuscular function
- Increased dead space (embolism, ARDS, emphysema)
- Increased carbon dioxide production ($\uparrow \dot{V}CO_2$, carbohydrate overfeeding, fever)

CARDIOVASCULAR PROBLEMS
- Left ventricular failure
- Hemodynamic instability

Modified from Marini J: Respir Care 40:233, 1995; Sharar S: Respir Care 40:239, 1995.

Inability to wean can sometimes be attributed to psychologic dependence, poor oxygenation status, or cardiovascular instability (congestive heart failure or ischemia).[2] However, the most common cause of inability to wean is an imbalance between ventilatory capability and ventilatory demand.[2] Inability to wean usually is caused by a concurrent pathological process that necessitates treatment.[2,3] Common causes of weaning failure are summarized in Box 44-17.

▶ CHRONICALLY VENTILATOR-DEPENDENT PATIENTS

Chronically ventilator-dependent patients present ethical, economic, and practical problems. From an economic point of view, long-term care of ventilator-dependent patients in an ICU is prohibitively expensive. Often, patients are transferred to subacute or long-term care facilities. In cases in which the family has adequate resources, the patient may be cared for in the home.

Table 44-8 ▶▶ Management of Problems Among Difficult-to-Wean Patients

Problem	Management Strategy
Anemia	Transfuse when hemoglobin level is ≤10 g/dL and hematocrit ≤30% if thought to be a factor in decreased tissue oxygenation.
Increased work of breathing	1. Tube-related a. Apply pressure support or ATC. b. Change size of small endotracheal tube. c. Cut length of endotracheal tube if 2 in (5 cm) past mouth. d. Deflate cuff if all breathing is spontaneous and risk of aspiration is minimal. e. Consider tracheotomy. 2. Secretion related (see later) 3. Bronchospasm related a. Administer bronchodilators • β_2-agonists with a nebulizer • Anticholinergics • Steroids • Methylxanthines b. Apply CPAP to reduce auto-PEEP. c. Manage cause. 4. Ventilator related a. Assure synchrony for machine breaths. b. Eliminate auto-PEEP. c. Use flow-by or flow trigger with or without pressure support.
Secretions, atelectasis, plugging	1. Systemically hydrate 2. Provide extra humidity (increase humidifier temperature to 35° C-37° C at airway connection) 3. Maximally bronchodilate when necessary. 4. Perform coughing exercises. 5. Perform chest physiotherapy. 6. Suction.
Dyspnea	1. Use positioning (out of bed, dangling, leaning forward). 2. Reassure and communicate with the patient. 3. Provide periodic bag insufflation while the patient is off the ventilator. 4. Increase endurance. a. Alternate weaning with rest to promote endurance. b. Consider providing inspiratory resistive training. 5. Provide distraction.
Malposition	1. Position to maximize diaphragmatic excursion and improve lung volume and gas exchange (sitting or dangling). 2. Use rocking chair. 3. Follow $\dot{V}_E$, V_T, rate, MIP, MVV, ABG values for optimum position.
Respiratory muscle fatigue	1. Direct management at cause. 2. Assure adequate oxygen transport and cardiac output. 3. Nourish patient. 4. Replace depleted electrolytes. 5. Decrease WOB. a. Administer supplemental oxygen. b. Clear secretions. c. Decrease airway resistance. d. Use mechanical ventilation to rest fatigued muscles; then rotate weaning and rest.
Hemodynamic and fluid problems	1. Administer volume replacement and drugs to increase contractility, increase or decrease preload, and decrease afterload. 2. Delay weaning until cardiovascular status is stable. 3. Use techniques and mode of ventilation to decrease mean airway pressure.
Infection	1. Identify potential sites of infection. 2. Remove lines early or replace periodically. 3. Control infection. 4. Wash hands and use gloves. 5. Nourish patient.
Metabolic problems	1. Control cause and postpone weaning if the patient has acidosis. 2. Keep carbon dioxide at baseline level if patient has COPD, or allow progressive renal compensation during long-term weaning. 3. Provide moderate carbohydrate loading with total parenteral nutrition.
Low magnesium level	4. Give supplements.

Table 44-8 ▶▶ Management of Problems Among Difficult-to-Wean Patients—cont'd

Problem	Management Strategy
High magnesium level	5. Provide dialysis or calcium chloride.
Low calcium level	6. Control cause before weaning.
Low phosphate level	7. Replace phosphate before weaning.
Nutrition	1. Assess weight, albumin, and total lymphocyte count at admission. 2. Label degree of malnutrition and calculate protein needs. 3. Nourish patient.
Exercise	1. Provide exercise therapy to increase muscle function, prevent contracture, and maintain joint integrity (passive-to-active range of motion and sitting to walking). 2. Increase strength during activities of daily living. 3. Secure physiotherapy consultation. 4. Consider use of exercise bicycle. 5. Encourage wheelchair rides or walks with portable ventilator. 6. Provide breathing retraining.
Psychological problems	1. Secure early psychiatric consultation. 2. Allow patient control. 3. Demonstrate staff accountability and honesty. 4. Provide communication method. 5. Decrease environmental stress. 6. Teach relaxation methods. 7. Provide mental stimulation. 8. Provide recreation. 9. Provide rewards for reaching short-term goals. 10. Encourage self-care. 11. Allow other patients to visit. 12. Provide flexible visiting hours. 13. Take patient out of ICU environment.
Sleep disturbances	1. Provide quiet environment (dim lights), reposition patient, give back rub, and administer sedation. 2. Provide for uninterrupted sleep. 3. Avoid weaning at night. 4. Provide relaxation method (hypnosis, biofeedback, progressive muscle relaxation). 5. Prescribe short-acting sedative hypnotics.
Pain	Administer minimal analgesia.

Modified from Norton LC, Neureuter A: Crit Care Nurse 9:42, 1989.

Regional weaning centers have been developed and have reported success in weaning most patients undergoing long-term mechanical ventilation.[3,11,12] Current guidelines suggest that unless there is clear evidence of an irreversible cause of ventilator dependency, such as a high spinal cord injury or amyotrophic lateral sclerosis, patients should not be considered permanently ventilator dependent until 3 months of weaning attempts have failed.[3] If the patient is unweanable, the goal should be to restore the patient to the highest level of independent function possible.[11] For example, portable, wheelchair-mounted ventilators have been effective in providing a surprising level of mobility and independence to persons quadriplegic owing to high cervical spinal injury. Table 44-8 describes the management of common problems among difficult-to-wean patients. Box 44-18 lists the goals of weaning of patients receiving long-term ventilation.

Box 44-18 • Goals for Weaning After Long-Term Mechanical Ventilation

- Reduce amount of support.
- Decrease invasiveness of support.
- Increase independence from mechanical devices.
- Preserve function.
- Maintain medical stability.

From Pierson DJ: Respir Care 40:289, 1995.

▶ TERMINAL WEANING

The term *terminal weaning* has been used to refer to the discontinuation of mechanical ventilatory support in the face of a catastrophic and irreversible illness.[63] The decision to proceed with disconnecting the ventilator when such an act is likely to cause the death of a patient is fraught with ethical, emotional, and practical problems. The decision should be made by the family in consultation with the patient's physician and in accordance with established ethical and legal guidelines.[63] Once the decision has been made, the process is generally one of ventilator disconnection rather than weaning. The respiratory therapist would be wise to allow the attending physician to perform the physical disconnection of the patient from the ventilator. The method of terminal weaning should be as humane and comfortable as possible and should not be done in a way that further burdens the family.[63]

KEY POINTS

- The most common cause of ventilator dependence is a ventilatory workload that exceeds the patient's ventilatory capabilities.
- Other common causes of ventilator dependence include oxygenation problems, cardiovascular instability, and psychological factors.
- The most important criterion in determining whether a patient is ready for ventilator discontinuation or weaning is significant improvement or reversal of the disease state or condition that caused the patient to need the ventilator in the first place.
- Traditional weaning criteria include a spontaneous respiratory rate less than 30 breaths/min, tidal volume greater than 5 mL/kg, vital capacity greater than 10 to 15 mL/kg, MIP less than –20 to –30 cm H_2O, minute ventilation less than 10 L/min, and an MVV more than twice minute ventilation.
- Newer weaning indices associated with patient success include f/V_T less than 105 and $P_{0.1}$/MIP less than 0.30.
- Factors that should be optimized before weaning include oxygenation, ventilation, acid-base balance and electrolyte levels, cardiovascular status, kidney function and fluid balance, sleep deprivation, psychological status, nutrition, and overall medical condition.
- Weaning techniques include use of a T tube alternating with full ventilatory support, SIMV, PSV, and a single, daily SBT.
- Spontaneous breathing trials or PSV may result in faster discontinuation of ventilatory support than does SIMV.

KEY POINTS—cont'd

- Monitoring of the patient during weaning should include physical assessment, respiratory rate and pattern, presence of dyspnea, pulse oximetry, use of a cardiac monitor for rhythm and rate, and blood pressure, as indicated.
- Before extubation, patients should be assessed for the ability to maintain and protect the natural airway and for the presence of upper airway edema, if suspected.
- Common causes of weaning failure include an excessive ventilatory workload in the presence of ventilatory muscle weakness or fatigue, oxygenation problems, cardiovascular instability, psychological dependence, and the presence of an underlying concurrent pathological condition necessitating treatment.
- Goals of weaning of long-term ventilator-dependent patients include reducing the amount of support, reducing the invasiveness of support, and increasing the patient's level of independent function.

References

1. MacIntyre N: Respiratory factors in weaning from mechanical ventilatory support, Resp Care 40:244, 1995.
2. Marini J: Weaning techniques and protocols, Resp Care 40:233, 1995.
3. Evidence-based guidelines for weaning and discontinuing ventilator support: a collective task force facilitated by the American College of Chest Physicians, the American Association for Respiratory Care, and the American College of Critical Care Medicine, Chest 120:375S, 2001.
4. Tobin M: Medical progress: advances in mechanical ventilation, N Engl J Med 344:1986,2001.
5. Clement JM, Buck EA: Weaning from mechanical ventilatory support, Dimens Crit Care Nurs 15:114, 1996.
6. Criteria for weaning from mechanical ventilation, evidence report/technology assessment no. 23, (AHRQ publication no. 01-E010), Rockville, MD, 2000, Agency for Healthcare Research and Quality.
7. American College of Chest Physicians: ACCP consensus conference: mechanical ventilation, Chest 104:1833, 1993.
8. Pierson DJ: Weaning from mechanical ventilation: why all the confusion? Resp Care 40:228, 1995.
9. Sassoon CSH, Machutte CK: What you need to know about the ventilator in weaning, Resp Care 40:249, 1995.
10. Meade MO, Guyalt H, Cook DJ: Weaning from mechanical ventilation: the evidence from clinical research, Resp Care 46:1408, 2001.

11. Pierson DJ: Long-term mechanical ventilation and weaning, Resp Care 40:289, 1995.
12. Pierson DJ: Nonrespiratory aspects of weaning from mechanical ventilation, Resp Care 40:263, 1995.
13. Marini JJ: The physiologic determinants of ventilator dependence, Respir Care 31:271, 1986.
14. Burns SM et al: Weaning from long-term mechanical ventilation, Am J Crit Care 4:4, 1995.
15. Goodnough Hanneman SK et al: Weaning from short term mechanical ventilation: a review, Am J Crit Care 3:421, 1994.
16. Yang KL: Reproducibility of weaning parameters: a need for specialization, Chest 102:1642, 1992.
17. Yang KL, Tobin MJ: A prospective study of indexes predicting the outcome of trials of weaning from mechanical ventilation, N Engl J Med 324:1445, 1991.
18. DeHaven CB et al: Breathing measurement reduces false-negative classification of tachypneic preextubation trial failures, Crit Care Med 24:976, 1996.
19. Pardee NE, Winterbauer RH, Allen JD: Bedside evaluation of respiratory distress, Chest 85:203, 1984.
20. Krieger BP, Isber J, Breitenbucher A, et al: Serial measurements of the rapid-shallow breathing index as a predictor of weaning outcome in elderly medical patients, Chest 112:1029, 1997.
21. Gandia F, Blanco J: Evaluation of indexes predicting outcome of ventilator weaning and value of adding supplemental inspiratory load, Intensive Care Med 18:327, 1992.
22. Sharar S: Weaning and extubation are not the same, Resp Care 40:239, 1995.
23. Levy MM, Miyasaki A, Langston D: Work of breathing as a weaning parameter in mechanically ventilated patients, Chest 109:1408, 1996.
24. Shikora PA, Benotti PN, Johannigman JA: The oxygen cost of breathing may predict weaning from mechanical ventilation better than respiratory rate to tidal volume ratio, Arch Surg 129:269, 1994.
25. Truwit J: Lung mechanics. In Dantzker DR, MacIntyre NR, Bakow ED, editors: Comprehensive respiratory care, Philadelphia, 1995, WB Saunders.
26. Kacmarek RM, Mack CW, Dimus S: Essentials of respiratory care, ed 3, St Louis, 1990, Mosby.
27. Bassili HR, Deitel M: Effect of nutritional support on weaning patients off mechanical ventilators, JPEN J Parenter Enteral Nutr 5:161, 1981.
28. Hess DR: Mechanical ventilation of the adult patient: initiation, management and weaning. In Burton GG, Hodgkin JE, Ward JJ, editors, Respiratory care: a guide to clinical practice, Philadelphia, 1997, Lippincott Williams & Wilkins.
29. Sassoon CSH: Noninvasive positive-pressure ventilation in acute respiratory failure: review of reported experience with special attention to use during weaning, Resp Care 40:282, 1995.
30. MacIntyre NR: Psychological factors in weaning from mechanical ventilatory support, Resp Care 40:277, 1995.
31. Esteban A, Frutos F, Tobin MJ, et al: A comparison of four methods of weaning patients from mechanical ventilation, N Engl J Med 332:345, 1995.
32. Peterson W et al: Two methods of weaning persons with quadriplegia from mechanical ventilation, Paraplegia 32:98, 1994.
33. Baily CR, Jones RM, Kelleher AA: The role of continuous positive airway pressure during weaning from mechanical ventilation in cardiac surgical patients, Anaesthesia 50:677, 1995.
34. Schachter EN, Tucker D, Beck GJ: Does intermittent mandatory ventilation accelerate weaning? JAMA 256:1210, 1981.
35. Esteban A et al: How is mechanical ventilation employed in the intensive care unit? An international utilization review, Am J Respir Crit Care Med 2000;161:1450,
36. Groeger JS, Levinson MR, Carlon GC: Assist control versus synchronized intermittent mandatory ventilation during acute respiratory failure, Crit Care Med 17:607, 1989.
37. Prakash O, Meij SH: Oxygen consumption and blood gas exchange during controlled and intermittent mandatory ventilation after cardiac surgery, Crit Care Med 13:556, 1985.
38. Savino JA et al: The metabolic cost of breathing in critical surgical patients, J Trauma 25:1126, 1985.
39. Shelledy DC, Mikles SP: Newer modes of mechanical ventilation, I: pressure support, Resp Manage 18:14, 1988.
40. Brochard L et al: Comparison of three methods of gradual withdrawal from ventilatory support during weaning from mechanical ventilation, Am J Respir Crit Care Med 150:896, 1994.
41. Shikora SA et al: Could the oxygen cost of breathing be used to optimize the application of pressure support? J Trauma 33:521, 1992.
42. Jounieaux V, Duran A, Levi-Valensi P: Synchronized intermittent mandatory ventilation with and without pressure support ventilation in weaning patients with COPD from mechanical ventilation, Chest 105:1204, 1994.
43. Shelledy DC, Mikles SP: Newer modes of mechanical ventilation: mandatory minute volume ventilation, II. Respir Manage 18:21, 1988.
44. Davis S, Potgieter PD, Linton DM: Mandatory minute volume weaning in patients with pulmonary pathology, Anaesth Intensive Care 17:170, 1989.
45. Campbell RS, Branson RD, Johannigman JA: Adaptive support ventilation, Respir Care Clin N Am 7:425, 2001.
46. Sulzer CF, Chiolero R, Chassot P, et al: Adaptive support ventilation for fast tracheal extubation after cardiac surgery: a randomized controlled study. Anesthesiology 95:1339, 2001.
47. Herschman Z et al: A comparison of the Puritan-Bennett 7200 a ventilator's flow-by mode to the T-piece mode prior to extubation in postsurgical patients, Resp Care 36:1119, 1991.
48. Guttmann J, Haberthur C, Mols G: Automatic tube compensation, Respir Care Clin N Am 7:475, 2001.
49. Shelledy DC, Lawson RW, Drumheller OJ: A comparison of the ventilatory efficiency of assisted ventilation with fixed inspiratory flow rates to volume supported ventilation with variable inspiratory flow, Resp Care 41:954, 1996.

50. Zarske R, Doring M: ATS and PPS: breathing support with optimum patient comfort, Lubeck, Germany, •, Drager Medizintechnik.
51. Grasso S, Ranieri VM: Proportional assist ventilation, Respir Care Clin N Am 7:465, 2001.
52. Wood G, MacLeod B, Moffatt S: Weaning from mechanical ventilation: physician-directed vs a respiratory-therapist-directed protocol, Resp Care 40:219, 1995.
53. Marini JJ: Dyspnea during weaning, Resp Care 40:271, 1995.
54. Morley TF et al: Use of capnography for assessment of the adequacy of alveolar ventilation during weaning, Am Rev Respir Dis 148:339, 1993.
55. Mohsenifar Z et al: Gastric intramural pH as a predictor of success or failure in weaning patients from mechanical ventilation, Ann Intern Med 119:794, 1993.
56. Stroetz RW, Hubmayr RD: Tidal volume maintenance during weaning with pressure support, Am J Respir Crit Care Med 152:1034, 1995.
57. Abalos A et al: Myocardial ischemia during the weaning period, Am J Crit Care 1:32, 1992.
58. Straus C et al: Contribution of the endotracheal tube and the upper airway to breathing workload, Am J Respir Crit Care Med 157:23, 1998.
59. Sharar S: The effects of artificial airways on airflow and ventilatory mechanics: basic concepts and clinical relevance, Resp Care 40:257, 1995.
60. Diehl J et al: Changes in the work of breathing induced by tracheotomy in ventilatory-dependent patients, Am J Respir Crit Care Med 159:383, 1999.
61. Hurford WE, Favorito F: Association of myocardial ischemia with failure to wean from mechanical ventilation, Crit Care Med 23:1475, 1995.
62. Hund EI et al: Critical illness polyneuropathy: clinical findings and outcomes of a frequent cause of neuromuscular weaning failure, Crit Care Med 24:1282, 1996.
63. Shekleton ME et al: Terminal weaning from mechanical ventilation: a review, AACN Clin Issues Crit Care Nurs 5:523, 1994.

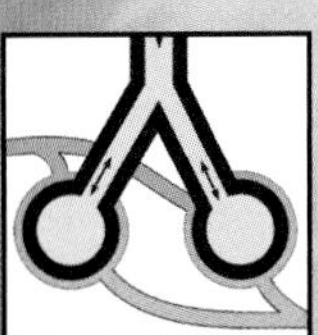

CHAPTER 45

Neonatal and Pediatric Respiratory Care

John Thompson, Cynthia Malinowski, and Barbara G. Wilson

In This Chapter You Will Learn:

- How to assess the fetus and newborn infant
- What maternal and fetal factors are associated with adverse outcomes
- How to apply respiratory care modalities to infants and children

Chapter Outline

Key Terms

ECMO
high-frequency ventilation
newborn/pediatric respiratory care
neutral thermal environment
sudden infant death syndrome

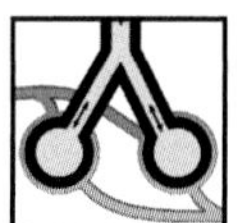

Caring for infants and children is one of the most challenging and rewarding aspects of respiratory care. Competent clinical practice in this area requires knowledge of the many pathophysiological differences among infants, children, and adults. Understanding the unique pathophysiology involved in neonatal and pediatric respiratory disorders (see Chapter 28) can assist the respiratory therapist in providing quality care to this patient population. A thorough understanding of how the respiratory system develops in the fetus is the first step towards acquiring the specialized knowledge needed to practice neonatal respiratory care (see Chapter 7). This chapter begins with an overview of neonatal patient assessment and then describes respiratory care modalities used to treat these patients.

▶ ASSESSMENT OF THE NEWBORN

Ideally, assessment of the newborn infant begins before birth. Consideration should be given to the maternal history and condition and the fetal and newborn status.

Maternal Factors

Maternal health and individual physiology, pregnancy complications, and maternal behaviors affect the health of the fetus. Any condition that leads to interference with placental blood flow or the transfer of oxygen to the fetus can cause an adverse outcome. The clinician must be prepared for the possibility of resuscitation at delivery. This is best anticipated by identifying risk factors that relate to neonatal compromise. Table 45-1 lists maternal conditions and specific anticipated fetal or neonatal outcomes related to the conditions.

Fetal Assessment

Fetal assessment is performed with ultrasonography, amniocentesis, fetal heart rate monitoring, and fetal blood gas analysis. Ultrasonography uses high-frequency sound waves to obtain a picture of the infant in utero. This allows the physician to: (1) view the position of the fetus and placenta, (2) measure fetal growth, (3) identify possible anatomical anomalies, and (4) qualitatively assess the amniotic fluid.

Amniocentesis involves direct sampling and quantitative assessment of amniotic fluid. Amniotic fluid may be inspected for meconium (fetal bowel contents) or blood. In addition, sloughed fetal cells can be analyzed for genetic normality. Lung maturation can be assessed with amniocentesis. The lethicin to sphingomyelin ratio (L/S ratio) involves measurement of two phospholipids, lethicin and sphingomyelin, synthesized by the fetus in utero. As shown in Figure 45-1, the L/S ratio rises with increasing gestational age. At approximately 34 to 35 weeks' gestation, this ratio abruptly rises above 2:1. An L/S ratio greater than 2:1 indicates stable surfactant production and mature lungs. Phosphatidylglycerol (PG) is another lipid found in the amniotic fluid that is used to assess fetal lung maturity. PG first appears at approximately 35 to 36 weeks' gestation. If the PG is more than 1% of the total phospholipids, then the risk of respiratory distress syndrome is less than 1%.

Fetal heart rate monitoring involves measurement of fetal heart rate and uterine contractions during labor. Examination of fetal heart rate changes related to uterine contractions identifies the fetus in distress. Fetal well-being is obtained by examining the variability and reactivity of the fetal heart rate. A normal fetal heart rate ranges between 120 to 160 beats/minute. Fetal tachycardia can be a sign of fetal hypoxemia, or could be related to more benign factors, such as prematurity or

Table 45-1 ▶ ▶ Maternal Condition and Neonatal Outcomes

Maternal Condition	Fetal or Neonatal Outcome
Previous pregnancy complication	Same outcome as previous fetus
Diabetes mellitus	LGA, congenital malformations, RDS, hypoglycemia
Pregnancy induced hypertension	Prematurity, SGA (preeclampsia)
Maternal age <17 years	Low birthweight, prematurity
Maternal age >35 years	Prematurity, chromosomal defects
Placenta previa	Prematurity, bleeding, SGA
Placenta abruptio	Fetal asphyxia, bleeding
Alcohol consumption	SGA, CNS dysfunction, mental retardation, facial dysmorphology
Smoking	SGA, prematurity, mental retardation, SIDS
Drug use	Placental abruption, IUGR, prematurity, CNS abnormalities, withdrawal disorders

IUGR, intrauterine growth retardation; *LGA*, large for gestational age; *RDS*, respiratory distress syndrome; *SGA*, small for gestational age; *SIDS*, sudden infant death syndrome.

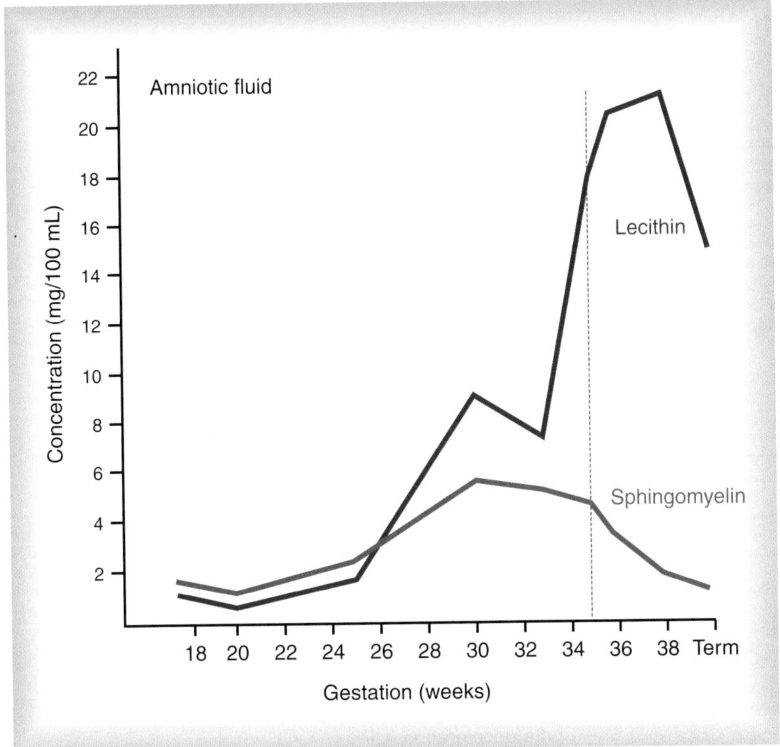

Figure 45-1
Lecithin *(broken line)* and sphingomyelin *(solid line)* concentrations plotted against gestational age. L/S ratio rises to 1.2 at 28 weeks and to 2 or more at 35 weeks, indicating maturation of the fetal lung. *(Modified from Gluck L et al: Am J Obstet Gynecol 109:440, 1971.)*

maternal fever. Temporary drops in fetal heart rate are called decelerations and can be mild (<15 beats/minute), moderate (15 to 45 beats/minute) or severe (>45 beats/minute). Decelerations are classified by their occurrence in the uterine contraction cycle. Figure 45-2 illustrates the three common patterns of early decelerations, late decelerations, and variable decelerations. Early decelerations occur when the fetal heart rates drops in the beginning of a contraction. This type of deceleration is benign and in most cases is caused by a vagal response related to compression of the fetal head in the birth canal. A late deceleration occurs when the heart rate drops 10 to 30 seconds after the onset of contractions. A late deceleration pattern indicates impaired maternal-placental blood flow, or uteroplacental insufficiency. With variable decelerations, there is no clear relationship between contractions and heart rate. This pattern is the most common of the three and probably related to umbilical cord compression. Short periods of cord compression are harmless. Longer periods of compression result in impaired umbilical blood flow and can lead to fetal distress. Fetal heart rate variability is the beat-to-beat variation in rate that occurs because of normal sympathetic or parasympathetic influences. A completely monotonous heart rate tracing may be indicative of fetal asphyxia. Fetal heart rate reactivity is the ability of the fetal heart rate to increase in response to movement or external stimuli. A healthy fetus will have two accelerations within a 20-minute period.

Fetal Blood Gas Analysis

When other factors indicate potential problems during labor and delivery, fetal blood pH can be used to determine severity. Normally, fetal blood is obtained from a capillary sample taken from the presenting body part, usually the scalp. Normal fetal capillary pH ranges from 7.35 to 7.25, with the lower values occurring late in labor. A pH below 7.20 may indicate that the fetus is experiencing asphyxia. There is no direct correlation between fetal scalp and arterial blood pH, therefore scalp pH should only be used to assist in interpreting clinical signs of fetal distress.

Evaluation of the Newborn

Assessment of the neonate begins immediately on delivery. The initial assessment includes performing a specific sequence of steps following delivery. These are: drying, warming, positioning, and suctioning. If the newborn has not begun breathing, lightly flicking the newborn's heel or vigorously rubbing the back provides physical stimulation. Decisions for further assessment and intervention are outlined by the American Academy of Pediatrics' Neonatal Resuscitation Program.

Assessment of the Apgar score is performed at one and five minutes postdelivery and should not be used to direct resuscitative efforts. Gestational age assessment and relationship of weight to gestational age are accomplished shortly after delivery.

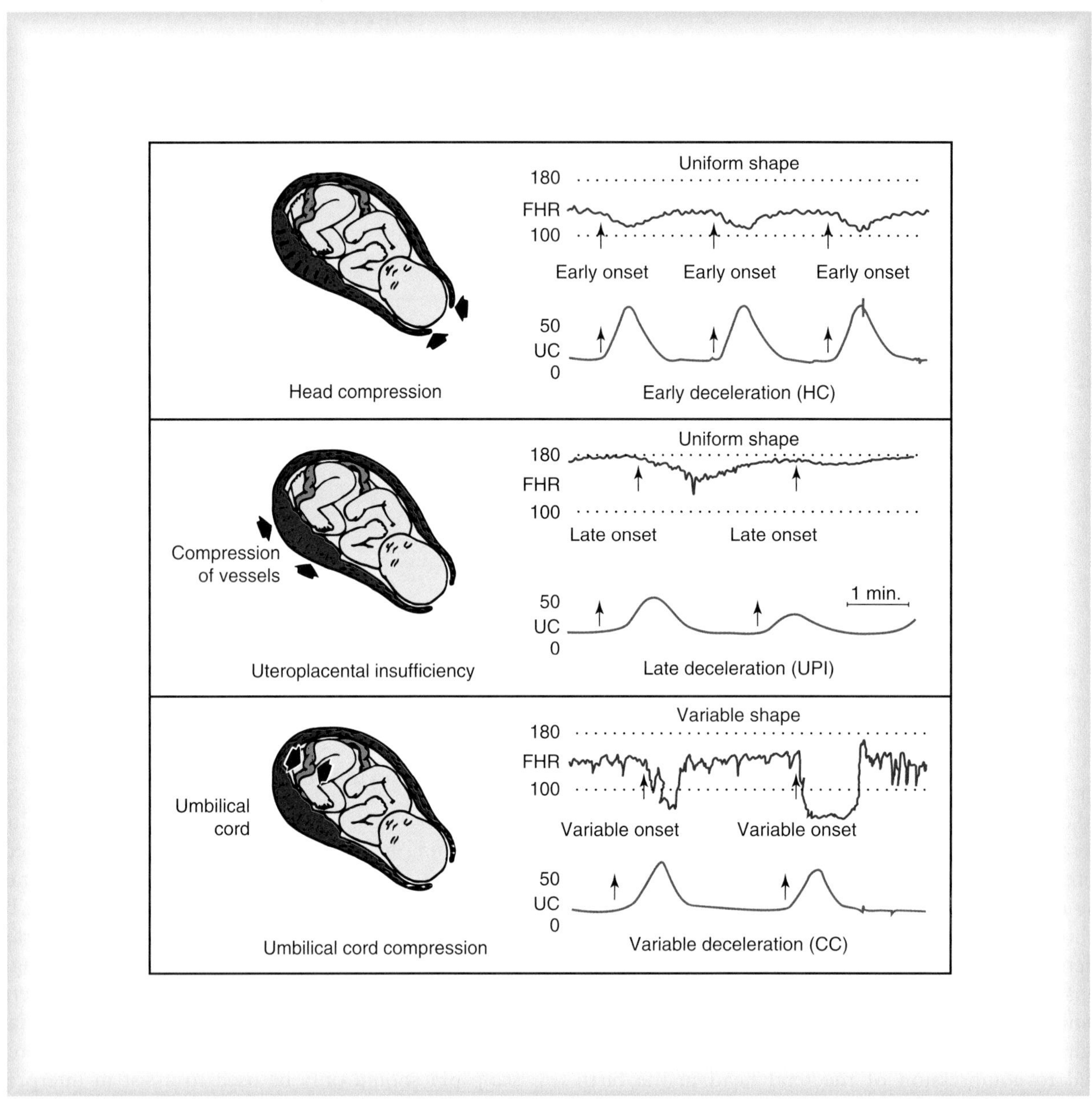

Figure 45-2

Fetal heart rate patterns. *(Modified from Avery GB, editor: Neonatology: pathophysiology and management of the newborn, ed 2, Philadelphia, 1981, JB Lippincott.)*

Apgar Score

The Apgar score is an objective scoring system used to rapidly evaluate the newborn. As shown in Table 45-2, the system has five components: heart rate, respiratory effort, muscle tone, reflex irritability, and skin color. Each component is rated according to standard definitions, resulting in a composite assessment score. In general, infants scoring 7 or higher at 1 minute are responding normally. An infant with a score of 7 may require supportive care, such as oxygen or stimulation to breathe. Infants with a 1-minute Apgar score of 6 or less may be receiving more aggressive care. The Apgar score may be influenced by gestational age, with lower gestational age newborns receiving lower scores. In this age-group, the Apgar score may not be an accurate indicator of the newborn's status.

Assessment of Gestational Age

Determination of gestational age involves assessment of multiple physical characteristics and neurological signs. Two common systems are used to determination gestational age: the Dubowitz scales and the Ballard scales. The Dubowitz scales involve assessment of 11 physical

Table 45-2 ▶ ▶ Apgar Scoring System for Newborn Assessment

	Score		
Sign	**0**	**1**	**2**
Heart rate	Absent	<100/min	>100/min
Respirations	Absent	Slow, irregular	Good, crying
Muscle tone	Limp	Some flexion	Active motion
Reflex irritability (catheter in nares, tactile stimulation)	No response	Grimace	Cough, sneeze, cry
Color	Blue or pale	Pink body with completely blue extremities	Pink

From Koff PB, Eitzman DV, Neu J: Neonatal and pediatric respiratory care, ed 2, St Louis, 1993, Mosby.

and 10 neurological signs.[1] Physical criteria include assessment of skin texture, skin color, and genitalia. Neurological criteria include posture and arm and leg recoil. The Ballard scales are a simplified version of the Dubowitz method and include six physical and six neurological signs as illustrated in Figure 45-3. Charts that describe each criterion for scoring can be found in other sources.[2] Soon after delivery, the newborn is stabilized, he or she is weighed, and gestational age is assessed. Infants born between 38 to 42 weeks are considered *term* gestation. Infants born before 38 weeks are *preterm*, while those born after 42 weeks are *postterm*.

All newborns weighing less than 2500 grams are called *low-birthweight (LBW)*. Newborns less than 1500 grams are called *very low-birthweight (VLBW)*. A newborn with a weight that is either too large or too small, or has been born preterm or postterm, has a higher risk of morbidity and mortality. As shown in Figure 45-4, by plotting the infant's gestational age against weight, the newborn's relative developmental status can be classified. Infants whose weight falls between the 10th and 90th percentiles are *appropriate for gestational age (AGA)*. Those above the 90th percentile are *large for gestational age (LGA)*, while those below the 10th percentile are *small for gestational age (SGA)*.

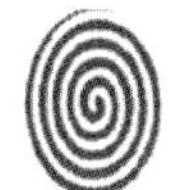

RULE OF THUMB

Infants weighing less than 2500 grams are considered low-birthweight neonates. Infants weighing less than 1500 g are considered very low-birthweight neonates.

By classifying infants into one of the combined categories, such as "preterm, AGA," the clinician can help identify those at highest risk and predict the nature of the risks involved and the likely mortality rate. Small, preterm infants are at highest risk. Compared with term babies, the lungs of these infants are not yet fully prepared for gas exchange. In addition, their digestive tracts cannot absorb fat as well, and their immune systems are not yet capable of warding off infection. Small, preterm infants also have a very large surface area to body weight ratio. This increases heat loss and impairs thermoregulation. Last, the vasculature of these small infants is less well developed, increasing the likelihood of hemorrhage (especially in the ventricles of the brain).

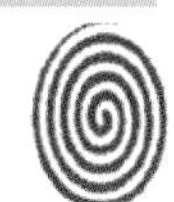

RULE OF THUMB

Infants born prior to 38 weeks of gestation are considered preterm.

Respiratory Assessment of the Infant

Not all respiratory problems occur at birth; many respiratory disorders develop after birth and may develop slowly or suddenly. Respiratory therapists are commonly called on to help assess and treat infants who develop respiratory distress after birth.

Physical Assessment

Infant physical assessment begins with measurement of vital signs. A normal newborn respiratory rate is 40 to 60 breaths/minute. The lower the gestational age of a newborn, the higher the normal respiratory rate. Although a 28-week gestational age infant may normally breath 60 times a minute, the rate more typical of the term newborn is 40 breaths/minute. Tachypnea (>60 breaths/minute) can occur because of hypoxemia, acidosis, anxiety, or pain. Respiratory rates below 40/minute should be interpreted with previous trends of the newborn's respiratory rate. A baseline respiratory rate of 36 breaths/minute in a term newborn is within normal

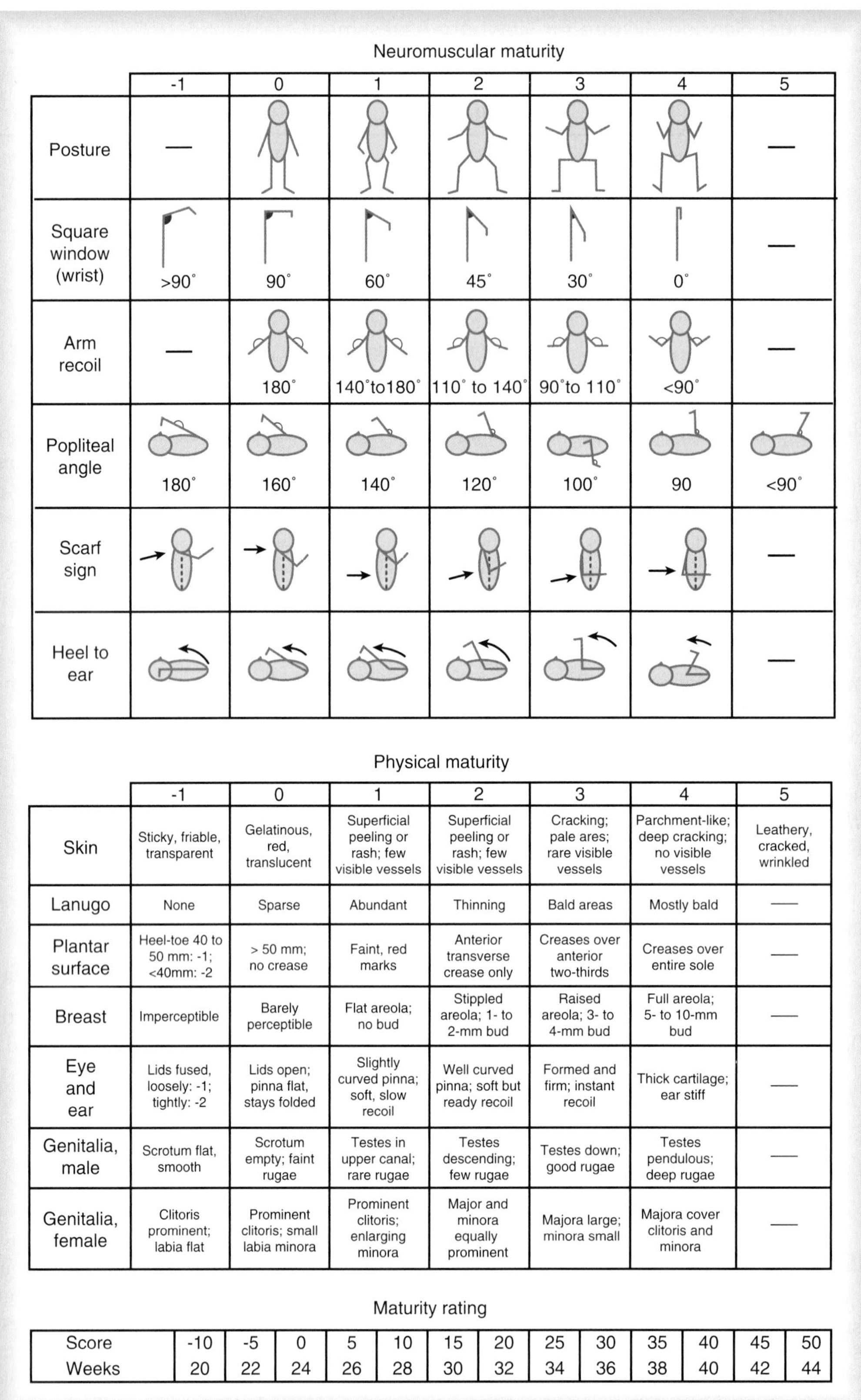

Neuromuscular maturity

	-1	0	1	2	3	4	5
Posture	—						—
Square window (wrist)	>90°	90°	60°	45°	30°	0°	—
Arm recoil	—	180°	140°to180°	110° to 140°	90°to 110°	<90°	—
Popliteal angle	180°	160°	140°	120°	100°	90	<90°
Scarf sign							—
Heel to ear							—

Physical maturity

	-1	0	1	2	3	4	5
Skin	Sticky, friable, transparent	Gelatinous, red, translucent	Superficial peeling or rash; few visible vessels	Superficial peeling or rash; few visible vessels	Cracking; pale ares; rare visible vessels	Parchment-like; deep cracking; no visible vessels	Leathery, cracked, wrinkled
Lanugo	None	Sparse	Abundant	Thinning	Bald areas	Mostly bald	—
Plantar surface	Heel-toe 40 to 50 mm: -1; <40mm: -2	> 50 mm; no crease	Faint, red marks	Anterior transverse crease only	Creases over anterior two-thirds	Creases over entire sole	—
Breast	Imperceptible	Barely perceptible	Flat areola; no bud	Stippled areola; 1- to 2-mm bud	Raised areola; 3- to 4-mm bud	Full areola; 5- to 10-mm bud	—
Eye and ear	Lids fused, loosely: -1; tightly: -2	Lids open; pinna flat, stays folded	Slightly curved pinna; soft, slow recoil	Well curved pinna; soft but ready recoil	Formed and firm; instant recoil	Thick cartilage; ear stiff	—
Genitalia, male	Scrotum flat, smooth	Scrotum empty; faint rugae	Testes in upper canal; rare rugae	Testes descending; few rugae	Testes down; good rugae	Testes pendulous; deep rugae	—
Genitalia, female	Clitoris prominent; labia flat	Prominent clitoris; small labia minora	Prominent clitoris; enlarging minora	Major and minora equally prominent	Majora large; minora small	Majora cover clitoris and minora	—

Maturity rating

Score	-10	-5	0	5	10	15	20	25	30	35	40	45	50
Weeks	20	22	24	26	28	30	32	34	36	38	40	42	44

Figure 45-3

The Ballard Gestational Age Assessment. *(Modified from Ballard JL et al: J Pediatr 95:769, 1979.)*

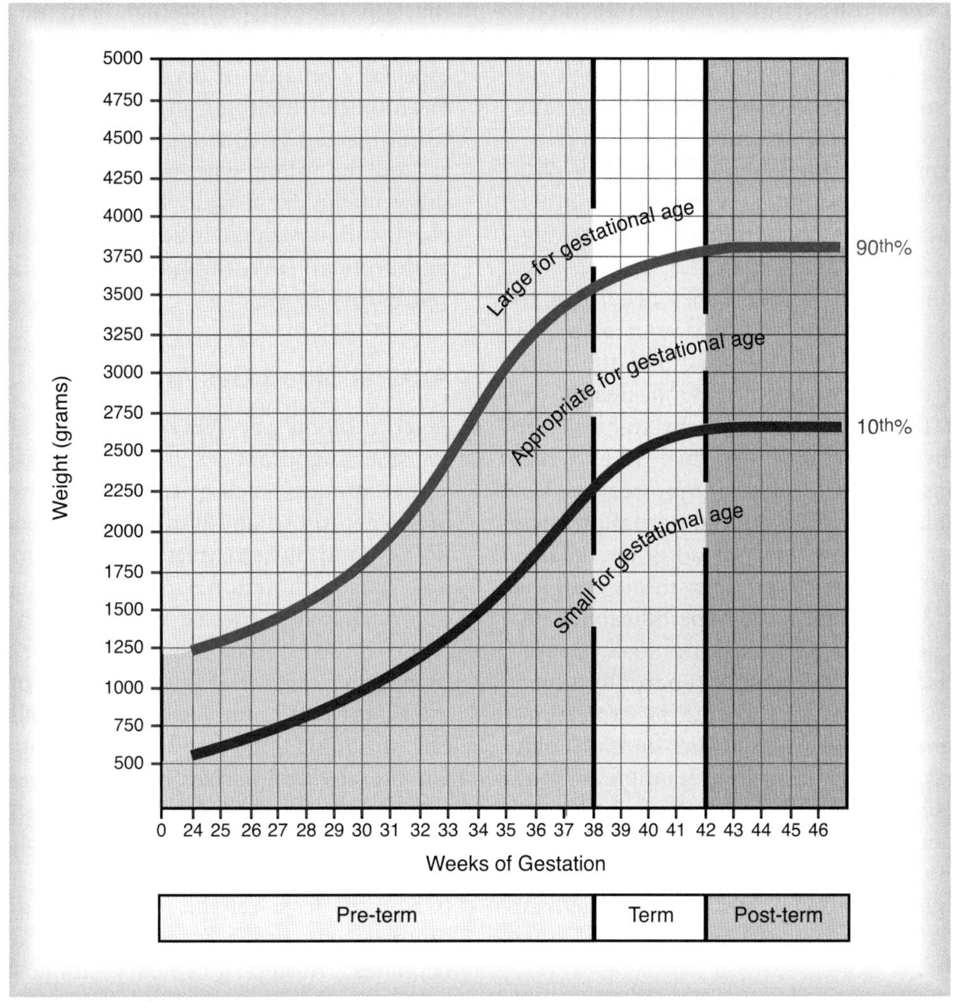

Figure 45-4
Colorado intrauterine growth chart. *(Modified from Avery GB, editor: Neonatology: pathophysiology and management of the newborn, ed 2, Philadelphia, 1981, JB Lippincott.)*

limits; however, a respiratory rate of 36 breaths/minute in a premature newborn previously breathing at 70 breaths/minute may indicate compromise. Causes of slow respiratory rates include medications, hypothermia, or neurological impairment. Normal infant heart rates vary between 100 to 160 beats/minute. Heart rate can be assessed by auscultation of the apical pulse, normally located at the fifth intercostal space, midclavicular line. Alternatively, the brachial and femoral pulse may be used. Weak pulses indicate hypotension, shock, or vasoconstriction. Bounding peripheral pulses occur with major left-to-right shunting through a patent ductus arteriosus (PDA).[3] A strong brachial pulse in the presence of a weak femoral pulse suggests either a PDA or coarctation of the aorta. Normal ranges of blood pressure are listed for various-sized neonates in Table 45-3.

Table 45-3 ▶ ▶ Normal Neonatal Blood Pressures

Weight (g)	Systolic (mm Hg)	Diastolic (mm Hg)
750	35-45	14-34
1000	39-59	16-36
1500	40-61	19-39
3000	51-72	27-46

From Whitaker K: Comprehensive perinatal and pediatric respiratory care, Albany, NY, 1992, Delmar.

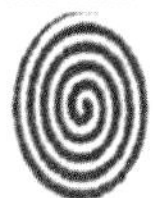

RULE OF THUMB

The normal respiratory rate for a full-term infant is 40 to 60 breaths per minute.

Thoracic assessment of infants is more difficult to perform and interpret than in adults, because of the small size and ease of sound transmission through the infant chest. Thorough observation of the infant greatly enhances the assessment data obtained. Infants in respiratory distress typically exhibit one or more key physical signs: nasal flaring, cyanosis, expiratory grunting, tachypnea, retractions, and paradoxical breathing. Nasal flaring is seen as dilation of the alar nasi on inspiration. The extent of flaring varies according to facial structure of the infant. Nasal flaring coincides with an increase in ventilatory demand and the work of breathing. In concept, nasal flaring decreases the resistance to air flow. It also may help stabilize the upper airway by minimizing negative pharyngeal pressure during inspiration.[4] Cyanosis may be absent in infants with anemia, even when arterial partial pressure of oxygen (PaO_2) levels are low. In addition, infants with high HbF levels may not become cyanotic until the PaO_2 falls below 30 mm Hg. Last, hyperbilirubinemia, common among newborns, can mask cyanosis. Grunting occurs when infants exhale against a partially closed glottis. By increasing airway pressure during expiration, grunting helps prevent airway closure and alveolar collapse. Grunting can vary from mild (audible only by stethoscope) to severe (audible with the naked ear). Grunting is most common in hyaline membrane disease, but is also seen in other respiratory disorders associated with alveolar collapse. Figure 45-5 illustrates the Silverman Score, which is a system of grading severity of lung disease.

Retractions represent the drawing in of chest wall skin between bony structures. Retractions can occur in the suprasternal, substernal, and intercostal regions. Retractions indicate an increase in work of breathing, especially because of decreased pulmonary compliance. Paradoxical breathing in infants differs from the adult form. Instead of drawing the abdomen in during inspiration, the infant with paradoxical breathing tends to draw in the chest wall. This inward movement of the chest wall may range in severity, as with retractions, and paradoxical breathing indicates an increase in ventilatory work.

Arterial Blood Gas Analysis

Arterial blood gas (ABG) analysis is an important tool for assessing infant respiratory distress. Many noninvasive techniques such as transcutaneous partial pressure of oxygen (PO_2) and partial pressure of carbon dioxide (PCO_2) and pulse oximetry are used to obtain comparable data, although ABG analysis remains the principle approach when precise results are critical. An infant ABG sample can be obtained by either arterial puncture or peripheral arterial line. Alternate means for obtaining infant ABG samples are: (1) umbilical artery catheterization and (2) capillary sampling or heel sticks. Chapter 16 summarizes the advantages, disadvantages, and complications of these sampling methods. Care must be taken in assessing the results of capillary sampling. The sampling method makes the capillary blood gas (CBG) the least reliable of all procedures as capillary samples may not accurately predict arterial values in neonates.[5] At best, a capillary sample can only be used to assess pH. It is important to remember that total blood volume of the infant is very small. Frequent blood

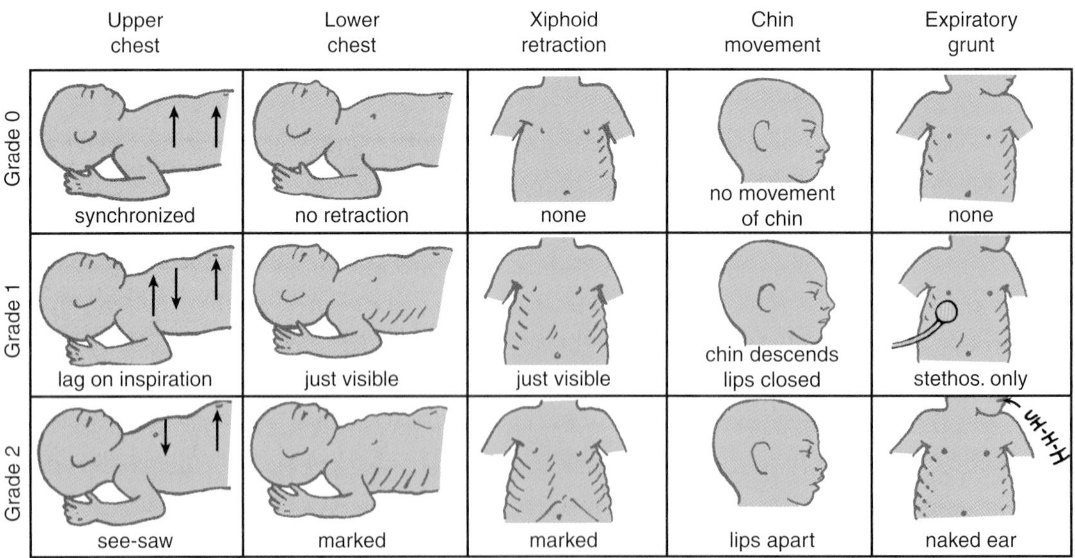

Figure 45-5
Silverman score—a system for grading severity of underlying lung disease. *(Modified from Silverman WA, Anderson DH: Pediatrics 17:1, 1956.)*

Table 45-4 ▶ ▶ Age-Related Values Commonly Reported for Normal Blood Gases

	Normal Preterm Infants (at 1 to 5 Hours)	Normal Term Infants (at 5 Hours)	Normal Preterm Infants (at 5 Days)	Children, Adolescents, and Adults
pH range	7.33	7.34	7.38	7.40
	7.29 to 7.37	7.31 to 7.37	7.34 to 7.42	7.35 to 7.45
Pco_2 range	47	35	36	40
	39 to 56	32 to 39	32 to 41	35 to 45
Po_2 range	60	74	76	95
	52 to 68	62 to 86	62 to 92	85 to 100
HCO_3^- range	25	19	21	24
	22 to 23	18 to 21	19 to 23	22 to 26
BE range	-4	-5	-3	0
	-5 to -2.2	-6 to -2	-5.8 to -1.2	-2 to +2

Modified from Orzalesi MM et al: Arch Dis Child 42:174, 1967; Koch G, Wendel H: Biol Neonate 12:136, 1968. From Koff PB, Eitzman DV, Neu J: Neonatal and pediatric respiratory care, St Louis, 1988, Mosby.
BE, Base excess; *HCO_3^-*, Bicarbonate.

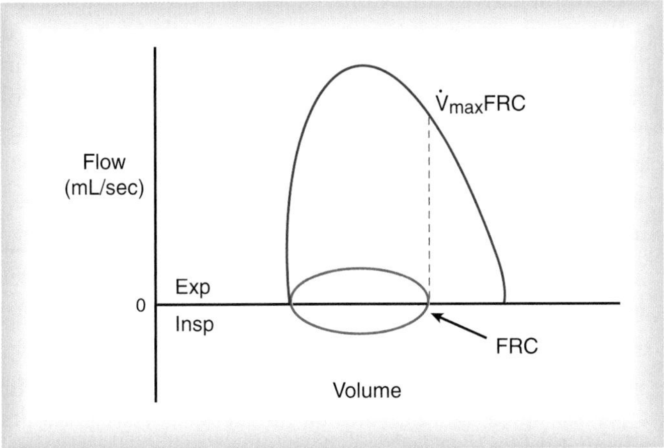

Figure 45-6
Ideal infant peak expiratory flow-volume (PEFV) curve obtained by thoracic compression. Note identification of $\dot{V}_{max}$FRC, the maximum flow at functional residual capacity.

sampling can critically deplete an infant's blood volume, therefore all blood "outs" must be recorded. Infant blood gas normal values are presented in Table 45-4.

Pulmonary Function Testing

In adults and older children, a voluntary forced exhalation is needed to produce maximum flow. Because infants and young children are unable to cooperate with instructions, they cannot perform the forced expiratory maneuver on command. To overcome this problem, a partial expiratory flow volume (PEFV) technique was developed and applied to young children.[6] The same method has been used to produce PEFV curves in infants. The maneuver is performed using a compressive cuff placed around the chest and abdomen of a sedated infant. The cuff is rapidly inflated to various pressures. This rapid external compression forces air out of the lungs, with the flow measured by a pneumotach attached to a mask. Volumes are integrated from the flow signal. Figure 45-6 depicts an ideal PEFV curve. Results are used to study normal lung growth and development, pathophysiology, and airway responsiveness.[7]

▶ GENERAL MANAGEMENT OF THE CRITICALLY ILL NEONATE

Many of the principles underlying the care of critically ill infants are similar to those for adults. However, neonatal intensive care involves several treatment differences such as temperature regulation, fluid and electrolyte balance, nutrition, and infection control.

Temperature Regulation

Newborns lose body heat faster than adults because of a low amount of subcutaneous fat and a large surface area-to-weight ratio. The smaller, more premature newborn has an even smaller amount of subcutaneous fat and a larger surface area-to-weight ratio than a term, larger newborn. Small infants cannot readily adapt to changing environmental temperatures, especially cold. Cold stress occurs when the newborn's skin temperature is less than 36° C, even if the newborn's core temperature is normal (usually because of the air temperature cooling the infant's skin). Cold stress or hypothermia in neonates increases oxygen consumption and can cause hypoglycemia, metabolic acidosis, apnea, pulmonary vascular hypertension, and increased right-to-left shunting through the ductus arteriosus and foramen ovale.

> **RULE OF THUMB**
>
> The smaller the infant, the higher the temperature needed to maintain the neutral thermal environment.

A neutral thermal environment (NTE) must be established for infants to maintain body temperature and prevent cold stress. An NTE is the ambient temperature at which the infant has the lowest oxygen consumption and metabolic rate while maintaining a normal body temperature. The ambient temperature needed to maintain an NTE varies between 32° and 35° C, depending on the infant's size. In general the smaller the infant, the higher the temperature needed for an NTE. The NTE requirements decrease over time. For example, the NTE for a 1500 to 2500 gram newborn infant is between 32.8° and 33.8° C. Six weeks later, the same infant can be kept in an NTE between 29.0° and 31.8° C. Either incubators or radiant warmers are used to achieve NTE conditions.

Fluid and Electrolyte Balance

It is difficult to maintain appropriate fluid balance in newborn infants because of the newborn's small total body fluid volume, larger body surface area-to-weight ratio, increased skin permeability, and immature renal function. Fluid balance must take into account gestational age, postpartum age, environmental temperature and humidity, and underlying pathology. The immaturity of the renal system not only may make fluid balance difficult, but it may make compensating for ventilatory acid-base imbalances impossible. Given the relatively large extracellular volume in infants, fluid and electrolyte shifts from one body compartment to another can occur readily, and the acid-base status of the blood can quickly fluctuate.

Nutrition

Infants require twice as many calories per kilogram as adults because of their high metabolic rates. Illnesses causing tissue damage and repair, infection, and fever greatly increase metabolic requirements.

Because sick infants generally cannot be fed orally, nutrition must be supplied parenterally. In most centers, 10% dextrose at the rate of 150 mL/kg/day is used initially to meet basic caloric needs. If oral feedings cannot start within 3 to 5 days, amino acids and fats must be given either orally or parenterally.

Infection Control

Because of their immature immune systems, critically ill newborn infants are highly susceptible to nosocomial infections.[8] Many begin as localized infections of areas such as the skin and conjunctiva. Any infection in a critically ill neonate can rapidly progress to more serious and life-threatening systemic infections. *Staphylococcus aureus* and group B β-hemolytic *Streptococcus* are the major gram-positive offenders. Colonization with these organisms occurs through caregiver hand transmission. Gram-negative infections, such as those caused by *Pseudomonas aeruginosa*, are more likely to be caused by contaminated equipment, particularly that used in respiratory care. Strict adherence to infection control procedures can minimize the likelihood of hospital-acquired newborn infections.

▶ BASIC RESPIRATORY CARE

Respiratory care of the infant and child incorporates approaches taken from adult practice. Important physiological and age-related differences between adults and children require variations in the provision of respiratory care. This section will focus on the equipment and techniques used in neonatal and pediatric oxygen therapy, bronchial hygiene, humidity and aerosol therapy, airway management, and resuscitation.

Oxygen Therapy

Goals and Indications

The goal of oxygen therapy is to provide adequate tissue oxygenation at the lowest inspired FIO_2. The primary indication for oxygen therapy in infants and children is documented hypoxemia. The definition of hypoxemia varies with the patient's age and disease state. In newborns older than 28 days, a PaO_2 <60 mm Hg or an SpO_2 <90% indicates hypoxemia.[9] Lower oxygenation levels are accepted in premature infants or children with congenital heart or chronic respiratory diseases.

Hazards and Precautions

Hyperoxia. Research suggests that the growing lung is more sensitive to oxygen toxicity than the adult lung.[10] Hyperoxia and its toxic effects may contribute to the development of bronchopulmonary dysplasia and retinopathy in the premature infant.[11] Retinopathy of prematurity (ROP) is a term used to describe hyperplasia of the retina. It affects neonates younger than one month of age who typically weigh less than 1500 grams.[12] Hyperoxia is not the only factor associated with ROP. Other factors linked with development of ROP are listed in Box 45-1. Hyperoxia may also have harmful cardiovascular effects. Increased PaO_2 levels in newborns promote constriction of the ductus arteriosus. Although this is normally a positive response, it can cause premature closure of the ductus arteriosus in infants with ductal dependent congenital heart defects. In addition, hyperoxia can increase aortic pressures and systemic vascular resistance, decreasing cardiac index and oxygen transport in children with acyanotic congenital heart disease.

Flip-Flop Mechanism

A potential complication in newborn oxygen therapy is the flip-flop phenomenon. Flip-flop refers to a larger than expected drop in the PaO_2 when the FIO_2 is lowered. When the FIO_2 is increased to original levels, the PaO_2 fails to improve, which is probably because of reactive pulmonary vasoconstriction. The pulmonary capillaries are sensitive to changes in PaO_2 and alter regional ratios and increase right-to-left shunting in response to these changes causing the PaO_2 to drop out of proportion to the reduction in FIO_2. Decreasing FIO_2 in small (1% to 2%) increments can usually prevent flip-flop.

Box 45-1 • Factors Other Than Oxygen Associated With Retinopathy of Prematurity[44-46]

- Immaturity
- Multiple episodes of bradycardia apnea
- Prolonged parenteral nutrition
- Number of blood transfusions
- Hypoxemia
- Hypercapnia
- Hypocapnia
- Hyperoxia
- Blood transfusions
- Intraventricular hemorrhage
- Infection
- Patent ductus arteriosus
- Prostaglandin synthetase inhibitors
- Vitamin E deficiency
- Lactic acidosis
- Respiratory distress syndrome
- Hyaline membrane disease
- Anemia of prematurity
- Hyperbilirubinemia
- Cardiovascular defects
- Hypocalcemia
- Hypothermia

Safe Levels of Oxygen Therapy

In view of these hazards and complications, oxygen therapy should be administered using a written care plan with specified clinical outcomes (i.e., titrate FIO_2 to maintain SpO_2 88% to 92%, notify physician if FIO_2 exceeds 0.40) and monitored continuously. There is little agreement on the safe upper limit for FIO_2, PaO_2, or SpO_2. In general, most clinicians keep the FIO_2 below 0.50 whenever possible with the PaO_2 60 to 80 mm Hg or the SpO_2 88% to 92% to minimize risk to the infant or child.[2,12]

Methods of Administration

The effectiveness of oxygen devices depends on the performance characteristics of the device (delivered FIO_2, flow rate, relative humidity, temperature) and the tolerance of the patient for using the device. Children are often frightened and combative. Selection of an oxygen device must be based on the degree of hypoxemia and the emotional and physical needs of the child and family. Oxygen can be administered to infants and children by mask, cannula, incubator, or oxyhood. Table 45-5 compares the advantages and disadvantages of standard oxygen delivery methods.

Monitoring

The risks of oxygen therapy in infants and children require that FIO_2, arterial oxygenation, and gas temperature be continuously monitored. FIO_2 should be monitored with an oxygen analyzer with low and high alarm limits set. Arterial oxygenation is most often assessed by noninvasive monitors such as pulse oximetry. Invasive measurement of PaO_2 may be required periodically to verify pH and $PaCO_2$. Temperature is monitored in-line with a target of an NTE of 33 +/-2° C for premature infants and newborns.

Bronchial Hygiene Therapy

Bronchial hygiene methods applicable to infants and children include postural drainage, percussion and vibration, directed coughing, and positive expiratory pressure (PEP) therapy.

Indications

Bronchial hygiene therapy is indicated when accumulated secretions impair pulmonary function and an infiltrate is visible on a chest radiograph.[13] Secretion retention is common in children who have pneumonia,

Table 45-5 ▶ ▶ Oxygen Delivery Devices

Device	Age	FDO_2	Advantages	Disadvantages
Air entrainment mask	≥ 3 years	High flow; 0.24-1.00	Precise FIO_2, good for transport, ease of application	Low relative humidity; pressure necrosis to face; difficult to fit and maintain on active child, not recommended for infants; risk of aspiration
Nasal cannula	Premature infants to adult	Low flow; 25 mL/min-6.0 LPM	Tolerated well by all ages	Inaccurate FIO_2; low relative humidity; excessive flows may cause inadvertent CPAP in infants, precise FIO_2 may be achieved with O_2 blender
Incubator	Newborns ≤ 28 days	< 0.40 FIO_2, combine use with cannula or hood for precise FIO_2	Low FIO_2 for stable infants, neutral thermal environment for premature infants	Varying FIO_2; long stabilization time; limits access to child for patient care
Oxyhood	Premature infants to ≤ 6 months of age	0.21-1.00 FIO_2 with oxygen blender maintained at 30-34° C	Warmed and humidified gas at stable FIO_2 during routine patient care	Overheating may cause apnea and dehydration; underheating may cause O_2 consumption; inadequate flow will cause CO_2 buildup; noise produced by humidification device may cause hearing loss
Mist tent	Infants to toddlers	High flow; 0.21-0.40 FIO_2	Allows child movement, high humidity, cool temperatures	Isolation of child from family; wet bedding and clothes; difficult to maintain stable FIO_2; risk of cross-contamination; limits patient care

bronchopulmonary dysplasia, cystic fibrosis, and bronchiectasis. Bronchial hygiene therapy can also be valuable in the initial management of aspirated foreign bodies.

Methods

Figure 45-7 shows positioning and percussion site differences for infants and children. Impact below the rib margins can damage abdominal viscera, and care must used when percussion and vibration are applied. This problem is greatest in small infants because of the relative size of the abdominal contents. Infants and small children cannot cough on command. For this reason, secretions mobilized with postural drainage and percussion often must be removed by suctioning. For larger children with excessive secretions, combining directed coughing with postural drainage and percussion may help improve pulmonary clearance. Adjunctive therapy devices such as PEP, flutter, or intermittent percussive ventilation (IPV) therapy have been effective in secretion clearance, especially in cystic fibrosis patients.[14]

Complications

Complications of bronchial hygiene therapy in infants and children may include regurgitation and possible aspiration, especially if postural drainage is done soon after feeding. This problem can be avoided if a nasogastric tube is in place or by timing therapy around feeding schedules (1 to 2 hours after feeding). Other complications of percussion and postural drainage in infants may include rib fractures, subperiosteal hemorrhages, and an increased risk of intraventricular hemorrhage. The rise in intracranial pressure (ICP) caused by any head-down positioning may precipitate intraventricular hemorrhage (IVH) in premature infants or children with brain injuries, therefore head-down positions are contraindicated in these children.[15]

Monitoring

Given the instability of most critically ill infants and children, a thorough initial assessment and ongoing patient evaluation during and after treatment are mandatory. Traditional assessment of vital signs, blood pressure, color, and breath sounds before, during, and after treatment should be supplemented with pulse oximetry monitoring if hypoxemia is suspected. If ICP monitoring is in use, ICP also should be assessed. Head-down positioning may cause hypoxemia in many critically ill infants and children. To offset hypoxemia in these patients, the FIO_2 may need to be increased during therapy to ensure that the SpO_2 is maintained at appropriate levels.

Humidity and Aerosol Therapy

Key differences in humidity and aerosol therapy in infants and children include assessment of patient response to therapy, age-related physiological changes, and equipment application.

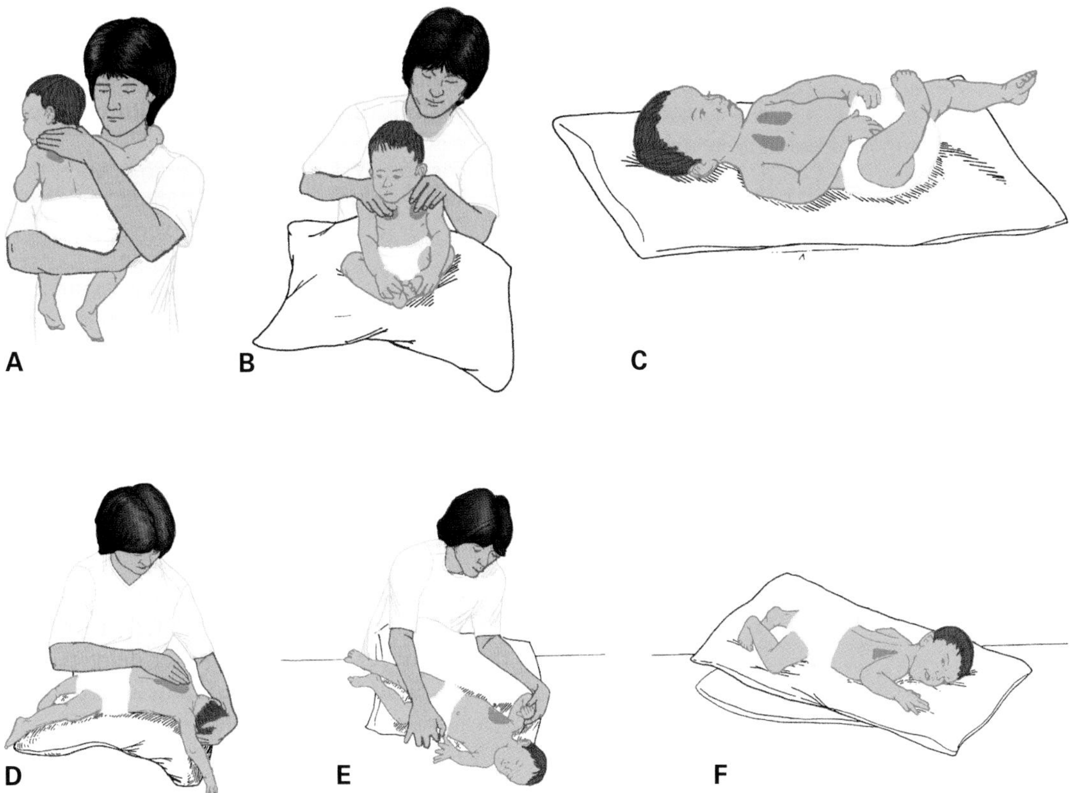

Figure 45-7
Postural drainage and percussion positions for infant and child. Angles of drainage for infant are not as obtuse as those for child. **A,** Posterior segments of right and left upper lobes are drained with patient in upright position at 30-degree angle forward. Percuss over upper posterior thorax. **B,** Apical segments of right and left upper lobes are drained with patient in upright position, leaning forward 30 degrees. Percuss over area between clavicle and tip of scapula on each side. **C,** Anterior segments of right and left upper lobes are drained with patient in flat, supine position. Percuss anterior side of chest directly under clavicles to around nipple area *(shaded)*. Avoid direct pressure on sternum. **D,** Right and left lateral basal segments of lower lobes are drained at 30 degrees Trendelenburg. Patient lies on appropriate side, rotated 30 degrees forward. Percuss over uppermost portions of lower ribs. **E,** Right and left anterior basal segments of lower lobes are drained at 30 degrees Trendelenburg. Patient lies on appropriate side with a 20-degree turn backward. Percuss above anterior lower margin of ribs. **F,** Right and left superior segments of lower lobes are drained at 15 degrees Trendelenburg, with patient in prone position. Percuss below scapula in midback area.

Humidity Therapy

Humidification of inspired gases for infants and children is based on the same principles presented in Chapter 32. In addition, high ambient humidity and temperature levels provided by environmental oxygen devices (oxyhoods, incubators) decrease evaporative heat and water loss in premature infants, minimizing temperature stress and fluid imbalances. Because of newborn thermoregulation, adjustment and monitoring of inspired gas are essential. Excessive gas temperature can result in hyperpyrexia and tachycardia. Inadequate gas temperature can cause hypothermia, apnea, acidosis, and stress.

Other oxygen devices, such as nasal cannulae, are dependent on less effective bubble humidifiers. The relatively low flows used in infants and children for nasal oxygen therapy make conventional bubble humidifiers generally acceptable. When the upper airway is bypassed by intubation, supplemental humidification must be provided using a heated humidifier or nebulizer. Because of problems with infection, fluid balance, and noise continuous nebulization is usually avoided in infants and toddlers. Humidification of inspired gases for infants and children receiving mechanical ventilation is commonly provided by a servocontrolled humidifier. Ideal features for these systems include the following: (1) low internal volume and constant water level to minimize compressed volume loss; (2) closed, continuous feed water supply to avoid contamination; (3) detachable hot plate heating; and (4) distal airway temperature sensor and high/low alarms. Common problems with humidifier systems include condensation in the tubing and inadequate humidification. Using heated wire circuits can prevent condensation. However, heated wire circuits are costly and can malfunction.[16,17] As an alternative, the inspiratory side of the circuit can be insulated with limited success (15% reduction in condensation). Inadequate humidification occurs in nonheated circuits when the humidifier temperature probe is placed too far upstream from the airway connector. Variable humidification problems occur when ventilator circuits pass through an environment and then into a warmed enclosure, such as an incubator or radiant warmer.

As an alternative to heated humidification systems, hygroscopic condenser humidifiers (HCH) have been developed and tested for neonatal mechanical ventilation.[18] With tidal volumes between 10 and 50 mL and at ambient temperatures of 24° and 38° C, these units meet or exceed the minimum of 30 mg/L, even with airway leaks up to 15% of the delivered volume. However, no guidelines exist for HCH application to infants. Until guidelines are developed, caution should be used in applying HCH devices to infants.

Box 45-2 • Guidelines for Aerosol Drug Delivery via SVN to Intubated Infants and Children Receiving Ventilatory Support

1. Position SVN in inspiratory limb of ventilator circuit 18 inches upstream from the patient Y adaptor
2. Dilute drug with 4 mL physiological saline (0.9%)
3. Set nebulizer flow to 6 to 8 L/min
4. Adjust ventilator flow to maintain pretreatment settings (TV, PIP, MAP)
5. %Tap sides of nebulizer to minimize dead volume
6. Continue treatment until no aerosol is produced
7. Remove equipment and return ventilator to pretreatment setting
8. Monitor patient for side effects

From Kacmarek RM, Hess D: Respir Care Clin N Am 36:952, 1991.

Aerosol Drug Therapy

Drug action in infants and children differs significantly from that in adults because of differences in physiology, which may include immature enzyme systems, immature receptors, and variable gastrointestinal (GI) absorption. Dosing may be imprecise and systemic effects hard to predict. For these reasons, topical administration by aerosol is a good alternative to systemic routes, especially for pulmonary disorders. The aerosol route is also safer and more comfortable than oral and parenteral approaches.

Small volume jet nebulizers (SVN), metered dose inhalers (MDI), and dry powder inhalers (DPI) can be used to deliver aerosolized drugs to infants and children.[19] Table 45-6 lists guidelines for using these devices among these age-groups. Continuous aerosol drug therapy is also utilized for patients unresponsive to intermittent SVN treatments and prior to intubation. Aerosol drug administration to intubated infants and children is challenging because of the decreased deposition from baffling of small endotracheal tubes in these patients, which prevents 90% of the drug from entering the lungs, regardless of delivery system. In addition, careful adjustments must be made to the ventilator so that nebulizer flows do not alter delivered tidal volumes and inspiratory pressures. Guidelines to ensure safe and effective aerosol drug delivery to intubated infants and children receiving ventilatory support using an SVN appear in Box 45-2.[20] Table 45-7 presents the dosage guidelines for commonly used medications in infants and children. Assessment of vital signs and breath sounds should be monitored during and after treatment to assess drug effects.

Table 45-6 ▶ ▶ Age Guidelines for Modes of Aerosol Drug Delivery

Mode	Minimum Age
SVN	Neonate (0-1 month)
MDI	5 years
With spacer	3 years
With spacer and mask	1-12 months
With endotracheal tube	Neonate
DPI	3-4 years

From Rau JL: Respir Care Clin N Am 36:514, 1991.

Airway Management

Airway management methods in infants and children are unique because of the anatomical differences between neonates and adults. Specifically, equipment and technique must be tailored to each child according to his or her size, weight, and postpartum age. A wide selection of infant- and pediatric-sized masks, oral airways, suction catheters, laryngoscope blades, and endotracheal tubes is needed to account for variations in patient age and weight. Table 45-8 provides recommendations regarding endotracheal tube and suction catheter sizes for infants and children.

Intubation

Endotracheal intubation is a generally safe method of airway management in infants and children, even when used for extended periods.[21] Complications and hazards associated with intubation in these age-groups are listed in Box 45-3. The infant's age or weight can be used to estimate proper endotracheal tube size and depth of insertion. If the tube is too small in diameter, a leak may result, decreasing delivered minute ventilation. Small endotracheal tubes have high inspiratory resistance, increasing the spontaneous work of breathing for the

Table 45-7 ▶ ▶ Commonly Used Aerosolized Medications

Medication Name	Dosage Form	Usual Child Dose	Comments
Bronchodilators			
β_2-Agonists			
Albuterol (Proventil, Ventolin)	MDI (90 mcg/puff)	1-2 puffs MDI q 15 min to q 6h ± PRN	May be used 15 minutes prior to exercise to prevent exercise-induced bronchospasm. Should be used as a rescue medication.
	Nebs (0.5%, 5 mg/mL)	0.01-0.05 mL/kg/dose (max 1 mL/dose) neb q 15min to q 6h ± PRN	
	Rotohaler (200 mcg caps)	1-2 caps inhaled q 15min to q 6h ± PRN	
Levalbuterol (Xopenex)	Nebs (0.63 mg/3 mL, 1.25 mg/3 mL)	0.32-1.25 mg neb q 6-8h ± PRN	May still cause extrapulmonary side effects including tachycardia and hypokalemia.
Salmeterol (Serevent)	MDI (21 mcg/puff)	2 puffs inhal q 12h	Not to be used as a rescue medication. Long-acting β_2-agonist.
	DPI–Diskus (50 mcg/inhal)	1 inhalation q 12h	QT_C prolongation has occurred in overdose.
Non-selective Bronchodilator			
Racemic epinephrine (Vaponefrin)	Nebs (2.25%)	0.25-0.5 mL neb q 1-4 h ± PRN	If shortage occurs, may use L-epinephrine (1:1000) 2.5-5 mL neb q 1-4h ± PRN
AntiCholinergic			
Ipratropium (Atrovent)	MDI (18 mcg/puff)	2 puffs inhal q 4-6 h ± PRN	MDI is contraindicated in patients with peanut allergy.
	Nebs (0.02%)	0.25-0.5 mg neb q 4-6 h ± PRN	For neonates, use 25 mcg/kg/dose neb tid. May cause mydriasis if aerosolized drug gets into the eye.
Anti-Inflammatory Agents			
Corticosteroids			
Beclomethasone (Beclovent, Vanceril)	MDI (42 mcg/puff)	1-2 puffs inhal qid or 2-4 puffs inhal bid	Start at lower end of dosing range if patient not previously on steroids.
	MDI double strength (84 mcg/puff)	2 puffs inhal bid	Titrate to lowest dose that is effective. Always rinse mouth after each treatment.
Budesonide (Pulmicort)	DPI-Turbuhaler (200 mcg/inhal)	1-2 puffs inhal bid	May take several weeks to see benefit. Not to be used as a rescue medication.
	Nebs-Respules (0.25 mg/2 mL, 0.5 mg/2 mL)	0.25-0.5 mg neb bid or 0.5-1 mg neb qd	
Flunisolide (Aerobid, Aerobid-M)	MDI (250 mcg/puff)	2-3 puffs inhal bid	
Fluticasone (Flovent)	MDI (44 mcg/puff, 110 mcg/puff, 220 mcg/puff)	2 puffs inhal bid (max 880 mcg/day)	
	Rotadisk (50 mcg/blister)	50-100 mcg inhal bid	
Triamcinolone (Azmacort)	MDI (100 mcg/puff)	1-2 puffs inhal qid	
Mast Cell Stabilizers			
Cromolyn (Intal)	MDI (800 mcg/puff)	2 puffs inhal qid	May take several weeks to see benefit. Not to be used as a rescue medication.
	Nebs (20 mg/2 mL)	20 mg neb qid	
Nedocromil (Tilade)	MDI (1.75 mg/puff)	2 puffs inhal qid	
Mucolytics			
N-acetylcysteine (Mucomyst)	Nebs (20%, 200 mg/mL)	3-5 mL neb qid	Consider pretreatment with albuterol 15 min prior to *N*-acetylcysteine secondary to bronchospasm.
Dornase alfa (Pulmozyme)	Nebs (2.5 mg/2.5 mL)	2.5 mg neb qid-bid	May cause hemoptysis.

Continued

Table 45-7 ▶ ▶ Commonly Used Aerosolized Medications—cont'd

Medication Name	Dosage Form	Usual Child Dose	Comments
Antiinfectives			
Pentamidine (Pentam)	Nebs (300 mg)	8 mg/kg/dose (max 300 mg/dose) neb Qmonth	Used for PCP prophylaxis.
Ribavirin (Virazole)	Powder (6 g vial)	2 g over 2 h neb q 8h x 3-7 days or 6 g over 12-18 h neb q 24 h x 3-7 days	Used for RSV treatment. Mutagenic, Teratogenic
Tobramycin (TOBI)	Nebs (300 mg/5 mL)	300 mg neb q 12 h	Used for pseudomonal infection of the lungs.

Table 45-8 ▶ ▶ Endotracheal Tube and Suction Catheter Sizes for Infants and Children

Age or Weight	Endotracheal tube ID (mm)	Tube length (cm) oral	Tube length (cm) nasal	Suction catheter (F)
Newborn				
Less than 1000 g	2.5	9-11	11-12	6
1000 to 2000 g	3.0	9-11	11-12	6
2000 to 3000 g	3.5	10-12	12-14	6
More than 3000 g	4.0	11-12	13-14	8
Children				
6 months	3.0-4.0	11-12	12-14	6-8
18 months	3.5-4.5	11-13	13-15	8
2 years	4.0-5.0	12-14	14-16	8-10
3-5 years	4.5-5.5	12-15	14-17	8-10
6 years	5.5-6.0	14-16	16-18	10
8 years	6.0-6.5	15-17	17-19	10-12
12 years	6.0-7.0	17-19	19-21	10-12
16 years	6.5-7.5	19-21	21-23	10-12

Estimating formula for tube internal diameter (ID) in mm:
Tube ID = (Age + 16)/4
Tube ID = Height (cm)/20
Estimating formula for tube length in cm:
Oral: 12 + (Age/2)
Nasal: 15 + (Age/2)

child. An inappropriately large endotracheal tube can cause mucosal and laryngeal damage that is evident after extubation, resulting in upper airway obstruction.[22]

Most neonatal and pediatric endotracheal tubes are uncuffed to eliminate cuff-related problems. However, the incidence of aspiration is increased with cuffless endotracheal tubes. Infant endotracheal tubes are small and can be easily kinked or obstructed. Proper head positioning and avoidance of cumbersome connecting apparatus are important in reducing these complications. Problems with tube position, infection, and inadvertent extubation are similar for oral and nasal routes.[23] Because the tongue is large and the epiglottis is anatomically high in infants and small children, practitioners generally find the Miller (straight) laryngoscope blade best for intubation. Care must be taken to avoid mucosal trauma during intubation because of the effect that upper airway swelling has on children with smaller anatomical airways. In addition, endotracheal tube movement can result in bronchial intubation.[24]

Box 45-3 • Complications and Hazards of Endotracheal Intubation in Infants and Children

- Palatal grooving (neonates)
- Incisal enamel hypoplasia (neonates)
- Accidental extubation
- Tube blockage
- Tracheal stenosis
- Esophageal perforation
- Tracheal perforation

Practitioners must confirm tube placement after each airway manipulation. Breath sounds may be of limited value in infants and small children for evaluation of tube position. Portable end tidal CO_2 monitoring devices may be utilized to determine proper tube placement. After proper endotracheal tube position is ensured, the tube must be carefully stabilized. Factors associated with accidental extubation of infants include patient agitation, suctioning, head-turning, chest physiotherapy, loose tape, too short a tube between lip and adapter, moving the patient during procedures, and endotracheal tube taping.[25]

Suctioning

Nasopharyngeal and tracheal suctioning help minimize aspiration, prevent endotracheal tube occlusion, and lower airway resistance in infants and children.[26] Suctioning may be a hazardous procedure and complications can occur. Box 45-4 lists the common complications and hazards associated with tracheal suctioning of infants and children. Of special concern in small infants are the cardiovascular and cerebrovascular changes that occur with suctioning.[27,28] Many of these effects are independent of changes in oxygenation and ventilation. Therefore tracheal suctioning of preterm infants and neonates should only be performed when clinical signs indicate a need.

Equipment. Oral and pharyngeal suctioning of infants can be done with a bulb syringe. A DeLee trap or a mechanical vacuum source with catheter may be used for nasopharyngeal and nasotracheal suctioning of neonates. Equipment for suctioning larger infants and children is similar to that used with adults with modifications in vacuum pressure and catheter size. Recommended suction pressures for neonates range from approximately -60 to -80 mm Hg. With large infants and children, pressures in the -80 to -100 mm Hg range are generally safe and effective. Catheter sizes are chosen according to the age of the patient and the size of the tracheal airway (see Table 45-8).

Box 45-4 • Complications and Hazards of Tracheal Suctioning in Infants and Small Children

- Infection
- Accidental extubation
- Atelectasis
- Blood pressure instability
- Increased intracranial pressure
- Cerebral vasodilation/increased blood volume
- Arterial hypoxemia
- Cerebral hypoxemia
- Hypercapnia
- Bradycardia
- Pneumothorax
- Mucosal damage

Procedure. To avoid hypoxemia during tracheobronchial aspiration, infants and children should be preoxygenated and ventilated before suctioning. Preoxygenation with 100% oxygen should be avoided in infants younger than 1 month because of the risk of hyperoxemia and retinopathies. Most clinicians recommend raising the FIO_2 by 10% to 15% for at least 1 minute before suctioning. This increase in FIO_2 is usually sufficient to prevent arterial and cerebral hypoxemia.[28] Older children can receive 100% oxygen without complication. With mechanically ventilated patients, manual inflation should always be done with an appropriate sized manual resuscitator with airway pressure manometer. Because desaturation in the arterial and cerebral circulations begins within 5 seconds of the onset of suctioning, limiting the duration of suctioning to 5 seconds or less can minimize hypoxemia. Other techniques for averting hypoxemia include use of endotracheal tube adapters that allow preoxygenation and suctioning without disconnection of the ventilator, and closed tracheal suction systems.[29]

Neonatal Resuscitation

Resuscitation procedures for infants and children are detailed in Chapter 31. Given the increasing frequency of respiratory therapists' involvement in the delivery room, a separate discussion of newborn resuscitation is presented here. The International Guidelines 2000 Conference on Cardiopulmonary Resuscitation (CPR) and Emergency Cardiac Care (ECC) established procedures for the resuscitation of the newborn. Figure 45-8 outlines the basic protocol. Immediately after delivery, the infant is assessed for presence of meconium, breathing or crying, muscle tone, color and term gestation. Efforts are directed at warming the infant as cold stress may increase oxygen consumption and impair all subsequent resuscitation efforts. Once the infant is dried and warmed, the airway is cleared by positioning and removal of secretions, if needed. The infant is positioned lying on its side or supine, with the head in a neutral position or slightly extended. A bulb syringe or 8-10 F suction catheter may be used for secretion removal; however, in the absence of blood or meconium, catheter suctioning should be limited, as aggressive pharyngeal suctioning may cause laryngospasm or bradycardia. Suction pressure should not exceed -100 mmHg.

In the presence of meconium, the mouth, nose, and pharynx should be suctioned as soon as the head is delivered using a 12-14 F catheter or bulb syringe. If the infant has absent or depressed respirations, a heart rate <100 beats/minutes or poor muscle tone, laryngoscopy

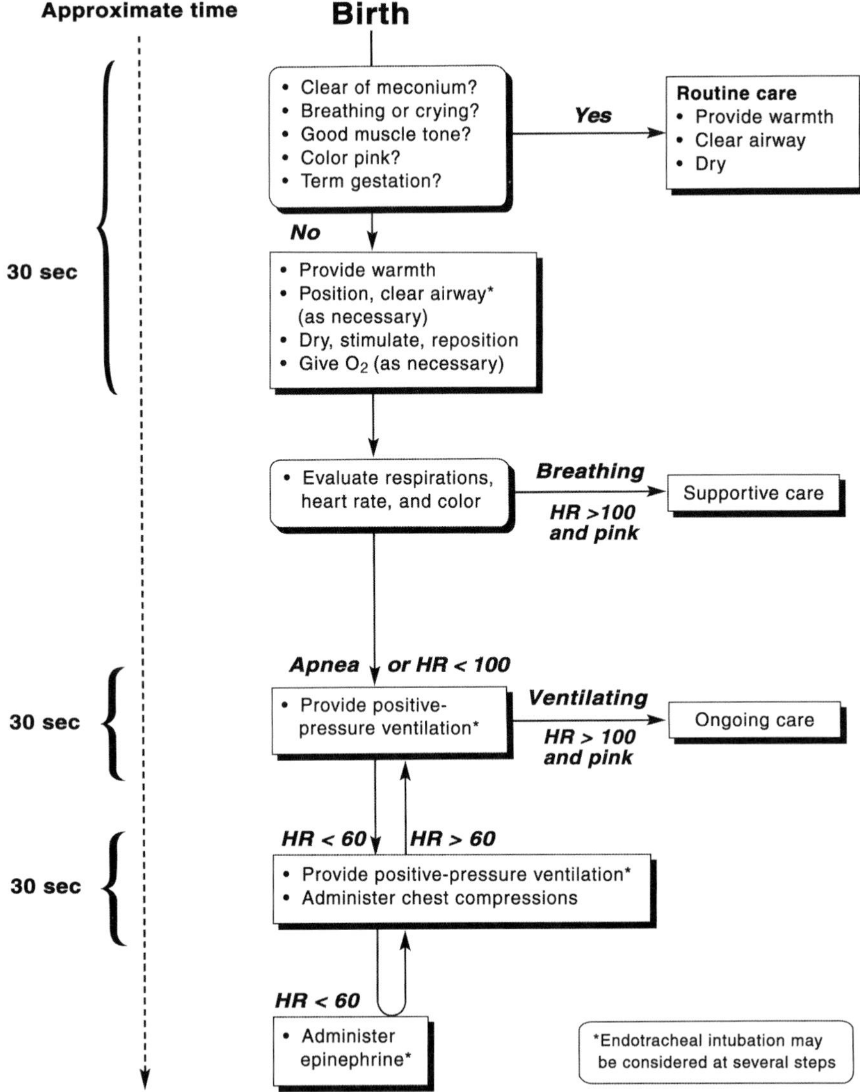

Figure 45-8

Algorithm for resuscitation of the newly born infant. *(Reproduced with permission from Pediatrics, Vol. 106, Page(s) e29, Copyright 2000.)*

and suctioning of the hypopharynx should be performed. If meconium is visible in the larynx, the trachea should also be suctioned, ideally through an endotracheal tube.

In the presence of apnea or inadequate respirations, tactile stimulation may be used to encourage spontaneous breathing. Oxygen should be administrated in the presence of cyanosis, bradycardia, or distress.

Respirations, heart rate and color are evaluated. If the infant is not breathing or the heart rate is below 100 beats/minute, positive pressure ventilation (PPV) with 100% oxygen is provided with a bag-valve-mask device. After application of PPV for 30 seconds, the heart rate is reassessed. If the heart rate is below 60 beats/minute, chest compressions are begun and PPV maintained. If, after adequate ventilation with 100% oxygen and chest compressions for 30 seconds the heart rate remains <60 beats/minute, appropriate medications are given. If spontaneous breathing is present and HR ≥100, PPVmay be gradually reduced and then discontinued. If spontaneous breathing remains inadequate or if HR remains <100 bpm, assisted ventilation is continued via bag-mask or endotracheal tube.

► CONTINUOUS POSITIVE AIRWAY PRESSURE

Spontaneous breathing may be supported with continuous positive airway pressure (CPAP), a breathing mode that maintains a constant pressure above baseline throughout inspiration and expiration. Raising the expiratory pressure above atmospheric pressure maintains a volume of gas in the lungs that is proportionate to the pressure applied and the total lung compliance. This gas volume augments the expiratory reserve volume (ERV)

Box 45-5 • Signs of Respiratory Distress Indicating a Need for Infant CPAP

- Tachycardia
- Severe retractions
- Grunting
- Periodic breathing
- Recurrent apnea
- Chest radiograph
- Nasal flaring
- Pale or cyanotic
- Tachypnea
- Low Spo_2
- Low lung volume

of the lung and increases functional residual capacity (FRC).

Continuous or demand flow during inspiration maintains airway pressure above the atmospheric pressure. CPAP is indicated when arterial oxygenation is inadequate despite a high FIO_2. This is usually accompanied by certain signs of respiratory distress (Box 45-5). For infants, CPAP is often needed when the Pao_2 is less than 50 mm Hg while the infant is breathing an $Fio_2 \geq 0.50$, providing the $Paco_2$ less than or equal to 50 mm Hg and the pH is greater than 7.25.

Methods of Administration

CPAP is commonly administered by nasal prongs for infants and positive pressure face masks for children. Infant CPAP levels are selected based on thorough clinical assessment of the patient. Levels are adjusted in small increments (1 to 2 cm H_2O), while carefully observing changes in Spo_2, respiratory rate, work of breathing, breath sounds, and blood pressure. When the appropriate CPAP level is identified, the respiratory rate usually drops toward normal and signs of respiratory distress decrease as Spo_2 rises. ABG analysis should be checked after 30 to 60 minutes to assess $Paco_2$ and pH. Fio_2 can then be weaned incrementally based on Spo_2 values >90%. Once the child is clinically stable and Fio_2 is being weaned, a chest radiograph should be obtained to assess adequacy of lung inflation. In general, CPAP levels should be raised if hypoxemia and respiratory distress persist. Worsening hypoxemia or hypercapnia, tachypnea, hypotension, and active abdominal muscle use during expiration indicate excessive CPAP settings.

CPAP should be decreased or discontinued when oxygenation is adequate at lower Fio_2 levels and chest radiograph and clinical assessment indicate resolution of the underlying disorder. The first step in weaning is to decrease the Fio_2 to nontoxic levels (<0.50), followed by lowering the CPAP pressure in 1 to 2 cm H_2O increments. All of these changes can be accomplished with pulse oximetry assessment and only periodic ABG sampling to verify an acceptable $Paco_2$ and pH. The CPAP appliance should be removed when the child can maintain adequate oxygenation without signs of respiratory distress on +2 to 3 cm H_2O and an Fio_2 of 0.40. On discontinuing CPAP, the child should be placed on an equivalent or slightly higher Fio_2.

▶ MECHANICAL VENTILATION

Effective neonatal-pediatric mechanical ventilation requires an understanding of developmental and age-related differences in pulmonary mechanics of children, such as respiratory rate, inspiratory flow, and tidal volume. The respiratory therapist must possess knowledge of the disease state and equipment performance to develop ventilatory strategies appropriate to the child's pulmonary pathophysiology and spontaneous breathing demands.

Basic Principles

Currently, there are two approaches to neonatal-pediatric mechanical ventilation: (1) conventional mechanical ventilation and (2) high-frequency ventilation. Another option, negative pressure ventilation, has been used with some success in managing refractory hypoxemia and pulmonary interstitial emphysema[30,31] but is limited in its scope and availability and will not be presented here.

Advanced technology has increased the available ventilator modes to include assist-control, synchronized intermittent mechanical ventilation (SIMV), and pressure support ventilation. Improvements in trigger sensitivity, ventilator response time, and ventilator monitoring facilitate patient-ventilator synchrony for the smallest premature infant, which may promote growth and weight gain during mechanical ventilation. The primary differences between neonatal/pediatric and adult ventilator performance are the precision and ranges of flow, volume, trigger sensitivity, and response time.

Patient-ventilator synchrony is defined as the matching of ventilator-delivered breaths to patient-demanded breaths during assisted or supported ventilation. Synchronous ventilation is a relatively new practice in neonatal and pediatric ventilatory care. To achieve truly synchronous ventilation in this population, the respiratory therapist must recognize ventilator parameter deficiencies in relation to the patient's spontaneous need and adjust the flow pattern, trigger, cycle, or limit to improve the interaction. Several methods of sensing spontaneous breathing efforts in small infants have been introduced to facilitate synchronous ventilatory support. Table 45-9 describes the characteristics of available patient-triggered systems.

APPLICATION OF CPAP TO NEONATES VIA NASAL PRONGS OR NASOPHARYNGEAL TUBE

AARC Clinical Practice Guideline (Excerpts)*

➤ INDICATIONS

Abnormalities on physical examination—tachypnea, substernal and suprasternal retractions, grunting, and nasal flaring; the presence of pale or cyanotic skin color and agitation

Inadequate oxygenation (Pao_2 <50 torr with FIO of ≤0.60, provided VE is adequate as indicated by a $Paco_2$ level of 50 torr and a pH ≥7.25)

The presence of poorly expanded and/or infiltrated lung fields on chest radiograph

The presence of a condition thought to be responsive to CPAP, including:

- Respiratory distress syndrome
- Pulmonary edema
- Atelectasis
- Tracheal malacia or other similar abnormality of the lower airways
- Recent extubation
- Transient tachypnea of the newborn
- Apnea of prematurity

➤ CONTRAINDICATIONS

- Although nasal CPAP has been used in bronchiolitis, this application may be contraindicated
- The need for intubation and/or mechanical ventilation as evidenced by the presence of:
  - Upper airway abnormalities that contraindicate nasal CPAP (e.g., choanal atresia, TE fistula)
  - Severe cardiovascular instability and impending arrest
  - Unstable respiratory drive with frequent apneic episodes resulting in desaturation and/or bradycardia
  - Ventilatory failure as indicated by the inability to maintain $Paco_2$ <60 torr and pH >7.25
- Application of nasal CPAP to patients with untreated congenital diaphragmatic hernia may lead to gastric distention and further compromise of thoracic organs

➤ HAZARDS AND COMPLICATIONS

Hazards and complications associated with equipment, including the following:

- Obstruction of nasal prongs from mucus plugging or kinking may interfere with delivery of CPAP and result in a decrease in Fio_2 through entrainment of room air via opposite naris or mouth.
- Inactivation of airway pressure alarms
  - High resistance through nasal appliances can maintain pressure in the system even after decannulation. This can result in failure of low airway pressure/disconnect alarms to respond
  - Complete obstruction of nasal prongs and nasopharyngeal tubes results in continued pressurization of the CPAP system without activation of low or high airway pressure alarms.
- Activation of a manual breath (commonly available on infant ventilators) may cause gastric insufflation and patient discomfort particularly if the peak pressure is set inappropriately high

Hazards and complications associated with the patient's clinical condition including the following:

- Lung overdistention causing barotrauma, $\dot{V}/\dot{Q}$ mismatch, hypercapnia, including work of breathing
- Impedance of pulmonary blood flow (increased pulmonary vascular resistance, decreased cardiac output)
- Gastric insufflation and abdominal distention potentially leading to aspiration
- Nasal irritation with septal distortion
- Skin irritation and pressure necrosis
- Nasal mucosal damage due to inadequate humidification

➤ ASSESSMENT OF NEED

ASSESSMENT OF NEED Determination that valid indications are present by physical, radiographic, and laboratory assessments

➤ ASSESSMENT OF OUTCOME

ASSESSMENT OF OUTCOME CPAP is initiated at levels of 4-5 cm H_2O and may be gradually increased up to 10 cm H_2O to provide the following:

- Stabilization of Fio_2 requirement ≤0.60 with Pao_2 levels >50 torr and/or the presence of clinically acceptable noninvasive monitoring of oxygen ($Ptco_2$), while maintaining an adequate VE as indicated by $Paco_2$ of 50-60 torr or less and pH ≥7.25
- Reduced work of breathing as indicated by decreased respiratory rate, retractions, grunting, nasal flaring
- Improvement in lung volumes and appearance of lung as indicated by chest radiograph
- Improvement in patient comfort as assessed by bedside caregiver

APPLICATION OF CPAP TO NEONATES VIA NASAL PRONGS OR NASOPHARYNGEAL TUBE—CONT'D

AARC Clinical Practice Guideline (Excerpts)*

➤ MONITORING

Patient-ventilator system checks should be performed at least every 2 to 4 hours and should include documentation of ventilator settings and patient assessments as recommended by the AARC CPG Patient-Ventilator System Checks (Chapter 43) and the CPG Humidification during Mechanical Ventilation (Chapter 32). Monitoring should include:

- Oxygen and carbon dioxide monitoring, including periodic sampling of ABG values and continuous noninvasive monitoring (e.g., transcutaneous O_2/CO_2 monitoring, pulse oximetry)
- Continuous monitoring of electrocardiogram and respiratory rate
- Continuous monitoring of proximal airway pressure, PEEP, and mean airway pressure (Paw)
- Continuous monitoring of FIO_2
- Periodic physical assessment of breath sounds and signs of increased work of breathing
- Periodic evaluation of chest radiographs

*For complete guideline see Respir Care 39 (8) :817-823, 1994.

Table 45-9 ▶ ▶ Characteristics of Patient-Triggered Ventilation System

	Sensor	V_T Measured at Airway	Features
Infrasonics Infant Star 500/950	Abdominal impedance capsule	No	Triggers inspiration by sensing inspiratory effort through abdominal movement
Bear 750 vs	Heated wire	Yes	Flow triggering Flow termination Volume assurance Inspiratory and bias flows Independently adjustable
Drager Babylog 8000 Plus	Heated wire	Yes	Volume guarantee Inspiratory and bias flows Independently adjustable
Sechrist IV 100B, IV 200 w/SAVI System	Chest ECG leads that measure change in thoracic impedance	No	Senses onset of inspiratory and expiratory effort Immediate termination of the positive pressure breath upon active exhalation to prevent a sudden increase in transpulmonary pressure
Bird VIP	Differential pressure	Yes	Adjustable flow termination Flow triggering Leak compensation
Bird VIP Gold	Differential pressure	Yes	Flow triggering Volume ensured pressure support PS and PC levels adjustable Independently in combined modes
Bird VIP Sterling	Differential pressure	Yes	Flow triggering PS and PC levels adjustable Independently in combined modes

PC, Pressure control; *PS*, pressure support.

Patient-ventilator asynchrony occurs when the patient's efforts to breathe go unmatched by ventilatory support. Ventilatory support below that demanded by the patient increases the imposed work of breathing and may result in worsening PaO_2 and $PaCO_2$ values because of increased oxygen consumption and carbon dioxide production. This interferes with gas exchange and ventilatory management causing poor weight gain and pulmonary air leak syndrome in infants.[32-34] Common problems with patient-triggering in infants and children include missed breaths and auto-triggering (Box 45-6). In assisted breathing modes, auto-triggering may result

Box 45-6 • Common Causes of Inappropriate Triggering

- Incorrect sensitivity setting
- Failed sensor
- Large endotracheal tube leak
- Misplaced sensor
- Cardiac oscillation
- Rainout in tubing

in an abnormally rapid ventilator rate. This may cause hyperventilation and/or render the infant apneic. When auto-triggering occurs during SIMV, the ventilator rate does not change, but asynchrony may occur.

Goals of Mechanical Ventilation

The goals of mechanical ventilation are to improve oxygen delivery to meet metabolic demand and eliminate

Neonatal Time Triggered, Pressure-Limited Time-Cycled Mechanical Ventilation

AARC Clinical Practice Guideline (Excerpts)*

INDICATIONS

- Apnea
- Hypoxemic (PaO_2 <50 torr) or hypercapnic (pH <7.20-7.25) respiratory despite the use of continuous positive airway pressure (CPAP) and supplemental oxygen (i.e., FIO_2 > or = to 0.60)
- Abnormalities on physical examination
  - Increased work of breathing demonstrated by grunting, nasal flaring, tachypnea, and sternal and intercostal retractions
  - The presence of pale or cyanotic skin and agitation
- Alterations in neurological status that compromise the central drive to breathe:
  - Apnea of prematurity
  - Intracranial hemorrhage
  - Congenital neuromuscular disorders
- Impaired respiratory function resulting in a compromised functional residual capacity (FRC) due to decreased lung compliance and/or increased airways resistance, including but not limited to:
  - Respiratory distress syndrome (RDS)
  - Meconium aspiration syndrome (MAS)
  - Pneumonia
  - Bronchopulmonary dysplasia
  - Bronchiolitis
  - Congenital diaphragmatic hernia
  - Sepsis
  - Radiographic evidence of decreased lung volume
- Impaired cardiovascular function
  - Persistent pulmonary hypertension of the newborn (PPHN)
  - Postresuscitation
  - Congenital heart disease
  - Shock
- Postoperative state characterized by impaired ventilatory function

CONTRAINDICATIONS

No specific contraindications when indications are judged to be present

HAZARDS AND COMPLICATIONS

- Air leak syndromes due to barotrauma and/or volume overinflation (i.e., volutrauma) including pneumothorax pneumomediastinum, pneumopericardium, pneumoperitoneum, subcutaneous emphysema, and pulmonary interstitial emphysema
- Chronic lung disease associated with prolonged positive pressure ventilation and oxygen toxicity (e.g., bronchopulmonary dysplasia)
- Airway complications associated with endotracheal intubation: Laryngotracheobronchomalacia
  - Laryngotracheobronchomalacia
  - Damage to upper airway structures
  - Malpositioning of ET tube
  - Obstruction of ETT with mucus
  - Kinking of ETT
  - Unplanned extubation
  - Air leak around uncuffed ETT
  - Subglottic stenosis
  - Main-stem intubation
  - Pressure necrosis

NEONATAL TIME TRIGGERED, PRESSURE-LIMITED TIME-CYCLED MECHANICAL VENTILATION—CONT'D

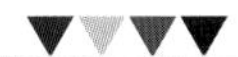

AARC Clinical Practice Guideline (Excerpts)*

Increased work of breathing (during spontaneous breaths) due to the high resistance of small ET tubes
Nosocomial pulmonary infectin (e.g., pneumonia)
Decreased venous return, decreased cardiac output, increased ICP leading to intraventricular hemorrhage
Supplemental oxygen may lead to an increased risk of retinopathy of prematurity (ROP)
Complications associated with endotracheal suctioning
Failure of the ventilator, alarms, circuit, humidifier; loss of or inadequate gas supply
Patient-ventilator asynchrony
Inappropriate ventilator settings leading to auto-PEEP, hypo- or hyperventilation, hypo- or hyperoxemia and increased work of breathing

➤ ASSESSMENT OF NEED

Determination that valid indications are present

➤ ASSESSMENT OF OUTCOME

- Establishment of neonatal assisted ventilation should result in improvement in patient condition and/or reversal of indications:
- Reduction in work of breathing as evidenced by decreases in respiratory rate, severity of retractions, nasal flaring and grunting
- Radiographic evidence of improved lung volume
- Subjective improvement in lung volume as indicated by increased chest excursion and aeration by chest auscultation
- Improved gas exchange
  - Ability to maintain a PaO_2 > or = 50 torr with FIO_2 <0.60
  - Ability to reverse respiratory acidosis and maintain a pH >7.23
- Subjective improvement as indicated by a decrease in grunting, nasal flaring, sternal and intercostal retraction, and respiratory rate

➤ MONITORING

- Patient-ventilator system checks should be performed every 2-4 hours and should include documentation of ventilator settings and patient assessments as recommended by the AARC CPG Patient-Ventilator System Checks (Chapter 43) and AARC CPG Humidification during Mechanical Ventilation (Chapter 32). Monitoring should include:
- Oxygen and CO_2 monitoring:
  - Periodic sampling of blood gas values; keep PaO_2 <80 torr in preterm infants to avoid ROP
  - The unstable infant should be monitored continuously by transcutaneous O_2 monitor or pulse oximeter
  - The unstable infant should be monitored continuously by transcutaneous or end-tidal CO_2 monitoring
  - Fractional concentration of oxygen delivered by the ventilator should be monitored continuously
- Continuous monitoring of cardiac activity (via electrocardiograph) and respiratory rate
- Monitoring of blood pressure by indwelling arterial line or by periodic cuff measurements
- Continuous monitoring of airway pressures including peak (PIP), PEEP, and mean pressure (Paw)
  - Higher Paw may improve oxygenation; however, Paw >12 cm H_2O may lead to barotrauma
  - The difference between PIP and PEEP (AP) in conjunction with patient mechanics determines VT. As the ΔP changes, VT will vary.
  - PIP should be adjusted initially to achieve adequate VT as reflected by chest excursion and adequate breath sounds and/or by VT measurement.
  - PEEP increases FRC and may improve oxygenation (PEEP is typically adjusted at 4-7 cm H_2O—higher levels may cause hyperinflation, particularly in obstructive airways disease [e.g., MAS or bronchiolitis]).
- Many neonatal ventilators provide continuous monitoring of ventilator rate, ti, and I : E. If only two of these variables are directly monitored, the third should be calculated
  - Lengthening ti increases Paw and should improve oxygenation
  - I : E in excess of 1 : 1 may lead to auto-PEEP and hyperinflation
  - Rates of 30-60/min with shorter ti (e.g., I : E of 1 : 2) are commonly used in patients with RDS

Continued

NEONATAL TIME TRIGGERED, PRESSURE-LIMITED TIME-CYCLED MECHANICAL VENTILATION—CONT'D

AARC Clinical Practice Guideline (Excerpts)*

- Depending on the internal diameter of the ventilator circuit, excessive flows can cause expiratory resistance that leads to increased work of breathing and increased PEEP. Some ventilators have demand-flow systems that permit the use of lower baseline flowrates but provide the patient with additional flow as needed
- Because of the possibility of complete obstruction or kinking of the ETT and the inadequacy of ventilator alarms in these situations, continuous tidal volume monitoring via an appropriately designed (minimum dead space) proximal airway flow sensor is recommended
- Periodic physical assessment of chest excursion and breath sounds and for signs of increased work of breathing and cyanosis
- Periodic evaluation of chest radiographs to follow the progress of the disease, identify possible complications, and verify ETT placement

*For complete guideline see Respir Care 39 (8) :808-816, 1994

carbon dioxide, while reducing the work of breathing for a patient. Ventilatory care should meet these goals while minimizing the deleterious effects of the interventions on the cardiorespiratory system. The ventilatory approach should be simple, meet the needs of the patient, and provide the greatest benefit at the lowest risk of complication.

Tidal Volume

Guidelines for individual ventilator parameters should be directed at restoring lung volume, specifically FRC. Tidal volume should be measured at the endotracheal tube to distinguish set from delivered tidal volume. Generally, tidal volumes of 6 to 8 mL/kg should be delivered at the endotracheal tube.

Modes of Mechanical Ventilation

Neonatal ventilation is evolving from the most common mode, time-cycled, pressure-limited, to volume-monitored and volume-targeted modes. Triggering and termination sensitivity have allowed the clinician to choose modes not previously available. Common adult modes are now incorporated in neonatal ventilators. Modes such as SIMV, pressure support, combined modes, and volume guarantees are new to mechanical ventilation. Clinical experience and research will help determine the roles of newer modes in the future.

Ventilator Rate

Ventilator rate is selected along with tidal volume to provide adequate alveolar ventilation for the patient. This is generally achieved by maintaining $Pa{CO_2}$ between 40 and 50 mm Hg for children. $Pa{CO_2}$ may be allowed to increase in children who are at risk for pulmonary barotrauma or who have chronic respiratory disease. Permissive hypercapnia is a valuable ventilator management strategy that may be tolerated by infants and children thereby allowing use of smaller tidal volumes and lower peak inspiratory pressures to prevent pulmonary barotrauma and volutrauma.[35-38]

$F{IO_2}$

The fraction of inspired oxygen should be adjusted to maintain the arterial oxygen saturation at $Sp{O_2}$ = 88% to 92%. $F{IO_2}$ should be analyzed continuously or frequently monitored to ensure the accuracy of set $F{IO_2}$. Efforts should be made to wean oxygen below 50% (or to maintain $Pa{O_2}$ <90 mm Hg in prematurity) to help prevent oxygen toxicity.

Positive End-Expiratory Pressure (PEEP)

The PEEP level in neonates is generally kept between 5 to 8 cm H_2O. The use of high-frequency ventilation (HFV) is instituted if an increase in FRC and recruitment is needed. In pediatric patients, the PEEP level is determined by performing a PEEP titration study. With this technique, PEEP is increased in 2 to 5 cm H_2O increments with 15 to 20 minutes of stability between increases. Lung compliance is measured along with indicators of cardiac output and oxygenation (pulse oximetry). The PEEP level that produces the best $Sp{O_2}$, lung compliance, and hemodynamics is the most appropriate PEEP for the patient. Daily assessment of lung

Table 45-10 ▶ ▶ Inspiratory Time Ranges By Age

Age	Time Range (seconds)
Low-birthweight infants	0.25-0.5
Term infants	0.50-0.6
Toddlers	0.50-0.75
Children	1.0-1.5

expansion by chest radiograph should include discussion of the level of PEEP. PEEP is often increased to the point that will allow the F_{IO_2} to be decreased to 60%. This may be considered the best PEEP level.

Inspiratory Time (T_i)

T_i is selected by the bedside clinician to facilitate patient comfort and synchronous breathing during mechanical ventilation. The patient's age, breathing pattern, and time constant of the lungs are considerations in the selection of T_i. Recommended initial T_i ranges by age-group are listed in Table 45-10.

Flow (Bias Flow Versus Inspiratory Flow)

Bias flow is the flow through the circuit that the child has available during a spontaneous breath. Bias flow should be high enough to meet the demands of a spontaneous breath but not so high as to impede exhalation. Inspiratory flow is the peak flow during a mechanical breath. Some neonatal ventilators allow the clinician to set the flow independently.

Equipment

Care must be taken to ensure that circuit dead space and compressible volume are minimal because of the small tidal volumes used in neonatal mechanical ventilation. Changes in the circuit's internal volume may interfere with alveolar ventilation. Humidifiers should have small internal volumes and continuous water feed systems to keep the water level and temperature constant. Condensation in infant ventilator circuits may result in aspiration of water or loss of tidal volume in pressure limited ventilation. Heated wire circuits or water traps in dependent portions of the ventilator circuit are helpful in eliminating these concerns.

Assessment of Mechanical Ventilation

Methods for monitoring patients receiving mechanical ventilation include physical assessment, direct observation, and continuous electronic surveillance of mechanical and physiological parameters. The respiratory therapist must incorporate all facets of ventilatory monitoring into a comprehensive, responsive care system focused on reducing morbidity and length of mechanical ventilation and improving patient outcomes. Physical examination of the chest is often the deciding factor between monitor error and true change in patient status, and its role is increasing as respiratory therapists use patient management protocols. Noninvasive techniques to assess gas exchange and pulmonary mechanics provide a continuous data stream with alarms to identify changes in ventilatory status and alert

MINI CLINI

Pediatric Mechanical Ventilation

PROBLEM

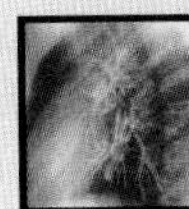

A 14-month-old child, who weighs 13 kg and has a history of chronic lung disease (BPD), requires mechanical ventilation after surgery for correction of gastric reflux. The surgeon requests that you select ventilator parameters and develop a weaning plan for this child. The child has an uncuffed 4.5 oral ETT in place. Sp_{O_2} is 100% with manual ventilation and 100% oxygen. Sedation is prescribed to keep the child comfortable but allow spontaneous breathing.

This child needs a ventilatory strategy that takes into account his age, disease process, amount of sedation and current ventilation needs. What would be the appropriate choices for his initial ventilator management in terms of mode, tidal volume, set rate, F_{IO_2}, and PEEP level?

SOLUTION

Mode—SIMV
Tidal volume—10 mL/kg or 130 mL in this case
F_{IO_2}—1.0 then titrated to an acceptable F_{IO_2}
PEEP—about 3 cm H_2O

If this child had previously been mechanically ventilated, reviewing the presurgery settings may be helpful in deciding a ventilator plan. If not, the following describes a rationale for the suggested parameters.

By using the mode of SIMV, patient-ventilator synchrony can be more easily achieved. This will reduce the need for sedation later, after the pain of surgery has dissipated. The initial tidal volume is based on current recommendations but should be modified based on P_{CO_2} levels. Because this child has chronic lung disease, a higher P_{CO_2} may be optimal at this time. Physical examination of the chest and measurement of the delivered tidal volume determine the effectiveness of the chosen volume and can be done at the bedside. The ventilator rate is determined by the normal respiratory rate for the age of the child, the desired P_{CO_2} level, and the number of spontaneous breaths the child is having. A younger child, with a higher P_{CO_2}, with a decreased respiratory drive (not contributing many spontaneous breaths) may have a higher set rate. The initial F_{IO_2} is usually reflective of the amount currently being delivered with hand ventilation but quickly titrated to maintain normal Sp_{O_2}. It would not be unusual for the child to be down to an F_{IO_2} of 0.40 after surgery.

caregivers. Integration of all assessment data is essential for efficient, cost-effective, high-quality ventilatory care.

Ventilator parameters should be measured routinely and recorded by personnel expert in neonatal-pediatric care. Spontaneous tidal volume and respiratory rate may be used as indicators of lung compliance, respiratory muscle strength, and work of breathing. Mechanical tidal volume and rate assessment ensure delivery of the prescribed alveolar ventilation and facilitate detection of airway or circuit leaks. Peak inspiratory pressures during volume ventilation reflect set tidal volume, inspiratory flow, airway resistance, lung compliance, and endotracheal tube size. Pressures should be measured at the airway to provide the most accurate values. Mean airway pressure ($\overline{P}_{aw}$) is an important indicator of the level of mechanical ventilation required to achieve adequate oxygenation. It is a function of tidal volume, inspiratory time, peak inspiratory pressure, peak flow, flow pattern, rate, and PEEP. Parameters should be adjusted to provide adequate alveolar ventilation and oxygenation at the lowest $\overline{P}_{aw}$.

Airway graphic analysis offers information for assessment of ventilator performance, breath type selection, patient pathophysiology, and a patient-ventilator interactions.[39-40] Waveforms help identify the characteristics of ventilator operation (trigger, cycle, limit, and flow pattern) and the cardiopulmonary status of the patient's lungs (decreased compliance, airway obstruction). Graphic analysis may be used to optimize patient-ventilator interactions, improve patient-ventilator synchrony, reduce work of breathing, and calculate a variety of physiological parameters related to respiratory mechanics. The most commonly displayed waveforms are flow, airway pressure, and volume (y-axis) plotted against time (x-axis). The timing sequence of ventilatory events can be determined through graphical analysis. Breath to breath comparison of all three waveforms simultaneously facilitates analysis of the patient-ventilator interface. Patient-ventilator abnormalities become evident when the timing and magnitude of flow, pressure, and volume are disproportionate or delayed. Additionally, each of these parameters (flow, pressure, volume) can be plotted against each other. Pressure-volume and flow-volume loops can be particularly helpful in assessing alterations in peak flow, work of breathing, overdistension of the lung, dynamic compliance, and premature termination of exhalation.

Optimal neonatal and pediatric ventilatory measurements are obtained when the pneumotachometer is positioned between the endotracheal tube and the ventilator circuit.[41] Volume is measured by integrating the flow signal from the pneumotachometer with measured inspiratory time. In this configuration, the pneumotachometer measures delivered, not set tidal volume. Inspiratory and expiratory volumes should be equal, but it is not uncommon in pediatric patients with uncuffed endotracheal tubes for the expiratory volume to be less than the inspiratory volume. An actual percentage leak can be calculated and may aid in the assessment of endotracheal tube size, adequacy of cuff inflation, or airway pathology.

Weaning From Mechanical Ventilation

The goals of mechanical ventilation change quickly as the patient's respiratory failure progresses to the resolution phase where successful weaning and extubation become essential components of the care plan. During the weaning phase of mechanical ventilation, lung volumes, compliance, and oxygenation are improving. The goal during the weaning phase is to facilitate effective spontaneous breathing as ventilatory support is reduced. Therefore patient-ventilator synchrony becomes an essential component of the weaning care plan. Clinicians must be able to manage rapidly changing pulmonary mechanics, patient demand/comfort, and ventilator performance to successfully reduce ventilatory support without increasing the work of breathing to a point of fatigue and failure.

The ventilator parameter most likely to have a deleterious effect on the patient should be weaned first. Typically, this is the FIO_2. Care plans should be focused on continuous noninvasive monitoring of oxygenation. Transcutaneous partial pressure of carbon dioxide ($P_{TC}CO_2$) or pulse oximetry (SpO_2) allows progressive oxygen weaning to maintain a $P_{TC}O_2$ of 60 to 80 mm Hg, or SpO_2 88% to 92%. FIO_2 may be decreased in increments of 2% to 5% to less toxic levels of FIO_2 <0.50. Premature infants often require small increases in FIO_2 as activity levels change, and FIO_2 may be titrated to maintain prescribed SpO_2 levels. Toxic effects of oxygen therapy include retinopathy of prematurity and bronchopulmonary dysplasia. PEEP levels should be reduced as FIO_2 decreases below 0.40 in 1 to 2 cm H_2O increments to approximately 5 cm H_2O. Patients are commonly extubated from this PEEP level to preserve the FRC of the lung.

Delivered tidal volume must be routinely measured as compliance improves to avoid over distension of the

Box 45-7 • Considerations for Extubation

- Spontaneous respiratory rate for age and weight
- Presence of apnea or periodic breathing
- Work of breathing
- Amount and consistency of respiratory secretions
- Vital signs
- Sedation needs
- SpO_2
- Spontaneous V_T

lung and reduce barotrauma. When adequacy of tidal volume is ensured at peak inspiratory pressure (PIP) <25 cm H_2O for term infants to children, the rate can be weaned in 2 to 4 breath increments to further reduce ventilatory support. When set rates approach <10 breaths per minute, F_{IO_2} <0.40, PEEP of 5 cm H_2O, and PIP <25 cm H_2O, the patient should be evaluated for extubation. Extubation to nasal CPAP is a common practice in neonates. Criteria to consider before extubation are listed in Box 45-7.

Upper airway edema from prolonged intubation should also be assessed measuring the amount of inspiratory pressure required to cause an air leak around the endotracheal tube. If pressure is >25 cm H_2O, a short course of intravenous steroid therapy may be indicated, as well as aerosolized racemic epinephrine postextubation. Patients are usually extubated from intermittent mandatory ventilation rates of 4 to 8 breaths/minute to minimize the work of breathing associated with small endotracheal tubes. Patients may be extubated to nasal CPAP, oxygen hood, or nasal cannula.

Assessment of expiratory synchrony is often overlooked as a factor in ventilator weaning. Expiratory synchrony is a function of FRC, auto-PEEP, and expiratory resistance. FRC is affected by the set PEEP and lung compliance. If FRC is too low, lung compliance and tidal volume decrease further, while respiratory rate increases to preserve minute ventilation. This creates a breathing pattern (inadequate V_T, increased respiratory rate) characteristic of the "failure to wean." If FRC is too high, pulmonary over distension occurs and alveolar dead space and Pa_{CO_2} increase, another characteristic of the "failure to wean." In either scenario, an inappropriate ventilator strategy (insufficient or excessive PEEP) contributed to the weaning failure.

Management of sedation in mechanically ventilated infants and children requires a uniform approach for all patients. Weaning patients should be maintained at a comfortable, but awake, level to facilitate spontaneous breathing. Sedation should be administered by continuous drip, instead of bolus, to prevent oversedation and maintain a consistent level of comfort. This approach individualizes the sedation to the needs of the patient throughout the day and night. It also reduces incidental agitation and somnolence because sedation is administered more consistently. It also decreases nursing and respiratory care time by maintaining the child in a predictable, consistent level of behavior as mechanical ventilation is decreased and optimizes opportunity to continuously wean across a 24-hour period.

High-Frequency Ventilation

High-frequency ventilation (HFV) is a widely accepted mode of mechanical ventilation in neonatal and pediatric critical care. Often considered nonconventional ventilation, HFV is a conventional mode of ventilation in many pediatric centers for severe respiratory failure and/or pulmonary barotrauma, respiratory distress syndrome (RDS), and air leak syndromes (Box 45-8). HFV has three common characteristics: (1) breathing rates in excess of 150 breaths/minute, (2) tidal volumes of 1 to 3 mL/kg, and (3) noncompliant ventilator circuitry. The three most common types of HFV are: (1) high-frequency jet (HFJV), (2) high-frequency flow interrupter (HFFIV), and (3) high-frequency oscillatory ventilation (HFOV).

HFJV provides a pulse of high-velocity blended gas through a side port. A background ventilator provides PEEP and intermittent bulk sigh volume breaths. Breath rates for HFJV are usually 100 to 600 breaths/minute, and exhalation is passive and facilitated by extremely short inspiratory times (20 to 40 milliseconds, or ms). HFFIVs deliver inspiratory flow to the patient in short bursts by a microprocessor-controlled solenoid valve. These ventilators produce breath rates of 2 to 22 Hz or 120 to 1320 breaths/minute (1 Hz = 60 breaths/minute). During HFFIV, inspiration and exhalation are both active processes. Active exhalation is defined as a drop in airway pressure during exhalation to accelerate exhaled gas flow. Conventional tidal volumes can also be administered intermittently as sigh breaths to prevent atelectasis and maintain end-expiratory lung volume. HFOV can produce breath rates in excess of 3000 breaths/minute with active inspiratory and expiratory phases and tidal volumes less than physiological dead space. This technology vibrates (oscillates) a volume of gas by a diaphragm to create a sinusoidal waveform throughout the conducting airways. A bias flow of fresh, humidified, and warmed gas intersects the oscillatory path to eliminate CO_2 from the circuit and prevent drying of the respiratory mucosa. No bulk sigh breaths are available in HFOV. Oxygenation is adjusted mainly by altering $\overline{P}_{aw}$ and F_{IO_2}. CO_2 elimination depends mainly on the pressure amplitude or gradient (PIP-PEEP).[42]

Box 45-8 • Clinical Indications for HFV

LOW VOLUME STRATEGY
- Air leak syndromes
- Pulmonary interstitial emphysema
- Bronchopleural fistula and pneumothorax
- Pneumomediastinum
- Pneumoperitoneum
- Impaired cardiac function

HIGH VOLUME STRATEGY
- Low lung volume
- High conventional mean airway pressure

Surfactant Replacement Therapy

AARC Clinical Practice Guideline (Excerpts)*

➤ INDICATIONS

- Prophylactic administration is indicated in (1) infants at high risk of developing RDS because of short gestation (<32 weeks) or low birthweight (<1300 g) and (2) infants with known surfactant deficiency
- Rescue therapy is indicated in preterm or full-term infants who (1) require intubation and mechanical ventilation due to increased work of breathing and O_2 requirements and (2) have clinical evidence of RDS

➤ CONTRAINDICATIONS

- Relative contraindications to surfactant administration are:
- The presence of congenital anomalies incompatible with life beyond the neonatal period
- Respiratory distress in infants with laboratory evidence of lung maturity

➤ HAZARDS AND COMPLICATIONS

- Procedural complications resulting from the administration of surfactant include:
  - Plugging of ET tube by surfactant
  - Hb desaturation/need for extra O_2
  - Bradycardia due to hypoxia
  - Pharyngeal deposition of surfactant
  - Administration of surfactant to only one lung
  - Drug dosing errors
  - Trachycardia due to agitation, with reflux of surfactant into ET tube
- Physiological complications of surfactant replacement therapy include:
  - Apnea
  - Pulmonary hemorrhage
  - Mucus plugs
  - Increased necessity for treatment for PDA
  - Marginal increase in ROP
  - Barotrauma with increased lung compliance

➤ ASSESSMENT OF NEED

Determine that valid indications are present:

- Assess lung immaturity prior to prophylactic administration of surfactant (see above)
- Establish the diagnosis of RDS in the presence of short gestation and/or low birthweight

➤ ASSESSMENT OF OUTCOME

- Reduction F_{IO_2} requirement and/or work of breathing
- mprovement in lung volumes and lung fields as indicated by chest radiograph
- Improvement in pulmonary mechanics (e.g., compliance, Raw, VT, VE, FRC, transpulmonary pressure
- Reduction in ventilator requirements (PIP, PEEP, Paw)
- Improvement in ratio of arterial to alveolar P_{O_2} (a/A P_{O_2}), oxygen index

➤ MONITORING

The following should be monitored as part of surfactant replacement therapy:

- Variables to be monitored during surfactant administration:
  - Proper placement of delivery device
  - F_{IO_2} and ventilator settings
  - Reflux of surfactant into ET tube
  - Heart/resp rate, chest expansion, skin color, and vigor
  - Position of patient (i.e., head direction)
  - Chest-wall movement
  - Oxygen saturation by pulse oximetry
- Variables to be monitored after surfactant administration:
  - Arterial blood gases
  - Chest radiography
  - Ventilator PIP, PEEP, Paw, F_{IO_2}
  - Heart/resp rate, chest expansion, skin color, and vigor
  - Pulmonary mechanics and volumes
  - Breath sounds
  - Blood pressure

*For complete guideline see Respir Care (8):824-829, 1994.

CO_2 Elimination During HFV

CO_2 elimination during HFV is determined by delivered alveolar ventilation. However, the minute ventilation delivered with HFV has a greater dependency on alterations in tidal volume rather than breath frequency, with tidal volume most affected by changes in PIP or amplitude (increase PIP or amplitude, increase tidal volume). Ventilator frequency should ideally be set to achieve the resonant frequency (best vibratory pattern) of the lung. The underlying lung structure and age of the patient determine resonant frequency (i.e., premature infants with surfactant depletion have decreased compliance and short time constants, and therefore a higher resonant frequency of the lung). Delivered HFV tidal volume is frequency dependent; as set frequency decreases and percent inspiratory (%I) time remains constant, tidal volume increases, resulting in increased CO_2 elimination and decreased $PaCO_2$. In pediatric patients, resonant frequency is lower; therefore a lower frequency is used. If breathing frequencies are increased for pediatric patients, delivered tidal volume and alveolar ventilation decrease, decreasing CO_2 elimination and increasing $PaCO_2$.

FRC

The delivered $\overline{P}_{aw}$ determines lung expansion during HFV. Because delivered tidal volumes are small, mean lung volume does not change dramatically during inspiration. Therefore FRC remains static around the volume produced by the $\overline{P}_{aw}$ and the compliance of the patient's lung. Set PEEP is the primary contributor to $\overline{P}_{aw}$ and FRC during HFV.

High-Frequency Strategies

Two strategies are used in HFV: (1) high volume strategy (recruitment) and (2) low volume strategy (air leak). The high volume is used to restore FRC by increasing $\overline{P}_{aw}$ until the critical opening pressures of the lung have been exceeded. Collapsed alveoli are then recruited and remain so throughout the ventilatory cycle. Adequate FRC may be determined clinically by observing incremental increases in arterial saturation (SpO_2) as FIO_2 is reduced and by evaluating the degree of lung expansion by chest radiograph. HFV patients should have a mean lung volume on chest radiograph that places the diaphragms at the eighth to ninth rib level.[43]

The low lung volume (air leak) is used to lower $\overline{P}_{aw}$ to the point of resolution of air leak. A higher FIO_2 may be needed to maintain adequate oxygenation.

Cardiovascular Effects

The cardiovascular effects of HFV vary with ventilatory strategy. Utilizing the high lung volume strategy, lung volume is recruited and $\overline{P}_{aw}$ can be slowly reduced while maintaining alveolar ventilation. This limits the adverse side effects of positive pressure ventilation on cardiovascular performance and may result in increased systemic blood flow. However, if mean airway pressures greater than those used during conventional ventilation are required during HFV, cardiovascular compromise may occur. Increases in intravascular volume and inotropic support (vasopressor) may preserve mean arterial blood pressure, cardiac output, and thus oxygen delivery. Increases in central venous pressure (CVP) or decreases in mean arterial pressure indicate decreases in systemic blood flow as a result of volume over distension of the lung and inappropriately high $\overline{P}_{aw}$, after adequate intravascular volume has been established.

Weaning From HFV

When the FIO_2 is equal to or less than 0.6, the $\overline{P}_{aw}$ is weaned slowly. When $\overline{P}_{aw}$ is less than 20 mm Hg, the patient may be trialed off or transitioned to conventional ventilation.

HFV with appropriate strategies has shortened the need for respiratory support and has improved the outcomes of VLBW infants.[44,45]

HFV in pediatric patients with respiratory failure has demonstrated significant improvement in oxygenation and a lower frequency of barotrauma.[46]

Complications of Mechanical Ventilation

Box 45-9 summarizes the most common complications associated with mechanical ventilation of infants.

Box 45-9 • Complications of Mechanical Ventilation in Infants and Children

- Ventilator-induced injuries
- Air leak syndromes
- Pneumothorax
- Pneumomediastinum
- Pneumopericardium
- Pneumoperitoneum
- Pulmonary interstitial emphysema
- Subcutaneous emphysema
- Parenchymal lung damage
- Bronchopulmonary dysplasia
- Cardiovascular complications
- Decreased venous return
- Decreased cardiac output
- Increased pulmonary vascular resistance
- Increased ICP
- Increased incidence of IVH
- Oxygen-induced injuries
- Oxygen toxicity
- Retrolental fibroplasia
- Airway complications
- Accidental extubation
- Atelectasis
- Inadequate humidification
- Endobronchial intubation
- Equipment contamination
- Postintubation stridor
- Endotracheal tube plugging/kinking
- Tracheal lesions
- Infection
- Ventilator-acquired pneumonia

▶ NITRIC OXIDE

Nitric oxide is an FDA-approved drug (gas) administered by inhalation (iNO). Nitric oxide is a selective pulmonary vasodilator. It has been investigated in term and near term newborns with persistent pulmonary hypertension from a variety of etiologies.[47,48] Nitric oxide improves oxygenation and reduces the need for extracorporeal membrane oxygenation (ECMO) by one third or more. Four primary precautions need to be considered when administering iNO.

1. Rebound: abrupt worsening of oxygenation when iNO is discontinued.
2. Methemoglobinemia: an increase in methemoglobin levels has been observed with high doses of iNO.
3. Elevated NO_2 (nitrogen dioxide) levels: these have been noted and need to be monitored.
4. iNO is contraindicated in patients with congenital heart disease who have a ductal dependent right-to-left shunt or pulmonary venous obstruction.

The recommended iNO dose is 20 parts per million (ppm) with optimal lung inflation.[49] A gradual weaning plan should be followed. iNO should be discontinued when 1 to 2 ppm is reached. The health care exposure limit for iNO is 25 ppm and 5 ppm for NO_2. The recommended dose is below the exposure limit and monitoring is generally the only safety precaution. iNO is an important drug for the treatment of pulmonary hypertension and an important responsibility of the respiratory therapist.

▶ EXTRACORPOREAL LIFE SUPPORT (ECLS)

The Extracorporeal Life Support Organization (ELSO) is an international registry of ECLS. As of July 2001, ELSO reported that more than 16,000 neonates have been treated with ECMO with a 78% survival rate. More than 4000 pediatric patients with cardiac or respiratory failure have been treated with ECMO with a 48% survival rate. In the adult population, more than 1000 patients required ECMO with a 45% survival rate. ECMO has become an important clinical adjunct for the complex patient.

ECMO describes a type of ECLS where cardiopulmonary bypass is used for prolonged gas exchange. There are two types of ECMO systems. Venoarterial (VA) bypass requires placement of a cannula into the right atrium by the right internal jugular vein (Figure 45-9). The blood is then oxygenated by the ECMO circuit using a membrane oxygenator, warmed, and returned to the aorta through a cannula placed into the right common carotid artery. Venovenous (VV) bypass is the preferred method and uses a double lumen catheter placed into the right atrium by the right internal jugular vein. The large outer lumen allows for venous drainage of blood, whereas the smaller inner lumen permits the return of oxygenated blood from the membrane oxygenator. Venovenous bypass is associated with fewer complications than the venoarterial route and is preferred when cardiovascular support is not required.[50,51]

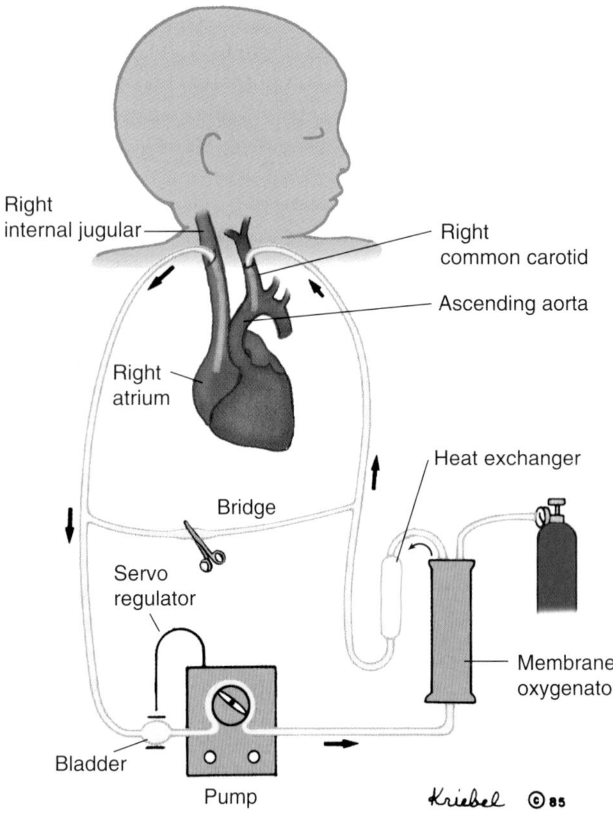

Figure 45-9
Venoarterial ECMO circuit. Venous blood is removed from the right atrium, oxygenated by passage by a diffusing membrane, and then returned to the patient. *(Modified from O'Rourke PP: Respir Care 36:7, 1991.)*

Box 45-10 • Inclusion Criteria for Neonatal ECMO

- Reversible lung disease
- Gestational age 35 weeks
- <Grade II IVH
- Significant shunting:
  - Oxygenation index >40
  - PaO_2 <50 torr with PIP >35 or $\bar{P}_{aw}$ >20
- Persistent acidosis
- Reversible anatomical shunting
- Reversible pulmonary hypertension
- Pulmonary barotrauma

Patients who are selected for ECMO are those who do not respond to maximal medical therapies. The most common disease states in the neonatal population where ECMO is used are persistent pulmonary hypertension (PPHN), meconium aspiration syndrome (MAS), sepsis, perinatal asphyxia, RDS, and congenital diaphragmatic hernia (CDH).[52] Criteria for patient selection are listed in Box 45-10. ECMO is being more widely used in the pediatric population in the treatment of acute respiratory distress syndrome (ARDS) and postoperative cardiac surgery support.

Neonatal-Pediatric Transport

Treatment of a critically ill infant or child is usually provided at a tertiary care facility. Such institutions have the trained staff and equipment needed to perform the complicated procedures that sustain life and aid in recovery. Institutions lacking these capabilities transport their critically ill infants or children to tertiary care facilities. Modes of transportation include ground ambulance, helicopter, or fixed wing aircraft. The transport team sets up an environment in the vehicle that is an extension of the receiving intensive care unit. The transport team is composed of experienced personnel specially trained to provide care for critically ill or injured children.[53] Typical team members include a registered nurse, respiratory therapist, and/or paramedic. Qualifications include one year of neonatal and pediatric critical care and completion of approved programs in pediatric advanced life support (PALS) and neonatal resuscitation (NRP). The role of the respiratory therapist during transport is changing rapidly to include respiratory assessment, airway management, and mechanical ventilation.[53] In addition, many respiratory therapists are cross trained to insert umbilical artery lines, start intravenous lines, and insert chest tubes. The respiratory therapist may be responsible for ensuring that the needed equipment and supplies are available. Box 45-11 lists the basic equipment and supplies needed to provide respiratory care during neonatal and pediatric transport.[54,55]

Box 45-11 • Equipment and Supplies Needed to Provide Respiratory Care During Neonatal and Pediatric Transport

EQUIPMENT

- Adequate supply of oxygen and compressed air
- Air-oxygen blender
- Mechanical ventilator with circuit
- Manual resuscitator capable of giving 100% O_2 with PEEP
- Noninvasive oxygen monitor (Sp_{O_2} or $P_{TC}O_2$)
- Oxygen analyzer
- Airway pressure monitor (electronic or mechanical)
- Electrocardiograph monitor
- Portable suction apparatus
- Laryngoscope handle
- Laryngoscope blades (sizes newborn to adult)
- Extra laryngoscope bulbs and batteries
- Stethoscope

SUPPLIES

- Supplies
- Resuscitation masks (sizes 0, 1, 2, 3, 4)
- Feeding tubes (size 6, 8, and 10 Fr)
- Disposable oxygen hood
- Oxygen connecting tubing
- Disposable hand-held nebulizer with tubing (for bronchodilators)
- Cloth adhesive tape for taping endotracheal tubes
- Tincture of benzoin for taping endotracheal tubes
- Pulse oximeter probes (at least two, in case one fails)
- Endotracheal tubes (sizes 2.5-7.0)
- Stylet
- Forceps
- Suction apparatus

KEY POINTS

- Neonatal and pediatric care is one of the most sophisticated specialty areas in the field of respiratory care. Competent practice in this area requires a firm understanding of the many anatomical and physiological differences between the infant, child, and adult.
- A critical component in the respiratory management of infants and children is thorough clinical assessment. Because of the significant anatomical and physiological differences between adults and infants, many of the assessment techniques useful with older patients do not apply to infants. Ideally, general assessment of the infant begins before birth and involves the maternal history, as well as the fetal and newborn status. As a child grows and develops, more of the assessment methods used with adults begin to apply.
- Respiratory care plan development is based on accurate patient information, detailed knowledge of the disease process, as well as current treatment guidelines and recommendations. Respiratory care modalities provide oxygen, aerosol and humidity, airway care, and mechanical ventilation to the neonate. CPAP is commonly employed in the neonatal patient to overcome atelectasis and oxygenation problems.

References

1. Dubowitz LMS, Dubowitz D, Goldberg C: Clinical assessment of gestational age in the newborn infant, J Pediatr 77:110, 1970.
2. Koff PB, Eitzman DV, Neu J: Neonatal and pediatric respiratory care, ed 2, St Louis, 1993, Mosby.
3. Shenoi A et al: Clinical profile and management of symptomatic patent ductus arteriosus in premature newborns, Indian J Pediatr 28:125, 1991.
4. Carlo WA: Alae nasi activation (nasal flaring) decreases nasal resistance in preterm infants, Pediatrics 72:338, 1983.
5. Courtney SE: Capillary blood gases in the neonate. A reassessment and review of the literature, Am J Dis Child 144:168, 1990.
6. Taussig LM: Determinants of forced expiratory flows in newborn infants, J Appl Physiol 53:1220, 1982.
7. American Thoracic Society: Respiratory mechanics in infants: physiological evaluation in health and disease, Am Rev Respir Dis 147:474, 1993.
8. Quie Pg: Lung defense against infection, J Pediatr 108:813, 1986.
9. American Association for Respiratory Care: Clinical practice guideline. Oxygen therapy in the acute care hospital, Respir Care Clin N Am 36:1410, 1991.
10. Coates AL: Oxygen therapy and long-term pulmonary outcome of respiratory distress syndrome in newborns, Am J Dis Child 13:892, 1982.
11. Flynn J et al: Retinopathy of prematurity. Diagnosis severity, and natural history, Ophthalmology 94:620, 1987.
12. American Academy of Pediatrics, American College of Obstetricians and Gynecologists: Guidelines for perinatal care, ed 2, Evanston, Illinois, 1988.
13. American Association for Respiratory Care: Clinical practice guideline: postural drainage therapy, Respir Care Clin N Am 36:1418, 1991.
14. Mahlmeister MJ et al: Positive expiratory pressure mask therapy: theoretical and practical considerations and a review of the literature, Respir Care Clin N Am 36:1218, 1991.
15. Emery JR, Peabody JL: Head position affects intracranial pressure in newborn infants, J Pediatr 103:950, 1983.
16. Emergency Care Research Institute: Heated wires can melt disposable breathing circuits, Health Devices 18:174, 1989.
17. Levy H, Simpson Q, Duval D: Hazards of humidifiers with heated wires, Crit Care Med 21:477,1993.
18. Gedeon A, Mebius C, Palmer K: Neonatal hygroscopic condenser humidifier, Crit Care Med 15:51, 1987.
19. Rau JL: Delivery of aerosolized drugs to neonatal and pediatric patients, Respir Care Clin N Am 36:514, 1991.
20. Kacmarek RM, Hess D: The interface between patient and aerosol generator, Respir Care Clin N Am 36:952, 1991.
21. Dankle SK, Schuller DE, McClead RE: Prolonged intubation of neonates, Arch Otolaryngol Head Neck Surg 113:841, 1987.
22. Black AE, Hatch DJ, Nauth-Misir N: Complications of tracheal intubation in neonates, infants and children: a review of 4 years' experience in a children's hospital, Br J Anaesth 65:461, 1990.
23. McMillan DD et al: Benefits of orotracheal and nasotracheal intubation in neonates requiring ventilatory assistance, Pediatrics 77:39, 1986.
24. Roopchand R et al: Instability of the tracheal tube in neonates: a postmortem study, Anaesthesia 44:107, 1989.
25. Brown MS: Prevention of accidental extubation in newborns, Am J Dis Child 142:1240, 1988.
26. Prendiville A, Thomson A, Silverman M: Effect of tracheobronchial suction on respiratory resistance in intubated preterm babies, Arch Dis Child 61:1178, 1986.
27. Durand M et al: Cardiopulmonary and intracranial pressure changes related to endotracheal suctioning in preterm infants, Crit Care Med 17:506, 1989.
28. Shah AR et al: Fluctuations in cerebral oxygenation and blood volume during endotracheal suctioning in premature infants, J Pediatr 120:769, 1992.
29. Monaco FJ, Meredith KS: A bench test evaluation of a neonatal closed tracheal suction system, Pediatr Pulmonol 13:121, 1992.
30. Cvetnic WG, Shoptaugh M, Sills JH: Intermittent mandatory ventilation with continuous negative pressure compared with positive end-expiratory pressure for neonatal hypoxemia, J Perinatol 12:316, 1992.
31. Cvetnic WG, Waffarn F, Martin JM: Continuous negative pressure and intermittent mandatory ventilation in the management of pulmonary interstitial emphysema: a preliminary study, J Perinatol 9:26, 1989.
32. Greenough A, Pool J: Neonatal patient triggered ventilation, Arch Dis Child 63:394, 1988.
33. Greenough A, Milner AD: Respiratory support using patient triggered ventilation in the neonatal period, Arch Dis Child 67:69, 1992.
34. Cleary JP et al: Improved oxygenation during synchronized vs. intermittent mandatory ventilation in VLBW infants with respiratory distress: A randomized crossover design, Pediatr Res 33:1226A, 1993.
35. Hickling KG, Walsh J, Henderson S, Jackson R: Low mortality rate in adult respiratory distress syndrome using low-volume, pressure-limited ventilation with permissive hypercapnia: a prospective study, Crit Care Med 22:1568, 1995.
36. Amato MBP et al. Effect of a protective-ventilation strategy on mortality in the acute respiratory distress syndrome, N Engl J Med 338:347, 1998.
37. Brochard L et al: Tidal volume reduction for prevention of ventilator-induced lung injury in acute respiratory distress syndrome, Am J Respir Crit Care Med 158:1831, 1998.
38. Stewart TE et al: Evaluation of a ventilation strategy to prevent barotrauma in patients at high risk for acute respiratory distress syndrome, N Engl J Med 338:355, 1998.
39. Wilson BG, Cheifetz IM, Meliones JN: The use of airway graphic analysis to optimize mechanical ventilation in small infants and children, Palm Springs, California, Bird Products Corporation, 1996.
40. Hess DR, Kacmarek R: Essentials of mechanical ventilation, ed 2, New York, McGraw-Hill, 2002, pp 271-283.
41. Cannon ML et al: Tidal volumes for ventilated infants should be determined with a pneumotachometer placed at the endotracheal tube, Am J Respir Crit Care Med 162:2109, 2000.

42. Coghill CH et al: Neonatal and pediatric high-frequency ventilation: principles and practice, Respir Care Clin N Am 36:596, 1991.
43. Minton S, Gertsman D et al: Early intervention in respiratory distress syndrome, Cardiopulmonary Review: Current Application and Economics, Yorba Linda, Calif, Sensomedics Critical Care, 1995.
44. Rimensberger PC et al: First intention high-frequency oscillation with early lung volume optimization improves pulmonary outcome in very low birth weight infants with respiratory distress syndrome, Pediatrics 105:1202, 2000.
45. Gerstmann DR et al: The Provo Multicenter Early High-frequency Oscillatory Ventilation Trial: improved pulmonary and clinical outcome in respiratory distress, Pediatrics 98:1044, 1996.
46. Arnold JH: Prospective, randomized comparison of high-frequency oscillatory ventilation and conventional mechanical ventilation in pediatric respiratory failure, Crit Care Med 22:1530, 1994.
47. The National Inhaled Nitric Oxide Study Group: Inhaled nitric oxide in full-term and nearly full-term infants with hypoxic respiratory failure, N Engl J Med 336:597, 1997.
48. Clark RH et al: Low dose nitric oxide therapy for persistent pulmonary hypertension of the newborn. Clinical Inhaled Nitric Oxide Research Group, N Engl J Med 342:469, 2000.
49. Package insert: INOmax® nitric oxide for inhalation, INO Therapeutics, Inc, Clinton, New Jersey.
50. O'Rourke PP: ECMO: where have we been? Where are we going? Respir Care 36(7):683-692, 1991.
51. O'Rourke PP: ECMO: current status, Neonatal Respir Dis 3:14, 911, 1993.
52. Thompson JE, Perlman N: Extracorporeal membrane oxygenation. In Koff PB, Eitzman DV, Neu J: Neonatal and pediatric respiratory care, ed 2, St Louis, 1993, Mosby.
53. Day SE: Intratransport, stabilization, and management of the pediatric patient, Pediatr Clin N Am 40:263, 1993.
54. American Academy of Pediatrics, Committee on Hospital Care: Guidelines for air and ground transportation of pediatric patients, Pediatrics 78:945, 1986.
55. Sayler JW: Transport of the critically ill and injured, Respir Care Clin N Am 36:720, 1991.

SECTION VII

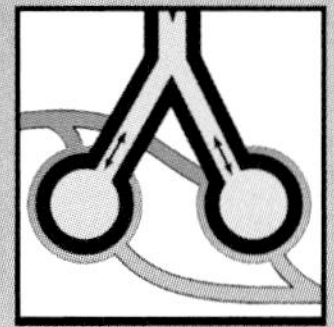

Preventative and Long-Term Care

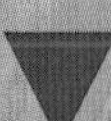
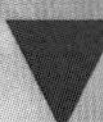
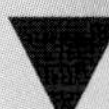

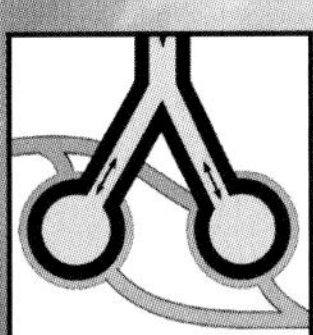

CHAPTER 46

Patient Education and Health Promotion

John A. Evans and Robert L. Wilkins

In This Chapter You Will Learn:

- How to write learning objectives in the cognitive, affective, and psychomotor domains
- How the adult and child learner are different
- How to evaluate patient education
- Why health education is important
- Which settings may be appropriate for implementation of health promotion activities
- How health promotion and disease prevention affect medical costs

Chapter Outline

Key Terms

affective domain
cognitive domain
disease prevention
health education
health promotion
psychomotor domain

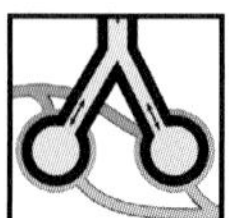

The role of the registered respiratory therapist (RRT) in patient education and health promotion is evolving. RRTs are frequently called on to educate patients about their cardiopulmonary diseases and techniques for treatment. In addition, RRTs may participate in health promotion programs such as smoking cessation classes. For these reasons, this chapter reviews important issues related to patient education and health promotion.

The top five causes of death in the United States are heart disease, cancer, cerebrovascular disease, chronic obstructive pulmonary disease (COPD), and accidents.[1] It should be noted that COPD has moved from the fifth cause of death to the fourth since 1998. It is believed by most experts in healthcare that the majority of these illnesses are preventable. Education of the public about the risk factors central to the prevention of these diseases probably has the greatest potential to make an impact on healthcare in our country. Thus, the emphasis in our current healthcare system should be on health promotion and disease prevention. RRTs will play a greater role in health promotion in the future.

▶ PATIENT EDUCATION

If we think of patient care as customer service, which it indeed should be, we cannot ignore education as a key component of that service. Whether we buy a car or a television set, we expect the salesperson to educate us about essential aspects of our purchase. We also expect this information to be provided to us in writing, and we even expect a guarantee. Likewise, education is an essential component of patient care. For patients to assume or resume control of their health, they must be educated. Because they rely on the healthcare practitioner to provide this education, every respiratory care curriculum should include didactic, laboratory, and clinical instruction on how to perform patient education. Knowledge is power. Education is an art.

Learning occurs in the following three domains: (1) cognitive, (2) affective, and (3) psychomotor. The *cognitive domain* involves helping a patient understand particular facts and/or concepts; the *affective domain* centers around the patient's attitude and motivational level; and the *psychomotor domain* refers to the patient's ability to perform a physical task. An effective RRT will provide patient education that encompasses all of these levels. Initially, it may be helpful for the RRT to develop written learning objectives for each domain, appropriate for the specific patient education topic that is to be addressed. These learning objectives will specify the teaching strategy for the patient education session. Objectives make clear what is to be accomplished and how, as well as providing direction and a method for evaluating the educational process. Just as it is essential for the classroom instructor to be prepared before each class session, it also is essential for the RRT to be prepared to provide high-quality patient education.

Cognitive Domain

The cognitive domain is probably the most recognizable to the RRT and may be the easiest to translate into learning objectives. These are facts and concepts that the RRT wants the patient to know and understand by the end of the education session. Objectives should be stated in measurable terms (operational) so that the RRT and the patient can recognize when the objective has been accomplished. To state an objective in behavioral terms, begin with a verb. Each objective should include a single patient behavior. For example, if the patient is to receive oxygen therapy, the RRT needs to convey certain factual information. Objectives for the cognitive domain might include the following: *identify* the indications for oxygen therapy; *state* the importance of using the prescribed liter flow; *explain* in writing the relationship between oxygen and combustion. Any factual information that you expect the patient to know, understand, or recognize falls under the cognitive domain.

Affective Domain

To convey cognitive information to the patient, the affective domain must first be evaluated. The patient's attitude and motivation to learn affect the other two learning domains. It is important to remember with patient education, timing is everything. Patients who have recently been given a poor prognosis or are in pain may not be in an optimal position to absorb the RRT's instruction. Maslow has suggested a hierarchy of needs, identifying physiological need as the most basic of human needs, followed by safety, love, esteem, and self-actualization.[2] Lower level needs must first be satisfied to move on to higher needs. For example, if a patient is dyspneic or in pain, he or she will probably not be receptive to learning the steps involved in cleaning a small-volume nebulizer (SVN). RRTs should assess a patient's readiness to learn by talking with the patient and his or her family, and by listening to the patient's concerns. It is important to develop a relationship of trust, and to be empathetic to the patient's concerns.

The RRT should begin with easy to master facts and skills. As the patient conquers these, motivation should increase as a feeling of accomplishment is fostered. Motivation is also enhanced by presenting material clearly, using a variety of teaching methods, and relating the facts and skills to practical applications. Getting patients to see "what's in it for them" is the key to motivation. Communicating to the patient that there is something they can do to maintain or improve their lifestyle is a necessary affective task.

Patients are best able to learn if they understand their disease process and what is expected of them; they accept their diagnosis; and they receive instruction both verbally and in writing.

Objectives in the affective domain, using the oxygen therapy example mentioned earlier, might include the following: *agree* that oxygen therapy is necessary; *verbalize* willingness to use it appropriately; and *follow* appropriate guidelines for its use.

Psychomotor Domain

Patients and their families exhibit a wide range of mechanical abilities, as do the therapists who are assigned to teach them. It is important to keep in mind that because a patient requires more time and repetition to become proficient at a given task, it does not mean that he or she is less intelligent or unmotivated. Relating skills that the patient uses on a daily basis (washing dishes) to skills necessary for performance of the psychomotor skill at hand (cleaning of equipment), patients may more readily associate everyday living tasks to those that are required for their treatment plan.

When teaching a psychomotor skill, repetition is key. Patients will remember 10% of what they hear, but more than 50% of what they do. Again, it is important to emphasize that the skill should have practical application.

MINI CLINI

Developing Learning Objectives for Using an Albuterol Metered-Dose Inhaler

PROBLEM

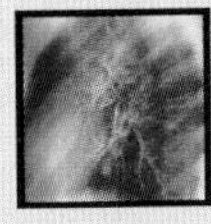

Your 31-year-old patient is newly diagnosed with asthma and is being discharged tomorrow. She requires instruction on how to properly use her albuterol metered-dose inhaler (MDI). Develop learning objectives for her, addressing each learning domain.

SOLUTION

Use a variety of learning objectives, including the following:

Cognitive domain: Describe the action of albuterol on bronchial smooth muscle; recognize when to seek medical attention.

Affective domain: Agree that it is important not to skip a dose; verbalize willingness to use the MDI; feel satisfaction by controlling the disease.

Psychomotor domain: Assemble the MDI and spacer; inhale slowly and deeply with inspiratory hold; shake the canister between puffs.

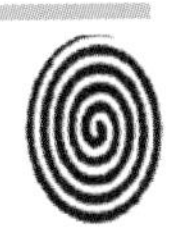

RULE OF THUMB

People learn by doing. Get the learner involved.

To confirm performance in the psychomotor domain, have your patients provide a return demonstration. During a return demonstration, patients show you what you taught them, repeating the steps in the procedure that you demonstrated. Be sure to provide help and encouragement as needed, and be patient—not everyone picks up skills at the same rate.

Learning objectives that may be categorized in the psychomotor domain under *oxygen therapy* include: *operate* an oxygen concentrator; *adjust* the flowmeter; and *change* the nasal cannula as necessary.

Teaching Tips

Following is a list of time-honored suggestions for improving patient education:

- Deal with the patient's immediate concerns first.
- Create a learning environment. Teach in a quiet and relaxed setting.
- Have patients use as many senses as possible during their learning session. Include hearing, seeing, touching, writing, and speaking whenever possible.
- Keep sessions short. If the material is complex, break it down into brief segments.
- Repeat, repeat, repeat!
- Provide many opportunities for the patient to practice psychomotor skills.
- Be prepared.
- Be organized.
- Demonstrate enthusiasm for what you are doing. The learner can always discern your level of motivation.
- Evaluate in a nonthreatening way and give good feedback.

Teaching Children Versus Adult Learners

Teaching children is often very different than teaching adults. Children are more motivated by external factors such as prizes as compared to adults who tend to have internal motivating factors. This suggests that adults will learn because they can easily see the intrinsic value of knowing more about their illness. Children, on the other hand, may need a more obvious reward system in place before learning can take place. Children have no problem taking instruction from adults because they are often dependent on such instruction. Adults, however, are more independent and do not like being dependent on others. This suggests that adults should be more involved in setting program goals and will readily learn skills that make them more independent. Other important issues related to differences between children and adult learners are listed in Box 46-1.

Box 46-1 • Learning Differences Between Children and Adults

CHILD
- Is motivated by external factors like grades
- Is directed by others
- Learning is big part of his or her life
- Trusts teacher
- Has limited experience
- Learns for the future
- Learns quickly
- Tends to learn according to developmental stage
- Has no problem with slow pace of learning
- Is subject oriented

ADULT
- Is motivated internally
- Is self directed
- Learning is only one part of his or her life
- Questions teacher
- Has rich experiences
- Learns for the present
- May learn more slowly
- Varies in learning ability
- Dislikes slow pace of learning
- Is problem oriented

MINI CLINI

MDI Instruction for a Pediatric Patient

PROBLEM

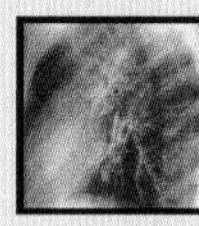

How would your approach to MDI instruction change if your patient was a 7-year-old boy suffering from asthma?

SOLUTION

Although the learning objectives may remain the same, the methods may be different. You may compare the slow, deep inspiration to getting ready to blow out the candles on a birthday cake. You may use swimming under water as an image to encourage breathholding. Use simple diagrams to show how the medication will act on his lungs. If he likes sports, tell him about athletes who compete well in spite of their asthma (you also can use this illustration to stress the importance of controlling the asthma). An abundance of resource material is available for the child with asthma—make use of it. Many local, state, and national lung associations offer such learning aids as age-appropriate books, coloring books, and puppets to make the learning process fun.

Evaluation of Patient Education

The critical question that remains when all of the education sessions are complete is, "Has the patient learned?" Evaluation is the process that answers that question. The method used to evaluate learning is determined by the learning objectives (i.e., cognitive, affective, psychomotor). Cognitive objectives are often evaluated through the use of a written examination. Objectives in the affective and psychomotor domains are evaluated through the use of performance check sheets.

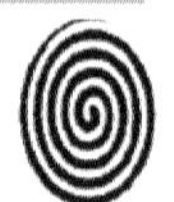

RULE OF THUMB

Evaluation results reflect the quality of instruction as much as the degree of learning.

Evaluation should occur both during and after the educational process. While the educational process is occurring, patients provide both positive and negative feedback to the therapist on many levels, for example, a puzzled look, a correct response to a question, or proper performance of a skill. Use these responses to either reinforce behavior or make adjustments to the education plan to achieve the desired results.

The Teachable Moment

The formal education process has been discussed previously. However, it is crucial for all healthcare practitioners to be alert for those "teachable moments," which often occur outside of a formal session. RRTs treat patients daily who have questions about their disease process and their care. It is very important to address these concerns with empathy and genuine concern, while listening to the patients' needs and responding to them appropriately and in a timely manner. Teachable moments are important, but they should not be the RRT's sole plan of action so far as education is concerned.

Practice Guidelines

Patient education is a key element of care. The American Association for Respiratory Care (AARC) has added two clinical practice guidelines addressing education, *Providing Patient and Caregiver Training* and *Training the Healthcare Professional for the Role of Patient and Caregiver Education*. For excerpts, see pp. 1195-1996.

▶ HEALTH EDUCATION

Health education may have been the earliest form of organized health promotion in the United States. In 1842, Horace Mann advocated health education in the

PROVIDING PATIENT AND CAREGIVER TRAINING

AARC Clinical Practice Guideline (Excerpts)*

➤ **INDICATIONS**
Patients who need to increase knowledge and understanding of health status and therapy; improve skills needed for safe and effective healthcare; and develop a positive attitude, strong motivation, and increased compliance.

➤ **CONTRAINDICATIONS**
None.

➤ **COMPLICATIONS**
Omission of essential steps concerning care, presentation of inconsistent information, or failure to validate the learning process can lead to unfavorable results.

➤ **LIMITATIONS**
- *For the patient:* Lack of motivation; impairment (physical, mental, or emotional); inability to understand instruction; illiteracy; language barriers; religious and/or cultural beliefs that are at odds with the material presented.
- *For the RCP:* Lack of a positive attitude or flexibility; limited knowledge of skill being taught; inadequate assessment of patient's readiness to learn; cultural or religious practices that may affect learning; inability to personalize the material; insufficient time; inadequate communication skills.
- *For the system:* Hospital stay too brief; lack of interdisciplinary communication and/or cooperation; inconsistent information presented; lack of an interpreter.
- *Other factors:* Lack of support system for the patient; reimbursement issues; interruptions, distractions, or noise; inadequate lighting, heat, or space; poorly chosen resources (e.g., incorrect reading level).

➤ **ASSESSMENT OF NEED**
Determine the gap between what the patient knows and what he or she needs to know. Apply this to cognitive, psychomotor, and affective domains.

➤ **ASSESSMENT OF OUTCOME**
Evaluate knowledge gained, skills mastered, and patient outlook and attitude.

➤ **MONITORING**
The monitoring of the training processes should include awareness of the patient's verbal and nonverbal responses, including eye contact, listening skills, and participation in discussion.

*For complete guideline see Respir Care 41:658, 1996.

public schools. It was not until 1875, however, that it became widespread. In that year, the Women's Christian Temperance Union lobbied for alcohol education in the schools. As a result of its efforts, 38 states passed legislation to require it. From that time, health education has been enhanced and expanded in our schools. We also now have public health agencies at the local, state, national, and international levels that provide health education and care for those who would otherwise have none.

Health education is a process of planned learning designed to enable individuals to make informed decisions and take responsible action regarding their health. The primary goal of health education is behavioral change. It is designed to promote, maintain, and improve both individual and community health. Health education covers the continuum between health and disease, between prevention and treatment.

As with health promotion, health education can occur on two levels, addressing both individuals and groups. It can occur in a variety of settings, from the home or school to the workplace or healthcare agency or institution. To be effective, health education must be combined with strategies for health promotion—the two are inextricably linked.

Although individuals must ultimately assume responsibility for their own health, promoting healthy behaviors through education is an important function of healthcare personnel. In this capacity, the RRT should serve as a role model for the public. Unless healthcare professionals

Training of the Healthcare Professional (HCP) for the Role of Patient and Caregiver Educator

AARC Clinical Practice Guideline (Excerpts)*

➤ INDICATIONS

- HCPs who must educate patients and caregivers about knowldege, skills, and motivation necessary to effectively participate in healthcare
- Evidence that HCPs lack the knowledge about educational principles and practices needed to:
  - Assess educational needs
  - Prepare educational objectives tailored to individuals or groups
  - Accomplish learning objectives
  - Prepare educational materials
  - Supervise practice of skills
  - Give feedback and assess outcomes
  - Modify educational efforts according to individual or group response

➤ CONTRAINDICATIONS

None.

➤ COMPLICATIONS

Inadequate training of the HCP may cause harm to the patient or inhibit the patient's ability to participate in the management of his or her own health.

➤ LIMITATIONS

- *Of the HCP:* Lack of educational preparation; unreceptive or inept; lack of interdisciplinary cooperation; inability to modify learning objectives based on age, culture, or religion; inability to communicate effectively
- *Of the system:*Inadequate time, space, or financial resources; insufficient faculty for training program; inconsistent information provided to the HCP
- *Of the patient or caregiver:* Negative attitude; lack of basic education; presence of a language barrier or perception of cultural conflict

➤ ASSESSMENT OF NEED

HCPs who provide education should be periodically assessed for adequate knowledge and skills by observation in a patient education setting and by a specialist.

➤ ASSESSMENT OF OUTCOME

Evaluate verbally and in writing; observe HCP in teaching setting; evaluate whether goals set concerning knowledge, skills, compliance, and attitude have been met; evaluate long-term through institutional quality improvement indicators.

➤ MONITORING

HCP training should include evidence of classes and in-service training; availability of written and audiovisual resources; and evaluation of training effectiveness.

*For complete guideline see Respir Care 41:654, 1996.

model healthy behaviors, successful health outcomes cannot be expected from the public. To this end, the AARC has created a role model statement to encourage RRTs to set a positive example for the public (Box 46-2).[3]

Providing a good example is not enough to ensure successful health education programming. For the desired outcomes to be achieved, certain conditions must first be met. The components are strikingly similar to patient education requirements. The essential components of effective health education are as follows:

1. Program participants must be actively engaged in the learning process.
2. Activities must incorporate the values and health beliefs of the learner. Familial, cultural, societal, and economic factors must be considered.

Box 46-2 • AARC Role Model Statement

As healthcare professionals engaged in the performance of cardiopulmonary care, RRTs must strive to maintain the highest personal and professional standards.

In addition to upholding the code of ethics, the RRT shall serve as a leader and advocate of public health.

The RRT shall participate in activities leading to awareness of the causes and prevention of pulmonary disease and the problems associated with the cardiopulmonary system. The RRT shall support the development and promotion of pulmonary disease awareness programs, to include smoking cessation programs, pulmonary function screenings, air pollution monitoring, allergy warnings, and other public education programs.

The RRT shall support research to improve health and prevent disease.

The RRT shall provide leadership in determining health promotion and disease prevention activities for students, faculty, practitioners, patients, and the general public.

The RRT shall serve as a physical example of cardiopulmonary health by abstaining from tobacco use and shall make a special personal effort to eliminate smoking and the use of other tobacco products from the home and work environment.

The RRT shall strive to be a model for all members of the healthcare team by demonstrating responsibility and cooperating with other healthcare professionals to meet the health needs of the public.

Effective 3/90
Revised 3/00

From American Association for Respiratory Care; Position Statement, 11030 Ables Lane, Dallas, TX 75229.

3. The role of the health educator is to facilitate behavioral change. Thus, the learning process should be approached cooperatively.
4. The development of predisposing, enabling, and reinforcing health attitudes requires effort, which will only reap results over time.
5. The healthcare practitioner must be willing to listen nonjudgmentally to the concerns of the learners. Empathy and understanding are necessary to foster a trusting relationship.
6. The level of learners' self-esteem and self-concept may either enhance or inhibit their ability to make decisions regarding their own health. The healthcare professional should be willing to provide emotional support as necessary.
7. The health educator's personal characteristics have a direct impact on the outcome of the educational program. Generally, successful outcomes occur as a result of confidence, without arrogance or an authoritative approach.

For RRTs to assist patients, caregivers, or the public in developing healthier life-styles, greater emphasis must be placed upon health promotion and disease prevention strategies.

▶ HEALTH PROMOTION AND DISEASE PREVENTION

In 1999, the United States spent $1.2 trillion on healthcare. Of this, $4.4 billion was allocated to government public health agencies designed for health promotion and disease prevention.[4] Four out of five of the major causes of death in the United States are heart disease, cancer, cerebrovascular disease, and COPD. These diseases have four central causes and are, in large part, preventable. Primary causes include a high-fat diet, excessive alcohol use, use of tobacco products, and inactivity.[5]

The standard medical practice in this country, based on the medical model, has been to diagnose and treat disease, rather than to prevent illness. Medical students learn to identify causes of disease and suggest treatments, rather than to identify risk factors present in their patients and suggest behavioral changes. High-risk individuals are counseled by these physicians and other healthcare professionals on a one-to-one basis in an effort to change their behavior.

Conversely, the public health model attempts to reduce disease in the nation as a whole through mass education campaigns. Examples include education about the hazards of drinking and driving, smoking, and food labeling to indicate fat and cholesterol content. RRTs are in the enviable position of having the potential to impact health on both of these levels (individual and population).

Prevention can occur on three levels: primary, secondary, and tertiary. The goal of *primary prevention* is to prevent occurrence of the disease, through immunization, for example. The goal of *secondary prevention* is early detection of disease, by PAP smears and mammograms, for example. The goal of *tertiary prevention* is to prevent acceleration of the disease process once it has occurred, with pulmonary rehabilitation being a good example. Certain diseases, such as breast cancer, must receive their focus at the secondary level. Others, where the causes have been identified and are preventable (acquired immunodeficiency syndrome [AIDS], hypertension, heart disease, COPD), should be approached as primary prevention. The public health approach attempts to reduce disease in the nation as a whole through mass education efforts. Who could have predicted the success of mass education in smoking cessation efforts over the past 30 years?

Other recent efforts, such as Healthy People 2010, have attempted to place the focus on the health of the population rather than on the individual.[6] The two broad goals of this plan are as follows: (1) to increase quality and years of healthy life; (2) to eliminate health disparities. These goals encompass the essential elements of health promotion and disease prevention, which are prevention of premature death, disease, and disability and improvement in the quality of life.

The recognition that allied health professionals play a vital role in these activities prompted professional organizations to develop policy statements about health promotion and disease prevention. The AARC policy statement appears in Box 46-3.[7]

RRTs can and should take an active role in developing educational materials to assist both the public and other health professionals in health promotion activities. "Peak Performance U.S.A." is a good example of one such project, developed by the AARC to improve the delivery of asthma care to children.[8] This project connects community school districts and local hospitals to educate school nurses about asthma management. Many medical manufacturers have also developed asthma kits of various types that include peak flowmeters, spacers, and educational materials. These are generally done with input from the medical community, in particular RRTs. Respiratory care educational programs need to be diligent in incorporating health promotion and disease prevention activities into all learning domains as part of their curricula.

Another specific area of health promotion that receives much attention in both the hospital and public health settings is nicotine intervention. Seventy percent of smokers report that they would like to quit but cannot.[9] Smoking cessation aids such as nicotine gum and nicotine patches are now available over-the-counter. But, these are far from a quick fix. Nicotine intervention is a progressive, comprehensive program incorporating a series of steps from risk identification to maintenance support. Coping strategies, withdrawal symptoms, weight, diet, exercise, support systems, and preparation/transformation of the home, are some of these steps. National, state, and local agencies, such as the American Cancer Society, American Lung Association, and American Heart Association, all offer educational materials and behavioral counseling. However, the RRT is in a unique position to influence the hospitalized patient or the patient receiving home healthcare. These patients may be suffering from nicotine withdrawal symptoms (the worst step for many) and may be more easily persuaded to attempt quitting. RRTs are well positioned in these settings, and it is important that they receive training as part of their educational preparation in nicotine intervention strategies.

Box 46-3 • Health Promotion and Disease Prevention

The AARC submits this paper to identify and illustrate the involvement of the RRT in the promotion of health and prevention of disease and supports these activities. The AARC realizes that RRTs are integral members of the healthcare team, in hospitals, home healthcare settings, pulmonary laboratories, rehabilitation programs, and all other environments where respiratory care is practiced.

The AARC recognizes that education and training of the RRT is the best method by which to instill the ability to improve the patient's quality and longevity of life, and that such information should be included in their formal education and training.

The AARC recognizes the RRT's responsibility to participate in pulmonary disease teaching, smoking cessation programs, pulmonary function studies for the public, air pollution alerts, allergy warnings, and sulfite warnings in restaurants, as well as research in those and other areas where efforts could promote improved health and disease prevention. Furthermore, the RRT is in a unique position to provide leadership in determining health promotion and disease prevention activities for students, faculty, practitioners, patients, and the general public.

The AARC recognizes the need to provide and promote consumer education related to the prevention and control of pulmonary disease and to establish a strong working relationship with other health agencies, educational institutions, federal and state government, businesses and other community organizations and to monitor such. Furthermore, the AARC supports efforts to develop personal and professional wellness models and action plans that will inspire and encourage all RRTs to cooperate on health promotion and disease prevention.

Effective 7/85
Revised 3/00

From American Association for Respiratory Care; Position Statement, 11030 Ables Lane, Dallas, TX 75229.

▶ IMPLICATIONS FOR RRTs

Because the RRT is able to function as both an individual counselor and a public health advocate, depending upon the setting and/or circumstance, it is useful to examine the most likely settings where the RRT's health promotion and disease prevention knowledge can be put to good use.

Healthcare Institutions

Healthcare institutions where RRTs provide both health education and promotion include in-patient facilities, such as hospitals and skilled nursing facilities, and ambulatory care centers, such as physicians' offices, clinics, or HMOs.

As primary prevention activists, RRTs may be involved with schools in their communities, educating children about the dangers of smoking. They may participate in wellness programs for staff and patients aimed at improving cardiopulmonary wellness through exercise.

In the area of secondary prevention, RRTs can perform blood pressure and pulmonary function screenings at local health fairs or other sites in their communities.

Tertiary prevention activities in healthcare institutions include pulmonary rehabilitation and asthma management education.

Work Site

Many studies have shown that healthier workers are absent from work less often, more satisfied with their job, and more productive. This all translates into a more cost-effective workplace. RRTs may find themselves involved in work site wellness by participating in the following: (1) performing pulmonary function and/or blood pressure screenings; (2) developing and implementing stress management or nicotine intervention programs; and (3) consulting on policies related to smoking and occupational or environmental exposure, such as asbestos, cotton, or silica dust.

Home

Home healthcare continues to be a rapidly growing segment of the healthcare industry. It has been proven time and again to be more cost-effective than hospital care. RRTs can perform a wide variety of services in the patient's home, from oxygen therapy to mechanical ventilation, on either a temporary or chronic basis. Generally, the focus is on tertiary prevention (preventing further decline). Patient education is of primary importance in the home in order for the patient to become as self-reliant as possible (see Chapter 47).

Community

Most of the health promotion activities described above pertain to the individual. At the community level, the focus is on the group. Community health promotion activities provided by the RRT may include the following: smoking cessation, family asthma management education, and COPD (better breathing) support groups. RRTs, who are BCLS certified instructors, also may volunteer to perform BCLS certification for various groups, or serve as educators and exhibitors at community health fairs.

Educational Institutions

Because many unhealthy behaviors begin in early childhood or adolescence, elementary, middle, and secondary schools are excellent places to begin health education activities. Education about smoking is one example.

Cigarette smoking is a primary risk factor associated with many of today's leading causes of death. Because most smoking begins in late childhood or early adolescence, schools provide the best setting in which to educate children about the dangers of tobacco. RRTs are well-equipped to provide these experiences. It is never too early to begin sending the antismoking message.

It is important to remember that among children, family members and their behaviors exert a strong influence on the children's knowledge level and attitudes about smoking, so plan on trying to reach the parents as well. Research shows that the more times individuals are approached about smoking cessation, the greater the likelihood that they will attempt to quit. The more times they try, the more likely they are to be successful. The RRT should also focus on the impact that peers and the media have on a child's decision to smoke.

RRTs also would do well to set a good example for the college and university students who may be completing clinical rotations under their tutelage.

▶ HEALTH PROMOTION, DISEASE PREVENTION, AND MEDICAL CARE COSTS

It is generally true that prevention of illness can reduce the cost of healthcare to society. However, primary prevention through mass public education is far more cost-effective than health education based on the current medical model, which seeks only to diagnose and then treat.[10] If methods known to decrease the incidence of coronary heart disease, cancer, and stroke (smoking cessation, reduced cholesterol levels, and decreased blood pressure) were intensified, healthcare costs associated with these illnesses could be reduced by 50%, or $1 billion per year.[11]

The goals of health promotion and disease prevention are to delay disability and death and maximize quality of life. Improvements in the standard of living, public health measures, and preventive medical care have made great strides toward that end. To a degree, individuals are increasingly accountable for their own health. Americans can choose to be healthy by avoiding tobacco, too much alcohol, inactivity, and foods high in fat. RRTs need to be at the center of health promotion and disease prevention activities. However, before this can occur, RRTs must be educated about educating. They need to understand and then practice the process of education. For patients, students, community, and peers to become as healthy as they can be, RRTs need to adopt an attitude of collaboration in a variety of settings, under many different circumstances. A patient's quality of life is directly linked to the quality of education he or she receives concerning his care. What better motivation to practice the art of education?

KEY POINTS

- Educators should use learning objectives from the cognitive, affective, and psychomotor domains when teaching most health-related knowledge and skills.
- Learning objectives should be written in operational terms.
- Review the teaching tips before you teach.
- Evaluate your teaching, so you can improve.
- The RRT has an impact on several areas of health education and health promotion, including nicotine intervention, asthma education, and community health screening.
- Health promotion and disease prevention activities, such as public education about smoking prevention and cessation and community and industrial PFT screening, can improve our nation's healthcare.

References

1. National Vital Statistics Report, Vol 49, No 3, June 26, 2001.
2. Maslow AH: A theory of human motivation, Psychology in Review 50:370, 1943.
3. AARC: Position statements: AARC Role Model Statement, March 2000, Dallas, AARC.
4. Internet source: Healthcare Financing Administration Office of the Actuary National Health Statistics Group; www.hcfa.gov/stats/NHE-0act/Lessons, 1999.
5. McGinnis JM, Foege WH: Actual causes of death in the United States, JAMA 270:2207, 1993.
6. Public Health Service, Office of Disease Prevention and Health Promotion: Healthy People 2010 (Stock No. 017-001-00547-9), Washington, DC, 1990, U.S. Government Printing Office.
7. AARC: Position Statements: Health promotion and disease prevention statement, March 2000, Dallas, Texas.
8. Bunch D: AARC launches nationwide "Peak performance U.S.A" project, AARC Times 17:39, 1993.
9. Fiore MC et al: Treating tobacco use and dependence. Quick reference guide for clinicians. Rockville, MD: U.S. Department of Health and Human Services. Public Health Service. October 2000.
10. Harvey B: Toward a national health policy, JAMA 264:252, 1990.
11. Terris M: Healthy lifestyles: the perspective of epidemiology, J Public Health Policy 13:186, 1992.

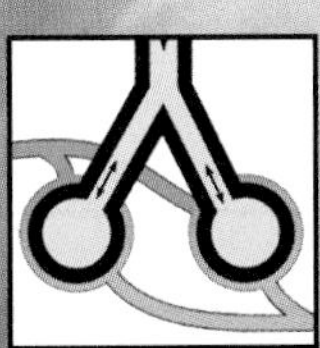

CHAPTER 47

Nutritional Aspects of Health and Disease

Georgia E. Hodgkin and Cynthia Ann Kwiatkowski

In This Chapter You Will Learn:

- What constitutes a healthful diet
- What dietary allowances are recommended for protein, vitamins, and key minerals
- How macronutrients supply the body's energy requirements
- What factors influence energy and macronutrient needs
- How to estimate daily resting energy expenditure (REE)
- What role vitamins, minerals, dietary fiber, and antioxidants play in good nutrition
- How starvation differs from hypercatabolic malnutrition
- How micronutrient deficiencies can impair function
- What effects malnutrition has on the respiratory system
- How a comprehensive nutrition assessment is conducted
- How to identify patients at high risk for malnutrition
- What indications, contraindications, hazards, and limitations apply to indirect calorimetry
- How to properly prepare a patient for indirect calorimetry
- How to interpret the results of indirect calorimetry
- How REE values are adjusted to reflect a patient's actual energy needs
- What effect too much protein, carbohydrate, or fat can have on a patient
- When enteral nutrition and parenteral nutrition are needed
- How to identify and minimize the common respiratory complications of enteral feedings
- What specific nutritional guidelines apply to patients frequently seen by respiratory therapists
- How common pulmonary medications affect nutrition

Chapter Outline

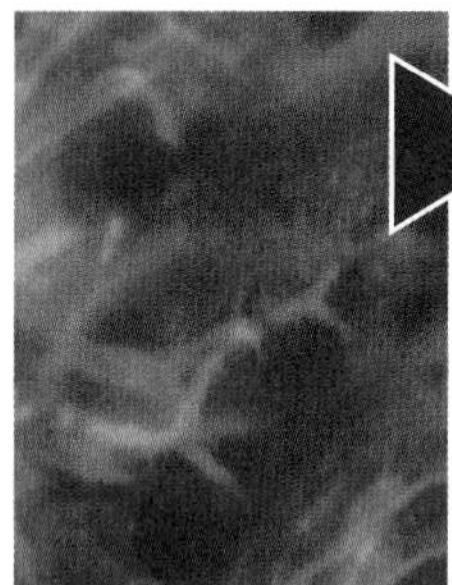

Key Terms

anergy
anthropometry
azotemia
basal metabolic rate
gluconeogenesis
indirect calorimetry
ketogenesis
kwashiorkor
marasmus
normometabolic
protein-energy malnutrition (PEM)
resting energy expenditure (REE)

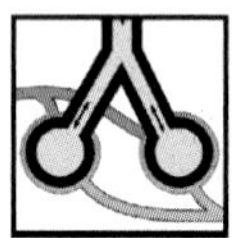

Adequate nutrition is essential for health. The relationship between nutrition and respiratory status is reciprocal. A balanced supply of nutrients is needed for proper respiratory function; oxygen is required for adenosine triphosphate (ATP) synthesis and muscle function, including the respiratory muscles. Poor or inadequate nutrient intake disrupts energy utilization and impairs normal organ function. Conversely, disease can either impair nutrient intake or alter metabolism, causing malnutrition.

▶ MAINTAINING HEALTH THROUGH GOOD NUTRITION

Dietary Guidelines

Over the past several years, numerous guidelines have been developed to assist both professionals and the public at large in planning an adequate diet to maintain health. These include the National Academy of Sciences' *Recommended Dietary Allowances* (RDAs),[1] the United States Department of Health and Human Services and Department of Agriculture's *Dietary Guidelines*,[2] the American Heart Association *Dietary Guidelines*,[3] the United States Department of Agriculture *Food Guide Pyramid*,[4] and the Food and Drug Administration's *Food Label*.[5] Table 47-1 provides a synthesis of the *Dietary Guidelines*.[2]

The RDAs set intake levels of essential nutrients judged adequate to meet the known nutrient needs of most healthy people. Individuals with acute and chronic diseases may require additional amounts of selected nutrients. As of 1997, the RDAs are being included as a component of a larger system, called Reference Daily Intakes (RDIs).

The Food Guide Pyramid (Figure 47-1) provides a simple framework for selecting a healthful diet. The pyramid graphically illustrates the number of portions of the five major food groups. Variety is important because no single food provides all the nutrients needed. To ensure intake of the wide range of nutrients, people should select food choices in the number and size of servings recommended in the pyramid. Those choosing meatless meals may select foods from the Vegetarian Food Pyramid (Figure 47-2).[6]

Foods are interchangeable within, not between, groups for similar nutrient values, except fruits and vegetables are often combined. The majority of daily calories should come from grains, fruits, and vegetables. Citrus fruits and dark green leafy and orange vegetables provide folate and the antioxidants, vitamin C and beta carotene. The broad spectrum of fruits and vegetables supplies trace minerals, many carotenoids, phytochemicals, and phytoestrogens.

The food guide pyramids have fats and oils at the apex, representing a small amount in the daily diet. Fats provide essential fatty acids and fat-soluble vitamins A, D, E, and K. However, selection of a diet low in fat, saturated fat, and cholesterol is important to control calorie intake and reduce risk of heart disease, hypertension, stroke, and diabetes, along with certain cancers.

Sodium has an essential role in regulation of fluid balance and blood pressure. Across populations, a high sodium intake is associated with high blood pressure. Sodium in the form of NaCl or salt is added during food processing to snack and convenience foods and also is found naturally in many foods, including dairy products. While the population as a whole may not be "sodium sensitive" or at risk of developing high blood pressure, moderation in sodium intake is not harmful.

Alcohol supplies calories with minimal nutrients. The risk of malnutrition rises in individuals consuming excess alcohol, which is consumed in lieu of a more nutritious diet. Excess alcohol can impair judgment and increase the risk of hypertension, stroke, certain cancers, and birth defects. The American Heart Association says that because of the relationship of ethanol "to a number of health hazards...there is little current justification to recommend alcohol (or wine specifically) as a cardioprotective strategy."[7]

Macronutrients and Energy Requirements

Macronutrients supply the body's energy requirements. The three macronutrients are protein, carbohydrate, and fat. Each contributes to calorie intake with four, four,

Table 47-1 ▶ ▶ Dietary Guidelines for Americans, 2000

Guideline	Recommendation
Aim for fitness	
Aim for healthy weight	Strive for a BMI between 18.5 and 25.
Be physically active each day	Be active at least 30 minutes (adults) or 60 minutes (children) most days.
Build a healthy base	
Let the pyramid guide your food choices	Build your meals on plants with smaller servings from the protein and dairy foods and minimal servings of fats and sweets.
Choose a variety of grains daily	Grains form the foundation of a healthy diet.
Choose a variety of fruits and vegetables daily	Include at least two servings of fruits and three of vegetables daily; Five-a-Day.
Keep food safe to eat	Wash hands prior to preparing food. Keep hot foods at 140° F or above and cold foods at 40° F or below. Dispose of food if outside this range for 2 hours.
Choose sensibly	
Choose a diet that is low in saturated fat and cholesterol and moderate in total fat	Keep saturated fat at <10% of calories and cholesterol at <300 mg/day.
Choose beverages and foods to moderate your intake of sugars	Added sugars by any name contribute to tooth decay and weight gain. Choose foods other than those with most of their calories from sugars.
Choose and prepare foods with less salt	Only $\frac{1}{4}$ teaspoon of salt is needed per day; choose <1 teaspoon or 2400 mg per day.
If you drink alcoholic beverages, do so in moderation.	No more than one drink per day for women and no more than two for men and then with meals to slow absorption. The reasons for not drinking are greater than the possible lowered risk for coronary heart disease.

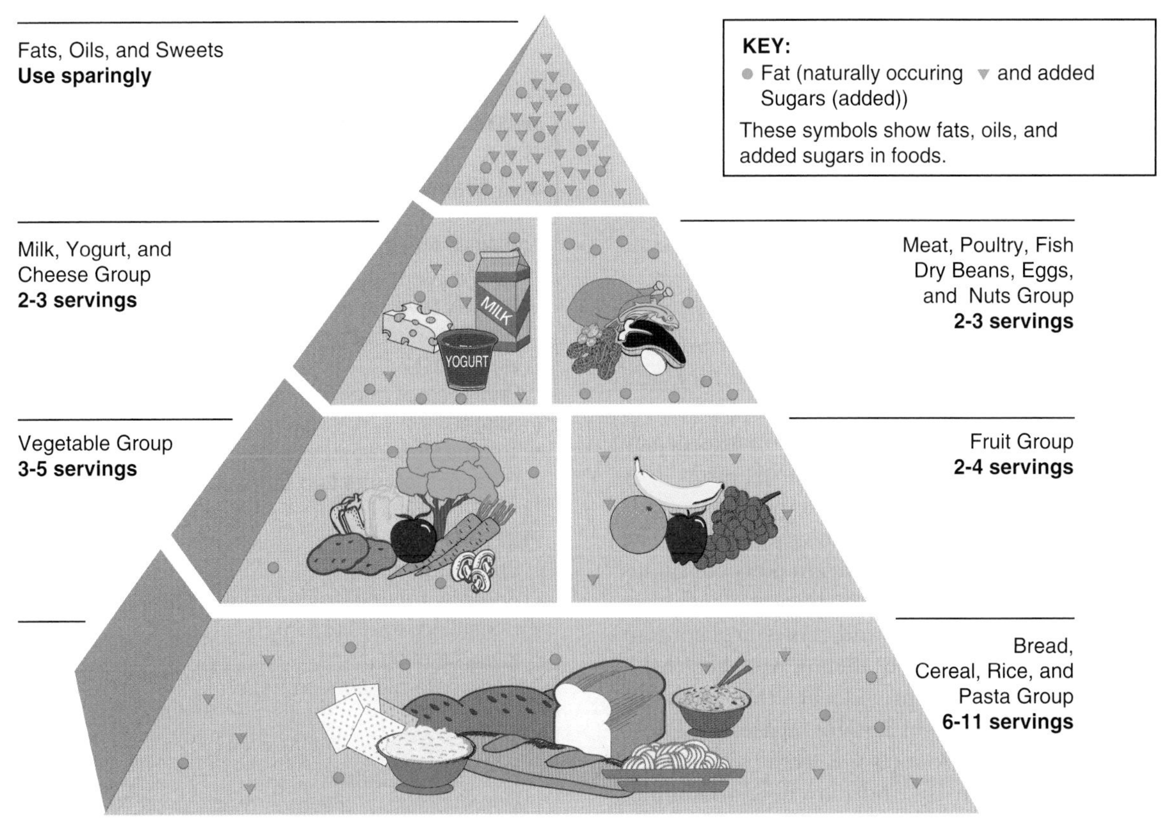

Figure 47-1
U.S. Department of Agriculture Food Guide Pyramid.

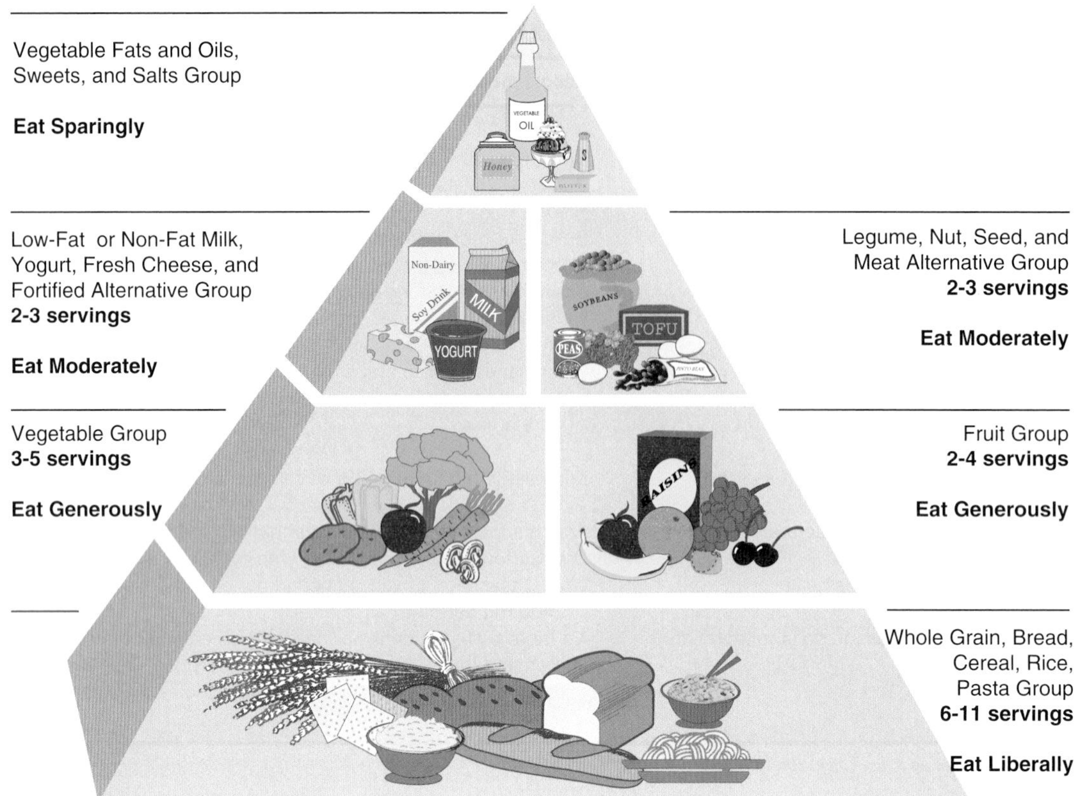

Figure 47-2
Vegetarian Food Pyramid.

and nine calories (kcal) per gram respectively. Alcohol is the only other calorie source with approximately seven calories per gram. Box 47-1 outlines the factors influencing energy and macronutrient needs.

Protein

Protein is composed of nine essential and 11 or so non-essential amino acids.[8] The amino acid ratios of proteins found in animal products (eggs, meat, fish, poultry, and dairy products) is slightly dissimilar from vegetable sources (nuts, beans, legumes, and grains). Soy protein is nearly equivalent. Consuming adequate calories each day within a mixed and varied diet provides the amino acids for building the proteins needed by the body.[9] The popularity of a multiplicity of vegetarian diets continues to grow as Americans chose more meatless meals in order to reduce the saturated fat and cholesterol content of their food choices. These diets "are healthful, nutritionally adequate, and provide health benefits in the prevention and treatment of certain diseases."[10] Those who eliminate all animal products (i.e., total vegetarians) must supplement vitamin B_{12} and may need to supplement calcium and vitamin D if they do not carefully choose foods rich in each. *Some* soy beverages will provide those three nutrients; read the label to be sure.

Box 47-1 • Factors Influencing Energy and Macronutrient Needs

ENERGY NEEDS
- Height, weight
- Activity level
- Growth state: infants through teens, pregnancy, lactation
- Presence of infection or fever
- Surgery
- Trauma, fractures
- Presence of infection or inflammation

PROTEIN NEEDS
- State of growth
- Surgery, trauma, fractures, infection
- Renal (kidney) function
- Liver function
- Corticosteroid administration

FAT NEEDS
- Total energy needs
- Hyperlipidemia, diabetes mellitus
- Liver, gallbladder, and pancreatic disorders
- Cardiovascular disease

The RDA for protein varies by age and sex, averaging approximately 0.8 g/kg/day for adults. There are approximately 7 grams of protein per ounce of meat, fish, poultry, or cheese. A 3-ounce portion (about the size of a deck of cards) of any of these foods has approximately 21 grams of protein. This is approximately half of the daily needs for a 50-kg individual. A serving of milk contains approximately 8 grams of protein. Most healthy adults, including vegetarians, consume more protein than recommended. Acute illnesses, trauma, infections, and surgery can increase protein needs up to 1 to 2 g/kg/day.

Carbohydrate

There are two major types of carbohydrates. Simple carbohydrates (monosaccharides and disaccharides) are found in sugars, candies, cakes, cookies, pies, pastries, milk, fruits, fruit juices and drinks, and other sweetened foods. Complex carbohydrates (polysaccharides and other indigestible dietary fibers) are found in whole grains, vegetables, beans, legumes, nuts, seeds, and fruits. The dietary guidelines and pyramid emphasize a high carbohydrate diet (50% to 60%), ideally from complex sources.

Fat

Dietary fat is the most concentrated source of calories (9 kcal/g). There are three types of fats: (1) saturated fatty acids (SFAs), (2) monounsaturated (MUFA) fatty acids, and (3) polyunsaturated (PUFA) fatty acids. SFAs are found in animal products, palm oil, and coconuts. They raise serum cholesterol levels more than MUFAs or PUFAs. MUFAs and PUFAs are widely distributed in foods. Olive, canola, and nut-based oils are rich in MUFAs. Ideally, no more than 25% to 30% of total dietary calories should come from fat, with approximately 10% PUFAs, 10% to 15% MUFAs, and less than 10% in the form of SFAs. Reducing the daily fat intake also reduces calorie intake.

Energy Expenditure and Energy Needs

An individual's energy requirements represent the ratio of energy intake to energy expenditure relative to body weight and activity level (see Box 47-1).

The classic measure of energy expenditure is the basal metabolic rate (BMR). Obtained after 10 hours of fasting, the BMR measures the number of calories (kcal) expended at rest per square meter of body surface per hour (kcal/m^2/hr). BMR varies by body size, age, and sex. Calorie needs for energy expenditure rise above the BMR based on activity level, stage of growth (pregnancy, lactation), and extent of injury.

In clinical practice, we are more interested in a patient's *daily* energy requirements (kcal/day). There are multiple methods for estimating daily energy needs. The "quick method" estimates daily energy needs based on a simple body weight factor. Alternatively, you can use the Harris-Benedict prediction equations to estimate daily resting energy expenditure (REE):[8]

$$\text{REE kcal/day (male): } 66 + [13.7 \times \text{weight (kg)}] + [5 \times \text{height (cm)}] - (6.8 \times \text{age})$$

$$\text{REE kcal/day (female): } 655 + [9.6 \times \text{weight (kg)}] + [1.8 \times \text{height (cm)}] - (4.7 \times \text{age})$$

Although the predicted REE averages approximately 10% higher than the BMR, it still tends to underestimate actual energy needs.

To overcome the limitations of estimating formulas, we can actually measure energy needs at the bedside. To do so, we use a procedure called *indirect calorimetry*. Indirect calorimetry involves measurement of a patient's oxygen consumption ($\dot{V}O_2$) and carbon dioxide production ($\dot{V}CO_2$). From these data, an actual REE can be quickly computed. Indirect calorimetry is described in more detail later in this chapter.

Of course, energy needs vary according to activity level and state of health. Energy needs of sick patients can be significantly higher than predicted normals. Energy needs for obese individuals are less because adipose tissue uses less energy than muscle. Energy needs should be reevaluated and adjusted whenever weight changes more than 5 to 10 pounds.

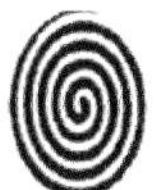

RULE OF THUMB

To estimate the energy needs of the average adult in kcal/day, identify the goal and multiply the individual's *actual* body weight in kilograms times the factor listed as follows:

Goal	Energy needs (kcal/kg)
Weight maintenance	25 to 30
Weight gain	30 to 35
Weight loss	20 to 25

Micronutrients and Dietary Supplements

Micronutrients provide no energy but are nonetheless essential to life. Micronutrients include vitamins, minerals, and other bioactive chemicals.

Most vitamins serve as coenzymes in the metabolism of protein, carbohydrate, and fat. Vitamins are either fat-soluble (A, D, E, K) or water-soluble (C, thiamin [B_1], riboflavin [B_2], pyridoxine [B_6], B_{12}, niacin, folacin, biotin, pantothenic acid). Minerals are essential structural components and play key roles in many vital processes, such as muscle contraction and fluid and acid-base balance.

Approximately half of the United States adult population use micronutrient supplements, mostly self-prescribed. Vitamin and mineral supplements may be beneficial for some persons (e.g., folic acid for women with child-bearing potential and vitamin B_{12} for persons 50 years of age and older). However, the best way to obtain the recommended levels of micronutrients is by eating a healthful diet, as previously outlined.[11] When the diet is optimal, routine use of nutritional supplements is of little benefit to most people. Moreover, unprescribed daily use of vitamin B_6, selenium, and the fat-soluble vitamins in amounts exceeding the RDAs should be avoided.[12]

Dietary Fiber

The two types of dietary fiber are soluble and insoluble. Soluble fibers (pectin, gums, hemicellulose, and mucilages) are found in fruits, fruit skins, oats, barley, and some vegetables, and insoluble fibers (cellulose, lignin) are found in whole grains, nuts, seeds, and some vegetables. The Daily Value recommendation for dietary fiber for healthy adults is 25 g/day.[5]

Dietary fiber is not a nutrient but has many important roles in the body. Soluble fibers help absorb water in the gastrointestinal (GI) tract; regulate GI transit time; and reduce the incidence of constipation, irritable bowel syndrome, and diverticular disease. Research has shown that populations consuming high-fiber diets, both soluble and insoluble, have reduced the incidence of colon cancer and diverticular disease. Soluble fiber has been shown to help regulate cholesterol and glucose metabolism.

Fluid Intake

Fluid intake is important to maintain hydration status. Healthy adults should ingest at least two liters of fluid per day or 1 mL/kcal/day.[13] Individuals who sweat heavily because of exercise need additional fluid to prevent dehydration. Sources of fluid include water, all beverages, gelatin, ices, ice cream, soup, and anything that is liquid at room temperature.

Thirst regulates the consumption of fluid usually, with the exception of the elderly, who tend to lose their sense of thirst. The elderly, athletes, and those performing heavy exercise should purposefully and intentionally consume fluids.

Antioxidants

Recently, there has been great interest in other bioactive chemicals that may have protective health roles. These include antioxidants and phytochemicals. The three most widely recognized antioxidants are vitamins C and E and beta-carotene. Antioxidants do help eliminate free radicals, but their role in immunity and cancer prevention is not yet fully understood.

Phytochemicals are substances found in edible fruits and vegetables that may play a role in cancer prevention.[11] Examples include indole (in broccoli), lycopene (abundant in tomato products), and allylic sulfides (in garlic and onions). As with antioxidants, conclusive knowledge of the protective effects of phytochemicals currently is lacking.

Those consuming diets rich in antioxidants tend to have better lung function than those who fail to include good sources of vitamins A (beta-carotene), C, and E.[14,15] Fruit and vegetable consumption appears to improve ventilatory function and decrease the risk of chronic obstructive pulmonary disease (COPD). Two antioxidants may be involved: flavonoids, such as quercetin, and vitamin C. The airway surface liquid of the lung contains considerable vitamin C where it may protect the body from harmful oxidants.[16] Roles for other antioxidants may be found for lung health in the future.

▶ MALNUTRITION

Malnutrition is a state of impaired metabolism in which the intake of essential nutrients falls short of the body's needs.

Protein-Energy Malnutrition

Protein-energy malnutrition (PEM) has adverse effects on respiratory musculature and the immune response.[17] PEM may be either primary or secondary. Primary PEM results from inadequate intake of calories and/or protein and is typically seen only in developing countries.[12]

Secondary PEM is due to underlying illness. Illness may cause (1) decreased caloric or protein intake (e.g., anorexia, dysphagia); (2) increased nutrient losses (e.g., malabsorption or diarrhea); and/or (3) increased nutrient demands (e.g., injury or infection).[18] As many as 50% of hospital patients may suffer from secondary PEM.

When PEM is due to inadequate nutrient intake or excessive loss, the body responds by *decreasing* its metabolic rate, ventilatory drive, thyroid function, and adrenergic activity.[19] As calorie intake decreases, energy for metabolic processes is initially supplied by converting liver glycogen stores into glucose (gluconeogenesis). However, liver reserves of glycogen are adequate for only approximately 12 to 18 hours.[20] Thereafter, endogenous fat stores are mobilized in the form of free fatty acids (ketogenesis). When fat stores are depleted, nutrient needs must be met by catabolizing skeletal muscle protein. This type of PEM usually manifests itself as a gradual wasting process, as seen in chronic diseases such as cancer and emphysema. The primary clinical sign is progressive weight loss.

Table 47-2 ▶ ▶ Comparison of Two Primary Forms of Protein-Energy Malnutrition

Parameter	Starvation (Marasmus)	Hypercatabolism (Kwashiorkor)
Etiology	Inadequate energy intake	Response to injury or infection
Examples	Cancer, pulmonary emphysema	Sepsis, burns
Body habitus	Thin, wasted, cachectic	May be normal, edematous
Rate of malnutrition	Slow	Rapid
Metabolic rate	Decreased	Increased
Fuel	Glucose/fat	Mixed
Catabolism	Decreased	Increased
Gluconeogenesis	Increased	Markedly increased
Glucagon	Increased	Markedly increased
Insulin	Decreased	Increased
Ketogenesis	Increased	Slightly increased
Catecholamines	Unchanged	Increased
Cortisol	Unchanged	Increased
Growth hormone	Increased	Increased
Visceral proteins	Normal	Decreased
Cytokines	Variable	Increased
Immune function	Normal	Impaired
Clinical course	Adequate responsiveness to short-term stress	Infections, poor wound healing, decubitus ulcers, skin breakdown
Mortality	Low unless related to underlying disease	High

When PEM is due to increased demand for nutrients, metabolism, thyroid function, and adrenergic activity all increase. Visceral protein levels tend to decrease early in the course of illness and are associated with impaired immunity.[19] This type of PEM typically occurs with acute catabolic disease, such as in sepsis, burns, or trauma. Weight loss and depletion of muscle and fat stores generally do not occur because of the rapidity of onset of the underlying disease.[18]

These two types of PEM are often referred to as *marasmus* and *kwashiorkor*. Marasmus is the form associated with inadequate nutrient intake (starvation), while kwashiorkor is the hypercatabolic form. Table 47-2 summarizes the key differences between these two forms of malnutrition.[12,18]

Micronutrient Malnutrition

The same problems that lead to PEM can produce deficiencies in micronutrients. Deficiencies of nutrients that are only stored in small amounts (e.g., the water-soluble vitamins) or are lost through external secretions (e.g., zinc in diarrhea fluid or burn exudate) are quite common.[12] Although the causes and results of micronutrient deficiencies are beyond the scope of this chapter, we describe a few of the most common problems.

Signs of scurvy (vitamin C deficiency) may be observed in chronically ill and/or patients with alcoholism hospitalized for acute illnesses. Low folic acid blood levels are common wherever illness, alcoholism, or poverty are present. Alcoholism is also associated with thiamin deficiency. Zinc deficiencies can impair clotting, slow wound healing, and impair immunity. Magnesium deficiencies can result in cardiac, vascular, neurological, and electrolyte abnormalities (hypocalcemia, hypokalemia), as well as decreases in respiratory muscle strength. Hypophosphatemia is seen frequently with cachexia or alcoholism, especially in patients receiving intravenous glucose or taking antacids. Severe hypophosphatemia can result in decreased muscle strength and contractility and acute cardiopulmonary failure.

Respiratory Consequences of Malnutrition

Malnutrition affects all organ systems. In addition, malnutrition appears to interact with disease processes to increase the morbidity and mortality of respiratory, cardiac, and renal failure.[19] Specific effects of malnutrition on the respiratory system are listed in Box 47-2.[12,18,21]

Box 47-2 • Respiratory Consequences of Malnutrition

RESPIRATORY MUSCLE DYSFUNCTION
- Loss of diaphragmatic mass and contractility
- Loss of accessory muscle mass and contractility

EFFECT ON CONTROL OF VENTILATION
- Decreased hypoxic and hypercapnic response

INCREASED INCIDENCE OF RESPIRATORY INFECTIONS
- Decreased lung clearance mechanisms
- Decreased secretory IgA
- Increased bacterial colonization

CHANGES IN LUNG PARENCHYMAL STRUCTURE
- Unopposed enzymatic digestion
- Loss of surfactant

Approximately a third of all patients with acute respiratory failure suffer from malnutrition. In these patients, the underlying diseases (e.g., sepsis, burns, trauma) increase energy expenditure and promote skeletal muscle catabolism. These patients are prone to hypercapnia and can be difficult to wean from ventilatory support. Malnourished patients who require mechanical ventilatory support also have higher mortality rates than those with normal nutritional status.[18]

Malnutrition also plays a role in COPD. The combined effect of increased energy expenditure (because of high work of breathing) and inadequate caloric intake contributes to a marasmus-type malnutrition. The resulting progressive muscle weakness and dyspnea can further limit caloric intake, as can several profound psychosocial factors. Box 47-3 summarizes the factors contributing to malnutrition in COPD patients.[21]

Box 47-3 • Underlying Causes of Malnutrition in Patients with COPD

INCREASED ENERGY EXPENDITURE
- Increased work of breathing

INADEQUATE CALORIC INTAKE
- Dyspnea while eating
- Gastrointestinal symptoms while eating
- Suppressed appetite from medications (e.g., theophylline)

POOR UTILIZATION OF CALORIES (MALABSORPTION)

PSYCHOSOCIAL FACTORS
- Depression
- Poverty
- Cigarette smoking

EATING AND LIVING ARRANGEMENTS

▶ NUTRITIONAL ASSESSMENT

A simple, brief nutrition screening tool may be used to identify patients who need a comprehensive nutritional assessment.[22] The assessment of nutritional status is challenging. A complete nutrition assessment involves in-depth review of clinical and historical data, measurement of physical and physiological parameters, and assessment of a variety of clinical laboratory tests.[23] Normally, a registered dietitian or clinical nutritionist plans and conducts the overall assessment. However, respiratory therapists may participate in selected elements of these assessments and must have general knowledge of the relevant procedures. Box 47-4 outlines the components of a comprehensive nutrition assessment for a patient with pulmonary disease.[23]

Box 47-4 • Components of a Comprehensive Nutritional Assessment

MEDICAL HISTORY AND PHYSICAL EXAMINATION
- Present diseases
- Current medications
- Activity level
- Physical assessment

ANTHROPOMETRICS
- Usual weight and height
- History of weight loss
- Actual versus ideal body weight (IBW)
- Percent IBW (height-weight index)
- Triceps skin fold
- Midarm muscle circumference

CLINICAL LABORATORY TESTS
- Visceral proteins
- Creatinine-height index
- Immune-related tests

DIETARY HISTORY
- Usual food intake
- Food likes and dislikes
- Appetite

TOTAL CALORIC REQUIREMENTS
- REE prediction (Harris-Benedict equations) x stress factor
- Indirect calorimetry

ACCESS TO FOOD
- Income
- Education
- Mobility
- Mechanical impediments

History and Physical Examination

A dietitian performs the nutrition assessment, the first step of which should be a review of the medical history and physical examination.[19] The patient's usual weight and amount and rate of recent loss should be determined. Also important to note is the patient's general appetite and any recent deviations from his or her normal diet. In this regard, a diet history, food diary, food frequency questionnaire, or calorie count may provide more accurate information. GI symptoms, such as dysphagia, nausea, vomiting, or abnormal stools should be recorded, as should the presence of any diseases associated with nutritional implications (e.g., diabetes, cardiovascular disease, nephropathies, cancer, cirrhosis). Additional considerations include medications, socioeconomic status, the ability to secure and prepare food, and food idiosyncrasies and intolerances.[23]

Simple physical assessment also can be useful. Tachycardia, tachypnea, or fever indicates high energy expenditure. Findings such as increased skin turgor (because of edema), glossitis (inflammation of the tongue), and cheilosis (cracking of lips caused by dehydration or riboflavin deficiency) indicate potential abnormalities associated with malnutrition. The skinfolds (triceps and others), upper arm circumference, and arm muscle area should also be measured and qualitatively assessed for subcutaneous fat stores and muscle bulk.[23]

Actual height and weight should be obtained during the physical examination. Based on these data, the clinician should compute the patient's height-weight index. The height-weight index is the ratio of actual body weight to ideal body weight (IBW), expressed as a percentage. IBW is determined using standard tables or simple formulas. The presence of a body weight less than 90% of predicted IBW is correlated with malnutrition and the increased risk of morbidity and mortality.[24] Likewise, recent weight loss in excess of 10% IBW also suggests malnutrition.[24]

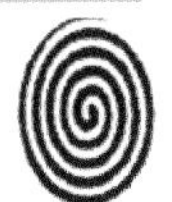

RULE OF THUMB

To estimate IBW in pounds, use the following simple formulas (Hamwi method):

Men	106 + 6 lbs for each inch height >60 inches
Women	100 + 5 lbs for each inch height >60 inches

Variations in weight occur throughout the day and may reflect changes in fluid status rather than nutritional status. It is important to measure weight at the same time each day and inspect the patient for signs of fluid retention when comparing height and weight. A bed scale is useful for weighing mechanically ventilated patients, however, the weight of ventilator tubing should be subtracted from the obtained weight. Unfortunately many critically ill patients are edematous and the measured weight may not reflect the real body cell mass.

Results of the history and physical can help identify patients at high risk for malnutrition (Box 47-5).[12] Respiratory therapists may notice changes in nutritional status that could lead to increased risk for malnutrition (Box 47-6).[23] Such patients should be referred promptly to their primary care provider or dietitian.

Anthropometry

Anthropometry is the technique of measuring body composition to determine the distribution of fat and muscle mass. The most commonly used measurements are triceps skinfold (fat reserves) and midarm muscle circumference (lean or skeletal muscle mass).

Box 47-5 • The Patient at High Risk for Malnutrition

- Underweight (% ideal body weight <90%) and/or recent loss of 10% or more of usual body weight
- Poor intake: anorexia, food avoidance (e.g., psychiatric condition), "nothing allowed by mouth" (NPO) status for more than approximately 5 days
- Protracted nutrient losses: malabsorption, enteric fistulae, draining abscesses or wounds, renal dialysis
- Hypermetabolic states: sepsis, protracted fever, extensive trauma, or burns
- Chronic use of alcohol or drugs with antinutrient or catabolic properties: steroids, antimetabolites (e.g., methotrexate), immunosuppressants, antitumor agents
- Impoverishment, isolation, advanced age, limited mobility

Box 47-6 • Nutritional Status Changes Observable by Respiratory Therapists

- Mechanics of breathing impacted by cachexia, obesity, pregnancy
- Increased coughing effort may indicate poor nutrition
- Viscosity of sputum, jugular venous pressure, ascites, edema suggest fluid imbalance
- Lung crackles relate to fluid overload or oncotic pressure changes (loss of blood protein)
- Wheezing may be associated with food intolerances, alcohol, aspirated food particles
- Late inspiratory crackles of atelectasis may result from decreased surfactant production from malnutrition
- S_3 heart sounds of congestive heart failure may indicate fluid imbalance
- S_4 heart sounds may be associated with severe anemia
- Pulmonary function measures may be related to:
  - FVC or FEV_1 decrease—severe malnutrition
  - FVC—excess fat weight
  - PEP and PIP decrease—poor nutrition
  - Lung compliance—fluid and serum albumin changes acutely, or chronic malnutrition
- Arterial blood gas values may be related to:
  - $PaCO_2$ increases—excess glucose, inadequate ventilation from lack of muscle energy
  - Oxygen saturation, oxygen content, hemoglobin—nutritional status
- Meal acceptance may be related to visible equipment—suction bottles, sputum specimens
- Lack of oxygen may increase difficulty of eating—ensure availability of oxygen via cannula if needed

Anthropometric techniques are well standardized; however, results are of limited value in acute care settings because of low sensitivity to short-term changes.[18,25] These measures are most useful for epidemiological surveys and in following the nutritional status of individual patients over long periods. For example, anthropometric measures could be useful in serial assessments of patients with COPD over the duration of a comprehensive rehabilitation and nutrition program.[21]

Clinical Laboratory Tests

Several laboratory tests can provide valuable information about a patient's nutritional status. However, numerous factors in addition to nutritional status affect all such test results. For this reason, clinicians must be careful not to assign nutritional significance to tests that may be abnormal for other reasons.[12]

Visceral Proteins

Visceral (or hepatic) proteins include albumin, transferrin, thyroxine-binding prealbumin, and retinol-binding protein. Blood levels of these markers indicate the level of protein synthesis and thus yield information on overall nutritional status. The general availability and stability of albumin levels from day to day make it one of the most useful tests for assessing long-term trends (Table 47-3). In combination with other findings, such as edema and poor wound healing, a serum albumin level less than 2.8 g/dL helps distinguish kwashiorkor from marasmus.[12]

The long half-lives of albumin (18 to 20 days) and transferrin (4 to 8 days) limit their usefulness in the acute care setting. With shorter half-lives, thyroxine-binding prealbumin (2 days) and retinol-binding protein (12 hours) are more sensitive indicators of nutritional deficiency.[23] Unfortunately, these two tests are not readily available in all settings and are extremely costly.

In interpreting test results, the clinician must understand that hepatic protein synthesis is altered by many factors other than nutritional status. Conditions altering visceral protein levels include liver disease, protein-losing disorders, and high-stress states such as acute infection or inflammation. Because these conditions are so common among the critically ill, visceral protein markers are of limited usefulness for assessing nutritional deficiency in the critical care setting.[25]

Table 47-3 ▶ ▶ Assessment of Serum Albumin

Level	Interpretation
3.5-5.0 g/dL	Normal
2.8-3.5 g/dL	Mild depletion
2.1-2.7 g/dL	Moderate depletion
<2.1 g/dL	Severe depletion

Creatinine-Height Index

Because the rate of creatinine formation in skeletal muscle is constant, the amount of creatinine excreted in the urine every 24 hours reflects skeletal muscle mass.[12] Predicted values are based on gender and height, with average normals ranging from approximately 18 mg/kg/day for women to approximately 23 mg/kg/day for men. Values less than 60% of predicted indicate a severe deficit of muscle mass. Factors that influence creatinine excretion, and thus complicate interpretation of this index, include age, diet, exercise, stress, and renal disease.[25]

Nitrogen Balance (Protein Catabolism)

Because urea nitrogen is a major by-product of protein catabolism, we can use its rate of urinary excretion to assess protein balance.[12] The rate of urea excretion in the urine is typically measured as the 24-hour urinary urea nitrogen (UUN). Using this value, catabolic protein loss is calculated as follows:

$$\text{Protein catabolic rate (g/day)} = [\text{24-hour UUN (g)} + 4] \times 6.25$$

The 4 g/day added to the 24-hr UUN is an estimate of the average daily unmeasured nitrogen lost through other sources (sweat, feces). This equation can provide misleading results in patients who exhibit rapid changes in blood urea nitrogen (BUN) levels (such as dialysis patients) or those undergoing rapid diuresis. Correction factors are available to account for these clinical situations.[12] Protein balance is then calculated using the following simple formula:

$$\text{Protein balance (g/day)} = \text{protein intake} - \text{protein catabolic rate}$$

Immune Status

Impaired immunity (anergy) is a common finding in malnutrition, especially the kwashiorkor-type. The result is often a reduction in lymphocytes, as measured by the total lymphocyte count or TLC (TLC = WBC × % lymphocytes). Unfortunately, the TLC is a rather nonspecific indicator that can fluctuate day to day, even in otherwise healthy people.

Malnourished patients also may exhibit signs of depressed immunity when challenged by certain hypersensitivity skin tests. Because a large number of disease states and drugs are associated with anergy, the value of this test also is limited.[25]

Pulmonary Function Parameters

Pulmonary function tests are most useful in tracking patients with chronic lung disease in whom malnutrition may play a role. Such tests can help determine the extent of physiological impairment present in these patients and the impact of comprehensive rehabilitation strategies, including exercise and nutrition (see Chapter 48). Tests can include routine spirometry and measures of respiratory muscle strength. Which tests are chosen depends on the patient's ability and what has been established as protocol by the pulmonary laboratory or rehabilitation program.[21]

Arterial blood gas (ABG) values can be altered by nutrition, and baseline values can influence the nutritional feeding regimen. An elevated Pa_{CO_2} may signal the need to modify carbohydrate intake or total caloric load.[26,27]

Total Caloric Requirements

Harris-Benedict Prediction Equations

As previously described, total caloric requirements can be estimated using the Harris-Benedict equations. These equations are multiplied by a "stress factor" of 1.20 to 1.50 to better estimate the caloric needs of acutely ill patients.[23] For patients with severe burns (>40% body surface area), a factor of 2.0 may be appropriate.[12] Alternatively, there are separate REE equations for both burn patients[28] and those with COPD.[21] More detail on adjusting REEs derived from the Harris-Benedict equations is provided later in this chapter.

Indirect Calorimetry

Indirect calorimetry is the estimation of energy expenditure by measurement of whole-body oxygen consumption and carbon dioxide production.[29] Data obtained can be used to assess a patient's metabolic state, determine nutritional needs, or assess response to nutrition therapy.[30]

To guide practitioners in using indirect calorimetry, the American Association for Respiratory Care (AARC) has published a *Clinical Practice Guideline: Metabolic Measurement Using Indirect Calorimetry During Mechanical Ventilation*. Excerpts appear on p. 1212.[29]

In regard to the indications for indirect calorimetry, the determination of energy and protein needs by empiric formula is sufficient for most patients. Given the cost and complexity of this procedure, its routine use cannot be justified.[19] Specific clinical conditions supporting the need for indirect calorimetry as a tool in nutrition assessment are listed in Box 47-7.[12,18,19,31]

Box 47-7 • Clinical Situations in Which Indirect Calorimetry May Be Indicated

- Patients with morbid obesity
- Patients who are difficult to wean from ventilatory support
- Patients for whom weight estimates are uncertain
- Patients with severe malnutrition
- Patients with high level of stress
- Patients at the extremes of weight and/or age
- Patients failing to respond to nutritional support

Equipment and Technique

Good calorimetry results require extensive preparation. Box 47-8 outlines the key preparatory steps to be taken in advance of testing.[12]

Box 47-8 • Preparation for Indirect Calorimetry

- 30 hours before test:
  - 24-hour urine urea nitrogen (UUN) collection (with sufficient time to receive result) if determination of carbohydrate, fat, and protein utilization desired
- 10 hours before test:
  - Patient fasting if measuring energy requirements; if feeding is continued results will reflect the patient's energy expenditure in response to feeding (may be spuriously high if the patient if being overfed)
- 4 hours before test:
  - Patient resting and avoiding physical activity, physical therapy, dressing changes
- 2 hours before test:
  - Endotracheal tube suctioned for the last time before test; further ventilator changes or suctioning avoided
- 1 hour before test:
  - Supine position, complete rest; analgesic or sedative administered if needed

Indirect calorimetry can be performed with a Douglas bag, a Tissot spirometer, and CO_2 and O_2 gas analyzers. The patient's expired gas is collected in the Douglas bag where it is sampled for O_2 and CO_2 concentrations; the Tissot spirometer measures expired volume. Commercially available metabolic carts are much easier to use. These automated systems either use a mixing chamber or perform breath-by-breath analysis. The breath-by-breath method provides real-time data, which may aid in ensuring optimal measurement conditions, particularly in mechanically ventilated patients.[30]

Figure 47-3 shows the basic configuration for open-circuit indirect calorimetry during mechanical ventilation using a metabolic cart with mixing chamber. Gas sampled from the inspiratory limb of the ventilator circuit is assessed for fractional inspired oxygen concentration (F_{IO_2}) using a paramagnetic or zirconium oxide oxygen analyzer. Volume exhaled by the patient is measured using a flow transducer. The patient's exhaled gas then

METABOLIC MEASUREMENT USING INDIRECT CALORIMETRY DURING MECHANICAL VENTILATION

AARC Clinical Practice Guideline (Excerpts)*

➤ INDICATIONS

Metabolic measurements may be indicated:

- In patients with known nutritional deficits or derangements.
- When the desire or perceived need is present to measure the O_2 cost of breathing in mechanically ventilated patients.
- When the need exists to assess the $\dot{V}O_2$ in order to evaluate the hemodynamic support of mechanically ventilated patients.

➤ CONTRAINDICATIONS

When a specific indication is present, there are no contraindications to performing a metabolic measurement using indirect calorimetry unless short-term disconnection of ventilatory support for connection of measurement lines results in hypoxemia, bradycardia, or other adverse effects.

➤ HAZARDS/COMPLICATIONS

Performing metabolic measurements using an indirect calorimeter is a safe, noninvasive procedure with few hazards or complications. Under certain circumstances and with particular equipment the following hazards/complications may be seen:

- Closed circuit calorimeters may cause a reduction in alveolar ventilation due to increased compressible volume of the breathing circuit.
- Closed circuit calorimeters may decrease the trigger sensitivity of the ventilator and result in increased patient work of breathing.
- Short-term disconnection of the patient from the ventilator for connection of the indirect calorimetry apparatus may result in hypoxemia, bradycardia, and patient discomfort.
- Inappropriate calibration or system setup may result in erroneous results causing incorrect patient management.

➤ ASSESSMENT OF NEED

Metabolic measurements should be performed only on the order of a physician after review of indications (above) and objectives.

➤ ASSESSMENT OF TEST QUALITY

- Test quality can be evaluated by determining whether:
  - RQ is consistent with the patient's nutritional intake.
  - RQ rests in the normal physiological range (0.67 to 1.3).
  - Measured $\dot{V}O_2$ is within ±10% of the mean value and measured $\dot{V}CO_2$ within ±6% of the mean value.
  - REE has been defined as the value obtained with the patient lying in bed, awake and aware of his/her surrounding.
- Outcome may be assessed by the interpretation and confirmation/manipulation of patient nutritional support regimen by a physician or nutritionist based on the measurement results.
- Outcome may be assessed by the successful manipulation of the mechanical ventilator settings and/or hemodynamic management based on the measurement of the $\dot{V}O_2$.

➤ MONITORING

- The following should be evaluated during the performance of a metabolic measurement to ascertain the validity of the results:
  - Clinical observation of the resting state
  - Patient comfort and movement during testing
  - Values in concert with the clinical situation
  - Equipment function
  - Results within the specifications of test quality (above)
- Measurement data should include a statement of test quality and list the current nutritional support, ventilator settings, and vital signs.

*For complete guidelines, see Respir Care 39:1170, 1994.

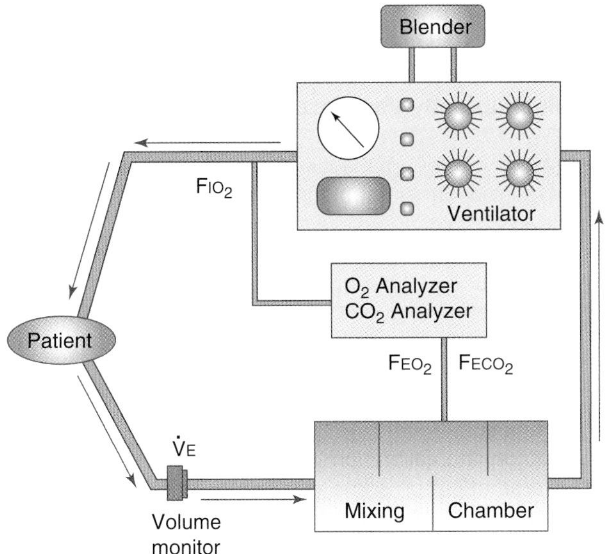

Figure 47-3
Open-circuit indirect calorimetry in a mechanically ventilated patient. Inspiratory gas is sampled for determination of FIO_2, volume is measured in the expiratory limb of the ventilator circuit, and mixed exhaled gas is drawn from the mixing chamber for analysis of FEO_2 and $FECO_2$. Bolded parameters are used to calculate oxygen consumption and carbon dioxide production. Arrows in figure indicate direction of gas flow. *(Modified from Witte MK: Metabolic measurements during mechanical ventilation in the pediatric intensive care unit, Respir Care Clin N Am 2:573, 1996.)*

Box 47.9 • Equations Used to Calculate $\dot{V}O_2$ and $\dot{V}CO_2$ Using the Gas Exchange Method

$$\dot{V}O_2 = \dot{V}E \times \left[\frac{1 - FEO_2 - FECO_2}{1 - FIO_2} \times FIO_2\right] - (\dot{V}E \times FEO_2)$$

$$\dot{V}CO_2 = \dot{V}E \times FECO_2$$

$$RQ = \frac{\dot{V}CO_2}{\dot{V}O_2}$$

enters a mixing chamber, from which a sample is drawn to measure $FECO_2$ (usually by infrared analysis) and fractional concentration of oxygen in expired gas (FEO_2). Exhaled gas is returned to the ventilator after volume and gas concentration measurements. Once all measurements are obtained, oxygen consumption ($\dot{V}O_2$), CO_2, and respiratory quotient (RQ) are computed using the equations in Box 47-9. *All measurements must be corrected to STPD conditions before computation.*[32]

The values are then used in the abbreviated Weir equation to determine REE:

$$REE = [(O_2 \times 3.9) + (CO_2 \times 1.1)] \times 1.44$$

Indirect calorimetry is more difficult to perform on spontaneously breathing patients, especially those breathing supplemental oxygen. Although a mouthpiece with noseclips or a mask can be used to collect expired gas, they tend to alter the patient's steady state and invalidate results.[30] Instead, most clinicians recommend using a plastic canopy that covers the patient's head. Expired gases are cleared from the canopy by a preset flow of air; expired gas concentrations are sampled and corrected for the air dilution.

Because standard modes of O_2 therapy do not deliver a consistent FIO_2 to spontaneously breathing patients, special delivery systems must be utilized. To overcome this problem, the clinician can substitute a precise oxygen mixture for the air used to clear the canopy. Alternatively, one can place a large gas reservoir (such as a Douglas bag) between an O_2 flow source and the subject.[30] This will ensure that the FIO_2 remains stable throughout the test procedure.

Problems and Limitations

Indirect calorimetry is a technically complex procedure that requires rigorous attention to both instrument and procedure quality control. Regarding instrumentation, small errors in measurements can result in large errors in calculated $\dot{V}O_2$, $\dot{V}CO_2$, and energy expenditure. For this reason, the calorimeter's gas analyzers and volume measurement device must be properly calibrated before each patient use. Gas analyzers should be accurate to the hundredth percent and linear over the clinical range of oxygen concentrations.[32,33]

Regarding procedure quality control, it is essential that measurements be made during steady state conditions. Although proper patient preparation (see Box 47-8) is helpful in this regard, steady state conditions can only be confirmed during the test procedure itself. A common standard for ensuring steady state conditions is five consecutive 1-minute averages with a variability of 5% or less.[30]

Perhaps the most significant problem in performing indirect calorimetry on mechanically ventilated patients is the presence of leaks (circuit, tracheal tube cuff, chest tubes).[29] Since any leak will invalidate test results, no procedure should commence until a leak-free patient-ventilator-calorimeter system is confirmed. Other sources of error during open-circuit indirect calorimetry of mechanically ventilated patients are listed in Box 47-10.[29]

Interpretation and Use of Results

Results obtained from indirect calorimetry are used both to assess metabolic status and plan nutritional support.

In regard to assessing metabolic status, the first step is to compare the REE obtained by calorimetry to that predicted by the Harris-Benedict equations. If the calorimetry REE is within 10% of the predicted value,

MINI CLINI

Metabolic Assessment Based on Indirect Calorimetry

PROBLEM

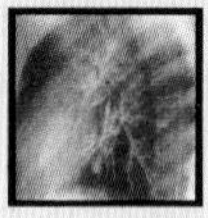

Interpret the following indirect calorimetry (IC) results obtained on four patients, each with a Harris-Benedict predicted REE of 1500 kcal/day receiving 1850 kcal/day of mixed substrate with an expected RQ of 0.85:

Patient	IC results	Interpretation
1	REE (IC) = 1500 RQ = 0.85	The patient is normometabolic and receiving the correct amount of kilocalories. RQ measured = RQ expected.
2	REE (IC) = 2000 RQ = 0.76	The patient is hypermetabolic and receiving an inadequate amount of kilocalories. The RQ is lower than expected because of metabolism of endogenous fat and protein sources.
3	REE (IC) = 1200 RQ = 0.95	The patient is hypometabolic and receiving too many kilocalories. The RQ is high, reflecting lipogenesis caused by overfeeding.
4	REE (IC) = 1500 RQ = 0.94	The subject is normometabolic and receiving the correct amount of kilocalories, but the RQ is higher than expected. Possible causes include: the subject is receiving more kilocalories from carbohydrates than expected, acute hyperventilation, acute metabolic acidosis, or inaccurate measurement.

From McArthur C: Indirect calorimetry, Respir Care Clin N Am 3:291, 1997.

the patient is considered *normometabolic*. Measured REEs greater than 10% above predicted values indicate a hypermetabolic state, whereas values below 90% of predicted indicate hypometabolism.

The second step in metabolic assessment is to interpret the respiratory quotient (RQ). Table 47-4 outlines the basic significance of the RQ relative to substrate utilization and general nutrition strategies.[30] Once a patient's predicted REE, actual REE, and RQ are known, you can provide a basis for energy needs.

Box 47-10 • Sources of Error During Open-Circuit Indirect Calorimetry of Mechanically Ventilated Patients

- Instability of FIO_2 because of changes in source gas pressure or ventilator/blender variability
- Delivery of high FIO_2 levels (>0.60)
- Inability to separate inspired and expired gases because of bias flow from flow-triggering systems, IMV systems, or specific ventilator characteristics
- The presence of anesthetic gases or gases other than O_2, CO_2, and nitrogen in the ventilation system
- The presence of water vapor resulting in sensor malfunction
- Inappropriate calibration
- Adverse effect on some ventilators' functions (triggering, expiratory resistance, pressure measurement)
- Total circuit flow exceeding internal calorimeter flow (if using dilutional principle)
- Concurrent peritoneal or hemodialysis

Table 47-4 ▶▶ Interpretation and Use of the Respiratory Quotient (RQ)

Value	Interpretation	General Nutrition Strategy
>1.00	Overfeeding	Decrease total kcal
0.9 to 1.00	Carbohydrate oxidation	Decrease carbohydrates or increase lipids
0.8 to 0.9	Fat, protein, and carbohydrate oxidation	Target range for mixed substrate
0.7 to 0.8	Fat and protein oxidation Starvation	Increase total kcal

Acute hyperventilation or acute metabolic acidosis will increase RQ and may lead to misinterpretation. Metabolism of ketones or ethyl alcohol will lower RQ below 0.7.

Alternative REE Measures

In patients with pulmonary artery catheters, REE can be measured using a modification of the Fick equation:

$$\text{REE (kcal/day)} = \text{Cardiac output} \times \text{Hemoglobin} \times (SaO_2 - S\bar{v}O_2) \times 95.18$$

As an example, in a patient with a cardiac output of 4.2 liters, a hemoglobin of 11 g/dL, an SaO_2 of 89% and an $S\bar{v}O_2$ of 69%, the REE would be computed as follows:

$$\text{REE} = 4.2 \times 11 \times (0.89 - 0.69) \times 95.18$$
$$\text{REE} = 4.2 \times 11 \times (0.20) \times 95.18$$
$$\text{REE} = 879 \text{ kcal/day}$$

▶ GENERAL ASPECTS OF NUTRITIONAL SUPPORT

The primary goal of nutritional support is the maintenance or restoration of lean body (skeletal muscle) mass. This is accomplished by (1) meeting the patient's overall energy needs and (2) providing the appropriate combination of substrates to do so. Also important is the route of administration used to provide the support.

Meeting Overall Energy Needs

Once the patient's REE is derived, it needs to be adjusted to account for variations in activity and/or stress levels. If using the Harris-Benedict equations, it is recommended that the predicted REE be corrected for both stress and activity levels (Box 47-11).[18] When the REE is derived from indirect calorimetry, only the activity factor need be used.

Box 47-11 • Adjustments of Harris-Benedict Predicted REE for Stress and Activity Levels

Instructions: Multiply REE times (1) the most relevant stress factor, then (2) the appropriate activity factor.

Condition	Factor
Stress Factors	
Malnutrition	0.7
Chronic renal failure, nondialyzed	1.00
Maintenance hemodialysis	1.00 to 1.05
Elective surgery, uncomplicated	1.0
Peritonitis	1.15
Soft-tissue trauma	1.15
Fracture	1.20
Infection, mild	1.00
Infection, moderate	1.20 to 1.30
Infection, severe	1.40 to 1.50
Burns, 0% to 20% BSA	1.00 to 1.50
Burns, 20% to 40% BSA	1.50 to 1.80
Burns, 40% to 100% BSA	1.80 to 2.00
Activity Factors	
Confined to bed	1.2
Out of bed	1.3

Example: A bedridden patient with a moderately severe infection has a Harris-Benedict predicted REE of 1100 kcal/day. Estimate this patient's actual energy needs.

Actual energy needs = predicted REE × stress factor × activity factor

Actual energy needs = 1100 k/cal × 1.25 × 1.2

Actual energy needs = 1650 k/cal

Providing the Appropriate Combination of Substrates

Once energy requirements are estimated, the patient's physician or registered dietitian determines the appropriate "mix" of macronutrients (protein, carbohydrate, fat) needed.

Protein

Amino acids or proteins are essential to maintaining or restoring lean body mass. Because illness usually increases protein catabolism and thereby protein requirements, the RDA of 0.8 g/kg/day is generally insufficient for sick patients. Based on the assessment of the protein catabolism rate (see p. 1210), protein intake may need to be doubled or even tripled above the RDA (1.5 to 3.0 g/kg/day).[13,26] Some recommend a cushion of approximately 10 g/kg/day above the estimated level of protein catabolism to ensure a positive protein balance.[12] Ideally, approximately 20% of a patient's estimated calorie needs should be provided by protein. Higher percentages of protein may be needed in cachectic patients, the elderly, and those suffering from severe infections. However, whenever high protein intakes are given, the patient should be monitored for progressive azotemia (rising BUN >100 mg/dL).

Too much protein is harmful, especially for patients with limited pulmonary reserves. Excess protein, especially by the parenteral route, can increase oxygen consumption, REE, minute ventilation ($\dot{V}_E$), and central ventilatory drive.[34] In addition, overzealous protein feeding may lead to symptoms such as dyspnea in patients with chronic pulmonary disease.

Carbohydrate

Nonprotein calorie sources (carbohydrates and fats) help prevent protein catabolism. Glucose (dextrose) is the most commonly administered intravenous carbohydrate. For critically ill patients, 50% to 60% of the total daily calories can be in the form of simple carbohydrate.[25,26,35] In the average-sized patient, daily glucose provision should be no greater than 300 to 400 g/day. Glucose blood levels should be monitored and kept below 225 mg/dL.

For the patient with pulmonary disease or those requiring mechanical ventilation, high carbohydrate loads can cause problems. High carbohydrate loads increase carbon dioxide production and the RQ, resulting in increased ventilatory demand, oxygen consumption, and work of breathing.[34] Although the observed effects are usually modest, some patients with limited functional reserves cannot tolerate these changes, resulting in development or worsening of ventilatory failure. Recent evidence indicates that this problem is probably more closely related to total calorie load (overfeeding) than to the proportion of carbohydrate in the diet.[12] Based on this knowledge, overfeeding should be carefully avoided in pulmonary disease or those requiring mechanical ventilation.

Fat

The remaining calories (20% to 30%) should be provided from fat.[26,35] In critically ill patients, omega-6 PUFAs should provide at least 7% of total calories.[25] Fat intakes in excess of 50% of energy needs have been associated with fever, impaired immune function, liver dysfunction, and hypotension.

Excess lipid administration can also have negative pulmonary effects, including decreased arterial oxygen saturation, decreased pulmonary diffusion capacity, and increased alveolar-arterial PO_2 gradient.[34] What causes these changes is not clear; current speculation relates to increased prostaglandin production. Likewise, the full clinical impact of excess lipid administration is not yet known.

Timing of Nutritional Support

The initiation of nutritional support is determined by the patient's nutritional status and the estimated length of time the patient will be unable to consume a diet by mouth to meet nutritional needs. To ensure a satisfactory nutritional and metabolic response, support should be started when nutrient and energy needs cannot be met with oral feedings.[36]

Routes of Administration

There are two primary routes for supplying nutrients to patients: enteral (oral and tube feeding) and parenteral (peripheral or central venous alimentation). Box 47-12 provides guidelines for initiating nutritional support as recommended by the American Society for Parenteral and Enteral Nutrition (ASPEN).[24,37]

Box 47-12 • Guidelines for the Initiation of Nutritional Support

Clinical settings where enteral nutrition should be part of routine care:

- Protein-Calorie Malnutrition (>10% loss of usual weight, or serum albumin <3.5 g/dL) with inadequate oral intake of nutrients for the previous 5 to 7 days
- Normal nutritional status with less than 50% of required nutrient intake orally for the previous 7 to 10 days
- Severe dysphagia
- Burns of >15% total BSA in infants and children and >25% total BSA in older children and adults
- Massive small bowel resection in combination with administration of total parenteral nutrition
- Low output (less than 500 mL/day) enterocutaneous fistulas

Clinical settings where parenteral nutrition should be part of routine care:

- Patients with inability to absorb nutrients by the GI tract
- Patients undergoing high-dose chemotherapy, radiation, and bone marrow transplantation
- Moderate to severe pancreatitis (bowel rest anticipated beyond 5 to 7 days)
- Severe malnutrition in the face of a nonfunctional GI tract (within 1 to 3 days)
- Severely catabolic patients with or without malnutrition when the GI tract is not usable within 7 to 10 days

From American Society for Parenteral and Enteral Nutrition (ASPEN), Silver spring, Md, 1998.

Enteral Feeding

Enteral feedings are the route of choice—"if the gut works, use it." The enteral route is safer and cheaper than the parenteral route. Enteral feeding stimulates gut hormones, subjects nutrients to the absorptive and metabolic controls of the intestinal tract and liver, and produces less hyperglycemia (providing for better immune function) than the parenteral route. In addition, the buffering capacity of enteral feeding can improve resistance against stress ulcers. Finally, enteral feeding maintains a more normal mucosa than the parenteral route (the intestinal mucosa may undergo atrophy during parenteral nutrition).[12]

Enteral Tube Routes. There are six primary sites for enteral tube feeding: nasogastric, nasoduodenal, nasojejunal, gastrostomy, jejunostomy, and esophagotomy. Site selection depends on GI function, respiratory status, surgical state, and anticipated length of time the patient will be on the tube feeding.

Gastric feedings are indicated if there are no physiological factors affecting the GI function such as gastroparesis, delayed gastric emptying, obstruction, or surgery in the upper GI tract.

Small bowel (duodenum and jejunal) feedings are indicated if the upper GI tract cannot be used. Intestinal feeding tube placement is often recommended to minimize the risk of aspiration because it is believed to decrease the risk of gastric distention and gastroesophageal reflux; however, this has not yet been convincingly demonstrated.[38]

Nasogastric and nasoenteric tubes are indicated if the duration of the enteral therapy is anticipated to be short term (<30 days). They can be placed at the bedside and generally have a large internal diameter, which helps deliver viscous feedings and medications. Nasoduodenal and nasojejunal tubes are placed through the nose past the pylorus.

Long-term feeding tubes can be placed endoscopically and surgically. Percutaneous endoscopic (PE) placement of a feeding tube can be done to establish gastric (PEG) or intestinal (PEJ) access. This method is generally preferred to surgical placement because it is associated with lower costs and lack of need for operating room time and anesthesia.[39] Surgical laparotomy is indicated if endoscopy is contraindicated.

Tube Feeding Administration. Three basic methods of tube feeding administration include: bolus, intermittent, and continuous drip. Bolus feedings involve the rapid infusion of 250 to 500 mL of feeding several times daily. Feedings are provided by a syringe into the feeding tube port. An increased risk of aspiration is associated with bolus feedings because of the rapid infusion of formula into the stomach. Nausea, vomiting, abdominal pain, and distention can develop in conjunction with this feeding route. This feeding method can only be used with gastric tubes and is primarily applied to patients who are stable and those on enteral nutritional support at home.

Intermittent feedings are also administered several times per day, but they are infused over at least a 30-minute period. Feedings can only be given into the gastric cavity. Intermittent feedings are associated with the same problems as bolus feedings.

Continuous drip infusion provides a constant, steady flow of formula at a predetermined rate for a set period, generally 12 to 24 hours per day. Drip regulators, roll clamps, or pumps are used to control rates. Because the small bowel lacks storage capacity, feedings delivered beyond the pylorus must be provided by the continuous drip method. This method is generally preferred for the critically ill patient because it is usually associated with less gastric residual volume, less abdominal distention, less gastroesophageal reflux, and a decreased incidence of aspiration.[38]

Enteral Formula Selection. Formula selection depends on the patient's medical and surgical state, GI function, energy and nutrient needs, and route of administration. There are eight broad categories of enteral formulas: oral supplements, blenderized, whole protein lactose-free, fiber containing, nutrient dense, elemental, disease specific, and modular. Table 47-5 describes the indications for these various formulas and lists some example commercial preparations.

Complications of Enteral Therapy. There are three categories of complications occurring in patients receiving enteral nutrition: gastrointestinal, mechanical, and metabolic. Complications may be avoided by careful selection of formulas, proper administration, and consistent monitoring of the patient.

Pulmonary aspiration is of particular concern in the critically ill respiratory patient. Aspiration can occur if

Table 47-5 ▶▶ Enteral Product Reference Guide

Category	Indications	Examples
Oral supplements	Given with an oral diet to increase calorie and protein intake	Boost,[1,2]Carnation Instant Breakfast[1]
Blenderized	Made from natural foods and usually lower in sucrose and corn syrup than other formulas. Beneficial if intolerance to synthetic formula exists.	Compleat,[1] Compleat Modified[1,2]
Fiber containing	Dietary fiber can increase stool bulk and transit time, decrease intraluminal pressure, and improve bowel motility.	Jevity,[1,2] FiberSource,[1,2] Nutren 1.0 with Fiber[1,2]
Nutrient dense	Increased calories in a limited volume. Useful in hypermetabolic states (burns, trauma, sepsis, major surgery), and congestive heart failure.	Two Cal HN,[1,2] Ensure Plus,[1,2] Deliver,[1,2] Nutren 2.0[1,2]
Elemental	Impaired GI function with an impaired ability to digest/absorb intact nutrients.	Peptamen,[2] Vital HN,[2] Criticare,[2] Vivonex TEN,[2] Subdue Plus,[2] Alitraq[2]
Disease specific	Liver disease	Nutrihep,[1,2] Deliver 2.0[1,2]
	Renal disease	Nepro,[1,2] Magnacal Renal,[1,2] NovaSource Renal[1,2]
	Pulmonary disease	Pulmocare,[1,2] NutriVent,[1,2] Respalor[1,2]
	Glucose intolerance	Diabetisource,[1,2] Glucerna,[1,2] Choice DMTF,[1,2] Glytrol[1,2]
	Fat modified	Travasorb MCT, Portagen, Advera,[1,2], Lipisorb[1,2]
	Trauma	TraumaCal[1,2]
	Immune-enhancing	Impact,[1,2] Advera,[1,2] Lipisorb[1,2]
Modular	Need to modify a single nutrient (carbohydrate, protein, fat)	Polycose, Promod, Microlipid, MCT oil

1, Intact nutrients; *2*, lactose free.

the patient is lying flat, has a depressed gag reflux, has delayed gastric emptying, or improper tube placement. The two most important ways to minimize the likelihood of aspiration are (1) to raise the head of the bed at least 45 degrees, and (2) to deliver the feeding beyond the pylorus using the continuous drip method. Tube placement always should be verified by radiographic examination before feeding.

Suspected aspiration can be confirmed by adding blue food coloring to the feeding and retrieving it by tracheobronchial suctioning. Aggressive suctioning of oropharyngeal secretions can help prevent aspiration. The greatest risk is in patients with endotracheal tubes. Endotracheal tubes increase aspiration risk because they alter sensation, impair glottic closure, increase secretion volume, and act as "wicks" for secretions to enter the airway.[38] The use of special endotracheal tubes that provide continuous aspiration of subglottic secretions may help overcome the leakage-type aspiration so common in tube-fed patients.[40]

Parenteral Nutritional Support

When it is not possible to provide nutritional support through the GI tract, intravenous or parenteral nutritional support may be needed. Parenteral nutritional support can be administered through a peripheral or central vein. Ideally, the vascular access line should be isolated and maintained as a sterile route and not used for any other purpose. Because the volume and concentration of nutrients given through a small vein is somewhat limited, peripheral parenteral nutrition is generally considered only for short-term support. Mechanical, infectious, and metabolic complications have been reported in patients parenterally fed.[41]

▶ NUTRITIONAL SUPPORT IN SPECIFIC CIRCUMSTANCES

Details on the appropriate nutritional support provided to all the various types of patients seen by respiratory therapists are beyond the scope of this chapter. Here we emphasize key points related to the nutritional support and management of the most common conditions encountered by practitioners.

General Guidelines for Critically Ill Patients

The general goals of nutritional support in critically ill patients are to (1) provide for energy needs; (2) maintain nitrogen balance; (3) provide adequate (not excessive) calories to preserve lean body mass (muscle); (4) provide a positive nitrogen balance; (5) provide adequate vitamins, minerals, and fat; and (6) provide appropriate fluid.[42] Table 47-6 outlines the general guidelines recommended to achieve these goals.[42]

Table 47-6 ▶▶ General Nutritional Guidelines for Chronically Critically Ill Patients

Category	Guideline
Energy need	Provide 25-30 kcal/kg/day for men and 20-25 kcal/kg/day for women in a volume consistent with the total fluid needs of the patient (approximately 1 mL H_2O/kcal); or, use the Harris-Benedict equations times a stress factor of 1.2-1.4.
Protein	20% of total calories/day; 1-2 g/kg/day and adjust by periodic monitoring of nitrogen balance.
Carbohydrate	60% to 70% total calories/day. Fat 20% to 30% total calories/day; provide essential fatty acids.
Micronutrients	Adequate vitamins and minerals, such as: vitamins A, B_6, C, E, potassium, magnesium, zinc, iron, selenium, and phosphate.
Fluid	Approximately 1 mL/kcal.
Specialized nutrients	Glutamine (may improve nitrogen stores), arginine (may improve immune system), and Omega-3 fatty acids (may reduce inflammatory processes).
Route of delivery	Use enteral nutrition unless the gut is not functioning, then choose total parenteral nutrition.

Compiled from Pingleton SK: Clin Chest Med 22:149, 2001.

Systemic Inflammatory Response Syndrome

The systemic inflammatory response syndrome (SIRS) underlies many critical illnesses, including sepsis and acute respiratory distress syndrome (ARDS). Metabolism in SIRS is characterized by increased total caloric requirements, hyperglycemia, triglyceride intolerance, increased net protein catabolism, and increased macronutrient and micronutrient requirements.[25] Caloric requirements may need to be increased by 10% to 20%. If blood glucose level exceeds 225 mg/dL, glucose intake must be reduced and/or insulin given. Because of the hypercatabolic state, protein administration may need to be increased to levels of 1.7 to 2.0 g/kg/day. If serum triglycerides exceed 500 mg/dL, total calories and/or the dose of PUFAs should be reduced.[25]

Requirements for micronutrients are also increased in SIRS. Because of the potential high losses of potassium, zinc, magnesium, calcium, and phosphorus serum levels of these minerals need to be closely monitored and maintained within the normal range.[25]

Mechanical Ventilation

Adequate nutritional support is crucial for the ventilator-dependent patient. During acute illness, proper nutrition helps prevent the loss of lean body mass. After the resolution of the acute phase of illness, good nutrition helps the muscles regain lost strength and improves the likelihood of successful ventilator weaning.[34]

For most patients requiring ventilatory support, following the general guidelines provided in Table 47-6 will suffice. As always, care must be taken to avoid overfeeding and the increased ventilatory demands that follow.

Patients with COPD present a special situation, both in terms of nutritional needs and ventilatory support. More detail on these patients is provided in the next section.

Nutritional support alone is not sufficient to ensure weaning of ventilator-dependent patients. For these patients, appropriate nutrition may need to be combined with a tailored exercise program designed to strengthen and retrain muscles. More detail on methods used to wean ventilator-dependent patients is provided in Chapter 44.

Chronic Obstructive Pulmonary Disease

Malnutrition occurs in as many as 70% of all patients with COPD,[43] and it is most evident in those with pulmonary emphysema. Progressive weight loss is common. The malnutrition seems to have two causes: an insufficient intake for a prolonged period and increased nutrient needs because of chronic increases in metabolism. The malnutrition and low body weight appear to be an independent factor associated with a poor prognosis.[44]

The degree of weight loss generally correlates with deterioration of pulmonary function values. Thus, COPD can create a cycle in which respiratory dysfunction promotes weight loss, and weight loss further hinders respiratory function.[12] Figure 47-4 illustrates the cycle.

Factors contributing to poor intake include fatigue, shortness of breath, frequent coughing, early fullness because of pressure on the abdominal cavity, increased dyspnea during eating, side effects from medications (nausea, vomiting, diarrhea, dry mouth), and depression. The increased metabolic rate is due to the added effort to breathe and frequent respiratory infections, both of which increase calorie and fluid needs.

The goal for the healthcare team is to carefully increase nutrient intake without overfeeding the patient. For most COPD patients, 1.2 to 1.5 times the REE is sufficient. If weight gain is desired and the patient is stable and ambulatory, intake can be increased to 2 times the REE, as long as it does not impair respiratory function. Cachectic patients with COPD should be refed

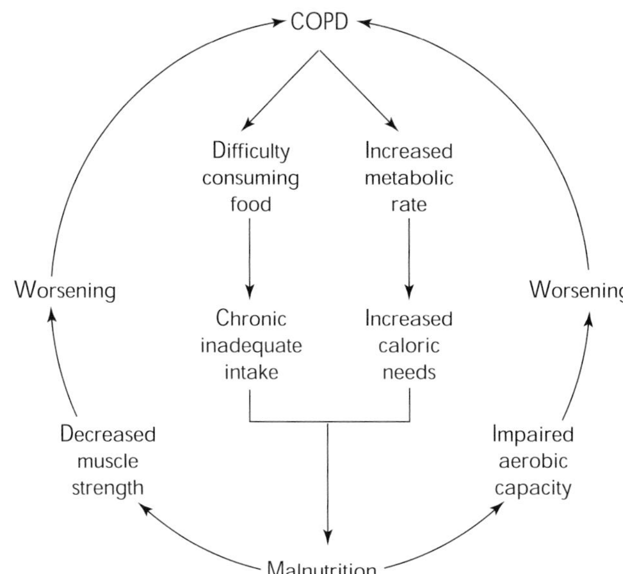

Figure 47-4
The vicious cycle of respiratory impairment and malnutrition in COPD.

cautiously.[13] Functional capacity, as well as the patient's overall health status, may improve with an anabolic stimulus, such as exercise, along with nutritional supplementation.[45]

In patients with COPD without hypercapnia, conventional macronutrient allocations are satisfactory (15% to 20% as protein, 50% to 60% carbohydrate, 20% to 30% fat). For patients with hypercapnia, the diet should be individually tailored to provide the lowest percentage of fat that maintains an acceptable Pa_{CO_2}.[12] However, as previously stated, setting an appropriate total calorie load is more important than fine-tuning the ratio of carbohydrate to fat.

Given the positive link between dietary intake and knowledge of diet and health, good patient education is critical.[46] Patients should be taught to select easy to consume, calorically dense foods (Box 47-13). Emphasis should be placed on small, frequent feedings with the use of high calorie, high protein nutritional supplements encouraged. Since many of the listed foods are not consistent with publicly disseminated guidelines, healthcare team members will need to explain and justify the differences. Other considerations in providing nutritional support to patients with COPD are listed in Box 47-14.[12] Medications prescribed for respiratory patients may influence food intake or interact with foods. Some of the common medications with their effects on nutrition are listed in Table 47-7.[47,48]

When patients with COPD are hospitalized for ventilatory failure, the clinical outcome is affected by nutritional support. Patients who receive adequate nutritional support are more readily weaned from

Box 47-13 • Sample Foods and Methods to Increase Nutrient Intake

- Dried fruits
- Whole milk or skim milk powder added to milk
- Nutritional supplements
- Rich desserts: cheesecake, sweet potato pie
- Puddings, custards, and ice creams
- Cream soups
- Added butter/margarine or cheese to vegetables
- Casseroles and egg dishes with sauces and gravies
- Fried foods
- Peanut butter or other nut butters
- Food preparation suggestions:
  - Pan fry in oil rather than broil
  - Use prepared meals for the microwave
  - Add skim milk powder or cheese to mashed potatoes

Box 47-14 • Nutritional Support for Patients With Pulmonary Disease

- Perform a complete nutritional assessment.
- Evaluate energy needs and provide an appropriate amount. (Do not overfeed or underfeed.)
- Ensure protein balance.
- Monitor fluids and electrolytes, especially phosphorus.
- Evaluate vitamin and mineral status as indicated.
- Consider high-fat, low-carbohydrate feedings in patients with hypercapnia.

Table 47-7 ▶▶ Common Respiratory Medication Interactions With Food

Medications	Interactions With Foods
β_2-Agonists	
*albuterol**	Peculiar taste, sore/dry throat, N/V, dyspepsia, diarrhea, increased appetite or anorexia, limit caffeine
Proventil	
Ventolin	
salmeterol	
Serevent	Dental pain, N/V, stomach ache, diarrhea
metaproterenol	Dry mouth/throat, N/V, dyspepsia, diarrhea, limit caffeine
Alupent	
Metaprel	
terbutaline	Dry mouth/throat and unusual taste (inhalant), N/V, dyspepsia, limit caffeine
Brethaire	
Brethine	
Bricanyl	
Anticholinergics	
ipratropium bromide	Dry mouth/throat, metallic/bitter taste, nausea, dyspepsia
Atrovent	
Mucolytic Agents	
dornase alfa	Sore throat, laryngitis
Pulmozyme	
Corticosteroids	
dexamethasone sodium phosphate	Increases appetite, increased weight, anorexia, esophagitis, N/V, dyspepsia, peptic ulcer, bloating, GI bleeding, GI perforation, protein catabolism, calcium wasting, increased folate requirement
Decadron	
Respihaler	
beclamethasone dipropionate	Dry mouth; decreased sense of taste, oral candidiasis; sore throat; N/V; rinse mouth after use and do not swallow rinse water
Beclovent	
Vanceril	
triamcinolone acetonide	Oral candidiasis, dry mouth, toothache, sore throat, pharyngitis with aerosol, nausea, abdominal pain, diarrhea, rinse mouth after use and do not swallow rinse water
Azmacort	
flunisolide	N/V, sore throat, unpleasant taste, loss of smell, abdominal pain, heartburn, constipation, gas
AeroBid	
fluticasone propionate	N/V, diarrhea, dyspepsia, and stomach disorder
Flovent	
budesonide	Oral candidiasis, dyspepsia, gastroenteritis, nausea
Pulmicort	

Table 47-7 ▶ ▶ Common Respiratory Medication Interactions With Food—cont'd

Medications	Interactions With Foods
Mediator Antagonists	
cromolyn sodium Intal	Take 30 minutes before meals and snacks. Open capsule and dissolve powder in 4 oz hot water; add 4 oz cold water (not juice, milk, or food). Unpleasant aftertaste, nausea. With aerosol/nebulizer: dry mouth/throat, sore throat. With oral capsule: abdominal pain, diarrhea.
zafirlukast Accolate	Take 1 hour before or 2 hours after food. N/V, dyspepsia, diarrhea, abdominal pain. Food decreased bioavailability of drug 40%.
zileuton Zyflo	Dyspepsia, N/V, abdominal pain, constipation, flatulence. Limit alcohol.
montelukast Singulaire	Chew tablet well. Caution with grapefruit juice, may increase side effects. Dyspepsia.

Compiled from the Physicians' Desk Reference, Montvale, NJ, Medical Economics, Inc, 2001 and Pronsky Z, Powers and Moore's Food Medication Interactions, ed 11, Birchrunville, PA, Food-Medication Interactions, 2000.
*The generic name is in italics, followed by brand names of the drug; N/V = nausea/vomiting.

mechanical ventilators than those whose diets are deficient in protein and energy. Moreover, in patients who are not catabolic, reducing energy intake to a level equal to or just below the REE may also aid weaning.[12]

Nutritional support may be ineffective in some patients.[49] Factors associated with such outcomes include aging, anorexia, and elevated inflammatory response.[50]

Cystic Fibrosis

The exocrine gland dysfunction seen in cystic fibrosis (CF) may cause chronic lung disease with recurrent infections. The same disturbance may cause pancreatic insufficiency. Metabolic problems in CF are similar to the patient with COPD, with reduced intake and increased metabolic needs. However, the pancreatic insufficiency causes malabsorption of all nutrients, especially fat. The administration of pancreatic enzyme supplements with meals enhances absorption but requires trial and error and intense education on how to balance the amount of food and the intake of enzymes. In addition, the time spent in various treatment programs reduces the ability to consume small frequent feedings.

The goals of nutrition management in CF are (1) to maximize a nutritional intake through calorically dense foods (see Box 47-13), (2) to balance intake with pancreatic enzymes to maximize absorption, and (3) to provide a nutrition plan that meets the changing clinical and psychosocial needs of the patient.[51] Use of calorically dense nutritional supplements (see Table 47-5) consumed throughout the day have proved useful in achieving weight gain.[52,53] Because of the malabsorption of micronutrients, vitamin and mineral supplementation is encouraged, especially the fat-soluble vitamins. Recent evidence suggests that the progressive pulmonary dysfunction seen in CF is partly attributable to nutritional deficiencies that can be readily corrected.[54] Thus helping CF patients achieve optimal nutritional health may minimize the decline in pulmonary function and improve their quality of life.[55]

KEY POINTS

- A healthy diet should combine foods from the five basic food groups; a majority of daily calories should come from grains, fruits, and vegetables.
- Macronutrients (protein, carbohydrate, and fat) supply the body's energy requirements.
- Micronutrients (vitamins, minerals, and other bioactive chemicals) provide no energy but play essential roles in normal metabolism and physiology.
- An individual's energy requirements represent the balance of energy intake to energy expenditure relative to body weight and activity level.
- The Harris-Benedict equations estimate daily REE; multiply by a stress or activity factor to determine total calorie needs.
- Malnutrition is a state of impaired metabolism in which the intake of essential nutrients falls short of the body's needs; marasmus is the form associated with inadequate nutrient intake (starvation), while kwashiorkor is the hypercatabolic form.
- Malnutrition can affect the respiratory system by causing loss of respiratory muscle mass and contractility, decreased ventilatory drive, impaired immune response, and alterations in lung parenchymal structure.

Continued

KEY POINTS—cont'd

- About a third of all patients with acute respiratory failure suffer from malnutrition, mainly the hypercatabolic form; these patients are prone to hypercapnia, can be difficult to wean from ventilatory support, and have higher mortality rates than those with a normal nutritional status.
- In chronic lung disease, the combined effect of increased energy expenditure (due to high work of breathing) and inadequate caloric intake contribute to a marasmus-type malnutrition.
- A complete nutritional assessment involves in-depth review of clinical and historical data, measurement of physical and physiological parameters, and assessment of a variety of clinical laboratory tests, as normally conducted by a registered dietitian.
- A body weight less than 90% of predicted IBW or recent weight loss in excess of 10% IBW is correlated with malnutrition.
- Indirect calorimetry involves measurement of whole-body $\dot{V}O_2$, $\dot{V}CO_2$ and RQ; results are used to assess a patient's metabolic state, determine nutritional needs, or assess response to nutrition therapy.
- Good calorimetry results require careful preparation of the patient over the prior 10 to 30 hours and careful calibration of the device prior to use on each patient.
- RQs >1.00 indicate overfeeding and the need to decrease total kcal; values between 0.7 to 0.8 indicate fat and protein oxidation due to starvation and the need to increase total kcal.
- The primary goal of nutritional support is to maintain or restore lean body (skeletal muscle) mass by (1) meeting the patient's overall energy needs and (2) providing the appropriate combination of macronutrients and micronutrients.
- Predicted REEs should be corrected for both stress and activity levels; typical factors range from 0.7 (for starvation) to 2.0 (for severe burns) of REE calories.
- For most patients, a balance of 20% of daily calorie needs from protein, 50% to 60% from simple carbohydrate, and 20% to 30% from fat is adequate.

KEY POINTS—cont'd

- For the patient with pulmonary disease, high carbohydrate loads can increase carbon dioxide production and the RQ, resulting in increased ventilatory demand, oxygen consumption, and work of breathing.
- Nutrients can be supplied enterally (oral and tube feeding) or parenterally (peripheral or central venous alimentation); whenever possible the enteral route should be used.
- The likelihood of aspiration during tube feedings can be minimized by delivering the feeding beyond the pylorus using the continuous drip method and raising the head of the bed at least 45 degrees.
- Nutritional support should be individualized according to patient needs and condition or disease process; follow accepted guidelines for SIRS, COPD, mechanical ventilation, and cystic fibrosis.

References

1. National Academy of Sciences: Recommended daily dietary allowances, ed 10, Washington, 1989, National Academy Press.
2. United States Department of Health and Human Services: Dietary guidelines for Americans, ed 5, Washington, D.C., 2000, U.S. Department of Agriculture; U.S. Department of Health and Human Services.
3. American Heart Association: Dietary guidelines, Dallas, 1993, American Heart Association.
4. United States Department of Agriculture: The food guide pyramid, Washington, 1992, U.S. Department of Agriculture.
5. Browne MB: Label facts for healthful eating, Dayton, The Mazer Corporation, 1993.
6. General Conference Nutrition Council: The vegetarian food pyramid, Hagerstown, MD, The Health Connection, 1994.
7. Goldberg IJ et al: Wine and your heart, Circ 103:472, 2001.
8. Whitney EN, Cataldo CB, Rolfes SR: Understanding normal and clinical nutrition, ed 5, Belmont, CA, West/Wadsworth, 1998.
9. Young VR, Pellett PL: Plant proteins in relation to human protein and amino acid nutrition, Am J Clin Nutr, 59(suppl):1203S, 1994.
10. Position of the American Dietetic Association on vegetarian diets, J Am Diet Assoc 97:1317, 1997.
11. American Dietetic Association: Position of the American Dietetic Association: phytochemicals and functional foods, J Am Diet Assoc 95:493, 1995.
12. Heimburger DC, Weinsier RL: Handbook of clinical nutrition, ed 3, St. Louis, 1997, Mosby.

13. Kleiner SM: Water: an essential but overlooked nutrient, J Am Diet Assoc 99:200, 1999.
14. Hu G, Cassano PA: Antioxidant nutrients and pulmonary function: the Third National Health and Nutrition Examination Survey (NHANES III), Am J Epidemiol 151:975, 2000.
15. Tabak C et al: Dietary factors and pulmonary function: a cross sectional study in middle-aged men from three European countries, Thorax 54:1021, 1999.
16. Van Duyn MAS, Pivonka A: Overview of the health benefits of fruit and vegetable consumption for the dietetics professional, J Am Diet Assoc 100:1511, 2000.
17. Donahoe M: Nutritional aspects of lung disease, Respir Care Clin N Am 4:85, 1998.
18. Mizock BA: Nutritional support of the hospitalized patient, Dis Mon 43:349, 1997.
19. Grossman GD: Nutritional assessment of critically ill patients, Respir Care Clin N Am 30:463, 1985.
20. Levine RJ: Carbohydrates. In Shils ME et al, editors: Modern nutrition in health and disease, ed 9, Baltimore, Williams & Wilkins, 1999.
21. Angelilleo VA: Nutrition and the pulmonary patient. In Hodgkin JE, Connors GL, Bell CW, editors: Pulmonary rehabilitation: guidelines to success, ed 2, Philadelphia, JB Lippincott, 1993.
22. Thorsdottir I, Gunnarsdottir I, Eriksen B: Screening method evaluated by nutritional status measurements can be used to detect malnourishment in chronic obstructive pulmonary disease, J Am Diet Assoc 1:648, 2001.
23. Peters JA: Nutritional assessment of patients with respiratory disease. In Wilkins RL, Krider SJ, Sheldon RL: Clinical assessment in respiratory care, ed 4, St. Louis, Mosby, 2000.
24. Gottschlich MM et al, editors: The science and practice of nutritional support, a case-based core curriculum, Dubuque, Kendall/Hunt, 2001.
25. American College of Chest Physicians: Applied nutrition in ICU patients (consensus statement), Chest 111:769, 1997.
26. Grant JP: Nutrition care of patients with acute and chronic respiratory failure, Nutr Clin Pract 9:11, 1994.
27. Ireton-Jones CS, Borman KR, Turner WW: Nutrition considerations in the management of ventilator-dependent patients, Nutr Clin Pract 8:60, 1993.
28. Ireton-Jones CS et al: Equations for estimating energy expenditures in burned patients with special reference to ventilatory status, J Burn Care and Rehabil 13:330, 1992.
29. American Association for Respiratory Care: Clinical practice guideline. Metabolic measurement using indirect calorimetry during mechanical ventilation, Respir Care Clin N Am 39:1170, 1994.
30. McArthur C: Indirect calorimetry, Respir Care Clin N Am 3:291, 1997.
31. McClave SA, McClain CJ, Snider HL: Should indirect calorimetry be used as part of nutritional assessment? J Clin Gastroenterol 33:14, 2001.
32. Witte MK: Metabolic measurements during mechanical ventilation in the pediatric intensive care unit, Respir Care Clin N Am 2:573, 1996.
33. Ritz R, Cunningham J: Indirect calorimetry. In Kacmarek RM, Hess DAY, Stoller JK, editors: Monitoring in respiratory care, St. Louis, Mosby, 1993.
34. Shikora SA, Benotti PN: Nutritional support of the mechanically ventilated patient, Respir Care Clin N Am 3:69, 1997.
35. Askanazi J: Nutrition for the patient with respiratory failure: glucose versus fat, Anesthesiology 54:373, 1981.
36. ASPEN: Standards of practice for nutrition support dieticians, Nutr Clin Prac 15:53, 2000.
37. Merritt RJ, editor: The A.S.P.E.N. nutritional support practice manual, Silver Spring, MD, ASPEN, 1998.
38. Elpern EH: Pulmonary aspiration in hospitalized adults, Nutr Clin Pract 12:5, 1997.
39. Lipman TO et al: Group I: choosing the appropriate method of placement of an enteral feeding tube in the high-risk population, Nutr Clin Pract 12:S54, 1997.
40. Valles J et al: Continuous aspiration of subglottic secretions in preventing ventilator-associated pneumonia, Ann Intern Med 122:179, 1995.
41. von Allmen DAY, Fischer JE: Metabolic complications. In Total parenteral nutrition, ed 2, New York, Little, Brown and Company, 1991.
42. Pingleton SK: Nutrition in chronic critical illness, Clin Chest Med 22:149, 2001.
43. Gray-Donald K et al: Nutritional status and mortality in chronic obstructive pulmonary disease, Am J Respir Crit Care Med 153:961, 1996.
44. Lando C et al: Prognostic value of nutritional status in chronic obstructive pulmonary disease, Am J Respir Crit Care Med 160:1856, 1999.
45. Schols AM: Nutritional abnormalities and supplementation in chronic obstructive pulmonary disease, Clin Chest Med 21:753, 2000.
46. Mackay L: Health education and COPD rehabilitation: a study, Nurs Stand 10:34, 1996.
47. Murray L: Physicians' desk reference, ed 55, Montvale, NJ, Medical Economics, 2001.
48. Pronsky Z: Powers and Moore's food medication interactions, ed 11, Birchrunville, PA, Food-Medication Interactions, 2000.
49. Ferreira IM et al: Nutritional support for individuals with COPD: a meta-analysis, Chest 117:672, 2000.
50. Creutzberg EC et al: Characterization of nonresponse to high caloric oral nutritional therapy in depleted patients with chronic obstructive pulmonary disease, Am J Respir Crit Care Med 161:745, 2000.
51. MacDonald A: Nutritional management of cystic fibrosis, Arch Dis Child 74:81, 1996.
52. Rettammel AL et al: Oral supplementation with a high-fat, high-energy product improves nutritional status and alters serum lipids in patients with cystic fibrosis, J Am Diet Assoc 95:454, 1995.
53. Mora-Gandarillas I et al: Nutritional status assessment in a group of cystic fibrosis patients, Am Esp Pediatr 44:40, 1996.
54. Thomson MA et al: Nutritional growth retardation is associated with defective lung growth in cystic fibrosis: a preventable determinant of progressive pulmonary dysfunction, Nutrition 11:350, 1995.
55. Zemel BS et al: Longitudinal relationship among growth, nutritional status, and pulmonary function in children with cystic fibrosis: analysis of the Cystic Fibrosis Foundation National CF Patient Registry, J Pediatr 137:374, 2000.

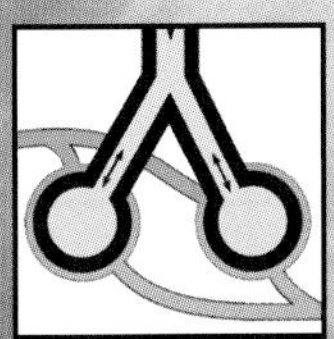

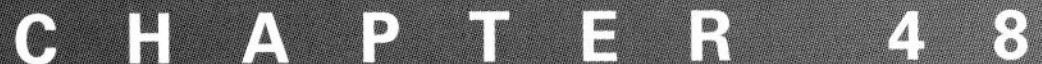

CHAPTER 48

Cardiopulmonary Rehabilitation

Kenneth A. Wyka

In This Chapter You Will Learn:

- What goals and objectives pulmonary rehabilitation aims to achieve
- What scientific evidence supports rehabilitation programming for patients with pulmonary disease
- How the body normally responds to exercise, and what factors limit maximum exercise levels
- Why psychosocial support is an essential component of pulmonary rehabilitation
- What specific benefits patients can expect from pulmonary rehabilitation activity
- What outcome measures can be used to evaluate pulmonary rehabilitation programs
- What indications, contraindications, and hazards are associated with pulmonary rehabilitation
- How to evaluate and select patients for pulmonary rehabilitation
- How to assist in exercise evaluation and distinguish between cardiac and ventilatory exercise limits
- What educational content needs to be addressed in a pulmonary rehabilitation program
- How to properly integrate exercise into a rehabilitation program
- Which health professionals make up the rehabilitation team
- What equipment and facilities are needed to run a pulmonary rehabilitation program
- How to cover the costs of a pulmonary rehabilitation program

Chapter Outline

Key Terms

12-minute walk
activities of daily living (ADL)
aerobic exercises
Borg dyspnea scale
cardiopulmonary exercise evaluation
comprehensive outpatient rehabilitative facilities (CORF)
contracture
hypoglycemia
inspiratory resistance
Karvonen's formula
metabolic equivalent of energy expenditure (METS)
O_2 pulse
onset of blood lactate accumulation (OBLA)

Continued

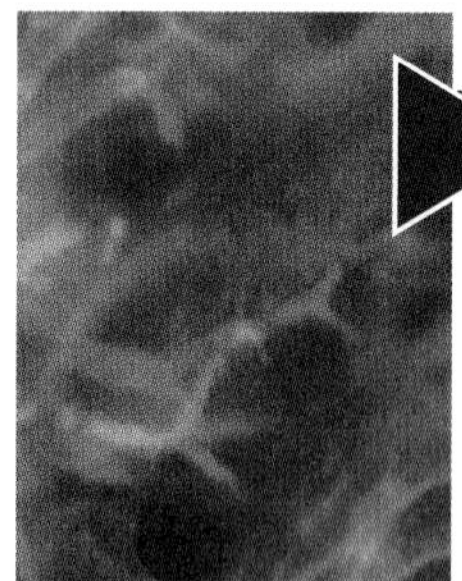

Key Terms — cont'd

progressive resistance
psychosocial support needs
reconditioning
respiratory quotient (RQ)
target heart rate
ventilatory muscle training
ventilatory threshold (VT)

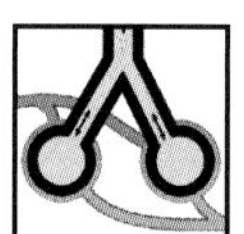

Steady improvements in acute care are presenting new medical and social problems. As more patients survive acute illnesses, there are increasing numbers of individuals with chronic disorders. These chronic disorders are associated with a wide spectrum of physiological, psychological, and social disabilities. Foremost among these groups are those with chronic cardiopulmonary disease. Although differences in diagnoses can impact treatment outcomes and survival, patients with chronic pulmonary disorders have much in common. All have difficulty coping with the physiological limitations of their diseases. Moreover, these physiological limitations result in many psychosocial problems. All too often, the end result is an unsatisfactory quality of life.

The high incidence of repeated hospitalizations and the progressive disability of these patients require well-organized programs of rehabilitative care. This chapter provides foundational knowledge on the goals, methods, and issues involved in providing planned programs of rehabilitation for individuals with chronic pulmonary disorders.

▶ DEFINITIONS AND GOALS

The Council on Rehabilitation defines *rehabilitation* as "the restoration of the individual to the fullest medical, mental, emotional, social, and vocational potential of which he or she is capable."[1] The overall goal is to maximize the functional ability and to minimize the impact the disability has on the individual, the family, and the community.

Pulmonary rehabilitation is the "art of medical practice wherein an individually tailored, multidisciplinary program is formulated, which through accurate diagnosis, therapy, emotional support, and education stabilizes or reverses both the physio- and psychopathology of pulmonary diseases and attempts to return the patient to the highest possible functional capacity allowed by his or her pulmonary handicap and overall life situation."[2]

The general goal of pulmonary rehabilitation is to improve the quality of life experienced by patients with a disabling pulmonary disease.[3] According to the American Thoracic Society, pulmonary rehabilitation has the following two specific objectives: (1) to control and alleviate the symptoms and pathophysiological complications of respiratory impairment and (2) to teach patients how to achieve optimal capability for carrying out their activities of daily living.[4]

▶ HISTORICAL PERSPECTIVE

Pulmonary rehabilitation is not a new concept. In 1951, Alvan Barach[5] recommended reconditioning programs for chronic lung patients to help improve their ability to walk without dyspnea. Unfortunately, decades passed before clinicians paid any attention to this concept. Instead of having their patients participate in reconditioning programs, most doctors simply prescribed O_2 therapy and bed rest. The result was a vicious cycle of skeletal muscle deterioration, progressive weakness and fatigue, and increasing levels of dyspnea, even at rest. Patients became homebound, then roombound and eventually bedbound. Clearly, improved avenues of therapy and rehabilitation were needed.

In 1962, Pierce and associates[6] published results confirming Barach's insight into the value of reconditioning. They observed that patients with chronic obstructive pulmonary disease (COPD) who participated in physical reconditioning exhibited lower pulse rates, respiratory rates, minute volumes, and CO_2 production during exercise. They also found, however, that these benefits occurred without significant changes in pulmonary function. Soon thereafter, Paez and associates[7] showed that reconditioning could improve both the efficiency of motion and oxygen utilization in patients with COPD. Subsequently, Christie[8] demonstrated that the benefits of reconditioning could be achieved on an outpatient basis with minimal supervision. Since Christie's work in 1968, other investigators have continued to research the benefits of pulmonary rehabilitation.

Today, the available evidence consistently indicates that pulmonary rehabilitation benefits patients with symptomatic COPD. When combined with smoking cessation, optimization of blood gases, and proper medication use, pulmonary rehabilitation offers the best treatment option for patients with symptomatic chronic airflow obstruction.[9] To provide this treatment option, comprehensive programs of pulmonary rehabilitation are being organized in a variety of settings. regardless of setting or design, such programs must be founded on the sound application of current knowledge in the clinical and social sciences.

▶ SCIENTIFIC BASES

Rehabilitation must focus on the patient as a whole and not solely on the underlying disease. For this reason, effective programming must combine knowledge from both the clinical and social sciences. Knowledge from the clinical sciences can help quantify the degree of physiological impairment and establish outcome expectations for reconditioning. Social sciences knowledge is helpful in determining the psychological, social, and vocational impact of the disability on the patient and family and in establishing ways to improve the patient's quality of life.

Physical Reconditioning

At rest, an individual maintains homeostasis by balancing external, internal, and cellular respiration. Physical activity, such as exercise, increases energy demands. To maintain homeostasis during exercise, the cardiorespiratory system must keep pace. Figure 48-1 shows how the body responds to exercise. Ventilation and circulation increase to supply tissues and cells with additional oxygen and eliminate the higher levels of carbon dioxide produced by metabolism. The ratio of carbon dioxide production ($\dot{V}CO_2$) to oxygen consumption ($\dot{V}O_2$) is referred to as the respiratory quotient, or RQ. Normally, at rest, an individual consumes about 250 mL of O_2 per minute and, in the process, produces approximately 200 mL of CO_2 per minute. The normal RQ is therefore about 0.8. Although the final pathway for carbohydrate, protein, and fat metabolism is shared, there are differences in the RQ for each. The RQ of carbohydrate is 1.0, that of protein is 0.8, and that of fat is 0.7.

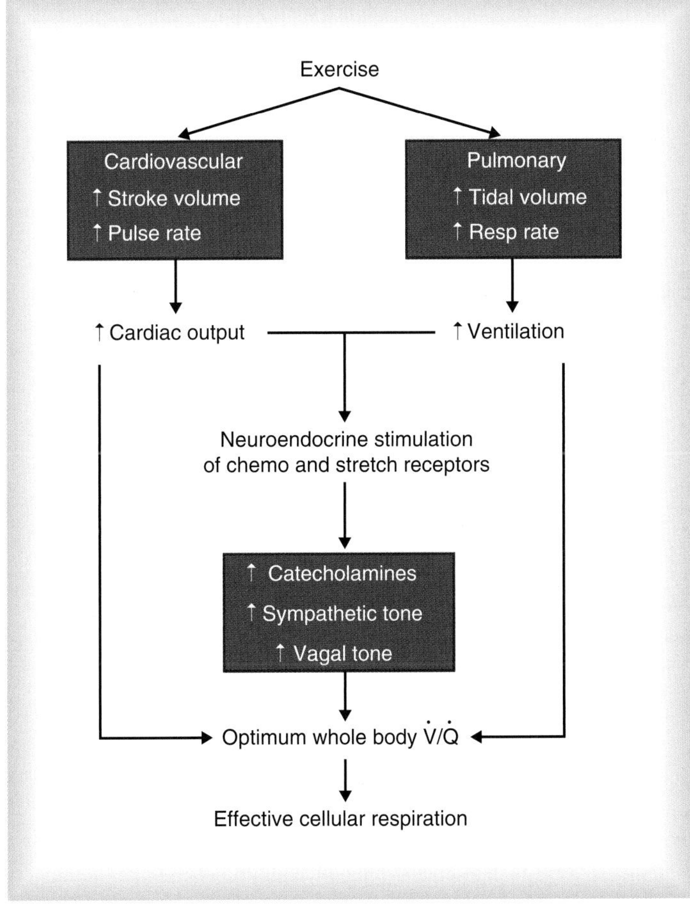

Figure 48-1
The body's response to increased levels of activity such as exercise.

As depicted in Figure 48-2, O_2 and CO_2 also increase in linear fashion as exercise intensity increases. If the body cannot deliver sufficient oxygen to meet the demands of energy metabolism, blood lactate levels increase above normal. In exercise physiology, this point is called the onset of blood lactate accumulation (OBLA). As this excess lactic acid is buffered, CO_2 levels rise and the stimulus to breathe increases. The result is an abrupt upswing in both CO_2 and $\dot{V}_E$ (referred to as the ventilatory threshold or VT). Beyond this point, metabolism becomes anaerobic, the efficiency of energy production decreases, lactic acid accumulates, and fatigue sets in.

The maximum voluntary ventilation (MVV) appears to be a good indicator of the respiratory system's ability to handle increased levels of physical activity. MVV can be measured directly or estimated (see accompanying Rule of Thumb). Normal individuals can achieve and maintain 60% to 70% of their MVV value on maximum exercise. This indicates that sufficient reserve still exists in the respiratory system and that ventilation is not the primary limiting factor for the termination of exercise.[10]

RULE OF THUMB

A good estimate of a patient's MVV is derived by multiplying the FEV_1 (forced expiratory volume in 1 second) by a factor of 35. As an example, to estimate the MVV of a patient with an FEV_1 of 1.5 L, simply multiply 1.5 L by 35:

MVV = FEV1 × 35

MVV = 1.5 L × 35 = 52.5 L/min

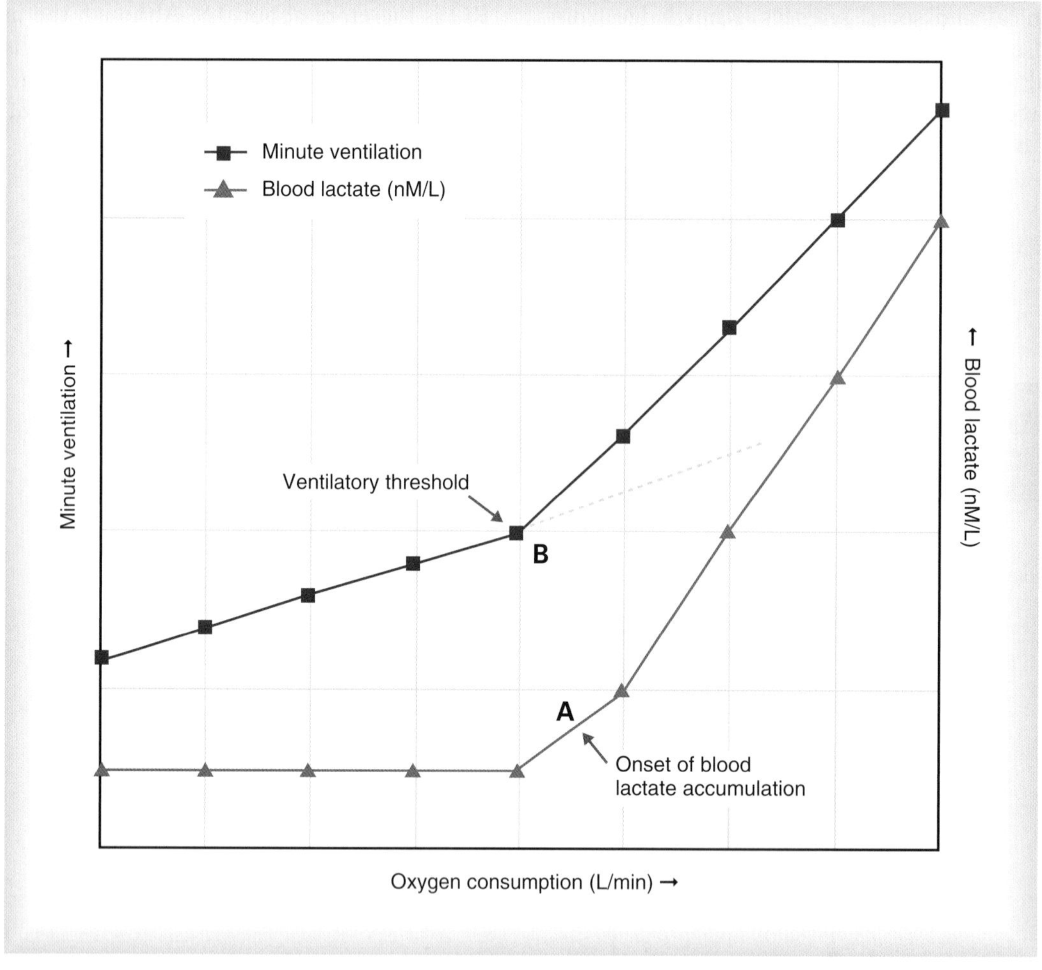

Figure 48-2

Minute ventilation, blood lactate, CO_2 production, and O_2 oxygen consumption during graded exercise to maximum. The dashed line represents the linear extrapolation between E and O_2 during submaximal exercise. Point A represents the onset of blood lactate accumulation or OBLA. At the same time, E and CO_2 "break" from their extrapolated rate of increase and abruptly rise *(Point B)*. This is referred to as the ventilatory threshold. *(Modified from McArdle WD, Katch FI, Katch VL: Exercise physiology: energy, nutrition and human performance, ed 4, Baltimore, 1996, Williams and Wilkins.)*

Patients with COPD who lack this reserve will have severe limitations to their exercise capabilities. Their high rate of CO_2 production during exercise results in respiratory acidosis and a shortness of breath out of proportion to the level of activity. In addition, as ventilation levels increase, a COPD patient's rate of oxygen consumption increases earlier and faster than normal (Figure 48-3). Together these factors limit patient tolerance for any significant increase in physical activity.

Pulmonary rehabilitation must therefore include efforts to physically recondition patients and increase their exercise tolerance. Reconditioning involves strengthening essential muscle groups, improving overall oxygen utilization, and enhancing the body's cardiovascular response to physical activity.

Psychosocial Support

If the overall goal of pulmonary rehabilitation is to improve the quality of patients' lives, then physical reconditioning alone is not sufficient. In fact, psychosocial indicators generally are better predictors of both the frequency and length of COPD patients' rehospitalization than are traditional measures of pulmonary function. Moreover, studies show that the relative success of reconditioning plays less of a role in determining whether patients complete a program than does meeting their psychosocial needs.[11]

There is a well-established relationship between our physical, mental, and social well-being. Everyday life is full of such relationships, such as the physical fatigue that follows a period of emotional tension. Many of these associations are part of normal human behavior. However, emotional states such as stress can cause or aggravate an existing physical problem. Likewise, physical manifestations of disease, such as recurrent dyspnea, can worsen stress.

Moreover, the progressive nature of COPD can negatively affect patients' overall outlook on their disease and reduce their motivation to adapt to its consequences. Respiratory therapists must realize that all their skilled technical services—as well as the best drug therapy—can be negated, and a patient can be driven on a progressively downhill course because of an unfavorable mental state.

Of course, emotional problems are not unique to patients with respiratory disease. Depression and hostility commonly occur with many acute and chronic diseases. In chronic respiratory disease, however, it may be a double-edged sword. Not only can emotional disturbances affect the general well-being of the patient, but they may also directly aggravate the very defects that are responsible for the underlying disability. The role of emotional and personality problems in the origin of childhood bronchial asthma is well known and has been extensively recorded in medical literature. It is quite probable that certain cases of adult (intrinsic) asthma, for which no specific allergic basis can be found, are attributable, in part, to psychological or emotional disorders. As compared to intrinsic asthma, however, psychological factors in chronic pulmonary disease are more a result of the disease rather than a

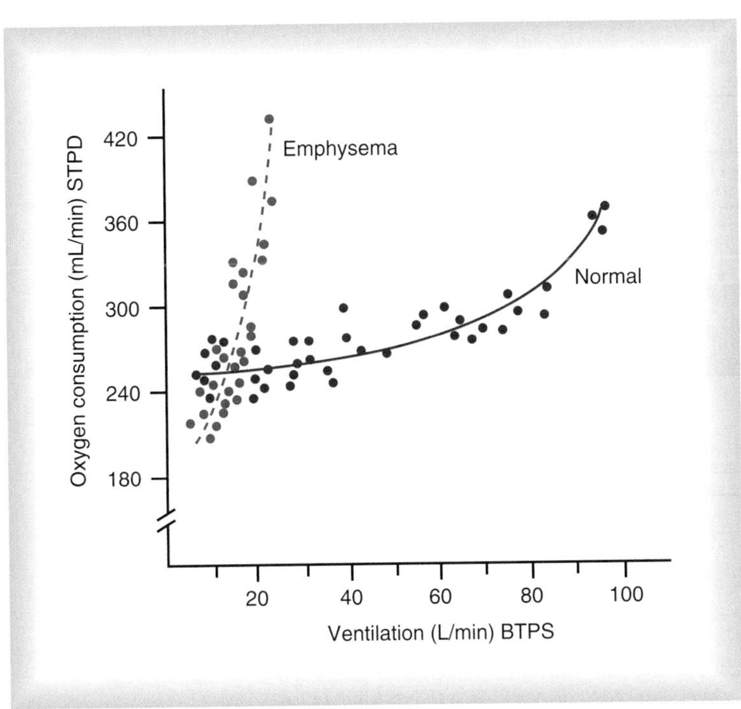

Figure 48-3

The changes in O_2 consumption with increasing ventilation in normal subject and in patient with emphysema. *BTPS*, Body temperature, body pressure saturated; *STPD*, volume of dry gas at 0° C and 760 mm Hg atmospheric pressure. *(Modified from Cherniack RM, Cherniack L, Naimark A: Respiration in health and disease, ed 3, Philadelphia, 1984, WB Saunders.)*

cause.[10] Often the patient with progressive emphysema develops severe anxiety, hostility, and stress as a direct consequence of the disability. Because patients are fearful of economic loss and death, they can also develop hostility toward the disease and often toward the people around them.

In regard to the social needs of patients with chronic lung disease, one commonly observes patients spontaneously receiving support and encouragement by simple association with each other. This informal observation suggests that the presence or absence of social support mechanisms may be a factor in determining how well patients adapt to their disability. Recent studies indicate that patients lacking a strong social support structure are at higher risk for rehospitalization than those with such networks. Clearly, well-designed pulmonary rehabilitation programming should take advantage of this knowledge and address the social support needs of participating patients.[12]

In terms of social function, the physiological impairment of chronic lung disease, in combination with other variables, can severely restrict a patient's ability to perform even the most routine tasks requiring physical exertion. Obviously, intolerance for physical exertion lessens the patient's social activity. More importantly, however, are the patients' potential loss of confidence in their ability to care for themselves that can accompany such impairments, and the resultant loss of feelings of dignity and self-worth. Labeling the patient as a pulmonary cripple only worsens the problem. Such factors can establish a cycle of further social withdrawal and intensify psychological depression and an increased frequency of acute exacerbations of the underlying disease.

Figure 48-4 presents elements of this cycle and shows how chronic lung disease and other variables can impact a patient's quality of life. It is here that the link between the physical reconditioning and psychosocial support components of rehabilitation becomes most evident. By reducing exercise intolerance and enhancing the body's cardiovascular response to physical activity, patients can develop a more independent and active lifestyle. For some, simply being able to walk to the market or play with their grandchildren will contribute to a greater feeling of social importance and self-worth. For others, physical conditioning may allow a return to near normal levels of activity, including vocational pursuits.

Many disabled pulmonary patients are in their economically productive years and are anxious to return to economic self-sufficiency. For them, occupational retraining and job placement are key ingredients in a good rehabilitation program. Such a program should be based on the individual needs and expectations of each patient. Not only must each patient's physical ability be considered but his or her education, past experience, aptitude, and personality as well. Evaluation and placement of the rehabilitation patient requires both the skills of vocational counselors and occupational therapists and the cooperation of business and industry. Whereas vocational rehabilitation efforts have succeeded for patients disabled by trauma or stroke, only recently have similar approaches been applied to patients with pulmonary disability.[13]

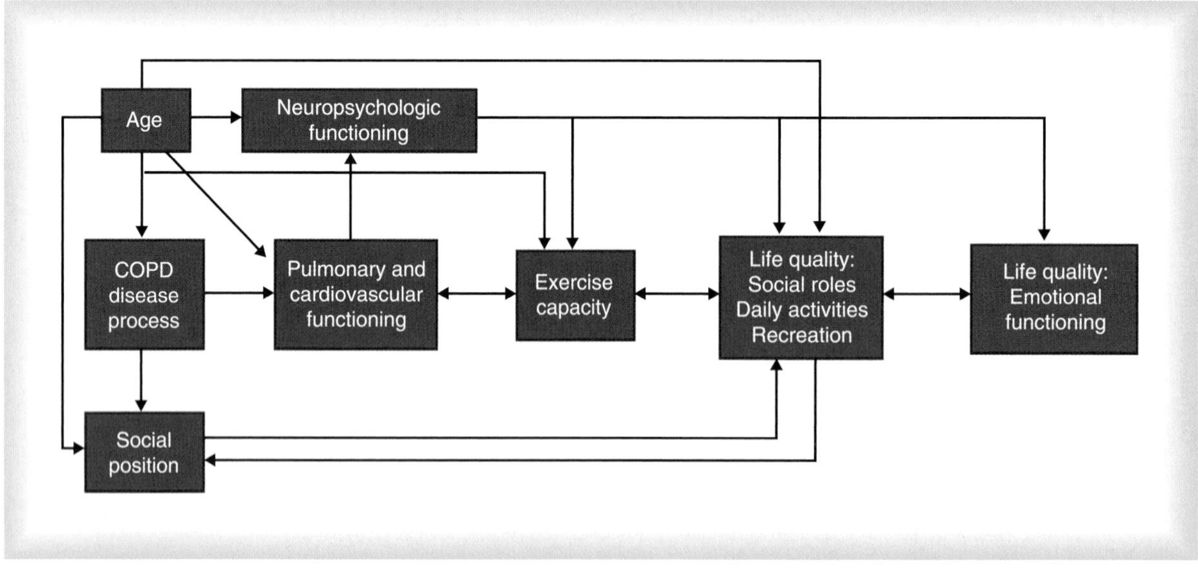

Figure 48-4
Model describing relationship between physical and psychological dysfunction in patients with chronic lung disease. *(Modified from McSweeney AJ et al: Life quality of patients with chronic obstructive pulmonary disease, Arch Intern Med 142:473, 1982.)*

▶ PULMONARY REHABILITATION PROGRAMMING

Program Goals and Objectives

Pulmonary rehabilitation programs vary in their design and implementation but generally share common goals. Examples of these common goals appear in Box 48-1.

These general goals assist planners in formulating more specific program objectives. When determining objectives, both patients and members of the rehabilitation team should have input. Depending on the specific needs of the participants, program objectives can include the following:

- Development of diaphragmatic breathing skills
- Development of stress management and relaxation techniques
- Involvement in a daily physical exercise regimen to condition both skeletal and respiratory-related muscles
- Adherence to proper hygiene, diet, and nutrition
- Proper use of medications, oxygen, and breathing equipment (if applicable)
- Application of airway clearance techniques (when indicated)
- Focus on group support
- Provisions for individual and family counseling

When program objectives are specifically defined and structured in a measurable way, strategies can be tailored to ensure the maximum results and benefit. Demonstration of program effectiveness also becomes easier and more acceptable by the medical community. However, benefits realized by participating patients are not always easy to identify and may be controversial.

Box 48-1 • Common Goals for Pulmonary Rehabilitation Programs

- Control of respiratory infections
- Basic airway management
- Improvement in ventilation and cardiac status
- Improvement in ambulation and other types of physical activity
- Reduction in overall medical costs
- Reduction in hospitalizations
- Psychosocial support
- Occupational retraining and placement (when and where possible)
- Family education, counseling, and support
- Patient education, counseling, and support
- Control of respiratory infections

Benefits and Potential Hazards

Benefits

An underlying assumption of all pulmonary rehabilitation programs designed for those with chronic lung disorders is that the disease process is progressive and irreversible. Based on this assumption, we cannot expect long-term improvements in objective indicators of pulmonary function such as those obtained by spirometry or blood gas analysis. The research literature clearly shows that rehabilitation does not alter the progressive deterioration in lung function that occurs with chronic pulmonary disorders.[14]

However, the evidence is just as convincing that properly implemented rehabilitation programs can improve a patient's overall utilization of oxygen by increasing the effectiveness of muscle use and by promoting more effective breathing techniques. We know that exercise ventilation in patients with COPD is inefficient in that the oxygen cost for a given amount of ventilation is excessive. We also know that training of specific skeletal muscle groups alone may not produce an improvement in exercise tolerance, but that training of respiratory-related muscles can improve exercise tolerance. Therefore to maximize rehabilitation outcomes, programs must have activities to recondition both the respiratory-related and skeletal muscles groups. Table 48-1 classifies the benefits of exercise reconditioning for chronic lung patients based on current knowledge of their acceptability and probability.[15]

Reconditioning provides more than just physiological benefits. However, achieving the related social, psychological, and vocational outcomes requires a complementary and multidisciplinary focus on psychosocial readaptation. For this reason, programs that attend solely to physical reconditioning efforts are not truly rehabilitative in nature. Only those that address *both* physical and psychosocial needs should be considered true rehabilitation programs.

Naturally, physiological benefits currently are more acceptable to the medical community and are easier to measure and document. Clinicians measure and document physiological benefits by performing periodic exercise evaluations on the patient. Psychosocial benefits, on the other hand, are more controversial and harder to substantiate. Nonetheless, participants in pulmonary rehabilitation tend to feel better, experience less dyspnea, and are able to lead more active and productive lives than those not involved in such activities.[16-18] Ultimately, these benefits may be the best indicators of program success.

In combination, these physiological and psychosocial benefits represent the desired outcomes of pulmonary rehabilitation. As shown in Box 48-2, these outcomes can be categorized and measured using both quantitative and qualitative methods. Results of these assess-

Table 48-1 ▶ ▶ Benefits From Exercise Reconditioning

Accepted Benefits	Potential Benefits	Unproven Benefits
Increased physical endurance	Increased sense of well-being	Prolonged survival
Increased max O_2 consumption	Improved secretion clearance	Improved PFT results
Increased activity levels with:	Increased hypoxic drive	Lowered pulmonary artery pressure
Decreased ventilation	Improved cardiac function	Improved blood gases
Decreased $\dot{V}O_2$		Improved blood lipids
Decreased heart rate		Change in muscle O_2 extraction
Increased VT		Change in step desaturation

From Hughes RL, Davison R: Limitations of exercise reconditioning in COPD, Chest 83:241, 1983.

MINI CLINI

What to Expect From Pulmonary Rehabilitation

PROBLEM

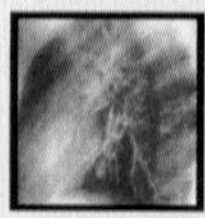

A respiratory therapist is asked to consult on a 63-year-old man hospitalized with severe COPD for possible participation in an outpatient pulmonary rehabilitation program. During the patient interview, the patient tells the therapist that if the program will not cure him, then he sees no reason to participate. How should the respiratory therapist respond to the patient keeping in mind his expectations of what pulmonary rehabilitation should accomplish?

SOLUTION

It is critical for all respiratory therapists and other caregivers involved in pulmonary rehabilitation to recognize that the focus of any program should attempt to treat the patient as a whole and not solely the underlying disease. A well-constructed pulmonary rehabilitation program should be able to both quantify the extent of physiological impairment and assist in establishing outcome expectations for physical reconditioning. Further, regardless of setting or design, such programs must address the psychological, social, and vocational impact of the disability on the patient and family and seek ways to improve the patient's quality of life. In this case, the respiratory therapist should speak to the benefits of pulmonary rehabilitation outside the traditional measures of pulmonary function. While pulmonary rehabilitation cannot affect the progressive deterioration in lung function that occurs with COPD, both education and exercise may improve his ability to perform activities of daily living and exercise tolerance. In addition, effective breathing techniques may lessen the frequency and severity of "panic breathing" episodes.

ments can then be used to evaluate patient outcomes and program effectiveness.

Potential Hazards

Although most patients with COPD can expect to realize benefits through physical reconditioning and pulmonary rehabilitation, certain potential hazards do exist. Potential hazards include the following:

I. Cardiovascular abnormalities
   A. Cardiac arrhythmias (can be reduced with supplemental oxygen during exercise)
   B. Systemic hypotension
II. Blood gas abnormalities
   A. Arterial desaturation
   B. Hypercapnia
   C. Acidosis
III. Muscular abnormalities
   A. Functional or structural injuries
   B. Diaphragmatic fatigue and failure
   C. Exercise-induced muscle contracture

Box 48-2 • Evaluation of Rehabilitation Program Outcomes

- Changes in exercise tolerance
- Before and after 6 or 12 minute walking distance
- Before and after pulmonary exercise stress test
- Review of patient home exercise logs
- Strength measurement
- Flexibility and posture
- Performance on specific exercises (e.g., ventilatory muscle, upper extremity)
- Changes in symptoms
- Dyspnea measurement comparison
- Frequency of cough, sputum production, or wheezing
- Weight loss or gain
- Psychological test instruments
- Other changes
- Activities of daily living (ADL) changes
- Postprogram follow-up questionnaires
- Preprogram and postprogram knowledge tests
- Compliance improvement with pulmonary rehabilitation medical regimen
- Frequency and duration of respiratory exacerbations
- Frequency and duration of hospitalizations
- Frequency of emergency department visits
- Return to productive employment

IV. Miscellaneous
  A. Exercise-induced asthma (more common in young patient with asthma than in patients with COPD)
  B. Hypoglycemia
  C. Dehydration

Proper patient selection, education, supervision, and monitoring are key factors in reducing possible hazards.

Patient Evaluation and Selection

Before beginning a pulmonary rehabilitation program, clinicians need to define and establish criteria for entry or selection. Patient selection requires comprehensive evaluation and testing.

Patient Evaluation

Patient evaluation should begin with a complete patient history: medical, psychological, vocational, and social. A well-designed patient questionnaire and interview form will assist with this step.

The patient's history should be followed by a complete physical examination (see Chapter 14). A recent chest film, resting electrocardiogram (ECG), complete blood count, serum electrolytes, and urinalysis will provide additional information on the patient's current medical status (see Chapter 15).

To determine the patient's cardiopulmonary status and exercise capacity, both pulmonary function testing and a cardiopulmonary exercise evaluation should be performed. The pulmonary function testing should include assessment of pulmonary ventilation, lung volume determinations, diffusing capacity (D_{LCO}), and prebronchodilator and postbronchodilator spirometry (see Chapter 17).

The cardiopulmonary exercise evaluation serves two key purposes in pulmonary rehabilitation. First, it quantifies the patient's initial exercise capacity. This provides the basis for the exercise prescription (including setting a target heart rate) and also yields the baseline data for assessing a patient's progress over time.[19] In addition, the evaluation helps clinicians determine the degree of hypoxemia or desaturation that can occur with exercise. This provides the objective basis for titrating O_2 therapy during the exercise program.

To guide practitioners in implementing exercise evaluation, the AARC has published *Clinical Practice Guideline: Exercise Testing for Evaluation of Hypoxemia and/or Desaturation.*[20] Excerpts appear on p. 1234.

The actual exercise evaluation procedure involves serial or continuous measurements of several physiological parameters during various graded levels of exercise on either an ergometer or treadmill (Box 48-3).

Box 48-3 • Common Physiological Parameters Measured During Exercise Evaluation

- Blood pressure
- Heart rate
- ECG
- Respiratory rate
- Arterial blood gases (ABGs)/O_2 saturation
- Maximum ventilation ($\dot{V}_E$max)
- O_2 consumption (either absolute $\dot{V}O_2$ or METS, the metabolic equivalent of energy expenditure)
- CO_2 production ($\dot{V}CO_2$)
- Respiratory quotient (RQ)
- O_2 pulse

To allow for steady state equilibration, these graded levels are usually spaced at 3-minute intervals. Work levels are increased progressively until either (1) the patient cannot tolerate a higher level, or (2) an abnormal or hazardous response occurs.

Regarding blood gas and arterial saturation measures, the clinician should obtain samples at rest and at peak exercise. Samples from single arterial punctures are as good as those drawn from indwelling cannulas. If the peak exercise puncture is unsuccessful, a sample drawn within 10 to 15 seconds of test termination will usually suffice. Due to its inherent problems, pulse oximetry has a limited but nonetheless important role in exercise evaluation. Its best use is as a monitor to warn clinicians of gross desaturation events during testing. In addition, the pulse oximeter also can be used to assess the patient's response to supplemental oxygen during exercise.[20]

Relative contraindications to exercise testing include (1) patients who cannot or will not perform the test; (2) severe pulmonary hypertension/cor pulmonale; (3) known electrolyte disturbances (hypokalemia, hypomagnesemia); (4) resting diastolic blood pressure >110 mm Hg or resting systolic blood pressure >200 mm Hg; (5) neuromuscular, musculoskeletal, or rheumatoid disorders exacerbated by exercise; (6) uncontrolled metabolic disease (e.g., diabetes); (7) SaO_2 or $SpO_2 < 85\%$ with the subject breathing room air; (8) untreated or unstable asthma.

Exercise evaluation also can help differentiate between patients with primary respiratory or cardiac limitations to increased work capacity. Table 48-2 summarizes these key similarities and differences. Obviously, besides helping to differentiate between the underlying cause of exercise intolerance, test results can assist clinicians in placing patients in the appropriate type of rehabilitation program.

To minimize patient risk during exercise evaluation, clinicians must adhere to certain safety measures. First, the patient should undergo a physical examination

Exercise Testing for Evaluation of Hypoxemia and/or Desaturation

AARC Clinical Practice Guideline (Excerpts)*

➤ INDICATIONS

- The need to assess/quantify arterial oxyhemoglobin (HbO_2) levels during exercise in patients suspected of desaturation
- The need to quantify the response to therapeutic intervention
- The need to titrate the optimum level of O_2 therapy during activity
- The need for preoperative assessment for lung resection or transplant
- The need to assess the degree of impairment for disability evaluation

➤ CONTRAINDICATIONS

Absolute contraindications include:

- Acute ECG changes indicating myocardial ischemia or serious cardiac dysrhythmias
- Unstable angina
- Acute pericarditis
- Aneurysm of the heart or aorta
- Uncontrolled systemic hypertension
- Recent (within prior 4 weeks) myocardial infarction or myocarditis
- Second- or third-degree heart block
- Recent systemic or pulmonary embolus
- Acute thrombophlebitis or deep venous thrombosis

Relative contraindications to exercise testing include:

- Patients who cannot or will not perform the test
- Severe pulmonary hypertension/cor pulmonale
- Known electrolyte disturbances (hypokalemia, hypomagnesemia)
- Resting diastolic blood pressure >110 torr or resting systolic blood pressure >200 torr
- Neuromuscular, musculoskeletal, or rheumatoid disorders exacerbated by exercise
- Uncontrolled metabolic disease (e.g., diabetes)
- Sao_2 or Spo_2 <85% with the subject breathing room air
- Untreated or unstable asthma

➤ PRECAUTIONS AND/OR POSSIBLE COMPLICATIONS

Indications for ending testing include:

- ECG abnormalities (e.g., dangerous dysrhythmias, ventricular tachycardia, ST-T wave changes)
- Severe desaturation (Sao_2 <80% or Spo_2 <83% and/or a 10% fall from baseline values)
- Angina
- Hypotensive responses
- A fall of >20 torr in systolic pressure, occurring after the normal exercise rise
- A fall in systolic blood pressure below the preexercise level
- Lightheadedness
- Request from patient to terminate test

Abnormal responses that may require discontinuation of exercise include (1) a rise in systolic blood pressure to >250 torr or of diastolic pressure to >120 torr; (2) a rise in systolic pressure of <20 torr from resting level; (3) mental confusion or headache; (4) cyanosis; (5) nausea or vomiting; (6) muscle cramping.

➤ ASSESSMENT OF NEED

Indications for exercise testing to evaluate hypoxemia and/or desaturation include:

- History and physical indicators suggesting hypoxemia and/or desaturation
- The presence of abnormal diagnostic test results (e.g., D_{LCO}, FEV_1, ABGs)
- The need to titrate or adjust a therapy

➤ MONITORING

The following should be monitored during testing:

- Physical assessment (chest pain, leg cramps, color, perceived exertion, dyspnea)

EXERCISE TESTING FOR EVALUATION OF HYPOXEMIA AND/OR DESATURATION—CONT'D

AARC Clinical Practice Guideline (Excerpts)*

- Respiratory rate
- Sp_{O_2}
- Cooperation and effort level
- Borg or modified Borg dyspnea scale
- Blood gas sampling site and technique
- Heart rate, rhythm, and ST-T wave changes
- Blood pressure

For the complete guidelines, see Respir Care 37:907, 1992.

Table 48-2 Exercise Parameters Distinguishing Cardiac and Ventilatory (COPD) Limitations

Parameter*	Cardiac+	COPD
Max $\dot{V}o_2$	↓	↓
Max HR	N or ↓	↓
O_2 pulse	↓	N
Max $\dot{Q}$	↓	↓
$\dot{Q}/\dot{V}o_2$	↓	N
Pa_{O_2}	N	↓
Pa_{CO_2}	↓	↑
$\dot{V}E/\dot{V}co_2$	↑	↑
VT	↓	N

Modified from Lane EE, Walker JF: Clinical arterial blood gas analysis, St Louis, 1987, Mosby.
*$\dot{V}O_2$, Oxygen consumption; HR, heart rate; Q, cardiac output; $\dot{V}E/\dot{V}co_2$, ratio of ventilation to CO_2 production; VT, ventilatory threshold.
+N, Normal; ↑, increased; ↓, decreased.

just before the test, including a resting ECG. Second, a qualified physician should be present throughout the entire test. Third, emergency resuscitation equipment (cardiac crash cart with monitor, defibrillator, oxygen, cardiac drugs, suction, and airway equipment) must be readily available. Fourth, staff conducting and assisting with the procedure should be certified in basic and advanced life support techniques. Last, the test should be terminated promptly whenever indicated.

With regard to test preparation, patients should fast 8 hours before the procedure. If the purpose of the test is to formulate an exercise prescription, the patient can take his or her regular medications. The patient should wear comfortable, loose-fitting clothing and footwear with adequate traction for treadmill or ergometer activity. The mouthpiece or face mask used during the test should be sized properly and fit comfortably with no leaks. Test conditions should be as standardized as possible to allow for comparison of both prerehabilitation and postrehabilitation results and periodically from year to year as the patient is treated and followed.

Patient Selection

Patients most likely to benefit from participation in pulmonary rehabilitation are those with persistent symptoms due to COPD. Other indications for pulmonary rehabilitation are listed in Box 48-4. Regardless of underlying conditions, patients also should be ex-smokers. Any patients who smokes should enroll in a smoking cessation program before starting pulmonary rehabilitation. Patients are excluded from pulmonary rehabilitation activities if (1) concurrent problems limit or preclude participation in exercise, or (2) their condition is complicated by malignant neoplasms, for example, lung cancer (Box 48-4).

Objectively, candidates considered for inclusion in a pulmonary rehabilitation program generally fall into one of the following groups:[21]

- Patients in whom there is a respiratory limitation to exercise resulting in termination at a level less than 75% of the predicted maximum oxygen consumption ($\dot{V}O_2max$)
- Patients in whom there is significant irreversible airway obstruction with a forced expiratory volume in one second (FEV_1) of less than 2 L or an $FEV_{1\%}$ (FEV_1/FVC) of less than 60%
- Patients in whom there is a significant restrictive lung disease with a total lung capacity (TLC) of less than 80% of predicted and single breath carbon monoxide diffusing capacity (D_{LCO}) of less than 80% of predicted

Box 48-4 • Indications and Contraindications for Pulmonary Rehabilitation

INDICATIONS

- Symptomatic patients with COPD
- Patients with bronchial asthma and associated bronchitis (asthmatic bronchitis)
- Patients with combined obstructive and restrictive ventilatory defects
- Patients with chronic mucocilliary clearance problems
- Patients having exercise limitations due to severe dyspnea

CONTRAINDICATIONS

- Cardiovascular instability requiring cardiac monitoring (consider cardiac rehabilitation)
- Malignant neoplasms involving the respiratory system
- Patients with severe arthritis or neuromuscular abnormalities (a relative contraindication—refer to physical therapy for case-by-case review)

- Patients with pulmonary vascular disease in whom the single breath carbon monoxide diffusing capacity (D_{LCO}) is less than 80% of predicted or in whom exercise is limited to less than 75% of maximum predicted oxygen consumption (predicted $\dot{V}O_2$ max).

Groups or classes for pulmonary rehabilitation should be kept homogeneous. Placing individuals in a program who are at different stages of cardiopulmonary disability can be very defeating. Those with mild to moderate impairment may become discouraged on how severe lung disease can become and those with severe impairment will feel they cannot keep up with or maintain the level of activity exhibited by those with less severe impairment. It is best to group patients together on the basis of severity and overall ability. In this way, patients can participate, compete, and progress together in the program without frustration, fear, or loss of motivation.

Program Design

Good design helps achieve specific programming objectives with the selected group of participating patients. Key design considerations involve both format and content, with emphasis on patient reconditioning and education.

Format

Programs can use either an open-ended or closed design, with or without planned follow-up sessions. With an open-ended format, patients enter the program and progress through it until they achieve certain predetermined objectives. There is no set time frame. Therefore depending on his or her condition, needs, motivation, and performance, an individual patient can complete an open-ended program over weeks or even months. This format is good for self-directed patients, or those with scheduling difficulties. It also may be the best format for patients requiring individual attention. The major drawback of the open-ended format is the lack of group support and involvement.

The more traditional closed design uses a set time period to cover program content. These programs usually run over 8 to 16 weeks, with classes meeting 1 to 3 times a week. However, insurance coverage may dictate exactly how many sessions a patient is qualified and covered for. Class sessions usually last 1 to 3 hours. Presentations are more formal and group support and involvement is encouraged. A major drawback to this format is that the schedule determines program completion, rather than the objectives. However, most programs allow patients to re-enroll if the anticipated improvements are not achieved. This format also may result in less individualized attention than the open-ended approach.[22]

MINI CLINI

Patient Selection for Pulmonary Rehabilitation

PROBLEM

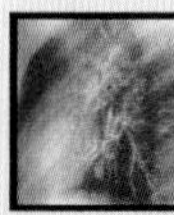

A patient is being evaluated for possible inclusion in a pulmonary rehabilitation program. The patient undergoes a complete history and physical, along with pulmonary function testing, arterial blood gas analysis, and exercise evaluation. During the exercise test, the patient develops severe hypertension and premature ventricular contractions. The physician recommends that the patient be admitted to pulmonary rehabilitation and prescribes a modified exercise routine. The respiratory therapist performing the test disagrees. How should the therapist proceed?

SOLUTION

The respiratory therapist should contact the department medical director for intervention. While this patient could possibly be admitted to pulmonary rehabilitation, there is a high risk that some type of adverse response might occur during the exercise component of the program. The best direction would be to treat the cardiac manifestations first. By identifying the causes of the exercise-induced hypertension and arrhythmia, these problems can be properly treated. Once under control, the patient may be admitted to pulmonary rehabilitation and safely participate in and complete the program. Any underlying condition should be treated and managed first before any pulmonary rehabilitation begins.

Table 48-3 ▶ ▶ Sample Pulmonary Rehabilitation Session

Component	Focus	Time Frame
Educational	Welcome (group interaction)	5 minutes
	Review of program diaries (past week's activities)	20 minutes
	Presentation of educational topic	20 minutes
	Questions, answers, and group discussion	15 minutes
Physical reconditioning	Physical activity and reconditioning	45 minutes
	Individual goal-setting and session summary	15 minutes
Total: 120 minutes (2 hours)		

Regardless of the format used, long-term improvements cannot be expected without planned follow-up.[16] Follow-up must be ongoing and available to all patients who complete the program. Frequently, this essential element of the process is difficult, especially when it is not covered by most insurance plans, but program coordinators must ensure that it is routinely scheduled. Follow-up or reinforcement could be open-ended (available during regular rehabilitation sessions and offering open attendance) or could be scheduled weekly, monthly, bimonthly, or quarterly. The important thing is to have some type of follow-up available.

Content

Rehabilitation program content usually combines physical reconditioning with education activities. Table 48-3 outlines a sample session incorporating these two complementary components. Programs providing reconditioning or education alone are unlikely to be effective.

As shown in Table 48-3, the ideal rehabilitation session should run for about 2 hours. Group size, available equipment, and group interaction will dictate session length. Patients should arrive 10 to 15 minutes before a scheduled session in order to allow for informal group interaction and support. Classes should begin on time and conclude promptly as scheduled. Educational presentations should be brief and to the point. The use of audio-visuals or demonstrations should be used to enhance understanding. In order to facilitate patient comprehension, the language should be simple, and unnecessary technical terms or concepts should be avoided. Handouts that enhance certain points made during a presentation are both useful and desirable. A folder or notebook in which program activities may be recorded and handout materials kept should be maintained by each patient.

Physical Reconditioning

The physical reconditioning component of the pulmonary rehabilitation program consists primarily of an exercise prescription with target heart rate based on the results of the patient's initial exercise evaluation. For most patients, an initial target heart rate is set using Karvonen's formula, or estimated as 20 beats/minute above resting. Due to the severity of their ventilatory impairment, some patients begin exercise reconditioning without a prescribed target heart rate.

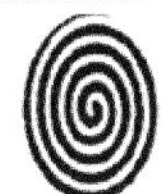

RULE OF THUMB

To set a target heart rate for patient exercise use Karvonen's formula:

Target heart rate = [(MHR – RHR) × (50% to 70%)] + RHR

Where MHR = maximum heart rate at limit of exercise tolerance and RHR = resting heart rate.

For example, a good target exercise heart rate for a patient with COPD with a MHR of 150 beats/minute and a RHR of 90 beats/minute would be [(150 – 90) × (0.60] + 90 = 126 beats/minute.

Typically, the exercise prescription includes the following four related components:[23,24]

1. Lower extremity (leg) aerobic exercises
2. Timed walking
3. Upper extremity (arm) aerobic exercises
4. Ventilatory muscle training

To ensure success with physical reconditioning, patients must actively participate both at the rehabilitation facility and at home. While exercising at the facility, patients should be monitored by pulse oximetry. Blood pressure measurements may also be made, but these are usually done at the start and end of each session. In addition, exercise sessions should be upbeat. Lively music helps to maintain a positive atmosphere. Clinicians must remember that these patients are ill and require a nurturing attitude from team members, family, and the group itself.

To ensure compliance with the program, a daily log or diary sheet must be completed. Figure 48-5 depicts a sample log sheet that makes up a section of the patient

Patient Log Week # ________

Day	PFlex	12-min Walk	Exercycle	Remarks
	No. ____ Duration ___	Distance ____ No. Stops ____	Distance ____ Duration ____	
	No. ____ Duration ___	Distance ____ No. Stops ____	Distance ____ Duration ____	
	No. ____ Duration ___	Distance ____ No. Stops ____	Distance ____ Duration ____	
	No. ____ Duration ___	Distance ____ No. Stops ____	Distance ____ Duration ____	
	No. ____ Duration ___	Distance ____ No. Stops ____	Distance ____ Duration ____	
	No. ____ Duration ___	Distance ____ No. Stops ____	Distance ____ Duration ____	
	No. ____ Duration ___	Distance ____ No. Stops ____	Distance ____ Duration ____	

Figure 48-5
Sample log or diary form on which patient in a pulmonary rehabilitation program records daily physical reconditioning activities and exercises.

manual. These log or diary forms are reviewed each time the patient attends a session. Based on this information, further individualized reconditioning goals are set.

Lower extremity exercises may include either walking or bicycling. Patients can walk on a stationary treadmill (with set goals for distance or time and grade), or on a flat, smooth surface. Patients can bicycle on an exercise cycle. With the treadmill or stationary bicycle, patients are required to cover a certain distance or duration every day that they are in the program. Commonly, the duration is set to 30 minutes daily, with patients encouraged to increase both their distance and equipment tension or resistance as tolerated. Patients with significant orthopedic deformities or disabilities should participate in aerobic aquatic exercises.

Walking also improves overall conditioning. This usually takes the form of a 12-minute walk performed once a day. The 12-minute walk is a convenient way for a patient to carry out a well-defined amount of activity with increasing vigor and results over a number of weeks. During the 12 minutes, patients should walk on flat ground for as far as possible. If severe dyspnea occurs, they should stop and rest, with the rest time included as part of the time interval. After resting briefly, they should try and continue walking at a comfortable pace. The objective is to walk as far as possible during the 12 minutes. Landmarks such as telephone poles, city blocks, or actual distance measures can be used to quantify progress. Under adverse weather conditions, the activity can be carried out indoors in shopping malls, stores, or long hallways. Patients should record their progress in their manuals or diaries.

Aerobic upper extremity exercises improve rehabilitation outcomes for patients whose regular activities involve lifting or raising the arms.[23,25] Arm ergometers or rowing machines are available for this purpose; however, simple calisthenics using either a broomstick or free weights (by prescription and with training) are a satisfactory alternative. Upper body endurance generally is more limited, with many patients capable of only 2 to 3 minutes of daily activity to start. Arm exercises should progressively get longer, up to 20 minutes if possible.[23] Upper body conditioning helps patients perform a number of useful activities at home and can also increase their overall physical endurance. As with other activity, patients should record daily results in their logs or manuals.

Although controversy exists, ventilatory muscle training probably can enhance the benefits of these more traditional exercises.[26] Ventilatory muscle training is based on the concept of progressive resistance. By imposing progressively greater loads on the inspiratory muscles (mainly the diaphragm) over time, both the patient's strength and endurance should increase. These improvements should, in turn, improve the patient's exercise tolerance.

Figure 48-6 shows a typical inspiratory resistance breathing device. The device is simply an adjustable flow resistor with a one-way breathing valve. The inspiratory load is created by forcing the patient to inhale through a restricted orifice. Varying the size of this orifice varies the inspiratory load, as do changes in the patient's inspiratory flow. During expiration, gas flows unimpeded out the one-way exhalation valve. Some models replace the variable size orifice with an adjustable spring-loaded valve. This ensures a relatively constant load regardless of how fast or slowly the patient breathes.

Because variations in breathing strategy during ventilatory muscle training can affect its outcomes, proper patient evaluation, training, and follow-up are a must. The respiratory therapist initially measures the patient's maximum inspiratory pressure (MIP, NIF or PI_{max}) using a calibrated pressure manometer. The respiratory therapist then compares the patient's maximum with established norms, as shown in Table 48-4. This preliminary measure of inspiratory pressure helps in establishing initial loads and provides the basis for the subsequent monitoring of patient progress.

Before beginning ventilatory muscle training, the patient should assume a position that relaxes the abdominal muscles, such as that used for cough training. If

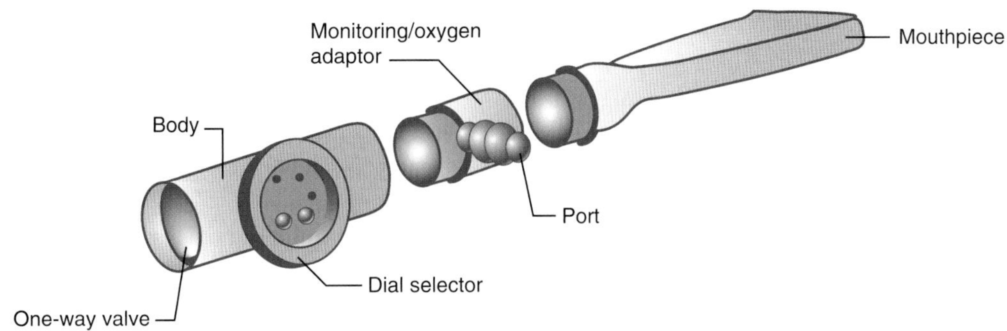

Figure 48-6
Flow-resistive breathing device.

Table 48-4 ▶▶ Normal Maximum Inspiratory Pressure (cm H_2O) by Age and Sex

	Mean (SD)	PI_{max} from Residual Volume
Age-group (years)	**Male**	**Female**
9 to 18	96 ± 35	90 ± 25
19 to 50	127 ± 28	91 ± 25
51 to 70	112 ± 20	77 ± 18
70	76 ± 27	66 ± 18

From Rochester DF, Hyatt RE: Respiratory muscle failure, Med Clin N Am 67:573, 1983.

using a flow resistive device, the respiratory therapist begins at the maximum orifice setting, while measuring the inspiratory pressure generated through the monitoring/oxygen adapter (a second adapter may be needed if the patient is receiving supplemental O_2). The respiratory therapist encourages the patient to breathe slowly through the device, at a rate no higher than 10 to 12 breaths/minute. If the patient's inspiratory pressure is less than 30% of the measured PI_{max}, the next smaller orifice is selected, with this procedure repeated until the 30% effort is consistently achieved.

At this point, the respiratory therapist instructs the patient to exercise with the device in one or two regular daily sessions of 10 to 15 minutes duration. As the level of resistance becomes more tolerable over time, the patient should progressively increase session duration up to 30 minutes. A self-maintained log of treatment times can help motivate the patient and assist the respiratory therapist in subsequent progress monitoring.

Educational Component

To complement the physical reconditioning aspect of the pulmonary rehabilitation effort, the educational portion of the program should cover topics that are both useful and necessary to the patient. Table 48-5 provides an example of topics covered during a 12-week rehabilitation program of the author's design. Included are recommendations regarding the best facilitators for each session. Naturally, other topics can be included, but in terms of relative importance, the ones mentioned generally have the highest priority.

Table 48-5 ▶▶ Typical Educational Topic Schedule for a 12-Week Pulmonary Rehabilitation Program

Session (Week)	Topic(s)	Recommended Facilitator(s)
1	Introduction and welcome; program orientation	Program administrator or rehabilitation team
2	Respiratory structure, function, and pathology	Physician or respiratory therapist
3	Breathing control methods	Physical therapist or respiratory therapist
4	Relaxation and stress management	Clinical psychologist
5	Proper exercise techniques and personal routines	Physical therapist or respiratory therapist
6	Methods to aid secretion clearance (bronchial hygiene)	Physical therapist or respiratory therapist
7	Home oxygen and aerosol therapy	Respiratory therapist
8	Medications: their use and abuse	Pharmacist, physician, or nurse practitioner
9	Medications: use of MDIs and spacers	Respiratory therapist
10	Dietary guidelines and good nutrition	Dietitian or nutritionist
11	Recreation and vocational counseling Activities of daily living	Occupational therapist
12	Follow-up planning and program evaluation Graduation	Rehabilitation team

The actual content of these sessions includes the following:

1. **Respiratory structure, function and pathology, including a discussion of dyspnea.** This presentation lays the groundwork for the program and gives each patient some basic information about the cardiorespiratory system and related disorders. The causes of shortness of breath are presented.
2. **Breathing control methods.** This serves as the cornerstone for the physical reconditioning effort. Patients must learn how to control their breathing efforts in order to ensure maximum result (ventilation) at a minimum of effort (energy expenditure). Diaphragmatic breathing with pursed-lips will help to accomplish this, but this technique will require daily practice on the part of the patient and continued reinforcement throughout the entire program by the group facilitator.
3. **Methods of relaxation and stress management.** Patients must learn to avoid aggravation and upsetting circumstances and to adopt, instead, a more relaxed attitude about their particular life circumstances. This will help to reduce unnecessary oxygen utilization, help to conserve energy, and help to avoid undesirable cardiovascular and nervous responses to stress.
4. **Exercise techniques and personal routines.** The rationale for and value of exercise should be covered and discussed along with suggestions for the adoption of personal exercise routines after the rehabilitation program is over.
5. **Secretion clearance and bronchial hygiene techniques.** This topic is especially helpful to those patients having secretion clearance problems associated with chronic bronchitis and bronchiectasis. Family members and friends may be invited to attend this session in order to acquire some basic skills with these procedures.
6. **Home oxygen and aerosol therapy.** A respiratory therapist with home care experience should provide this session. The focus should be on the care and use of home care equipment and self-administration of therapy. Those patients not yet on this type of therapeutic regimen may have questions or fears and be unreceptive to the concept. Presenting the modalities available and having patients discuss their positive experiences with respiratory home care personnel will help alleviate the fears and anxieties of nonusers.
7. **Medications.** This is another topic where patients have numerous questions and concerns. Content should emphasize proper use of medications, along with possible abuses and adverse effects. Participants' current prescriptions should dictate which specific drugs to cover. Common categories include β-adrenergics, anticholinergics, steroids, diuretics, and xanthines. The session leader should demonstrate proper use of metered dose inhalers (MDIs), including spacers/holding chambers. Sufficient time should be provided for questions and answers. Two sessions should be allotted for this topic.
8. **Dietary guidelines.** This subject focuses on weight management and good nutrition as it relates to cardiopulmonary health. Emphasis should be on the importance of a sound high-protein, low-carbohydrate diet (see Chapter 45). The facilitator also should cover proper eating habits, methods of gaining and losing weight, foods to avoid, ways to increase appetite, and daily menu planning. This session will stimulate patients to eat better and thus supply their bodies with the necessary fuel for increased energy production.
9. **Recreation and vocational counseling.** This session should motivate participants to participate in recreational activities and, according to ability, return to work. The topic is often presented at the end of the program when patients have increased their physical endurance and are preparing for a more active and productive life-style. The class may brainstorm ideas for recreational or physical activities, from which members can generate action plans. Ideally, the group facilitator will perceive changes in group members' attitudes toward physical activity. Patients should be more confident in their ability to walk, exercise, and get out of the home. Their overall psychological outlook can definitely change for the better if they have been successful in the program.

These topics should be presented in an orderly, coherent fashion using supplementary audiovisual tools and demonstrations, where appropriate. Team members should allocate sufficient time both for the class sessions themselves and for setup and breakdown of equipment.

The program facilitator or leader must ensure that sessions begin on time and encourage maximum participation by each patient. In addition to technical knowledge, session leaders must possess group facilitation skills and be able to motivate patients to participate both in class and at home and to adhere to program guidelines. This task is not an easy one, but with patience and persistence it can be accomplished. The desired end result is to help patients lead more productive lives with decreased hospitalizations.

Program Implementation

This section explores various aspects of program implementation. In 1987, the AARC and the American Association of Cardiovascular and Pulmonary Rehabilitation (AACVPR) jointly conducted the first national survey of pulmonary rehabilitation programs. This National Pulmonary Rehabilitation Survey was published in 1988 and demonstrated the variation existing in program structure, content, staffing, and cost throughout the United States.[27]

Staffing

With regard to staffing and necessary personnel, pulmonary rehabilitation should be a multidisciplinary endeavor. Team care is enhanced by involving a variety of health care professionals in the planning, implementation, and evaluation components of the program (Figure 48-7). In addition to professional involvement, family members are needed to provide feedback and ensure that instructions and the exercise prescription are carried out at home.[28]

Facilities

Because both the location and quality of facilities can directly affect patient attendance, rehabilitation personnel must pay careful attention to this important program resource. For example, patients will be less likely to attend programs that are inaccessible to public transportation, have poor parking arrangements, or are physically difficult to reach. Clearly, the facility must be wheelchair accessible. For elderly patients who do not drive, arrangements can be made with community organizations to provide transportation to and from the program. Ideally, the facility should provide two separate rooms for the program—one room for the educational activities and one room for physical reconditioning. Rooms should be spacious and comfortable with adequate lighting, ventilation, and temperature control. Chairs should be comfortable with good back support. Restroom facilities should be readily accessible. A room for individual counseling is helpful, but any private office will suffice. It is also preferable to have pulmonary function testing and blood gas analysis capabilities on site. If this space is used by other departments for other functions, then proper scheduling of rehabilitation sessions needs to be considered.

Scheduling

Another aspect of program implementation involves timely scheduling of the rehabilitation sessions. With the open-ended format, patients can more or less attend rehabilitation at any time convenient to them as long as the facility is open and staffed accordingly. With the

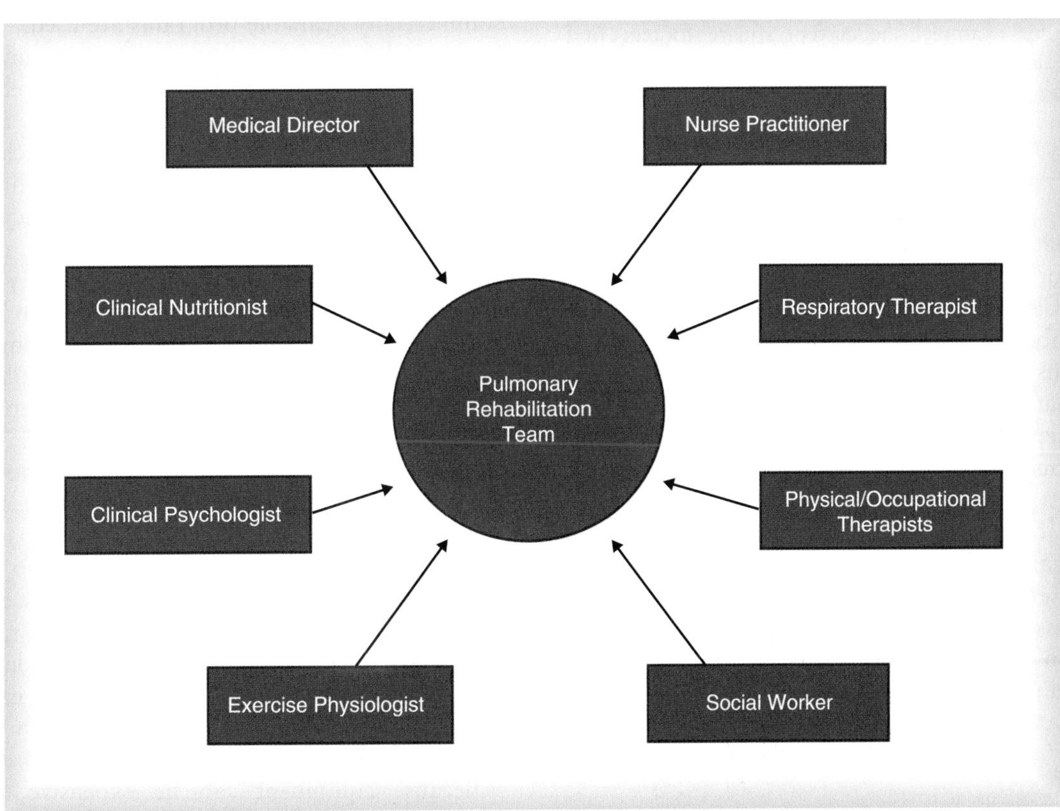

Figure 48-7
The multidisciplinary nature of pulmonary rehabilitation.

MINI CLINI

Facilities Planning for Pulmonary Rehabilitation

PROBLEM

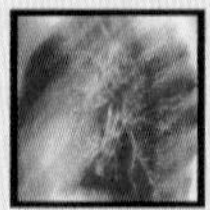

A respiratory therapist has been asked to assist in the planning process for starting a pulmonary rehabilitation program to support a 350-bed, full-service hospital. According to the strategic plan, the physical location of the rehabilitation center is about three blocks away from the hospital. The therapist has not seen the proposed site but was asked to approve a recommendation that the facility be used. What factors should the respiratory therapist take into account before making a decision on site selection?

SOLUTION

Because the hospital is currently in the planning process for starting a pulmonary rehabilitation program and has not made final facilities selection, the respiratory therapist is in a key position to assess, among other areas, issues related to the proposed site. Patient attendance and participation will be adversely affected if the facility is unreachable, such as at the top of a hill. If the location is in a high crime or unsafe area with little or no security, this too would discourage patients from attending. As true with any program, public transportation that does not permit accessibility to the proposed facility would be a limiting factor, as would little or no available parking. There are numerous other facility considerations outside the actual physical location of the rehabilitation center that would then need to be addressed. For example, the current square footage of available space and room for future expansion would need to be evaluated relative to anticipated needs, as would whether the facility itself is wheelchair accessible with no barriers present.

closed format, sessions are scheduled one to three times per week, for 1 to 3 hours, with programs running 8 to 16 weeks. Class times need to be scheduled when the largest number of patients are able to attend. Traffic patterns, bus schedules, and availability of rides are concerns that need to be discussed. The ideal situation involves a separate area set totally aside for pulmonary rehabilitation with a dedicated staff of professionals conducting the program. Then scheduling for either open-ended or closed-design programs becomes easier and more manageable. Sessions can be conducted in the morning, afternoon, or evening hours and even on weekends if necessary. Proper scheduling helps to encourage participation and removes potential stumbling blocks, which could undermine the rehabilitation process.

Class Size

Class size is another issue that must be addressed. Theoretically, a rehabilitation program could be conducted with as few as one participant or up to 15 or more, depending on available space, equipment, and staff. However, to foster group identity, interaction, and support, small group discussions are encouraged. The ideal class size should range from three to 10 participants. Keeping the class size manageable facilitates vital group interaction processes and allows for more individualized attention. These factors help sustain motivation, thereby reducing the likelihood of participant attrition.

Naturally, economic concerns surface when class size is considered. Although it is clear that program quality must be the first priority, program viability realistically depends on the number of participants. As a general guideline, programs should be conducted with a class size that is comfortable with regards to space and staffing and one that is also economically feasible. Such an approach will help ensure that programs produce meaningful patient outcomes.

Equipment

Both the instruction and reconditioning component of the program require equipment. To meet the educational needs of the program, a blackboard or flipchart along with a 35 mm slide or power point projector, screen, overhead projector, and cassette tape player are needed. A videotape player with monitor may also be helpful, especially if individualized instruction or commercially available programs are used. Also, slides, tapes, and formal learning packages dealing with the educational topics covered during the rehabilitation program should be available for group and individualized presentation. These can be purchased from outside sources or designed and developed in-house.

For physical reconditioning, stationary bicycles, treadmills, rowing machines, upper extremity ergometers, weights, pulse oximeters, and inspiratory resistance breathing devices represent the minimum equipment requirements. The actual quantity of equipment needed depends on class size, scheduling, and available space. Enough equipment should be on hand to keep all patients exercising and to monitor their activity. Emergency oxygen and bronchodilator medications should also be maintained in the rehabilitation area. Equipment guidelines for a class of six to 10 participants include the following: five stationary bicycles, two treadmills, two rowing machines, two upper extremity ergometers, five pulse oximeters for monitoring heart rate and O_2 saturation, one emergency oxygen cylinder (E), and bronchodilator medications. In addition, each patient should be supplied with an inspiratory resistance breathing device.

Because equipment can be expensive, care must be taken in its selection and purchase. Devices and appliances should be durable, easy and safe to use, simple to maintain, and not overly expensive. Initially, basic items are purchased. As a program develops and expands, equipment resources can be enhanced. Other program needs include the following:

- Maintaining individual patient manuals, including daily log forms or activity diaries
- Providing light refreshments for program participants
- Developing a communication network to announce schedule changes due to emergencies or cancellation of class sessions due to illness or weather
- Identifying available durable medical equipment (DME) providers for those in need of specialized home care equipment
- Developing a system of charges and mechanism for patient payment

By considering all of the factors needed for effective implementation of pulmonary rehabilitation, programs will have lower patient attrition and a greater chance for overall success. As programs are conducted, regular evaluations by both patient and staff must be made. Needed changes should be implemented on an ongoing basis. Only in this manner can one expect continued refinement of the process and improvement in patient outcomes.

Cost, Fees, and Reimbursement

Rehabilitation programs usually project their fees based on the average cost per participant. According to regional labor and material prices, costs vary throughout the country.

Several factors must be considered when projecting program costs (Box 48-5). Obviously, the larger the class size and the more participants involved in the overall program, the lower the cost will be per patient. The aim should be to offer and conduct the highest quality program possible at a reasonable cost that meets any existing budgetary constraints.

Box 48-5 • Factors Affecting Pulmonary Rehabilitation Program Costs

- Marketing and program promotion
- Number of personnel involved in program facilitation and administration
- Space and utility expenses
- Audio-visual, exercise, and monitoring equipment (purchase and maintenance)
- Production and duplication of course materials
- Patient supplies
- Office supplies
- Refreshments
- Miscellaneous expenses

When determining patient charges, consideration must also be given to the type and amount of funding that has been received to offset program expenses and available insurance reimbursement. Preprogram and postprogram testing and evaluations will naturally generate revenues but should not be included in the formulation of program charges. However, payments for pulmonary function testing, exercise testing, arterial blood gas analysis, and other evaluations may help to keep a pulmonary rehabilitation program financially viable.

Charges for an entire program or for each session must be structured in a way that does not deter patient attendance. Many pulmonary patients are on a fixed income and have other living and medical expenses to account for. A happy medium between a patient's ability to pay and program expenses must be identified. Any scholarships or funding from local charitable organizations, foundations, or agencies, such as the American Lung Association, will help ease the financial burden. The most comprehensive and effective program available will have no impact if patients are unwilling or unable to attend and participate because of financial limitations.

The cost of providing pulmonary rehabilitation has increased over the years, as have health care costs in general. Nationwide charges for pulmonary rehabilitation vary, depending on program length and most importantly, insurance coverage. With most insurance plans reimbursing programs at 80% after a deductible, each patient would be responsible for the remaining 20% or copayment. Additional or supplemental medical coverage may cover this balance.

Inpatient rehabilitation reimbursement policies vary throughout the country, as do charges for participation in these programs. In 1982, the Centers for Medicare and Medicaid Services or CMMS (formerly the Health Care Financing Administration or HCFA) published the final rules for Medicare reimbursement guidelines for comprehensive outpatient rehabilitative facilities (CORFs). Under Part B of Medicare, the scope of services of a CORF now includes reimbursement for outpatient activities and one home visit. Reimbursement requires that the CORF meet the conditions of participation established in section 933 of Public Law 96-499. This also includes provisions for certification of the program. Each CORF must present its program description and anticipated results to local third-party payers to establish reimbursement mechanisms.

By following these guidelines, Medicare will establish an allowable charge for the program and reimburse 80% of this rate after the patient meets the annual prescribed deductible. Other programs, both inpatient and outpatient in nature, have obtained reimbursement from third-party payers by charging for rehabilitation sessions as physical therapy exercises for COPD,

MINI CLINI

Obtaining Insurance Payment for Pulmonary Rehabilitation

PROBLEM

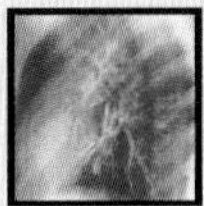

A respiratory therapist is asked to design and implement a pulmonary rehabilitation program on an outpatient basis at her hospital. After completing the first class that ran for 12 weeks, the hospital scheduled another one. However, even though the institution had been submitting bills on a timely basis to a number of insurance providers, including Medicare, no payment had been received. What is the problem and how can it be corrected?

SOLUTION

Apparently, the insurance companies have either denied claims or have not responded to those being submitted. This problem is often associated with either improper or inaccurate claim filing. The respiratory therapist should work closely with the billing department at the hospital to ensure that all information is complete for each patient (e.g., correct patient identification numbers), that the hospital has the correct addresses to submit claims, and that diagnosis and procedures have been properly coded. Some insurance companies have their own coding schemes and these must be followed accordingly. Managed care companies also require preauthorization and this must be obtained before entering any patient with a managed care plan into pulmonary rehabilitation. Finally, follow-up telephone calls are always helpful and should be conducted if payment is not received in a timely fashion.

reconditioning exercise sessions, office visits with therapeutic exercises, serial pulse oximetry determinations, and/or physician office visits. The goal is to obtain as much insurance reimbursement as possible, thereby decreasing the financial burden on the patient. Box 48-6 provides a listing of all possible sources of reimbursement.[28,29]

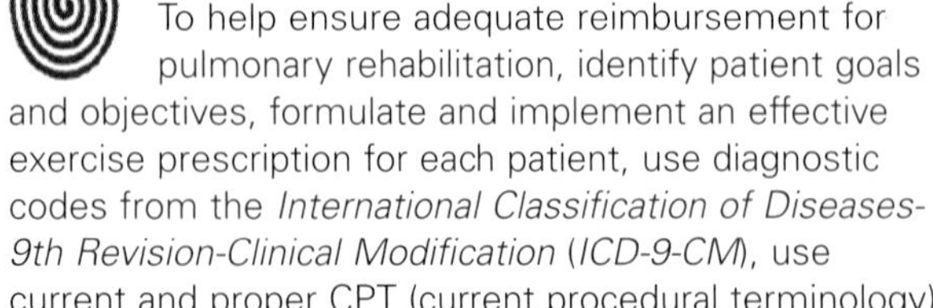

RULE OF THUMB

To help ensure adequate reimbursement for pulmonary rehabilitation, identify patient goals and objectives, formulate and implement an effective exercise prescription for each patient, use diagnostic codes from the *International Classification of Diseases-9th Revision-Clinical Modification* (*ICD-9-CM*), use current and proper CPT (current procedural terminology) coding and document, document, document!

Until there is either a blanket code or payment for pulmonary rehabilitation under a prospective payment system (PPS), programs will have to continue to obtain reimbursement following the currently accepted plans, policies, and provisions of each individual insurance carrier.

Box 48-6 • Sources of Reimbursement for Pulmonary Rehabilitation Programs

NONGOVERNMENTAL HEALTH INSURANCE PROGRAMS

PRIVATE, SINGLE, OR GROUP HEALTH INSURANCE PLANS
- Health maintenance organizations (HMOs)
- Preferred provider organizations (PPOs)

MEDICARE SUPPLEMENT

FEDERAL AND STATE HEALTH INSURANCE PROGRAMS
- Medicare
- Medicaid
- Uncompensated services (Hill-Burton)
- Comprehensive outpatient rehabilitation facility (CORF)
- Veteran's administration benefits
- Civilian health and medical programs of the uniformed services (CHAMPUS)
- Federal workers insurance

ANCILLARY LIABILITY AND CASUALTY INSURANCE PROGRAMS
- Automobile insurance, related to auto accidents
- Worker's compensation, related to accidents on the job
- Business insurance coverage, related to injuries sustained on business premises
- Homeowner's insurance, related to injuries sustained on the owner's premises
- Malpractice insurance on providers of health care
- Product and service liability insurance related to product or service-cased injuries

OTHER OPTIONS OF REIMBURSEMENT
- Senior care
- Rehabilitation hospitals
- Grants

Program Results

Patient and program outcomes must be evaluated at the conclusion of the program and periodically thereafter. Evaluation results must compare preprogram and current patient status and should include physiological, psychological, and sociological data. Results of pulmonary rehabilitation must be communicated to the patient, family, referring physician, and home care company, if appropriate. From here, further goals and objectives for continued improvement may be established to provide the basis for follow-up and reinforcement activities.

If no improvements in physical or psychosocial measures occur within a class or group, program deficiencies are the most likely cause. Specifically, insufficient professional training in rehabilitation methods, a lack of uniformity in approach, inadequate program length, and/or lack of follow-up are the major reasons for unsatisfactory outcomes.

National Emphysema Treatment Trial

In 1996, the National Heart, Lung, and Blood Institute (NHLBI) and Health Care Financing Administration or HCFA (now the Centers for Medicare and Medicaid Services) announced the start of a scientific study to evaluate the effectiveness of lung volume reduction surgery (LVRS). This scientific study was called the National Emphysema Treatment Trial (NETT) and created 18 clinical centers along with a coordination center with the purpose of comparing medical and surgical approaches in the treatment of emphysema. Pulmonary rehabilitation played and continues to play a major role in this study. Hopefully, the importance of pulmonary rehabilitation will be recognized, both in the treatment of COPD and before any patient with COPD undergoes LVRS, resulting in a blanket code for pulmonary rehabilitation.[30]

KEY POINTS

- Pulmonary rehabilitation has two major aims: (1) to control and alleviate disease symptoms and (2) to help patients achieve optimal levels of activity.
- Patients best able to benefit from pulmonary rehabilitation are those with symptomatic COPD; those with unstable cardiovascular disorders should be referred for cardiac rehabilitation.
- Effective rehabilitation programming requires a multidisciplinary approach and combines physical reconditioning with education and psychosocial support.
- Rehabilitation does not alter the progressive deterioration in pulmonary function that occurs with chronic lung disease.
- Increased exercise tolerance, decreased intensity of symptoms, and improved activity levels are the best documented benefits of pulmonary rehabilitation.
- Exercise capacity is limited by the body's ability to deliver sufficient oxygen to meet the demands of energy metabolism; work levels above this limit abruptly increase both lactic acid and carbon dioxide production.
- The exercise evaluation (1) provides the basis for the exercise prescription, (2) yields the baseline data needed to assess a patient's progress, and (3) helps determine the degree of hypoxemia/need for supplemental O_2 during exercise.
- Reconditioning should combine both lower and upper extremity aerobic exercises with ventilatory muscle training.
- The educational portion of a rehabilitation program should provide patients with knowledge they can use to help cope with their disease and better manage symptoms.
- Decisions regarding facilities, scheduling, class size, and equipment can all affect rehabilitation program outcomes.
- Patient charges should be based on projected costs, as offset by external funding and/or available insurance reimbursement.

References

1. Council on Rehabilitation: Definition of rehabilitation, Chicago, 1942, Council on Rehabilitation.
2. Petty TL: Pulmonary rehabilitation, Basics of RD 4:1, 1975.
3. Harris PL: A guide to prescribing pulmonary rehabilitation, Prim Care 12:253, 1985.
4. American Thoracic Society: Pulmonary rehabilitation [official statement], Am Rev Respir Dis 124:663, 1981.
5. Barach AL, Bickerman HA, Beck G: Advances in the treatment of nontuberculous pulmonary disease, Bull N Y Acad Med 28:353, 1952.
6. Pierce AK et al: Responses to exercise training in patients with emphysema, Arch Intern Med 113:28, 1964.
7. Paez PN et al: The physiological basis of training patients with emphysema, Am Rev Respir Dis 95:944, 1967.
8. Christie D: Physical training in chronic obstructive lung disease, Br Med J 2:150, 1968.
9. Celli BR: Pulmonary rehabilitation in patients with COPD, Am J Respir Crit Care Med 152:861, 1995.
10. Shenkman B: Factors contributing to attrition rates in a pulmonary rehabilitation program, Heart Lung 14:53, 1985.
11. Dudley DL et al: Psychosocial concomitants to rehabilitation in chronic obstructive pulmonary disease. Part 1. Psychosocial and psychological considerations, Chest 77:413, 1980.

12. Dudley DL et al: Psychosocial concomitants to rehabilitation in chronic obstructive pulmonary disease. Part 2. Psychosocial treatment, Chest 77:544, 1980.
13. Dyksterhuis JE: Vocational rehabilitation of chronic obstructive pulmonary disease patients, Rehabil Lit 33:136, 1972.
14. Niederman MS et al: Benefits of a multidisciplinary pulmonary rehabilitation program. Improvements are independent of lung function, Chest 99:798, 1991.
15. Hughes RL, Davison R: Limitations of exercise reconditioning in COLD, Chest 83:241, 1983.
16. Wijkstra PJ et al: Long-term benefits of rehabilitation at home on quality of life and exercise tolerance in patients with chronic obstructive pulmonary disease, Thorax 50:824, 1995.
17. Lacasse Y et al: Meta-analysis of respiratory rehabilitation in chronic obstructive pulmonary disease, Lancet 348:1115, 1996.
18. Ojanen M et al: Psychosocial changes in patients participating in a chronic obstructive pulmonary disease rehabilitation program, Respiration 60:96, 1993.
19. Ries AL: The importance of exercise in pulmonary rehabilitation, Clin Chest Med 15:327, 1994.
20. American Association for Respiratory Care: AARC clinical practice guideline: Exercise testing for evaluation of hypoxemia and/or desaturation, Respir Care Clin N Am 37:907, 1992.
21. Wasserman K et al: Selection criteria for exercise training in pulmonary rehabilitation, Eur Respir J Suppl 7:604, 1989.
22. Hodgkin JE: Organization of a pulmonary rehabilitation program, Clin Chest Med 7:541, 1986.
23. Celli BR: Physical reconditioning of patients with respiratory diseases: legs, arms, and breathing retraining, Respir Care Clin N Am 39:481, 1994.
24. Zu Wallack RL et al: Predictors of improvement in the 12-minute walking distance following a six-week outpatient pulmonary rehabilitation program, Chest 99:805, 1991.
25. Lake FR et al: Upper-limb and lower-limb exercise training in patients with chronic airflow obstruction, Chest 97:1077, 1990.
26. Weiner P, Azgad Y, Ganam R: Inspiratory muscle training combined with general exercise reconditioning in patients with COPD, Chest102:1351, 1992.
27. Bickford LS, Hodgkin JE: National pulmonary rehabilitation survey, Respir Care Clin N Am 33:1030, 1988.
28. Bunch D: Obtaining reimbursement for your pulmonary rehabilitation program, AARC Times 14:38, 1990.
29. Connors G et al: Obtaining third-party reimbursement for pulmonary rehabilitation, AARC Times 16:50, 1992.
30. Foss CM: Lung volume reduction surgery: what's up with "NETT"? AARC Times 25:42, 2001.

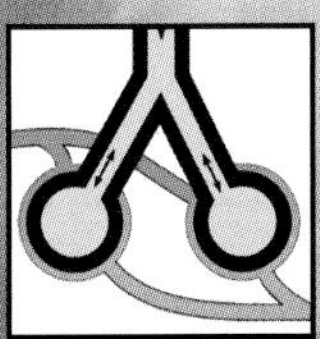

CHAPTER 49

Respiratory Care in Alternative Settings

Albert J. Heuer and Craig L. Scanlan

In This Chapter You Will Learn:

- What constitutes the alternative or postacute care setting
- What are the recent developments and trends in alternative site respiratory care
- Who regulates postacute care
- What standards apply to the delivery of postacute respiratory care
- How to help formulate an effective discharge plan
- What factors to evaluate when assessing alternative care sites and support services
- How to justify, provide, evaluate, and modify oxygen (O_2) therapy in postacute care settings
- How to select, assemble, monitor, and maintain O_2 therapy equipment in alternative settings
- What special challenges exist in providing ventilatory support outside the acute care hospital
- How to instruct patients or caregivers and confirm their ability to provide postacute care
- Which patients can most benefit from ventilatory support outside acute care hospitals
- How to select, assemble, monitor, and maintain portable ventilatory support and continuous positive airway pressure (CPAP) equipment, including applicable interfaces or appliances
- How to properly document and evaluate patient progress in the postacute care setting
- How to ensure safety and infection control in alternative patient care settings

Chapter Outline

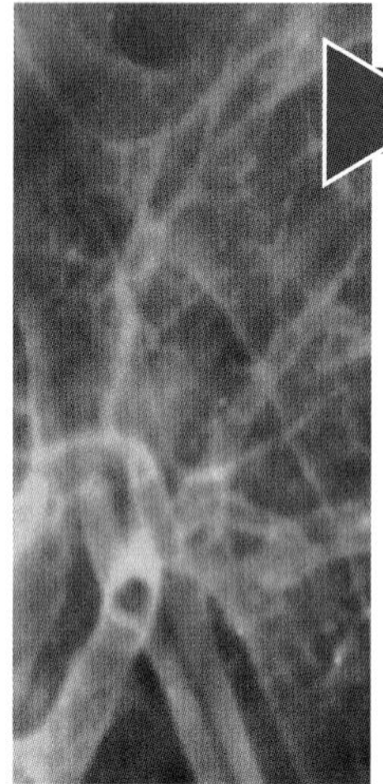

Key Terms

apnea-hypopnea index (AHI)
air stacking
Centers for Medicare and Medicaid Services (CMS)
conditions of participation
conjunctivitis
durable medical equipment (DME) company
in-exsufflator
molecular sieve
noninvasive positive pressure ventilation (NIPPV)
oxygen-conserving devices
postacute care
skilled nursing facility (SNF)
sleep apnea-hypopnea syndrome (SAHS)
subacute care
sudden infant death syndrome (SIDS)
transtracheal oxygen therapy (TTOT)

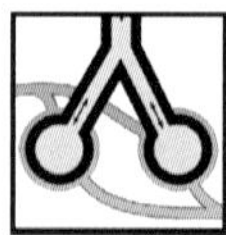

With the introduction of Medicare in 1965, the cost savings and patient welfare benefits associated with home care and other nonacute care settings was finally recognized. Accordingly, this legislation established a reimbursement structure for healthcare services in alternative settings, including those provided at home. Since its adoption, Medicare is credited with substantial increases in the number of patients cared for at home. From 1967 to 1985, the number of home care agencies certified to participate in Medicare tripled to almost six thousand. More recently, the number of home care agencies has leveled off mainly due to reimbursement cuts due to managed care and Medicare reductions resulting from the Balanced Budget Act of 1997. Despite this, however, over eight million Americans continued to receive healthcare at home in 1999 at an estimated cost of $36 million.[1]

Although home care remains by far the most common alternative site for providing healthcare, a host of other postacute care settings, including subacute, rehabilitation, and skilled nursing facilities (SNFs), provide respiratory care to patients. Many of these patients in alternative settings require respiratory services including supplemental O_2, assisted ventilation, aerosol therapy, respiratory monitoring, pulmonary rehabilitation, and patient/caregiver education for asthma and other respiratory disorders.

Although respiratory care in alternative settings offers advantages over acute care facilities such as lower cost and greater patient well-being and comfort, it is not without challenges. Improper or premature discharging of patients to alternative settings and poor care plan implementation can erase these benefits and result in short-term readmission to acute care settings, worsening of patient condition, or even death.[2,3] However, these risks can be minimized through proper patient screening and evaluation, appropriate discharge planning, including a multidisciplinary care plan, proper care plan implementation, and patient follow-up.[4]

This chapter provides relevant definitions, discusses recent policy developments, covers aspects of optimal discharge and patient care planning, and reviews various therapeutic respiratory modalities in the alternative site.

▶ RECENT DEVELOPMENTS AND TRENDS

Over the past several years, there have been several developments in the area of respiratory care in alternative sites. These and other changes illustrate the dynamic nature of healthcare policy as it affects respiratory care in alternative settings.

One of the most notable changes is the introduction of Medicare's prospective payment system (PPS). Until the introduction of the PPS, Medicare mainly reimbursed providers such as home care agencies on a monthly or one-time, fee-for-service basis for each therapeutic modality. However, under the PPS, a much greater emphasis is placed on the reimbursement for respiratory services in alternative sites on a predetermined base amount for each patient, adjusted for factors such as the health condition and care needs. Additionally, legislation related to the introduction of the PPS also reduced the fee-for-service monthly reimbursement for respiratory equipment used at home, such as O_2 concentrators. The net effect is an overall reduction in the reimbursement for respiratory care services provided in alternate settings.[5]

It should be noted that at the writing of this chapter, the appropriateness and precise implementation of the

PPS is still under review. Since the PPS was initially introduced, government has recognized potential inequities in this system and modified its implementation. One example of this is a temporary exemption of SNFs from the PPS until a more equitable reimbursement system could be adopted. It is expected that the PPS will continue to be reviewed and modified appropriately to help ensure that proper patient care can be efficiently provided in alternative sites.[6]

Another major change involves the reimbursement for respiratory therapists' time for administering care and patient education in alternative care settings such as the home. Until this time, reimbursements under federal Medicare and state Medicaid programs applied to respiratory equipment, such as home O_2 and mechanical ventilators, and respiratory therapists' time was not covered under federal Medicare and state Medicaid programs. However, a few states have adopted pilot programs to reimburse providers for certain therapies and education done by respiratory therapists within such settings. Beyond this, reimbursement for programs aimed at educating patients and caregivers regarding respiratory diseases' management, such as asthma, are also being reviewed. Finally, the PPS may actually open doors for respiratory therapists working at home. Prospectively paying an all-inclusive amount, which is adjusted for the severity of a patient's condition and needs such as home ventilation, may eliminate past concerns that respiratory therapy would be an additional cost to Medicare.

As a result of the delicate balance between cost and appropriate patent care, it appears that the PPS and other related policy will continue to be reviewed and modified appropriately by governmental agencies such as the Centers for Medicare and Medicaid Services (CMS), formerly the Health Care Financing Agency (HCFA).[7]

A further development is a significant increase in the popularity of another form of alternative site known as assisted living facilities. These facilities permit residents, who are generally elderly and/or disabled, to live in their own unit either alone or with a companion. Generally, routine healthcare and other support services are available through an on-site nursing and health aide staff. These arrangements permit residents to live relatively independently with the convenience and safety of routine health services nearby. As a result of this trend , a growing number of home care and other alternative site respiratory therapists are providing care to patients at such locations.

An additional development entails a research study done at the request of the American Association for Respiratory Care (AARC) by Muse and associates[8] to investigate the value of respiratory therapists in skilled nursing facilities. Published in 1999, this study found that Medicare beneficiaries treated by respiratory therapists had better outcomes and lower cost. It is hoped that The Muse Report and other similar projects will help public agencies and private healthcare payers recognize the value of respiratory therapists in alternative care settings and hence shape the payment policies accordingly.

▶ DEFINITIONS AND GOALS

With the healthcare system in a constant state of flux, applying firm definitions to any one of its elements is difficult. Nonetheless, there is an evolving consensus on the scope and purpose of both subacute and home care.

As the elderly population grows and managed care becomes the dominant delivery model, more and more health services are being provided outside the acute care hospital.[9] These alternative, or *postacute care*, settings include subacute, rehabilitation, and SNFs, and the home. Rather than representing distinct entities, however, these approaches are just part of a large and evolving continuum of care that aims to provide services at a level, cost, and in a setting appropriate to the patient's condition.

The delivery of respiratory services outside the acute care hospital is undergoing rapid growth. Because these services typically are provided after an acute episode of hospitalization, good discharge planning is critical. Moreover, because this type of care focuses on the whole person rather than simply a disease process, coordinated team effort among many disciplines is essential. The most common respiratory care services provided in these alternative settings are continuous OXYGEN therapy, long-term mechanical ventilation, aerosol drug administration, airway care, sleep apnea treatment, sleep/apnea home monitoring, and pulmonary rehabilitation. All areas incorporate an emphasis on patient and family education.

Subacute Care

According to the National Subacute Care Association, *subacute care* is a comprehensive level of inpatient care for stable patients who (1) have experienced an acute event resulting from injury, illness, or exacerbation of a disease process; (2) have a determined course of treatment, and (3) require diagnostics or invasive procedures but not those requiring acute care.[10] Typically, the severity of the patient's condition requires active physician direction with frequent on-site visits, professional nursing care, significant ancillary services, and an outcomes-focused interdisciplinary approach using a professional team.

Whereas the goal of acute care is to apply intensive resources to stabilize patients after severe episodic illness, subacute care aims to restore the *whole* patient back to the highest practical level of function, ideally that of self-care. This holistic approach requires goal-oriented interdisciplinary team care, with frequent assessment of progress and a time-limited plan of care.[11]

Although most patients receiving subacute care are elderly, all age-groups can be found at these sites. Pediatric, adolescent, and adult patient populations requiring ventilatory support or extensive care, depending on their diagnosis, are also cared for at these sites. Some of the patient conditions include neurological disorders or injuries, musculoskeletal deformities, genetic defects, and any type of chronic pulmonary disease.

Home Care

Currently, most postacute respiratory care is provided in the home. Home care should always be the first choice, but when patients have multiple ailments and are unable to care for themselves, when adequate patient support is unavailable, or when the home environment is unsuitable, an alternative care site must be selected.

The AARC defines respiratory home care as those specific forms of respiratory care provided in the patient's place of residence by personnel trained in respiratory care working under medical supervision.[12]

The primary goal of home care is to provide quality healthcare services to clients in their home setting, thus minimizing their dependence on institutional care. In regard to respiratory home care, several specific objectives are evident. Respiratory home care can contribute to the following:

- Supporting and maintaining life
- Improving patients' physical, emotional, and social well-being
- Promoting patient and family self-sufficiency
- Ensuring cost-effective delivery of care
- Maximizing patient comfort near the end of life

Most patients for whom respiratory home care is considered are those with chronic respiratory diseases. Applicable categories of disorders include the following:

- Chronic obstructive pulmonary disease (COPD)
- Cystic fibrosis (CF)
- Chronic neuromuscular disorders
- Chronic restrictive conditions
- Carcinomas of the lung

Although not all aspects of respiratory home care have proven effective, various studies have shown that carefully selected treatment regimens can be of significant benefit to patients. These benefits include increased longevity, improved quality of life, increased functional performance, and a reduction in the individual and societal costs associated with hospitalization.[13,14]

▶ STANDARDS

Standards for the delivery of healthcare in the subacute and home setting derive from several different sources. These include federal and state laws and private-sector accreditation.

Governmental Laws and Regulations

The majority of reimbursement for postacute care is through either the federal Medicare or federal/state Medicaid programs. As a result, government plays a major role in setting standards.

The Medicare Provider Certification Program ensures that institutional providers that serve Medicare beneficiaries, for example, hospitals, SNFs, and home health agencies, meet minimum health and safety requirements. These requirements are called *conditions of participation*. Current conditions of participation emphasize quality indicators, outcome measures, and cost efficiency designed to improve the quality and effectiveness of care provided to beneficiaries. Institutions undergo certification surveys to determine their compliance with the applicable conditions of participation. These surveys are conducted by either state survey agencies or private accrediting organizations such as the Joint Commission on Accreditation of Health Care Organizations (JCAHO).

State survey agencies are the federal government's partners and principal agents in performing institutional certification. Typically, a state survey agency is either the state health department or state licensing authority for healthcare facilities. The main function of the state survey agency is to ensure that facilities providing Medicare or Medicaid services comply with state and federal health, safety, and quality standards. Compliance is determined by periodic on-site inspections. Inspection reports are public information and can be obtained by contacting the applicable state survey agency.

In addition to federal Medicare/Medicaid conditions of participation, most states set additional regulations that govern licensing of postacute and home healthcare providers. Because these regulations are different in each state, readers should contact their state health department for details.

Private Sector Accreditation

The primary agency responsible for standard setting and voluntary accreditation of postacute care providers is JCAHO. JCAHO develops and publishes standards for both long-term/subacute care and home care.[15,16] Both standards share a basic organizational framework of several functional categories relating to patient care and the organization. These categories include patient rights, ethics, and assessment, as well as organizational leadership, management of information, and control of infection.

Currently, there are several categories of accreditation, ranging from "Full Accreditation" to "Not Accredited." A provider's accreditation status depends on the level of compliance with the applicable standards. Insufficient or unsatisfactory compliance with a standard in a specific critical area of performance results in a Type I recommendation, which requires formal follow-up to ensure correction. Supplemental recommendation requires resolution but no formal follow-up.

In regard to home care, the JCAHO provides different protocols for different types of home care agencies. The home equipment management protocol pertains only to those companies that rent or sell home medical equipment. In most cases, this type of provider is involved only with basic oxygen and aerosol therapy set-ups and does not provide in-depth visits for patient assessment or evaluation. On the other hand, agencies involved with clinical respiratory services render periodic home visits with patient assessment. Agencies applying for accreditation at this level are involved with more sophisticated forms of home care that require routine follow-up visits, such as management of artificial airways and ventilator-dependent patients. The standards for this type of home care accreditation are more extensive and rigorous.

▶ TRADITIONAL ACUTE CARE VERSUS POSTACUTE CARE

For the registered respiratory therapist (RRT), working in the postacute care setting is distinctly different from working in an acute care hospital. Key differences involve resource availability, supervision and work schedules, documentation and assessment, and professional/patient interaction (Table 49-1).[17] Although some practitioners find the alternative work settings not to their liking, many find the greater independence, professional team orientation, creativity, and higher level of patient and family interaction quite rewarding. In addition, most RRTs working in the postacute care environment argue that only in these settings is their full scope of training really used.

▶ DISCHARGE PLANNING

Effective discharge planning provides the foundation for quality postacute care. A properly designed and implemented discharge plan guides the multidisciplinary team in successfully transferring the respiratory care patient from the healthcare facility to an alternative site of care.[18] Effective implementation of the discharge plan also ensures the safety and efficacy of the patient's continuing care.

To guide practitioners in providing quality care, the AARC has published *Clinical Practice Guideline: Discharge Planning for the Respiratory Care Patient.*[19] Excerpts appear on p. 1252.

Multidisciplinary Team

Although a physician normally initiates an order to discharge a patient to a postacute care site, many other healthcare professionals are involved in the discharge process. Table 49-2 identifies these key professionals, along with their major responsibilities. As with pulmonary rehabilitation (Chapter 48), a team approach

Table 49-1 ▶▶ Some Major Differences Between the Traditional Acute Care Setting and Alternative Settings for Delivery of Respiratory Care Services

Area	Traditional Setting (Acute Care Hospital)	Alternative Settings (Subacute, Long-term, Home Care)
Diagnostic resources	In-house laboratory, x-ray, ABG, PFT	Must rely on outside vendors to provide diagnostic tests
Equipment support	Extensive; supported by piped-in O_2 and suctioning	Limited availability; must use portable O_2 and suctioning systems
Travel requirements	None; remain in one facility	Must travel between facilities or residences
Level of supervision	Direct supervision	RCP works independently with minimal supervision
Patient assessment	Moderate—primarily provided by attending physician/residents	Heavy—core responsibility related to care planning
Documentation requirements	Moderate—limited to medical recordkeeping	Heavy—includes initial justification, ongoing follow-up, and often detailed financial recordkeeping
Work schedule	Specific hours	Varied work schedule, often including "on-call" off hours coverage
Time constraints	More than one shift to deliver therapy	Must complete all therapy during shift/visit
Patient-family interaction	Limited treatment time available; little family interaction	One-on-one therapy; intensive family interaction
Professional interaction	Primarily attending physicians and patient's nurse(s)	Continuous interaction with all members of professional team

Discharge Planning for the Respiratory Care Patient

AARC Clinical Practice Guideline (Excerpts)*

➤ INDICATIONS

Discharge planning is indicated for all respiratory care patients being considered for discharge or transfer to alternative sites. The plan should be developed/implemented as early as possible prior to transfer.

➤ CONTRAINDICATIONS

There are no contraindications to the development of a discharge plan.

➤ PRECAUTIONS AND/OR POSSIBLE COMPLICATIONS

Undesirable and/or unexpected outcomes may occur if the patient is discharged prior to the full implementation of the plan. Undesirable or unexpected patient outcomes may also occur due to (1) the natural course of the disease or (2) other factors beyond the control of the discharge planning process.

➤ METHOD

Discharge planning and implementation should begin as early as possible. The complexity of the plan is determined by the patient's medical condition, needs, and goals. The steps in the planning process are:

- Patient evaluation
  - The patient's medical condition
  - The respiratory and ventilatory support required
  - The patient's physical and functional ability and activities of daily living
  - The patient and family's psychosocial condition
  - The patient and family's desires for medical and ventilator care
  - The goalss of care (patient/family, physician, the health-care professionals, bedside caregivers)
- Site evaluation for continuing care
  - Personnel
  - Equipment and supplies
  - Physical environment (safety and suitability)
- Financial resources
- Development of the multidisciplinary plan of care based on the patient's needs and goals, to include:
  - Plan for integration into the community
  - Plan for patient self-care as appropriate
  - Roles and responsibilities of team members for daily care management
  - Documented mechanism for securing and training additional caregivers
  - Alternative emergency and contingency plans
  - Plan for use, maintenance, and troubleshooting of equipment
  - Time frame for implementation
  - Medication administration
  - Method for ongoing assessment of outcomes
  - Method to assess growth and development of pediatric patients
  - Mechanism for communication among all members of healthcare team
  - Follow-up (e.g., medical, respiratory care)
  - Plan for monitoring and appropriately responding to changes in the patient's medical condition
- Education and training with clear demonstration and documentation of competencies must occur prior to discharge and address key elements of the plan of care.

➤ ASSESSMENT OF NEED

All patients with a respiratory diagnosis should be assessed for a discharge plan.

➤ ASSESSMENT OF OUTCOME

The desired outcome of the discharge plan is determined by:

- No readmission due to discharge plan failure
- Satisfactory performance of all treatments and modalities by caregivers as instructed
- The treatment's meeting the patients's needs/goals
- The site's providing the necessary services
- The equipment's meeting the patient's needs
- Caregivers' ability to assess the patient, troubleshoot, and solve problems as they arise
- The patient and family's satisfaction

➤ MONITORING

The discharge plan coordinator and the physician should monitor the progress of the discharge plan. Each team member should participate in regularly scheduled team conferences to assess the progress of the discharge plan. Modifications may be made according to the individual patient's goals and needs.

For the complete guideline, see Respir Care 40:1308, 1995.

Table 49-2 ▶▶▶ Members of the Postacute Care Team

Discipline	Responsibilities
Utilization review	Advises and/or recommends consideration of patient discharge. Documents patient's in-hospital care.
Discharge planning (social service or community/ public health)	Brings all the needed elements together and ensures that a patient can be discharged to postacute care setting. Makes contacts with outside agencies that may assist with patient care.
Physician	Writes order for patient discharge. Evalutes patient's condition and prescribes needed care. Establishes therapeutic objectives.
Respiratory care	Evalutes patient and recommends appropriate respiratory care; provides care and follow-up accordingly.
Nursing	Writes/implements nursing care plan for patient; assesses patient's status and provides necessary follow-up.
Dietary/nutrition	Assesses patient's nutritional needs and writes dietary plan for patient. Makes arrangements for meals as may be necessary.
Physical/occupational therapy	Provides necessary physical therapy and recommends any additional modalities or procedures.
Psychiatry/psychology	Assesses patient's emotional status and provides any needed counselling or support.
DME supplier/home care company	Provides needed equipment and supplies and handles any emergency situations involving delivery or equipment operation.

produces the best patient results. Communication and mutual respect for each team member's talents and abilities are two key elements in making subacute care work. Any breakdown in the system may delay or adversely affect patient discharge, as well as the patient's physical health and mental well-being.

Site and Support Service Evaluation

The primary factors determining the appropriate site for discharge are the goals and needs of the patient. These goals and needs should be met in an optimal and cost-effective manner using the resources available at the proposed site. In terms of institutional personnel, the staff of the selected facility must clearly have all the competencies required to meet the patient's ventilatory and respiratory needs, be able to provide other needed healthcare services (e.g., physical therapy), and provide adequate 24-hour coverage.[19]

For discharge to the home, it is essential that caregivers' abilities to learn and perform the required care be evaluated before transfer. Caregivers must clearly demonstrate and have documented the competencies required to care for the specific patient and, in combination, provide 24-hour coverage.[19]

RULE OF THUMB

To confirm that a nonprofessional caregiver can perform a particular skill, you must go beyond demonstration and verbal confirmation of his or her understanding. The RRT must *observe* a return demonstration, whereby the caregiver properly performs the same procedural steps you demonstrated. Providing the caregiver with a checklist of procedure steps is useful for both teaching and documentation of caregiver mastery of the competency.

Beyond performing a particular skill, it is imperative for the discharge team to ensure that an adequate number of professional and nonprofessional caregivers are part of the care plan to provide appropriate patient care coverage. This is particularly true when more complicated modes, such as mechanical ventilation, or multiple therapies are required by the patient. An unfortunate, but all to common discharge planing mistake is the reliance on too few individuals and or overestimation of caregiver capabilities in alternative settings. Generally there is substantial caregiver strain associated with overseeing such patients. Proper assessment of the capabilities and number of potential caregiver capabilities in light of the therapy needed at home and appropriate training of such individuals can help address this concern.

Equipment support and selected clinical services for respiratory home care patients are often provided by a durable medical equipment (DME) supplier. DME suppliers range in size from multimillion dollar national corporations offering a broad range of services, to small local companies. These companies, both large and small, usually provide the following services:

- 24-hour, 7 days-a-week service
- Third-party insurance processing
- Home instruction and follow-up by an RRT
- Most forms of respiratory care

When selecting a DME supplier, the discharge planning team, including the patient and family members, should consider the company's accreditation status, cost and scope of services, dependability, location, personnel, past track record, and availability. To ensure a basic level of quality, one should select a DME supplier that is JCAHO accredited. In addition, the service should be problem-free and provided by a reliable, experienced, professional, and courteous staff. Charges should be

Box 49-1 • Assessing the Home Environment

ACCESSIBILITY
- In and out of home/apartment
- Accessibility between rooms
- Doorway width/threshold heights
- Stairways
- Wheelchair mobility
- Bathroom
- Kitchen
- Carpeting

EQUIPMENT
- Available space
- Electrical power supply
- Amperage
- Grounded outlets
- Presence of hazardous appliances

ENVIRONMENT
- Heating/ventilation
- Humidity
- Lighting
- Living space

MINI CLINI

Assessing the Home Environment

PROBLEM

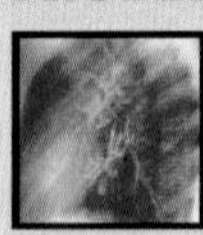

A wheelchair-bound patient with a tracheostomy who requires mechanical ventilation is being discharged to the home care setting. Inspection of the two-story home reveals front and rear elevated porch entrances with all bedrooms upstairs. All room floors (except the kitchen and bathrooms) are covered with high pile carpeting. The largest bedroom is 12 ft × 14 ft. The electrical service is rated at 75 amps, and the only grounded outlets are in the kitchen and garage. Heating is provided by a forced hot-air system; there is a single window air conditioner in the patient's bedroom. What problems do you see and what changes would you recommend to provide the proper home environment for this patient?

SOLUTION

Although wheelchair bound, this patient is still mobile. Both the elevated porch entrances and the high pile carpeting will restrict mobility. A ramp entrance will need to be constructed, and the carpeting removed or covered with a flat, hard surface material. Given the size of the patient's upstairs room and the obstacle of the stairwell, it would be best to identify a large first-story room for conversion to a bedroom. Because the patient will probably need at least an electric bed, ventilator, and suction machine, the electrical service capacity is inadequate and needs upgrading to ensure at least 15-20 amps in the patient area, with 200 amps overall. Appliance, counter, sink, and toilet heights need to be assessed for easy patient access.

reasonable and competitive, and clinical respiratory services should be provided by credentialed RRTs.

Finally, the selected site must meet basic safety standards and be suitable for managing the patient's specific condition. It should be free of fire, health, and safety hazards; provide adequate heating, cooling, and ventilation; provide adequate electrical service; provide for patient access and mobility with adequate patient space (room to house medical and adaptive equipment) and storage facilities. Further, the selected site must be capable of operating, maintaining, and supporting all equipment needed by the patient. This should include both respiratory and ancillary equipment and supplies as needed, such as the ventilator, suction, O_2, intravenous therapy, nutritional therapy, and adaptive equipment.[19] Box 49-1 lists some key factors one should assess in planning the discharge of a respiratory care patient to the home environment.

▶ OXYGEN THERAPY IN ALTERNATIVE SETTINGS

O_2 therapy is by far the most common mode of respiratory care in postacute care settings. This high usage is based on the fact that O_2 therapy improves both survival and quality of life in selected patient groups, especially those with advanced COPD.[20,21] In particular, studies have shown improved nocturnal O_2 saturation, reduced pulmonary artery pressure, and lower pulmonary vascular resistance with appropriate out-patient O_2 therapy.[22,23]

To guide practitioners in providing quality care, the AARC has published a *Practice Guideline on Oxygen Therapy in the Home or Extended Care Facility*.[24] Excerpts from the AARC guideline, including the indications, contraindications, precautions and possible complications, method, assessment of need, assessment of outcome and monitoring appear on p. 1255.

The Oxygen Therapy Prescription

As indicated in the practice guideline, O_2 prescriptions must be based on documented hypoxemia, as determined by either blood gas analysis or oximetry. Prescriptions for O_2 no longer can be based simply on patient diagnosis or signs and symptoms. In addition, prn O_2 is no longer acceptable in the postacute care setting.

Once the need for O_2 therapy is established, the physician writes a prescription. A prescription for O_2 therapy in the postacute care setting must include the following elements:[25]

OXYGEN THERAPY IN THE HOME OR EXTENED CARE FACILITY

AARC Clinical Practice Guideline (Excerpts)*

➤ INDICATIONS

- Documented hypoxemia
- Adults, children, and infants >28 days old: Pa_{O_2} ≤55 torr or Sa_{O_2} <88% (room air)
- Pa_{O_2} of 56-59 torr or Sa_{O_2} ≤89% in association with specific clinical conditions (e.g., cor pulmonale, congestive heart failure, or erythrocythemia with hematocrit ≥56%)
- Patients who do not qualify for O_2 therapy at rest may qualify during ambulation, sleep, or exercise if their Sa_{O_2} falls below 89% during these specific activities

➤ CONTRAINDICATIONS

No absolute contraindications to O_2 therapy exist when indications are present.

➤ PRECAUTIONS AND/OR POSSIBLE COMPLICATIONS

- In spontaneously breathing hypoxemic patients with COPD, O_2 therapy may increase the Pa_{CO_2}
- Problems may occur if the patient fails to comply with the doctor's orders or receives inadequate instruction
- Complications may result from use of nasal cannulae or transtracheal catheters
- Fire hazard is increased in the presence of increased oxygen concentrations
- Bacterial contamination associated with certain nebulizers and humidifers may occur
- Physical hazards include unsecured cylinders, ungrounded equipment, and liquid oxygen burns
- Power or equipment failure can lead to an inadequate oxygen supply

➤ ASSESSMENT OF NEED

- Initial need is determined by documented hypoxemia at rest or during activity (above)
- Additional blood gas analysis is indicated whenever there is a major change in cardiopulmonary status
- Blood gases should be repeated after 1-3 months to determine the need for long-term O_2 therapy (LTOT)
- Once the need for LTOT has been documented, repeated measures are needed only to follow the course of the disease, to assess changes in clinical status, or to facilitate changes in the oxygen prescription

➤ ASSESSMENT OF OUTCOME

Outcome is determined by clinical and physiological assessment to establish adequacy of patient response to therapy.

➤ MONITORING

- Patient
  - The patient/caregiver should routinely assess for changes in status (e.g., use of dyspnea scales/diaries)
  - Patients should be visited/monitored at least monthly by credentiated personnel
  - Pa_{O_2} and/or SO_2 measurement should be repeated when indicated or to follow the disease course
  - SO_2 measurements also may used to determine appropriate O_2 flow for ambulation, exercise, or sleep
- Equipment
  - All O_2 equipment should be checked at least daily by the patient or caregiver for proper function, prescribed flow, F_{IO_2}, remaining liquid or gas content, and backup supply
  - During visits, the RRT should reinforce proper patient/caregiver practices and ensure that equipment is being maintained as per manufacturers's recommendations
  - Liquid systems need to be checked to ensure adequate delivery
  - O_2 concentrators should be checked regularly to ensure at least 85% O_2 at 4 L/min

*For the complete guideline, see Respir Care 37:918, 1992.

- Flow rate in liters/minute and/or concentration
- Frequency of use in hours/day and minutes/hour (if applicable)
- Duration of need (up to a maximum of 12 months in the home)
- Diagnosis (severe primary lung disease, secondary conditions related to lung disease and hypoxia, related conditions or symptoms that may improve with O_2)
- Laboratory evidence (arterial blood gas [ABG] analysis or oximetry under the appropriate testing conditions). Home care companies cannot provide this testing.

Department of Health and Human Services
Health Care Financing Administration

Form Approved
OMB No. 0938-0534

ATTENDING PHYSICIAN'S CERTIFICATION OF MEDICAL NECESSITY FOR HOME OXYGEN THERAPY *(Legible handwritten entries acceptable)*

Public reporting burden for this collection of information is estimated to average 15 minutes per response, including the time for reviewing instructions, searching existing data sources, gathering and maintaining the data needed, and completing and reviewing the collection of information. Send comments regarding this burden estimate or any other aspect of this collection of information, including suggestions for reducing this burden, to HCFA, P.O. Box 26684, Baltimore, MD 21207; and to the Office of Information and Regulatory Affairs, Office of Management and Budget, Washington, DC 20503.

Patient's Name, Address, and HIC No.	Supplier's Name, Address, and Identification No.

Certification: ☐ Initial ☐ Revised ☐ Renewed

INFORMATION BELOW TO BE ENTERED ONLY BY PHYSICIAN OR PHYSICIAN'S EMPLOYEE

1. Pertinent Diagnoses, ICD-9-CM Codes, and Findings - CHECK ALL THAT APPLY:

☐ Emphysema (492.8) ☐ Chronic Obstructive Bronchitis (491.2)
☐ COPD (496) ☐ Chronic Obstructive Asthma (493.20)
☐ Cor Pulmonale (416.9) ☐ Congestive Heart Failure (428.0)
☐ Interstitial Disease (515) ☐ Secondary Polycythemia (289.0)
☐ Other ____________ ☐ Hematocrit 57% or more Yes☐ No☐
Specify Code

2.A. I last examined this patient for this condition on: ____/____/____ Month Day Year

2.B. Home oxygen prescribed: ____/____/____ Month Day Year

2.C. Estimated length of need: ☐ 1-3 months ☐ 4-12 months ☐ Lifetime

3.A. Results of Most Recent Arterial Blood Gas and/or Oxygen Saturation Tests (Patient Breathing Room Air)

	PO2	02 Saturation	Date
(1) At Rest			
(2) Walking			
(3) Sleeping			
(4) Exercising			
(5) Other :			

3.C. Physician/Provider Performing Test(s) *(Printed/Typed Name and Address)*:

3.B. If performed under conditions other than room air, explain:

NOTE: If PO2 Level exceeds 59 mm Hg or the arterial blood saturation exceeds 89% at rest on room air, the claim will be disallowed withc compelling medical evidence. Check block ☐ if you have attached a separate statement on your letterhead of additional documentation.

4. Oxygen Flow Rate : _____ Liters per minute ☐ Continuous (24 hrs/day)

☐ Noncontinuous (Enter hrs/day): _____ Walking _____Sleeping _____Exercise Program _____Other (specify) _______

5. Oxygen Equipment Prescribed If you have prescribed a particular form of delivery, check applicable block(s). Otherwise leave blank.

A. Supply System

(1) Stationary Source ☐ Concentrator ☐ Liquid Oxygen ☐ Compressed Gas ☐ Other

(2) Portable or Ambulatory Source ☐ Liquid Oxygen ☐ Compressed Gas ☐ Other ________

B. Delivery System

☐ (1) Nasal Cannula
☐ (2) 02 Conserving Device
☐ Pulse 02 System
☐ Reservoir System
☐ Other ________
☐ (3) Transtracheal Catheter
☐ (4) Other ________

6. If you have prescribed a portable or ambulatory system, describe activities/exercise that patient regularly pursues which require this sys in the home and which cannot be met by a stationary system (e.g., amount and frequency of ambulation).

CERTIFICATION

THE PATIENT HAS APPROPRIATELY TRIED OTHER TREATMENT MEASURES WITHOUT SUCCESS. OXYGEN THERAPY AND OXYGEN EQUIPMENT AS PRESCRIBED IS MEDICALLY INDICATED AND IS REASONABLE AND NECESSARY FOR THE TREATMENT OF THIS PATIENT. THIS FORM AND ANY STATEMENT ON MY LETTERHEAD ATTACHED HERETO HAS BEEN COMPLETED BY ME, OR BY MY EMPLOYEE AND REVIEWED BY ME. THE FOREGOING INFORMATION IS TRUE, ACCURATE, AND COMPLETE, AND I UNDERSTAND THAT ANY FALSIFICATION, OMISSION, OR CONCEALMENT OF MATERIAL FACT MAY SUBJECT ME TO CIVIL OR CRIMINAL LIABILITY.

Attending Physician's Signature: *(A STAMPED SIGNATURE IS NOT ACCEPTABLE)*	Date:

Physician's Name, Address, Telephone No., and Identification No.:

HCFA-484 (5-90)

*U S GPO 1990 261 1'4 13580

Figure 49-1

Form from the Centers for Medical and Medicad Services (CMS) used to certify the medical necessity for home oxygen therapy.

- Additional medical documentation (no acceptable alternatives to home O_2 therapy).

For home use, the ordering physician must authorize O_2 therapy using the HCFA Certification of Medical Necessity for Home Oxygen Therapy form (Figure 49-1). When O_2 therapy starts in the hospital but continues in the home, analysis of arterial blood O_2 should be repeated after 1 to 3 months to determine the need for long-term O_2 therapy.[26] Once the need for long-term therapy is documented, repeat ABGs or SpO_2 measurements are not needed. However, blood O_2 levels may still be measured when the need arises to assess changes in the patient's condition or to adjust the O_2 prescription.

Supply Methods

Most alternative care sites do not have bulk O_2 storage or delivery systems. In these settings, O_2 normally is supplied from one of the following three sources:[27] (1) compressed O_2 cylinders, (2) liquid O_2 systems, or (3) O_2 concentrators. Table 49-3 summarizes the major advantages and disadvantages of each system.

Compressed Oxygen Cylinders

The primary use of compressed O_2 cylinders in alternative settings is for either ambulation (small cylinders) or as a backup to liquid or concentrator supply systems (H/K cylinders). Safety measures for cylinder O_2 are the same as those covered in Chapter 34. For home use, you should thoroughly review these safety measures with both the patient and family. After instruction, you should always confirm and document caregivers' actual abilities to safely use the delivery system.

In addition to the cylinder gas, a pressure reducing valve with flowmeter is needed to deliver O_2 at the prescribed flow. Standard clinical flowmeters deliver flows up to 15 L/minute; flows used in alternative settings are typically in the 0.25 to 5.0 L/minute range. For this reason, you should select a calibrated low-flow flowmeter whenever possible. Alternatively, you can use a preset flow restrictor (see Chapter 34).

As in the hospital, there is usually no need to humidify nasal O_2 at flows of 4 L/minute or less.[24] If humidification is needed, you can use a simple unheated bubble humidifier. Because the mineral content of tap water may be high (hard water), water used in these humidifiers should be distilled. Otherwise, the porous diffusing element may become occluded. Although complete blockage is unlikely, occlusion of the diffusing element can impair humidification and alter flow.

Liquid Oxygen Systems

Because 1 cubic foot of liquid O_2 equals 860 cubic feet of gas, liquid O_2 systems can store large quantities of O_2 in small spaces. This is ideal for the high-volume user. As shown in Figure 49-2, a typical personal liquid O_2 system is a miniature version of a hospital stand tank.

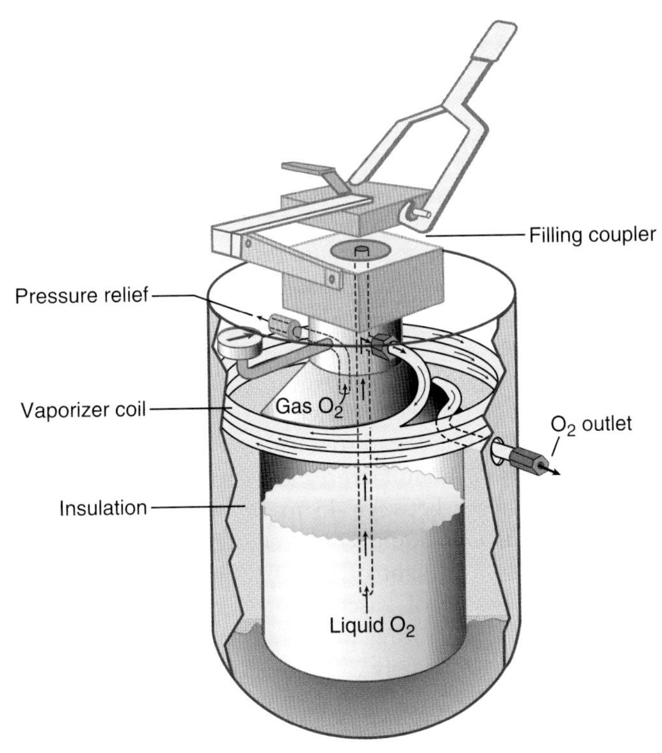

Figure 49-2
Diagram of a personal liquid oxygen supply system. *(Modified from Lampton LM: Home and outpatient oxygen therapy. In Brashear RE, Rhodes ML, editors: Chronic obstructive lung disease, St Louis, 1978, Mosby.)*

Table 49-3 ▶▶ Advantages and Disadvantages of the Major Alternative Oxygen Supply Systems

System	Advantages	Disadvantages
Compressed oxygen	Good for small-volume user No waste or loss Stores oxygen indefinitely Widespread availability Portability (small cylinders)	Large cylinders are heavy and bulky High-pressure safety hazard Provides limited volume Requires frequent deliveries Tight valves can be a problem
Liquid oxygen system	Provides large volumes Low-pressure system (20-25 psi) Portable units can be refilled from reservoir (up to 8-hour supply at 2 L/min) Valuable for rehabilitation	Must be delivered as needed Loss of O_2 because of venting of system when not in use Low temperature safety hazard Cannot operate ventilators or other high-pressure devices Some difficulty in filling portable unit
Oxygen concentrator	No waste or loss Low-pressure system (15 psi) Cost-effective when continual supply of oxygen is needed Eliminates need for deliveries	Disruption in electrical service renders system inoperable Backup oxygen is needed Cannot operate ventilators or other high-pressure devices FIO_2 decreases with increasing flow High electrical costs possible

Like its larger counterpart, this system consists of a reservoir unit similar in design to a thermos bottle. The inner container of liquid O_2 is suspended in an outer container, with a vacuum in between. The liquid O_2 is kept at approximately -300° F. Because of constant vaporization, gaseous O_2 always exists above the liquid. When the cylinder is not in use, this vaporization maintains pressures between 20 and 25 psi. When pressures rise above this level, gas vents out the pressure relief valve.

When flow is turned on, gaseous O_2 passes through a vaporizing coil, where it is warmed by exposure to room temperature. It then leaves the system through an outlet, where it is metered by a flow control valve. With low-flow O_2 being so common in the postacute care setting, these metering devices are usually calibrated in 0.5 L/minute units, and limited to a maximum flow of 5 to 8 L/minute.

If the cylinder pressure drops below a preset level during use (usually 20 psi), an economizer valve closes, causing the liquid O_2 to move up the center tube and into the vaporizing coil. When in the vaporizing coil, the liquid O_2 is converted to a gas.

Depending on manufacturer and model, small liquid O_2 cylinders hold between 45 to 100 pounds of liquid O_2. To calculate a liquid O_2 system's duration of flow, first convert the weight of liquid O_2 in pounds to the equivalent volume of gaseous O_2 in liters. At normal liquid cylinder operating pressures, 1 pound of liquid O_2 equals approximately 344 liters of gaseous O_2. See the accompanying Mini Clini for an example of how you can compute a liquid O_2 system's duration of flow.

To help avoid these computations, many manufacturers provide simple conversion charts for this purpose. Table 49-4 is an example of a conversion chart for a typical 100-pound personal liquid O_2 system.

Many personal liquid O_2 systems also come with smaller portable units (Figure 49-3). This system is ideal for the ambulatory patient who is capable of physical activity. Typical portable units weigh between 5 to 14 pounds and can be refilled directly from the stationary reservoir. Most portable units come with a carrying case or small cart, and can provide 5 to 8 hours of O_2 at a flow of 2 L/minute. Either an adjustable flow restrictor

Table 49-4 ▶▶ Conversion Chart for Computing the Duration of Flow for a 100-lb (40 L) Liquid Oxygen Reservoir

Gauge reading	1	2	3	4	4
Weight (lb)	12.5	25	50	75	100
Liquid liters	5	10	20	30	40
Gaseous liters	4,303	8,606	17,212	25,818	34,424
Duration of Flow (Hours)					
Flow (L/minute)					
1	72	143	287	430	574
2	36	72	143	215	287
3	24	48	96	143	191
4	18	36	72	108	143
5	14	29	57	86	115

MINI CLINI

Computing a Liquid Oxygen System's Duration of Flow

PROBLEM

A home care patient receives nasal oxygen at 2 L/min from a 100-lb liquid oxygen system. The system gauge indicates that the cylinder is half full. Approximately how long will this system last until empty?

SOLUTION

Step 1: Compute the available liquid oxygen (in lb)

$$100 \times 0.5 = 50 \text{ lb}$$

Step 2: Compute the available gaseous oxygen

Weight (lb) remaining × factor

$$50 \text{ lb} \times 344 \text{ L/lb} = 17{,}200 \text{ L}$$

Step 3: Divide the available volume of gaseous oxygen by the prescribed liter flow

$$\text{Duration of flow (min)} = \frac{\text{Volume of gaseous } O_2 \text{ (L)}}{\text{Liter flow (L/min)}}$$

$$\text{Duration of flow (min)} = \frac{17{,}200 \text{ L}}{2 \text{ L/min}} = 8{,}600 \text{ min} = 143.3 \text{ hr} \approx 6 \text{ days}$$

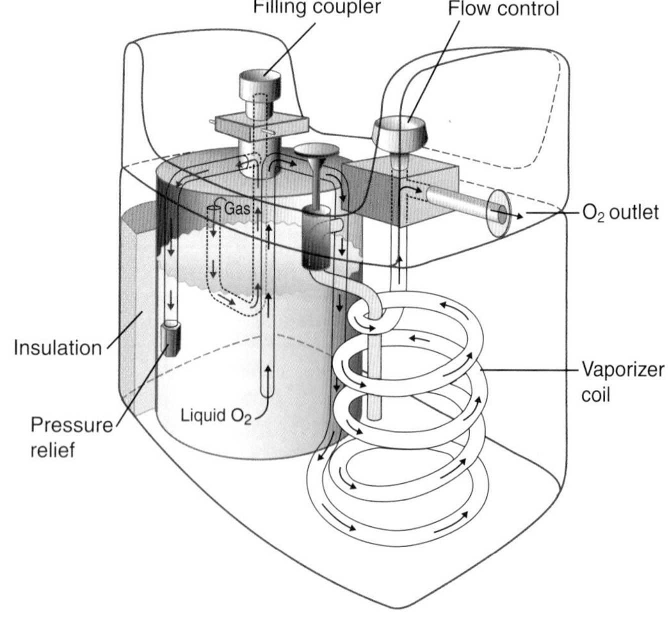

Figure 49-3
Diagram of a portable liquid oxygen unit. *(Modified from Lampton LM: Home and outpatient oxygen therapy. In Brashear RE, Rhodes ML, editors: Chronic obstructive lung disease, St Louis, 1978, Mosby.)*

or Bourdon-type gauge is used to meter flow, with a weight gauge used to indicate O_2 contents. The functional use time of portable liquid O_2 units can be extended with O_2-conserving devices.

Because of the extremely low temperature of liquid O_2, patients and caregivers must be extremely careful when refilling these portable systems. Box 49-2 lists the steps needed to fill a portable liquid O_2 unit from a reservoir.[27] The procedure takes approximately one to two minutes, depending on the size of the portable tank. Wearing gloves can help prevent liquid O_2 skin burns.

Box 49-2 • Steps for Filling a Portable Liquid Oxygen Unit From the Reservoir

1. Make sure there is enough liquid oxygen in the reservoir to fill the portable unit.
2. Check the connectors on both units to make sure that they are clean and dry. Moisture on these connectors could cause the connectors to freeze together.
3. Connect the portable unit to the reservoir according to the manufacturer's instructions. The flow-rate controller should be turned off.
4. Open the portable unit vent. Allow the portable unit to fill until the vent begins to pass liquid oxygen instead of gas. Close the vent valve.
5. Disengage the portable unit according to the manufacturer's instructions.

From Sleeper G: Home oxygen therapy equipment. In Lucus J et al, editors: Home respiratory care, Norwalk, Conn., 1988, Appleton & Lange.

Oxygen Concentrators

An O_2 concentrator is an electrically-powered device that physically separates the O_2 in room air from nitrogen. The most common type of concentrator uses a *molecular sieve* to extract O_2. Concentrators using membrane technology also exist, but they are not in common use.

The molecular sieve concentrator uses a pump to compress and deliver filtered room air to one of two sets of sieves (Figure 49-4). These sieves contain sodium-aluminum silicate pellets that absorb nitrogen, carbon dioxide, and water vapor. To remove these unwanted gases from the pellets, an automatic pressure swing cycle switches back and forth between the sieve sets. Whereas one set is pressurized to produce O_2, the other is depressurized to purge N_2, CO_2, and water vapor.

Gas leaving the sieves is stored in a small accumulator. At flows of 1 to 2 L/minute, the typical molecular sieve concentrator provides between 92% and 95% O_2. At 3 to 5 L/minute, O_2 concentrations fall to between 85% and 93%. With most concentrator outputs limited to 5 L/minute, higher flows can only be achieved by running two systems together in parallel.

O_2 concentrators are the most cost-efficient supply method for patients in alternative settings who need continuous low-flow O_2. For home use, a concentrator running 24 hours per day will increase the average monthly electrical bill by only 5% to 10%. Depending on the season, heat given off by the concentrator's compressor can also affect energy usage by raising room temperature.

When used with patients receiving low-flow O_2, O_2 concentrators are just as effective in raising blood O_2 levels as more traditional supply systems (such as 100% cylinder gas with a cannula). Moreover, current home care reimbursement regulations favor the use of cost-

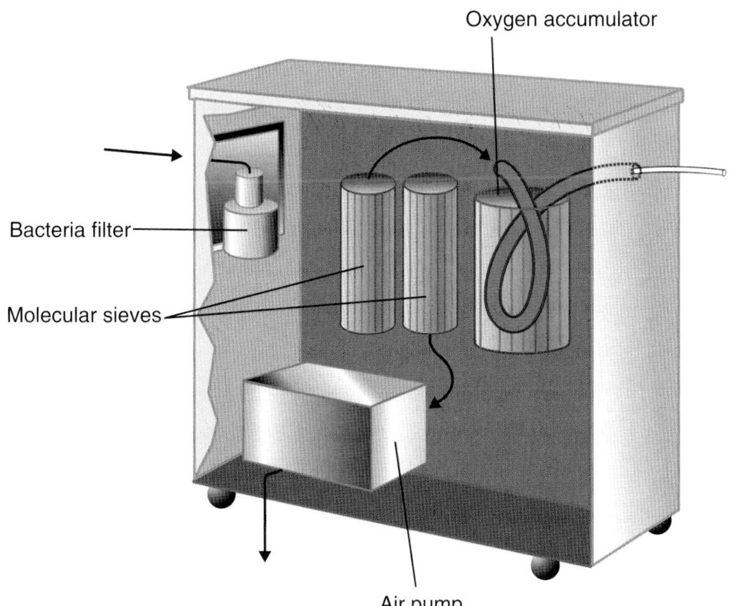

Figure 49-4
A molecular sieve oxygen concentration.

efficient O_2 systems. As a result, the use of O_2 concentrators and conserving systems is becoming increasingly popular.

Problem-Solving and Troubleshooting

Technical problems with O_2 supply systems in alternative settings are similar to those encountered in the acute care hospital (see Chapter 34). In addition to these technical problems, situations can arise when patients or caregivers fail to properly follow instructions or respond as needed to simple incidents. To avoid communication problems, always reinforce verbal instruction by providing simple written instructions for subsequent reference. In addition, you should always confirm and document caregivers' actual abilities to use the delivery system safely, including how to troubleshoot simple problems.[24]

To avoid problems before they occur, have the patient or caregiver check all O_2 delivery equipment at least once a day.[18] The proper function of all equipment, including liter flow and concentration, should be confirmed. In addition, the remaining liquid or compressed gas content of the supply system should be checked. Last, concentrator air inlet filters must be cleaned weekly. In the home setting, providing the patient or caregiver with a simple checklist or log diary form can help ensure that these important tasks are performed regularly.

Unlike the hospital setting, O_2 supply problems in the postacute care setting cannot always be addressed immediately. For this reason, you must ensure that all such systems have an emergency backup supply. This is normally provided by a large H/K cylinder. If a home care patient's primary O_2 supply is by concentrator, you should also notify the local power company in writing that life support equipment is in use at that location. In the event of an outage, the company will try to restore power to that location first. Alternatively, an emergency gasoline electrical generator can provide backup power for a concentrator.

Possible physical hazards to patients and caregivers include unsecured cylinders, ungrounded equipment, mishandling of liquid (resulting in burns), and fire.[24] Careful preliminary instruction, followed by ongoing assessment of the environment, can help minimize these problems. Bacterial contamination of nebulizer or humidification systems is another problem.[24] Infection control procedures designed to minimize this problem are discussed in detail on p. 1280.

Inaccurate O_2 flows or concentrations can also occur. Accurate flow output of O_2 systems should be confirmed by the supplier (using calibrated laboratory meters) before equipment is placed in alternative settings.[28] In the home, O_2 concentrator fractional inspired oxygen concentration (F_{IO_2}) levels should be checked and confirmed as part of a routine monthly maintenance visit.[29] Routine maintenance of these devices should include cleaning and replacing filters, checking the alarm system, and confirming the F_{IO_2} levels using either the unit's O_2 sensor or a separate calibrated O_2 analyzer. If the concentration is less than the manufacturer's specification at the given flow, the pellet canisters are probably exhausted and should be replaced.

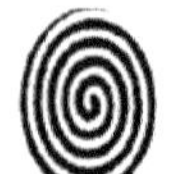

RULE OF THUMB

If an O_2 concentrator cannot supply at least 85% O_2 at 5 L/minute, the pellet canisters are probably exhausted and should be replaced.

Because both concentrators and personal liquid O_2 systems operate at low pressures, they cannot be used to drive equipment needing 50 psi, such as pneumatically powered ventilators and large-volume jet nebulizers. However, because the typical postacute care ventilator is electrically powered and uses a flowmeter to provide supplementary O_2, this limitation is generally not a problem. Nonetheless, when 50 psi O_2 is needed, large gas cylinders are the storage system of choice. Many patients using liquid O_2 express concern when they hear gas venting from their system. The RRT should explain to patients that venting is a normal feature of liquid O_2 systems. Venting does not occur during continual use, because system pressures never build up to activate the relief valve.

Delivery Methods

The most common O_2 delivery system for long-term care is the nasal cannula. Simple O_2 masks and air entrainment masks (AEMs) may also be used but are much less common. Also rare in alternative settings are nasal catheters and reservoir masks. To decrease O_2 use and costs, a number of O_2-conserving devices has been developed. These include the transtracheal O_2 catheter, the reservoir cannula, and the demand or pulse-flow O_2 delivery system.

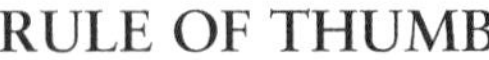

RULE OF THUMB

O_2-conserving devices exhibit performance comparable to a nasal cannula at approximately one third to one half the flow. Based on this knowledge, when switching a patient from a nasal cannula at 2 L/minute to an O_2-conserving device, you would start out at half the original flow, in this case 1 L/minute. You would then assess the response using a pulse oximeter and adjust the flow accordingly.

The performance characteristics, advantages, and disadvantages of the transtracheal O_2 catheter and reservoir cannula were detailed in Chapter 35. Here we focus on the application of the transtracheal O_2 catheter and the technical aspects of demand-flow systems.

Transtracheal Oxygen Therapy

Not all patients requiring long-term O_2 therapy are good candidates for transtracheal O_2 therapy (TTOT). TTOT is indicated only for those patients who meet one or more of the following criteria: (1) they cannot be adequately oxygenated with standard approaches; (2) they do not comply well when using other devices; (3) they exhibit complications from nasal cannula use; (4) they prefer TTOT for cosmetic reasons; and (5) they have need for increased mobility.[30] TTOT may also be a treatment alternative for some patients with sleep apnea when nasal CPAP is not tolerated or when combined O_2 and nasal CPAP are required.

As with most postacute care modalities, the success of TTOT depends mainly on effective patient education and ongoing self-care with professional follow-up. Key patient responsibilities include routine catheter cleaning and recognizing and troubleshooting common problems. Box 49-3 describes key self-care guidelines for patients with transtracheal O_2 catheters.

Box 49-3 • Self-care Guidelines for Patients With Transtracheal Oxygen Catheters

- The catheter should never be out of your tract for more than a few minutes or your tract may close. If you cannot reinsert the catheter, put on a nasal cannula and call your doctor.
- Always keep the catheter clean to ensure proper function.
- If you believe the catheter is not working properly, first clean it. If you still believe that the catheter isn't working, put on a nasal cannula and call your doctor.
- If your humidifier pop-off is making noise, clear any hose blockage and clean the catheter.
- The catheter must never be removed or inserted while oxygen is flowing through it.
- Always keep your tract opening clean and dry. Do not use antibiotics or other ointments.
- Always keep the oxygen hose under your shirt, blouse, T-shirt, or pajama-top and clipped to the top of your pants, skirt, or pajama bottom.
- Do not pull, twist, crush, cut, glue, boil, or abuse the catheter. Treat it as your lifeline.
- Any product that is cracked, broken, develops a permanent kink or foul odor should be immediately discarded and replaced. Catheters and hoses should be routinely replaced every 3 months.
- When traveling, always take catheter cleaning supplies, a nasal cannula, and a spare catheter.

From Spofford B et al: Transtracheal oxygen therapy: a guide from the respiratory therapist, Respir Care Clin N Am 32:345, 1987.

Demand Flow Oxygen Systems

A demand flow O_2 delivery device uses a flow sensor and valve to synchronize gas delivery with the beginning of inspiration.[31] As indicated in Figure 49-5, *A*, with continuous O_2 flow, most of the effective O_2 delivery occurs during the first half of inspiration. All the O_2 delivered during the latter half of inspiration and throughout most of expiration is wasted. Figure 49-5, *B*, shows the effect of a synchronized pulse of O_2 delivered at the beginning of inspiration. Ideally, this O_2 pulse should occur during the first quarter of inspiration. Under these conditions, a pulsed O_2 system can produce SaO_2 levels equal to those seen with continuous flow, while using 60% less O_2.[32]

In theory, demand-flow O_2 systems provide the greatest savings in O_2 usage for a given level of arterial saturation. In addition, there is no need for humidification. Demand-flow systems also have been successfully adapted for use with transtracheal catheters, resulting in even more efficient O_2 delivery. Unfortunately, current Medicare reimbursement guidelines provide no additional payments to cover the additional cost of demand delivery systems. Moreover, some patients receiving demand-flow O_2 desaturate during exercise. For this reason, all patients recommended for long-term O_2 therapy should be tested for desaturation with the same system they will use outside the hospital.

Selecting a Long-Term Oxygen Delivery System

As when selecting hospital-based O_2 therapy systems, always consider the following "three Ps" when selecting a long-term O_2 system: *P*urpose, *P*atient and *P*erformance. The goal is always to match the performance of the equipment to both the objectives of therapy (purpose) and the patient's special needs.

Problem-Solving and Troubleshooting

Most problems with long-term O_2 delivery systems are people problems. Patients and caregivers often fail to follow instructions or comply with the prescribed therapeutic regimen.[24] As a general rule, caregivers should be allowed to operate and maintain O_2 delivery devices only after they have been instructed by credentialed RRTs and have demonstrated the appropriate level of skill.[24] In no case should the patient or caregiver be allowed or instructed to alter flow settings. Instead, when in doubt, they should be taught to switch to the backup supply at the same liter flow.

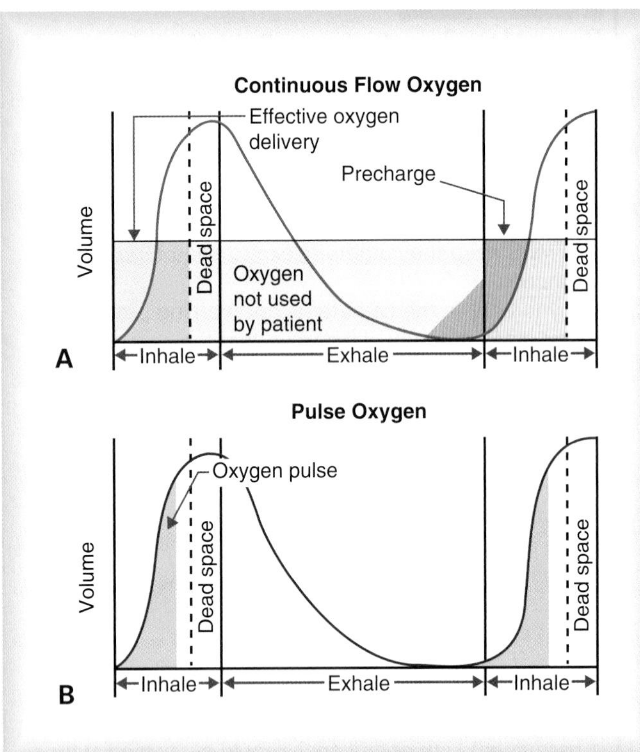

Figure 49-5
Demand flow oxygen delivery. With continuous flow **(A)**, most oxygen is delivered during the first half of inhalation, with the remainder wasted. With a coordinated pulse **(B)**, most oxygen is delivered during the first 25% of inspiration, and no waste occurs. *(Modified from O'Donohue WJ: The future of home oxygen therapy, Respir Care 33:1125, 1988.)*

Technical problems are most common with TTOT and demand-flow systems. Most problems with TTOT are related to initial catheter insertion or ongoing maintenance. Most problems with demand-flow systems are based on the current limits of this technology.

The most common complications of TTOT are listed in Box 49-4. Although these problems occur infrequently, you must be on constant guard for their occurrence. In particular, you should immediately report any evidence of tract tenderness, fever, excessive cough, increased

MINI CLINI

Selecting a Long-term Oxygen Delivery System

PROBLEM

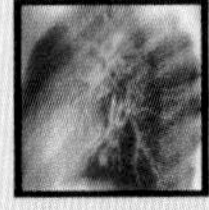

The following three patients require long-term oxygen: (1) a stable home care patient with restricted activity needing a low FIO_2; (2) an active home care patient with low FIO_2 needs who desires increased mobility; and (3) a patient in a long-term care facility with a tracheostomy who needs moderate levels of oxygen and high humidity. Select the best oxygen delivery system for each patient.

SOLUTION

Patient 1: Because the majority of home care patients who need oxygen are relatively stable, and because the FIO_2 needs are minimal, traditional low-flow therapy by nasal cannula (using either a concentrator or liquid reservoir) is the most common and accepted approach. When combined with a portable gas cylinder (for backup and limited walking), this combination is ideal for patients with restricted activity.

Patient 2: For an active patient with low FIO_2 needs who desires increased mobility, a conserving device used in conjunction with a portable liquid oxygen system (with the large reservoir used inside the home) is the ideal choice. For example, while a portable liquid oxygen unit can provide 5 to 8 hours of oxygen at 2 L/minute by standard nasal cannula, use of a conserving device can double or even triple this time frame. Given that reservoir cannulas are poorly accepted by most patients, and that demand-flow systems are somewhat bulky and unreliable, the choice of device usually narrows to a transtracheal catheter or pendant reservoir cannula. Patients who meet the criteria for TTOT and can provide meticulous self-care should receive TTOT. When TTOT is not indicated or fails, the pendant reservoir cannula is an acceptable alternative.

Patient 3: Postacute care patients with artificial airways who need oxygen present a special problem. Because of both high oxygen usage and infection concerns, an oxygen-powered air entrainment nebulizer is not satisfactory. Instead, a compressor-driven humidifier with supplemental oxygen, bled in at low flows from a concentrator should be used. In this case, the RRT must compute the proper flows for air and oxygen (Chapter 34) and confirm the FIO_2 by calibrated analyzer.

dyspnea, or subcutaneous emphysema to the patient's physician.

To avoid complications or product failure, catheters and their tubing should be replaced every 3 months, at which time a check-up by the physician is also recommended. The patient or caregiver should clean the catheter every day, per the self-care guidelines listed on p. 1261. Always instruct patients to put on a nasal cannula and call their doctor if any major problem occurs.

Because transtracheal catheters normally are used with humidifiers, you also must be prepared to troubleshoot this equipment. Guidelines for dealing with leaks and obstructions in O_2 delivery systems using humidifiers are provided in Chapter 35. Given the small bore of transtracheal catheters, you should generally use a humidifier with a high pressure (2 psi) relief valve, otherwise, the pop-off will constantly sound. As previously discussed, distilled water is satisfactory for airway humidification in alternative settings. Because nondisposable humidifiers are often used at these sites, you should teach patients and caregivers proper techniques for cleaning and disinfecting this equipment. Common problems with demand-flow O_2 delivery systems are listed in Box 49-5.[33]

Box 49-4 • Complication of Transtracheal Oxygen Therapy

- Bleeding*
- Pneumothorax*
- Bronchospasm*
- Subcutaneous emphysema
- Catheter dislodgment/lost tract
- Increased sputum production
- Blockage by inspissated mucus
- Infection or abscess
- Cephalad position
- Tract tenderness

From Spofford B et al: Transtracheal oxygen therapy: a guide for the respiratory therapist, *Respir Care Clin N Am* 32:345, 1987.
*Complications associated mainly with insertion.

Box 49-5 • Major Problems With Demand Oxygen Delivery Systems

- Devices are cumbersome and cosmetically unattractive.
- The initial and maintenance costs of equipment are high and not fully reimbursed.
- Devices may possess poor response times and delays in valve opening or closing.
- Clinical studies of efficacy have been mostly short-term in scope.
- The catheters and sensors may frequently malfunction because of either sensor dislodgment or plugging or changes in breathing problems.

From O'Donohue WJ: Oxygen conserving devices, Respir Care Clin N Am 32:37, 1987.

▶ VENTILATORY SUPPORT IN ALTERNATIVE SETTINGS

Providing successful ventilatory support outside the acute care hospital requires careful patient selection and good discharge planning.[34] Key factors include an interdisciplinary team approach, effective caregiver and family education, thorough assessment and preparation of the environment, and careful selection of needed equipment and supplies. Properly planned ventilatory support delivered in alternative settings can provide major benefits for both patient and family, with substantial savings in healthcare costs.[35]

Patient Selection

Most patients needing ventilatory support outside the acute care hospital fall into one of the following three broad categories:[36]

1. Patients unable to maintain adequate ventilation over prolonged periods (noninvasive nocturnal or intermittent use in particular)
2. Patients requiring continuous mechanical ventilation for long-term survival
3. Patients who are terminally ill with short life expectancies

Table 49-5 provides more detailed profiles of these patient groups. In addition to adults, a growing number of ventilator-assisted children are being managed in alternative settings. The same basic principles of discharge planning and patient care for adult patients should be followed for ventilator-assisted children.[37]

Regardless of diagnosis, patients being considered for ventilatory support in alternative settings must be medically and psychologically stable. In regard to assessing patient stability, Box 49-6 outlines the criteria developed by the American College of Chest Physicians (ACCP).[38]

Settings and Approaches

The most common setting for ventilatory support outside the acute care is the home. Additional sites include subacute care and long-term care facilities, including specialized long-term units designed specifically for ventilator patients.[38,39]

Table 49-5 ▶▶ Profiles of Patient Groups Requiring Ventilatory Support in Alternative Settings

Group Description	Diseases Involved
Profile 1	
Mainly composed of neuromuscular and thoracic wall disorder; particular stage of disease process allows patient certain periods of spontaneous breathing time during day; generally requires only nocturnal mechanical support	Amyotrophic lateral sclerosis Multiple sclerosis Kyphoscoliosis and related chest wall deformities Diaphragmatic paralysis Myasthenia gravis
Profile 2	
Requires continuous mechanical ventilatory support associated with long-term survival rates	High spinal cord injuries Apneic encephalopathies Severe COPD Late-stage muscular dystrophy
Profile 3	
Usually returns home at request of patient and family; patient's condition is terminal, life expectancy is short, and patient and family wish to spend remaining time at home; patients usually pose management problems in the home because of their rapidly deteriorating conditions	Lung cancer End-stage COPD Cystic fibrosis

Box 49-6 • Criteria to Determine Patient Stability for Ventilatory Support in Alternative Settings

- Absence of severe dyspnea while on a ventilator
- Acceptable arterial blood gas results
- Inspired oxygen concentrations that are relatively low
- Psychological stability
- Evidence of developmental progress (for pediatric/adolescent candidates)
- Absence of life-limiting cardiac dysfunction and arrhythmias
- If possible, no PEEP or if needed, PEEP should not exceed 10 cm H_2O
- Ability to clear airway secretions either by cough or suction
- A tracheostomy tube as opposed to an endotracheal tube
- No readmissions expected for more than 1 month

From O'Donohue WJ et al: Long-term mechanical ventilation:guidelines for management in the home and at alternate community sites—report of the Ad Hoc Committee, Respiratory Care Section, American College of Chest Physicians, Chest 90(suppl):1S, 1986.

Based on individual evaluation of patient need, one of the following two major support approaches may be considered: (1) invasive or (2) noninvasive support. In alternative settings, invasive ventilatory support always involves application of positive pressure ventilation by tracheotomy. Noninvasive approaches include positive and negative pressure ventilation via an intact upper airway or abdominal displacement methods.[40,41]

Standards and Guidelines

Standards and guidelines for ventilatory support outside the acute care hospital are evolving. In the late 1980s, both the ACCP and the AARC developed and published recommendations for the care of ventilator-assisted individuals in the home and alternative care sites.[38,42] The original AARC standards appear in Box 49-7.

More recently, the AARC has developed a clinical practice guideline on long-term invasive mechanical ventilation in the home.[43] Excerpts appear on p. 1266.

Special Challenges in Providing Home Ventilatory Support

Postacute care institutions that provide ventilatory support differ from acute care facilities mainly in their level of technology support. The home setting not only lacks this support, but also must depend extensively on nontechnical, nonprofessional caregivers. For these reasons, providing ventilatory support in the home presents many special challenges.

Prerequisites

For home ventilatory support to be successful, several prerequisites must be met.[44] These include the following:

- Willingness of family to accept responsibility
- Adequacy of family and professional support
- Overall viability of the home care plan
- Stability of patient
- Adequacy of home setting

Box 49-7 • American Association for Respiratory Care Students for the Provision of Care to Ventilator-Assisted Patients in an Alternative Site

STANDARD I
The provision of care to a ventilator-assisted patient located in an alternative site shall be defined and guided by established written policies and procedures accepted by both the discharging institution and the alternative care site.

STANDARD II
The services provided to ventilator-assisted patients shall be dispensed in accordance with a prescription written by the physician responsible for the care of that particular patient.

STANDARD III
Participants shall be prepared for their responsibilities in the provision of services through appropriate training and education.

STANDARD IV
The ventilator-assisted patient shall be provided with safe and effective equipment appropriate for that patient's physiological needs.

STANDARD V
There shall be established recording and reporting mechanisms for the program.

STANDARD VI
The quality and appropriateness of care provided under the auspices of the program must be monitored and evaluated by the program's medical director and identified problems must be resolved.

From American Association for Respiratory Care: Standards for the provision of care to ventilator-assisted patient in alternative site, AARC Times 11:45, 1987.

In regard to the home setting, the same factors listed in Box 49-1 should be evaluated for patients being considered for home ventilatory support.

Planning

Successful home ventilatory support requires extensive planning, education, and follow-up by all members of the home care team. Basic steps in the discharge process for a ventilator-dependent patient include the following:

1. Family is consulted regarding feasibility.
2. Physician writes appropriate orders.
3. Discharge planner coordinates efforts of team members and discharge plan is formulated.
4. Physician and other team members discuss plan with family and/or caregivers.
5. Education and training are initiated and completed.
6. Patient and family are prepared for discharge.
7. Home layout is assessed with necessary changes made.
8. Equipment and supplies are readied.
9. Discharge planner meets with team and makes final preparations.
10. Patient is discharged (with trial period, if necessary).
11. Local power company is notified regarding the presence of life support equipment; appropriate backup power (battery or compressed gas source) is made available.
12. Ongoing and follow-up care provided by visiting nurse, RRT, and other healthcare professionals (as necessary).

Caregiver Education

To properly prepare patients, family, and other caregivers for home discharge, a comprehensive educational program must be undertaken and completed. Essential skills that must be taught include the following:[34]

- Simple patient assessment
- Airway management, including tracheostomy and stoma care, cuff care, suctioning, changing tubes/ties
- Chest physical therapy techniques, including percussion, vibration, coughing
- Medication administration, including oral and aerosol
- Patient movement and ambulation
- Equipment operation and maintenance
- Equipment troubleshooting
- Cleaning and disinfection
- Emergency procedures

Emergency situations that caregivers must be trained to recognize and properly deal with include:

- Ventilator or power failure
- Ventilator circuit problems
- Airway emergencies
- Cardiac arrest

All caregivers should successfully complete this educational process. The specific timeframe for this varies depending upon caregiver ability and availability for training sessions. Training generally requires a minimum of 1 to 2 weeks over which time several education sessions can take place and cover instruction, demonstration, caregiver practice, and evaluation. Ideally, the patient should be placed on the actual ventilator that

Long-Term Invasive Mechanical Ventilation in the Home

AARC Clinical Practice Guideline (Excerpts)*

➤ INDICATIONS

- Patients requiring invasive long-term ventilatory support have demonstrated:
  - An inability to be completely weaned from invasive ventilatory support or
  - A progression of disease etiology that requires increasing ventilatory support
- Conditions that meet these criteria may include but are not limited to:
  - Ventilatory muscle disorders
  - Alveolar hypoventilatory syndrome
  - Primary respiratory disorders
  - Obstructive diseases
  - Restrictive diseases
  - Cardiac disorders including congenital anomalies

➤ CONTRAINDICATIONS

Contraindications to long-term home mechanical ventilation include:

- An unstable condition that requires a level of care or resources not available in the home, as indicated by:
  - FIO_2 requirement >0.40
  - PEEP >10 cm H_2O
  - Need for continuous invasive monitoring (adults)
  - Lack of mature tracheostomy
- Patient's choice not to receive home mechanical ventilation
- Lack of an appropriate discharge plan
- Unsafe physical environment as determined by the patient's discharge planning team
  - Presence of fire, health, or safety hazards, including unsanitary conditions
  - Inadequate basic utilities (such as heat, air conditioning, electricity)
- Inadequate resources for care in the home:
  - Financial
  - Personnel (e.g., inadequate medical follow-up, inability of patient to care for self, inadequate respite care for caregivers, inadequate numbers of competence caregivers)

➤ PRECAUTIONS AND/OR POSSIBLE COMPLICATIONS

Deterioration or acute change in clinical status of patient. The following may cause death or require rehospitalization for acute treatment:

- *Medical*: Respiratory alkalosis, respiratory acidosis, hypoxemia, barotrauma, seizures, hemodynamic instability, airway complications, respiratory infection, bronchospasm, exacerbation of underlying disese, or natural course of the disease
- *Equipment-related*: failure of the ventilator, malfunction of equipment, inadequate warming and humidification of the inspired gases, inadvertent changes in ventilator settings, accidental disconnetion from ventilator, accidental decannulation
- *Psychosocial*: depression, anxiety, loss of resources—caregiver or financial, detrimental change in family structure or coping capacity

➤ ASSESSMENT OF NEED

Long-term invasive mechanical ventilation in the home is needed when one or more documentable indications exist in the absence of any contraindications. There must not be any need for higher level of services or frequent changes in the care plan. Further, it must be shown that the strategy will be cost effective and likely either to (1) sustain and extend or enhance the quality of life, (2) reduce morbidity, or (3) improve or sustain physical and psychological function.

➤ ASSESSMENT OF OUTCOME

At least the following aspects of patient management and condition should be evaluated periodically as long as the patient receives mechanical ventilation in the home:

- Implementation and adherence to the plan of care
- Quality of life

Long-Term Invasive Mechanical Ventilation in the Home—Cont'd

AARC Clinical Practice Guideline (Excerpts)*

- Patient satisfaction
- Resource utilization
- Growth and development in the pediatric patient
- Unanticipated morbidity, including need for higher level site of care
- Unanticipated mortality

➤ MONITORING

The frequency of monitoring should be determined by the ongoing individualized care plan and be based upon the patient's current medical condition. The ventilator settings, proper function of equipment, and the patient's physical condition should be monitored and verified: (1) with each initiation of invasive ventilation to the patient, including altering the source of ventilation, as from one ventilator or resuscitation bag to another ventilator; (2) with each ventilator setting change; (3) on a regular basis as specified by individualized plan of care.

All appropriately trained caregivers should follow the care plan and implement the monitoring that has been prescribed. These caregivers may operate, maintain and monitor all equipment, and perform all aspects of care required by the patient after having been trained and evaluate on their level of knowledge for that equipment and the patient's clinical response to each of the interventions.

Lay caregivers should monitor the following regularly:

- Patient's physical condition: respiratory rate, heart rate, color changes, chest excursion, diaphoresis, lethargy, blood pressure, body temperature
- Ventilator settings (frequency should be specified in the plan of care):
  - Peak pressures
  - Preset tidal volume
  - Frequency of ventilator breaths
  - Verification of F_{IO_2}
  - PEEP level (if applicable)
  - Appropriate humidification of inspired gases
  - Temperature of inspired gases (if applicable)
  - Heat and moisture exchanger function
- Equipment function (frequency should be specified in the plan of care):
  - Appropriate configuration of ventilator circuit
  - Alarm function
  - Cleanliness of filter(s)—according to manufacturer's recommendation
  - Internal and external battery power level(s)
  - Overall condition of all equipment
  - Self-inflating bag-valve–mask—cleanliness and function

A properly trained credentialed healthcare professional should perform a thorough, comprehensive assessment of the patient and the patient-ventilator system on a regular basis as prescribed by the plan of care. In addition to the above, the practitioner should implement, monitor, and assess results of other interventions as indicated by the clinical situation and anticipated in the care plan.

- Pulse oximetry—for patients requiring a change in F_{IO_2} or those with a suspected change in condition
- End-tidal CO_2—may be useful for establishing trends in CO_2 levels during weaning
- Specimen collection (and analysis as applicable) as prescribed by physician—including but not limited to sputum and blood work (e.g., arterial blood gas analysis and complete blood counts)
- Cardiorespiratory monitoring (electrocardiogram, heart-rate trending)
- Pulmonary function testing
- Ventilator settings
- Exhaled tidal volume
- Analysis of fraction of inspired oxygen

Properly trained and credentialed healthcare professionals are also responsible for maintaining interdisciplinary communication concerning the plan of care.

Properly trained and credentialed healthcare professionals should integrate the respiratory plan of care into the patient's total care plan. The plan of care should include:

- All aspects of patient's respiratory care
- Ongoing assessment and education of the caregivers involved

*For the complete guideline, see Respir Care 40:1313, 1995.

will be used in the home setting *before* discharge. In the early stages after discharge, patient follow-up by a RRT may need to occur every day. As patient and family become more familiar with the equipment and procedures, follow-up visitations can decrease to weekly or biweekly, as needed.[45,46]

Invasive Versus Noninvasive Ventilatory Support

Until recently, invasive positive pressure ventilation by tracheostomy was the de facto standard for long-term mechanical ventilation, especially for patients requiring 24-hour support. However, long-term tracheostomy is associated with many serious complications, including secretion retention, infection, and aspiration. In addition, a permanent tracheostomy poses significant communication problems between caregivers and patients. Moreover, because many long-term care facilities treat a tracheostomy as an open wound, patient placement at certain sites is prohibited.[47] Last, invasive ventilation by tracheostomy poses significant limits on the quality of life patients can experience.

For these reasons, noninvasive support is becoming increasingly popular. Noninvasive ventilatory support involves any method designed to augment alveolar ventilation without an endotracheal airway. Noninvasive positive pressure ventilation (NIPPV) is usually the first choice. Any individual requiring mechanical ventilation can be supported with NIPPV if:[47]

1. The patient is mentally competent, cooperative, and not using heavy sedation or narcotics.
2. Supplemental O_2 therapy is unnecessary or minimal.
3. SaO_2 can be maintained above 90% by aggressive airway clearance techniques.
4. Bulbar muscle function is adequate for swallowing without potentially dangerous aspiration.
5. No history exists of substance abuse or uncontrollable seizures.
6. Unassisted or manually assisted peak expiratory flows during coughing exceed 3 L/second.
7. No conditions are present that interfere with NIPPV interfaces (e.g., facial trauma, inadequate bite for mouthpiece, presence of nasogastric tube, or facial hair that can hamper airtight seal).

Patients who can benefit from NIPPV generally fall into one of two categories or types.[48] Type 1 patients have conditions in which cessation of ventilation could lead to imminent death. This category includes both acutely ill patients (asthma, acute exacerbation of COPD, pulmonary edema) and those requiring long-term, 24-hour support (some patients with quadriplegia, idiopathic hypoventilation syndrome). Type 2 patients have conditions in which NIPPV may offer clinical benefit, but cessation is not life-threatening. Type 2 patients generally require only intermittent support. Examples of patients in this category include those with chronic neuromuscular and chest wall diseases, such as muscular dystrophy and kyphoscoliosis. The application of long-term NIPPV for patients with obstructive disorders such as end-stage COPD or CF is less well documented, although some favorable results have been reported.[48]

Relative contraindications to NIPPV include severe upper airway dysfunction, copious secretions that cannot be cleared by spontaneous or assisted cough, or O_2 concentration requirements exceeding 40%.[48]

Once popular in alternative settings, negative pressure ventilation is now considered a second-line strategy for noninvasive ventilatory support. Compared to NIPPV, negative pressure ventilation is harder to apply, more cumbersome, and less well tolerated (because of poor breath synchronization). Moreover, negative pressure ventilation tends to limit patient mobility and can worsen upper airway obstruction in susceptible patients.

Nonetheless, negative pressure ventilation may be appropriate in those patients who are unable to use NIPPV or who have failed NIPPV trials.[41] Negative pressure ventilation may also be considered for patients who require frequent airway access for suctioning or those with severe nasal congestion.[47]

Equipment

Box 49-8 lists the essential equipment and supplies needed for ventilator-dependent patients in alternative settings.[34,36]

Selecting the Appropriate Ventilator

The choice of ventilator for a patient in an alternative care setting should be based on the patient's clinical need and the available support resources. In some cases, patient needs may dictate that more than one ventilator be provided.[43] A second back-up ventilator should be provided for patients who cannot maintain spontaneous ventilation for more than 4 consecutive hours; for patients living in an area where a replacement ventilator cannot be secured within 2 hours; and for patients whose care plan requires mechanical ventilation during mobility.

In general, ventilators chosen for care in alternative settings must be dependable and easy for caregivers to operate. If mobility is an essential element of the patient's care plan, the ventilator system selected should be portable.[43] For these reasons, electrically powered devices (that run on both AC and DC battery power) are the best choice for ventilatory support in alternative settings. If the patient is receiving ventilatory support in

Box 49-8 • Essential Equipment and Supplies Needed for Ventilator-Dependent Patients in Alternative Settings

EQUIPMENT
- Ventilator(s)
- Manual resuscitator (bag-valve-mask unit)
- Heated ventilator humidifier with thermostat or HME
- Monitoring/alarm devices (including remote where necessary)
- 12-volt battery and battery charger
- Air compressor
- Oxygen source
- Power strip/surge protector
- Suction machine with backup (manual or battery)
- Stethoscope/sphygmomanometer
- Oxygen analyzer
- Pulse oximeter
- Hospital bed with table
- Patient lift
- Bedside commode, urinal, or bedpan
- Wheelchair

SUPPLIES
- Oxygen
- Oxygen appliances
- Airway appliances (masks, mouthpieces, or tracheostomy tubes)
- Tracheostomy care kits
- Ventilator circuits
- Bacterial filters
- HMEs
- Connecting tubing (aerosol, oxygen, suction)
- Suction catheters
- Gloves
- Distilled water
- SVN/MDI with ventilator adapters
- **Cleaning/disinfection supplies:**
  - 10-cc syringe
  - 15-22 mm tubing adapter
  - Extra tracheostomy tubes including one a size smaller

a postacute care facility, emergency AC power should be available.

If invasive ventilation by tracheostomy is the selected approach, the best choice is a positive-pressure ventilator. The invasive route also requires a humidification system, preferably a servocontrolled heated humidifier with temperature probes and alarms. Tracheostomy patients may also use a heat-moisturizer exchanger (HME) during transport or to enhance their mobility.[43] For patients with intact upper airways, a device capable of NIPPV is the first choice, unless contraindicated (Box 49-9 lists the absolute contraindications against using NIPPV).[49] In patients with intact upper airways for whom NIPPV is contraindicated or unsuccessful, a negative pressure ventilator should be considered.

Box 49-9 • Absolute Contraindications Against Using NIPPV

- Need for immediate intubation
- Hemodynamic instability
- Uncooperative patient
- Facial burns or trauma
- Need for airway protection

Table 49-6 ▶▶ Essential, Recommended, and Optional Features of a Positive Pressure Ventilator for Use in an Alternative Care Setting

Feature	Necessity
Positive pressure tidal breaths	Essential
Mandatory rate	Essential
Flow or I:E or inspiratory time	Recommended*
Expiratory pressure (PEEP)	Optional
FIO_2 to 1.0	Optional
Patient spontaneous breath (e.g., CPAP, IMV)	Optional
Breath-triggering mechanism (flow or pressure sensors to initiate a ventilator breath)	Recommended*
Flow-timing interaction (e.g., pressure support)	Optional
Feedback control (e.g., mandatory minute ventilation)	Optional

*Essential if the patient has intact ventilatory drive and respiratory muscles or if the possibility of partial or complete ventilator independence is anticipated.

Positive-Pressure Ventilators

Table 49-6 lists the essential, recommended, and optional features needed on positive-pressure ventilators used in alternative care settings.[50] An essential feature is basic to safe and effective operation in most patient care settings. A recommended feature helps provide optimal patient management. An optional feature is possibly useful in limited situations but not needed for most patients.

As in the acute care setting, debate exists over the use of volume-cycled versus pressure-limited ventilators in alternative settings. Whereas volume-cycled ventilation has been the predominant mode of support in these settings, pressure-limited ventilation is gaining popularity for use in selected patients.

Figure 49-6 shows a common volume-cycled ventilator used in alternative settings, the Nellcor Puritan Bennett LP10 Plus. Like most of these devices, the LP10 is time- or patient-triggered, flow- or pressure-limited, and volume-cycled. As shown in Figure 49-7, these devices typically use an electric motor to power a rotary-drive piston, which generates a sine-wave flow

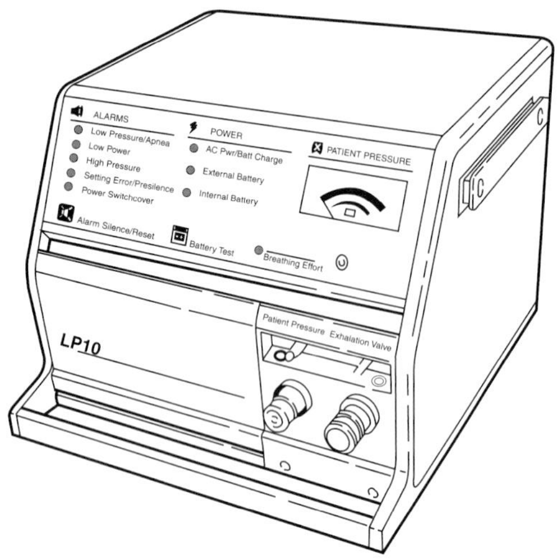

Figure 49-6
Nellcor Puritan Bennett LP10 Plus. *(Courtesy Nellcor Puritan Bennett, Minneapolis, Minn.)*

pattern. Depending on the manufacturer and model, these, devices can provide volumes from 50 to 3,000 mL, and rates from 1 to 69 breaths/minute.[51]

Most positive-pressure ventilators designed for post-acute care have an internal battery, which can provide up to an hour of use should AC line power fail. For longer periods of use away from AC line power, many of these devices can run for as long as 10 to 12 hours using a 12 V deep-cell (marine) battery.

Although intermittent mandatory ventilation (IMV)/ synchronized intermittent mandatory ventilation (SIMV) is now available on most portable volume-cycled ventilators, this mode should be avoided on patients with poor inspiratory muscle strength. This is because of the high imposed work of breathing that characterizes these systems.[52] A continuous flow H-valve circuit can provide IMV with minimal work of breathing, but this approach reduces portability.[43]

Recently, a host of compact ventilators with extensive capabilities, such as pressure support with SIMV, have been introduced for use in transport and at alternate sites of care. One such ventilator, the microprocessor controlled PulmoneticSystems LTV 1000, which is approximately the size and weight of a laptop computer and has many of the capabilities of much larger mechanical ventilators used in alternate sites and in acute care. This and other similar models offer ventilator-dependent patients the advantages of greater mobility and space conservation.[53]

Additionally, time- or patient-triggered, pressure-limited, flow-cycled devices (pressure support with timed backup) have been successfully applied in alternative settings.[54,55] Units such as the Respironics bi-level positive airway pressure (BiPAP) S/T-D (Figure 49-8), Healthdyne Quantum PSV, and Puritan-Bennett 335 are specifically designed to provide this type of support, usually noninvasively by nasal or oronasal masks.[56]

Table 49-7 compares the advantages and disadvantages of current generation portable volume-cycled and pressure-limited ventilators for use in alternative settings.[56,57]

Any existing positive-pressure ventilator can be used to provide NIPPV.[48,58] Most patients, especially those with COPD, prefer pressure-limited over volume-cycled ventilation. However, those with neuromuscular or neurological disorders often favor the consistent high inflations provided by volume ventilation, which enhance

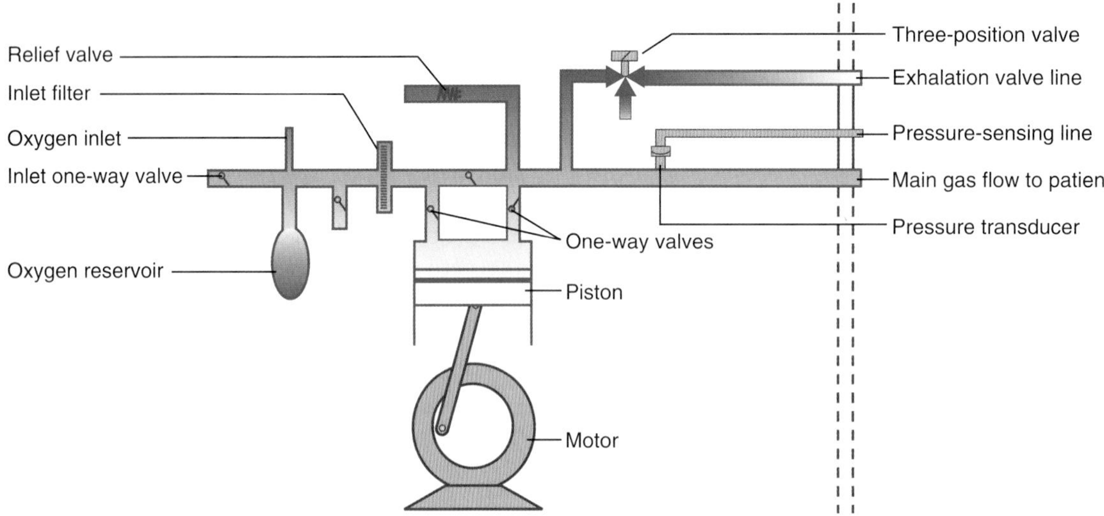

Figure 49-7
Functional diagram of Nellcor Puritan Bennett LP10 Plus. *(Modified from image courtesy Nellcor Puritan Bennett, Minneapolis, Minn.)*

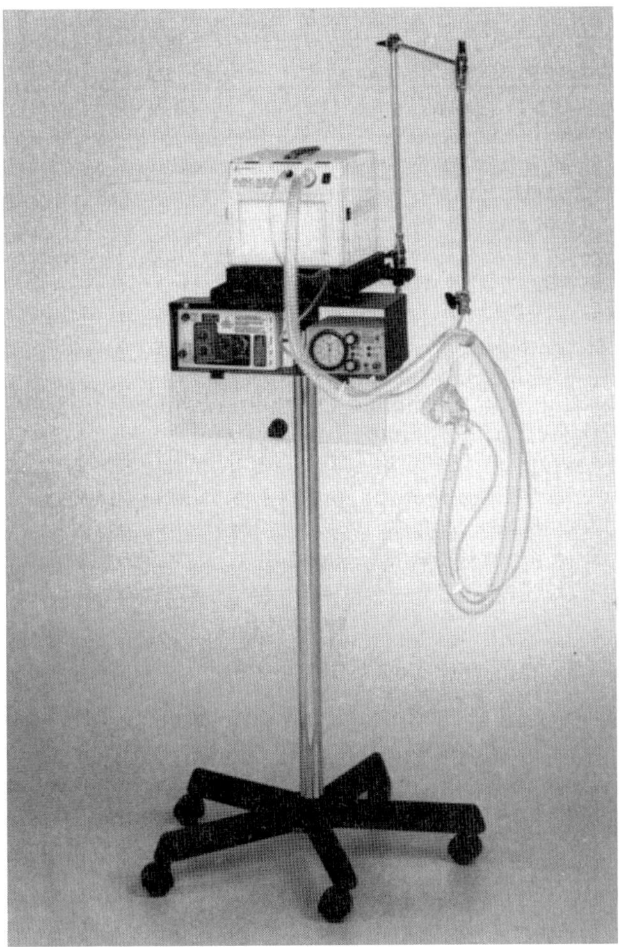

Figure 49-8
Respironics BiPAP S/T-D. *(Courtesy Respironics, Inc., Murrysville, Penn.)*

coughing and phonation. In addition, the alarm capabilities and internal battery backup provided with current portable volume ventilators make them the best choice for patients who cannot sustain any spontaneous breathing at all.[56]

The biggest challenge with NIPPV is not selecting the right ventilator, but getting a good, comfortable, leak-free interface. Available interfaces include oronasal (full) masks, nasal masks, and simple, flanged, or custom mouthpieces. For long-term use, some patients prefer alternating between devices. For example, the patient may prefer a simple mouthpiece for easy accessibility during the day, with a nasal mask providing leak-free support at night.[48] Table 49-8 summarizes some of the common problems associated with NIPPV interfaces and how to correct them.[59]

All positive pressure ventilators used in alternative settings must have an alarm to indicate loss of power (pneumatic and/or electrical). Portable volume-cycled ventilators should also incorporate a high pressure alarm/cycle override. For patients with conditions in which cessation of ventilation would cause death, a patient-disconnect alarm (low-pressure or low-exhaled volume) must be provided.[43,48] In some settings, a remote alarm and/or secondary disconnect alarm may be needed. A secondary alarm may be based on chest-wall impedance and cardiac activity, exhaled volume, end-tidal CO_2, or pulse oximetry with alarm capabilities.[43] For postacute care patients who require only intermittent NIPPV, a loss of power alarm is sufficient.[48]

Negative-Pressure Ventilators

With the increased popularity of NIPPV, negative-pressure ventilators are now a second-line choice for ventilatory support in postacute care settings.[41,60] Although much less popular than in the past, negative-pressure ventilators that are sometimes still used in postacute care include the iron lung (Figure 49-9); chest cuirass; and wrap, or "pneumosuit."

A typical iron lung has its own electrical motor and drive system to generate negative pressure. The chest cuirass (a rigid shell) and wrap-type systems (Nylon fabric surrounding a semicylindrical tent-like support) are simply enclosures that allow application of negative pressure to the thorax. Thus, these devices require a separate electrically powered negative-pressure generator. Examples of negative-pressure generators used to power cuirass or wrap-type systems include the Emerson 33-CRE, the Puritan-Bennett (Thompson) Maxivent, and the LifeCare NEV-100.[60]

Evaluation and Follow-up

Patient parameters to be monitored during positive-pressure ventilation are essentially the same as those assessed in the acute care setting, with an emphasis on simplicity.[61] For example, while the caregiver should be assessing the patient's vital signs, lung sounds, and sputum production on a daily basis, ABG analysis (by the RRT) may be conducted only monthly, or only when changes in the care plan are needed. Likewise, compliance and resistance measures will be performed only when other evidence indicates the need.

Routine follow-up visits by an RRT help ensure the success of patient management within the home. Equipment must be checked and cleaned as necessary. The patient's status should be carefully assessed and appropriate recommendations for change should be made to the primary or prescribing physician. Any prescribed respiratory therapy should be administered during the visit and all necessary supply items left with the patient's caregivers. After each visit, a report form must be completed and kept on record as part of the documentation process. Subsequent follow-up visits should take place regularly (weekly or biweekly) and whenever needed.

Table 49-7 ▶▶▶ Advantages and Disadvantages of Portable Volume-Cycled and Pressure-Limited Ventilators for Use in Alternative Settings

Approach	Advantages	Disadvantages
Volume-cycled ventilators	Can deliver higher volumes and at higher pressures as needed for patients with poor lung compliance Flows can be adjusted for comfort Consume less electricity, permitting greater mobility on batteries Quiet Lower mean pleural pressure for the same peak airway pressure Permit air stacking* Can be used to operate intermittent abdominal pressure ventilators Have alarms that can increase safety and help with nocturnal ventilation	Heavy weight Alarms can be annoying Some models are complicated Low and inaccurate FIO_2 High imposed spontaneous work of breathing (SIMV mode) Not responsive to changing flow demands
Pressure-limited ventilators	Very responsive to changing flow demands No annoying alarms Lightweight Less expensive Can compensate for small leaks	Not all can provide volumes needed for coughing/preventing atelectasis Do not allow air stacking* High initial flows can cause mouth drying/gagging and sleep arousal High power consumption (limits patient mobility) Discomfort and increased thoracic pressures from expiratory positive airway pressure (EPAP) Peak pressure provides less useful feedback than on volume ventilator Absence of alarms decreases safety Noisy Higher mean pleural pressure CO_2 rebeathing can be a problem EPAP can make eating difficult or hazardous for 24-hour users Low and inaccurate FIO_2 No internal batteries

* *Air stacking* refers to multiple, consecutive machine breaths designed to (1) maximize insufflation, (2) increase lung compliance, (3) raise voice volume, or (4) increase expiratory cough flows.

Table 49-8 ▶▶▶ Adverse Effects of NIPPV Interfaces and Possible Corrective Actions

Interface	Adverse Effect	Remedy
Nasal and oronasal masks	Discomfort	Proper fit, adjust strap tension, change mask type
	Nasal bridge redness, pressure sores, conjunctivitis	Reduce strap tension, use forehead spacer, try nasal "pillow," use artificial skin
	Acneiform rash	Cortisone cream, alternative (gel) mask
Oronasal masks	Impede speech and eating	Permit periodic removal if tolerated by the patient
	Claustrophobia	Choose clear masks with minimal bulk
	Aspiration	Exclude patients unable to protect airway; nasogastric tubes for patient with nausea and abdominal distention
Mouthpieces/lip seals	Interference with swallowing, salivary retention	Coaching, adaptation
	Pressure on lips, cheeks	Proper fit, strap adjustment
	Dental deformity	Orthodontic consultation
	Aerophagia	Simethicone, coaching
	Allergic reactions	Change prosthetic materials
	Nasal air leaking	Nose clips, pledgets
	Accidental disconnection	Appropriate alarms in ventilator-dependent patients

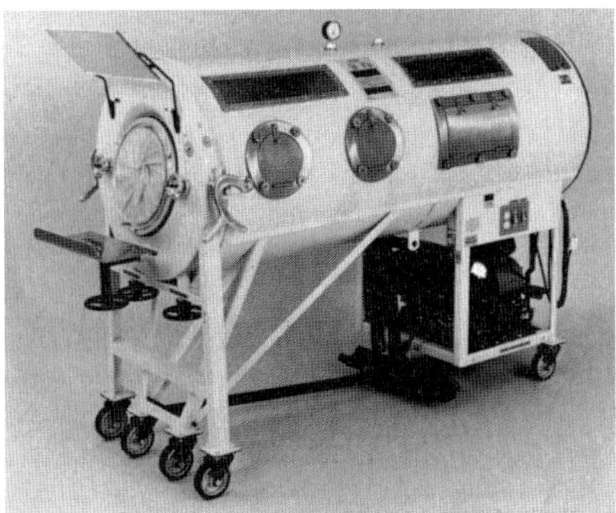

Figure 49-9
Emerson iron lung negative pressure ventilator. *(Courtesy J.H. Emerson Co., Cambridge, Mass.)*

▶ OTHER MODES OF POSTACUTE RESPIRATORY CARE

In addition to O_2 therapy and ventilatory support, other modes of respiratory care are now common in the postacute care setting. These may represent the primary therapy or may be used to supplement other modes of care. Included for discussion here are bland aerosol therapy, aerosol drug administration, airway care and clearance methods, nasal CPAP/BiPAP, and apnea monitoring.

Bland Aerosol Therapy

The delivery of bland aerosols has been a common postacute care practice for many years. According to the AARC's Clinical Practice Guideline, bland aerosol therapy includes the delivery of sterile water or various concentrations of saline solution in aerosol form.[62] The aerosol can be produced by either an ultrasonic or jet nebulizer. If using a jet nebulizer, a 50-psi air compressor is also required. Supplemental O_2 is provided by either a concentrator or liquid supply system.

Depending on patient condition and therapeutic objectives, bland aerosol therapy may be either continuous or intermittent. Historically, this approach has been used for patients with tracheostomies or those with difficulty clearing thick secretions, as in CF. Current knowledge, however, suggests that bland aerosol therapy alone has little effect on the properties of mucus or its clearance.[62] It may, however, be useful as an adjunct to airway clearance procedures in patients who regularly produce large amounts of sputum.[63]

The major problem is infection from contaminated equipment. To reduce the incidence of infection, equipment and patient delivery systems must be cleaned and changed every 24 hours. Disinfection procedures are discussed on p. 1280.

Aerosol Drug Administration

As in the acute care setting, the aerosol route is popular for drug administration to respiratory patients undergoing postacute care (see Chapter 33). Drug categories commonly administered by the aerosol route include β-adrenergic bronchodilators, anticholinergic agents, and antiinflammatory drugs. Recently, the aerosol drug route has also been used to treat upper airway disorders (such as laryngotracheobronchitis and rhinitis) and even to deliver insulin to patients with diabetes.[64]

Most pulmonary drug agents are available in either metered dose inhaler (MDI) or dry powder inhaler (DPI) form. Alternatively, the caregiver can use a small-volume nebulizer (SVN) powered by a low-output diaphragm compressor. Guidelines on selecting the best delivery method for aerosolized drugs are outline in the AARC clinical practice guideline.[65] In regard to home use of SVN/compressor systems, Medicare now limits reimbursement by (1) requiring a certificate of medical necessity and (2) capping rental costs. Coverage will only be provided if (1) the patient has tried but failed to effectively use an MDI with a spacer, (2) spirometry shows at least a 12% improvement in either FEV_1 or peak expiratory flow, and (3) evidence exists that the nebulizer can help prevent hospitalization.

Airway Care and Clearance Methods

Postacute care patients with tracheostomies require both daily stoma care and tracheobronchial suctioning. Tracheostomy care can be provided by any trained caregiver, but tube changes should only be performed by the patient's nurse, physician, or RRT.

In most postacute care settings, tracheobronchial suctioning is accomplished using a portable electrically powered suction pump with collection bottle and suction tubing. Caregivers should be taught proper suctioning methods before patient discharge from the acute care setting, with reinforcement and follow-up as needed. Because many of these systems measure pressure in inches of mercury (in Hg), care must be taken to teach proper adjustment according to patient age. Daily maintenance and cleaning are a must. In the postacute care setting, it is not uncommon for a single suction catheter to be used for 24 hours and then discarded. This measure helps control supply costs. To prevent bacterial growth, catheters are placed in a disinfecting solution such as hydrogen peroxide or 2.5% acetic acid between suctioning attempts.

RULE OF THUMB

For portable suction units calibrated in inches of mercury (in Hg), the following vacuum ranges are recommended (adjustment may be needed based on volume and viscosity of secretions):

Patient category	Vacuum setting (in Hg)
Infants	5 to 7
Children	7 to 12
Adults	12 to 15

For postacute care patients with intact upper airways who need help with secretion clearance, numerous methods are available. These include both patient-independent and caregiver-dependent techniques.[66] Patients can be taught to independently apply coughing, forced exhalation, active cycle of breathing, and autogenic drainage methods. Caregiver assistance will be required with traditional postural drainage, percussion and vibration, and directed or assisted cough. Additional assistance can be provided by mechanical devices such as the positive expiratory pressure (PEP) mask, the in-exsufflator, the flutter valve, the intrapulmonary percussive ventilator, and the high-frequency chest compression vest, which are routinely used for patients with CF. Application of any independent method or any technique performed by nonprofessional caregivers must involve good preliminary instruction and ongoing follow-up to confirm proper performance.

Nasal CPAP

Nasal CPAP has become an accepted form of home care used to treat the sleep apnea-hypopnea syndrome (SAHS). For Medicare reimbursement of home nasal CPAP equipment, the sleep apnea diagnosis must be confirmed by polysomnography. With proper application and patient compliance, CPAP can dramatically lessen or resolve the many problems associated with SAHS (morning headaches, daytime hypersomnolence, cognitive impairment). This, in turn, can enhance the patient's quality of life and may also lessen the incidence of more severe complications, such as systemic and pulmonary hypertension.[67]

Equipment

A typical nasal CPAP apparatus consists of a flow-generator or blower, one-way valve or reservoir bag, nasal mask, and PEEP/CPAP valve (Figure 49-10). Most systems provided manually adjustable pressures in the 2.5 to 30 cm H_2O range. Some newer units have a ramp feature that gradually raises the pressure to the prescribed level over a time interval. This helps some patients fall asleep and may increase therapy compliance.

A variation of nasal CPAP is BiPAP. Whereas CPAP uses a single pressure level, BiPAP uses two: (1) IPAP (inspiratory positive airway pressure) and (2) EPAP (expiratory positive airway pressure). In some patients, independent adjustment of IPAP and EPAP achieves the

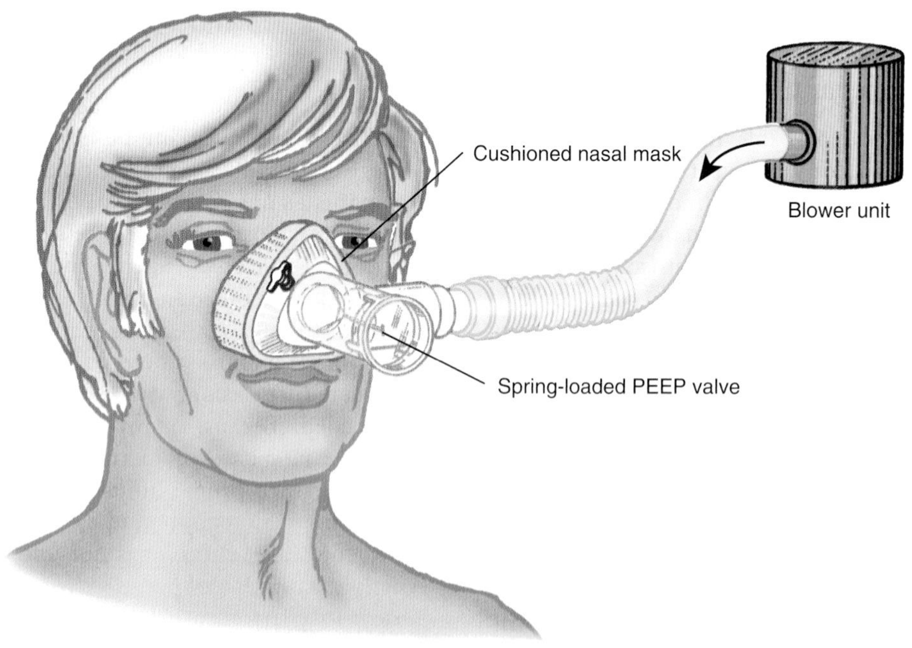

Figure 49-10
Simple nasal CPAP apparatus.

same results as conventional nasal CPAP, but at lower levels of expiratory pressure. This may aid in patient ventilation and reduce the adverse effects associated with nasal CPAP therapy and improve long-term therapeutic compliance.[68]

Determining the Proper CPAP Level

The proper CPAP level for a given patient is determined by one of several methods. The most common method is to conduct the sleep study, titrating different levels of CPAP. Observed changes in the apnea-hypopnea index (AHI) are then correlated with the various CPAP pressures. The prescribed level of CPAP is the lowest pressure at which apneic episodes are reduced to an acceptable frequency and duration.

Recently, CPAP units have been developed that automatically adjust the airway pressure in response to apnea, hypopnea, airflow limitation, or snoring. This auto-CPAP may result in lower effective pressures and better patient compliance, while eliminating the need for sleep-study titration.[69]

Alternatively, CPAP may be titrated against pulse oximetry data (Figure 49-11). In this case, the goal is to use the lowest CPAP pressure that will prevent arterial desaturation (SpO_2<90%).

Use and Maintenance

Once the proper CPAP pressure is determined, the patient is fitted for a mask and trained in the proper use, cleaning, and maintenance of the equipment. Typical patient instructions for self-administration of nasal CPAP therapy are provided in Box 49-10.

Problem-Solving and Troubleshooting

Patient problems associated with nasal CPAP include reversible upper airway obstruction, skin irritation, conjunctivitis, epistaxis, and nasal discomfort (dryness, burning, and congestion). Reversible upper airway obstruction (usually because of a flaccid epiglottis) is a rare problem that contraindicates nasal CPAP. Skin irritation is usually because of tight mask straps or a dirty mask. Persistent redness on the face or around the nose is the primary sign. Adjusting the straps (while maintaining a good mask seal) can help prevent irritation. In addition, the mask should be cleaned daily to remove dirt and facial oils. Even with proper care, most masks harden over time, causing problems with irritation and leaks. For this reason, nasal masks should be replaced at least every 3 months, or sooner if leakage or discomfort occur.

Conjunctivitis probably is the result of mask leakage around the bridge of the nose, which is easily corrected by ensuring a good seal in this area. Epistaxis and nasal discomfort are associated with drying of the nasal mucosa—a particular problem in cold, dry winter climates. Methods used to overcome excessive drying include in-line humidifiers, room vaporizers, HMEs, chin straps (to decrease loss of upper airway moisture), and saline nasal sprays.[70] Because none of these methods

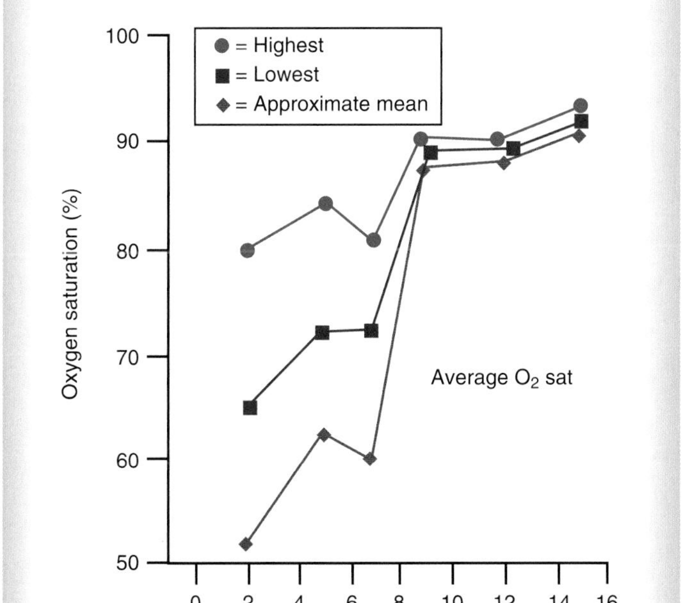

Figure 49-11

Titrated CPAP levels and corresponding oxygen saturations taken while the patient was asleep and using nasal CPAP. *(Modified from Sleeper GP, Strohl KP, Armeni MA: Nasal CPAP for at-home treatment of obstructive sleep apnea: a case report, Respir Care Clin N Am 30:90, 1985.)*

Box 49-10 • Typical Patient Instructions for Self-Administration of Nasal CPAP Therapy

EQUIPMENT PREPARATION

1. Place blower unit on a level surface (table or nightstand) close to where you sleep.
2. Make sure that the air exhaust and inlet vents are not obstructed.
3. Plug machine into a standard grounded (3 prong) electrical outlet.
4. Check air inlet filter to be sure it is in place and free of dust.
5. Connect one end of the tubing to the mask. Then place the mask over the nose.
6. Adjust strap tightness to seat mask firmly over nose.
7. Turn on the blower and verify a flow of air.
8. Ensure proper fit and adjustment of mask and headgear. Air should not be leaking out around the bridge of the nose into the eyes or from the mask to upper lip.
9. You are now ready to sleep with mask on.

IN THE MORNING

1. Remove mask by slipping strap off back of head (you may leave the head-strap connected between cleaning).
2. Turn off blower.
3. Wash the mask every morning with a mild detergent, then rinse with water. This keeps the mask soft and airtight.
4. Store the mask in plastic bag to keep free of dust and dirt.

WEEKLY

1. Wipe off the blower unit with a clean, damp cloth.
2. Wash the head-strap and circuit tubing.
3. Service the filters according to the instructions in your patient manual.

have proved satisfactory for all patients, selection should be based on individual patient acceptance and observed improvement in comfort.

The most common problem with the actual CPAP apparatus is an inability to reach or maintain the set pressure. This is usually because of either inadequate flow or system leaks. As part of their initial training, patients and caregivers should be taught how to recognize and correct these common problems. Box 49-11 outlines the procedures patients or caregivers can use to troubleshoot both inadequate flows and system leaks.

It is important to follow-up with these patients soon after they begin CPAP therapy to promptly resolve these complications. If left unresolved, these issues often discourage the patient and result in decreased compliance and a return of original symptoms.[71]

MINI CLINI

Troubleshooting Nasal Dryness With CPAP

PROBLEM

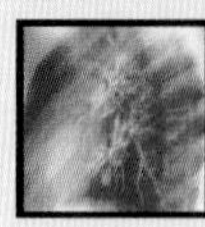

A 43-year-old obese man with documented obstructive sleep apnea has been advised by his attending physician that home CPAP therapy at night will be needed. The home care RRT makes an appointment with the patient to assess his tolerance to the CPAP unit. During the visit, the patient notes that he has been experiencing nasal discomfort. How can the RRT assist in problem-solving with this specific complaint and what are some of the other potential patient problems associated with CPAP therapy that the clinician should be alerted to?

SOLUTION

CPAP devices use some type of nasal mask with supporting headgear. Complaints of nasal discomfort are common and most likely because of the effects of dry airflow through the CPAP unit blower. However, other factors may aggravate the sensation of nasal irritation. For example, poor systemic hydration could worsen nasal mucosal drying. In addition, environmental humidity may be a factor. Cold, dry, winter climates can aggravate symptoms, as can dry, forced-air heating systems. In these cases, the RRT might recommend increasing oral intake of fluids (if no restrictions on fluid intake) or installation of a room or heating system humidifier. Alternatively, saline nasal spray may be used prn, or an in-line humidifier or HME might be tried.

Box 49-11 • Patient-Caregiver Instructions for Troubleshooting CPAP Equipment

INADEQUATE FLOW

1. Make sure that the unit is plugged into a working electrical outlet.
2. Confirm that the unit is turned on.
3. Make sure all connections are tight.
4. Confirm that airflow is coming from blower.
5. Make sure that the intake/exhaust vents are not obstructed.
6. Check the blower inlet filter to confirm that air can easily enter unit. If the filter appears obstructed, wash it.
7. If there is still no flow, contact your home care provider.

AIR LEAKS

1. Check mask fit, and readjust mask or headgear if necessary.
2. Contact your home care provider for a replacement mask if adjustments do not resolve the problem.

Apnea Monitoring

Sudden infant death syndrome (SIDS) is another disorder with which the RRT working in the postacute care setting may become involved. Hospitalized infants at risk for SIDS are frequently set up on apnea monitors. After extensive family instruction in both equipment use and resuscitation, some of these infants may be discharged to the home with this equipment.[72]

Most apnea monitors detect both respirations and heart rate and activate audio and visual alarms when preset high or low limits are reached. Follow-up visits by an RRT or nurse are usually frequent at first, but become less needed as the family becomes skilled with the equipment and monitoring routine. Apnea monitors are usually discontinued after an infant demonstrates negative pneumocardiograms. In general, apnea monitors are needed for a period of two to four months for many of these patients.[73]

▶ PATIENT ASSESSMENT AND DOCUMENTATION

Postacute care settings demand extensive patient assessment and documentation. These requirements are based on both stringent reimbursement criteria and the rehabilitation orientation characterizing these settings.

Institutional Subacute and Long-Term Care

In the institutions providing subacute or long-term care, the assessment and documentation process involves four key components: screening, treatment planning, ongoing assessment, and discharge (Figure 49-12).[17]

Screening

On admission to a postacute care facility, all patients with a respiratory-related admitting diagnosis should be screened by an RRT.[17] This screening is accomplished solely by chart review, without direct contact with the newly admitted patient or resident. During screening, the RRT reviews the pertinent respiratory diagnosis, onset and severity of symptoms (including the impressions of the resident's nurse), current radiograph results, pulmonary function tests, arterial blood gases, and other nonrespiratory treatment orders (such as physical therapy).

Should this review indicate the need for a more in-depth assessment, the RRT would then recommend a more complete evaluation. On receipt of the appropriate orders, the RRT would interview the resident and conduct a physical assessment, including inspection, palpation, auscultation, and percussion. Key observations would include description of breath sounds; rate, depth, and pattern of respirations; heart rate; signs of dyspnea; cough; sputum production; level of consciousness; and ability of the resident to understand and follow commands. Also noteworthy would be the resident's prior respiratory status, use of supplemental O_2, skin turgor, and medications. Where indicated, a pulse oximetry test is also performed during the evaluation.[17]

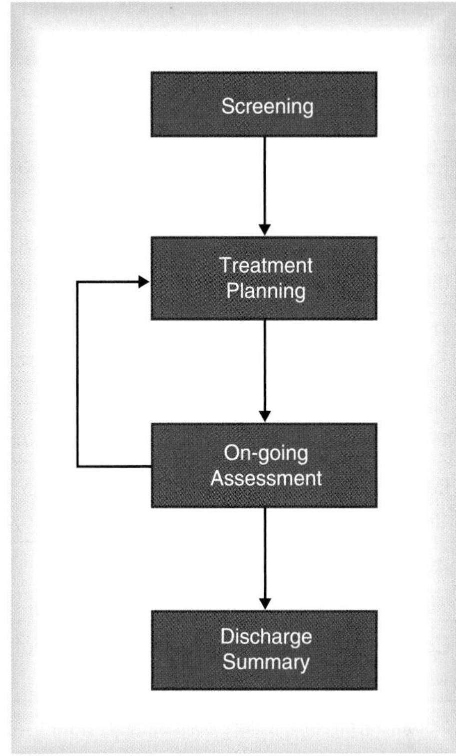

Figure 49-12
The assessment and documentation process in institutional subacute or long-term care.

Treatment Planning

Based on the information obtained, the RRT would then design a specific treatment plan for the resident. Short- and long-term goals to address the rehabilitation potential are also determined at that time. Figure 49-13 provides an example of a treatment plan for a resident admitted with a history of COPD and congestive heart failure (CHF), and pulmonary fibrosis.[17]

Ongoing Assessment

Once therapy has been initiated, the RRT uses several other tools to monitor a resident's progress. In addition to regular treatment documentation, the RRT must provide a weekly summary on each resident (Figure 49-14). The weekly summary provides a synopsis of residents' progress, including any changes in their respi-

Respiratory Care Evaluation		
1. Facility Name and Number Atlantic Nursing	2. HIC Number 532-34-7656A	3. Resident Number 33456932
4. Resident Sara Jones	5. Room Number 314B	6. Physician Dr. Parish
7. Diagnosis/Condition Bilateral pneumonia	8. ICD-9 Code 486	9. Date of Birth 11/20/10
10. Prior Respiratory Status Resident denies prior history of pulmonary problems		
11. Pertinent Medical/Surgical Information 7/14/03: admitted to facility for CVA; history of diabetes		
12. Respirations (depth, pattern, rhythm, rate) 24/min; symmetrical and unlabored		
13. Auscultation good airflow at apexes; decreased bilaterally; bronchial sounds at bases		
14. Cough (frequency, strength, productivity, pattern, etc.) weak and nonproductive		
15. Sputum (amount, color, consistency, odor) None		
16. Dyspnea (circle one)	(Class 1:) If SOB consistent with activity Class 2: If SOB climbing hills or stairs	Class 3: Can walk at own pace but not at normal pace without SOB Class 4: SOB walking 100 yards on level ground
17. Vital Signs (heart rate, pulse quality) 84/min regular but faint		
18. Cognition Answers appropriately; oriented ×3		
19. Diagnostic Tests (CXR, oximetry, lab, spirometry, etc.) 7/19/03: CXP – bilateral infiltrates at bases; small right effusion 7/20/03: SpO_2 = 87% air		
20. Additional Information (drugs, allergies, etc.) Lasix -40 mg/d resident C/O inspiratory pain-lower right side		
21. Rehabilitation Potential (for stated goals) Good for stated goals		
22. Short Term Goals 1. Correct hypoxemia with low flow O_2; 2. improve aeration with bronchodilator; 3. promote cough and mobilize secretions		
23. Long Term Goals 1. improve CXR; return patient to prior respiratory status		
24. Plan 1. add Dx pneumonia; 2. start nasal O_2 @ 2 L/min via concentrator; 3. albuterol via MDI/mask 2 puffs qid 7 days; 4. follow up on CXR to R/O pneumonia in 7 days		
25. Respiratory Therapist S. Mason, RRT		26. Date: 7/20/03

Figure 49-13

Example of a respiratory care treatment plan for a resident admitted to a subacute care facility with a history of COPD and CHF and pulmonary fibrosis. *(Modified from Rubenstein B, O'Nale S, Dalton M: Long-term care offers opportunities for RCPs, AARC Times 18:42, 1994.)*

Respiratory Care Weekly Summary

1. Facility Name and Number Atlantic Nursing	2. HIC Number 532-34-7656A	3. Resident Number 33456932
4. Resident Sara Jones	5. Room Number 314B	6. Physician Dr. Parish
7. Diagnosis/Condition Bilateral pneumonia	8. ICD-9 Code 486	9. Date of Birth 11/20/10
10. Date Therapy Initiated 7/20/03	11. Week of (Inclusive Dates) 7/20/03-7/27/03	

12. Current Respiratory Status

Resident is an alert 92 YO white female admitted to facility on 7/14/03 for CVA; history of diabetes but no history of pulmonary problems.

Resident was evaluated by RT on 7/20/03 and found to have decreased breath sounds bilaterally; bronchial sounds at bases with a weak and nonproductive cough, class 1 dyspnea, and an SpO_2 of 87% on room air. Resident C/O inspiratory pain-lower right side. A CXR on 7/19/03 indicated bilateral inflitrates at bases; small right effusion. Sputum culture positive for pseudomonas on 7/23/03.

On 7/20/03, resident started on nasal O_2 @ 2 L/min via concentrator and albuterol via MDI/mask 2 puffs qid 7 days. Resident placed on Cefazidime 1 gm IM q12h ×10 days on 7/23/03. SpO_2 is now 95% and cough productive of 5-10 mL mucopurulent sputum per treatment session. RT has instructed resident in use of deep breathing and coughing techniques.

RT will continue with present course of therapy at this time. Follow up CXR needed to assess progress. Care plan has been addressed with goals reflecting treatment plan.

13. Recommendations

1. Continue nasal O_2 @ 2 L/min
2. Continue albuterol via MDI/mask 2 puffs qid 7 days
3. Obtain follow up CXR 7/27/04

14. Respiratory Therapist S. Mason, RRT	15. Date of Summary: 7/27/03

Figure 49-14

Example of a weekly summary for a resident of a subacute care facility receiving respiratory care. *(Modified from Rubenstein B, O'Nale S, Dalton M: Long-term care offers opportunities for RCPs, AARC Times 18:42, 1994.)*

ratory status, results of any additional tests, explanation of any patient education, and recommendations for additional therapy. These summaries become part of the resident's permanent record, with a copy going to the attending physician.[17]

Discharge Summary

When a resident reaches his or her maximum potential, has attained all set goals, or is discharged, the RRT must complete a discharge summary. The discharge summary describes the complete course of respiratory therapy, including its success or failure.

Home Care

A home care plan must specify not only the types of care provided, but also a clear strategy for follow-up visitation. The individual making the follow-up visits could be the attending physician, the visiting nurse, a physical therapist, or an RRT. For patients receiving respiratory care at home, follow-up evaluation by a home care team member should occur at least monthly.[12] Some patients may require more frequent follow-up, especially those recently discharged or those requiring ventilatory support. Factors to consider when deciding on the frequency of home visits include the following:

- The patient's condition and therapeutic needs (objectives)
- The level of family or caregiver support available
- The type and complexity of home care equipment
- The overall home environment
- The ability of the patient to provide self-care

When a visit is made by an RRT, a number of functions must be performed. These include the following:

- Patient assessment (objective and subjective data), including pretreatment and posttreatment measurements of pulse, respiratory rate, blood pressure, and expiratory flows (FEV_1, PEFR)
- Patient's compliance with prescribed respiratory home care
- Equipment assessment (operation, cleanliness, and need for related supplies)
- Identification of any problem areas or patient concerns
- Statement related to patient goals and therapeutic plan

A standard written report, consistent with the care plan, should be completed by the visiting RRT. Copies should be sent to the patient's physician, the home care referral source, and any other member of the team requiring this information. The report should become part of the patient's medical record and should be referred to when following the patient's course and overall progress.

▶ EQUIPMENT DISINFECTION AND MAINTENANCE

With more and more patients receiving respiratory care outside the hospital, the danger of infection caused by contaminated articles and equipment has grown. To help minimize home-related infection, the American Respiratory Care Foundation (ARCF) has developed guidelines for disinfecting home respiratory care equipment.[74] Comparable guidelines for infection control in long-term care facilities have been published.[75] Emphasis in these guidelines is on the sources of infection, basic principles of infection control, patients at high risk, disinfection methods, equipment processing, and care of solutions and medications. These guidelines complement JCAHO accreditation standards, which devote a whole section just to surveillance, prevention, and control of infection.[15,16]

In regard to the principles of infection control, the ARCF recommends proper handwashing technique by all caregivers. In addition, visits to the patient by friends or relatives with respiratory infections are discouraged. In regard to medical equipment suppliers, the ARCF guidelines require that all permanent equipment (such as ventilator circuits, O_2 delivery equipment, and aerosol systems) be sterilized or receive high-level disinfection before being supplied to another patient. Disposable or single-patient use equipment must be used by one patient only. In terms of cleaning, the ARCF recommends that all equipment be completely disassembled and washed first in cool water to soften and loosen dried material. This initial wash should be followed by a soak in warm soapy water for several minutes, with equipment scrubbed as needed to remove any remaining organic material. Following this step, the equipment must be thoroughly rinsed to remove any residual soap and drained of excess water.

According to the ARCF guidelines, neither quaternary ammonium compounds (quats) or acetic acid should be used to disinfect home care equipment. Instead, high-level disinfection with glutaraldehyde is recommended. In our opinion, this guideline is too stringent for many home care settings. It fails to account for both individual differences in patient risk and the broader bactericidal activity exhibited by some new disinfectants. Issues such as infection risk, cost, and safety must be considered by both the provider and patient before selecting the best disinfectant.

In regard to using water for humidification or nebulization, the ARCF recommends that it be boiled, stored in the refrigerator, and discarded after 24 hours. The ARCF also recommends that manufacturers' guidelines for the proper handling of specific medications be strictly followed. In addition to these general guidelines, the ARCF provides detailed instructions for patients and caregivers on how to clean and disinfect selected respiratory care equipment. Box 49-12 provides an example of patient instructions for cleaning and disinfecting a ventilator circuit.[74]

Where appropriate and applicable, the clinical practice guidelines adopted by the AARC also contain an infection control section outlining accepted techniques for proper disposal and/or disinfection of contaminated equipment and supplies along with precautions for infection control.

▶ PALLIATIVE CARE

This chapter would not be complete without some discussion of palliative respiratory care in alternative settings. Though the primary goal of home care involves minimizing a patient's dependence on institutional care, an additional goal is to maximize the comfort and well-being of the terminally ill patient near the end of life.

The World Health Organization's definition of palliative care involves the control of pain and other symptoms such as dyspnea of terminally ill patients and maximizing the psychological, social, and spiritual well-being of family members and patients nearing the end of life.[76] Many terminally ill patients suffer from respiratory dysfunction directly or indirectly resulting from their terminal illness. Some of these patients choose to experience the remainder of their life at home. Hospice is a philosophy of care, which helps support the efforts of such patients by providing clinician coverage and equipment to these patients at home.[77]

Respiratory modalities, such as O_2 therapy and mechanical ventilation of aerosol drug administration, can be combined with other therapies, such as pain management, to increase patients' comfort and permit them to die at home with their family and friends nearby.

The RRT can help such patients and families by providing training on the proper use and maintenance of such equipment. The presence of the RRT can also be a supportive influence for such patients and their families. Though such cases can place a psychological strain on the RRT, maximizing the comfort of terminally ill patients can be rewarding, and such experiences rarely go unforgotten.

Box 49-12 • Patient and Caregiver Instructions for Cleaning and Disinfection of Ventilator Circuits

Before you start to clean and disinfect your equipment, be sure that:

- Your work area is clear and clean
- You have all of your supplies out and ready for use
- Your hands are clean
- Clean gloves are available in case you need them
- You have a clean apron or a clean old shirt to put over your clothes to protect them from splashes and spills of dirty water that may contain germs

CONSIDERATIONS

- The outer surface of the ventilator may be wiped off as necessary with a clean, damp (not wet) cloth. You do not need to worry about cleaning the inside of the machine, but it should be checked and necessary maintenance should be done according to manufacturer's recommendations by someone from the company that supplied the machine.
- The patient circuit must be taken completely apart, cleaned, and disinfected every 48 to 72 hours.

PROCEDURE

1. Take the circuit completely apart. Wipe the outer surface of the small tubes with a damp, clean cloth. Hang from line with clips or clothes pins. Take large-bore tubings, connectors, nebulizer or humidifier, and exhalation valve apart, wash first in cool water to soften and loosen dried material. Then soak in warm soapy water for several minutes. Scrub with brush to remove any phlegm or secretions or other material that should not be there. Rinse until all soap is gone. Drain off as much water as you can.
2. Place the parts in the disinfectant solution. Be certain that all of the inside and outside surfaces of the parts are covered with the disinfectant. Leave the parts in the disinfectant for at least 15 minutes or the manufacturer's recommended length of time. Check the clock or use a timer.
3. Be sure that your hands or gloves are clean. Rinse all of the parts thoroughly under running water.
4. Drain off as much water as you can and hang tubings to dry. Put small parts on a clean, dry surface.
5. When all parts are completely dry, put the exhalation valve and nebulizer back together, then put the circuit back together ready for use. Be sure that your hands are clean before you start to put the circuit back together. Store the circuit in a clean plastic bag.
6. It is best to have at least three complete ventilatory circuits, one in use, one being cleaned or drying, and one in reserve.

KEY POINTS

- More and more health services are being provided in postacute care settings (i.e., subacute, rehabilitation, and skilled nursing facilities and the home).
- Subacute care aims to restore the *whole* patient back to the highest level of function, ideally that of self care.
- Standards for subacute and home healthcare derive from federal and state laws and private-sector accreditation, mainly JCAHO.
- The acute and postacute care settings differ in regard to resource availability, supervision and work schedules, documentation and assessment, and professional/patient interaction.
- Effective discharge planning (1) guides the multidisciplinary team in transferring patients from acute care facilities to alternative sites of care and (2) ensures the safety and efficacy of the patient's continuing care.
- Whether in an institution or the home, caregivers must have all the competencies required to meet the patient's ventilatory and respiratory needs and provide adequate 24-hour coverage. The selected site also must meet basic safety standards and be suitable for managing the patient's specific condition.
- O_2 prescriptions for patients in alternative settings must be based on documented hypoxemia, as determined by either blood gas analysis or oximetry.
- In most alternative care sites, O_2 normally is supplied using either liquid O_2 systems or concentrators. Gaseous cylinders serve as backup supplies for portable use.
- Most postacute care patients needing O_2 use a nasal cannula; conserving devices such as the transtracheal catheter, reservoir cannula, and the demand-flow O_2 system can decrease O_2 use and costs and provide greater patient mobility.
- Because most problems with long-term O_2 therapy are "people" problems, caregivers should be allowed to operate and maintain O_2 delivery devices only after they have been instructed by credentialed RRTs and have demonstrated the appropriate skill level.
- Key factors needed for successful postacute ventilatory support include (1) careful patient selection, (2) effective discharge planning, (3) an interdisciplinary team approach, (4) effective caregiver and/or family education, (5) thorough assessment and preparation of the environment, and (6) careful selection of needed equipment and supplies.
- Patients being considered for ventilatory support in alternative settings must be medically and psychologically stable.
- Most postacute care patients requiring mechanical ventilation can be supported with noninvasive positive pressure ventilation if they are alert and cooperative, can maintain acceptable oxygenation without high F_{IO_2}, have intact airway reflexes and adequate clearance mechanisms, and can be fitted with an appropriate NIPPV interface.
- Positive pressure ventilators used in alternative settings should be electrically powered, dependable, easy to operate, and portable (run on both AC and DC power). Loss of power alarms are essential, high-pressure alarms are needed on volume-cycled ventilators, and patient-disconnect alarms must be provided for any patients who cannot breath on their own.
- Negative-pressure ventilators, such as the iron lung, chest cuirass, and "pneumosuit," are now a second-line choice for ventilatory support in postacute care settings.
- Bland aerosols may aid airway clearance in patients who produce large amounts of sputum; delivery is usually by an ultrasonic nebulizer or a jet nebulizer driven by an air compressor; supplemental O_2 is provided by either a concentrator or liquid supply system; infection control with these systems is a must.
- Postacute care patients with tracheostomies require both daily stoma care and tracheobronchial suctioning; tube changes should only be performed by a qualified health professional.
- Postacute care patients with intact upper airways may use either independent methods (such as coughing) or caregiver-assisted techniques (such as postural drainage, percussion, and vibration) to facilitate secretion removal.
- A typical nasal CPAP system consists of a blower, PEEP/CPAP valve and nasal mask; some units can raise pressure to the

KEY POINTS—cont'd

prescribed level over time (ramping); others can autoadjust the CPAP level in response to apnea, hypopnea, airflow limitation, or snoring.

- The proper CPAP level can be determined by polysomnography, continuous monitoring of hemoglobin saturation, or by an autoCPAP system.
- The most common problem with nasal CPAP systems is an inability to reach or maintain the set pressure, usually because of either inadequate flow or system leaks.
- In the institutions providing subacute or long-term care, the assessment and documentation process involves four key components: screening, treatment planning, ongoing assessment, and discharge.
- Proper caregiver handwashing, limiting visits by those with respiratory infections, providing sterile or disposable clean equipment, and proper equipment processing are the keys to infection control in the postacute care setting.
- Providing palliative care to keep terminally ill patients as comfortable as possible is an important aspect of respiratory care in alternative sites.

References

1. U.S. Department of Health and Human Services: Basic statistics about home care, 1-25, 2000.
2. Sin DD, Tu JV: Are elderly patients with airway obstruction being prematurely discharged?, Am J of Respir Crit Care 161:1513, 2000.
3. Ramsey SD: Suboptimal medical therapy in COPD, Chest 117:33, 2000.
4. American Association for Respiratory Care: Clinical practice guideline: discharge planning for the respiratory care patient, Respir Care Clin N Am 40:1308, 1995.
5. U. S. Department of Health and Huuan Services: Medicare fact sheet, 1-4, 1999.
6. Bunch D: Mercy Medical subacute unit gets BBRA '99 exception, AARC Times, 24:54, 2000.
7. Bunch D: Home health agency PPS overview: how the new system could affect RRTs in home health, AARC Times 24:28, 2000.
8. Muse and associates: A comparison of Medicare nursing home residents who receive services from a respiratory therapist with those who do not: executive summary, 1999.
9. Bunch D: Managed care drives healthcare systems to integrate services outside of hospitals, AARC Times 20:22, 1996.
10. National Subacute Care Association: New definition of subacute care: NSCA redefines what subacute care really is, NSCA News 2:22-26, 1996.
11. Bunch D: Subacute care: The clinical approach, AARC Times, 21:36, 1997.
12. American Association for Respiratory Care: Home respiratory care services. An official position statement by the American Association for Respiratory Care, 2000.
13. Dunne PJ: The demographics and economics of long-term oxygen therapy, Respir Care Clin N Am 45:223, 2000.
14. Fields AI et al: Home care cost-effectiveness for respiratory technology-dependent children, Am J Dis Child 145:729, 1991.
15. Joint Commission on Accreditation of Healthcare Organizations:1996 Comprehensive Accreditation Manual for Long Term Care, Oakbrook Terrace, Ill, 1996, JCAHO.
16. Joint Commission on Accreditation of Healthcare Organizations:1997-1998 Comprehensive Accreditation Manual for Home Care, Oakbrook Terrace, Ill, 1996, JCAHO.
17. Rubenstein B, O'Nale S, Dalton M: Long-term care offers opportunities for RCPs, AARC Times 18:42, 1994.
18. Gilmartin ME: Transition from the intensive care unit to home: patient selection and discharge planning, Respir Care Clin N Am 39:456, 1994.
19. American Association for Respiratory Care: Clinical practice guideline: discharge planning for the respiratory care patient, Respir Care Clin N Am 40:1308, 1995.
20. Anthonisen NR: Home oxygen therapy in chronic obstructive pulmonary disease, Clin Chest Med 7:673, 1986.
21. Baudouin SV et al: Long-term domiciliary oxygen treatment for chronic respiratory failure reviewed, Thorax 45:195, 1990.
22. Christopher KL: Long-term oxygen therapy. In Pierson DJ, Kacmarek RM, editors: Foundations of respiratory care, New York, 1992, Churchill-Livingstone.
23. Tiep BL: Long-term home oxygen therapy, Clin Chest Med 11:505, 1990.
24. American Association for Respiratory Care: Clinical practice guideline: oxygen therapy in the home or extended care facility, Respir Care Clin N Am 37:918, 1992.
25. O'Donohue WJ: Home oxygen therapy. Why, when and how to write a proper prescription, Postgrad Med 87:59, 1990.
26. Conference Report: New problems in supply, reimbursement and certification of medical necessity for long-term oxygen therapy, Am Rev Respir Dis 142:721, 1990.
27. Kacmarek RM: Delivery systems for long-term oxygen therapy, Respir Care Clin N Am 45:84, 2000.
28. Lucas J: Selecting the optimum oxygen system. In Lucas J et al, editors: Home respiratory care, Norwalk, Conn., 1988, Appleton & Lange.
29. Conference Report: Problems in prescribing and supplying oxygen for Medicare patients, Am Rev Respir Dis 134:340, 1986.

30. Spofford B et al: Transtracheal oxygen therapy: a guide for the respiratory therapist, Respir Care Clin N Am 32:345, 1987.
31. Franco MA et al: Pulse dose oxygen delivery system, Respir Care Clin N Am 29:1034, 1985.
32. O'Donohue WJ: The future of home oxygen therapy, Respir Care Clin N Am 33:1125, 1988.
33. O'Donohue WJ: Oxygen conserving devices, Respir Care Clin N Am 32: 37, 1987.
34. Gilmartin ME: Transition from the intensive care unit to home: patient selection and discharge planning, Respir Care Clin N Am 39:456, 1994.
35. Bach JR et al: The ventilator-assisted individual: cost analysis of institutionalization vs. rehabilitation and in-home management, Chest 101:26, 1992.
36. Lucas J: Ventilator care at home. In Lucas J et al editors: Home respiratory care, Norwalk, Conn., 1988, Appleton & Lange.
37. Eigen H, Zander J: Home mechanical ventilation of pediatric patients: American Thoracic Society, Am Rev Respir Dis 141:258, 1990.
38. O'Donohue WJ et al: Long-term mechanical ventilation: guidelines for management in the home and at alternate community sites. Report of the Ad Hoc Committee, Respiratory Care Section, American College of Chest Physicians, Chest 90 (suppl):1S, 1986.
39. Baldwin DK: Long-term ventilator-dependent care in nursing homes, Geriatr Nurs 17:20, 1996.
40. Hill NS, Bach JR, editors: Noninvasive mechanical ventilation, Respir Care Clin N Am 2:161, 1996.
41. Hill NS: Use of negative pressure ventilation, rocking beds, and pneumobelts, Respir Care Clin N Am 39:532,1994.
42. American Association for Respiratory Care: Standards for the provision of care to ventilator-assisted patients in an alternative site, AARC Times 11:45, 1987.
43. American Association for Respiratory Care: Clinical practice guideline: long-term invasive mechanical ventilation in the home, Respir Care Clin N Am 40:1313, 1995.
44. Pierson DJ, George RB: Mechanical ventilation in the home: possibilities and prerequisites, Respir Care Clin N Am 31:266, 1986.
45. Smith CE et al: Adaptation in families with a member requiring mechanical ventilation at home, Heart Lung 20:349, 1991.
46. Thomas VM et al: Caring for the person receiving ventilatory support at home: caregivers' needs and involvement, Heart Lung 21:180, 1992.
47. Bach JR, Saporito LR: Indications and criteria for decannulation and transition from invasive to noninvasive long-term ventilatory support, Respir Care Clin N Am 39:515, 1994.
48. American Association for Respiratory Care and American Respiratory Care Foundation: Consensus statement—noninvasive positive pressure ventilation, Respir Care Clin N Am 2:364, 1997.
49. Wunderink RG, Hill NS: Continuous and periodic application of noninvasive ventilation in respiratory failure, Respir Care Clin N Am 42:394, 1997.
50. American Association for Respiratory Care: Consensus statement on the essentials of mechanical ventilators—1992, Respir Care Clin N Am 37:1000, 1992.
51. Kacmarek RM, Spearman CB: Equipment used for ventilatory support in the home, Respir Care Clin N Am 31:310, 1986.
52. Kacmarek RM et al: Imposed work of breathing during synchronous intermittent mandatory ventilation provided by five home care ventilators, Respir Care Clin N Am 35:405, 1990.
53. Pulmonetics Systems, Inc.: LTV 900 Ventilator User Manual, 1999.
54. Waldhorn RE: Nocturnal nasal intermittent positive pressure ventilation with bi-level positive airway pressure (BiPAP) in respiratory failure, Chest 101:516, 1992.
55. Robertson PL, Roloff DW: Chronic respiratory failure in limb-girdle muscular dystrophy: successful long-term therapy with nasal bilevel positive airway pressure, Pediatr Neurol 10:328, 1994.
56. Drinkwine J, Kacmarek RM: Noninvasive positive pressure ventilation: equipment and techniques, Respir Care Clin N Am 2:183, 1996.
57. Bach JR: The prevention of ventilatory failure because of inadequate pump function, Respir Care Clin N Am 42:403, 1997.
58. Meecham-Jones DJ, Wedzicha JA: Comparison of pressure and volume preset nasal ventilator systems in stable chronic respiratory failure, Eur Respir J 6:1060, 1993.
59. Hill NS: Complications of noninvasive positive pressure ventilation, Respir Care Clin N Am 42:432, 1997.
60. Gilmartin ME: Body ventilators: equipment and techniques, Respir Care Clin N Am 2:195, 1996.
61. Gilmartin ME: Monitoring in the home and outpatient setting. In Kacmarek RM, Hess D, Stoller JK, editors: Monitoring in respiratory care, St Louis, 1993, Mosby.
62. American Association for Respiratory Care: Clinical practice guideline: bland aerosol administration, Respir Care Clin N Am 38:1196, 1993.
63. Conway JH et al: Humidification as an adjunct to chest physiotherapy in aiding tracheobronchial clearance in patients with bronchiectasis, Respir Med 86:109, 1992.
64. American Association for Respiratory Care: Clinical practice guideline: delivery of aerosols to the upper airway, Respir Care Clin N Am 39:803, 1994.
65. American Association for Respiratory Care: Clinical practice guideline: selection of aerosol delivery device, Respir Care Clin N Am 37:891, 1992.
66. Hardy KA, Anderson BD. Noninvasive clearance of airway secretions, Respir Care Clin N Am 2:323, 1996.
67. Kryger MH: Management of obstructive sleep apnea, Clin Chest Med 13:481, 1992.
68. Sanders MH, Kern N: Obstructive sleep apnea treated by independently adjusted inspiratory and expiratory positive airway pressures by nasal mask: physiological and clinical implications, Chest 98:317, 1990.
69. Series F: Auto-CPAP in the treatment of sleep apnea hypopnea syndrome, Sleep 19:S281, 1996.
70. Strumpf DA et al: Alternative methods of humidification during use of nasal CPAP, Respir Care Clin N Am 35:217, 1990.

71. Pepin JL et al: Effective compliance during the first 3 months of continuous positive airway pressure, Am J Respir Crit Care, 160:1124, 1999.
72. Orlowski JP: Infant apnea monitoring. In Lucas J et al, editors: Home respiratory care, Norwalk, Conn., 1988, Appleton & Lange.
73. Sivan TR: Duration of home monitoring for infants discharged with apnea of prematurity, Biol Neonate, 78:168, 2000.
74. American Respiratory Care Foundation: Guidelines for disinfection of respiratory care equipment used in the home, Respir Care Clin N Am 33:801, 1988.
75. Nicolle LE, Garibaldi RA: Infection control in long-term care facilities, Infect Control Hosp Epidemiol 16:348, 1995.
76. Fins JJ: Principles of palliative care: an overview, Resp Care Clin N Am 45:1320, 2000.
77. Curtis JR: Communicating with patients and their families about advance planning and end-of-life care, Resp Care Clin N Am 45:1385, 2000.

APPENDIX 1

Temperature Correction of Barometric Reading

Temperature (° C)	730 mm Hg	740	750	760	770	780
15.0	1.78	1.81	1.83	1.86	1.88	1.91
16.0	1.90	1.93	1.96	1.98	2.01	2.03
17.0	2.02	2.05	2.08	2.10	2.13	2.16
18.0	2.14	2.17	2.20	2.23	2.26	2.29
19.0	2.26	2.29	2.32	2.35	2.38	2.41
20.0	2.38	2.41	2.44	2.47	2.51	2.54
21.0	2.50	2.53	2.56	2.60	2.63	2.67
22.0	2.61	2.65	2.69	2.72	2.76	2.79
23.0	2.73	2.77	2.81	2.84	2.88	2.92
24.0	2.85	2.89	2.93	2.97	3.01	3.05
25.0	2.97	3.01	3.05	3.09	3.13	3.17
26.0	3.09	3.13	3.17	3.21	3.26	3.30
27.0	3.20	3.25	3.29	3.34	3.38	3.42
28.0	3.32	3.37	3.41	3.46	3.51	3.55
29.0	3.44	3.49	3.54	3.58	3.63	3.68
30.0	3.56	3.61	3.66	3.71	3.75	3.80
31.0	3.68	3.73	3.78	3.83	3.88	3.93
32.0	3.79	3.85	3.90	3.95	4.00	4.05
33.0	3.91	3.97	4.02	4.07	4.13	4.18
34.0	4.03	4.09	4.14	4.20	4.25	4.31
35.0	4.15	4.21	4.26	4.32	4.38	4.43

From U.S. Department of Commerce, Weather Bureau; Barometers and the measurements of atmospheric pressure, Washington, DC, 1941, U.S. Government Printing Office.

APPENDIX 2

Factors to Convert Gas Volumes from ATPS to STPD

Observed Pa	15°	16°	17°	18°	19°	20°	21°	22°	23°	24°	25°	26°	27°	28°	29°	30°	31°	32°
700	0.855	851	847	842	838	834	829	825	821	816	812	807	802	797	793	788	783	778
702	857	853	849	845	840	836	832	827	823	818	814	809	805	800	795	790	785	780
704	860	856	852	847	843	839	834	830	825	821	816	812	807	802	797	792	787	783
706	862	858	854	850	845	841	837	832	828	823	819	814	810	804	800	795	790	785
708	865	861	856	852	848	843	839	834	830	825	821	816	812	807	802	797	792	787
710	867	863	859	855	850	846	842	837	833	828	824	819	814	809	804	799	795	790
712	870	866	861	857	853	848	844	839	836	830	826	821	817	812	807	802	797	792
714	872	868	864	859	855	851	846	842	837	833	828	824	819	814	809	804	799	794
716	875	871	866	862	858	853	849	844	840	835	831	826	822	816	812	807	802	797
718	877	873	869	864	860	856	851	847	842	838	833	828	824	819	814	809	804	799
720	880	876	871	867	863	858	854	849	845	840	836	831	826	821	816	812	807	802
722	882	878	874	869	865	861	856	852	847	843	838	833	829	824	819	814	809	804
724	885	880	876	872	867	863	858	854	849	845	840	835	831	826	821	816	811	806
726	887	883	879	874	870	866	861	856	852	847	843	838	833	829	825	818	813	808
728	890	886	881	877	872	868	863	859	854	850	845	840	836	831	826	821	816	811
730	892	888	884	879	875	870	866	861	857	852	847	843	838	833	828	823	818	813
732	895	891	886	882	877	873	868	864	859	854	850	845	840	836	831	825	820	815
734	897	893	889	884	880	875	871	866	862	857	852	847	843	838	833	828	823	818
736	900	895	891	887	882	878	873	869	864	859	855	850	845	840	835	830	825	820
738	902	898	894	889	885	880	876	871	866	862	857	852	848	843	838	833	828	822
740	905	900	896	892	887	883	878	874	869	864	860	855	850	845	840	835	830	825
742	907	903	898	894	890	885	881	876	871	867	862	857	852	847	842	837	832	827
744	910	906	901	897	892	888	883	878	874	869	864	859	855	850	845	840	834	829
746	912	908	903	899	895	890	886	881	876	872	867	862	857	852	847	842	837	832
748	915	910	906	901	897	892	888	883	879	874	869	864	860	854	850	845	839	834
750	917	913	908	904	900	895	890	886	881	876	872	867	862	857	852	847	842	837
752	920	915	911	906	902	897	893	888	883	879	874	869	864	859	854	849	844	839
754	922	918	913	909	904	900	895	891	886	881	876	872	867	862	857	852	846	841
756	925	920	916	911	907	902	898	893	888	883	879	874	869	864	859	854	849	844
758	927	923	918	914	909	905	900	896	891	886	881	876	872	866	861	856	851	846
760	930	925	921	916	912	907	902	898	893	888	883	879	874	869	864	859	854	848
762	932	928	923	919	914	910	905	900	896	891	886	881	876	871	866	861	856	851
764	934	930	926	921	916	912	907	903	898	893	888	884	879	874	869	864	858	853
766	937	933	928	925	919	915	910	905	900	896	891	886	881	876	871	866	861	855
768	940	935	931	926	922	917	912	908	903	898	893	888	883	878	873	868	863	858
770	942	938	933	928	924	919	915	910	905	901	896	891	886	881	876	871	865	860
772	945	940	936	931	926	922	917	912	908	903	898	893	888	883	878	873	868	862
774	947	943	938	933	929	924	920	915	910	905	901	896	891	886	880	875	870	865
776	950	945	941	936	931	927	922	917	912	908	903	898	893	888	883	878	872	867
778	952	948	943	938	934	929	924	920	915	910	905	900	895	890	885	880	875	869
780	955	950	945	941	936	932	927	922	917	912	908	903	898	892	887	882	877	872

$$\text{Factor} = \frac{[PB_{abs} \text{ corrected for } t_{amb} - P_{H_2O}) \text{ at } t_{amb}] \times 0.359}{[t_{amb} + 273]}$$

APPENDIX 3

Factors to Convert Gas Volumes From STPD to BTPS at Given Barometric Pressures

Pressure	Factor	Pressure	Factor
740	1.245	760	1.211
742	1.241	762	1.208
744	1.238	764	1.203
746	1.235	766	1.200
748	1.232	768	1.196
750	1.227	770	1.193
752	1.224	772	1.190
754	1.221	774	1.188
756	1.217	776	1.183
758	1.214	778	1.181

$$\text{Factor} = \frac{863}{[P_{B_{amb}} - 47]}$$

APPENDIX 4

Table of Normal Values*

Test	Normal Value/Range*
Vital Signs	
Temperature	
Oral	97.0°-99.5° F (36.5°-37.5° C)
Axillary	96.7°-98.5° F (35.9°-36.9° C)
Rectal/ear	98.7°-100.5° F (37.1°-38.1° C)
Pulse	
Newborn	90-170/min
1 year old	80-160/min
Preschool	80-120/min
10 year old	70-110/min
Adult	60-100/min
Respirations	
Newborn	35-45/min (70 with stimulus)
1 year old	25-35/min
Preschool	20-25/min
10 year old	15-20/min
Adult	12-20/min
Blood Pressure (mean systolic/diastolic mm Hg)	
<1 month old (3000 g)	80/46
3-6 years	94/52
6-10 years	98/62
11-13 years	106/66
14-19 years	108/64 (girls) 116/68 (boys)
20+ years	120/80
Blood Gases and Related Parameters	
Arterial Blood Gases	
pH	7.35-7.45
$Paco_2$	35-45 mm Hg
HCO_3	22-26 mEq/L
BE	±2 mEq/L
Pao_2	80-100 mm Hg
Sao_2	93%-97%
COHb	<3%
Mixed Venous Blood Gases (Hb = 15 gm/dL)	
$C\bar{v}O_2$	12-15 mL/dL
$P\bar{v}O_2$	35-40 torr
$S\bar{v}O_2$	70%-75%
Oxygenation Parameters	
$P(A - a)o_2$ (A – a gradient)	25-65 mm Hg (100% O_2)
$Pao_2 \div PAO_2$ (a/A ratio)	>0.74
$Pao_2 \div FIO_2$ (P/F ratio)	>200
$\dot{Q}s \div \dot{Q}t$ (percent shunt)	<5%
$C(a - \bar{v})O_2$	4-6 mL/dL
Ventilation Parameters	
$\dot{V}E$	5-10 L/min
$PtcCO_2$	35-45 torr; normal pH
$P_{ET}CO_2$	35-43 torr; 4.6%-5.6%
VDS/VT	0.25-0.40
Hematology	
Red blood cells	M 4.6-6.2 × 10^6/mm^3 F 4.2-5.4 × 10^6/mm^3
Reticulocytes	0.5%-1.5%
Hemoglobin	M 13.5-16.5 g/dL F 12.0-15.0 g/dL
Hematocrit	M 42%-54% F 38%-47%

Table of Normal Values*—cont'd

Test	Normal Value/Range*
White Blood Cells	4500-11,500/mm^3
Neutrophils	40%-75%
Eosinophils	0%-6%
Basophils	0%-1%
Lymphocytes	20%-45%
Monocytes	2%-10%
Platelets	150,000-400,000/mm^3
Prothrombin time (PT)	12-14 sec
Partial Thromboplastin Time (PTT)	25-37 sec
Clinical Chemistry	
Acid phosphatase (ACP)	0.11-0.60 U/L
Alanine aminotransferase (ALT; SGPT)	5-35 U/L
Albumin	3.5-5.0 g/dL
Alkaline phosphatase (ALP)	30-85 ImU/mL
Alpha$_1$-antitrypsin	>250 mg/dL
Ammonia	15-110 µg/dL
Amylase	25-125 U/L
Aspartate aminotransferase (AST; SGOT)	10-40 U/L
Bilirubin (total)	Adult: 0.1-1.0 mg/dL Newborn: 1.0-12.0 mg/dL
Calcium	9.0-10.5 mg/dL (total) 4.5-5.6 mg/dL (ionized)
Chloride	98-105 mEq/L
Cholesterol	150-200 mg/dL
CO_2 content	23-30 mEq/L
Creatinine phosphokinase (CPK, CK)	55-170 U/L (SI)
Creatinine	0.5-1.2 mg/dL
Glucose (fasting blood sugar)	70-150 mg/dL
Lactic dehydrogenase (LDH)	45-90 U/L
Lypase (values method dependent)	0-417 U/L
Magnesium	1.8-2.4 mg/dL
Osmolarity	285-295 mOsm/kg H_2O
Phosphorus	3.0-4.5 mg/dL
Potassium	3.5-4.8 mEq/L
Sodium	137-147 mEq/L
Total protein	6.3-7.9 g/dL
Urea Nitrogen (BUN)	7-20 mg/dL
Pulmonary Function (70 Kg Male)	
V_T	500 mL (5-8 mL/kg)
IRV	3600 mL
ERV	1200 mL
RV	1200 mL
IC	3600 mL
FRC	2400 mL
TLC	6000 mL
FVC	4800 mL
FEV_1	4200 mL
FEV_1/FVC (%)	>70%
$FEF_{200-1200}$	8.5 L/sec
FEF_{25-75}	4.5 L/sec
PEFR	9.5 L/sec
$FEF_{25\%}$	9.0 L/sec
$FEF_{50\%}$	6.5 L/sec
$FEF_{75\%}$	3.5 L/sec
MVV	120-180 L/min
D_LCOsb	40 mL/min/mm Hg
D_LCOsb/V_A	6.6 mL/min/mm Hg/L
Beside Pulmonary Mechanics	
R_{aw}	5-15 cm H_2O/L/sec (ET tube)
C_{LT}	60-100 mL/cm H_2O

Table of Normal Values*—cont'd

Test	Normal Value/Range*
Beside Pulmonary Mechanics—cont'd	
Work (P × V)	0.03-0.05 kg • m/L
VC	65-75 mL/kg
NIF	Male: 100-150 (negative) cm H_2O Female: 115-65 (negative) cm H_2O
Hemodynamics	
Systolic blood pressure	100-140 mm Hg
Diastolic blood pressure	60-90 mm Hg
Mean arterial blood pressure	70-105 mm Hg
Central venous pressure	<6 mm Hg
Right artrial pressure	2-6 mm Hg
Right ventricular pressure, systolic	20-30 mm Hg
Right ventricular pressure, diastolic	2-6 mm Hg
Pulmonary artery pressure, systolic	20-30 mm Hg
Pulmonary artery pressure, diastolic	6-15 mm Hg
Pulmonary artery pressure, mean	10-20 mm Hg
Pulmonary artery wedge pressure, mean	4-12 mm Hg
Cardiac output	4.0-8.0 L/min
Cardiac index (CI)	2.5-4.0 L/min/m^2
Stroke volume (SV)	60-130 mL/beat
Stroke index (SI)	30-50 mL/beat/m^2
Left ventricular stroke work	50-62 gm • meters/m^2
Right ventricular stroke work	8-10 gm • meters/m^2
Systemic vascular resistance (SVR)[†]	15-20 mm Hg/L/min
Pulmonary vascular resistance (PVR)[†]	1.5-3.0 mm Hg/L/min

*Unless otherwise specified, all normals cited are for adults. Normal values and ranges vary by laboratory, norms used and/or reference text; values here are derived from multiple sources. Consult your lab and/or reference manual(s) for normals used in your institution or agency.

[†]To convert resistance measures to dynes • sec • cm^{-5} multiply by 80.

Glossary

A

12-minute walk usually a part of a pulmonary rehabilitation program, performed once a day for the duration of the program. The objective is for each patient to walk on a flat, smooth surface as far as possible during the 12 minutes, stopping as necessary and quantifying the total distance covered

a/A ratio the ratio of arterial-to-alveolar oxygen partial pressures (PaO_2/PAO_2); a measure of the efficiency of oxygen transfer across the lung

AARC abbreviation for the American Association for Respiratory Care, which is the primary voluntary professional association for respiratory care practitioners

abdominal paradox an abnormal breathing pattern seen as a sinking inward motion of the abdomen with each inspiratory effort; a sign of diaphragm fatigue

abduct to move a limb away from the body

absolute humidity the actual mass or content of water in a measured volume of air. It is usually expressed in grams per cubic meter or pounds

absorption atelectasis atelectasis due to the absorption of oxygen from obstructed or partially obstructed alveoli with high oxygen concentrations

A/C alternative abbreviation for assist/control ventilation; see assist/control

ACCP abbreviation for the American College of Chest Physicians

accreditation the process by which a private, nongovernmental agency recognizes that an institution or organization meets prespecified standards of quality; commonly applies to educational institutions or programs and healthcare agencies such as hospitals and nursing homes

acetazolamide a carbonic anhydrase inhibitor with diuretic properties; inhibits formation of carbonic acid in the proximal tubules of the kidneys, thereby promoting elimination of sodium, potassium, bicarbonate, and water; prolonged use can cause an alkaline diuresis leading to metabolic acidosis

acetylcholinesterase an enzyme that inactivates the neurotransmitter acetylcholine by hydrolyzing the substance to choline and acetate

acetylcysteine a mucolytic agent that lowers the viscosity of mucoid secretions by chemically disrupting the sulfhydryl bonds of mucopolysaccharides

acid compound that yields hydrogen ions (H^+) when dissolved in an aqueous solution

acidemia the state in which arterial blood is more acidic than normal (pH < 7.35)

acid-fast of or pertaining to a bacterial stain that does not decolorize easily when washed with an acid solution; also refers to certain bacteria (especially Mycobacteria), which retain red dyes after an acid wash

acidosis an abnormal physiological process resulting in an increase in the hydrogen ion concentration in the body; may be caused by either an excess accumulation of an acid or the loss of base

aciduria the presence of a greater-than-normal hydrogen ion concentration in the urine (normal urine pH ranges from 4.6 to 8.0, with an average value of 6.0)

acquired immune deficiency syndrome (AIDS) an immune disorder caused by infection with the human immunodeficiency virus (HIV); HIV directly attacks the T-lymphocytes and T-helper cells of the immune system, thereby compromising both cell-mediated and humoral (antibody) immunity

acromegaly a chronic metabolic condition characterized by a gradual, marked enlargement and elongation of the bones of the face, jaw, and extremities

acronym a word formed by the initial letters of each major part of a multiword term; for example, "PEEP" is the acronym for positive end-expiratory pressure

ACTH abbreviation for adrenocorticotropic hormone; a pituitary hormone that stimulates the adrenal cortex

actinomycosis a chronic, systemic fungal disease caused by infection with organisms of the genus Actinomyces; most commonly affects the skin but can involve the lungs and other organ systems

action potential a rapid reversal in the membrane potential occurring in certain nerve and muscle cells, caused by a change in the membrane permeability for sodium ions, which rapidly diffuse into the cell, thereby reversing its charge

active cycle of breathing (ACB) an airway clearance strategy consisting of repeated cycles of breathing control and thoracic expansion, followed by the forced expiratory technique

active transport the movement of molecules across membranes in a direction opposite that expected due to diffusion or osmotic pressure

activities of daily living (ADL) a quantifiable measure of an individual's ability to perform common tasks associated with independent functioning

acute lung injury (ALI) a condition characterized by alveolar flooding caused by an acute insult (for example, sepsis) and accompanied by dysfunction in other nonpulmonary organs. Acute lung injury is distinguished from ARDS by a lower lung injury score

acute respiratory distress syndrome (ARDS) a respiratory disorder characterized by respiratory insufficiency and hypoxemia. Triggers include gram-negative sepsis, oxygen toxicity, trauma, pneumonia, and systemic inflammatory responses

ACV alternative abbreviation for assist/control ventilation; see assist/control

Addison's disease a life-threatening condition caused by partial or complete failure of adrenocortical function, often resulting from autoimmune processes, infection (especially tubercular or fungal), neoplasm, or hemorrhage in the gland

adduct to move a limb toward the axis of the body

adenopathy any enlargement of a gland, especially a lymphatic gland

adenovirus any one of the 33 medium-sized viruses of the Adenoviridae family, pathogenic to humans, that cause conjunctivitis, upper respiratory infection, or gastrointestinal infection

ADH abbreviation for antidiuretic hormone; a hormone stored and released by the posterior lobe of the pituitary gland that stimulates the reabsorption of water by the renal tubular epithelial cells; due to mild vasopressor effects ADH is also called *vasopressin*

ADL abbreviation for activities of daily living; a quantifiable measure of an individual's ability to perform common tasks associated with independent functioning

adrenergic of or pertaining to the sympathetic nerve fibers of the autonomic nervous system that use epinephrine or epinephrine-like substances as neurotransmitters; any chemical or drug that mimics the effect of these neurotransmitters. Also called *sympathomimetic drug*; catecholamine

adrenocorticosteroid (also *corticosteroid*) a broad term referring to any of the steroid hormones produced by the adrenal cortex, including their synthetic equivalents; major categories include the glucocorticoids (for example, hydrocortisone), the mineralocorticoids (for example aldosterone), and the androgens

adult respiratory distress syndrome (ARDS) a pattern of clinical physiological and pathological features characterizing the lung's response to a variety of injuries and resulting in diffuse damage to the alveolar-capillary membrane

advanced cardiac life support (ACLS) emergency medical procedures beyond basic life support; includes intravenous fluid line establishment, possible defibrillation, drug administration, control of cardiac arrhythmias, and use of ventilation equipment. ACLS usually requires direct or indirect supervision by a physician

adventitious lung sounds abnormal lung sounds superimposed on the basic underlying breath sounds

aerobic living only in the presence of oxygen

aerobic exercise any physical activity that requires increased cardiac output and ventilation to meet the increased oxygen demands of the skeletal muscles

aerosol a suspension of solid or liquid particles in a gas

aerosol density (particulate) the number of aerosol particles per unit of carrier gas

aerosol density (weight) the actual weight of aerosol carried in a given volume of gas in milligrams of aerosol per liter (mg/L)

aerosol output the weight or mass of aerosol particles produced by a nebulizer per unit time or volume

AFB abbreviation for acid-fast bacillus, especially Mycobacteria that retain red dyes after an acid wash

affective domain the area of emotion, mood, or feeling

afferent carrying or conducting impulses toward the central nervous system; opposite of efferent

affidavit a written statement of facts given voluntarily under oath

affinity (in pharmacology) the tendency a drug has to combine with a receptor; refer to agonist

afterload the load against which an activated muscle must try to shorten; greater afterloads result in lower velocities

agammaglobulinemia a rare disorder characterized by the absence of the serum immunoglobulin, gamma globulin, associated with an increased susceptibility to infection

agglomeration the process of gathering together into a mass, as when many small aerosol particles come together to form a single large particle

aging (aerosol) the process in which aerosol particles change size due to evaporation or hygroscopic properties

agonist of or pertaining to a chemical substance or drug that has affinity and exerts a desired or expected effect (as opposed to an antagonist)

AHI abbreviation for the apnea-hypopnea index, used to quantify the severity of obstructive sleep apnea (OSA) and its response to treatment with CPAP

AIDS abbreviation for acquired immune deficiency syndrome

air stacking a technique used by some chronic neuromuscular disease patients to maximize lung insufflation, increase lung compliance, raise voice volume, or increase expiratory cough flows; performed by taking multiple consecutive breaths from a positive pressure ventilator

airborne precautions safeguards designed to reduce the risk of airborne transmission of infectious agents

airborne transmission transmission of infectious organisms via dissemination of the infectious agent in the air either by aerosol droplets, droplet nuclei, or dust particles

airway conductance a measure of the ease with which gas flows through the respiratory tract; abbreviated as G, conductance is the reciprocal of airway resistance, that is, G = flow/change in pressure

airway occlusion pressure ($P_{0.1}$) the inspiratory pressure generated 100 milliseconds after airway occlusion. $P_{0.1}$ is effort independent and is thought to be a good measure of central respiratory drive

airway pressure release ventilation (APRV) a form of pressure-controlled synchronized intermittent mandatory ventilation (SIMV)

airway resistance a measure of the impedance to ventilation caused by the movement of gas through the airways; abbreviated as Raw, airway resistance is computed as the change in pressure along a tube divided by the flow

alar nasi the wing-like lateral projections of the nose

algorithm a predetermined group of directions to solve a problem in a finite number of steps

ALI abbreviation for acute lung injury

alkalemia a combining form meaning a decreased hydrogen-ion concentration in the blood; as applied to arterial blood, denotes a pH>7.45

alkaloid any one of a large group of alkaline organic chemicals found in plants that exert powerful physiological activity; examples include morphine, cocaine, nicotine, and atropine

alkalosis an abnormal physiological process resulting in a decrease in the hydrogen ion concentration in the body; may be caused by either an excess accumulation of base or the loss of acid

allegation a written statement by a party to a suit concerning what the party expects to prove

allographic of or pertaining to a tissue graft or organ transplant between individuals of different genetic makeup

allopathic referring to the system of medicine whereby disease is treated by antagonistic therapy, such as an antibiotic to treat infection; more generally, the predominant system of medicine education in the United States

alpha-1 antitrypsin a chemical substance that inhibits the action of the proteolytic enzyme trypsin; associated with a form of destructive emphysema

alveolar air equation an equation used in computing the efficiency of oxygen transfer in clinical practice; $P_{AO_2} = F_{IO_2}(P_B - P_{H_2O}) - (Pa_{CO_2} \div R)$

alveolar-capillary membrane the tissue that separates air from blood in the lung; consists of alveolar epithelium, basement membrane, and capillary endothelium, along with their associated structures

alveolar macrophage a phagocytic cell commonly found in alveoli. These cells clear bacteria and other debris from the alveolar spaces

alveolarization the process of alveolar development from epithelial tissue

ambient of or referring to the surrounding environmental conditions

American Standard Safety System (ASSS) specifications adopted in the United States and Canada for threaded high-pressure connections between compressed gas cylinders and their attachments

American Society for Testing and Materials (ASTM) a nongovernmental agency that establishes performance standards for various equipment and materials

amino acid one of a large class of organic compounds containing both an amino (NH_2^-) and carboxyl ($COOH^-$) group

amniocentesis the process of direct sampling and quantitative assessment of the amniotic fluid

ampere the basic unit of electrical energy current; equivalent to the amount of electrons flowing when 1 volt of electromotive force is applied to a circuit with 1 ohm of resistance

amyotrophic lateral sclerosis (ALS) a degenerative disease of the motor neurons often characterized by atrophy of the muscles of the hands, forearms, and legs and eventually involving most of the body, including the muscles of respiration

anaerobe a microorganism that grows and lives in the complete or almost complete absence of oxygen

anaerobic of or referring to the ability to live without oxygen

anaerobic threshold during exercise, the point where increased levels of lactic acid result in an increased CO_2 production and minute ventilation; the RQ equals or exceeds 1.0, indicating that CO_2 production equals or exceeds O_2 consumption; at this point metabolism becomes anaerobic, thereby decreasing energy production and increasing muscle fatigue

analog a representation of numerical quantities by an output signal that measures continuous physical variables (such as voltage, length, pressure, flow) proportionate to the input

analog-to-digital converter (ADC) an instrument measuring an analog signal and converting it to digital form, thus enabling the data to be fed to a computer

analyte any substance that is measured; the term is usually applied to a component of blood or other body fluid

analyzer a mechanical device used to measure delivered oxygen concentrations. The three most common are the physical analyzer, the electrical analyzer, and the electrochemical analyzer

anaphylaxis an exaggerated hypersensitivity reaction to a previously encountered antigen

anastomosis a communication between two ducts or blood vessels that allows flow from one to another

anemia an abnormal condition characterized by a reduction in the number of circulating red blood cells or the amount of normal hemoglobin available to carry oxygen

anergy lack of activity; an immunodeficient condition characterized by a lack of or diminished reaction to an antigen or group of antigens. This state may be seen in advanced tuberculosis and other serious infections, acquired immunodeficiency syndrome, and some malignancies

anesthesiology the science of anesthesia; using drugs or chemical substances to cause partial or complete loss of sensation, particularly pain

anesthetic a drug or chemical substance that causes partial or complete loss of sensation

aneurysm a localized dilatation of the wall of a blood vessel, usually caused by atherosclerosis and hypertension, or, less frequently, by trauma, infection, or a congenital weakness in the vessel wall

angina pectoris a paroxysmal attack of severe chest pain associated with coronary insufficiency; commonly radiates from the heart to the shoulders and arms

angiography the x-ray visualization of the internal anatomy of the heart and blood vessels after the intravascular introduction of radiopaque contrast medium

angiotensin a blood polypeptide formed by the action of renin and angiotensinogen; the active form (angiotensin II) causes vasoconstriction and stimulates aldosterone secretion by the adrenal cortex

angle of Louis a slightly oblique angle where the manubrium articulates with the body of the sternum

anion an ion that migrates to the anode (positive electrode) in an electrolytic solution; a negative ion

anion gap the difference in concentration between the major serum electrolyte cations and anions; used to help diagnose the cause of metabolic acidosis

ankylosing spondylitis a chronic inflammatory disease of unknown origin, first affecting the spine and adjacent structures and commonly leading to eventual fusion (ankylosis) of the involved joints

anode the electrode to which anions migrate in an electrolytic reaction; the positive electrode

anomaly a broad term denoting any deviation from what is regarded as normal

anorexia lack or loss of appetite, resulting in the inability to eat

antagonist (in pharmacology) a drug that has affinity but produces no effect; an antagonist can be competitive (forms reversible bond with receptor) or noncompetitive (forms irreversible bond)

antecubital fossa the triangular area at the bend of the elbow; frequently used as the site for venipuncture and brachial artery blood sampling

anterior nares the opening to the nose

anterolateral situated in front and to one side or the other

anteroposterior from the front to the back of the body, commonly associated with the direction of the roentgenographic or x-ray beam (an "AP" exposure)

anthropometry the science of measuring the human body as to height, weight, and size of component parts, including skin folds, to study and compare the relative proportions under normal and abnormal conditions. Also called *anthropometric measurement*

antiarrhythmic of or pertaining to a procedure or substance that prevents, alleviates, or corrects an abnormal cardiac rhythm

antibiotic therapy treatment of infections with an antimicrobial agent, such as the penicillins

antibody a soluble protein synthesized by plasma cells in response to a specific antigen with which it interacts; in conjunction with the activation of complement, antibody production represents a key component of the humoral immunity

anticholinergic of or pertaining to a blockade of acetylcholine receptors that results in the inhibition of the transmission of parasympathetic nerve impulses

antigen a substance, usually a protein, that causes the formation of an antibody and reacts specifically with that antibody; see antibody

antiinflammatory of or pertaining to a substance or procedure that counteracts or reduces inflammation

antisepsis the destruction of pathogenic microorganisms existing in their vegetative state on living tissue

antiseptic tending to inhibit the growth and reproduction of microorganisms

antitoxin an antibody capable of neutralizing a specific toxin, for example, tetanus antitoxin

anxiolytic a drug or chemical agent capable of reducing anxiety, apprehension, or restlessness

aortic regurgitation backflow of blood from the aorta into the left ventricle; indicates an incompetent valve

aPEEP abbreviation for auto-PEEP (also iPEEP for intrinsic PEEP)

Apgar score the evaluation of an infant's physical condition, usually performed 1 minute and 5 minutes after birth, based on a rating of five factors that reflect the infant's ability to adjust to extrauterine life

aphagia a condition characterized by the loss of the ability to swallow as a result of organic or psychological causes

aphasia an abnormal neurological condition in which language function is defective or absent because of an injury to certain areas of the cerebral cortex

apical of or pertaining to the summit or apex

apices the uppermost portions of the lungs

apnea an absence of spontaneous breathing

apnea-hypopnea index (AHI) a measure of the incidence of apneic episodes used to quantify the severity of obstructive sleep apnea (OSA) and its response to treatment with CPAP

apnea of prematurity a disorder of preterm infants, probably of CNS origin, characterized by frequent apneic pauses lasting more than 20 seconds and often associated with cyanosis, pallor, hypotonia, or bradycardia

apneustic breathing a pattern of respirations characterized by a prolonged inspiratory phase followed by expiratory apnea

apneustic center a localized collection of neurons in the pons located at the level of the area vestibularis that moderates the rhythmic activity of the medullary respiratory centers

APRV abbreviation for airway pressure release ventilation; a form of pressure-controlled synchronized intermittent mandatory ventilation (SIMV)

ARCF abbreviation for the American Respiratory Care Foundation; a philanthropic agency that promotes the field of respiratory care through grants and awards

ARDS abbreviation for acute respiratory distress syndrome

arrhythmia any deviation from the normal pattern of the heartbeat

arteriography a method of radiologic visualization of arteries performed after a radiopaque contrast medium is introduced into the bloodstream or into a specific vessel by injection or through a catheter

arteriole one of the blood vessels of the smallest branch of the arterial circulation

arteriolized blood blood that has been fully oxygenated by passage through the lungs

arteriovenous anastomosis a communication between an artery and a vein, either as a congenital anomaly or as a surgically produced link between vessels

asbestosis a restrictive lung disease caused by prolonged exposure to asbestosis fibers; associated with a high incidence of malignant lung tumors and pleural abnormalities

ascites accumulation of fluid in the abdomen

asepsis the absence of pathogenic microorganisms; the removal of pathogenic microorganisms or infected material

aspergillosis an infection caused by a fungus of the genus Aspergillus, capable of causing inflammatory, granulomatous lesions on or in any organ

asphyxia cessation of ventilation leading to acute hypoxia and hypercapnia

aspirate (verb) to withdraw fluid by negative pressure; (noun) the fluid so withdrawn

aspiration the act of inhaling, especially in reference to the pathological aspiration of vomitus or material foreign to the respiratory tract (see aspiration pneumonia); also the process of withdrawing fluid by negative pressure

aspiration pneumonia an inflammatory condition of the lungs and bronchi caused by the inhalation of foreign material or vomitus containing acid gastric contents

assault any conduct that creates a reasonable apprehension of being touched in an injurious manner; no actual touching is required to prove assault

assist/control (A/C or ACV) continuous mandatory ventilation (CMV) in which the minimum breathing rate is predetermined, but the patient can initiate ventilation at an increased rate

ASSS abbreviation for American Standard Safety System; specifications adopted in the United States and Canada for threaded high-pressure connections between compressed gas cylinders and their attachments

asthma a respiratory disorder characterized by recurring episodes of paroxysmal dyspnea, wheezing on expiration/inspiration caused by constriction of the bronchi, coughing, and viscous mucoid bronchial secretions. The episodes may be precipitated by inhalation of allergens or pollutants, infection, cold air, vigorous exercise, or emotional stress. Also called *bronchial asthma*

ASTM abbreviation for American Society for Testing and Materials, a nongovernmental agency that establishes performance standards for various equipment and materials

asymptomatic literally means 'without symptoms'

asynchronous (of an event or device) a computer operation in one command performed in response to a signal that the previous command has been completed. One operation is completed before the next is initiated

asynchronous breathing an abnormal breathing pattern in which the rib cage and abdomen do not move outward together, indicating that the respiratory muscles are not working in synchrony; an early indicator of an excessive respiratory muscle load

asynchrony pertaining to ventilatory support, a situation in which interaction between the patient and machine is poorly coordinated, causing extra patient effort and discomfort

asystole the absence of a heartbeat, as distinguished from fibrillation, in which electric activity persists but contraction ceases

ATA abbreviation for atmospheric pressure absolute; a measure of pressure used in hyperbaric medicine; 1 ATA equals 760 mm Hg or 101.32 kPa

atelectasis abnormal collapse of distal lung parenchyma

atelectrauma alveolar collapse due to inappropriate mechanical ventilation settings

atherosclerosis an arterial disorder characterized by the deposit of plaques of cholesterol, lipids, and cellular debris in the inner layers of the walls or arteries

atmospheric pressure absolute (ATA) a measure of pressure used in hyperbaric medicine; 1 ATA equals 760 mm Hg or 101.32 kPa

atomizer a device that produces an aerosol suspension of liquid particles without using baffles to control particle size

atopy a hereditary tendency to develop immediate allergic reactions, as in asthma, atopic dermatitis, or vasomotor rhinitis, because of the presence of an antibody

ATPS abbreviation for ambient temperature, ambient pressure, saturated (with water vapor)

atrial myxoma a benign tumor that originates in the intratrial septum of the heart

atrial natriuretic hormone a hormone that inhibits sodium reabsorption by the kidneys, thus increasing sodium and water excretion in the urine

atrioventricular of or pertaining to the area between the atria and ventricles of the heart

atrophy a wasting or diminution of size or physiological activity of a part of the body because of disease or other influences, especially muscle tissue

ATS abbreviation for the American Thoracic Society

atypical pneumonia a group of relatively mild symptoms of chills, headache, muscular pains, moderate fever, and coughing but without evidence of a bacterial infection. Chest x-ray film may show mottling at the bases. Eaton agent, or *Mycoplasma pneumoniae*, may be the cause of the symptoms

auditory pertaining to the sense of hearing

auscultation the act of listening for sounds within the body to evaluate the condition of the heart, lungs, pleura, intestines, or other organs or to detect the fetal heart sound

authoritarian of or pertaining to the principle of blind obedience of one to another

autoclave apparatus that uses steam under pressure to sterilize articles and equipment

autogenic drainage (AD) a modification of directed coughing, beginning with low-lung-volume breathing, inspiratory breath holds, and controlled exhalation, and progressing to increased inspired volumes and expiratory flows

autogenous infection an infection originating within the organism affected

autoimmune disease one of a large group of diseases characterized by the subversion or alteration of the function of the immune system of the body

automaticity a term denoting the heart's ability to generate its own intrinsic electrical rhythm

auto-PEEP abnormal and usually undetected residual pressure above atmospheric remaining in the alveoli at end-exhalation due to dynamic air trapping. Also called *intrinsic PEEP*

autoregulation automatic control of a mechanical or physiological system; necessitates both a sensing mechanism (to measure what is regulated) and a feedback 'loop' (to respond to changes)

autosomal inheritance a pattern of inheritance in which the transmission of a recessive gene on an autosome results in a carrier state if the person is heterozygous for the trait and in the affect state if the person is homozygous for the trait

avirulent the inability of a microorganism to cause a pathological effect

Avogadro's law a law in physics stating that equal volumes of all gases at a given temperature and pressure contain the identical number of molecules

axilla a pyramid-shaped space forming the underside of the shoulder between the upper part of the arm and the side of the chest; that is, the 'armpit'

axillary of or pertaining to the axilla

azotemia the buildup of excess nitrogenous waste products in the blood, usually due to renal failure

B

Babinski's reflex dorsiflexion of the big toe with extension and fanning of the other toes elicited by firmly stroking the lateral aspect of the sole of the foot

bacteremia the presence of bacteria in the blood

bactericidal destructive to bacteria

bacteriostatic tending to restrain bacterial growth

baffle a surface in a nebulizer designed specifically to cause impaction of large aerosol particles, causing either further fragmentation or removal from the suspension via condensation back into the reservoir

baffling the process of removing large water particles from suspension in a jet nebulizer so that the particles entering the patient's airways are of a uniform therapeutic size

bagassosis a self-limited lung disease caused by an allergic response to bagasse, the fungi-laden, dusty debris left after the syrup has been extracted from sugar cane

BAL abbreviation; see bronchoalveolar lavage

bandwidth the rate of digital data transmission over a transmission line or channel, expressed in bits (kilobits, megabits) per second

barbiturate any one of a group of organic compounds derived from barbituric acid, which have the capacity to cause depression of the central nervous system; examples include Amytal, phenobarbitol, and sodium pentothal

baroreceptor one of the pressure-sensitive nerve endings in the walls of the atria of the heart, the vena cava, the aortic arch, and the carotid sinus

barotrauma physical injury sustained as a result of exposure to ambient pressures above normal, most commonly secondary to positive pressure ventilation, for example, pneumothorax, pneumomediastinum

barrel chest an abnormal increase in the anterior-posterior diameter of the chest due to hyperinflation of the lungs

basal metabolic rate (BMR) the amount of energy used in a unit of time by a fasting, resting subject. The rate, determined by the amount of oxygen used, is expressed in calories consumed per hour per square meter of body surface area or per kilogram of body weight. Also called *basal energy expenditure (BEE)*

base a compound that yields hydroxyl ions [OH^-] when dissolved in an aqueous solution

base excess (BE) the difference between the normal buffer base (NBB) and the actual buffer base (BB) in a whole blood sample, expressed in mEq/L; a normal BE is + 2 mEq/L

basic life support (BLS) cardiopulmonary resuscitation designed to reinstitute either circulatory or respiratory function without equipment or drugs

battery (legal) an unconsented actual touching that causes injury

BCG vaccine an active immunizing agent against tuberculosis prepared from Bacille Calmette-Guerin

benevolent deception actions in which the truth is withheld from the patient for his or her own good

beneficence the principle that requires that health providers go beyond doing no harm and actively contribute to the health and well being of their patients

benign not malignant or recurrent; characterized by mild symptoms or effect

bigeminy literally 'an association in pairs'; commonly refers to the cardiac arrhythmia characterized by paired premature ventricular contractions

bi-level positive airway pressure (BiPAP) a spontaneous breath mode of ventilatory support, which allows separate regulation of the inspiratory and expiratory pressures

bilirubin the orange-yellow pigment of bile, formed principally by the breakdown of hemoglobin in red blood cells after termination of their normal life span

biofeedback a process providing a person with visual or auditory information about the autonomic-physiological functions of his or her body, as blood pressure

biopsy the procedure whereby tissues are excised for microscopic examination and diagnosis

biotrauma inflammation of the lungs in response to inappropriate mechanical ventilation that promotes alveolar overdistension in inspiration and derecruitment on exhalation

Biot's respiration breathing characterized by irregular periods of apnea alternating with periods in which four or five breaths of identical depth are taken

BiPAP abbreviation for bi-level positive airway pressure

biphasic consisting of two phases

bit Binary digIT, a quantum of data in computer storage corresponding to a 1 or 0

blood-brain barrier an anatomic-physiological feature of the brain thought to consist of walls of capillaries in the central nervous system and surrounding astrocytic glial membranes. The barrier separates the parenchyma of the central nervous system from blood. The blood-brain barrier prevents or slows the passage of some drugs and other chemical compounds, radioactive ions, and disease-causing organisms such as viruses from the blood into the central nervous system

board certified holding certification in a medical specialty; usually obtained by passing one or more examinations offered by a specialty society or credentialing agency

body humidity the absolute humidity in a volume of gas saturated at a body temperature of 37° C; equivalent to 43.8 mg/L

Bohr effect the effect of variations in blood pH on the affinity of hemoglobin for oxygen

boiling point the temperature at which the vapor pressure of a liquid equals the ambient pressure exerted on the liquid

BOMA abbreviation for the Board of Medical Advisors, the medical advisory group for the American Association for Respiratory Care

bore the internal diameter of a tube

Borg dyspnea scale a validated scale used by patients to quantify the severity of their dyspnea

botulism an often fatal form of food poisoning caused by an endotoxin produced by the bacillus *Clostridium botulinum*

Bourdon gauge a fixed orifice, variable pressure flow metering device

BPF abbreviation for bronchopleural fistula

brachial of or pertaining to the arm

brachiocephalic trunk the short branch of the aortic arch giving rise to the right common carotid and right subclavian arteries; also called the *innominate artery*

brachytherapy treatment of malignant neoplasms by implanting radioactive materials directly into the tumor

bradycardia an abnormally decreased heart rate

bradykinin a polypeptide cellular mediator responsible for provoking smooth muscle contraction

bradypnea an abnormal decrease in breathing rate

breach of contract failure, without legal excuse, to carry out the terms of a legal agreement

breach of duty failure to complete an assignment that is legal and agreed upon

breathing exercises a broad category of physical activities designed to increase the strength and endurance of the respiratory muscles and to promote their more efficient use

bronchi larger branching airways dividing into the lobes and segments of the lung

bronchiectasis an abnormal condition of the bronchial tree characterized by irreversible dilatation and destruction of the bronchial walls

bronchioles branching airways beginning 5 to 14 divisions below the segmental bronchi; usually 2 mm in diameter or less

bronchiolitis an acute infection of the lower respiratory tract causing expiratory wheezing, respiratory distress, inflammation, and obstruction of the bronchioles; bronchiolitis is usually caused by the respiratory syncytial virus (RSV) and is most common in infants under 2 years of age

bronchitis an acute or chronic inflammation of the mucous membranes of the tracheobronchial tree

bronchoalveolar lavage (BAL) the instillation and aspiration of fluids into the lungs in order to diagnose or treat certain conditions

bronchoconstriction narrowing of the bronchi due to contraction of their smooth muscle

bronchodilation the reversal of bronchoconstriction, usually via sympathetic stimulation

bronchodilator a substance, especially a drug, that relaxes contractions of the smooth muscle of the bronchioles to improve ventilation to the lungs. Pharmacologic bronchodilators are prescribed to improve aeration in asthma, bronchiectasis, bronchitis, and emphysema

bronchogenic carcinoma the most common malignant lung tumor originating in bronchi

bronchography an x-ray examination of the bronchi after they have been coated with a radiopaque substance

bronchophony abnormal voice sounds heard over lung consolidation

bronchopleural fistula any air communication from the lung to the pleural space

bronchopneumonia an acute inflammation of the lungs and bronchioles, characterized by chills, fever, high pulse and respirator rates, bronchial breathing, cough with purulent bloody sputum, severe chest pain, and abdominal extension

bronchopulmonary dysplasia (BPD) a chronic respiratory disorder characterized by scarring of lung tissue, thickened pulmonary arterial walls, and mismatch between lung ventilation and perfusion. It often occurs in infants who have been dependent on long-term artificial pulmonary ventilation

bronchorrhea the excessive discharge of respiratory tract secretions

bronchospasm an abnormal contraction of the smooth muscle of the bronchi, resulting in an acute narrowing and obstruction

bronchovesicular breath sounds sharing the characteristics of those heard over the trachea (bronchial sounds) and those arising from the more distal alveolar region (vesicular sounds)

Brownian diffusion a primary mechanism for deposition of inhaled particles less than 3 mm in diameter into the lung parenchyma

bruit an abnormal sound heard on auscultation of the heart or large vessels, caused by turbulence or obstruction

BTPS abbreviation for body temperature, ambient pressure, saturated (with water vapor)

BTU abbreviation for British Thermal Unit, the fps unit of heat energy; a BTU is the amount of heat required to raise the temperature of 1 lb of water 1° F; 1 BTU equals 252 calories (cgs)

buccal of or pertaining to the inside of the cheek or the gum next to the cheek

buffer a chemical substance that, when added to a solution, minimizes fluctuations in pH

buffer base the total blood buffer capable of binding hydrogen ions. Normal buffer base (NBB) ranges from 48 to 52 mEq/L

buffer system a chemical solution consisting of a weak acid and its salt, which has the ability to minimize changes in pH when adding acid or alkali

bulla a thin-walled blister of the skin, mucous membranes, or lung greater than 1 cm in diameter

BUN abbreviation for blood urea nitrogen, a major by-product of protein metabolism that normally is excreted by the kidneys

byte (kilo-, mega-, giga-) a collection of eight data bits that function as one; one byte can represent a character, and several bytes together can represent a word

C

cachexia general ill health and malnutrition characterized by weakness and emaciation

canals of Lambert intercommunicating channels between terminal bronchioles and the alveoli that are about 30 mm in size and appear to remain open even when bronchiolar smooth muscle is contracted

candidiasis infection of the skin or mucous membranes caused chiefly by the yeastlike fungus Candida albicans; commonly referred to as *thrush* when localized to the mouth and pharynx; can spread systemically in immunocompromised hosts

cannula any flexible tube that is inserted into the body

cannulation the insertion of a cannula into a body duct or cavity, as into the nose, trachea, bladder, or a blood vessel

capnography the process of obtaining a tracing of the proportion of carbon dioxide in expired air using a capnograph

capnometer an instrument used in anesthesia, respiratory physiology, and respiratory care to measure the proportion of carbon dioxide in expired air

capnometry the measurement of carbon dioxide in a volume of gas, usually by methods of infrared absorption or mass spectrometry

carboxyhemoglobin a compound produced by the chemical combination of hemoglobin with carbon monoxide

carboxyhemoglobinemia a decrease in the oxygen carrying capacity of the blood due to the saturation of hemoglobin with carbon monoxide instead of oxygen

carcinogenic of or pertaining to the ability to cause the development of a cancer

cardiac index a standardized measure of cardiac performance equal to a patient's cardiac output in L/min divided by the body surface area in square meters

cardiac output the volume of blood pumped per minute by the heart

cardiac tamponade compression of the heart due to the collection of blood, fluid, or gas under pressure in the pericardium

cardiogenic originating in or caused by the heart; as in cardiogenic shock

cardiomegaly hypertrophy of the heart caused most frequently by pulmonary hypertension; also occurring in arteriovenous fistula, congenital aortic stenosis, ventricular septal defect, patent ductus arteriosus, and Paget's disease

cardiomyopathy any disease that affects the myocardium, as alcoholic cardiomyopathy

cardiopulmonary exercise evaluation an exercise-based assessment of the pulmonary rehabilitation patient designed to determine the patient's exercise capacity and risk for desaturation

cardiopulmonary resuscitation (CPR) a basic emergency procedure for life support, consisting of artificial respiration and manual external cardiac massage

cardioversion the restoration of the heart's normal sinus rhythm by delivery of a synchronized electric shock through two metal paddles placed on the patient's chest

carina the sharp pointed cartilage at the bifurcation of the right and left mainstem bronchi

carotid sinus reflex the decrease in the heat rate as a reflex reaction from pressure on or within the carotid artery at the level of its bifurcation

catabolism the destructive phase of metabolism whereby complex substances are broken down into simpler ones, with the concurrent release of energy

catecholamine any one of a group of sympathomimetic compounds composed of a catechol molecule and the aliphatic portion of an amine

catheterization the introduction of a catheter into a body cavity or organ to inject or remove a fluid

cathode the negative pole or electrode of an electrical source

cavitation the formation of cavities within the body, as those formed in the lungs by tuberculosis

CBC abbreviation for complete blood count

CC abbreviation for chief complaint

CDC abbreviation for Centers for Disease Control and Prevention, a federal agency of the U.S. government that provides facilities and services for the investigation, identification, prevention, and control of disease

CD-ROM computer disk read-only memory; similar to audio disks that are read by laser, CD-ROMs are used for access to large unchanging reference databases

Central Processing Unit (CPU) the primary component of the computer; the CPU houses the core memory, the control component to manage computer system operations, and the arithmetic and logic unit (ALU)

central sleep apnea absence of breathing as the result of medullary depression that inhibits respiratory movement, which becomes more pronounced during sleep

cephalad toward the head

cerebral aneurysm an abnormal localized dilatation of a cerebral artery, most commonly the result of congenital weakness of the media or muscle layer of the vessel wall

cerebral hemorrhage a hemorrhage from a blood vessel in the brain; sometimes called a *cerebrovascular accident* or *CVA*

cerebral palsy a motor function disorder caused by a permanent, nonprogressive brain defect or lesion present at birth or shortly thereafter

cerebrospinal pertaining to or involving the brain and the spinal cord

cerebrovascular of or pertaining to the vascular system of the brain

certification a voluntary process whereby a nongovernmental or private agency or association grants recognition to an individual who has met certain predetermined qualifications for recognition in a given field of study or practice

certified pulmonary function technician (CPFT) an individual, qualified by education and/or experience, who has successfully completed the pulmonary function certification examination of the NBRC

certified respiratory therapist (CRT) a respiratory therapist who has successfully completed the technician (entry-level) certification examination of the NBRC

cervical of or pertaining to the neck or the region of the neck

chemoreceptor a sensory nerve cell activated by changes in the chemical environment surrounding it, as the chemoreceptors in the carotid artery that are sensitive to the P_{CO_2} in the blood, signaling the respiratory center in the brain to increase or decrease ventilation

chest physical therapy (CPT) a collection of therapeutic techniques designed to aid clearance of secretion, improve ventilation, and enhance the conditioning of the respiratory muscles; includes positioning techniques; chest percussion and vibration; directed coughing; and various breathing and conditioning exercises

chest radiograph an x-ray image of the chest. Both a posterior to anterior, or P-A, view and a lateral, or side, view routinely are obtained

Cheyne-Stokes respiration an abnormal, repeating pattern of breathing characterized by alternating progressive hypopnea and hypoventilation, ending in a brief apnea

CHF abbreviation for congestive heart failure; an abnormal condition that reflects impaired cardiac pumping. It is caused by myocardial infarction, ischemic heart disease, or cardiomyopathy

choanal atresia a congenital anomaly in which a bony or membranous occlusion blocks the passageway between the nose and pharynx

cholinergic of or pertaining to nerve fibers that elaborate acetylcholine at the myoneural junctions

chronic bronchitis a very common debilitating pulmonary disease, characterized by greatly increased production of mucus by the glands of the trachea and bronchi and resulting in a cough with expectoration for at least 3 months of the year for more than 2 consecutive years

chylothorax a pleural fluid collection that is high in triglycerides, usually from disruption of the thoracic duct

civil action action brought to enforce, redress, or protect private rights, including all types of actions other than criminal proceedings

civil law the body of law that every particular nation, state, or city establishes to provide civil or private rights and remedies

clearance removal; in aerosol therapy, the process whereby deposited particles are removed from the site of deposition, or the removal of still suspended particles in the exhaled air

closed buffer system a buffer system in which all components of acid-base reactions remain in the system. Products accumulate and reach equilibrium with reactants, and chemical activity ceases (no further buffering activity can take place). Examples of closed buffer systems in the body are nonbicarbonate buffers (for example, plasma proteins, Hb, phosphates)

clubbing bulbous swelling of the terminal phalanges of the fingers and toes, often associated with certain chronic lung diseases

CMN abbreviation for a certificate of medical necessity; the documentation needed for a patient to receive reimbursement for home O_2 therapy

CMV abbreviation for continuous mandatory ventilation; the application of pressure greater than atmospheric at the airway opening during every inspiration, used to support ventilation; during expiration, pressure returns to atmospheric; CMV may be applied in either the control or assist/control mode

CNS abbreviation for central nervous system

coalescence the growing together of two or more objects, as in the coalescence of water vapor molecules into water droplets

Coanda effect a phenomenon in hydrodynamics whereby a fluid in motion may be attracted or held to a wall

CoARC acronym for Committee on Accreditation for Respiratory Care; establishes standards and oversees approval of educational programs in respiratory care

coarctation of the aorta a congenital cardiac anomaly characterized by a localized narrowing of the aorta, which results in increased pressure proximal to the defect and decreased pressure distal to it

coccidioidomycosis an infectious fungal disease caused by the inhalation of spores of the organism Coccidioides immitis, which is carried on windborne dust particles

cognitive domain the area of the mental processes of comprehension, judgment, memory, and reasoning

cohesion the attractive force between like molecules

cohort a collection or sampling of individuals who share a common characteristic, as members of the same age or the same sex

cohorting grouping individuals who share a common characteristic, as members of the same age or the same sex, or those sharing a common infection

collateral circulation a redundant blood pathway developed through enlargement of secondary vessels after obstruction of a main channel

colloid a substance that contains large molecules that attract and hold water; also a dispersion or a gel

colonization the process by which microorganisms establish a presence and grow in or on the human body; does not necessarily indicate a pathological response

community-acquired pneumonia an acute inflammation of the lungs contracted from the environment (as distinguished from nosocomial, or hospital-acquired, pneumonia)

compliance volume change per unit in applied pressure

Comprehensive Out-Patient Rehabilitation Facility (CORF) a Medicare-approved facility that provides a broad scope of ambulatory rehabilitation services as defined in section 933 of Public Law 96-499

compressed volume the volume of gas compressed in the ventilator circuit and not delivered to the patient during a positive pressure breath

computerized tomography a radiographic technique that produces a film that represents a detailed cross section of tissue structure

CON abbreviation for Certificate of Need, a verification made by a regulatory group that a major capital improvement, such as the addition of a wing to a hospital or the purchase of a MRI device, is needed

concave curved or rounded inward like a bowl

condensation change of state from gas to liquid, as with water vapor condensation

conduction the transfer of heat by the direct interaction of atoms or molecules in a hot area that contact atoms or molecules in a cooler area

conductivity the ability of myocardial tissue to propagate electrical impulses

confidentiality the nondisclosure of certain information except to another authorized person

congenital present at birth, as a congenital anomaly or defect

congenital diaphragmatic hernia an abnormality in the development of the diaphragm resulting in a persistent opening between the abdominal and thoracic cavities; due to displacement of the abdominal contents into the thorax, this condition may impede lung growth and development on the affected side

congestive heart failure (CHF) an abnormal condition that reflects impaired cardiac pumping. It is caused by myocardial infarction, ischemic heart disease, or cardiomyopathy

conjunctivitis inflammation of the conjunctiva, caused by bacterial or viral infection, allergy, or environmental factors

connective tissue disease any of a group of acquired disorders that have in common diffuse immunologic and inflammatory changes in small blood vessels and connective tissue. The cause of most of these diseases is unknown. Also called *collagen vascular disease*

consolidation the process of becoming solid; especially applies to the loss of aeration of the terminal respiratory units due to fluid extravasation and the collection of exudate, as in certain forms of pneumonia

constriction a narrowing or squeezing together

constrictive pericarditis an inflammation of the pericardium (usually chronic) in which calcium and fibrous deposits surround the heart and restrict its normal filling

contact precautions safeguards designed to reduce the risk of transmission of epidemiologically important microorganisms by direct or indirect contact

contact transmission transmission of infectious organisms between an infected individual and host via direct contact, indirect contact, or droplet contact

continuing education educational activity designed to upgrade, enhance, or expand a professional's knowledge or skills that are conducted after completion of formal entry-level educational preparation

continuous positive airway pressure (CPAP) a method of ventilatory support whereby the patient breathes spontaneously without mechanical assistance against threshold resistance, with pressure above atmospheric maintained at the airway throughout breathing

Continuous Quality Improvement (CQI) a management strategy designed to enhance organization performance

contract, expressed an actual agreement between parties whose terms are stated orally or written, at the time the agreement is made

contract, implied a contract not created or evidenced by the explicit agreement of the parties, but inferred by the law, as a matter of reason and justice form their acts or conducts, making it a reasonable assumption that a contract existed between them by tacit understanding

contractility the property of muscle tissue to shorten in response to a stimulus, usually electrical

contracture an abnormal, usually permanent condition of a joint, characterized by flexion and fixation and caused by atrophy and shortening of muscle fibers or by loss of the normal elasticity of the skin, as from the formation of extensive scar tissue over a joint

contractile force the ratio of diaphragmatic pressure to maximum diaphragmatic pressure

contractility the property of muscle tissue to shorten, thereby generating force

contraindication any circumstance that renders a particular treatment or treatment approach inadvisable or improper

control mode continuous mandatory ventilation (CMV) in which the frequency of breathing is determined by the ventilator according to a preset cycling pattern without initiation by the patient (time-triggered ventilatory support)

convalescence the period of recovery from an illness, operation, or injury

convection heat transfer through the mixing of fluid molecules at different temperature states via thermal currents

COPD abbreviation for chronic obstructive pulmonary disease; COPD is a broad term used to describe generalized airway obstruction that is not fully reversible with treatment; almost always a mixture of emphysema and chronic bronchitis, with, at times, elements of asthma

cor pulmonale right ventricular hypertrophy/failure and pulmonary hypertension due to certain parenchymal or vascular lung disorders

CORF abbreviation for Comprehensive Out-Patient Rehabilitation Facility; a Medicare-approved facility that provides a broad scope of ambulatory rehabilitation services as defined in section 933 of Public Law 96-499

corticosteroid any one of the natural or the synthetic hormones associated with the adrenal cortex, which influences or controls key processes of the body, as carbohydrate and protein metabolism, electrolyte and water balance, and the function of the cardiovascular system and kidneys

costal cartilages the fibrous tissues that connect the ribs to the sternum and to each other anteriorly

costochondral of or pertaining to a rib and its cartilage

costophrenic pertaining to the ribs and diaphragm; especially the angle formed by the lower ribs' intersection with the diaphragm

costophrenic angle the acute angle where the costal pleura meets the diaphragm

costovertebral of or relating to a rib and the vertebral column

cough forceful expiratory effort designed to expel mucus and other foreign material from the upper airway

countershock a high-intensity, short-duration electric shock applied to the heart, resulting in total depolarization

CPAP abbreviation for continuous positive airway pressure; a method of ventilatory support whereby the patient breathes spontaneously without mechanical assistance against threshold resistance, with pressure above atmospheric maintained at the airway throughout breathing

CPFT abbreviation for certified pulmonary function technician

CQI abbreviation for Continuous Quality Improvement; a management strategy designed to enhance organization performance

crackles a discontinuous type of adventitious lung sound

creatinine a substance formed from the metabolism of creatine, commonly found in blood, urine, and muscle tissue

credentialing a broad term referring to the recognition of individuals who have met certain predetermined standards attesting to their occupational skill or competence; includes both licensure and certification

crepitus a dry crackling sound or sensation; may apply to breath sounds, that is 'a crepitant rale' or to the sensation felt when palpating an area of subcutaneous emphysema

cricoid cartilage a ring of cartilage that forms the lower border of the larynx

cricothyrotomy an emergency incision into the larynx between the cricoid and thyroid cartilages, performed to open the airway in a person choking

criteria for hospitalization conditions to be met to admit the patient to the hospital

critical pressure the pressure exerted by a vapor in an evacuated container at its critical temperature

critical temperature the highest temperature at which a substance can exist as a liquid, regardless of pressure

cross-training the process of providing healthcare professionals with multiple skills in areas that span single disciplines, for example, training a respiratory care practitioner to take chest x-rays

croup an infectious disorder of the upper airway occurring chiefly in infants and children that normally results in subglottic swelling and obstruction

CRT abbreviation for certified respiratory therapist; a respiratory therapist who has successfully completed the technician (entry-level) certification examination of the NBRC

CSF abbreviation for cerebrospinal fluid

Cushing's disease a metabolic disorder characterized by the abnormally increased secretion of adrenocortical steroids caused by increased amounts of adrenocorticotropic hormone (ACTH)

CVA abbreviation for cerebrovascular accident

CVP abbreviation for central venous pressure; the blood pressure measured in or near the right atrium

CWP abbreviation for coal-workers' pneumoconiosis; CWP is due to chronic exposure to coal dust, which consists mainly of carbon; pathological changes are similar to silicosis

cyanosis an abnormal bluish discoloration of the skin or mucous membranes

cyanotic heart disease of or pertaining to anatomical congenital heart defects that cause large right-to-left shunting; such 'venous admixture' results in the characteristic cyanosis

cycling mechanism (ventilator) the means by which a ventilator ends the inspiratory phase of mechanical ventilation, either pressure, volume flow, or time

cystic fibrosis an autosomal recessive disease characterized by pancreatic insufficiency, abnormally thick secretions from the exocrine glands, and an increased concentration of sodium and chloride in the sweat glands; known in Europe as *mucoviscidosis*

cystoscopy the direct visualization of the urinary tract by means of a cystoscope inserted in the urethra

cytochrome oxidase system the major intracellular pathway for oxidative metabolism and energy production

cytokine a chemical or humoral factor that influences cellular proliferation and immune responses; also called *peptide regulatory factors*

cytomegalovirus a member of a group of large species-specific herpes-type viruses with a wide variety of disease effects

cytotoxic of or pertaining to chemical or biological substances that are lethal to living cells

cytotoxic agent a chemical or biological substance that is lethal to living cells

D

Dalton's law (in physics) a law stating that the total pressure exerted by a mixture of gases is equal to the sum of the pressures that could be exerted by the gases if they were present alone in the container

damped referring to an analog waveform in which oscillations have a diminished (and erroneous) amplitude

data any information or arrangement of a character set meant to represent information

database a group of related records and files on a direct access storage device, stored in such a way to allow appending, manipulating, and retrieving data

DBMS abbreviation for database management system, a software program used to organize, store, retrieve, and manipulate text, numeric data, and/or graphical data

deadspace respired gas volume that does not participate in gas exchange; may be anatomic, alveolar, or mechanical

debilitated weakness, especially to the extent of being unable to participate in care

debridement the removal of foreign material and dead tissue from an infected or traumatized area in order to expose healthy tissue

decongestant of or pertaining to a substance or procedure that eliminates or reduces congestion or swelling

decontamination the process whereby contaminants are removed from objects, usually by simple physical means, such as washing

decubitus ulcer an inflammation, sore, or ulcer in the skin over a bony prominence

defendant the person denying the party against whom relief or recovery is sought in an action or suit; also, the accused in a criminal case

defibrillation the termination of ventricular fibrillation by delivering a direct electric countershock to the patient's precordium

Department of Health and Human Services (DHHS) a department of the U.S. federal government that has many agencies involved in health delivery, for example, the Food and Drug Administration is an agency that requires a certain level of purity for medical gases

dependent (gravity) being bottom-most relative to the earth's gravitational field

depolarization the reduction of a membrane potential to a less negative value; in cardiac fibers, this results in the release of calcium ions into the myofibrils and activates the contractile process

deposition the testimony of a witness taken upon interrogatories, either oral or in writing

deponent one who testifies to the truth of certain facts; one whose deposition is given

detoxify the process of removing toxic agents or poisons
dew point the temperature at which water vapor condenses back to its liquid form
diabetic ketoacidosis an acute, life-threatening complication of uncontrolled diabetes mellitus in which urinary loss of water, potassium, ammonium, and sodium results in hypovolemia, electrolyte imbalance, extremely high blood glucose levels, and the breakdown of free fatty acids, causing a severe metabolic acidosis, often with coma
dialysis the process of separating colloids and crystalline substances in solution by the difference in their rate of diffusion through a semipermeable membrane
diameter-indexed safety system (DISS) specifications established to prevent accidental interchange of low pressure (less than 200 psig) medical gas connectors. The DISS is used in respiratory care to connect equipment to a low pressure gas source
diaphoresis the secretion of sweat, especially the profuse secretion associated with an elevated body temperature, physical exertion, exposure to heat, and mental or emotional stress
diaphragm the large dome-shaped muscle that separates the thorax from the abdomen; the primary muscle of ventilation
diaphragmatic hernia the protrusion of part of the stomach through an opening in the diaphragm, most commonly an abnormally enlarged esophageal hiatus
diastolic blood pressure the baseline blood pressure in the arteries during ventricular relaxation
DIC abbreviation for disseminated intravascular coagulation; DIC is a thrombohemorrhagic disorder that accompanies a variety of clinical conditions and involves activation of the clotting cascade, the generation of excess thrombin, intravascular coagulation, occlusion of capillaries and arterioles with fibrin, and tissue ischemia
dicrotic notch a notch on the descending limb of a pulse tracing; especially that seen in the tracing of arterial blood pressure due to closure of the mitral valve
diffusing capacity of the lung (DL) the number of milliliters of gas that transfer from the lungs to the pulmonary blood per minute for each torr partial pressure difference between the alveoli and pulmonary capillary blood
diffusing capacity of the lung to alveolar volume ratio (DLCO/VA) an index of the diffusing capacity for each liter of lung volume and an index of the functional alveolar surface area available for diffusion
diffusion the physical process whereby atoms or molecules tend to move from an area of higher concentration or pressure to an area of lower concentration or pressure
diffusion coefficient the rate of diffusion of a gas; in cgs units, the diffusion coefficient is defined as the number of milliliters of a gas at 1 atmosphere of pressure that will diffuse a distance of 1 mm over a square centimeter surface area per minute
diffusion deposition the deposition of aerosol particles on a surface due to their random bombardment by carrier gas molecules
diplegia bilateral paralysis of both sides of any part of the body or of like parts on the opposite sides of the body
diplopia double vision
disability the lack of ability to perform normal mental or physical tasks; especially the loss of mental or physical powers due to injury or disease
disease prevention activities designed to protect patients or other members of the public from actual or potential health threats and their harmful consequences
disinfectant a chemical agent capable of destroying at least the vegetative phase of pathogenic microorganisms; there are five major categories of disinfectants used in clinical practice: the alcohols, the phenols and their derivatives, the halogens, the aldehydes, and the quaternary ammonium compounds
disinfection the process of destroying at least the vegetative phase of pathogenic microorganisms by physical or chemical means
DISS abbreviation for diameter-indexed safety system; specifications established to prevent accidental interchange of low pressure (less than 200 psig) medical gas connectors. The DISS is used in respiratory care to connect equipment to a low-pressure gas source
distensibility of or pertaining to the ease of inflation or compliance
distensible capable of being enlarged or expanded under pressure
distillation the condensation of a vapor obtained by heating a liquid; commonly used to separate out liquids with different boiling points as in the production of oxygen by fractional distillation
distributive justice refers to the proper allotment of the benefits and burdens in a society, such as taxes and subsidies
diuresis increased formation and secretion of urine
diuretic a chemical substance that causes diuresis
DME company a company that manufactures, sells, or rents durable medical equipment
Do_2 common abbreviation for delivery of oxygen to the tissues (the product of cardiac output × arterial oxygen content)
downstream a relative reference to a point more distal from the source in a stream of flowing fluid
droplet nuclei the residue of evaporated water droplets; due to their small size (0.5 to 12 mm) droplet nuclei can remain suspended in the air for long periods of time
droplet precautions safeguards designed to reduce the risk of droplet transmission of infectious agents
drug-related lung disease lung disease caused by a drug
drug signaling the mechanism by which a drug exerts its effect on receptors
dual-control a mode of ventilation in which the control variable (pressure, volume, flow) switches during a breath
ductus arteriosus a vascular channel in the fetus that joins the pulmonary artery directly to the descending aorta; it normally closes after birth
due process of law law in its regular course of administration through courts of justice
duodenum the shortest, widest, and most fixed portion of the small intestine, taking an almost circular course from the pyloric valve of the stomach so that its termination is close to its starting point
duty cycle during breathing, the ratio of inspiratory time to the total time for a complete breathing cycle

dynamic hyperinflation an increase in functional residual capacity (FRC) above the elastic equilibrium volume of the respiratory system. Causes include increased flow resistance, short inspiratory time, and increased postinspiratory muscle activity (see also auto-PEEP)
dysarthria difficult, poorly articulated speech, resulting from interference in the control over the muscles of speech, usually because of damage to a central or peripheral motor nerve
dysphagia difficulty in swallowing
dysphasia impaired speech
dysphonia same as *dysphasia*; impaired speech
dyspnea difficult or labored breathing as perceived by the patient
dysoxia an abnormal metabolic state in which the tissues are unable to properly use the oxygen made available to them
dyssynchrony pertaining to ventilatory support, a situation in which interaction between the patient and machine is poorly coordinated, causing extra patient effort and discomfort

E

$ECCO_2R$ abbreviation for extracorporeal carbon dioxide removal
ECG abbreviation for electrocardiogram
echocardiography a diagnostic procedure for studying the structure and motion of the heart
eclampsia the gravest form of toxemia of pregnancy, characterized by grand mal convulsion, coma, hypertension, proteinuria, and edema
ECMO abbreviation for extracorporeal membrane oxygenation; the procedure whereby venous blood is pumped outside the body to a heart-lung machine for oxygenation and returned to the body through an artery
ectopic situated in an unusual place, away from its normal location; for example, an ectopic pregnancy is a pregnancy that occurs outside the uterus
ectopic focus the origination of a heart beat from some place in the heart other than the SA node
edema excess fluid in the interstitial spaces between cells; in the lungs edema fluid may also be present in the airways and alveolar spaces
efferent carrying or conduction impulses away from the central nervous system; opposite of afferent
efficacy (of a drug) the peak or maximum biological effect
effort-dependent of or pertaining to a test or procedure the accuracy or success of which depends on patient effort
effort-independent of or pertaining to a test or procedure the accuracy or success of which does not depend on patient effort
effusion the escape of fluid from blood vessels because of rupture or seepage, usually into a body cavity
egophony the sound of normal voice tones as heard through the chest wall during auscultation
EGTA abbreviation for the esophageal gastric tube airway; a modification of the esophageal obturator airway (EOA), which includes a gastric tube that can be extended beyond the distal tip into the stomach in order to remove air or gastric contents
EIP abbreviation for end-inspiratory pause; a technique whereby a specific inflation volume is momentarily held at the end of inspiration during mechanical ventilation, for either therapeutic or diagnostic purposes
ejection fraction (EF) the ratio of cardiac stroke volume to end-diastolic volume
ejection volume the ratio of cardiac stroke volume to end-diastolic volume
elastance (also elasticity) the tendency of matter to resist a stretching force and recoil or return to its original size or form after deformation or expansion; the reciprocal of compliance
elastin a protein that forms the principal substance of yellow elastic tissue fibers
electrocardiography the process of obtaining a tracing of the electrical activity of the heart (an electrocardiogram) for purposes of identifying abnormalities
electrochemical pertaining to the electrical effects that accompany chemical action and the chemical activity produced by electrical influence
electrolysis the process of applying an electrical current across an anode and cathode in a solution, usually to create or enhance a chemical reaction
electrolyte a chemical substance that dissociates into ions when placed into a solution, thus becoming capable of conducting electricity
electromyography the recording and study of the electrical properties of muscle
electrooculogram a recording of the electrical activity of the eye muscles, indicating type and magnitude of eye movements
electrophysiology the recording and study of the electrical properties of living tissue
ELISA abbreviation for enzyme-linked immunosorbent assay, a test commonly used to detect the presence of antibodies to specific infectious agents, such as the HIV virus
embolectomy a surgical incision into an artery for the removal of an embolus or clot, performed as emergency treatment for arterial embolization
embolism the condition in which an object (often a blood clot) travels from its origin and becomes lodged in a smaller blood vessel, causing partial or complete blockage
embolization the process by which an embolus forms and lodges in a branch of the vasculature
embolus a foreign object, a quantity of air or gas, a bit of tissue or tumor, or a piece of a thrombus that circulates in the bloodstream until it becomes lodged in a vessel
emetic a substance that causes vomiting
emphysema a destructive process of the lung parenchyma leading to permanent enlargement of the distal air spaces; classified as either centrilobular (CLE), which mainly involves the respiratory bronchioles or panlobular (PLE), which can involve the entire terminal respiratory unit
empirical ascertained or discovered by observation
emulsification the process of mixing two or more substances that are not mutually soluble into a uniform dispersion; specifically applies to the breakdown of fat globules in the intestines via the action of bile acids

empyema pus within the pleural space. A pleural fluid Gram stain that shows bacteria also qualifies

end diastolic volume the volume of blood remaining in the left ventricle after the ventricle has contracted

endobronchial within a bronchus

endocarditis inflammation of endocardium and the heart valves, as caused by a variety of diseases

endocrine system the network of ductless glands and other structure that elaborate and secrete hormones directly into the bloodstream, affecting the function of specific target organs

endogenous growing within or arising from the body

endorphin any one of the neuropeptides composed of many amino acids, elaborated by the pituitary gland and acting on the central and peripheral nervous systems to reduce pain

endoscopy the visualization of the interior of organs and cavities of the body with an endoscope

endothelium the layer of squamous epithelial cells that lines the heart, the blood and the lymph vessels, and the serous cavities of the body

endotracheal referring to the lumen of the trachea; as in a tube that is inserted into the trachea

enteric of or pertaining to the intestinal tract

Enterobacteriaceae a family of aerobic and anaerobic bacteria that includes both normal and pathogenic enteric microorganisms

entitlement a right or claim; alternatively the process of granting or providing a right, such as the right to adequate healthcare

enzyme an organic catalyst produced by living cells

EOA abbreviation for esophageal obturator airway; the EOA consists of a cuffed hollow tube tipped with a soft plastic obturator at its tip; the tube passes through a mask and has several holes in its upper portion; once passed into the esophagus, the cuff is inflated, thereby preventing aspiration and allowing ventilation with positive pressure

eosinophilia an increase in the number of eosinophils in the blood, accompanying many inflammatory conditions

eosinophilic granuloma a simple or multiple growth in the bone or lung characterized by numerous eosinophils and histiocytes. Eosinophilic granulomas occur most frequently in children and adolescents

EPAP abbreviation for expiratory positive airway pressure, or the application of positive pressure to the airway during expiration only (as opposed to continuous positive airway pressure)

epidemiology the study of the relationships among various factors and the distribution and frequency of diseases in the population

epigastric of or pertaining to the epigastrium

epigastrium the part of the abdomen in the upper zone between the right and left hypochondriac regions

epiglottis a flat cartilage that extends from the base of the tongue backward and upward

epiglottitis an acute and often life-threatening infection of the upper airway, which causes severe obstruction secondary to supraglottic swelling; caused primarily by Haemophilus influenzae, type B, and affecting mainly children under the age of 5

epinephrine an adrenal hormone and synthetic adrenergic vasoconstrictor

epistaxis bleeding from the nose caused by local irritation of mucous membranes, violent sneezing, fragility of the mucous membrane or of the arterial walls, chronic infection, trauma, hypertension, leukemia, vitamin K deficiency, or most often, picking of the nose

epithelium the covering of the internal and external organs of the body, including the lining of vessels

Epstein-Barr virus the herpesvirus associated with infectious mononucleosis

equal pressure point (EPP) during forced exhalation, the point along an airway where the pressure inside its wall equals the intrapleural pressure; upstream beyond this point, the pleural pressure exceeds the pressure inside the airway, tending to promote bronchiolar collapse

equilibrate to bring into balance

equilibration the process of bringing into balance

ergometer an apparatus designed to measure the amount of work performed by an animal or human subject

erythema a redness of the skin due to capillary congestion; caused by injury, inflammation, or infection

erythema nodosum a hypersensitivity vasculitis characterized by tender red subcutaneous nodules on the shins and associated with strep infections, TB, and sarcoidosis

erythrocyte a red blood cell

erythrocythemia an increase in the number of erythrocytes circulating in the blood

erythrocytosis the process resulting in an abnormal increase in the number of circulating red cells

erythropoiesis the process of erythrocyte production involving the maturation of a nucleated precursor into a hemoglobin-filled, nucleus-free erythrocyte that is regulated by erythropoietin, a hormone produced by the kidney

esophageal obturator airway a cuffed hollow tube tipped with a soft plastic obturator at its tip; the tube passes through a mask and has several holes in its upper portion; once passed into the esophagus, the cuff is inflated, thereby preventing aspiration and allowing ventilation with positive pressure

esophageal opening pressure the oral pressure at which the esophagus distends and opens, allowing gas to insufflate the stomach; estimated to range from 20 to 25 cm H_2O

ethylene oxide a gas used to sterilize surgical instruments and other supplies

EtO common abbreviation for ethylene oxide

Eustachian tubes bilateral tubes that connect the nasopharynx to the middle ear and mastoid sinus

evacuate to remove or withdraw from, especially to empty of air and create a vacuum

evaporation the change in state of substance from its liquid to its gaseous form occurring below its boiling point

evaporation/condensation the reciprocal change of state between water vapor and liquid water occurring below its boiling point

ex vivo outside the body

exacerbate to worsen

exacerbation a worsening of a condition, usually acutely

excitability a property of myocardial tissue, shared with other muscle and nerve tissues and representing a responsiveness to stimulation caused by electrical, chemical, or mechanical factors in the cell or in its surrounding environment

expectorant a chemical agent that promotes the expectoration of respiratory tract secretions, usually by increasing their production or by lowering their viscosity

expiratory reserve volume (ERV) the total amount of gas that can be exhaled from the lung following a quiet exhalation

expiratory resistance (retard) a modification of the expiratory phase of positive pressure ventilation in which a restricted orifice, or flow resistor, is used to slow the flow of exhaled gases from the patient

exponential a nonlinear relationship between two variables in which one varies with a power of the other, for example, $x = y^2$

external oblique abdominal muscle group that functions as an accessory muscle of ventilation

extracellular occurring outside a cell or cell tissue or in cavities or spaces between cell layers or groups of cells

extracorporeal something that is outside the body, as extracorporeal circulation, in which venous blood is diverted outside the body to a heart-lung machine and returned to the body through a femoral or other artery

extracorporeal carbon dioxide removal ($ECCO_2R$) the procedure whereby blood is passed from the patient through an external membrane, which filters carbon dioxide in order to support ventilation

extracorporeal membrane oxygenation (ECMO) the procedure whereby venous blood is pumped outside the body to a heart-lung machine for oxygenation and returned to the body

extrasystole cardiac contraction that is abnormal in timing or in origin of impulse with respect to the fundamental rhythm of the heart

extrathoracic outside the thorax

extrinsic allergic alveolitis an inflammatory form of interstitial pneumonia that results from a Type III or immune complex antigen-antibody reactions to certain organic dusts

extubate withdrawing a tube from an orifice or cavity of the body

exudate a fluid with a high protein content that escapes into the extracellular space; usually due to inflammation or infection

exudative relating to the oozing of fluid and other materials from cells and tissues, usually as a result of inflammation or injury

exudative pleural effusion any pleural effusion high in protein or LDH that implies inflammation or vascular injury on the pleural surface

F

false imprisonment the unlawful arrest or detention of a person without warrant, by an illegal warrant, or by an illegally executed warrant

fasciculation a small involuntary muscular contraction visible under the skin

FDA abbreviation for Food and Drug Administration; sets standards for drug safety and purity

febrile to have a fever

fenestrated open like a window; from the Latin *fenestra*, meaning window

fenestrated tracheotomy tube a double cannulated tracheotomy tube that has an opening in the posterior wall of the outer cannula above the cuff; removal of the inner cannula allows free breathing through the tube

fetal hemoglobin (HbF) a hemoglobin variant that has a greater affinity for oxygen than does adult hemoglobin; HbF is gradually replaced over the first year of life by HbA

fetid foul smelling

fever abnormal elevation of body temperature due to disease

FFB abbreviation for flexible fiberoptic bronchoscope

fiberoptic pertaining to the technical process by which an internal organ or cavity can be viewed, using glass or plastic fibers to transmit light through a specially designed tube

fibrinolysis a continual process of fibrin decomposition by fibrinolysin that is the normal mechanism for the removal of small fibrin clots

fibrinoplasia the formation of fibrous tissue

fibrosis synonym for fibroplasia

Fick formula (cardiac output) a formula for computing cardiac output based on knowledge of oxygen consumption and the arterial-venous oxygen content difference

Fick's law of diffusion a law for determining the rate of gaseous diffusion across biological membranes

fissures narrow clefts or slits; the lines that divide or separate the lobes of the lung glottis

fistula any tube-like passageway between two organs or between an organ and the body surface

fixed acid a titratable, nonvolatile acid representing the byproduct of protein catabolism; examples include phosphoric or sulfuric acid

fixed performance device oxygen therapy equipment that supplies inspired gases at a consistent preset oxygen concentration. Also called *high flow system*

flaccid weak or flabby; especially as applied to muscles lacking normal tone

flail chest a traumatic chest injury in which a portion of the rib cage becomes unstable due to multiple rib fractures or costochondral separation; typically, the flail region exhibits paradoxical movement during inspiration, contributing to a maldistribution of ventilation

flange a rim used to strengthen an object, to help guide it, to facilitate its attachment to another object

floppy disk a thin plastic disk, usually 3.5 inches in diameter, used for magnetic storage of computer files; also called a *diskette*

flow generator a ventilator that delivers a flow pattern that is independent of the patient's respiratory mechanics or effort

flow resistance the difference in pressure between the two points along the tube, divided by the actual flow

flow restrictor a fixed orifice; constant pressure flow metering device

flowmeter a device operated by a needle valve that controls and measures gas flow according to the principles of viscosity and density

fluid entrainment the use of the Bernoulli effect to draw a second fluid into a stream of flow

fluidics a branch of engineering in which hydrodynamic principles are incorporated into flow circuits for such purposes as switching, pressure and flow sensing, and amplification

fomite nonliving material, such as bed linens or equipment, which may transmit pathogenic organisms

Food and Drug Administration (FDA) an agency of the U.S. Department of Health and Human Services. The FDA sets standards for medical gases

foramen ovale an opening in the septum between the right and the left atria in the fetal heart. This opening provides a bypass for blood that would otherwise flow to the fetal lungs. After birth the foramen ovale functionally closes

forced expiration technique (FET) a modification of the normal cough sequence designed to facilitate clearance of bronchial secretions while minimizing the likelihood of bronchiolar collapse

forced expiratory flow at 25% ($FEF_{25\%}$ or V_{max25}) the maximum expiratory flow after 25% of the forced vital capacity has been exhaled

forced expiratory flow at 50% ($FEF_{50\%}$ or V_{max50}) the maximum expiratory flow after 50% of the forced vital capacity has been exhaled

forced expiratory flow at 75% ($FEF_{75\%}$ or V_{max75}) the maximum expiratory flow after 75% of the forced vital capacity has been exhaled

forced expiratory flow between 200 mL and 1200 mL ($FEF_{200\text{-}1200}$) a measure of the average expiratory flow during the early phase of exhalation. Specifically, it is a measure of the flow rate for the 1000 mL of expired gas immediately following the first 200 mL of expired gas. Formerly called the *maximum expiratory flow rate (MEFR)*

forced expiratory flow between 75% and 85% of the forced vital capacity ($FEF_{75\%\text{-}85\%}$) a measure of the average expiratory flow during the end of the forced vital capacity

forced expiratory flow between 25% and 75% of the forced vital capacity ($FEF_{25\%\text{-}75\%}$) a measure of the average expiratory flow during the middle half of the forced vital capacity

forced expiratory volume, half second ($FEV_{0.5}$) the maximum volume of gas that the patient can exhale during the first half of a forced vital capacity maneuver

forced expiratory volume, 1 second (FEV_1) the maximum volume of gas that the patient can exhale during the first second of the forced vital capacity maneuver

forced expiratory volume, 3 seconds (FEV_3) the maximum volume of gas that the patient can exhale during the first 3 seconds of the forced vital capacity maneuver

forced expiratory volume in 1 second ratio (%FEV_1/FVC) the percent of the measured forced vital capacity that can be exhaled in 1 second

forced inspiratory flow at 50% ($FIF_{50\%}$) the maximum inspiratory flow after 50% of the forced vital capacity has been inspired

forced vital capacity (FVC) the maximum volume of gas that the subject can exhale as forcefully and as quickly as possible

formalism the ethical viewpoint that relies on rules and principles

fractional distillation the process of separating the components of a liquid mixture according to their boiling points via the application of heat; the primary commercial process used to produce oxygen

Frank-Starling principle as a muscle fiber is stretched, the greater will be the tension the muscle fiber generates when contracted

FRC abbreviation for functional residual capacity

fremitus a tremulous vibration of the chest wall that can be auscultated or palpated during physical examination

French scale a measurement scale used commonly to size the diameter of catheters; 1 French unit equals approximately 0.33 mm

FTE abbreviation for full-time equivalent, a unit corresponding to the number of hours per week (or month or year) worked by a normal full-time employee

full ventilatory support ventilatory support modes in which the ventilator provides all the minute ventilation requirements of the patient

functional residual capacity (FRC) the total amount of gas left in the lungs after a resting expiration

fungicide an agent destructive to fungi

furosemide (Lasix) a rapid acting sulfonamide diuretic and antihypertensive agent; inhibits reabsorption of sodium and chloride in the loop of Henle, and the proximal and distal tubules; also enhances the excretion of potassium, calcium, hydrogen and bicarbonate ions; can cause hypokalemic metabolic alkalosis and hypocalcemic tetany

FVC abbreviation for forced vital capacity; the maximum volume of gas that the subject can exhale as forcefully and as quickly as possible

G

galvanometer an instrument that measures the flow of electrical current by electromagnetic action

gastric distention swelling or extension of the stomach

gastrointestinal of or pertaining to the organs of the gastrointestinal tract, from mouth to anus

gestation the period of development of the embryo and fetus from fertilization of the ovum to birth

globin the protein component of hemoglobin

glomerulonephritis an inflammation of the glomerulus of the kidney, characterized by proteinuria, hematuria, decreased urine production, and edema

glomerulus the network of vascular tufts in the nephron responsible for filtration of plasma

glossopharyngeal of or pertaining to the tongue and pharynx

glottis the variable opening between the vocal cords

glossopharyngeal of or pertaining to the tongue and pharynx

glucocorticoid an adrenocortical steroid hormone that increases glyconeogenesis, exerts an antiinflammatory effect, and influences many body functions

glutaraldehyde a high level disinfectant solution that can also be used as a sterilant

goblet cells mucus producing cells, shaped like goblets, found among the epithelial cells lining the airways

goiter a hypertrophic thyroid gland associated with abnormal thyroid function

Goodpasture's syndrome a chronic relapsing pulmonary hemosiderosis, usually associated with glomerulonephritis and characterized by a cough with hemoptysis, dyspnea, anemia, and progressive renal failure

Graham's law the law stating that the rate of diffusion of a gas through a liquid (or the alveolar-capillary membrane) is directly proportional to its solubility coefficient and inversely proportional to the square root of its density

granulocytopenia an abnormal condition of the blood, characterized by a decrease in the total number of granulocytes

granuloma a circumscribed mass of cells (mainly histiocytes) normally associated with the presence of chronic infection or inflammation

granulomatous composed of or having the characteristics of a granuloma

gravida a combining form indicating number of pregnancies, for example, gravida 2 indicates two pregnancies

ground a connection between the electrical circuit and the ground, which becomes a part of the circuit

grunting abnormal short, deep hoarse sounds in exhalation. The grunt occurs because the glottis briefly stops the flow of air, increasing intrapulmonary pressure. Grunting is most common in RDS infants where it probably helps prevent alveolar collapse

Guillain-Barré syndrome an idiopathic, peripheral polyneuritis characterized by lower extremity weakness that progresses to the upper extremities and face; may lead to flaccid paraplegia and marked respiratory muscle weakness

gynecology the branch of medicine involved in the diagnosis and treatment of diseases of the female genital tract

H

Haldane effect the influence of hemoglobin saturation with oxygen on CO_2 dissociation

half-life (in pharmacology) the time taken by the body to decrease a given concentration of a drug to half its initial level

hard copy computer output that is physically represented on paper such as graphs or printed material

hard disk a magnetic disk for storing data that can store more data than a floppy disk and access that data much more quickly; also called a *fixed disk*

Hb common abbreviation for hemoglobin

HbA abbreviation for hemoglobin A, or normal adult hemoglobin

HbCO abbreviation for carboxyhemoglobin, hemoglobin saturated with carbon monoxide

HbF abbreviation for fetal hemoglobin

health education a process of planned learning opportunities designed to enable individuals to make informed decisions about and act to promote his or her health

health maintenance organization (HMO) an organized system providing a comprehensive range of healthcare services to a voluntarily enrolled consumer population; in return for a prepaid, fixed fee, the enrollee is guaranteed a defined set of benefits

health promotion the combination of educational, organizational, economic, and environmental support necessary for behavior conducive to health; includes both disease prevention and wellness activities

health services activities designed to maintain or improve health. Includes public health services (for example, communicable disease control); environmental health services (for example, air pollution control); and personal health services (for example, diagnosis, treatment, and rehabilitation)

heat capacity the number of calories required to raise the temperature of 1 g of a substance 1° C (cgs) or 1 lb of a substance 1° F (fps); by definition, the heat capacity of water is 1 cal in the cgs system and 1 BTU in the fps system

Heimlich maneuver an emergency procedure for dislodging a bolus of food or other obstruction from the trachea to prevent asphyxiation

heliox a low density therapeutic mixture of helium with at least 20% oxygen; used in some centers to treat large airway obstruction

hematocrit a measure of the packed cell blood volume, obtained by centrifugation of a blood sample

hematogenous originating or transported in the blood

hematology the branch of medicine involved in the study of blood morphology, physiology, and pathology

hematopoiesis the normal formation and development of blood cells in the bone marrow

heme the pigmented iron-containing, nonprotein portion of the hemoglobin molecule

hemidiaphragm pertaining to the left or right dome of the diaphragm

hemithorax either the left or right side of the thorax

hemizygous vein a large vein of the lower left thoracic wall that empties into the azygous vein (trunk connecting the superior and inferior vena cavae)

hemorrhage the escape of blood from the vascular system

hemodialysis a procedure in which impurities or wastes are removed from the blood, used in treating renal insufficiency and various toxic conditions

hemodynamic monitoring the bedside collection of data on the performance of the cardiovascular system, including the assessment of both cardiac and vascular parameters

hemolysis rupture of the red blood cells

hemoptysis coughing up blood from the respiratory tract

hemostasis the termination of bleeding by mechanical or chemical means or by the complex coagulation process of the body, consisting of vasoconstriction, platelet aggregation, and thrombin and fibrin synthesis

hemothorax an accumulation of blood and fluid in the pleural space, between the parietal and visceral pleura, usually the result of trauma. Hematocrit should be greater than 50% of the serum value

Henderson-Hasselbalch equation the relationship among pH, the pKa of a buffer system, and the ratio of the concentrations of bicarbonate to dissolved CO_2

Henry's law (in physics) a law stating that the solubility of a gas in a liquid is proportional to the pressure of the gas if the temperature is constant and if the gas does not chemically react with the liquid

HEPA abbreviation for high efficiency particulate air, usually applied to air filtration devices capable of 99.99% efficacy on particulate matter down to 0.3 μm in size

HEPA filter a 'high efficiency particulate air' filtration device, usually capable of 99.99% efficacy on particulate matter down to 0.3 μm in size

hepatomegaly an abnormal enlargement of the liver that is usually a sign of disease

Hering-Breuer inflation reflex a parasympathetic inflation reflex mediated via the lung's stretch receptors that appears to influence the duration of the expiratory pause occurring between breaths

herniation a protrusion of a body organ or portion of an organ through an abnormal opening in a membrane

herpes any inflammatory disease caused by a herpesvirus, especially herpes zoster or herpes simplex

heterodisperse referring to an aerosol consisting of particles of varying diameters and sizes

hexachlorophene a topical bacteriocide and detergent

HFJV abbreviation for *high frequency jet ventilation*; a mode of ventilatory support in which small pulses of pressurized gas are delivered through a catheter at rates between 100-200/minute

HFO abbreviation for *high frequency oscillation*; a mode of ventilatory support characterized by very high rates (up to 3600/minute)

HFPPV abbreviation for *high frequency positive pressure* ventilation

HFV abbreviation for *high frequency ventilation*

HHA abbreviation for home health agency; a public or private provider of home healthcare services, usually regulated by state departments of health; HHAs can provide a broad range of services, including the provision of home health aids, nursing care, and rehabilitative personnel

HHb symbol for reduced (deoxygenated) hemoglobin

high flow system oxygen therapy equipment that supplies inspired gases at a consistent preset oxygen concentration (see also fixed performance device)

high frequency chest wall compression (HFCC) a mechanical technique for augmenting secretion clearance; small gas volumes are alternately injected into and withdrawn from a vest by an air-pulse generator at a fast rate, creating an oscillatory motion against the patient's thorax

high frequency jet ventilation (HFJV) a mode of ventilatory support in which small pulses of pressurized gas are delivered through a catheter at rates between 100-200/minute

high frequency oscillation (HFO) a mode of ventilatory support characterized by very high rates (up to 3600/minute or 60 Hz)

high frequency positive pressure ventilation (HFPPV) a mode of ventilatory support with rates between 60-100/minute and small tidal volumes often approaching anatomic dead space

high frequency ventilation (HFV) ventilatory support provided at rates significantly higher than normal breathing frequencies. See also HFPPV, HFJV, HFO

hilum the vertical opening(s) on either side of the mediastinum through which all the airways and pulmonary vessels pass

histoplasmosis an infection caused by inhalation of spores of the fungus Histoplasma capsulatum

histotoxic hypoxia hypoxia due to chemical poisoning of the cells, as by cyanide, which occurs in the presence of normal oxygen delivery to the tissues

HIV abbreviation for the *human immunodeficiency virus*, the cause of AIDS

HME abbreviation for *heat and moisture exchanger*; a passive device used to humidify and warm the inspired air of patients receiving ventilatory support

HMO abbreviation for *health maintenance organization*; an organized system providing a comprehensive range of healthcare services to a voluntarily enrolled consumer population; in return for a prepaid, fixed fee, the enrollee is guaranteed a defined set of benefits

holistic of or pertaining to the whole; in healthcare, a philosophy whereby the person is viewed in totality as a mental, physical, and emotional being interacting with the environment

home healthcare the provision of health services in the home setting to aged, disabled, sick, or convalescent individuals who do not need institutional care

homeostasis a relative constancy in the internal environment of the body, naturally maintained by adaptive responses that promote healthy survival

homogenous of uniform structure or composition

host (computer) the primary or controlling computer that directs the operations of a group of other computers; or a central information system or database that can be accessed by multiple users

HTML abbreviation for *hypertext markup language*, the text-based language used to construct Web pages and interpreted by Web browsers

HTTP abbreviation for *hypertext transmission protocol*, the Internet protocol used to transmit Web pages

huff cough a type of forced expiration with an open glottis to replace coughing when pain limits normal coughing

humidifier a device that adds molecular water to gas

humidity water in molecular vapor form; absolute humidity is a measure of the actual content or weight of water present in a given volume of air; relative humidity is the ratio of actual water vapor present in a gas to the capacity of the gas to hold the vapor at a given temperature

humidity deficit the difference in water vapor content between inspired air and the saturated gas conditions present in the lungs

humoral of or pertaining to the body fluids; used especially to denote physiological activity occurring via chemical or biological mediators in the body fluids (as opposed to neurological stimulation)

hydrostatic relating to the pressure of fluids or to their properties when in equilibrium

hydrostatic pressure pressure due to the weight of fluid; related to the volume of fluid in a container and the effects of gravity

hydrothorax a noninflammatory accumulation of serous fluid in one or both pleural cavities

hygrometer an instrument that directly measures relative humidity of the atmosphere or the proportion of water in a specific gas or gas mixture, without extracting the moisture

hygroscopic attracting or absorbing moisture from the air

hyperalimentation overfeeding or the ingestion or administration of a greater-than-optimal amount of nutrients in excess of the demands of the appetite

hyperbaric oxygen therapy the therapeutic application of oxygen at pressures greater than 1 atmosphere (1 atm or 760 torr). Also called *hyperbaric oxygenation*

hyperbasemia the abnormal presence of an excess of total buffer base in the blood; a base excess (BE)> +2.0

hyperbilirubinemia greater-than-normal amounts of the bile pigment bilirubin in the blood, often characterized by jaundice, anorexia, and malaise

hypercalcemia greater-than-normal amounts of calcium in the blood, most often resulting from excessive bone resorption and release of calcium, as occurs in hyperparathyroidism, metastatic tumors of bone, Paget's disease, and osteoporosis

hypercapnia the abnormal presence of excess amounts of carbon dioxide in the blood (in arterial blood, a P_{CO_2} greater than 45 torr)

hypercapnic respiratory failure the inability to maintain the normal removal of carbon dioxide from the tissues. It may be indicated by a Pa_{CO_2} of more than 50 torr in an otherwise healthy individual (also called *ventilatory failure*)

hyperchloremia an excessive level of chloride in the blood

hyperextension a position of maximum extension

hyperglycemia an abnormal increase in serum glucose

hyperinflation a condition of maximum inflation; as pertaining to artificial ventilatory support, the application of volumes greater than normal to reinflate collapsed alveoli

hyperkalemia greater-than-normal amounts of potassium in the blood

hyperlucent extremely clear or transparent; as applied to x-rays, allowing easy x-ray penetration and thus appearing black on the negative film

hypermagnesemia an elevated level of magnesium ($Mg^{+}+$) in the blood

hypernatremia greater-than-normal concentration of sodium in the blood, caused by excessive loss of water and electrolytes owing to polyuria, diarrhea, excessive sweating, or inadequate water intake

hyperosmolarity a state of condition of abnormally increased osmolarity in the blood or body fluids

hyperoxia a condition of abnormally high oxygen tension in the blood

hyperoxygenation the application of oxygen concentrations in excess of those needed to maintain adequate oxygenation in order to prevent hypoxemia during certain procedures such as suctioning

hyperphosphatemia greater-than-normal concentration of phosphate ions in the blood

hyperplastic of or pertaining to a condition of hyperplasia

hyperpnea deep breathing

hyperpyrexia an extremely elevated temperature sometimes occurring in acute infectious diseases, especially in young children

hypersensitivity of or pertaining to a tendency of the immune system to exhibit an excessive or exaggerated response against environmental antigens that are not normally harmful

hypersensitivity pneumonitis an inflammatory form of interstitial pneumonia that results from an immunologic reaction in a hypersensitive person. The reaction may be provoked by a variety of inhaled organic dusts, often those containing fungal spores. The disease can be prevented by avoiding contact with the causative agents. Also called *extrinsic allergic alveolitis*

hypersomnolence a condition characterized by pathologically excessive drowsiness or sleep

hypertension persistently high blood pressure

hyperthyroidism a condition characterized by hyperactivity of the thyroid gland

hypertonic having a greater concentration of solute than another solution, hence exerting more osmotic pressure than that solution, as a hypertonic saline solution that contains more salt than is found in body fluids

hypertrophy an increase in the size of a tissue or organ due to a growth in the size of cells present

hyperventilation ventilation in excess of that necessary to meet metabolic needs; signified by a P_{CO_2} less than 35 torr in the arterial blood

hypervolemia an increase in the amount of extracellular fluid, particularly in the volume of circulating blood or its components

hypnotic a drug or chemical agent that induces sleep

hypobasemia the abnormal presence of a deficit of total buffer base in the blood; a negative base excess (BE) < −2.0

hypocalcemia a deficiency of calcium in the serum that may be caused by hypoparathyroidism, vitamin D deficiency, kidney failure, acute pancreatitis, or inadequate plasma magnesium and protein

hypocapnia the presence of lower-than-normal amounts of carbon dioxide in the blood (in arterial blood, a P_{CO_2} < 35 torr)

hypochloremia a decrease in the chloride level in the blood serum below the normal range

hypoglycemia a less-than-normal amount of glucose in the blood, usually caused by administration of too much insulin, excessive secretion of insulin by the islet cells of the pancreas, or by dietary deficiency (normal blood glucose levels range from 70 to 105 mg/dL)

hypokalemia a condition in which an inadequate amount of potassium, the major intracellular cation, is found in the circulating bloodstream

hypomagnesia a low level of magnesium ($Mg^{+}+$) in the blood

hyponatremia a less-than-normal concentration of sodium in the blood, caused by inadequate excretion of water or by excessive water in the circulating bloodstream

hypopharynx the lower portion of the airway between the epiglottis and larynx

hypophosphatemia a low level of phosphate ion in the blood

hypopnea shallow breathing

hypotension an abnormal condition in which the blood pressure is not adequate for normal perfusion and oxygenation of the tissues

hypothalamus a portion of the brain lying beneath the thalamus and at the base of the cerebrum; responsible for temperature regulation, certain behavioral functions, and the secretory activities of the pituitary gland

hypothermia an abnormal and dangerous condition in which the temperature of the body is below 32° C, usually caused by prolonged exposure to cold

hypothyroidism a condition characterized by decreased activity of the thyroid gland

hypotonia a condition characterized by decreased muscle tone or strength

hypotonic having a tonicity less than normal saline (0.9% NaCl)

hypoventilation ventilation less than that necessary to meet metabolic needs; signified by a P_{CO_2} greater 45 mm Hg in the arterial blood

hypovolemia an abnormally low circulating blood volume

hypoxemia an abnormal deficiency of oxygen in the arterial blood

hypoxemic respiratory failure the inability to maintain the normal delivery of oxygen to the tissues. It may be indicated by a Pa_{O_2} of less than 60 mm Hg in an otherwise healthy individual breathing supplemental oxygen

hypoxia an abnormal condition in which the oxygen available to the body cells is inadequate to meet their metabolic needs

hysteresis the failure of two associated phenomena to coincide, as in the observed difference between the inflation and deflation volume-pressure curves of the lung

Hz symbol for Hertz, a physical term meaning cycles per second

I

iatrogenic caused by treatment of diagnostic procedures

ICP abbreviation for intracranial pressure

idiopathic without known cause

idiopathic pulmonary fibrosis the formation of scar tissue in the connective tissue of the lungs without known cause

I:E ratio inspiratory-expiratory time ratio; the relationship between the inspiratory and expiratory time provided during positive pressure ventilation. Also symbolized as $t_I{:}t_E$

IEEE abbreviation for the Institute of Electrical and Electronic Engineers, a voluntary group responsible, in part, for developing standards related to electrical devices and equipment, including those used in respiratory care

ileus an obstruction of the intestines, as a dynamic ileus caused by immobility of the bowel, or a mechanical ileus in which the intestine is blocked by mechanical means

ILV abbreviation for independent lung ventilation, a mode of ventilation in which each lung receives a different level or type of support

immunocompromised immunodeficient

immunocompromised host an immunodeficient patient highly susceptible to infection

immunodeficient pertaining to conditions in which a patient's cellular or humoral immunity is inadequate and resistance to infection is decreased

immunoglobulin (immunoglobin) any five structurally and antigenically distinct antibodies present in the serum and external secretions of the body and formed in response to specific antigens

immunosuppressed of or pertaining to the purposeful administration of agents designed to interfere with the ability of the immune system to respond to antigenic stimulation

impedance (electrical) a form of electrical resistance observed in an alternating circuit expressed as the ratio of voltage applied to current produced

impedance (mechanical) the force opposing movement in a mechanical system; as applied to ventilatory mechanics, the sum of the resistive and elastic forces opposing inflation

IMV abbreviation for intermittent mandatory ventilation; periodic ventilation with positive pressure, with the patient breathing spontaneously between breaths. These periodic breaths may be either time-triggered (control mode IMV) or patient-triggered (synchronous intermittent mandatory ventilation, or SIMV)

in situ in the natural or usual place

incisura a cut, notch, indentation, or depression; often used to refer to the dicrotic notch observed on the tracing of arterial blood pressure

indirect calorimetry the measurement of the amount of energy a body consumes (in kcal) by determining the consumption of oxygen and production of carbon dioxide

induration hardening of tissue, particularly the skin

indwelling located inside the body; commonly refers to invasive diagnostic or therapeutic devices

inert not taking part in chemical reactions; not pharmacologically active

inertial impaction the deposition of particles by collision with a surface; the primary mechanism for pulmonary deposition of particles over 5 mm in diameter

in-exsufflator a mechanical device that provides an artificial cough by alternately applying positive pressure and negative pressure to the airway

infarction the development and formation of a localized area of tissue necrosis

infiltrate a fluid that passes through body tissues

inflammable the property of igniting and burning easily and rapidly. Also called *flammable*

inflation hold maneuver a mechanical breath maneuver that momentarily holds the delivered volume in the lungs under static conditions. An inflation hold may also be used to estimate total compliance and inspiration airway resistance

inflation reflex a vagal response that limits or modulates the pattern of breathing

influenza an acute, usually self-limiting infectious viral disorder that produces fever, myalgia, headache, and malaise

informed consent a general principle of law that states that health professionals have a duty to disclose what a reasonably prudent health professional in the medical community in the exercise of reasonable care would disclose to a patient as to whatever grave risks of injury might be incurred from a proposed course of treatment

infrared light electromagnetic radiation with wavelengths between 10^{-5} and 10^{-4} m; infrared radiation is perceived as heat when it strikes the body

infrastructure pertaining to physical facilities and associated structures; for example, buildings, parking decks, and power-generating stations

inguinal of or pertaining to the groin

inherent rhythmicity the unique ability of cardiac muscle to spontaneously originate an electrical impulse; also called *automaticity*

innominate without a name; commonly refers to the innominate artery, also called the *brachiocephalic trunk*

inotropic pertaining to the force or energy of muscular contractions, particularly contractions of the heart muscle

insensible water loss the loss of body fluids by means other than through the urinary system, gastrointestinal tract, or sweating; includes evaporative water loss through the lungs and skin

insomnia inability to sleep

inspiratory capacity (IC) the maximum amount of air that can be inhaled from the resting end-expiratory level or FRC; the sum of the tidal volume and inspiratory reserve volume

inspiratory-expiratory (I:E) time ratio the relationship between the inspiratory and expiratory time provided during positive pressure ventilation. Also symbolized as t_I:t_E

inspiratory reserve volume (IRV) the maximum volume of air that can be inhaled following a normal quiet inspiration

inspiratory resistance inhalation against some type of resisting force, such as abdominal breathing practice with the Pflex or threshold inspiratory muscle trainer

inspissated (of a fluid) thickened or hardened through the absorption or evaporation of the liquid portion, as can occur with respiratory secretion when the upper airway is bypassed

instill to introduce a fluid into a body cavity or passage

insufflation blowing of a gas or powder into a tube, cavity, or organ to allow visual examination, to remove an obstruction, or to apply medication

intercostal of or pertaining to the space between two ribs

intercostals referring to the muscle groups between the ribs

interface the means of connection between electronic devices or between an electronic device and a human

intermittent mandatory ventilation (IMV) a mode of mechanical ventilatory support in which the patient receives a preset number of machine breaths per minute set by time. The patient is allowed to breath spontaneously as often as desired in between machine breaths. Depending on the base rate, IMV can provide partial or full ventilatory support

internal oblique abdominal muscle group that functions as an accessory muscle of ventilation

International Standards Organization (ISO) a nongovernmental agency that sets standards for various technical equipment and procedures

Internet a global network of computer networks using TCP/IP protocols to communicate with each other

interstitial of or pertaining to the interstitium

interstitial fluid fluid between cells but outside of the vascular spaces

interstitial lung disease a respiratory disorder characterized by a dry, unproductive cough and dyspnea on exertion. X-ray films usually show fibrotic infiltrates in the lung tissue, usually in the lower lobes

interstitium the extracellular space

interventricular of or pertaining to the space between the ventricles of the heart

intervertebral of or pertaining to the space between any two vertebrae, as the fibrocartilaginous discs

intraabdominal within the abdomen

intraalveolar within the alveoli

intraaortic balloon counterpulsation a circulatory support technique in which a balloon placed in the aorta is synchronously inflated during diastole in order to increase mean aortic pressures and coronary blood flow to the myocardium

intracardiac within the heart

intracellular within cells

intracranial with the cranium

intractable having no relief, as a symptom or disease that remains unrelieved despite the application of therapeutic measures

intramuscular within a muscle; used commonly to refer to an injection method whereby a hypodermic needle is introduced into a muscle to administer a medication

intraoperative within or during a surgical procedure

intrapartum of or pertaining to the period commencing from the onset of labor to the completion of the third stage of labor (expulsion of the placenta)

intrapleural within the pleural 'space'

intrapulmonary within the lungs; often used to refer to alveolar pressure (Palv)

intrapulmonary percussive ventilation (IPV) an airway clearance technique that uses a pneumatic device to deliver a series of pressurized gas minibursts at high rates (1.6 to 3.75 Hz) to the respiratory tract, usually via a mouthpiece; usually combined with aerosolized bronchodilator therapy

intrathoracic within the thorax

intrauterine within the uterus

intravascular within a blood vessel or in the vascular fluid compartment

intravenous (IV) within a vein; usually describing a method for infusing fluids and drugs

intubation the passage of a tube into a body aperture; commonly refers to the insertion of an endotracheal tube within the trachea

intrinsic PEEP (iPEEP) the inadvertent build up of positive pressure in the alveoli due to incomplete exhalation of the inhaled volume. Also called *auto-PEEP*

in utero in the uterus

invasive characterized by a tendency to spread or infiltrate; also refers to the use of diagnostic or therapeutic methods requiring access to the inside of the body

in vitro (of a biological reaction) occurring in a laboratory apparatus

in vivo (of a biological reaction) occurring in a living organism

I/O abbreviation for intake and output; the recording of a patient's fluid intake and output; may also refer to computer input/output

iodophor an antiseptic or disinfectant that combines iodine with another agent

IPPB abbreviation for intermittent positive pressure breathing; the application of inspiratory positive pressure, usually with accompanying humidity or aerosol therapy, to a spontaneously breathing patient as a short-term treatment modality, usually for periods of time not exceeding 15 to 20 minutes

IPPV common abbreviation for intermittent positive pressure ventilation, a general term for ventilatory support using positive pressure

irritant receptors vagal sensory sites that respond to irritation of the airways

ischemia a localized reduction in perfusion to a body organ or part, often marked by pain and organ dysfunction, as in ischemic heart disease

isolation precautions safeguards designed to prevent the spread of infectious agents among patients, personnel, and visitors. Isolation precautions may be disease-specific or categorical (grouping diseases that require similar isolation precautions)

isolation protocols infection control measures that combine barrier-type precautions (include handwashing and the use of gloves, masks, and/or gowns) with the physical separation of infected patients in specific disease categories in order to disrupt transmission of pathogenic microorganisms

isothermal a process of gas compression or expansion in which the gas temperature remains constant; heat energy must be either added (during expansion) or taken away (during compression) to maintain the energy equilibrium; compare with adiabatic

isothermic saturation boundary (ISB) the point at which inspired gas becomes fully saturated to 100% relative humidity at body temperature

isotonic (of a solution) having the same concentration of solute as another solution, hence exerting the same amount of osmotic pressure as that solution, as an isotonic saline solution that contains an amount of salt equal to that found in the extracellular fluid

isovolumic having the same volume

IT abbreviation for implantation tested; as applied to invasive devices, indicates that the materials used have been shown nontoxic to living tissue

IV abbreviation for intravenous; within a vein

J

J receptors vagal sensory sites that are located in the alveolar units; so named because they are found primarily in 'juxtaposition' to the pulmonary capillaries

jargon the special technical language and terms of a particular field or profession

jaundice a yellow discoloration of the skin, mucous membranes, and eyes due to high tissue level of bilirubin

JCAHO abbreviation for Joint Commission on Accreditation of Health Care Organizations, a private, voluntary association that establishes standards for accrediting institutions and agencies responsible for healthcare delivery

Joint Commission on Accreditation of Health Care Organizations (JCAHO) a private nongovernmental agency that establishes guidelines for the operation of hospitals and other healthcare facilities, conducts accreditation programs and surveys, and encourages the attainment of high standards of institutional medical care in the United States

justice a principle of fair and equal treatment for all, with due reward and honor

juxtamedullary situated near the medulla

K

Karvonen's formula a simple formula used to set a target heart rate for patient exercise

ketoacidosis a metabolic acidosis due to the accumulation of excess ketones in the body, resulting from faulty carbohydrate metabolism, as can occur in certain forms of diabetes

kilobyte (Kb) a unit of computer data equal to 1024 bytes

kinetic energy the energy a body possesses by virtue of its motion

Korotkoff sound sounds heard during the taking of blood pressure using a sphygmomanometer and stethoscope

Kussmaul's respiration hyperpnea associated with diabetic ketoacidosis

kwashiorkor protein-energy malnutrition due to the stress of disease and the resulting increase in catabolic rate

kyphoscoliosis an abnormal condition characterized by an anteroposterior and lateral curvature of the spine

kyphosis an abnormal condition of the vertebral column, characterized by increased anteroposterior convex curvature of the thoracic spine

L

lactate an anion of lactic acid

Lambert-Eaton syndrome a disorder of neuromuscular conduction commonly associated with an underlying malignancy that leads to muscle weakness often with sensory deficits that can often be improved by repetitive muscle contraction against pressure

laminar flow a pattern of flow consisting of concentric layers of fluid flowing parallel to the tube wall at linear velocities that increase toward the center

LAN abbreviation for local area network

LaPlace formula a principle of physics that the tension on the wall of a sphere is the product of the pressure times the radius of the chamber

laryngectomy a surgical removal of the larynx, performed to treat cancer of the larynx

laryngitis inflammation of the larynx

laryngoscope an endoscope for examining the larynx

laryngoscopy the process of viewing the larynx with a laryngoscope

laryngospasm an involuntary contraction of the laryngeal muscles resulting in complete or partial closure of the glottis

laryngotracheobronchitis an inflammation of the larynx, trachea, and large bronchi that can result in hoarseness, a nonproductive cough, and dyspnea. Also referred to as croup.

laryngotracheitis inflammation of the larynx and trachea

lateral away from the body midline; situated on the side

lateral decubitus a side-lying position (either left or right)

lavage the washing or irrigation of an organ, such as the stomach or lung

law of continuity the velocity of a fluid moving through a tube and constant flow varies inversely with the available cross-sectional area

LED abbreviation for light-emitting diode; an electronic component that emits light when exposed to current flow

length of stay (LOS) a measure pertaining to the number of elapsed days between a patient's admission and their discharge from an inpatient healthcare facility

lesion a general term referring to any injury or pathological change in body tissue

leukocyte a white blood cell, one of the formed elements of the circulating blood system

leukocytosis an abnormal increase in the number of circulating white blood cells

leukocytopenia an abnormal decrease in white blood cells

LGA abbreviation for large for gestational age; pertaining to newborn infants whose body weight falls above the 90th percentile for their gestational age

liability a legal obligation or responsibility

libel a false accusation written, printed, or typewritten, or presented in a picture or a sign that is made with malicious intent to defame the reputation of a person who is living or the memory of a person who is dead, resulting in public embarrassment, contempt, ridicule, or hatred

licensure the granting of permission by a competent authority (usually a governmental agency) to an organization or individual to engage in a specific practice or activity

lingula the lower division of the left upper lobe that corresponds developmentally to the right middle lobe

LFPPV-ECCO$_2$R acronym for *low-frequency positive-pressure ventilation with extracorporeal carbon dioxide removal;* a mode of ventilatory support designed to minimize the harmful effects of conventional mechanical ventilation

lobectomy a type of chest surgery in which a lobe of a lung is excised, performed to remove a malignant tumor and to treat uncontrolled bronchiectasis, trauma with hemorrhage, or intractable tuberculosis

lobes the major divisions of the lungs; the right lung has three lobes and the left lung two lobes

lobule literally a small lobe; in pulmonary anatomy may refer to the primary lobule or terminal respiratory unit of the lung (also called the *acinus*), or the secondary lobule; the secondary lobule is the smallest gross anatomical unit of lung tissue set apart by true connective tissue septa and corresponds to clusters of from three to five primary lobules

logarithm a number system founded on exponential relationships using a base value such as 10 or e (the natural log)

long-term care the provision of medical, social, and/or personal care services on a recurring or continuing basis to persons with chronic physical or mental disorders

lordotic pertaining to a radiographic position in which the patient stands with his or her back toward the film and leans backward, such that only the shoulders, neck, and head touch the film; this positions the x-ray beam at an angle ideal for viewing the lung apices without obstruction by the normally superimposed shadows of the clavicles

low-flow system a variable performance oxygen therapy device that delivers oxygen at a flow that provides only a portion of the patient's inspired gas needs. Also called *variable performance system*

lower respiratory tract infection any infectious disease of the left and right bronchi and the alveoli

lumen a cavity within any organ or structure of the body, or a channel in a tube or catheter

lung abscess an inflammatory lesion resulting in necrosis of lung tissue and associated with one or more of the following: suppression of the cough reflex, aspiration of infected material, bronchial obstruction, pneumonias, ischemia, as with pulmonary infarction, or blood sepsis

lung cancer a pulmonary malignancy attributable in the majority of cases to cigarette smoking. Epidermoid cancers and adenocarcinomas each account for approximately 30% of lung tumors, about 25% are small or oat-cell carcinomas, and 15% are large-cell anaplastic cancers

lupus erythematosus a chronic, superficial inflammation of the skin in which reddish lesions or macules up to 3 to 4 cm in size spread over the body

LVEDP abbreviation for left ventricular end-diastolic pressure

lymphadenopathy of or pertaining to a disease of the lymph nodes; refers also to the visualization of enlarged lymph nodes on x-ray

lymphocytosis an increase in blood lymphocytes

M

macrophage any phagocytic cell of the reticuloendothelial system

macroshock a shock from an electrical current of 1 mA or greater that is applied externally to the skin

malignant tending to become worse; as applied to tumors, having the property of metastasis

malpractice (in law) professional negligence that is the proximate cause of injury or harm to a patient, resulting from a lack of professional knowledge, experience, or skill that can be expected in others in the profession or from a failure to exercise reasonable care or judgment in the application of professional knowledge, experience, or skill

mandatory breath a ventilatory support breath either initiated or ended by the machine

mandatory minute volume ventilation (MMV) a variation of the IMV mode of ventilatory support in which the ventilator keeps the total minute volume constant

manifold a pipe with many connections; in medical gas storage, a collection of gas cylinders linked together for purposes of bulk storage, and usually including at least one reserve bank and other safety systems, such as low pressure alarms

MAO abbreviation for monoamine oxidase, an enzyme that catalyzes the oxidation of amines

MAO inhibitor any of a chemically heterogeneous group of drugs used primarily in the treatment of depression or anxiety, and sometimes hypertension; MAO inhibitors may interact with a variety of foods and indirect acting adrenergics such as ephedrine, causing severe hypertensive episodes

manubrium the upper triangular portion of the sternum

marasmus protein-energy malnutrition due to starvation

mass spectrometry an analytic method for assessing the concentration of gas mixtures based on their separation by molecular weight

mast cells cells located in the airways that release potent vasoactive substances when stimulated

maxillary of or pertaining to the maxilla, or upper jaw

maxillofacial of or pertaining to the upper jaw, nose, and cheek

maximum expiratory pressure (MEP) a measure of the output of the expiratory muscles against a maximum stimulus, measured in cm H_2O positive pressure

maximum inspiratory pressure (MIP) a measure of the output of the inspiratory muscles against a maximum stimulus, measured in cm H_2O negative pressure. Also known as *negative inspiratory force (NIF)* or *maximum inspiratory force (MIF)*

maximum voluntary ventilation (MVV) the maximum volume of air in liters per minute that a subject can breathe during a 12 to 15 second period. It is a very patient-dependent test. Formerly called the *maximum breathing capacity (MBC)*

MDI abbreviation for metered dose inhaler; a pressurized cartridge used for self-administration of exact dosages of aerosolized drugs

MDR-TB acronym for multiple drug resistant tuberculosis

meconium a material that collects in the intestines of a fetus and forms the first stools of a newborn

meconium aspiration syndrome the inhalation of meconium by the fetus or newborn. It can block the air passages and cause failure of the lungs to expand

medial situated or oriented toward the midline of the body

mediastinoscopy a diagnostic procedure whereby a device is inserted into the mediastinum for purposes of visualization or biopsy

mediastinum a portion of the thoracic cavity lying in the middle of the thorax (between the two pleural cavities). It extends from the vertebral column to the sternum and contains the trachea, esophagus, heart, and great vessels of the circulatory system

medulla the most internal part of an organ or structure; for example, medulla oblongata, the bulbous portion of the spinal cord just above the foramen magnum that contains the cardiac, respiratory, and vasomotor 'centers'

megabyte (Mb) a unit of computer data equivalent to 1024 kilobytes, or approximately 1 million bytes

megahertz (MHz) a measure of the frequency of wave cycles; 1 million cycles per second

MEP abbreviation for maximum expiratory pressure; a measure of the output of the expiratory muscles against a maximum stimulus, as measured in cm H_2O positive pressure

mesothelioma a rare malignant tumor of the mesothelium of the pleura or peritoneum, associated with earlier exposure to asbestos

metabolic acidosis nonrespiratory processes resulting in acidemia

metabolic alkalosis nonrespiratory processes resulting in alkalemia

metastasis the process by which tumor cells are spread to distant parts of the body

metered dose inhaler (MDI) a pressurized cartridge used for self-administration of exact dosages of aerosolized drugs

methemoglobin an abnormal form of hemoglobin in which the iron component has been oxidized from the ferrous to the ferric state

methemoglobinemia an abnormal condition characterized by high levels of methemoglobin in the blood and thus a reduction in oxygen-carrying capacity; may be caused by nitrite poisoning or ingestion of a certain oxidizing agent or a genetic defect in the enzyme NADH methemoglobin reductase (an autosomal dominant trait)

methylxanthine a category of naturally occurring drug agents (including caffeine and theophylline) that exert a broad range of physiological effects, including CNS and myocardial stimulation, smooth muscle relaxation, and diuresis; used commonly in respiratory care as bronchodilators or respiratory stimulants

METS abbreviation for the multiple equivalents of resting O_2 consumption, an indirect measure of physiological work performed during exercise and stress testing

microaerosol an extremely fine aerosol of uniform and small particle size produced by sequential baffling and characterized by mass median diameters that are generally less than 1.0 μm

microampere (μA) a unit of electrical current equivalent to 1 millionth (10^{-6}) ampere (an ampere in the current produced by 1 volt applied across a resistance of 1 ohm)

microatelectasis localized or focal atelectasis that may not manifest itself on radiographic examination

microembolization embolization due to extremely small bloodborne particles, usually smaller than that visible with the naked eye

micrognathia underdevelopment of the jaw, especially the mandible

microshock a shock from a usually imperceptible electrical current (< 1 milliampere) that is allowed to bypass the skin and follow a direct, low-resistance pathway into the body

midaxillary of or pertaining to the imaginary line drawn vertically downward from the middle of the axilla

midclavicular of or pertaining to the imaginary line drawn vertically downward from the middle of the clavicle

midline an imaginary line that divides the body into right and left halves

midscapular of or pertaining to the imaginary line draw vertically downward from the middle of the scapula

midsternal of or pertaining to the imaginary line vertically bisecting the sternum

milliequivalent (mEq) a quantitative amount of a reacting substance that has a specific chemical combining power; 1 mEq equals the gram atomic weight of a substance divided by its valence × 0.001

millimole an SI unit of matter equal to one-thousandth of a mole (a mole is any quantity of matter that contains 6.023×10^{23} atoms, molecules, or ions)

millivolt (mV) one-thousandth of a volt

MIP abbreviation for maximum inspiratory pressure, the negative pressure generated during a maximally forced inspiratory effort against an obstruction to flow; also called *negative inspiratory force (NIF)* and *PImax*

misallocation the process of prescribing diagnostic or treatment services when not indicated, consisting both of "over-ordering" and "under-ordering" services

mitosis the process whereby a cell normally replicates itself, forming two daughter cells, each with the same number of chromosomes as the parent cell

MLT abbreviation for minimal leak technique, a method for determining the cuff inflation volume on endotracheal tubes; during MLT, air is slowly injected into the cuff until the leak stops; once a seal is obtained, a small amount of air is removed, allowing a slight leak at peak inflation pressure

MMV abbreviation for mandatory minute ventilation; a mode of ventilatory support. MMV ensures delivery of a preset minimum minute volume, with the patient allowed to breathe spontaneously

modem MOdulator-DEMolulator, a device that uses modulation to convert a digital signal to an analog signal for transmission across a standard telephone line

modified Allen test the most common technique to determine the adequacy of ulnar circulation

MODS abbreviation for multiple organ dysfunction syndrome

mole the SI unit of matter containing 6.023×10^{23} atoms, molecules, or ions

molecular sieve a crystalline chemical separation device with molecular size pores that adsorbs small but not large molecules

monodisperse referring to an aerosol in which particles are of uniform size

morbidity the state of being ill; in statistics, the ratio of those ill to those who are well

morphology the study of structures and forms in living things

mortality the number of deaths per unit population in any specific age group, disease category, region, or other classification, usually expressed as deaths per 1000, 10,000, or 100,000

mottling a condition of spotting with patches of color

MOV abbreviation for minimal occluding volume; the minimum endotracheal tube cuff pressure needed to prevent gas leakage during a positive pressure inspiration

MSVC abbreviation for maximum sustainable ventilatory capacity

mucociliary of or pertaining to ciliated mucosa

mucoid resembling mucus

mucokinesis the process of moving mucus, that is, therapeutic methods designed to aid in removal of excess or abnormal secretion of the respiratory tract

mucolysis the breaking down of mucus; usually refers to chemical degradation of mucopolysaccharide by certain drug agents called *mucolytics*

mucolytic a drug agent capable of mucolysis

mucopolysaccharide any one of a group of polysaccharides containing hexosamine and being the chief constituent of normal mucus

mucoprotein a compound, present in all connective and supporting tissue, that contains polysaccharides combined with protein and is relatively resistant to denaturation

mucopurulent characteristic of a combination of mucus and pus

mucosa the upper layer of tissue lining the airways, including the mucous blanket, epithelium, and lamina propria

multiple equivalents of resting O_2 consumption (METS) an indirect measure of physiological work performed during exercise and stress testing

multiple organ dysfunction syndrome (MODS) a condition in which dysfunction of many different organs occurs, usually accompanying acute lung injury

muscle fatigue condition involving a loss of the capacity to develop force and/or velocity of a muscle resulting from muscle activity overload, which is reversible by rest

myasthenia gravis a disorder of neuromuscular conduction that leads to muscle weakness of the skeletal muscles, particularly those of the face, throat, and respiratory system. Weakness and respiratory failure can occur rapidly as muscle strength decreases with repetitive contraction against a load

Mycobacteria acid-fast microorganisms belonging to the genus *Mycobacterium*

Mycoplasma a genus of ultramicroscopic pleomorphic organisms that lack rigid cell walls, grow on artificial media but do not retain the Gram stain, and are able to pass through bacterial filters; a cause of atypical pneumonia

mycoses any disease caused by fungi

mydriasis dilation of the pupil of the eye

myocardial infarction occlusion of a coronary artery resulting in distal myocardial tissue necrosis, often accompanied by significant complications

myocarditis an inflammatory condition of the myocardium caused by viral, bacterial, or fungal infection, serum sickness, rheumatic fever, or chemical agents, or as a complication of a collagen disease

myopathy an abnormal condition of skeletal muscle leading to muscle weakness, wasting, and histologic changes in the muscle tissue, as seen in any of the muscular dystrophies

myxedema a severe form of hypothyroidism characterized by dry swelling and abnormal deposits of mucin in the tissues

myxoma a connective tissue neoplasm that often grows to enormous size

N

nano (n) the prefix used in the metric system for billionths. A nanosecond is one billionth of a second

narcolepsy an idiopathic syndrome characterized by sudden sleep attacks

nasal flaring dilation of the alar nasi on inspiration; an early sign of an increase in ventilatory demands and the work of breathing, especially in infants

nasogastric of or pertaining to the passageway from the nose to the stomach; usually applied to tubes or catheters placed in the stomach through the nose

nasopharynx the upper portion of the airway behind the nasal and oral cavities

nasotracheal of or pertaining to the passageway from the nose to the trachea; usually applied to tubes or catheters placed in the trachea through the nose, such as a nasotracheal tube, or nasotracheal suctioning

National Board of Respiratory Care (NBRC) the national credentialing agency for respiratory care practitioners and pulmonary function technologists

National Fire Protection Agency (NFPA) an agency involved in improved methods of fire protection and prevention, including creating standards for the storage of flammable and oxidizing gases

NBRC abbreviation for the *National Board of Respiratory Care;* the national credentialing agency for respiratory care practitioners and pulmonary function technologists

nebulization the production of an aerosol suspension of liquid particles in a gaseous medium using baffling to control particle size

nebulizer a device that produces an aerosol suspension of liquid particles in a gaseous medium using baffling to control particle size

necrosis local tissue death due to disease or injury

necrotizing pertaining to a process that produces necrosis

needle-capping device a safety device used to prevent or minimize needle stick injuries when capping a syringe needle (as required after blood gas sampling)

NEEP acronym for negative end-expiratory pressure

negative end-expiratory pressure (NEEP) the application of subatmospheric pressure to the airway during the expiratory phase of positive pressure ventilation

negative inotropism a decrease in the contractility of the heart

negligence the omission to do something that a reasonable person, guided by those ordinary considerations, would do

neonatal pertaining to the period between birth and 28 days of age

neoplasia the new and abnormal development of cells that may be benign or malignant

neoplasm an abnormal growth of new tissue, either benign or malignant

nephron a structural and functional unit of the kidney, resembling a microscopic funnel with a long stem and two convoluted sections

neurologic pertaining to neurology or the nervous system

neuromuscular pertaining to the muscle and nerves

neuropathy any of a number of abnormal conditions characterized by inflammation and/or degeneration of the nerves

neurosurgery any surgery involving the brain, spinal cord, or peripheral nerves

neutral thermal environment (NTE) an ambient environment that prevents or minimizes the loss of body heat

neutropenia an abnormal decrease in the number of neutrophils in the blood

neutrophil a polymorphonuclear granular leukocyte that stains well with neutral dyes; the circulating white blood cells essential for phagocytosis

NFPA abbreviation for National Fire Protection Agency

nicotinic pertaining to the effect of acetylcholine at the parasympathetic and sympathetic ganglionic or somatic skeletal muscles receptor sites

NIPPV abbreviation for noninvasive positive pressure ventilation

noninvasive pertaining to a diagnostic or therapeutic technique that does not require the skin to be broken or a cavity or organ of the body to be entered, as obtaining a blood pressure reading by auscultation with a stethoscope and sphygmomanometer

noninvasive positive pressure ventilation (NIPPV) positive pressure ventilation without endotracheal intubation or tracheotomy, usually via a form-fitting nasal mask

noninvasive ventilation mechanical ventilation performed without intubation or tracheostomy, usually with mask ventilation

nonmaleficence the principle that obligates healthcare providers to avoid harming patients and to actively prevent harm where possible

nonresectable not removable by surgery

normocapnia a state characterized by a normal partial pressure of carbon dioxide in the arterial blood (35 to 45 torr)

normovolemic a state characterized by normal fluid volumes

nosocomial pertaining to or originating in a hospital, as a nosocomial infection

nosocomial infection an infection acquired after hospitalization. Also called *hospital-acquired infection*

nosocomial pneumonia an infectious inflammatory process of the lung parenchyma that originates in the hospital

O

O_2ER abbreviation for oxygen extraction ratio; the ratio of oxygen consumption to oxygen delivery

O_2 pulse the ratio of oxygen consumption to heart rate (mL oxygen consumed per beat); a measure of the heart's efficiency in delivering oxygen

obesity hypoventilation syndrome a general syndrome involving chronic hypercapnia and hypoxemia, sleep apnea, and decreased respiratory center responsiveness to carbon dioxide. Complications, due primarily to chronic hypoxemia, include polycythemia, pulmonary hypertension, and cor pulmonale

oblique slanting; not perfectly vertical or horizontal

obliterate to remove or destroy

obstetrics the branch of medicine concerned with pregnancy and childbirth

obstructive sleep apnea (OSA) a condition in which five or more apneic periods (of at least 10 seconds each) occur per hour of sleep and characterized by occlusion of the oropharyngeal airway with continued efforts to breathe

obtunded insensitive to pain or other stimuli due to a reduced level of consciousness

obturator a device used to block a passage or a canal or to fill in a space, as the obturator used to insert a tracheostomy tube

ocular of or pertaining to the eye; also an eyepiece in any instrument

oliguria a diminished capacity to form and pass urine; for adults, generally defined as < 500 mL/day

oncotic marked by or associated with swelling; often used as a synonym for osmotic forces

Ondine's curse apnea caused by loss of automatic control of respiration (derived from the name of a fabled water nymph)

opacification the process of becoming opaque (less able to transmit light or penetrating radiation); used commonly to refer to the development of areas of increased density on the x-ray, as occurs in ARDS

opiate a narcotic drug that contains opium, derivatives of opium, or any of several synthetic chemicals with opium-like activity; morphine is the model in this category

opportunistic referring to an infection caused by normally nonpathogenic organisms in a host whose resistance has been decreased by disorders such as diabetes mellitus, human immunodeficiency virus (HIV), or cancer; a surgical procedure; or immunosuppressive drugs

optimum PEEP the ideal level of PEEP, balancing benefits and risks

orifice an entrance or outlet to a body cavity or tube

oropharynx the three anatomical divisions of the pharynx lying behind the oral cavity and midway between the nasopharynx and laryngopharynx

orotracheal of or pertaining to the passageway from the mouth to the trachea; usually applied to tubes or catheters placed in the trachea through the mouth, such as an orotracheal tube or orotracheal suctioning

orthopnea labored breathing in the reclining position

orthostatic pertaining to or caused by standing upright, as with orthostatic hypotension

oscillation a back-and-forth motion; vibration or the effects of mechanical or electrical vibration

OSA abbreviation for obstructive sleep apnea; a condition in which five or more apneic periods (of at least 10 seconds each) occur per hour of sleep and characterized by occlusion of the oropharyngeal airway with continued efforts to breathe

OSHA abbreviation for the Occupational Safety and Health Administration, a branch of the U.S. Department of Labor responsible for regulation pertaining to on-the-job safety

osmolarity the osmotic pressure of a solution expressed in osmols or milliosmols per kilogram of the solution

osmotic pressure the force produced by solvent particles across semipermeable membranes

osteoporosis a disorder characterized by abnormal rarefaction of bone, occurring most frequently in postmenopausal women, in sedentary or immobilized individuals, and in patients on long-term steroid therapy

otitis inflammation or infection of the ear, such as otitis media or otitis externa

outflow resistance the force against which the ventricles must pump to move blood into the arteries

output data produced via a computer program from available input; for example, if a program adds 4 to an input value, and the input is 5, the resulting output would be 9

overdistention a state of stretch or expansion beyond the normal limits

overhydration a state characterized by an excess of body fluids

oximeter a photoelectric device (usually noninvasive) used to determine the saturation of blood hemoglobin with oxygen with an oximeter

oximetry the process of determining the saturation of hemoglobin with oxygen with an oximeter

oxygen-conserving devices special low-flow delivery systems modified to reduce the oxygen waste that occurs during patient exhalation

oxygen toxicity the pathological response of the body and its tissues resulting from long-term exposure to high partial pressures of oxygen; pulmonary manifestations include cellular changes causing congestion, inflammation, and edema

oxyhemoglobin the chemical combination resulting from the covalent bonding of oxygen to the ferrous iron pigment in hemoglobin

P

$P_{0.1}$ the mouth pressure 100 ms after the start of an occluded inspiration; a measure of the output of the respiratory center

P_{50} the partial pressure of oxygen at which hemoglobin is 50% saturated with oxygen, standardized to a pH of 7.40; used as a measure of hemoglobin affinity for oxygen; with a normal value of 26.6 mm Hg

PAC abbreviation for premature atrial contraction

palate the bony plate that separates the nasal cavity from the oral cavity

pallor an unnatural paleness or absence of color in the skin

palmar pertaining to the palm

palpitation a pounding or racing of the heart

pandemic (of a disease) occurring throughout the population of a country, a people, or the world

paradox something contrary to common sense, logic, or experience

paradoxical breathing a pattern of breathing in which the abdomen is observed to move outward while the lower rib cage moves inward during an inspiratory effort. This pattern can indicate excessive respiratory muscle loading, diaphragmatic weakness, or impending respiratory failure. Also called *abdominal paradox*

paranasal situated near or alongside the nose, as the paranasal sinuses

parasympathetic pertaining to the craniosacral component of the autonomic nervous system, consisting of the oculomotor, facial, glossopharyngeal, vagus, and pelvic nerves; any physiological action mediated by or mimicking that of acetylcholine

parasympathomimetic denoting a pharmacologic agent that mimics the effects of stimulation of organs and structures by the parasympathetic nervous system by occupying cholinergic receptor sites and acting as an agonist or by increasing the release of the neurotransmitter acetylcholine

parenchyma the essential or distinctive tissue of an organ

parenteral not in or through the digestive system

paresis slight or incomplete paralysis

paresthesia any subjective sensation, experienced as numbness, tingling, or a 'pins and needles' feeling

parietal pleura a thin membrane covering the surface of the chest wall, mediastinum, and diaphragm that is continuous with the visceral pleura around the lung hilum

paroxysmal nocturnal dyspnea (PND) attacks of dyspnea commonly occurring at night, especially in the recumbent position, and associated with congestive heart failure and cardiac pulmonary edema

partial pressure the pressure exerted by a single gas in a gas mixture

partial thromboplastin time (PTT) a test for detecting coagulation defects of the intrinsic clotting system by adding activated partial thromboplastin to a sample of test plasma and comparing it with a control of normal plasma; normal is 60 to 80 seconds

partial ventilatory support modes of ventilatory support in which the patient must contribute to the total minute volume with spontaneous breathing

Pascal's principle a law stating that a confined liquid transmits pressure equally in all directions

passive atelectasis collapse of distal lung units due to persistent ventilation with small tidal volumes

pasteurization the process of applying heat, usually to milk or cheese, for a specified period for the purpose of killing or retarding the development of pathogenic bacteria

patent open and unblocked, as a patent airway

pathological indicative of or caused by a disease

pathophysiology the study of the biological and physical manifestations of disease as they correlate with the underlying abnormalities and physiological disturbances

patient-focused care a nontraditional organization of services that emphasizes a team approach to service delivery using cross-trained providers, as well as simplification of processes required to provide patient care

patient-physician privilege the right of patients to refuse to divulge or have divulged by their physician, the communications made between them and their physician

PAV abbreviation for proportional assist ventilation, a mode of ventilatory support in which the level of mechanical assistance varies with patient demand

PAWP abbreviation for pulmonary arterial wedge pressure (also called the *pulmonary capillary wedge pressure [PCWP]* or *occluded pulmonary artery pressure [PAo]*); reflects downstream pressure in the pulmonary circulation; under optimum conditions PAWP indicates left ventricular end-diastolic pressure (LVEDP), or left ventricular preload

PCIRV abbreviation for pressure controlled inverse ratio ventilation; equivalent to time-triggered, pressure-limited, time-cycled ventilation with I:E ratios greater than 1:1

PCP abbreviation for *Pneumocystis carinii* pneumonia; caused by *Pneumocystis carinii* (probably a fungi), PCP causes an acute interstitial pneumonia with high mortality (50%); PCP is most common among patients with an abnormal or altered immunologic status, particularly those suffering from AIDS; current treatment is with co-trimoxazole or pentamidine isethionate

PCV abbreviation for *pressure control ventilation*

PCWP abbreviation for pulmonary capillary wedge pressure; see PAWP

PDA abbreviation for patent ductus arteriosus, a common cardiovascular anomaly of infants in which the ductus arteriosus either fails to close or reopens after birth

peak expiratory flow rate (PEFR) the maximum, greatest expiratory flow rate in L/sec

pectoralis major the large fan-shaped muscle that arises from the sternum and clavicle and inserts into the upper arm; accessory muscle of ventilation

pectoriloquy the transmission of the sounds of speech through the chest wall

pectus carinatum chicken breasted; undue protrusion of the sternum

pectus excavatum funnel breasted; undue concavity of the sternum

pediatrics the branch of medicine concerned with the treatment and prevention of disorders of childhood

PEEP abbreviation for positive end-expiratory pressure; the application and maintenance of pressure above atmospheric at the airway throughout the expiratory phase of positive pressure mechanical ventilation

pendelluft movement of gas from 'fast' to 'slow' filling spaces during breathing; alternatively, the ineffective movement of gas back and forth (accompanied by mediastinal shifting) between a healthy lung and one with a flail segment caused by a crushing chest injury

penicillinase resistant a descriptive term applied to certain antibiotics resistant to the action of penicillinase, an enzyme produced by some bacteria that activates penicillin

percent body humidity (%BH) referring to the amount of water vapor in a volume of gas as the percent of the water in gas saturated at a body temperature of 37° C (43.8 mg/L)

percutaneous through the skin

perfuse the passage of fluid (usually blood) through the body

peribronchial around the bronchi

pericarditis an inflammation of the pericardium associated with trauma, malignant neoplastic disease, infection, uremia, myocardial infarction, collagen disease, or idiopathic causes

pericardium a fibrous, serous sac that surrounds the heart and roots of the great vessels

peripheral any of a variety of devices that can be attached to a computer and directed by the CPU, including printers, display devices, external data storage, instrument interfaces, and communication devices

perinatal of or pertaining to the time and process of giving birth or to being born

perioperative of or pertaining to the period of time immediately before, during, and after surgery

periosteum a fibrous vascular membrane covering the bones, except at their extremities

peritoneal dialysis a dialysis procedure in which the peritoneum is used as the diffusible membrane, with a dialysate fluid infused and removed directly into the peritoneal cavity

peritubular around the tubules; specifically around the proximal or distal tubules of the nephron

permanent gas the gaseous phase of a substance with a critical temperature so low that it cannot be compressed into a liquid under ambient conditions

permissive hypercapnia during ventilatory support, the use of subnormal volumes to protect the lung against barotrauma; the $PaCO_2$ is allowed to rise as long as the pH remains in a safe range

PERRLA acronym indicating pupils equal, round, react to light, accommodation; a normal physical examination finding

persistent pulmonary hypertension of the newborn (PPHN) a clinical syndrome seen in infants soon after birth and characterized by abnormally increased pulmonary vascular resistance

pertussis an acute, highly contagious respiratory disease characterized by paroxysmal coughing that ends in a loud whooping inspiration

petechia a tiny purple or red spot that appears on the skin as a result of minute hemorrhages within the dermal or submucosal layers

P/F ratio a ratio of the arterial partial pressure of oxygen to the inspired fractional concentration of oxygen (PaO_2/FIO_2); a measure of the efficiency of oxygen transfer across the lung

phagocytosis the process by which certain cells engulf and dispose of microorganisms and cell debris

pharyngitis inflammation or infection of the pharynx, usually causing symptoms of a sore throat

phlegm mucus from the tracheobronchial tree

phonocardiography the analog recording of heart sounds, usually on a strip chart recorder; useful in the diagnosis of certain valvular abnormalities that produce heart murmurs

phospholipid one of a class of compounds, widely distributed in living cells, containing phosphoric acid, fatty acids, and a nitrogenous base

photoplethysmography the use of light waves to detect changes in the volume of an organ or tissue; pulse oximeters use the principle of photoplethysmography to measure the arterial pulse

phrenic nerves paired nerves that originate as branches of spinal nerves C3-C5, pass down along the mediastinum, and innervate the diaphragm

Pickwickian syndrome an abnormal condition characterized by severe obesity, decreased responsiveness to carbon dioxide, a restrictive pulmonary function pattern, hypersomnolence, and polycythemia

PIE abbreviation for *pulmonary interstitial emphysema;* a form of pulmonary barotrauma due to air leakage into lung tissue

piezoelectric crystal a transducer capable of converting electrical energy in the physical energy of high frequency vibrations

piezoelectric transducer a transducer capable of converting electrical energy in the physical energy of high frequency vibrations

PImax abbreviation for maximum inspiratory pressure, or the negative pressure generated during a maximally forced inspiratory effort against an obstruction to flow; also called *maximum inspiratory force (MIF)* and *negative inspiratory force (NIF)*

pin-indexed safety system (PISS) part of the American standard safety system, these specifications apply only to the valve outlets of small cylinders, up to and including size E, which use a yoke-type connection

PISS abbreviation for pin-indexed safety system

pK the negative log of the ionization constant of a solution; the buffering power of a buffer system is greatest when its pH and pK values are equal; pKa is the negative log of the acid component of a buffer

placenta the highly vascular organ through which the fetus absorbs oxygen and vital nutrients, and excrete carbon dioxide and other waste products of metabolism

placenta abruptio (also abruptio placentae) separation of a normally implanted placenta in a pregnancy of 20 weeks or more duration or during labor but before delivery; a significant cause of maternal and fetal mortality

placenta previa an abnormal condition of pregnancy in which the placenta is implanted low in the uterus, such that it impinges or covers the internal os of the cervix

plaintiff a person who brings an action; a person who seeks remedial relief for an injury to his rights

plasma the watery, colorless fluid portion of the blood and lymph in which cellular elements are suspended

plasmapheresis a laboratory procedure in which the plasma proteins are separated by electrophoresis for identification and evaluation of the proportion of the various proteins

platypnea the opposite of orthopnea; that is, an abnormal condition characterized by difficult breathing in the standing position, which is relieved in the lying or recumbent position

plethysmograph a device for measuring pressure; in pulmonary physiology, a chamber in which the subject sits in order to measure lung pressures and volumes

plethysmography the process of measuring and recording variations in the volume of an organ or body part with a plethysmograph

pleura a thin layer of mesothelium that covers the lungs and lines the inside of the thoracic cavities

pleural effusion the abnormal collection of fluid in the pleural space

pleural empyema a pleural effusion in which the fluid is purulent or contains pyogenic organisms

pleural space the space between the visceral pleura covering the lung and the parietal pleura covering the chest wall

pleurisy pain that comes from the pleural surface usually a direct result of viral infections but has been generalized to any condition (for example, pulmonary embolism) causing pleural pain. Synonymous with pleurodynia

pleurodesis the procedure of fusing the parietal and visceral pleura to prevent formation of pleural fluid or recurrence of pneumothorax

PMI abbreviation for point of maximum impulse

PND abbreviation for paroxysmal nocturnal dyspnea

pneumatocele a thin-walled, air-filled cyst occurring in lung tissue

pneumocardiography the recording of variations in cardiac function through sensors that monitor respiratory changes, such as pressure changes in the bronchi or changes in thoracic dimensions

pneumocephalus a condition in which gas or air is inside the cranium

pneumography recording of respiratory movements on a graph

pneumoconiosis any disease of the lung caused by chronic inhalation of inorganic dusts, usually mineral dusts of occupational or environmental origin

pneumocyte (also pneumonocyte) a general term applied to the cells constituting the alveolar region of the lungs

pneumomediastinum a presence of air or gas in the mediastinal tissues, which may lead to pneumothorax or pneumopericardium

pneumonectomy the surgical removal or all or part of a lung

pneumonia an inflammatory process of the lung parenchyma, usually infectious in origin

pneumonitis inflammation of the lung

pneumopericardium a presence of air or gas in the pericardium

pneumoperitoneum a presence of air or gas in the peritoneal cavity; may occur as the result of disease, or may be induced for diagnostic visualization

pneumotachometer any device for measuring gas flow

pneumotachygraph an instrument that incorporates a pneumotachometer to recording variations in the flow of respiratory gases

pneumotaxic center a center in the upper part of the pons that rhythmically inhibits inspiration independently of the vagi

pneumothorax the presence of air or gas in the pleural space of the thorax; if this air or gas is trapped under pressure, a tension pneumothorax exists

point-of-care (POC) testing analysis at the bedside, as opposed to conventional laboratory testing

Poiseuille's law the law relating pressure difference needed for laminar flow through a tube to the viscosity of the fluid, the length of the tube, the rate of flow, and the tube radius

poliomyelitis an infectious disease caused by one of three small RNA viruses, which can impair anterior horn cell and produce a clinical picture ranging from asymptomatic to severe paralysis

polycythemia an abnormal increase in the number of erythrocytes in the blood; termed secondary if attributable to defined causes other than direct stimulation of the bone marrow, such as occurs in chronic hypoxemia

polymorphonuclear having a nucleus with a number of lobules or segments connected by a fine thread

polyp a small, tumor-like growth that projects from the surface of a mucous membrane

polysomnography the measurement and recording of variations in airflow and diaphragmatic activity during sleep; used in the diagnosis of sleep apnea

POMR abbreviation for problem oriented medical record, a method of recording data about the health status of a patient

pons the prominence on the ventral surface of the brainstem, between the medulla oblongata and the cerebral pedicles of the midbrain

pores of Kohn openings between adjacent alveoli

positive end-expiratory pressure (PEEP) the application and maintenance of pressure above atmospheric at the airway throughout the expiratory phase of positive pressure mechanical ventilation

positive expiratory pressure (PEP) an airway clearance technique in which the patient exhales against a fixed-orifice flow resistor in order to help move secretions into the larger airways for expectoration via coughing or swallowing

positive inotropism an increase in the contractility of muscle tissue

positive pressure ventilation the application of positive pressure to the lungs in order to improve gas exchange

postacute care health services provided outside the acute care hospital; includes subacute care, rehabilitation, skilled nursing facilities (SNFs), and home care

posterolateral situated behind and to one side or the other

posteromedial situated behind and toward the middle

postterm of or pertaining to an infant born after 42 weeks gestation, regardless of weight

postural drainage the therapeutic use of patient positioning and gravity to facilitate the mobilization of respiratory tract secretions

potency (in pharmacology) the biological activity of a drug per unit weight, or the amount a drug required to produce a given effect

power of attorney an instrument authorizing another to act as one's agent or attorney

PPD abbreviation for purified protein derivative, a material used in testing for tuberculin sensitivity

ppm abbreviation for parts per million, a common ratio measure for dilute solution or gas mixtures

PPO abbreviation for preferred provider organization, a healthcare service organization that negotiates special rates for its services with selected groups or organizations

precordium the external anterior anatomical region over the heart and lower thorax

precursor something that comes before or precedes; in chemistry and pharmacology, a substance from which another is formed or synthesized; in clinical diagnosis, a symptom or sign that precedes another

preeclampsia an abnormal condition of pregnancy characterized by the onset of acute hypertension after the twenty fourth week of gestation, usually accompanied by proteinuria and edema

preload the pressure stretching the ventricular walls at the onset of ventricular contraction

preoperative of or pertaining to the period of time preceding a surgical procedure

pressure control ventilation (PCV) a mode of ventilatory support in which mandatory support breaths are delivered to the patient at a set inspiratory pressure

pressure generator a ventilator that delivers a pressure pattern that is independent of the patient's respiratory mechanics

pressure support ventilation (PSV) a mode of ventilatory support designed to augment spontaneous breathing; patient-triggered, pressure-limited, flow-cycled ventilation

pressure-time index (PTI) the ratio of the mean-to-maximum transdiaphragmatic pressure difference times the inspiratory duty cycle; a measure of load that correlates highly with oxygen consumption of the ventilatory muscles

pressure-time product the product of pressure over a time interval, usually pleural pressure times inspiratory time during breathing

preterm pertaining to an infant born prior to 38 weeks gestation, regardless of weight

prevention any action directed to preventing illness and promoting health to eliminate the need for secondary or tertiary healthcare

preventive maintenance the regularly scheduled testing and service of in-use equipment, designed to prevent failure or malfunction

primary pulmonary hypertension a form of pulmonary hypertension that occurs in the absence of other heart or lung diseases and is characterized by diffuse narrowing of the pulmonary arterioles without obvious reason

primary spontaneous pneumothorax a pneumothorax that occurs without underlying lung disease

problem oriented medical record (POMR) a method of recording data about the health status of a patient in a problem system

prognostic referring to a finding that is diagnostic or predictive

programming language a special type of software application designed to help create computer programs using a particular set of instructions, such as BASIC or C++

progressive resistance a method of increasing the strength of a weak or injured muscle by gradually increasing the resistance against which the muscle works, such as by using graduated weights over a period. Also called *graduated resistance*

prolapsed cord an umbilical cord that protrudes beside or ahead of the presenting part of the fetus

propellant something that propels or provides thrust, as the propellant in a metered dose inhaler

prophylactic preventing the spread of disease; preventive

proprioceptor any sensory nerve ending, as those located in muscles, tendons, and joints, that responds to stimuli arising from movement or spatial position

prospective payment a system of healthcare cost reimbursement in which the amount paid to a provider is determined in advance and irrespective of actual costs incurred

protein-energy malnutrition (PEM) a wasting condition resulting from a diet deficient in either protein or energy (calories) or both

prothrombin a plasma protein synthesized in the liver that, when exposed to thromboplastin and calcium, forms the thrombin component of a blood clot

prothrombin time (PT) a one-stage test for detecting certain plasma coagulation defects caused by deficiencies in factors V, VII, or X

protocol a written plan specifying the procedures to be followed in a given activity; as applied to electronic communications, a collection of rules that determine how two or more computers 'talk' to each other

pseudocolumnar literally, 'column-like'; used to describe a type of epithelial cell that appears columnar in shape

pseudostratified of or pertaining to an epithelial cell type that appears to be organized in layers, but in which each cell actually contacts the basement membrane

psig abbreviation for pounds per square inch-gauge; that is, the pressure above atmospheric registered on a meter or gauge

PSV abbreviation for *pressure support ventilation*

PSVmax the pressure support level needed to provide tidal volumes of 10-15 mL/kg

psychomotor domain the area of observable performance of skills that require some degree of neuromuscular coordination

psychosis any major medical disorder characterized by extreme derangement of personality; for example, severe depression, agitation, regressive behavior

psychosocial of or pertaining to the mental, emotional, and social aspects of human existence or development

psychosomatic of or pertaining to the relationship between the emotional state or outlook of an individual (psyche) and the physical responses of the individual's body (soma)

PTI abbreviation for pressure-time index

ptosis an abnormal condition of one or both upper eyelids in which the eyelid droops owing to a congenital or acquired weakness of the levator muscle or paralysis of the third cranial nerve

pulmonary alveolar proteinosis a chronic lung disease characterized by deposition of an eosinophilic proteinaceous material in the alveolar region, which severely impairs gas exchange

pulmonary edema a condition in which excessive amounts of plasma enter the pulmonary interstitium and alveoli; usually accompanied by severe respiratory distress, tachypnea, and hypoxemia

pulmonary embolism the blockage of a pulmonary artery by foreign matter. The obstruction may be fat, air, tumor tissue, or a thrombus that usually arises from a peripheral vein (most frequently arising from the deep veins of the legs). Pulmonary embolism is detected by chest radiographic films, pulmonary angiography, and radioscanning of the lung fields

pulmonary fibrosis scarring of lung tissue involving the formation of fibrous tissue or lesions

pulmonary hemosiderosis a pulmonary disorder characterized by the deposition of abnormal quantities of hemosiderin (an insoluble form of ferric oxide) in the lung parenchyma

pulmonary hypertension a condition characterized by abnormally high pulmonary artery pressures, that is, mean pulmonary artery pressures in excess of 22 mmHg

pulmonary infiltrate a fluid that passes through the lungs

pulmonary surfactant a detergent-like substance secreted into the alveoli that reduces surface tension and stabilizes alveoli

pulmonary vasculitis an inflammatory condition of the blood vessels of the lungs

pulmonologist a medical doctor who specializes in the treatment of disorders of the respiratory system and holds certification in pulmonary diseases through the American Board of Internal Medicine

pulse deficit the discrepancy between the ventricular rate auscultated at the apex of the heart and the arterial rate of the radial pulse

pulse oximetry the noninvasive estimation of arterial oxyhemoglobin saturation based on the combined principles of photoplethysmography and spectrophotometry

pulse pressure the difference between systolic and diastolic blood pressure

pulsus alternans alternating between strong and weak heart beats

pulsus paradoxus an abnormal decrease in pulse pressure with each inspiratory effort

purulent consisting of or containing pus

PVC abbreviation for premature ventricular contraction; also used as an abbreviation for polyvinyl chloride

pyogenic pus-producing

Q

quality assurance any evaluation of services provided and the results achieved as compared with accepted standards

quality control a planned, systematic approach to designing, measuring, assessing, and improving performance

R

racemic pertaining to a compound made up of optical isomers

radiation therapy the treatment of neoplastic disease by using x-rays or gamma rays, usually from a cobalt source, to deter the proliferation of malignant cells by decreasing the rate of mitosis or impairing deoxyribonucleic acid synthesis

radioaerosol an aerosol with particles that have been labeled with a radioactive isotope; used to assist researchers in analyzing pulmonary aerosol deposition and clearance

radiolucent pertaining to a substance or tissue that readily permits the passage of x-rays or other radiant energy; compare with radiopaque

radiopaque of or pertaining to a substance or tissue that does not readily permit the passage of x-rays or other radiant energy; compare with radiolucent

rale discontinuous types of lung sounds heard on auscultation of the chest, usually during inspiration; the term *crackle* is now preferred

random access memory (RAM) a volatile memory storage system in which specific storage locations can be addressed directly, without the need for sequential searching

rapid shallow breathing index (f/V_T) the patient's spontaneous respiratory rate (f) in breaths per minute divided by the spontaneous tidal volume in liters. Values above 100 are associated with poor weaning outcomes

read only memory (ROM) unalterable computer memory from which data can be read but not written or modified; typically, ROM holds permanent sets of instructions such as those used repetitively by the system hardware; compare with random access memory (RAM)

rebreathe to inhale expired gas (high in carbon dioxide content)

rebreathed volume the volume of any breathing apparatus that results in previously expired gas being inhaled; equivalent to the mechanical deadspace

reconditioning physical activity to strengthen essential muscle groups, improve overall oxygen use, and enhance the body's cardiovascular response to physical activity

recontamination the process by which articles previously contaminated and cleaned or sterilized become contaminated again

recredentialing the process by which an individual who already holds a credential in a given profession demonstrates ongoing competency by successfully completing current credentialing requirements

rectus abdominis abdominal muscle group that functions as an accessory muscle of ventilation

recurrent laryngeal nerves branches of vagus nerves that innervate the larynx

REDOX an acronym pertaining to any REDuction-OXidation chemical reaction

reducing valve a valve that reduces gas pressure

REE abbreviation for resting energy expenditure; a measure of caloric outlays at rest

reexpansion pulmonary edema pulmonary edema that forms following rapid reexpansion of a lung that has been compressed with pleural fluid or pneumothorax

referred pain pain occurring at a site distal to its origin

refractory pertaining to a disorder that is resistant to treatment

refractory hypoxemia an abnormal deficiency of oxygen in the arterial blood that is resistant to treatment; usually indicates the presence of right-to-left shunting

refractory period the period of time during the depolarization stage of the action potential in which cardiac tissue fibers cannot respond to additional electrical stimulation

registered pulmonary function technologist (RPFT) an individual, qualified by education and/or experience and previously certified in pulmonary function technology, who has successfully completed the pulmonary function registry examination of the NBRC

registered respiratory therapist (RRT) a respiratory therapist who has successfully completed the registry (therapist) examination of the NBRC

regulator a device that controls both pressure and flow

regurgitation the backward flow of blood through an incompetent valve of the heart

rehabilitation the restoration of the individual to the fullest medical, mental, emotional, social, and vocational potential of which he/she is capable

rehabilitation (pulmonary) a multidisciplinary program designed to help stabilize or reverse both the physiopathology and psychopathology of pulmonary diseases and return patients to the highest possible functional capacity allowed

reliability pertaining to equipment, the consistency of fault-free operation, often measured as the mean time between failures; in statistics, the repeatability of a test or measure

repolarization the process by which the cell is restored to its resting potential

resect to remove surgically

reservoir system an oxygen delivery system that provides a reservoir oxygen volume that the patient taps into when the patient's inspiratory flow exceeds the device flow

residual volume (RV) the volume of gas remaining in the lungs after a complete exhalation

res ipsa loquitur 'the thing speaks for itself;' rule of evidence whereby negligence of alleged wrongdoer may be inferred from the mere fact that the accident happened

resistance impedance to flow in a tube or conduit; quantified as ratio of the difference in pressure between the two points

resorption atelectasis collapse of distal lung units due to mucus plugging of airways

respirator a mask-like apparatus used to filter inspired air for breathing

respiratory acidosis hypoventilation resulting in acidemia

respiratory alkalosis hypoventilation resulting in alkalemia

respiratory alterans alternating between use of the diaphragm for short periods and use of the accessory muscles to breathe. It is indicative of end-stage respiratory muscle fatigue

respiratory bronchiolitis edema and airway narrowing caused by infection in the small bronchi and bronchioles

respiratory care protocol a specification of actions that allows respiratory care practitioners to independently initiate and adjust therapy, within guidelines previously established by medical staff; also called *therapist-driven* protocol

respiratory exchange ratio (R) the ratio of the amount of carbon dioxide moving into the alveoli per minute and the amount of oxygen leaving the alveoli per minute; for the lung as a whole, R is normally 0.8

respiratory failure a condition in which the exchange of oxygen and/or carbon dioxide between the alveoli and the pulmonary capillaries is inadequate

Respiratory Index (RI) the ratio of the alveolar-arterial oxygen tension gradient to the arterial partial pressure of oxygen ($P(A\text{-}a)O_2/\ PaO_2$); a measure of the efficiency of oxygen transfer across the lung

respiratory insufficiency a condition in which breathing is accompanied by abnormal signs or symptoms, such as dyspnea or paradoxical breathing

respiratory quotient (RQ) the body's total exchange of oxygen for carbon dioxide, expressed as the ratio of the volume of carbon dioxide produced to the volume of oxygen consumed per unit of time at steady-state conditions. Depending on the net metabolic needs of all parts of the body at a given moment, the ratio ranges from 0.7 to 1 and averages around 0.8. The values of RQ change according to the fuel being metabolized; the RQ of fat is lower than that of glucose, whereas the RQ of protein is between that of glucose and fat

respiratory therapist a graduate of a CAAHEP/CoARC accredited school designed to qualify the graduate for the registry examination of the National Board for Respiratory Care (NBRC)

respiratory therapy consult service a program in which respiratory care services are determined by respiratory care practitioners based on prescribed guidelines or algorithms, otherwise known as an *evaluate-and-treat* program

respirometer a device used to measure the volume of respired air or gas

respondeat superior 'let the master answer'; it means that the master is liable in certain cases for the wrongful acts of his servant; for example, a doctor may be liable for the wrongful acts of his assistant. The doctrine is inapplicable where injury occurs while the servant is acting outside the legitimate scope of authority

response time a measure (usually in msec) of the speed with which a mechanical ventilator can respond to a patient's inspiratory effort and cycle into the inspiratory phase

resting potential a difference in charge, or negative electrical potential, that exists between the inside and outside of a nerve or cardiac tissue cell in the resting state due to concentration differences of potassium and sodium ions across the cell membrane

restrictive lung disease a broad category of disorders with widely variable etiologies, but all resulting in a reduction in lung volumes, particularly the inspiratory and vital capacities; categorized according to origin; that is, skeletal/thoracic, neuromuscular, pleural, interstitial, and alveolar

retention as applied to aerosol therapy, the proportion of particles deposited within the respiratory tract, either at a specific location or as a whole

retinopathy a noninflammatory eye disorder resulting from changes in the retinal blood vessels

retinopathy of prematurity (ROP) an abnormal ocular condition that occurs in some premature or low birth-weight infants who receive oxygen. Previously called *retrolental fibroplasia*

retractions the sinking inward of the skin around the chest cage with each inspiratory effort

retrolental fibroplasia a formation of fibrous tissue behind the lens of the eye, resulting in blindness

retrosternal behind the sternum

rhinitis inflammation of the mucous membranes of the nose, usually accompanied by swelling of the mucosa and a nasal discharge

rhinorrhea the free discharge of a thin nasal mucus

rhinovirus any of about 100 serologically distinct, small RNA viruses that cause about 40% of acute respiratory illnesses

rhonchi abnormal sounds heard on auscultation of a respiratory airway obstructed by thick secretions, muscular spasm, neoplasm, or external pressure

rhonchial fremitus an abnormal vibration felt on the chest wall as air passes through a narrowed airway

right-to-left shunt an anatomical bypass in which blood flows from the venous to the arterial side of the circulation, bypassing the lungs. This lowers both the oxygen content and the PO_2 of the arterial blood

rise-time the rate of increase in a parameter; in ventilatory support, the rate at which airway pressure rises during early inspiration (a function of flow)

role fidelity the concept that practitioners in each specialty have a duty to understand the limits of their role and to practice with fidelity

ROS abbreviation for review of symptoms, a component of the medical history

RSV abbreviation for *respiratory syncytial virus*

rule utilitarianism a moral reasoning approach based not on which act has the greatest utility but on which rule would promote the greatest good if it were generally followed

S

SAHS acronym for the sleep apnea/hypopnea syndrome

sarcoidosis a chronic disorder of unknown origin characterized by the formation of tubercles of non-necrotizing epithelioid tissue

scalenes referring to the three muscles arising from the cervical vertebrae, inserting into the first and second ribs; accessory muscles of ventilation

sclera the tough white outer layer of the eye

scleroderma a relatively rare autoimmune disease that results in chronic thickening of connective tissues

scoliosis an abnormal lateral curvature of the spine. Severe scoliosis can be accompanied by respiratory compromise

scope of practice general guidelines and parameters for the clinician's practice; deviation could be a source of legal problems

secondary lobules the minor divisions of the pulmonary segments

secondary spontaneous pneumothorax a pneumothorax that occurs because of underlying lung disease

sedimentation the primary mechanism for deposition of particles 1 to 5 mm in diameter in the central airways, when particles slow and settle out of suspension

segments the minor divisions of the lung; each segment is associated with a major branch of the airway

semipermeable a biological or synthetic membrane that permits the passage of molecules of solvent only but not solute

sensitivity a measure of the amount of effort (pressure, flow) that must be generated by a patient in order to trigger a mechanical ventilator into the inspiratory phase; alternatively, the mechanism used to set or control this level; also called the *trigger level*

sensitivity (of a test) the ratio of true positive test results to all patients having the condition being tested for

sensitivity control in ventilatory support, pressure-triggering or flow-triggering for initiating breaths; the ventilator must 'sense' the patient's effort

sensorium a general term referring to the relative state of a patient's consciousness or alertness

sepsis a toxic condition resulting from infection

septicemia systemic infection in which pathogens are present in the circulating blood stream, having spread from an infection in any part of the body; also called *bacteremia*

septic shock shock due to bacteria in the blood stream (bacteremia), especially Gram-negative organisms associated with nosocomial infections

septum a wall or division; the nasal septum divides the internal nasal passages

sequela any abnormal condition that follows and is the result of a disease, treatment, or injury, as paralysis following poliomyelitis, deafness following treatment with an ototoxic drug, or a scar following a laceration

servo-control closed-loop control of a process based on a measurement parameter

servo-controlled heating system in a humidifier, a heating unit that monitors the temperature of gas delivered to the patient, adjusting the power to the heater based on the difference between the temperature setting and the temperature monitored by a thermistor probe placed downstream from the humidifier, at or near the patient airway connection

SGA abbreviation for small for gestational age; of or pertaining to newborn infants whose body weight falls below the 10th percentile for their gestational age

shock a condition in which perfusion to vital organs is inadequate to meet their metabolic needs; includes hypovolemic, cardiogenic, septic, anaphylactic, and neurogenic forms

shunt as applied in pulmonary medicine, a bypass between the venous (right) and arterial (left) sides of the circulation; if 'right-to-left,' dilution of arterial blood oxygen content occurs; if 'left-to-right,' oxygen content of the arterial blood is not affected, however, cardiac workload is significantly increased

side effect (in pharmacology) any effect produced by a drug other than its desired effect

SIDS abbreviation for *sudden infant death syndrome*, commonly called *crib death*; the leading cause of death in infants less than 1 year old in the United States

silicosis a lung disorder caused by continued, long-term exposure to the dust of an inorganic compound, silicon dioxide, which is found in sands, quartzes, and in many other stones; chronic silicosis is marked by widespread fibrotic nodular lesions in both lungs

sigmoid pertaining to an S shape

SIMV abbreviation for synchronous intermittent mandatory ventilation

singultus hiccup

sinusitis an inflammation of one or more paranasal sinuses

sinusoidal of or pertaining to the shape of a sine wave

situs inversus lateral transposition of the organs of the abdomen and thorax; one of the features of Kartagener's syndrome

slander any words spoken with malice that are untrue and prejudicial to the reputation, professional practice, commercial trade, office, or business of another person

sleep-disordered breathing periods of an absence of attempts to breathe during sleep

small cell cancer a malignant, usually bronchogenic epithelial neoplasm consisting of small tightly packed round, oval, or spindle-shaped epithelial cells that stain darkly and contain neurosecretory granules and little or no cytoplasm. Many malignant tumors of the lung are of this type. Also called *oat cell carcinoma* or *small cell carcinoma*

SNF abbreviation for *skilled nursing facility*

SOAP (in a problem-oriented medical record) abbreviation for *subjective*, *objective*, *assessment*, and *plan*, the four parts of a written account of the health problem

software programs or ROM-based instructions that control the computer

solenoid an electronically powered actuator or switch

solubility coefficient (gas) the volume of that gas that can be dissolved in 1 mL of a given liquid at standard pressure and specified temperature

somnolence sleepiness

sonography the process of imaging deep structures of the body by measuring and recording the reflection of pulsed or continuous high-frequency sound waves

specific compliance the absolute compliance value of the lung divided by the lung volume at FRC and expressed in units of mL/cm H_2O/L

specificity (of a test) the ratio of true negative test results to all patients not having the condition being tested for

spectrophotometry the measurement of color in a solution by determining the amount of light absorbed in the ultraviolet, infrared, or visible spectrum, widely used in clinical chemistry to calculate the concentration of substances in solution

sphygmomanometer an instrument for measuring the force of the pulse (from which the blood pressure is estimated)

spinal shock a form of shock associated with acute injury to the spinal cord

spirometer a device for measuring lung volumes or flows

spirometry laboratory evaluation of lung function using a spirometer

splinting the process of immobilizing, restraining, or supporting a body part

Spo_2 abbreviation for oxyhemoglobin saturation, as measured by pulse oximetry

spontaneous breath ventilatory support breaths initiated and ended by the patient

sporicidal destructive to the spore form of bacteria

sporicide any agent effective in destroying spores, as compounds of chlorine and formaldehyde, and the glutaraldehydes

spurious false

sputum mucus from the respiratory tract that has passed through the mouth

squamous appearing like plates or scales; a type of epithelial tissue

stability in aerosol therapy, a measure of the ability of an aerosol to remain in suspension over time

standard bicarbonate the plasma concentration of HCO_3^- in mEq/L that would exist if the Pco_2 were normal (40 torr)

standard precautions guidelines recommended by the Centers for Disease Control and Prevention to reduce the risk of transmission of blood-borne and other pathogens in hospitals. Standard precautions apply to (1) blood; (2) all body fluids, secretions, and excretions, *excluding sweat*, regardless of whether they contain blood; (3) nonintact skin; and (4) mucous membranes

stasis a disorder in which the normal flow of a fluid through a vessel of the body is slowed or halted

status asthmaticus an acute, severe, and prolonged asthma attack that does not respond to normal treatment approaches

statute an act of the legislature declaring, commanding, or prohibiting something

statute of limitations a statute declaring that no suit shall be maintained nor any criminal charge be made unless brought about within a specified period of time after the right accrued

statutory imposed by legal authority

stenosis a narrowing of one of the cardiac valves

sterile free from any living microorganisms

sterilization the complete destruction of all microorganisms, usually by heat or chemical means

sternoclavicular of or pertaining to the sternum and clavicle

sternomastoids referring to the muscles that arise from the sternum and clavicle and insert into the jaw; accessory muscles of ventilation

sternum the elongated flattened bone forming the middle portion of the anterior thorax

Stokes-Adams syncope episodes of syncope due to heart block

stretch receptors vagal sensory sites that respond to deformation of smooth muscle tissues in the airways

strict liability a theory in tort law that can be used to impose liability without fault, even in situations where injury occurs under conditions of reasonable care; the most common cases of strict liability involve the use of dangerous products or techniques

stridor a high-pitched, continuous type of adventitious lung sound heard from the upper airway

stroke volume volume of blood ejected by the left ventricle during each contraction

subacute care a level of treatment that is between chronic and acute

subatmospheric below atmospheric; used to describe pressures below ambient; see hypobarism

subcostal below the ribs

subcutaneous beneath the skin

subcutaneous emphysema an accumulation of air in the subcutaneous tissues due to leakage from the lung

subglottic below the glottis

sublingual beneath the tongue

submicronic pertaining to a particle (particularly colloid particles) less than 10^{-5} cm in size and not visible with a standard light microscope

submucosa beneath the mucosa

subphrenic below the diaphragm

sulfhemoglobin a form of hemoglobin containing an irreversibly bound sulfur molecule that prevents normal oxygen binding

sudden infant death syndrome (SIDS) the leading cause of death in infants less than 1 year old in the United States. Commonly called *crib death*

supplemental oxygen oxygen delivered at concentrations exceeding 21% to increase the amount circulating in the blood

supraclavicular the area of the body above the clavicle, or collar bone

supraglottic above the glottis

suprasternal above the sternum

supraventricular above the ventricles

surfactant a surface-acting agent that forms a monomolecular layer over pulmonary alveolar surfaces. These agents prevent alveolar collapse at lower lung volumes by reducing alveolar surface tension

surveillance (bacteriologic) an ongoing process designed to ensure that infection control procedures are working; generally involves equipment, microbiological identification, and epidemiological investigation

suspension a dispersion of large particles suspended in a fluid medium; without physical agitation, the particles will eventually settle out

sustained maximal inspiration (SMI) a therapeutic breathing maneuver in which patients are coached to inspire from the resting expiratory level up to their inspiratory capacity (IC), with an end-inspiratory pause

sympathetic pertaining to the thoracolumbar component of the autonomic nervous system, for which norepinephrine serves as the postganglionic neurotransmitter; also used to describe any physiological action mediated by or mimicking that of norepinephrine or epinephrine; see adrenergic

sympathomimetic denoting a pharmacologic agent that mimics the effects of stimulation of organs and structures by the sympathetic nervous system by occupying adrenergic receptor sites and acting as an agonist or by increasing the release of the neurotransmitter norepinephrine at postganglionic nerve endings

syncope temporary unconsciousness; fainting

synchronous intermittent mandatory ventilation (SIMV) a mode of ventilatory support using periodic assisted ventilation with spontaneous breathing in between. Assisted breaths are responsive to patient demand

synergistic acting together; more specifically, having the characteristics of synergism, the phenomenon whereby two agents acting together have an effect greater than their algebraic sum

systemic of or pertaining to the body as a whole

systolic blood pressure the peak blood pressure occurring in the arteries during ventricular contraction

T

tachycardia an abnormally elevated heart rate

tachyphylaxis a phenomenon in which the repeated administration of some drugs results in a marked decrease in effectiveness

tachypnea an abnormal elevation of breathing rate

tamponade stoppage of the flow of blood to an organ or a part of the body by pressure, as by a tampon or a pressure dressing applied to stop a hemorrhage or by compression of a part by an accumulation of fluid, as in cardiac tamponade

tangent a line drawn perpendicular to a given point in a curve

target heart rate the heart rate achieved at 65% of a patient's maximum oxygen consumption during the exercise evaluation, used for aerobic conditioning

taxonomy an orderly classification, as a taxonomy of organisms

TDP abbreviation for therapist-driven protocol, a specification of actions that allow RCPs to independently initiate and adjust therapy, within guidelines previously established by medical staff

tension pneumothorax air in the pleural space that exceeds atmospheric pressure causing outward expansion of the ribs, downward depression of the diaphragm, mediastinal shift, and hypotension

tension-time index the product of contractile force (ratio of diaphragmatic pressure to maximum diaphragmatic pressure) and contractile duration (ratio of inspiratory time to total breathing cycle time)

term pertaining to an infant born between 38 to 42 weeks gestation

tetany a condition characterized by cramps, convulsions, twitching of the muscles, and sharp flexion of the wrist and ankle joints

tetralogy of Fallot a congenital cardiac anomaly that consists of four defects: pulmonic stenosis, ventricular septal defect, malposition of the aorta so that it arises from the septal defect or the right ventricle, and right ventricular hypertrophy

therapeutic index the difference between the minimum therapeutic and minimum toxic concentrations of a drug

therapeutic positioning application of gravity to achieve specific clinical objectives, including mobilization of secretions (postural drainage), improving the distribution of ventilation (dependent positioning), and relieving dyspnea (relaxation positioning)

therapist-driven protocol a specification of actions that allow respiratory care practitioners to independently initiate and adjust therapy, within guidelines previously established by medical staff; also called *respiratory care protocol*

thermistor an electric thermometer the impedance of which varies with temperature; used for detecting flow at the mouth and nose during sleep studies

thoracentesis the surgical perforation of the chest wall and pleural space with a needle for diagnostic or therapeutic purposes or for the removal of a specimen for biopsy

thoracic computed tomography a radiographic technique that produces a cross-sectional view of the chest structures, with the ability to detect subtle changes in density

thoracotomy a surgical opening into the thoracic cavity

Thorpe tube a variable orifice, constant pressure flow metering device

threshold potential membrane potential or voltage difference in cardiac tissue fibers at which spontaneous depolarization occurs

threshold resistor in positive airway pressure therapy, a device against which a patient exhales; the pressure generated by a threshold resistor can be set to provide specific expiratory pressures independent of flow

threshold response pertaining to a physiological action caused by the minimum stimulus needed to provoke it

thrill a fine palpable vibration felt accompanying a cardiac or vascular murmur

thrombocytopenia an abnormal condition in which the number of blood platelets is reduced, usually associated with neoplastic diseases or an immune response to a drug

thrombolysis the process by which thrombi are dissolved

thrombolytic pertaining to a drug or other agent that dissolves thrombi

thrombophlebitis inflammation of a vein, often accompanied by formation of a clot

thrombosis an abnormal vascular condition in which thrombus develops within a blood vessel of the body

thrombus an aggregation of platelets, fibrin, and cellular blood components that can cause obstruction of a blood vessel

tibial of or pertaining to the tibia

tidal volume (V_T) the volume of air that is inhaled or exhaled from the lungs during effortless breath

time constant a mathematical expression describing the relative efficacy of lung unit filling and emptying, and computed as the product of compliance times resistance (measured in seconds)

tomography an x-ray technique that produces a film representing a detailed cross-section of tissue structure at a predetermined depth

torr a unit of pressure equivalent to 1/760 atmosphere at STPD; 1 mm Hg

tort a legal wrong committed upon a person or property independent of contract

tortfeasor a wrong doer; the individual who commits or is guilty of a tort

total buffer base (BB) the total quantity of all blood buffers capable of binding hydrogen ions, normally ranges from 48 to 52 mEq/L

total lung capacity (TLC) the total amount of gas in the lungs after a maximum inspiration

tourniquet a device applied around an extremity that is designed to compress blood vessels and thereby prevent blood flow to or from the distal area

trachea the large main intrathoracic airway

tracheitis any inflammatory condition of the trachea

tracheobronchial of or pertaining to the trachea and large bronchi

tracheobronchomegaly a rare congenital condition in which the size of the large airways are greatly enlarged

tracheoesophageal of or pertaining to the trachea and esophagus, as with a tracheoesophageal fistula

tracheomalacia softening of the tracheal cartilages

tracheostomy an opening through the neck into the trachea, through which an indwelling tube may be inserted

tracheotomy the procedure by which an incision is made into the trachea through the neck below the larynx, in order to gain access to the lower airways

transaction any human interaction; in human communication, denotes a two-way process, in which participants are mutually influenced by the interaction

transbronchial across the bronchi or bronchial wall, as a transbronchial biopsy

transcutaneous across the skin, as a transcutaneous PO_2 electrode

transducer a device capable of converting one form of energy into another and commonly used for measurement of physical events; for example, a pressure transducer may convert the physical phenomenon of force per unit area into an analog electrical signal

transect to sever or cut across, as in preparing a cross-section of tissue

transfusion the direct introduction of blood or blood products from another source into the blood stream

transmural across the wall; usually pertains to the pressure difference between inside and outside a vessel or conducting tube

transplacental across or through the placenta, specifically in reference to the exchange of nutrients, waste products, and other material between the developing fetus and the mother

transpulmonary across the lung; of or pertaining to the difference in a parameter (such as pressure) between the alveoli and pleural space

transrespiratory across the respiratory system; of or pertaining to the difference in a parameter (such as pressure) between the alveoli and the body surface

transrespiratory pressure gradient the pressure differential between the mouth and the alveoli that causes gas to flow in and out of the lungs

transthoracic across the thorax; of or pertaining to the difference in a parameter (such as pressure) between the pleural space and body surface

transudate a fluid passed through a membrane or squeezed through a tissue or into the space between the cells of a tissue

transudative pleural effusion a pleural effusion low in protein and LDH, usually caused by congestive heart failure, nephrosis, or cirrhosis

traumatic brain injury a general term referring to any class of either focal or diffuse lesions that can result from head trauma. These lesions can include injury to the nerve body (axon), hypoxic brain damage, swelling, hemorrhage, contusions, laceration, or infection

treatment regimen a comprehensive plan of various treatments designed to combat a certain disease or disorder

Trendelenburg position a position in which the head is low and the body and legs are on an inclined plane

trepopnea labored breathing in the upright position

triage a classification of casualties of war and other disasters according to the gravity of injuries, urgency of treatment, and place for treatment

trigeminy occurring in groups of threes; used frequently to describe certain cardiac arrhythmias, especially three premature ventricular contractions in a row

trigger sensitivity in ventilatory support, the change in pressure or flow the patient must produce to initiate a breath

triple point that combination of temperature and pressure that allows the solid, liquid, and vapor forms of a given substance to exist in equilibrium with one another

TTOT abbreviation for *transtracheal oxygen therapy*

tuberculosis a chronic granulomatous infection caused by an acid-fast bacillus, *Mycobacterium tuberculosis.* It is generally transmitted by the inhalation or ingestion of infected droplets and usually affects the lungs, although infection of multiple organ systems occurs

turbinates bony structures that extend from the lateral walls of the interior nasal passages

turgor the normal resiliency of the skin caused by the outward pressure of the cells and interstitial fluid

U

ulnar of or pertaining to the ulnar bone or the area around it

ultrasonic nebulizer (USN) a humidifier in which an electric signal is used to produce high-frequency vibrations in a container of fluid. The vibrations break up the fluid into aerosol particles

ultrasonography the diagnostic use of ultrasound to provide visualization of internal organs and structures

ultrasound sound waves that occur at frequency beyond that which humans can normally discern (over 20,000 vibrations per second)

unperfused lacking blood flow

upstream a relative reference to a point closer to the source in a stream of flowing fluid

uremia the presence of excessive amounts of urea and other nitrogenous waste products in the blood, as occurs in renal failure

urinalysis a physical, microscopic, or chemical examination of urine

URL abbreviation for uniform resource locator, the Web address of a document

urticaria a pruritic skin eruption characterized by transient wheals of varying shapes and sizes with well-defined erythematous margins and pale centers

USN abbreviation for ultrasonic nebulizer

USP abbreviation for the United States Pharmacopeia, an officially recognized compendium of drug uses, strengths, and purity standards

uteroplacental insufficiency a general term describing any physiological or anatomical abnormality of the placental system that impairs normal exchange across the placenta and threatens the viability of the fetus

uvulopalatopharyngoplasty (UVPPP) a surgical procedure used in treating severe obstructive sleep apnea, which involves shortening of the soft palate and removal of the uvula and tonsils

V

vacuum an absence of pressure

vagolytic of or pertaining to an action or agent that antagonizes or blocks parasympathetic activity

vagotomy a cutting of certain branches of the vagus nerve, performed with gastric surgery, to reduce the amount of gastric acid secreted and lessen the chance of recurrence of gastric ulcer

vagovagal reflexes reflexes caused by stimulation of parasympathetic receptors in the airways that can result in laryngospasm, bronchoconstriction, hyperpnea, and bradycardia; often associated with mechanical stimulation, as during procedures such as tracheobronchial aspiration, intubation, or bronchoscopy

vagus nerves paired nerves that provide autonomic innervation to the lungs

validity the degree to which the results of a given test actually reveal what the test intends to measure

Valsalva maneuver any forced expiratory effort against a closed glottis, as when an individual holds the breath and tightens the muscles in a concerted, strenuous effort to move a heavy object or to change position in bed

Van der Waals forces the mutual attractive forces exerted between atoms or molecules in proximity to each other

vaporization the process whereby matter in its liquid form is changed into its vapor or gaseous form

vaporizer a device that converts a liquid into a vapor; more specifically, an apparatus designed to increase ambient humidity using the principles of either evaporation or boiling

VAPS abbreviation for variable assist pressure support, a form of pressure support ventilation that assures a minimum tidal volume

variable performance device an oxygen therapy device that delivers oxygen at a flow that provides only a portion of the patient's inspired gas needs. Also called *low flow system*

vascularization the process by which body tissue becomes vascular and develops proliferating capillaries

vasculitis a narrowing of the lumen of any blood vessel, especially the arterioles and the veins in the blood reservoirs of the skin and the abdominal viscera

vasoconstriction narrowing of the blood vessels

vasodilation widening or distention of blood vessels, particularly arterioles, usually caused by nerve impulses or certain drugs that relax smooth muscle in the walls of the blood vessels

vasomotor pertaining to the nerves and muscles that control the caliber of the lumen of the blood vessels

vasopressin see ADH (antidiuretic hormone)

vasopressor pertaining to a process, condition, or substance that causes the constriction of blood vessels. Also called *vasoconstrictor*

VCV acronym for volume controlled ventilation, a mode of ventilatory support in which volume (or flow × time) serves as the cycle variable

vectorborne transmission of infectious organisms from one host to another via an animal carrier, especially an insect

venous admixture the mixing of venous blood with arterial blood, resulting in a decrease in the oxygen content of the latter; occurs in anatomical and physiological shunting

venostasis a disorder in which the normal flow of blood through a vein is slowed or halted

ventilation/perfusion (/) ratio the ratio of pulmonary alveolar ventilation to pulmonary capillary perfusion, both measured quantities being expressed in the same units

ventilator-associated pneumonia pneumonia that develops in the hospital in a patient on mechanical ventilation

ventilator asynchrony a complication of mechanical ventilation in which the patient's spontaneous pattern of breathing is not synchronous with the pattern offered by the ventilator. This results in an increase in the work of breathing

ventilatory muscle training exercises designed to improve the strength and/or endurance of the muscles of breathing

ventilatory threshold (VT) during exercise, the point where increased levels of lactic acid result in an increased CO_2 production and minute ventilation; the RQ equals or exceeds 1.0, indicating that CO_2 production equals or exceeds O_2 consumption; at this point metabolism becomes anaerobic, thereby decreasing energy production and increasing muscle fatigue

ventricular fibrillation sustained, chaotic depolarization of the ventricular myocardium resulting in discoordinated and ineffective contraction

ventrolateral positioned or located toward the back and side

venule any one of the small blood vessels that gather blood from the capillary plexuses and anastomose to form the veins

veracity the principle that binds the health provider and the patient to tell the truth, creating an environment of trust and mutual sharing of information

vertebra any of the 33 bones of the spinal column, composed of a body, a spinous process, and pairs of pedicles and processes between the vertebral column and sternum

vestibule a space or a cavity that serves as the entrance to a passageway, as the vestibule of the nose

virtue ethics the viewpoint that asks what a virtuous person would do in a similar circumstance; it is based on personal attributes of character or virtue, rather than on rules or consequences

virulence the power of microorganisms to produce disease

visceral pleura a thin membrane covered by mesothelial cells that covers the entire surface of the lung, dipping into the lobar fissures

viscosity the internal force that opposes flow of a fluid, either liquids or gases

viscous resistance impedance to motion caused by frictional forces among molecules, especially in fluids

vital capacity (VC) the total amount of air that can be exhaled after a maximum inspiration; the sum of the inspiratory reserve volume, the tidal volume, and the expiratory reserve volume

vocational of or pertaining to work

volatile acid an acid that can be excreted in its gaseous form; physiologically, carbonic acid is a volatile acid; some 24,000 mM of CO_2 are eliminated from the body daily via normal ventilation

volutrauma alveolar overdistension and damage due to ventilation with high peak inflation pressures

$\dot{V}/\dot{Q}$ imbalance any abnormal deviation in the distribution of ventilation to perfusion among the lung's alveolar-capillary units

VQI abbreviation for ventilation-perfusion index, an estimate of the venous admixture or physiologic shunt occurring in the lungs

V_T/t_I the mean spontaneous inspiratory flow, used to assess respiratory drive

W

watt a unit of power, equivalent to work done at the rate of 1 joule per second

wellness a dynamic state of health in which an individual progresses toward a higher level of functioning, achieving an optimum balance between internal and external environment

wheezes a continuous type of adventitious lung sound

word processor a computer program for handling text; includes text entry and display, editing, formatting, and printing of the final output

work of breathing the amount of force needed to move a given volume into the lung with a relaxed chest wall. Mathematically work is the integral of pressure times volume

X

xanthine a nitrogenous byproduct of the metabolism of nucleoproteins

xiphisternal of or pertaining to junction of the xiphoid process with the body of the sternum

xiphoid of or pertaining to the xiphoid process of the sternum

xiphoid process the pointed lower portion of the sternum

Z

ZEEP abbreviation for zero end-expiratory pressure

zero end-expiratory pressure (ZEEP) the default baseline value during positive pressure ventilation; it is normally in effect unless purposely changed

Ziehl-Neelsen test one of the most widely used methods of acid-fast staining, commonly used in the microscopic examination of a smear of sputum suspected of containing *Mycobacterium tuberculosis*

zone valve an on/off piping valve that controls medical gas distribution to a prespecified zone of a building

Index

Page numbers followed by *f* indicate figures; *t*, tables; *b*, boxes.

C

F

G

I

T

U

V